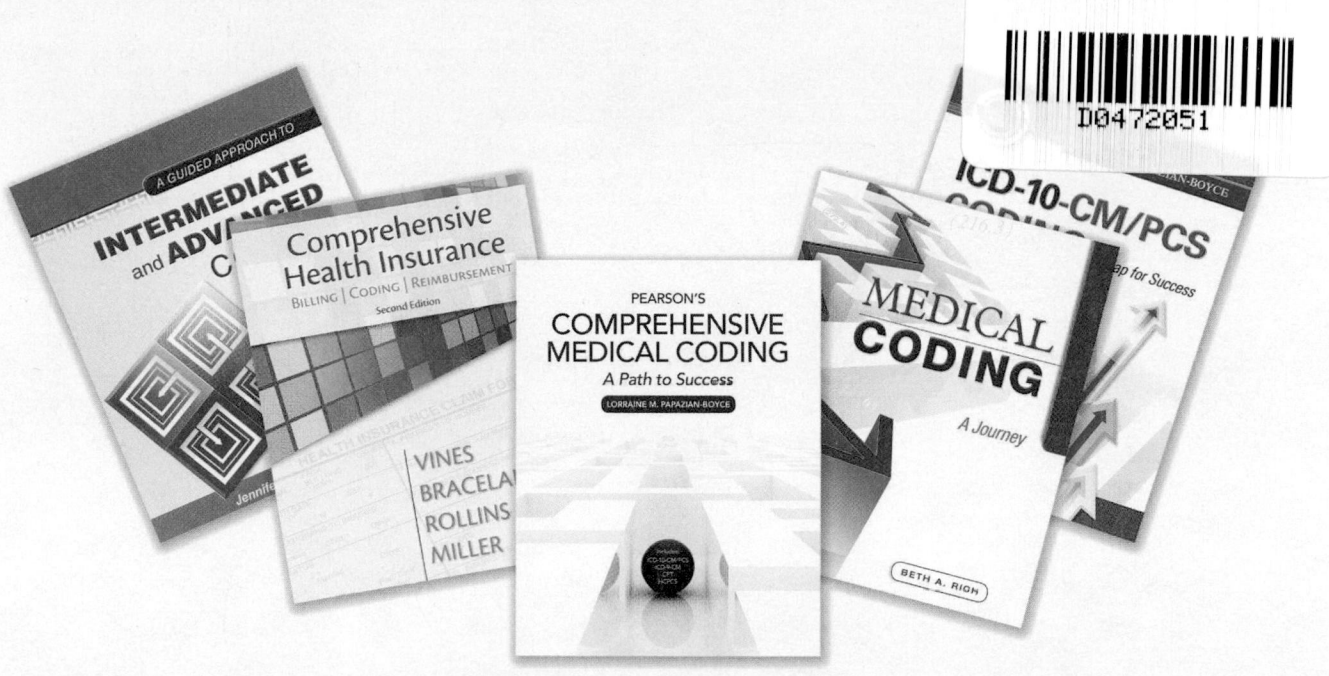

PEARSON'S COMPREHENSIVE MEDICAL CODING
A PATH TO SUCCESS

Lorraine M. Papazian-Boyce, MS, CPC

AHIMA-Approved ICD-10-CM/PCS Trainer

Educator of the Year—Instruction, 2011,
Career Education Corporation

Most Promising New Textbook Excellence Award, 2013,
Textbook and Academic Authors Association

PEARSON

Boston • Columbus • Indianapolis • New York • San Francisco
Amsterdam • Cape Town • Dubai • London • Madrid • Milan • Munich • Paris • Montréal • Toronto
Delhi • Mexico City • São Paulo • Sydney • Hong Kong • Seoul • Singapore • Taipei • Tokyo

Publisher: Julie Levin Alexander
Publisher's Assistant: Sarah Henrich
Acquisitions Editor: Marlene Pratt
Program Manager: Faye Gemmellaro
Program Management, Team Lead:
  Melissa Bashe
Project Management, Team Lead:
  Cindy Zonneveld
Project Manager: Yagnesh Jani
Editorial Assistant: Lauren Bonilla
Development Editor: Alexis Ferraro,
  iD8-TripleSSS Media Development, LLC
Marketing Manager: Brittany Hammond
Senior Marketing Coordinator: Alicia Wozniak
Marketing Specialist: Michael Sirinides
Full-Service Project Management:
  Dennis Free, Aptara

Associate Product Strategy Manager:
  Michael Gonclaves
Senior Operations Specialist: Mary Ann
  Gloriande
Digital Program Manager: Amy Peltier
Media Project Manager: William Johnson
Creative Director: Andrea Nix
Art Director: Maria Guglielmo Walsh
Cover Designer: Wanda España
Cover Image: Morena/Fotolia
Composition: iEnergizer Aptara®, Ltd.
Printing and Binding: RR Donnelley/Willard
Cover Printer: Phoenix Color/Hagerstown
Text Font: 11/13.5 Adobe Garamond Pro

Notice: The authors and the publisher of this volume have taken care that the information and technical recommendations contained herein are based on research and expert consultation and are accurate and compatible with the standards generally accepted at the time of publication. Nevertheless, as new information becomes available, changes in clinical and technical practices become necessary. The reader is advised to carefully consult manufacturers' instructions and information material for all supplies and equipment before use, and to consult with a health care professional as necessary. This advice is especially important when using new supplies or equipment for clinical purposes. The authors and publisher disclaim all responsibility for any liability, loss, injury, or damage incurred as a consequence, directly or indirectly, of the use and application of any of the contents of this volume.

Credits and acknowledgments borrowed from other sources and reproduced, with permission, in this textbook appear on page. CPT copyright 2014 American Medical Association. All rights reserved. CPT is a registered trademark of the American Medical Association.

Library of Congress Cataloging-in-Publication Data

Papazian-Boyce, Lorraine, author.
  Pearson's comprehensive medical coding / Lorraine M. Papazian-Boyce.
        p. ; cm.
  Comprehensive medical coding
  Includes index.
  ISBN 978-0-13-379778-7   ISBN 0-13-379778-3
  I. Title.   II. Title: Comprehensive medical coding.
  [DNLM: 1. International statistical classification of diseases and related health problems. 10th revision. Clinical modification.   2. International statistical classification of diseases and related health problems. 10th revision. Procedure coding system.   3. Current procedural terminology (Standard ed.: 1998)   4. Clinical Coding—Problems and Exercises.   5. Disease—classification—Problems and Exercises.   6. International Classification Diseases—Problems and Exercises. WX 18.2]
  R728.8
  616.001'2—dc23
                                                                    2014012415

3   16

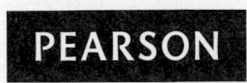

ISBN-10:   0-13-379778-3
ISBN-13:   978-0-13-379778-7

To Dave: You are my first, last, and never-failing supporter. I love you.

To my fellow coding instructors and virtual colleagues: You give me the passion to write. I appreciate your enthusiasm more than you know. You can do this!

Preface

Pearson's Comprehensive Medical Coding: A Path to Success is a comprehensive text on the healthcare industry's coding systems: ICD-10-CM/PCS, ICD-9-CM, CPT, and HCPCS. It is intended for students studying coding at career colleges, community colleges, and universities. Students might be planning to become dedicated coders or be preparing for a related role, such as health information specialist, clinician, or administrator. The book is also useful for professional coders and providers, as well as billers, claims examiners, and medical assistants.

The text is written to be friendly to those with basic exposure to, but not mastery of, medical terminology and limited or no experience in the medical field. The flexibility of the organization allows the text to be used for a single comprehensive coding course or divided among separate courses on diagnosis coding, physician procedure coding, and inpatient hospital procedure coding. The Instructor's Resource Manual provides suggested outlines for various types and lengths of course configurations. Experienced professionals can skim the basics and concentrate on new information.

More than 6,200 exercise questions give students ample opportunity to develop and fine-tune their skills. Progressively challenging exercises embedded within the text of each chapter build on one another and guide students through coding principles. End-of-chapter review questions further challenge students and reinforce key concepts.

CONCEPTUAL APPROACH

The goal of this text is not only to create a comprehensive coding text but to approach coding in a way that gives instructors new tools to communicate successfully and gives students new skills to learn effectively. This approach was proven successful in my award-winning first text, *ICD-10-CM/PCS Coding: A Map for Success*, and is applied to all code sets in this text. Four concepts are the focus of each chapter.

Abstracting, Assigning, and Arranging Codes

Students need a simple and methodical approach to the complex coding process. This text organizes coding around the learning mnemonic for an Ace Coder: "Abstract, Assign, and Arrange (Sequence)" codes. Each coding chapter includes a section of the chapter for each concept, complete with a Guided Example and exercises.

The Abstracting section of each chapter focuses on how to read and interpret documentation and identify key pieces of information without assigning any codes. A unique and original table, Key Criteria for Abstracting, appears for each body system to guide students through details specific to each body system.

The Assigning section of each chapter focuses on the mechanics of navigating the coding manuals and determining the correct code. Annotated and color-coded illustrations of pages from the indices and tabular lists of each coding manual visually guide students through what can sometimes be a dizzying array of Main Terms, subterms, and code options.

The Arranging section of each chapter focuses on identifying when multiple codes are required and how to sequence them, as well as how to apply modifiers.

The Official Guidelines for Coding and Reporting (OGCR) and CPT Guidelines are integrated into each chapter's discussion, rather than being reprinted in their entirety with minimal explanation. Guided Examples walk students through the three steps of coding and reveal the critical thinking process of applying guidelines and negotiating the intricacies of the coding manuals. By consistently and repeatedly focusing on these basic skills, the outcome is students who can tackle a variety of coding scenarios with confidence.

Application of Medical Terminology

Students need to apply what they learned in medical terminology and anatomy courses to coding. Each chapter begins with a review of medical terminology applicable to the body system being discussed. To support the increased emphasis on anatomy in ICD-10-CM/PCS, the body system diagrams are dually labeled with the English word and the medical combining form, such as *stomach* and *gastr/o*. This helps students make both visual and verbal connections with medical terms. Commonly used prefixes and suffixes, as well as easily confused medical terms, are presented within each body system. Terminology exercises and examples in each chapter show students how to continue building terminology skills and apply them to coding. The outcome is students who understand the terminology they encounter in coding exercises and, as a result, code more accurately.

Relationship of Diagnoses and Procedures

Students need to understand how diagnoses and procedures relate to each other. Every chapter highlights diagnoses and the related treatments together so students learn the relationship between the two. Exercises describe both diagnoses and services, even though the coding focus is on one or the other. End-of-chapter exercises in the procedure coding chapters require both diagnosis and procedure codes. The outcome is students who comprehend the full coding picture and, as a result, make a smooth transition into coding cases.

Context of the Patient Encounter

Students need to abstract information from a patient encounter rather than code solely from isolated statements that are five to ten words in length. In this text, exercises use an original "mini-medical-record," which presents excerpts of patient, diagnostic, and procedural information. "Tips" accompany difficult exercises to help students interpret the information. The outcome is students who learn abstracting skills in every exercise and are better prepared for advanced coding courses and the workplace.

ORGANIZATION OF THE TEXT

Students are motivated and confident when they understand why they are studying a subject and where they are going before they begin. The organization of this text gives students a context and framework for coding, covers the technical coding topics for each code set in detail, then wraps up the content with a look ahead.

Section I, "Foundations of Coding," establishes the basis of the coding career, the reimbursement process, and the ICD-10-CM/PCS transition. Students enter coding class with many questions about their future careers, so those questions are addressed up front. Then, by walking students through the claims and reimbursement process, they gain a contextual understanding of how codes are used and how they affect an organization's success. An overview of the transition from ICD-9-CM to ICD-10-CM/PCS helps students understand the context in which they enter this field.

Section II, "ICD-10-CM Coding," arranges chapters based on ease of student learning, rather than following the strict order of the manual itself. Four chapters that apply across all body systems appear before the individual body system chapters: neoplasms, symptoms, Z-codes, and external cause codes. The Instructor's Resource Manual provides a crosswalk for those who wish to teach chapters in the traditional order of the coding manual.

Each ICD-10-CM chapter is covered in one textbook chapter. No chapters are combined or split, which allows great flexibility to adapt the book to any curriculum format. The chapters can be taught in any order that best suits the curriculum. A variety of crosswalks appear in the accompanying Instructor's Resource Manual.

Section III, "ICD-9-CM Coding," includes two chapters that provide an overview of the legacy coding system.

Section IV, "CPT/HCPCS Coding," presents procedure coding for body systems in the same order as presented in Section II, again with one body system per chapter. This is convenient for programs that wish to pair diagnosis and procedure coding.

Evaluation and Management (E/M) coding is presented in a unique way. Chapter 31 provides a basic overview of E/M rather than presenting an overwhelming amount of information in a single chapter. Subsequent chapters build on this foundation by presenting an E/M case, documentation guidelines, and Guided Example at the end of each CPT body system chapter. This helps students to develop their understanding of E/M throughout the course and to appreciate the total context of a given medical specialty.

A similar approach is taken with CPT modifiers. Chapter 30 provides a basic overview of modifiers, with additional details and examples given throughout the body system chapters.

Section V, "ICD-10-PCS Coding," provides an introduction to coding for inpatient hospitals. ICD-10-PCS was developed based on the type of Root Operation rather than body system, so the emphasis is on helping students understand the characteristics of and differences between Root Operations. Medical and Surgical Root Operations, which account for 85% of all PCS codes, are covered in greatest detail to help students learn the structure and use of ICD-10-PCS. These skills then are applied to the other Sections of PCS in subsequent chapters.

Section VI, "Putting It All Together," appears in the online content and consists of two chapters. Chapter 59 introduces students to coding from chart notes and operative reports, as well as using electronic coding tools. Chapter 60 discusses professionalism in depth to bring students full circle from where they started in Chapter 1 with an introduction to careers.

FEATURES

Consistent pedagogical elements appear in each chapter to facilitate instruction and learning.

Learning Objectives—Each chapter begins with a list of the primary skills students should have after completing the chapter.

Key Terms and Abbreviations—A list of the important terms students need to know but may not have learned in previous classes is provided at the beginning of each chapter. These terms are set in blue boldface type and are defined upon first appearance in the chapter. They also are included in the Glossary at the end of the book. Supplemental terms are set in black boldface type and are defined in the Glossary.

Chapter Outline—A list of the major topics covered in the chapter appears at the beginning.

Introduction—The text uses analogies at the beginning of chapters to create a "hook" with a common frame of reference and provides a familiar perspective for relating to new information.

Success Step—Short tips help students abstract, assign, and arrange (sequence) codes.

Coding Caution—Short warnings alert students to coding situations that can be tricky or confusing.

Coding Practice—Coding exercises throughout the chapter consist of three to six patient scenarios related to a specific chapter topic. The first exercise in the coding chapters reviews medical terms related to the body system or type of procedure and introduces students to simple coding for the body system. Subsequent exercises walk students through the skills of abstracting, assigning, and sequencing codes. Exercises increase in difficulty as the chapter progresses, while remaining appropriate for an introductory course.

Guided Examples—Step-by-step demonstrations allow students to experience the thinking process of a seasoned coder as they observe a coder abstract, assign, and sequence codes from a mini-medical-record.

Figures—Anatomic illustrations show English names and medical terms for major body parts and organs. Illustrations annotate sample pages from the coding manuals to guide students' understanding of layout and appropriate use. Photographs and diagrams portray key points and clarify new information.

Tables—Tables provide definitions of terms, conditions, and treatments, as well as comparative information that highlights key concepts.

Summary—Each chapter ends with a brief restatement of key points in the chapter.

Typefaces and Punctuation

Distinct fonts and color-coding enable student to visually identify various types of information. Typefaces are intermixed in the
narrative to highlight information taken directly from a medical
record or the coding manual. Four fonts are used as follows:

- Key terms and abbreviations
- Simulated content in a patient's medical record
- **Codes, code titles, and instructional notes from
  the ICD-10-CM/PCS coding manuals**
- **Supplemental terms and abbreviations** (Sections I, II,
  and III)

The names of chapters, sections, and selected features in the
coding manuals are treated as proper nouns and therefore are
capitalized. This use is to be distinguished from the common
use of a term. For example, the Digestive System subsection of
the CPT manual is treated as a proper noun and capitalized. The
organ system known as digestive system is a common noun and
not capitalized. In Section V, "ICD-10-PCS," the term *Character*
is capitalized when referring to the positions in a PCS code. The
features of PCS such as coding Tables and the name of each PCS
Character, such as Section, Body System, and so on, are treated
as proper nouns and capitalized. When a body system, body
part, or approach is referenced as a common noun, it is not capitalized. This variation is capitalization is intentional for the
sake of clarity and not a copyediting or proofreading error.

End-of-Chapter Material

The review at the end of each chapter reinforces key concepts,
provides opportunity for additional skills practice, and offers
resources for additional learning.

Concept Quiz —Definitions and key concepts are reviewed
using ten completion and ten multiple-choice questions.

Coding Challenge —Ten coding scenarios drawn from all
sections of the chapter review coding skills learned in the
chapter. The Coding Challenge in procedure coding chapters
requires both diagnosis and procedure codes.

Keep on Coding —Twenty-five coding exercises in a one-line
statement format provide additional student practice.

End-of-Book Material

The following material at the end of the text provides reference
information for students.

Glossary —The Glossary defines key terms, supplemental
terms, and abbreviations and indicates the chapter in which
the term was introduced.

Index —An alphabetic crosswalk identifies page references for
major topics discussed in this text.

Online Content

The following content of the text appears online:

Section VI, "Putting It All Together" —Two chapters provide
a wrap-up for the course and a look ahead to advanced coding,
health information technology, and professionalism in the
workplace.

Coder's Toolbox —A list of Internet resources related to
chapter content provides students a starting point for additional
information or instructor-assigned research projects.

Resources

- Textbook
- Student Workbook (available separately) contains even more
  practice and reinforcement opportunities and helps you
  prepare for quizzes and exams.

The Instructor Package:

- Instructor's Resource Manual contains a wealth of information
  to help faculty plan and manage the Medical Coding course.
  Answers to Coding Practice Exercises can be found here.
- PowerPoint® Slides
- Testgen® computerized test bank

Interactive Media

Visit our new MyHealthProfessions Lab to accompany Pearson's Comprehensive Medical Coding. Here you'll find extensive resources, including:

- A pre-/post-test homework engine, which enables students
  to learn and master concepts as homework, preparing them
  for classroom work.
- Access your free trial of SpeedECoder® online medical
  coding software at http://sec.pearsonhighered.com

ABOUT THE AUTHOR

Lorraine M. Papazian-Boyce, MS, CPC
AHIMA-Approved ICD-10-CM/PCS Trainer

Lorraine M. Papazian-Boyce is an award-winning author
and instructor. She authored the Pearson text *ICD-10-CM/
PCS Coding: A Map for Success*, which received the Most
Promising New Textbook Award—2013 from the Textbook
and Academic Authors Association. She was named Educator of the Year - Instruction in 2011 by Career Education
Corporation (CEC).

Lorraine holds an M.S. in Health Systems Management and
the Certified Professional Coder (CPC) credential. She is an
AHIMA-Approved ICD-10-CM/PCS Trainer and Ambassador
and is an appointee on the Faculty Development Workgroup of
the American Health Information Management Association
(AHIMA)—Council for Excellence in Education.

Lorraine has over 30 years of experience in healthcare administration as a college instructor, in both traditional and online
settings; owner of a medical billing service; office manager; consultant to hospitals, nursing homes, and physicians; and board of
directors officer. She is a frequent speaker in this field. She has
taught most aspects of healthcare operations and reimbursement both to practicing professionals and in a formal academic
career college setting. She is known as someone who is thorough
in covering material and effective in communicating it to learn-
ers, in both oral and written formats. She knows exactly where in
the curriculum college students struggle, what their questions
are, and what techniques best clarify information for them. As a
former employer and as an externship coordinator, she also

knows what today's students need to succeed in the medical workplace. Her driving passion is taking complex technical subjects and breaking them down into practical, understandable pieces that others can implement.

She is a contributor and/or subject matter expert to several Pearson texts, including *Pearson's Comprehensive Medical Assisting*, 3rd ed., by Nina M. Beaman, et al.; *Medical Coding: A Journey*, by Beth A. Rich; *Administrative Medical Assisting: Foundations and Practices*, 2nd ed., by Christine Malone; *Guide to Medical Billing and Coding*, 3rd edition, by Sarah Brown and Lori Tyler; *Comprehensive Health Insurance: Billing, Coding, and Reimbursement*, by Deborah Vines, Ann Braceland, Elizabeth Rollins, and Susan H. Miller; *A Guided Approach to Intermediate and Advanced Coding*, by Jennifer Lame and Glenna Young; *Mastering Medisoft*, by Bonnie J. Flom; *Medical Assisting: Foundations and Practices*, by Margaret Frazier, et al; and *Medical Insurance Billing Course Connect*.

ACKNOWLEDGEMENTS

Developing this text has been a long, challenging, exciting, and rewarding experience. I am deeply appreciative to those who walked with me on this journey. Marlene Pratt, Acquisitions Editor, recognized my unique approach to coding and supported my vision to create a comprehensive coding solution using the framework of my successful first text, *ICD-10-CM/PCS Coding: A Map for Success*. She assembled a development and production team who worked tirelessly through the ups and downs of the project: Alexis Breen Ferraro, Developmental Editor, and Susan Simpfenderfer, Principal, of iD8-TripleSSS Media Development; Faye Gemmellaro, Yagnesh Jani, and Lauren Bonilla of Pearson; Dennis Free and his team from Aptara; and many others unknown to me who finessed the details of this book.

Subject Matter Experts

A special thank you goes to my team of subject matter experts who wrote exercises, reviewed content for accuracy, and otherwise performed tasks that would have been impossible for me to do while maintaining a rigorous writing schedule. The professionalism and enthusiasm demonstrated by each individual made working with them my pleasure.

- **Angela R. Campbell, RHIA,** *AHIMA Approved ICD-10-CM/PCS Trainer; Medical Insurance Manager, Eastern Illinois University; Curriculum Designer/Adjunct Instructor, Northwestern College; Lead Faculty Member/Adjunct Instructor, Ultimate Medical Academy; Adjunct Instructor, The College of Health Care Professions*, who, in addition to writing exercises and performing accuracy checks, reviewed hundreds of chapter files as they made their way through the production process. Without her unceasing effort, this book could not have been finished within the desired time frame.

- **Kate Gabriel-Jones, CPC,** *author, Medical Coding: Evaluation and Management*, who lent her expertise on CPT Evaluation and Management coding to enhance students' understanding of this complex topic.

- **Mary Lou Hilbert, MBA, RHIT, CCS,** *Program Manager, Health Information Technology and Medical Coding and Billing, Seminole State College of Florida;* whose keen eye and commitment to this project from beginning to end helped ensure attention to detail.

- **Krystal S. Phillips, RHIA, CHTS-IS,** *AHIMA ICD-10-CM/PCS Ambassador; Adjunct Instructor, Columbus State Community College*, whose hard work on the CPT chapters and endless enthusiasm are much appreciated.

- **Christine Tufts-Maher, MSHI, MS, RHIA,** *Professor, Seminole State College of Florida*, whose expertise on ICD-10-PCS helped us put the finishing touches on the project.

REVIEWERS

The following educators and healthcare professionals provided invaluable feedback during development:

Geanetta Johnson Agbona CPC, CPC-I, CBCS
Instructor, Medical Coding
South Piedmont Community College
Charlotte, North Carolina

Felecia Calloway, MBA, CCA, CBCS
Instructional Systems Designer
Virginia College
Montgomery, Alabama

Ora Clark, RHIT, AHIMA, CPC, AAPC
Medical Insurance/Billing & Coding Adjunct Faculty
Oconee Fall Line Technical College
Dublin, Georgia

Michelle Cranney, DHSc, RHIA, CCS-P, CPC
Assistant Professor, Health Information Management
Ashford University
Seattle, Washington

Janet A. Evans, RN, MBA, MS, CCS, CPC-I
Instructor, Introduction to HCPCS (CPT) Coding
Burlington County College
Pemberton, New Jersey

Chemo Faustino, CPC
Program Director, Medical Billing & Coding
Sanford-Brown College
Ft. Lauderdale, Florida

Michelle Griggs, CPC, CPC-I, CPMA
Program Director, Medical Insurance/Billing & Coding
Virginia College
Richmond, Virginia

Wahiyda Harding, RHIA, CCS, CTR,
Program Chair, Medical Insurance/Billing & Coding
Westwood College
Atlanta, Georgia

Kerry Heinecke, MS, RHIA
Program Director, HIM
Mid-State Technical College
Marshfield, Wisconsin

Susan Herzberg, RHIA, CCS, CCS-P
Adjunct Professor, Medical Coding
Westchester Community College
Valhalla, New York

Mary Anita Kahler, RHIT, ICD 10-CM Trainer
Instructor, Medical Insurance/Billing & Coding
Coastal Carolina Community College
Jacksonville, North Carolina

Bobbie J. Lautenschlager, CCA, CMRS, CPC
Program Director, Medical Billing & Coding
American School of Technology
Columbus, Ohio

Robin Maddalena, CMT, CEHRS
Adjunct Professor, Medical Insurance/Billing & Coding,
  Electronic Health Records
Tunxis Community College
Farmington, Connecticut

Kim S. Norris, MBA, CPC
Program Director, Medical Billing & Coding
Carrington College
Tucson, Arizona

Lakisha Parker, AAS, CPC, CPC-I, ACPAR
Program Director, Medical Billing & Coding/Healthcare
  Reimbursement
Virginia College
Birmingham, Alabama

Elizabeth Roberts, CPC, CBCS, ICD-10 CM/PCS Trainer
Former Instructor, Medical Billing & Coding at Virginia
  College
Current Independent ICD-10 Consultant
Las Cruces, New Mexico

Gerald Robinson, CPC, ICD-10-CM/PCS Trainer
HIM Director & Adjunct Instructor
Ultimate Medical Academy
Tampa, Florida

Rolando Russell, MBA/HCM, CPC, CPAR
Program Director
Ultimate Medical Academy
Tampa, Florida

Jennifer J. Talbot, RHIA, CCS-P, ICD-10-CM/PCS Trainer
Program Director, HIT
Kirtland Community College
Roscommon, Michigan

Jeanette Thomas, RHIA, RHIT, CPC-H, CPC
Instructor, Health Information Systems
Clayton State University
Morrow, Georgia

Lydia Wikoff
Instructor, Billing & Coding
Southeastern College
Jacksonville, Florida

Contents in Brief

(continued)

SECTION FIVE

ICD-10-PCS Procedure Coding 975

Online Chapters

SECTION SIX

Putting It All Together

Contents

SECTION THREE

ICD-9-CM Coding   441

SECTION FOUR

CPT/HCPCS Procedure Coding   469

SECTION FIVE

ICD-10-PCS Procedure Coding 975

Online Chapters

Guide to Key Features

This Guide to Key Features acquaints users with the text and shows them how to use the pedagogical features to their greatest advantage.

Chapter Opener Features

Learning Objectives—Each chapter begins with a list of the primary skills students should have after completing the chapter.

Learning Objectives

After completing this chapter, you should have the skills to:

16.1 Spell and define the key words, medical terms, and abbreviations related to the respiratory system.

16.2 Discuss the structure, function, and common conditions of the respiratory system.

16.3 Identify the main characteristics of coding for respiratory system conditions.

Key Terms and Abbreviations—A list of the important terms students need to know but may not have learned in previous classes is provided at the beginning of each chapter. These terms are set in **blue** boldface type and are defined upon first appearance in the chapter. They also are included in the Glossary at the end of the book. Supplemental terms are set in black boldface type and are defined in the Glossary.

Key Terms and Abbreviations

acute exacerbation	chronic bronchitis
acute rhinitis	chronic obstructive pulmonary
aerosol therapy	disease (COPD)
airway obstruction	culture and sensitivity
allergic rhinitis	emphysema
alveolus	endotracheal intubation
atopic	exchange
bronchodilator	extrinsic
bronchogenic	hospital-acquired condition
bronchus	(HAC)
bronchial tree	hypercapnia
bronchiole	hypoxemia

Introduction—The text uses analogies at the beginning of chapters to create a "hook" with a common frame of reference and provides a familiar perspective for relating to new information.

INTRODUCTION

As you travel to a higher elevation than what you're accustomed to, breathing becomes more difficult. This is not because there is less oxygen in the air but because a decrease in air pressure causes us to inhale less air with each breath.

A pulmonologist specializes in diagnosing and treating conditions of the lungs and lower respiratory system. An otolaryngologist specializes in diagnosing and treating conditions of the upper respiratory system. Primary care physicians treat uncomplicated conditions of the respiratory system and refer more complicated cases to specialists.

Chapter Outline—A list of the major topics covered in the chapter appears at the beginning. A consistent framework across all coding chapters makes it easy to transition among body systems.

Chapter Outline

- **Respiratory System Refresher**
- **Coding Overview of the Respiratory System**
- **Abstracting for Respiratory System Conditions**
- **Assigning Codes for Respiratory System Conditions**

In-Chapter Features

Success Step—Short tips throughout the chapter help students abstract, assign, and arrange (sequence) codes.

Coding Caution—Short warnings throughout the chapter alert students to coding situations that can be tricky or confusing.

SUCCESS STEP

ICD-9-CM provided a chapter-wide note to assign an additional code to identify the infectious organism. Because ICD-10-CM has many combination codes that describe the condition and the organism, this chapter-wide note was eliminated. However, you still see a similar note in certain categories that do not provide a combination code.

CODING CAUTION

In ICD-9-CM asthma codes were divided based on whether asthma was extrinsic or intrinsic. In ICD-10-CM, these terms lead you to default codes for unspecified asthma. Instead, you need to locate asthma based on the severity level as mild intermittent, moderate intermittent, moderate persistent, and severe persistent.

Coding Practice—Coding exercises at multiple points throughout the chapter consist of three to six patient scenarios related to a specific chapter topic. The first exercise in the coding chapters reviews medical terms related to the body system or type of procedure and introduces students to simple coding for the body system.

CODING PRACTICE

Exercise 16.1 Respiratory System Refresher

Instructions: Use your medical terminology skills and resources to define the following conditions related to the respiratory system, then assign the diagnosis code. Follow these steps:

• Use slash marks "/" to break down each term into its root(s) and suffix.

• Define the meaning of the word, based on the meaning of each word part.

• Assign the default ICD-10-CM diagnosis code for the condition using the Index and Tabular List.

Example: tonsillitis tonsil/itis   Meaning: *inflammation of the tonsils*   ICD-10-CM Code: *J03.90*

1. pneumatocele   Meaning _____

2. bronchiolitis   Meaning _____

3. pneumohemothorax   Meaning _____

4. rhinorrhea   Meaning _____

5. nasopharyngitis   Meaning _____

CODING PRACTICE

Exercise 16.5 Coding Neoplasms of the Respiratory System

Instructions: Read the mini-medical-record of each patient's encounter, then abstract, assign, and sequence ICD-10-CM diagnosis codes using the Index and Tabular List. Write the code(s) on the line provided.

1. INPATIENT HOSPITAL Gender: F Age: 51
Reason for encounter: radiotherapy for lung cancer due to cigarette smoking
Assessment: NSCLC, upper left lobe
Plan: return for daily treatments
3 ICD-10-CM Codes _____

2. INPATIENT HOSPITAL Gender: F Age: 56
Reason for encounter: lung biopsy of mass found on X-ray when patient was treated for pneumonia, CT scan was inconclusive
Assessment: benign neoplasm in right inferior lobe
Plan: Patient has been asymptomatic so there is no need to do a resection at this time.
1 ICD-10-CM Code _____

Subsequent exercises walk students through the skills of abstracting, assigning, and sequencing codes. Exercises increase in difficulty as the chapter progresses, while remaining appropriate for an introductory course.

Tables—Tables throughout the text provide definitions of terms, conditions, and treatments, as well as comparative information that highlights key concepts.

End of Chapter Features

The review at the end of each chapter reinforces key concepts and provides opportunity for additional skills practice.

Concept Quiz—Definitions and key concepts are reviewed using ten completion and ten multiple-choice questions.

Coding Challenge—Ten coding scenarios are drawn from all sections of the chapter review coding skills learned in the chapter. The Coding Challenge in procedure coding chapters requires both diagnosis and procedure codes.

Keep on Coding—Twenty-five coding exercises in a one-line statement format provide additional student practice.

SECTION ONE

Foundations of Coding

Welcome to your new career in coding! You are in for the trip of a lifetime, one that is sure to take you to new and unknown places, a few familiar ones, and perhaps some that seem a little scary. This text is your road map, complete with success steps and caution signs.

Section One: Foundations of Coding acquaints you with the medical coding field, potential career opportunities, how coding relates to reimbursement and payment, and provides an overview of the transition to ICD-10-CM/PCS.

PROFESSIONAL PROFILE

MEET...

Kristy Rodecker, CPC, CPC-H, CMA
Home-Based Medical Coder

I have been in the medical billing and coding field for ten years. I was certified as a CPC five years ago and have been coding from home since then. I started out as a front desk receptionist in a busy, multi-physician neurology office and worked my way through school to be an administrative medical assistant.

When the opportunity arose, I took a data entry position at a small billing company that was a one-and-a-half hour drive (one way) and paid peanuts! The experience I gained was priceless and it was the stepping stone for the rest of my career. The company allowed coders to work from home once they worked at the facility for six to twelve months. They wanted coders to understand the way the company worked to make sure the coders knew what they were doing before they worked independently. Once I could pass all of their milestones I began to code remotely. Eventually, I took on assignments for other coding companies as well, including Nicka, MRSI, Med Data, and Summit—sometimes coding for several companies at once. For some companies I am a regular employee and for others I work as an independent contractor.

As a home-based medical coder, I log in remotely to the customer's database to access the medical records, code them, and submit the claims to insurance companies. I enjoy reading the interesting medical records, learning about new procedures, and the challenge of finding an accurate code. I also enjoy the flexibility of setting my own hours.

The most challenging aspect of my job is isolation. Working from home can give you a good dose of cabin fever. I find it important to attend my local AAPC chapter meetings and I also volunteer at the hospital so that I can stay involved in our local medical community.

I am frequently asked by aspiring coders how to work from home, so I created a free, informational website (**www. medicalbillingandmedicalcoding.com**) to help them avoid unscrupulous get-rich-quick schemes and find ways to be successful.

My advice to coding students is to set an achievable goal and go for it! Be willing to take an entry-level position, ask lots of questions, and go the extra mile to prove you are an asset.

Chapter 1

Your Career and Coding

Chapter Outline

- **What Is Coding?**
- **Understanding Patient Encounters**
- **Certification**
- **Coding Careers**

Learning Objectives

After completing this chapter, you should have the skills to:

1.1 Spell and define the key words, medical terms, and abbreviations related to your career and coding.

1.2 Define coding, HIPAA-mandated code sets, and coding skills.

1.3 Describe how patient encounters relate to coding.

1.4 Identify the types of coding certification.

1.5 Understand the career path and performance expectations for a coding career.

Key Terms and Abbreviations

AAPC	ancillary	code set	inpatient encounter
abstract	attending physician	coding	midlevel job
admitting privileges	assign	diagnosis	outpatient encounter
advanced-level job	arrange	document	payers
amend	career path	encounter	procedure
American Health Information Management Association (AHIMA)	case production	entry-level job	query
	certification	Health Insurance Portability and Accountability Act (HIPAA)	sequence
	code		

In addition to the key terms listed here, students should know the terms defined within tables in this chapter.

INTRODUCTION

When starting on a trip, you are more likely to get where you want to go when you have a destination in mind. In this chapter you will learn about your ultimate destination: the coding profession. By understanding what coding is, the relationship between physicians and coders, and potential career opportunities, you will formulate ideas on your career goals and the steps needed to reach them.

Many jobs in the healthcare field work with codes even though they may not have a job title of Coder. For example, medical assistants, billers, schedulers, and medical secretaries may use codes as part of their jobs. This text uses the term *coder* to refer to anyone who assigns, reads, or uses codes as part of their job.

A wide variety of healthcare professionals provides patient services and uses codes to bill for their services in addition to medical doctors (MDs). For example, dentists (DDSs or DMDs), osteopaths (DOs), chiropractors (DCs), and nurse practitioners (NPs) also bill their services with the same codes as physicians. This text uses the terms *physician* and *provider* interchangeably to refer to any healthcare professional who provides services that are billed with codes.

WHAT IS CODING?

Coding is the process of accurately assigning codes to verbal descriptions of patients' conditions and the healthcare services provided to treat those conditions. Medical **codes** are a combination of letters and numbers, three to seven characters in length. **Diagnosis** codes describe patient illnesses, diseases, conditions, injuries, or other reasons for seeking healthcare services. **Procedure** codes describe the services healthcare professionals provide to patients, such as evaluation, consultation, testing, treatments, and surgery.

Code Sets

The healthcare system in the United States uses several distinct systems of medical codes, called **code sets**, for different purposes. The various systems were developed by different organizations and follow different guidelines for their use. The **Health Insurance Portability and Accountability Act (HIPAA)**, a federal law passed in 1996, has numerous provisions relating to consumer health insurance and electronic health transactions. HIPAA defines the code sets that **covered entities** must use for electronic health transactions and the purpose of each (■ TABLE 1-1).

Table 1-1   ■   HIPAA-MANDATED CODE SETS

Code Set Name	Purpose	Developed By	Code Format/Examples
CDT Codes on Dental Procedures and Nomenclature	Dental services (occupies section D of HCPCS codes)	American Dental Association (ADA)	Letter D + 4 numbers • D7230
CPT Current Procedural Terminology	Hospital outpatient and physician procedure coding	American Medical Association (AMA)	5 numbers • 99213 • 36415
HCPCS Healthcare Common Procedure Coding System	Supplies, items, and services not covered by CPT, physician and nonphysician services, Medicare services, supplies	Centers for Medicare and Medicaid Services (CMS)	1 letter + 4 numbers • A1234 • G9874
ICD-10-CM International Classification of Diseases, 10th Revision, Clinical Modification	Diagnosis coding (replacement system for ICD-9-CM)	National Center for Health Statistics (NCHS) based on ICD-10 from the World Health Organization (WHO)	3 to 7 alphanumeric characters • I10 • A52.15 • T50.A11D
ICD-10-PCS International Classification of Diseases, 10th Revision, Procedure Coding System	Hospital inpatient procedure coding (replacement system for ICD-9-CM, Volume 3)	CMS	7 alphanumeric characters • 0B7B8DZ • 4A04XB1 • 01500ZZ
ICD-9-CM International Classification of Diseases, 9th Revision, Clinical Modification	Diagnosis coding, implemented 1979 (replaced by ICD-10-CM)	NCHS	3 to 5 numbers; supplemental codes that begin with V or E • 123 • 123.45 • V10.23 • E987.4
ICD-9-CM procedure codes	Hospital inpatient procedure coding, implemented 1979 (replaced by ICD-10-PCS)	NCHS	3 or 4 numbers • 12.3 • 12.34
NDC National Drug Codes	Identifies the manufacturer, product, and package size of all drugs and biologics recognized by the Food and Drug Administration (FDA)	Department of Health and Human Services (HHS)	10 numbers divided into 3 segments • 1234-5678-90 • 12345-678-90 • 12345-6789-0

Three Skills of an Ace Coder

Coding is more than looking up numbers in a manual or software program. Accurate coding requires three major skills, which are described next: abstracting, assigning, and arranging (sequencing).

Abstracting

Before coders can assign codes, they **abstract** information from the medical record. To abstract, coders read the medical record and determine which elements of the encounter require codes. They identify the reason for the encounter, diagnostic statements from the physician, complications and coexisting conditions, and the services provided. If the medical record is not properly abstracted, it is impossible to assign the correct codes. Each code set has various rules for abstracting, and some rules are specific to a particular condition or procedure.

SUCCESS STEP

The term *abstract* also describes a task in health information management in which inpatient coders review the medical record and cull data required for reporting, such as patient demographics and length of stay.

Assigning

The codes a coder selects or **assigns** must accurately describe both the information documented in the medical record and the patient's condition and services. Each character of the code must be correct. Diagnosis and procedure codes must reflect the highest level of specificity possible and contain the correct number of characters for that code. The official guidelines on how to assign codes vary among code sets because each has slightly different requirements.

Arranging

When more than one diagnosis or procedure code is required for an encounter, coders must **arrange**, or **sequence**, the codes in a specific order. Official coding guidelines dictate the proper sequencing, which varies depending on the codes assigned and the circumstances of the patient encounter. Codes that are not sequenced properly are not considered to be correct.

SUCCESS STEP

Memorize the definitions of the three coding skills: abstracting, assigning, and arranging. Remind yourself of these each time you sit down to code.

CODING PRACTICE

Exercise 1.1 What Is Coding?

Instructions: Write the answers to the following questions in the space provided.

1. Define coding. _____

_____

_____

_____

2. What is the difference between diagnosis coding and procedure coding? _____

_____

_____

3. List and briefly define the three skills of an "ace" coder. _____

_____

_____

_____

UNDERSTANDING PATIENT ENCOUNTERS

Coders assign diagnosis and procedure codes to a patient **encounter** (*a specific interaction between a patient and healthcare provider*) after an encounter has been completed. The provider documents the reason(s) for the encounter and the services provided in the patient's medical record. Coders read the medical record and other information the physician provides to identify the main reason for the encounter, any additional reasons for the service, the main service provided, and any additional services provided. The following sections provide an overview of patient encounters with the healthcare system, including the types of encounters and the process of an encounter. This helps coders better understand their role.

Types of Encounters

Patient encounters are generally classified by the location of the encounter because different coding and billing rules apply to each. The two basic types of locations are outpatient and inpatient, which are described next.

Outpatient Encounters

Outpatient encounters are physician interactions with patients who receive services and have not been formally admitted to a healthcare institution, such as an acute-care hospital, long-term care facility, or rehabilitation facility. Patients request outpatient encounters when they have particular health problems, need preventive services, or for follow-up or ongoing treatment for known problems. ■ TABLE 1-2 lists examples of outpatient encounters.

Table 1-2 ■ **EXAMPLES OF OUTPATIENT ENCOUNTERS**

Setting	Purpose	Examples
Ambulatory surgery	Surgical procedure that does not require an overnight stay in the hospital	Tonsillectomy, cataract removal
Cardiology lab	Testing to evaluate a heart problem	EKG, echocardiogram, cardiac catheterization
Diagnostic radiology	Imaging study to evaluate or diagnose a health problem	X-ray, MRI, CT, PET
Emergency department	Treatment of an injury or health problem that cannot be delayed without harm to the patient	Broken leg, chest pain
Laboratory	Specimen collection	Blood draw
Observation	Extended monitoring which may require an overnight stay but does not meet the requirements for a formal inpatient admission	Chest pain
Physical therapy	Treatment of a musculoskeletal problem	Therapeutic exercises, electrical muscle stimulation
Physician office	Evaluation and management of a new or existing health problem; preventive care services	Back pain, diabetes check-up, immunization
Therapeutic radiology	Receive a treatment using radiation	Anticancer radiation therapy

Inpatient Encounters

Inpatient encounters are physician interactions with patients who have been formally admitted to a healthcare facility, such as an acute-care hospital, long-term care facility, or rehabilitation facility. Patients cannot admit themselves to a facility; a physician must admit a patient for a specific medical reason, which is to either diagnose or treat a health problem. Physicians contract with hospitals for **admitting privileges**, meaning they have authority to admit patients and care for them in a specific hospital. They write admitting orders, conduct an admitting history and physical, and complete paperwork required by the institution. One physician, usually the one who admits the patient, is the **attending physician** who oversees and coordinates all aspects of the patient's care while an inpatient. Other physicians also may be involved in the diagnosis or treatment of the patient. A patient may also receive **ancillary** services, such as laboratory, radiology, or physical therapy, as an inpatient.

The facility codes and bills for the room, board, nursing care, use of the operating room, and most ancillary services. Physicians code and bill for services they personally provide, such as hospital visits, surgical procedures, and interpretation of laboratory or radiology tests. A third-party company may contract with the facility to provide services such as radiology or physical therapy, in which case that company codes and bills its own services to the patient.

Therefore, coders do not code for everything pertaining to a specific patient. They code for the services provided by their employer, such as the hospital, the surgeon, or the physical therapist. They also code for the diagnoses that describe why the patient received these particular services, but they do not code for unrelated diagnoses.

Steps in the Encounter

While each encounter is unique to the patient's situation, it generally involves three steps: diagnosis, treatment, and documentation.

Diagnosis

When a patient presents to a physician with a health problem, the physician needs to establish a diagnosis. If a diagnosis was established in a previous encounter, the physician reviews the patient's progress and updates the diagnosis. Establishing or updating a diagnosis involves a history, a physical examination, and testing.

History. A physician takes a patient's medical history, which includes questions about current symptoms and past medical problems. Because most symptoms can be caused by several different conditions, the physician asks a series of questions to narrow the possibilities. If a diagnosis was established in a previous encounter, the physician updates the history based on what has happened since the last encounter.

Physical Examination. The physician conducts a physical examination to further identify and evaluate abnormalities. The examination may focus on a specific body system or it may cover the entire body. Examinations include visual inspection, palpation (*physical touching*), and auscultation (*listening to various parts of the body*).

Testing. A physician performs or orders diagnostic tests, such as blood tests, imaging, biopsies, and physical function tests, such as EKGs, based on the patient's situation. In some cases, the patient's condition does not require any tests.

Based on the findings from these sources, the physician identifies the most likely diagnosis and the rationale for it. Depending on the complexity of the problem, the physician may determine the diagnosis in a single encounter or it may take multiple patient encounters and multiple rounds of testing to arrive at a conclusion.

Guided Example of Physician Diagnosis. Refer to the following example throughout this chapter to learn more about patient encounters. The first portion of the example demonstrates how physicians diagnose conditions.

▶ Patient Norman Markowitz, age 41, schedules an office appointment to see Dr. Kristen Conover, a family practice physician, on January 5, due to back pain.

  ❑ Dr. Conover takes a history by asking Mr. Markowitz when the pain started, how severe it is, what makes it better or worse, and if it has occurred before.

  ❑ She performs a physical examination to see if she can detect abnormalities such as tightness, lumps, knots, or protrusions.

  ❑ She asks Mr. Markowitz to perform specific maneuvers, such as standing, sitting, and leaning forward or backward, to determine his physical abilities.

  ❑ She uses a reflex hammer to test his reflexes.

  ❑ She takes an X-ray in the office, which is negative for a fracture.

  ❑ She orders blood tests, which come back negative for arthritis on January 12.

  ❑ She then schedules Mr. Markowitz for an MRI examination on January 17, which reveals a displaced intervertebral disc.

▶ Next, Dr. Conover will provide a treatment plan.

Treatment Plan

After establishing the diagnosis, the physician formulates a treatment plan. The treatment plan may include medication, surgery, lifestyle changes, or therapy. For complicated problems that take time to diagnose, the physician may treat symptoms to provide relief to the patient until the underlying cause is determined.

Guided Example of a Treatment Plan. Continue with the example of patient Norman Markowitz, who saw Dr. Conover due to back pain, to learn more about the treatment plan.

▶ Dr. Conover prescribes medication to relieve Mr. Markowitz's back pain while waiting for results of the blood tests and MRI.

  ❑ After she receives the MRI results of a displaced disc, she asks Mr. Markowitz to schedule another appointment for follow-up.

  ❑ On January 24, they discuss treatment options and decide to continue medication and refer Mr. Markowitz for physical therapy.

  ❑ They also discuss the possibility of surgery if physical therapy does not provide adequate relief.

▶ Next, Dr. Conover will document the encounter.

Documentation

After each patient encounter, the physician **documents** the encounter, recording the reason for the encounter, the diagnostic techniques used, tests or treatments planned, and the overall assessment of the patient. This documentation is the basis from

which coders assign diagnostic and procedure codes for each encounter. Coders do not do the following:

- determine what is wrong with the patient
- determine what condition(s) the patient has based on the symptoms
- code for services provided prior to the current encounter
- code for services planned but not provided during the current encounter
- code for services delivered by other providers
- code for past conditions that are resolved
- code for current conditions that the physician does not document as relevant to the current encounter

When the documentation is unclear, coders do not make assumptions about missing information. They **query** (*ask*) the physician for clarification and the physician **amends** (*adds information to*) the medical record, if necessary.

Guided Example of Documentation. Continue with the example of Norman Markowitz, who saw Dr. Conover due to back pain, to learn more about documentation. Sherry Whittle, CPC, is a fictitious certified coder who guides you through documentation and coding.

▶ Sherry Whittle, CPC, codes for two outpatient encounters for Mr. Markowitz, January 5 and January 24, because those were the two dates that Dr. Conover saw him in the office.

  ❑ For the January 5 encounter, Sherry assigns the ICD-10-CM diagnosis code **M54.5, Low back pain** (or ICD-9-CM code **724.2 Lumbago**), because Dr. Conover had not yet determined the cause of the back pain.

  ❑ She assigns CPT procedure codes for the office visit and the X-ray that was performed in the office.

  ❑ She does not assign procedure codes for the blood test or the MRI because Dr. Conover did not provide those services. These services will be billed by the organization that provides the service.

▶ For the January 24 encounter, Sherry assigns the ICD-10-CM diagnosis code **M51.26, Other intervertebral disc displacement, lumbar region** (or ICD-9-CM code **722.10 Displacement of lumbar intervertebral disc without myelopathy**), because Dr. Conover established the diagnosis based on the MRI results.

  ❑ She also assigns a CPT code for the office visit.

  ❑ She does not assign procedure codes for physical therapy because Mr. Markowitz will go to a physical therapy clinic for the service. The physical therapy clinic will bill for the services it provides.

  ❑ She does not assign procedure codes for surgery because surgery was not performed.

▶ Finally, the codes and billing information will be entered into the computer and submitted to the patient's insurance company for payment.

CODING PRACTICE

Exercise 1.2   Understanding Patient Encounters

Instructions: Write the answers to the following questions in the space provided.

1. When do coders assign codes to patient encounters?

_____

_____

_____

2. What are the three steps in a patient encounter?

_____

_____

_____

3. What are the three elements involved in establishing a diagnosis?

_____

_____

CERTIFICATION

Certification is a voluntary achievement that documents that a coder has attained a certain level of proficiency by passing a rigorous examination. Certification is offered by professional organizations and is an additional step beyond a formal educational degree. It does not replace a degree and a degree is not required in order to become certified. Certification began as a form of recognition before there were many educational degrees in this area. Today, certification plus education enhances a coder's professional standing and often results in higher compensation.

Certification is not mandated by the government and is not a legal requirement. Whether or not certification is required, and which certification is acceptable, is determined by individual employers.

Most large clinics and hospitals require coders to be nationally certified. Two primary organizations offer coding certifications that are recognized by most employers: **AAPC** (formerly known as the American Academy of Professional Coders) and the **American Health Information Management Association** (AHIMA). Both organizations offer several certification credentials, each with a unique focus.

AAPC

Founded in 1988, AAPC has historically focused on physician-based and outpatient coders (■ FIGURE 1-1). Current membership is approximately 126,000, with more than 95,000 holding certification. AAPC has local chapters in many cities that hold

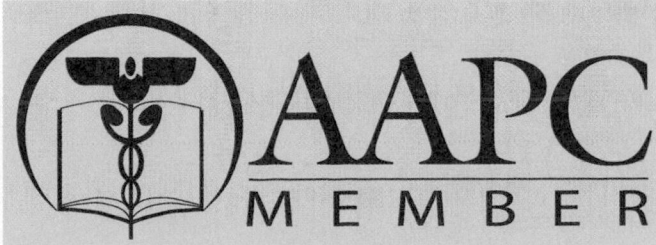

Figure 1-1 ■ AAPC offers several coding certifications.
Source: AAPC. Reprinted with permission.

monthly meetings, workshops, and provide networking opportunities for members.

The primary certification is Certified Professional Coder (CPC), which focuses on coding of services, procedures, and diagnoses for physician offices. The Certified Professional Coder-Hospital (CPC-H) certification focuses on outpatient hospital services, while the Certified Professional Coder-Payer (CPC-P) focuses on coding and reimbursement skills needed by **payers** (*insurance companies or public programs that pay for healthcare services*). The Certified Professional Coder-Apprentice (CPC-A) is earned by coders with less than two years' professional experience. AAPC also offers specialty coding certifications that enable coders to demonstrate superior levels of expertise in a medical specialty, such as orthopedics, obstetrics, or cardiology. Coders take a separate examination to achieve each type of certification.

AHIMA

Founded in 1928, AHIMA has historically focused on hospital coders and has more than 71,000 members. AHIMA has 52 Component State Associations (CSAs) that provide professional education and networking opportunities for members.

The primary certification is Certified Coding Specialist (CCS), which focuses on hospital inpatient and outpatient coding. The Certified Coding Specialist-Physician (CCS-P) certification focuses on physician-based coding. The Certified Coding Apprentice (CCA) credential is geared toward entry-level coders with little or no job experience. Additional certifications are offered in more specialized functions such as the administration of privacy and security programs in healthcare organizations; data analysis; and medical records administration. Each type of certification requires coders to take a separate examination.

AHIMA and AAPC certifications are accepted in all states. When considering which certification to pursue, it is helpful to know if one particular credential is preferred over another in the local geographic area. Research this information by reviewing job postings, talking to the human resources department at area employers, and asking experienced coders in the community. As their careers progress, some coders choose to obtain certification in more than one area of expertise, such as physician and inpatient, and may become certified by both AAPC and AHIMA. Refer to the organizations' websites, **www. aapc.com** and **www.ahima.org**, to determine the current requirements for earning each certification.

SUCCESS STEP

When you become a member of a local AAPC or AHIMA chapter, you have the opportunity to meet coders in other companies, share helpful information, and potentially learn about job openings.

CODING PRACTICE

Exercise 1.3 Certification

Instructions: Write the answers to the following questions in the space provided.

1. What is certification?

_____

_____

_____

2. List and define three certifications offered by AAPC.

_____

_____

_____

3. List and define three certifications offered by AHIMA.

_____

_____

_____

CODING CAREERS

Most coding students are seeking a long-term coding career. In addition to learning the mechanics of coding, students are wise to begin learning about their career path and job performance expectations for accuracy and productivity.

Career Path

A **career path** is the progression of jobs and responsibilities throughout one's working life. In coding, like most careers, new graduates do not start at the top; they start at a basic level and work their way up with greater responsibility and more skills at each level. The career options, compensation, and benefits generally increase at each level of advancement. Advancement may come from within the same organization or it may come by moving to a new organization. In order to plan a possible career path, coding students want to learn about the job market, levels of advancement, and internal and external jobs.

Understanding the Job Market

Coders have many career options regarding where they work and what type of job they perform. While many students imagine themselves working in a hospital, the healthcare field offers many other types of organizations as well. Potential employers include all types of healthcare providers, payers, and third-party service organizations such as medical billing services. Sometimes it is best to start out in a small medical or dental office to get basic experience and then move to a larger organization later in your career. Working for a health insurance company or medical billing service can give coders a broad range of experience that will open up many career options later on. ■ TABLE 1-3 lists examples of various types of healthcare employers.

Table 1-3 ■ EXAMPLES OF TYPES OF ORGANIZATIONS THAT MAY REQUIRE CODING SKILLS

❏ Acupuncturist	❏ Medical billing service
❏ Ambulance service	❏ Naturopathic office (ND)
❏ Ambulatory surgery center (ASC)	❏ Nursing facility (NF)
❏ Chiropractic office (DC)	❏ Optometrist (OD)
❏ Clearinghouse	❏ Osteopath (DO)
❏ Consulting firm	❏ Pharmacy
❏ Dental office	❏ Physician office (medical, surgical, all specialties) (MD)
❏ Durable Medical Equipment supplier (DME)	❏ Physical therapy clinic
❏ Health insurance company	❏ Self-insured employer
❏ Home healthcare	❏ Temporary staffing agency
❏ Hospital	❏ Third Party Administrator (TPA)
❏ Laboratory	❏ Workers' Compensation (WC)

Table 1-4 ■ EXAMPLES OF JOB TITLES THAT MAY REQUIRE CODING SKILLS

❑ Accounts Receivable (A/R) Specialist	❑ Insurance Follow-up Specialist
❑ Admitting Clerk	❑ Insurance Verifier
❑ Billing Clerk	❑ Intake Specialist
❑ Charge Entry Specialist	❑ Medical Biller
❑ Claims Analyst	❑ Medical Receptionist
❑ Claims Processor	❑ Medical Records Clerk
❑ Coder I/Coder II	❑ Patient Account Specialist
❑ Coding Assistant	❑ Patient Financial Services Clerk
❑ Electronic Claims Processor	❑ Patient Service Representative
❑ Health Information Analyst	❑ Refund Specialist
❑ Insurance Biller	❑ Scheduler

There are many job titles in the field of medical coding (■ TABLE 1-4). The same job might be called by different titles in two different organizations, so it is good to be open minded about potential job titles.

SUCCESS STEP

Some job titles, such as Accounts Receivable or Biller, are also used by nonmedical businesses. Even the job title Coder can apply to a computer engineer. When searching job postings, remember to specify a search for the healthcare field.

Levels of Advancement

Most coders look for an **entry-level job** upon graduation in order to gain basic skills, become familiar with the healthcare field, and establish excellent work habits. When possible, coders can look for a job in healthcare that builds on previous experience in a call center, bookkeeping, customer service, or patient care. Some companies offer internships (*paid training programs for those new to the field*), but this is not the norm.

After a few years of experience at entry level, coders potentially become eligible for advancement to a **midlevel job**. A midlevel job allows coders to expand their skills, learn new specialties, assume more independence, and take on more responsibility.

After five or so years of proven experience, coders can progress to an **advanced-level job**. Advanced-level jobs require a solid track record of good performance in a related area. Advanced-level jobs often include management of others but may also focus on a specialized area of expertise, such as chart auditing. Technical specialization is an excellent career path for coders who are not interested in supervision or management of others. ■ TABLE 1-5 shows examples of a coding career path in a physician office, a hospital, and an insurance company.

Table 1-5 ■ EXAMPLES OF A CODING CAREER PATH

	Years of Experience	Physician Office	Hospital	Insurance Company
Entry Level	0–2 years	Front office receptionist Medical records file clerk Charge data entry operator	Admissions representative Cashier Billing office data entry clerk Patient account representative	Member services representative Claims representative trainee Sales assistant
Midlevel	3–5 years	Coding specialist Insurance verifier Referral coordinator Billing specialist Home-based coder	Outpatient billing clerk Medical documentation researcher Patient accounts team leader Coding assistant	Claims analyst Provider services representative Member services team leader Hospital claims specialist
Advanced Level	More than 5 years	Billing manager Coding manager Chart auditor Collections manager	Chart auditor Medical records manager Inpatient coding specialist Home-based coder Cancer registrar Patient accounts manager	Supervisor, member services Supervisor, claims processing Claims auditor Legal researcher
		Consulting - Freelance coder - Business owner - Trainer - Author - Instructor		

Internal and External Job Openings

When coders are ready to change jobs and advance their careers, they may seek a new job internally within their current organization, or they may choose to look externally for a job with a different company.

Many organizations post their job openings internally, available only to current employees, for a period of time before they are advertised to the public. This means that established employees can apply for a promotion or transfer to another department but stay with the same company and keep their benefits. Companies like to promote from within because they are already familiar with the employee's personality and work ethic. Therefore, one good career strategy for a coder is to identify a desired employer, secure an entry-level job in that company, perform at a high level, and take advantage of opportunities to move to another job in the same company when ready.

Coders can also move between types of organizations, such as from an insurance company to a doctor's office or hospital. When coders start in a small office that has limited advancement opportunities, they can progress by moving to a larger organization or another small one that has an opening at a more advanced level. When they want to gain experience in another aspect of the healthcare industry, they can seek employment with a different type of organization. If an ultimate career goal, such as a hospital coding position, cannot be achieved in the first job, then coders can plan a career path to help get there.

SUCCESS STEP

Joining your local chapter of AAPC or AHIMA will give you the chance to get to know coders in other companies and can potentially lead to future job opportunities. Networking in this manner is an important part of your career path.

Performance Expectations

Whatever career path coders choose, or even if they are not sure where they want to end up, it is always important to demonstrate excellent job attendance, follow directions, and meet the employer's expectations for quantity and quality of work. Every job task is an opportunity to earn a good reference, and it is those recommendations that help coders get to the next step in their careers.

Performance expectations are the outcomes employers need coders to achieve in order to demonstrate competence in the job. Coding jobs have high expectations because securing payment for services from insurance companies requires a high degree of accuracy and productivity by coders. Most employers have expectations related to coding accuracy and productivity.

Coding Accuracy

Coding accuracy involves the three coding skills discussed earlier in this chapter: abstracting, assigning, and arranging (sequencing). The average expectation for coding accuracy in these three areas is 95% to 98%. New coders' work is reviewed by a mentor or supervisor until they achieve the required level of accuracy. Samples of all coders' work are reviewed by supervisors and peers on an ongoing basis to ensure that everyone maintains a high level of accuracy. High accuracy is required to be eligible for greater responsibility, advancement, or special benefits such as working from home.

Productivity

Not only is accuracy critical to a coder's job, high productivity (*the amount of work accomplished in a specified time frame*) is also necessary. Productivity skills include keyboarding and case production, which are discussed next.

Keyboarding. Most coders use computers to determine or enter the codes. Therefore, high levels of speed and accuracy in keyboarding are essential. Coders must be proficient in alphanumeric (*a combination of letters and numbers*) keyboarding because most codes contain both letters and numbers. Many employers require that coders pass a keyboarding test before they schedule a job interview. Each employer sets its own speed requirement; 30 to 40 words per minute (wpm) or 9,000 to 12,000 keystrokes per hour (ksph) are common minimums. In keyboarding, any errors are deducted from the overall speed, so it is best to work on accuracy first, and then build up speed after the basics are mastered. With daily keyboarding drills, most students can achieve this minimum level in six months or less.

Case Production. Most coders are expected to meet a **case production** standard to code a specific number of cases each day, while maintaining high accuracy. The specific production standard is based on the type of record being coded; whether coders are assigning diagnosis codes, procedure codes, or both; whether coders work from paper or electronic charts; and what other responsibilities, such as billing, coders do at the same time. For example, coders who specialize in radiology coding generally code more encounters per hour than coders who specialize in complex surgical procedures because the records they are coding from are far less complicated. ■ TABLE 1-6 provides examples of case production standards. Students do not achieve these production standards while learning, but such standards are common in the workplace.

Table 1-6 ■ **EXAMPLES OF CASE PRODUCTION STANDARDS**

Specialty	Charts per Hour
Emergency Department	10–30
Inpatient Hospital	4–10
Laboratory	100–200
Radiology	100–200
Surgery	1–8

CODING PRACTICE

Exercise 1.4 Coding Careers

Instructions: Write the answers to the following questions in the space provided.

1. List five types of organizations that may require coding skills.

_____

_____

_____

_____

_____

2. Why do coding jobs have high performance expectations?

_____

_____

_____

_____

_____

3. What keyboarding speed rate is commonly required by employers? _____

_____

CHAPTER SUMMARY

In this chapter you learned that:

- Coding is the process of accurately assigning codes to verbal descriptions of patients' conditions and the healthcare services provided to treat those conditions.
- The three skills of an ace coder are abstracting, assigning, and arranging (sequencing).
- Coders assign diagnosis and procedure codes to patient encounters after an encounter is completed.

- Certification is a voluntary achievement that documents a coder having attained a certain level of proficiency by passing a rigorous examination offered by AAPC or AHIMA.
- Students are wise to learn about their career path and job performance expectations for accuracy and productivity.

CONCEPT QUIZ

Take a moment to look back through this chapter and solidify your skills. This is your opportunity to pull together everything you have learned.

Completion

Instructions: Write the term that answers each question based on the information you learned in this chapter. Choose from the following list. Some choices may be used more than once, and some choices may not be used at all.

abstract	diagnosis
accuracy	inpatient
amend	keyboarding
ancillary	outpatient
arrange	procedure
assign	production
assume	query
attending	testing
career path	treatment
code	

1. _____ codes describe patient illnesses, diseases, conditions, injuries, or other reasons for seeking healthcare services.

2. The three skills of an "ace" coder are to _____ information from the medical record; _____ the accurate code number; and _____ the codes in proper order.

3. _____ encounters are physician interactions with patients who have not been formally admitted to a healthcare institution, such as an acute care hospital, long-term care facility, or rehabilitation facility.

4. _____ encounters are physician interactions with patients who have been formally admitted to a healthcare facility, such as an acute care hospital, long-term care facility, or rehabilitation facility.

5. _____ services include laboratory, radiology, or physical therapy.

6. The _____ physician oversees and coordinates all aspects of the patient's care.

7. A _____ is the progression of jobs and responsibilities throughout one's working life.

(continued)

(continued from page 11)

8. The _____ plan may include medication, surgery, lifestyle changes, or therapy.

9. When the documentation is unclear, coders _____ the physician for clarification.

10. Most coders are expected to meet a case _____ standard to code a specific number of cases each day, while maintaining high _____.

Multiple Choice

Instructions: Circle the letter of the best answer to each question based on the information you learned in this chapter.

1. The replacement code set used for diagnosis coding is
   A. HCPCS.
   B. ICD-9-CM Volume 2.
   C. ICD-10-CM.
   D. ICD-10-PCS.

2. _____ is the replacement code set that is used for hospital inpatient procedure coding.
   A. CDT
   B. CPT
   C. ICD-9-CM Volume 1
   D. ICD-10-PCS

3. Which of the following is NOT a HIPAA-mandated code set?
   A. ICD-10-CM
   B. DSM-V
   C. CDT
   D. NDC

4. What is a specific interaction between a patient and healthcare provider?
   A. Admission
   B. Office visit
   C. Observation
   D. Encounter

5. Which of the following is NOT an example of an outpatient encounter?
   A. Ambulatory surgery
   B. Hospital admission
   C. Emergency department
   D. Observation

6. Coders do which of the following tasks?
   A. Determine what condition(s) the patient has based on the symptoms.
   B. Assign diagnostic and procedure codes for patient encounters after an encounter is completed.
   C. Code for services planned, but not provided, during the current encounter.
   D. Code for past conditions that are resolved.

7. Which statement about certification is NOT true?
   A. All states legally mandate coder certification.
   B. Certification is a voluntary achievement.
   C. Professional organizations offer certification.
   D. Coders have a choice of which certification to pursue.

8. What kind of job do most coders seek upon graduation in order to gain basic skills, become familiar with the healthcare field, and establish excellent work habits?
   A. Hospital
   B. Entry-level
   C. Midlevel
   D. Advanced-level

9. Which of the following is an example of an entry-level job?
   A. Data Entry Clerk
   B. Insurance Verifier
   C. Inpatient Coding Specialist
   D. Coding Assistant

10. How do organizations post their job openings to make them available only to current employees for a period of time before they are advertised to the public?
    A. Internally
    B. Externally
    C. Online
    D. Word of mouth

Coding and Reimbursement

Chapter 2

Learning Objectives

After completing this chapter, you should have the skills to:

2.1 Spell and define the key words, medical terms, and abbreviations relating to reimbursement.

2.2 Define the types of healthcare payers.

2.3 Discuss the importance and content of documentation.

2.4 Describe the life cycle of an insurance claim.

2.5 Explain the federal compliance initiatives.

Chapter Outline

- **Healthcare Payers**
- **Documentation**
- **Life Cycle of an Insurance Claim**
- **Federal Compliance**

Key Terms and Abbreviations

abuse
audit
automatic adjudication
beneficiary
Centers for Medicare and Medicaid Services (CMS)
Children's Health Insurance Program (CHIP)
clean claim
compliance
denied
Department of Health and Human Services (HHS)
documentation
entitlement program
explanation of benefits (EOB)

False Claims Act (FCA)
fraud
front-end edit check
group health plan
individual health insurance
managed care plan
manual review
Medicaid
medical necessity
medical payment
medical record
medical review
Medicare
Medicare Administrative Contractor (MAC)

Medicare Advantage
Medigap
Office of the Inspector General (OIG)
Original Medicare
overcoding
Part A
Part B
Part C
Part D
personal injury protection (PIP)
preferred provider
private health insurance
progress note
prompt pay

Qui Tam
reconcile
Recovery Audit Contractor (RAC)
rejected claim
remittance advice (RA)
self-insured health plan
suspended
third-party administrator (TPA)
third-party payer
Tricare (TC)
Veterans Health Administration (VHA)
whistleblower
workers' compensation (WC)

In addition to the key terms listed here, students should know the terms defined within tables in this chapter.

INTRODUCTION

When driving, you know that you need to obey the laws and that some laws, such as the speed limit, vary from town to town and state to state. If you miss seeing a speed limit sign, you know the state police will not accept that as an excuse. In healthcare, you also need to understand the rules of different entities, such as different payers. Even if your ultimate job does not directly involve billing, you still want to have a basic understanding of how your work as coder impacts reimbursement so you can become a valuable team member.

HEALTHCARE PAYERS

Third-party payers are entities other than the patient or physician who pay for healthcare services. They reimburse physicians and hospitals for 86% of all healthcare services in the United States. Patients pay the remaining 14% of services directly. Third-party payers include several government programs, over 1,300 private insurance companies, workers' compensation, and automobile medical payments insurance. Coders need to understand the various types of third-party payers because each has separate, and sometimes conflicting, rules about coding and billing.

All healthcare payments to hospitals, physicians, and other providers are based on coding. Procedure codes describe the services provided to patients. Physicians and hospitals assign money charges to each procedure code. Diagnosis codes justify why the services were needed. When the diagnosis code(s) does not adequately explain why the services were provided, payment may be denied or delayed.

Government Programs

Health benefit plans funded by federal or state governments pay for 47% of healthcare services. These are **entitlement programs** for which **beneficiaries** (*recipients of services*) qualify based on specific criteria. The various types of government and private insurance programs are summarized in the following sections.

Medicare

Medicare, sometimes abbreviated as MCR, established in 1965, is funded by the federal government and is the single largest payer of healthcare services in the United States, accounting for 24% of healthcare payments. Medicare is administered by the **Centers for Medicare and Medicaid Services (CMS)**, which is a division of the **Department of Health and Human Services (HHS)**. Medicare pays for healthcare services for most people age 65 and over, people of any age with end-stage renal disease, and people with disabilities. Because it is so large, Medicare has a tremendous impact on healthcare policy and payment trends and, by extension, on coding. Other government programs and private health insurance are not required to follow Medicare rules, but it is not unusual for them to follow Medicare's lead to a considerable extent. The Medicare program has four parts, each of which also has separate rules and coding guidelines.

Part A. Medicare **Part A**, also called **Original Medicare** or traditional Medicare, is hospital insurance that covers a specific list of services for inpatient hospital care, skilled nursing facilities, hospice, and home healthcare. Most Americans who have worked as an adult, or are married to someone who has, are automatically eligible for Part A and do not pay a premium to receive benefits. They do pay deductibles and coinsurance.

Part B. Medicare **Part B** covers a specific list of physician services, outpatient hospital care, and home healthcare. It was created to provide medical coverage in addition to the hospital coverage of Part A. Part B is optional and most people are required to pay a premium to enroll, as well as deductibles and coinsurance.

Medicare Part A and Part B claims are processed by private companies called **Medicare Administrative Contractors (MACs)**. Many Medicare coding and billing rules are the same across the country, but MACs have latitude in how certain policies are interpreted and applied. Therefore, coders need to keep up to date on the national rules, as well as the MAC rules.

Part C. Medicare **Part C**, also called **Medicare Advantage**, is an optional replacement of Part A and Part B that is offered by private health insurance companies. Many Part C plans are managed care and often have a preferred or required network of providers. Private insurance companies are paid through contracts with Medicare and believe they can provide care more cost effectively than traditional Medicare, thus making a profit. Patients choose Part C when they believe they can receive more benefits for the same or slightly more cost. The amount of premium, deductible, and coinsurance varies with each plan offered by a private company.

Part D. Medicare **Part D**, also called prescription drug coverage, is offered by private insurance companies through contracts with Medicare and provides limited benefits for prescription drugs. Patients choose from a variety of private plans, each of which may cover different medications, and select the one that covers the majority of their most costly prescriptions. Patients pay premiums, deductibles, and coinsurance. According to Medicare, most Part C plans also include Part D.

Medigap. Medigap is a Medicare supplement insurance policy sold by private insurance companies to fill gaps in Part A and Part B coverage. In most states, patients choose from ten standardized plans labeled Plan A through Plan J. Medigap policies apply only to Original Medicare, not Part C.

Medicaid

Medicaid, sometimes abbreviated as MCD, also established in 1965, is a program for low-income families that is funded jointly by the federal government and state governments. It accounts for 18% of national healthcare payments. CMS establishes the general plan requirements, but states have considerable latitude in determining eligibility and coverage rules. Billing and coding requirements are also determined and administered by each state.

Other Government Programs

Other government programs include:

- Tricare (TC)—health insurance coverage for family members of active duty personnel and for retired military personnel and their families.

- Children's Health Insurance Program (CHIP)—established in 1997 by the federal government to provide health insurance to children in families with incomes below 200% of the federal poverty level.
- Veterans Health Administration (VHA)—an integrated healthcare delivery system with more than 1,400 sites of care, including hospitals, community clinics, community living centers, and various other facilities to provide health services to veterans with service-connected disabilities.

Private Health Insurance

Private health insurance is coverage for healthcare services offered by private corporations, such as Aetna, Cigna, or UnitedHealthcare, and not-for-profit organizations, such as Blue Cross and Blue Shield. Private health insurance pays for 39% of national healthcare expenses. The three major sources of private health insurance are group health plans, self-insured plans, and individual insurance. Each insurance company and each plan offered by a company may have different requirements for coding and billing. Typically, the provider's coding and billing departments maintain files on the requirements of each plan. Most laws regarding private health insurance companies are determined by each state's legislature and implemented by the state Department of Insurance.

Group Health Plans

Approximately 60% of Americans are covered by a **group health plan** offered through their employer or union. The employer or union contracts with a private insurance company to provide a specific list of benefits to its employees. Often, they negotiate more than one option, each with a different set of benefits and different costs. The advantage of a group health plan is that the risk, or cost of medical care, is shared by a large number of people, resulting in lower premiums.

Employees choose which plan they want to enroll in based on its benefits and costs. Typically the employer pays the majority of the monthly premium and deducts a smaller portion of the premium, such as 10% or 20%, from employees' paychecks. Usually employees can cover their family members for an additional cost. In addition, employees pay deductibles and coinsurance or copays for the actual services they receive.

Self-Insured Health Plans

Self-insured health plans are offered by large employers or unions who, rather than purchasing group health insurance, set aside money in a reserve fund and pay for employees' medical expenses from the fund. States regulate how much money employers must set aside in order to ensure that they will have enough money to pay catastrophic (high cost) medical expenses.

In all other respects, a self-insured plan works similarly to a group health plan in that a specific list of benefits is covered, and, typically, employees pay a small monthly premium, deductibles, coinsurance, and copayments for medical care received. Often claims are processed by a private company called a **third-party administrator (TPA)**.

Individual Health Insurance

Individual health insurance is a plan that people purchase directly from a health insurance company, such as those who are self-employed or do not have benefits through an employer or government program. Approximately 9% of Americans are covered by individual health insurance.

Workers' Compensation

Workers' compensation (WC) plans pay for medical costs due to employment-related injuries or illnesses. Each state establishes its own requirements for WC insurance, but must comply with federal minimums. WC may be offered by private insurance companies approved by the state, large companies who self-insure, or a statewide insurance pool. Employers pay insurance premiums to cover the costs of care injured employees receive. Federal government employees are covered by federal WC plans.

WC programs are not subject to HIPAA regulations because they do not qualify as a health insurance plan. However, states have separate privacy and security rules that govern WC. WC plans may have unique coding and billing requirements, such as their own private code sets. Coding departments need to maintain a file containing these unique requirements.

Automobile Insurance

Automobile insurance policies often include **medical payments**, also called med pay, coverage or **personal injury protection (PIP)**, which pays for medical expenses incurred during an automobile accident. Automobile insurance is regulated by each state's Department of Insurance, not by federal or HIPAA laws that govern health insurance companies. Auto insurance companies often contract with external bill review companies to review medical claims and recommend payment amounts. Coders need to be aware of any special requirements for patients being treated for automobile accident injuries. Typically the coding or billing department maintains a file detailing these requirements for each company.

Managed Care Plans

Managed care plans are companies that attempt to control the cost of healthcare while providing better outcomes. There are many different forms of managed care, but, in general, managed care plans contract with physicians, hospitals, and other providers to offer services for a lower fee than health plans; then they contract with private health insurance companies and self-insured plans to promote an exclusive network of **preferred providers**. When patients use preferred providers, they are responsible for lower out-of-pocket costs for deductibles, coinsurance, and copayments than if they select a provider not on the preferred list. Managed care plans are not a separate type of insurance, but rather a way of offering services to patients who are enrolled in a group health plan, self-insured plan, or individual health plan. Managed care plans also offer services to Medicare Part C programs, Medicaid, and even WC. Managed care companies are regulated primarily by federal laws. Well-known managed care plans include Kaiser Permanente, Group Health Cooperative, WellPoint, and Humana.

CODING PRACTICE

Exercise 2.1 **Healthcare Payers**

Instructions: Write the answers to the following questions in the space provided.

1. Medicare pays for healthcare services for whom?

2. Medicaid pays for healthcare services for whom?

3. What are the three types of private health insurance plans?

DOCUMENTATION

Payers have freedom to determine what services they will include in an insurance policy based on state and federal requirements, but they also have a contractual obligation to pay for these services. To fulfill this obligation they may request information to determine whether the service is covered, including the site (location) of service; the medical need for and appropriateness of the diagnostic and therapeutic services provided; and the accuracy of codes for services billed based on the medical record.

Medical Necessity

The fact that a physician determines a patient needs a particular service or supply item does not mean that the insurance company or payer will agree. **Medical necessity** (*establishing the medical need for services*) is one of several criteria payers use to determine if, and how much, they will pay for a particular service. One of the reasons that payers establish medical necessity rules is to avoid paying unscrupulous providers who might provide a service just so they could receive payments, not because the patient actually needs the service or would benefit from it. It also helps prevent patients from demanding services they do not need, such as expensive tests or cosmetic surgery.

Each of the payers discussed earlier in this chapter establishes its own definition of medical necessity and writes it into each insurance policy. ■ Table 2-1 lists common criteria for medical necessity and examples of each. By law, Medicare can pay only for services that are medically necessary, which is defined as services and supplies that

- are needed to diagnose or treat a medical condition or improve the functioning of a malformed body member;
- meet the standards of good medical practice in the local area; and
- are not mainly for the convenience of the patient or physician.

In addition to a general definition of medical necessity, payers may also establish criteria for specific conditions, such as limiting the number of physical therapy visits for back pain; requiring an X-ray before ordering more expensive magnetic resonance imaging (MRI); or restricting the age and frequency of preventive screening, such as a screening mammogram every two years for women over age 50. When providers recommend a treatment that varies from the insurance company's standard list, they may need to obtain preauthorization and provide special reports to justify the service. For some conditions, specific medical necessity criteria are not public information, and patients may learn of them only after a claim is **denied** (*the claim was processed and found to be ineligible for payment*).

Coders should not manipulate codes in a way that distorts or alters the diagnoses and procedures as documented in the medical record. This is unethical and fraudulent. Coders do need to be certain they are accurately describing everything that was done for the patient and the reasons for which the services were provided.

Table 2-1 ■ **EXAMPLES OF MEDICAL NECESSITY CRITERIA**

Criterion	Appropriate Example	Inappropriate Example
Improve a patient's condition	Physical therapy to treat an acute back injury	Ongoing physical therapy to maintain general back comfort
Evidence-based practice	Medications proven to benefit patients based on scientific studies	Experimental drugs or treatments
Rendered by appropriate provider	Patient going to internal medicine or family practice physician to diagnose an initial symptom (e.g., stomach pain)	Patient going directly to gastroenterologist and having many expensive tests performed to diagnose an initial symptom of stomach pain
Least-restrictive setting	Suture removal in physician office; outpatient cataract surgery	Suture removal in the emergency department; inpatient cataract surgery without a medical reason
Not for patient or physician convenience	Liposuction for medical reasons	Liposuction for cosmetic reasons

The Medical Record

The **medical record** is the comprehensive collection of all information on a patient at a particular facility. A medical record may be paper based or electronic and provides a written, chronological record of the patient's care, including important facts, findings, and observations about an individual's health history and health status (■ FIGURE 2-1 and ■ FIGURE 2-2). It reports past and present illnesses, examinations, tests, treatments, and outcomes and is a legal document that verifies the care provided. The diagnosis and procedure codes reported on the health insurance claim form or billing statement must be supported by information in the medical record for each encounter. Patients have separate medical records with each physician they see and each facility to which they are admitted.

> ### SUCCESS STEP
>
> The medical record is admissible in a court of law as evidence and must be handled with the same care as any legal document.

Documentation is the written or electronic record of medical care and services provided. The word *documentation* is used to refer to the overall medical record as well as to **progress notes** (*the record of a specific patient encounter*). Thorough documentation is necessary, not only because it is the basis for delivering high-quality patient care but also because it helps improve reimbursement. Excellent documentation can reduce the amount of time needed to code a claim, result in more accurate and complete coding, and minimize common problems associated with claims processing. ■ TABLE 2-2 (page 18) shows

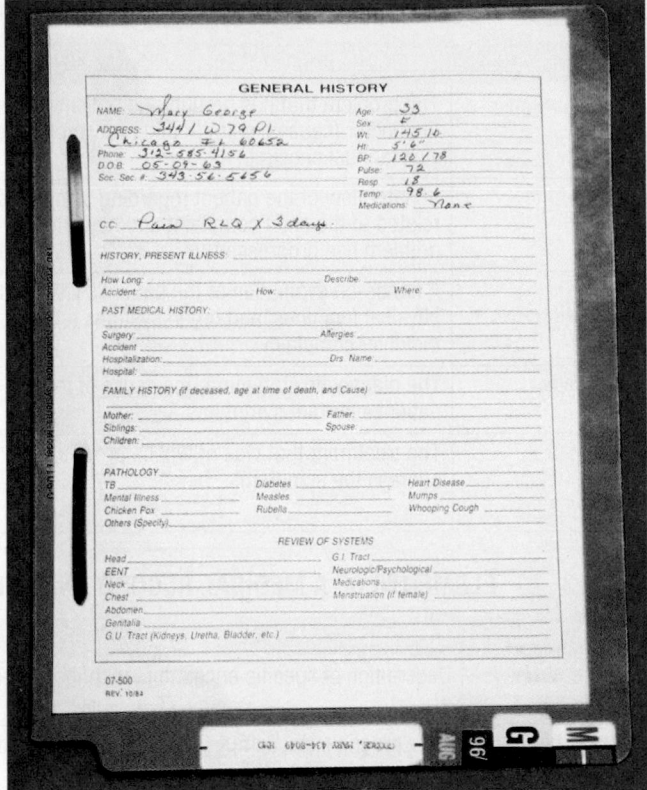

Figure 2-1 ■ Example of a Paper-Based Medical Record

major elements of a progress note and how coders use each type of information.

■ TABLE 2-3 (page 18) shows major elements of a medical record and how coders use each type of information.

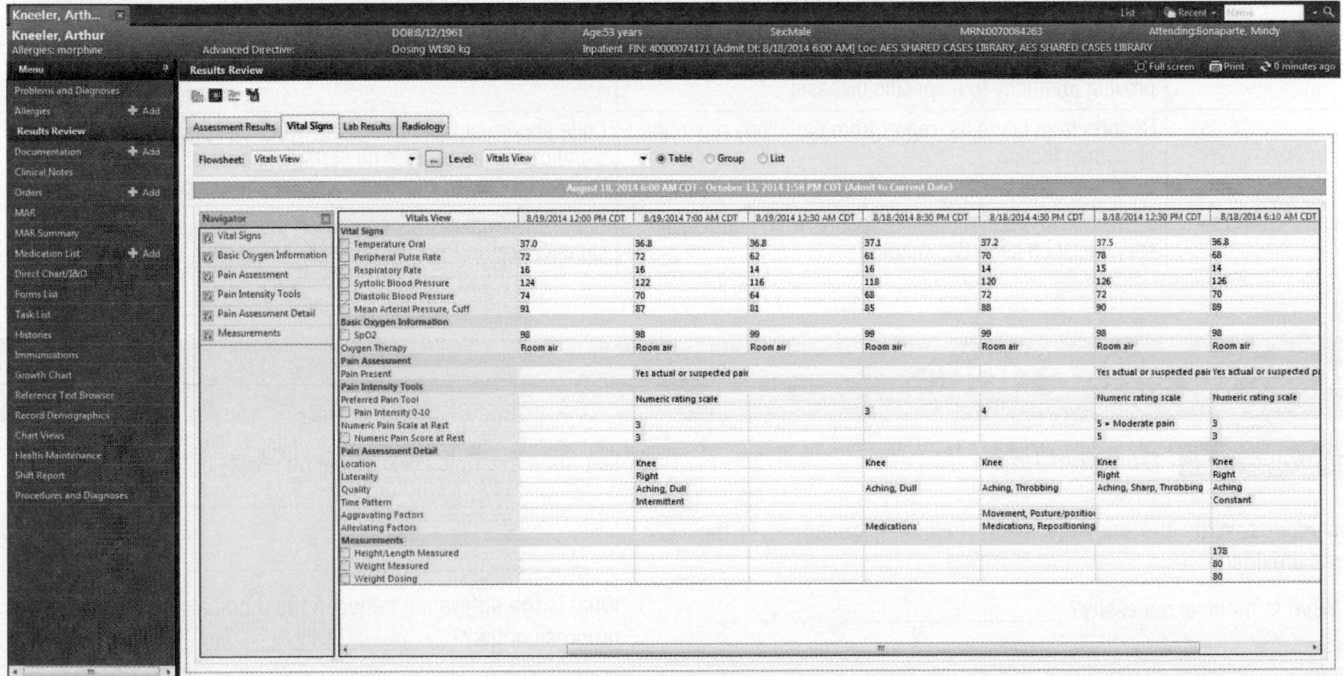

Figure 2-2 ■ Example of an Electronic Medical Record.
Source: © by Cerner Corporation. Used by permission of Cerner Corporation.

Table 2-2 ■ **ELEMENTS OF A PROGRESS NOTE AND THEIR USE IN CODING**

Element	Description	Coding Application
Chief complaint (CC)	The problem that has brought the patient to see the doctor (nausea, pain) or other reason for the visit (annual checkup)	Code for symptoms if the physician does not make a definitive diagnosis for an outpatient encounter.
History of the present illness (HPI)	An interview of the patient regarding symptoms related to the chief complaint and how the problem has progressed	May add details to the diagnostic statement.
Physical examination (PE)	A hands-on evaluation of the patient's vital signs, physical functions, and organ systems relevant to the chief complaint	May add details to the diagnostic statement.
Assessment	The diagnostic statement; the cause of the patient's current symptoms	This is the starting point for assigning diagnosis codes. Verify the details using other areas of the medical record when necessary.
Plan	The treatment that was or will be provided to address the symptoms	Inpatient hospitals code for procedures performed during the stay. Outpatient hospitals and physicians code for services provided during the encounter. Do not code for future planned treatments.

Table 2-3 ■ **ELEMENTS OF A MEDICAL RECORD AND THEIR USE IN CODING**

Element	Description	Coding Application
Progress notes	Description of specific encounters with the patient	Code each patient encounter based on the progress notes for that visit.
Obstetric history	Prior pregnancies, complications, and their outcomes	Use specific codes for first pregnancy, previous multiple pregnancies, and history of certain complications.
Surgical history	Date and type of past operations, operative reports (a narrative of exactly how the surgeon performed the procedure)	Assign codes for acquired absence (*surgical removal*) of certain organs. When an operation is performed during the current encounter, review the operative report to determine the exact procedure performed and the postoperative diagnosis.
Medications and medical allergies	Current and past medications; allergies to specific medications	Code for long-term use of certain medications.
Family history	The health status of immediate family members, causes of death (if known), diseases common in the family	Assign codes for family history of certain conditions.
Social history	Education, occupation, religious affiliation, natural support network, lifestyle habits (tobacco, alcohol, illicit drug use, sexual activity)	Assign codes for certain lifestyle habits.
Immunization history	Date and type of past vaccinations, titers (blood tests proving immunity to a specific disease)	Do not code for past vaccinations.
Lab test/ pathology results	Reports from lab tests; report from pathology regarding specimen testing	Code abnormal test results only when the physician indicates significance and makes no certain diagnosis. Review pathology reports for biopsy results (e.g., malignant neoplasm).
Ancillary reports	Narrative reports or copies of reports from additional services such as EKGs, imaging	Code abnormal results only when the physician indicates significance and makes no certain diagnosis.

CODING PRACTICE

Exercise 2.2 Documentation

Instructions: Write the answers to the following questions in the space provided.

1. What is medical necessity? _____
_____
_____

2. List three examples of medical necessity criteria.
_____
_____
_____

3. What is the difference between the medical record and progress notes? _____
_____
_____

LIFE CYCLE OF AN INSURANCE CLAIM

There are many steps involved in converting a patient encounter into a paid insurance claim. Each step needs to be completed in a timely and accurate manner in order for providers to receive correct payment for their services. The exact procedures are not the same in every office and every hospital, but the general process is similar.

Before the Encounter

The life cycle of an insurance claim begins when the patient calls the physician to make an appointment, a patient arrives at the emergency department, or a physician admits a patient to the hospital. Although providers do not code or bill for scheduling an appointment, the appointment begins when providers begin collecting insurance information. When time allows, patients preregister by completing paperwork regarding their health condition and insurance prior to the appointment. The provider verifies eligibility with the insurance company through a telephone call or secure website in order to determine if the patient is covered by insurance and what services are covered and/or require preauthorization.

During the Encounter

When patients arrive for their appointment or hospital admission, they complete registration forms or confirm the preregistration information, provide a copy of their insurance card, and possibly make a payment, if required by the insurance. They see the physician and/or receive the treatments and procedures needed. The physician documents the patient's problem in a progress note and may check off services and diagnoses on an encounter form or charge slip. Finally, patients check out, schedule the next appointment, if needed, and may make a payment if they did not pay before they saw the physician.

After the Encounter

After the encounter is complete, the specific steps for coding and billing depend on how the encounter is recorded. In a physician's office that uses encounter forms, the physician will have already checked off the services and diagnoses for the visit. The encounter form is given to the billing department for data entry into the computer. If no encounter form is used, the chart is given to the coding department, where a coder reviews the progress note, assigns diagnosis and procedure codes, and enters the codes into the computer. The billing department verifies that all information for the encounter is complete. Usually the computer system automatically inserts the charges for each procedure entered by the coder, so billers also verify that all charges are present and accurate. When they have completed their verifications, billers flag the claim in the computer as ready to be submitted to the insurance company. Most offices transmit claims electronically, usually daily or weekly depending on the volume of claims. Small offices with 10 or fewer employees may print out claims on paper billing forms and mail them, but this is becoming less common.

At the Insurance Company

When payers receive electronic claims, the computer system first performs a **front-end edit check**, which scans the claims for valid data including the policy number, patient name, provider number, diagnosis codes, and procedure codes. If any data was entered incorrectly by the biller or coder, such as a nonexistent code number or policy number, the computer automatically rejects the claim. A **rejected claim** is one that is not accepted into the insurance company's computer system for processing due to missing or invalid data. Providers may learn of rejected claims through an electronic or paper report. However, sometimes they may not know the claim was rejected until they notice that payment was never received. When paper claims are submitted, the insurance company either scans them or enters data manually, then runs the front-end edit.

Clean claims are those that pass the front-end edit checks and have no missing or invalid information. Most clean claims are processed using **automatic adjudication**, a process in which the computer automatically determines which procedure codes are covered, calculates how much the insurance company is obligated to pay, then triggers the payment. Medicare is required to pay clean claims within 14 days of receipt. Many private payers also pay clean claims within a few days of receipt.

The payment may be sent to the provider either electronically or by a paper check. The insurance company also sends a **remittance advice (RA)** or **explanation of benefits (EOB)**, a statement that lists all the services the provider billed, which ones were accepted for payment, how much the insurance company will pay, how much the patient owes, and how much will not be paid. If there are any services that are not eligible to be paid, the statement lists the reasons. Although the terms RA and EOB often are used interchangeably, the RA is the statement sent to the provider and the EOB is the statement sent to the patient. The EOB contains information similar to the RA, but it may be formatted differently and contain fewer details, such as no diagnosis or procedure codes.

Some claims are **suspended** from the automatic process for **manual review**. Reasons that claims are suspended include the following:

- high dollar amounts
- specific diagnoses and procedures that the payer may wish to monitor
- medical necessity review
- illogical information, such as a patient gender or age that does not match the codes
- questions about the patient's enrollment status
- any other reason the payer may want to research.

A claims analyst reviews the claim, determines if more information is needed from the provider or patient, and sends a letter if needed. Sometimes the claims analyst may have medical questions about the claim, such as if the procedure was appropriate for the diagnosis or if all of the services were medically necessary. These claims are sent to the **medical review** department, where a nurse, physician, or other clinician investigates the situation. They also may send a letter to the provider or patient requesting additional information or copies of documentation.

Clean claims may be processed within a few days of receipt, but claims that require manual review may take several weeks. Most states have **prompt pay** laws that require insurance companies to process claims within a specific period of time, such as 30 or 45 days. If the claim cannot be processed because of missing or incorrect information, insurance companies must issue any inquiry letters to providers or patients within this timeframe.

Table 2-4 ■ **CODING PROBLEMS CAUSING REJECTED OR DENIED CLAIMS**

Problem	Example
Characters in a code are mistyped, creating an invalid code.	Diagnosis code **007.0** instead of **O07.0** (number *zero* instead of letter *Oh*) PCS code **0J533ZZ** instead of **0J553ZZ**
Codes have too many or too few characters.	Diagnosis code **T20.511** instead of **T20.511A** Diagnosis code **Q68.10** instead of **Q68.1**
Diagnosis does not match the procedure.	Diagnosis code **K28.0 Acute gastrojejunal ulcer with hemorrhage** with a procedure code for removal of gallbladder. This may happen when the code was mistyped and should have been **K82.0 Obstruction of gallbladder.**
Codes are sequenced incorrectly.	Diagnosis codes **M36.1 Arthroplasty in neoplastic disease** and **C91.A0 Mature B-cell leukemia Burkitt type not having achieved remission.** An instructional note with code M36.1 instructs the coder to "Code first underlying neoplasm."
Additional codes are required.	Diagnosis code **I69.891 Dysphagia following other cerebrovascular disease** instructs coder to "Use additional code to identify the type of dysphagia."
The services described in one code are included (bundled) into another code.	CPT procedure code **58150** includes removal of uterus, ovaries, and fallopian tubes, so these should not be billed separately.
Patient age or gender does not match the diagnosis or procedure.	Diagnosis code **O09.611 Supervision of young primigravida, first trimester** used for 18 year old, but the code is defined as younger than age 16 at expected date of delivery.
A CPT procedure code requires a modifier in order to be paid.	Two lesions of the same size on the same site are removed. Append CPT modifier **−59** to the second lesion to identify it as a separate lesion and not a duplicate line item.

After Insurance Processing

After the payer has processed the claim, the provider receives a check or electronic deposit and an RA. Depending on the sophistication of the provider's computer system, the payment may be automatically posted to the patient's account or a person may need to manually enter it into the computer or manual bookkeeping system. The biller or payment poster **reconciles** the RA. They compare the RA to the original bill to verify that each service billed was paid in the amount expected.

If payment was denied for one service or for the entire claim, an accounts receivable specialist needs to investigate the reason. Usually the reason is stated on the RA, but the specialist may need to call the insurance company for clarification. Solutions may involve obtaining additional information from the patient, asking the coding department to review the documentation and the codes assigned, or providing copies of documentation. ■ TABLE 2-4 gives examples of coding problems that may cause

claim rejections or denials. The provider needs to respond to insurance company inquiries quickly because any delay by the provider adds to the time it takes to receive payment. A new prompt payment period begins when the payer receives the requested information.

After all insurance payments are received and follow-up is complete, the office sends the patient a bill for any deductible, coinsurance, or patient-responsibility amounts that have not been paid.

SUCCESS STEP

A student intern or new coder can bring immense value to an organization by offering to follow up on problem and unpaid claims. Positive financial results are almost always seen for neglected claims that are reactivated. In addition, new coders can learn a tremendous amount about coding and the payment process by doing insurance follow-up.

CODING PRACTICE

Exercise 2.3 Life Cycle of an Insurance Claim

Instructions: Write the answers to the following questions in the space provided.

1. Why does the life cycle of an insurance claim begin when the patient calls the physician to make an appointment?

_____
_____
_____
_____
_____

2. Define automatic adjudication.

_____
_____
_____
_____
_____

3. List three coding problems that cause rejected or denied claims.

_____
_____
_____
_____
_____

FEDERAL COMPLIANCE

Not getting paid or being underpaid is not the worst impact of improper coding or billing on a provider. The worst impact is being overpaid. When providers are overpaid they are legally obligated to report the overpayment to Medicare, to refund the money, and possibly even pay interest on it.

In this era of electronic transmissions, it is much easier for payers to track patterns of billing, compare a physician to the average or norm, and target providers who deviate from the norm. If an insurance company or Medicare detects a pattern of overpayments due to **overcoding** (*coding for a more complex diagnosis or procedure than is documented*) or improper billing, they can conduct an **audit** (*an investigation of the provider's billing and coding practices*). Going through an audit is time consuming and costly, but if violations are found, severe financial penalties, loss of Medicare privileges, and even imprisonment are possible.

This should not scare coders but make them aware of the importance of their role and the need for accuracy. Medicare places the responsibility for knowing the rules on providers (and by extension their coders). Medicare's stance is that once they publish a rule, providers should know about it and follow it.

CODING CAUTION

You already know that if an officer stops you for speeding, the excuse "I didn't see the sign" will not get you very far. It is the same with Medicare. They expect you to know and follow a multitude of rules, and the rules are usually less clear and less obvious than a speed limit sign on the side of the road.

Violating coding and billing rules can be classified as fraud or abuse. **Fraud** is knowingly billing for services that were never given or billing for a service that has a higher reimbursement than the service actually provided. **Abuse** is mistakenly accepting payment for items or services that should not be paid for by Medicare, due to improper coding and billing practices. Examples are billing for a noncovered service, assigning a more costly code to a lesser service, or coding in a way that does not follow national or local coding guidelines.

Compliance simply means following the rules. Healthcare providers must follow rules established by multiple federal, state, and county government agencies. Some rules are specific to healthcare and others pertain to any type of business. Companies and organizations establish compliance programs to actively keep informed about regulations, educate employees, and make sure that everyone in the company is cooperating. Investigation of fraud and abuse is primarily the responsibility of the Office of the Inspector General (OIG) and Recovery Audit Contractors (RACs).

Office of the Inspector General

Although HIPAA is best known for its privacy rules and healthcare transaction standards, it also created several programs to further control fraud and abuse in healthcare. One of these provisions increased the amount of money the **Office of the Inspector General (OIG)** can spend to investigate fraud

and abuse. It also increased the penalties for violations. The OIG is a division of HHS that investigates fraud, abuse, and other noncompliance matters in the Medicare and Medicaid programs. As a result, healthcare fraud and abuse investigations have become a major focus, and a highly profitable one, for the government. The Health Care Fraud and Abuse Control (HCFAC) program's *Annual Report for Fiscal Year 2012* reports a three-year rolling average return on investment of $7.90 recouped for every dollar spent on enforcement activities. Over three billion dollars was recouped during fiscal year 2012 alone. OIG accomplishes its mission through the False Claims Act (FCA) and compliance programs, which are discussed next.

False Claims Act

OIG uses the **False Claims Act (FCA)** as the basis for much of its investigation and prosecution. The FCA imposes penalties on individuals and companies who defraud government programs. It was passed in 1863, during the Civil War, to combat widespread fraud in which contractors sold the government faulty rifles and ammunition, rotten food, and sick horses. The **Qui Tam** provision of the FCA includes a financial reward to **whistleblowers**, those who turn in violators. The FCA has been updated several times, including 1986, 2009, and 2010.

Knowingly submitting a bill to a government healthcare program, such as Medicare, that contains incorrect codes is considered to be presenting a false claim for payment because the provider is requesting payment for a service that was not provided. If the same coding or billing error is made repeatedly, it can be considered fraud because the provider is responsible to know all the rules about how services should be billed and coded. The FCA is interpreted in a broad sense to include not only intentional misrepresentation but also errors made from ignorance. Medicare providers and their staff are obligated to know all the Medicare rules.

Compliance Programs

Also as a result of HIPAA, the OIG began promoting voluntary compliance programs for the healthcare industry. The OIG provided guidance to assist healthcare entities in developing effective internal controls to help them be aware of and follow the requirements of federal, state, and private health plans. The OIG believes that healthcare institutions that adopt and implement compliance programs significantly reduce fraud, abuse, and waste. Therefore, investigators tend to be more lenient with organizations that have implemented a voluntary compliance plan. The OIG issued sample compliance programs, which include seven major characteristics:

1. Develop and distribute written standards of conduct, policies, and procedures that address specific areas of potential fraud.
2. Designate a high-level manager to be the chief compliance officer who oversees compliance activities.
3. Develop and implement education and training for employees.
4. Establish a process for reporting exceptions.

5. Develop an internal system to respond to accusations or reports of improper activities and implement disciplinary measures when appropriate.

6. Develop an audit and monitoring system.

7. Investigate and correct system-wide problems and develop policies regarding employment or retention of sanctioned individuals.

The Patient Protection and Affordable Care Act (PPACA), passed in 2010, mandates compliance programs for providers who contract with Medicare, Medicaid, and CHIP. The timeline for defining and implementing compliance programs has not yet been established. This rule places the greatest burden on smaller healthcare providers who never established a voluntary compliance program because now they will have to establish one in order to continue serving Medicare patients.

Recovery Audit Contractor

In the Tax Relief and Health Care Act of 2006, Congress required a permanent and national **Recovery Audit Contractor (RAC)** program, which was implemented in 2010. The RAC program uses independent contractors to identify improper Medicare payments to healthcare providers and suppliers made on claims of healthcare services provided to Medicare beneficiaries. Improper payments may be overpayments or underpayments. Overpayments can occur when healthcare providers submit claims that do not meet Medicare's coding or medical necessity policies. Underpayments can occur when healthcare providers submit claims for a simple procedure but the medical record reveals that a more complicated procedure was actually performed. Healthcare providers that might be reviewed include hospitals, physician practices, nursing homes, home health agencies, durable medical equipment suppliers, and any other provider or supplier that bills Medicare Parts A and B.

CODING PRACTICE

Exercise 2.4   Federal Compliance

Instructions: Write the answers to the following questions in the space provided.

1. What are the potential consequences of receiving an overpayment from Medicare? _____

_____

_____

_____

2. Define overcoding. _____

_____

_____

3. What law, passed in 1863, is the basis for much of the OIG's investigation and prosecution? _____

_____

_____

CHAPTER SUMMARY

In this chapter you learned that:

- Third-party payers reimburse physicians and hospitals for 86% of all healthcare services in the United States. Coders need to understand the different types of third-party payers because each has separate, and sometimes conflicting, rules about coding and billing.

- To fulfill their contractual obligations, payers may request information to verify whether the service is covered, including the site (location) of service; the medical need for and

appropriateness of the diagnostic and therapeutic services provided; and the accuracy of codes for services billed on the claim based on the medical record.

- Each step in the life cycle of an insurance claim must be completed in a timely and accurate manner in order for providers to receive correct payment for their services.

- When providers are overpaid they are legally obligated to report the overpayment to Medicare, to refund the money, and possibly even pay interest on it.

CONCEPT QUIZ

Take a moment to look back through this chapter and solidify your skills. This is your opportunity to pull together everything you have learned.

Completion

Instructions: Write the term that answers each question based on the information you learned in this chapter. Choose from the following list. Some choices may be used more than once and some choices may not be used at all.

abuse	medical record	progress notes
compliance	Medigap	RA
RA/EOB	OIG	RCA
family history	Part A	social history
FCA	Part B	TC
fraud	Part C	VHA
medical necessity	Part D	

1. Medicare _____ is hospital insurance that covers a specific list of services for inpatient hospital care, skilled nursing facilities, hospice, and home healthcare.

2. _____ is a Medicare supplement insurance policy sold by private insurance companies to fill gaps in Part A and Part B coverage.

3. _____ is health insurance coverage for family members of active duty personnel and for retired military personnel and their families.

4. _____ is the health status of immediate family members, causes of death (if known), and diseases common in the family.

5. Each patient encounter is coded based on the _____ for that visit.

6. The _____ is a statement that lists all the services the provider billed, which ones were accepted for payment, how much the insurance company will pay, how much the patient owes, and how much will not be paid.

7. _____ is knowingly billing for services that were never given or billing for a service that has a higher reimbursement than the service provided.

8. _____ is mistakenly accepting payment for items or services that should not be paid for by Medicare.

9. _____ investigates fraud, abuse, and other noncompliance matters in the Medicare and Medicaid programs.

10. The OIG issued sample _____ programs, which include seven major characteristics.

Multiple Choice

Instructions: Circle the letter of the best answer to each question based on the information you learned in this chapter.

1. Who regulates med pay or personal injury protection from automobile insurance policies?
   A. each state's Department of Insurance
   B. HIPAA
   C. CMS
   D. each state's Department of Transportation

2. What program is funded jointly by the federal and state governments?
   A. Medicare
   B. Medicaid
   C. Workers' compensation
   D. Self-insured health plan

3. An example of the medical necessity criterion evidence-based practice is
   A. suture removal in the emergency department.
   B. liposuction for medical reasons.
   C. a patient going to an internal medicine or family practice physician to diagnose an initial symptom of stomach pain.
   D. medications proven to benefit patients based on scientific studies.

4. When should the provider verify eligibility with the insurance company?
   A. Before the encounter
   B. During the encounter
   C. After the encounter
   D. After insurance company processing

5. When is the patient chart given to the coding department to review the progress note, assign diagnosis and procedure codes, and enter the codes into the computer?
   A. During the encounter
   B. After the encounter
   C. At the insurance company
   D. After insurance company processing

6. When does the computer system perform a front-end edit check?
   A. During the encounter
   B. After the encounter
   C. At the insurance company
   D. After insurance company processing

7. Which of the following is NOT a coding problem that causes rejected or denied claims?
   A. The patient's insurance has expired.
   B. Characters in a code are mistyped, creating an invalid code.
   C. The diagnosis does not match the procedure.
   D. Additional codes are missing.

8. Knowingly submitting a bill to a government healthcare program, such as Medicare, that contains incorrect codes is considered to be presenting a/an
   A. medical necessity.
   B. denial.
   C. false claim.
   D. RA.

9. The Patient Protection and Affordable Care Act (PPACA), passed in 2010, mandates _____ for providers who contract with Medicare, Medicaid, and CHIP.
   A. front-end edit checks
   B. independent contractors
   C. compliance programs
   D. fraud and abuse

10. The RAC program uses _____ to identify Medicare overpayments and underpayments to healthcare providers and suppliers.
   A. front-end edit checks
   B. independent contractors
   C. compliance programs
   D. HIPAA

Chapter 3

The Transition to ICD-10-CM/PCS

Chapter Outline

- **History of ICD-10-CM/PCS**
- **Overview of the Transition Process**
- **Impact on Healthcare Information Systems**
- **Impact on Medical Providers**
- **Impact on Medical Coders**

Learning Objectives

After completing this chapter, you should have the skills to:

3.1 Spell and define the key words, medical terms, and abbreviations related to the transition to ICD-10-CM/PCS.

3.2 Describe the history of ICD-10-CM/PCS.

3.3 Provide an overview of the transition process.

3.4 Discuss the impact of ICD-10-CM/PCS on healthcare information systems.

3.5 Discuss the impact of ICD-10-CM/PCS on medical providers.

3.6 Discuss the impact of ICD-10-CM/PCS on medical coders.

Key Terms and Abbreviations

Accredited Standards Committee (ASC) X12N Version 4010

Accredited Standards Committee (ASC) X12N Version 5010

final rule

General Equivalence Mapping (GEM)

granular

healthcare administrator

International Classification of Diseases, 10th Revision (ICD-10)

morbidity

mortality

National Center for Health Statistics (NCHS)

PCS

transaction standards

underdosing

In addition to the key terms listed here, students should know the terms defined within tables in this chapter.

For updates and corrections, visit our student resource site at

www.pearsonhighered.com/healthprofessionsresources

INTRODUCTION

Have you ever driven down a road you have been on hundreds of times, only to find out that the route has changed and now you have to go a new way? As disconcerting as this may be, you soon learn the new route and come to appreciate the improvements. The healthcare industry is facing its own "rerouting" with the implementation of ICD-10-CM/PCS. For those who have worked with the old system for years, this transition may be disruptive and unnerving; those new to coding may wonder what all the fuss is about. This chapter helps you understand the reasons the change is being made, the enormity of its impact, and how to adapt to the new environment.

HISTORY OF ICD-10-CM/PCS

The International Classification of Diseases, 10th Revision, Clinical Modification (ICD-10-CM), used for diagnosis coding, and the International Classification of Diseases, 10th Revision, Procedure Coding System (ICD-10-PCS, or **PCS**), used for procedure coding, are two separate and distinct systems that were developed by different groups. ICD-10-CM is based on ICD-10, developed by the World Health Organization (WHO) for worldwide use. ICD-10-PCS was developed by the Centers for Medicare and Medicaid (CMS) for use in the United States only. As a result, even though both code sets are called "ICD-10" and are implemented at the same time in the United States, they serve different purposes, use different and sometimes opposite conventions, and follow different guidelines. Understanding the differences in how the systems developed will help clarify their different purposes.

> ## SUCCESS STEP
>
> When speaking of ICD-10-CM/PCS, coding professionals often use the shorthand CM to refer to ICD-10-CM and the shorthand PCS to refer to ICD-10-PCS.

Background of ICD-10-CM

ICD-10-CM is an update and major revision to the ICD-9-CM, which has been used for diagnosis reporting in the United States since 1979. The **International Classification of Diseases, 10th Revision (ICD-10)**, without the Clinical Modification (CM) designation, is a worldwide reporting system developed by WHO for classifying epidemiological (*study of diseases in large populations*) and **mortality** (*causes of death*) data. After its first full release in 1994, the system was gradually adopted by over 130 countries internationally.

The United States **National Center for Health Statistics (NCHS)** adapted and expanded ICD-10 to focus on **morbidity** (*causes of disease and illness*) in the United States. This adaptation has the phrase Clinical Modification attached to the name, creating the full name International Classification of Diseases, 10th Revision, Clinical Modification (ICD-10-CM). The code set provides diagnoses for tracking and billing patient encounters and uses terminology and detail consistent with medical practice in the United States. All modifications in ICD-10-CM must conform to WHO conventions for ICD-10. The United

States has used ICD-10-CM for coding and classifying mortality data from death certificates since January 1, 1999.

Countries such as Canada and Australia have already successfully implemented ICD-10 in hospitals, but these countries do not use it in outpatient settings as the United States does. The United States' version of ICD-10 diagnosis codes is much more **granular** (*detailed*) than it is in other nations. The United States' version contains approximately 70,000 codes, compared to about 16,000 codes in the Canadian version and about 22,000 in the Australian version. ICD-10-CM is also more detailed than ICD-9-CM, which contained approximately 16,000 codes.

ICD-10-CM applies to all providers, such as hospitals, physicians, skilled nursing facilities, rehabilitation facilities, and home health agencies; payers, such as private insurance companies and government Medicare and Medicaid programs; and other HIPAA-covered entities, such as software vendors, clearinghouses, and third-party billing services.

In January 2009, CMS issued two **final rules** (*a legally required notice of final regulations which is published in the* **Federal Register**) for replacing the 30-year-old ICD-9-CM code set with ICD-10-CM/PCS. The first rule specified the compliance date for mandatory use of ICD-10-CM/PCS as October 1, 2013. In 2012, HHS extended the implementation date to October 1, 2014. In April 2014, Congress passed legislation that extended the implementation date to October 1, 2015, or later. (As this text went to press, the exact implementation date was unknown. Refer to **www.cms.gov/Medicare/ICD10** for current details.)

The second rule updated the HIPAA **transaction standards** (*programming specifications*) so software accommodates the use of the ICD-10-CM/PCS code sets. The compliance date for the second rule was January 1, 2012. Transaction standards are discussed in detail later in this chapter.

The coding process for ICD-10-CM is very similar to that of ICD-9-CM, although the organization of the manual, the format of codes, and some guidelines are different.

Background of ICD-10-PCS

ICD-10-PCS was developed by CMS for use in the United States in inpatient hospital settings only and is not used in other countries. ICD-10-PCS replaces ICD-9-CM Volume 3 procedure codes hospitals used since 1979. HIPAA requires that outpatient hospitals and physicians use Current Procedural Terminology (CPT) codes for billing. Some states may require that hospitals use ICD-10-PCS in outpatient settings, such as the emergency department, outpatient radiology, and outpatient surgery, for tracking and statistical purposes only.

ICD-9-CM contained Volume 3 for inpatient procedure codes, but ICD-10-CM does not contain any procedure codes. ICD-10-PCS is a separate system that CMS developed through a contract with 3M Health Information Systems. PCS was initially published in 1998 and has been updated annually since then. ICD-10-PCS contains over 72,000 codes compared to approximately 3,000 codes in ICD-9-CM Volume 3. ICD-10-PCS coding manual organization, code format, definitions, and guidelines are completely different from ICD-9-CM Volume 3 procedure codes and from CPT procedure codes.

PCS applies to all inpatient hospitals, including acute care hospitals, psychiatric facilities, and rehabilitation facilities; payers, such as private insurance companies and government Medicare and Medicaid programs; and other HIPAA-covered entities, such as software vendors, clearinghouses, and third-party billing services.

Benefits of ICD-10-CM/PCS

CMS and the American Health Information Management Association (AHIMA) identify numerous benefits that are expected to result from ICD-10-CM/PCS:

- Codes more accurately describe patient conditions and procedures, reducing the need for attachments to claims.

- Codes provide more detailed and higher-quality data for tracking the quality, safety, and effectiveness of health services.

- After users become familiar with the new system, it is expected to save time and money.

- Consistency across codes and more specific code descriptions help reduce coding errors.

- Combined with the increased use of electronic medical records, the new code sets provide more consistent and more detailed data for physician use.

- Advancements in technology and medical practice are reflected in the organization and description of codes.

- The coding system in the United States becomes more consistent with that used in other countries.

- Public officials can better track and respond to domestic and international public health threats.

- The structure of the new code sets allows room to add codes, as needed, in the future.

CODING PRACTICE

Exercise 3.1 **History of ICD-10-CM/PCS**

Instructions: Write the answers to the following questions in the space provided.

1. What organization adapted ICD-10 for use in the United States?

_____

_____

2. Name three benefits of ICD-10-CM/PCS.

_____

_____

_____

3. ICD-10-PCS was developed for use by what type of provider?

_____

_____

OVERVIEW OF THE TRANSITION PROCESS

The transition to convert from ICD-9-CM to ICD-10-CM/PCS is one of healthcare's top priorities and expenditures. Coding changes impact many more parts of organizations than other recent changes, such as implementation of the national provider identifier (NPI) in 2005. While previous changes primarily affected transactions with external partners, the ICD-10-CM/PCS transition impacts providers' internal operations as well.

All covered entities are affected. Everyone who is part of the healthcare system or uses its data is impacted, including providers, payers, regulators, vendors, claims clearinghouses, medical billing services, researchers, educational institutions, and support staff in each of these settings. All computer systems that collect, transmit, receive, or store diagnostic data need updating because of the expanded length, format, and structure of codes. These changes further impact the budgets of organizations and the productivity of workers.

Fortunately, patients are minimally affected because the code set is generally transparent to (*unseen by*) them. However, it is likely that overall processing times may be longer at the beginning of the transition as users get used to the new systems and work out all the bugs. This may affect patients indirectly because others are taking longer to send bills, make payments, and answer questions.

Reasons for Change

The reason that the transition from ICD-9-CM to ICD-10-CM/PCS is such a major undertaking is because of the many differences between the two systems. This chapter discusses overall differences between the code sets. Some of the major differences include the following:

- ICD-10-CM/PCS contain many times the number of codes as their ICD-9-CM counterparts. This requires established coders to learn a more detailed coding process. It also requires that computer system capacity be upgraded.

- The length of diagnosis codes increased from three to five characters in ICD-9-CM to a length of three to seven characters in ICD-10-CM. Procedure codes increased from three or four characters in ICD-9-CM Volume 3 to seven characters in ICD-10-PCS. This required changes to all computer software that uses codes to accommodate a longer field size.

- Code structure changed from primarily numeric in ICD-9-CM (except for V and E codes) to all codes being alphanumeric in ICD-10-CM. This required changes to all computer software that uses codes to accept both numbers and letters for every code.

- Code formats were added in ICD-10-CM to include seventh characters to describe a particular circumstance. This requires established coders to learn new skills.
- ICD-10-CM terminology and disease classifications were updated to be consistent with current clinical practice. ICD-10-PCS provides unique definitions for procedures. This requires coders to learn and apply new terminology.
- ICD-10-CM codes describe greater levels of clinical detail and specificity that may have been described by a single code in ICD-9-CM. This requires established coders to learn a more detailed coding process.
- ICD-10-CM contains more combination codes that describe multiple related conditions with a single code. ICD-10-PCS requires more multiple coding than ICD-9-CM Volume 3 because most procedural combination codes were eliminated. Both of these changes require that established coders relearn certain coding rules and guidelines.

Preparing for the Change

When ICD-10 was implemented in countries such as Canada and Australia, the national, provincial, and local governments paid for software upgrades and staff training. In the United States, the costs are borne individually by each hospital, physician, and health plan. Experience in other countries demonstrated that the change requires a significant investment of time and money. Healthcare providers in other countries experienced decreased productivity for many months following the change. It became critical that healthcare organizations prepare with the information and tools they need to streamline the change process.

Healthcare administrators are the individuals in each healthcare organization responsible for managing the organization, including the transition to ICD-10-CM/PCS. This includes physicians who own their own practices as well as their managers. Administrators also include hospital and health plan managers. Others responsible for the ICD-10-CM/PCS transition include managers of clinical areas such as laboratory, radiology, and pharmacy; information systems; finance, including billing and coding; quality assurance; compliance; and public health. CMS and professional organizations published numerous rules and time schedules to aid providers in the transition. Administrators must adapt these guidelines to their own organization to ensure that the organization is able to make the transition to ICD-10-CM/PCS in a timely manner.

Planning for ICD-10-CM/PCS transition began several years in advance of implementation, in order to analyze systems; update administrative processes; coordinate activities with clearinghouses, billing services, and payers; reprint encounter forms; train staff; and establish budgets for these activities. The overall process to plan for, implement, and monitor the ICD-10-CM/PCS transition requires approximately five years.

The remainder of this chapter discusses specific impacts on information systems, providers, and coders.

CODING PRACTICE

Exercise 3.2 Overview of the Transition Process

Instructions: Write the answers to the following questions in the space provided.

1. List five examples of HIPAA-covered entities affected by the transition to ICD-10-CM/PCS. _____

_____

_____

2. List three examples of healthcare administrators.

_____

_____

_____

3. Name three major differences between ICD-9-CM and ICD-10-CM/PCS. _____

_____

_____

IMPACT ON HEALTHCARE INFORMATION SYSTEMS

One of the greatest impacts of ICD-10-CM/PCS within a healthcare organization is the effect on healthcare information systems. Typically an organization has more than one electronic information system that is affected. These may include scheduling, patient registration, medical records, billing, coding, payment posting, quality, and compliance reporting. In large organizations, multiple departments are affected, including laboratory, pharmacy, radiology, medical records, quality assurance, and finance. Reporting to external federal and state regulators is affected, including reporting of adverse drug events, medical devices, pay for performance, research, public health, and newborn screening. Contracts with health plans and payers with provisions related to specific diagnoses or inpatient procedures also need to be reviewed and modified to incorporate the new diagnosis codes.

Prior to ICD-10-CM/PCS the healthcare industry used an electronic transaction standard called **Accredited Standards Committee (ASC) X12N Version 4010**. This standard lacked all the functions needed, so **Accredited Standards Committee (ASC) X12N Version 5010** was developed. Version 5010 is the revised set of HIPAA transaction standards adopted to replace the current Version 4010 standards. Five types of transaction standards required updating:

- claims, encounter, and payment information
- coordination of benefits
- eligibility for a health plan
- referrals
- non-HIPAA-mandated formats for Medicare Fee-for-Service (FFS)

The overall transition process from Version 4010 to Version 5010 required three years to accomplish. Providers were required to use Version 5010 on or after January 1, 2012, for HIPAA-mandated transactions. After a short grace period, electronic transactions not compliant with Version 5010 were subject to rejection. Each type of transaction required separate complex programming changes in Version 5010, such as the following:

- Modify field sizes to accommodate the longer codes.
- Change data type of fields from primarily numeric to completely alphanumeric for every character.
- Add a new field as a version indicator to distinguish between ICD-9-CM and ICD-10-CM/PCS codes.
- Increase the number of diagnosis codes allowed on a claim.
- Implement detailed rules to improve the explanations of claim corrections, reversals, recoupment of payments, and the processing of refunds.

These changes affected providers, payers, and vendors such as software companies, clearinghouses, and third-party billing services. All of these organizations needed to update their systems. In addition, they needed to communicate and work together to ensure that all parties were making the needed changes on schedule.

CODING PRACTICE

Exercise 3.3 Impact on Healthcare Information Systems

Instructions: Write the answers to the following questions in the space provided.

1. Name the five types of electronic transactions that required updating in the Version 5010 standard.

   _____
   _____
   _____
   _____
   _____

2. What is Version 5010 and when was it mandatory?

   _____
   _____
   _____
   _____
   _____
   _____

3. Name three programming changes implemented in Version 5010.

   _____
   _____
   _____
   _____

IMPACT ON MEDICAL PROVIDERS

Physicians who own their own practices experience all the impacts on operations and budgets described earlier in this chapter:

- They are responsible for implementing the impacts on information systems.
- They need to make sure the coders they employ receive adequate training.
- They need to ensure that their own medical documentation provides the additional level of specificity needed under ICD-10-CM/PCS.
- Providers who personally assign some or all diagnostic codes themselves also need to learn the coding guidelines for ICD-10-CM.
- They must accomplish all of these changes while continuing to maintain a high patient load.

This section focuses on the specific impacts on providers' internal operations in three areas: documentation, scheduling, and treatment plans.

Impact on Documentation

One of the most concerning aspects of ICD-10-CM/PCS implementation that directly affects all clinical providers is the potential for increased quantity and detail of documentation. Because ICD-10-CM/PCS provides for a greater level of granularity and specificity, providers are responsible to ensure that their documentation provides the required information. Certainly a change of this magnitude is expected to cause a temporary loss of productivity while physicians and other clinical staff adjust to the new requirements. However, many effects on productivity may be permanent, such as the requirement for increased detail. This requirement never disappears because it consumes additional time each and every time a provider documents a patient encounter, even after the provider has adjusted to the initial changes.

To determine the need for documentation improvements, hospitals as well as physician practices conduct studies that evaluate random samples of various types of medical records. They determine if the documentation contains the required level of detail in new coding systems. Then they identify documentation weaknesses in order to develop a priority list of specific diagnoses and procedures that require more detail or other changes.

Physicians who perform inpatient hospital procedures have needed to learn about new documentation requirements for PCS in addition to CM. Recall that hospitals use PCS codes to report the facility portion of inpatient procedures that physicians perform. Even though physician offices do not report PCS codes, physicians' hospital documentation must provide the required information for hospital PCS coders. ■ TABLE 3-1 provides examples of documentation changes needed for ICD-10-CM/PCS.

Impact on Scheduling

Coders do not assign codes until the insurance claim is prepared, but the impact on coding begins as soon as the patient encounter is scheduled. Schedulers often select the reason or purpose for patients' planned visits from a list that is ultimately tied to diagnosis codes. When providers need to check eligibility, make a referral, or obtain pre-authorization from the patient's health plan, diagnosis codes are usually required. When the patient presents for the visit, the coinsurance, copayment, or deductible payment may be affected by the expected diagnosis or visit type.

Impact on Treatment

The effect on examinations and treatment decisions is a critical and sensitive area for providers. Health plans may update coverage policies to reflect the greater specificity in ICD-10-CM/PCS coding. For example, the diagnostic criteria for coverage of

Table 3-1 ■ **EXAMPLES OF DOCUMENTATION CHANGES UNDER ICD-10-CM/PCS**

Category	Example
Laterality	Conditions and procedures that relate to paired body parts, such as eyes, ears, and all extremities, contain laterality in both ICD-10-CM and PCS.
Genetic diagnoses	ICD-9-CM has one code for Down syndrome, but in ICD-10-CM, the codes for Down syndrome require genetic testing results to identify the specific type of Down (meiotic nondisjunction, mitotic nondisjunction, or translocation).
Medical history	Lifestyle habits such as alcohol, tobacco, and drug abuse and dependence are required as additional codes with many diagnoses. Postmenopausal osteoporosis requires documentation of current pathological fractures.
Anatomic specificity	Throughout PCS more details regarding anatomic site are required. For example, release of a shoulder ligament requires that the specific ligament be identified.

a particular treatment could become more specific and, therefore, more limited. Providers may need to document additional details to support a patient's treatment plan. Providers may need to alter past treatment protocols or explain to patients why their course of treatment may change, or not be fully covered, due to new insurance company requirements. The extent of this impact will not be known until health plans review their ICD-10-CM/PCS implementation activities and determine what changes to make in their policies.

CODING PRACTICE

Exercise 3.4   Impact on Medical Providers

Instructions: Write the answers to the following questions in the space provided.

1. Name three impacts on physicians who own their own practices. _____

_____

_____

_____

2. List four examples of changes needed in physician documentation under ICD-10-CM/PCS.

_____

_____

_____

_____

3. How does ICD-10-CM/PCS potentially impact scheduling?

_____

_____

_____

IMPACT ON MEDICAL CODERS

Medical coders are affected by ICD-10-CM/PCS on a daily basis. Any delays or errors in using the new code set directly impact the revenue of the organization. Therefore, coders must

be trained and proficient well before the "Go Live" date so they can be immediately effective. This involves learning the new code set, new coding guidelines, and new or updated software and updating professional certifications.

New Terminology

The detail added to ICD-10-CM/PCS codes requires additional knowledge of medical terminology, anatomy and physiology, pathophysiology, and pharmacology. Terminology used in ICD-9-CM is replaced with more current clinical terminology. ■ TABLE 3-2 shows examples of terminology differences between ICD-9-CM and ICD-10-CM.

ICD-10-PCS has numerous terminology changes because standard definitions are an integral part of the code set. ■ TABLE 3-3 shows examples of terminology differences between ICD-9-CM Volume 3 procedure codes and ICD-10-PCS.

New Abstracting Challenges

Just as providers identify areas where ICD-10-CM/PCS requires additional documentation details, coders working for those providers learn what details to abstract in order to code the case completely and accurately. ■ TABLE 3-4 provides examples of changes in abstracting diagnoses. ■ TABLE 3-5 provides examples of changes in abstracting procedures.

New Coding Challenges

ICD-10-CM introduces several new coding challenges, including new coding concepts, increased use of combination codes, and new guidelines. In addition, ICD-10-CM/PCS more clearly distinguishes between diagnostic and procedural descriptors for codes. Examples of each follow.

New Coding Concepts

New coding concepts are introduced in ICD-10-CM/PCS that did not exist in ICD-9-CM. Coders must identify and understand the new concepts in order to assign the correct code. Examples include the following:

- Blood type is a coding criterion in ICD-10-CM but not in ICD-9-CM.

Table 3-2 ■ EXAMPLES OF TERMINOLOGY DIFFERENCES BETWEEN ICD-9-CM AND ICD-10-CM

ICD-9-CM Classification	ICD-10-CM Classification
Status asthmaticus	Mild intermittent
	Mild persistent
	Moderate persistent
	Severe persistent
Bleeding/Hemorrhage	Hemorrhage used when referring to ulcers
	Bleeding used for diseases such as gastritis, duodenitis, diverticulitis, and diverticulosis
Burns	Burns that come from a heat source, electricity, or radiation
	The term *corrosion* is used to describe chemical burns.
Diabetes Type I or Type II; not stated as uncontrolled or stated as uncontrolled	Diabetes Type 1 or Type 2

Table 3-3 ■ EXAMPLES OF TERMINOLOGY DIFFERENCES BETWEEN ICD-9-CM VOLUME 3 AND ICD-10-PCS

ICD-9-CM Volume 3 Classification	ICD-10-PCS Classification
Number of vessels treated	Number of sites treated
Excision, resection, removal used interchangeably	Excision, resection, removal each has unique and specific definition and cannot be used interchangeably.
Ligament	Indicate the specific ligament involved

Table 3-4 ■ EXAMPLES OF CHANGES IN DIAGNOSIS ABSTRACTING

Topic	Change	Impact
Complications	**ICD-9-CM:** Limited codes for surgical complications. **ICD-10-CM:** Codes for complications are expanded. Makes a distinction between intraoperative complications and postoperative disorders.	Coders become familiar with the expanded range of code choices and the new terminology.
External cause episode of care	**ICD-9-CM:** No codes for external cause episode of care. **ICD-10-CM:** External cause codes and injury codes require a seventh-character indicating if the episode of care is initial, subsequent, or for sequela.	This information should be easily determined from the medical record. Requires an additional step in code assignment.
Falls	**ICD-9-CM:** Falls, one of the leading external causes of injury, are described by about 40 codes. **ICD-10-CM:** Has codes for approximately 100 types of falls. Uses the 7th character to identify the episode of care as initial, subsequent, or sequela.	Changes result in approximately 300 codes for falls. Coders become familiar with the expanded range of code choices and applications of the 7th character.
Laterality	**ICD-9-CM:** Codes do not distinguish laterality (right or left side) for injuries or conditions of bilateral sites such as eyes, ears, and extremities. **ICD-10-CM:** Most bilateral sites have codes for laterality.	Physicians who are not accustomed to documenting this information must be educated to document the laterality. Laterality presents an added step in code selection.
Obstetrics	**ICD-9-CM:** Assign a fifth digit for the episode of care—delivered, antepartum, or postpartum—and the presence of a complication. **ICD-10-CM:** Code the trimester of pregnancy and weeks of gestation.	Easily determined from the medical record. Does not require additional documentation by physicians. Requires that coders develop a new methodology.

Table 3-5 ■ **EXAMPLES OF CHANGES IN PROCEDURE ABSTRACTING**

Topic	Change	Impact
Coronary bypass	**ICD-9-CM Vol. 3:** Defines codes based on the number of arteries bypassed. **ICD-10-PCS:** Defines codes based on the number of sites bypassed to and site bypassed from.	Coders must learn the new definitions. Coders must learn more detailed anatomy of the heart vessels.
Eponyms	**ICD-9-CM Vol. 3:** Eponyms are commonly used as the only description of a procedure. **ICD-10-PCS:** PCS does not use procedure eponyms because they can be performed with numerous variations.	When surgeons describe procedures using eponyms, coders must read the detailed operative report to determine the exact nature of what was done and assign the corresponding code.
Joint replacements	**ICD-9-CM Vol. 3:** One code for many joint replacements. **ICD-10-PCS:** As many as 18 possible codes for a joint replacement based on laterality, the surface treated, and the type of tissue substitute.	Physicians need to document additional details. Coders must learn to locate the details.
Laterality	**ICD-9-CM Vol. 3:** Codes do not distinguish laterality. **ICD-10-PCS:** Most bilateral sites have codes for laterality.	Physicians who are not accustomed to documenting this information must be educated to document laterality. Laterality presents an added step in code selection.
Procedural terms	**ICD-9-CM Vol. 3:** No standard definition of procedural terms. Many terms can be used interchangeably. **ICD-10-PCS:** ICD-10-PCS applies specific and unique definitions to terms such as *excision*, *resection*, and *extraction*.	Physicians are not expected to adopt PCS definitions in their documentation. Coders must read the procedural documentation carefully and apply the correct PCS definitions, regardless of the terms physicians use.

- Injury by **underdosing** (*taking too little*) of a medication is new in ICD-10-CM.

Changes in Combination Codes

Some conditions that required multiple coding in ICD-9-CM are identified with a combination code in ICD-10-CM. Coders learn what situations are combined into a single code and what situations require separate coding.

- For example, diabetes type 2 with diabetic cataract is identified with two codes in ICD-9-CM, one for diabetes and a second for cataracts in diseases classified elsewhere. ICD-10-CM uses a combination code that includes both the type of diabetes and the specific complication.

The opposite is true in PCS. ICD-9-CM procedure codes include many combination codes for procedures commonly performed together. In ICD-10-PCS, most combination codes are eliminated and multiple coding is more common. This preserves the purity and integrity of the system.

New Guidelines

While many of the Official Guidelines for Coding and Reporting for diagnosis coding are similar between ICD-9-CM and ICD-10-CM, coders must be alert for those that are different. Examples include the following:

- When coding for anemia in cancer (neoplastic disease) ICD-9-CM directs coders to sequence the codes according to the reason for the encounter. Anemia is sequenced first when it is the primary reason for the encounter.
  - ICD-10-CM guidelines direct coders to always sequence the neoplasm code first.

- ICD-9-CM defines acute myocardial infarction (AMI) as one occurring within the past eight weeks.
  - ICD-10-CM defines AMI as one occurring within the past four weeks or less.

For procedure coding, ICD-9-CM Volume 3 does not have guidelines, but ICD-10-PCS does have coding guidelines that coders must learn and follow.

Separation of Diagnostic and Procedural Descriptors

ICD-9-CM sometimes provided multiple diagnosis codes for a condition based on the procedure that was performed. ICD-9-CM Volume 3 sometimes has multiple procedure codes based on the reason the procedure was performed. ICD-10-CM/PCS attempts to eliminate this blurring between diagnosis and procedure codes. An example of each follows.

- ICD-9-CM provides approximately 36 separate V-codes for encounters for immunization based on the type of immunization to be administered.
  - ICD-10-CM has one code for an immunization encounter (**Z23**) with the instructional note to use a procedure code to describe the specific type of immunization given.
- ICD-9-CM Volume 3 provides separate procedure codes for uterine repair based on whether the repair was for a laceration, fistula, an old obstetric laceration, or a current obstetric laceration.
  - ICD-10-PCS codes only for the type of repair. The problem requiring repair is described using the diagnosis code. Only current obstetric lacerations receive a separate repair code.

Coder Training and Certification

Coders need to update their coding skills and their professional certification for ICD-10-CM/PCS. Coding professionals recommend that full training of all staff take place approximately three to six months prior to the compliance date. However, training must be continued after the implementation date as providers learn by experience the details that must be fine-tuned.

Professional organizations such as AAPC and AHIMA offer training in a variety of formats including distance education courses, audio seminars, web-based in-services, self-directed learning using printed materials or electronic tools, off-site workshops in a traditional classroom setting with a certified trainer, or in-house classes with a certified trainer.

Established coders need to demonstrate their proficiency in ICD-10-CM/PCS to maintain certification. AHIMA and AAPC have specific requirements for coders to upgrade their skills to ICD-10-CM/PCS. Coders already certified through AHIMA for ICD-9-CM must complete a specified amount of continuing education based on their specialty and coding credential. Coders certified by AAPC must take an ICD-10-CM proficiency assessment.

Coders should also upgrade keyboarding skills from what were primarily numeric data entry skills to full alphanumeric keyboarding because all ICD-10-CM/PCS codes have a random sequencing of alphabetic and numeric characters.

CODING CAUTION

Because of the large amount of code set training that is needed, there are few formal programs that focus on upgrading coders' keyboarding skills. Smart coders will take the initiative to address this skill on their own because alphanumeric keyboarding is considerably more time consuming than largely numeric keyboarding.

Table 3-6 ■ **EXAMPLE OF GEM ONE-TO-MANY FORWARD MAPPING**

ICD-9-CM	ICD-10-CM
424.1 Aortic valve disorders	I35.0 Nonrheumatic aortic (valve) stenosis
	I35.1 Nonrheumatic aortic (valve) insufficiency
	I35.2 Nonrheumatic aortic (valve) stenosis with insufficiency
	I35.8 Other nonrheumatic aortic valve disorders
	I35.9 Nonrheumatic aortic valve disorder, unspecified

Appropriate Use of GEMs

CMS and the Centers for Disease Control and Prevention (CDC) needed to create a way to compare data between ICD-9-CM and ICD-10-CM/PCS and analyze long-term trends. They developed **General Equivalence Mappings (GEMs)** to be the authoritative source for comparing codes between the two code sets. Because there are more ICD-10-CM codes than ICD-9-CM codes, GEMs do not provide an exact one-to-one match between code sets but, rather, provide a general approximation of the relationship (■ TABLE 3-6). CMS publishes GEMs as public domain electronic files available on its website. Researchers use GEMs to analyze large volumes of data over a time span that includes data both before and after ICD-10-CM/PCS. Without GEMs, it would be nearly impossible to establish healthcare trends.

Coders should not use GEMs to assign codes for specific patient encounters. This means that they should not look up the ICD-9-CM code first, then use GEMs to select the ICD-10-CM/PCS code. Doing so would be misuse of data and a potentially fraudulent coding practice. All ICD-10-CM/PCS codes should be assigned using the ICD-10-CM/PCS Index and Tabular List.

CODING PRACTICE

Exercise 3.5   Impact on Medical Coders

Instructions: Write the answers to the following questions in the space provided.

1. Briefly describe how abstracting will change for each of the following conditions.
   a. obstetrics_____
   b. falls_____
   c. laterality_____

2. Name three examples of medical terms that have new definitions under ICD-10-CM/PCS.

   _____
   _____
   _____

3. Describe an inappropriate use of GEMs by a coder.

   _____
   _____
   _____

CHAPTER SUMMARY

In this chapter you learned that:

- ICD-10-CM, used for diagnosis coding, and ICD-10-PCS, used for procedure coding, are two separate and distinct systems that were developed by different groups.
- The transition to convert from ICD-9-CM to ICD-10-CM/PCS is one of healthcare's top priorities and expenditures.
- One of the greatest impacts of ICD-10-CM/PCS within a healthcare organization is the effect on healthcare information systems.

- Providers are impacted by ICD-10-CM/PCS in the areas of documentation, scheduling, and treatment plans.
- Coders must learn the new code set, new coding guidelines, and new or updated software, and they must update professional certifications.

CONCEPT QUIZ

Take a moment to look back at the transition to ICD-10-CM/PCS and solidify your skills. This is your opportunity to pull together everything you have learned.

Completion

Instructions: Write the term that answers each question based on the information you learned in this chapter. Choose from the following list. Some choices may be used more than once and some choices may not be used at all.

AAPC	ICD-10-PCS
AHIMA	ICD-9-CM
CDC	January 1, 2012
CMS	morbidity
complicated	mortality
five	October 1, 2014
GEMs	seven
granular	three
ICD-10	transaction standards
ICD-10-CM	Version 5010

1. ICD-10-CM codes contain _____ to _____ characters.
2. ICD-10-PCS codes contain _____ characters.
3. _____ is causes of disease and illness.
4. Version 5010 is mandatory on the date _____.
5. The U.S. version of ICD-10 diagnosis codes is much more _____ than it is in other nations.
6. The code set _____ was developed by WHO for worldwide use.
7. The code set _____ is used only by inpatient hospitals.
8. Coders already certified through _____ for ICD-9-CM must complete a specified amount of continuing education based on their specialty and coding credential.

9. _____ uses more combination codes than ICD-9-CM.
10. Researchers use _____ to analyze large volumes of data, but coders should not use them for code assignment.

Multiple Choice

Instructions: Circle the letter of the best answer to each question based on the information you learned in this chapter.

1. Which of the following is NOT a benefit of ICD-10-CM?
   A. Codes more accurately describe patient conditions and procedures, reducing the need for attachments to claims.
   B. Advancements in technology and medical practice are reflected in the organization and description of codes.
   C. The structure of the new code set allows physicians to create new codes whenever they need to if an appropriate code is not already available.
   D. Public officials can better track and respond to domestic and international public health threats.

2. Which of the following conditions does NOT require updated terminology in ICD-10-CM?
   A. Diabetes
   B. Influenza
   C. Asthma
   D. Burns

3. Who is required to use ICD-10-CM?
   A. All physicians
   B. HIPAA-covered entities
   C. Inpatient hospitals only
   D. Patients

4. Which of the following is NOT a requirement that impacts health information systems?
   A. Create separate fields for ICD-9-CM and ICD-10-CM codes.
   B. Modify field sizes to accommodate the longer codes.
   C. Change data type of fields from primarily numeric to completely alphanumeric for every character.
   D. Add a new field as a version indicator to distinguish between ICD-9-CM and ICD-10-CM/PCS codes.

(continued)

(continued from page 33)

5. Which of the following is NOT an example of provider documentation changes under ICD-10-CM/PCS?
   A. Laterality
   B. Genetic diagnoses
   C. Acute vs. chronic
   D. Anatomic specificity

6. Changes in procedure abstracting under ICD-10-PCS include all of the following EXCEPT
   A. eponyms.
   B. coronary bypass.
   C. joint replacements.
   D. external causes.

7. Which code set provides separate procedure codes for a uterine repair based on the diagnosis?
   A. ICD-9-CM Volume 1
   B. ICD-9-CM Volume 3
   C. ICD-10-CM
   D. ICD-10-PCS

8. GEMs do not provide an exact one-to-one match between ICD-9-CM and ICD-10-CM because
   A. there are more ICD-9-CM codes than ICD-10-CM codes.
   B. there are more ICD-10-CM codes than ICD-9-CM codes.
   C. there is no way to compare ICD-9-CM and ICD-10-CM.
   D. all of the above.

9. Which of the following areas impact coders?
   A. Learning new software
   B. Enhanced data entry skills
   C. Expanded medical terminology
   D. All of the above

10. Which is the most accurate description of GEMs?
    A. An exact one-to-one matching of the ICD-9-CM and ICD-10-CM codes
    B. An authoritative guide to assign ICD-10-CM codes to patient records for billing
    C. The authoritative source for comparing codes between ICD-10-CM/PCS and ICD-9-CM
    D. Electronic software that provides a definitive translation of ICD-9-CM codes to ICD-10-CM codes

SECTION TWO

ICD-10-CM Diagnosis Coding

Section Two: ICD-10-CM Diagnosis Coding guides you through the steps of diagnosis coding for each body system. You will learn how to apply the three skills of an ace coder—Abstract, Assign, and Arrange—for a broad variety of patient encounters.

PROFESSIONAL PROFILE
MEET...

Pauline T. Newton, Patient Financial Services
Director
Carlisle Regional Medical Center, an HMA Facility

I have been in the billing and coding field for the past 34 years and I am continually learning something new. Even though I have a Bachelors of Arts in Business Management, I recently went back to school and earned an Associate of Science degree in medical records, coding, and billing from an accredited college to enhance my career skills. I am now working toward a Bachelor of Science in Healthcare Administration.

I went back to school in order to gain skills to address the challenges of Recovery Audit Contractor (RAC) audits I was facing in my job. I wanted to understand what the auditors are looking at and where our hospital could be lacking in documentation. Now I am able to work more closely with clinicians to conduct random audits on medical records. Internal chart reviews help ensure that we are capturing all the revenue for services rendered and that the documentation supports what we bill. I also have a new understanding of insurance claims and reasons for denials. I worked with the case management and health information management (HIM) departments to create a proactive approach to potential denials as well as improve our presentation of Medicare appeals to the review board and judge advocate.

I currently participate on several committees in the hospital that directly use the knowledge I gained through my formal education: Denials Management Committee, Revenue Cycle Committee, RAC Audit Committee, and Corporate Compliance Committee.

I am involved with the professional organization Healthcare Financial Management Association (HFMA), including serving as an officer of our local chapter. I was awarded the HFMA Follmer Bronze Award in 2007 for my presentations and workshops related to Revenue Cycle presented for our chapter.

My advice to new coders would be the two most important things I have learned during my career: embrace change and continue to learn and grow.

Chapter 4

Introduction to ICD-10-CM Diagnosis Coding

Chapter Outline

- **Organization of ICD-10-CM**
- **ICD-10-CM Guidelines and Conventions**
- **How to Code Diagnoses**

Learning Objectives

After completing this chapter, you should have the skills to:

4.1 Spell and define the key words, medical terms, and abbreviations related to ICD-10-CM coding.

4.2 Identify the organization of the ICD-10-CM manual.

4.3 Discuss ICD-10-CM Official Guidelines for Coding and Reporting.

4.4 Name ICD-10-CM conventions.

4.5 Demonstrate the diagnosis coding process including abstracting, assigning, and arranging codes.

Key Terms and Abbreviations

abstract
arrange
assign
block (ICD-10-CM)
category (ICD-10-CM)
chapter (ICD-10-CM)
circumstances of admission
clinically significant condition
code (ICD-10-CM)
coding path

combination code
convention
Coordination and Maintenance Committee
default code (ICD-10-CM)
eponym
etiology
first-listed diagnosis
four cooperating parties
initial encounter (ICD-10-CM)

instructional note
late effect
Main Term
manifestation
multiple coding
nonessential modifier (ICD-10-CM)
Official Guidelines for Coding and Reporting (OGCR)
principal diagnosis

relevant
sequela (ICD-10-CM)
sequence
subcategory (ICD-10-CM)
subchapter (ICD-10-CM)
subsequent encounter (ICD-10-CM)
subterm
uncertain diagnosis

In addition to the key terms listed here, students should know the terms defined within tables in this chapter.

INTRODUCTION

As much as we would like, no vehicle is without difficulties or breakdowns. When you take your vehicle to a mechanic for service, the mechanic needs to figure out what is wrong before he or she can fix it. They need to diagnose the problem. Similarly, when patients see physicians, physicians must diagnose the condition before they know what services to provide. In this chapter you will learn how to code for the conditions that physicians diagnose.

This chapter provides an introduction to ICD-10-CM diagnosis coding and lays the foundation for the next 21 chapters in this section. You will become acquainted with the organization of the ICD-10-CM coding manual and learn the official guidelines and conventions. Finally, you will follow a guided example of the three skills of an ace coder: how to abstract, assign, and arrange diagnosis codes.

ORGANIZATION OF ICD-10-CM

The International Classification of Diseases, 10th Revision, Clinical Modification (ICD-10-CM) is used to code diagnoses that describe patient illnesses, diseases, conditions, injuries, or other reasons for seeking healthcare services. ICD-10-CM is the United States' clinical modification of the World Health Organization's (WHO) International Classification of Diseases, 10th Revision (ICD-10). The inclusion of the term *clinical modification* in the United States' ICD-10-CM emphasizes the intent of the modification to classify and manage data related to the actual examination and treatment of patients. Uses in the United States include tracking morbidity, indexing medical records, reporting ambulatory as well as inpatient care, and reflecting advances in medical care.

Accurate coding of diagnoses is necessary in order to explain why services were provided. To code accurately, coders need to be familiar with the process for updating ICD-10-CM as well as the overall organization of the manual, the distinct sublevels of organization, and the significance of each.

Updates in ICD-10-CM

Because medical knowledge is constantly expanding and improving, the system for diagnosis coding must keep pace with those changes. ICD-10-CM replaces ICD-9-CM, which was used for diagnosis coding in the United States since 1979. ■ TABLE 4-1 summarizes the major differences between ICD-9-CM and ICD-10-CM.

Many of the **Official Guidelines for Coding and Reporting (OGCR)** (*rules that provide information and direction in identifying the diagnoses to be reported*) are similar between the two code sets. OGCR Section I.A reflects new and updated conventions. Sections I.B, II, III, and IV reflect changes related to differences in code structure, such as additional characters, seventh characters, and laterality. Guidelines in Section C reflect changes in chapter organization and updated clinical terminology, definitions, and practice.

CODING CAUTION

Coders who are familiar with ICD-9-CM OGCR must be especially alert to learn which guidelines in ICD-10-CM OGCR are similar to ICD-9-CM and which are different.

Table 4-1 ■ COMPARISON OF CODES IN ICD-9-CM AND ICD-10-CM

Feature	ICD-9-CM	ICD-10-CM
Number of codes	16,000	70,000+
Code length	3 to 5 digits	3 to 7 characters
Code structure	3-digit category 4th and 5th digits for etiology, anatomic site, manifestation	3-character category 4th, 5th, 6th characters for etiology, anatomic site, severity 7th character for additional information
First character	Always numeric, except E codes and V codes	1st character is always alphabetic.
Subsequent characters	All numeric	2nd character is always numeric; all other characters may be alphabetic or numeric.
Decimal point	Mandatory after 3rd character, except E codes, where decimal point is after 4th character	Mandatory after 3rd character on all codes
7th Character	None	Some codes use a 7th character to provide additional information.
Placeholders	None	Character **X** is used as a placeholder in certain 6- and 7-character codes.

In addition to the major conversion from ICD-9-CM to ICD-10-CM, the code set is updated annually. Code definitions are revised, new codes are added, and outdated codes are deleted. Updates are effective each year on October 1 to coincide with the beginning of the federal fiscal year. Each HIPAA-covered entity must update its systems and paperwork to incorporate the changes. The ICD-10-CM **Coordination and Maintenance Committee** oversees all changes, which must be consistent with WHO's ICD-10. The Coordination and Maintenance Committee is a federal interdepartmental committee comprised of representatives from the **four cooperating parties:** the Centers for Medicare and Medicaid Services (CMS), the National Center for Health Statistics (NCHS; part of the Centers for Disease Control and Prevention [CDC]), the American Hospital Association (AHA), and the American Health Information Management Association (AHIMA).

Overall Organization

The ICD-10-CM manual is a single volume and is not separated into three volumes as the ICD-9-CM is. Locate the Contents page near the front of the manual and become familiar with the contents and organization of the ICD-10-CM manual listed in ■ TABLE 4-2, page 38. The purpose of each of these Contents topics is discussed later in this chapter.

Table 4-2 ■ **OVERVIEW OF THE ICD-10-CM MANUAL**

Type of Information	Name of Section	Purpose
Introductory material	Preface Introduction How to Use the ICD-10-CM ICD-10-CM Official Conventions Additional Conventions ICD-10-CM Official Guidelines for Coding and Reporting	Information and rules on how to use the manual.
Index	ICD-10-CM Index to Diseases and Injuries (Index) ICD-10-CM Table of Neoplasms ICD-10-CM Table of Drugs and Chemicals ICD-10-CM Index to External Causes	Alphabetical list of diseases and injuries, reasons for encounters, and external causes. Two tables provide quick look-ups, one for neoplasms and one for drugs and chemicals causing injury. Coders must always reference one of these indices or tables when searching for a code.
Tabular List	ICD-10-CM Tabular List of Diseases and Injuries	Alphanumerical list of diseases and injuries, reasons for encounters, and external causes. Provides additional instruction on how to use, assign, and sequence codes. Coders must always reference the Tabular List to verify a code, after consulting the Index, and before assigning the final code.

Chapter Structure

The last section of the Contents page, ICD-10-CM Tabular List of Diseases and Injuries, is further subdivided into 21 chapters. Each chapter contains codes for a body system or related conditions. Coders must become acquainted with the chapter topics within ICD-10-CM as well as the internal structure within each chapter in order to locate information and follow instructional notes. Instructional notes are official coding directions throughout the ICD-10-CM manual. Coders are required to follow instructional notes in order to abstract, assign, and arrange codes accurately. The various types of instructional notes are discussed later in this chapter.

The location within the ICD-10-CM chapter structure where instructional notes appear dictates what codes they apply to. Each chapter is subdivided into blocks, categories, subcategories, and codes (■ TABLE 4-3) as described below:

• A **block** or **subchapter** is a contiguous range of codes within a chapter. It is comparable to a section in ICD-9-CM.

• A **category** is three characters in length. A three-character category that has no further subdivisions is called a code.

• A **subcategory** is either four or five characters. Each level of subdivision after a category and before a code is a subcategory. A four- or five-character subcategory that has no further subdivisions is called a code.

• A **code** is the final level of subdivision. Codes may be three, four, five, six, or seven characters in length (■ TABLE 4-4). All codes in the Tabular List of the official version of the ICD-10-CM appear in boldface type. Entries that require a seventh character are referred to as codes, not subcategories, even though they are not complete without the seventh character.

Any instructional notes listed at the beginning of the chapter apply to all codes within that chapter. Instructional notes at the beginning of a block apply to all codes within that block but not to other blocks. Instructional notes at the beginning

Table 4-3 ■ **ORGANIZATIONAL STRUCTURE OF ICD-10-CM CHAPTERS**

Level	Example
Chapter	Chapter 15. Pregnancy, Childbirth and the Puerperium (O00-O9A)
Block	Pregnancy with abortive outcome (O00-O08)
Category	O03 Spontaneous abortion
Subcategory	O03.3 Other and unspecified complications following incomplete spontaneous abortion
Code	O03.31 Shock following incomplete spontaneous abortion

Table 4-4 ■ **EXAMPLES OF ICD-10-CM CODES WITH VARYING NUMBER OF CHARACTERS**

Code Length	Example
3-character code	I10
4-character code	F52.8
5-character code	K70.30
6-character code	L89.511
7-character code	T22.761A
7-character code with placeholder X	T51.0X1D V52.0XXS O33.4XX0

of the category apply to all codes within that category but not to previous or subsequent categories. Instructional notes at the beginning of the subcategory apply to all codes within that subcategory but not to previous or subsequent subcategories. Instructional notes that appear under a specific code apply only to that code.

CODING CAUTION

Be on the watch for letters that can be easily confused with numbers. The letter capital **I** can be confused with the number **1**. The letter **S** can be confused with the number **5**. The letter capital **O** can be confused with the number **0**. In the ICD-10-CM manual, the number zero might be written as **Ø** to help distinguish it from the capital letter **O**.

CODING PRACTICE

Exercise 4.1   Organization of ICD-10-CM

Instructions: Look up the following entries in the ICD-10-CM manual. Determine if each entry is a block, category, subcategory, or code and write the answer next to each entry.

Example: F01 Vascular dementia   *category*

1. **D56** Thalassemia _____

2. **F20.0** Paranoid schizophrenia _____

3. Diseases of esophagus, stomach and duodenum **(K20-K31)** _____

4. **O60.12** Preterm labor second trimester with preterm delivery second trimester _____

5. **O48.1** Prolonged pregnancy _____

6. **S37.0** Injury of kidney _____

7. **S67** Crushing injury of wrists, hand and fingers

_____

8. **T28.1XXS** Burn of esophagus, sequela

_____

9. Visual disturbances and blindness **(H53-H54)**

_____

10. **F01.5** Vascular dementia

_____

ICD-10-CM GUIDELINES AND CONVENTIONS

ICD-10-CM is accompanied by OGCR and Conventions, both of which direct the coder how to use the manual.

Official Guidelines for Coding and Reporting

Refer to the Contents page of the ICD-10-CM manual to locate the sections and *ICD-10-CM Official Guidelines for Coding and Reporting (OGCR)* and *ICD-10-CM Conventions.*

- OGCR are rules that complement the conventions and instructional notes to provide additional information and direction in identifying the diagnoses to be reported. The Health Insurance Portability and Accountability Act (HIPAA) requires that coders adhere to OGCR when assigning ICD-10-CM diagnosis codes.

- **Conventions** are the use of symbols, typeface, and layout features to succinctly convey interpretive information. Conventions appear in the section *ICD-10-CM Official Conventions.* Most conventions also appear in OGCR, Section I.A.

SUCCESS STEP

Conventions help you to avoid costly errors and point you in the right direction. Just as new drivers need to memorize the meaning of traffic signs, such as Stop, Yield, Do Not Enter, and Speed Limit, coders need to memorize the conventions.

Refer to the ICD-10-CM manual and locate the first page of ICD-10-CM Official Guidelines for Coding and Reporting (OGCR), which contains a detailed list of contents. The topics are referenced by an alphanumeric numbering system and page numbers. An overview of each OGCR section is provided next.

Section I

Section I Conventions, General Coding Guidelines and Chapter Specific Guidelines, contains the following major divisions:

A. Conventions for the ICD-10-CM: the general rules for the use of the coding manual independent of the guidelines. Most, but not all, of the conventions listed here also appear in the separate preceding section, ICD-10-CM Official Conventions.

B. General Coding Guidelines: overall rules that apply to all chapters in ICD-10-CM.

C. Chapter-Specific Coding Guidelines: guidelines for specific diagnoses and/or conditions, divided by ICD-10-CM chapter. Unless otherwise indicated within a specific guideline, these apply to all healthcare settings.

Section II

Section II, Selection of Principal Diagnosis, describes rules for abstracting the main diagnosis for inpatient settings. The guidelines for inpatient settings are different than for outpatient settings. **Principal diagnosis** applies only to inpatient settings. It is the "condition established after study to be chiefly responsible for occasioning the admission of the patient to the hospital for care," as defined by the **Uniform Hospital Data Discharge Set (UHDDS)**. Refer to the coding manual to review the topics in this section.

Section III

Section III, Reporting **Additional Diagnoses**, describes rules for abstracting **secondary** or extra diagnoses, in addition to the principal diagnosis, for inpatient settings. Refer to the coding manual to review the topics in this section.

Section IV

Section IV, Diagnostic Coding and Reporting Guidelines for Outpatient Services, describes rules for abstracting diagnoses in outpatient settings. Coding guidelines for outpatient diagnoses vary in several ways from those for inpatient diagnoses. The two most notable differences are the following:

- In the outpatient setting, the **first-listed diagnosis** is the diagnosis, condition, problem, or other reason for the encounter shown in the medical record to be chiefly responsible for the services provided. First-listed diagnosis applies only to outpatient settings; principal diagnosis applies only to inpatient settings. Secondary or additional diagnoses apply to all healthcare settings.

- Coding guidelines for inconclusive or **uncertain diagnoses** (*diagnoses preceded by the words* probable, possible, *suspected, questionable, rule out, working diagnosis, or a similar word*) were developed for inpatient reporting and do not apply to outpatients.

Refer to the coding manual to review the topics in this section.

SUCCESS STEP

The OGCR is updated each year after the coding manual is published. Although the coding manual is updated in October, the OGCR may not be updated until after the physical manual is published. Refer to the websites of the Center for Medicare and Medicaid Services (CMS) at **www.cms.gov** or the Centers for Disease Control and Prevention (CDC) at www.cdc.gov to download the most current guidelines.

Conventions

Coders' skills to recognize and interpret the conventions are crucial to interpreting ICD-10-CM instructions and assigning the accurate codes. Many ICD-10-CM conventions are the same as those used by ICD-9-CM, shown in ■ TABLE 4-5. Conventions that are new in ICD-10-CM are summarized in ■ TABLE 4-6. The tables that follow also identify where each convention is discussed in OGCR. Examples appear later in this chapter as well as throughout this text.

In addition to the official ICD-10-CM conventions, many publishers include proprietary symbols and colorcoding that

alert the user to special rules, warnings, and guidelines. The key to publisher-specific conventions usually appears in the introductory portion of the coding manual as well as at the bottom of each page.

Several of the most important conventions are discussed next. Refer to the ICD-10-CM manual and look up the examples that follow.

Exclusion Notes

ICD-10-CM Tabular List utilizes two exclusion notes: Excludes1 and Excludes2. Exclusion notes may appear at the beginning of a block, category, subcategory, or after a code. Notes at the category or subcategory level apply to all codes that follow, so it is important to check for these notes not only under the code, but also under the preceding block, category, and subcategory headings. For example, refer to category **K55 Vascular disorder of intestine** in the Tabular List and notice the note **Excludes1: necrotizing enterocolitis of newborn (P77.–)**. This note applies to all the subsequent codes, **K55.0** through **K55.9**. If coders read only the notes for one code, such as **K55.1**, they would miss the added instruction at the beginning of the category **K55**.

Excludes1 indicates that the condition represented by the code and the condition listed as excluded are mutually exclusive and should not be coded together. When an Excludes1 note appears under a code, none of the codes that appear after it should be used with the code where the note appears. For example, the Excludes1 note under **K55** means that **necrotizing enterocolitis of newborn (P77.-)** should not be reported with any of the codes within the **K55** category.

Excludes2 indicates that the condition excluded is not part of the condition represented by the code, but the patient may have both conditions at the same time. These conditions are not mutually exclusive. When an Excludes2 note appears under a code, it is acceptable to use the main code and the excluded code if the patient is documented to have both conditions. For example, refer to the Tabular List entry **K86.0 Alcohol induced chronic pancreatitis** and notice the note **Excludes2: alcohol induced acute pancreatitis (K85.2)**. The second condition, alcohol induced acute pancreatitis, is not included in code **K86.0** but may be reported together with it if the documentation states that the patient has both conditions.

Some codes may have both Excludes1 and Excludes2 notes. For example, the block **Diseases of liver (K70-K77)** has an Excludes1 note for **Jaundice NOS (R17)**, meaning that **R17** should not be reported with any of the codes from **K70** through **K77**. The same block also has several Excludes2 notes. The conditions listed under Excludes2 are not included in any of the codes **K70** through **K77** but may be reported together with them if the patient is documented to have both conditions. **K77** may appear on a different physical page than the block heading, so the coder who fails to review the beginning of the category will not be aware of these important instructions.

If a code does not have any exclusion notes, then it can be used with any other code that is supported by the medical record and the OGCR.

Table 4-5 ■ **CONVENTIONS THAT ARE THE SAME FOR ICD-9-CM AND ICD-10-CM**

Convention	Meaning/Use	OGCR Reference
( ) **Parentheses**	Index and Tabular: Nonessential modifiers that describe the default variations of a term. These words are not required to appear in the documentation in order to use the code.	I. A. 7
: **Colon**	Tabular: Appears after an incomplete term that requires one or more modifiers following the colon to be classified to that code or category.	I. A. 7
[ ] **Square brackets**	Index: Indicates sequencing on etiology/manifestation codes or other paired codes. The code in square brackets [ ] should be sequenced second. Tabular: Synonyms, alternative wording, explanatory phrases.	I. A. 7
And	Tabular: Means *and/or*.	I. A. 8 I. A. 14
Boldface (heavy type)	Index: Main terms. Tabular: Code titles.	Appears in Conventions, not OGCR
Code Also	Tabular: More than one code may be required to fully describe the condition.	I. A. 17
Code First/Use Additional Code	Tabular: Provides sequencing instructions for conditions that have both an underlying etiology and multiple body system manifestations and certain other codes that have sequencing requirements.	I. A. 13
Includes notes	Tabular: Begin with the word **Includes** and further define, clarify, or give examples.	I. A. 10
Inclusion terms	Tabular: A list of synonyms or conditions included within a classification.	I. A. 11
Italics (slanted type)	Tabular: Exclusion notes, manifestation codes.	Appears in Conventions, not OGCR
NEC	Index and Tabular: Not Elsewhere Classifiable. The medical record contains additional details about the condition, but there is not a more specific code available to use.	I. A. 6. a & b
NOS	Tabular: Not Otherwise Specified. Information to assign a more specific code is not available in the medical record.	I. A. 6. a & b
See	Index: It is necessary to reference another Main Term or condition to locate the correct code.	I. A. 16
See Also	Index: Coder may refer to an alternative or additional Main Term if the desired entry is not found under the original Main Term.	I. A. 16
With	Tabular: In a code title, means *both* or *together*.	I. A. 15

Table 4-6 ■ **NEW CONVENTIONS IN ICD-10-CM**

Convention	Meaning/Use	Reference
Excludes1	Tabular: Mutually exclusive codes. None of the codes that appear after it should be used with the original code itself.	OGCR I. A. 12. a
Excludes2	Tabular: The condition excluded is not part of the condition represented by the code but may be reported together if documented.	OGCR I. A. 12. b
X	Tabular: A placeholder in codes with fewer than six characters that require a seventh character. The **X** itself has no meaning and is not replaced with an actual number or letter. In some codes, the **X** is used to reserve room for future expansion.	OGCR I. A. 4 OGCR I. A. 5
– **Short dash**	Tabular and Index: Additional characters should be assigned in place of the -. The additional characters may be number or letters.	This symbol is used but not explained in OGCR or Conventions.
With/Without	Tabular: Within a set of alternative codes, describe options for final character.	Conventions
4th 5th **6th 7th**	Tabular: Some publishers place a symbol in front of a code to indicate that an additional character is needed for the code to be complete. This text uses the symbols shown here.	Publisher-specific convention

CODING PRACTICE

Exercise 4.2　Conventions: Exclusion Notes

Instructions: For each pair of codes, indicate whether they can be used together based on the exclusion notes. Look up the first code listed in each question. Read the **Excludes1** and **Excludes2** note(s) and determine whether the second code can be reported together with the first code. Circle the correct answer.

1. **G43.001** and **G43.709**	OK	Do not use together
2. **D56.1** and **D57.411**	OK	Do not use together
3. **H71.00** and **H60.410**	OK	Do not use together
4. **M21.532** and **M21.721**	OK	Do not use together
5. **O07.0** and **O04.84**	OK	Do not use together
6. **R22.2** and **R19.01**	OK	Do not use together
7. **R29.890** and **N63**	OK	Do not use together
8. **M80.012** and **M89.712**	OK	Do not use together
9. **S83.015A** and **M23.204**	OK	Do not use together
10. **T38.0X5D** and **T49.0X5D**	OK	Do not use together

Use Additional Characters

ICD-10-CM alerts coders to use additional characters on a code in two ways:

- a symbol in front of a code
- a short dash (-) at the end of a code number.

When coders see one of these conventions, it means a subcategory needs additional characters and the coder should look down to the next level for more specificity. In ICD-10-CM the additional values for characters 4 through 6 are listed below the subcategory. ■ FIGURE 4-1 illustrates the symbol to use additional characters.

SUCCESS STEP

Many publishing companies print the ICD-10-CM coding manual and each company may use different symbols to alert coders to the need for additional characters. If you do not see symbols such as **4th**, **5th**, **6th**, or **7th** in your edition of the coding manual, check the introductory material at the beginning of the manual to learn what symbols the publisher uses.

For example, OGCR C.12.a.2) for Chapter 12, Diseases of Skin and Subcutaneous Tissue (L00-L99), states, **Assignment of the code for Unstageable pressure ulcer (L89.- - 0) should**

be based on the clinical documentation. The use of two short dashes (- -) means that this guideline applies to all codes beginning with **L89** and ending in **0**, such as **L89.000, L89.010, L89.130**, etc. In the earlier example, **Excludes1: necrotizing enterocolitis of newborn (P77.-)**, the designation **P77.-** uses the short dash (-) to indicate all codes beginning with **P77**.

Seventh Characters and Placeholders

Some codes require a seventh character that reports special information. The seventh character must appear in the seventh position, regardless of the length of the code. The need for a seventh character may be indicated by a symbol, such as **7th**, preceding a code. When a three-, four-, or five-character code requires a seventh character, the placeholder **X** must fill any empty positions preceding the seventh position. The **X** itself has no meaning and is not replaced with an actual number or letter. Definitions for the seventh character may appear immediately above the code entry, or at a preceding block, category, or subcategory level.

The range of codes the seventh characters apply to is dictated by where the characters and definitions appear within the organizational hierarchy. Codes that require a seventh character are invalid if the seventh character is omitted; therefore, the claim may be rejected by the payer. ■ FIGURE 4-2 illustrates an example entry in the Tabular List that requires both a seventh character and a placeholder. To assign a code for *unspecified open wound of scalp, initial encounter,* follow these steps in the Tabular List:

- Select code **S01.00**.
- Because the code is only five characters in length, the **7th** symbol reminds you to add the placeholder **X** for the sixth character, before adding the seventh character.
- Finally, add the seventh character **A** to designate the initial episode of care.
- The final code is **S01.00XA**.

5th　K94.2　Gastrostomy complications
　　　　　K94.20　Gastrostomy complication, unspecified
　　　　　K94.21　Gastrostomy hemorrhage
　　　　　K94.20　Gastrostomy infection
　　　　　K94.20　Gastrostomy malfunction

Figure 4-1　■　Example of a Symbol to Use Additional Characters

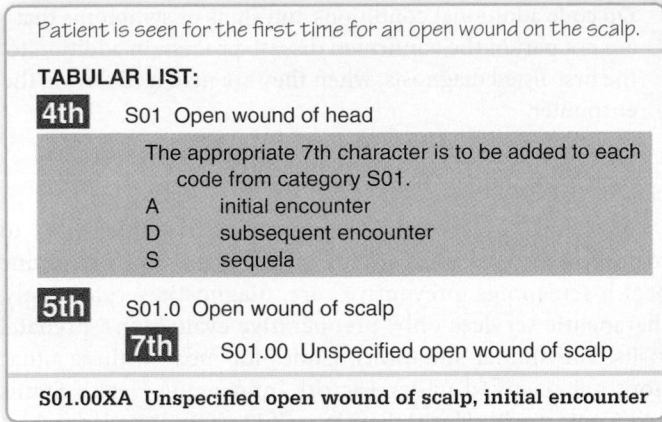

Patient is seen for the first time for an open wound on the scalp.

TABULAR LIST:

4th   S01   Open wound of head

The appropriate 7th character is to be added to each code from category S01.
A   initial encounter
D   subsequent encounter
S   sequela

5th   S01.0   Open wound of scalp

7th   S01.00   Unspecified open wound of scalp

S01.00XA   Unspecified open wound of scalp, initial encounter

Figure 4-2 ■ Example Use of a Placeholder (X) and a 7th character (A)

Laterality

ICD-10-CM contains a new OGCR, Section I.B.13, Laterality. For conditions that affect bilateral sites, such as eyes, ears, arms, and legs, the fifth or sixth character indicates whether the condition affects the right or left side. Approximately 28% of ICD-10-CM codes include a designation for laterality. A limited

number of these codes also provide an option for bilateral (*both sides affected*). If there is no designation for bilateral, assign separate codes for the right side and the left side. If laterality is unspecified, assign the code for **unspecified** side. The implementation of laterality is one example of why ICD-10-CM has many times the number of codes as ICD-9-CM does. In ICD-9-CM a condition such as *Marginal corneal ulcer* has one code number, 370.01, whereas ICD-10-CM has four codes plus a subcategory heading (five entries total) for the same condition (■ FIGURE 4-3).

SUCCESS STEP

It is important to notice exactly where a set of seventh character definitions appears within the organizational hierarchy. When the seventh characters and definitions appear at the beginning of a chapter, they are used with all subsequent codes in the chapter; when they appear at the beginning of a block, they are used with all codes in the block; when they appear at the beginning of a category or subcategory, they are used with all codes in the category or subcategory, respectively.

ICD-10-CM code	Description	Level of organization
H16.04	Marginal corneal ulcer	Subcategory
H16.041	Marginal corneal ulcer, right eye	Code
H16.042	Marginal corneal ulcer, left eye	Code
H16.043	Marginal corneal ulcer, bilateral	Code
H16.049	Marginal corneal ulcer, unspecified eye	Code

Figure 4-3 ■ Example of Laterality in ICD-10-CM

CODING PRACTICE

Exercise 4.3   Conventions: Use Additional Characters, Seventh Characters, and Placeholders

Instructions: Look up the following codes in the Tabular List and determine whether each is correct, needs additional characters, needs a placeholder, and/or needs a seventh character. Some codes may need more than one of these items. If the code is correct, write *Correct* in the space provided. If the code is incorrect, write the correct code for the stated condition in the space provided.

1. **E65** Localized adiposity _____

2. **E66** Morbid obesity due to excess calories _____

3. **G43.1** Migraine with aura, not intractable, with status migrainosus _____

4. **I48.9** Unspecified atrial fibrillation _____

5. **O31.00** Papyraceous fetus, first trimester, fetus 1

_____

6. **O29.8X2** Other complications of anesthesia during pregnancy, second trimester _____

7. **S71.151** Bite, right thigh, sequela _____

8. **S84.22** Injury of cutaneous sensory nerve at lower leg level, left leg, initial encounter _____

9. **S72.02** Displaced fracture of epiphysis, left femur, subsequent encounter for closed fracture with nonunion _____

10. **T59.6X** Toxic effect of hydrogen sulfide, accidental, subsequent encounter _____

HOW TO CODE DIAGNOSES

Diagnosis coding requires three skills of an ace coder:

- **Abstract**—read the medical record and determine which elements of the encounter require codes.

- **Assign**—determine codes that accurately describe the patient's condition, reflect the highest level of specificity possible, and contain the correct number of characters for each code.

- **Arrange (sequence)**—place codes in the order dictated by the OGCR and instructional notes.

Although coders do not need to memorize specific codes, they do need to memorize the skills and steps of the coding process.

When coders begin the process of assigning diagnosis codes, they do not necessarily know how many codes will be required. In some cases, a **combination code** is available, which describes two or more conditions in a single code. Other times, **multiple coding** is required, which means that two or more codes are needed to fully describe a condition. Coders learn how many codes are needed by following the guidelines, conventions, and instructional notes in the Index, Tabular List, and OGCR.

Abstracting Diagnoses

The first step in coding is to identify the diagnosis(es) to be coded based on the documentation. The OGCR provide guidelines for this task in Section I.B, as well as Section IV for outpatient services and Sections II and III for inpatient services. Chapter-specific guidelines in Section I.C provide more detailed guidance for selected conditions. This section provides an overview of abstracting outpatient and inpatient diagnoses.

Abstracting Outpatient Diagnoses

For outpatient coding, the coder needs to identify the main reason for the services provided, which is the first-listed diagnosis. Recall that this is the diagnosis, condition, problem, or other reason for the encounter shown in the medical record to be chiefly responsible for the services provided (OGCR IV.A). Coding conventions and the general (OGCR I.B) and chapter-specific (OCGR I.C) guidelines take precedence over Section IV outpatient guidelines if there is a conflict. Key rules for abstracting outpatient diagnoses follow:

- Do **not** code **signs** or **symptoms** that are an integral part of the disease process when the diagnosis has been established.

- Do **not** code an uncertain diagnosis, which is indicated in the medical record by words such as *probable, possible, suspected, questionable, rule out,* or *working diagnosis.*

- **Do** code the presenting signs and symptoms when the diagnosis is uncertain. This guideline for outpatient services is different than the guideline for uncertain diagnoses for inpatient services.

- **Do** code additional conditions and signs or symptoms that are not part of the confirmed disease process, in addition to the first-listed diagnosis, when they are managed during the encounter.

- Do **not** code conditions that are resolved, not treated, or have no bearing on the current encounter.

ICD-10-CM also provides codes for encounters due to reasons other than a disease or injury. These may be routine health screenings, preventive care, diagnostic services only, therapeutic services only, preoperative evaluations, prenatal visits, and similar situations. Codes for most of these situations are classified under Factors Influencing Health Status and Contact with Health Services (Z00-Z99). Detailed guidelines appear in OGCR IV and codes are indexed in the Index to Diseases and Injuries.

Abstracting Using the Mini-Medical-Record

This text uses a mini-medical-record format for examples and exercises, which extracts the most essential information from a patient's medical record. Refer to ■ FIGURE 4-4 to become acquainted with this format and to learn how to interpret it.

Guided Example of Abstracting Diagnoses

■ TABLE 4-7 provides general guidance on how to abstract diagnoses. These abstracting criteria are general questions to ask regarding most conditions. Abstracting questions are a guide, and not every question applies to, or can be answered for, every case. For example, age and gender are not relevant for every diagnosis. Not every case includes signs and symptoms. More detailed abstracting criteria are presented for each body system throughout this text.

Table 4-7 ■ **KEY CRITERIA FOR ABSTRACTING DIAGNOSES (GENERAL GUIDELINES)**

- ❑ What are the gender and age of the patient?
- ❑ What is the patient's chief complaint or reason for the encounter or inpatient admission?
- ❑ Is the encounter inpatient or outpatient?
- ❑ What symptoms and signs are described?
- ❑ Does the physician provide a definitive diagnosis?
- ❑ Does the physician provide a diagnosis that is uncertain, probable, possible, qualified, or rule out?
- ❑ Which symptoms and signs are integral to the definitive diagnosis?
- ❑ Which symptoms and signs are related, but not integral, to the definitive diagnosis?
- ❑ What unrelated conditions, symptoms, or signs are managed during the encounter?
- ❑ What conditions, symptoms, or signs are not managed during the encounter?
- ❑ What is the laterality, if any, of the condition?
- ❑ What is the treatment plan or procedure? Is it consistent with the diagnosis?
- ❑ Is the condition the result of an injury or external cause?

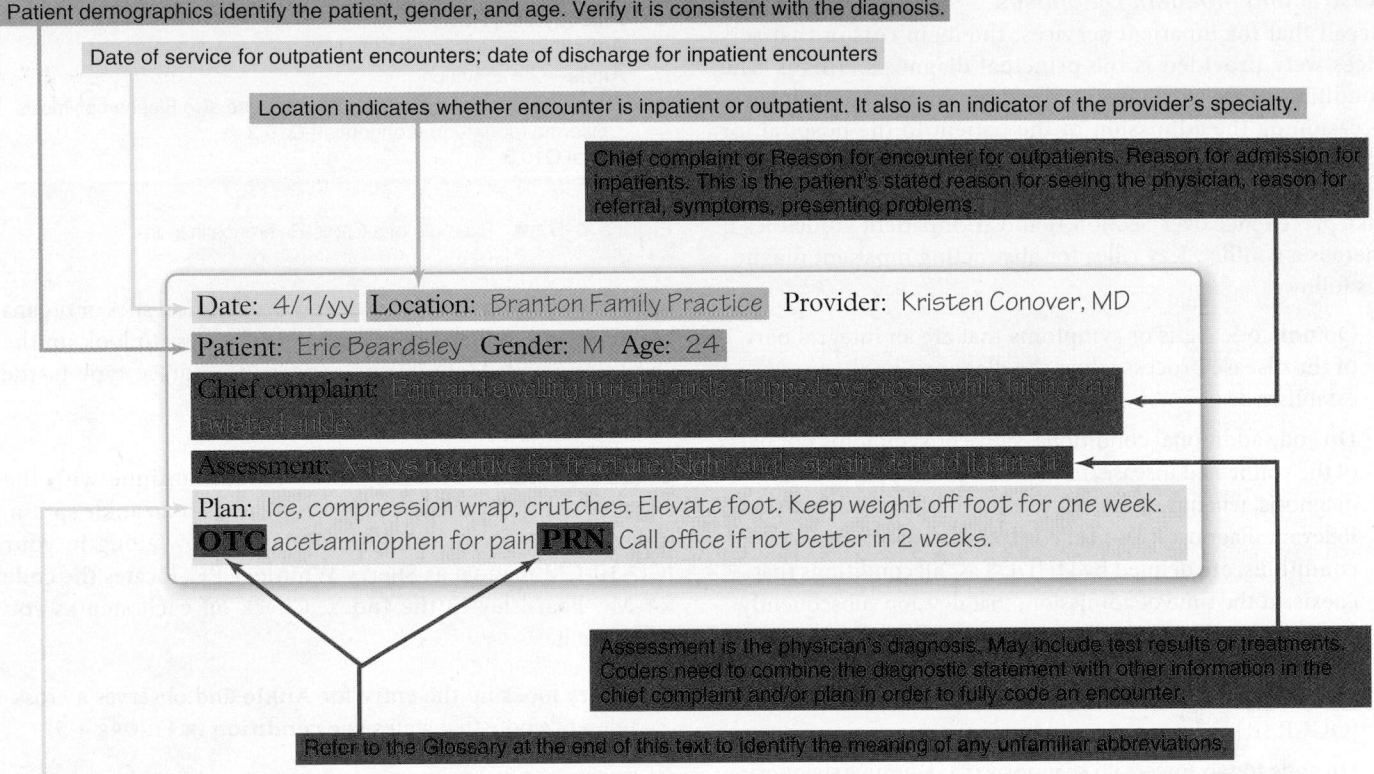

Patient demographics identify the patient, gender, and age. Verify it is consistent with the diagnosis.

Date of service for outpatient encounters; date of discharge for inpatient encounters

Location indicates whether encounter is inpatient or outpatient. It also is an indicator of the provider's specialty.

Chief complaint or Reason for encounter for outpatients. Reason for admission for inpatients. This is the patient's stated reason for seeing the physician, reason for referral, symptoms, presenting problems.

Date: 4/1/yy Location: Branton Family Practice Provider: Kristen Conover, MD

Patient: Eric Beardsley Gender: M Age: 24

Chief complaint: Pain and swelling in right ankle. Tripped over rocks while hiking and twisted ankle.

Assessment: X-rays negative for fracture. Right ankle sprain, deltoid ligament.

Plan: Ice, compression wrap, crutches. Elevate foot. Keep weight off foot for one week. **OTC** acetaminophen for pain **PRN**. Call office if not better in 2 weeks.

Assessment is the physician's diagnosis. May include test results or treatments. Coders need to combine the diagnostic statement with other information in the chief complaint and/or plan in order to fully code an encounter.

Refer to the Glossary at the end of this text to identify the meaning of any unfamiliar abbreviations.

Plan is the treatment plan after the conclusion of the encounter or after-discharge. May mention treatment provided during the encounter.

Figure 4-4 ■ Key to Interpreting the Mini-Medical-Record

Refer to the following example, which begins here and continues throughout the chapter, to learn more about abstracting a diagnosis for an outpatient visit. Follow along with fictitious coder Sherry Whittle, CPC, as she reads the progress notes from the patient Eric Beardsley's office visit (Figure 4-4). Check off each step as you complete it.

▶ First, Sherry reviews the demographic information and reads Mr. Beardsley's chief complaint. Then she refers to Table 4-7, Key Criteria for Abstracting Diagnoses, and answers each question from the medical record. (*Questions from the Key Criteria table appear in italics.* Answers taken directly from the medical record appear in this special font. Any other comments or observations appear in a normal font.)

❑ *What are the gender and age of the patient?* Male, age 24

❑ *What is the patient's chief complaint or reason for the encounter?* Pain and swelling in the right ankle

❑ *Is the encounter inpatient or outpatient?* Outpatient (office)

❑ *What symptoms and signs are described?* Pain and swelling

❑ *Does the physician provide a definitive diagnosis?* Yes. Right ankle sprain, deltoid ligament

❑ *Does the physician provide a diagnosis that is uncertain, probable, possible, qualified, or rule out?* No

❑ *Which symptoms and signs are integral to the definitive diagnosis?* Pain and swelling

❑ *Which symptoms and signs are related, but not integral, to the definitive diagnosis?* None

❑ *What unrelated conditions, symptoms, or signs are managed during the encounter?* None

❑ *What conditions, symptoms, or signs are not managed during the encounter?* No other conditions, symptoms, or signs were documented.

❑ *What is the laterality, if any, of the condition?* Right

❑ *What is the treatment plan or procedure?* Ice, compression wrap, crutches. *Is it consistent with the diagnosis?* Yes

❑ *Is the condition the result of an injury or external cause?* Yes. Tripped over rocks while hiking and twisted ankle.

▶ Sherry will code the diagnosis Right ankle sprain, deltoid ligament. Next, she needs to assign the codes.

SUCCESS STEP

You do not always know how many codes you will end up with, or even exactly which conditions require a code, at the time of abstracting. You abstract *potential* conditions and elements to be coded. OGCR and instructional notes in the Tabular List provide further direction about how many and what codes are needed in a specific situation.

Abstracting Inpatient Diagnoses

Recall that for inpatient services, the main reason that services were provided is the principal diagnosis. This is "the condition established after study to be chiefly responsible for occasioning the admission of the patient to the hospital for care" (OGCR Section II). Coding conventions and the general (OGCR I.B) and chapter-specific (OGCR I.C) guidelines take precedence over Section II and III inpatient guidelines if there is a conflict. Key rules for abstracting inpatient diagnoses follow:

- Do **not** code signs or symptoms that are an integral part of the disease process when the diagnosis has been established.

- **Do** code additional conditions, signs, or symptoms not part of the confirmed disease, in addition to the principal diagnosis, when they are **relevant** to the current admission. Relevant diagnoses, also called **clinically significant conditions**, are defined by UHDDS as "all conditions that coexist at the time of admission, that develop subsequently, or that affect the treatment received and/or the length of stay. Diagnoses that relate to an earlier episode which have no bearing on the current hospital stay are to be excluded" (OGCR III).

- **Do** code for an uncertain diagnosis if a definitive diagnosis is not available at the time of discharge and/or after all test results are reported. This guideline is different for inpatient services than outpatient. For inpatient, code an uncertain diagnosis as if it exists because it is the reason for the hospital admission and any diagnostic and therapeutic services provided (OGCR II.H).

CODING CAUTION

Coding sounds simple to the casual observer, but as you are about to learn, it is an extended research process that involves many comparisons and cross-checks. Learning the detailed steps of coding will make you a more accurate coder. Unfortunately, there are no shortcuts.

Assigning Diagnosis Codes

After identifying the first-listed diagnosis or principal diagnosis in the medical record, the next step is to assign the most specific code possible that describes the condition. To assign a diagnosis code, first look up the condition in the Index to Diseases and Injuries (Index), then verify the code in the Tabular List.

Locate the Main Term in the Index

The first step in assigning the code is to locate the **Main Term** (*the primary index entry*) in the ICD-10-CM Index to Diseases and Injuries. The Main Term is the name of the condition or reason for the visit, usually presented as a noun. Coders need to be knowledgeable about several details regarding the organization of the Index, which are discussed next.

> Anisocytosis R71.8
> Anisometropia (congenital) H52.31
> Ankle—*see condition*
> Ankyloblepharon (eyelid) (acquired)—*see also* Blepharophimosis
>   filiforme (adnatum) (congential) Q10.3
>   total Q10.3

Figure 4-5 ■ Example of a Cross-Reference in Index

Anatomical Sites Are Not Indexed. Anatomical sites or organs are rarely indexed as Main Terms, so it is best to look up the condition itself. Main Terms appear in boldface type in the index.

Guided Example of Using the Index. Continue with the example of Eric Beardsley, who was treated for an ankle sprain, to learn more about using the Index. Follow along in your ICD-10-CM manual as Sherry Whittle, CPC, locates the code for Mr. Beardsley in the Index. Check off each step as you complete it.

▶ Sherry looks up the entry for **Ankle** and observes a cross-reference note that states *see* condition (■ FIGURE 4-5).

   ❑ She recalls that this is a cross-reference directing her to look up the term that describes the *condition affecting the ankle*, which in this case is a sprain.

   ❑ She does not look up the word *condition*.

   ❑ Sherry will look up the Main Term **Sprain** because that is the condition that affects the ankle.

Subterms. Subterms are words indented under each Main Term that further describe the Main Term in greater detail, such as anatomical location or other disease variation. Subterms appear in roman type (*not boldface*) and are indented three spaces under the Main Term. Many subterms have additional subterms indented under them. Each subterm is an expansion of the Main Term or previous subterm it is indented under. In some editions of the coding manual, the ICD-10-CM Index provides shading, guidelines, or dashes to help align the various levels of indentation. Refer to ■ FIGURE 4-6 for the layout and compare the figure to the actual coding manual.

Guided Example of Locating the Main Term. Continue to follow along in your ICD-10-CM manual as Sherry Whittle, CPC, looks up the Main Term **Sprain** for Mr. Beardsley's case. Check off each step as you complete it.

▶ Sherry locates the Main Term **Sprain** in the Index to Diseases and Injuries.

   ❑ She scans the entire entry for **Sprain**, which continues onto the next several columns on the next page. At the top of each column is a heading **Sprain – continued**, telling her which Main Term is being continued.

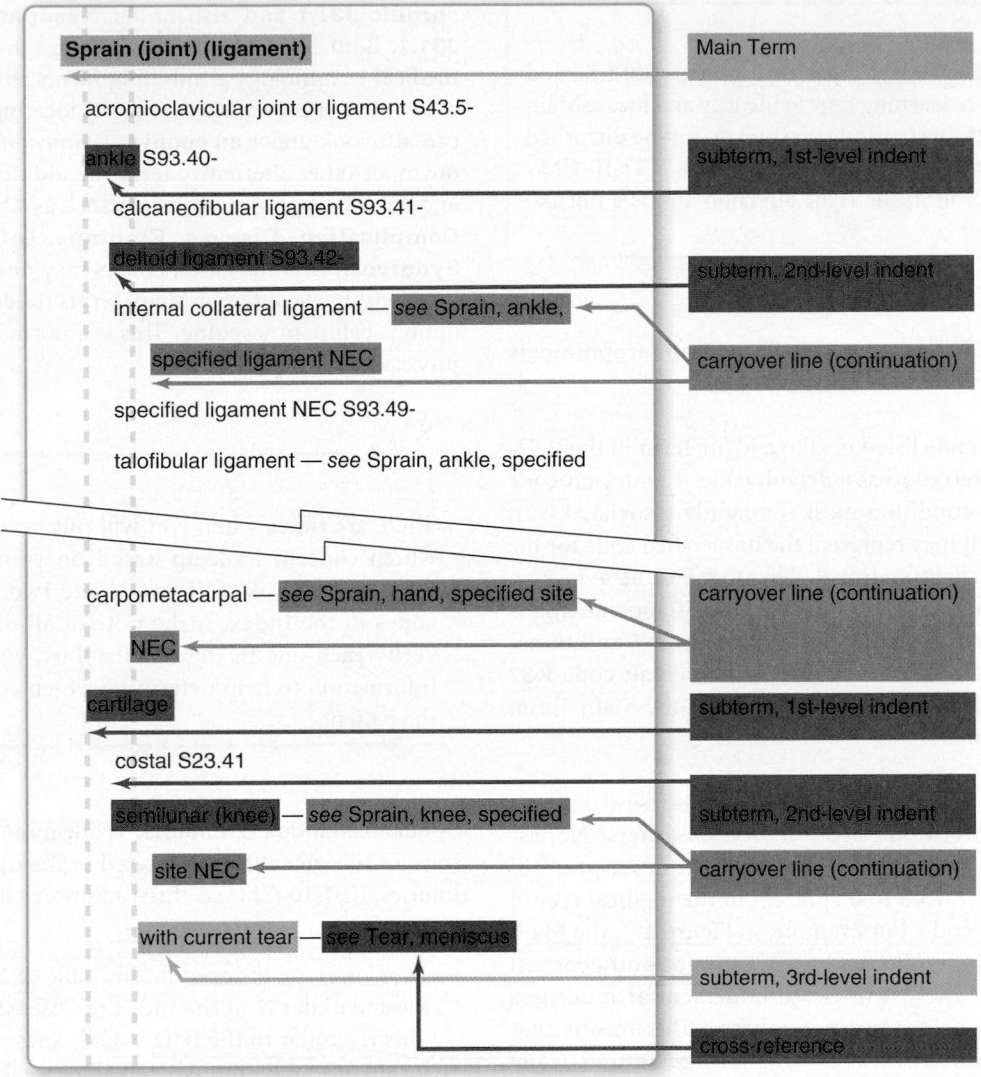

Figure 4-6 ■ Example of Main Term and Subterm Indents in the Index

❑ She notices that all the subterms describe anatomical sites of a sprain.

❑ She locates the subterm **ankle**, for the anatomical site.

❑ She notices that additional subterms further describe the anatomical site within the ankle, such as **calcaneofibular ligament S93.41-** and **deltoid ligament S93.42-**. These subterms are second-level indents. Both of these entries are part of the overall entry for ankle because they are indented under the subterm **ankle**.

❑ Sherry identifies the second-level subterm **deltoid ligament S93.42-** as the best match for Mr. Beardsley's case.

❑ The full name of this entry combines the Main Term and each indented subterm: **Sprain + ankle + deltoid ligament** (Figure 4-6).

Also notice in Figure 4-6 that a third-level indent appears further down in the entry for **Sprain**. The subterm **cartilage** is a first-level indent, so it is parallel to the subterm **ankle**. These two subterms are mutually exclusive. **Cartilage** has a second-level indented subterm for the sites **costal** and **semilunar**. **Semilunar** has a third-level indented subterm, **with current tear**. The full entry for this subterm is **Sprain, cartilage, semilunar, with current tear**.

Cross-References. As previously mentioned, some subterms provide cross-referencing instructions, which begin with the word *see* or *see also*. When the instruction following the word *see* or *see also* is capitalized, the coder should look under the word listed to find the correct code. For example, under **Sprain, cartilage, semilunar, with current tear**, the subterm **with current tear** provides cross-referencing instructions to *see* **Tear, meniscus**. This means the coder should look up the Main Term **Tear** and the subterm **meniscus** in order to locate the code.

Refer to Figure 4-5 for an example of a *see also* cross-reference. Notice that the Main Term **Ankyloblepharon** has two subterms. In addition to reviewing these subterms, coders

SUCCESS STEP

In the beginning, you may experience a process of trial and error while you are learning how to identify and locate Main Terms. Do not let this frustrate you and do not be disturbed by cross-reference notes in the Index. This is ICD-10-CM's way of pointing you in the right direction and is a normal part of coding.

should also cross-reference the Main Term **Blepharophimosis** for additional codes.

Default Codes. A code listed next to a Main Term in the ICD-10-CM Index is referred to as a **default code**. The default code may represent the condition most commonly associated with the Main Term, or it may represent the unspecified code for the condition, which usually ends in 9. Refer to ■ FIGURE 4-7 for an example of a default code. In this example, if appendicitis is documented in the medical record without any additional information, such as acute or chronic, the default code **K37** should be assigned because it appears next to the Main Term, **Appendicitis**.

Nonessential Modifiers. The words in parentheses ( ) after a Main Term or subterm are **nonessential modifiers**. Nonessential modifiers are included in the default description of the code and do not need to be present in the medical record in order to use the code. For example, in Figure 4-7, the Main Term **Appendicitis** is followed by the terms **(pneumococcal)** and **(retrocecal)**. These words are nonessential modifiers because they are enclosed in parentheses. This means that pneumococcal and retrocecal appendicitis are automatically included in the default appendicitis code **K37**. However, these words do not need to be present in the medical record in order to assign this code because they are nonessential modifiers. The conditions appendicitis, pneumococcal appendicitis, and retrocecal appendicitis are all classified with the same code, **K37**.

Also notice that in the ICD-10-CM Index, the entry **Appendicitis** has numerous subterms with different codes. Coders must review all the subterms and locate the most specific one before selecting a code to verify. Do not automatically select the default code without reviewing the subterms.

Multiple Coding Paths. Conditions may have multiple **coding paths**, which means they can be indexed under more than one Main Term. For example, chronic rhinopharyngitis (*inflammation of the nose and throat*) appears under **Rhinopharyngitis, chronic J31.1** and also under **Nasopharyngitis, chronic J31.1**. Both Main Terms lead to the same code because the medical terminology combining forms rhin/o and nas/o both mean nose. If coders have difficulty locating a Main Term, they can also look under an **eponym** (*named after a person*), a synonym, or other alternative term. In addition, coders can reference broad-ranging Main Terms, such as **Abnormal**, **Anomaly**, **Complication**, **Disease**, **Findings**, **Infection**, **Injury**, or **Syndrome**. In some cases, coders may need to look in several locations under different Main Terms to identify multiple code options before proceeding. This is a normal part of the coding process.

Appendicitis (pneumococcal) (retrocecal) K37

Figure 4-7 ■ Example of Index Entry for a Default Code with Nonessential Modifiers

SUCCESS STEP

There are times when you will not be completely sure of which code to look up based on your research in the Index. That is okay. If you locate two or three possible codes in the Index, make note of all of them. After you verify each one in the Tabular List, you will have more information to help determine which code best describes the patient.

Specialized Index Locations. While most conditions and reasons for the encounter are located in the Index to Diseases and Injuries, ICD-10-CM has three additional locations for specialized codes.

- *Neoplasms* are indexed in the Table of Neoplasms, located under **N** in the Index to Diseases and Injuries. This is similar to the ICD-9-CM. Some publishers may locate this table immediately after the Index to Diseases and Injuries.
- *Poisonings, adverse effects, and underdosing caused by drugs and chemicals* are indexed in the ICD-10-CM Table of Drugs and Chemicals, which is located following the Index to Diseases and Injuries. This is similar to the ICD-9-CM.
- *External causes of illness and injury* are located in a separate index, the ICD-10-CM Index to External Causes, which follows the Table of Drugs and Chemicals. This is similar to the **E** code index in ICD-9-CM. External causes reported under "E codes" in ICD-9-CM are generally reported using codes beginning with the letters **V**, **W**, **X**, and **Y** in ICD-10-CM and appear within the Tabular List.

SUCCESS STEP

Just as some publishers use different symbols to alert coders to special situations, some may organize the sections of the coding manual in a different order. Refer to the Table of Contents at the beginning of your coding manual to learn how it is organized.

CODING PRACTICE

Exercise 4.4   Locating the Main Term

Instructions: Underline the Main Term in each of these diagnoses. Then look up the Main Term in the Index to confirm that you chose the correct term. If the Index cross-references another entry, write the name of the cross-reference in the space provided. Then look up the cross-referenced entry.

Example: <u>Short</u> arm   <u>Deformity, limb, unequal length</u>

1. Complicated open wound of left ear, initial encounter

   _____

2. Deprivation of water, subsequent encounter

   _____

3. Urinary tract infection _____

4. Chickenpox _____

5. Blackwater fever _____

6. Gallbladder infection _____

7. Quartan malaria _____

8. Cerebrovascular disease _____

9. Congestive heart failure _____

10. Type 1 diabetes _____

Verify Codes in the Tabular List

After identifying the potential code(s) in the Index, the next step in assigning a code is to verify it in the Tabular List. This is an essential step because the Index is not designed to provide the full code or full information about how to use the code. Verifying codes requires cross-referencing information at several points.

A short dash (-) at the end of an Index entry indicates that additional characters are required. Even when a dash is not included at the Index entry, it is necessary to refer to the Tabular List to verify that no seventh character is required and to review the instructional notes. Characters for laterality and the seventh character can only be assigned in the Tabular List. The Tabular List also includes instructional notes that must be followed, such as those for sequencing, multiple coding, and inclusion and exclusion notes discussed earlier in the chapter.

To verify a code, look up the code number in the Tabular List and follow these steps:

1. Read the code title to confirm that the code accurately describes the intended condition.

2. Read the instructional notes under the code.

3. Check for symbols preceding the entry indicating that additional characters are required.

4. Cross-reference the titles of the subcategory and the three-character category and read any instructional notes under those titles.

5. Cross-reference the titles of the block and the chapter headings and read any instructional notes under those titles.

6. Compare and contrast any other codes being considered for first-listed or principal diagnosis.

7. Assign all required characters and write down the code, taking time to double check for transcription or typographical errors.

8. Repeat this process for each code required.

Guided Example of Verifying Codes in the Tabular List

Continue with the example of Eric Beardsley, who has a right ankle sprain of the deltoid ligament, to learn more about verifying codes in the Tabular List.

Follow along in your ICD-10-CM manual as Sherry Whittle, CPC, verifies the diagnosis code. Check off each step after you complete it.

▶ Recall that Sherry located the entry **S93.42-** in the Index.

   ❏ Sherry notices the entry ends with a short dash (-). She knows this means that she will need to assign additional digits when she verifies the code in the Tabular List.

▶ Sherry looks up the entry **S93.42** in the Tabular List.

   ❏ She notices that this is a subcategory, not a code, because additional characters are required. The symbol **6th** in front of the entry tells her that a sixth character is required.

   ❏ She confirms the title of the category **Sprain of deltoid ligament** is consistent with the progress note.

▶ She reads the code choices listed and notices that the sixth character defines laterality with choices for right ankle, left ankle, and unspecified ankle.

   ❏ She refers back to the progress note to confirm which ankle was affected.

   ❏ She selects code **S93.421** for the right ankle.

▶ Sherry notices that the symbol **7th** appears in front of the code **S93.421**. This tells her that a seventh character is required to complete the code.

   ❏ The seventh character is not listed under the code, so she knows she needs to review the previous subcategory, category, and block headings to locate the seventh character options. She knows she needs to review these headings anyway in order to locate any possible instructional notes.

S93 Dislocation and sprain of joints and ligaments at ankle, foot and toe level
Includes:
avulsion of joint or ligament of ankle, foot and toe
laceration of cartilage, joint or ligament of ankle, foot and toe
sprain of cartilage, joint or ligament of ankle, foot and toe
traumatic hemarthrosis of joint or ligament of ankle, foot and toe
traumatic rupture of joint or ligament of ankle, foot and toe
traumatic subluxation of joint or ligament of ankle, foot and toe
traumatic tear of joint or ligament of ankle, foot and toe
Excludes2: strain of muscle and tendon of ankle and foot (S96.-)
Code also any associated open wound
The appropriate 7th character is to be added to each code from category S93
A - initial encounter
D - subsequent encounter
S - sequela

Figure 4-8 ■ Tabular List Entry for Category Heading S93

▶ Sherry confirms the subcategory title **S93.4, Sprain of ankle** is the correct anatomic site because other joints, such as the shoulder, also have a **deltoid** muscle or ligament.

❑ She reads the note **Excludes2: injury of Achilles tendon (S86.0-)** under the subcategory title and verifies that does not apply to her case because the Achilles tendon was not documented.

▶ Next she works back up the organizational hierarchy of the Tabular List until she locates the three-character category heading **S93, Dislocation and sprain of joints and ligaments at ankle, foot and toe level** (■ FIGURE 4-8).

❑ Sherry reads the entries for the **Includes** note under the category heading. She observes that one of entries is **sprain of cartilage, joint or ligament of ankle, foot and toe**, which is consistent with the Mr. Beardsley's progress note.

❑ Sherry notices the instructional note **Code also any associated open wound** following the Includes list. She understands that if Dr. Conover had documented an open wound in addition to the sprain, she would need an additional code for the wound. Because a wound was not documented, she knows she can bypass this note.

❑ Sherry reads the note **Excludes2: strain of muscle and tendon of ankle and foot (S96.-)** and understands that if Dr. Conover had also documented a muscle or tendon strain, she would need an additional code because **Excludes2** means that **strain of muscle and tendon of ankle and foot (S96.-)** is not included in this category.

❑ Sherry identifies the list of seventh characters for this category.

▶ Next, Sherry reviews the seventh character assignments that apply to all codes in category **S93**.

❑ She reviews the progress note to determine if this episode of care was the **initial encounter** (*active treatment*), **subsequent encounter** (*treatment during the healing phase*), or a **sequela** (*late effect or problem after active healing is completed*).

❑ The progress note does not specifically use any of these words, but Sherry determines from the context that this

was Mr. Beardsley's first encounter for treatment of the sprain. If this had been a follow-up visit or later problem, Dr. Conover would have explicitly stated that.

❑ The seventh character for initial encounter is **A**, so Sherry assigns **A** at the end of the code, to arrive at **S93.421A**.

▶ Sherry knows she is not quite done. She still needs to check the block and chapter headings for any possible instructional notes.

❑ She is not sure where the block begins, so she refers to the beginning of the entries for codes beginning with **S** in the Tabular List, which coincides with the beginning of the chapter (■ FIGURE 4-9).

❑ She finds an instructional note with the word **NOTE:** which instructs her to **Use secondary code(s) from Chapter 20, External causes of morbidity, to indicate cause of injury**. (External cause codes are discussed in Chapter 8 of this text.)

❑ She reads the other instructional notes under the chapter heading and finds no other notes that apply to this case.

❑ She scans the list of block headings in this chapter and locates the block for **S90-S99 Injuries to the ankle and foot**.

▶ Sherry turns to the beginning of the block **S90-S99** (■ FIGURE 4-10).

❑ She reads the **Excludes2** notes and determines that they do not apply to this case because none of these conditions are documented.

❑ Sherry is tempted to think it was a waste of time to cross-reference the beginning of the chapter and block for additional instructions because none were found. However, she knows from experience that as soon as she tries to take a shortcut, it backfires on her and causes her to miss important information or instructions.

▶ Sherry assigns diagnosis code **S93.421A** to this encounter. She will also assign external cause codes for tripping while hiking.

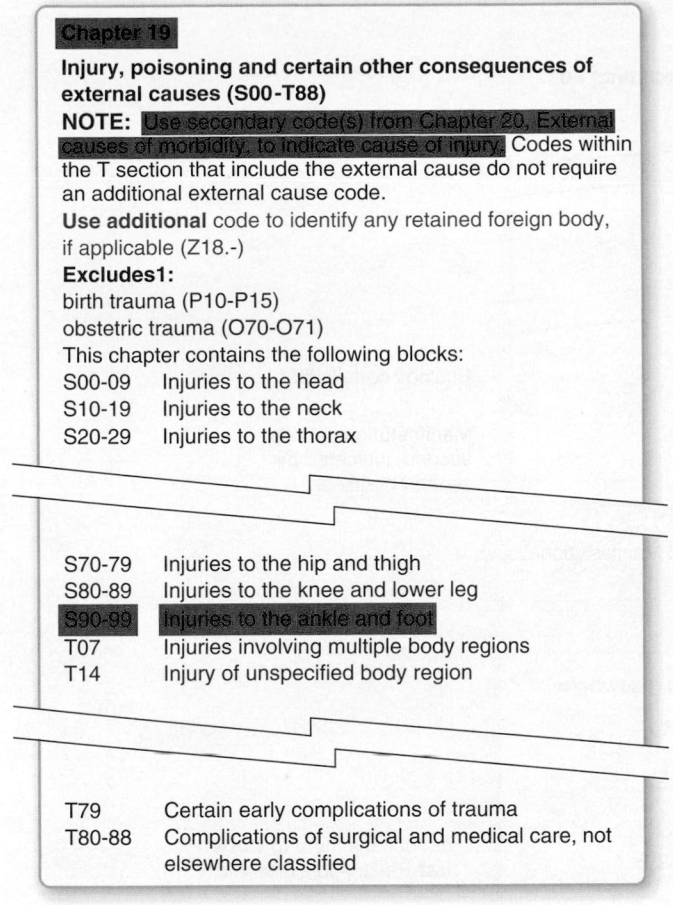

Injuries to the ankle and foot (S90-S99)

Excludes2:
burns and corrosions (T20-T32)
fracture of ankle and malleolus (S82.-)
frostbite (T33-T34)
insect bite or sting, venomous (T63.4)

Figure 4-10 ■ Tabular List Entry for Block Heading S90-S99

Arranging Diagnosis Codes

The final step in diagnosis coding is to arrange, or sequence, codes in the correct order when there is more than one diagnosis code. Coders may need to assign more than one diagnosis code when patients have more than one condition that is being treated or managed during an encounter; there is an etiology/manifestation relationship; multiple coding is required; or instructional notes in the Tabular List direct the coder to additional codes needed. Each of these situations is discussed below. In addition, the OGCR discusses requirements for multiple coding related to specific diseases.

SUCCESS STEP

This text uses the term *arrange* as a learning mnemonic for *sequence* in order to remind you of the coding skills of **A**bstract, **A**ssign, and **A**rrange. In the workplace, most professional coders simply use the term *sequence*.

More Than One Condition Treated

When more than one condition is treated or managed during an encounter, sequence the principal or first-listed diagnosis first. When it is difficult to determine which condition is the principal diagnosis, refer to the following guidelines:

- When two or more interrelated conditions each potentially meet the definition for principal diagnosis, either condition may be sequenced first if the **circumstances of admission** (*facts, signs, and symptoms that require the admission*), the Index, or the Tabular List provide no further guidance (OGCR II.B).

- When two or more distinct conditions equally meet the definition for principal diagnosis, either condition may be sequenced first if the circumstances of admission, the Index, or the Tabular List provide no further guidance (OGCR II.C).

When the principal or first-listed diagnosis is clear, sequence the additional conditions in order of importance to the encounter or in order of severity or risk to the patient's health and well-being.

Etiology/Manifestation

Etiology/manifestation is an ICD-10-CM convention for certain conditions that have both an underlying **etiology** (*cause*) and **manifestations** (*signs and symptoms*) in multiple body systems (OGCR I.A.13). Sequence the etiology first and the manifestation second. Coders may not always know in advance if a particular combination of diseases is an etiology/manifestation relationship, so the ICD-10-CM manual alerts coders with sequencing instructions.

CODING CAUTION

Do not apply etiology/manifestation rules if ICD-10-CM does not list instructional notes or other conventions indicating this relationship.

Refer to the following example of dementia in Parkinson's disease, where Parkinson's disease is the etiology and dementia is a manifestation. Common sequencing instructions for etiology/manifestation follow with examples:

- The Index lists both conditions and both codes together. The etiology code is first; the manifestation code is second and appears in [brackets]. Always sequence the code in brackets second (■ FIGURE 4-11, page 52).

- In the Tabular List entry for the manifestation code, the manual provides an instructional note **Code first** and lists codes for possible etiologies. The condition listed after this note should be sequenced second (■ FIGURE 4-12, page 52).

- The manifestation code title often includes the phrase **in diseases classified elsewhere**. Code titles with this phrase may be highlighted in the Tabular List as a reminder that manifestation codes may never be the first-listed or principal diagnosis.

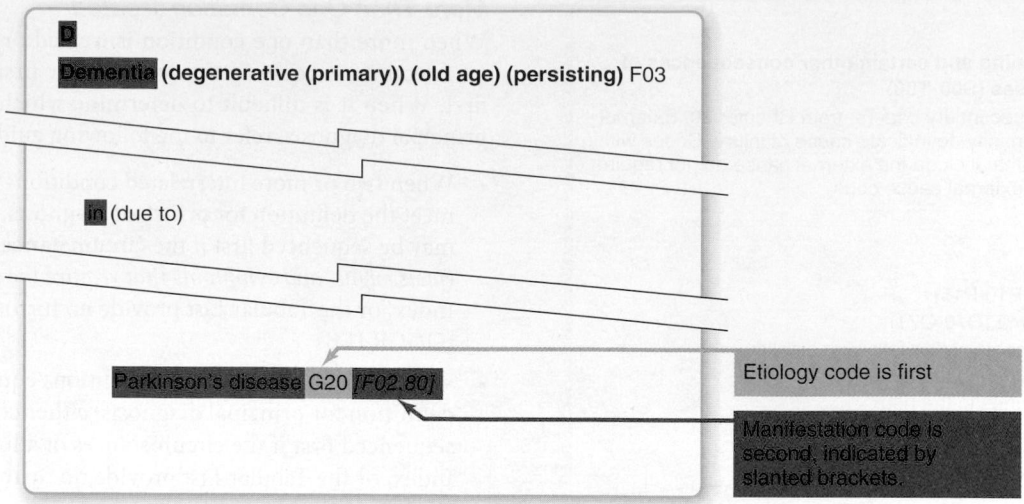

Figure 4-11 ■ Example of Index Entry for Etiology and Manifestation Codes

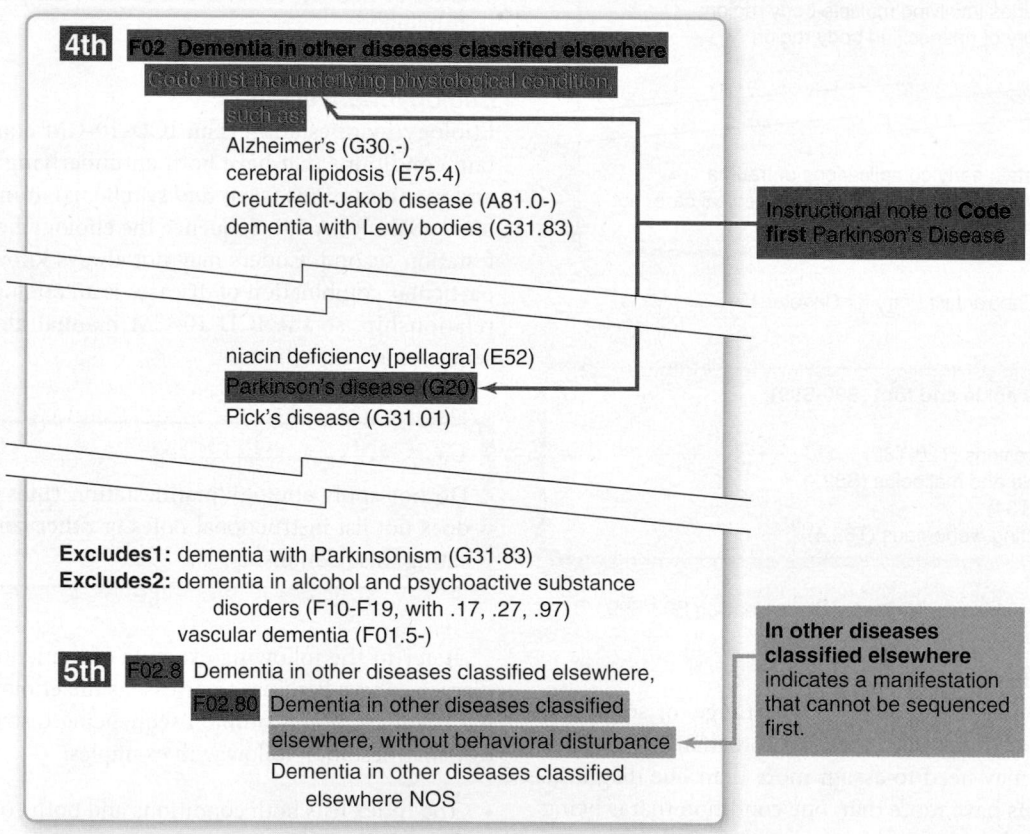

Figure 4-12 ■ Example of Tabular List Entry for Code First Instructions

CODING CAUTION

Do not assign a code from the **Use additional code** list for any condition that is not documented in the medical record. If the etiology documented in the medical record does not appear in the list, you should refer to the Index and locate the code for the specific etiology you need.

CODING CAUTION

Notice that Figure 4-13 has an **Excludes1** note for **dementia with Parkinsonism** and cross-references the coder to **G31.83**. When you cross-reference **G31.83**, you see the code title is **Dementia with Lewy bodies**, which is a specific kind of dementia. Since this condition is not documented in the medical record, use the original code **G20**.

> **G20 Parkinson's disease**
> Hemiparkinsonism
> Idiopathic Parkinsonism or Parkinson's disease
> Paralysis agitans
> Parkinsonism or Parkinson's disease NOS
> Primary Parkinsonism or Parkinson's disease
> **Excludes1:** dementia with Parkinsonism (G31.83)

Figure 4-13 ■ Example of Tabular List Entry for an Etiology Code (G20)

- When two codes are listed in the Index, remember to verify both codes in the Tabular List. ■ Figure 4-13 shows the Tabular List entry for the etiology code **G20**.

- In some instances, the etiology code in the Tabular List provides the instructional note **Use additional code** and lists common manifestations. Refer to ■ Figure 4-14 to see how this note is used for **Alzheimer's disease, late onset, and dementia with behavioral disturbance**. Assign and arrange the codes as follows:

  (1) **G30.0 Alzheimer's disease with early onset**

  (2) **F02.81 Dementia with behavioral disturbance**

Use Additional Code

The Tabular List also lists the instructional note **Use additional code** in other situations besides etiology/manifestation. The note may appear under code, subcategory, category, block, or chapter titles, so the coder must always review these headings for instructions. Refer to the ICD-10-CM manual Chapter 10, Diseases of the Respiratory System (J00-J99), and locate the note **Use additional code** under the chapter title. This instructional note applies to all codes in the chapter (OGCR I.A.13).

Code First

Code first notes also appear under certain codes that are not specifically manifestation codes but may be due to an underlying cause. When there is a **Code first** note and an underlying condition is present, the underlying condition should be sequenced first (OGCR I.A.13 and I.B.7).

Code, if Applicable, Any Causal Condition First

Code, if applicable, any causal condition first notes indicate that this code may be assigned as a principal diagnosis when the causal condition is unknown or not applicable. If a causal condition is known, then the code for that condition should be sequenced as the principal or first-listed diagnosis (OGCR I.B.7).

> ## CODING CAUTION
> Do not automatically assign additional codes when you see an instructional note. The condition must be documented in the medical record in order to assign a code.

Code Also

A **Code also** note instructs that two codes may be required to fully describe a condition, but this note does not provide sequencing direction (OGCR I.A.17).

Acute and Chronic

Providers may document that a patient has both acute and chronic forms of the same condition, such as bronchitis or cholecystitis. The sequencing is determined by how the Index presents the acute and chronic conditions. The Index lists acute and chronic conditions in one of two ways:

- The Index may list subterms for both acute and chronic at the same level of indentation.

  When this occurs, sequence the code for acute first and the code for chronic second (OGCR I.B.8) (■ Figure 4-15, page 54).

- The Index may list **chronic** as a subterm of **acute**, or vice versa, which leads to a combination code (■ Figure 4-16, page 54). When this occurs, assign one code, the combination code, that describes both conditions: **K81.2 Acute cholecystitis with chronic cholecystitis**

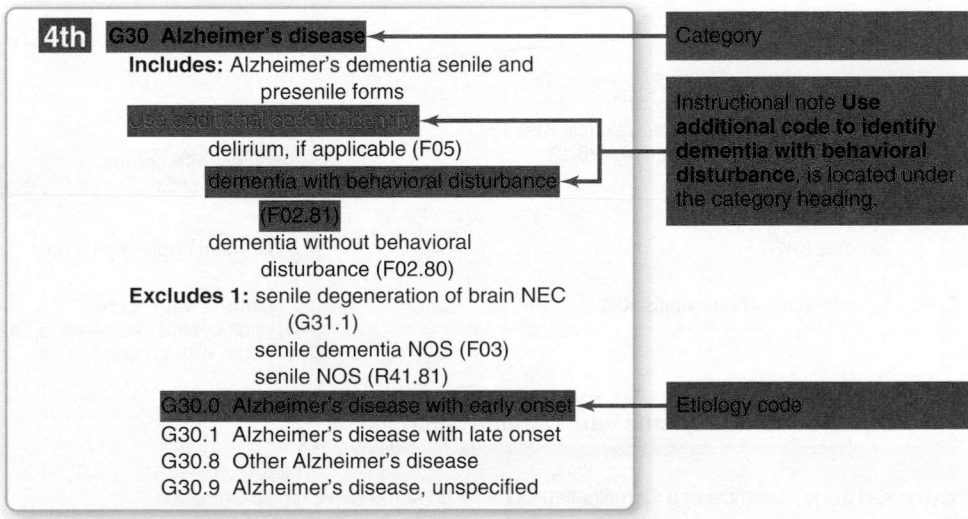

Figure 4-14 ■ Tabular List Entry with the Instructional Note Use Additional Code

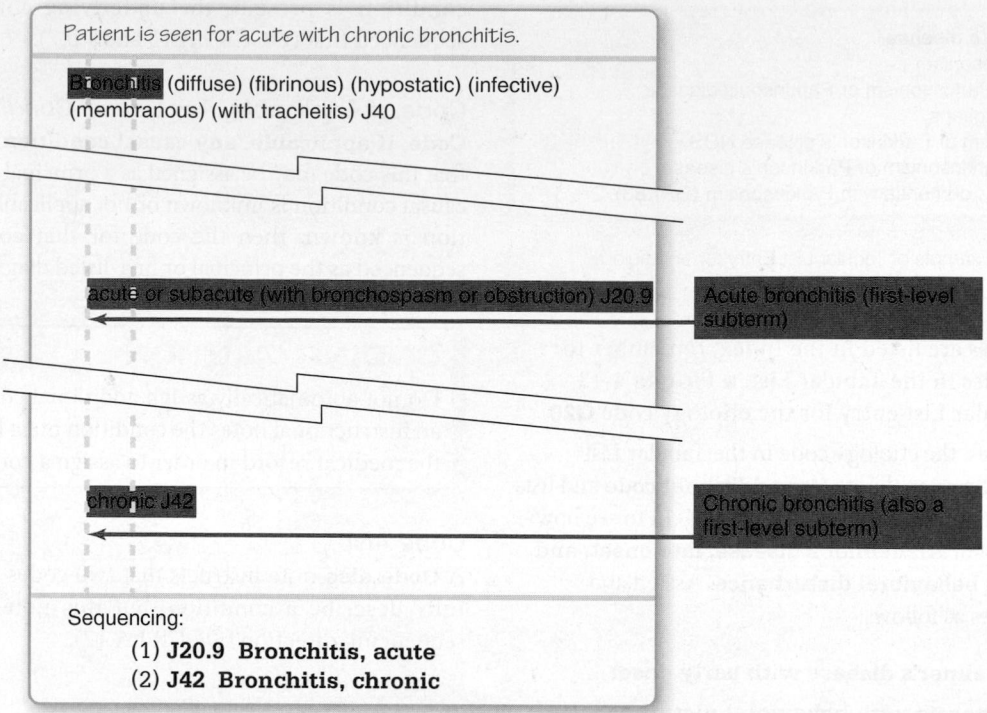

Figure 4-15 ■ Example of Multiple Coding for an Acute and Chronic Condition

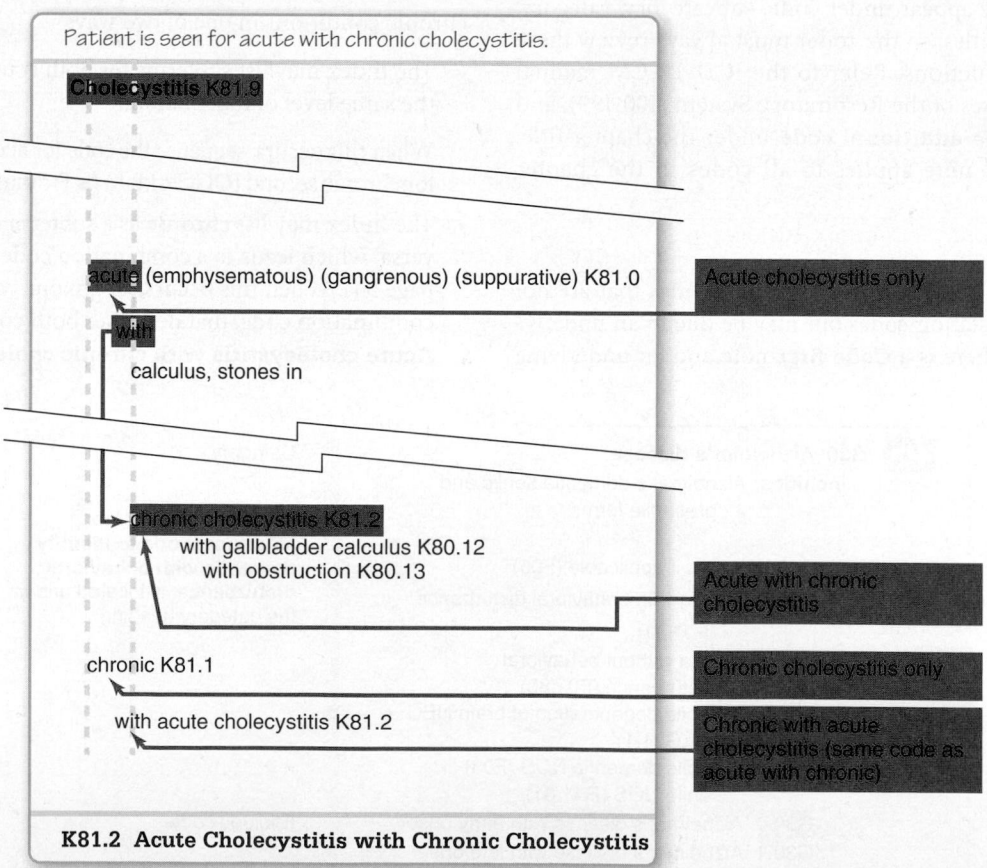

Figure 4-16 ■ Example of a Combination Code for an Acute with Chronic Condition

Regardless of how the Index lists the entries, always verify the codes in the Tabular List and follow any instructional notes.

Other Multiple Code Situations

In addition to the general guidelines for sequencing multiple codes, multiple codes may be needed in many specific situations such as obstetrics, injuries, surgical or procedural complications, and late effects. OGCR Section I.C, Chapter Specific-Coding Guidelines, defines these rules.

> **SUCCESS STEP**
>
> As you have seen, there is not one simple rule that tells you how to sequence multiple codes. Your knowledge of OGCR and ability to read all instructional notes in the Tabular List guide you in each situation.

CODING PRACTICE

Exercise 4.5   How to Code Diagnoses

Instructions: Read the diagnostic statement below, then answer the questions that follow to assign the correct codes. Sequence multiple codes in the correct order.

1. Toxic shock syndrome due to *Streptococcus* A

   a. Underline the Main Term, then look it up in the Index.

   b. What is the subterm? _____

   c. Locate the subterm. What code is listed? _____
   _____

   d. Locate the code listed in step c in the Tabular List. Is there a symbol indicating that an additional digit is required?
   _____

   e. What instructional note appears under the code?
   _____
   _____

   f. What is the name of the organism? _____
   _____
   _____

   g. Cross-reference the block heading **A30-A49**. Do any instructional notes appear? _____

   h. Cross-reference the title for ICD-10-CM Chapter 1. What does the Includes note say? _____
   _____

   i. Read the other notes under the Chapter title. Do any of these notes apply to this case? _____
   _____

   j. Refer back to the code you looked up in steps c and d. Cross-reference the categories listed in the instructional note. Which category do you need? _____
   _____

   k. Which code in this category do you assign for the organism?
   _____

   l. Cross-reference the block title B95-B97. Is there an instructional note? _____ Read the note.

   m. You have identified two codes for this case. Which code is sequenced first? _____

   n. Which code is sequenced second? _____
   _____

CHAPTER SUMMARY

In this chapter you learned that:

- The ICD-10-CM manual is a single volume and is not separated into three volumes as the ICD-9-CM is.
- ICD-10-CM is accompanied by Official Guidelines for Coding and Reporting (OGCR) and Conventions, both of which direct the coder in how to use the manual.
- Diagnosis coding involves the three skills of an ace coder:

- Abstract—read the medical record and determine which elements of the encounter require codes
- Assign—determine codes that accurately describe the patient's condition, reflect the highest level of specificity possible, and contain the correct number of characters for that code
- Arrange—place codes in the order dictated by the guidelines and instructional notes (sequence).

CONCEPT QUIZ

Take a moment to look back at diagnosis coding and solidify your new skills. This is your opportunity to pull together everything you have learned.

Completion

Instructions: Write the term that answers each question based on the information you learned in this chapter. Choose from the list below. Some choices may be used more than once and some choices may not be used at all.

-	Code Also
( )	Code First
4th	Excludes1
5th	Excludes2
6th	Includes
7th	*See*
*	Use Additional Code
:	X
[ ]	

1. The convention _____ identifies nonessential modifiers that describe the default variations of a term.

2. The convention _____ identifies mutually exclusive codes that should not be used together.

3. The convention _____ appears after the code number and tells the coder to assign additional characters.

4. A code that appears in _____ in the Index should be sequenced second.

5. The convention _____ appears in front of a four-character code to indicate that a fifth character is required.

6. The convention _____ is a placeholder in codes with less than six characters that require a seventh character.

7. The convention _____ indicates that the condition excluded is not part of the condition represented by the code, but the patient may have both conditions at the same time.

8. The convention _____ instructs the coder to sequence the etiology first.

9. The convention _____ instructs the coder to sequence the manifestation second.

10. The convention _____ instructs the coder to reference another Main Term or condition to locate the correct code.

Multiple Choice

Instructions: Circle the letter of the best answer to each question based on the information you learned in this chapter.

1. Signs and symptoms should be coded in the inpatient setting when
   A. they are relevant to the current admission and are not integral to the confirmed diagnosis.
   B. the diagnosis is uncertain.
   C. they are an integral part of the confirmed diagnosis.
   D. they related to a previous, resolved condition.

2. In the outpatient setting, the _____ diagnosis is the diagnosis, condition, problem, or other reason for the encounter shown in the medical record to be chiefly responsible for the services provided.
   A. principal
   B. uncertain
   C. first-listed
   D. Main Term

3. _____ diagnoses are preceded by the words *probable, possible, suspected, questionable, rule out, working diagnosis,* or a similar word.
   A. Principal
   B. Uncertain
   C. First-listed
   D. Main Term

4. In an inpatient setting, the _____ diagnosis is the condition established after study to be chiefly responsible for occasioning the admission of the patient to the hospital for care.
   A. principal
   B. uncertain
   C. first-listed
   D. Main Term

5. _____ are rules that complement the conventions and instructional notes to provide additional information and direction in identifying the diagnoses to be reported.
   A. OGCR
   B. Conventions
   C. Exclusions
   D. Instructional notes

6. _____ are the use of symbols, typeface, and layout features to succinctly convey interpretive information.
   A. OGCR
   B. Conventions
   C. Exclusions
   D. Instructional notes

7. _____ means to read the medical record and determine which elements of the encounter require codes.
   A. Abstracting
   B. Assigning
   C. Arranging
   D. Cross-referencing

8. A _____ is a contiguous range of codes within a chapter in ICD-10-CM.
   A. block
   B. category
   C. section
   D. subcategory

9. _____ is a new OGCR that defines separate codes for the right and left sides of the body.
   A. Bilateral
   B. Multiple coding
   C. Arranging
   D. Laterality

10. Do not code signs or symptoms that are a/an _____ part of the disease process when the diagnosis has been established.
   A. uncertain
   B. nonessential
   C. etiology
   D. integral

CODING CHALLENGE

Instructions: Read the mini-medical-record, then answer the questions that follow to abstract, assign, and arrange (sequence) the correct codes.

OFFICE   Gender: M   Age: 75

Chief complaint: *Visit to monitor hypertension and* **CHF. C/o** *increased* **SOB**.

Assessment: *Chronic combined systolic and diastolic heart failure, due to hypertension. Patient is a current and long-term tobacco user. Change diuretic. Use supplemental O$_2$ PRN.*

Part 1: Abstract

1. Read through the mini-medical-record. Observe the patient demographics. Compare the chief complaint to the final assessment.
   a. What symptom did the patient report in the chief complaint?

   _____

   b. What two conditions are stated in the assessment?

   _____
   _____

2. a. Is the symptom integral to one of the conditions stated in the assessment? _____

   b. Should you code for the symptom? _____

   c. Why or why not? _____

   d. What is the first condition due to? _____

   _____

Part 2: Assign

3. You can look up the conditions in any order you wish, as long as you sequence them correctly in the end based on the instructional notes you find during this exercise.

Today, begin by coding the underlying condition, the condition that the heart failure is *due to*.

a. Look up the Main Term **Hypertension** in the Index, then the subterm **heart, with, heart failure**. What code is listed? _____

b. Verify this code in the Tabular List. Is there a symbol In front of this code indicating that you need additional characters?

_____

4. a. What does the instructional note under the code say?

   _____

   b. Based on this instructional note, should the code for **Hypertension** be sequenced first or second?

   _____

5. a. Locate the beginning of this block for **Hypertensive diseases**. Read the instructional notes. Now refer back to the mini-medical-record. What lifestyle habit is documented? _____

   b. Which instructional note applies to this patient? (Tip: *history* describes a past condition that no longer exists.)

   _____

   You will verify this code later in this exercise.

   c. Review the instructional notes at the beginning of ICD-10-CM Chapter 9. Do any of these notes apply to this patient? _____

6. a. Now determine the code for heart failure. Look again at the instructional note under the code for **Hypertension**. What code is listed in the instructional note? _____

   b. What does the - at the end of the code mean?

   _____

7. a. Verify the code listed in the instructional note. Review the four-character subcategories under this heading and locate the one that describes **Combined systolic and diastolic heart failure**. Write down the subcategory code.

   _____

(continued)

(continued from page 57)

b. Now review the five-character codes under this subcategory. What code describes **Chronic combined systolic and diastolic heart failure?** _____
_____

8. Cross-reference the three-character category heading for **Heart failure.** Read through the instructional notes. What condition should be coded first that applies to this patient?

_____

This code should match the one you assigned in step 3.a. The instructional note confirms that you assigned the correct first code or alerts you to the fact that the first code was not correct.

9. Now you need to assign a third code for the lifestyle habit you listed in step 5.a above. List the code here. _____
Verify the code. (This code is sequenced last.)

Part 3: Arrange

10. You have identified three codes for this case. Review your answers in the previous questions to determine the correct sequencing.

a. What code is sequenced first based on the instructional notes in steps 4.b and 8?

_____

b. What code is sequenced second? _____

c. What code is sequenced third? _____

KEEP ON CODING

Instructions: Read the diagnostic statement, then use the Index and Tabular List to assign and sequence ICD-10-CM diagnosis codes. Write the code(s) on the line provided.

1. Acquired flat foot, left: ICD-10-CM Code(s) _____

2. Encounter for immunotherapy: ICD-10-CM Code(s) _____

3. Stage 3 pressure ulcer, left buttock: ICD-10-CM Code(s) _____

4. Alcohol dependence: ICD-10-CM Code(s) _____

5. Fistula, left elbow: ICD-10-CM Code(s) _____

6. Family history of alcohol abuse: ICD-10-CM Code(s) _____

7. Body mass index of 38 in an adult: ICD-10-CM Code(s) _____

8. Benign hypertension: ICD-10-CM Code(s) _____

9. Dysphagia following a cerebral infarction with difficulty swallowing: ICD-10-CM Code(s) _____

10. Severe abdominal pain with abdominal rigidity: ICD-10-CM Code(s) _____

11. Repeated falls: ICD-10-CM Code(s) _____

12. Merkel cell carcinoma of the right eyelid: ICD-10-CM Code(s) _____

13. Pain due to malignant neoplasm: ICD-10-CM Code(s) _____

14. Type 2 diabetes mellitus with moderate diabetic retinopathy with macular edema: ICD-10-CM Code(s) _____

15. Insect bite, left ankle, subsequent encounter: ICD-10-CM Code(s) _____

16. Second and third degree chemical burns, right ankle, initial encounter: ICD-10-CM Code(s) _____

17. Fused toes, bilateral: ICD-10-CM Code(s) _____

18. Chronic cystitis with hematuria: ICD-10-CM Code(s) _____

19. Pneumocystis pneumonia: ICD-10-CM Code(s) _____

20. Anemia: ICD-10-CM Code(s) _____

21. Encounter for blood typing: ICD-10-CM Code(s) _____

22. Ventilator associated pneumonia: ICD-10-CM Code(s) _____

23. Head lice: ICD-10-CM Code(s) _____

24. Polyhydramnios, second trimester, fetus 3: ICD-10-CM Code(s) _____

25. Acute otitis externa, right ear: ICD-10-CM Code(s) _____

Chapter 5

Neoplasms (C00-D49)

Chapter Outline

- **Neoplasm Refresher**
- **Coding Overview of Neoplasms**
- **Abstracting for Neoplasms**
- **Assigning Codes for Neoplasms**
- **Arranging Codes for Neoplasms**

Learning Objectives

After completing this chapter, you should have the skills to:

5.1 Spell and define the key words, medical terms, and abbreviations related to neoplasms.

5.2 Discuss the behavior and common types of neoplasms.

5.3 Identify the main characteristics of coding for neoplasms.

5.4 Abstract diagnostic information from the medical record for coding neoplasms.

5.5 Assign codes for neoplasms and related conditions.

5.6 Arrange codes for neoplasms and related conditions.

5.7 Discuss the Official Guidelines for Coding and Reporting related to neoplasms.

Key Terms and Abbreviations

adenocarcinoma	carcinoma of unknown primary (CUP)	leukemia	primary (malignant neoplasm)
adjuvant therapy		malignant	prognosis
behavior	cell type	metastasize	secondary (malignant neoplasm)
benign	external radiotherapy	neoplasm	site of origin
CA in situ	family history	oncologist	staging
cancer	histology	overlapping lesion	topography
carcinoma (CA)	internal radiotherapy	personal history	

In addition to the key terms listed here, students should know the terms defined within tables in this chapter.

For updates and corrections, visit our student resource site at

www.pearsonhighered.com/healthprofessionsresources

INTRODUCTION

Driving into a pothole can be quite a jolt to the system. When potholes are not repaired quickly, they grow bigger and more dangerous each day. The medical field has its own potholes. One of them is cancer, a collection of diseases that affects nearly every person either directly or indirectly.

An oncologist is a physician who specializes in diagnosing and treating tumors. Medical oncologists specialize in medical treatments such as chemotherapy. Surgical oncologists specialize in surgical treatment, such as the surgical excision of malignant tumors (*cancer*). Radiation oncologists specialize in treating malignant tumors with radiation therapy. Physician specialists of a particular body system may also be involved in treating patients with tumors and cancer affecting that body system.

NEOPLASM REFRESHER

Neoplasms are abnormal growth of new tissue, which may be **malignant** (*life threatening*) or **benign** (*not life threatening*). Malignant neoplasms are commonly referred to as cancer. Neoplasms can occur in any body system and at any anatomical site. **Oncologists** are physicians who specialize in the diagnosis and treatment of tumors. In order to code neoplasms, coders need to be familiar with neoplasm-related terminology, benign neoplasm behavior, and malignant neoplasm behavior.

Neoplasm-Related Terminology

Neoplasms are classified based on the **behavior** (*malignant or benign*), **topography** or **site of origin** (*anatomic site where the growth begins*), **histology** (*type of tissue*), and **cell type** (*characteristics or appearance of the cell*) of the growth. As you learn about different types of neoplasms, remember to put together the root or combining form for body parts you already know with suffixes and prefixes to define new terms for conditions and procedures related to neoplasms.

For example, the suffix -oma means tumor, and gastr/o means stomach, so gastroma refers to a neoplasm in the stomach (gastr/oma). Sarc/o refers to connective tissue, so sarcoma refers to a neoplasm of connective tissue (sarc/oma) and is nearly always malignant.

Terms for neoplasms frequently contain more than one root to fully describe the tumor. For example, **adenocarcinoma** (adeno/carcin/oma) has two roots to describe a cancerous (carcin/o) tumor in a gland (aden/o). Refer to ■ TABLE 5-1 for a refresher on how to build medical terms related to neoplasms.

CODING CAUTION

Be alert for medical word terms that are spelled similarly and have different meanings.

adenoma (*tumor of a gland*) and
　　adenocarcinoma (*cancerous tumor of a gland*)

diagnosis (*complete knowledge—determining the nature of a disease*) and **prognosis** (*future knowledge—the expected course of the disease*)

Benign Neoplasm Behavior

A benign neoplasm does not have the ability to invade surrounding tissue or spread to other parts of the body. Types of benign neoplasms are tumors, warts, moles, polyps, and fibroids. In some cases, physicians can determine if a neoplasm is benign or malignant through visual inspection. If they believe the growth could be malignant or are unsure of its behavior, they perform a **biopsy** to obtain a specimen. They send the specimen to the laboratory where a **pathologist** examines it microscopically.

Many benign neoplasms present no health problems and require no treatment. However, a large benign neoplasm can apply pressure to or interfere with surrounding organs or structures, and this can create health problems. For example, a benign brain tumor is not cancerous, but it can compress cranial nerves or apply pressure to areas of the brain and may need to be removed to protect brain function. ■ TABLE 5-2 (page 62) outlines the differences between benign and malignant neoplasms.

Malignant Neoplasm Behavior

The ability of malignant neoplasms to **metastasize** (*spread and invade organs*) makes them life threatening. When tumors invade vital organs, they cause organ malfunction, leading to death if not treated. It is important to distinguish between the common term **cancer** and the medical terms malignant neoplasm and **carcinoma** (CA). Refer to the following to review the similarities and differences in these terms:

- Carcinoma is a malignant tumor of epithelial cells, which line body cavities and organs. Not all areas of the body have epithelial cells, so true carcinoma only occurs in structures that contain epithelial cells.

- Carcinoma in situ (CA in situ) refers to cells that have begun to change but are contained within the epithelial layer. When malignant cells break through the epithelial

---

Table 5-1 ■ **EXAMPLE OF CONSTRUCTING MEDICAL TERMS FOR NEOPLASMS**

Prefix/Combining Form	Suffix	Complete Medical Term
neo- (*new*)	**-plasm** (*growth*)	**neo + plasm** (*new growth*)
sarc/o (*connective tissue*)	**-oma** (*tumor*)	**sarc + oma** (*tumor of connective tissue*)
my/o (*muscle*)		**aden + oma** (*tumor of a gland*)
carcin/o (*cancerous*)		**myo + sarc + oma** (*tumor of connective tissue and muscle*)
aden/o (*gland*)		**adeno + carcin + oma** (*cancerous tumor of a gland*)

Table 5-2 ■ **COMPARISON OF BENIGN AND MALIGNANT NEOPLASM CHARACTERISTICS**

Characteristic	Benign Neoplasm	Malignant Neoplasm
Rate of growth	Grows slowly	Grows rapidly
Encapsulation	Is encapsulated	Is not encapsulated
Differentiation	Has cells that resemble the normal cells from which they arose (well-differentiated)	Has cells that undergo permanent change, abnormal rapid proliferation (anaplastic and undifferentiated)
Growth pattern	Grows by expansion and causes pressure on surrounding tissue	Has invasive growth and metastasis
Metastasis	Remains localized (nonmetastatic)	Spreads through bloodstream and lymphatic system Causes extensive tissue destruction due to invasiveness
Recurrence	Does not recur when surgically removed	Can recur when surgically removed if invasive growth has occurred
Cachexia	Produces no cachexia (*extreme weakness, fatigue, wasting, and malnutrition*)	Produces cachexia

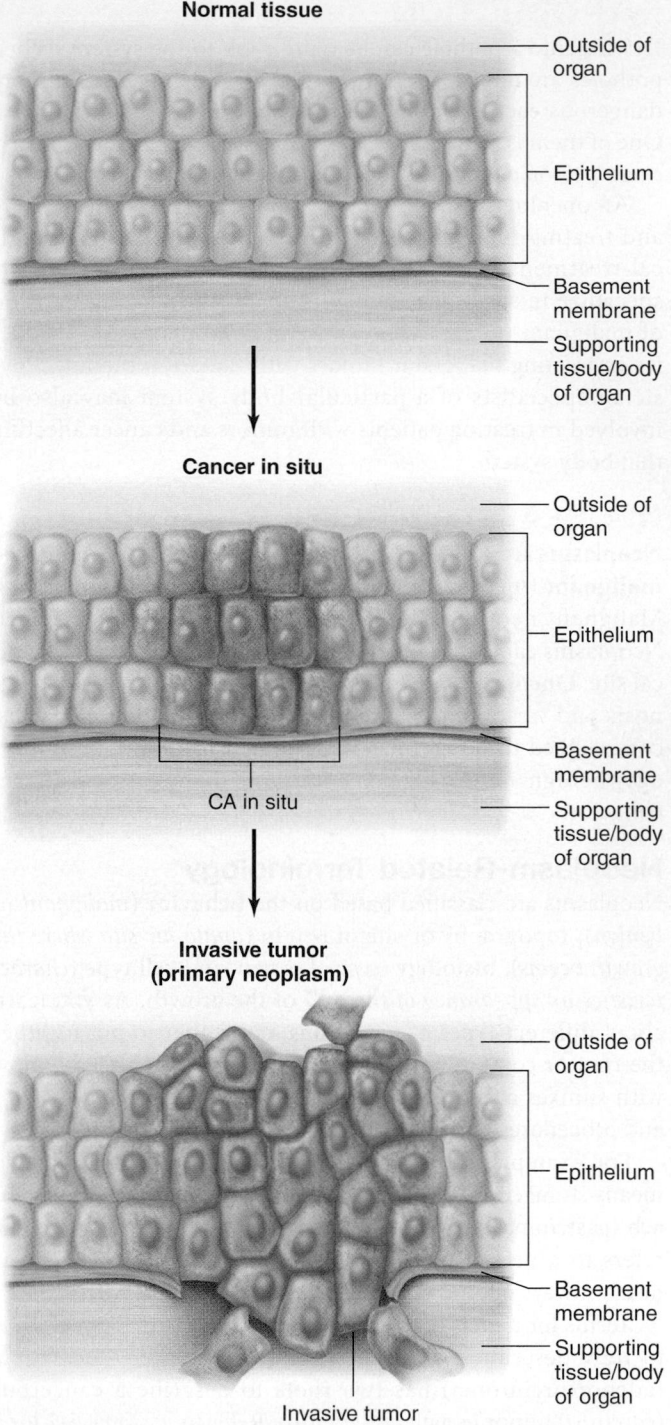

Figure 5-1 ■ Progression of CA in Situ to Primary Neoplasm

membrane into the organ, they become a **primary malignant neoplasm** (■ FIGURE 5-1).

- Malignant neoplasm is a life-threatening new growth of any type of tissue. Although malignant neoplasms are cancerous, not all are classified as carcinoma. Malignant neoplasms can also occur in other types of cells such as bone, muscle, and fat.

- Cancer, in its most limited meaning, is synonymous with carcinoma. However, our language uses cancer loosely to refer to many types of malignancies, including ones that are not tumors. For example, cancer is often used to describe **leukemia**, which is a malignant disease of the blood-forming organs but does not produce tumors.

SUCCESS STEP

Be aware of different forms of the word metastasize, which literally means *beyond control*. Metasta**size** (verb) means to transform or spread diseased cells. Metasta**sis** (noun) is the process of spreading or the condition resulting from the spread of diseased cells. Metasta**ses** (plural) refer to multiple secondary tumors or sites. Metasta**tic** (adjective) means pertaining to having spread.

Cancer is not one disease but, rather, a group of over 100 diseases in which cells in one part of the body begin to mutate and grow out of control. The American Cancer Society (ACS) estimates that one-half of all men and one-third of all women will develop cancer at some point in their lives. The most common sites of cancer are the prostate for men, breast for women, lung, and colon/rectum (■ FIGURE 5-2). The most common childhood cancers are leukemia and

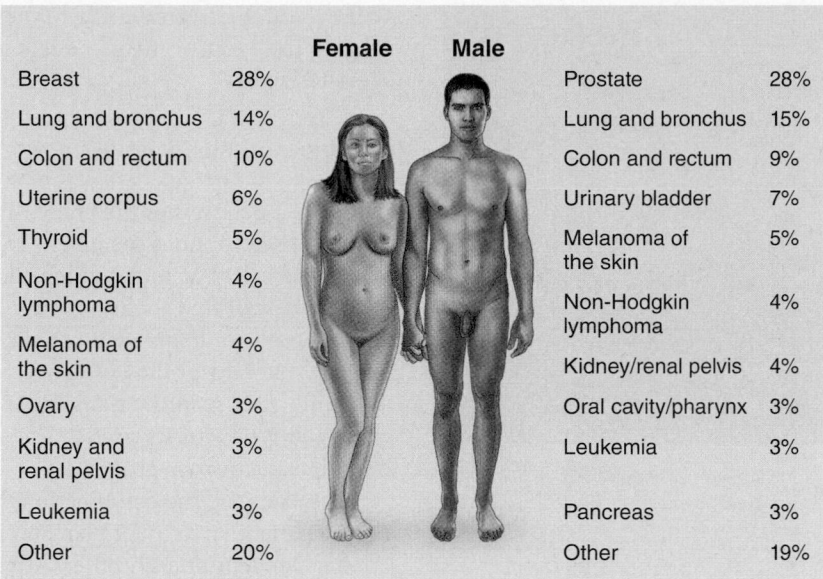

Female		Male	
Breast	28%	Prostate	28%
Lung and bronchus	14%	Lung and bronchus	15%
Colon and rectum	10%	Colon and rectum	9%
Uterine corpus	6%	Urinary bladder	7%
Thyroid	5%	Melanoma of the skin	5%
Non-Hodgkin lymphoma	4%	Non-Hodgkin lymphoma	4%
Melanoma of the skin	4%	Kidney/renal pelvis	4%
Ovary	3%	Oral cavity/pharynx	3%
Kidney and renal pelvis	3%	Leukemia	3%
Leukemia	3%	Pancreas	3%
Other	20%	Other	19%

Figure 5-2 ■ Most Frequent Sites of New Cancer Cases

medulloblastoma, a cancer that affects the cerebellum, brain, and spinal cord.

Cells become cancerous due to damaged DNA that is not repaired as it is in normal cells. The damaged cells do not die as they normally should but, rather, replicate and make new damaged cells. Cancer spreads when the damaged cells invade nearby tissues and when damaged cells move into the bloodstream or lymphatic system, which carry them to other areas of the body. The anatomic site where the neoplasm begins is the primary site. The sites it spreads to are the **secondary sites** or metastases. The most common sites for metastases are the liver, lungs, and bone. Cancer cells that have metastasized retain the characteristics of the organ in which they originated. For example, breast cancer cells that have spread to the lung still look like breast cells under the microscope. Breast cancer that has spread to the lung is called metastatic breast cancer (■ FIGURE 5-3).

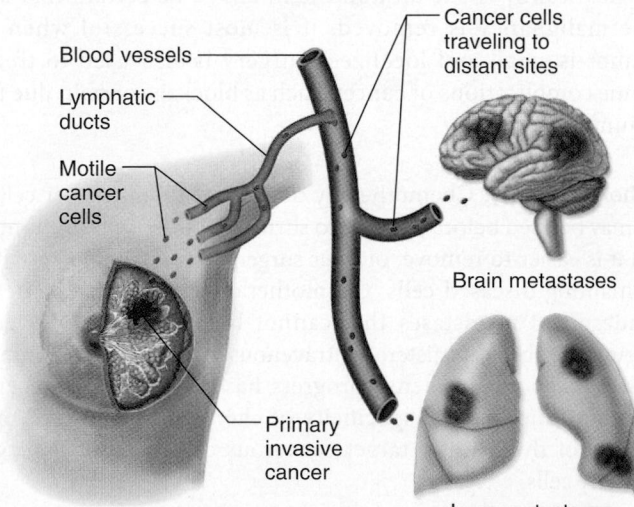

Figure 5-3 ■ Metastasis of Breast Cancer to the Brain and Lung

Topography is the anatomic site where the neoplasm begins. Many histological and cell types of malignant neoplasms and cancers can affect any given site. For example, colorectal cancer includes the following histological types, each of which originates from a different type of tissue:

- adenocarcinoma, which originates in the glands
- leiomyosarcoma, which originates in smooth muscle tissue
- lymphoma, which originates in the lymph nodes
- malignant melanoma, which originates in pigment cells of the skin
- neuroendocrine, which originates in hormone-producing cells that are a cross between nerve cells and endocrine cells

Each of these histological types can appear in many different organs. For example, adenocarcinoma may appear in the colon, prostate, lungs, breast, stomach, pancreas, and cervix. Each histological type may have a variety of cell subtypes, which are often named based on their appearance. For example, adenocarcinoma of the colon has a mucinous cell subtype (*comprised of at least 60% mucus*) and a signet ring cell subtype (*looks like a ring when viewed microscopically*). Physicians must identify the specific subtype of cell in order to determine the behavior, the patient's **prognosis** (*expected outcome*), and treatment plan. Hundreds of different cell subtypes are known for various topographical and histological types of cancer.

Coders need to know how malignant neoplasms and other cancers are diagnosed and treated in order to abstract, assign, and sequence codes.

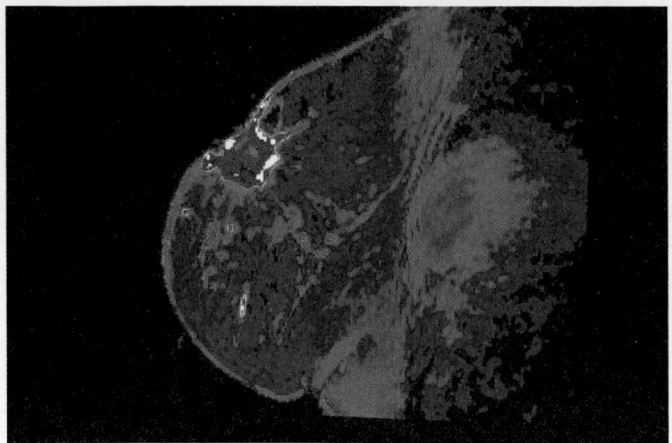

Figure 5-4 ■ MRI Image of the Breast. *Source: © Dr. Steven Harmes/National Cancer Institute (NCI).*

Diagnosis

Physicians diagnose cancer through **screening** examinations or in response to patient symptoms. Screening examinations detect certain types of cancer at an early stage. Cancer that is detected during an early stage is more likely to respond to treatment. Examples of screening tests include the following:

- colonoscopy—colon cancer
- mammogram—breast cancer
- papanicolaou (PAP) test—cervical cancer
- prostate-specific antigen (PSA) blood test—prostate cancer
- digital rectal examination (DRE)—prostate cancer

When patients present with symptoms, physicians may diagnose cancer with blood tests, biopsies, and imaging, such as computed tomography (CT), magnetic resonance imaging (MRI), or positron emission tomography (PET) (■ FIGURE 5-4). After making a diagnosis of cancer, physicians determine the stage and grade of the disease in order to help determine the best course of treatment.

Staging. Staging is the process of determining how far the cancer has spread. Several staging systems exist and various systems are used for specific types of cancers. Two common staging systems are TNM and stage grouping. TNM staging assigns numbers to describe how far the primary tumor (T) has grown in its original site; extent of spread to regional (nearby) lymph nodes (N), and whether the cancer has metastasized (M) to other organs of the body. The results of TNM staging are then combined into stage grouping. Stage grouping uses numbers to designate the malignancy from the least advanced (stage 0) to the most advanced (IV). The specific criteria for each stage of TNM and stage grouping are unique to each anatomical site. For example, the definition of stage II colon cancer is different than stage II breast cancer. Physicians state the diagnosis by referencing the stage of cancer at the time it is discovered. However, all cancers will eventually become the highest stage if left untreated. Staging information helps coders confirm if the disease has metastasized.

Grading. Grading describes how closely the cancer cell type looks like a normal cell when viewed microscopically. A pathologist determines the grade through microscopic inspection of a tissue or fluid specimen. The grade is rated from G1, a low-grade cell that looks much like normal tissue, to G4, a high-grade cell that looks very abnormal. Low-grade cancers tend to grow and spread more slowly than high-grade cells. Several different grades of cancer cells can affect any given anatomic site, so physicians must determine each patient's exact cell type and its grade. The grade of the cell does not change as the disease progresses.

Physicians use the combination of stage and grade to determine a patient's treatment plan and prognosis. Stage and grade are independent of each other. A patient can have a low stage and high grade, a high stage and a low grade, or any combination in between. For example, a patient with a lymphoma type that is stage IV (widespread) and grade G1 (slow growing), such as follicular cell lymphoma, may have a better outcome than a patient with a type of carcinoma of the uterus that is stage I (localized) but grade G4 (rapidly growing and spreading), such as clear cell carcinoma.

Treatment

Physicians recommend treatment plans based on topography, stage, and grade of cancer as well as the patient's age and health condition. The three primary types of treatment are surgery, chemotherapy, and radiotherapy. They may be used alone or in conjunction with each other. When more than one type of treatment is used, the additional treatments are referred to as **adjuvant therapies.** Some malignancies are more responsive to one type of treatment than another. Which treatments are used, and in what order, is unique to each type of cancer and each patient.

Surgery. Surgery is used to remove the tumor and a portion of the healthy tissue around the tumor to be certain that all the malignancy is removed. It is most successful when a tumor is small and localized. Surgery is also used to treat some complications of cancer, such as blockage or pain due to a tumor.

Chemotherapy. Chemotherapy uses drugs to kill cancer cells. It may be used before surgery, to shrink the size of a large tumor so it is easier to remove, or after surgery, to kill any potentially remaining diseased cells. Chemotherapy is also used to treat widespread metastases that cannot be surgically removed. Drugs may be administered intravenously or orally, or a combination of both. Immense progress has been made in recent years to improve the specificity of chemotherapy drugs, the ability of the drug to target cancerous cells but not damage healthy cells.

Radiotherapy. Radiotherapy can be external or internal. **External radiotherapy** directs precise doses of X-ray beams at specific sites in order to kill or shrink tumors and cancerous cells. **Internal radiotherapy** uses radioactive pellets or containers within a body cavity to target the malignant area. Radiotherapy may be used before surgery to shrink the size of a tumor or after surgery to slow potential metastasis.

Each treatment method has its advantages and drawbacks. Unfortunately, treatments aimed at killing cancer cells also kill healthy cells, resulting in side effects for patients. Patients, their families, and their physicians make difficult and personal decisions regarding what is best in any given situation.

CODING PRACTICE

Exercise 5.1   Neoplasm Refresher

Instructions: Use your medical terminology skills and resources to define the following neoplasms. Do not assign codes. Follow these steps:

- Use slash marks "/" to break down each term into its root(s) and suffix.
- Define the meaning of the word, based on the meaning of each word part.

Example: sarcoma   Meaning: *neoplasm of connective*
       sarc/oma   *tissue*

1. osteosarcoma _____
2. leiomyoma _____
3. lipoma _____
4. liposarcoma _____
5. adenoma _____
6. adenocarcinoma _____
7. osteoma _____
8. melanoma _____
9. neuroblastoma _____
10. lymphoma _____

CODING OVERVIEW OF NEOPLASMS

ICD-10-CM Chapter 2, Neoplasms (C00-D49), contains 21 blocks or subchapters that are divided by anatomical site. Review the block names and code ranges listed at the beginning of Chapter 2 in the ICD-10-CM manual to become familiar with the content and organization. This chapter classifies all malignant and most benign neoplasms. Some benign neoplasms are classified in the specific body system chapter. For example, adenomas of the prostate are classified in ICD-10-CM Chapter 14, Diseases of the Genitourinary System (N00-N99).

Notice the following characteristics of codes in the neoplasm chapter:

- Codes beginning with C classify malignant neoplasms.
- Codes beginning with D classify neoplasms in situ, benign, and of uncertain or unspecified behavior.
- Some codes contain an alphabetic character in the third position of the code, such as C7A, C7B, D3A.

This ICD-10-CM chapter compares to Chapter 2 in ICD-9-CM and reflects numerous category expansions. Characters have been added to code for laterality and more specific sites. Codes for leukemia contain characters to identify whether the disease is in remission or relapse. OGCR I.C.2.c.1), Anemia associated with malignancy, has been updated.

Instructional notes at the beginning of ICD-10-CM Chapter 2 address functional activity, morphology, overlapping sites, and malignant neoplasm of ectopic tissue.

CODING CAUTION

When diagnosis codes have a letter for other than the first or last character, they can be tricky to locate because they do not appear in a manner consistent with alphanumeric rules. For example, category **C7A** is sequenced after **C75** and before **C76**, but category **D3A** appears after **D36** and before **D37**. Be aware of this inconsistency and know that you may need to take a few moments to locate the code.

ICD-10-CM provides Official Guidelines for Coding and Reporting (OGCR) for neoplasms in OGCR section I.C.2. OGCR provides specific direction for sequencing codes for multiple neoplasms, complications, adjuvant therapies, and other situations. In addition, frequent instructional notes throughout the chapter direct coders to use multiple codes to describe harmful lifestyle habits that contribute to neoplasms.

ABSTRACTING FOR NEOPLASMS

When abstracting patient cases with neoplasms, coders must look for several pieces of information that will help determine the first-listed or principal diagnosis and the sequencing of any additional diagnoses. Refer to OGCR I.C.2 for detailed guidance on abstracting neoplasms. ■ TABLE 5-3 (page 66) highlights key questions to answer when reviewing the medical record. Coders use answers to these questions when assigning and sequencing codes. Remember that the abstracting questions are a guide and

Table 5-3 ■ **KEY CRITERIA FOR ABSTRACTING NEOPLASMS**

- ❑ What is the histologic description of the neoplasm or cancer?
- ❑ What is the anatomic site of the neoplasm?
- ❑ Is the neoplasm stated as malignant or benign?
- ❑ If malignant, is the neoplasm primary, secondary, in situ, or of unknown histologic origin?
- ❑ Has the malignant neoplasm metastasized? If so, to what sites?
- ❑ What complications are documented, such as anemia, dehydration, or a surgical complication?
- ❑ If anemia is present, is it due to the malignancy itself or due to a treatment such as chemotherapy, radiotherapy, or immunotherapy?
- ❑ Is the reason for the encounter or admission the malignancy or an unrelated condition?
- ❑ If the reason for the encounter is the malignancy, what is the specific purpose?
  - treatment of the primary site
  - treatment of a metastatic site(s)
  - treatment of a complication
  - chemotherapy
  - radiotherapy
  - immunotherapy
  - pain management
  - determination of the extent of malignancy
  - aftercare
  - follow-up care
- ❑ Is the patient in remission from leukemia, multiple myeloma, or malignant plasma neoplasm?
- ❑ If the primary malignancy was previously excised, is there any remaining evidence of primary malignancy, metastasis, or any related treatment?
- ❑ Does the patient have a personal history or family history of malignant neoplasm?

that not every question applies to, or can be answered for, every case. For example, complications of cancer may not be present in every patient.

Abstracting Metastases

An important task in abstracting is determining the sites of the primary and any secondary neoplasms. Coders must give special attention to the specific wording used to describe various neoplasm sites. In particular, take note of the prepositions *from*, *to*, and *in* because they describe the direction in which the neoplasm has spread. Refer to ■ TABLE 5-4 to better understand how metastases are documented.

Guided Example of Abstracting Neoplasms

Refer to the following example here and throughout the chapter to learn more about coding for neoplasms. Karla Destefano, CPC, is a fictitious certified coder who guides you through the coding process.

Table 5-4 ■ **ALTERNATIVE DESCRIPTIONS OF METASTASES**

Statement	Primary Site	Secondary Site(s)
Colon cancer with metastasis *to* the liver	Colon	Liver
Metastatic liver cancer *from* the colon	Colon	Liver
Metastatic colon cancer	Colon	Unknown
Metastatic cancer *in* lung, liver, and bone	Unknown	Lung, liver, and bone
Liver metastases	Unknown	Liver

Date: 5/1/yy Location: East Side Oncology

Provider: Richard Blackford, MD

Patient: Anthony Payne Gender: M Age: 68

Reason for encounter: review test results to determine extent of prostate cancer

Assessment: adenocarcinoma of prostate with metastasis to colon

Plan: surgery to be followed with radiotherapy

Follow along in your ICD-10-CM manual as Karla abstracts the diagnosis. Check off each step after you complete it.

▶ Karla begins by reviewing the medical record to abstract the diagnosis. She refers to the Key Criteria for Abstracting Neoplasms (Table 5-3).

- ❑ *What is the histologic description of the neoplasm or cancer?* adenocarcinoma
- ❑ *What is the anatomic site of the neoplasm?* prostate
- ❑ *Is the neoplasm stated as malignant or benign?* Adeno-carcinoma by definition is malignant. In addition, the fact that it has spread indicates it is malignant.
- ❑ *If malignant, is the neoplasm primary, secondary, in situ, or of unknown histologic origin?* The prostate is primary because it is not stated as secondary.
- ❑ *Has the malignant neoplasm metastasized? If so, to what sites?* She notes that the secondary site is the colon.
- ❑ *What complications are documented?* None
- ❑ *Is the reason for the encounter or admission the malignancy or an unrelated condition?* The malignancy
- ❑ *Does the patient have a personal history or family history of malignant neoplasm?* None stated

▶ Next, Karla will assign the codes.

CODING PRACTICE

Exercise 5.2   **Abstracting Diagnoses for Neoplasms**

Instructions: Read the mini-medical-record of each patient's encounter and answer the abstracting questions. Write the answer on the line provided. Do not assign any codes.

1. OFFICE   Gender: F   Age: 59

Reason for encounter: chemotherapy

Assessment: adenocarcinoma of the right breast, lower outer quadrant, with metastasis to the brain

Plan: return for next treatment in 3 weeks

a. What is the primary site? _____

b. Is metastasis documented? Where? _____

c. Are any complications documented? _____

d. What is the specific purpose of the visit? _____
_____

2. INPATIENT HOSPITAL   Gender: F   Age: 44

Procedure: embolization of uterine fibroids

Postprocedural diagnosis: intramural (*within the muscle wall*) leiomyoma, uterus

Plan: FU in office in 4 weeks

a. What is embolization? _____
_____

b. What is a leiomyoma? _____
_____

c. What is the anatomic site? _____
_____

d. Is the neoplasm malignant or benign? _____
_____

3. OFFICE   Gender: M   Age: 43

Reason for encounter: review results of biopsy and CT scan

Assessment: gastric adenocarcinoma, fundus

Plan: surgery to be followed by radiotherapy

a. What is the primary site? _____
_____

b. What part of the stomach is the fundus? _____
_____

(continued)

3. (continued)

c. Is metastasis documented? Where? _____
_____

d. Are any complications documented? _____
_____

e. What is the specific purpose of the visit? _____
_____

4. INPATIENT HOSPITAL   Gender: F   Age: 15

Reason for admission: limb-salvage surgery after chemotherapy to shrink tumor

Procedure description: successfully cut out tumor from left thigh

Postprocedural assessment: osteosarcoma in the left thigh

Plan: discharge in 1–2 days

a. What is the primary site? _____
_____

b. Is metastasis documented? _____
_____

c. Are any complications documented? _____
_____

d. What is the specific purpose of the encounter?
_____

e. What is the medical term for the bone in the thigh?
_____

5. INPATIENT HOSPITAL   Gender: M   Age: 67

Reason for admission: anemia

Assessment: anemia due to classical lymphocyte depleted Hodgkin lymphoma

Plan: administer IV iron supplements

a. What is the primary neoplasm? _____
_____

b. Is metastasis documented? _____
_____

c. What complication is documented? _____
_____

d. What is the reason for the admission? _____

(continued)

CODING PRACTICE *(continued)*

6. INPATIENT HOSPITAL Gender: M Age: 61

Reason for procedure: brain stem tumor

Procedure description: used Gamma Knife surgery to destroy tumor

Postprocedural diagnosis: squamous cell carcinoma of the lung with brain stem metastases

Plan: FU in office 1 week, evaluate for chemotherapy

Tip: Look up unfamiliar terms in a medical dictionary or on the Internet.

(continued)

6. *(continued)*

a. What is the primary neoplasm? _____

_____

b. Is metastasis documented? What site? _____

_____

c. Which site is the reason for the procedure?

_____

d. What is Gamma Knife surgery? _____

_____

ASSIGNING CODES FOR NEOPLASMS

Assigning codes for neoplasms involves three steps:

1. Search for the histological term in the Index to Diseases and Injuries.
2. Locate the anatomical site and behavior in the Table of Neoplasms.
3. Verify the code(s) in the Tabular List.

Search for the Histological Term in the Index

Coders use both the Index to Diseases and Injuries and the Table of Neoplasms to locate codes for neoplasms. Careful abstracting and attention to the terms in the documentation determine how to locate the code.

When the histological type is documented, search for that term in the Index. The histological term identifies the tissue type of a neoplasm, such as carcinoma, melanoma, sarcoma, or leukemia. When the Index lists a code for the histological type, coders may proceed to the Tabular List to verify the code (■ FIGURE 5-5).

In many cases, the Index lists a cross-reference note to the Table of Neoplasms, such as **specified site - *see* Neoplasm, malignant.** In this situation, coders need to refer to the Table of Neoplasms, locate the column for Malignant Primary, then locate the anatomic site in the left-hand column (■ FIGURE 5-6). Recall that the Table of Neoplasms appears in the Index to Diseases and Injuries under the letter **N** in most editions of the ICD-10-CM manual.

SUCCESS STEP

To help remember where the Table of Neoplasms is located and to find it quickly, place an adhesive tab along the top edge of the first page of the Table of Neoplasms. By placing it on the top edge, it will not be obscured by other tabs for the Index to Diseases and Injuries and the Tabular List.

Personal or Family History

When physicians document that patients are at risk due to a personal or family history of malignant neoplasm, assign a code for the history. **Personal history** is a condition the patient had in the past, was removed or resolved, and is no longer being treated, but has the potential for recurrence and therefore may require continued monitoring. To locate codes for personal history, search the Index for **History, personal, malignant neoplasm**, then locate the subterm for the anatomic site.

Family history is a condition that a patient's family member had in the past or currently has that causes the patient to be at higher risk of also contracting or developing the disease. The family member may be alive or deceased. The family member's malignancy may have been removed and/or may still be undergoing treatment. To locate codes for family history, search the Index for **History, family, malignant neoplasm,** then locate the subterm for the body system.

SUCCESS STEP

The significance of personal or family history must be documented by the physician as relevant to the current condition or encounter. Patients must have a blood relationship to the family member, such as a parent or sibling. The history of grandparents, aunts, and uncles may be relevant for certain cancers with proven genetic links, such as breast cancer.

Melanoma (malignant) C43.9

    skin C43.9
      abdominal wall C43.59

Figure 5-5 ■ Example of Index Entry for a Histological Type of Neoplasm

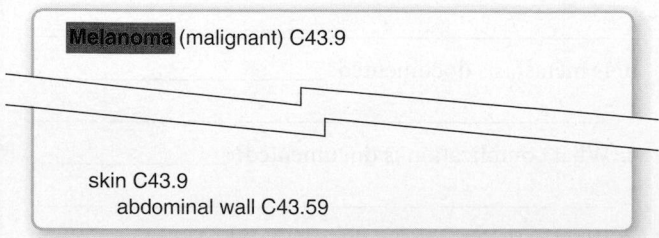

Carcinoma (malignant) — *see also* Neoplasm, by site, malignant
   acidophil
     specified site — *see* Neoplasm, malignant, by site

Figure 5-6 ■ Example of Cross-Reference to Table of Neoplasms

	Malignant Primary	Malignant Secondary	Ca in situ	Benign	Uncertain Behavior	Unspecified Behavior
Neoplasm, neoplastic	C80.1	C79.9	D09.9	D36.9	D48.9	D49.9
abdomen, abdominal	C76.2	C79.8-	D09.8	D36.7	D48.7	D49.89
cavity	C76.2	C79.8-	D09.8	D36.7	D48.7	D49.89
organ	C76.2	C79.8-	D09.8	D36.7	D48.7	D49.89
viscera	C76.2	C79.8-	D09.8	D36.7	D48.7	D49.89
wall	C44.59	C79.2-	D04.5	D23.5	D48.5	D49.2
connective tissue	C49.4	C79.8-	-	D21.4	D48.1	D49.2
abdominopelvic	C76.8	C79.8-	-	D36.7	D48.7	D49.89

Figure 5-7 ■ Example of the Table of Neoplasms

Locate Site and Behavior in the Table of Neoplasms

The Table of Neoplasms lists the codes for neoplasms by anatomical site. Anatomical sites appear in the left column of the table in alphabetical order (■ FIGURE 5-7). Many sites have indented subterms, similar to indentations in the Index to Diseases and Injuries. Subterms in the Table of Neoplasms describe specific locations within a large anatomical site. For example, the anatomic site **abdomen, abdominal** has subterms for **cavity**, **organ**, **viscera**, and **wall**. **Abdominal wall** has a second-level subterm for **connective tissue**.

The Table of Neoplasms has six columns, one for each anatomic site, that describe the possible behavior of the neoplasm: Malignant Primary, Malignant Secondary, CA in situ, Benign, Uncertain Behavior (*the physician documents that he/she has not determined whether the neoplasm is malignant or benign*), or Unspecified Nature (*the physician does not document whether the neoplasm is malignant or benign*). The description of the neoplasm will often indicate which of the six columns to use. For example, benign fibroadenoma of breast is coded using the Benign column; carcinoma in situ of cervix uteri is coded using the CA in situ column. Some sites do not have codes in all six columns because some behaviors do not occur in certain sites. For example, cancer in situ does not occur in bone, muscle, or connective tissue. Cancer in situ occurs only in epithelial cells, and these sites do not have epithelial cells.

SUCCESS STEP

When a malignant neoplasm is not specified as primary, secondary, or in situ, you should code it as primary. Secondary and CA in situ must be stated in the medical record in order to assign codes from those columns.

Unknown Anatomic Site

When the anatomic site of the primary or secondary neoplasm is not known, assign a code from the first line of the Table of Neoplasms, which is labeled **Neoplasm, neoplastic**. The same codes also appear under the subterm **Neoplasm, unknown site or unspecified**. There are two common situations when this may occur:

- **Carcinoma of unknown primary (CUP)** occurs when the neoplasm is diagnosed at a late stage after it has metastasized and the physician is unable to determine the site of origin.

- The secondary site may not be specified when the neoplasm has metastasized to multiple areas throughout the body, and treatment is directed at the overall body rather than one specific site.

The subterm for **unknown site** provides codes in all six columns, so coders should select the appropriate column. For example, it is possible for the primary site to be specified but not the secondary; for the secondary site to be specified but not the primary; or for neither to be specified. In all cases, coders should query the physician and review all information in the medical record before assigning a code for unspecified site.

Overlapping Lesions

Some anatomic sites provide a listing for **overlapping lesions**. Overlapping lesions are contiguous sites where the tumor continues from one site to an adjacent one without interruption. Refer to ■ FIGURE 5-8 (page 70) and review the entries for **lung** in the Table of Neoplasms. Separate entries describe distinct sites within the lung with separate codes. Use the entry for overlapping lesion when the physician documents that two contiguous sites within the lung are affected and the lesions have overlapping boundaries.

Patients may also have multiple tumors in contiguous sites that are not overlapping. For example, distinct tumors in two different lobes of the same lung that do not meet or overlap should be assigned two separate codes for primary malignant neoplasm of each lobe. Coders must review the

	Malignant Primary	Malignant Secondary	Ca in situ	Benign	Uncertain Behavior	Unspecified Behavior
lung	C34.9-	C78.0-	D02.2-	D14.3-	D38.1	D49.1
azygos lobe	C34.1-	C78.0-	D02.2-	D14.3-	D38.1	D49.1
carina	C34.0-	C78.0-	D02.2-	D14.3-	D38.1	D49.1
hilus	C34.0-	C78.0-	D02.2-	D14.3-	D38.1	D49.1
linqula	C34.1-	C78.0-	D02.2-	D14.3-	D38.1	D49.1
lobe NEC	C34.9-	C78.0-	D02.2-	D14.3-	D38.1	D49.1
lower lobe	C34.3-	C78.0-	D02.2-	D14.3-	D38.1	D49.1
main bronchus	C34.0-	C78.0-	D02.2-	D14.3-	D38.1	D49.1
middle lobe	C34.2-	C78.0-	D02.21	D14.31	D38.1	D49.1
overlapping lesion	C34.8-	-	-	-	-	-
upper lobe	C34.1-	C78.0-	D02.2-	D14.3-	D38.1	D49.1

Figure 5-8 ■ Example of Entry in Table of Neoplasms for an Overlapping Lesion

documentation carefully to determine if the sites are overlapping or distinct.

Malignant Neoplasm of the Liver

The liver is a common site for metastasis because it filters the blood, which is a route through which cancer spreads. Primary liver cancer is rare but does occur as the result of cirrhosis and alcoholism. When abstracting and assigning codes for malignant neoplasms of the liver, coders must take extra care to determine if it is primary or secondary.

Verify Codes in the Tabular List

All codes in the Table of Neoplasms must be verified in the Tabular List. Codes listed with a short dash (-) at the end require an additional character for laterality, which must be determined from the Tabular List. The Tabular List also provides instructional notes directing coders when additional codes are required and what sequencing is required. The beginning of ICD-10-CM Chapter 2 (C00-D49) provides several instructional notes that apply to all codes in the chapter.

Guided Example of Assigning Neoplasm Codes

Continue with the example from earlier in this chapter of Anthony Payne, who saw Dr. Blackford for prostate cancer. Follow along in your ICD-10-CM manual as Karla Destefano, CPC, assigns the codes for the conditions she abstracted. Check off each step after you complete it.

▶ Karla reviews the conditions she abstracted.

❑ adenocarcinoma of prostate

❑ metastasis to colon

▶ Karla locates the Main Term for the primary neoplasm in the Index.

❑ She looks up **A, adenocarcinoma**.

❑ The Main Term entry contains an instructional note (*see also* **Neoplasm, malignant, by site**).

❑ She searches the subterms for **prostate** but cannot find it (■ FIGURE 5-9).

- Therefore, she knows she needs to refer to the Table of Neoplasms as directed in the instructional note.

❑ Karla searches for **N** in the Index to Diseases and Injuries and locates the Table of Neoplasms.

❑ She searches the left column for the subterm **prostate** and locates the entry.

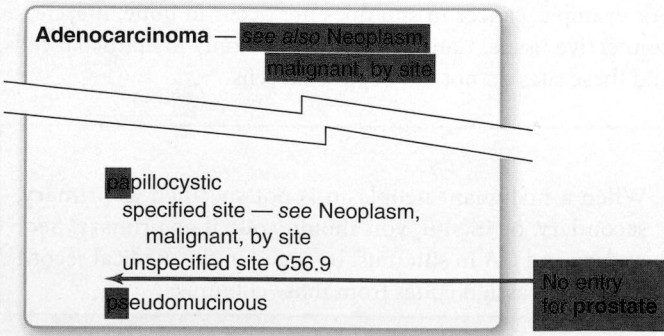

Adenocarcinoma — *see also* Neoplasm, malignant, by site

papillocystic
  specified site — *see* Neoplasm, malignant, by site
  unspecified site C56.9

pseudomucinous

No entry for prostate

Figure 5-9 ■ Index Entry for Adenocarcinoma, Subterms Beginning with p

❑ She checks the medical record to confirm that prostate cancer is primary.

❑ She refers to the first code column of the Table of Neoplasms, **Malignant Primary**, and selects the code **C61**.

▶ Next, Karla proceeds to verify the code in the Tabular List.

❑ Karla locates **C61** in the Tabular List and verifies the code title, **Malignant neoplasm of prostate**.

❑ She reviews the **Excludes1** note under the code and sees that **Malignant neoplasm of seminal vesicles** should not be coded here. She double-checks the medical record to be certain that seminal vesicles are not documented.

❑ Karla confirms that the block title **Malignant neoplasms of male genital organs (C60-C63)** contains no additional instructional notes.

❑ Karla reviews the instructional notes at the beginning of **Chapter 2 Neoplasms (C00-D49)**. She determines that they do not apply to this case because she has no functional activity to report (first note); morphology codes are not required for billing (second note); there are no overlapping boundaries (third note); and the neoplasm does not involve ectopic tissue (fourth note).

▶ Karla assigns code **C61, Malignant neoplasm of prostate** for the primary neoplasm.

▶ Karla reviews the medical record and identifies the metastatic site is the colon.

❑ She returns to the Table of Neoplasms and locates the subterm for **intestine**.

❑ Under **intestine** she locates the subterm for **large**, then **colon** (■ FIGURE 5-10).

❑ She refers to the column **Malignant Secondary** and locates the code **C78.5**.

▶ Karla locates the code in the Tabular List and verifies the title, **C78.5, Secondary malignant neoplasm of large intestine and rectum**.

❑ She reviews the category heading **C78, Secondary malignant neoplasm of respiratory and digestive organs** and confirms this case does not include any of the conditions listed under the **Excludes1** note.

CODING CAUTION

Although the Table of Neoplasms provides an entry for **C, colon**, it cross-references you to **C79.89 Secondary malignant neoplasm of other specified sites**, which is less specific than **C78.5**. Therefore, it is best to search for colon under the subterms **intestine, large** in order to locate the most specific code.

❑ She reviews the block heading **Malignant neoplasms of ill-defined, other secondary and unspecified sites (C76-C80)** and notes that there are no instructional notes.

❑ She already checked the notes at the beginning of **Chapter 2** so she does not need to do so again.

▶ Karla double-checks the medical record one last time to be sure she did not overlook anything. She has assigned the codes:

❑ **C61 Malignant neoplasm of prostate** for the primary neoplasm

❑ **C78.5 Secondary malignant neoplasm of large intestine and rectum** for the metastatic site

▶ Next, Karla needs to sequence the codes.

	Malignant Primary	Malignant Secondary	Ca in situ	Benign	Uncertain Behavior	Unspecified Behavior
intestine, intestinal	C26.0	C78.80	D01.40	D13.9	D37.8	D49.0
large	C18.9	C78.5	D01.0	D12.6	D37.4	D49.0
appendix	C18.1	C78.5	D01.0	D12.1	D37.3	D49.0
caput coli	C18.0	C78.5	D01.0	D12.0	D37.4	D49.0
cecum	C18.0	C78.5	D01.0	D12.0	D37.4	D49.0
colon	C18.9	C78.5	D01.0	D12.6	D37.4	D49.0
and rectum	C19	C78.5	D01.1	D12.7	D37.5	D49.0

Figure 5-10 ■ Table of Neoplasms Entry for Large Intestine, Colon

CODING PRACTICE

Exercise 5.3 Assigning Codes for Neoplasms

Instructions: Read the mini-medical-record of each patient's encounter, review the information abstracted in Exercise 5.2, and assign ICD-10-CM diagnosis codes using the Index and Tabular List. Write the code(s) on the line provided.

---

1. INPATIENT HOSPITAL   Gender: F   Age: 44

Reason for procedure: uterine fibroids

Procedure description: inserted catheter through femoral artery to uterus and injected polyvinyl alcohol (PVA) to block arteries leading to tumor

Postprocedural diagnosis: intramural (*within the muscle wall*) leiomyoma, uterus

Plan: FU in office in 4 weeks

Tip: The Main Term is the name of the tumor, not its site.

1 ICD-10-CM Code _____

---

2. INPATIENT HOSPITAL   Gender: F   Age: 15

Reason for admission: limb-salvage surgery after chemotherapy to shrink tumor

Procedure description: successfully cut out tumor from left thigh

Postprocedural assessment: osteosarcoma in the left thigh

Plan: discharge in 1–2 days

Tip: Remember to identify the medical term for the thigh bone.

1 ICD-10-CM Code _____

---

3. OFFICE   Gender: M   Age: 43

Reason for encounter: review results of biopsy and CT scan

Assessment: gastric adenocarcinoma, fundus

Plan: surgery to be followed by radiotherapy

Tip: Under the subterm stomach, search for the specific location within the stomach.

1 ICD-10-CM Code _____

ARRANGING CODES FOR NEOPLASMS

Sequencing of neoplasm codes is determined by the circumstances of the encounter or admission. The findings from abstracting (Table 5-3) help coders determine how to sequence multiple codes. In particular, be alert for the following circumstances that call for specific sequencing:

- evaluation or treatment directed at the primary neoplasm
- evaluation or treatment directed at the metastasis
- encounter solely for chemotherapy, radiotherapy, or immunotherapy
- evaluation or treatment for a complication
- personal or family history of malignant neoplasm

Refer to ■ TABLE 5-5 for a summary of sequencing rules for neoplasms, then read the more detailed instructions that follow.

Evaluation or Treatment Directed at the Primary Malignancy

When the reason for the encounter is evaluation or treatment of the malignancy, sequence the primary neoplasm first, followed by codes for metastatic sites, complications, or any other relevant conditions (OGCR I.C.2.a and OGCR I.C.2.l.1)). Treatment of the malignancy includes surgical removal of the neoplasm, diagnostic testing to determine the location or extent of the malignancy, and therapies such as **paracentesis** or **thoracentesis**.

When *both* the primary and secondary sites are being treated or evaluated, sequence the primary malignancy first, followed by the code(s) for the secondary site(s). Use a code for the primary malignancy as long as the patient is receiving treatment for it, even if the tumor has been surgically removed (OGCR I.C.2.l.1)).

CODING CAUTION

Be careful to understand the difference between primary or secondary malignant neoplasm and principal or first-listed diagnosis. The terms *primary* and *secondary* refer to the progression of the malignancy: where it started and where it spread to. Principal and first-listed diagnoses refer to the sequencing of codes. A code for primary neoplasm is not always sequenced first and a code for secondary neoplasm is not always sequenced second.

Evaluation or Treatment of the Metastasis

When the reason for the encounter is evaluation or treatment of the secondary malignancy or metastasis *only*, sequence the code for the secondary site as the principal or first-listed diagnosis; sequence the code for the primary malignancy as an additional code (OGCR I.C.2.b and OGCR I.C.2.l.2)).

When *both* the primary and secondary sites are evaluated or treated, sequence the primary site first.

Table 5-5 ■ SUMMARY OF COMMONLY USED SEQUENCING RULES FOR NEOPLASMS

Reason for Encounter	Sequencing
Evaluation or treatment of primary neoplasm or *both* primary and secondary sites	1. Primary neoplasm 2. Secondary neoplasm
Evaluation or treatment of metastasis	1. Secondary neoplasm 2. Primary neoplasm
Evaluation or treatment *only* for complication of neoplasm (except anemia)	1. Complication 2. Primary neoplasm 3. Secondary neoplasm
Evaluation or treatment of anemia due to neoplasm	1. Neoplasm 2. Anemia
Encounter solely for chemotherapy, radiotherapy, or immunotherapy	1. Encounter for chemotherapy, radiotherapy, or immunotherapy 2. Complications during the therapy, if any 3. Primary neoplasm 4. Secondary neoplasm
Treatment, such as surgery, followed by chemotherapy, radiotherapy, or immunotherapy	1. The neoplasm that was the objective of the treatment. 2. Any additional neoplasms.
Screening due to family history of malignant neoplasm	1. Screening 2. Family history of malignant neoplasm
Follow-up after completing treatment for a malignant neoplasm that no longer exists	1. Follow-up 2. Personal history of malignant neoplasm
Evaluation or treatment for an unrelated condition	1. Unrelated condition 2. Neoplasm, if documented as relevant

Encounter Solely for Chemo-, Radio-, or Immunotherapy

When the reason for the encounter or admission is *only* for administration of chemotherapy, radiotherapy, or immunotherapy, assign the principal or first-listed diagnosis for **Encounter for**, followed by the name of the therapy (OGCR I.C.2.e.2)). To locate the code in the Index, search for the Main Term **Chemotherapy**, **Radiotherapy**, or **Immunotherapy**, as appropriate. Sequence codes for the primary and/or secondary neoplasms as additional codes.

CODING CAUTION

The codes titled **Encounter for** are diagnosis codes that describe the *reason* for the encounter. They are not procedure codes. You must also assign procedure codes that describe the service(s) provided using ICD-10-PCS codes for inpatient hospitals or CPT codes for physician office and outpatient services.

When the primary malignancy has been surgically removed but the patient is still receiving treatment, assign the code for **Encounter for** the therapy first, followed by the code for malignant neoplasm. Do not assign a code for personal history of malignant neoplasm when the patient is still receiving treatment, even when it has been surgically removed.

When an episode of care involves surgical removal of the neoplasm followed by chemotherapy or radiation therapy during the *same* episode of care, sequence the neoplasm code first, followed by the **Encounter for** therapy code(s) (OGCR I.C.2.e.1)).

Evaluation or Treatment for a Complication

When an encounter is for management of a complication associated with a neoplasm, such as dehydration, and the treatment is *only* for the complication, sequence the complication first, followed by the appropriate code(s) for the neoplasm (OGCR I.C.2.l)). However, if treatment is directed at the neoplasm and the complication is *also* treated, sequence the appropriate neoplasm code first, followed by the codes for the complications.

The exception to these sequencing rules is when the complication is anemia. When the encounter is for management of an anemia associated with the malignancy and the treatment is *only* for anemia, sequence the appropriate code for the *malignancy* as the principal or first-listed diagnosis followed by code **D63.0, Anemia in neoplastic disease** (OGCR I.C.2.l.4)).

SUCCESS STEP

To locate the code for anemia due to cancer in the Index, search for **Anemia**, then the subterm **in**, then the subterm **neoplastic disease**.

CODING CAUTION

Coders familiar with ICD-9-CM should note that the OGCR for sequencing of anemia in neoplastic disease is different in ICD-10-CM.

Personal or Family History of Malignant Neoplasm

When a physician documents that family history of malignant neoplasm contributes to a patient's health risk, sequence the diagnosis code for screening first, followed by the history code. For example, a patient with a history of colonic polyps and a family history of colorectal cancer may need a colonoscopy more frequently than the general population. Sequence the codes as follows:

1. Screening for malignant neoplasm of colon
2. Personal history of colon polyps (benign neoplasm)
3. Family history, malignant neoplasm of digestive organs

When a physician sees a patient for follow-up after cancer treatment has been completed and the disease no longer exists, assign a code for follow-up first, followed by the appropriate personal history code (OGCR I.C.21.c.8)).

SUCCESS STEP

Although it takes a lot of experience to memorize every OGCR for the coding of neoplasms, even new coders can memorize the *fact* that this ICD-10-CM chapter has many guidelines. This serves as a reminder to refer to the OGCR for specific guidance.

The circumstances discussed here are the most common that coders encounter. Refer to the OGCR I.C.2.c for additional detailed guidance on sequencing related to neoplasms.

Guided Example of Arranging Neoplasm Codes

Continue with the example from earlier in this chapter of Anthony Payne, who saw Dr. Blackford for prostate cancer. Follow along in your ICD-10-CM manual as Karla Destefano, CPC, sequences the codes. Check off each step after you complete it.

▶ Karla reviews the codes she assigned.

❑ **C61 Malignant neoplasm of prostate**

❑ **C78.5 Secondary malignant neoplasm of large intestine and rectum**

▶ She reviews the reason for the encounter in the medical record: review test results to determine extent of prostate cancer

❑ Therefore, she sequences the primary neoplasm as the first-listed diagnosis, followed by the metastatic site:

(1) **C61 Malignant neoplasm of prostate**

(2) **C78.5 Secondary malignant neoplasm of large intestine and rectum**

CODING PRACTICE

Exercise 5.4 **Arranging Codes for Neoplasms**

Instructions: Read the mini-medical-record of each patient's encounter, review the information abstracted in Exercise 5.2, assign ICD-10-CM diagnosis codes using the Index and Tabular List, and sequence the codes correctly. Write the code(s) on the line provided.

1. OFFICE Gender: F Age: 59

Reason for encounter: chemotherapy

Assessment: adenocarcinoma of the right breast, lower outer quadrant, which metastasized to multiple overlapping sites in the brain

Plan: return for next treatment in 3 weeks

Tip: Refer to OGCR I.C.2.e.2) for a reminder on how to sequence these codes. Remember to verify all codes in the Tabular List.

3 ICD-10-CM Codes _____

_____

2. INPATIENT HOSPITAL Gender: M Age: 61

Reason for procedure: brain stem tumor

Procedure description: used Gamma Knife surgery to destroy tumor

Postprocedural diagnosis: squamous cell carcinoma of the lung with brain stem metastases

Plan: FU in office 1 week, evaluate for chemotherapy

Tip: The site that is the reason for surgery should be sequenced first.

2 ICD-10-CM Codes _____

3. INPATIENT HOSPITAL Gender: M Age: 67

Reason for admission: anemia

Assessment: anemia due to classical lymphocyte depleted Hodgkin lymphoma

Plan: administer IV iron supplements

Tip: Refer to OGCR I.C.2.l.4) for sequencing guidance.

2 ICD-10-CM Codes _____

CHAPTER SUMMARY

In this chapter you learned that:

- Neoplasms are abnormal growth of new tissue, which may be malignant or benign.
- ICD-10-CM Chapter 2, Neoplasms (C00-D49), contains 21 blocks or subchapters that are divided by anatomical site.
- When abstracting patient cases with neoplasms, coders must look for several pieces of information that will help determine the first-listed or principal diagnosis and the sequencing of any additional diagnoses.

- Coders use both the Index to Diseases and Injuries and the Table of Neoplasms to locate codes for neoplasms.
- Sequencing of neoplasm codes is determined by the circumstances of the encounter or admission. OGCR provides detailed guidance on sequencing.
- ICD-10-CM provides Official Guidelines for Coding and Reporting (OGCR) for neoplasms in OGCR section I.C.2, which provide specific direction for sequencing codes for multiple neoplasms, complications, adjuvant therapies, and other situations.

CONCEPT QUIZ

Take a moment to look back through neoplasms and solidify your skills. This is your opportunity to pull together everything you have learned.

Completion

Instructions: Write the term that answers each question based on the information you learned in this chapter. Choose from the following list. Some choices may be used more than once and some choices may not be used at all.

adjuvant	malignant
behavior	metastasis
benign	overlapping
CA in situ	primary neoplasm
carcinoma	radiotherapy
chemotherapy	sarcoma
CUP	secondary neoplasm
grading	staging
histology	topography
immunotherapy	

1. _____ describes the anatomical site where the neoplasm begins.

2. _____ describes the tissue type.

3. _____ describes a neoplasm that has spread to other sites.

4. _____ is the process of determining how far the cancer has spread.

5. Chemotherapy, radiotherapy, and immunotherapy are examples of _____ therapy.

6. _____ uses drugs to kill cancer cells.

7. _____ occurs only in epithelial cells.

8. _____ tumors are contiguous sites where the neoplasm continues from one site to the adjacent one without interruption.

9. _____ describes how closely the cancer cell looks like a normal cell when viewed microscopically.

10. _____ means life threatening.

Multiple Choice

Instructions: Circle the letter of the best answer to each question based on the information you learned in this chapter.

1. Which of the following is NOT a characteristic of malignant neoplasms?
   A. Are not encapsulated
   B. Have invasive growth and metastasis
   C. Produce no cachexia
   D. Can recur when surgically removed

2. Malignant neoplasms metastasize through
   A. exchange of bodily fluids.
   B. the bloodstream and lymphatic system.
   C. genetic transmission.
   D. bacteria.

3. Personal history of malignant neoplasm is
   A. a condition that a patient's family member had in the past or currently has that causes the patient to be at higher risk of also contracting or developing the disease.
   B. a primary neoplasm that has metastasized.
   C. a condition the patient currently has and is receiving treatment for.
   D. a condition the patient had in the past, was removed or resolved, and is no longer being treated, but has the potential for recurrence.

4. Which of the following is NOT a column on the Table of Neoplasms?
   A. Personal History
   B. Malignant Primary
   C. Benign
   D. Uncertain Behavior

5. Which of the following statements about the Table of Neoplasms is TRUE?
   A. Coders always should consult the Table of Neoplasms instead of the Index to Diseases and Injuries.
   B. Codes in the Table of Neoplasms must always be verified in the Tabular List.
   C. The Table of Neoplasms classifies only malignant neoplasms.
   D. The Table of Neoplasms combines the Index and Tabular list into one document.

(continued)

(continued from page 75)

6. When a patient is seen for evaluation or treatment of metastasis, which code should be sequenced first?
   A. Primary neoplasm
   B. Secondary neoplasm
   C. CA in situ
   D. Complication

7. When a patient is seen for dehydration due to colon cancer that has metastasized to multiple sites, which code should be sequenced first?
   A. Colon cancer
   B. Metastatic site
   C. Dehydration
   D. Encounter for chemotherapy

8. When a patient is admitted for surgery to remove a tumor from the breast then receives chemotherapy while still in the hospital, which code should be sequenced first?
   A. Breast cancer
   B. Encounter for surgery
   C. Encounter for chemotherapy
   D. Aftercare

9. When a patient receives a colonoscopy more frequently than normal because of a family history of colon cancer, which code should be sequenced first?
   A. Screening
   B. Family history of malignant neoplasm
   C. Personal history of malignant neoplasm
   D. Colon cancer

10. When a patient who previously had surgery to remove a malignant neoplasm of the lung has an encounter only for radiotherapy, which code(s) should be assigned?
    A. Malignant neoplasm only
    B. Encounter for radiotherapy only
    C. Malignant neoplasm first and encounter for radiotherapy second
    D. Encounter for radiotherapy first and malignant neoplasm second

CODING CHALLENGE

Instructions: Read the mini-medical-record of each patient's encounter, then abstract, assign, and sequence ICD-10-CM diagnosis codes using the Index and Tabular List. Write the code(s) on the line provided.

---

1. OFFICE   Gender: F   Age: 32

Chief complaint: management of multiple myeloma

Assessment: multiple myeloma in remission

Plan: recheck in 6 months

Tip: The fifth character in the code specifies remission.

1 ICD-10-CM Code _____

---

2. OUTPATIENT SURGERY   Gender: M   Age: 67

Reason for procedure: removal of tumor in left cheek

Procedure description: removed one lesion, 0.5 cm

Postprocedural diagnosis: basal cell adenoma left parotid salivary gland

Plan: recheck in 6 months

Tip: The parotid salivary gland is located in the cheek.

1 ICD-10-CM Code _____

---

3. OFFICE   Gender: F   Age: 57

Chief complaint: review colon biopsy results

Assessment: adenocarcinoma in situ in sigmoid colon

(continued)

---

3. (continued)

Plan: schedule surgery

Tip: What is another term for the colon? Search for this term to find the code you need.

1 ICD-10-CM Code _____

---

4. OFFICE   Gender: M   Age: 27

Chief complaint: evaluate unusual mole on forehead

Assessment: malignant melanoma

Plan: schedule removal next week

Tip: Remember to search for the subterm **skin**.

1 ICD-10-CM Code _____

---

5. OFFICE   Gender: F   Age: 35

Chief complaint: review pathology results of lesion removed from skin of left breast 1 week ago

Assessment: CA in situ, completely removed

Plan: self-check entire skin once a month to watch for any additional lesions. Schedule a re-check appointment with office in 6 months.

1 ICD-10-CM Code _____

6. OUTPATIENT HOSPITAL   Gender: F   Age: 71

Reason for encounter: *radiotherapy to lung*

Assessment: *metastatic cancer in the right lung, CUP*

Plan: *5 treatments per week for 6 weeks*

Tip: The site being treated is the first-listed diagnosis.

3 ICD-10-CM Codes _____

_____

7. OFFICE   Gender: F   Age: 63

Chief complaint: *monitoring of benign neoplasm*

Assessment: *benign Islet cell neoplasm of the pancreas*

Plan: *return visit if any new problems arise*

1 ICD-10-CM Code _____

8. OUTPATIENT HOSPITAL   Gender: F   Age: 66

Reason for encounter: *screening colonoscopy*

Assessment: *personal history of carcinoma of the colon which was successfully removed five years ago, no new findings today*

Plan: *colonoscopy in 5 years*

Tip: Refer to OGCR I.C.21.c.8) for coding and sequencing guidance.

2 ICD-10-CM Codes _____

9. INPATIENT HOSPITAL   Gender: M   Age: 48

Reason for admission: *Surgery for widespread metastases from pancreatic cancer.*

Assessment: *Surgery was performed, followed by inpatient chemotherapy.*

Plan: *begin weekly regimen of outpatient chemotherapy*

Tip: Refer to OGCR I.C.2.e.1).

2 ICD-10-CM Codes _____

10. INPATIENT HOSPITAL   Gender: F   Age: 81

Reason for admission: *admitted from Emergency Department after collapsing at home, arrived by ambulance*

Assessment: *dehydration and hyponatremia (sodium deficiency) due to chemotherapy for metastatic bilateral ovarian cancer*

Tip: The code for the complication is a combination code. Metastatic ovarian cancer means that the ovary is the primary site and the secondary site is unknown. Refer to OGCR I.B.13 to review rules for coding bilateral conditions. Refer to OGCR I.C.2.e.4) for sequencing guidance.

4 ICD-10-CM Codes _____

_____

KEEP ON CODING

Instructions: Read the diagnostic statement, then use the Index and Tabular List to assign and sequence ICD-10-CM diagnosis codes. Write the code(s) on the line provided.

1. Carcinoma in situ of false vocal cord: ICD-10-CM Code(s) _____

2. Benign neoplasm of the mouth: ICD-10-CM Code(s) _____

3. Benign carcinoid tumor of the right kidney: ICD-10-CM Code(s) _____

4. Mesothelioma of lung: ICD-10-CM Code(s) _____

5. Metastatic carcinoma of the parietal lobe of the brain: ICD-10-CM Code(s) _____

6. Benign adenomatous polyps of colon: ICD-10-CM Code(s) _____

7. Chief cell adenoma: ICD-10-CM Code(s) _____

8. Kaposi sarcoma with HIV of stomach: ICD-10-CM Code(s) _____

9. Basal cell carcinoma of right hand: ICD-10-CM Code(s) _____

10. Malignant melanoma of skin of abdominal wall: ICD-10-CM Code(s) _____

(continued)

(continued from page 77)

11. Malignant neoplasm of nipple of the right breast: ICD-10-CM Code(s) _____

12. Follicular lymphoma, Grade IIIb, inguinal region: ICD-10-CM Code(s) _____

13. Acute leukemia, in relapse: ICD-10-CM Code(s) _____

14. Melanoma of left forearm: ICD-10-CM Code(s) _____

15. Carcinoma in situ, cervical stump: ICD-10-CM Code(s) _____

16. Family history of breast cancer: ICD-10-CM Code(s) _____

17. Personal history of brain cancer: ICD-10-CM Code(s) _____

18. Malignant neoplasm of the right upper and lower lobes of the lung, primary: ICD-10-CM Code(s) _____

19. Admission for chemotherapy for ovarian cancer: ICD-10-CM Code(s) _____

20. Malignant primary cancer of the body of the pancreas: ICD-10-CM Code(s) _____

21. Metastatic cancer to the rib: ICD-10-CM Code(s) _____

22. Anemia due to left intraocular cancer: ICD-10-CM Code(s) _____

23. Metastatic cancer of the liver, with unknown primary site: ICD-10-CM Code(s) _____

24. Invasive hydatidiform mole: ICD-10-CM Code(s) _____

25. Adenocarcinoma of the parotid gland with metastasis to the spine: ICD-10-CM Code(s) _____

Symptoms, Signs, and Abnormal Clinical and Laboratory Findings, Not Elsewhere Classified (R00-R99)

Chapter 6

Learning Objectives

After completing this chapter, you should have the skills to:

6.1 Spell and define the key words, medical terms, and abbreviations in this chapter.

6.2 Distinguish between symptoms, signs, abnormal clinical findings and abnormal laboratory findings, and confirmed diagnoses.

6.3 Identify the main characteristics of coding symptoms, signs, and abnormal findings.

6.4 Abstract symptoms, signs, abnormal findings, and confirmed diagnoses from the medical record.

6.5 Assign codes for symptoms, signs, abnormal findings, and confirmed diagnoses.

6.6 Arrange codes for symptoms, signs, abnormal findings, and confirmed diagnoses.

6.7 Discuss the Official Guidelines for Coding and Reporting related to symptoms, signs, and abnormal findings.

Chapter Outline

- **Symptoms and Signs Refresher**
- **Coding Overview of Symptoms and Signs**
- **Abstracting Symptoms and Signs**
- **Assigning Codes for Symptoms and Signs**
- **Arranging Codes for Symptoms and Signs**

Key Terms and Abbreviations

abnormal
confirmed
impression
integral
modifier
qualified
qualifier
related
unrelated

In addition to the key terms listed here, students should know the terms defined within tables in this chapter.

For updates and corrections, visit our student resource site at

www.pearsonhighered.com/healthprofessionsresources

INTRODUCTION

While on a road trip, you hope never to feel the car suddenly vibrate or to hear an unknown clanging or hissing sound. You know you need to get to the nearest mechanic quickly because these are symptoms and signs of an underlying problem. The mechanic may perform a visual inspection or conduct diagnostic testing to determine the source of the problem and repair it.

Patients experience a symptom or notice a change in their health, so they go to the doctor to have it checked out. The physician interviews the patient, conducts a physical examination, and orders any necessary tests. At times, physicians can make a diagnosis quickly and, other times, they must order further testing or consult with a specialist.

Coders must learn to distinguish patient symptoms, signs, abnormal findings, and test results from the underlying diagnosis. Physicians of all specialties evaluate symptoms, signs, and abnormal findings.

As you read this chapter, open your medical terminology book and keep a medical dictionary handy to refresh your memory of any unfamiliar terms. Also bookmark reliable Internet sites. These resources are especially important to help you learn what symptoms or signs are common with various conditions.

SYMPTOMS AND SIGNS REFRESHER

To determine a patient's diagnosis, a physician evaluates numerous sources of information: the patient's chief complaint and description of the problem, a visual observation of the patient, a physical examination, and results of laboratory tests, imaging, and other evaluations. The physician's goal is to establish a definitive diagnosis and prescribe a treatment plan to cure the problem and/or alleviate the symptoms. An **abnormal** test result or clinical finding is one in which the readings are not within the normal average range established for that particular test. Sometimes a confirmed diagnosis is not possible because the physician needs multiple encounters, extended testing, evaluation by specialists, surgery, or other procedures to arrive at a diagnosis.

Refer to ■ TABLE 6-1 to review the meanings of various types of diagnostic data.

Symptoms and signs are often identified with prefixes or suffixes that are applied to word roots from specific body systems. Refer to ■ TABLE 6-2 for a refresher on how to build medical terms related to symptoms, signs, and abnormal findings.

CODING CAUTION

Be aware of easily confused medical terms that have similar spellings and different meanings, such as:

dysphagia (*difficulty swallowing*) and **dysphasia** (*difficulty speaking*)

hem/e (*blood*) and **hemi-** (*half, side*)

hypo- (*low, below*) and **hyper-** (*high, excessive*)

Table 6-1 ■ **DEFINITION AND EXAMPLES OF DIAGNOSTIC DATA SOURCES**

Data	Definition	Example
Symptom	Subjective evidence of a disease or condition, usually reported by the patient	Pain, anxiety, fatigue, nausea
Sign	Objective evidence of a disease or condition that can be observed by the physician	Fever, limp, crying, bleeding, vomiting
Abnormal clinical finding	Evidence of a disease or condition discovered through physical examination or testing	Palpation of a lump or mass, irregular EKG, X-ray showing a fracture
Abnormal laboratory test	Result of a chemistry test, blood test, biological culture that is outside of (higher or lower than) the normal numerical range, or microscopic specimen examination that differs from the standard visual features	Elevated or low blood glucose, high or low complete blood count, microscopic dysplasia

Table 6-2 ■ **EXAMPLE OF CONSTRUCTING MEDICAL TERMS FOR SYMPTOMS, SIGNS, AND ABNORMAL FINDINGS**

Prefix/Combining Form	Suffix	Complete Medical Term
dys- (*abnormal, painful*)		dys + uria (*difficulty urinating*) dys + phagia (*difficulty swallowing*) dys + meno + rrhea (*difficulty or painful menstrual flow*)
hem/e (*blood*)	-uria (*condition of urine*) -ptysis (*to spit, cough*) meno + rrhea (*menstrual flow*)	hemat + uria (*blood in urine*) hemo + ptysis (*coughing up blood*)
poly- (*many*)		poly + uria (*frequent urination*) poly + meno + rrhea (*frequent menstrual flow*)

CODING PRACTICE

Exercise 6.1   Symptoms and Signs Refresher

Instructions: Define the following symptoms, signs, and abnormal findings, then assign the diagnosis code.

Follow these steps:

- Use slash marks "/" to break down each term into its root(s) and suffix.
- Define the meaning of the word, based on the meaning of each word part.
- Assign the default ICD-10-CM diagnosis code for the condition using the Index and Tabular List.

Example: dysuria dys/ur/ia   Meaning: *condition of painful urination*   ICD-10-CM Code: *R30.0*

1. dyspnea   Meaning _____   ICD-10-CM Code _____
2. nocturia   Meaning _____   ICD-10-CM Code _____
3. aphagia   Meaning _____   ICD-10-CM Code _____
4. epistaxis   Meaning _____   ICD-10-CM Code _____
5. lymphadenopathy   Meaning _____   ICD-10-CM Code _____
6. hyperemesis   Meaning _____   ICD-10-CM Code _____
7. hypoxemia   Meaning _____   ICD-10-CM Code _____
8. cyanosis   Meaning _____   ICD-10-CM Code _____
9. glycosuria   Meaning _____   ICD-10-CM Code _____
10. tachycardia   Meaning _____   ICD-10-CM Code _____

CODING OVERVIEW OF SYMPTOMS AND SIGNS

ICD-10-CM Chapter 18, Symptoms, Signs, and Abnormal Clinical and Laboratory Findings, Not Elsewhere Classified (R00-R99), contains 14 blocks or subchapters that are divided by anatomical site. Review the block names and code ranges listed at the beginning of Chapter 18 in the ICD-10-CM manual to become familiar with the content and organization.

This chapter includes symptoms, signs, and abnormal results of clinical and laboratory procedures. It also includes ill-defined conditions that do not fit anywhere else in ICD-10-CM or that can be indicative of multiple conditions. Signs and symptoms that point to a specific diagnosis appear in other chapters of the classification. For example, fevers of unknown origin or that are drug induced appear in this chapter, but fevers with a known cause, such as a fever due to heat or a specific organism, appear in other chapters. An abnormal blood culture appears in this chapter, but an abnormal white blood cell count is classified to ICD-10-CM Chapter 3, Diseases of the Blood and Blood Forming Organs.

This chapter is comparable to ICD-9-CM Chapter 16 (780-799). Codes have been added, deleted, and expanded for clarity and specificity. Significant expansions have been made to codes in the block **Abnormal findings on examination of other body fluids, substances and tissues, without diagnosis (R83-R89)** in order to further specify the type of finding. Coding for **Coma (R40.2-)** has been expanded from a single code in ICD-9-CM (780.01) to 16 codes, each with one of five extensions to reflect the Glasgow Coma Scale ratings. Review the

instructional notes at the beginning of the chapter that discuss how coders should report codes in this chapter. Also review the **Excludes2** note, which lists several conditions not classified to this chapter. Frequent instructional notes throughout the chapter direct coders to use multiple codes to describe related or underlying conditions associated with various symptoms.

ICD-10-CM provides Official Guidelines for Coding and Reporting (OGCR) for symptoms, signs, and abnormal clinical and laboratory findings in OGCR section I.C.18. OGCR provides a detailed discussion of when to report and not report codes from this chapter. OGCR also discusses coding of symptoms and signs related to several specific conditions: repeated falls, coma, **functional quadriplegia**, **systemic inflammatory response syndrome (SIRS)**, and death not otherwise specified (NOS). Additional OGCR related to symptoms, signs, and abnormal findings appear in OGCR I.B.4, 5, and 6; II.A, II.E; IV.D and IV.H.

ABSTRACTING SYMPTOMS AND SIGNS

Abstracting requires coders to be knowledgeable of disease processes and the related symptoms, signs, abnormal clinical findings, and abnormal laboratory test results so they can distinguish which elements should be coded and which should not. They also must distinguish when a physician makes a confirmed diagnosis, in contrast to when the diagnosis is uncertain, because different coding rules apply to these situations. ■ TABLE 6-3 (page 82) highlights key questions to answer when reviewing the medical record. Coders use answers to these questions when assigning and sequencing codes. Remember that the

Table 6-3 ■ KEY CRITERIA FOR ABSTRACTING SYMPTOMS, SIGNS, ABNORMAL FINDINGS, AND CONFIRMED CONDITIONS

❏ What symptoms does the patient report?

❏ What signs does the physician document?

❏ What abnormal laboratory findings are reviewed?

❏ What confirmed diagnoses are documented?

❏ What diagnoses are identified as uncertain with words such as *possible, probable, rule out, suspected*?

❏ Which symptoms, signs, and abnormal findings are integral to the condition?

❏ Which symptoms, signs, and abnormal findings are related but not integral to the condition?

❏ Which symptoms, signs, and abnormal findings are unrelated to the condition?

abstracting questions are a guide and that not every question applies to, or can be answered for, every case. For example, not all patients have abnormal laboratory findings. Details that will help answer these questions follow in the remainder of this section of the chapter.

Integral, Related, and Unrelated Findings

Coders must distinguish between symptoms, signs, and abnormal findings that are an **integral** (*routine*) part of a disease process, those that are **related** but not integral, and those that are **unrelated**. They need a solid understanding of common conditions and their symptoms so they can make these distinctions. Refer to ■ TABLE 6-4 to review symptoms, signs, and abnormal findings for commonly diagnosed conditions.

Integral Symptoms

When a diagnosis is confirmed, assign codes to the named condition, but do *not* assign codes for the symptoms, signs, and abnormal findings that are integral to the condition

Table 6-4 ■ SYMPTOMS, SIGNS, AND ABNORMAL FINDINGS FOR COMMONLY DIAGNOSED CONDITIONS

Condition	Symptoms and Signs	Abnormal Findings
Allergic contact dermatitis	Rash, erythema, pruritus, burning	
Anemia	Fatigue, **SOB**, decreased exercise tolerance	Folic acid
Asthma	Dyspnea, difficulty exhaling, wheezing	
Appendicitis	**RLQ** pain, fever, nausea, vomiting	
Benign prostatic hyperplasia (BPH)	Nocturia, polyuria, dysuria, oliguria	
Cerebrovascular accident (CVA)	Headache, muscular weakness, speech disturbance, loss of consciousness	Angiography, CT scan, MRI
Colorectal cancer	Melena, change in bowel habits, lower abdominal pain	Biopsy, colonoscopy
Congestive heart failure (CHF)	SOB, fatigue, edema	EKG, echocardiogram, **BP**, X-ray
Dementia	Language, memory, and mood deficits	
Depression	Prolonged sadness, sleep and appetite changes, feelings of guilt and anxiety	
Diabetes mellitus (DM)	Polyuria, polydipsia	Hyperglycemia, elevated glucose, elevated **HbA1C**
Endometriosis	Pelvic pain, diarrhea, constipation, menorrhagia, fatigue	
Epilepsy	Convulsions, seizures	**EEG**
Gastroenteritis	Nausea, vomiting, diarrhea, abdominal pain	Stool culture
Gout	Joint pain, heat, swelling, redness	
Hiatal hernia	Indigestion, heartburn, acid reflux, esophagitis	
Hypercholesterolemia	**Asymptomatic**	Elevated serum cholesterol
Hypertension (HTN)	Asymptomatic	Elevated blood pressure
Leukemia	Fatigue, weight loss, fever, hemorrhages	Blood tests
Osteoarthritis (OA)	Joint pain and stiffness, muscle weakness, enlarged joints	X-ray
Pneumonia	Chest pain, fluid in lungs, fever, productive cough	X-ray
Rosacea	Flushing, persistent erythema, papules pustules, telangiectasia	
Urinary tract infection (UTI)	Polyuria, dysuria, hematuria	Urinalysis

(OGCR I.B.4 and 5; I.C.18.a). Integral or routine symptoms are those that most patients with the condition experience. For example:

- The physician documents *Fever and RLQ pain due to acute ruptured appendicitis.* Fever and pain are symptoms integral to a ruptured appendix, so the coder assigns a code only for the appendicitis. Do *not* assign codes for fever and pain.

SUCCESS STEP

Be proactive and keep a reference book on diseases on your desk so you can consult it when you are unsure if a symptom is integral, related, or unrelated. Consider creating "cheat sheets" with notes on conditions commonly coded in your office to guide you through the learning process. If you are unsure about a symptom, consult a colleague or supervisor; do not guess.

Do not code clinical findings that are integral to the condition. For example:

- The physician documents *Three elevated BP readings over the past three months. Hypertension.* The coder assigns a code for hypertension, but not for elevated blood pressure, because a series of elevated blood pressure readings is the definition of hypertension.

Do not code laboratory test results that are integral to the condition. For example:

- The physician documents *Elevated glucose HbA1C results, type 2 diabetes.* The coder assigns a code for type 2 diabetes, but not for elevated glucose or HbA1C because those tests are used to establish the diagnosis.

Do code for the symptoms, signs, abnormal clinical findings, or abnormal test results when a diagnosis is not stated. For example:

- The physician documents *Three elevated BP readings over the past three months.* The coder assigns a code for elevated blood pressure, but not hypertension, because the physician did not document hypertension as a diagnosis.
- The physician documents *Elevated glucose HbA1C results. Refer to dietician for meal plan.* The coder assigns a code for elevated glucose, but not diabetes, because the physician did not document diabetes as a diagnosis. Coders should not assign a diagnosis that is not documented.

CODING CAUTION

The physician's diagnosis stands on its own. Coders do not assign codes to symptoms to justify *why* the physician arrived at the diagnosis. Assign codes for the symptoms *only* if the diagnosis is not confirmed. When the diagnosis is confirmed, code *only* the diagnosis, not the symptoms.

Related Symptoms

Do code for symptoms that are related to the disease process but not integral to it (OGCR I.B.6). Related symptoms are those

that patients occasionally experience with the confirmed diagnosis but are not common or routine. For example:

- The physician documents *RLQ pain, fever, vomiting, dehydration due to acute ruptured appendicitis.* Administered IV fluids. Dehydration is the result of the fever and vomiting associated with appendicitis but is not a routine part of the condition. Additional treatment was provided for the dehydration. Therefore, assign a code for dehydration in addition to ruptured appendicitis.

Unrelated Symptoms

Do code for symptoms that are unrelated to the confirmed diagnosis (OGCR I.C.18.b). Unrelated symptoms are those that are not associated with the confirmed diagnosis and may indicate an additional problem or condition. For example:

- The physician documents *Fever, difficulty breathing, hemoptysis, X-ray positive for pneumonia, sputum culture for hemoptysis.* Fever and difficulty breathing are integral to pneumonia, which the physician confirmed with a chest X-ray. Hemoptysis is not a symptom associated with pneumonia, so it should be coded in addition to pneumonia.

Uncertain Diagnoses

When physicians cannot establish a definite diagnosis, outpatient coders assign codes for the symptoms, signs, and abnormal findings until a diagnosis is established (OGCR IV.H). Coders must interpret the terms physicians use in documentation in order to understand whether a diagnosis is confirmed or uncertain. An uncertain diagnosis is one that the physician is not completely confident of. Particularly in the outpatient setting, physicians may require multiple visits, consultation with a specialist, and test results in order to determine a diagnosis. Coders assign codes for symptoms until the diagnosis is established. After the diagnosis is established, they no longer code the symptoms that are integral to the condition.

By default, interpret any diagnostic statement as **confirmed**, one the physician is confident of, *unless* the physician indicates it is uncertain. A diagnosis may be uncertain when a patient has symptoms and signs that can be attributed to many different conditions or when test results do not provide clear data. An uncertain diagnostic statement contains **qualifiers** or **modifiers** (*word(s) that limit the meaning of another*) before the name of the condition (■ TABLE 6-5).

An uncertain diagnosis is also called a **qualified** diagnosis. The words *qualified* and *qualifier* have two opposite meanings. One common meaning is *meeting a standard or set of criteria.* An alternative meaning is one of *limiting or restricting.* When

Table 6-5   ■   **TERMS INDICATING UNCERTAIN DIAGNOSES**

❑ likely	❑ rule out (R/O)
❑ possible	❑ still to be ruled out
❑ probable	❑ suspected
❑ questionable	

coders and physicians use the expression *qualified diagnosis*, they are using the second meaning of the word, a *diagnosis that is limited or uncertain.*

Physicians may use the heading **Impression** in their progress notes for the diagnostic statement. This word also carries multiple meanings, which sometimes causes confusion for new coders. One meaning is *an idea or belief that is vague or unclear.* Physicians use an alternate meaning, *an effect produced on the mind by outside stimuli.* Therefore, use of the word *impression* does not describe an uncertain diagnosis.

In the outpatient setting, do not assign a code to an uncertain diagnosis. Instead, code the symptoms, signs, and abnormal test results documented by the physician (OGCR IV.D and H). In the inpatient setting, when the diagnosis documented at the time of discharge is stated as uncertain, code the condition as if it existed (OGCR III.A and IV.H). The rationale for this guideline is that the diagnostic workup, arrangements for further workups, and initial treatments provided must relate to the principal diagnosis.

SUCCESS STEP

When you code for an uncertain diagnosis in an inpatient setting, assign the usual code for the condition. You do not assign any additional codes to indicate it is uncertain.

Abnormal Clinical and Laboratory Findings

When coding inpatient services, abstract abnormal clinical and laboratory findings *only* when the provider documents their clinical significance. Do not automatically abstract and code all findings that are outside the normal range. In rare cases, the provider may order additional tests to further evaluate abnormal findings, or prescribe a treatment, but not document their clinical significance. In this situation, coders should query the provider regarding the possible significance of the findings (OGCR III.B).

Guided Example of Abstracting Symptoms and Signs

Refer to the following example to learn more about abstracting symptoms, signs, and abnormal findings. Sherry Whittle, CPC, is a fictitious coder who guides you through this case.

Date: 6/1/yy Location: Branton Family Practice
Provider: Kristen Conover, MD
Patient: Chad Wang Gender: M Age: 6
Chief Complaint: nausea, vomiting, and diarrhea
Assessment: gastroenteritis
Plan: bed rest and plenty of fluids

Follow along as Sherry Whittle, CPC, reviews the medical record and abstracts the diagnosis. Check off each step after you complete it.

▶ Sherry begins by referring to Key Criteria for Abstracting Symptoms, Signs, Abnormal Findings, and Confirmed Conditions (Table 6-3).

❑ *What symptoms does the patient report?* nausea, vomiting, and diarrhea

❑ *What signs does the physician document?* None

❑ *What abnormal laboratory findings are reviewed?* None

❑ *What confirmed diagnoses are documented?* gastroenteritis

❑ *What diagnoses are identified as uncertain with words such as possible, probable, rule out, suspected?* None

❑ *Which symptoms, signs, and abnormal findings are integral to the condition?* All

❑ *Which symptoms, signs, and abnormal findings are related but not integral to the condition?* None

❑ *Which symptoms, signs, and abnormal findings are unrelated to the condition?* None

▶ Because the symptoms of nausea, vomiting, and diarrhea are all integral to gastroenteritis, Sherry does not abstract these items to code.

❑ The only diagnosis code to be assigned is gastroenteritis. (You will learn how to do this when you study the digestive system.)

CODING PRACTICE

Exercise 6.2 Abstracting Symptoms and Signs

Instructions: Read the mini-medical-record of each patient's encounter and answer the abstracting questions. Write the answer on the line provided. Do not assign any codes.

---

1. OFFICE Gender: M Age: 61

Reason for encounter: review result of liver function study

Assessment: abnormal liver function test

(continued)

---

1. (continued)

Plan: biopsy

a. Does the physician state a confirmed diagnosis?

_____

b. Is this a sign, a symptom, an abnormal clinical finding, or an abnormal laboratory test?

_____

c. What Main Term will you look up in the Index?

_____

2. INPATIENT HOSPITAL   Gender: M   **Age:** 74

Reason for admission: irregular heartbeat, chest pain, and lightheadedness

Assessment: atrial fibrillation

Plan: cardiologist evaluation

Tip: Do not code symptoms that are integral to a confirmed condition.

a. What symptoms and signs are mentioned?

_____

b. Does the physician state a confirmed diagnosis?

_____

c. Are all of the symptoms and signs integral to the diagnosis? _____

d. Which symptoms and signs should be coded?

_____

e. What condition will you code? _____

_____

---

3. INPATIENT HOSPITAL   Gender: F   **Age:** 16

Reason for admission: repeated seizures

Assessment: seizures of unknown cause

Plan: continued follow-up with neurologist, medication

a. Does the physician state a confirmed diagnosis?

_____

b. What symptom should be coded? _____

_____

c. What is the Main Term? _____

_____

---

4. OFFICE   Gender: F   **Age:** 45

Chief complaint: polydipsia, polyuria, and difficulty sleeping, most recent blood test showed hyperglycemia

Assessment: type 2 diabetes, possible sleep apnea

Plan: evaluate for sleep apnea

a. What symptoms and signs are mentioned?

_____

b. Does the physician state a confirmed diagnosis? _____ What is it? _____

c. Does the physician state an uncertain diagnosis? _____ What is it? _____

(*continued*)

---

4. (continued)

d. Should you code an uncertain diagnosis for an outpatient encounter? _____ What should you code instead? _____

e. Which symptoms and signs are integral to the confirmed diagnosis? _____

f. Which symptoms and signs relate to the unconfirmed diagnosis? _____

g. What two conditions/symptoms will you code?

_____

---

5. OFFICE   Gender: M   **Age:** 29

Chief complaint: extreme nervousness and irritability

Assessment: R/O hyperthyroidism

Plan: thyroid workup

a. What symptoms and signs are mentioned?

_____

b. What does R/O (rule out) mean? _____

_____

c. Does the physician state a confirmed diagnosis?

_____

d. Does the physician state an uncertain diagnosis? _____ What is it? _____

e. What two conditions/symptoms will you code?

_____

---

6. INPATIENT HOSPITAL   Gender: M   **Age:** 52

Reason for admission: abdominal pain

Discharge diagnosis: epigastric pain due to acute pancreatitis or cholangitis (*inflammation of the common bile duct*)

Plan: pain medication, antibiotics as precaution, further imaging

Tip: This is a hospital discharge, so inpatient OGCR apply.

a. What symptoms and signs are mentioned? _____

_____

b. Does the physician state a confirmed diagnosis?

_____

c. What alternative or comparative diagnoses does the physician document? _____

ASSIGNING CODES FOR SYMPTOMS AND SIGNS

The most challenging aspect of coding for symptoms, signs, and abnormal findings is distinguishing integral, related, and unrelated symptoms and distinguishing confirmed and uncertain diagnoses. After this is accomplished, assigning codes is relatively straightforward. The Main Term for many symptoms and signs codes is the name of the symptom or sign. Combination codes also exist for definitive diagnoses and certain related symptoms. Coding for abnormal test results can be more challenging and is discussed later in this section.

Codes for Symptoms and Signs

Main Term entries for most symptoms and signs in the Index often are the name of the symptom or sign, such as pain, fever, vomiting, or weakness. Review the subterms carefully for anatomic sites or other descriptions of the condition. If none of the specific subterms apply, use the default code immediately following the Main Term.

Refer to the Main Term **Fever** in the ICD-10-CM Index (■ FIGURE 6-1). The default code is **R50.9**. More than 200 subterms describe specific types or causes of fever. When a subterm applies, verify and assign the code listed with the subterm. When no subterm applies, verify and assign the default code.

Combination Codes

Do use combination codes when available. ICD-10-CM contains combination codes that identify both the definitive diagnosis and certain related symptoms. When using this kind of combination code, do not assign an additional code for the related symptom. For example:

- The physician documents Type 2 diabetes with gastroparesis. ICD-10-CM provides an entry in the Index for **Diabetes, with gastroparesis E11.43**. Use the combination code and do not assign a separate code for gastroparesis.

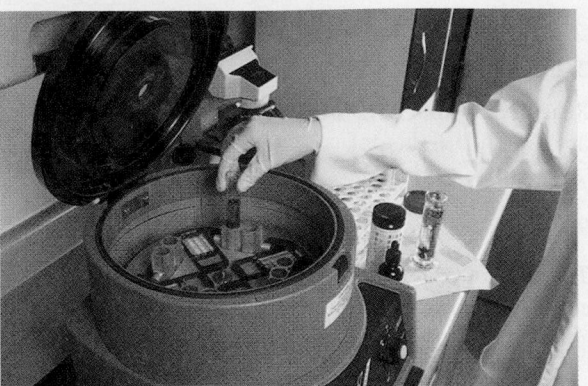

Figure 6-2 ■ Laboratory Technician Performing a Urinalysis Test. *Source: Michal Heron/Pearson Education/PH College.*

Codes for Abnormal Findings

Physicians may receive test results from the laboratory that are abnormal, but they are still unable to establish a firm diagnosis. In this situation, coders assign codes for the abnormal test result (■ FIGURE 6-2). To locate the Main Term for abnormal clinical and laboratory findings, identify the word in the diagnostic statement that describes how the result *differs* from normal. Refer to ■ TABLE 6-6 for commonly used Main Terms and examples of subterm entries. Also be alert for instructional notes and cross-references in the Index that may lead to alternative entries.

Guided Example of Assigning Symptoms and Signs Codes

Refer to the following example to learn how to assign codes for symptoms. This case is similar to the earlier example of Chad Wang, who was seen for nausea, vomiting, and diarrhea and was diagnosed with gastroenteritis. However, notice how this example should be coded differently based on the wording of the Assessment.

Date: 6/1/yy   Location: Branton Family Practice

Provider: Kristen Conover, MD

Patient: Charlene Winger   Gender: F   Age: 15

Chief Complaint: nausea, vomiting, and diarrhea

Assessment: suspected gastroenteritis

Plan: stool culture, bed rest, and plenty of fluids

Follow along as Sherry Whittle, CPC, assigns codes for nausea, vomiting, and diarrhea. Check off each step as you complete it.

▶ First, Sherry abstracts the case.

  ❑ She reads the presenting symptoms nausea, vomiting, and diarrhea.

Fever (inanition) (of unknown origin) (persistent) (with chills) (with rigor) **R50.9**
  abortus A23.1
  Aden (dengue) A90
  African tick-borne A68.1
  American
      mountain (tick) A93.2
      spotted A77.0
  aphthous B08.8
  arbovirus, arboviral A94

Figure 6-1 ■ Example of Index Entry for a Sign (Fever) with Subterms

Table 6-6 ■ **COMMONLY USED MAIN TERMS FOR ABNORMAL FINDINGS**

Main Term	Diagnostic Statement Examples	Index Entry Examples
Abnormal	Abnormal liver function test	Abnormal, function studies, liver
	Abnormal hemoglobin in urine	Abnormal, urine, hemoglobin
Anomaly	Heart auricle anomaly	Anomaly, heart, auricle
	Hip anomaly	Anomaly, hip, NEC
Deficiency	Low growth hormone	Deficiency, hormone, growth
	Vitamin D deficiency	Deficiency, vitamin D
Elevated	High fasting glucose	Elevated, fasting glucose
	Elevated blood pressure	Elevated, blood pressure
Findings, abnormal, inconclusive, without diagnosis	Lead in blood	Findings, in blood, lead
	Abnormal urine glucose	Findings, urine, glucose
Loss	Transient loss of consciousness	Loss, consciousness, transient

❏ She reads the Assessment *suspected gastroenteritis*.

❏ She notes that "suspected" makes gastroenteritis an uncertain diagnosis.

❏ As a result, she identifies the three symptoms—nausea, vomiting, and diarrhea—to code and does not code gastroenteritis.

▶ Sherry searches the Index for the Main Term **Nausea** (■ FIGURE 6-3).

❏ She reads the nonessential modifier **(without vomiting)** which is the default for code R11.0.

❏ She locates the subterm **with vomiting, R11.2**, which provides a combination code for two of the symptoms of this patient.

▶ Sherry verifies code **R11.2** in the Tabular List.

❏ She reads the code title for **R11.2, Nausea with vomiting, unspecified** and confirms that this accurately describes the symptoms.

▶ Sherry checks for instructional notes in the Tabular List.

❏ She cross-references the beginning of category **R11** and reads the **Excludes1** instructional note. None of the conditions listed describe the patient, so she may proceed.

❏ She cross-references the beginning of the block **R10-R19** and reads the **Excludes1** instructional note.

None of the conditions listed describe the patient, so she may proceed.

❏ She cross-references the beginning of **Chapter 18 (R00-R99)** and reads the detailed instructional notes. She determines that note **(e) cases in which a more precise diagnosis was not available** describes this case and that she is coding correctly.

▶ Next, Sherry searches the Index for the Main Term **Diarrhea**.

❏ She reads through all of the available subterms but finds none that apply. She checks the documentation to confirm that the diarrhea is not stated as either viral or bacterial. It is not and that is likely the reason a stool culture was obtained.

❏ She selects the default entry **Diarrhea, diarrheal (disease) (infantile) (inflammatory) R19.7**.

▶ Sherry verifies code **R19.7** in the Tabular List.

❏ She reads the code title for **R19.7, Diarrhea, unspecified** and confirms that this accurately describes the symptom because more detailed information is not provided in the medical record.

▶ Sherry checks for instructional notes in the Tabular List.

❏ She cross-references the beginning of category **R19** and identifies the instructional note **Excludes1: acute abdomen (R10.0)**. This does not describe the patient's symptoms so she knows she can proceed.

❏ She cross-references the beginning of the block **R10-R19** and chapter in the previous step and recalls that there are no notes that would change the code she selected.

▶ Sherry reviews the codes she has assigned for this case.

❏ **R11.2 Nausea with vomiting, unspecified**

❏ **R19.7 Diarrhea, unspecified**

Nausea (without vomiting) R11.0
   with vomiting R11.2
     gravidarum — *see* Hyperemesis, gravidarum
     marina T75.3
     navalis T75.3

Figure 6-3 ■ Index Entry for Nausea, with Vomiting

▶ Next, Sherry must determine how to sequence the codes.

CODING PRACTICE

Exercise 6.3 Assigning Codes for Symptoms and Signs

Instructions: Read the mini-medical-record of each patient's encounter, review the information abstracted in Exercise 6.2, and assign ICD-10-CM diagnosis codes using the Index and Tabular List. Write the code(s) on the line provided.

1. OFFICE   Gender: M   Age: 61

Reason for encounter: *review result of liver function study*

Assessment: *abnormal liver function test*

Plan: *biopsy*

1 ICD-10-CM Code _____

2. INPATIENT HOSPITAL   Gender: M   Age: 74

Reason for admission: *irregular heartbeat, chest pain, and lightheadedness*

Assessment: *atrial fibrillation*

Plan: *cardiologist evaluation*

Tip: Do not code symptoms that are integral to a confirmed condition.

1 ICD-10-CM Code _____

3. INPATIENT HOSPITAL   Gender: F   Age: 16

Reason for admission: *repeated seizures*

Assessment: *seizures of unknown cause*

Plan: *continued follow-up with neurologist, medication*

1 ICD-10-CM Code _____

ARRANGING CODES FOR SYMPTOMS AND SIGNS

In general, multiple codes for symptoms, signs, and abnormal findings are sequenced using the same guidelines as any other codes. Special situations include coding for a confirmed diagnosis and related symptoms, coding a confirmed diagnosis and unrelated symptoms, coding symptoms followed by a diagnosis, and coding symptoms with no confirmed diagnosis. These are discussed next.

Confirmed Diagnosis and Related Symptoms

The physician may document a confirmed diagnosis and a symptom, sign, or abnormal finding that is related but not integral. Sequence the confirmed diagnosis first, followed by the related symptom (■ FIGURE 6-4).

Confirmed Diagnosis and Unrelated Symptoms

The physician may document a confirmed diagnosis and an unrelated symptom, sign, or abnormal finding. Sequence the code chiefly responsible for the services provided first. When both the confirmed diagnosis and the unrelated symptom are equally responsible, sequence either code first (■ FIGURE 6-5).

Symptom Followed by Diagnoses

Occasionally, the physician may document a symptom, sign, or abnormal finding followed by two contrasting or comparative diagnoses. Sequence the symptom code first. Code all the contrasting or comparative diagnoses as additional diagnoses (OGCR II.E) (■ FIGURE 6-6).

Patient seen for RLQ pain, fever, vomiting, dehydration due to acute ruptured appendicitis. Administered IV fluids.

(1) **K35.2 Acute ruptured appendicitis with generalized peritonitis**
(2) **E86.0 Dehydration**

Figure 6-4 ■ Example of Sequencing for Confirmed Diagnosis and Related Symptom

---

Patient c/o of fever, difficulty breathing, hemoptysis. X-ray is positive for pneumonia. Sputum culture is ordered for hemoptysis.

(1) **J18.9 Pneumonia**
(2) **R04.2 Hemoptysis**

Figure 6-5 ■ Example of Sequencing for a Confirmed Diagnosis and Unrelated Symptom

> Patient is seen for right shoulder pain due to rotator cuff syndrome or loose body in shoulder joint.
>
> (1) **M25.511 Pain in right shoulder**
> (2) **M75.111 Incomplete rotator cuff tear or rupture of right shoulder, not specified as traumatic**
> (3) **M24.011 Loose body in right shoulder**

Figure 6-6 ■ Example of Sequencing for Symptom Followed by Contrasting or Comparative Diagnoses

Symptoms with No Confirmed Diagnosis

The physician may document only symptoms, signs, and abnormal findings and no confirmed diagnosis. Assign the main reason for the encounter as the principal or first-listed diagnosis. When more than one symptom is equally responsible for the encounter, sequence either code first.

Guided Example of Arranging Symptoms and Signs Codes

To practice skills for sequencing codes for symptoms and signs, continue with the example from earlier in the chapter about patient Charlene Winger, who was seen for symptoms of nausea, vomiting, and diarrhea, with no confirmed diagnosis.

Follow along in your ICD-10-CM manual as Sherry Whittle, CPC, sequences the codes. Check off each step after you complete it.

▶ First, Sherry confirms the diagnosis codes she assigned.

❑ **R11.2 Nausea with vomiting, unspecified**

❑ **R19.7 Diarrhea, unspecified**

▶ Sherry determines that the physician documented only symptoms but no confirmed diagnosis.

❑ The documentation does not state that one symptom was chiefly responsible for the encounter.

❑ Therefore, either diagnosis may be sequenced first.

▶ Sherry finalizes the codes and sequencing for this case:

❑ **R11.2 Nausea with vomiting, unspecified**

❑ **R19.7 Diarrhea, unspecified**

CODING PRACTICE

Exercise 6.4   Arranging Codes for Symptoms and Signs

Instructions: Read the mini-medical-record of each patient's encounter, review the information abstracted in Exercise 6.2, assign ICD-10-CM diagnosis codes using the Index and Tabular List, and arrange the codes in proper sequence. Write the code(s) on the line provided.

1. OFFICE   Gender: F   Age: 45

Chief complaint: polydipsia, polyuria, and difficulty sleeping, most recent blood test showed hyperglycemia

Assessment: type 2 diabetes, possible sleep apnea

Plan: evaluate for sleep apnea

Tip: Determine which symptoms are integral to diabetes and which one is unrelated.

2 ICD-10-CM Codes _____

2. OFFICE   Gender: M   Age: 29

Chief complaint: extreme nervousness and irritability

Assessment: R/O hyperthyroidism

Plan: thyroid workup

Tip: A condition described as "rule out" means it is uncertain.

2 ICD-10-CM Codes _____

3. INPATIENT HOSPITAL   Gender: M   Age: 52

Reason for admission: abdominal pain

Discharge diagnosis: epigastric pain due to acute pancreatitis or cholangitis (*inflammation or infection of the common bile duct*)

Plan: pain medication, antibiotics as precaution, further imaging

Tip: Because this is a hospital discharge, follow inpatient OCGR.

3 ICD-10-CM Codes _____

_____

CHAPTER SUMMARY

In this chapter you learned that:

- Sometimes a confirmed diagnosis is not possible because the physician needs multiple encounters, extended testing, evaluation by specialists, surgery, or other procedures to arrive at a diagnosis.

- ICD-10-CM Chapter 18, Symptoms, Signs, and Abnormal Clinical and Laboratory Findings, Not Elsewhere Classified (R00-R99), contains 14 blocks or subchapters that are divided by anatomical site.

- Abstracting requires coders to be knowledgeable of disease processes and the related symptoms, signs, abnormal clinical

findings, and abnormal laboratory test results so they can distinguish which elements should be coded and which should not.

- The Main Term for many symptoms and signs codes is the name of the symptom or sign. Coding for abnormal test results can be more challenging.

- In general, multiple codes for symptoms, signs, and abnormal findings are sequenced using the same guidelines as any other codes, but a few special situations exist.

- ICD-10-CM provides Official Guidelines for Coding and Reporting (OGCR) for symptoms, signs, and abnormal clinical and laboratory findings in OGCR section I.C.18.

CONCEPT QUIZ

Take a moment to look back at symptoms, signs, and abnormal findings and solidify your skills. This is your opportunity to pull together everything you have learned.

Completion

Instructions: Write the term that answers each question based on the information you learned in this chapter. Choose from the following list. Some choices may be used more than once and some choices may not be used at all.

abnormal	outpatient
clinical	related
confirmed	sign
finding	symptom
inpatient	uncertain
integral	unrelated
laboratory	

1. A (an) _____ is the subjective evidence of a disease or condition, usually reported by the patient.

2. A symptom that is _____ is a routine part of the disease process.

3. A qualified diagnosis is _____.

4. An abnormal _____ finding is evidence of a disease or condition discovered through physical examination.

5. A (an) _____ is objective evidence of a disease or condition that can be observed by the physician.

6. _____ symptoms are those that patients occasionally experience with the confirmed diagnosis but are not common or routine.

7. *Rule out, suspected,* and *likely* are words physicians use to describe a (an) _____ diagnosis.

8. _____ symptoms are those that are not caused by the confirmed diagnosis and may indicate an additional problem or condition.

9. A laboratory test result that is outside of the normal numerical range is _____.

10. In the _____ setting, if the diagnosis documented at the time of discharge is uncertain, code the condition as if it existed.

Multiple Choice

Instructions: Circle the letter of the best answer to each question based on the information you learned in this chapter.

1. Which of the following is an example of a symptom?
   A. Nausea
   B. Vomiting
   C. Bleeding
   D. Fever

2. Which of the following is an example of an abnormal clinical finding?
   A. Elevated glucose
   B. Bleeding
   C. Irregular EKG
   D. Microscopic dysplasia

3. All of the following are integral to a CVA EXCEPT
   A. headache.
   B. muscular weakness.
   C. speech disturbance.
   D. dysuria.

4. Which of the following conditions are asymptomatic?
   A. Osteoarthritis
   B. Hypertension
   C. Gastroenteritis
   D. Anemia

5. _____ symptoms should NOT be coded when the physician provides a confirmed diagnosis.
   A. Integral
   B. Related
   C. Unrelated
   D. All

6. When should an uncertain diagnosis be coded as though it existed?
   A. Inpatient setting
   B. Outpatient setting
   C. Emergency department
   D. Never

7. All of the following Main Terms can be used to locate abnormal findings in the Index EXCEPT
   A. Abnormal.
   B. Deficiency.
   C. Findings.
   D. Uncertain.

8. Physicians may use all of the following terms EXCEPT
   _____ to indicate an uncertain diagnosis.
   A. possible
   B. integral
   C. suspected
   D. rule out

9. A physician may not be able to document a confirmed diagnosis because
   A. additional testing is necessary.
   B. the code is difficult to locate.
   C. the patient has multiple symptoms.
   D. the OGCR is unclear.

10. Which of the following statements is TRUE?
    A. Coders should assign codes for all symptoms and all conditions documented.
    B. Coders should assign codes for symptoms that are related but not integral to the diagnosis.
    C. Coders should never assign codes for uncertain diagnoses.
    D. Coders should assign a rule out code when coding for uncertain diagnoses.

CODING CHALLENGE

Instructions: Read the mini-medical-record of each patient's encounter, then abstract, assign, and sequence ICD-10-CM diagnosis codes using the Index and Tabular List. Write the code(s) on the line provided.

1. OFFICE   Gender: F   Age: 41

Reason for visit: review abnormal mammogram results

Assessment: microcalcifications in right breast

Plan: mammogram with magnification to r/o ca

1 ICD-10-CM Code _____

2. OFFICE   Gender: F   Age: 31

Reason for encounter: review lung X-ray

Assessment: abnormal shadow, right lung, inferior lobe

Plan: refer to pulmonologist

Tip: An X-ray is classified as diagnostic imaging.

1 ICD-10-CM Code _____

3. OFFICE   Gender: F   Age: 23

Chief complaint: review results of blood test performed last week because patient was concerned she had been exposed to HIV

Assessment: Nonconclusive HIV test

Plan: further testing needed

Tip: Search for the Main Term **HIV** or **Test**.

1 ICD-10-CM Code _____

4. OFFICE   Gender: M   Age: 24

Chief complaint: sneezing, scratchy throat, postnasal drip

Assessment: suspected seasonal allergies

Plan: OTC antihistamine

3 ICD-10-CM Codes _____
_____

5. INPATIENT HOSPITAL   Gender: M   Age: 27

Reason for admission: lumbar pain, weakness in left leg

Discharge diagnosis: probable herniated intervertebral lumbar disc, sciatica

Plan: refer to physical therapy

Tip: The description of the admission and discharge indicates that this was an inpatient stay so follow the OCGR for inpatient settings.

1 ICD-10-CM Code _____

6. OFFICE   Gender: F   Age: 24

Reason for encounter: repeat PAP test

Assessment: abnormal cervical PAP test result, cytologic (*cellular*) evidence of malignancy

Plan: possible colposcopy based on repeat test results

1 ICD-10-CM Code _____

(*continued*)

(continued from page 91)

7. OFFICE   Gender: M   Age: 56

Chief complaint: review blood work results

Assessment: glucose reading of 107, insulin resistant

Plan: HbA1c in 3 months to check long-term glucose levels

1 ICD-10-CM Code _____

8. OFFICE   Gender: F   Age: 36

Chief complaint: daily headaches

Assessment: likely migraines

Plan: refer to neurologist for further testing and evaluation

1 ICD-10-CM Code _____

9. INPATIENT HOSPITAL   Gender: F   Age: 62

Reason for admission: shortness of breath

Assessment: increased edema, congestive heart failure

Discharge instructions: begin new diuretic, follow up with cardiologist

1 ICD-10-CM Code _____

10. OFFICE   Gender: F   Age: 50

Chief complaint: review recent lab work

Assessment: Everything was normal except for low Vitamin D.

Plan: Rx 50,000 IU of Vitamin D once a week for 8 weeks; recheck in 8 weeks

Tip: A "low" test result is indexed as a deficiency.

1 ICD-10-CM Code _____

KEEP ON CODING

Instructions: Read the diagnostic statement, then use the Index and Tabular List to assign and sequence ICD-10-CM diagnosis codes. Write the code(s) on the line provided.

1. Right lower quadrant rebound abdominal tenderness: ICD-10-CM Code(s) _____

2. Nonvisualization of gallbladder: ICD-10-CM Code(s) _____

3. Heartburn: ICD-10-CM Code(s) _____

4. Absent bowel sounds: ICD-10-CM Code(s) _____

5. Slow heart beat: ICD-10-CM Code(s) _____

6. Overactivity: ICD-10-CM Code(s) _____

7. Auditory hallucinations: ICD-10-CM Code(s) _____

8. Nosebleed: ICD-10-CM Code(s) _____

9. Shortness of breath: ICD-10-CM Code(s) _____

10. Severe sepsis with septic shock: ICD-10-CM Code(s) _____

11. Excessive sweating: ICD-10-CM Code(s) _____

12. Late walker: ICD-10-CM Code(s) _____

13. Change in bowel habits: ICD-10-CM Code(s) _____

14. Heart murmur: ICD-10-CM Code(s) _____

15. Hiccough: ICD-10-CM Code(s) _____

16. Finding of cocaine in blood: ICD-10-CM Code(s) _____

17. Age-related cognitive decline: ICD-10-CM Code(s) _____

18. Intermittent urinary stream: ICD-10-CM Code(s) _____

19. Hoarseness: ICD-10-CM Code(s) _____

20. Abnormal blood-gas level: ICD-10-CM Code(s) _____

21. Respiratory arrest: ICD-10-CM Code(s) _____

22. Unsteadiness on feet: ICD-10-CM Code(s) _____

23. Abnormal liver scan: ICD-10-CM Code(s) _____

24. Failure to gain weight: ICD-10-CM Code(s) _____

25. Febrile seizures, simple: ICD-10-CM Code(s) _____

Chapter 7

Factors Influencing Health Status and Contact with Health Services (Z00-Z99)

Chapter Outline

- **Introduction to Z Codes**
- **Coding Overview of Z Codes**
- **Abstracting Z Codes**
- **Assigning Z Codes**
- **Arranging Z Codes**

Learning Objectives

After completing this chapter, you should have the skills to:

7.1 Spell and define the key words, medical terms, and abbreviations related to factors influencing health status and contact with health services.

7.2 Describe when to report codes for factors influencing health status and contact with health services.

7.3 Discuss the main characteristics of coding for factors influencing health status and contact with health services.

7.4 Abstract information required for coding factors influencing health status and contact with health services from the medical record.

7.5 Assign codes for factors influencing health status and contact with health services.

7.6 Sequence codes for factors influencing health status and contact with health services and related conditions.

7.7 Discuss the Official Guidelines for Coding and Reporting related to factors influencing health status and contact with health services.

Key Terms and Abbreviations

ostomy
Z codes

In addition to the key terms listed here, students should know the terms defined within tables in this chapter.

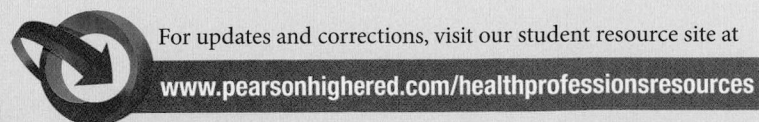
For updates and corrections, visit our student resource site at

www.pearsonhighered.com/healthprofessionsresources

INTRODUCTION

Car owners sometimes visit or call the mechanic although they have not experienced a breakdown. They may seek an oil change, periodic preventive maintenance, winterization, tightening of some loose screws, tire rotation, or a variety of other types of information. Mechanics may apply a windshield sticker or send a postcard to remind owners of the next scheduled maintenance, important tips, or other information they need to know about the car.

In healthcare, patients receive services even though they are not ill or injured. They may seek annual physical examinations, vaccinations, screening examinations, follow-up care, or maternity care. Physicians need to track information about patients' health status, health history, and health risks that do not present current problems but could in the future. In this chapter you will learn how to use ICD-10-CM for patient encounters when patients receive healthcare services even though they are not ill or injured.

INTRODUCTION TO Z CODES

ICD-10-CM Chapter 21 classifies factors influencing health status and contact with health services. For the sake of brevity, this text refers to these codes as **Z codes**. Z codes represent reasons for encounters and may be used in any healthcare setting when the reason for the encounter is not a disease, injury, or external cause that is classified in the preceding ICD-10-CM chapters for body systems (A00 to Y99). Z codes are used in two general types of circumstances:

- A person encounters the health services for some specific purpose that, in itself, is not a disease or injury. Examples are receiving limited care or service for a current condition, donating an organ or tissue, receiving **prophylactic** vaccination, or discussing a problem.

- A circumstance or problem exists that influences the person's health status, but is not, in itself, a current illness or injury. Examples are being a carrier of a communicable disease, having a family history of certain conditions, and wearing a prosthetic device such as a pacemaker or an artificial limb.

Z codes are classified into 15 categories, which are defined in ■ TABLE 7-1. Acquaint yourself with these definitions and examples, as they are the foundation for learning to abstract, assign, and sequence Z codes. Refer to the specific Official Guidelines for Coding and Reporting (OGCR) listed for a full discussion of how to use each category.

> ### SUCCESS STEP
>
> Although you do not need to memorize specific codes, it is helpful to memorize the Z code categories and definitions. By knowing the circumstances in which Z codes are required, you will become more accurate when abstracting.

Table 7-1   ■   DEFINITIONS AND EXAMPLES OF Z CODE CATEGORIES

Z Code Category/OGCR	Definition	Example Codes
Contact/Exposure (OGCR I.C.21.c.1))	Patient does not show any sign or symptom of a disease but is suspected to have been exposed to it by close personal contact with an infected individual or is in an area where a disease is epidemic.	Z20.5 Contact with and (suspected) exposure to viral hepatitis Z20.820 Contact with and (suspected) exposure to varicella
Inoculations and vaccinations (OGCR I.C.21.c.2))	Reported for encounters for prophylactic inoculations and vaccinations against a disease.	Z23 Encounter for immunization
Status (OGCR I.C.21.c.3))	A patient is either a carrier of a disease or has the sequela or residual of a past disease or condition.	Z21 Asymptomatic HIV infection status Z67.10 Type A blood, Rh positive Z68.23 Body mass index (BMI) 23.0-23.9, adult Z94.1 Heart transplant status
History (of) (OGCR I.C.21.c.4))	Personal history codes explain a patient's past medical condition that no longer exists and is not receiving any treatment, but that has the potential for recurrence, and therefore may require continued monitoring. Family history codes are for a patient who has a family member(s) who has had a particular disease, which causes the patient to be at higher risk of also contracting the disease.	Z86.11 Personal history of tuberculosis Z80.3 Family history of malignant neoplasm of breast
Screening (OGCR I.C.21.c.5))	Seemingly well individuals receive testing for disease or disease precursors so that early detection and treatment can be provided for those who test positive for the disease.	Z12.31 Encounter for screening mammogram for malignant neoplasm of breast Z13.1 Encounter for screening for diabetes mellitus
Observation (OGCR I.C.21.c.6))	A person is being observed for a suspected condition that is ruled out. This category is rarely used.	Z03.73 Encounter for suspected fetal anomaly ruled out
Aftercare (OGCR I.C.21.c.7))	The initial treatment of a disease has been performed and the patient requires continued care during the healing or recovery phase or for the long-term consequences of the disease.	Z44.002 Encounter for fitting and adjustment of unspecified left artificial arm Z51.11 Encounter for antineoplastic chemotherapy

(*continued*)

Table 7-1 ■ (*continued*)

Z Code Category/OGCR	Definition	Example Codes
Follow-up (OGCR I.C.21.c.8))	Continuing surveillance following completed treatment of a disease, condition, or injury when the condition has been fully treated and no longer exists.	Z08 Encounter for follow-up examination after completed treatment for malignant neoplasm Z39.2 Encounter for routine postpartum follow-up
Donor (OGCR I.C.21.c.9))	Living individuals are donating blood or other body tissue.	Z52.4 Kidney donor
Counseling (OGCR I.C.21.c.10))	A patient or family member receives assistance in the aftermath of an illness or injury, or when support is required in coping with family or social problems.	Z31.5 Encounter for genetic counseling Z69.010 Encounter for mental health services for victim of parental child abuse
Encounters for Obstetrical and Reproductive Services (OGCR I.C.21.c.11))	A patient receives obstetric or reproductive encounters when none of the problems or complications included in the codes from the obstetrics chapter (ICD-10-CM Chapter 15 (**O00-O9A**)) exist.	Z34.01 Encounter for supervision of normal first pregnancy, first trimester Z37.0 Single live birth Z3A.17 (Pregnancy, weeks of gestation, 17 weeks)
Newborns and Infants (OGCR I.C.21.c.12))	Reports the health supervision and care of foundling, routine child health examination, and classification of birth status of liveborn infants.	Z00.110 Health examination for newborn under 8 days old
Routine and Administrative Examinations (OGCR I.C.21.c.13))	Used for encounters for routine examinations or administrative purposes.	Z00.00 Encounter for general adult medical examination without abnormal findings Z02.1 Encounter for pre-employment examination Z32.01 Encounter for pregnancy test, result positive
Miscellaneous (OGCR I.C.21.c.14))	Additional codes provide useful information on circumstances that may affect a patient's care and treatment.	Z28.01 Immunization not carried out because of acute illness of patient Z53.09 Procedure and treatment not carried out because of other contraindication Z76.0 Encounter for issue of repeat prescription
Nonspecific (OGCR I.C.21.c.15))	Used primarily in inpatient settings when there is no further documentation to permit more precise coding.	Z86.59 Personal history of other mental and behavioral disorders Z92.23 Personal history of estrogen therapy

CODING PRACTICE

Exercise 7.1   **Introduction to Z Codes**

Instructions: Write your answer to each question in the space provided.

1. Give three examples of Z codes that describe the main reason for the encounter. _____

   _____

2. What is the OGCR location of guidelines for each of the following Z code categories?

   Example: History *OGCR I.C.21.c.4)*

   a. Contact/Exposure _____

   b. Status _____

   c. Aftercare _____

   d. Routine and Administrative Examinations

   _____

3. Identify the Z code category for each of the following codes:

   Example: Z67.10 Type A blood, Rh positive *Status*

   a. Z12.31 Encounter for screening mammogram for malignant neoplasm of breast _____

   b. Z52.4 Kidney donor _____

   c. Z86.59 Personal history of other mental and behavioral disorders _____

   d. Z86.11 Personal history of tuberculosis

   _____

Tip: Refer to Table 7-1.

Tip: Refer to Table 7-1.

CODING OVERVIEW OF Z CODES

ICD-10-CM Chapter 21, Factors Influencing Health Status and Contact with Health Services (Z00-Z99), contains 14 blocks or subchapters. Review the block names and code ranges listed at the beginning of Chapter 21 in the ICD-10-CM manual to become familiar with the content and organization. This chapter is used to report reasons for encounters that are not due to a current illness or injury or to report health status or risk factors documented as significant by the physician.

ICD-10-CM Z codes are comparable to the ICD-9-CM Supplementary Classification of Factors influencing Health Status and Contact with Health Services (V01-V91). In ICD-10-CM, the codes are part of the regular classification rather than being a supplementary classification.

Some ICD-10-CM Z codes are directly comparable to ICD-9-CM V codes, such as those in the category **Outcome of delivery (Z37)**.

Some ICD-9-CM categories were significantly expanded in ICD-10-CM, including those for examinations (**Z02**), encounters for other specific health care (**Z40-Z53**), health hazards related to socioeconomic and psychosocial circumstances (**Z55 to Z65**), and counseling (**Z70**). For example, ICD-9-CM **V70.3 Other medical examination for administrative purposes**, a single code, is replaced with ICD-10-CM category **Z02 Encounter for administrative examination**, which contains more than 10 codes.

Some ICD-9-CM V codes were reduced in specificity or eliminated. For example, ICD-9-CM subcategory **V64.4x Closed procedures converted to open procedures** does not have a corresponding category in ICD-10-CM. ICD-9-CM categories V03-V06 for immunizations were reduced to a single ICD-10-CM code, **Z23**.

ICD-10-CM provides OGCR Z codes in OGCR section I.C.21. OGCR contains a detailed discussion of the categories of Z codes, when to report them, and which codes may only be sequenced as the principal or first-listed diagnosis. Additional OGCR related to Z codes appear throughout the guidelines, particularly in OGCR I.B.3, I.C.1.a (HIV), I.C.2 (neoplasms), I.C.4 (endocrine), I.C.15 (obstetrics), I.C.19 (injuries), I.C.20 (external causes), and IV.B. In the Tabular List, instructional notes throughout all chapters alert coders to many circumstances that require Z codes.

ABSTRACTING FOR Z CODES

Because Z codes are applicable to a wide variety of situations, there is not one concise rule that guides coders when Z codes are needed. Refer to ■ TABLE 7-2 for guidance on how to abstract for the most commonly used Z codes. Locate the patient situation in the left column, then refer to the appropriate Main Term in the right column. Remember that the abstracting questions are a guide and that not every encounter requires a Z code. In addition, some situations not in this table also require Z codes, which are discussed later in this chapter.

In addition to using Z codes when they describe the reason for the encounter, coders receive direction to abstract for Z codes from two sources:

- Instructional notes in the Tabular List
- OGCR I.C.21

Reason for the Encounter

When a Z code(s) describes the main reason for the encounter, abstracting is fairly straightforward. Coders identify the main

Table 7-2   ■   **KEY CRITERIA FOR ABSTRACTING Z CODES**

Patient Situation	Main Term
❑ Is the reason for the encounter a routine examination?	Examination
❑ Is the reason for the encounter to receive an inoculation or vaccination against a disease?	Inoculation
❑ Does the physician document a past medical condition that no longer exists and is not receiving any treatment but has the potential for recurrence?	History, personal
❑ Does the physician document that the patient has a family member(s) who has had a particular disease, which causes the patient to be at higher risk of also contracting the disease?	History, family
❑ Is the reason for the encounter testing for disease or disease precursors in seemingly well individuals so that early detection and treatment can be provided?	Screening
❑ Does the physician document a lifestyle habit that poses a risk factor?	Use
❑ Is the reason for the encounter continued care during the healing or recovery phase after initial treatment has been completed?	Aftercare
❑ Is the reason for the encounter continuing surveillance following completed treatment of a disease, condition, or injury when the condition has been fully treated and no longer exists?	Follow-up
❑ Is the reason for the encounter to receive assistance in the aftermath of an illness or injury or for support in coping with family or social problems?	Counseling
❑ Did a woman give birth during the encounter?	Outcome of delivery
❑ Is the patient a newborn who was born during the current admission?	Newborn, born

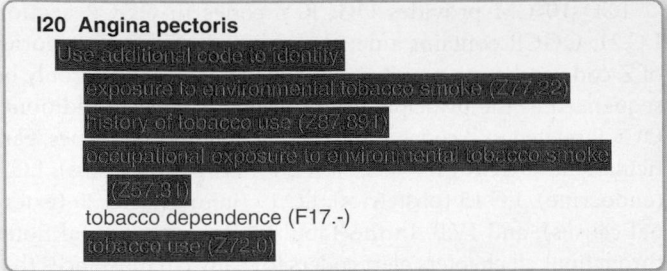

I20 Angina pectoris
   Use additional code to identify:
       exposure to environmental tobacco smoke (Z77.22)
       history of tobacco use (Z87.891)
       occupational exposure to environmental tobacco smoke
           (Z57.31)
       tobacco dependence (F17.-)
       tobacco use (Z72.0)

Figure 7-1 ■ Example of Instructional Notes in Tabular List Requiring Z Codes (Category I20)

reason for the encounter, then search for the Main Term in the Index to Diseases and Injuries (Index) to locate the Z code. Examples of Z codes describing the main reason for the encounter include the following:

- aftercare
- counseling
- follow-up
- immunizations
- observation
- routine pregnancy
- routine or administrative examinations (pre-employment, annual check-up)
- screening examinations (colonoscopy, mammogram)

Instructional Notes

In many circumstances, the Tabular List provides instructional notes directing the coder to assign certain types of Z codes (■ FIGURE 7-1). Examples of Z codes required by instructional notes include the following:

- birth status of newborn
- long-term use of medication
- occupational risk factors
- outcome of delivery (following pregnancy)
- tobacco, alcohol, drug use

Coders must distinguish between codes for history and current use. As shown in Figure 7-1, report **history of tobacco use (Z87.891)** when tobacco use occurred in the past, but the patient is not currently using tobacco. Report **tobacco use (Z72.0)** when the patient currently uses tobacco. Report **tobacco dependence (F17.-)** rather than **tobacco use (Z72.0)** when the medical record documents the dependence.

CODING CAUTION

Remember that codes in instructional notes should be reported only when they apply to the patient. For example, do not report **Z87.891 History of nicotine dependence** if the patient does not have a history of tobacco use or dependence.

Official Guidelines

The most challenging situation is when OGCR require Z codes to describe supplemental information related to the encounter but the Tabular List does not provide instructional notes. The Tabular List cannot anticipate every patient circumstance for every diagnosis in which a Z code is needed. This is when coders' knowledge of OGCR guides them to abstract the information. Examples of Z codes that may be required by the OGCR and rely on coders' knowledge include the following:

- acquired absence of organ or body part
- artificial opening status
- blood type
- BMI
- carrier
- do not resuscitate (DNR) status
- internal or external prosthetics, functional implements, or enabling devices
- personal or family history
- postprocedural states
- problems related to life circumstances such as education, literacy, employment, unemployment, housing, family situation
- transplant waiting list, recipient, or donor

Guided Example of Abstracting Z Codes

Refer to the following example here and throughout the chapter to learn more about using Z codes. Sherry Whittle, CPC, is a fictitious coder who guides you through coding this case.

Date: 7/1/yy   Location: Branton Medical Center Outpatient Procedure Clinic

Provider: Stanley Garrett, MD

Patient: Angela Holmes   Gender: F   Age: 50

Procedure: screening colonoscopy

Findings: none

Plan: next colonoscopy in 10 years

Follow along as Sherry abstracts the Z code. Check off each step as you complete it.

▶ Sherry refers to Key Criteria for Abstracting Z Codes (Table 7-2) and looks for questions that may apply to this patient.

❏ *Is the reason for the encounter a routine examination?* While this is a routine colonoscopy, a colonoscopy is not considered to be an examination.

❏ *Does the physician document a past medical condition that no longer exists and is not receiving any treatment but that has the potential for recurrence?* No. If the patient were receiving the colonoscopy because of previous colon cancer, then Sherry would answer "yes" and be directed to a different Z code category and a different Main Term.

❑ *Does the physician document that the patient has a family member(s) who has had a particular disease, which causes the patient to be at higher risk of also contracting the disease? No. If the colonoscopy were being done at a more-frequent-than-normal interval because of having family members with colon cancer, Sherry would answer "yes" and would assign a code for family history of colon cancer.*

❑ *Is the reason for the encounter testing for disease or disease precursors in seemingly well individuals so that early detection and treatment can be provided? Yes, this is the definition of a screening.*

▶ Next, Sherry will assign the code.

CODING PRACTICE

Exercise 7.2   Abstracting for Z Codes

Instructions: Read the mini-medical-record of each patient's encounter and answer the abstracting questions. Write the answer on the line provided. Do not assign any codes.

1. OFFICE   Gender: M   Age: 52

Reason for encounter: annual medical examination

Assessment: comprehensive metabolic panel test results are normal, no new problems

Plan: **RTO** 1 year

a. What is the reason for the encounter? _____

_____

b. Were there any abnormal findings? _____

   If yes, what are they? _____

_____

2. OFFICE   Gender: F   Age: 24

Reason for encounter: supervision of normal second pregnancy, third trimester, 34 weeks

Assessment: Estimated Date of Delivery (EDD) 8/3/yy

Plan: RTO 1 week

a. What is the reason for the encounter? _____

_____

b. Were there any abnormal findings? _____

   If yes, what are they? _____

_____

3. OFFICE   Gender: M   Age: 76

Reason for encounter: adjustment of cardiac pacemaker

Assessment: reprogrammed pacemaker, no problems

Plan: RTO 6 months

a. What is the reason for the encounter? _____

b. Were there any abnormal findings? _____

   If yes, what are they? _____

_____

4. OUTPATIENT HOSPITAL   Gender: F   Age: 47

Reason for encounter: screening mammogram

Assessment: normal mammogram, both breasts

Plan: repeat screening 6 months due to personal history of breast cancer

Tip: The National Cancer Institute recommends mammograms every one to two years for women over age 50.

a. What is the reason for the encounter? _____

_____

b. Were there any abnormal findings? _____

   If yes, what are they? _____

_____

c. Why is this patient receiving a mammogram more frequently than normal? _____

_____

5. OFFICE   Gender: M   Age: 61

Reason for encounter: 6-month follow-up after removal of prostate due to malignant neoplasm of prostate

Assessment: no new findings, no recurrence of disease, no current treatment

Plan: next FU 6 months

a. What is the reason for the encounter? _____

_____

b. Were there any abnormal findings? _____

   If yes, what are they? _____

c. What past condition is documented? _____

_____

d. A condition that no longer exists but presents potential for recurrence is classified as what? _____

_____

e. What gland was previously removed? _____

_____

(continued)

CODING PRACTICE *(continued)*

6. INPATIENT HOSPITAL   Gender: M   Age: 48

Reason for admission: *unresolved angina pectoris, current tobacco use*

Assessment: *EKG negative for AMI,* **ECC** *normal, angiogram normal*

Discharge Plan: *Rx nitroglycerin, follow up in office 1 week*

(continued)

6. (continued)

a. What is the reason for the encounter? _____

_____

b. Were there any abnormal findings? _____

   If yes, what are they? _____

   _____

c. What lifestyle habit is documented? _____

_____

ASSIGNING Z CODES

When assigning Z codes, coders need to know what Main Terms to search for in the Index, how to distinguish between diagnosis codes and procedure codes, and when to *not* use a Z code.

Locating Main Terms

Coders normally search for the name of a condition or disease in the Index in order to locate codes. Because Z codes are not conditions, new coders may be puzzled about what Main Term to search for. Remember to identify the noun that describes the reason or purpose of the encounter. Refer to ■ TABLE 7-3 for commonly used Main Terms.

Diagnosis vs. Procedure Codes

When the reason for the encounter is a screening examination or specific health service, the title of the Z code may *look like* a procedure code, but it is a diagnosis code—the reason for the encounter. Coders assign a Z code for the diagnosis and an ICD-10-PCS or CPT code for the procedure. (This chapter discusses only Z codes.) Examples when confusion may occur include the following:

- Persons encountering health services for examinations. For the diagnosis, assign a Z code (**Z00-Z13**) as the reason for the encounter, then assign a procedure code to identify the complexity of the examination.

- Persons encountering health services in circumstances related to reproduction. For the diagnosis, assign a Z code (**Z30-Z39**) to describe the reason for the encounter, then assign a procedure code to identify the service(s) provided.

- Encounters for other specific health procedures, such as fitting or adjustment of a prosthetic device, prophylactic or cosmetic surgery, or care of an **ostomy** (*artificial opening between a hollow organ and the skin*). For the diagnosis, assign a Z code (**Z40-Z53**) to describe the reason for the encounter, then assign a procedure code to identify the service(s) provided.

When Not to Use Z Codes

In some cases, diagnosis codes from body system chapters may include information that coders would otherwise report with a status Z code. When this is the case, do not assign a Z code that repeats the same information. In addition, do not assign aftercare codes when the patient has a current condition that is coded from a body system chapter. Aftercare codes are used only after the initial treatment of a disease has been performed and the patient requires continued care during healing or recovery. Refer to ■ FIGURE 7-2 to learn more about body system chapter codes that override the need for Z codes.

In the example in Figure 7-2, because the diagnosis code is specific to a colostomy, do not also assign **Z93.9 Colostomy status**. In addition, because the colostomy malfunction is a

Table 7-3   ■   COMMONLY USED MAIN TERMS FOR Z CODES

❑ Absence, acquired	❑ History, family
❑ Admission (for)	❑ History, personal
❑ Aftercare	❑ Immunization
❑ Contact	❑ Newborn, born
❑ Counseling	❑ Newborn, twin, triplet, quadruplet
❑ Donor	❑ Outcome of delivery
❑ Encounter (for)	❑ Pregnancy
❑ Examination	❑ Status
❑ Exposure	❑ Supervision (of)
❑ Fitting (and adjustment of)	
❑ Follow-up	

Patient is seen for a hernia at the site of a colostomy.

CORRECT:

K94.03 Colostomy malfunction
   Mechanical complication of colostomy

INCORRECT:

Z43.3 Encounter for attention to colostomy
Z93.3 Colostomy Status

Figure 7-2 ■ Example of a Diagnosis Code That Overrides the Need for a Z Code

current condition, do not assign code **Z43.3 Encounter for attention to colostomy**.

Guided Example of Assigning Z Codes

To learn more about assigning Z codes and procedure codes, continue with the example about Angela Holmes who was seen at Branton Medical Center Outpatient Procedure Clinic for a screening colonoscopy.

Follow along as Sherry Whittle, CPC, assigns the Z code. Check off each step as you complete it.

▶ Sherry searches the Index for the Main Term **Screening** (■ Figure 7-3).

 ❑ She locates the subterm **Colonoscopy, Z12.11**.

 ❑ She reviews the rest of the subterms and also locates **neoplasm (malignant)**, which has a second-level subterm **colon Z12.11**.

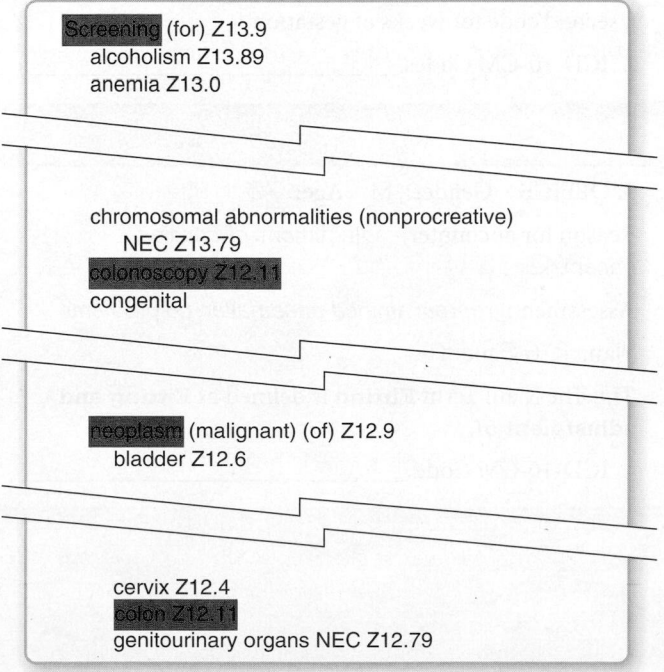

Screening (for) Z13.9
 alcoholism Z13.89
 anemia Z13.0

 chromosomal abnormalities (nonprocreative)
  NEC Z13.79
 colonoscopy Z12.11
 congenital

 neoplasm (malignant) (of) Z12.9
  bladder Z12.6

  cervix Z12.4
  colon Z12.11
  genitourinary organs NEC Z12.79

Figure 7-3 ■ Index Entry for the Main Term Screening

 ❑ She determines that both entries point to the same code because the purpose of a screening colonoscopy is to identify any benign polyps or sign of malignant neoplasm.

▶ Next, Sherry verifies code **Z12.11** in the Tabular List.

 ❑ She reads the code title for **Z12.11, Encounter for screening for malignant neoplasm of colon** and confirms that this accurately describes the reason for the encounter.

▶ Sherry checks for instructional notes in the Tabular List.

 ❑ She cross-references the beginning of category **Z12, Encounter for screening for malignant neoplasms** and reads the instructional notes (■ Figure 7-4, page 102).

 ❑ The first instructional note defines what this category is used for. She determines that the patient's encounter meets this definition.

 ❑ The second instructional note states **Use additional code to identify any family history of malignant neoplasm (Z80.-)**. She checks the medical record for documentation of a family history of colon cancer and finds none, so she does not assign a code from **Z80**.

 ❑ The third instructional note is an **Excludes1** note that tells her to NOT use this category for an encounter for diagnostic examination. A diagnostic colonoscopy would be one performed because the patient presented with specific symptoms or signs, such as rectal bleeding, which the physician investigates. This patient did not present with any symptoms, so this note does not change the coding.

▶ Next, Sherry cross-references the beginning of the block **(Z00-Z13)** and reads the instructional notes, which apply to all codes in the block. The **NOTE:** does not apply because there were no abnormal findings of the colonoscopy. The **Excludes1** note does not apply because this encounter was unrelated to pregnancy and reproduction.

▶ She cross-references the beginning of **Chapter 21 (Z00-Z99)** and reads the instructional notes, which describe the use of Z codes.

 ❑ She notices the statement **A corresponding procedure code must accompany a Z code if a procedure is performed**. This confirms her thinking that she should assign a Z code for the diagnosis and a procedure code for the service performed.

▶ Sherry confirms the diagnosis code she has assigned for this case.

 ❑ **Z12.11 Encounter for screening for malignant neoplasm of colon**

▶ Next, Sherry will assign a CPT code to describe the physician's service of performing the colonoscopy. (CPT coding is covered elsewhere in this text.)

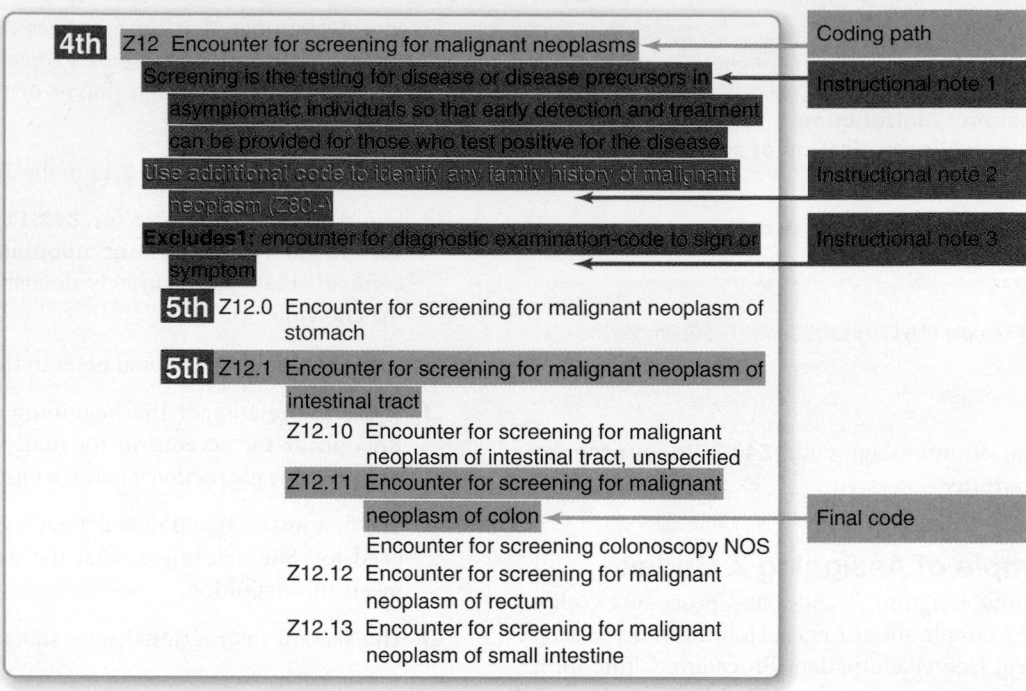

Figure 7-4 ■ Tabular List Entry for Category Z12 and Code Z12.11

CODING PRACTICE

Exercise 7.3 **Assigning Z Codes**

Instructions: Read the mini-medical-record of each patient's encounter, review the information abstracted in Exercise 7.2, and assign ICD-10-CM diagnosis codes using the Index and Tabular List. Write the code(s) on the line provided.

---

1. OFFICE   Gender: M   Age: 52

Reason for encounter: *annual medical examination*

Assessment: *comprehensive metabolic panel test results are normal, no new problems*

Plan: **RTO** 1 year

1 ICD-10-CM Code _____

---

2. OFFICE   Gender: F   Age: 24

Reason for encounter: *supervision of normal second pregnancy, third trimester, 34 weeks*

Assessment: *Estimated Date of Delivery (EDD) 8/3/yy*

Plan: RTO 1 week

(continued)

---

2. (continued)

Tip: The subterm for a second pregnancy is classified as "specified NEC." Assign one code for the supervision and a second code for weeks of gestation.

2 ICD-10-CM Codes _____

---

3. OFFICE   Gender: M   Age: 76

Reason for encounter: *adjustment of cardiac pacemaker*

Assessment: *reprogrammed pacemaker, no problems*

Plan: RTO 6 months

Tip: The Main Term **Fitting** is defined as **Fitting and adjustment of**.

1 ICD-10-CM Code _____

ARRANGING Z CODES

Instructional notes in the Tabular List and the OGCR provide sequencing guidance regarding which Z codes are permitted only as the principal or first-listed diagnosis code and which may be the sole diagnosis code or additional (secondary) diagnosis codes.

Principal or First-Listed Diagnosis

OGCR I.C.21.c.16) lists the Z codes and categories that may *only* be reported as the principal or first-listed diagnosis. The exception is when patients have multiple encounters on the same day and the medical records for the encounters are combined, as may be the case for inpatient records.

Instructional notes in the Tabular List and OGCR from other chapters may also provide direction for Z code sequencing. For example, OGCR I.C.21.c.16) lists the following categories as principal or first-listed diagnosis only:

- **Z51.0 Encounter for antineoplastic radiation therapy**
- **Z51.1- Encounter for antineoplastic chemotherapy and immunotherapy**

OGCR I.C.2.e provides additional guidelines, which state the following:

- When an episode of care involves the surgical removal of a neoplasm, followed by adjunct chemotherapy or radiation therapy during the same episode of care, sequence the *neoplasm* code *first*, then assign any additional diagnoses.

When more than one type of antineoplastic therapy is provided during the same encounter, either may be sequenced first.

Therefore, coders must review all the OGCR related to an encounter and apply critical thinking skills to compare and contrast the guidelines.

Sole Diagnosis Code

Any code listed in OGCR I.C.21.c.16) may also be assigned as the only diagnosis code for an encounter. This is often the case when patients seek specific health services, such as routine and administrative medical examinations or supervision of a normal pregnancy, and have no other problems or conditions.

> ### CODING CAUTION
>
> Category **Z38 Liveborn infants according to place of birth and type of delivery** must always be sequenced *first* on *newborn* records that include the birth encounter. However, category **Z37 Outcome of delivery** must always be a *secondary* code on records of *mothers* that include the delivery encounter.

Status codes and history codes are rarely used as the sole diagnosis code because they do not represent the sole reason for an encounter. For example, codes for family history, BMI, blood type, or DNR describe supplemental information and are used in conjunction with other Z codes or codes from the body system chapters.

Additional Diagnosis Codes

Any code not listed in OGCR I.C.21.c.16) may be used as a secondary, or additional, diagnosis code. When no specific OGCR exists for sequencing a Z code, follow OGCR that apply to sequencing all diagnosis codes.

CODING PRACTICE

Exercise 7.4 Arranging Z Codes

Instructions: Read the mini-medical-record of each patient's encounter, review the information abstracted in Exercise 7.2, assign ICD-10-CM diagnosis codes using the Index and Tabular List, and sequence them correctly.

---

1. OUTPATIENT HOSPITAL   Gender: F   Age: 47

Reason for encounter: screening mammogram

Assessment: normal mammogram, both breasts

Plan: repeat screening 6 months due to personal history of breast cancer

2 ICD-10-CM Codes _____

---

2. OFFICE   Gender: M   Age: 61

Reason for encounter: 6-month follow-up after removal of prostate due to malignant neoplasm of prostate

Assessment: no new findings, no recurrence of disease, no current treatment

Plan: next FU 6 months

Tip: Assign codes for the examination, acquired absence of organ, and history of malignant neoplasm.

3 ICD-10-CM Codes _____

_____

(continued)

CODING PRACTICE (continued)

3. INPATIENT HOSPITAL   Gender: M   Age: 48

Reason for admission: unstable angina pectoris, current tobacco use

Assessment: EKG negative for AMI, **ECC** normal, angiogram normal

(continued)

3. (continued)

Discharge Plan: Rx nitroglycerin, follow up in office 1 week

Tip: Remember to read the instructional notes at the beginning of the three-digit category.

2 ICD-10-CM Codes _____

CHAPTER SUMMARY

In this chapter you learned that:

- Z codes represent reasons for encounters and may be used in any healthcare setting when the reason for the encounter is not a disease, injury, or external cause that is classified in the preceding ICD-10-CM chapters for body systems (A00 to Y89).

- ICD-10-CM Chapter 21, Factors Influencing Health Status and Contact with Health Services (Z00-Z99), contains 14 blocks or subchapters.

- Coders abstract information described by Z codes in three different types of circumstances: Z codes describe the reason for the encounter; instructional notes in the Tabular List direct coders to use Z codes; Z codes are required by the OGCR only.

- When assigning Z codes, coders need to know what Main Terms to search for in the Index, how to distinguish between diagnosis codes and procedure codes, and when to not use a Z code.

- Instructional notes in the Tabular List and the OGCR provide sequencing guidance regarding which Z codes are permitted only as the principal or first-listed diagnosis code and which may be the sole diagnosis code or additional (secondary) diagnosis codes.

- ICD-10-CM provides OGCR Z codes in OGCR section I.C.2, which contains a detailed discussion of the categories of Z codes, when to report them, and which codes may only be sequenced as the principal or first-listed diagnosis.

CONCEPT QUIZ

Take a moment to look back at health status and health services and solidify your skills. This is your opportunity to pull together everything you have learned.

Completion

Instructions: Write the term that answers each question based on the information you learned in this chapter. Choose from the following list. Some choices may be used more than once and some choices may not be used at all.

aftercare	newborns and infants
contact/exposure	observation
counseling	obstetrical and reproductive
donor	routine and administrative examinations
follow-up	screening
personal history	status
family history	miscellaneous
inoculations and vaccinations	

1. _____ Z codes describe testing for disease or disease precursors in seemingly well individuals so that early detection and treatment can be provided for those who test positive for the disease.

2. _____ Z codes describe a patient's past medical condition that no longer exists and is not receiving any treatment but that has the potential for recurrence and therefore may require continued monitoring.

3. _____ Z codes describe a person who is being observed for a suspected condition that is ruled out.

4. _____ Z codes describe when a patient or family member receives assistance in the aftermath of an illness or injury.

5. Z00.00 Encounter for general adult medical examination is an example of the Z code category _____.

6. _____ Z codes describe when the initial treatment of a disease has been performed and the patient requires continued care during the healing or recovery phase or for the long-term consequences of the disease.

7. _____ Z codes describe a patient who has a family member(s) who has had a particular disease that causes the patient to be at higher risk of also contracting the disease.

8. Z53.09 Procedure and treatment not carried out because of other contraindication is an example of the Z code category for _____.

9. _____ Z codes describe continuing surveillance following completed treatment of a disease, condition, or injury when the condition has been fully treated and no longer exists.

10. Z37.0 Single live birth is an example of the Z code category for _____ services.

Multiple Choice

Instructions: Circle the letter of the best answer to each question based on the information you learned in this chapter.

1. The formal name for Z codes is
   A. Supplemental Reasons for Health Service Encounters.
   B. Personal and Family History of Certain Diseases.
   C. Factors Influencing Health Status and Health Behavior.
   D. Factors Influencing Health Status and Contact with Health Services.

2. Which of the following is NOT a situation that requires Z codes?
   A. Tobacco, alcohol, drug use
   B. Tobacco dependence
   C. Acquired absence of organ
   D. Transplant waiting list, recipient, or donor

3. A category of Z code that is rarely used is
   A. observation.
   B. history.
   C. outcome of delivery.
   D. screening.

4. All of the following Main Terms lead to Z codes EXCEPT
   A. Absence
   B. Encounter
   C. Abnormal
   D. Follow-up

5. When should you assign a procedure code in addition to a Z code?
   A. Always
   B. When both codes are listed together in the Index
   C. When an instructional note in the Tabular List instructs you to do so
   D. Never

6. Do not assign a Z code when
   A. the initial treatment of a disease has been performed and the patient requires continued care during healing or recovery.
   B. diagnosis codes from body system chapters include the same information.
   C. a CPT code is required.
   D. more than one service is provided during the same encounter.

7. Z codes may be used in what healthcare setting(s)?
   A. Inpatient settings only
   B. Outpatient settings only
   C. Preventive care settings only
   D. Any healthcare setting

8. The code Z23 Encounter for immunization is an example of what category of Z code?
   A. Inoculations and vaccinations
   B. Newborns and infants
   C. Preventive care encounters
   D. Routine and administrative examinations

9. The Z code category Encounters for Obstetrical and Reproductive Services includes which of the following codes?
   A. Z32.01 Encounter for pregnancy test, result positive
   B. Z20.4 Contact with and suspected exposure to rubella
   C. Z38.01 Single liveborn infant, delivered by cesarean
   D. Z34.01 Encounter for supervision of normal first pregnancy, first trimester

10. The Z code category Aftercare includes which of the following codes?
    A. Z03.73 Encounter for suspected fetal anomaly ruled out
    B. Z08 Encounter for follow-up examination after completed treatment for malignant neoplasm
    C. Z44.002 Encounter for fitting and adjustment of unspecified left artificial arm
    D. Z69.010 Encounter for mental health services for victim of parental child abuse

CODING CHALLENGE

Instructions: Read the mini-medical-record of each patient's encounter, then abstract, assign, and sequence ICD-10-CM diagnosis codes using the Index and Tabular List. Write the code(s) on the line provided.

1. INPATIENT HOSPITAL Gender: M Age: 1 day

Assessment: normal healthy newborn after cesarean delivery here yesterday

Discharge Plan: FU with pediatrician in 2 weeks

Tip: Search under the Main Term *Newborn* and subterm *born*.

1 ICD-10-CM Code _____

2. INPATIENT HOSPITAL Gender: M Age: 67

Reason for admission: initial antineoplastic chemotherapy, risk of **tumor lysis syndrome** and dehydration

Assessment: small cell carcinoma in both lungs, dehydration due to chemotherapy

Discharge Plan: RTO 1 week

Tip: Refer to OGCR I.C.2.e for guidance on code assignment and sequencing. Remember to code for laterality.

4 ICD-10-CM Codes _____

_____

(continued)

(continued from page 105)

3. OFFICE   Gender: F   Age: 45

Reason for encounter: follow-up exam after completing treatment for surgical removal of uterus due to **endometrial** cancer

Assessment: no new findings

Plan: FU 6 months

Tip: Remember to read all instructional notes in the Tabular List.

3 ICD-10-CM Codes _____

_____

4. INPATIENT HOSPITAL   Gender: F   Age: 62

Reason for admission: radical cystectomy followed by inpatient radiotherapy

Assessment: stage III carcinoma of the bladder, invasive into bladder, no metastasis found

Plan: continue radiotherapy as outpatient

1 ICD-10-CM Code _____

5. OFFICE   Gender: M   Age: 15

Reason for encounter: school sports physical

Assessment: cleared for football

Plan: discussed safety precautions and conditioning

1 ICD-10-CM Code _____

6. OFFICE   Gender: M   Age: 12 months

Reason for encounter: Hepatitis B, **MMR**, and **varicella** immunizations

Assessment: child has a heavy cold today, so immunization was not carried out

Plan: reschedule when he is healthy

2 ICD-10-CM Codes _____

7. INPATIENT HOSPITAL   Gender: M   Age: 29

Reason for admission: Patient is a donor match for brother who has end-stage renal disease (ESRD).

Assessment: removal of kidney for transplantation to brother

Plan: FU in office, 4 weeks

1 ICD-10-CM Code _____

8. OFFICE   Gender: F   Age: 4

Reason for encounter: routine 4-year-old exam

Assessment: no new findings, MMR and varicella immunizations administered

Plan: RTO 1 year, call if any new problems

2 ICD-10-CM Codes _____

9. INPATIENT HOSPITAL   Gender: F   Age: 23

Reason for admission: normal delivery, 39 weeks' gestation

Outcome: single liveborn infant

Discharge Plan: FU in office, 2 weeks

Tip: Locate the delivery under the Main Term **Delivery** and subterm **normal**. Remember to read the instructional notes in the Tabular List.

3 ICD-10-CM Codes _____

_____

10. OFFICE   Gender: F   Age: 65

Reason for encounter: management of coronary artery disease (CAD)

Assessment: chronic CAD, BP well controlled

Plan: renew Rx for **anticoagulant** (warfarin) which patient has used successfully for 5 years, discussed eating habits due to borderline cholesterol and the need to quit smoking

Tip: The first code is the disease. Read the instructional notes at the beginning of the category for the second code. The third code is for long-term drug therapy.

3 ICD-10-CM Codes _____

_____

KEEP ON CODING

Instructions: Read the diagnostic statement, then use the Index and Tabular List to assign and sequence ICD-10-CM diagnosis codes. Write the code(s) on the line provided.

1. Encounter for pregnancy test with a negative result: ICD-10-CM Code(s) _____

2. Blood type AB, Rh positive: ICD-10-CM Code(s) _____

3. Dental examination and cleaning: ICD-10-CM Code(s) _____

4. Surgical procedure canceled per patient decision: ICD-10-CM Code(s) _____

5. Status post heart transplant without complications: ICD-10-CM Code(s) _____

6. Renal dialysis status: ICD-10-CM Code(s) _____

7. Encounter for removal of breast implant: ICD-10-CM Code(s) _____

8. Status post coronary angioplasty: ICD-10-CM Code(s) _____

9. Family history of diabetes mellitus: ICD-10-CM Code(s) _____

10. History of tobacco use: ICD-10-CM Code(s) _____

11. Encounter for paternity testing: ICD-10-CM Code(s) _____

12. Encounter for supervision of high-risk pregnancy in the 20th week (second trimester): ICD-10-CM Code(s) _____

13. Liveborn single female, delivered vaginally in the hospital: ICD-10-CM Code(s) _____

14. Lack of physical exercise: ICD-10-CM Code(s) _____

15. Long-term use of nonsteroidal anti-inflammatory drug (NSAID): ICD-10-CM Code(s) _____

16. Allergy to seafood: ICD-10-CM Code(s) _____

17. Presence of a cerebrospinal shunt: ICD-10-CM Code(s) _____

18. Physical restraint status: ICD-10-CM Code(s) _____

19. Do not resuscitate (DNR) status: ICD-10-CM Code(s) _____

20. Homelessness: ICD-10-CM Code(s) _____

21. Pregnant state incidental to encounter: ICD-10-CM Code(s) _____

22. Personal history of kidney stones: ICD-10-CM Code(s) _____

23. Cystic fibrosis carrier: ICD-10-CM Code(s) _____

24. History of adult neglect: ICD-10-CM Code(s) _____

25. Routine well-child exam, age six months, with abnormal findings: ICD-10-CM Code(s) _____

Chapter 8

External Causes of Morbidity (V00-Y99)

Chapter Outline

- **Introduction to External Causes**
- **Coding Overview of External Causes**
- **Abstracting for External Causes**
- **Assigning Codes for External Causes**
- **Arranging Codes for External Causes**

Learning Objectives

After completing this chapter, you should have the skills to:

8.1 Spell and define the key words, medical terms, and abbreviations related to external causes of morbidity.

8.2 Describe the purpose of external cause codes.

8.3 Discuss the main characteristics of coding external causes of morbidity.

8.4 Abstract information required for coding external causes of morbidity and related conditions from the medical record.

8.5 Assign codes for external causes of morbidity and related conditions.

8.6 Arrange codes for external causes of morbidity and related conditions.

8.7 Discuss the Official Guidelines for Coding and Reporting related to external causes of morbidity.

Key Terms and Abbreviations

activity	causal event	intent	status
adverse effect	complication	misadventure	terrorism
cause	external cause	place of occurrence	

In addition to the key terms listed here, students should know the terms defined within tables in this chapter.

For updates and corrections, visit our student resource site at

www.pearsonhighered.com/healthprofessionsresources

INTRODUCTION

When your tire fails because the treads are worn down or the retread delaminates, you know the problem is inherent to the tire. When your tire goes flat because you pick up a nail or someone slashes your tires, the cause is external to the tire. In either case, you still need to repair the tire.

In healthcare, some medical problems develop because of the internal failure of an organ system or biological function; other medical problems are due to external causes, such as an accident or assault. These special circumstances require you to identify and code for external causes of illness and injuries.

Physicians of any specialty may use external cause codes, but they are often used in the emergency department, family practice, orthopedics, and ophthalmology because these physicians specialize in circumstances or body systems frequently affected by external causes.

INTRODUCTION TO EXTERNAL CAUSES

External cause codes describe the event or circumstances that caused an injury or medical problem. Diagnosis codes from the body system chapters describe the actual injury or condition that results. External cause codes may be used in any healthcare setting and with any diagnosis code, but they are secondary codes and should *never* be used as a principal or first-listed diagnosis (OGCR I.C.20.a.1) and 6)).

An **external cause** is an event such as an accident, force of nature, assault, or situation that causes an injury or **adverse effect** (*negative physical reaction*), **complication** (*an abnormal medical reaction that results from a medical or surgical procedure*), or **misadventure** (*an error during a medical or surgical procedure*). Examples of external causes include floods, automobile accidents, falls, prescribed or illegal drugs, and medical or surgical procedures.

Many states require the reporting of external cause codes to track statistics. External cause codes assist third-party payers in tracking the liability (*who is at fault*) for medical costs and enable health researchers to collect standardized data for injury research and injury prevention strategies.

CODING OVERVIEW OF EXTERNAL CAUSES

ICD-10-CM Chapter 20 External Causes of Morbidity (V00-Y99) contains 33 blocks or subchapters. Review the block names and code ranges listed at the beginning of Chapter 20 in the ICD-10-CM manual to become familiar with the content and organization. Also review the instructional note at the beginning of the chapter that discusses how to use external cause codes.

ICD-10-CM Chapter 20 corresponds with ICD-9-CM Supplementary Classification of External Causes of Injury and Poisoning (E000-E999), commonly referred to as E codes. ICD-10-CM includes external cause codes as part of the main classification rather than as a supplementary classification as ICD-9-CM did. However, ICD-10-CM provides a separate Index to External Causes. Numerous title changes, expansions, and reorganization appear in ICD-10-CM. Nearly all external cause codes require a seventh character. Many external cause events that were a single code in ICD-9-CM are categories in ICD-10-CM, with expansion at the subcategory level in order to add specificity. Transport accidents are reorganized based on the mode of transportation. Codes for complications of medical and surgical care are greatly expanded. Place of occurrence codes have greater specificity, including the type of dwelling and room of the house in which the injury occurred. Late effect of external cause codes are eliminated because late effects are reported with a seventh character in ICD-10-CM.

ICD-10-CM provides Official Guidelines for Coding and Reporting (OGCR) external causes in OGCR section I.C.20. OGCR provides detailed discussion of when to report codes from this chapter and how they are to be used. Additional OGCR for using external cause codes in conjunction with specific conditions appear throughout the OGCR and as instructional notes throughout the Tabular List.

CODING CAUTION

There is no national requirement for mandatory reporting of external cause codes. Providers are encouraged to voluntarily report external cause codes because they provide valuable data for injury research and the evaluation of injury prevention strategies (OGCR I.C.20).

ABSTRACTING FOR EXTERNAL CAUSES

Whenever patients are treated for injuries, adverse effects, or complications from procedures, coders abstract information related to the external cause of the condition. Multiple external cause codes are required, each describing a different aspect of the event, if the documentation provides the required information. In addition to the clinical diagnosis, external cause information that must be abstracted appears in ■ TABLE 8-1.

Place of occurrence, Activity, and Status codes are in the block **Supplementary factors related to causes of morbidity classified elsewhere (Y90-Y99)**. An instructional note in the Tabular List instructs coders that these categories may be used to provide supplementary information concerning causes of morbidity. They are not to be used as the only external cause code.

Intent and Cause

Combination codes report both intent and cause. **Intent** describes whether the event was accidental or intentional. **Cause**

Table 8-1 ■ KEY CRITERIA FOR ABSTRACTING EXTERNAL CAUSES

❑ **Diagnosis:** What physical injury(ies) or health condition did the patient sustain?

❑ **Intent:** What is the purpose or intent of the injury: accidental, self-harm, assault, legal intervention, military operation, or medical procedure?

❑ **Cause/causal event:** How did the injury or health condition happen?

❑ **Place:** Where did the event occur?

❑ **Activity:** What was the patient doing at the time of the event?

❑ **Status:** What was the patient's employment status at the time the event occurred: civilian employment, military, volunteer, or recreational/leisure?

or **causal event** describes the event or action that resulted in the injury. Code(s) for intent and cause are reported *every* time the patient receives treatment for the injury (OGCR I.C.20.a.2)).

Because intent and cause are described in a combination code, determine the intent first. Doing so helps to locate the Main Term in the Index to External Causes. Options for intent include the following:

- accidental
- self-harm
- assault
- result of legal, military, or terrorist activity
- undetermined

The cause or event code is based on the intent. For example, separate codes exist for an accidental fall, a fall that is a suicide attempt, and a fall that is due to an assault. The vast majority of cause codes are for accidental intent, so accident codes are the most specific. The most common causes of accidents are traffic accidents and falls.

When the intent of the cause of an injury or other condition is unknown or unspecified, code the intent as **accidental**. All transport accident categories assume **accidental** intent (OGCR I.C.20.h)). When the documentation states that the intent cannot be determined, then abstract the intent as **undetermined**.

SUCCESS STEP

Always abstract before you attempt to assign codes. Write down notes with key information to help keep the details organized. When you begin to assign codes, you may need to refer back to the medical record and abstract additional details based on the specificity of information the code requires.

SUCCESS STEP

Coders also need to abstract the episode of care, which describes the phase of treatment. Identifying the episode of care is necessary in order to assign the seventh character of an external cause code. Options for the episode of care are:

- **initial** episode, which identifies that the patient received active treatment for the injury during the encounter;
- **subsequent** episode, which identifies that the patient received routine care during the healing phase at the encounter; and
- **sequela** episode, which identifies an encounter at which the patient was treated for a complication after the healing phase is complete.

CODING CAUTION

The seventh character for the **initial** episode of care does not refer only to the *first* encounter but to any encounter during *active treatment*, such as initial stabilization of fracture, initial surgery, and cast application. Use the character for **subsequent** care during the healing phase, such as for a cast change, an X-ray to monitor healing, or removal of a fixation device.

Place of Occurrence (Y92.-)

The **place of occurrence** code describes where the injury occurred, such as a public street or a single-family home. Report only *one* place per injury and *only* at the initial encounter for treatment (OGCR I.C.20.b and d). Review the category **Y92.-** to familiarize yourself with the various types of settings. Within each setting, such as single-family residence, codes designate the specific room or area where the injury occurred.

Activity (Y93.-)

An **activity** code describes what the person was doing when the injury occurred, such as running, playing sports, or preparing food. Report *one* activity code per injury when it provides additional information about the event. Report the activity code *only* at the initial encounter for treatment (OGCR I.C.20.c and d). Review the category **Y93.-** to familiarize yourself with the various types of activities. Activity codes are not applicable to poisonings, adverse effects, medical misadventures, complications, or late effects.

Be careful to differentiate the activity from the causal event. The causal event, such as a fall, may occur while doing any number of activities, such as running, walking, or working in the yard. When a person is engaged in an activity, such as walking, an injury could occur as a result of a variety of events, such as falling, tripping, or being struck by an object or vehicle. Every injury should be coded with a causal event, but not every injury requires an activity code. Assign an activity code when it provides additional information.

Status (Y99.-)

Status codes describe the person's employment status in relation to the event that caused the injury (OGCR I.C.20.d and k). Report *one* status code per injury event and *only* at the initial encounter for treatment. The status code indicates whether the event occurred during military activity or whether a civilian was at work or engaged in a volunteer activity.

Guided Example of Abstracting External Causes

Refer to the following example throughout this chapter in order to practice your abstracting, assigning, and arranging external cause code skills. Marcy Elwood, CCS, is a fictitious coder who guides you through coding this case.

Date: 8/1/yy   Location: Branton Medical Center Emergency Department Provider: Cynthia Hiatt, MD

Patient: Charles Fink   Gender: M   Age: 24

Reason for encounter: Patient had an accident on his day off. He was painting the outside of his single family home when he fell off a ladder.

Assessment: fractured left tibia

Plan: Applied long leg cast. Use crutches to keep weight off. Follow-up with orthopedic clinic.

Follow along as Marcy abstracts the diagnosis. Check off each step after you complete it.

▶ Marcy begins by reading the medical record. She refers to the Key Criteria for Abstracting External Causes (Table 8-1) to abstract the diagnosis. She will abstract all the information first, then assign the actual codes later in this chapter.

❑ *Diagnosis: What physical injury(ies) or health condition did the patient sustain?* She notes that the diagnosis is fractured left tibia because it describes the injury the patient experienced and writes this down.

❑ *Intent: What is the purpose or intent of the injury: accidental, self-harm, assault, legal intervention, military operation, or medical procedure?* She notes that the intent is stated as an accident and writes this down.

❑ *Causal event: How did the injury or health condition happen?* She notes that the causal event is a fall. Specifically, the fall was from a ladder. She writes this down.

❑ *Place of occurrence: Where did the event occur?* She notes that the fall occurred outside of a single-family home. She writes this down.

❑ *Activity: What was the patient doing at the time of the event?* Marcy notes that the patient was painting the outside of his house and writes this down.

❑ *Status: What was the employment status at the time the event occurred: civilian employment, military, volunteer, or recreational/leisure?* Marcy determines the patient was doing the work for personal purposes on his day off. Even though he is employed, the accident was not related to his employment.

▶ Marcy reviews all the data she abstracted for this case and verifies it against the medical record.

❑ Diagnosis: fractured left tibia, initial encounter

❑ Intent and cause: accidental fall from ladder, initial encounter

❑ Place: outside of single-family home

❑ Activity: painting outside of house

❑ Status: personal

▶ Next, Marcy will assign the codes.

CODING PRACTICE

Exercise 8.1   Abstracting for External Causes

Instructions: Read the mini-medical-record of each patient's encounter and answer the abstracting questions. Write the answer on the line provided. Do not assign any codes.

---

1. INPATIENT HOSPITAL   Gender: F   Age: 85

Chief complaint: Laceration on the forehead. Fell off toilet and hit her head on the sink.

Assessment: 3-cm laceration

Plan: see family physician for suture removal in 10 days

a. What is the diagnosis? _____

_____

b. What event caused the injury? _____

_____

c. Was this an initial, subsequent, or sequela episode of care? _____

_____

---

2. EMERGENCY DEPT   Gender: F   Age: 5

Reason for encounter: burn due to accidentally touching hot stove

Assessment: second-degree burn to the right hand

(continued)

---

2. (continued)

Plan: Dressed wound. Instructed parent on wound care. Follow up with family physician in 2 weeks. Call if any problems develop.

a. What is the diagnosis? _____

_____

b. What event caused the injury? _____

_____

c. Was this an initial, subsequent, or sequela episode of care? _____

_____

---

3. INPATIENT HOSPITAL   Gender: M   Age: 25

Reason for admission: assault by handgun to leg 6 weeks ago. Patient was treated for fracture to femur caused by a bullet. Bullet was removed but fracture has not healed properly so surgery is needed.

Discharge diagnosis: malunion of nondisplaced comminuted (*bone broken into fragments*) fracture, left femur shaft

Plan: FU in office in 3 weeks

a. What is the diagnosis? _____

_____

b. What event caused the injury? _____

_____

(continued)

CODING PRACTICE (continued)

3. (continued)

c. Was this an initial, subsequent, or sequela episode of care? _____

_____

4. INPATIENT HOSPITAL   Gender: M   Age: 47

Reason for admission: heart attack due to overexertion while shoveling snow in driveway of his single-family home.

Discharge diagnosis: acute myocardial infarction (AMI)

Plan: FU in office in 2 weeks

a. What is the diagnosis? _____

_____

b. What event caused the injury? _____

_____

c. Was this an initial, subsequent, or sequela episode of care? _____

_____

d. Where did the injury occur? _____

_____

e. What was the patient doing at the time of the injury?

_____

_____

f. Was the activity done for civilian work, leisure, volunteer service, or military operations? _____

_____

5. INPATIENT HOSPITAL   Gender: F   Age: 41

Reason for admission: second surgery for fractured scapula, which was the result of a traffic accident. She was driving a van as a volunteer for the swim team and collided with a pickup truck.

Assessment: displaced fracture of body of left scapula, malunion

a. What is the diagnosis? _____

_____

b. What event caused the injury? _____

_____

(continued)

5. (continued)

c. Was this an initial, subsequent, or sequela episode of care? _____

_____

d. Where did the injury occur? _____

_____

e. What was the patient doing at the time of the injury?

_____

_____

f. What kind of vehicle was the patient in? _____

_____

g. Was she the driver or a passenger? _____

_____

h. What kind of vehicle did she collide with? _____

i. What is the external cause status? _____

_____

6. EMERGENCY DEPT   Gender: M   Age: 53

Reason for encounter: Patient was walking on a public sidewalk while making a delivery as part of his job when he was bit on the leg by a German shepherd dog that was running free in the neighborhood.

Assessment: puncture wound, left calf

Plan: follow up with orthopedic physician in 2 weeks

a. What is the diagnosis? _____

_____

b. What event caused the injury? _____

_____

c. Was this an initial, subsequent, or sequela episode of care? _____

_____

d. Where did the injury occur? _____

_____

e. What was the patient doing at the time of the injury?

_____

_____

f. Was the activity done for civilian work, leisure, volunteer service, or military operations? _____

_____

ASSIGNING CODES FOR EXTERNAL CAUSES

To assign codes to cases involving external causes, coders use a separate Index to External Causes and verify the codes in the Tabular List.

> ## SUCCESS STEP
>
> Coders familiar with ICD-9-CM will notice that although ICD-10-CM has a separate Index to External Causes, it does *not* have a separate Tabular List as ICD-9-CM did. External cause codes appear in Chapter 20 (V00 to Y99) of the Tabular List.

Index to External Causes

The Index to External Causes is separate from the Index to Diseases and Injuries (Index) and appears immediately before the Tabular List. When coding cases that involve external causes, use both indices, as follows:

- Use the Index to Diseases and Injuries to locate the diagnosis code(s) for the injury or condition.
- Use the Index to External Causes to locate external cause codes for intent and cause, place of occurrence, activity, and employment status.

In order to use the Index to External Causes successfully, coders must locate Main Terms for each type of external cause code. Coders should also learn how to locate codes specifically for traffic accidents, the most commonly used and largest block in the external cause chapter.

> ## SUCCESS STEP
>
> If you have not already done so, apply an adhesive index tab to the first page of the Index to External Causes to help you remember where to find it. This index is not long enough that you need alphabetic tabs for every letter in the index, but it is helpful to insert a few tabs to make it easier to navigate. Good places to mark with tabs are A-B, C-O, and P-Z.

Main Terms

Main Terms for external cause codes for intent and causal event can be located in two ways: search for the intent or search for the event. Regardless of which way coders search for Main Terms, they must be attentive to multiple levels of indented subterms in order to locate the correct code, as follows:

- When searching for intent, the Main Term is the intent, such as **Accident** or **Assault**. Causal events are subterms indented under each Main Term.
- When searching for the causal event, the event is the Main Term, such as **Fall** or **Bite**. Each indent is a subterm under each causal event.

Main Terms for place, activity, and status are located under entries that carry those names: **Place**, **Activity**, and **Status**. Refer to ■ TABLE 8-2 for a list of commonly used Main Terms in

Table 8-2 ■ COMMONLY USED MAIN TERMS IN THE INDEX TO EXTERNAL CAUSES

❑ Accident	❑ Incident
❑ Activity	❑ Jump
❑ Assault	❑ Legal
❑ Bite	❑ Military operations
❑ Burn	❑ Misadventure
❑ Complication	❑ Place
❑ Contact	❑ Radiation
❑ Drowning	❑ Status
❑ Explosion	❑ Striking against
❑ Exposure to	❑ Struck by
❑ Failure	❑ Suicide
❑ Fall	❑ War operations
❑ Forces of nature	

the Index to External Causes. As in the Index to Diseases and Injuries, Main Terms have indented subterms that further define the specifics of entry. Remember to carefully review all available subterms in order to locate the most specific code.

> ## SUCCESS STEP
>
> Three specific status codes exist for Status: (1) **civilian activity done for pay, Y99.0**, (2) **military activity, Y99.1**, and (3) **volunteer activity, Y99.2**. All other status descriptions such as student, hobby, or leisure activity are grouped together under one nonspecific code, **Other external cause status, Y99.8**.

> ## SUCCESS STEP
>
> When burns are caused by contact with a hot object, such as a stove or iron, search under the Main Term **Burn**. When burns are caused by a fire with flames, such as a campfire or house fire, search under the Main Term **Exposure (to)** and subterm **fire, flames**.

Motor Vehicle Accidents

The Index entry for motor vehicle accidents is several pages long and has numerous levels of subterms (■ FIGURE 8-1, page 114). The most common types of accidents can be located as follows:

1. Locate the Main Term **Accident**.
2. Locate the subterm **transport**.
3. Locate the next level of subterm for the type of vehicle the patient was riding in, such as **bus**, **car**, or **motorcycle**.
4. Locate the next subterm to identify the patient as the **driver** or **passenger**.
5. Locate the next level of subterm that identifies what object the vehicle collided with, such as **animal**, **car**, or **pedal cycle**.

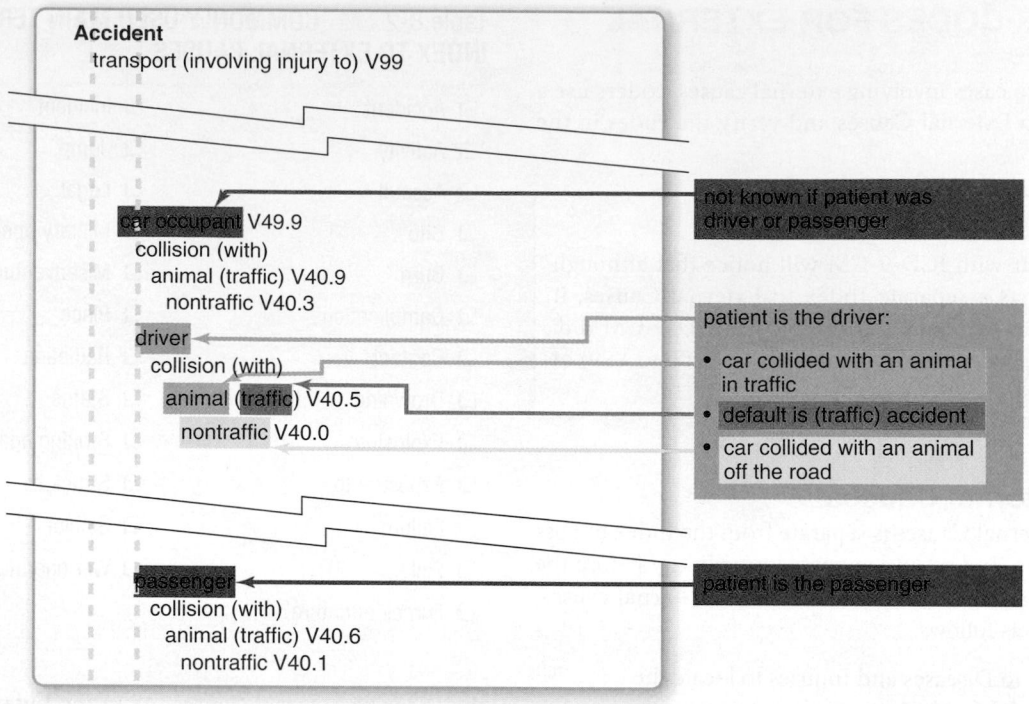

Figure 8-1 ■ Example of Index to External Causes, Main Term and Subterms for an Automobile Accident

6. The default code for motor vehicle accidents is for a traffic accident, as indicated by the parentheses for a nonessential modifier, **(traffic)**. When a vehicle accident occurs anywhere except a public highway, use the subterm **nontraffic**. The Tabular List provides definitions for the various types of accidents.

7. When the patient was a pedestrian or bicyclist who was hit by a vehicle, search under **Accident, transport, pedestrian** or **Accident, transport, pedal cyclist**.

Review the extensive instructional notes in the Tabular List at the beginning of the block **V00 to V99, Transport Accidents**. These notes provide definitions of transport vehicles, types of collisions, and vehicle occupants so that all coders use the codes in a consistent manner. A note also instructs coders to **Use additional code to identify** an airbag injury, type of street or road, or use of cellular telephone or electronic device at time of accident.

Verify in Tabular List

Coders should verify all external cause codes in the Tabular List. Doing so can help catch mistakes that are easily made when navigating multiple levels of indented subterms in the Index to External Causes. In addition, seventh characters can be assigned only from the Tabular List.

Most external cause codes for intent and cause from **V00** to **Y38** require a seventh character to describe the episode of care. Seventh characters for external causes appear under each three-digit category heading in the Tabular List (■ FIGURE 8-2). Refer to ■ TABLE 8-3 to learn when to use each character (OGCR I.C.19.a).

> ### CODING CAUTION
> External cause codes for place, activity, and status do NOT use seventh characters for the episode of care.

Recall that the convention **7th** means that the final character must be in the seventh position, and coders should assign the placeholder **X** in any unused positions. Because the code **W50.01 Bitten by alligator** is only five characters, add the character **X** in the sixth position, before adding the seventh character. For example, **Bitten by alligator, initial encounter** is written as **W58.01XA**.

When the external cause and intent are included in a combination code from another chapter, do not report an additional code from Chapter 20 (OGCR I.C.20.a.8)). For example, **Poisoning by penicillin, accidental** is reported with code **T36.0X1-**. Because the diagnosis code describes both cause and intent, an external cause code is not reported. In addition, do not report place, activity, and status codes with poisonings. Poisonings are discussed in detail in Chapter 13 of this text.

Some external cause codes are combination codes that identify two or more related or sequential events that result in an

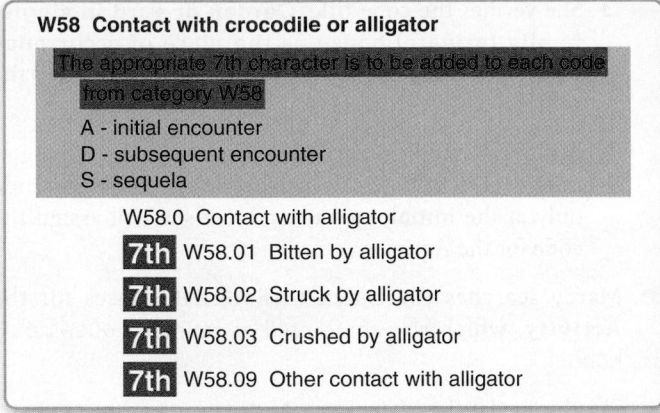

Figure 8-2 ■ Example of the Location of Seventh Characters Under Category Titles in Index to External Causes

injury, such as a fall that results in striking against an object. Such a code may be used when the injury is due to either the event alone or both at the same time. Assign the combination code that describes the full sequence of events, regardless of whether the most serious injury was from the fall itself or from striking the object (OGCR I.C.20.a.7)).

Assign as many external cause event codes as necessary to fully explain each cause. If only one external cause code can be recorded, assign the code most related to the principal diagnosis (OGCR I.C.20.a.4)). However, assign only one code each for place, activity, and status, and report these codes only for the initial encounter.

Guided Example of Assigning External Cause Codes

Continue with the example from earlier in the chapter about patient Charles Fink, who fell off a ladder while painting his house, to learn more about using the Index to External Causes.

Follow along in your ICD-10-CM manual as Marcy Elwood, CCS, assigns codes. Check off each step after you complete it.

▶ Marcy reviews the information she abstracted:

❑ Diagnosis: *fractured left tibia, initial encounter*

❑ Intent and cause: *accidental fall from ladder, initial encounter*

❑ Place: *outside of single-family home*

❑ Activity: *painting outside of house*

❑ Status: *personal*

▶ The first code Marcy will assign is the diagnosis code for the injury.

❑ She searches the Index to Diseases and Injuries for the diagnosis that she abstracted, *fractured left tibia, initial encounter.*

❑ She locates the Main Term **Fracture** and subterm **tibia S82.20-**.

▶ Marcy verifies the diagnosis code **S82.20-** in the Tabular List.

❑ She locates the subcategory title, **S82.20-, Unspecified fracture of shaft of tibia**.

❑ The symbol **6th** tells her to assign a sixth character, located below the subcategory title. She assigns the sixth character, **2**, for the left tibia.

❑ The symbol **7th** tells her to assign a seventh character located at the beginning of the category **S82**. She assigns the seventh character, **A**, for the initial encounter for closed fracture.

❑ The diagnosis code is **S82.202A, Unspecified fracture of shaft of left tibia, initial encounter for closed fracture**.

Table 8-3 ■ SEVENTH-CHARACTER DEFINITIONS AND EXAMPLES

7th Character	Definition	Example
A Initial Encounter	Use while the patient is receiving active treatment for the injury.	Surgical treatment Emergency department encounter Evaluation and treatment by a new physician
D Subsequent Encounter	Use for encounters after the patient has received active treatment for the injury and is receiving routine care for the injury during the healing or recovery phase.	Cast change or removal Removal of external or internal fixation device Medication adjustment Visits following injury treatment
S Sequela	Use for complications or conditions that arise as a direct result of an injury after the healing phase is complete.	Scar formation after a burn

▶ Marcy turns her attention to the external cause codes. She locates the Index to External Causes, located immediately before the Tabular List. First, she will code the intent and cause.

▶ Marcy searches the Index to External Causes for the intent and cause of the injury, which she abstracted as *accidental fall from ladder*.

- ❑ She locates the Main Term **Fall** and notes that the default intent is **(accidental)**, so she knows she is in the right place.

- ❑ She locates the subterm **from, off, out of**.

- ❑ She locates the second-level subterm, **ladder W11**.

▶ Marcy verifies the first external cause code for **accidental fall off ladder**.

- ❑ She locates the Tabular List entry **W11**. She verifies the external cause code title, **Fall on and from ladder**, which accurately describes the situation.

- ❑ She cross-references the subchapter title **Other External Causes of Accidental Injury (W00-X58)** to verify that the fall code relates to an accidental intent.

- ❑ She notices the symbol 7th in front of the code, which tells her a seventh character is required.

- ❑ She reviews the seventh character options, which are listed under the code, and identifies that **A** represents **the initial encounter**.

- ❑ She also notices that the **X** in the symbol means that because the code is three digits long, she must use the placeholder holder **X** to fill out the fourth, fifth, and sixth characters of the code.

- ❑ She assigns the code **W11.XXXA** for **Accidental fall from ladder, initial encounter**. Next she will assign the code for Place of occurrence.

▶ Marcy searches the Index to External Causes for the **Place of occurrence**, which she abstracted as *outside of single-family home*.

- ❑ She locates the Main Term **Place** and the **subterm residence (non-institutional) (private) Y92.009**. She notices there are more subterms for the type of residence, so she does not assign this code.

- ❑ She locates the next level of subterm, **house, single family Y92.019**. She notices there are more subterms for the specific location at the house, so she does not assign this code.

- ❑ She selects the subterm **yard Y92.017** because the accident occurred outside.

▶ Marcy verifies the second external cause code for place of occurrence, **house, single family, yard**.

- ❑ She locates the Tabular List entry for **Y92.017**.

❑ She verifies the code title, **Garden or yard in single-family (private) house as the place of occurrence of the external cause**, which accurately describes the situation.

❑ She reviews the instructional notes at the beginning of the category **Y92**, which instruct her to report this code only at the initial encounter. Next she will assign the code for the Activity.

▶ Marcy searches the Index to External Causes for the **Activity**, which she abstracted as *painting outside of house*.

- ❑ She locates the Main Term **Activity**.

- ❑ She searches for a subterm that describes *painting outside of house*, but cannot find anything that specific.

- ❑ She reviews the subterms again, searching for a broader term that would include *painting outside of house*.

- ❑ She locates the subterm **maintenance**, then the subterm **exterior building NEC Y93.H9**.

▶ Marcy verifies the external cause code for activity, **maintenance, exterior building NEC**.

- ❑ She searches for the Tabular List entry for **Y93.H9**.

- ❑ She locates the category **Y93** and observes that alphabetic characters for the fourth character of the code begin after **Y93.7** and before **Y93.8**.

- ❑ She verifies the code title, **Y93.H9 Activity, other involving exterior property and land maintenance, building and construction**, which accurately describes the situation. Next, Marcy will assign a code for the Status.

▶ Marcy searches the Index to External Causes for the **Status**, which she abstracted as *personal*.

- ❑ She locates the Main Term **Status of external cause** and reviews the subterms.

- ❑ She notices that there is no entry for personal, but there is an entry for **leisure activity Y99.8**.

▶ Marcy verifies the final external cause code for status, **leisure activity**.

- ❑ She locates the Tabular List entry for **Y99.8**.

- ❑ She verifies the code title, **Other external cause status**, which accurately describes the situation

▶ Marcy reviews the information she located in the Index to External Causes.

- ❑ Intent and cause: **accidental fall off ladder W11.XXXA**

- ❑ Place: **house, single family, yard Y92.017**

❑ Activity: **maintenance, exterior building NEC Y93.H9**

❑ Status: **leisure activity Y99.8**

▶ Marcy reviews the diagnosis code, **S82.202A Unspecified fracture of shaft of left tibia, initial encounter**.

▶ Next, Marcy needs to determine how to sequence the codes.

CODING CAUTION

When place of occurrence, activity, or status are not documented, omit the code. Do not use place of occurrence code **Y92.9** if the place is not stated or is not applicable (OGCR I.C.20.b). Do not assign **Y93.9 Unspecified activity** if the activity is not stated (OGCR I.C.20.c). Do not assign code **Y99.9 Unspecified external cause status** if the status is not stated (OGCR I.C.20.k). Use these codes only when the *documentation specifically states* that the information is not known or available.

CODING PRACTICE

Exercise 8.2 Assigning Codes for External Causes

Instructions: Read the mini-medical-record of each patient's encounter, review the information abstracted in Exercise 8.1, and assign ICD-10-CM diagnosis codes using the Index to Diseases and Injuries, the Index to External Causes, and the Tabular List. Write the code(s) on the line provided.

1. EMERGENCY DEPT   Gender: F   Age: 85

Chief complaint: Laceration on the forehead. Fell off toilet and hit her head on the sink.

Assessment: 3-cm laceration

Plan: see family physician for suture removal in 10 days

Tip: Code the diagnosis and the external cause event. This medical record does not give you information for place, activity, or status codes.

2 ICD-10-CM Codes _____

2. EMERGENCY DEPT   Gender: F   Age: 5

Reason for encounter: burn due to accidentally touching hot stove

Assessment: second-degree burn to the right hand

(continued)

2. (continued)

Plan: Dressed wound. Instructed parent on wound care. Follow up with family physician in 2 weeks. Call if any problems develop.

Tip: Code the diagnosis and the external cause event. This medical record does not give you information for place, activity, or status codes.

2 ICD-10-CM Codes _____

3. INPATIENT HOSPITAL   Gender: M   Age: 25

Reason for admission: assault by handgun to leg 6 weeks ago. Patient was treated for fracture to femur caused by a bullet. Bullet was removed but fracture has not healed properly so additional surgery is needed.

Discharge diagnosis: malunion of nondisplaced comminuted (*bone broken into fragments*) fracture, left femur shaft

Plan: FU in office in 3 weeks

Tip: Code the diagnosis and the external cause event. This medical record does not give you information for place, activity, or status codes. On the fracture code, assign the seventh character for **subsequent encounter for closed fracture with malunion**.

2 ICD-10-CM Codes _____

ARRANGING CODES FOR EXTERNAL CAUSES

External cause codes are always secondary codes; they can *never* be the principal or first-listed diagnosis. Sequence external cause codes as follows:

1. The principal or first-listed diagnosis.

2. Secondary diagnosis codes from the body system chapters.

3. External cause combination code for the intent and causal event code that most closely supports the principal or first-listed diagnosis. If more than one intent and causal event code applies, sequence them as follows (OGCR I.C.20.b to f):

1) Child and adult abuse

2) **Terrorism** events (*events designated by the FBI as terrorism*)

3) Cataclysmic events

4) Transport accidents

4. Place of occurrence code, if required.

5. Activity code, if required.

6. Status code, if required.

If the reporting format (the claim form or computer screen) limits the number of external cause codes that can be used in reporting clinical data, report the combination code for the intent and causal event most related to the principal diagnosis. If the format permits capture of additional external cause codes, report intent/cause codes of any additional causal events, including misadventures, before reporting the codes for place, activity, or external status (OGCR I.C.20.b to e)).

CODING CAUTION

Recall that external cause, place, activity, and status codes are not applicable to poisonings, adverse effects, misadventures, or late effects. When these three types of codes apply, assign them only for the initial encounter.

Guided Example of Arranging External Cause Codes

Continue with the example about Charles Fink, who fell off a ladder while painting his house, in order to practice skills for arranging external cause codes.

▶ Follow along as Marcy Elwood, CCS, sequences the codes she verified earlier. Check off each step after you complete it.

❑ Marcy sequences the diagnosis code **S82.202A, Unspecified fracture of shaft of left tibia, initial**

encounter for closed fracture first because it meets the criteria for the first-listed diagnosis.

❑ The second code is the external cause code for intent and causal event, **W11.XXXA, Accidental fall from ladder, initial encounter.**

❑ The third code is the external cause code for place, **Y92.017, Garden or yard in single-family (private) house as the place of occurrence of the external cause.**

❑ The fourth code is the external cause code for activity, **Y93.H9, Activity, other involving exterior property and land maintenance, building and construction.**

❑ The fifth code is the external cause code for status, **Y99.8, Other external cause status.**

▶ Finally, Marcy cross-references each code against the medical record to be certain that she did not overlook anything.

▶ The final code assignment and sequencing is

(1) **S82.202A Unspecified fracture of shaft of left tibia, initial encounter for closed fracture**

(2) **W11.XXXA Accidental fall from ladder, initial encounter**

(3) **Y92.017 Garden or yard in single-family (private) house as the place of occurrence of the external cause**

(4) **Y93.H9 Activity, other involving exterior property and land maintenance, building and construction**

(5) **Y99.8 Other external cause status**

CODING PRACTICE

Exercise 8.3   Arranging Codes for External Causes

Instructions: Read the mini-medical-record of each patient's encounter, review the information abstracted in Exercise 8.1, assign ICD-10-CM diagnosis codes using the Index to Diseases and Injuries, the Index to External Causes, and the Tabular List, and sequence them correctly.

1. INPATIENT HOSPITAL   Gender: M   Age: 47

Reason for admission: heart attack due to overexertion while shoveling snow in driveway of his single-family home.

Discharge diagnosis: AMI

(continued)

1. (continued)

Plan: FU in office in 2 weeks

Tip: You need one diagnosis code and three external cause codes.

4 ICD-10-CM Codes _____

_____

2. INPATIENT HOSPITAL   Gender: F   Age: 41

Reason for admission: second surgery for fractured scapula, which was the result of a traffic accident. She was driving a van as a volunteer for the swim team and collided with a pickup truck.

(continued)

2. (continued)

Assessment: *displaced fracture of body of left scapula, malunion*

Plan: *follow up in office in 3 weeks*

Tip: Report place, activity, and status only for the initial encounter.

2 ICD-10-CM Codes _____

3. EMERGENCY DEPT   Gender: M   Age: 53

Reason for encounter: *Patient was walking on a public sidewalk while making a delivery as part of his job when he was bit on the leg by a German shepherd dog that was running free in the neighborhood.*

Assessment: *puncture wound, left calf*

Plan: *follow up with orthopedic physician in 2 weeks*

Tip: This is the initial encounter, so provide the full range of four external cause codes.

5 ICD-10-CM Codes _____

_____

CHAPTER SUMMARY

In this chapter you learned that:

- External cause codes describe the event that created an injury or medical problem.
- ICD-10-CM Chapter 20 External Causes of Morbidity (V00–Y99) contains 33 blocks or subchapters.
- Whenever patients are treated for injuries, adverse effects, or complications from procedures, coders must abstract multiple external cause codes, each describing different aspects of the event.

- Coders use a separate Index to External Causes to locate codes then verify them in the Tabular List.
- External cause codes are always secondary codes and must be sequenced in a specific order.
- ICD-10-CM provides Official Guidelines for Coding and Reporting (OGCR) in OGCR I.C.20, which discusses when to report codes from ICD-10-CM Chapter 20 and how they are to be used.

CONCEPT QUIZ

Take a moment to look back at external causes and solidify your skills. This is your opportunity to pull together everything you have learned.

Completion

Instructions: Write the term that answers each question based on the information you learned in this chapter. Choose from the following list. Some choices may be used more than once and some choices may not be used at all.

activity	military operations
adverse effect	misadventure
causal event	place
complication	principal
external cause	secondary
falls	status
first-listed	suicide
intent	traffic accident

1. _____ codes describe the purpose of the injury as accidental or intentional.

2. _____ is a negative physical reaction.

3. _____ codes describe what the person was doing at the time of the event.

4. Reporting of _____ codes allows third-party payers to determine liability for medical costs.

5. _____ codes describe employment status at the time the event occurred.

6. _____ and _____ are reported with a combination code.

7. _____ is an error during a medical or surgical procedure.

8. External cause codes are always _____ codes.

9. _____, _____, and _____ codes are NOT applicable to poisonings, adverse effects, misadventures, complications, or late effects.

10. The most commonly used and largest block in the external cause chapter is _____.

(continued)

(continued from page 119)

Multiple Choice

Instructions: Circle the letter of the best answer to each question based on the information you learned in this chapter.

1. What healthcare setting uses external cause codes?
   A. Outpatient setting only
   B. Emergency department only
   C. Inpatient setting only
   D. All healthcare settings

2. Which of the following does NOT describe an intent?
   A. Accidental
   B. Military operation
   C. Assault
   D. Intentional

3. How should the intent be coded when the intent of the cause of an injury or other condition is unknown or unspecified?
   A. Undetermined
   B. Accidental
   C. Assault
   D. External

4. What type of intent is assumed for all transport accident categories?
   A. Assault
   B. Accidental
   C. Undetermined
   D. External

5. Which of the following is NOT an option for episode of care?
   A. Initial
   B. Subsequent
   C. Final
   D. Sequela

6. Which type of external cause code is reported at every encounter related to the injury?
   A. Intent and cause
   B. Place
   C. Activity
   D. Status

7. Where are external cause codes indexed?
   A. Index to Diseases and Injuries
   B. Index to External Causes
   C. Table of Drugs and Chemicals
   D. Tabular List

8. Which of the following is NOT a Main Term in the Index to External Causes?
   A. Fracture
   B. Failure
   C. Fall
   D. Military operations

9. Which of the following is NOT a status code?
   A. Civilian activity done for pay
   B. Military activity
   C. Volunteer activity
   D. Vacation activity

10. Which code is sequenced first?
    A. Diagnosis code
    B. Causal event code
    C. Place of occurrence code
    D. Status code

CODING CHALLENGE

Instructions: Read the mini-medical-record of each patient's encounter and assign diagnosis codes using the Index to Diseases and Injuries, the Index to External Causes, and Tabular List, and sequence them correctly. Write the code(s) on the line provided.

1. INPATIENT HOSPITAL   Gender: F   Age: 20

Reason for admission: Admitted through ED. Patient was on her way home from work and was walking on a local street because there was no sidewalk. It was after dark and a car struck her when the driver did not see her.

Discharge diagnosis: Concussion without loss of consciousness, fracture in the lower end of radius, right arm.

(continued)

1. (continued)

Discharge plan: FU in office 3 weeks. Call if any symptoms such as dizziness or headache.

Tip: Assign a diagnosis code for each injury and assign four external codes. Sequence the concussion as the principal diagnosis.

6 ICD-10-CM Codes _____

_____

2. INPATIENT HOSPITAL   Gender: M   Age: 19

Reason for admission: Admitted from ED after fall from canoe and submersion in cold water in Branton Lake. He was instructing a class as part of his job.

(continued)

2. (continued)

Discharge diagnosis: bradycardia (*slow heart rate*) due to **hypothermia**, hypoxemia (*oxygen depletion*)

Discharge plan: FU in office, 1 week

Tip: Assign three diagnosis codes and five external cause codes. Instructional notes in the Tabular List for hypothermia direct you to one of the external cause codes.

8 ICD-10-CM Codes _____

_____

_____

3. INPATIENT HOSPITAL   Gender: M   Age: 20

Reason for admission: Admitted from ED for dislocated shoulder. He was texting his girlfriend while driving on the freeway and ran his motorcycle into a sign post.

Discharge diagnosis: dislocated right acromioclavicular (*shoulder*) joint, 100% displacement

Discharge plan: Immobilize joint for 2 weeks. FU in office 2 weeks. Recommended course on motorcycle safety.

Tip: The patient's status is not identified.

4 ICD-10-CM Codes _____

_____

4. INPATIENT HOSPITAL   Gender: F   Age: 80

Planned procedure: scheduled for total knee replacement, left knee, due to primary osteoarthritis

Postprocedural diagnosis: procedure performed in error on right knee, which also had degeneration due to osteoarthritis

Discharge plan: Physical therapy and rehab.

Tip: External cause codes for place, activity, and status are not required because this is a misadventure. In the Index to External Causes, under the entry for **Misadventure, performance of inappropriate operation**, you will see a cross-reference to a different Main Term.

2 ICD-10-CM Codes _____

5. INPATIENT HOSPITAL   Gender: M   Age: 21

Reason for admission: knife stab wounds to the chest after a gang fight in a public park

Discharge diagnosis: Intrathoracic wound with laceration of right lung.

Tip: External cause codes for activity and status are not needed.

3 ICD-10-CM Codes _____

_____

6. INPATIENT HOSPITAL   Gender: M   Age: 22

Reason for admission: Admitted from ED. Patient was riding his bicycle for recreation through a parking lot and was hit by a bus. He impacted the handlebar and appears to have internal injuries.

Assessment: stomach laceration

Tip: The Index to External Causes classifies *bicyclist* using the term **pedal cyclist**.

5 ICD-10-CM Codes _____

_____

7. EMERGENCY DEPT   Gender: M   Age: 27

Chief complaint: State police officer arrived by ambulance after being struck in the head by a baton while taking down a suspect. Loss of consciousness for 15 minutes.

Assessment: concussion to head

Tip: The causal event is legal intervention. Do not assign an activity code because there is none that adds information to the encounter.

3 ICD-10-CM Codes _____

_____

8. INPATIENT HOSPITAL   Gender: F   Age: 18

Reason for admission: stupor, vomiting, muscle cramps, **anhidrosis**, dyspnea, elevated pulse after being outside in the sun all day at the beach where she was working as a lifeguard, body temperature 104 degrees.

Assessment: heat stroke with stupor

Tip: Distinguish integral symptoms of heat stroke from complications that the Tabular List instructional notes direct you to code.

5 ICD-10-CM Codes _____

_____

(*continued*)

(continued from page 121)

9. OFFICE   Gender: M   Age: 35

Reason for encounter: *second visit for sore back after slipping while playing golf*

Assessment: *MRI negative for disc damage, lumbar sprain*

Plan: *Refer to physical therapy*

2 ICD-10-CM Codes _____

10. EMERGENCY DEPT   Gender: M   Age: 28

Chief complaint: *put nail through thumb with nail gun while performing his construction job as a carpenter*

Assessment: *puncture wound, right thumb*

5 ICD-10-CM Codes _____

_____

KEEP ON CODING

Instructions: Read the diagnostic statement, then use the Index to External Causes and Tabular List to assign and sequence ICD-10-CM diagnosis codes. Write the code(s) on the line provided.

1. Burn of the hand while onboard a sailboat, initial encounter: ICD-10-CM Code(s) _____

2. Injury occurred while cheerleading (activity code): ICD-10-CM Code(s) _____

3. Injury while using a chainsaw, subsequent encounter: ICD-10-CM Code(s) _____

4. Late effect of being struck by golf ball: ICD-10-CM Code(s) _____

5. Electrocution by a toaster, suicide attempt, initial encounter: ICD-10-CM Code(s) _____

6. Bitten by a raccoon, initial encounter: ICD-10-CM Code(s) _____

7. Overexposure in a tanning bed, sequela: ICD-10-CM Code(s) _____

8. Incorrect procedure performed on correct patient: ICD-10-CM Code(s) _____

9. Pellet gun injury, intent undetermined, initial encounter: ICD-10-CM Code(s) _____

10. Overexposure to sound waves, subsequent encounter: ICD-10-CM Code(s) _____

11. Burned by a hot toaster, initial encounter: ICD-10-CM Code(s) _____

12. Hunting rifle discharge, unknown intent, initial encounter: ICD-10-CM Code(s) _____

13. Excessive fluid administered during a transfusion: ICD-10-CM Code(s) _____

14. Human bite during an assault, initial encounter: ICD-10-CM Code(s) _____

15. Drowning of undetermined intent after a fall in the swimming pool, initial encounter: ICD-10-CM Code(s) _____

16. Blood alcohol level 65 mg/100 mL: ICD-10-CM Code(s) _____

17. Fall into a well, subsequent encounter: ICD-10-CM Code(s) _____

18. Fall from the steps due to ice, initial encounter: ICD-10-CM Code(s) _____

19. Pecked by a macaw, initial encounter: ICD-10-CM Code(s) _____

20. Fall from a motorcycle, driver, in a nontraffic accident, initial encounter: ICD-10-CM Code(s) _____

21. Fall from scaffolding, initial encounter: ICD-10-CM Code(s) _____

22. Subsequent encounter from being stranded in a snow blizzard: ICD-10-CM Code(s) _____

23. Fall from inline roller skates, subsequent encounter: ICD-10-CM Code(s) _____

24. Injured in the garden of a private house (place of occurrence): ICD-10-CM Code(s) _____

25. Failure of sterile precautions during an injection, initial encounter: ICD-10-CM Code(s) _____

Diseases of the Digestive System (K00-K95)

Chapter 9

Learning Objectives

After completing this chapter, you should have the skills to:

9.1 Spell and define the key words, medical terms, and abbreviations related to the digestive system.

9.2 Discuss the structure, function, and common conditions of the digestive system.

9.3 Identify the main characteristics of coding for digestive system conditions.

9.4 Abstract diagnostic information from the medical record for coding diseases of the digestive system.

9.5 Assign diagnosis codes to patient encounters related to the digestive system.

9.6 Arrange multiple diagnosis codes for patient encounters related to the digestive system.

9.7 Abstract, assign, and sequence codes for neoplasms of the digestive system.

9.8 Discuss the Official Guidelines for Coding and Reporting for the digestive system.

Chapter Outline

- **Digestive System Refresher**
- **Coding Overview of the Digestive System**
- **Abstracting for Digestive System Conditions**
- **Assigning Codes for Digestive System Diagnoses**
- **Arranging Codes for Digestive System Diagnoses**
- **Coding Neoplasms of the Digestive System**

Key Terms and Abbreviations

accessory organs
alimentary canal
barium enema
comorbidity
digestive system
diverticulosis
diverticula
diverticulitis
gastrointestinal (GI) system
Helicobacter pylori (H. pylori)

In addition to the key terms listed here, students should know the terms defined within tables in this chapter.

INTRODUCTION

Your automobile takes in gasoline, utilizes certain components to power the vehicle, and expels the byproducts through the exhaust system. A problem at any point in the complicated process affects the way the vehicle functions. The digestive system serves a similar function for your body.

In this chapter you will learn more about how the digestive system works, why sometimes it does not work as it should, and how physicians treat these conditions. Gastroenterologists are physicians who specialize in the study, diagnosis, and treatment of digestive system diseases. Dentists specialize in the study, diagnosis, and treatment of disorders of the oral cavity,

which is part of the digestive system. Primary care physicians and internal medicine physicians treat many common digestive system disorders. They refer complex cases to a gastroenterologist or dentist.

DIGESTIVE SYSTEM REFRESHER

The function of the **digestive system**, also called the **gastrointestinal (GI) system**, is to receive nutrients, break them down, absorb them into the blood to be used by the body, and eliminate solid waste products. The digestive system consists of the **alimentary canal** and **accessory organs** (■ FIGURE 9-1). The alimentary canal is a continuous tube, approximately 30 feet in

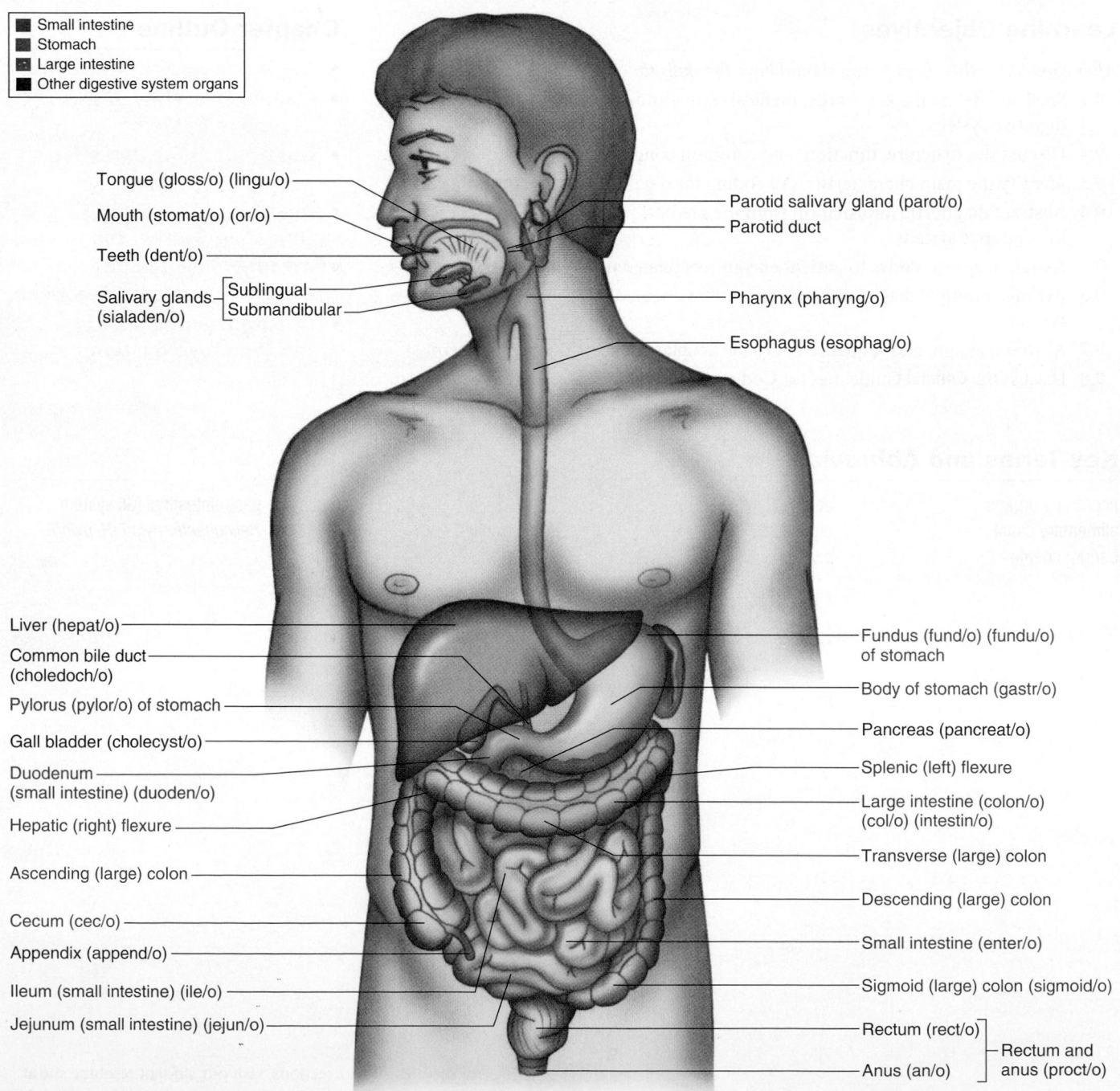

■ Small intestine
■ Stomach
■ Large intestine
■ Other digestive system organs

Tongue (gloss/o) (lingu/o)
Mouth (stomat/o) (or/o)
Teeth (dent/o)
Salivary glands (sialaden/o) — Sublingual / Submandibular

Parotid salivary gland (parot/o)
Parotid duct
Pharynx (pharyng/o)
Esophagus (esophag/o)

Liver (hepat/o)
Common bile duct (choledoch/o)
Pylorus (pylor/o) of stomach
Gall bladder (cholecyst/o)
Duodenum (small intestine) (duoden/o)
Hepatic (right) flexure
Ascending (large) colon
Cecum (cec/o)
Appendix (append/o)
Ileum (small intestine) (ile/o)
Jejunum (small intestine) (jejun/o)

Fundus (fund/o) (fundu/o) of stomach
Body of stomach (gastr/o)
Pancreas (pancreat/o)
Splenic (left) flexure
Large intestine (colon/o) (col/o) (intestin/o)
Transverse (large) colon
Descending (large) colon
Small intestine (enter/o)
Sigmoid (large) colon (sigmoid/o)
Rectum (rect/o)
Anus (an/o) — Rectum and anus (proct/o)

Figure 9-1 ■ The Digestive (Gastrointestinal) System

Table 9-1 ■ **EXAMPLE OF CONSTRUCTING MEDICAL TERMS FOR THE DIGESTIVE SYSTEM**

Combining Form	Suffix	Complete Medical Term
gastr/o (*stomach*) **enter/o** (*intestines*) **colon/o** (*large intestine*)	**-logy** (*study of*)	**gastro + entero + logy** (*the study of the stomach and intestines*)
	-itis (*inflammation*)	**gastr + itis** (*inflammation of the stomach*) **enter + itis** (*inflammation of the intestines*)
	-scopy (*visual examination*)	**gastro + scopy** (*visual examination of the stomach*) **colono + scopy** (*visual examination of the large intestine*)

length, which begins at the mouth; continues through the esophagus, stomach, small intestine, and large intestine; and exits the body at the rectum and anus. The accessory organs assist in digestion, but are not directly connected to the alimentary canal. They are the salivary glands, liver, gall bladder, and pancreas.

Each structure in the digestive system is labeled with its name as well as its medical terminology root/combining form in Figure 9-1. Remember to apply medical terminology skills to combine the root or combining form for the body part with suffixes to define new terms for conditions and procedures, as shown in ■ TABLE 9-1.

CODING CAUTION

Be alert for medical word roots with similar spellings but different meanings:

chole/o (*bile or gall*), **col/o** (*colon*), and **colp/o** (*vagina*)

cholecyst/o (*gall bladder*) and **cyst/o** (*bladder or sac, often used in reference to the urinary bladder*)

ile/o (*ileum, part of the small intestine*) and **ili/o** (*ilium, the pelvic bone*)

ileum (*small intestine*) and **ileus** (*a paralytic condition of the small intestine*)

Conditions of the Digestive System

The functions of the digestive system are:

- ingestion—taking in food (mouth, esophagus; aided by the salivary glands)
- digestion—breaking down food (stomach, small intestine; aided by the liver, gall bladder, and pancreas)

- absorption—transferring nutrients to the body (small intestine, large intestine)
- elimination—removing solid waste from the body (large intestine, rectum, anus)

SUCCESS STEP

Remember the difference between an organ system and a body region or cavity. Do not confuse the digestive system (an organ system) with the abdomen (a body region or cavity). Digestive system organs are located in the head, neck, thoracic cavity, abdominal cavity, and pelvic cavity.

Digestive system conditions account for approximately 12% of all inpatient procedures and 31% of all ambulatory procedures, according to the National Digestive Diseases Information Clearinghouse (NDDIC). Treating these conditions costs about $98 billion per year. Over 236,000 people die each year from digestive system conditions. Diseases and conditions of the digestive system can be caused by heredity, the type and amount of food consumed, substance abuse, particularly alcohol and tobacco, or mental health conditions. Diseases are diagnosed through a combination of physical examination, medical history, signs and symptoms, blood tests, imaging, endoscopy, and biopsy. Common treatments include dietary changes, alcohol and tobacco abstinence, medication, and/or surgery.

■ TABLE 9-2 highlights common conditions affecting the digestive system and common diagnostic methods. This table provides a general reference to help understand where a particular diagnosis or procedure fits into the overall picture of the digestive system, but it does not list everything you need to know. Refer to medical resources to learn more about conditions affecting the digestive system.

Table 9-2 ■ **COMMON CONDITIONS AFFECTING THE DIGESTIVE SYSTEM**

Condition	Description	Diagnostic Methods
Appendicitis	Inflammation and possible rupture of the appendix	Blood count, physical examination
Celiac disease	An abnormal immune reaction to gluten and poor absorption of nutrients	Blood tests, intestinal biopsy, presence of **dermatitis herpetiformis (DH)**
Cholecystitis	Inflammation of the gall bladder	Ultrasound (US), computerized axial tomography (CT), fecal fat test

(*continued*)

Table 9-2 ■ (continued)

Condition	Description	Diagnostic Methods
Choledocholithiasis	**Calculi** in the common bile duct	US, CT, fecal fat test
Cholelithiasis	Calculi in the gall bladder	US, CT, fecal fat test
Cirrhosis	Scarring of liver tissue that blocks the normal flow of blood through the liver	Blood tests, imaging tests, liver biopsy
Crohn's disease	An **inflammatory bowel disease (IBD)** with inflammation and ulcers in the alimentary tract characterized by a thickening of the mucous membrane	Blood tests, stool test, endoscopy, biopsy
Diverticular disease	Diverticulosis: the presence of diverticula (*pouches formed when the lining of the intestine pushes through the intestinal muscle layer*) Diverticulitis: a bacterial infection of diverticula	Blood tests, stool sample, **digital rectal examination (DRE)** colonoscopy, barium enema (*injection of a chalky substance into the colon through the anus and viewing the organs on an X-ray; also called* **lower GI series**)
Esophagitis	Irritation of the esophagus caused by acid reflux and a weak **cardiac sphincter**	Physical examination, symptoms of **heartburn**
Gastritis	Inflammation of the stomach lining	Gastroscopy blood test, stool test, test for *Helicobacter pylori,* or *H. pylori* (*bacteria that causes ulcers*)
Gastroenteritis	Bacterial or viral infection of the stomach and intestines	Stool culture, symptoms of vomiting, nausea, and/or abdominal pain
Gastroesophageal reflux disease (GERD)	Backward flow of stomach contents (food or liquid) into the esophagus	**Barium swallow** or **upper GI series, esophagogastroduodenoscopy (EGD),** esophageal **manometry**
Hepatitis	Inflammation of the liver due to viruses named A, B, or C	Blood tests, liver biopsy
Hernia	Protrusion of an organ through a weakened area in a muscle, such as the diaphragm (hiatal hernia) or groin muscle (inguinal hernia)	X-ray
Intestinal obstruction	A physical blockage of the intestine that prevents waste from passing through	CT, X-ray, barium enema, barium swallow
Irritable bowel syndrome (IBS)	A combination of symptoms such as cramping, abdominal pain, bloating, constipation, diarrhea	Medical history, symptoms, examination, rule out other problems
Pancreatitis	Inflammation of the pancreas	US, CT, **endoscopic ultrasound (EUS), magnetic resonance cholangiopancreatography (MRCP)**
Stomatitis	Redness, ulcers, and/or bleeding of the mouth due to bacteria, viruses, or fungi	Physical examination, immunological tests, cultures
Ulcer	A sore on the lining of the stomach (gastric ulcer) or duodenum (peptic ulcer)	Blood test for *H. pylori*, urea breath test, stool antigen test, endoscopy, barium swallow
Ulcerative colitis	An IBD with inflammation and sores, called ulcers, in the lining of the rectum and colon	Physical examination, medical history, blood tests, stool sample, colonoscopy, sigmoidoscopy
Volvulus	Twisting of a portion of the small or large intestine or stomach into a loop that obstructs the passage of digestive material	CT, X-ray, barium enema, barium swallow, endoscopy blood tests

CODING PRACTICE

Exercise 9.1 Digestive System Refresher

Instructions: Use your medical terminology skills and resources to define the following conditions of the digestive system, then assign the ICD-10-CM diagnosis code.

Follow these steps:

- Use slash marks "/" to break down each term into its root(s) and suffix.
- Define the meaning of the word, based on the meaning of each word part.
- Assign the default diagnosis code for the condition using the Index and Tabular List.

Example: gastritis gastr/itis   Meaning: _inflammation of the stomach_   Code: _K29.70_

1. ileus   Meaning _____   ICD-10-CM Code _____
2. hematemesis   Meaning _____   ICD-10-CM Code _____
3. gingivitis   Meaning _____   ICD-10-CM Code _____
4. volvulus   Meaning _____   ICD-10-CM Code _____
5. stomatitis   Meaning _____   ICD-10-CM Code _____
6. hepatoma   Meaning _____   ICD-10-CM Code _____
7. diverticulitis   Meaning _____   ICD-10-CM Code _____
8. diverticulosis   Meaning _____   ICD-10-CM Code _____
9. proctitis   Meaning _____   ICD-10-CM Code _____
10. cholangitis   Meaning _____   ICD-10-CM Code _____

CODING OVERVIEW OF THE DIGESTIVE SYSTEM

Chapter 11 of ICD-10-CM, Diseases of the Digestive System (K00-K95), contains 10 blocks or subchapters that are divided by anatomical site. Review the block names and code ranges listed at the beginning of Chapter 11 in the ICD-10-CM manual to become familiar with the content and organization. Review the **Excludes2** note that lists several conditions not classified to this chapter, such as digestive conditions that are perinatal, congenital, pregnancy-related, injuries, symptoms, or neoplasms. Each of these conditions will be discussed in the corresponding chapter of ICD-10-CM, with the exception of neoplasms, which are discussed at the end of this chapter.

ICD-10-CM Chapter 11 corresponds with ICD-9-CM Chapter 9 (520-579). Extensive instructional notes direct coders to assign additional codes to identify certain lifestyle habits involving use or exposure to tobacco and alcohol. Crohn's disease has been expanded from a single code in ICD-9-CM to multiple subcategories and codes, which identify site and complications. Classification of ulcers does not include the presence or absence of an obstruction in ICD-10-CM. Hemorrhoids have been moved from the circulatory system in ICD-9-CM to the digestive system in ICD-10-CM.

ICD-10-CM provides no Official Guidelines for Coding and Reporting (OGCR) for the digestive system. Combination codes that describe complications of digestive system conditions are common. In addition, frequent instructional notes direct coders to use multiple codes to describe the underlying cause or harmful lifestyle habits that contribute to gastrointestinal conditions. Review OGCR sections I.B.7 and I.B.9 of the General Coding Guidelines to review the use of multiple coding and combination codes, respectively.

ABSTRACTING FOR DIGESTIVE SYSTEM CONDITIONS

When abstracting for the digestive system, coders need to look for manifestations, complications, and lifestyle habits associated with digestive system conditions. Key factors to review for coding cases that involve the digestive system appear in ■ TABLE 9-3. Remember that the abstracting questions are a guide and that

not every question applies to, or can be answered for, every case. For example, lifestyle habits may not be present for every patient.

Manifestations are symptoms and signs that occur as a result of the underlying condition. Certain digestive system diseases can exist alone or as a manifestation of another condition. For example, liver disorders can be a manifestation of congenital syphilis or congenital **toxoplasmosis**.

Common complications in the digestive system are bleeding, obstruction, and infection. Ulcers, enteritis, colitis, and gastritis may occur with or without bleeding. An obstruction is a blockage of an organ and can be caused by calculi (_stones_), tumors, organic matter, or volvulus. Gall bladder and intestinal diseases may occur with or without an obstruction. When an infection is present, coders need to abstract the infectious agent, such as _Streptococcus_, _Escherichia coli_ (_E. coli_), or _Staphylococcus_.

Lifestyle habits are patient behaviors that cause or contribute to a condition. Lifestyle habits that contribute to many digestive system conditions include use, history of use, dependence, and exposure to tobacco or tobacco smoke and alcohol.

Many digestive system codes are combination codes that include the complication or **comorbidity** (_two diseases occurring together_). Multiple coding is needed for lifestyle habits and for complications and comorbidities that do not have a combination code. When abstracting, coders do not necessarily know

Table 9-3 ■ KEY CRITERIA FOR ABSTRACTING DIGESTIVE SYSTEM CONDITIONS

- ❑ What is the condition?
- ❑ What is the anatomic site?
- ❑ What is the laterality, if any?
- ❑ Is bleeding or hemorrhaging documented?
- ❑ What other manifestations or complications are documented?
- ❑ What comorbidities are documented?
- ❑ What lifestyle habits are documented as current or with a history of, such as alcohol use or abuse and tobacco exposure, use, or abuse?

which complications and comorbidities will be assigned a combination code and which will require multiple coding.

Guided Example of Abstracting for Digestive System Conditions

Refer to the following example throughout this chapter to practice skills for abstracting, assigning, and sequencing codes for digestive system conditions. Jill Hynes, CPC, is a fictitious coder who guides you through this case.

Date: 9/1/yy   Location: Branton Gastroenterology

Provider: Stanley Garrett, MD

Patient: Gina Addington   Gender: F   Age: 28

Chief complaint: rectal bleeding, Crohn's disease since age 10

Assessment: Crohn's disease, colon, new complication of rectal bleeding

Plan: liquid diet 1 week, FU if not improved

Follow along as Jill Hynes, CPC, abstracts the diagnosis. Check off each step after you complete it.

▶ Jill refers to the Key Criteria for Abstracting Digestive System Conditions (Table 9-3).

❑ *What is the condition?* Crohn's disease

❑ *What is the anatomic site?* colon

❑ *Is bleeding or hemorrhaging documented?* Yes, rectal bleeding, which is a new complication.

❑ *What other manifestations or complications are documented?* None

❑ *What comorbidities are documented?* None

❑ *What lifestyle habits are documented as current or with a history of?* None

▶ Until Jill researches this condition in the ICD-10-CM manual to assign codes, she does not know if Crohn's disease with rectal bleeding will require one or two codes.

CODING PRACTICE

Exercise 9.2   **Abstracting for Digestive System Conditions**

Instructions: Read the mini-medical-record of each patient's encounter and answer the abstracting questions. Write the answer on the line provided. Do not assign any codes.

1. OFFICE   Gender: M   Age: 54

Chief complaint: indigestion

Assessment: chronic perforated peptic ulcer in stomach with bleeding

Plan: change diet, change Rx

a. What symptom is documented? _____

_____

b. Where is the ulcer located? _____

_____

c. What signs or complications are present? _____

_____

d. Is the ulcer acute or chronic? _____

_____

e. Will you code for the symptoms? _____

   Why or why not? _____

f. What is the diagnosis to be coded? _____

_____

2. OUTPATIENT SURGERY   Gender: F   Age: 61

Procedure: repair, right inguinal hernia

Postprocedural diagnosis: recurrent right inguinal hernia

Plan: FU in office

a. Where is an inguinal hernia located? _____

_____

b. Is the hernia unilateral or bilateral? _____

_____

c. Is the hernia documented as recurrent? _____

_____

d. Is an obstruction documented? _____

_____

e. Is gangrene documented? _____

_____

3. OFFICE   Gender: M   Age: 67

Reason for visit: FU on lower GI series

Assessment: ulcerative colitis with fistula (*an abnormal connection between an organ, vessel, or intestine and another structure*)

Plan: begin liquid diet, Rx antibiotics, FU 2 weeks

a. What test is the follow-up visit for? _____

_____

b. Should you code for the test? _____

   Why or why not? _____

c. What type of colitis is documented? _____

_____

d. What complication is documented? _____

_____

e. What diagnosis will you code? _____

_____

4. OFFICE   Gender: M   Age: 56

Chief complaint: abdominal pain and bloating, fatigue, vomiting

Assessment: alcoholic liver cirrhosis with ascites due to alcohol addiction

Plan: counseled patient regarding abstinence from alcohol, reduce salt intake

a. What symptoms are documented? _____

_____

b. What is the anatomic site of the cirrhosis? _____

_____

c. What complication is present? _____

_____

d. What is the cause of the cirrhosis? _____

_____

e. What lifestyle habit is documented? _____

_____

f. Will you code the symptoms? _____

   Why or why not? _____

g. What diagnosis will you code? _____

_____

5. OFFICE   Gender: M   Age: 59

Chief complaint: hematemesis, history of cirrhosis

Assessment: portal hypertension (*increase in blood pressure in the portal vein*) with portal hypertensive gastropathy

Plan: endoscopic therapy, drug therapy, and dietary changes

a. What symptom(s) are documented? _____

_____

b. Is cirrhosis past or present? _____

   Why? _____

c. What is the primary condition diagnosed? _____

_____

d. What is the complication? _____

_____

e. Will you code the symptoms? _____

   Why or why not? _____

f. Will you code the cirrhosis? _____

   Why? _____

g. What is the first-listed diagnosis? _____

_____

6. OFFICE   Gender: M   Age: 33

Chief complaint: redness and tenderness around colostomy site

Assessment: colostomy infection, cellulitis of abdominal wall due to methicillin-susceptible *Staphylococcus aureus* (MSSA)

a. What symptom(s) are documented? _____

_____

b. What two conditions are documented? _____

_____

c. What is the infectious agent? _____

_____

d. Will you code the symptoms? _____

   Why or why not? _____

ASSIGNING CODES FOR DIGESTIVE SYSTEM DIAGNOSES

Coders frequently assign combination codes to describe common complications or manifestations of digestive system conditions. As a result, the digestive system chapter in ICD-10-CM has more codes and more detail than ICD-9-CM. For example, the category **K50 Crohn's disease** contains more than 25 codes, many of which are combination codes that describe common complications of Crohn's disease. This is in contrast to ICD-9-CM, which contained only four codes, to identify the anatomical site, in the category **555 Regional enteritis**. Crohn is an eponym for Burrill Bernard Crohn, a gastroenterologist who identified the condition in 1932. Most codes in category **K50 Crohn's disease** contain six characters:

- Characters 1 to 3 classify Crohn's disease in general.
- Character 4 identifies the site as the small intestine, large intestine, both, or unspecified.
- Character 5 indicates whether a complication is present.
- Character 6 describes the specific complication.

Index entries for conditions with combination codes can be rather long and involved, with many subterms and many levels of indentation, in order to identify all the possible combinations of conditions. Be thorough when searching these entries to be certain to locate the correct item. When verifying the code in the Tabular List, read the description carefully to be sure it matches the combination of conditions in the scenario. Many wrong turns can be caught when verifying.

Guided Example of Assigning Digestive System Diagnosis Codes

Continue with the example from earlier in the chapter about patient Gina Addington, who had Crohn's disease, to practice skills for assigning digestive system codes.

Follow along in your ICD-10-CM manual as Jill Hynes, CPC, assigns codes to the diagnosis. Check off each step after you complete it.

▶ Jill begins by locating the Main Term in the Index.

❏ Jill looks up **C, Crohn's disease**.

❏ She reviews the cross-reference note that directs her to **E, Enteritis, regional** (■ FIGURE 9-2). (With experience, you will learn to go directly to the entry for **Enteritis, regional**.)

❏ Under the entry for **E, Enteritis, regional** Jill reviews the subterms that describe the various sites within the intestinal tract.

❏ She locates the subterm for **colon**.

❏ Jill reviews the instruction to cross-reference the subterm **Enteritis, regional, large intestine**.

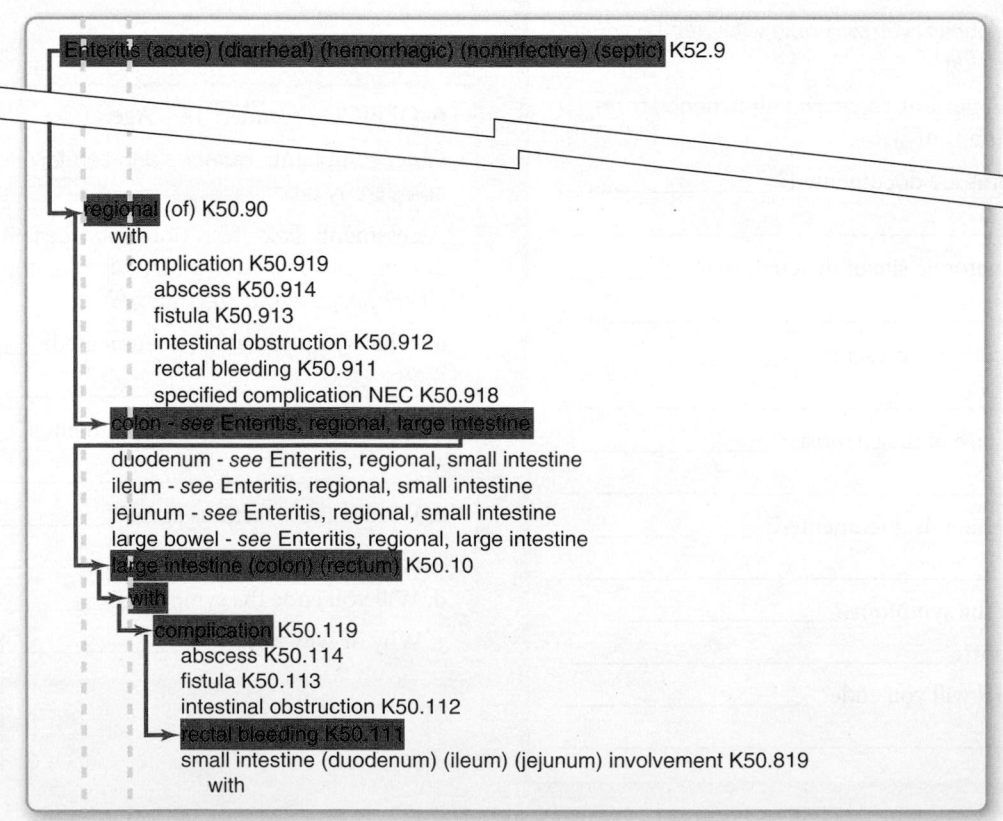

Enteritis (acute) (diarrheal) (hemorrhagic) (noninfective) (septic) K52.9

    regional (of) K50.90
      with
        complication K50.919
          abscess K50.914
          fistula K50.913
          intestinal obstruction K50.912
          rectal bleeding K50.911
          specified complication NEC K50.918
      colon - *see* Enteritis, regional, large intestine
      duodenum - *see* Enteritis, regional, small intestine
      ileum - *see* Enteritis, regional, small intestine
      jejunum - *see* Enteritis, regional, small intestine
      large bowel - *see* Enteritis, regional, large intestine
      large intestine (colon) (rectum) K50.10
        with
          complication K50.119
            abscess K50.114
            fistula K50.113
            intestinal obstruction K50.112
            rectal bleeding K50.111
        small intestine (duodenum) (ileum) (jejunum) involvement K50.819
          with

Figure 9-2 ■ Index Entry for Enteritis, Regional

- ❑ Under the subterm for **large intestine**, Jill reviews the additional subterms that describe various associated conditions and complications.

- ❑ She refers back to the medical record and identifies the complication of rectal bleeding.

- ❑ She locates the subentry for **with**, then **rectal bleeding**.

- ❑ Jill confirms that there are no further subentries under **rectal bleeding** and identifies the code **K50.111** that she will verify in the Tabular List.

▶ Now Jill verifies the code in the Tabular List. She locates the entry for code **K50.111**.

- ❑ Jill confirms that the code description **Crohn's disease of large intestine with rectal bleeding** accurately describes the diagnosis (■ FIGURE 9-3).

- ❑ She notes that a seventh character is not required because there is not a **7th** symbol next to it and there are no additional codes under it.

- ❑ Jill reviews the instructional notes at the beginning of the subclassification **K50.1** that state which sites are included. She sees that Crohn's disease of both the colon and rectum are included in this subcategory. The **Excludes1** note reminds her that this entry *excludes* Crohn's disease that affects *both* the large and small intestines and she should cross-reference subcategory

K50.8 if that is what she were coding. She makes a mental note of this for future reference.

- ❑ She reviews the instructional notes at the beginning of the category **K50**. She notes there is an instruction to **Use additional code to identify manifestations.** Jill checks the chart note to be certain that it does not mention any manifestations, which it does not. If Dr. Garrett had listed more manifestations, this is how she would know they should be coded in addition to Crohn's disease. She also reads the **Includes** and **Excludes** notes and concludes that she is on the right track.

SUCCESS STEP

Do not become frustrated by multiple cross-references. When driving, you may see a detour sign that redirects your course. Sometimes part way through the detour the signs seem to stop and you wonder if you are still on the right path or if you missed a sign that directs you to an important turn. When that happens, it can take awhile to get back on the right street. You do not want to let this happen when coding! Cross-references are ICD-10-CM's way of making sure you get to the right place.

- ❑ Next, Jill reviews the instructional notes at the beginning of the block **Noninfective enteritis and colitis (K50-K52)**. None of these exclusions apply to the current case.

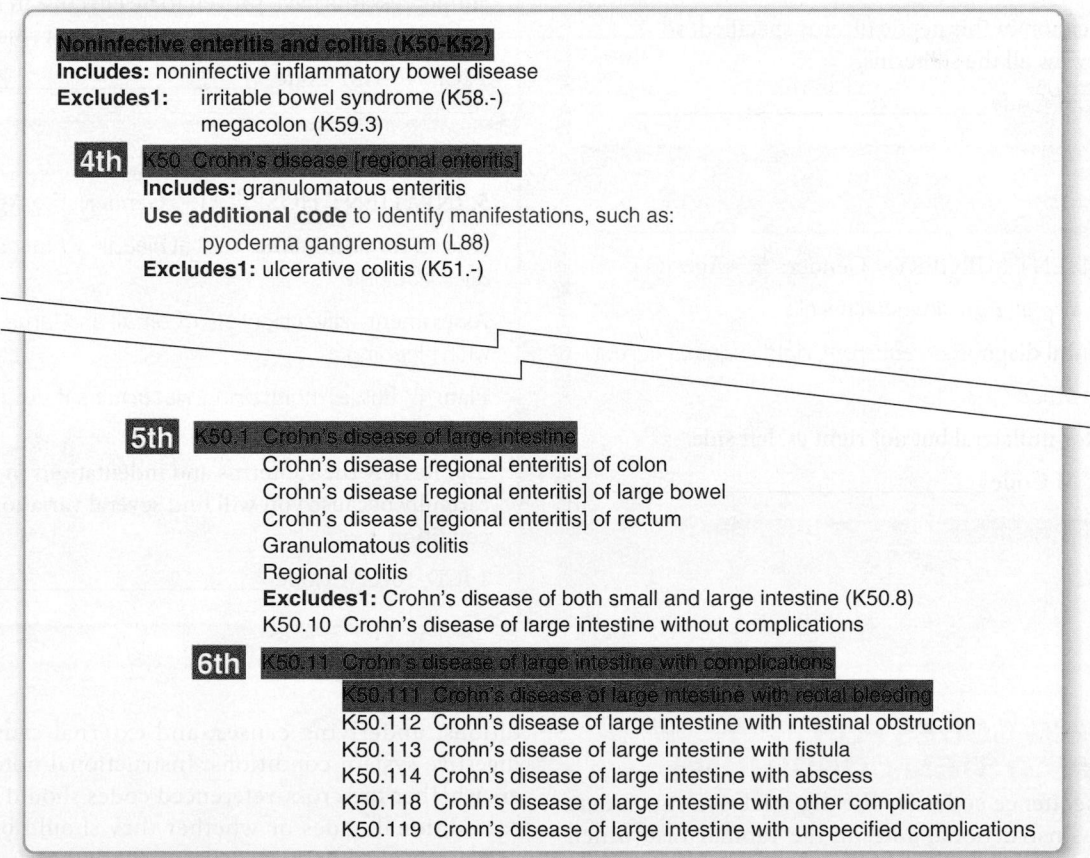

Noninfective enteritis and colitis (K50-K52)
Includes: noninfective inflammatory bowel disease
Excludes1:   irritable bowel syndrome (K58.-)
                  megacolon (K59.3)

4th   K50   Crohn's disease [regional enteritis]
Includes: granulomatous enteritis
Use additional code to identify manifestations, such as:
        pyoderma gangrenosum (L88)
Excludes1: ulcerative colitis (K51.-)

5th   K50.1   Crohn's disease of large intestine
        Crohn's disease [regional enteritis] of colon
        Crohn's disease [regional enteritis] of large bowel
        Crohn's disease [regional enteritis] of rectum
        Granulomatous colitis
        Regional colitis
        Excludes1: Crohn's disease of both small and large intestine (K50.8)
        K50.10   Crohn's disease of large intestine without complications
6th   K50.11   Crohn's disease of large intestine with complications
        K50.111   Crohn's disease of large intestine with rectal bleeding
        K50.112   Crohn's disease of large intestine with intestinal obstruction
        K50.113   Crohn's disease of large intestine with fistula
        K50.114   Crohn's disease of large intestine with abscess
        K50.118   Crohn's disease of large intestine with other complication
        K50.119   Crohn's disease of large intestine with unspecified complications

Figure 9-3 ■ Tabular List Entry for Crohn's Disease

❏ Finally, she refers to the beginning of ICD-10-CM Chapter 11 and reviews the **Excludes** notes to be sure that none of these exclusions apply to her current case.

▶ Jill is confident that she completed all verifications and cross-checks, so she assigns code **K50.111 Crohn's disease of large intestine with rectal bleeding**.

CODING PRACTICE

Exercise 9.3 Assigning Codes for Digestive System Diagnoses

Instructions: Read the mini-medical-record of each patient's encounter, review the information abstracted in Exercise 9.2 for questions 1, 2, and 3, and assign ICD-10-CM diagnosis codes using the Index and Tabular List. For questions 4 and 5, abstract the cases on your own before assigning codes. Write the code(s) on the line provided.

1. OFFICE   Gender: M   Age: 54

Chief complaint: indigestion

Assessment: chronic perforated peptic ulcer in stomach with bleeding

Plan: change diet, change Rx

Tip: The location of this peptic ulcer is specified, so carefully review all the subterms.

1 ICD-10-CM Code _____

2. OUTPATIENT SURGERY   Gender: F   Age: 61

Procedure: repair, right inguinal hernia

Postprocedural diagnosis: recurrent right inguinal hernia

Plan: FU in office

Tip: Code for unilateral but not right vs. left side.

1 ICD-10-CM Code _____

3. OFFICE   Gender: M   Age: 67

Reason for visit: FU on lower GI series

Assessment: ulcerative colitis with fistula

Plan: begin liquid diet, Rx antibiotics, FU 2 weeks

1 ICD-10-CM Code _____

4. OFFICE   Gender: M   Age: 31

Chief complaint: cramping and diarrhea for 3 days, not helped with OTC antidiarrheals

Assessment: irritable bowel syndrome with diarrhea

Plan: modify diet, Rx antidepressant

Tip: The doctor prescribed an antidepressant not because the patient was depressed, but because tricyclic antidepressants have proven to be effective in relieving stomach pain in IBS, according to current research.

1 ICD-10-CM Code _____

5. INPATIENT HOSPITAL   Gender: F   Age: 47

Reason for admission: rectal bleeding, history of diverticulosis

Assessment: diverticulitis of small and large intestines with bleeding

Plan: IV fluids, monitoring, determine if surgery is needed

Tip: Review the subterms and indentations in the Index carefully because you will find several variations of this condition.

1 ICD-10-CM Code _____

ARRANGING CODES FOR DIGESTIVE SYSTEM CONDITIONS

To correctly sequence codes for the digestive system, coders need to follow instructional notes in the Tabular List, which directs coders to assign additional codes for associated conditions, underlying causes, and external causes related to digestive system conditions. Instructional notes direct coders whether the cross-referenced codes should be sequenced as additional codes or whether they should be coded first.

■ TABLE 9-4 highlights the most common instructional notes in

Table 9-4   ■   **COMMON INSTRUCTIONAL NOTES FOR THE DIGESTIVE SYSTEM**

Use Additional Code to Identify:	Location of Note
Alcohol abuse and dependence (F10.-)	K20 Esophagitis
	K25 Gastric ulcer
	K26 Duodenal ulcer
	K27 Peptic ulcer
	K28 Gastrojejunal ulcer
	K29.0 Acute gastritis
	K29.2 Alcoholic gastritis
	K70 Alcoholic liver disease
	K86.0 Alcohol-induced chronic pancreatitis
Alcohol abuse and dependence (F10.-)	K11 Diseases of salivary glands
Exposure to environmental tobacco smoke (Z77.22)	K05 Gingivitis and periodontal diseases
Exposure to tobacco smoke in the perinatal period (P96.81)	K12 Stomatitis and related lesions
History of tobacco use (Z87.891)	K13 Other diseases of lip and oral mucosa
Occupational exposure to environmental tobacco smoke (Z57.31)	K14 Diseases of tongue
Tobacco dependence (F17.-)	
Tobacco use (Z72.0)	
Specify type of infection	K94.02 Colostomy infection
	K94.12 Enterostomy infection
	K94.22 Gastrostomy infection
	K94.32 Esophagostomy infection

the digestive system chapter and the categories where they appear. Notice that multiple coding is often required to describe lifestyle habits, such as alcohol abuse or tobacco abuse, that may contribute to digestive system conditions.

Instructional notes may appear at the beginning of the chapter, the beginning of a block or subchapter, the beginning of a three-character category, the beginning of a subcategory, or under the final code. Therefore, it is important to search for information not only directly under the code, but also at the previous levels of the classification hierarchy.

Guided Example of Arranging Digestive System Diagnosis Codes

Refer to the following new example to practice skills for sequencing codes for the digestive system. Jill Hynes, CPC, is a fictitious coder who guides you through this case. Assume that the abstracting identified an abscess of the submandibular salivary gland and current heavy tobacco use.

Date: 9/2/yy   Location: *Branton Gastroenterology*

Provider: *Stanley Garrett, MD*

Patient: *Gary Spates*   Gender: M   Age: 52

Chief complaint: *"lump and tenderness in my jaw"*

Assessment: *abscess, submandibular salivary gland, heavy current tobacco use*

Plan: *drain abscess, Rx antibiotics*

Follow along in your ICD-10-CM manual as Jill Hynes, CPC, assigns and sequences codes for this case. Check off each step after you complete it.

▶ Jill begins by locating the Main Term in the Index.

❑ Jill looks up **A, Abscess**.

❑ She locates the subterm for **salivary (duct) (gland)**.

❑ Jill confirms that there are no further subentries under **salivary** and identifies the code **K11.3** that she will verify in the Tabular List.

▶ Jill locates code **K11.3** in the Tabular List.

❑ She confirms that the code description **Abscess of salivary gland** accurately describes the diagnosis. She notes that there are no further breakdowns for the specific salivary gland affected.

❑ She reviews the instructional note at the beginning of the category **K11** (■ FIGURE 9-4), which states to **Use additional code**. As she reads the items listed, she observes that they relate to certain lifestyle habits. She knows that an instructional note at the beginning of a category applies to all of the codes in that category, so this instructional note applies to all codes from **K11.0** to **K11.9**. The fact that the tobacco use is to be an *additional* code tells her that the abscess should be sequenced first and the tobacco use should be sequenced second.

> **K11 Diseases of salivary glands**
> **Use additional code** to identify:
> alcohol abuse and dependence (F10.-)
> exposure to environmental tobacco smoke (Z77.22)
> exposure to tobacco smoke in the perinatal period (P96.81)
> history of tobacco use (Z87.891)
> occupational exposure to environmental tobacco smoke (Z57.31)
> tobacco dependence (F17.-)
> tobacco use (Z72.0)

Figure 9-4   ■   Instructional Notes for Category K11 Diseases of the Salivary Glands

► Next, Jill codes for *heavy current tobacco use*.

❑ She notices several possible code options in the instructional note:

  ▪ **history of tobacco use (Z87.891)**

  ▪ **tobacco dependence (F17.-)**

  ▪ **tobacco use (Z72.0)**

Jill recalls that even though tobacco use is part of Mr. Spates' medical history, OGCR I.C.21.c.4) states she should use **history (of)** codes only to describe a past medical condition that no longer exists. Because Mr. Spates' tobacco use is documented as *current*, she eliminates code **Z87.891, History of tobacco use**.

❑ She checks the medical record to see if Dr. Garrett stated tobacco dependence. He did not, so she eliminates code **F17.- tobacco dependence**. She knows she cannot interpret the word *heavy* to mean dependence.

❑ She identifies **Z72.0, Tobacco use** as the most appropriate code.

❑ She verifies **Z72.0** in the Tabular List and notes there are no further codes. She reviews the **Excludes1** conditions and verifies that she is on the right path because none of the conditions listed in the note were documented by Dr. Garrett.

❑ Next, Jill goes back to the original code and checks for instructional notes at the beginning of the block **Diseases of the oral cavity and salivary glands (K00-K14)**. This block has no further notes.

❑ Finally, she refers to the beginning of ICD-10-CM Chapter 11 and reviews the **Excludes** notes to be sure that none of these exclusions apply to her current case.

► Jill is confident that she completed all verifications and cross-checks. She sequences **Z72.0** second because the instructional note described it as an additional code.

► Jill finalizes the code assignment and sequencing for this case.

(1) **K11.3 Abscess of salivary gland**

(2) **Z72.0 Tobacco use**

CODING PRACTICE

Exercise 9.4 Arranging Codes for Digestive System Diagnoses

Instructions: Read the mini-medical-record of each patient's encounter, review the information abstracted in Exercise 9.2 for questions 1, 2, and 3, assign ICD-10-CM diagnosis codes using the Index and Tabular List, and sequence them correctly.

---

1. OFFICE Gender: M Age: 56

Chief complaint: *abdominal pain and bloating, fatigue, vomiting*

Assessment: *alcoholic liver cirrhosis with ascites due to alcohol addiction*

Plan: *counseled patient regarding abstinence from alcohol, reduce salt intake*

Tip: Read the instructional note at the beginning of the category to use an additional code.

2 ICD-10-CM Codes _____

---

2. OFFICE Gender: M Age: 59

Chief complaint: *hematemesis, history of cirrhosis*

Assessment: *portal hypertension (increase in blood pressure in the portal vein) with portal hypertensive gastropathy*

(continued)

---

2. (continued)

Plan: *endoscopic therapy, drug therapy, and dietary changes*

Tip: Code portal hypertension first, then follow the instructional notes to code gastropathy.

3 ICD-10-CM Codes _____

_____

---

3. OFFICE Gender: M Age: 33

Chief complaint: *redness and tenderness around colostomy site*

Assessment: *colostomy infection, cellulitis of abdominal wall due to methicillin-susceptible Staphylococcus aureus (MSSA)*

Plan: *Rx antibiotics*

Tip: Sometimes coding is like a treasure hunt. You never know where it will take you. Read the instructional notes under the code for colostomy infection to identify the second code. Read the instructional notes under the block heading for cellulitis to identify the third code.

3 ICD-10-CM Codes _____

_____

4. OFFICE Gender: M Age: 38

Chief complaint: fecal incontinence that has not improved

Assessment: nontraumatic anal sphincter tear

Plan: sphincteroplasty

Tip: Read the instructional notes under the code for nontraumatic anal sphincter tear to identify the second code.

2 ICD-10-CM Codes _____

5. OFFICE Gender: M Age: 14

Procedure: 2 dental fillings

Postprocedural diagnosis: caries (*cavities*), tooth 2 pit and fissure surface, enamel only; tooth 3 pit and fissure surface, penetrating dentin

Plan: 6-month check-up

Tip: Assign separate codes for each tooth because the depth of the caries was different on each one. Dentists identify each tooth with a number, beginning at the right rear molar on the top of the mouth.

2 ICD-10-CM Codes _____

CODING NEOPLASMS OF THE DIGESTIVE SYSTEM

Neoplasms of the digestive system do not appear in ICD-10-CM Chapter 11 (K00-K95); they appear in Chapter 02 (C00-D49). Codes for neoplasms of the digestive system appear in two different blocks within the neoplasm chapter:

- Malignant neoplasm of lip, oral cavity and pharynx (C00-C14)
- Malignant neoplasm of digestive organs (C15-C26)

Review these two blocks in the ICD-10-CM manual to become familiar with the content.

According to the Centers for Disease Control and Prevention, the most common sites for cancer in the digestive system are the colon and rectum; cancer of these sites is referred to as colorectal cancer. Colorectal cancer is the third most common cancer in the United States and, in most cases, develops slowly over many years. The number of deaths due to colorectal cancer has declined over the past 15 years, largely because fewer cases are being diagnosed. Colorectal cancer, which most often begins as a polyp, can be detected early through a colonoscopy. Cancer that is detected early is more easily treated. Colorectal cancer can be prevented through removal of polyps during a

SUCCESS STEP

Refer to the entry **intestine, large** in the Table of Neoplasms to identify more codes for colon cancer.

colonoscopy, before they have time to turn into cancer. When coding for colon cancer, determine whether the disease affects only the colon or both the colon and rectum because there are different codes, as shown in ■ FIGURE 9-5.

The liver is also a common site of cancer in the digestive system because many types of cancer metastasize to the liver. The liver filters the blood, which is one of the main ways that cancer cells move throughout the body. Most cancer found in the liver is metastatic. Primary liver cancer occurs most often in patients with cirrhosis and alcoholic liver disease. When coding for cancer in the liver, verify whether it is primary or is a metastasis.

Patients with malignant neoplasms of the esophagus, stomach, and pancreas have low survival rates because they have few symptoms and are usually not diagnosed until a late stage, when the neoplasms have already metastasized. Cancer of the gall bladder and small intestine are relatively rare.

	Malignant Primary	Malignant Secondary	Ca in situ	Benign	Uncertain Behavior	Unspecified Behavior
colon	C18.9	C78.5	-	-	-	-
- with rectum	C19	C78.5	D01.1	D12.7	D37.5	D49.0

Figure 9-5 ■ Table of Neoplasms Entry for Colon

CODING PRACTICE

Exercise 9.5 Coding Neoplasms of the Digestive System

Instructions: Read the mini-medical-record of each patient's encounter, then abstract, assign, and sequence ICD-10-CM diagnosis codes using the Index and Tabular List. Write the code(s) on the line provided.

---

1. OUTPATIENT SURGERY Gender: F Age: 57

Procedure: *screening colonoscopy due to finding of polyps 5 years ago and family history of colon cancer*

Finding: *3 new adenomatous polyps were found at the sigmoid flexure and removed*

Plan: *5-year follow-up*

Tip: Identify where the sigmoid flexure is located. Code the patient's personal history as well as the family history because both present risk factors for the patient.

3 ICD-10-CM Codes _____

_____

---

2. OFFICE Gender: F Age: 61

Reason for visit: *FU on CT scan*

Assessment: *adenocarcinoma of overlapping sites (rectum and sigmoid) of the large intestine*

Plan: *refer to oncologist*

Tip: A tumor in two sites that are adjacent (*immediately next to each other*) is considered to be overlapping.

1 ICD-10-CM Code _____

---

3. OFFICE Gender: M Age: 54

Reason for visit: *FU on liver biopsy*

Assessment: *hepatocellular cancer due to alcohol dependence and chronic hepatitis C*

Plan: *refer to oncologist for evaluation of treatment options*

Tip: Read the instructional notes in the Tabular List under the first code to identify the additional conditions that need to be coded.

3 ICD-10-CM Codes _____

_____

---

4. OFFICE Gender: F Age: 70

Reason for visit: *FU on colonoscopy results*

Assessment: *cancer in situ, rectum*

Plan: *schedule surgery, refer to oncologist for adjuvant therapy*

1 ICD-10-CM Code _____

---

5. OFFICE Gender: M Age: 68

Reason for visit: *FU on biopsy and imaging*

Assessment: *adenocarcinoma of the pancreas with liver and lymph gland metastases*

Plan: *chemotherapy, palliative care*

Tip: Code for the primary cancer and both metastatic sites.

3 ICD-10-CM Codes _____

_____

CHAPTER SUMMARY

In this chapter you learned that:

- The digestive system consists of the alimentary canal and accessory organs, which provide for ingestion, digestion, absorption, and elimination of food.
- Chapter 11 of ICD-10-CM, Diseases of the Digestive System (K00-K95), contains 10 blocks or subchapters that are divided by anatomical site.
- When abstracting for digestive system conditions, coders need to look for manifestations, complications, and associated lifestyle habits.

- Coders frequently assign combination codes to describe complications of digestive system conditions.
- To sequence codes for the digestive system, follow instructional notes in the Tabular List, which direct coders to assign additional codes for associated conditions, underlying causes, and external causes related to digestive system conditions.
- Colorectal cancer is the third most common cancer in the United States; the liver is a common site of metastases.
- There are no OGCR for the digestive system, but there are many instructional notes in the Tabular List.

CONCEPT QUIZ

Take a moment to look back at the digestive system and solidify your skills. Try to answer the questions from memory first, then refer to the discussion in this chapter and the Glossary at the end of this book if you need a little extra help.

Completion

Instructions: Write the term that answers each question based on the information you learned in this chapter. Choose from the following list. Some choices may be used more than once and some choices may not be used at all.

calculi	liver
colon	multiple coding
combination coding	pancreas
gall bladder	small intestine
instructional notes	stomach
large intestine	

1. Col/o is the combining form for _____ or
   _____.
2. Cholecyst/o is the combining form for _____.
3. Hepat/o is the combining form for _____.
4. Enter/o and ile/o are combining forms for
   _____.
5. Fund/o is the combining form for the top portion of the
   _____.
6. _____ describes more than one aspect of a condition, or multiple conditions, in a single code.
7. _____ requires that more than one code be assigned to fully describe a patient's condition.
8. _____ may appear at the beginning of the chapter, the beginning of a block or subchapter, the beginning of a three-character category, the beginning of a subcategory, or under the final code.
9. Most cancer found in the _____ is metastatic.
10. _____ is often required to describe lifestyle habits, such as alcohol abuse or tobacco use, which may contribute to digestive system conditions.

Multiple Choice

Instructions: Circle the letter of the best answer to each question based on the information you learned in this chapter.

1. All of the following are functions of the digestive system EXCEPT
   A. ingestion.
   B. absorption.
   C. circulation.
   D. elimination.

2. What structures assist in digestion but are not directly connected to the alimentary canal?
   A. Large and small intestines
   B. Accessory organs
   C. Rectum and anus
   D. Teeth

3. What condition is an abnormal immune reaction to gluten and poor absorption of nutrients?
   A. Celiac disease
   B. Crohn's disease
   C. Diverticular disease
   D. Gastroesophageal reflux disease

4. What is a barium enema?
   A. Swallowing a chalky substance and viewing it on an X-ray
   B. A group of disorders in which the intestines become red and swollen
   C. Endoscopic examination of the esophagus, stomach, and duodenum
   D. Injecting a chalky substance into the colon through the anus and viewing the organs on an X-ray

5. To what term does the Index entry for Crohn's disease cross-reference the coder?
   A. Colonitis, large
   B. Diverticulitis
   C. Intestinal obstruction
   D. Enteritis, regional

6. What does the word root chole/o mean?
   A. Colon
   B. Gall bladder
   C. Bile
   D. Vagina

7. Category K11 provides instructional notes to code which of the following?
   A. History of tobacco use
   B. Specific type of allergy
   C. Any associated fecal incontinence
   D. Viral hepatitis

8. What is MRCP?
   A. Endoscopic Ultrasound
   B. Magnetic Resonance Cholangiopancreatography
   C. Esophagogastroduodenoscopy
   D. Magnetic Resonance Imaging of Colon and Pancreas

9. Which condition is NOT classified as a disease of the digestive system?
   A. Ileus
   B. Obesity
   C. Stomatitis
   D. Hematemesis

10. What is diverticulitis?
    A. Pouches formed when the lining of the intestine pushes through the intestinal muscle layer
    B. The presence of diverticula
    C. Diversion of the colon
    D. A bacterial infection of diverticula

CODING CHALLENGE

Instructions: Read the mini-medical-record of each patient's encounter, then abstract, assign, and sequence ICD-10-CM diagnosis codes using the Index and Tabular List. Write the code(s) on the line provided.

1. EMERGENCY DEPT   Gender: M   Age: 15

Chief complaint: vomiting, acute abdominal pain, RLQ tenderness, T 101°

Assessment: acute appendicitis with rupture

Plan: laparoscopic appendectomy

1 ICD-10-CM Code _____

2. OFFICE   Gender: F   Age: 41

Reason for visit: referred by her oncologist for mouth ulcers due to chemotherapy for metastatic colon cancer (*primary colon cancer that has spread*)

Assessment: oral mucositis, side effect from chemotherapy for metastatic colon cancer

Plan: oral debridement, pain relief

Tip: First, code for the condition being treated. For the second code, read the instructional note in the Tabular List after you verify the first code. Then, code the colon cancer to identify the reason for the chemotherapy. Finally, code for unspecified metastatic sites.

4 ICD-10-CM Codes _____

_____

3. OFFICE   Gender: M   Age: 43

Chief complaint: "My hiatal hernia seems worse than usual"

Assessment: strangulated hiatal hernia

Plan: schedule hernia repair

Tip: Strangulation is classified as an obstruction.

1 ICD-10-CM Code _____

4. OFFICE   Gender: M   Age: 36

Chief complaint: "I've been having problems with my GERD"

Assessment: GERD

Plan: adjust Rx, call if problems continue

1 ICD-10-CM Code _____

5. INPATIENT HOSPITAL   Gender: F   Age: 52

Reason for admission: pain RUQ, T 102 degrees, vomiting

Procedure: laparoscopic cholecystectomy

Discharge diagnosis: acute cholecystitis with calculi in the common bile duct causing obstruction

Tip: When you search for the Main Term **Cholecystitis**, follow the cross-reference listed in the Index.

1 ICD-10-CM Code _____

6. OUTPATIENT SURGERY   Gender: M   Age: 56

Chief complaint: nausea, vomiting, constipation

Assessment: inflammatory colon polyps, intestinal obstruction

Plan: high-fiber diet and increased liquids, Rx corticosteroid to reduce inflammation, FU 2 weeks

Tip: Main Term is polyps. Thoroughly review all available subterms to locate the correct combination code.

1 ICD-10-CM Code _____

7. OFFICE   Gender: M   Age: 26

Chief complaint: yellow teeth

Assessment: amelogenesis imperfecta (*a tooth development disorder in which the teeth are covered with thin, abnormally formed enamel and are easily damaged*)

Plan: apply crowns

1 ICD-10-CM Code _____

8. EMERGENCY DEPT   Gender: M   Age: 12

Chief complaint: "My son forgot that he isn't supposed to eat eggs and ate a hardboiled egg at his friend's house. He has had diarrhea and vomiting for 4 hours and I'm getting worried."

Assessment: allergic gastroenteritis due to eggs

Plan: Rx antiemetic, antidiarrheal

2 ICD-10-CM Codes _____

9. INPATIENT HOSPITAL   Gender: F   Age: 30

Reason for admission: LUQ pain and swelling increasing over the past 3 days, indigestion

Treatment: IV fluids, pain control, nasogastric suctioning

Discharge diagnosis: acute pancreatitis due to opioid dependence and intoxication

2 ICD-10-CM Codes _____

10. INPATIENT HOSPITAL   Gender: F   Age: 41

Reason for admission: admitted from ED with severe and steady abdominal pain, fever, excessive perspiration, T 101°

Treatment: IV antibiotics, fluids, colectomy

Discharge diagnosis: generalized peritonitis due to E. coli, irritable bowel syndrome

3 ICD-10-CM Codes _____
_____

KEEP ON CODING

Instructions: Read the diagnostic statement, then use the Index and Tabular List to assign and sequence ICD-10-CM diagnosis codes. Write the code(s) on the line provided.

1. Carcinoma of the buccal mucosa: ICD-10-CM Code(s) _____

2. Erosion of teeth due to diet: ICD-10-CM Code(s) _____

3. Enterostomy hemorrhage: ICD-10-CM Code(s) _____

4. Cyst of pancreas: ICD-10-CM Code(s) _____

5. Mucous retention cyst of salivary gland: ICD-10-CM Code(s) _____

6. Cardiospasm: ICD-10-CM Code(s) _____

7. Malignant neoplasm of tongue with a history of tobacco use: ICD-10-CM Code(s) _____

8. Hydrops of the gall bladder: ICD-10-CM Code(s) _____

9. Acute gingivitis, plaque induced: ICD-10-CM Code(s) _____

10. Eosinophilic esophagitis: ICD-10-CM Code(s) _____

11. Hairy leukoplakia: ICD-10-CM Code(s) _____

12. Incisional hernia without obstruction or gangrene: ICD-10-CM Code(s) _____

13. Acute appendicitis with localized peritonitis: ICD-10-CM Code(s) _____

14. Ulcerative pancolitis and abscess: ICD-10-CM Code(s) _____

15. Stage 3 hemorrhoids: ICD-10-CM Code(s) _____

(*continued*)

(continued from page 139)

16. Slow-transit constipation: ICD-10-CM Code(s) _____

17. Chronic cholecystitis with cholelithiasis without obstruction: ICD-10-CM Code(s) _____

18. Postprocedural liver failure: ICD-10-CM Code(s) _____

19. Cheilosis: ICD-10-CM Code(s) _____

20. Esophageal ulcer with bleeding: ICD-10-CM Code(s) _____

21. Retained dental root: ICD-10-CM Code(s) _____

22. Glossodynia: ICD-10-CM Code(s) _____

23. Alcoholic cirrhosis of liver with ascites: ICD-10-CM Code(s) _____

24. Malignant neoplasm of overlapping sections of the esophagus: ICD-10-CM Code(s) _____

25. Hemoperitoneum: ICD-10-CM Code(s) _____

Endocrine, Nutritional, and Metabolic Diseases (E00-E89)

Chapter 10

Learning Objectives

After completing this chapter, you should have the skills to:

10.1 Spell and define the key words, medical terms, and abbreviations related to endocrine, nutritional, and metabolic diseases.

10.2 Discuss the structure, function, and common conditions of the endocrine system.

10.3 Identify the main characteristics of coding for endocrine, nutritional, and metabolic diseases.

10.4 Abstract diagnostic information from the medical record for coding endocrine, nutritional, and metabolic diseases.

10.5 Assign codes for endocrine, nutritional, and metabolic diseases and related conditions.

10.6 Arrange codes for endocrine, nutritional, and metabolic diseases and related conditions.

10.7 Code neoplasms of the endocrine system.

10.8 Discuss the Official Guidelines for Coding and Reporting related to endocrine, nutritional, and metabolic diseases.

Chapter Outline

- **Endocrine System Refresher**
- **Coding Overview of the Endocrine System**
- **Abstracting for Endocrine System Conditions**
- **Assigning Codes for Endocrine System Conditions**
- **Arranging Codes for Endocrine System Conditions**
- **Coding Neoplasms of the Endocrine System**

Key Terms and Abbreviations

causal relationship	hormones	hypoglycemia	target organ
diabetes mellitus (DM)	hyperglycemia	metabolism	trachea
diabetic ketoacidosis (DKA)	hyperosmolarity hyperglycemic nonketotic syndrome (HHNS)	serum assay	
endocrine system			
HbA1c			

In addition to the key terms listed here, students should know the terms defined within tables in this chapter.

INTRODUCTION

When your vehicle gets a little sluggish, you may decide to use a fuel additive to boost its performance. Your body's hormones are, in a sense, like fuel additives for your car. They perform a variety of tasks that keep other organ systems and structures working smoothly. It is the endocrine system's job to produce, store, and release hormones.

An endocrinologist is a physician who specializes in endocrine, nutritional, and metabolic diseases. When primary care physicians (PCPs) are unable to diagnose or manage a complex endocrine, nutritional, or metabolic condition, they refer the patient to an endocrinologist.

As you read this chapter, open up your medical terminology book and keep a medical dictionary handy to refresh your memory of any unfamiliar terms.

ENDOCRINE SYSTEM REFRESHER

The function of the **endocrine system** is to produce, store, and release **hormones**, which are chemical messengers. Hormones regulate many body functions including growth, development, **metabolism** (*the processes of digestion, elimination, breathing, blood circulation, and maintaining body temperature*), sexual function, reproduction, and mood. The endocrine system consists of several ductless glands that are not directly connected to each other (■ FIGURE 10-1). The function of each gland is summarized in ■ TABLE 10-1. The ovaries and testes function as part of the reproductive system in addition to their endocrine function; the pancreas has an **exocrine** function in the digestive system in addition to its endocrine function.

In Figure 10-1, each structure in the endocrine system is labeled with its name, as well as its medical terminology root/combining form. Refer to ■ TABLE 10-2 for a refresher on how to build medical terms related to the endocrine system.

CODING CAUTION

Be alert for medical terms that are spelled similarly and have different meanings.

ne<u>phr</u>opathy (*kidney disease*) and **ne<u>ur</u>opathy** (*nerve disease*)

hyp<u>o</u>thyroidism (*state of low thyroid function*) and **hyp<u>er</u>thyroidism** (*state of high thyroid function*)

thyr/o (*thyroid*), **thy<u>m</u>/o** (*thymus gland*), and **th<u>al</u>am/o** (*thalamus, a portion of the brain*)

Conditions of the Endocrine System

Endocrine, nutritional, and metabolic disorders tend to have gradual onsets and generalized symptoms such as fatigue, weakness, weight change, hair loss, muscle weakness, nervousness, appetite change, and irritability, making them difficult to diagnose. When a structure in the endocrine system malfunctions, the result is either hypofunction or hyperfunction of a gland, a hormone, or a **target organ** (*the organ receiving hormones*).

Endocrine disorders are best diagnosed through **serum assays** (*lab tests that measure the presence and quantity of a substance in the blood*). Common treatments include injection of

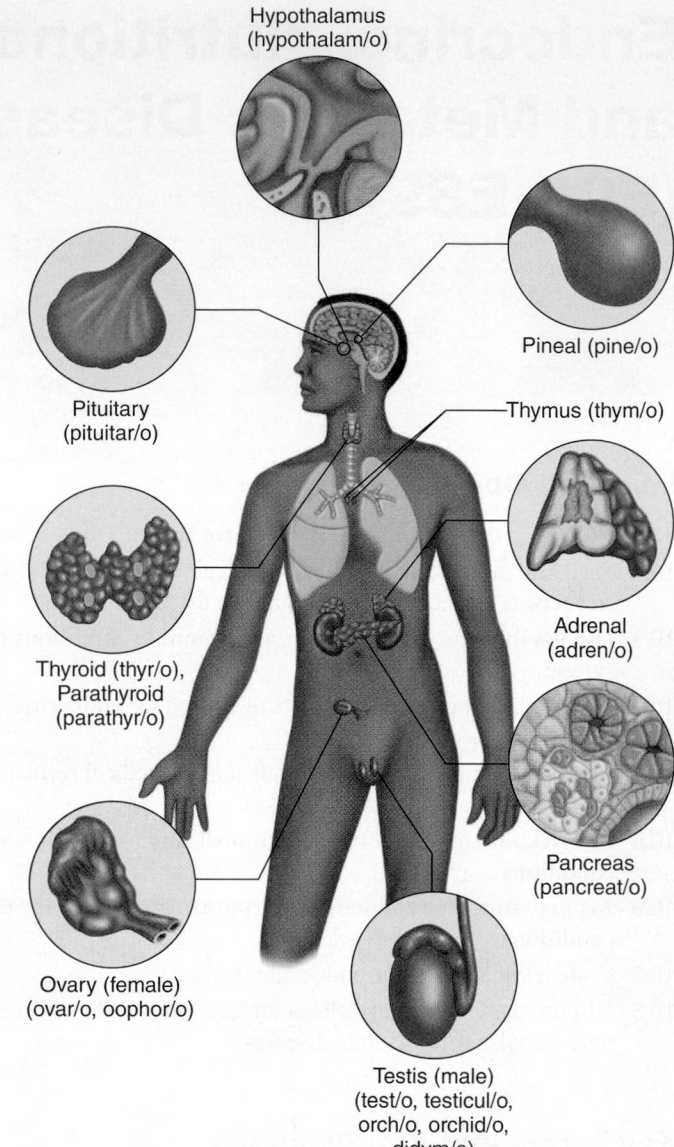

Figure 10-1 ■ The Endocrine System

Table 10-1 ■ FUNCTION OF ENDOCRINE GLANDS

Gland	Endocrine Function
Pituitary	Controls most activity in the endocrine system
Hypothalamus	Controls the pituitary gland
Pineal	Regulates waking/sleeping functions
Thymus	Produces T-cells used by the immune system
Thyroid	Regulates metabolism
Parathyroid	Regulates the level of circulating calcium
Pancreas (Islets of Langerhans)	Synthesis, storage, and release of **glucagon** and **insulin**
Adrenal	Secretes steroid hormones
Ovaries/testes (gonads)	Secrete estrogen and testosterone

Table 10-2 ■ EXAMPLE OF CONSTRUCTING MEDICAL TERMS FOR THE ENDOCRINE SYSTEM

Prefix	Combining Form	Suffix	Complete Medical Term
hypo- (below, low) **hyper-** (above, high)	**glyc/o** (sugar)	**-emia** (condition of the blood) **-uria** (condition of the urine) **-ism** (state of)	**hypo + glyc + emia** (low sugar in the blood) **hyper + glyc + emia** (excessive sugar in the blood) **glyco + uria** (sugar in the urine)
	thyr/o (thyroid)		**hypo + thyroid + ism** (state of low thyroid function) **hyper + thyroid + ism** (state of high thyroid function)
	protein/o (protein)		**protein + emia** (protein in the blood) **protein + uria** (protein in the urine)

hormones, surgical removal of all or part of a gland, and surgical removal of a tumor that is causing the problem.

The most common diseases of the endocrine system are **diabetes mellitus (DM)** and thyroid disorders. These conditions present concepts and terminology that coders must be familiar with.

Diabetes Mellitus

Diabetes mellitus is a condition resulting in elevated glucose levels over an extended period of time and excess excretion of urine, usually due to malfunction of the pancreas. Coders need to be familiar with several types of diabetes, which are highlighted in ■ TABLE 10-3. According to the National Diabetes Association, diabetes affects more than 8% of the population or nearly 26 million people, and an additional 79 million people are estimated to have **prediabetes**.

Diabetes causes both acute and chronic complications. Acute complications consist of the following:

- **Hyperglycemia** is the condition of severely elevated blood glucose levels, usually occurring in type 1 diabetics, due to a lack or deficiency of insulin. Hyperglycemia can cause **diabetic ketoacidosis (DKA)** in which a high level of ketones (*a chemical made when the body breaks down fat into energy*) accumulate in the blood, turning it acidic. Symptoms include nausea, vomiting, abdominal pain, shock, coma, and death, if it is not treated immediately.

- **Hyperosmolarity hyperglycemic nonketotic syndrome (HHNS)** is elevated glucose without ketoacidosis, usually occurring in elderly type 2 diabetics with other conditions, and can result in hyperosmolar coma and death.

- **Hypoglycemia** is abnormally low blood glucose, often due to excessive use of insulin or other glucose-lowering medications. Symptoms are dizziness, confusion, weakness, tremors, seizures, coma, and brain death.

SUCCESS STEP

Diabetes mellitus literally means *sweet urine disease*. The word *diabetes* is based on the Greek word meaning *siphon*. Aretus the Cappadocian, a second-century physician, described patients as having polyuria and passing water like a siphon. In 1675, Thomas Willis, the father of modern neuroscience, added *mellitus* because *mel* is the Latin word for *honey* or *sweetness*.

Table 10-3 ■ OVERVIEW OF DIABETES MELLITUS

Type of Diabetes	Description	Treatment	Frequency
Type 1 Diabetes Mellitus (previously called insulin-dependent diabetes mellitus [IDDM] or juvenile-onset diabetes)	Body's immune system attacks pancreatic beta cells so that the pancreas does not produce insulin.	No prevention or cure known. Patients *must* receive insulin, delivered through injection or pump, to survive.	5% of all diagnosed cases of diabetes
Type 2 Diabetes Mellitus (previously called non–insulin-dependent diabetes mellitus [NIDDM] or adult-onset diabetes)	Pancreas produces insulin, but the body does not use it properly. In some cases, insulin production is decreased also.	Prevent, delay, or reverse the onset of type 2 diabetes with weight loss, increased physical activity, and the medication metformin. Some people *may* need insulin.	90% to 95% of all diagnosed cases of diabetes
Secondary Diabetes Mellitus	Elevated glucose is caused by an external factor, such as medication, surgery, pancreatic disease, or other illness.	Treat underlying cause if possible. Manage with diet, exercise, medication, and insulin, as needed.	1% to 5% of all diagnosed cases of diabetes
Gestational Diabetes Mellitus (GDM) (Note: Gestational diabetes is coded under the reproductive system, not the endocrine system.)	Elevated glucose is diagnosed during pregnancy in women with no history of diabetes.	Must control the condition quickly to prevent adverse effects on baby. Manage with diet, exercise, and sometimes insulin.	2% to 10% of pregnant women. Using recently updated diagnostic criteria, the rate is expected to increase to 18% of pregnancies.

Table 10-4 ■ **COMMON THYROID DISORDERS**

Condition	Description	Treatment
Graves disease (diffuse toxic goiter)	Overproduction by the thyroid gland due to an **autoimmune** condition in which autoantibodies are directed against the thyroid-stimulating hormone (TSH) receptor.	Disable the thyroid gland's ability to produce hormones through radioactive iodine and/or antithyroid drugs, beta blockers, thyroidectomy.
Hyperthyroidism	Inappropriately elevated thyroid function.	Antithyroid medications (methimazole and propylthiouracil [PTU])
Hypothyroidism	Deficiency of thyroid hormone, usually due to lack of production of the hormone by the thyroid or inadequate secretion of hormones by the pituitary gland or hypothalamus.	Administer supplemental TSH and thyroxine (T4).
Nontoxic goiter	Enlargement of the thyroid that is not associated with overproduction of thyroid hormone or malignancy.	Supplemental thyroid hormone, thyroidectomy
Thyrotoxicosis (thyroid storm)	Excessive quantities of circulating thyroid hormone due to overproduction by the thyroid gland, overproduction originating outside the thyroid, or loss of storage function and leakage from the gland.	Cardiac monitor, supplemental oxygen, aggressive hydration, cooling measures, electrolyte replacement, antithyroid medications

Chronic complications of diabetes can affect nearly every organ system. The most frequent organ systems affected are the following:

- eye (cataracts, blindness)
- urinary (**nephropathy**, kidney failure)
- nervous (**neuropathy**)
- circulatory (**gangrene**, stroke, hypertension, **peripheral artery disease [PAD]**).

Thyroid Disorders

The thyroid is a butterfly-shaped gland in front of the **trachea** (*windpipe*) that produces two hormones, tri-iodothyronine (T3) and thyroxine (T4), that regulate how the body breaks down food and uses or stores energy.

■ TABLE 10-4 summarizes the most common thyroid disorders with which coders need to be familiar.

CODING PRACTICE

Exercise 10.1 Endocrine System Refresher

Instructions: Use your medical terminology skills and resources to define the following terms related to the endocrine system, then assign the diagnosis code.

Follow these steps:

- Use slash marks "/" to break down each term into its root(s) and suffix.
- Define the meaning of the word, based on the meaning of each word part.
- Assign the default ICD-10-CM diagnosis code for the condition using the Index and Tabular List.

Example: hyperthyroidism hyper/thyroid/ism   Meaning: *pertaining to excessive thyroid*   ICD-10-CM Code: *E05.90*

1. thyrotoxicosis   Meaning _____   ICD-10-CM Code _____
2. adrenalitis   Meaning _____   ICD-10-CM Code _____
3. thyromegaly   Meaning _____   ICD-10-CM Code _____
4. thyroiditis   Meaning _____   ICD-10-CM Code _____
5. hyperglycemia   Meaning _____   ICD-10-CM Code _____
6. hyperlipidemia   Meaning _____   ICD-10-CM Code _____
7. panhypopituitarism   Meaning _____   ICD-10-CM Code _____
8. parathyroid tetany   Meaning _____   ICD-10-CM Code _____
9. hypoparathyroidism   Meaning _____   ICD-10-CM Code _____
10. acromegaly   Meaning _____   ICD-10-CM Code _____

CODING OVERVIEW OF THE ENDOCRINE SYSTEM

ICD-10-CM Chapter 4, Endocrine, Nutritional, and Metabolic Diseases (E00-E89), contains 10 blocks or subchapters that are divided by anatomical site and type of disorder. Review the block names and code ranges listed at the beginning of Chapter 4 in the ICD-10-CM manual to become familiar with the content and organization.

ICD-10-CM Chapter 4 corresponds with ICD-9-CM Chapter 3 (240–279). Diabetes mellitus occupies five categories divided by etiology, including a new category for drug-induced diabetes. In ICD-10-CM, combination codes identify the type of diabetes and manifestations, reducing the need for multiple coding of this common condition, as required in ICD-9-CM.

In addition to the most common conditions of diabetes and thyroid disorders, this ICD-10-CM chapter also classifies other endocrine system conditions, including the following:

- dysfunction of other endocrine glands, such as adrenal, pituitary, and parathyroid
- endocrine-related disorders of glands that serve multiple systems, such as the pancreas, ovaries, and testes
- nutritional disorders, such as malnutrition and deficiencies of specific vitamins and nutrients
- obesity
- disorders of metabolism, such as electrolyte imbalances and the body's inability to properly utilize sugar, fat, or copper

ICD-10-CM provides Official Guidelines for Coding and Reporting (OGCR) for endocrine, nutritional, and metabolic diseases in OGCR section I.C.4. OGCR provides detailed guidance regarding assigning and sequencing codes for diabetes mellitus and secondary diabetes mellitus.

SUCCESS STEP

ICD-9-CM classified gout and osteomalacia with diseases of the endocrine system. However, medical science now considers them to be musculoskeletal diseases, so codes for gout and osteomalacia now appear in ICD-10-CM Chapter 13, Diseases of the Musculoskeletal System.

ABSTRACTING FOR ENDOCRINE SYSTEM CONDITIONS

To abstract diagnoses for endocrine system conditions, coders must distinguish between integral symptoms and signs as opposed to the conditions, complications, and manifestations.

Keep in mind that any diagnosis must be documented by the physician; do not assign a diagnosis based only on test results. Physicians consider a variety of factors, in addition to test results, to establish a diagnosis. They may evaluate a trend of test results over a period of time, order other tests or imaging, or

Table 10-5 ■ KEY CRITERIA FOR ABSTRACTING DIABETES MELLITUS

- ❑ What type of diabetes is documented?
- ❑ Are coexisting conditions documented as related to diabetes?
- ❑ What acute complications are documented?
- ❑ What chronic complications are documented?
- ❑ If secondary DM is documented, what is the cause?
- ❑ If either type 2 or secondary DM is documented, is insulin used on a long-term basis?
- ❑ Is a family history of DM documented?
- ❑ Which problem or complication is the reason for the encounter?

---

receive an evaluation from a specialist. For example, a patient may have a test result of hyperglycemia but not be diagnosed as diabetic until the result recurs several times over a period of months and additional tests, such as HbA1c (*a blood test that measures glucose attached to hemoglobin*) or a **glucose tolerance test (GTT)**, are evaluated.

Abstracting for Diabetes Mellitus

When coders learn how to accurately abstract for diabetes mellitus, they learn detailed skills that serve them well when abstracting many other conditions as well. In addition, diabetes is a commonly coded condition because patients with diabetes tend to have complications necessitating frequent medical care. ■ TABLE 10-5 lists key criteria for abstracting diabetes. Remember that abstracting questions are a general guide and that not all questions apply to every case. For example, not every patient has both acute and chronic complications.

Do not assume that all conditions documented are complications of diabetes. The specific words the physician uses in documentation indicate whether there is a **causal relationship** (*one disease being caused by another*). For example, cataracts may be a complication of diabetes or they may be unrelated. When physicians document *diabetic cataracts*, where *diabetic* is a modifier of cataract, they mean that the cataracts are *caused by* diabetes. When they document *age-related cataracts*, the cataracts are a result of aging and should not be identified as a complication of diabetes, even if the patient also has diabetes.

Similarly, physicians document a condition with the use of *secondary to, due to, with,* or *in,* when they are indicating causality. When physicians document a condition with the use of *and,* the conditions are unrelated. When a physician's documentation is unclear, it is important to query the physician for clarification.

These distinctions are critical when assigning codes. Conditions that arise due to diabetes usually are assigned a combination code describing both conditions. Conditions that are unrelated are assigned separate codes. Refer to ■ TABLE 10-6 (page 146) for examples of how physicians document related and unrelated conditions and how they are coded differently.

Table 10-6 ■ **EXAMPLES OF DOCUMENTATION AND CODING FOR RELATED AND UNRELATED CONDITIONS**

Related Conditions	Unrelated Conditions
Diabetes type 1 with cataract **E10.36 Type 1 diabetes mellitus with diabetic cataract**	Age-related cataracts. Diabetes type 1 **H25.9 Unspecified age-related cataract** **E10.9 Type 1 diabetes mellitus without complications**
Diabetic peripheral neuropathy **E11.40 Type 2 diabetes mellitus with diabetic neuropathy, unspecified**	Diabetes type 2. Peripheral neuropathy **E11.9 Type 2 diabetes mellitus without complications** **G62.9 Polyneuropathy, unspecified**
Secondary diabetes due to chronic pancreatitis with diabetic gastroparesis **K86.1 Other chronic pancreatitis** **E08.43 Diabetes mellitus due to underlying condition with diabetic autonomic (poly)neuropathy** **K31.84 Gastroparesis**	Diabetes type 2 and gastroparesis **E11.9 Type 2 diabetes mellitus without complications** **K31.84 Gastroparesis**

CODING CAUTION

Remember that *type 2* diabetes and *secondary* diabetes are different conditions. In type 2 diabetes, elevated glucose is due to the body's inability to store or release insulin. In secondary diabetes, elevated glucose is caused by an underlying condition or medication. Type 2 and secondary diabetes are identified with different codes.

Abstracting for Thyroid Disorders

When abstracting for thyroid disorders, coders must identify the cause of the condition and whether **goiter** or thyrotoxicosis is documented. The presence of these complications will affect code assignment later. Some thyroid conditions are **congenital**, so this information should also be noted. ■ TABLE 10-7 lists key criteria for abstracting thyroid disorders.

Guided Example of Abstracting Diagnoses for the Endocrine System

Refer to the following example throughout the chapter to practice skills for abstracting and assigning codes for the endocrine system. Tamara Brownlee, CCS-P, is a fictitious coder who guides you through the coding process.

Table 10-7 ■ **KEY CRITERIA FOR ABSTRACTING THYROID DISORDERS**

❑ Is the condition hyperthyroidism or hypothyroidism?

❑ What is the cause of the condition?

❑ Is the condition congenital?

❑ Is goiter documented?

❑ Is thyrotoxicosis crisis documented?

Date: 10/1/yy   Location: Branton Medical Center

Provider: Ann Trull, MD

Patient: Justin Kraft   Gender: M   Age: 12

Reason for admission: hyperglycemia, ketoacidosis, glycosuria, family history (mother and grandmother) of type 1 diabetes

Tests: glucose tolerance test (GTT) positive for diabetes. Abdominal x-ray and CT of pancreas are normal.

Discharge diagnosis: new-onset type 1 diabetes

Discharge plan: insulin injections bid (twice a day), FU office 2 weeks

---

Follow along in your ICD-10-CM manual as Tamara Brownlee, CCS-P, abstracts the diagnosis. Check off each step after you complete it.

▶ Tamara reads the entire medical record and refers to Key Criteria for Abstracting Diabetes Mellitus (Table 10-5).

❑ *What type of diabetes is documented?* new-onset type 1 diabetes

❑ *Are coexisting conditions documented as related to diabetes?* Tamara notes the symptoms documented under Reason for admission.
- She identifies that hyperglycemia and glycosuria are integral to type 1 diabetes and should not be coded in addition to the disease (OGCR II.A).

❑ *What acute complications are documented?* She identifies that ketoacidosis is an acute complication that should be coded in addition to type 1 diabetes.

❑ *Is a family history of DM documented?* She identifies that family history of type 1 diabetes is significant because it poses a risk factor for the patient (OGCR I.C.21.c.4)).

❑ *Which problem or complication is the reason for the encounter?* She identifies that type 1 diabetes is the principal diagnosis, the **condition established after study to be chiefly responsible for occasioning the admission of the patient to the hospital for care** (OGCR II).

▶ Next, Tamara needs to assign codes.

CODING PRACTICE

Exercise 10.2 Abstracting for Endocrine System Conditions

Instructions: Read the mini-medical-record of each patient's encounter and answer the abstracting questions. Write the answer on the line provided. Do not assign any codes.

---

1. OFFICE   Gender: M   **Age:** 56

Reason for encounter: monitoring of diabetes

Assessment: type 2 diabetes

Plan: HbA1c level is a little high. Discussed further diet management and exercise to better manage glucose

a. What is the reason for the encounter? _____

_____

b. What type of diabetes does the patient have?

_____

c. What complications are documented? _____

_____

d. What other conditions exist? _____

_____

---

2. OFFICE   Gender: M   **Age:** 62

Chief complaint: open sore on right heel

Assessment: Patient has developed a foot ulcer with skin breakdown due to type 2 diabetes.

Plan: Refer to wound care.

a. What is the reason for the encounter? _____

_____

b. What type of diabetes does the patient have?

_____

c. What complications are documented? _____

_____

d. Where is the ulcer located? _____

_____

e. What is the extent of damage due to the ulcer?

_____

---

3. INPATIENT HOSPITAL   Gender: F   **Age:** 58

Reason for admission: Admitted from emergency department due to weakness, shortness of breath, and severe abdominal pain with vomiting. Patient forgot to take insulin before going out to dinner.

(continued)

---

3. (continued)

Assessment: DKA, type 1 DM

a. What is the reason for the encounter? _____

_____

b. What type of diabetes does the patient have?

_____

c. What complications are documented? _____

_____

d. What symptoms did the patient present with?

_____

e. Should the symptoms be coded? _____

   Why or why not? _____

f. Should long-term use of insulin be coded? _____

   Why or why not? _____

_____

---

4. INPATIENT HOSPITAL   Gender: F   **Age:** 36

Reason for admission: insulin-induced hypoglycemia

Assessment: Patient has chronic pancreatitis for 2 years with secondary diabetes. Patient has struggled to monitor and self-administer insulin correctly.

Plan: Prescribe insulin pump. FU in office.

a. What is the reason for the encounter? _____

_____

b. What type of diabetes does the patient have?

_____

c. What complications are documented? _____

_____

d. What other conditions exist? _____

_____

e. Should long-term use of insulin be coded? Why or why not? _____

f. What Main Term should you look under in the Index to locate long-term use of insulin?

_____

g. What is the principal diagnosis? _____

   Why? _____

(continued)

CODING PRACTICE *(continued)*

5. OFFICE Gender: F Age: 65

Reason for encounter: *management of longstanding neuropathy*

Assessment: *peripheral autonomic neuropathy, type 2 diabetes*

Plan: *FU 6 months*

a. What is the reason for the encounter? _____
_____

b. What type of diabetes does the patient have?
_____

c. Is the neuropathy related to the diabetes?
_____

   Why or why not? _____

d. What is the first-listed diagnosis? _____

e. What is the additional diagnosis? _____

6. OFFICE Gender: M Age: 25

Reason for encounter: *follow up on test results after evaluation of proximal muscle weakness, easy bruising, weight gain*

Assessment: *endogenous Cushing syndrome due to pituitary adenoma*

Plan: *evaluate for surgery to remove tumor*

a. What is the reason for the encounter? _____
_____

b. What are the symptoms? _____
_____

c. Should the symptoms be coded? _____
   Why or why not? _____

d. Is the adenoma malignant or benign? _____
   Why? _____

e. What is the first-listed diagnosis? _____

f. What is the cause of the first-listed diagnosis?
_____

g. What is the additional diagnosis? _____

ASSIGNING CODES FOR ENDOCRINE SYSTEM CONDITIONS

When assigning codes for the endocrine system, carefully review the information abstracted from the medical record and determine whether the condition is the primary condition or the result of a disease or condition in another body system. This information will affect what codes to assign and how to sequence them. Special attention to the Index is required. Diabetes is used as an example of assigning codes to endocrine system disorders.

Because diabetes has many variations and complications, coders must be especially careful to follow indented subterms in the Index. The Main Term **Diabetes** has only a few first-level subterm entries, each of which have second- and third-level indented subterms that are used as follows:

- First-level subterms identify the type of diabetes.
- Second-level subterms identify that complications are present through the word **with**.
- Third-level subterms identify the specific complication(s) with each type of diabetes.

The exception is when the type of diabetes is not specified. In this case, the complications are listed directly under the Main Term entry, following the indented subterm **with**. Notice that these are the same codes as **Diabetes, type 2**

because OGCR directs coders to assign **type 2 diabetes** when the specific type is not documented in the medical record (OGCR I.C.4.a.2)). When the type of diabetes is specified, search for the corresponding first-level subterm before locating the complication.

CODING CAUTION

Selecting the correct *first-level subterm* is critical in order to arrive at the correct code because each type of diabetes can have similar complications. Consequently, the same second- and third-level indented terms appear under each different type of diabetes, but with different codes, which are determined by the first-level subterm.

Refer to ■ FIGURE 10-2 for an abbreviated view of the Index entry **Diabetes**. Selected subterms are shown. Review the first-level subterms and notice that each identifies a different type of diabetes, such as **due to drug or chemical** or **due to underlying condition**. All first-level subterms have the same second- and third-level subterms, **amyotrophy** and **arthropathy**. Each instance of **amyotrophy** and **arthropathy** has a different code because it is a combination code of the manifestation *and* the type of diabetes it is indented under.

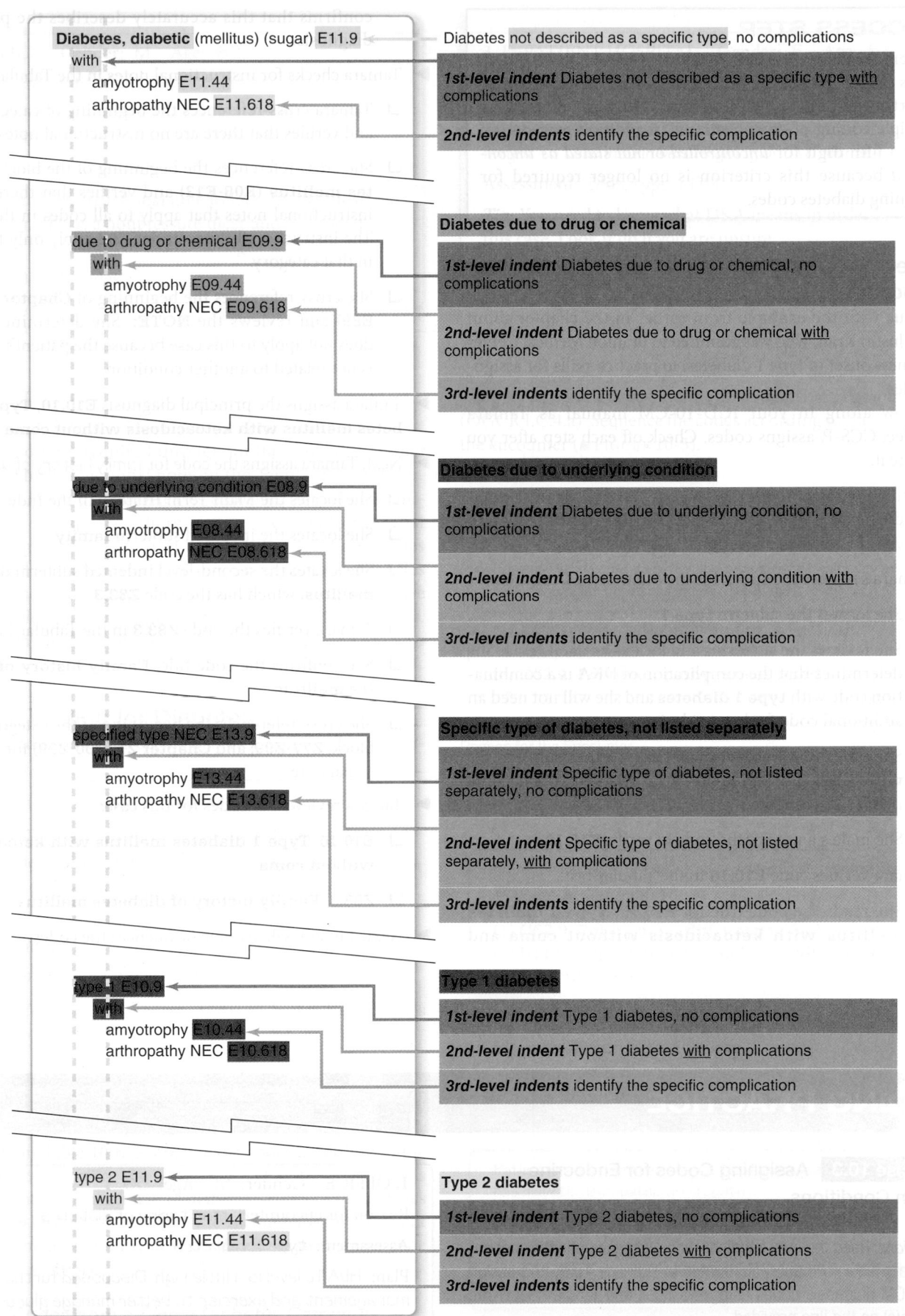

Figure 10-2 ■ Index Entry for Diabetes Showing Structure of Subterms

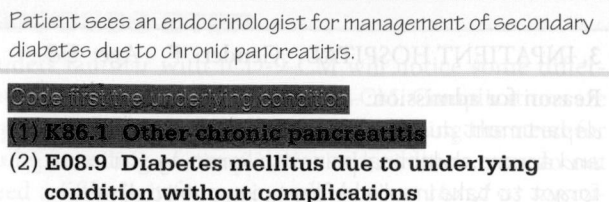

Patient sees an endocrinologist for management of secondary diabetes due to chronic pancreatitis.

Code first the underlying condition

(1) **K86.1 Other chronic pancreatitis**

(2) **E08.9 Diabetes mellitus due to underlying condition without complications**

Figure 10-6 ■ Example of Sequencing the Underlying Condition

Patient with type 2 diabetes and diabetic nephropathy sees a nephrologist for management of kidney disease. Patient uses insulin to manage the diabetes.

Use additional code to identify any insulin use (Z79.4)

(1) **E11.21 Type 2 diabetes mellitus with diabetic nephropathy**

(2) **Z79.4 Long term (current) use of insulin**

Figure 10-8 ■ Example of Sequencing Long-Term Use of Insulin

Multiple Codes for Complications

Although all diabetic complications are assigned combination codes from the block **Diabetes mellitus (E00-E13)**, some complications also require codes from other body system chapters to provide additional details. Instructional notes at the beginning of the three-digit category direct the coder and include the following:

- Code first the underlying condition for secondary diabetes.
- Code first the drug or chemical causing secondary diabetes.
- Use an additional code to identify the stage of chronic kidney disease.
- Use an additional code to identify the site of skin ulcer.
- Use an additional code to identify a complication not listed.

For secondary diabetes, sequence the underlying cause first, such as the underlying condition or the drug causing the diabetic reaction. Sequence the code for secondary diabetes as an additional code (OGCR I.C.4.a.6)(b)). The instructional note in the Tabular List indicates this with the words **Code first underlying condition** or **Code first drug or chemical** (■ Figure 10-6).

When assigning multiple codes to describe additional details about a complication, sequence the code for diabetes first and the additional codes for the details about the complication second. The instructional note in the Tabular List indicates this with the words **Use additional code to identify** (■ Figure 10-7).

Multiple Codes for Long-term Use of Insulin

Multiple coding is required to identify long-term insulin use by type 2 diabetics and patients with secondary diabetes. According to the American Diabetic Association, approximately 20% to 25% of type 2 and secondary diabetics require insulin on a continuing basis. Instructional notes in the Tabular List direct coders to use **Z79.4 Long term (current) use of insulin** to identify long-term insulin use by these patients. Do not assign this code if insulin is given temporarily to bring a type 2 patient's blood glucose under control during an encounter (OGCR I.C.4.a.3)) and (OGCR I.C.4.a.6)(a)). Sequence the diabetes code first and the **Z** code second (■ Figure 10-8).

SUCCESS STEP

Because all type 1 diabetics must use insulin, **Z79.4** is not required and should not be reported with a diagnosis of type 1 diabetes.

Multiple Coding for Complications Due to Insulin Pump Malfunction

Diabetic patients may wear an insulin pump to regulate insulin evenly and avoid self-administering injections. Underdosing or overdosing of insulin due to insulin pump failure is reported with two codes from ICD-10-CM Chapter 19 Injury, Poisoning and Certain Other Consequences of External Causes (S00-T88) to describe the pump failure and the resulting problem (OGCR I.C.4.a.5)). Also assign codes for the type of diabetes and any related complications (■ Figure 10-9).

Multiple Conditions with Multiple Codes

Because diabetes is such a complicated disease, it is not uncommon for coders to encounter cases where several multiple coding situations must be addressed at the same time (■ Figure 10-10).

Multiple Coding for Other Endocrine System Conditions

Coders must always be alert for instructional notes in the Tabular List that direct them to assign more than one code.

Patient with type 1 diabetes sees wound care for a diabetic foot ulcer with muscle necrosis on the heel of the left foot.

(1) **E10.621 Type 1 diabetes mellitus with foot ulcer**

Use additional code to identify site of ulcer (L97.4-, L97.5-)

(2) **L97.423 Non-pressure chronic ulcer of left heel and midfoot with necrosis of muscle**

Figure 10-7 ■ Example of Sequencing Details of a Complication

> Patient is seen in the emergency department for ketoacidosis due to the failure of her insulin pump and underdosing. She has type 1 diabetes and moderate nonproliferative diabetic retinopathy.
>
> (1) **T85.614A Breakdown (mechanical) of insulin pump, initial encounter**
> (2) **T38.3X6A, Underdosing of insulin and oral hypoglycemic [antidiabetic] drugs, initial encounter**
> (3) **E10.10 Type 1 diabetes mellitus with ketoacidosis without coma**
> (4) **E10.339 Type 1 diabetes mellitus with moderate nonproliferative diabetic retinopathy without macular edema**

Figure 10-9 ■ Example of Sequencing Complications from Insulin Pump Failure

Remember to refer to the beginning of the category and block for instructions when assigning codes from the endocrine system. Common situations in this chapter include the following examples and instructional notes.

1. Assign applicable codes from ICD-10-CM Chapter 4 for complications related to neoplasms or other conditions. Example:

   See NOTE: at beginning of Chapter 4.

2. Sequence codes from this chapter as additional codes when they are a manifestation of a disease in a different body system. Example:

   1) **A50.59 Other late congenital syphilis, symptomatic**

   2) **E35 Disorders of endocrine glands in diseases classified elsewhere**

3. Assign an additional code to identify the infectious agent in acute infections. Example:

   E06.0 Acute thyroiditis

   Use additional code (B95-B97) to identify infectious agent.

4. Assign an additional code to identify intellectual disabilities associated with congenital conditions. Example:

E00 Congenital iodine-deficiency syndrome

Use additional code (F70-F79) to identify associated intellectual disabilities.

5. Assign a code for body mass index (BMI), if known, with codes for obesity. Example:

E66 Overweight and obesity

Use additional code to identify body mass index (BMI), if known (Z68.-).

6. Sequence first any drug causing an endocrine condition. Example:

E06.4 Drug-induced thyroiditis

Code for adverse effect, if applicable, to identify drug (T36-T50 with fifth or sixth character 5)

Guided Example of Arranging Endocrine System Diagnosis Codes

To learn more about sequencing codes for the endocrine system, continue with the example about patient Justin Kraft, who was admitted to Branton Medical Center due to new onset of type 1 diabetes. Follow along as Tamara Brownlee, CCS-P, sequences the codes.

▶ Tamara reviews the codes for this case:

   ❑ **E10.10 Type 1 diabetes mellitus with ketoacidosis without coma**

   ❑ **Z83.3 Family history of diabetes mellitus**

▶ She identifies that type 1 diabetes is the principal diagnosis, the **condition established after study to be chiefly responsible for occasioning the admission of the patient to the hospital for care** (OGCR II).

   ❑ A code for family history of a disease is rarely a principal diagnosis.

▶ Tamara finalizes the codes and sequencing for this case.

   (1) **E10.10 Type 1 diabetes mellitus with ketoacidosis without coma**

   (2) **Z83.3 Family history of diabetes mellitus**

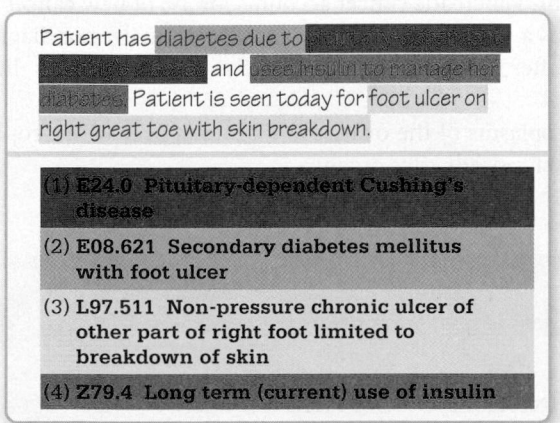

Patient has diabetes due to ████████████████ ██████ ███████ and uses insulin to manage her diabetes. Patient is seen today for foot ulcer on right great toe with skin breakdown.

(1) **E24.0 Pituitary-dependent Cushing's disease**
(2) **E08.621 Secondary diabetes mellitus with foot ulcer**
(3) **L97.511 Non-pressure chronic ulcer of other part of right foot limited to breakdown of skin**
(4) **Z79.4 Long term (current) use of insulin**

Figure 10-10 ■ Example of Sequencing Multiple Conditions with Multiple Codes

CODING PRACTICE

Exercise 10.4 **Arranging Codes for Endocrine System Conditions**

Instructions: Read the mini-medical-record of each patient's encounter, review the information abstracted in Exercise 10.2, assign ICD-10-CM diagnosis codes using the Index and Tabular List, and sequence them correctly.

1. INPATIENT HOSPITAL   Gender: F   Age: 36

Reason for admission: insulin-induced hypoglycemia

Assessment: Patient has chronic pancreatitis for 2 years and associated diabetes. Patient has struggled to monitor and self-administer insulin correctly.

Plan: Prescribe insulin pump. FU in office.

Tip: Refer to OGCR for secondary diabetes.

3 ICD-10-CM Codes _____

_____

2. OFFICE   Gender: F   Age: 65

Reason for encounter: management of longstanding neuropathy

Assessment: peripheral autonomic neuropathy, type 2 diabetes

Plan: FU 6 months

Tip: The neuropathy is not stated as "due to" or "in" the diabetes.

2 ICD-10-CM Codes _____

3. OFFICE   Gender: M   Age: 25

Reason for encounter: follow up on test results after evaluation of proximal muscle weakness, easy bruising, weight gain

Assessment: endogenous Cushing syndrome due to pituitary adenoma

Plan: evaluate for surgery to remove tumor.

Tip: An adenoma is benign, an adenocarcinoma is malignant.

2 ICD-10-CM Codes _____

CODING NEOPLASMS OF THE ENDOCRINE SYSTEM

Neoplasms of the endocrine system do not appear in ICD-10-CM Chapter 4 Endocrine, Nutritional, and Metabolic Diseases (E00-E89); they appear in Chapter 2 (C00-D49). Codes for neoplasms of the endocrine system appear in the following blocks within the neoplasm chapter:

- C73-C75 Malignant neoplasm of thyroid and other endocrine glands
- C7A Malignant neuroendocrine tumors
- C7B Secondary neuroendocrine tumors
- D3A Benign neuroendocrine tumors

Review these blocks in the ICD-10-CM manual to become familiar with the content.

The most common sites for cancer in the endocrine system are the thyroid and pancreas. Thyroid cancer is the fifth most common cancer in women and accounts for 5% of new cancer cases, according to the American Cancer Society (ACS). Most types of thyroid cancer are treatable, and most patients are cured and have a normal life expectancy. The American Society of Clinical Oncologists (ASCO) reports that the incidence rates of thyroid cancer in both women and men have been increasing in recent years, and researchers are working to learn the reasons. Pancreatic cancer accounts for 3% of new cancer cases but has a poor survival rate because it is usually not diagnosed until after it has metastasized widely and, therefore, is difficult to treat.

Neoplasms of the ovaries and testes appear with neoplasms of other reproductive organs.

CODING PRACTICE

Exercise 10.5 **Coding Neoplasms of the Endocrine System**

Instructions: Read the mini-medical-record of each patient's encounter, then abstract, assign, and sequence ICD-10-CM diagnosis codes using the Index and Tabular List. Write the code(s) on the line provided.

1. INPATIENT HOSPITAL   Gender: F   Age: 35

Reason for encounter: thyroidectomy

Assessment: serous papillary carcinoma of the thyroid

Plan: thyroid hormone replacement

1 ICD-10-CM Code _____

2. OFFICE   Gender: M   Age: 7

Reason for encounter: *follow up on a solitary nodule discovered during a routine check-up 10 days ago*

Assessment: Follicular adenoma of the thyroid

Plan: *partial thyroidectomy*

1 ICD-10-CM Code _____

3. OUTPATIENT HOSPITAL   Gender: M   Age: 5

Chief complaint: *review X-ray and CT performed for dyspnea and cough*

Assessment: *thymoma*

Tip: According to Medscape, the most common location for mediastinal tumors in children is near the trachea, resulting in respiratory symptoms.

1 ICD-10-CM Code _____

4. INPATIENT HOSPITAL   Gender: M   Age: 51

Reason for Admission: *surgical removal of carcinoid tumor*

Diagnosis: *malignant carcinoid tumor of small intestine* with **carcinoid syndrome**

Plan: *FU in office*

Tip: Look up **carcinoid** tumor, not cancer or carcinoma.

2 ICD-10-CM Codes _____

5. INPATIENT HOSPITAL   Gender: F   Age: 45

Reason for encounter: *chemotherapy*

Assessment: *adenocarcinoma of pancreas with metastases to liver, lung, and colon*

Tip: Review OGCR I.C.2.e.2) for coding and sequencing reminders.

5 ICD-10-CM Codes _____

_____

CHAPTER SUMMARY

In this chapter you learned the following:

- The function of the endocrine system is to produce, store, and release hormones, which are chemical messengers that regulate body functions including growth, development, metabolism, sexual function, reproduction, and mood.

- ICD-10-CM Chapter 4, Endocrine, Nutritional, and Metabolic Diseases (E00-E89), contains 10 blocks or subchapters that are divided by anatomical site and type of disorder.

- To abstract endocrine system conditions, coders must distinguish between integral symptoms and signs as opposed to the conditions, complications, and manifestations.

- When assigning codes for the endocrine system, carefully review the information abstracted from the medical record and determine whether the condition is the primary condition or the result of a disease or condition in another body system.

- Multiple coding is required throughout the endocrine system as directed by instructional notes in the Tabular List and conventions in the Index to Diseases and Injuries.

- The most common sites for cancer in the endocrine system are the thyroid and pancreas.

CONCEPT QUIZ

Take a moment to look back through endocrine, nutritional, and metabolic diseases and solidify your skills. Try to answer the questions from memory first, then refer to the discussion in this chapter and the Glossary at the end of this book if you need a little extra help.

Completion

Instructions: Write the term that answers each question based on the information you learned in this chapter. Choose from the following list. Some choices may be used more than once and some choices may not be used at all.

body mass index (BMI)

diabetic ketoacidosis (DKA)

Graves disease

hyperglycemia

hyperosmolarity hyperglycemic nonketotic syndrome (HHNS)

hyperthyroidism

hypoglycemia

hypothalamus

hypothyroidism

metabolism

ovaries

pancreas

pituitary

testes

thyroid

thyrotoxicosis

(continued)

(continued from page 155)

1. The _____ gland controls most activity in the endocrine system.

2. The _____ and _____ support both the endocrine system and reproductive system.

3. _____ includes the processes of digestion, elimination, breathing, blood circulation, and maintaining body temperature.

4. _____ is elevated glucose without ketoacidosis, usually occurring in elderly type 2 diabetics with other conditions.

5. The _____ is a butterfly-shaped gland in front of the trachea that produces two hormones, tri-iodothyronine (T3) and thyroxine (T4).

6. _____ is excessive quantities of circulating thyroid hormone due to overproduction by the thyroid gland, overproduction originating outside the thyroid, or loss of storage function and leakage from the gland.

7. _____ is a deficiency of thyroid hormone, usually due to lack of production of the hormone by the thyroid or inadequate secretion of hormones.

8. Assign a code for _____ , if known, with codes for obesity.

9. _____ is overproduction by the thyroid gland due to an autoimmune condition.

10. Cancer of the _____ accounts for 3% of new cancer cases but has a poor survival rate because it is usually not diagnosed until after it has metastasized widely.

Multiple Choice

Instructions: Circle the letter of the best answer to each question based on the information you learned in this chapter.

1. The type of diabetes in which the body's immune system attacks pancreatic beta cells so that the pancreas does not produce insulin is
   A. type 1 diabetes.
   B. type 2 diabetes.
   C. secondary diabetes.
   D. ketoacidosis.

2. The type of diabetes in which elevated glucose is caused by an external factor, such as medication, surgery, pancreatic disease, or other illness, is
   A. type 1 diabetes.
   B. type 2 diabetes.
   C. secondary diabetes.
   D. ketoacidosis.

3. _____ accounts for 90% to 95% of all diagnosed cases of diabetes.
   A. Type 1 diabetes
   B. Type 2 diabetes
   C. Secondary diabetes
   D. Gestational diabetes

4. In _____ a high level of ketones accumulate in the blood, turning it acidic, and it can be life threatening if not treated immediately.
   A. hyperglycemia
   B. diabetic ketoacidosis
   C. hyperosmolarity hyperglycemic nonketotic syndrome
   D. hypoglycemia

5. Which of the following disorders is not classified in ICD-10-CM Chapter 4, Endocrine, Nutritional, and Metabolic Diseases (E00-E89)?
   A. DKA
   B. HHNS
   C. DM
   D. GDM

6. Which of the following word choices does NOT establish a causal relationship in physician documentation?
   A. due to
   B. in
   C. with
   D. and

7. Which of the following is NOT a key criterion for abstracting thyroid disorders?
   A. Is the condition congenital?
   B. Is goiter documented?
   C. Is insulin used on a long-term basis?
   D. Is thyrotoxicosis crisis documented?

8. Multiple coding may be required in all of the following situations EXCEPT when
   A. a patient has an unrelated condition, in addition to diabetes.
   B. a patient has a diabetic complication.
   C. a type 2 diabetic uses insulin on a long-term basis.
   D. a patient experiences complications due to the malfunction of an insulin pump.

9. Under the Main Term Diabetes in the Index, first-level subterms identify
   A. the type of diabetes.
   B. that complications are present.
   C. the specific complication(s) with each type.
   D. long-term use of insulin.

10. The most frequent sites of cancer in the endocrine system are the
   A. thyroid and lung.
   B. thyroid and pancreas.
   C. ovaries and pancreas.
   D. thyroid and parathyroid.

CODING CHALLENGE

Instructions: Read the mini-medical-record of each patient's encounter, then abstract, assign, and sequence ICD-10-CM diagnosis codes using the Index and Tabular List. Write the code(s) on the line provided.

1. INPATIENT HOSPITAL Gender: F Age: 35

Reason for admission: T 102 F, tachycardia, extreme anxiety, nausea, diarrhea

Assessment: thyrotoxicosis with goiter and thyroid storm

Plan: Rx PTU (propylthiouracil) for thyroid and beta blocker propranolol to control heart rate

1 ICD-10-CM Code _____

2. INPATIENT HOSPITAL Gender: M Age: 42

Reason for admission: Patient found non-responsive. Family reports patient being on a fast.

Assessment: nondiabetic hypoglycemic coma

Plan: instructed on diet and glucometer, FU 1 week

1 ICD-10-CM Code _____

3. OFFICE Gender: F Age: 25

Chief complaint: weight loss, decreased appetite, decreased sexual drive, and increased sensitivity to cold

Assessment: hypopituitarism

Plan: hormone replacement therapy, FU 4 wk

1 ICD-10-CM Code _____

4. OFFICE Gender: M Age: 40

Reason for encounter: FU on lab test results of 24-hour aldosterone excretion rate 18 mcg; 24-h urine sodium above 400 mEq (*milliequivalent*) after presenting with severe hypokalemia, fatigue, muscle weakness, cramping, and hypertension

Assessment: primary hyperaldosteronism (*Conn syndrome*) with secondary hypertension

Plan: medication to normalize BP, Na (*sodium*), electrolytes, and aldosterone

2 ICD-10-CM Codes _____

5. OFFICE Gender: F Age: 32

Chief complaint: irregular and infrequent menstrual periods, recent weight gain, noticeable loss of body hair under arms and pubic area

Assessment: polycystic ovarian syndrome

Plan: Rx hormones, FU 1 month

1 ICD-10-CM Code _____

6. OFFICE Gender: F Age: 51

Reason for encounter: Annual check-up

Assessment: Test results show abnormally low vitamin D level. Patient is obese due to excess calories and has a BMI of 30.5.

Plan: Rx vitamin D 50,000 IU/week for 8 weeks, then recheck.

Tip: Remember that you need a Z code for the annual checkup.

4 ICD-10-CM Codes _____
_____

7. OFFICE Gender: M Age: 48

Chief complaint: insomnia, hand tremor, hyperactivity, excessive sweating, weight loss

Assessment: Graves' disease with uninodular goiter

Plan: radioiodine therapy

1 ICD-10-CM Code _____

8. INPATIENT HOSPITAL Gender: M Age: 57

Reason for admission: cold clammy skin and pallor, rapid breathing & heart rate

Assessment: hypovolemia

Plan: FU 1 wk

1 ICD-10-CM Code _____

(continued)

INTRODUCTION

A new car's finish consists of a primer layer that helps the paint adhere to the structure of the car, several layers of paint, and a clear coat on top that serves as a protective finish. A scratch in the clear coat can easily be buffed out, but a scratch through to the underlying metal can be costly to restore to new condition.

Your skin is the protective covering of your body and also consists of several layers, each with its own function. Repairing damage to the skin can be easy or difficult, depending on how far the damage penetrates.

A dermatologist is a physician who specializes in diagnosing and treating conditions of the skin and subcutaneous tissues. Primary care physicians treat uncomplicated conditions of the skin and subcutaneous tissues. They refer patients with more complex conditions to dermatologists.

INTEGUMENTARY SYSTEM REFRESHER

The **integumentary** (*pertaining to a covering*) system consists of the skin and accessory structures: hair, nails, **sebaceous** (*pertaining to oil*) glands, and **sudoriferous** (*pertaining to sweat*) glands (■ FIGURE 11-1). It is the largest organ in the body, weighing approximately 6 pounds and covering approximately 20 square feet, which is the size of a 4- by 5-foot rug. The integumentary system has four primary functions:

- **protection**—helps prevent invasion by pathogens, mechanical harm, and loss of fluids and electrolytes.

- **regulation**—increases and decreases body temperature through constriction and dilation of blood vessels and sweat glands.

- **sensation**—contains sensory receptors for pain, touch, heat, cold, and pressure.

- **secretion**—gives off perspiration (*water and salt*) to control temperature and sebum (*oil*) to protect from dehydration and penetration by harmful substances.

In Figure 11-1, each structure in the integumentary system is labeled with its name as well as its medical terminology root/combining form. As you learn about conditions and procedures that affect the skin and **subcutaneous** (*under the skin*) structures, remember to apply medical terminology skills to combine word roots, prefixes, and suffixes you already know to define new terms. Refer to ■ TABLE 11-1 for a refresher on how to build medical terms related to the integumentary system.

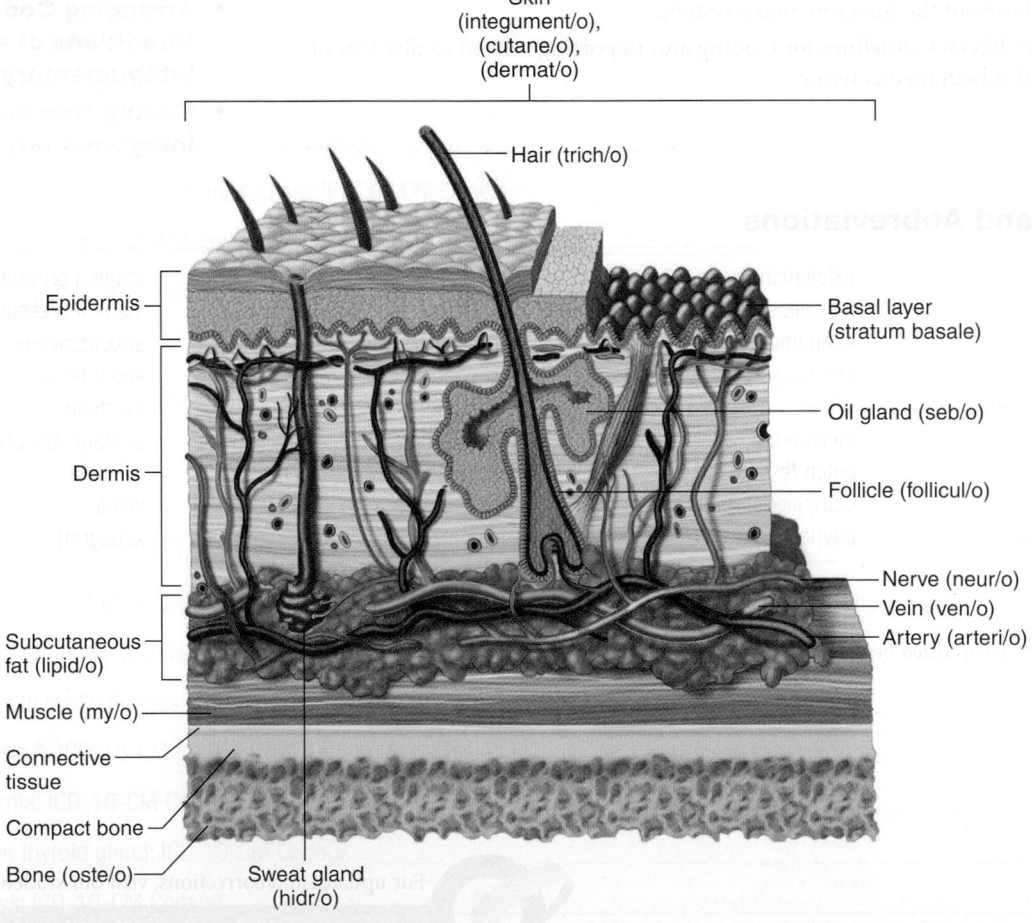

Skin
(integument/o),
(cutane/o),
(dermat/o)

Hair (trich/o)

Epidermis

Basal layer
(stratum basale)

Oil gland (seb/o)

Dermis

Follicle (follicul/o)

Nerve (neur/o)
Vein (ven/o)
Artery (arteri/o)

Subcutaneous
fat (lipid/o)

Muscle (my/o)

Connective
tissue

Compact bone

Bone (oste/o)

Sweat gland
(hidr/o)

Figure 11-1 ■ The Integumentary System

Table 11-1 ■ **EXAMPLE OF CONSTRUCTING MEDICAL TERMS FOR THE INTEGUMENTARY SYSTEM**

Combining Form/Prefix	Suffix	Complete Medical Term
derm/o, dermat/o (*skin*) cutane/o (*skin*) myc/o (*fungus*) erythr/o (*redness*)	-itis (*inflammation*) -osis (*condition*) -al (*pertaining to*) -plasty (*surgical repair*)	dermat + itis (*inflammation of the skin*) intra + derm + al (*pertaining to within the skin*) erythro + derma (*red skin*) dermo + myc + osis (*skin condition related to fungus*) dermo + plasty (*surgical repair of the skin*)
pachy- (*thick*) intra- (*within*) sub- (*below*)		sub + derm + al (*pertaining to under the skin*) sub + cutane + ous (*pertaining to under the skin*)

CODING CAUTION

Be alert for medical terms that are spelled similarly and have different meanings.

myc/o (*fungus*) and **my/o** (*muscle*)

urticaria (*hives*) and **-uresis** (*urination*)

onych/o (*nail*) and **onc/o** (*tumor*)

Conditions of the Integumentary System

Common conditions of the integumentary system are summarized in ■ TABLE 11-2. Physicians diagnose problems through visual inspection, **patch testing** (*applying an aller-*

gen to the skin to observe the reaction), **biopsy** (*scraping, punching, or cutting a piece of skin and examining it under a microscope*), and **culture** (*performing a test to identify the microorganism that is causing an infection*). Treatments include the following:

- medication to treat the underlying condition
- incision and drainage of fluid
- surgical removal of the lesion or damaged skin
- applying replacement tissue using an **autograft** (*tissue from the patient*), **allograft** (*tissue from another person*), **xenograft** (*tissue from an animal*), or a **synthetic** (*manmade tissue*) substitute.

Table 11-2 ■ **COMMON CONDITIONS OF THE INTEGUMENTARY SYSTEM**

Condition	Description	Examples
Bacterial infection	Infection caused by bacteria and treatable with antibiotics	Abscess, **furuncle, carbuncle**, cellulitis (*inflammation under the skin*) due to *Staphylococcus* or *Streptococcus*
Bulla (blister)	Raised area of epidermis filled with fluid	Pemphigus (*autoimmune disease that erupts in blisters*)
Dermatitis	A flat or raised eruption that can be caused by irritation, allergy, or infection	Eczema, atopic dermatitis, contact dermatitis, urticaria (*hives*), keratosis (*overgrowth of horny tissue*), erythema multiforme (*red fluid-filled lesions that can cause layers of skin to fall off*)
Papulosquamous disorders	Papules (*firm bumps*) and scales	Psoriasis (*round red patches covered with white scales*), pityriasis (*rough, dry scales*), lichen (*eruption of flat papules*)
Radiation disorders	Damage to the skin resulting from exposure to radiation	Sunburn, actinic keratosis (*a precancerous lesion*), radiodermatitis
Skin appendages	Nails, hair, sweat glands	Ingrowing nail, misshaped nails, alopecia (*baldness*), folliculitis (*inflammation of space around the hair root*), acne, sweat disorders
Nonpressure ulcers	Breakdown of skin that is not the result of prolonged pressure	Diabetic ulcer, ulcers due to poor circulation or clots (postphlebitic, postthrombotic, venostasis)
Decubitus ulcer (pressure ulcer, bed sore)	Breakdown of the skin, usually over bony parts of body, caused by continuous pressure, friction, moistness, and heat	Stage 1—redness that does not go away Stage 2—damage to epidermis that extends into the dermis Stage 3—damage through the full thickness of the dermis and into the subcutaneous tissue (fat) Stage 4—damage extending into the muscle, tendon, or bone Unstageable—ulcers covered with dead cells, **eschar**, or wound exudate that cannot be visually assessed
Pigmentation disorder	Damage to or unhealthy melanin cells that give color to the skin	Age spots, freckles, vitiligo (*loss of pigmentation*)

CODING PRACTICE

Exercise 11.1 Integumentary System Refresher

Instructions: Use your medical terminology skills and resources to define the following terms related to the integumentary system, then assign the diagnosis code.

Follow these steps:

- Use slash marks "/" to break down each term into its root(s) and suffix.
- Define the meaning of the word, based on the meaning of each word part.
- Assign the default ICD-10-CM diagnosis code for the condition using the Index and Tabular List.

Example: dermatitis dermat/itis   Meaning: *inflammation of the skin*   ICD-10-CM Code: *L30.9*

1. pachyderma   Meaning _____   ICD-10-CM Code _____
2. hypertrichosis   Meaning _____   ICD-10-CM Code _____
3. perifolliculitis   Meaning _____   ICD-10-CM Code _____
4. cellulitis   Meaning _____   ICD-10-CM Code _____
5. erythroderma   Meaning _____   ICD-10-CM Code _____
6. pyoderma   Meaning _____   ICD-10-CM Code _____
7. onychocryptosis   Meaning _____   ICD-10-CM Code _____
8. hyperkeratosis   Meaning _____   ICD-10-CM Code _____
9. hidraenitis   Meaning _____   ICD-10-CM Code _____
10. onychodystrophy   Meaning _____   ICD-10-CM Code _____

CODING OVERVIEW OF THE SKIN AND SUBCUTANEOUS TISSUE

ICD-10-CM Chapter 12, Diseases of the Skin and Subcutaneous Tissue (L00-L99), contains nine blocks or subchapters that are divided by anatomic site and type of condition. This chapter includes skin disorders and infections other than neoplasms and injuries. Review the block names and code ranges listed at the beginning of Chapter 12 in the ICD-10-CM manual to become familiar with the content and organization.

ICD-10-CM Chapter 12 corresponds with ICD-9-CM Chapter 12 (680-709). Many categories have been expanded to reflect the greater specificity available in ICD-10-CM. Examples are pemphigus, pemphigoid, alopecia areata, carbuncle and furuncle of the trunk, impetigo, and psoriasis. Pressure ulcer codes are combination codes that identify the stage, site, and laterality in a single code, whereas ICD-9-CM requires multiple codes.

Take note of the **Excludes2** note, which lists skin conditions not classified in this chapter. The following types of skin disorders are classified in other ICD-10-CM chapters:

- Burns (Chapter 19, Injury and Poisoning)
- Neoplasms (Chapter 2, Neoplasms)
- Viral, bacterial, and fungal infections (Chapter 1, Certain Infectious and Parasitic Diseases)
- Parasites (Chapter 1, Certain Infectious and Parasitic Diseases)

ICD-10-CM provides Official Guidelines for Coding and Reporting (OGCR) for Diseases of the Skin and Subcutaneous Tissue in OGCR section I.C.12. OGCR provides detailed discussion of assigning codes for pressure ulcer stages. Additional guidelines related to skin infections appear in OGCR I.C.1.b. Guidelines related to burns and other skin injuries appear in OGCR I.C.19.d. Instructional notes throughout the chapter provide information on multiple coding and sequencing.

ABSTRACTING FOR CONDITIONS OF THE INTEGUMENTARY SYSTEM

When abstracting for diseases of the integumentary system, coders need to be familiar with the various types of lesions and complications, as well as the systems used to describe the extent of damage to the skin (■ TABLE 11-3). Remember that the

Table 11-3 ■ **KEY CRITERIA FOR ABSTRACTING CONDITIONS OF THE INTEGUMENTARY SYSTEM**

- ❏ What is the type of lesion (carbuncle, abscess, urticaria, mole, corn)?
- ❏ What is the anatomic site (face, back, hand)?
- ❏ What is the laterality (right or left side)?
- ❏ Is there an underlying cause (another condition, exposure to a drug, or environmental substance)?
- ❏ What is the infectious agent, if any?
- ❏ Are there complications or manifestations (gangrene)?
- ❏ What is the depth or extent of damage?

Table 11-4 ■ CLASSIFICATION OF BURNS

Degree	Name	Description
1st	Superficial	Damage to the epidermis
2nd	Partial thickness	Damage to the epidermis and part of the dermis
3rd	Full thickness	Damage to the entire depth of the dermis

CODING CAUTION

ICD-10-CM uses the Arabic numerals 1, 2, 3, and 4 to identify pressure ulcer stages. The National Pressure Ulcer Advisory Panel, and many physicians, use the Roman numerals I, II, III, and IV. Coders need to be familiar with both ways of writing and reading numbers.

abstracting questions are a guide and that not every question applies to, or can be answered for, every case. For example, not every case has an infectious agent.

Depth of damage is described based on documentation of what layers of tissue are affected. The description varies based on the condition, such as the following:

- Conditions confined to the epidermis by definition, such as contact dermatitis or superficial lesions, do not require depth descriptions.
- Sunburns are classified by the degree of the burn (■ TABLE 11-4).
- Pressure ulcers are assigned a numerical stage from 1 to 4, based on depth (■ FIGURE 11-2).

- Nonpressure ulcers are classified as follows:
  - limited to breakdown of skin
  - fat layer exposed
  - necrosis of muscle
  - necrosis of bone

Guided Example of Abstracting Diagnoses for the Integumentary System

Refer to the following example throughout this chapter to practice skills for abstracting and assigning codes for the integumentary system. Joshua Grider, CPC, is a fictitious coder who guides you through this case.

Stage 1: Skin discolored but intact

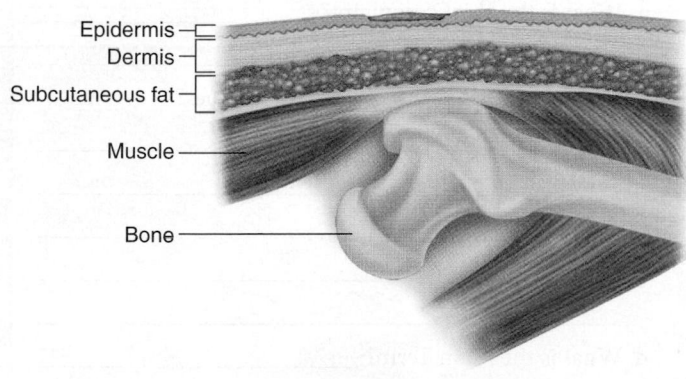

Stage 2: Shallow open ulcer through part of the dermis

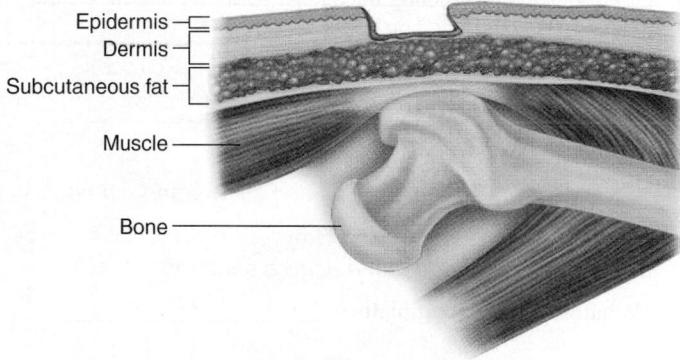

Stage 3: Full-thickness loss of dermis with exposure of subcutaneous fat

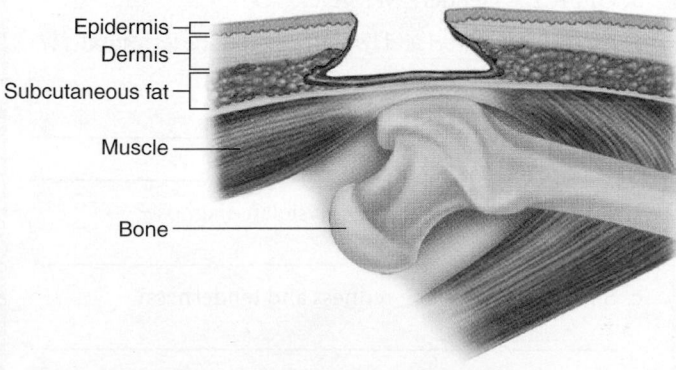

Stage 4: Exposed bone, muscle, or tendon

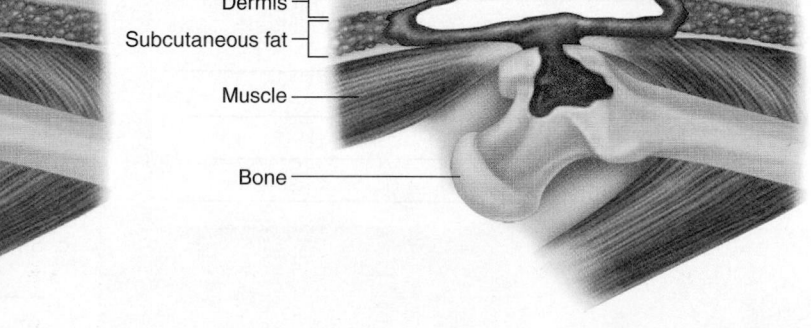

Figure 11-2 ■ Classification of Pressure Ulcer Stages

Date: 11/1/yy   Location: Dermatology Associates

Provider: Lawrence Staton, MD

Patient: Naomi Vargas   Gender: F   Age: 84

Reason for encounter: debride and change dressing on pressure ulcer per referral from home health care nurse

Assessment: damage through the full thickness of the dermis and into the subcutaneous (SC) tissue; stage 3 pressure ulcer, right buttock

Plan: FU visits from home health care

Follow along as Joshua Grider, CPC, abstracts the diagnosis. Check off each step after you complete it.

▶ Joshua reads through the entire record, paying special attention to the reason for the encounter and the final assessment.

❏ He notes that the procedure of debriding the wound is consistent with a stage 3 ulcer. He refers to Key Criteria

for Abstracting Conditions of the Integumentary System (Table 11-3).

❏ *What is the type of lesion?* pressure ulcer

❏ *What is the anatomic site?* buttock

❏ *What is the laterality?* right

❏ *Is there an underlying cause?* No

❏ *What is the infectious agent, if any?* None

❏ *Are there complications or manifestations?* No

❏ *What is the depth or extent of damage?* stage 3

❏ He refers to the definition of pressure ulcer stages and confirms that the description damage through the full thickness of the dermis and into the subcutaneous tissue is consistent with a stage 3 ulcer.

▶ Next, Joshua needs to assign the codes.

CODING PRACTICE

Exercise 11.2   **Abstracting for Conditions of the Integumentary System**

Instructions: Read the mini-medical-record of each patient's encounter and answer the abstracting questions. Write the answer on the line provided. Do not assign any codes.

1. OFFICE   Gender: F   Age: 5

Chief complaint: was at the beach all day and did not have sunscreen applied

Assessment: a severe second degree sunburn

a. What is the chief complaint? _____

_____

b. What is the source of the sunburn? _____

_____

c. What degree is the sunburn? _____

_____

d. What is the definition of a second-degree sunburn? _____

_____

_____

_____

2. OFFICE   Gender: F   Age: 17

Chief complaint: red itchy patches after hiking

Assessment: contact dermatitis due to poison ivy

a. What is the chief complaint? _____

_____

b. Should you code for the red itchy patches?

_____

Why or why not? _____

_____

c. What is the diagnosis? _____

_____

d. What is the Main Term? _____

_____

3. OFFICE   Gender: M   Age: 15

Chief complaint: red and tender area on the left great toe

Assessment: ingrown nail

a. What is the reason for the visit? _____

_____

b. What condition does the physician diagnose?

_____

c. Should you code the redness and tenderness?

_____

Why or why not? _____

_____

2. OFFICE Gender: F Age: 17

Chief complaint: red itchy patches after hiking

Assessment: contact dermatitis due to poison ivy

Tip: Recall that external cause codes for activity are not applicable to poisonings, so you do not need any additional codes.

1 ICD-10-CM Code _____

3. OFFICE Gender: M Age: 15

Chief complaint: red and tender area on the left great toe

Assessment: ingrown nail

1 ICD-10-CM Code _____

ARRANGING CODES FOR CONDITIONS OF THE INTEGUMENTARY SYSTEM

Sequencing of codes for the integumentary system follows the general coding guidelines OGCR III and IV as well as instructional notes in the Tabular List. In some cases, coders must apply multiple instructional notes for one code. A single category may include notes for **Code first** instructions as well as one or more **Use additional code** instructions. **Code first** means that the code listed should be sequenced before the code from the category in which it appears. **Use additional code** means that the code listed should be sequenced after the code from the category in which it appears.

Guided Example of Arranging Integumentary System Diagnosis Codes

Refer to the following new example of a patient with Stevens-Johnson syndrome to learn how to arrange codes when there are multiple instructional notes. Joshua Grider, CPC, guides you through this case. Review the following mini-medical-record to learn what information Joshua abstracted for each code.

Follow along in your ICD-10-CM manual as Joshua Grider, CPC, assigns and arranges codes. Check off each step after you complete it.

▶ Joshua first assigns the code for Stevens-Johnson syndrome. He locates the Main Term **Stevens-Johnson syndrome**

L51.1 in the Index then refers to the Tabular List to verify the code.

❑ He reads through the instructional notes at the beginning of category **L51** in the Tabular List (■ FIGURE 11-3, page 168).

▶ Joshua reads the first instructional note, which states **Use additional code to identify drug, (T36-T50 with fifth or sixth character 5)**.

❑ The documentation states that the condition is the result of taking a prescribed sulfonamide.

❑ Joshua sequences code **T37.0X5A Adverse effect of sulfonamides, initial encounter** as the second code because the instructional note states **Use additional code**, which means the drug code should appear *after* the code from this category (**L51**) for the condition.

▶ Joshua sequences the condition code first, **L51.1 Stevens-Johnson syndrome**.

▶ Joshua reads the second instructional note, which states **Use additional code to identify associated manifestations: stomatitis (K12.-)**.

❑ He refers to the documentation and confirms the manifestation, mouth sores.

❑ He sequences the third code as **K12.32 Oral mucositis (ulcerative) due to other drugs** because the instructional

---

Date: 11/2/yy Location: Branton Medical Center Provider: Lawrence Staton, MD

Patient: Ralph Wray Gender: M Age: 2

Reason for admission: Sudden outbreak of lesions on face, bilaterally on arms and legs, groin after taking a prescribed sulfonamide. Fever.

Assessment: Stevens-Johnson syndrome, 64% exfoliation

(1) **L51.1 Stevens-Johnson syndrome**
(2) **T37.0X5A Adverse effect of sulfonamides, initial encounter**
(3) **K12.32 Oral mucositis (ulcerative) due to other drugs**
(4) **L49.6 Exfoliation due to erythematous condition involving 60-69 percent of body surface**

---

4. OFFICE Gender: F Age: 64

Chief complaint: evaluation of cellulitis on her right leg

Assessment: lab results show the cellulitis to be due to Streptococcus A

Plan: Rx oral antibiotics. If it does not improve within 3 days or gets worse, she will need to be admitted for IV antibiotics.

a. What condition is being evaluated? _____

_____

b. What is the anatomic site? _____

_____

c. What is the laterality? _____

_____

d. What is the infectious agent? _____

_____

5. OFFICE Gender: M Age: 25

Reason for encounter: follow-up on erythema multiforme minor with stomatitis due to herpes simplex virus

Assessment: Stomatitis showing improvement. 15% of his skin is exfoliated.

a. What condition is being treated? _____

_____

b. What is the manifestation? _____

_____

(continued)

5. (continued)

c. What virus caused the condition? _____

_____

d. What does exfoliation mean? _____

_____

e. What is the percentage of exfoliation? _____

6. OFFICE Gender: M Age: 73

Reason for encounter: debride and dress chronic ulcer on right calf

Assessment: chronic ulcer due to postphlebitic syndrome. Healing is progressing. At last visit some muscle necrosis was visible. Today only the fat layer is exposed.

a. What condition is being treated? _____

_____

b. What is the anatomic site? _____

_____

c. What is the laterality? _____

_____

d. Is this a pressure ulcer or a nonpressure ulcer? _____

_____

e. What is the underlying condition? _____

ASSIGNING CODES FOR CONDITIONS OF THE INTEGUMENTARY SYSTEM

When assigning codes for the integumentary system, coders need to be alert for easily confused Index entries and must use the information abstracted regarding the depth or extent of skin damage, when applicable.

Skin ulcers are classified into separate categories based on whether they are pressure (decubitus) ulcers or nonpressure ulcers. Pressure ulcers are caused by prolonged pressure on an area, usually a bony prominence, such as the heel, elbow, or hip. Pressure ulcers are indexed under the Main Term **Ulcer**, then the subterm **pressure**, then a second-level subterm for the anatomic site. The most common causes of nonpressure skin ulcers are diabetes and circulatory problems. Nonpressure skin ulcers are indexed under the Main Term **Ulcer** and a subterm for the anatomic site.

The stage or depth of a pressure ulcer changes as the wound heals or worsens. Assign a code based on the stage documented during the encounter. For an ulcer that worsens during the course of an inpatient admission, assign a code for the highest stage (OGCR I.C.12.a.6)). When patients have more than one pressure ulcer, assign separate codes for each ulcer (OGCR I.C.12.a.1)).

Some skin conditions cause **exfoliation** (*falling off in scales or layers*) of the skin. These codes provide the instructional note **Use additional code to identify percentage of skin exfoliation (L49-)**.

Guided Example of Assigning Integumentary System Diagnosis Codes

To practice skills for assigning codes for conditions of the integumentary system, continue with the example from earlier in the chapter about patient Naomi Vargas, who was seen by Dr. Stanton due to a stage 3 pressure ulcer on the right buttock.

Follow along in your ICD-10-CM manual as Joshua Grider, CPC, assigns codes. Check off each step after you complete it.

▶ First, Joshua confirms the diagnosis stage 3 pressure ulcer on the right buttock.

▶ Joshua searches the Index for the Main Term **Ulcer.**

- ❑ He reviews the subterms and notes that many types of ulcers are indexed here, including ulcers in internal organs.

- ❑ He locates a subterm for **buttock.**

- ❑ He locates the second-level subterm for **exposed fat layer L98.412.**

▶ Joshua verifies the code in the Tabular List.

- ❑ He reads the code title **L98.412 Non-pressure chronic ulcer of buttock with fat layer exposed.**

- ❑ Joshua notices that this code is for a *nonpressure* ulcer, which is *not* the diagnosis for this patient.

CODING CAUTION

Remember to distinguish the *cause* of the skin ulcer. A pressure ulcer is caused by continuous pressure on an area, often found in patients with limited mobility. A nonpressure ulcer is due to another cause, such as venous insufficiency or diabetes, not pressure.

▶ Joshua realizes he selected an incorrect subterm in the Index, so **he returns to the Index** entry for the Main Term **Ulcer** to search for a different subterm.

- ❑ He locates the subterm **pressure.**

- ❑ He locates the second-level subterm **buttock L89.3.**

▶ Joshua returns to the Tabular List to verify code **L89.3.**

- ❑ He reads the category title **L89.3, Pressure ulcer of buttock.**

- ❑ He notices the convention **5th** instructing him to assign a fifth character.

- ❑ He reads the titles of the fifth-character categories and notes that they indicate laterality.

- ❑ He locates **L89.31 Pressure ulcer of right buttock.**

- ❑ He notices the convention **6th** instructing him to assign a sixth character.

- ❑ He reads the titles of the sixth-character codes and notes that they indicate stage.

- ❑ He locates **L89.313, Pressure ulcer of right buttock, stage 3.**

- ❑ He confirms that this accurately describes the diagnosis in the medical record.

▶ Joshua checks for instructional notes in the Tabular List.

- ❑ He cross-references the beginning of category **L89** and reads the instructional notes.

  - ▪ The inclusion notes confirm that this category classifies pressure or decubitus ulcers. The **Excludes2** note confirms that other types of ulcers are not coded here.

  - ▪ He reads the note to **Code first any associated gangrene (I96).**

  - ▪ He cross-references the medical record to confirm that gangrene is not documented. Because it is not documented, he does *not* assign a code for gangrene.

- ❑ Next, Joshua cross-references the beginning of the block **Other Disorders of the Skin and Subcutaneous Tissue (L80-L99)** and verifies that there are no instructional notes.

- ❑ Finally, he cross-references the beginning of Chapter 12 Diseases of the Skin and Subcutaneous Tissue (L00-L99) and reviews the instructional notes.

  - ▪ The only instructional note is an **Excludes2** note indicating what conditions are not classified in this chapter.

  - ▪ He determines that the **Excludes2** does not apply to this case because the patient's condition does not fit the description of any of the listed conditions.

▶ Joshua cross-references the medical record and finalizes the code for this case:

- ❑ **L89.313 Pressure ulcer of right buttock, stage 3.**

CODING PRACTICE

Exercise 11.3 Assigning Codes for Conditions of the Integumentary System

Instructions: Read the mini-medical-record of each patient's encounter, review the information abstracted in Exercise 11.2, and assign ICD-10-CM diagnosis codes using the Index and Tabular List. Write the code(s) on the line provided.

---

1. OFFICE   Gender: F   Age: 5

Chief complaint: was at the beach all day and did not have sunscreen applied

Assessment: a severe second degree sunburn

1 ICD-10-CM Code _____

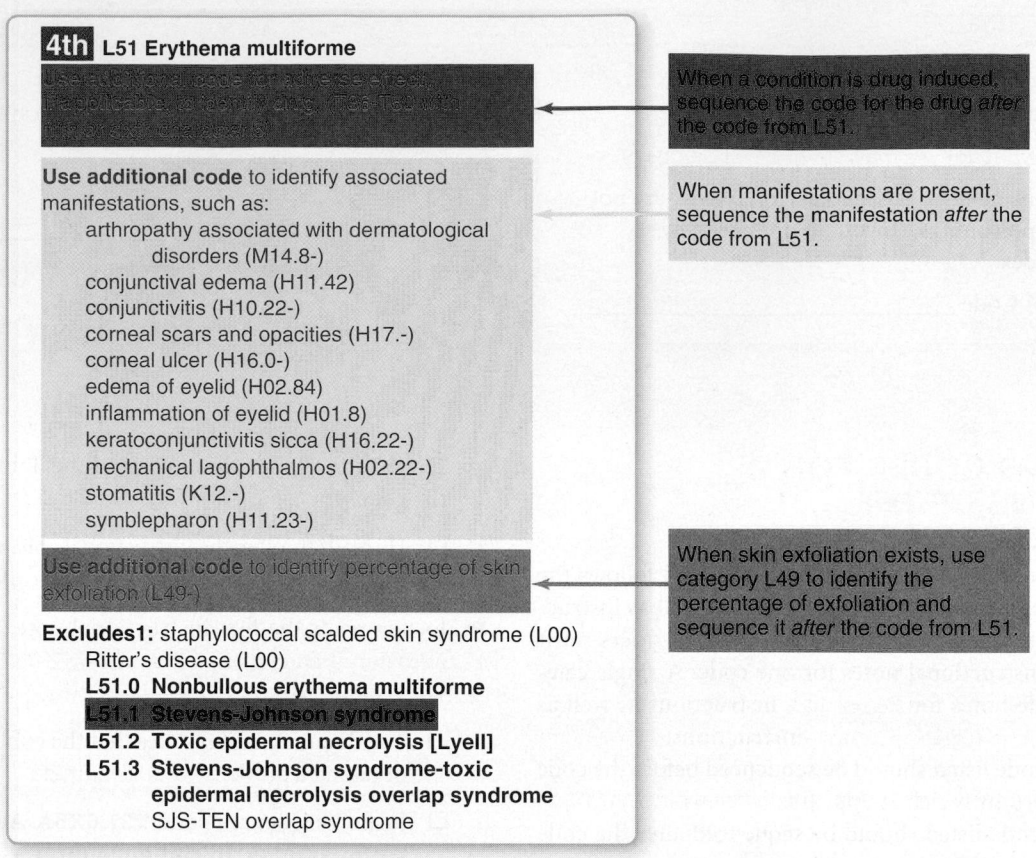

Figure 11-3 ■ Multiple Coding and Sequencing Instructions for All Codes within a Category

note **Use additional code** means the manifestation code should be sequenced *after* the code from this category **(L51)** for the condition.

▶ Joshua reads the third instructional note, which states **Use additional code to identify percentage of skin exfoliation (L49-).**

- ❑ He refers to the documentation and confirms 64% exfoliation.

- ❑ He sequences the fourth code as **L49.6 Exfoliation due to erythematous condition involving 60-69 percent of body surface** because this is also stated to be an *additional* code.

CODING PRACTICE

Exercise 11.4 Arranging Codes for Conditions of the Integumentary System

Instructions: Read the mini-medical-record of each patient's encounter, review the information abstracted in Exercise 11.2, assign ICD-10-CM diagnosis codes using the Index and Tabular List, and arrange them correctly.

---

1. OFFICE   Gender: F   Age: 64

Chief complaint: evaluation of cellulitis on her right leg

Assessment: lab results show the cellulitis to be due to *Streptococcus A*

(continued)

---

1. (continued)

Plan: Rx oral antibiotics. If it does not improve within 3 days or gets worse, she will need to be admitted for IV antibiotics.

Tip: Read the instructional notes at the beginning of the three-character category to learn whether the code for the infectious organism should be sequenced first or as an additional code.

2 ICD-10-CM Codes _____

2. OFFICE   Gender: M   Age: 25

Reason for encounter: follow-up on erythema multiforme and stomatitis minor due to herpes simplex virus

Assessment: Stomatitis showing improvement. 15% of his skin is exfoliated.

Tip: Sequence the condition first, the manifestation second, and the exfoliation third.

3 ICD-10-CM Codes _____

_____

3. OFFICE   Gender: M   Age: 73

Reason for encounter: debride and dress chronic ulcer on right calf

Assessment: chronic ulcer due to postphlebitic syndrome. Healing is progressing. At last visit some muscle necrosis was visible. Today only the fat layer is exposed.

Tip: Sequencing is indicated in the instructional notes.

2 ICD-10-CM Codes _____

CODING NEOPLASMS OF THE INTEGUMENTARY SYSTEM

Neoplasms of the integumentary system do not appear in ICD-10-CM Chapter 12, Diseases of the Skin and Subcutaneous Tissue (L00-L99). Codes for neoplasms of the integumentary system appear in block C43-C44 in the neoplasm chapter.

Skin cancers are named after the type of cell in which they start. The most common cancer in the integumentary system is basal cell (*lowest layer of the epidermis*) carcinoma (BCC),

which accounts for 75% of new skin cancer cases, according to the American Cancer Society. **Squamous cell carcinoma** (SCC), named after the flat squamous cells in which it begins, is also common. BCC and SCC, while malignant, tend to spread slowly and are usually treated with a high degree of success.

The most serious neoplasm of the integumentary system is malignant **melanoma**, a tumor of melanocytes, which causes 75% of deaths due to skin cancer. If found early, melanoma is treatable, but it can metastasize to other areas of the body, in which case it is difficult to treat and usually fatal.

CODING PRACTICE

Exercise 11.5   Coding Neoplasms of the Integumentary System

Instructions: Read the mini-medical-record of each patient's encounter, then abstract, assign, and arrange ICD-10-CM diagnosis codes using the Index and Tabular List. Write the code(s) on the line provided.

1. OFFICE   Gender: F   Age: 45

Reason for encounter: removal of lesions from eyebrow, chin, and lip

Assessment: removed three lesions, basal cell carcinoma

Plan: instructed patient to perform skin check monthly

Tip: Remember that you should not report the same diagnosis code twice for the same encounter (OGCR I.B.12).

2 ICD-10-CM Codes _____

2. OFFICE   Gender: M   Age: 42

Reason for encounter: unusual mole on nose

Assessment: melanoma in situ

(continued)

2. (continued)

Plan: schedule outpatient surgery to remove

Tip: Remember to look up **Melanoma** before deciding whether you should go to the Table of Neoplasms.

1 ICD-10-CM Code _____

3. INPATIENT HOSPITAL   Gender: F   Age: 51

Reason for admission: immunotherapy

Assessment: metastatic melanoma which started on the back

3 ICD-10-CM Codes _____

_____

4. OFFICE   Gender: F   Age: 36

Reason for encounter: suspicious mole between nose and lip

Assessment: nevus nasolabial groove

Plan: no treatment necessary

1 ICD-10-CM Code _____

(continued)

CODING PRACTICE (continued)

5. OFFICE Gender: M Age: 68

Reason for encounter: referred by family physician for areas on left arm where skin is breaking down

Assessment: Merkel cell carcinoma in kidney transplant recipient

(continued)

5. (continued)

Plan: schedule removal in one week

Tip: Chronic immune suppression is a risk factor for the rare Merkel cell carcinoma. Therefore, code the patient's organ transplant status.

2 ICD-10-CM Codes _____

CHAPTER SUMMARY

In this chapter you learned that:

- The integumentary system consists of the skin and accessory structures: hair, nails, sebaceous glands, and sudoriferous glands.

- ICD-10-CM Chapter 12, Diseases of the Skin and Subcutaneous Tissue (L00-L99), contains nine blocks or subchapters that are divided by anatomic site and type of condition.

- When abstracting for diseases of the integumentary system, coders need to be familiar with the various types of lesions and complications, as well as the systems used to describe the extent of damage to the skin.

- When assigning codes for the integumentary system, coders need to be alert for easily confused Index entries and must use

the information abstracted regarding the depth or extent of skin damage for certain conditions.

- Sequencing of codes for the integumentary system follows the general coding guidelines OGCR III and IV as well as instructional notes in the Tabular List.

- Skin cancers are named after the type of cell in which they start, with the most common being basal cell carcinoma (BCC).

- ICD-10-CM provides OGCR for Diseases of the Skin and Subcutaneous Tissue in OGCR section I.C.12, which provides detailed discussion of assigning codes for pressure ulcer stages.

CONCEPT QUIZ

Take a moment to look back at diseases of the skin and subcutaneous tissue and solidify your skills. This is your opportunity to pull together everything you have learned.

Completion

Instructions: Write the term that answers each question based on the information you learned in this chapter. Choose from the following list. Some choices may be used more than once and some choices may not be used at all.

allograft	folliculitis
autograft	hair
BCC	melanoma
cellulitis	nails
decubitus	protection
erythema multiforme	regulation
exfoliation	SCC

secretion	stage 3
sensation	stage 4
skin	urticaria
stage 1	xenograft
stage 2	

1. The skin's _____ function increases and decreases body temperature through constriction and dilation of blood vessels and sweat glands.

2. _____ is an inflammation of space around the hair root.

3. _____ is an inflammation under the skin.

4. A _____ ulcer is a breakdown of the skin, usually over bony parts of body, caused by continuous pressure, friction, moistness, and heat.

5. _____ is the medical term for hives.

6. _____ is the most common cancer in the integumentary system and accounts for 75% of new skin cancer cases.

7. _____ occurs when skin falls off in layers.

8. Trich/o is the combining form for _____.

9. Replacement skin tissue from another person is a/an _____.

10. The skin's _____ function helps prevent invasion by pathogens, mechanical harm, and loss of fluids and electrolytes.

Multiple Choice

Instructions: Circle the letter of the best answer to each question based on the information you learned in this chapter.

1. Which of the following is NOT a common method used to diagnose skin conditions?
   A. Patch testing
   B. Biopsy
   C. X-ray
   D. Visual inspection

2. Psoriasis, pityriasis, and lichen are examples of _____ disorders.
   A. papulosquamous
   B. decubitus
   C. pigmentation
   D. dermatitis

3. Pressure ulcers are classified into _____ stages.
   A. two
   B. three
   C. four
   D. five

4. An unstageable pressure ulcer is one that
   A. extends into the muscle, tendon, or bone.
   B. has metastasized to other areas of the body.
   C. is not documented by a physician.
   D. cannot be visually assessed because of dead cells, eschar, or exudate.

5. Which of the following disorders is classified in ICD-10-CM Chapter 12?
   A. Burns
   B. Viral infections
   C. Parasites
   D. Radiation exposure

6. All of the following are nonpressure ulcers of the skin EXCEPT
   A. diabetic ulcer.
   B. peptic ulcer.
   C. venostasis ulcer.
   D. postphlebitic ulcer.

7. Coders should locate a code for a pressure ulcer on the right buttock by searching the Index for what Main Term and subterm?
   A. Pressure, buttock
   B. Buttock, ulcer
   C. Ulcer, buttock
   D. Ulcer, pressure

8. For an ulcer that worsens during the course of an inpatient admission, assign a code for
   A. the highest stage.
   B. the lowest stage.
   C. the stage at admission.
   D. each stage that occurred during the hospital stay.

9. If skin exfoliation exists, use category L49 to identify the percentage of
   A. healthy skin.
   B. lesions.
   C. exfoliation.
   D. dermatitis.

10. Skin cancers are named after
    A. the anatomic site where they start.
    B. the type of cell in which they start.
    C. the rate at which they spread.
    D. the site they metastasize to.

CODING CHALLENGE

Instructions: Read the mini-medical-record of each patient's encounter, then abstract, assign, and sequence ICD-10-CM diagnosis codes using the Index and Tabular List. Write the code(s) on the line provided.

1. OFFICE   Gender: F   Age: 27

Reason for encounter: localized pain in the tail bone area

Assessment: abscessed pilonidal cyst

Plan: use depilatory cream and antibiotic, call office if symptoms do not subside

1 ICD-10-CM Code _____

(continued)

(continued from page 171)

2. OFFICE Gender: F Age: 3

Reason for admission: body covered with blisters, child appears to be in pain

Assessment: Ritter's disease, involving 68 % of body surface

Plan: Rx pain medication, return to burn center for skin debridement

2 ICD-10-CM Codes _____

3. INPATIENT HOSPITAL Gender: F Age: 24

Reason for admission: painful blisters on the skin and mucous membrane of the mouth

Assessment: pemphigus vulgaris

Plan: Rx steroids, FU PCP 2 wk

1 ICD-10-CM Code _____

4. OFFICE Gender: M Age: 47

Reason for encounter: referred by PCP for red, sore skin lesion

Assessment: inflamed seborrheic keratosis

Plan: local anesthetic provided and lesion removed, call office if any redness occurs

1 ICD-10-CM Code _____

5. OFFICE Gender: M Age: 89

Reason for encounter: Red open skin area in sacral region

Assessment: pressure ulcer, stage 3, sacral region

Plan: Debrided wound and applied dressing. Refer to wound care clinic for FU.

1 ICD-10-CM Code _____

6. OFFICE Gender: F Age: 52

Reason for encounter: redness on the central face across the cheeks, nose, and forehead

Assessment: rosacea

Plan: Rx oral antibiotics. FU 6 weeks. Advised on diet and lifestyle changes to minimize symptoms.

1 ICD-10-CM Code _____

7. OUTPATIENT SURGERY Gender: M Age: 44

Reason for encounter: repair of scar

Assessment: keloid scar

Plan: repaired scar, monitor for infection

1 ICD-10-CM Code _____

8. OFFICE Gender: M Age: 41

Reason for encounter: swollen lump under skin in right armpit for 2 weeks, fever

Assessment: carbuncle due to methicillin-susceptible Staphylococcus aureus (MSSA)

Plan: antibiotic, call if no improvement within 1 week

2 ICD-10-CM Codes _____

9. INPATIENT HOSPITAL Gender: F Age: 70

Reason for admission: swelling in left leg with apparent infection

Assessment: cellulitis, left leg, Streptococcus A

Plan: Rx antibiotics, topical medication, call office if symptoms worsen after discharge

2 ICD-10-CM Codes _____

10. OFFICE Gender: M Age: 6 months

Reason for encounter: Mother is concerned about severe rash and blistering in child's perinanal area, hips, and buttocks that seems to be getting worse.

Assessment: diaper dermatitis

Plan: Reviewed diaper hygiene. Rx ointment.

1 ICD-10-CM Code _____

KEEP ON CODING

Instructions: Read the diagnostic statement, then use the Index and Tabular List to assign and sequence ICD-10-CM diagnosis codes. Write the code(s) on the line provided.

1. Infantile eczema: ICD-10-CM Code(s) _____

2. Retiform parapsoriasis: ICD-10-CM Code(s) _____

3. Café au lait spots: ICD-10-CM Code(s) _____

4. Discoid lupus erythematosus: ICD-10-CM Code(s) _____

5. Eosinophilic cellulitis: ICD-10-CM Code(s) _____

6. Stage 3 decubitus ulcer of the right lower back: ICD-10-CM Code(s) _____

7. Trichorrhexis nodusa: ICD-10-CM Code(s) _____

8. Allergic urticaria: ICD-10-CM Code(s) _____

9. Carbuncle of the face: ICD-10-CM Code(s) _____

10. Basal cell carcinoma of skin of right calf: ICD-10-CM Code(s) _____

11. Allergic contact dermatitis due to cosmetics: ICD-10-CM Code(s) _____

12. Solar urticaria: ICD-10-CM Code(s) _____

13. Acne keloid: ICD-10-CM Code(s) _____

14. Nonpressure ulcer of the back with necrosis of the bone: ICD-10-CM Code(s) _____

15. Neurodermatitis: ICD-10-CM Code(s) _____

16. Bockhart impetigo: ICD-10-CM Code(s) _____

17. Anetoderma of Jadassohn-Pellizzari: ICD-10-CM Code(s) _____

18. Nonbullous erythema multiforme with 45% skin exfoliation: ICD-10-CM Code(s) _____

19. Infantile acne: ICD-10-CM Code(s) _____

20. Vitiligo: ICD-10-CM Code(s) _____

21. Alopecia mucinosa: ICD-10-CM Code(s) _____

22. Onychogryphosis: ICD-10-CM Code(s) _____

23. Malignant melanoma in situ of the right eyelid: ICD-10-CM Code(s) _____

24. Postprocedural hemorrhage of skin following dermatologic procedure: ICD-10-CM Code(s) _____

25. Omphalitis in an adult: ICD-10-CM Code(s) _____

Chapter 12

Diseases of the Musculoskeletal System and Connective Tissue (M00-M99)

Chapter Outline

- **Musculoskeletal System Refresher**
- **Coding Overview of the Musculoskeletal System**
- **Abstracting for Conditions of the Musculoskeletal System**
- **Assigning Codes for Conditions of the Musculoskeletal System**
- **Arranging Codes for Conditions of the Musculoskeletal System**
- **Coding Neoplasms of the Musculoskeletal System**

Learning Objectives

After completing this chapter, you should have the skills to:

12.1 Spell and define the key words, medical terms, and abbreviations related to diseases of the musculoskeletal system and connective tissue.

12.2 Discuss the structure, function, and common conditions of the musculoskeletal system.

12.3 Identify the main characteristics of coding for diseases of the musculoskeletal system and connective tissue.

12.4 Abstract information from the medical record required for coding diseases of the musculoskeletal system and connective tissue.

12.5 Assign codes for diseases of the musculoskeletal system and connective tissue.

12.6 Arrange codes for diseases of the musculoskeletal system and connective tissue.

12.7 Code neoplasms of the musculoskeletal system.

12.8 Discuss the Official Guidelines for Coding and Reporting related to diseases of the musculoskeletal system and connective tissue.

Key Terms and Abbreviations

appendicular skeleton	fatigue fracture	march fracture	pathologic fracture
axial skeleton	femur	metastatic bone disease (MBD)	proximal epiphysis
body	fragility fracture	muscular system	shaft
cartilage	insertion	musculoskeletal (MS) system	skeletal system
delayed	involuntary	neck	tendon
diaphysis	joint	nonunion	traumatic
distal epiphysis	ligament	origin	vertebra
fascia	malunion	osseous	voluntary

In addition to the key terms listed here, students should know the terms defined within tables in this chapter.

INTRODUCTION

Automotive engineers spend thousands of hours designing an amazing chassis that supports and protects you and also allows you to drive in comfort. In the human body, the musculoskeletal system is the chassis that everything else is built on.

Orthopedic physicians specialize in diagnosing and treating conditions of the musculoskeletal system. Orthopedic surgeons may be subspecialists in a particular anatomic site, such as the spine or the knee. Rheumatologists specialize in diagnosing and treating arthritis and other diseases of the joints, muscles, and bones. Physical therapists, or physiotherapists, are non-physician practitioners who hold a master's or doctorate degree and use various physical treatments and exercises to help patients with musculoskeletal conditions or injuries restore function, improve mobility, and reduce pain. Primary care physicians treat uncomplicated conditions of the musculoskeletal system. They refer patients in need of rehabilitation to physical therapists and refer patients with more complex conditions to orthopedic specialists.

As you read this chapter, open up your medical terminology book to the musculoskeletal system and keep a medical dictionary handy to refresh your memory of any unfamiliar terms. The musculoskeletal system has hundreds of structures with scientific names, and no one can remember all of them. Resources ensure that you have the information you need at your fingertips.

MUSCULOSKELETAL SYSTEM REFRESHER

The **musculoskeletal (MS) system** consists of the **skeletal system** and the **muscular system**. The function of the skeletal system is to support the body, protect internal organs, produce blood cells, store minerals, and serve as a point of attachment for the skeletal muscles. The function of the muscular system is to provide for movement of the body as well as the operation of individual organs, maintain body posture, and help produce heat.

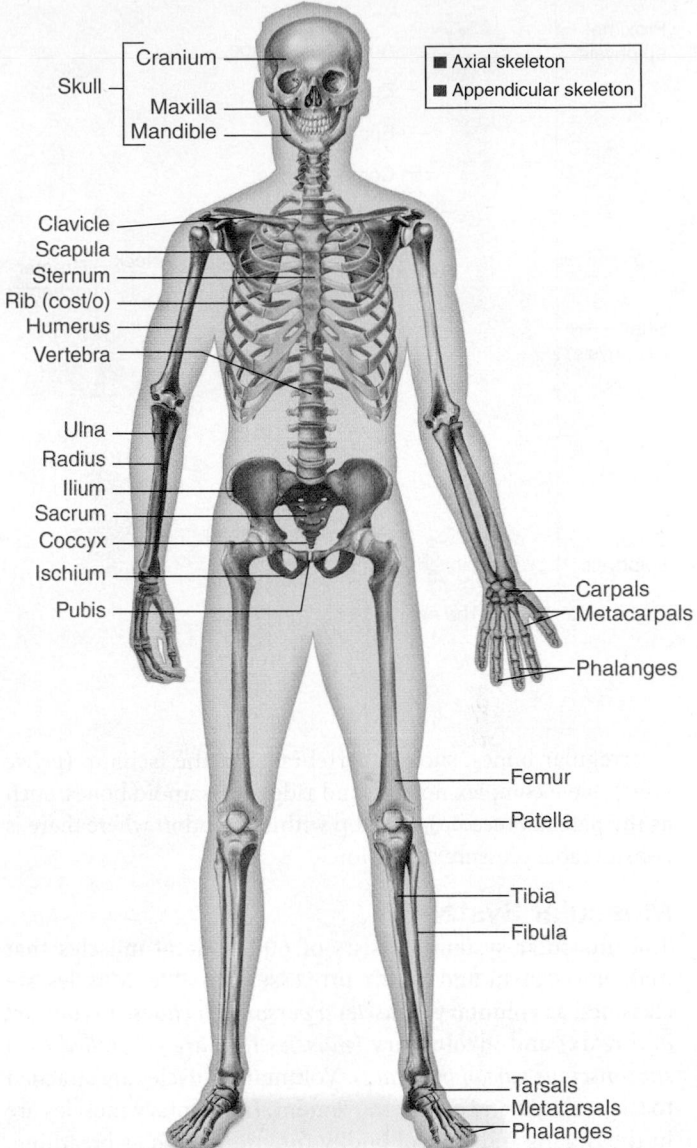

Figure 12-1 ■   The Skeletal System

Skeletal System

The skeletal system consists of 206 bones, as well as **cartilage** (*fibrous tissue found at the ends of bones*), **ligaments** (*fibrous tissue that connects bones to bones*), **tendons** (*fibrous tissue that connects bones to muscles*), and **fascia** (*fibrous tissue that connects muscle to muscle*). **Joints** are where two or more bones meet (■ FIGURE 12-1). The skeleton has two divisions: the axial skeleton and the appendicular skeleton. The **axial skeleton** contains 80 bones that are basically stationary and make up the skull, sternum, ribs, and **vertebrae** (*bony segments of the spine*). The **appendicular skeleton** contains 126 bones and consists of the arms, shoulders, wrists, hands, legs, hips, ankles, and feet.

Bones are also described by their shapes: long, short, flat, irregular, and sesamoid. Long bones comprise the arms and

legs and have three major parts: the **proximal epiphysis**, the rounded end of the bone closest to the trunk; the **diaphysis** or shaft, the long narrow part of the bone; and the **distal epiphysis**, the rounded end of the bone furthest from the trunk. The area between the proximal epiphysis and the shaft is the **neck**. The **femur** (*thigh bone*) is an example of a long bone and is the largest bone in the body (■ FIGURE 12-2, page 176).

Short bones are cubical in shape, being of nearly equal length and width. The carpals (*wrist bones*) and tarsals (*ankle bones*) are examples of short bones.

Flat bones are thin, broad, and usually curved. They consist of two parallel layers of compact bone with a layer of spongy bone in between, and they lack the marrow cavity. The ribs, scapulae (*shoulder blades*), and cranium are examples of flat bones.

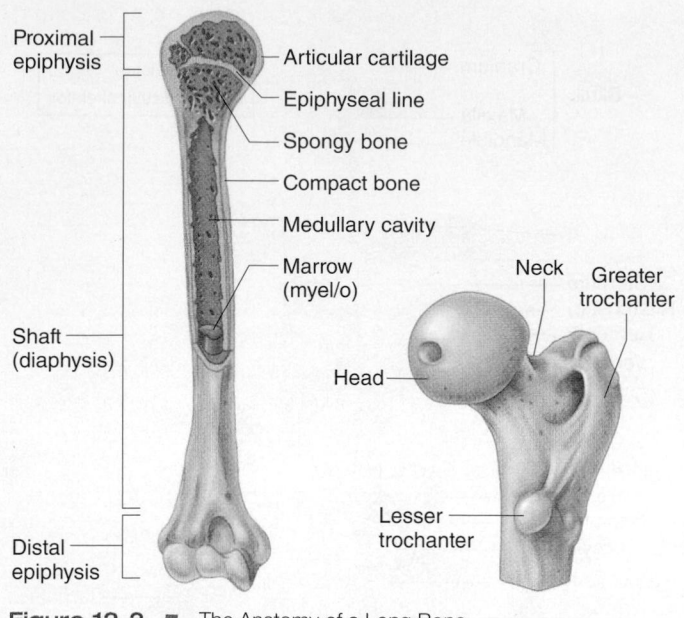

Figure 12-2 ■ The Anatomy of a Long Bone

tion of the muscle; and the **insertion**, where the muscle attaches to a bone that moves.

Remember to apply medical terminology skills to combine word roots, prefixes, and suffixes you already know to define new terms related to the musculoskeletal system. Refer to ■ TABLE 12-1 for a refresher on how to build medical terms related to the musculoskeletal system.

> ### CODING CAUTION
>
> Remember to distinguish between medical terms with similar spellings but different meanings:
>
> **cost/o** (*rib*) and **chondr/o** (*cartilage*)
>
> **ilium** (*pelvic bone*) and **ileum** (*small intestine*)
>
> **my/o** (*muscle*) and **myel/o** (*bone marrow*)
>
> **sacr/o** (*sacrum, lowest part of back*) and **sarc/o** (*flesh, connective tissue*)

Irregular bones, such as vertebrae and the ischium (*pelvic bone*), have complex notches and ridges. Sesamoid bones, such as the patella (*kneecap*), develop within a tendon where there is considerable pressure or tension.

Muscular System

The muscular system consists of 600 skeletal muscles that make movement and bodily processes possible. Muscles are classified as **voluntary** (*muscles a person can choose to contract and relax*) and **involuntary** (*muscles that are controlled by a subconscious part of the brain*). Voluntary muscles are attached to the skeleton and enable movement. Involuntary muscles are in the organs and control bodily functions such as breathing, digestion, and the heartbeat. Muscles are named based on their location and function. Muscles have three distinct parts: the **origin**, where the muscle is fixed; the **body**, or main por-

Conditions of the Musculoskeletal System

Coders use medical resources, such as a reference book on diseases, to understand conditions of the musculoskeletal system, diagnostic methods, and common treatments. Common conditions of the musculoskeletal system are highlighted in ■ TABLE 12-2. Conditions are diagnosed through physical examination, imaging, biopsy, and lab tests. X-rays are used to evaluate conditions of the bone because they clearly show the difference between hard tissue and soft tissue. Computerized tomography (CT) and magnetic resonance imaging (MRI) are used to evaluate muscle and other soft-tissue disorders because they show more contrast between different types of soft tissue. Blood tests are used for conditions such as rheumatoid arthritis, which is detected by the presence of Rh factor, and infections, which elevate the

Table 12-1 ■ **EXAMPLE OF CONSTRUCTING MEDICAL TERMS FOR THE MUSCULOSKELETAL SYSTEM**

Combining Form	Suffix	Complete Medical Term
my/o (*muscle*)		**myo + sitis** (*muscle inflammation*)
		my + asthenia (*muscle weakness*)
	-algia (*pain*)	**my + algia** (*muscle pain*)
	-asthenia (*weakness*)	**myo + sarc + oma** (*malignant tumor in the muscle*)
arthr/o (*joint*)	**-itis** (*inflammation*)	**arthr + itis** (*inflammation of a joint*)
	sarc + oma (*malignant tumor*)	**arthr + algia** (*pain in a joint*)
oste/o (*bone*)		**osteo + arthr + itis** (*inflammation of a bone and joint*)
		osteo + sarc + oma (*malignant tumor in the bone*)

Table 12-2 ■ COMMON CONDITIONS OF THE MUSCULOSKELETAL SYSTEM

Condition	Description
Arthritis	Damage or inflammation of the joints
Bursitis	Inflammation of fluid around a joint
Degeneration	Breakdown of bone or tissue
Dislocation	Two bones out of place at the joint
Fracture	Broken bone
Infection	Muscle or bone inflammation due to an infectious agent
Osteoporosis	Thinning of bone tissue and loss of bone density
Sprain	Overstretching, bruising, or tearing of a ligament
Strain	Overstretching, bruising, or tearing of a bone or tendon
Subluxation	Partial dislocation of bones in a joint
Tendonitis	Inflammation of a tendon, often caused by overuse

white blood cell count. Noninvasive treatments are pain medication, antibiotics for infections, and physical therapy to improve or restore function. Surgery may be performed to reshape a structure, remove an abnormal growth, or repair and stabilize a bone by inserting orthopedic hardware such as rods, pins, or screws.

SUCCESS STEP

The shoulder is the most frequently dislocated joint in the body because its shallow socket allows it to move in many directions. As a result, it can slip out of place when force is applied. You may have seen an athlete dislocate a shoulder during a sporting event, "pop" it back into place, and continue participating in the event.

CODING PRACTICE

Exercise 12.1   Musculoskeletal System Refresher

Instructions: Use your medical terminology skills and resources to define the following conditions related to the musculoskeletal system, then assign the diagnosis code.

Follow these steps:

- Use slash marks "/" to break down each term into its root(s) and suffix.

- Define the meaning of the word, based on the meaning of each word part.
- Assign the default ICD-10-CM diagnosis code for the condition using the Index and Tabular List.

Example: arthritis arthr/itis   Meaning: *inflammation of a joint*   ICD-10-CM Code: *M19.90*

1. arthropathy   Meaning _____   ICD-10-CM Code _____
2. osteomyelitis   Meaning _____   ICD-10-CM Code _____
3. fibromyalgia   Meaning _____   ICD-10-CM Code _____
4. lordosis   Meaning _____   ICD-10-CM Code _____
5. chondrocalcinosis   Meaning _____   ICD-10-CM Code _____
6. spondylolisthesis   Meaning _____   ICD-10-CM Code _____
7. chondromalacia   Meaning _____   ICD-10-CM Code _____
8. osteolysis   Meaning _____   ICD-10-CM Code _____
9. tenosynovitis   Meaning _____   ICD-10-CM Code _____
10. fasciitis   Meaning _____   ICD-10-CM Code _____

CODING OVERVIEW OF THE MUSCULOSKELETAL SYSTEM

ICD-10-CM Chapter 13, Diseases of the Musculoskeletal System and Connective Tissue (M00-M99), contains 18 blocks or subchapters that are divided by type of condition and type of tissue. Review the block names and code ranges listed at the

beginning of Chapter 13 in the ICD-10-CM manual to become familiar with the content and organization.

ICD-10-CM Chapter 13 corresponds with ICD-9-CM Chapter 13 (710-739). ICD-10-CM has expanded a majority of codes in this chapter, including laterality, specificity of site, and/or episode of care. Expanded instructional notes in the ICD-10-CM Tabular List direct coders to assign additional codes for underlying and associated conditions. New codes appear for osteoporosis with and without a current pathological fracture, as well as for osteoarthritis and rheumatoid arthritis.

This chapter includes chronic or recurrent conditions of the joint, bone, and soft tissue, including those of the jaw. It does not include codes for traumatic (*acute current injury that results from an accident*) fractures, injuries, congenital and perinatal conditions, neoplasms, or symptoms and signs, which are classified in other ICD-10-CM chapters. Review the **Excludes2** note at the beginning of the chapter to cross-reference the locations of these codes.

ICD-10-CM provides Official Guidelines for Coding and Reporting (OGCR) for the musculoskeletal system in OGCR section I.C.13. OGCR discusses coding for site and laterality, pathologic fractures, and osteoporosis. Additional OGCR related to conditions of the musculoskeletal system appear in OGCR I.C.19 and I.C.20.

ABSTRACTING FOR CONDITIONS OF THE MUSCULOSKELETAL SYSTEM

The keys to abstracting diagnoses for the MS system are familiarity with the anatomy, knowledge of medical terms, and careful attention to the details of the documented condition. ■ TABLE 12-3 highlights key questions to ask when abstracting MS conditions. Pathologic fractures require additional abstracting, shown in ■ TABLE 12-4. Remember that abstracting questions are a general guide and all questions may not apply to every patient. For example, not all conditions have laterality. When there is a traumatic injury, also abstract the external cause.

Guided Example of Abstracting Diagnoses for the Musculoskeletal System

Refer to the following example throughout this chapter to learn skills for abstracting and assigning codes for conditions affecting the musculoskeletal system. Jacob Bates, CCS, is a fictitious coder who guides you through this case.

Table 12-3 ■ KEY CRITERIA FOR ABSTRACTING MUSCULOSKELETAL CONDITIONS

- ❑ What type of condition is documented: fracture, dislocation, subluxation, sprain, infection, inflammation, or degeneration?
- ❑ What type of tissue or structure is affected: bone, joint, cartilage, muscle, tendon, or ligament?
- ❑ What is the specific subtype of condition (e.g., osteoarthritis vs. rheumatoid arthritis)?
- ❑ What is the anatomic site?
- ❑ What is the laterality?
- ❑ For osteoporosis: Does the patient have a pathologic fracture? Does the patient have a history of healed pathologic fractures?
- ❑ Is the condition acute, chronic, or a late effect?
- ❑ Is the encounter for active treatment?
- ❑ Is the encounter for aftercare during the healing phase?
- ❑ Is the encounter for follow-up after active healing is complete?

Table 12-4 ■ KEY CRITERIA FOR ABSTRACTING PATHOLOGIC FRACTURES

- ❑ Is the fracture traumatic or pathologic?
- ❑ What type of pathologic fracture is it?
- ❑ What is the underlying disease?
- ❑ What bone is fractured?
- ❑ What is the laterality?
- ❑ Were any additional bones fractured?
- ❑ Is the healing routine, **delayed** (*patient waited to seek care*), **nonunion** (*failure of the ends of the fractured bone segments to reunite*), or **malunion** (*ends of fractured bone segments did not heal with proper alignment*)?
- ❑ Is the encounter for active treatment?
- ❑ Is the encounter for aftercare during the healing phase?
- ❑ Is the encounter for follow-up after active healing is complete?

Date: 3/1/yy   Location: Valley Hospital

Provider: Bruce Prentice, MD

Patient: Nadine Tubbs   Gender: F   Age: 80

Reason for admission: admitted from physician office where she was seen for hip pain. X-rays showed fracture.

Procedure performed: repair of fracture with a metal rod

Discharge plan: pathologic fracture of right femoral neck due to osteoporosis. Referred to rehab for 6 weeks.

Follow along as Jacob Bates, CCS, abstracts the diagnosis. Check off each step after you complete it.

▶ Jacob reads through the entire record, paying special attention to the reason for the admission and the discharge plan. He refers to the Key Criteria for Abstracting Pathologic Fractures (Table 12-4).

- ❑ *Is the fracture traumatic or pathologic?* pathologic
- ❑ *What is the underlying disease?* osteoporosis
- ❑ *What bone is fractured?* femur
- ❑ *What site on the bone is fractured?* neck
- ❑ *What is the laterality?* right
- ❑ *Is the encounter for active treatment?* Yes, the episode of care is the initial encounter because the fracture was repaired and there is no mention of previous treatment for it.
- ❑ Jacob will not abstract pain because pain is a symptom integral to the condition.

▶ Jacob has completed abstracting. Next, he will assign the codes.

CODING PRACTICE

Exercise 12.2   Abstracting for Conditions of the Musculoskeletal System

Instructions: Read the mini-medical-record of each patient's encounter and answer the abstracting questions. Write the answer on the line provided. Do not assign any codes.

---

1. OFFICE   Gender: F   Age: 48

Chief complaint: *Patient came in for management of fibromyalgia which was diagnosed last year. C/o increased pain in lower back and hips.*

Assessment: *fibromyalgia*

Plan: *Refer to physical therapy for modified exercise program and pain relief. Adjusted medication.*

a. What are the presenting symptoms? _____

_____

b. What is the underlying condition? _____

_____

c. Should you code the symptoms? _____

   Why or why not? _____

_____

d. Should you code an encounter for physical therapy?
   _____ Why or why not? _____

_____

---

2. OFFICE   Gender: F   Age: 66

Reason for encounter: *management and monitoring of osteoarthritis*

Assessment: *degenerative osteoarthritis of the right knee*

a. What type of arthritis does the patient have?

_____

b. What is the anatomic site? _____

_____

c. What is the laterality? _____

_____

d. Is the arthritis described as generalized? _____

_____

e. Is the arthritis posttraumatic? _____

---

3. OFFICE   Gender: M   Age: 72

Chief complaint: *acute hip pain*

Assessment: *X-rays show a fracture of the ilium due to age-related osteoporosis*

a. What is the presenting symptom? _____

_____

b. What is the diagnosis of the cause of the pain?

_____

c. What is the underlying condition? _____

_____

d. What type of fracture is this? _____

_____

e. Should the symptom be coded? _____

   Why or why not? _____

_____

---

4. OUTPATIENT SURGERY   Gender: M   Age: 56

Reason for encounter: *vertebroplasty (injection of acrylic cement into a fractured vertebra to stabilize it) to correct compression fracture*

Assessment: *collapsed vertebrae L3 and L4 due to bone metastasis from prostate cancer*

a. What procedure was performed? _____

_____

b. What is the reason for the procedure? _____

_____

c. What is the anatomic site? _____

_____

d. What type of fracture is this? _____

_____

e. What additional diagnoses exist? _____

_____

f. What is the principal diagnosis? _____

_____

g. What is the second diagnosis? _____

_____

h. What is the third diagnosis? _____

_____

(continued)

CODING PRACTICE *(continued)*

5. OFFICE Gender: M Age: 36

Reason for encounter: *left knee pain*

Assessment: *chronic knee derangement due to an old injury of the anterior horn of the medial meniscus. Injury was sustained during a tackle in a college football game 15 years ago.*

a. What is the symptom? _____

_____

b. Should you code the symptom? _____

Why or why not? _____

_____

c. What is the episode of care? _____

_____

d. What is the site within the knee where the original injury occurred? _____

_____

e. What is the laterality? _____

_____

f. What external cause event caused the injury? _____

_____

g. Should you code for the activity? _____

Why or why not? _____

_____

6. OFFICE Gender: F Age: 70

Reason for encounter: *follow-up on test results after complaints of hand pain*

Assessment: *elevated WBC count, calcification evident on X-rays. Arthritis in crystal arthropathy (presence of calcification within soft tissues) of the right hand due to dicalcium phosphate crystals. Patient previously diagnosed with primary hyperparathyroidism which is associated with this condition.*

Plan: *corticosteroid injection, RTO 4 wk*

a. What condition is newly diagnosed? _____

_____

b. What is the cause of the condition? _____

_____

c. What is the anatomic site? _____

_____

d. What is the laterality? _____

_____

e. What is the previously existing condition? _____

_____

f. Should the previously existing condition be coded? _____ Why or why not? _____

_____

ASSIGNING CODES FOR CONDITIONS OF THE MUSCULOSKELETAL SYSTEM

Assigning codes for MS disorders may require coders to cross-reference the medical record multiple times to accurately capture the details of the disorder. This serves as a cross-check for abstracting because it is easy to overlook one or more details. Coders may not know exactly what information is required until they assign the code, review the subterms in the Index, and read the instructional notes in the Tabular List. In addition, careful attention to the spelling of medical terms is necessary to locate the correct term in the Index. Conventions in the Index and Tabular List indicate when multiple coding is required for infections, underlying conditions, and complications. The Tabular List conventions also notify coders when a seventh character is required and what the seventh-character choices are for any given code.

SUCCESS STEP

Because there are 206 bones and 600 muscles, it is common to encounter terms you may be unfamiliar with when coding the MS system. Just as you keep a map or global positioning navigator handy when driving in unfamiliar areas, a quick check in a medical terminology or anatomy book will help smooth out the bumps in the road.

Most of the codes within Chapter 13 have site and laterality designations. The site represents the bone, joint, or muscle involved. For some conditions where more than one bone, joint, or muscle is usually involved in the same type of injury, the Index provides a combination for multiple sites available (OGCR I.C.13.a) (■ FIGURE 12-3).

Patient has osteochondropathy of ankles, knees, and hip.

Osteochondropathy M93.90
   ankle M93.97-
   elbow M93.92-
   foot M93.97-
   hand M93.94-
   hip M93.95-
   Kienböck's disease of adults M93.1
   knee M93.96-
   multiple joints M93.99

Figure 12-3 ■ Example of a Combination Code for Multiple Sites

For some conditions, such as **avascular necrosis of bone** and osteoporosis, the bone may be affected at the upper or lower end. Although the portion of the bone affected may be at the joint, code the site as the bone, not the joint (OGCR I.C.13.a.1)) (■ FIGURE 12-4). Code the joint when the joint capsule itself is affected, as in arthritis.

Guided Example of Assigning Musculoskeletal System Diagnosis Codes

Continue with the example from earlier in the chapter about patient Nadine Tubbs, who was admitted to Valley Hospital because of a pathologic fracture, to practice skills for assigning codes for the MS system.

Follow along in your ICD-10-CM manual as Jacob Bates, CCS, assigns codes. Check off each step after you complete it.

▶ First, Jacob confirms that the diagnosis is pathologic fracture of the right femoral neck due to osteoporosis.

❑ Jacob searches the Index for the Main Term **Fracture, pathological**. He notes that this is a separate Main Term from **Fracture, traumatic**.

❑ He locates the subterm **due to**.

❑ He locates the second-level subterm **osteoporosis M80.00**.

❑ He notes that there are no further subterms for anatomic site.

❑ However, he does notice a cross-reference for **postmenopausal** *see* **Osteoporosis, postmenopausal, with pathological fracture**.

Patient has avascular necrosis at the proximal epiphysis of the left radius.

Index:
Necrosis, bone *see also* **Osteonecrosis**
Osteonecrosis, idiopathic, radius M87.03-
Tabular List:
M87.032 Idiopathic aseptic necrosis of left radius

Figure 12-4 ■ Example of Coding the Site as Bone, Not Joint 1

❑ He cross-references the Main Term **Osteoporosis** and the subterm **postmenopausal**.

❑ Now he sees a second-level subterm **with pathological fracture**.

❑ Under this entry he notices no entry for femur, but does see additional subterms for **ilium, ischium**, and **pelvis**, all of which point to **M80.05**. He decides to research this option because these bones are adjacent to the femoral joint and he knows that the ICD-10-CM often classifies them together.

CODING CAUTION

If Jacob does not follow the cross-reference **Osteoporosis, postmenopausal, with pathological fracture**, he will verify **M80.00 Age-related osteoporosis with current pathological fracture, unspecified site**. The words **unspecified site** should be a red flag and cause him to either return to the Index or review the Tabular List to locate a more specific code for the **femur**.

▶ Jacob verifies code **pelvis M80.05** in the Tabular List.

❑ He reads the code title for **M80.05, Age-related osteoporosis with current pathological fracture, femur** and confirms that this accurately describes the principal diagnosis and identifies the anatomic site of the femur.

❑ Jacob looks for any conventions or instructional notes with the code.

❑ He notices the convention **6th** that directs him to use a sixth character with **M80.05** for laterality.

❑ He double-checks the medical record to verify the laterality as **right**.

❑ The code for right femur is **M80.051**.

❑ He notices the convention **7th** that tells him a seventh character is required with **M80.051**.

❑ He refers to the beginning of category **M80** to locate the seventh character.

❑ He selects the seventh character **A, initial encounter** because the episode of care is for active treatment. Even though the patient was previously seen in the physician's office, there was no treatment, so seventh character **D, subsequent encounter for fracture with routine healing** is not appropriate.

❑ Jacob verifies that the complete code is **M80.051A**.

▶ Jacob checks for any additional instructional notes in the Tabular List.

❑ Since he is already at the beginning of the three-digit category, he reviews the notes that appear, including the definition of a fragility fracture.

❑ He reviews the note **Use additional code to identify major osseous defect, if applicable** and double-checks the medical record to be certain no defects are documented.

❑ He also double-checks the medical record to see whether there is a personal history of a (healed) osteoporosis fracture, which there is not. If there were, he would need to assign code **Z87.310** for the history.

❑ He cross-references the beginning of the block **M80-M94** and verifies that there are no instructional notes.

❑ He cross-references the beginning of **Chapter 12 (M00-M99)** and reviews the instructional notes. He determines he does not need to assign an external cause code because the patient's fracture was not due to an external cause, but was due to a disease.

▶ Jacob finalizes the code for this case:

❑ **M80.051A Age-related osteoporosis with current pathological fracture, right femur, initial encounter.**

CODING PRACTICE

Exercise 12.3 Assigning Codes for Conditions of the Musculoskeletal System

Instructions: Read the mini-medical-record of each patient's encounter, review the information abstracted in Exercise 12.2, and assign ICD-10-CM diagnosis codes using the Index and Tabular List. Write the code(s) on the line provided.

1. OFFICE Gender: F Age: 48

Chief complaint: *Patient came in for management of fibromyalgia which was diagnosed last year. C/o increased pain in lower back and hips.*

Assessment: *fibromyalgia*

Plan: *Refer to physical therapy for modified exercise program and pain relief. Adjusted medication.*

1 ICD-10-CM Code _____

2. OFFICE Gender: F Age: 66

Reason for encounter: *management and monitoring of osteoarthritis*

Assessment: *degenerative osteoarthritis of the right knee*

1 ICD-10-CM Code _____

3. OFFICE Gender: M Age: 72

Chief complaint: *acute hip pain*

Assessment: *X-rays show a fracture of the ilium due to age-related osteoporosis*

Tip: The ilium is classified with the femur in the Tabular List, so do not be confused when you read the code title.

1 ICD-10-CM Code _____

ARRANGING CODES FOR CONDITIONS OF THE MUSCULOSKELETAL SYSTEM

When MS disorders require multiple coding, coders must be attentive to the sequencing indicated in the instructional notes. Because there is a wide variety of code sequencing situations, this section provides several short examples rather than a single guided example of arranging codes. Examples of the most commonly encountered situations follow, including pathologic fracture, infectious conditions, osseous defects, and external causes.

Pathologic Fractures

Pathologic fractures, also called **fragility fractures**, are fractures caused by disease rather than trauma (OGCR I.C.13.d.2)). They result from a fall from a standing height or less and would not cause a fracture in a normal healthy bone. ICD-10-CM classifies four types of pathologic fractures and provides instructional notes for sequencing codes (■ Table 12-5).

Infectious Conditions

Infectious conditions, such as **pyogenic arthritis** and myositis, require coders to use an additional code for the infectious agent (■ Figure 12-5).

Osseous Defects

Pathologic fractures, osteomyelitis, and osteonecrosis require coders to use an additional code to describe any major bone defects. Pathologic fractures also require an additional code for a history of healed pathologic fractures (■ Figure 12-6).

Table 12-5 ■ **DEFINITIONS AND SEQUENCING INSTRUCTIONS FOR PATHOLOGIC FRACTURES**

Type of Fracture	Definition	Instructional Note
Osteoporotic	A fragility fracture in person with osteoporosis.	Use additional code to identify major osseous (*bone*) defect, if applicable (**M89.7-**). Use additional code to identify personal history of (healed) osteoporosis fracture, if applicable (**Z87.310**).
Neoplastic	A fragility fracture due to neoplastic disease.	Code also underlying neoplasm.
Stress	Fracture of a bone that has been subjected to repeated use or impact. Also called a **march fracture** or **fatigue fracture**.	Use additional external cause code(s) to identify the cause of the stress fracture.
Other	A fragility fracture caused by a disease other than osteoporosis or neoplasm. Any other type of pathological fracture.	Code also underlying condition.

External Cause

Stress fractures and soft-tissue disorders, which are caused by overuse or pressure, require coders to assign and sequence an external cause code as a secondary code. In many cases, the only external cause code will be an activity code because there is not an applicable event code. This is an exception to the general rule that requires that activity codes be assigned only in conjunction with external cause event codes (■ FIGURE 12-7).

Patient is seen for pyogenic arthritis in the right elbow due to methicillin-susceptible *Staphylococcus aureus*.

(1) **M00.021 Staphylococcal arthritis, right elbow**
(2) **B95.61 Methicillin susceptible staphylococcus aureus as the cause of diseases classified elsewhere**

Figure 12-5 ■ Sequencing for an Infectious Condition

Patient is seen for chronic osteomyelitis of left scapula due to methicillin-susceptible *Staphylococcus aureus* with major osseous defect.

(1) **M86.612 Other chronic osteomyelitis, left shoulder**
(2) **B95.61 Methicillin susceptible staphylococcus aureus as the cause of diseases classified elsewhere**
(3) **M89.712 Major osseous defect, left shoulder region**

Figure 12-6 ■ Example of Sequencing for Osseous Defects

Patient is seen for tendonitis of the left forearm due to overuse in baseball.

Index Entry for Main Term, Tendonitis:
Tendinitis, tendonitis — *see also* Enthesopathy
  Achilles M76.6-

due to use, overuse, pressure — *see also* Disorder, soft tissue, due to use
  specified NEC — *see* Disorder, soft tissue, due to use, specified NEC

Index Entry for Cross-referenced Main Term, Disorder:
Disorder
  soft tissue M79.9
    ankle M79.9
    due to use, overuse and pressure M70.90
      ankle M70.97-
      bursitis — *see* Bursitis
      foot M70.97-
      forearm M70.93-
      hand M70.94-
      lower leg M70.96-

Tabular List for Category M70:
  Other soft tissue disorders (M70-M79)
M70 Soft tissue disorders related to use, overuse and pressure
    Includes: soft tissue disorders of occupational origin
    Use additional external cause code to identify activity causing disorder (Y93.-)

Final Code Assignment and Sequencing:
(1) **M70.932 Unspecified soft tissue disorder related to use, overuse and pressure, left forearm**
(2) **Y93.64 Activity, baseball**

Figure 12-7 ■ Example of Sequencing of External Causes

Multiple Sites

Earlier in the chapter, Figure 12-3 demonstrated how to assign a combination code for multiple sites, rather than coding each site separately, when more than one bone, joint, or muscle is involved. However, not all categories provide a combination code for multiple sites. When the Index does not provide a code for multiple sites, assign separate codes to indicate each of the sites involved, as shown in ■ FIGURE 12-8 (OGCR I.C.13.a). When each site is equally responsible for the encounter, sequence any of the codes first (OGCR II.C and IV).

CODING CAUTION

When the Index does not provide a subterm for **multiple sites**, it is helpful also to review the Tabular List entries to be certain that no code for multiple sites exists. In some cases, a multiple site code exists even though it is not listed as a subterm in the Index. The code for **multiple sites** usually appears at the end of a category and ends in the number 8.

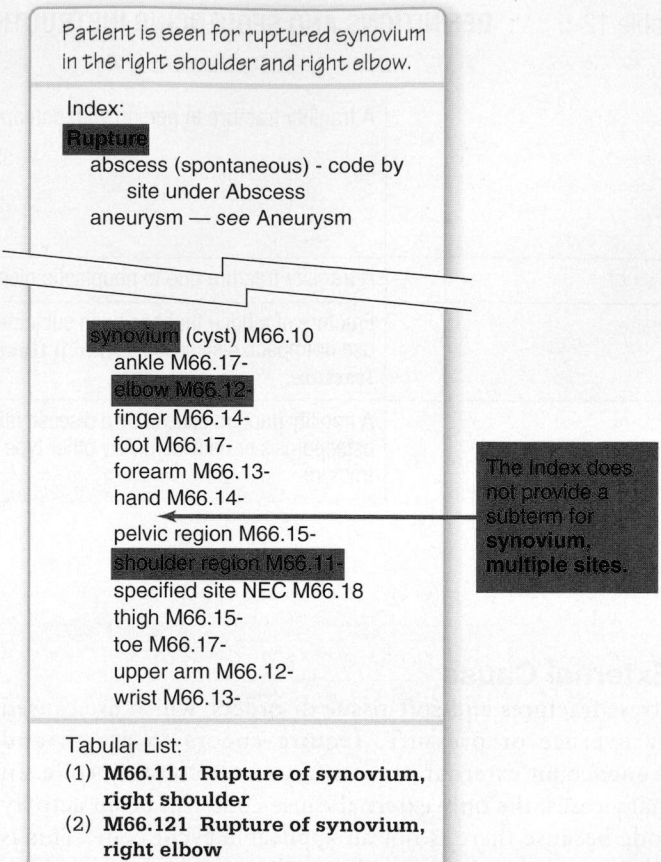

Patient is seen for ruptured synovium in the right shoulder and right elbow.

Index:

Rupture
  abscess (spontaneous) - code by site under Abscess
  aneurysm — *see* Aneurysm

synovium (cyst) M66.10
  ankle M66.17-
  elbow M66.12-
  finger M66.14-
  foot M66.17-
  forearm M66.13-
  hand M66.14-
  pelvic region M66.15-
  shoulder region M66.11-
  specified site NEC M66.18
  thigh M66.15-
  toe M66.17-
  upper arm M66.12-
  wrist M66.13-

The Index does not provide a subterm for synovium, multiple sites.

Tabular List:
(1) **M66.111 Rupture of synovium, right shoulder**
(2) **M66.121 Rupture of synovium, right elbow**

Figure 12-8 ■ Example of Assigning Separate Codes for Multiple Sites

CODING PRACTICE

Exercise 12.4 **Arranging Codes for Conditions of the Musculoskeletal System**

Instructions: Read the mini-medical-record of each patient's encounter, review the information abstracted in Exercise 12.2, assign ICD-10-CM diagnosis codes using the Index and Tabular List, and sequence them correctly.

1. OUTPATIENT SURGERY   Gender: M   Age: 56

Reason for encounter: vertebroplasty (*injection of acrylic cement into a fractured vertebra to stabilize it*) to correct compression fracture

Assessment: collapsed vertebrae L3 and L4 due to bone metastasis from prostate cancer

Tip: The reason for the vertebroplasty is the principal diagnosis. Sequence metastasis second because it caused
(*continued*)

1. (continued)

the compression fracture. Sequence the primary neoplasm third.

3 ICD-10-CM Codes _____
_____

2. OFFICE   Gender: M   Age: 36

Reason for encounter: left knee pain

Assessment: chronic knee derangement due to an old injury of the anterior horn of the medial meniscus. Injury was sustained during a tackle in a college football game 15 years ago.

Tip: The fact that this is due to an "old injury" makes it a sequela. Remember to use the Index of External Causes to locate the external cause (event) code.

2 ICD-10-CM Codes _____

(*continued*)

3. OFFICE   Gender: F   Age: 70

Reason for encounter: follow-up on test results after complaints of hand pain

Assessment: elevated WBC count, calcification evident on X-rays. Impression: arthritis in crystal arthropathy (*presence of crystal-like deposits in the joints*) of the right hand due to dicalcium phosphate crystals.

(continued)

3. (continued)

Patient previously diagnosed with primary hyperparathyroidism which is associated with this condition.

Plan: corticosteroid injection, RTO 4 wk

Tip: You may start with the Main Term **Arthritis** or **Arthropathy**.

2 ICD-10-CM Codes _____

CODING NEOPLASMS OF THE MUSCULOSKELETAL SYSTEM

Neoplasms of the musculoskeletal system do not appear in ICD-10-CM Chapter 12, Diseases of the Musculoskeletal System and Connective Tissue (M00-M99). Codes for neoplasms of the musculoskeletal system appear in the block C40-C41 within the neoplasm chapter. Codes for leukemia, which originates in the bone marrow, appear in categories C90-C96.

The most common cancer in the musculoskeletal system is **metastatic bone disease (MBD)** because the bone is a frequent site of metastasis from primary neoplasms in other organs, including the breast, lung, prostate, kidney, and thyroid. According to the American Academy of Orthopaedic Surgeons, approximately 50% of tumors can metastasize to the bone.

Cancer that begins in the bone is called primary bone cancer, or sarcoma, and is named after the specific type of tissue in which it originates, such as osteosarcoma (*sarcoma of bone*) or chondrosarcoma (*sarcoma of cartilage*). Ewing sarcoma forms in the shaft of long bones, the hip, and ribs. Children and young people are more likely than adults to have bone cancers. Soft-tissue sarcomas are relatively rare but are quite aggressive and dangerous, particularly when they occur in adults.

Leukemia is a cancer that starts in the bone marrow and affects the cells that form new blood cells. About one-third of childhood cancers are leukemias, the most common of which is acute lymphoblastic leukemia.

All malignant neoplasms in the musculoskeletal system are either primary or secondary. CA in situ does not exist because bone and connective tissue do not have the epithelial cells that give rise to CA in situ.

CODING PRACTICE

Exercise 12.5   Coding Neoplasms of the Musculoskeletal System

Instructions: Read the mini-medical-record of each patient's encounter, then abstract, assign, and sequence ICD-10-CM diagnosis codes using the Index and Tabular List. Write the code(s) on the line provided.

1. INPATIENT HOSPITAL   Gender: M   Age: 14

Reason for admission: surgical removal of tumor

Assessment: osteosarcoma in the right tibia

1 ICD-10-CM Code _____

2. INPATIENT HOSPITAL   Gender: F   Age: 48

Reason for encounter: pain management for MBD

Assessment: left breast cancer with metastasis to bone

Tip: The code for neoplasm-related pain may be assigned as the principal or first-listed code when the stated reason for the admission/encounter is documented as pain control/pain management. The underlying neoplasm should be reported as an additional diagnosis (OGCR I.C.6.b.5)).

3 ICD-10-CM Codes _____

_____

(continued)

CODING PRACTICE *(continued)*

3. INPATIENT HOSPITAL   Gender: F   Age: 13

Reason for admission: *induction chemotherapy with a goal of remission*

Assessment: *acute lymphoblastic leukemia*

2 ICD-10-CM Codes _____

4. OFFICE   Gender: F   Age: 63

Reason for encounter: *pain and lump on diaphysis of humerus*

Assessment: *possible chondrosarcoma*

Plan: *CT, MRI*

(continued)

4. *(continued)*

Tip: Remember the guidelines about coding uncertain conditions (OGCR II.H, IV.D, and IV.H). You need to determine whether this is an inpatient or outpatient encounter based on the location stated. You also need to identify where the humerus is.

2 ICD-10-CM Codes _____

5. INPATIENT HOSPITAL   Gender: M   Age: 16

Reason for admission: *surgical removal of tumor, followed by chemotherapy*

Assessment: *Ewing sarcoma, left femur*

Tip: Refer to OGCR I.C.2.a and I.C.2.e.1) for sequencing guidance.

2 ICD-10-CM Codes _____

CHAPTER SUMMARY

In this chapter you learned that:

- The musculoskeletal (MS) system consists of the skeletal system, which supports the body, protects internal organs, produces blood cells, stores minerals, and serves as a point of attachment for the skeletal muscles; and the muscular system, which provides for movement of the body, operates individual organs, maintains body posture, and helps produce heat.

- ICD-10-CM Chapter 13, Diseases of the Musculoskeletal System and Connective Tissue (M00-M99), contains 18 blocks or subchapters that are divided by type of tissue, such as bone, joint, spine, vertebrae, cartilage, and tendon.

- The keys to abstracting for the MS system are familiarity with the anatomy, knowledge of medical terms, and careful attention to the details of the documented condition.

- Assigning codes for MS disorders may require coders to cross-reference the medical record multiple times to accurately capture the details of the disorder.

- When codes for MS disorders require multiple coding, coders must be attentive to the sequencing indicated in the instructional notes.

- The most common cancer in the musculoskeletal system is metastatic bone disease (MBD) because the bone is a frequent site of metastasis from primary neoplasms in other organs, including the breast, lung, prostate, kidney, and thyroid.

- ICD-10-CM provides Official Guidelines for Coding and Reporting (OGCR) for the musculoskeletal system in section I.C.13, which discusses coding for site and laterality, pathologic fractures, and osteoporosis.

CONCEPT QUIZ

Take a moment to look back at diseases of the musculoskeletal system and connective tissue and solidify your skills. This is your opportunity to pull together everything you have learned.

Completion

Instructions: Write the term that answers each question based on the information you learned in this chapter. Choose from the following list. Some choices may be used more than once and some choices may not be used at all.

appendicular
axial
cartilage
delayed
diaphysis
distal epiphysis
involuntary
joints
ligaments

malunion
nonunion
osteoporosis
pathologic
proximal epiphysis
stress
tendons
traumatic
voluntary

1. A _____ fracture is an acute current injury that results from an accident.

2. A _____ fracture is a fracture of a bone that has been subjected to repeated use or impact.

3. _____ are fibrous tissue that join muscles to bones.

4. _____ healing occurs when a patient waits to seek care for a fracture.

5. _____ is when the ends of fractured bone segments do not heal with proper alignment.

6. The _____ is the shaft, or long narrow portion of a long bone.

7. The _____ is the rounded end of the bone closest to the trunk.

8. The _____ consists of the arms, shoulders, wrists, hands, legs, hips, ankles, and feet.

9. _____ are fibrous tissue that connect bones to bones.

10. _____ muscles are controlled by a subconscious part of the brain and control bodily functions such as breathing and digestion.

Multiple Choice

Instructions: Circle the letter of the best answer to each question based on the information you learned in this chapter.

1. A fracture that occurs as the result of a disease process is a _____ fracture.
   A. neoplastic
   B. traumatic
   C. pathologic
   D. stress

2. All of the following are key criteria for abstracting pathologic fractures EXCEPT
   A. What is the underlying disease?
   B. Is the fracture open or closed?
   C. What is the laterality?
   D. Is the encounter for aftercare during the healing phase?

3. When more than one bone, joint, or muscle has the same condition, how should the coder assign codes?
   A. Assign individual codes for each site.
   B. Assign a code for the most serious injury only.
   C. Assign a seventh character that indicates the number of sites.
   D. Assign a code for multiple sites.

4. When a bone is affected by osteoporosis at the end near the joint, coders should
   A. assign a code for the bone.
   B. assign a code for the joint.
   C. assign a combination code for both the bone and the joint.
   D. assign a not elsewhere classified (NEC) code.

5. Arthritis that is due to another disease requires coders to
   A. sequence the underlying condition first and the arthritis second.
   B. sequence the arthritis first and the underlying condition second.
   C. sequence either first, based on the main reason for the encounter.
   D. None of the above.

6. X-rays are used to evaluate conditions of the _____ because they clearly show the difference between hard tissue and soft tissue.
   A. tendons
   B. ligaments
   C. muscles
   D. bones

7. The presence of Rh factor in the blood allows physicians to use blood tests to diagnose
   A. infections.
   B. rheumatoid arthritis.
   C. osteoarthritis.
   D. fractures.

8. _____ is the failure of the ends of fractured bone segments to reunite.
   A. Delayed healing
   B. Malunion
   C. Nonunion
   D. Pathologic fracture

9. A frequent site for metastatic cancer is
   A. muscle.
   B. joints.
   C. tendons.
   D. bone.

10. Leukemia starts in
   A. blood.
   B. joints.
   C. bone marrow.
   D. tendons.

CODING CHALLENGE

Instructions: Read the mini-medical-record of each patient's encounter, then abstract, assign, and sequence ICD-10-CM diagnosis codes using the Index to Diseases and Injuries, the Index to External Causes, and the Tabular List. Write the code(s) on the line provided.

1. OFFICE   Gender: F   Age: 61

Reason for encounter: pain, redness, and swelling in left knee

Assessment: abscess of bursa, left knee, due to *Streptococcus A*

Plan: Reapply dressing as directed. Take antibiotic as instructed.

2 ICD-10-CM Codes _____

2. INPATIENT HOSPITAL   Gender: F   Age: 32

Reason for admission: repair of C5 and C6 disc

Assessment: acute and chronic pain due to herniated cervical disc at C5-C6

Plan: FU with rehab, FU with surgeon 1 wk

1 ICD-10-CM Code _____

3. INPATIENT HOSPITAL   Gender: F   Age: 28

Reason for admission: admitted for lumbar spinal fusion. She was previously diagnosed with spinal stenosis in her lumbar region. I told her that if the pain could not be controlled, she could opt for surgery. After ongoing efforts to manage the pain unsuccessfully, she decided to have surgery.

Assessment: osseous stenosis at L3-L4-L5

Plan: FU 1 wk

1 ICD-10-CM Code _____

4. OFFICE   Gender: M   Age: 15

Reason for encounter: Swollen glands and high fever with pain in right shoulder, right elbow, and right hand. Abdominal spasmodic pain and diarrhea

Assessment: juvenile arthritis with systemic onset (Still disease), shoulder, elbow, hand, and ulcerative colitis

Plan: Rx anti-inflammatory. RTO 3 wk

2 ICD-10-CM Codes _____

5. INPATIENT HOSPITAL   Gender: F   Age: 21

Reason for admission: continuing pain in right shoulder after ineffective physical therapy (PT)

Assessment: frozen right shoulder

Plan: Manipulation under anesthesia for shoulder. Return to PT. FU office 1 wk.

1 ICD-10-CM Code _____

6. OFFICE   Gender: F   Age: 57

Reason for encounter: pain on left big toe area when walking

Assessment: hallux valgus, left

Plan: Referred to orthopedic surgeon following unsuccessful treatment with orthotics

1 ICD-10-CM Code _____

7. OFFICE   Gender: M   Age: 47

Reason for encounter: weakness in the right forefoot

Assessment: drop foot

Plan: Refer to PT for fitting of lightweight orthoses

1 ICD-10-CM Code _____

8. INPATIENT HOSPITAL   Gender: F   Age: 23

Reason for admission: rotator cuff repair

Assessment: recurrent rotator cuff syndrome

Plan: PT, RTO 1 wk

1 ICD-10-CM Code _____

9. INPATIENT HOSPITAL   Gender: M   Age: 1 year

Reason for encounter: Repair of clubfoot

Assessment: acquired right talipes equinovarus (clubfoot)

Plan: PT, RTO 1 wk

1 ICD-10-CM Code _____

10. INPATIENT HOSPITAL   Gender: M   Age: 45

Reason for admission: *sudden onset of pain and swelling in left hip, fever*

Testing: arthrocentesis (*removing fluid from a joint with a needle*), blood culture, X-ray

(continued)

10. (continued)

Assessment: *bacterial pyogenic arthritis due to Pseudomonas aeruginosa, likely due to patient's intravenous drug abuse*

3 ICD-10-CM Codes _____

_____

KEEP ON CODING

Instructions: Read the diagnostic statement, then use the Index and Tabular List to assign and sequence ICD-10-CM diagnosis codes. Write the code(s) on the line provided.

1. Pneumococcal arthritis of left ankle: ICD-10-CM Code(s) _____

2. Felty syndrome, left hip: ICD-10-CM Code(s) _____

3. Dysplastic osteoarthritis of right hip: ICD-10-CM Code(s) _____

4. Lead-induced chronic gout, vertebrae: ICD-10-CM Code(s) _____

5. Panarteritis nodosa: ICD-10-CM Code(s) _____

6. Low-back pain: ICD-10-CM Code(s) _____

7. Rheumatoid nodule, right wrist: ICD-10-CM Code(s) _____

8. Stress fracture, right foot, initial encounter: ICD-10-CM Code(s) _____

9. Plica syndrome, left knee: ICD-10-CM Code(s) _____

10. Psoas tendinitis, right hip: ICD-10-CM Code(s) _____

11. Subacute osteomyelitis, right humerus: ICD-10-CM Code(s) _____

12. Sicca syndrome with myopathy: ICD-10-CM Code(s) _____

13. Rhabdomyosarcoma of the hip, left: ICD-10-CM Code(s) _____

14. Relapsing polychondritis: ICD-10-CM Code(s) _____

15. Spondylolysis, lumbar region: ICD-10-CM Code(s) _____

16. Postsurgical lordosis: ICD-10-CM Code(s) _____

17. Arthralgia of temporomandibular joint: ICD-10-CM Code(s) _____

18. Rheumatoid bursitis, left hand: ICD-10-CM Code(s) _____

19. Age-related osteoporosis with current pathologic fracture of the right ankle, initial encounter: ICD-10-CM Code(s) _____

20. Achilles tendinitis, right leg: ICD-10-CM Code(s) _____

21. Spinal stenosis, cervical region: ICD-10-CM Code(s) _____

22. Diastasis of muscle of the left shoulder: ICD-10-CM Code(s) _____

23. Spontaneous rupture of the flexor tendon, lower leg: ICD-10-CM Code(s) _____

24. Fibromyalgia: ICD-10-CM Code(s) _____

25. Osteitis deformans of skull: ICD-10-CM Code(s) _____

Chapter 13

Injury, Poisoning, and Certain Other Consequences of External Causes (S00-T88)

Chapter Outline

- **Injury and Poisoning Refresher**
- **Coding Overview of Injury and Poisoning**
- **Abstracting Diagnoses for Injury and Poisoning**
- **Assigning Diagnosis Codes for Injury and Poisoning**
- **Arranging Diagnosis Codes for Injury and Poisoning**

Learning Objectives

After completing this chapter, you should have the skills to:

13.1 Spell and define the key words, medical terms, and abbreviations related to injury, poisoning, and certain other consequences of external causes.

13.2 Discuss the common forms of injury and poisoning.

13.3 Identify the main characteristics of diagnosis coding for injury, poisoning, and certain other consequences of external causes.

13.4 Abstract information from the medical record required for diagnosis coding for injury, poisoning, and certain other consequences of external causes.

13.5 Assign diagnosis codes for injury, poisoning, and certain other consequences of external causes.

13.6 Arrange multiple diagnosis codes for injury, poisoning, and certain other consequences of external causes.

13.7 Discuss the Official Guidelines for Coding and Reporting related to injury, poisoning, and certain other consequences of external causes.

Key Terms and Abbreviations

burn	contusion	Gustilo classification system	physis
circumstances of admission	corrosion	nondisplaced	Rule of Nines
clavicle	degree	open (fracture)	total body surface area (TBSA)
closed	displaced	Salter-Harris classification	

In addition to the key terms listed here, students should know the terms defined within tables in this chapter.

For updates and corrections, visit our student resource site at
www.pearsonhighered.com/healthprofessionsresources

INTRODUCTION

As you are driving down the road, you occasionally need to pull over to let an ambulance pass. Your heart may pause for a moment as you wonder, "What happened? Who is in it? Who are their loved ones?" You never learn the answers, but you always send a prayer and good energy their way. Unfortunately, accidents and injuries are part of life, and coders follow special requirements to code these situations. In this chapter you will learn about different types of injuries and poisonings and how physicians treat these conditions.

Any physician may treat injuries and poisonings because they can affect any body system. Physician specialties that most commonly treat these conditions are emergency medicine, primary care, orthopedics, and dermatology.

As you read this chapter, refer to anatomic resources on the integumentary system and musculoskeletal systems, both of which are frequently affected by injuries.

INJURY AND POISONING REFRESHER

Injury and poisoning can encompass a wide variety of conditions and a range of definitions, so it is critical that coders understand how ICD-10-CM defines terms, rather than rely on how they might use the words in everyday conversation. Coders use medical resources, such as a reference book on diseases, to understand injuries, diagnostic methods, and common treatments. In particular, coders must be familiar with specific terminology related to burns, traumatic fractures, and poisoning and adverse effects, which are reviewed in detail. Other types of injuries are summarized in ■ TABLE 13-1. Also refer to Table 12-2, Common Conditions of the Musculoskeletal System, for a refresher on dislocations, subluxations, sprains, and strains.

Table 13-1 ■ TYPES OF INJURIES

Injury	Description
Abuse	Physical, emotional, or sexual mistreatment by one person toward another
Complications of care	Unanticipated results of a medical or surgical procedure
Foreign body	An object that does not belong in the body
Laceration	A torn or jagged wound
Open wound	A wound in which underlying tissue is exposed to the air
Penetrating wound Puncture wound	A wound caused by a sharp pointed object passing through the skin into the underlying tissues
Perforation	Cutting or puncturing the wall or membrane of an internal organ or structure
Superficial injury	An injury to the surface of the skin, such as an abrasion, blister, contusion (*bruise*), constriction, insect bite, or superficial foreign body
Traumatic amputation	Severing a body part accidentally
Wound	A cut or opening in the skin or mucous membrane

Burns

Burns are damage to skin by heat, electricity, or radiation. In ICD-10-CM, **corrosions** are damage to skin due to chemicals. Both burns and corrosions are described by the **degree** (*depth*) of the burn (■ FIGURE 13-1, page 192). Burns of the eye and internal organs are *not* assigned degrees (OGCR I.C.19.d).

Traumatic Fractures

Traumatic fractures result from an accident rather than a disease. The most frequently broken bone in the body is the **clavicle** (*collar bone*), often caused by a direct blow to the shoulder, such as during a fall, as the result of an automobile collision, or by an outstretched arm that is attempting to break a fall. In babies, clavicle fractures can occur during a difficult delivery. Traumatic fractures are described based on combinations of several criteria:

- body region
- specific bone
- site on the bone
- line of break (■ FIGURE 13-2, page 192)
- **open** (*the bone breaks through the skin*) or **closed** (*the bone does not break the skin*)
- **displaced** (*the fragments of bone move out of alignment*) or **nondisplaced** (*the fragments of bone remain properly aligned*)

SUCCESS STEP

The classification of fractures as displaced or nondisplaced is a new concept in ICD-10-CM that did not exist in ICD-9-CM.

Physicians further classify fractures using specially developed classification systems based on the type of fracture. Two such systems that are incorporated into ICD-10-CM are the Gustilo system for open fractures and the Salter-Harris system for epiphysis fractures. Coders must refer to the documentation to determine how the fracture is classified then assign the corresponding diagnosis code.

Gustilo Open Fracture Classification

Open fractures are classified using the **Gustilo classification system** (■ TABLE 13-2, page 193), which organizes open fractures into three major types depending on the method of injury, soft-tissue damage, and degree of skeletal involvement. Progression from type I to IIIC describes a higher degree of force involved in the injury, increased soft-tissue and bone damage, and greater potential for complications.

Salter-Harris Epiphysis Fracture Classification

Epiphysis fractures are classified using the **Salter-Harris classification** to identify the involvement of the growth plate (■ FIGURE 13-3, page 193). Fracture of the growth plate is an injury unique to childhood and usually heals without permanent deformity. A small percentage, however, are complicated by growth arrest and subsequent deformity. The Salter-Harris classification aids in estimating both the prognosis and the potential for growth disturbance (■ TABLE 13-3, page 193).

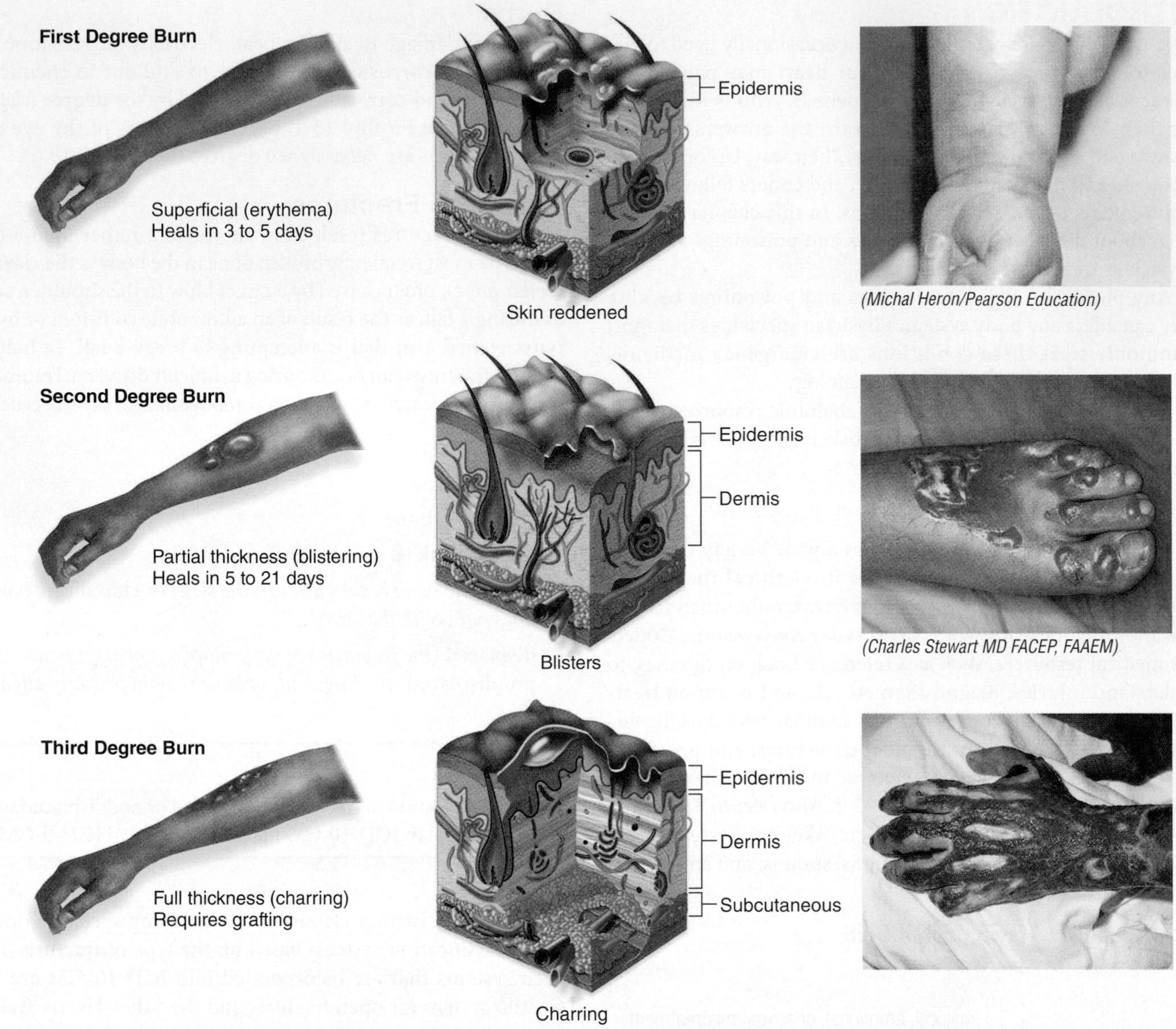

First Degree Burn

Superficial (erythema)
Heals in 3 to 5 days

— Epidermis

Skin reddened

(Michal Heron/Pearson Education)

Second Degree Burn

Partial thickness (blistering)
Heals in 5 to 21 days

— Epidermis

— Dermis

Blisters

(Charles Stewart MD FACEP, FAAEM)

Third Degree Burn

Full thickness (charring)
Requires grafting

— Epidermis

— Dermis

— Subcutaneous

Charring

Figure 13-1 ■ Comparison of Burn Depth. *Source: Pearson Education/PH College.*

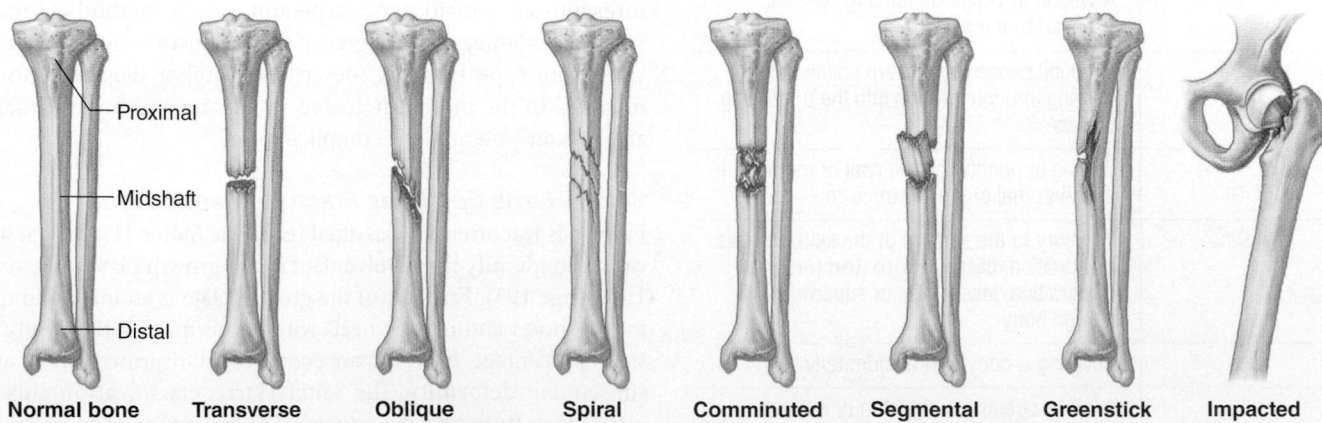

— Proximal

— Midshaft

— Distal

Normal bone   **Transverse**   **Oblique**   **Spiral**   **Comminuted**   **Segmental**   **Greenstick**   **Impacted**

Figure 13-2 ■ Common Break Lines of Fractures

Table 13-2 ■ GUSTILO CLASSIFICATION OF OPEN FRACTURES

Type		Description
I		Wound smaller than 1 cm with minimal soft-tissue injury and clean wound bed. Fracture is usually a simple transverse, short oblique fracture, with minimal comminution (fragmentation).
II		Wound larger than 1 cm with moderate soft-tissue damage, without flaps, avulsions. Fracture is usually a simple transverse, short oblique fracture, with minimal comminution.
III		Fractures that involve extensive damage to the soft tissues, including muscle, skin, and neurovascular structures. The injury is often accompanied by a high-velocity injury or a severe crushing component.
S U B T Y P E	IIIA	Adequate soft-tissue coverage despite soft-tissue laceration regardless of the size of the wound. This includes segmental fractures or severely comminuted fractures.
	IIIB	Extensive soft tissue lost and bony exposure. This is usually associated with massive contamination.
	IIIC	Fracture in which there is a major arterial injury requiring repair for limb salvage.

Poisoning, Adverse Effects, and Underdosing

ICD-10-CM provides specific definitions for injuries from drugs, chemicals, and biological substances (■ TABLE 13-4). Coders need to learn how ICD-10-CM uses these terms and not rely on the common language definition. The use of these definitions when assigning codes is discussed later in this chapter.

Over 50% of all exposures to poisoning occur in children age five and younger, but this age group accounts for less than 2% of fatalities. Nearly 40% of fatalities occur in persons age 40 to 59. Intentional poisonings account for nearly 14% of all exposures (American Association of Poison Control Centers).

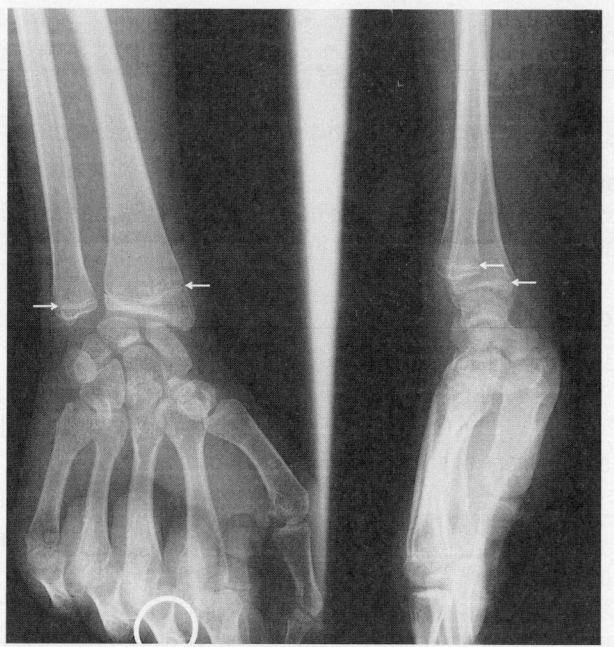

Figure 13-3 ■ X-ray Showing the Epiphysis (Growth Plate). *Source: Courtesy of Teresa Resch.*

Table 13-3 ■ SALTER-HARRIS CLASSIFICATION OF EPIPHYSIS FRACTURES

Type	Description
I	A transverse fracture through the physis (*growth plate*)
II	A fracture through the physis and the metaphysis, sparing the epiphysis
III	A fracture through the physis and epiphysis, sparing the metaphysis
IV	A fracture through all three elements of the bone, the physis, metaphysis, and epiphysis
V	A crush or compression fracture of the physis

Table 13-4 ■ DEFINITIONS FOR INJURIES FROM DRUGS, CHEMICALS, AND BIOLOGICAL SUBSTANCES

Injury	Definition	Example
Adverse effect	A medication that was correctly prescribed and properly administered causes an undesired physical response.	Allergic reaction to an initial dose of penicillin Interaction between prescribed lithium and Diuril, both taken correctly
Poisoning	The improper use of a medication that causes an undesired physical response: • overdose of any drug, whether intentional or accidental • error made in prescription, wrong drug given or taken in error • interaction of drugs and alcohol • nonprescribed drugs taken with correctly prescribed and administered drug	Administering penicillin to someone known to be allergic Nausea, vomiting, and tachycardia from drinking alcohol while taking metformin
Underdosing	Taking less of a medication than is prescribed by a provider or a manufacturer's instruction causes an undesired physical response.	Diabetic ketoacidosis due to taking too little insulin
Toxic effect	A harmful substance is ingested, or comes in contact with a person, and causes an undesired physical response.	Swallowing bleach Rash from wearing latex gloves

CODING PRACTICE

Exercise 13.1 Injury and Poisoning Refresher

Part A

Instructions: Read the following definitions presented in this section. Write the term being defined in the space provided.

1. _____ the fragments of bone move out of alignment

2. _____ unanticipated results of a medical or surgical procedure

3. _____ cutting or puncturing the wall or membrane of an internal organ or structure

4. _____ skin damage due to chemicals

5. _____ a classification system used for open fractures

Part B

Instructions: Read each of the following patient situations and determine whether it is an **adverse effect**, **poisoning**, **underdosing**, or **toxic effect**. Write the answer in the space provided.

6. _____ A patient sees her doctor when she breaks out in hives and has shortness of breath after taking prescribed sulfa for an infection. She has never taken sulfa or had this reaction to any medication before.

7. _____ A diabetic patient who takes prescribed metformin drinks alcohol at a party. He experiences severe nausea, vomiting, and tachycardia and is taken to the emergency department.

8. _____ A two-year-old gets into rubbing alcohol while his mother's back is turned. She does not think he drank any of it, but he did rub it in his eyes and is screaming. She calls Poison Control, then rushes him to the emergency department.

9. _____ An elderly woman is seen in the emergency department for an electrolyte imbalance after having taken a newly prescribed diuretic with lithium, which had been prescribed for her last year.

10. _____ A type 1 diabetic is seen in the emergency department for ketoacidosis after getting confused and taking too little insulin.

CODING OVERVIEW OF INJURY AND POISONING

ICD-10-CM Chapter 19, Injury, Poisoning, and Certain Other Consequences of External Causes (S00-T88), contains 22 blocks or subchapters that are divided by anatomic site and type of injury. Review the block names and code ranges listed at the beginning of Chapter 19 in the ICD-10-CM manual to become familiar with the content and organization.

ICD-10-CM Chapter 19 compares to ICD-9-CM Chapter 17 (800-999). The ICD-10-CM chapter is reorganized, grouping together all types of injuries for each anatomic region. Codes have been expanded due to additional details and laterality. Most codes also require seventh characters to identify the episode of care. The Table of Drugs and Chemicals has also been reorganized and expanded.

This ICD-10-CM chapter includes traumatic injuries to all body systems. The **S** section classifies injuries related to single body regions, such as the head, neck, and hip/thigh. The **T** section classifies injuries to unspecified body regions, effects of foreign bodies, burns, frostbite, poisonings, and other complications and consequences of external causes.

This chapter does not include obstetric trauma, which is classified in categories **O70** and **O71**, or birth trauma, which is classified in categories **P10** through **P15**. It also does not include conditions that arise from a disease process, even though the resulting condition may be similar to a traumatic injury. For example, a pathologic fracture is classified in ICD-10-CM Chapter 13, Diseases of the Musculoskeletal System and Connective Tissue (M00-M99), but a traumatic fracture is classified in ICD-10-CM Chapter 19, Injury, Poisoning, and Certain Other Consequences of External Causes (S00-T88).

ICD-10-CM Official Guidelines for Coding and Reporting (OGCR) for injury and poisoning appear in section I.C.19, which is divided into the following topics:

a. Application of 7th Characters in Chapter 19

b. Coding of Injuries

c. Coding of Traumatic Fractures

d. Coding of Burns and Corrosions

e. Adverse Effects, Poisoning, Underdosing and Toxic Effects

f. Adult and child abuse, neglect and other maltreatment

g. Complications of care

Instructional notes at the beginning of ICD-10-CM Chapter 19 direct coders to use secondary codes from ICD-10-CM Chapter 20, External Causes of Morbidity, to indicate the cause of injury. Many codes within section **T** already include the external cause, so those codes do not require an additional external cause code. When a retained foreign body is involved, use an additional code from category **Z18 Retained foreign body fragments** to identify the object.

ABSTRACTING DIAGNOSES FOR INJURY AND POISONING

Each type of injury has unique criteria for abstracting. Most conditions in ICD-10-CM Chapter 19 also require information on

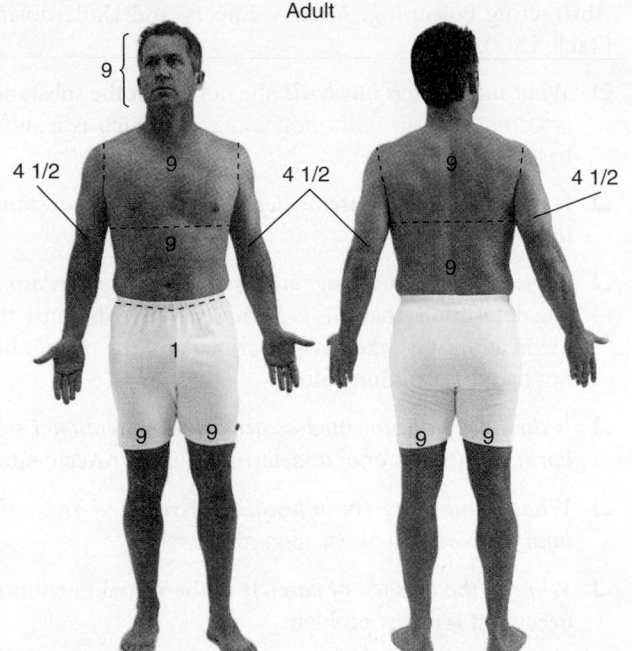

Figure 13-4 ■ Rule of Nines for Reporting Burns (All numbers are percentages of total body surface area.) *Source: Michal Heron/Pearson Education.*

the external cause. Refer to Table 8-1, Key Criteria for Abstracting External Causes, as a refresher on how to abstract data for external causes, and remember to abstract for external causes in addition to the injury. Key criteria for abstracting burns, traumatic fractures, and poisoning and adverse effects follow.

Abstracting Burns
Because burns often involve multiple body areas, specific anatomic sites may not be documented. When that is the case, report the percentage of the **total body surface area (TBSA)** affected by second- and third-degree burns. In addition, when a death occurs or more than 20% of the body is affected by third-degree burns, OGCR recommends, but does not require, reporting the percentage of TBSA involved (OGCR I.C.19.d.6)). Physicians estimate the percentage of TBSA using the Rule of Nines, which divides the body into areas, each of which comprises 9% of the total body surface area (■ FIGURE 13-4). The percentages vary slightly among adults, children, infants, obese patients, and pregnant women. Key criteria for abstracting burns appear in ■ TABLE 13-5.

Table 13-5 ■ KEY CRITERIA FOR ABSTRACTING BURNS
- ❑ Is the burn due to heat or a chemical (corrosion)?
- ❑ What is the anatomic site?
- ❑ What is the laterality?
- ❑ What is the greatest depth (degree) of burn on each site?
- ❑ Are any burns nonhealing?
- ❑ Are any burns infected?
- ❑ What is the episode of care?
- ❑ What percentage of the body surface involves third-degree burns?

Table 13-6 ■ KEY CRITERIA FOR ABSTRACTING TRAUMATIC FRACTURES
- ❑ Is the fracture traumatic or pathologic?
- ❑ Does the patient have osteoporosis?
- ❑ What bone is fractured?
- ❑ What is the laterality?
- ❑ Were any additional bones fractured?
- ❑ Where on the bone is the fracture located?
- ❑ What type of fracture occurred?
- ❑ Is the fracture displaced or nondisplaced? (*Default is displaced.*)
- ❑ Is the fracture open or closed? (*Default is closed.*)
- ❑ For open fractures, what is the Gustilo classification?
- ❑ For epiphysis fractures, what is the Salter-Harris classification?
- ❑ What is the episode of care?
- ❑ Is the healing routine, delayed, nonunion, or malunion?
- ❑ Is the encounter for follow-up after active healing is complete?

Abstracting Traumatic Fractures
Criteria for abstracting traumatic fractures are more detailed than criteria for pathologic fractures. Knowledge of the anatomy of the skeletal system is essential because fractures are identified by their anatomic location. Knowledge of different types of fracture lines is also critical (Figure 13-2). Key criteria for abstracting traumatic fractures appear in ■ TABLE 13-6.

Abstracting Poisoning
When abstracting poisoning, adverse effects, and underdosing, coders must identify the name of the drug or substance involved. Careful attention to spelling is required because drug names may have similar spelling but belong to a different class of drugs. Key criteria for abstracting poisoning and adverse effects appear in ■ TABLE 13-7.

Guided Example of Abstracting Diagnoses for Injury and Poisoning
Refer to the following example throughout this chapter to practice skills for abstracting, assigning, and sequencing injury and poisoning codes. Chelsea Kutcher, CPC-H, is a fictitious coder who guides you through this case.

Table 13-7 ■ KEY CRITERIA FOR ABSTRACTING POISONING, ADVERSE EFFECTS, AND UNDERDOSING
- ❑ What substance is involved?
- ❑ Is a diagnosis of abuse or dependence on the substance documented?
- ❑ Is the injury a poisoning, adverse effect, or underdosing?
- ❑ Is the injury documented as accidental, intentional self-harm, an assault, or of undetermined intent? (The default intent *is accidental.*)
- ❑ What conditions (manifestations) resulted from the injury?
- ❑ What is the episode of care?

Date: 03/1/yy   Location: Branton Medical Center Emergency Department   Provider: Cynthia Hiatt, MD

Patient: Gwen Beene   Gender: F   Age: 23

Reason for encounter: hives and has shortness of breath

Assessment: Patient has allergic reaction to Trimethoprim-Sulfamethoxazole prescribed two days ago by her family physician, Dr. Conover, for a urinary tract infection (UTI). She has never taken sulfa or had this reaction to any medication before.

Plan: d/c Trimethoprim-Sulfamethoxazole, notify PCP

Follow along as Chelsea Kutcher, CPC-H, abstracts the diagnosis. Check off each step after you complete it.

▶ Chelsea reads through the entire record, paying special attention to the reason for the encounter and the final assessment. She notes that the patient has a new allergic reaction to a medication, so she refers to the Key Criteria for

Abstracting Poisoning, Adverse Effects, and Underdosing (Table 13-7).

❏ *What substance is involved?* She notes that the substance is trimethoprim-sulfamethoxazole, which is a sulfa-based anti-infective.

❏ *Is a diagnosis of abuse or dependence on the substance documented?* No.

❏ *Is the injury a poisoning, adverse effect, or underdosing?* She determines that this is an adverse effect because the medication was taken as prescribed and the patient has not had this reaction before.

❏ *Is the injury documented as accidental, intentional self-harm, an assault, or of undetermined intent?* Accidental.

❏ *What conditions (manifestations) resulted from the injury?* Hives and shortness of breath.

❏ *What is the episode of care?* It is the initial encounter because it is a new problem.

▶ Next, Chelsea needs to assign the codes.

CODING PRACTICE

Exercise 13.2 Abstracting Diagnoses for Injury and Poisoning

Instructions: Read the mini-medical-record of each patient's encounter and answer the abstracting questions. Write the answer on the line provided. Do not assign any codes.

1. EMERGENCY DEPT   Gender: M   Age: 8

Chief complaint: pain, tenderness, swelling, and distortion on right knee after being tackled while playing football at school

Assessment: X-ray shows type III fracture of growth plate at the upper end of the tibia

Plan: surgery and internal fixation to ensure proper alignment of the growth plate and the joint surface

a. What bone is fractured? _____

   What is the laterality? _____

b. What site on the bone is injured? _____

   _____

c. How are fractures to the growth plate classified?

   _____

d. What is the type (classification system level) of this fracture? _____

e. What are the symptoms? _____

f. Should the symptoms be coded? _____

   _____

(continued)

1. (continued)

   Why or why not? _____

g. What is the episode of care? _____

h. What is the causal event? _____

i. What is the intent? _____

j. What is the location? _____

k. What is the external cause status? _____

   _____

l. What activity was he engaged in? _____

   _____

2. INPATIENT HOSPITAL   Gender: M   Age: 23

Reason for admission: patient arrived by ambulance after a barn fire that occurred on his own farm which is his job

Assessment: third degree burns to left forearm, second degree burns to left upper arm and shoulder, smoke inhalation

a. Is the burn due to a controlled flame or an uncontrolled fire? _____

b. What is the degree, site, and laterality of the most serious burn? _____

(continued)

2. (continued)

c. What is the degree, site, and laterality of other burns? _____

d. What does OGCR I.C.19.d.2) instruct regarding burns of the same local site (three-digit category)? _____

e. What other problems does the patient have? _____

f. What is the episode of care? _____

g. What is the causal event? _____

h. What is the intent? _____

i. What is the location? _____

j. What is the external cause status? _____

_____

k. What activity was he engaged in? _____

_____

3. OFFICE   Gender: F   Age: 35

Reason for encounter: suture removal from wound to right index finger, sustained when she accidentally cut her finger with a butcher knife while preparing dinner

Assessment: Wound is healed. Removed sutures.

a. What is the injury? _____

b. What is the anatomic site and laterality? _____

_____

c. What is the reason for the encounter? _____

_____

d. What is the episode of care? _____

e. What is the causal event? _____

f. Should you assign an aftercare code for removal of sutures? _____

Why or why not? _____

4. EMERGENCY DEPT   Gender: M   Age: 67

Chief complaint: irregular pulse, palpitations, confusion

Assessment: Cumulative intoxication effect (*a buildup in the body*) from digitalis which had been taken as prescribed for atrial fibrillation. Patient also has stage 2 chronic kidney disease which put him at risk for intoxication.

(continued)

4. (continued)

a. What are the symptoms? _____

Should they be coded? _____

Why or why not? _____

b. Is this an adverse effect or accidental poisoning? _____

Please give the reason for your answer. _____

_____

c. What is the substance? _____

d. What condition was the medication prescribed for? _____

e. What condition raised the patient's risk for intoxication? _____

f. What is the episode of care? _____

5. EMERGENCY DEPT   Gender: F   Age: 19

Chief complaint: examination after alleged date rape by her boyfriend

Assessment: Conducted physical examination and urine test. Flunitrazepam was found in a urine test. The injury was determined to be sexual assault.

a. What is the substance? _____

b. What is the intent? _____

c. What is the reason for the encounter? _____

_____

d. What event occurred? _____

e. What is the episode of care? _____

f. Who is the perpetrator? _____

g. Should you assign a code to identify the perpetrator? _____

Why or why not? _____

6. OFFICE   Gender: M   Age: 31

Chief complaint: accident in which automobile battery exploded and something got in his eyes while he was working on his car in the driveway at his single family home

Assessment: sulfuric acid burn on both eyelids and right cornea, second degree sulfuric acid burn to forehead and right cheek

(continued)

CODING PRACTICE *(continued)*

6. *(continued)*

a. Is the burn due to heat or a chemical? _____

_____

b. What is the coding term for this type of burn?

_____

c. What is the substance? _____

d. What is the anatomic site? _____

e. What is the laterality? _____

f. What is the greatest depth (degree) of burn on each site? _____

(continued)

6. *(continued)*

g. What is the episode of care? _____

h. What is the causal event? _____

i. What is the intent? _____

j. What is the location? _____

k. What is the external cause status? _____

_____

l. What is the activity? _____

ASSIGNING DIAGNOSIS CODES FOR INJURY AND POISONING

Each type of injury has unique coding guidelines, so coders need to become familiar with a variety of situations. Because the most severe injuries are often accompanied by less serious injuries, the OGCR instruct coders *not* to assign codes for superficial injuries, such as abrasions or contusions, when more severe injuries, such as an open wound or fracture of the *same* site, are present. Assign codes for the more severe injuries (OGCR I.C.19.b.1)).

Most codes in ICD-10-CM Chapter 19 require a seventh character for the episode of care. In addition to the most common seventh characters for the episode of care—**A Initial encounter**, **D Subsequent encounter**, and **S Sequela**—codes for traumatic fractures often provide additional options within each. Use seventh characters for an **Initial encounter** while the patient is receiving active treatment for the injury. Use seventh characters for a **Subsequent encounter** after the active treatment has been completed and the patient is in the healing phase. Use seventh characters for a **Sequela** for late effects of the injury. A patient may be seen by a new or different provider over the course of treatment for an injury. Assign the seventh character based on whether the patient is undergoing active treatment and not whether the provider is seeing the patient for the first time (OGCR I.C.19.a). ■ FIGURE 13-5 portrays how the seventh character changes throughout the treatment cycle.

This section of the chapter demonstrates how to assign codes for the three major types of injuries—burns, traumatic fractures, and poisoning—then also discusses two special topics: child or adult abuse and complications of care.

Assigning Codes for Burns

Burns are classified by anatomic site, depth (degree), extent, and causal event or agent (source). Burns of the eye and internal organs are classified by site and causal event or agent but not by degree. Event and agent codes are external cause codes that are located in the Index to External Causes. The following information summarizes key guidelines to keep in mind when assigning codes for burns (■ FIGURE 13-6, page 200):

- Assign separate codes for each burn site (OGCR I.C.19.d.5)). Search the Index for the Main Term **Burn** and a subterm for the anatomic site.

- When the same local site (three-character category level, **T20-T28**) has multiple burns of different degrees, assign a code only for highest degree recorded in the diagnosis (OGCR I.C.19.d.2)).

- Assign additional codes for any infection of the burn site (OGCR I.C.19.d.4)) and for other related conditions, such as smoke inhalation or respiratory failure (OGCR I.C.19.d.1)c)).

- Assign a code for the percentage of TBSA involved from categories **T31 Burns classified according to extent of body surface involved** or **T32 Corrosions classified according to extent of body surface involved** in the following situations (OGCR I.C.19.d.6)):

  - when the site of the burn is not specified

  - when there is a need for additional data, such as that required by the state health department

  - to provide data for evaluating burn mortality, such as that needed by burn units

  - when a third-degree burn involves 20% or more of TBSA

CODING CAUTION

Use character **D subsequent encounter** for all follow-up and aftercare of injuries. Do not report aftercare **Z** codes with injuries (OGCR I.C.21.c.7) and I.C.19.a.)

SUCCESS STEP

Nonhealing burns and necrosis of burned skin are coded in the same way as an acute burn (OGCR I.C.19.d.3)).

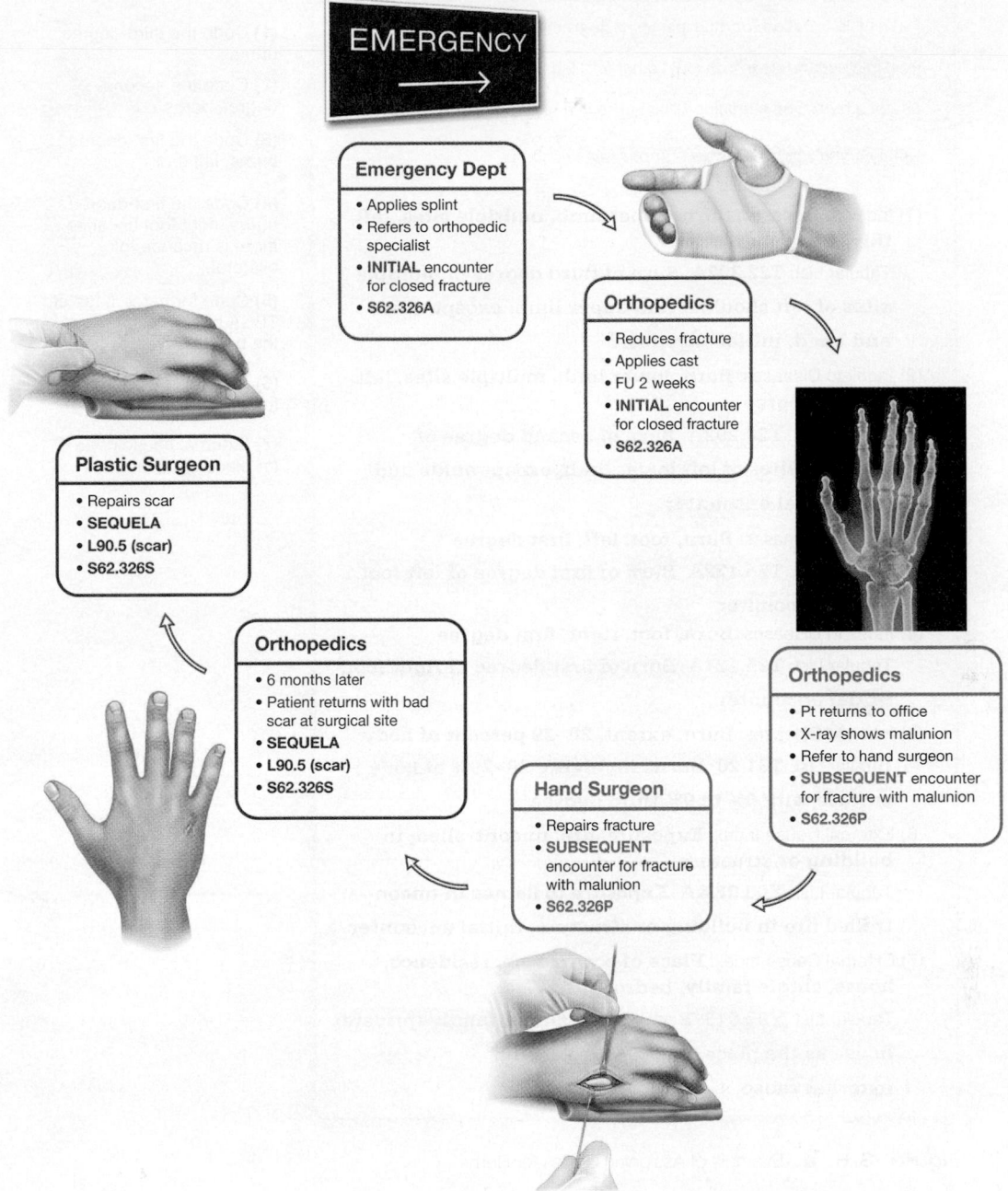

Figure 13-5 ■ Episode of Care for S62.326 Displaced fracture of shaft of fifth metacarpal bone, right hand.

Assigning Codes for Traumatic Fractures

In addition to the seventh characters **A**, **D**, and **S** used for most injury and poisoning codes, traumatic fracture codes use several additional seventh characters that describe combinations of the following criteria:

- open or closed
- Gustilo classification for open fractures (■ FIGURE 13-7, page 200)
- routine or delayed healing
- normal union, malunion, or nonunion

Seventh character options appear at the beginning of each three-digit category and are summarized in ■ TABLE 13-8.

The details of code selection vary with the type of fracture. For example, some categories provide separate codes for displaced and nondisplaced fractures. Categories **S49**, **S59**, **S79**, and **S89** classify epiphysis fractures using the Salter-Harris system.

OGCR I.C.19.c provides guidance on the default coding of fractures when certain details are not documented, as follows:

- When a fracture is not documented as open or closed, assign a code for closed.
- When a fracture is not documented as displaced or not displaced, assign a code for displaced.

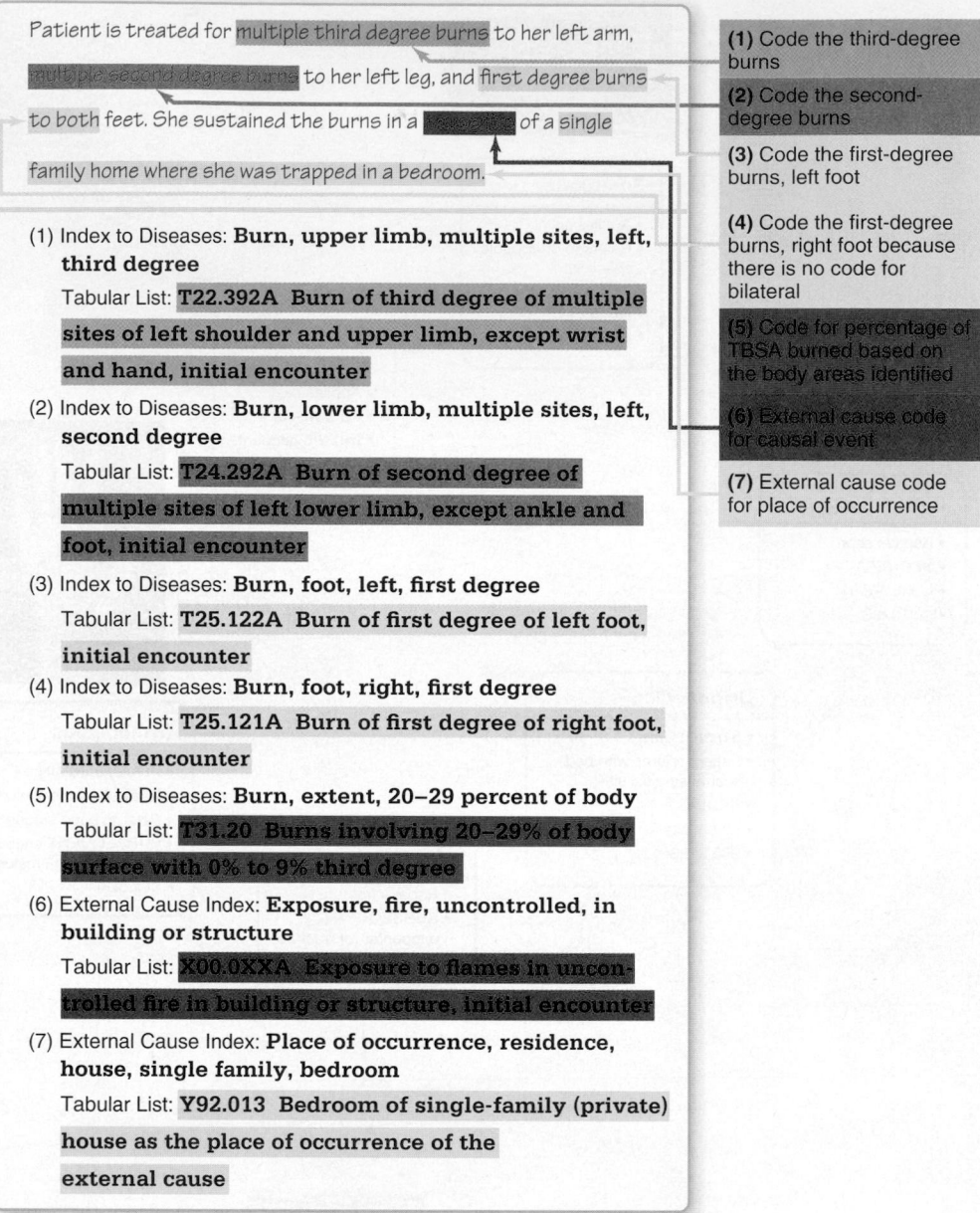

Patient is treated for multiple third degree burns to her left arm, multiple second degree burns to her left leg, and first degree burns to both feet. She sustained the burns in a ▮▮▮▮▮▮▮ of a single family home where she was trapped in a bedroom.

(1) Code the third-degree burns

(2) Code the second-degree burns

(3) Code the first-degree burns, left foot

(4) Code the first-degree burns, right foot because there is no code for bilateral

(5) Code for percentage of TBSA burned based on the body areas identified

(6) External cause code for causal event

(7) External cause code for place of occurrence

(1) Index to Diseases: **Burn, upper limb, multiple sites, left, third degree**
Tabular List: **T22.392A Burn of third degree of multiple sites of left shoulder and upper limb, except wrist and hand, initial encounter**

(2) Index to Diseases: **Burn, lower limb, multiple sites, left, second degree**
Tabular List: **T24.292A Burn of second degree of multiple sites of left lower limb, except ankle and foot, initial encounter**

(3) Index to Diseases: **Burn, foot, left, first degree**
Tabular List: **T25.122A Burn of first degree of left foot, initial encounter**

(4) Index to Diseases: **Burn, foot, right, first degree**
Tabular List: **T25.121A Burn of first degree of right foot, initial encounter**

(5) Index to Diseases: **Burn, extent, 20–29 percent of body**
Tabular List: **T31.20 Burns involving 20–29% of body surface with 0% to 9% third degree**

(6) External Cause Index: **Exposure, fire, uncontrolled, in building or structure**
Tabular List: **X00.0XXA Exposure to flames in uncontrolled fire in building or structure, initial encounter**

(7) External Cause Index: **Place of occurrence, residence, house, single family, bedroom**
Tabular List: **Y92.013 Bedroom of single-family (private) house as the place of occurrence of the external cause**

Figure 13-6 ■ Example of Assigning Codes for Burns

Patient is seen for follow-up on an open fracture of the right tibia plateau. The fracture occurred at the lateral condyle. The physician classifies the fracture as Type II using the Gustilo scale. X-rays show that the fracture is healing well.

Index: **Fracture, tibia, plateau, *see* upper end, bicondylar**
Tabular List:
S82.14 Bicondylar fracture of tibia
   1 sixth digit for **right tibia, displaced**
      E seventh character for **subsequent encounter for open fracture type I or II with routine healing**
Final code: **S82.141E Displaced bicondylar fracture of right tibia, subsequent encounter for open fracture type I or II with routine healing**

Figure 13-7 ■ Example of Coding a Gustilo Fracture

Table 13-8 ■ **MATRIX OF SEVENTH CHARACTERS FOR TRAUMATIC FRACTURES OF LONG BONES**

Treatment Phase	Closed	Open Type I or II	Open Type IIIA, B, or C
Initial	A	B	C
Routine healing	D	E	F
Delayed healing	G	H	J
Nonunion healing	K	M	N
Malunion healing	P	Q	R
Sequela	S	S	S

SUCCESS STEP

When a patient with known osteoporosis suffers a fracture, remember to assign a code from category **M80 Osteoporosis with current pathological fracture**, NOT a traumatic fracture code. Do this even when the patient has a minor fall or trauma. If the fall or trauma would not usually break a normal, healthy bone, you should assign a code for pathologic fracture due to osteoporosis (OGCR I.C.19.c.1)).

Assigning Codes for Poisoning

To assign codes for poisoning, adverse effects, toxic effects, and underdosing, use the Table of Drugs and Chemicals (■ FIGURE 13-8). Assign as many codes as necessary to describe completely all drugs or medicinal or biological substances (OGCR I.C.19.e.2)). When two or more drugs or medicinal or biological substances are reported, code each individually unless a combination code is listed in the Table of Drugs and Chemicals (OGCR I.C.19.e.4)). Do not assign an additional external cause code because the external cause is included in the injury code.

SUCCESS STEP

The Table of Drugs and Chemicals is located at the end of the Index to Diseases and before the Index to External Causes. If you haven't already done so, place a red self-adhesive tab along the top edge of the page to make it easier to find.

To use the Table of Drugs and Chemicals follow these steps:

1. Locate the name of the substance in the left-hand column. Some substances have subterms indented below them on the next line.
2. Select the substance code in the column that corresponds to the intent determined during abstracting. When the intent is not stated, code it as accidental. When the intent is underdosing, assign codes as follows:
   a. If underdosing exacerbates the condition for which the medication was prescribed, assign a code for the condition.
   b. Assign a code for noncompliance or complication of care to further indicate intent, if known.
3. Verify the code in the Tabular List. Do not code directly from the Table of Drugs and Chemicals.
4. Confirm that the code title reflects the intent.
5. Assign the seventh character for the episode of care.
6. When more than one substance is involved, repeat the steps for each substance.
7. Assign additional codes to identify the condition(s) or manifestation(s) that resulted.

Substance	Poisoning, Accidental (unintentional)	Poisoning, Intentional self-harm	Poisoning, Assault	Poisoning, Undetermined	Adverse effect	Underdosing
Trimethobenzamide	T45.0X1	T45.0X2	T45.0X3	T45.0X4	T45.0X5	T45.0X6
Trimethoprim	T37.8X1	T37.8X2	T37.8X3	T37.8X4	T37.8X5	T37.8X6
with sulfamethoxazole	T36.8X1	T36.8X2	T36.8X3	T36.8X4	T36.8X5	T36.8X6
Trimethylcarbinol	T51.3X1	T51.3X2	T51.3X3	T51.3X4	-	-
Trimethylpsoralen	T49.3X1	T49.3X2	T49.3X3	T49.3X4	T49.3X5	T49.3X6
Trimeton	T45.0X1	T45.0X2	T45.0X3	T45.0X4	T45.0X5	T45.0X6
Trimetrexate	T45.1X1	T45.1X2	T45.1X3	T45.1X4	T45.1X5	T45.1X6

Figure 13-8 ■ Table of Drugs and Chemicals

SUCCESS STEP

ICD-10-CM introduces some changes to the Table of Drugs and Chemicals. Underdosing is a new concept not present in ICD-9-CM and has a separate column on the table. Poisonings are reported with a combination code that describes both the substance and intent. A separate external cause code for intent is no longer required. The Therapeutic Use column from ICD-9-CM is renamed Adverse Effect and appears as the fifth column.

Guided Example of Assigning Injury and Poisoning Diagnosis Codes

To practice skills for using the Table of Drugs and Chemicals, continue with the example from earlier in the chapter about patient Gwen Beene, who was seen in the Branton Medical Center Emergency Department due to an allergic reaction to trimethoprim-sulfamethoxazole.

Follow along in your ICD-10-CM manual as Chelsea assigns codes. Check off each step after you complete it.

▶ First, Chelsea confirms the diagnosis of hives and shortness of breath due to adverse effect of trimethoprim-sulfamethoxazole.

▶ Chelsea locates the Table of Drugs and Chemicals at the end of the Index to Diseases.

❑ She searches for the Main Term **Trimethoprim** in the left-hand column of the table (Figure 13-8).

❑ She locates the subterm **with Sulfamethoxazole** on the next line.

❑ She locates the column for **Adverse Effects**.

❑ She locates code where the column for **Adverse Effects** crosses the row for **with Sulfamethoxazole**.

❑ She identifies the code **T36.8X5**.

▶ Chelsea verifies code **T36.8X5** in the Tabular List.

❑ She reads the code title for **T36.8X5, Adverse effect of other systemic antibiotics** and confirms that this accurately describes the diagnosis.

❑ She notes the convention **7th** that directs her to assign a seventh character.

❑ She refers to the beginning of category **T36** to review the seventh characters available for episode of care.

❑ The episode of care is **A, initial encounter** because this is the first encounter for the problem.

❑ She assigns code **T36.8X5A**.

▶ Chelsea checks for instructional notes in the Tabular List.

❑ She cross-references the beginning of the block **Poisoning by, adverse effects of and underdosing of drugs, medicaments and biological substances (T36-T50)** and sees several instructional notes.

❑ She reviews the **Includes** notes that give the definition of poisoning and adverse effect and concludes that she chose the correct category of adverse effect because the medication was properly administered.

❑ She reads another instructional note that says **Code first for adverse effects, the nature of the adverse effect**. Therefore, she knows that she should code for hives and shortness of breath.

❑ She cross-references the beginning of **Chapter 19 (S00-T88)** and reviews the instructional notes. She reads the note that says **Use secondary code(s) from Chapter 20, External causes of morbidity, to indicate cause of injury. Codes within the T section that include the external cause do not require an additional external cause code**. She determines she does not need an additional code for external cause because the code from section **T** includes the cause, which is an adverse effect to a medication.

▶ Chelsea assigns the codes for the manifestations.

❑ She searches the Index for the Main Term **Hives**, which cross-references her to **Urticaria**.

▪ She searches for the Main Term **Urticaria** and the subterm **due to drug**, which directs her to code **L50.0**.

▪ She verifies the code in the Tabular List and confirms the code title **L50.0, Allergic urticaria**.

▪ She cross-references the beginning of the category, block, and chapter for any applicable instructional notes.

❑ She searches the Index for the Main Term **Shortness** and subterm **breath**, which directs her to code **R06.02**.

▪ She verifies the code in the Tabular List and confirms the code title **R06.02, Shortness of breath**.

▪ After cross-referencing the beginning of the category, block, and chapter for any applicable instructional notes, she returns to the Index to locate the code for hives.

▶ Chelsea identifies the codes for this case:

❑ **T36.8X5A** Adverse effect of other systemic antibiotics, initial encounter

❑ **L50.0** Allergic urticaria

❑ **R06.02** Shortness of breath

CODING CAUTION

Use the Table of Drugs and Chemicals only for poisoning, adverse effects, and underdosing. Do *not* use this table to report the fact that a patient is taking, or has been prescribed, a medication when no injury is involved.

Special Topics

OGCR provide guidelines for adult and child abuse and complications of care. Coding for these topics is summarized next.

Adult and Child Abuse, Neglect, and Other Maltreatment

Coding of adult and child abuse or neglect is based on whether the medical record documents the abuse as confirmed or suspected (OGCR I.C.19.f)). To learn how to code for abuse, neglect, and other maltreatment, review the following guidelines:

- When the medical record documents abuse or neglect, assign a code for confirmed maltreatment from category **T74.-**.

  1. Search the Index for the Main Term **Maltreatment**.
     - Select a subterm that identifies the victim as **adult** or **child**.
     - Select a second-level subterm for **confirmed**.

  2. Assign an external cause code from the assault section **(X92-Y08)** to identify the cause of any physical injuries.
     - Search the External Cause Index for the Main Term **Assault**, then select the applicable subterm to identify the method of assault.

  3. Assign a perpetrator code **(Y07)** when the perpetrator of the abuse is known.
     - Search the External Cause Index for the Main Term **Perpetrator**, then select the applicable subterm to identify the relationship of the perpetrator to the victim.

- When the medical record documents suspected abuse, assign a code for suspected maltreatment from category **T76.-**.

  1. Search the Index for the Main Term **Maltreatment**.
     - Select a second-level subterm for **suspected**.

  2. For suspected cases of abuse or neglect, *do not* report external cause or perpetrator code.

  3. If a suspected case of abuse, neglect, or mistreatment is ruled out during an encounter, assign code **Z04.71, Encounter for examination and observation following alleged adult physical abuse**, or code **Z04.72, Encounter for examination and observation following alleged child physical abuse**, *not* a code from **T76**. The inclusion notes under **Z04.71** and **Z04.72** state **Suspected . . . physical and sexual abuse, ruled out**.

- Sequence the codes as follows (■ FIGURE 13-9):

  1. The code from category **T74.-** or **T76.-** to identify confirmed or suspected abuse, neglect, and other maltreatment.

  2. Additional codes to identify any associated mental health condition or injury (OGCR I.C.19.f).

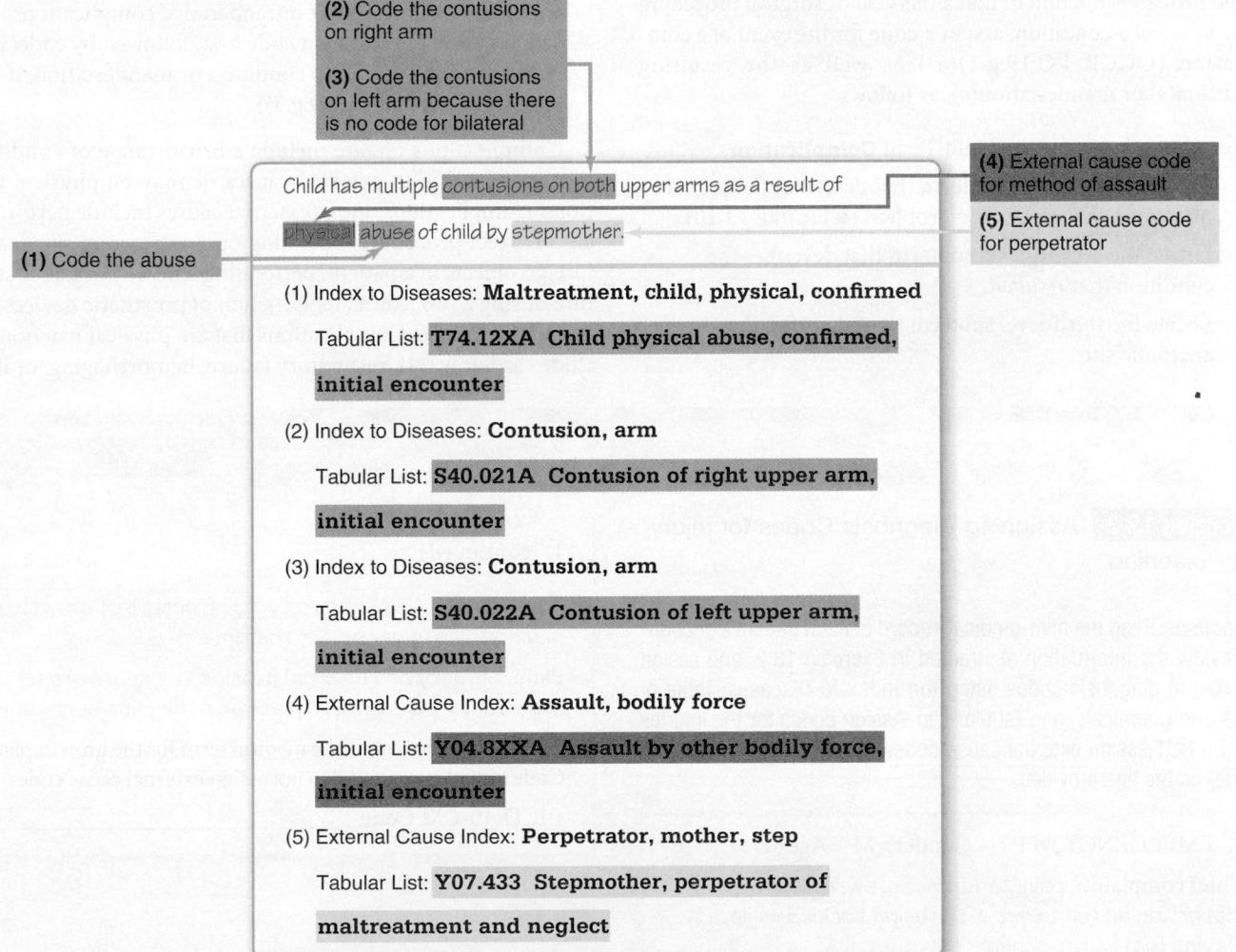

(2) Code the contusions on right arm

(3) Code the contusions on left arm because there is no code for bilateral

(4) External cause code for method of assault

(5) External cause code for perpetrator

Child has multiple contusions on both upper arms as a result of physical abuse of child by stepmother.

(1) Code the abuse

(1) Index to Diseases: **Maltreatment, child, physical, confirmed**

Tabular List: **T74.12XA Child physical abuse, confirmed, initial encounter**

(2) Index to Diseases: **Contusion, arm**

Tabular List: **S40.021A Contusion of right upper arm, initial encounter**

(3) Index to Diseases: **Contusion, arm**

Tabular List: **S40.022A Contusion of left upper arm, initial encounter**

(4) External Cause Index: **Assault, bodily force**

Tabular List: **Y04.8XXA Assault by other bodily force, initial encounter**

(5) External Cause Index: **Perpetrator, mother, step**

Tabular List: **Y07.433 Stepmother, perpetrator of maltreatment and neglect**

Figure 13-9 ■ Example of Code Assignment and Sequencing for Child Abuse

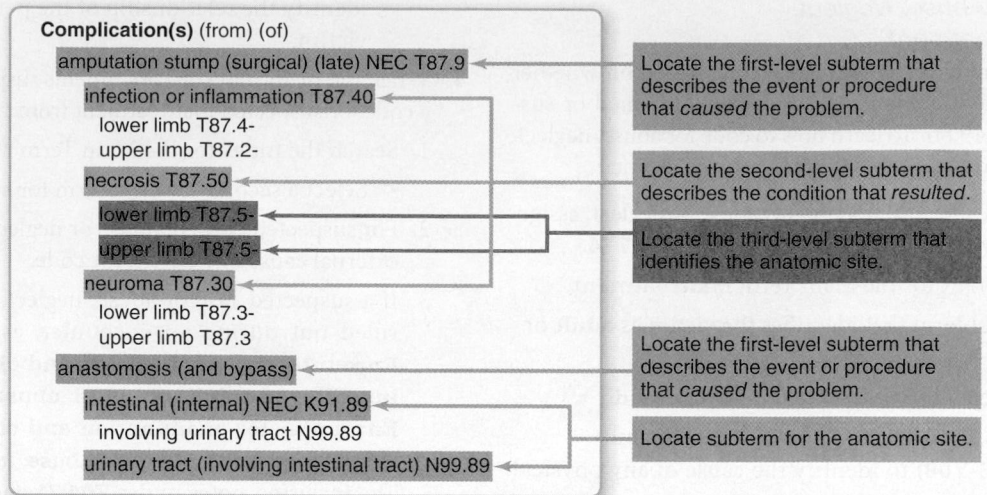

Figure 13-10 ■ Example of Index Entry for the Main Term Complication

3. An external cause code to identify the method of assault.

4. An external cause code to identify the perpetrator (for confirmed abuse only).

Complications of Care

When providers document that a medical or surgical procedure is the cause of a condition, assign a code for the event of a complication (OGCR I.C.19.g.1)(a)) as well as the resulting condition(s) or manifestation(s), as follows:

- Search the Index for the Main Term **Complication**.
  - Locate the first-level subterm that describes the event or procedure that *caused* the problem (■ FIGURE 13-10).
  - Locate the second-level subterm that describes the condition that *resulted*.
  - Locate the third-level subterm that identifies the anatomic site.

- Some complications of care codes are combination codes that describe the nature of the complication as well as the type of procedure that caused the complication.
  - When the external cause is included in a combination code, do not assign an additional external cause code.
- When a complication code is available from a body system chapter, such as those for intraoperative complications, sequence the body system code first, followed by code(s) for the specific complication condition or manifestation, if applicable (OGCR I.C.19.g.5)).

Complications of care include a broad range of conditions that may be due to external causes or may be physical reactions. Complications due to external causes include performing an incorrect procedure, operating on an incorrect site, leaving foreign objects in a patient, perforating a nearby organ or structure during a procedure, malfunction of prosthetic devices, and certain infections. Complications that are physical reactions include cardiac arrest, respiratory failure, hemorrhaging, or **ileus**.

CODING PRACTICE

Exercise 13.3   Assigning Diagnosis Codes for Injury and Poisoning

Instructions: Read the mini-medical-record of each patient's encounter, review the information abstracted in Exercise 13.2, and assign ICD-10-CM diagnosis codes using the Index to Diseases, Table of Drugs and Chemicals, and Tabular List. Assign codes for the injuries only. Do NOT assign external cause codes in this exercise. Write the code(s) on the line provided.

1. EMERGENCY DEPT   Gender: M   Age: 8

Chief complaint: *pain, tenderness, swelling, and distortion on right knee after being tackled while playing football at school*

(continued)

1. (continued)

Assessment: *X-ray shows type III fracture of growth plate at the upper end of the tibia*

Plan: *surgery and internal fixation to ensure proper alignment of the growth plate and the joint surface*

Tip: Physis (physeal) is the medical term for the growth plate. Code only the fracture. Do not assign external cause codes.

1 ICD-10-CM Code _____

2. INPATIENT HOSPITAL Gender: M Age: 23

Reason for admission: patient arrived by ambulance after a barn fire that occurred on his own farm which is his job

Assessment: third degree burns to left forearm, second degree burns to left upper arm and shoulder, smoke inhalation

Tip: Assign a code for the burns and a code for the smoke. Do not code activity, status, or location external cause codes.

2 ICD-10-CM Codes _____

3. OFFICE Gender: F Age: 35

Reason for encounter: suture removal from wound to right index finger, sustained when she accidentally cut her finger with a butcher knife while preparing dinner

Assessment: Wound is healed. Removed sutures.

Tip: Assign a code for the injury with the appropriate seventh character for care provided during the healing phase. Do not assign external cause codes.

1 ICD-10-CM Code _____

ARRANGING DIAGNOSIS CODES FOR INJURY AND POISONING

Patients with injuries and poisoning often present with multiple problems. The general rule is to sequence the code for the most serious injury first, as determined by the provider and the focus of treatment (OGCR I.C.19.b).

Injuries often involve peripheral nerves or blood vessels. When the *primary* injury is to the blood vessels or nerves, that injury should be sequenced first. When a primary injury results in *minor* damage to peripheral nerves or blood vessels, sequence the primary injury first, with additional codes for injuries to nerves, spinal cord, or blood vessels (OGCR I.C.19.b.2)).

Patients may be treated for sequelae or after-effects after the primary injury has healed, such as scars. Sequence first code(s) that describe the after-effect conditions or manifestations. Then report the code that identifies the original injury, with the seventh character **S Sequela** (OGCR I.C.19.a). Refer to ■ FIGURE 13-11 to learn more about sequencing injury codes and sequelae.

CODING CAUTION

Remember to assign the seventh character to the injury code only. Do not assign a seventh character to the code for the condition that resulted unless directed to do so by instructional notes in the Tabular List, as occurs with traumatic fractures.

Arranging Codes for Burns

When more than one burn is present, the first code should reflect the highest degree of burn (OGCR I.C.19.d.1)). The size of the damaged area is *not* a factor in sequencing burn codes.

The OGCR state that **circumstances of admission** govern the selection of the principal diagnosis or first-listed diagnosis in certain situations. This means that sequencing is based on

A patient is treated for a keloid scar that forms following a third degree burn on the right cheek.

(1) **L91.0 Hypertrophic disorders of the skin**
(2) **T20.36XS Burn of third degree of forehead and cheek, sequela**

Figure 13-11 ■ Example of Coding the Sequelae of an Injury

the specific reason for admission and which injuries are most serious. The circumstances of admission apply when a patient has both internal and external burns (OGCR I.C.19.d.1)(b)) or has other related conditions, such as smoke inhalation and/or respiratory failure (OGCR I.C.19.d.1)(c)).

For example, consider a patient with second-degree burns and life-threatening respiratory failure due to smoke inhalation. Sequence respiratory failure first because it is more serious than second-degree burns.

Arranging Codes for Traumatic Fractures

Sequence multiple fractures based on the severity of the fracture (OGCR I.C.19.c.2)). The severity may be determined by either the location of the fracture or the type of fracture. Review the following examples to learn more about sequencing multiple fractures:

- A fracture to the skull is more serious than a fracture to a finger.
- An open fracture is more serious than a closed fracture.
- A fracture that causes damage to another organ, such as a fractured rib that punctures a lung, is more serious than one that does not, such as a fractured arm.

If coders cannot determine the relative severity of multiple fractures based on the documentation, they should consult with their supervisor or query the physician.

Arranging Codes for Poisoning

The OGCR are different for sequencing poisonings, adverse effects, and underdosings (OGCR I.C.19.e). When coding poisonings, the first code should be from categories **T36** through **T50** to identify the type and intent of injury. Next, report the codes that identify all resulting conditions or manifestations.

When coding for adverse effects, sequence first the code(s) for the manifestations or resulting conditions. Then, sequence the **T** code, which is a combination code for the drug and the intent (adverse effect). Sequence codes for underdosing encounters as follows:

1. The principal or first-listed diagnosis should be the resulting condition or manifestation.
2. Sequence the underdosing **T** code as an additional code.
3. Sequence a code for complication of care or a **Z** code for noncompliance, as applicable.

Guided Example of Arranging Injury and Poisoning Diagnosis Codes

To practice skills for sequencing codes for adverse effects, continue with the example from earlier in the chapter about patient Gwen Beene, who was seen at Branton Medical Center Emergency Department due to an allergic reaction to trimethoprim-sulfamethoxazole.

Follow along in your ICD-10-CM manual as Chelsea sequences the codes. Check off each step after you complete it.

▶ First, Chelsea confirms the three diagnoses:

❑ **T36.8X5A Adverse effect of other systemic antibiotics, initial encounter**

❑ **R06.02 Shortness of breath**

❑ **L50.0 Allergic urticaria**

▶ Chelsea reviews the instructional notes she found at the beginning of the block **T36-T50** that said **Code first for adverse effects, the nature of the adverse effect.**

❑ The words **Code first** mean that the manifestations should be sequenced before the **T** code for the drug that caused the adverse effect.

▶ Chelsea also reviews OGCR I.C.19.5)(a) that states

When coding an adverse effect of a drug that has been correctly prescribed and properly administered, assign the appropriate code for the nature of the adverse effect followed by the appropriate code for the adverse effect of the drug (T36-T50).

❑ This confirms that the the manifestation codes should be sequenced first, followed by the **T** code.

❑ She sequences **R06.02, Shortness of breath** first because it is a more serious condition than hives.

▶ Chelsea finalizes the sequencing for this case:

1. **R06.02 Shortness of breath**
2. **L50.0 Allergic urticaria**
3. **T36.8X5A Adverse effect of other systemic antibiotics, initial encounter**

CODING PRACTICE

Exercise 13.4 Arranging Diagnosis Codes for Injury and Poisoning

Instructions: Read the mini-medical-record of each patient's encounter, review the information abstracted in Exercise 13.2, assign ICD-10-CM diagnosis codes using the Index to Diseases, the Index to External Causes, the Table of Drugs and Chemicals, and the Tabular List, and sequence them correctly. DO assign external cause codes in this exercise.

---

1. EMERGENCY DEPT   Gender: M   Age: 67

Chief complaint: irregular pulse, palpitations, confusion

Assessment: Cumulative intoxication effect (*a buildup in the body*) from digitalis which had been taken as prescribed for atrial fibrillation. Patient also has stage 2 chronic kidney disease which put him at risk for intoxication.

Tip: Sequence codes as follows: 1) the condition that describes the adverse effect, 2) the drug that caused the adverse effect, 3) reason he was at risk.

3 ICD-10-CM Codes _____

_____

---

2. EMERGENCY DEPT   Gender: F   Age: 19

Chief complaint: examination after alleged date rape by her boyfriend

Assessment: Conducted physical examination and urine test. Flunitrazepam was found in a urine test.

(continued)

---

2. (continued)

The injury was determined to be sexual assault.

Tip: Assign a code from the Table of Drugs and Chemicals, a code for the examination as the reason for the encounter, and two external causes codes for the type of assault and the perpetrator.

4 ICD-10-CM Codes _____

_____

---

3. OFFICE   Gender: M   Age: 31

Chief complaint: accident in which automobile battery exploded and something got in his eyes while he was working on his car in the driveway at his single family home

Assessment: sulfuric acid burn on both eyelids and right cornea, second degree sulfuric acid burn to forehead and right cheek

Tip: Assign a code from the Table of Drugs and Chemicals, four codes for the injuries, and two external cause codes for place and status. Read the instructional notes in the Tabular List for help on sequencing. Recall that burns to the eye are not rated by degree. The burn to the cornea is the most serious and the burns to the cheek and forehead are the least serious.

7 ICD-10-CM Codes _____

_____

CHAPTER SUMMARY

In this chapter you learned that:

- Injury and poisoning can encompass a wide variety of conditions and a range of definitions, so it is critical that coders understand how ICD-10-CM defines terms.

- ICD-10-CM Chapter 19, Injury, Poisoning, and Certain Other Consequences of External Causes (S00-T88), contains 22 blocks or subchapters that are divided by anatomic site and type of injury.

- The most common injuries are burns, fractures, and poisonings, each of which has unique criteria for abstracting.

- Each type of injury has unique coding guidelines, so coders need to become familiar with a variety of situations.

- In general, sequence the code for the most serious injury first, as determined by the provider and the focus of treatment.

- ICD-10-CM Official Guidelines for Coding and Reporting (OGCR) for injury and poisoning appear in section I.C.19, which is divided into sections based on the type of injury.

CONCEPT QUIZ

Take a moment to look back at injury and poisoning and solidify your skills. This is your opportunity to pull together everything you have learned.

Completion

Instructions: Refer to category **S72 Fracture of femur** in the ICD-10-CM manual. Read the descriptions of the seventh characters. Write the letter that matches each definition in the space provided. Some choices may be used more than once and some choices may not be used at all.

A	J
B	K
C	M
D	N
E	P
F	Q
G	R
H	S

1. The character _____ describes a subsequent encounter for closed fracture with malunion.

2. The character _____ describes a subsequent encounter for open fracture type IIIA, IIIB, or IIIC with routine healing.

3. The character _____ describes a subsequent encounter for closed fracture with nonunion.

4. The character _____ describes an initial encounter for closed fracture.

5. The character _____ describes an initial encounter for open fracture type IIIA, IIIB, or IIIC.

6. The character _____ describes a subsequent encounter for open fracture type I or II with delayed healing.

7. The character _____ describes sequelae.

8. The character _____ describes an initial encounter for open fracture type I or II.

9. The character _____ describes a subsequent encounter for closed fracture with routine healing.

10. The character _____ describes a subsequent encounter for open fracture type I or II with routine healing.

Multiple Choice

Instructions: Circle the letter of the best answer to each question based on the information you learned in this chapter.

1. Which is NOT a criteria used in assigning codes for burns?
   A. Depth
   B. Anatomic site
   C. Open or closed
   D. Extent

2. Traumatic fracture codes have seventh characters for all of the following EXCEPT
   A. displaced or nondisplaced.
   B. open or closed.
   C. routine or delayed healing.
   D. sequelae.

3. When a patient with osteoporosis has a minor fall, coders should assign
   A. a code for a traumatic fracture only.
   B. a code for osteoporosis fracture only.
   C. a code for a traumatic fracture AND a code for osteoporosis fracture.
   D. a code for external cause only.

4. Which of the following is NOT true regarding the Table of Drugs and Chemicals?
   A. Locate the name of the substance in the left-hand column.
   B. Select the substance code in the column that corresponds to the intent.
   C. Assign codes directly from the table without verifying in the Tabular List.
   D. Assign additional codes to identify the condition(s) or manifestation(s) that resulted.

(continued)

(continued from page 207)

5. To assign a code for adult or child abuse, search the Index for the Main Term
   A. Abuse.
   B. Maltreatment.
   C. Child.
   D. Confirmed.

6. When the medical record documents suspected abuse,
   A. assign a code to identify the suspected perpetrator.
   B. search the Index for the Main Term Suspected.
   C. assign a code only for the injuries, but not the abuse.
   D. search the Index for the Main Term Maltreatment and subterm suspected.

7. Assign a complications of care code when
   A. patients have more than one condition.
   B. providers document that a medical or surgical procedure is the cause of a condition.
   C. providers perform complicated procedures.
   D. physician documentation is unclear.

8. When a patient has multiple injuries, how should codes be sequenced?
   A. Sequence the codes in numerical order.
   B. Sequence conditions in the order the physician mentions them in the medical record.
   C. Sequence burns first, fractures second, and wounds third.
   D. Sequence the code for the most serious injury first.

9. When patients are treated for a sequela or after-effects after the primary injury has healed, how should codes be sequenced?
   A. Sequence the code that identifies the original injury first and the after-effect second.
   B. Sequence the after-effect condition first and the primary injury second.
   C. Assign codes for the after-effect but not the original injury.
   D. Sequence according to the circumstances of admission.

10. When coding adverse effects, how should codes be sequenced?
    A. Sequence according to the circumstances of admission.
    B. Sequence the external cause code first.
    C. Sequence the code for the resulting condition or manifestation first.
    D. Sequence the code for type and intent of injury first.

CODING CHALLENGE

Instructions: Read the mini-medical-record of each patient's encounter, then abstract, assign, and sequence ICD-10-CM diagnosis codes using the Index to Diseases, the Index to External Causes, and the Tabular List. Write the code(s) on the line provided.

---

1. OFFICE   Gender: F   Age: 71

Chief complaint: swollen and painful right wrist and large bruises on right calf after she tripped and fell in the living room of her apartment yesterday.

Assessment: Colles fracture. Extensive hematoma on the calf is due to her long term Coumadin (*anticoagulant/blood thinner*) therapy. Patient was previously diagnosed with age-related osteoporosis.

Plan: Arm casted, **INR** (*international normalized ratio blood clotting test*) performed, RTO to access healing of fracture and cast removal

Tip: Assign four diagnosis codes and two external cause codes.

6 ICD-10-CM Codes _____

_____

---

2. OFFICE   Gender: M   Age: 21

Reason for encounter: follow-up on shoulder dislocation sustained when the motorcycle he was driving collided with an automobile three weeks ago.

Current status: Patient continues to have persistent pain and is unable to work

Assessment: dislocated right shoulder, acromioclavicular joint, 150% displacement

Plan: Outpatient surgery scheduled for reducing dislocation. This will be performed under IV sedation. Preop instructions provided to the patient.

Tip: Assign a code for the injury and an external cause code for the accident.

2 ICD-10-CM Codes _____

---

3. EMERGENCY DEPT   Gender: F   Age: 19

Reason for encounter: infected wound where she stepped on nail last week

Assessment: puncture wound left foot

Plan: Continue antibiotic ointment, begin 10 day regime of antibiotics, review status of tetanus immunization. Redress wound. RTO in 3 days

(continued)

3. (continued)

Tip: Assign a code for the injury and an external cause code. Read the instructional notes for the category.

3 ICD-10-CM Codes _____

_____

4. INPATIENT HOSPITAL   Gender: M   Age: 45

Reason for admission: Admitted from emergency department due to skull fracture. He was unconscious for 90 minutes, but returned to his normal state of consciousness.

Assessment: open occipital condylar fracture (Type I) of base of skull with subarachnoid hemorrhage.

Plan: Craniotomy performed based on CT results which showed bleeding. Vessel occlusion performed. Patient in ICU following surg. RTO 4 days post discharge and weekly thereafter for two weeks.

Tip: A combination code describes the injury and the loss of consciousness. The external cause is not documented. Do not assign external cause codes.

2 ICD-10-CM Codes _____

5. EMERGENCY DEPT   Gender: M   Age: 37

Reason for encounter: ketoacidosis with coma. Admit for observation. Stat blood chemistry and insulin administration.

Assessment: Type 1 diabetic forgot to take insulin. He is here on vacation and got confused due to the time zone change and an erratic schedule.

Plan: FU with endocrinologist when returns home. 1 week.

Tip: Follow the guidelines for underdosing. OGCR I.C. 19.e.5.(c)

3 ICD-10-CM Codes _____

_____

6. OFFICE   Gender: M   Age: 34

Reason for encounter: removal of cast

Assessment: X-rays show full healing of oblique fracture of left radius shaft. Cast removed.

Tip: Do not assign aftercare **Z** codes with injury codes. OGCR I.C.19.a.

1 ICD-10-CM Code _____

7. EMERGENCY DEPT   Gender: F   Age: 28

Chief complaint: Patient was brought in by her neighbor. She was at home stripping wood furniture inside on a rainy day. She got a severe headache and nausea due to the fumes and began vomiting.

Assessment: acetone toxicity

Plan: OTC medication for headache, restore fluids orally, postpone furniture finishing until it is possible to have better ventilation

Tip: Assign three diagnosis codes for the poisoning and manifestations and three external cause codes.

6 ICD-10-CM Codes _____

_____

8. OFFICE   Gender: M   Age: 48

Reason for admission: Admitted from emergency department, where he was seen after an accident while riding as a passenger in an off-road recreational vehicle

Assessment: transverse fracture right tibia shaft, notified patient's oncologist, who is currently treating him for prostate cancer

Plan: FU with oncologist and orthopedic surgeon in office

Tip: Refer to OGCR I.C.2.

3 ICD-10-CM Codes _____

_____

9. INPATIENT HOSPITAL   Gender: M
Age: 18 months

Reason for admission: Child got into some open whiskey and was found unconscious. He had been left alone by his stepfather who ran out to the corner store. Admit for overnight observation.

Assessment: Child neglect and abandonment. Alcohol toxicity. Blood alcohol level (BAC) of .360 (360 mg per 100 ml of blood)

Plan: Stabilized with oxygen and IV fluids. Social service evaluation of home, mandatory report to dept of human services

Tip: Assign three diagnosis codes and three external cause codes for BAC, perpetrator, and place of occurrence. (Do not assign codes for the coma scale.)

6 ICD-10-CM Codes _____

_____

(continued)

(continued from page 209)

10. INPATIENT HOSPITAL Gender: F Age: 22

Chief complaint: admitted from physician's office after complaining of fast heart beat

Assessment: supraventricular tachycardia that is a late effect of a heroin overdose during a suicide attempt 3 months ago

(*continued*)

10. (continued)

Plan: Stabilized rhythm with vagal maneuvers. Discharged on regime of antiarrhythmic med. Referral for substance addiction.

Tip: Assign codes for the injury and the current manifestation.

2 ICD-10-CM Codes _____

KEEP ON CODING

Instructions: Read the diagnostic statement, then use the Index and Tabular List to assign and sequence ICD-10-CM diagnosis codes. Write the code(s) on the line provided.

1. Abrasion of the scalp, initial encounter: ICD-10-CM Code(s) _____

2. Fracture of the mandible, subsequent encounter: ICD-10-CM Code(s) _____

3. Laceration of the left carotid artery, initial encounter: ICD-10-CM Code(s) _____

4. Muscle strain of the lower back, initial encounter: ICD-10-CM Code(s) _____

5. Accidental ingestion of toxic mushrooms, initial encounter: ICD-10-CM Code(s) _____

6. Bone marrow transplant failure: ICD-10-CM Code(s) _____

7. Crushing injury of the left upper arm, initial encounter: ICD-10-CM Code(s) _____

8. Heat collapse, initial encounter: ICD-10-CM Code(s) _____

9. Fracture of the left sacrum, type 3, subsequent encounter: ICD-10-CM Code(s) _____

10. Complete amputation of right breast, traumatic injury, late effect: ICD-10-CM Code(s) _____

11. Late effect of a moderate laceration of the spleen: ICD-10-CM Code(s) _____

12. Nonunion of fracture of femoral neck, right: ICD-10-CM Code(s) _____

13. Acute transfusion reaction due to Rh incompatibility, initial encounter: ICD-10-CM Code(s) _____

14. Traumatic compartment syndrome of the left hip, initial encounter: ICD-10-CM Code(s) _____

15. Partial traumatic amputation, left leg, subsequent encounter: ICD-10-CM Code(s) _____

16. Blast injury of right ear, initial encounter: ICD-10-CM Code(s) _____

17. Traumatic hemopneumothorax, subsequent encounter: ICD-10-CM Code(s) _____

18. Foreign body in nostril, initial encounter: ICD-10-CM Code(s) _____

19. Late effect of a third-degree burn of the left ankle: ICD-10-CM Code(s) _____

20. Displaced avulsion fracture of the right ischium, initial encounter: ICD-10-CM Code(s) _____

21. Major contusion of left kidney, traumatic, initial encounter: ICD-10-CM Code(s) _____

22. Displaced longitudinal fracture of right patella, initial encounter: ICD-10-CM Code(s) _____

23. Open bite of the right buttock, subsequent encounter: ICD-10-CM Code(s) _____

24. Sprain of right ankle, initial encounter: ICD-10-CM Code(s) _____

25. Adverse effect of overuse of laxatives, subsequent encounter: ICD-10-CM Code(s) _____

Diseases of the Circulatory System (I00-I99)

Chapter 14

Learning Objectives

After completing this chapter, you should have the skills to:

14.1 Spell and define the key words, medical terms, and abbreviations related to diseases of the circulatory system.

14.2 Discuss the structure, function, and common conditions of the circulatory system.

14.3 Identify the main characteristics of coding for diseases of the circulatory system.

14.4 Abstract diagnostic information from the medical record for coding diseases of the circulatory system.

14.5 Assign codes for diseases of the circulatory system.

14.6 Arrange multiple diagnosis codes for diseases of the circulatory system.

14.7 Discuss the Official Guidelines for Coding and Reporting related to diseases of the circulatory system.

Chapter Outline

- **Circulatory System Refresher**
- **Conditions of the Circulatory System**
- **Coding Overview of the Circulatory System**
- **Abstracting for Circulatory System Conditions**
- **Assigning Codes for Circulatory System Conditions**
- **Arranging Codes for Circulatory System Conditions**

Key Terms and Abbreviations

acute myocardial infarction (AMI)	cardiovascular (CV) system	mitral valve	right atrium
angiography	cerebral	mitral valve prolapse (MVP)	right ventricle
angioplasty	circulatory system	mitral valve stenosis	sinoatrial (SA) node
aorta	click murmur syndrome	myocardial infarction (MI)	ST elevation MI (STEMI)
aortic valve	coronary artery bypass graft (CABG)	myocardium	stent insertion
arrhythmia		native	stress testing
artery	coronary circulation	nonautologous	subendocardial
arteriole	current MI	nonbiological	subsequent MI
atrioventricular bundle (bundle of His)	diastole	non-ST elevation MI (NSTEMI)	superior vena cava
	Doppler ultrasonography	nontransmural	systemic circulation
atrioventricular (AV) node	echocardiography	occlusion	systole
atrioventricular (AV) valve	electrocardiography (ECG, EKG)	old (healed) MI	transmural MI
atrium/atria	embolectomy	pacemaker	tricuspid valve
autologous	endarterectomy	parietal pericardium	valve repair
Barlow syndrome	endocardium	pericardium	valve replacement
bundle branch	epicardium	plaque	vein
bypass graft	Holter monitor	precerebral	venography
capillary	inferior vena cava	pulmonary circulation	ventricle
cardiac catheterization	internal mammary artery (IMA)	pulmonary valve	venule
cardiac function test	left atrium	Purkinje fiber	visceral pericardium
cardiac scan	left ventricle	regurgitation	

In addition to the key terms listed here, students should know the terms defined within tables in this chapter.

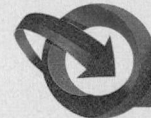

For updates and corrections, visit our student resource site at

INTRODUCTION

You probably do not give much thought to your vehicle's fuel pump as long as it is working properly. But when it is not, your vehicle may stall when the accelerator is pressed or not start at all. Mechanics listen to hear the pump running and test the fuel pressure with a gauge on their way to diagnosing the problem. Just as the fuel pump is responsible for circulating gas throughout the engine, the human heart is also a pump with the job of circulating blood. Physicians listen to the heart with a stethoscope and measure blood pressure as part of their diagnostic methods.

In this chapter you will learn more about how the circulatory system works, why sometimes it does not work as it should, and how physicians treat these conditions. Cardiologists are physicians who specialize in diagnosing and treating diseases of the circulatory system. Subspecialities in cardiology include pediatric cardiology and cardiothoracic surgery. Primary care physicians diagnose and treat common conditions of the circulatory systems and refer complex cases to cardiologists.

CIRCULATORY SYSTEM REFRESHER

The function of the **circulatory system**, also called the **cardiovascular (CV) system**, is to distribute blood throughout the body. It consists of the heart, which is the pump, and blood vessels, which are the tubes that carry blood. The distribution or transportation task provides three functions:

- carries oxygen and nutrients to body tissues for metabolism
- carries waste products of metabolism to the kidneys and other excretory organs
- circulates electrolytes and hormones needed to regulate body functions

The circulatory system consists of pulmonary circulation, systemic circulation, and coronary circulation. **Pulmonary circulation**, which occurs between the heart and the lungs, carries deoxygenated blood from the heart to the lungs, where it is replenished with oxygen, then back to the heart. **Systemic circulation**, which occurs between the heart and the rest of the body, carries oxygenated blood away from the heart to the tissues and cells of the body, then carries oxygen-depleted blood back to the heart. **Coronary circulation**, which occurs within the heart, carries blood from the aorta to the tissues of the heart to maintain the function of the heart itself (■ FIGURE 14-1).

According to the Centers for Disease Control and Prevention, heart disease is the leading cause of death in the United States for both men and women, accounting for over 25% of all deaths each year. Every year about 785,000 people have a first heart attack and another 470,000, who previously had a heart attack, have another one. In the United States, health care services, medications, and lost productivity related to heart disease cost more than $315 billion per year.

To understand disorders of the circulatory system, coders need to understand the structure and operation of the heart muscle, the conduction system, and the blood vessels.

The Heart Muscle

The heart is a muscular organ that contains four chambers: two **atria**, which receive blood from the body (**right atrium**) and the

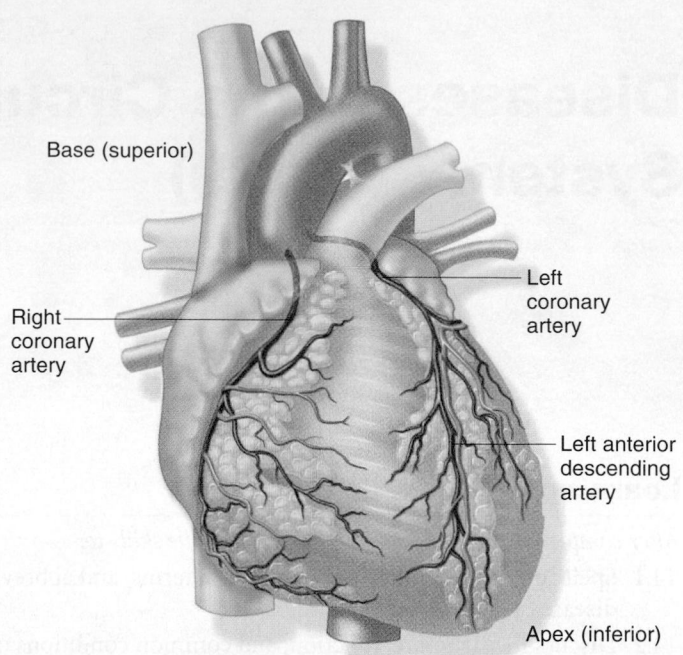

Base (superior)

Right coronary artery

Left coronary artery

Left anterior descending artery

Apex (inferior)

Figure 14-1 ■ The Major Arteries and Vessels of Coronary Circulation

lungs (**left atrium**), and two **ventricles**, which eject blood to the lungs (**right ventricle**) and the body (**left ventricle**) (■ FIGURE 14-2). Four valves control the one-way flow of blood into, through, and out of the heart: the **tricuspid** (*right atrium to right ventricle*), **mitral** (*left atrium to left ventricle*), **pulmonary** (*right ventricle to pulmonary artery*), and **aortic** (*left ventricle to aorta*) valves. The mitral and tricuspid valves are **atrioventricular (AV) valves** because they control the flow of blood from atria to ventricles. During every heart cycle, each chamber relaxes as it fills with blood during **diastole** and contracts as it ejects blood during **systole**.

The heart wall is a thick muscle consisting of three layers:

- the **endocardium**, the smooth inner layer that reduces friction as the blood flows through the heart;
- the **myocardium**, the thick muscular inner layers that contract to pump blood; and
- the **pericardium**, a double-walled sac filled with fluid, which is the outer layer.

The pericardium consists of the **epicardium** or **visceral pericardium** (*inner layer*) and the **parietal pericardium** (*outer layer*).

Disorders of the Heart Muscle

Myocardial infarction (MI), commonly known as a heart attack, is the death of heart tissue caused by an interruption to the blood supply. The most common cause of MI is **occlusion** (*blockage*) of a coronary artery by **plaque** (*a buildup of cholesterol inside the wall of blood vessels*). MIs are described by the heart wall that is affected: anterior, posterior, or inferior. A **transmural MI** extends through the entire thickness of the heart muscle. A **subendocardial** or **nontransmural** infarction affects only a small portion of the heart wall, usually due to a decreased, but not totally occluded, blood supply.

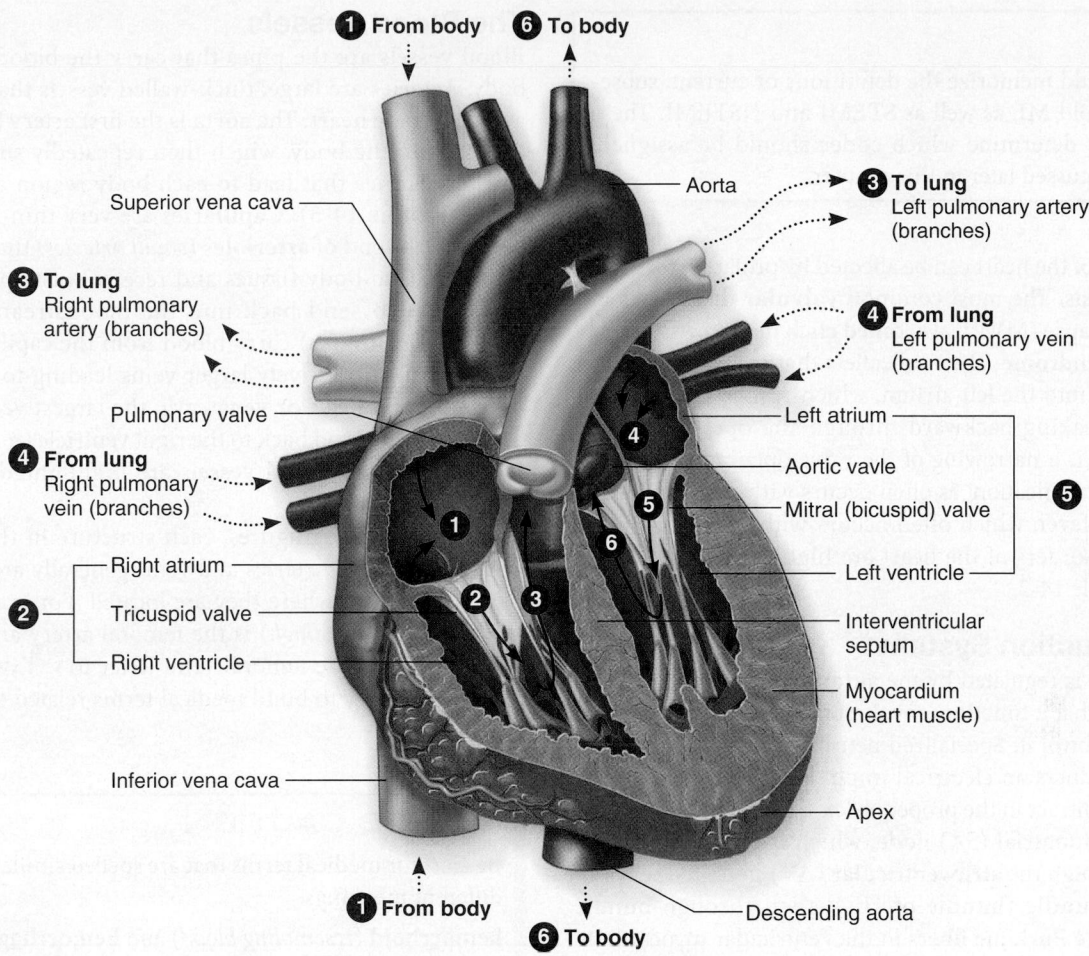

Figure 14-2 ■ The Path of Blood Flow Through the Heart

❶ From body

❻ To body

Aorta

❸ **To lung**
Left pulmonary artery
(branches)

❹ **From lung**
Left pulmonary vein
(branches)

Left atrium

Aortic vavle

Mitral (bicuspid) valve

❺

Left ventricle

Interventricular
septum

Myocardium
(heart muscle)

Apex

Descending aorta

❻ To body

❶ From body

Superior vena cava

❸ **To lung**
Right pulmonary
artery (branches)

Pulmonary valve

❹ **From lung**
Right pulmonary
vein (branches)

Right atrium

❷ Tricuspid valve

Right ventricle

Inferior vena cava

An MI that has occurred within the past four weeks is an **acute myocardial infarction (AMI)**, also referred to as a **current MI**. An MI that occurs within four weeks of a previous AMI is also clinically acute but is referred to as a **subsequent MI** to distinguish it from the original MI. An MI more than four weeks old is an **old (healed) MI**.

CODING CAUTION

If you are familiar with ICD-9-CM, it is important to note that the time frame for acute MI has changed. Under ICD-9-CM, an acute MI was eight weeks, but in ICD-10-CM, an acute MI is only four weeks.

MIs are further described based on the results of an electrocardiogram (ECG, EKG) (■ FIGURE 14-3). Each part of the EKG is labeled with a letter denoting a specific phase of the heart's electrical activity. The ST segment is elevated in an MI that completely occludes a vessel, known as **ST elevation MI (STEMI)**. When the vessel is partially blocked, the ST segment is not elevated, resulting in a **non-ST elevation MI (NSTEMI)**.

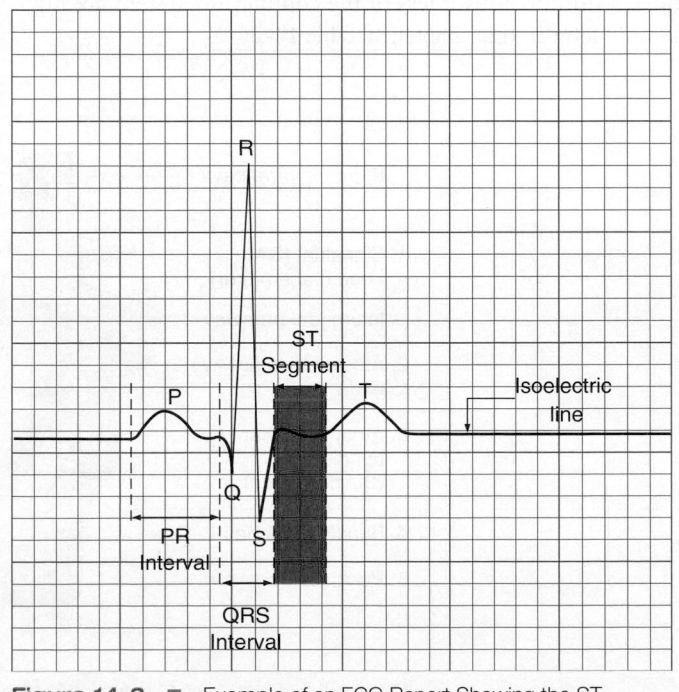

Figure 14-3 ■ Example of an ECG Report Showing the ST Segment

The valves of the heart can be affected by prolapse, regurgitation, or stenosis. The most common **valvular** disorder is **mitral valve prolapse (MVP)**, also called **click murmur syndrome** and **Barlow syndrome**. The two leaflets that comprise the valve fall backward into the left atrium, which results in **regurgitation**, blood leaking backward through the opening. **Mitral valve stenosis** is a narrowing of the valve opening, which may be caused by calcification, as often occurs with the aortic valve, or rheumatic fever, which often occurs with the mitral valve. Additional disorders of the heart are highlighted later in this chapter in Table 14-2.

The Conduction System

The heart rate is regulated by the **autonomic nervous system**, which means that it functions involuntarily and humans cannot voluntarily control it. Specialized neuromuscular tissue within the heart conducts an electrical impulse that stimulates each chamber to contract in the proper order. The electrical impulses begin in the **sinoatrial (SA) node**, which is the pacemaker of the heart, through the **atrioventricular (AV) node** to the **atrioventricular bundle (bundle of His)**, then through **bundle branches** to the **Purkinje fibers** in the ventricular myocardium (■ Figure 14-4).

Faulty electrical signaling in the heart causes **arrhythmia** (*an abnormal heartbeat*). A **pacemaker** is a small electronic device that is implanted in the chest to correct arrhythmia by speeding up, slowing down, smoothing out, or coordinating the heartbeat. Additional disorders of the conduction system are highlighted later in this chapter in Table 14-2.

The Blood Vessels

Blood vessels are the pipes that carry the blood through the body. **Arteries** are large, thick-walled vessels that carry blood away from the heart. The **aorta** is the first artery leading out of the heart to the body, which then repeatedly subdivides into smaller arteries that lead to each body region and anatomic site (■ Figure 14-5). **Capillaries** are very thin-walled membranes at the end of **arterioles** (*small arteries*) that allow blood to diffuse into body tissues and receive waste products from the tissues to send back into the bloodstream. **Veins** and **venules** (*small veins*) carry blood from the capillaries back to the heart in successively larger veins leading to the **superior vena cava** and **inferior vena cava**, the largest veins that carry deoxygenated blood back to the right ventricle (■ Figure 14-6). Disorders of the blood vessels are highlighted later in this chapter in Table 14-2.

In the preceding figures, each structure in the circulatory system is labeled. Arteries and veins generally are named after the anatomic site where they are located. For example, the artery in the femur (*thigh*) is the femoral artery and the vein in the upper leg is the femoral vein. Refer to ■ Table 14-1 for a refresher on how to build medical terms related to the circulatory system.

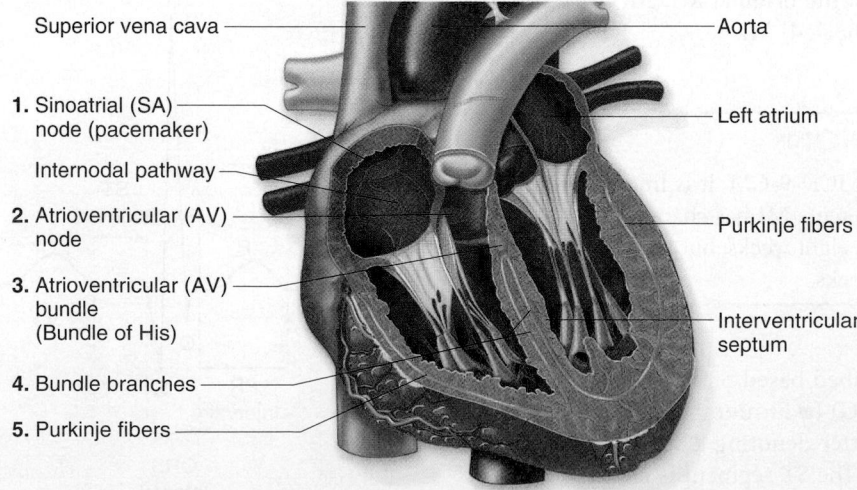

Figure 14-4 ■ The Conduction System of the Heart

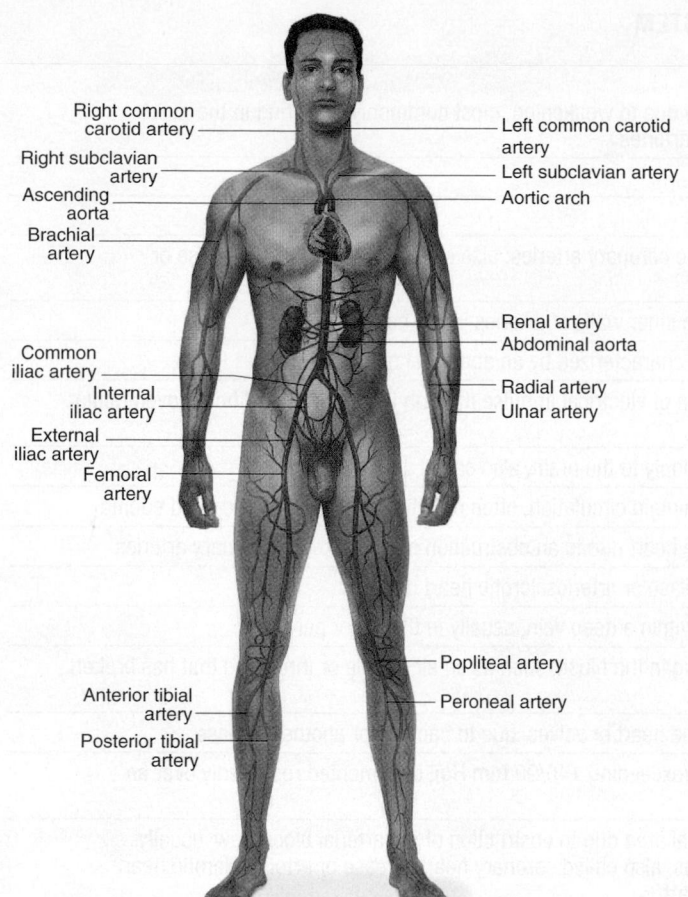

Figure 14-5 ■ The Major Arteries of Systemic Circulation

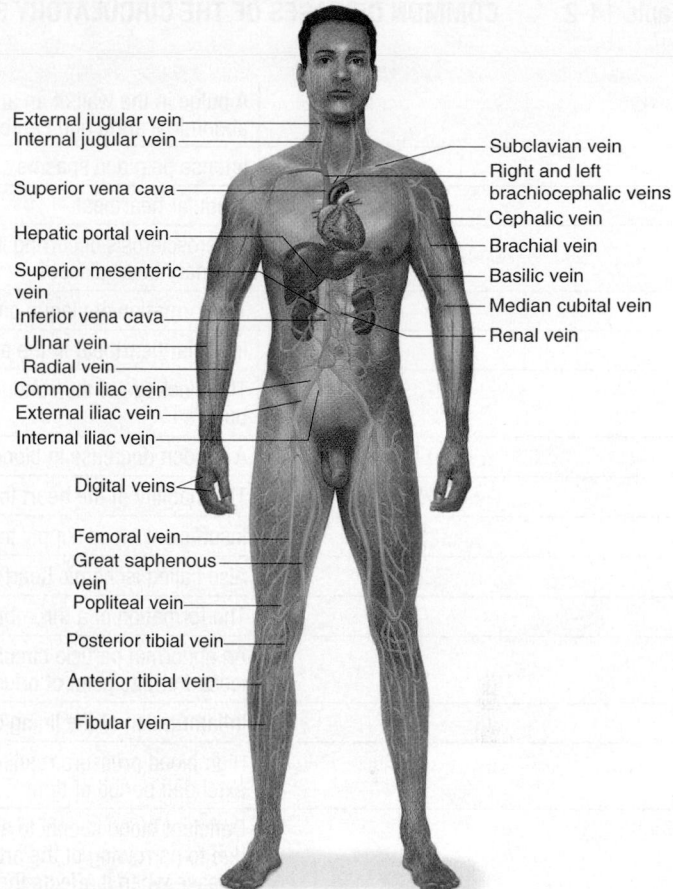

Figure 14-6 ■ The Major Veins of Systemic Circulation

Conditions of the Circulatory System

Diseases and disorders of the circulatory system can affect the heart muscle, the conduction system of the heart, coronary circulation, or systemic (peripheral) circulation. Diseases of the heart structure generally are caused by a weakness or looseness in one or more components. Diseases of coronary circulation affect the veins and arteries that feed the heart. The most common is the blockage of a coronary artery, which diminishes blood flow to the heart. Diseases of the conduction system result in cardiac arrhythmias, irregularities of the heartbeat. Diseases of systemic circulation include an abnormality in a vein or artery in the arms and legs, such as hardening of the arteries and blockages. Refer to ■ TABLE 14-2 (page 216) for a summary of diseases affecting the circulatory system.

This section provides a general reference to help understand the most common diagnoses of the circulatory system but does not list everything you need to know. Use medical terminology skills discussed earlier in this chapter to learn the meaning of unfamiliar words. Remember to keep standard reference books handy in case you get stuck.

Neoplasms of the Circulatory System

Neoplasms of the cardiovascular system are rare, and when they do occur, most are benign. Secondary or metastatic neoplasms of the heart occur in 1% of the population; primary neoplasms are even more infrequent.

Table 14-1 ■ EXAMPLE OF CONSTRUCTING MEDICAL TERMS FOR THE CIRCULATORY SYSTEM

Combining Form	Suffix	Complete Medical Term
my/o (*muscle*)		**endo + cardi + itis** (*inflammation of the lining inside the heart*) **myo + cardi + itis** (*inflammation of the heart muscle*)
angi/o (*vessel*)	**-gram** (*recording*) **-itis** (*inflammation*) **-plasty** (*repair*)	**angio + gram** (*recording of the vessels*)
cardi/o (*heart*)		**electro + cardio + gram** (*electrical recording of the heart*) **echo + cardio + gram** (*recording of the sound of the heart*)
end/o (*within*)		**angio + plasty** (*repair of a blood vessel*)

Table 14-2 ■ **COMMON DISEASES OF THE CIRCULATORY SYSTEM**

Condition	Definition
Aneurysm	A bulge in the wall of an artery due to weakening, most commonly occurring in the abdominal aorta and cerebral arteries
Angina	Intense pain and spasms
Arrhythmia	Irregular heartbeat
Arteriosclerotic heart disease (ASHD)	Atherosclerosis occurring in the coronary arteries; also called ischemic heart disease or coronary heart disease
Atherosclerosis	The formation of plaque on the inner walls of arteries in the heart
Atrial fibrillation (A-fib)	Irregular heartbeat in the atria characterized by an abnormal quivering of heart fibers
Bundle branch block (BBB)	The blockage of the conduction of electrical impulse through the branches of the atrioventricular bundle
Cerebrovascular accident (CVA)	A sudden decrease in blood supply to the brain; also called stroke
Congestive heart failure (CHF)	The inability of the heart to maintain circulation, often resulting in water retention and edema
Coronary artery disease (CAD)	Insufficient blood supply to the heart due to an obstruction of one or more coronary arteries
Coronary heart disease (CHD)	Also called ischemic heart disease or arteriosclerotic heart disease
Deep vein thrombosis (DVT)	The formation of a thrombus within a deep vein, usually in the leg or pelvis
Embolus	An abnormal particle circulating in the blood, such as an air bubble or thrombus that has broken loose from its point of origin
Endocarditis	Inflammation of the lining of the heart or valves, due to bacteria or another disease
Hypertension (HTN)	High blood pressure readings (exceeding 140/90 mm Hg), documented repeatedly over an extended period of time
Ischemia	Deficient blood supply to a local area due to obstruction of the arterial blood flow, usually due to narrowing of the arteries; also called coronary heart disease or arteriosclerotic heart disease when it affects the heart
Mitral valve prolapse (MVP)	Weakness in the flaps of the mitral valve, which allows blood to flow backward from the right ventricle into the right atrium
Myocardial infarction (MI)	The death of heart tissue due to a blockage of the blood supply
Pericarditis	Inflammation of the pericardial sac that surrounds the heart
Peripheral artery disease (PAD)	Damage to arteries outside the heart resulting in decreased blood flow
Stenosis	A narrowing of a valve or vessel
Thrombus	A clot of blood formed within a blood vessel that remains attached to its point of origin
Transient ischemic attack (TIA)	A brief episode of cerebral ischemia
Ventricular fibrillation (V-fib)	Irregular heartbeat in the ventricles, characterized by an abnormal quivering of heart fibers, which can result in cardiac arrest

Diagnostic Methods

Diseases of the circulatory system are diagnosed with laboratory tests, imaging studies, and cardiac function studies, which are described as follows:

- Laboratory tests measure the levels of substances in the blood, such as the following:
  - cardiac enzymes
    - creatine phosphokinase (CPK)
    - lactate dehydrogenase (LDH)
    - glutamic oxaloacetic transaminase (GOT)
  - cholesterol
  - triglycerides

- Imaging studies are visualizations of the circulatory system using X-ray and ultrasound techniques, including the following:
  - **angiography** (*X-ray taken after an opaque dye is injected into a blood vessel*)
  - **cardiac scan** (*a scan of the heart after the patient receives radioactive thallium intravenously*)
  - **Doppler ultrasonography** (*an image created by measuring sound-wave echoes off of tissues and organs*)
  - **echocardiography** (*noninvasive ultrasound to visualize internal cardiac structures*)
  - **venography** (*X-ray of the veins by tracing the venous pulse*)

- **Cardiac function tests** measure the capacity of the heart in real time, including the following:
  - **cardiac catheterization** (*passage of a thin tube through a blood vessel to the heart to visualize the structure, collect blood samples, and determine the blood pressure of the heart*)
  - **electrocardiography** (**ECG, EKG**) (*a graphical recording of the electrical activity of the heart*)
  - **Holter monitor** (*a portable EKG worn by the patient for an extended period of hours or days to measure heart activity in a variety of situations*)
  - **stress testing** (*measuring EKG and oxygen levels as a patient performs an increasing level of exercise on a treadmill or stationary bicycle*)

Treatment Methods

Heart disease is treated with a wide range of medications that regulate circulatory system functions, medical procedures such as a pacemaker or **implantable cardioverter-defibrillator** to regulate heart activity, and surgery to repair defects. Common procedures include the following:

- **angioplasty** (*insertion of an inflatable catheter in a blood vessel that expands to compress plaque against the walls of the vessel*)

- **bypass graft** (*creation of a new route around a blockage in a blood vessel using a vessel from another part of the body, another person, or a synthetic substitute*)
- **coronary artery bypass graft** (**CABG**) (*open-heart surgery to create a bypass around a blocked coronary artery, usually using the* **internal mammary artery** [**IMA**] *or a vein from the leg*)
- **embolectomy** (*removal of a clot from a blood vessel*)
- **endarterectomy** (*removal of the diseased or damaged inner lining of an artery*)
- **stent insertion** (*placement of a mesh tube in a blood vessel to keep it open; necessary in atherosclerosis*)
- **valve repair** (*correction of a physical defect*)
- **valve replacement** (*replacement of a heart valve with an synthetic or porcine [pig] valve*)

Heart transplants, first done in 1967, are the third most common organ transplant in the United States and are performed in extreme cases of heart failure when other treatments have failed. According to the American Heart Association, approximately 2,100 heart transplants are performed each year in the United States. However, the need is far greater than that but cannot be met, due to a shortage of available donor organs.

CODING PRACTICE

Exercise 14.1 Circulatory System Refresher

Instructions: Use your medical terminology skills and resources to define the following conditions related to the circulatory system, then assign the diagnosis code.

Follow these steps:

- Use slash marks "/" to break down each term into its root(s) and suffix.
- Define the meaning of the word, based on the meaning of each word part.
- Assign the default ICD-10-CM diagnosis code for the condition using the Index and Tabular List.

Example: endocarditis endo/card/itis   Meaning: *inflammation of the lining of the heart*   ICD-10-CM Code: *I38*

1. hypertension   Meaning _____   ICD-10-CM Code _____

2. myocarditis   Meaning _____   ICD-10-CM Code _____

3. cardiomyopathy   Meaning _____   ICD-10-CM Code _____

4. atheroma   Meaning _____   ICD-10-CM Code _____

5. arteriosclerosis   Meaning _____   ICD-10-CM Code _____

6. arrhythmia   Meaning _____   ICD-10-CM Code _____

7. lymphocele   Meaning _____   ICD-10-CM Code _____

8. thrombophlebitis   Meaning _____   ICD-10-CM Code _____

9. thromboangiitis   Meaning _____   ICD-10-CM Code _____

10. pyopneumopericardium   Meaning _____   ICD-10-CM Code _____

CODING OVERVIEW OF THE CIRCULATORY SYSTEM

ICD-10-CM Chapter 9, Diseases of the Circulatory System (I00-I99), contains 11 blocks or subchapters that are divided by the type of disease. Review the block names and code ranges listed at the beginning of Chapter 9 in the ICD-10-CM manual to become familiar with the content and organization.

ICD-10-CM Chapter 9 corresponds with ICD-9-CM Chapter 7 (390-459). Many codes have been expanded to identify specific anatomic sites and laterality. Terminology has been updated for angina pectoris, myocardial infarction, atherosclerosis, pulmonary embolism, cardiac arrest, and nontraumatic subarachnoid hemorrhage to be consistent with current clinical practice. ICD-9-CM category 438, Late effects of cerebrovascular disease, has been significantly expanded in ICD-10-CM category I69, Sequelae of cerebrovascular disease. OGCR for myocardial infarction and hypertensive heart disease have also been updated.

This chapter includes disorders that affect the heart and the pulmonary, systemic, and coronary circulatory systems. Conditions may consist of acquired physical dysfunctions or infections.

This chapter does not include congenital diseases of the circulatory system, which are classified in ICD-10-CM Chapter 17, Congenital Malformations, Deformations, and Chromosomal Abnormalities (Q00-Q99), or diseases of the blood, which are classified in ICD-10-CM Chapter 3, Diseases of the Blood and Blood-Forming Organs and Certain Disorders Involving the Immune Mechanism (D50-D89).

ICD-10-CM provides Official Guidelines for Coding and Reporting (OGCR) for the circulatory system in OGCR section I.C.9. OGCR provide detailed discussion regarding hypertension, atherosclerotic coronary artery disease and angina, cerebrovascular accident and disease, and acute myocardial infarction. The Tabular List contains no instructional notes at the beginning of the chapter but does provide many instructional notes throughout the chapter regarding additional codes that are required to identify related conditions and lifestyle habits related to tobacco use.

ABSTRACTING FOR CIRCULATORY SYSTEM CONDITIONS

Coders need to pay close attention to detail when abstracting for the CV system because codes must be specific to anatomic site, nature of the disease, and comorbidities. Coders rely on their knowledge of anatomy to identify the exact site of the disorder and their knowledge of diseases to identify the specific form of the disease and coexisting conditions. They also must identify circumstances that require Z codes. Key factors to review when coding cases that involve the circulatory system appear in ■ TABLE 14-3. Remember that the abstracting questions are a guide and that not every question applies to, or can be answered for, every case. For example, the questions about myocardial infarction do not apply to patients who have not had this condition.

Table 14-3 ■ KEY CRITERIA FOR ABSTRACTING CONDITIONS OF THE CIRCULATORY SYSTEM

- ❑ What part of the circulatory system is affected?
- ❑ What is the specific anatomic site?
- ❑ What type of disorder is present?
- ❑ Is the condition further specified as complete, partial, current, or old?
- ❑ What is the underlying cause?
- ❑ What symptoms are documented that are not integral to the condition?
- ❑ Is the condition acquired or congenital?
- ❑ Is the condition related to pregnancy?
- ❑ Does the patient have a current, subsequent, or old MI?
- ❑ Has the patient had more than one AMI in the past four weeks?
- ❑ What other CV conditions coexist?
- ❑ What conditions exist in other organ systems?
- ❑ Which conditions are documented as being related to the CV condition?
- ❑ What is the patient's exposure to or use of tobacco?
- ❑ Does the patient use anticoagulants or antithrombotics on a long-term basis?
- ❑ Does the patient have a family history of CV disease?
- ❑ Does the patient wear a pacemaker?
- ❑ Has the patient had a CABG?
- ❑ If a vessel is blocked or diseased, is it an artery or vein? Is it native (*the patient's original vessel*) or a graft?
- ❑ If a grafted vessel is blocked, is the grafted vessel autologous (*from the patient*), biological nonautologous (*from a source other than the patient, such as a cadaver or animal*), or nonbiological (*synthetic*)?
- ❑ Is the patient waiting for or a recipient of a heart transplant?

Guided Example of Abstracting for Circulatory System Conditions

Refer to the following example throughout this chapter to learn skills for abstracting, assigning, and sequencing circulatory system codes. Tanisha Riemann, CCS-P, is a fictitious coder who guides you through the coding process.

Date: 4/1/yy   Location: Branton Medical Center

Provider: Matthew Bunker, MD

Patient: Gordon Rothe   Gender: M   Age: 76

Reason for admission: admitted from emergency department due to unstable angina, patient has been on warfarin since a CABG of the left anterior descending coronary artery (LAD) 11 years ago using the left saphenous vein, continues to use tobacco although he states that his usage has decreased

Assessment: atherosclerosis of grafted vessel

Plan: balloon angioplasty to clear the partially blocked graft, Rx atorvastatin to address lipid rich plaque

Follow along as Tanisha Riemann, CCS-P, abstracts the diagnosis. Check off each step after you complete it.

► Tanisha reads through the entire record, paying special attention to the reason for the encounter and the final assessment. She refers to the Key Criteria for Abstracting Conditions of the Circulatory System (Table 14-3) to guide her review.

❏ She notes the presenting symptom of unstable angina.

❏ *What part of the circulatory system is affected?* grafted vessel

❏ *What is the specific anatomic site?* The heart, near the left anterior descending coronary artery

❏ *What type of disorder is present?* blocked graft and atherosclerosis

❏ Is the condition further specified as complete, partial, current, or old? partially blocked

❏ *Does the patient have a current, subsequent, or old MI?* No

❏ *What other CV conditions coexist?* lipid rich plaque

❏ *What is the patient's exposure to or use of tobacco?* The patient continues to use tobacco although he states that his usage has decreased.

❏ Does the patient use anticoagulants or antithrombotics on a long-term basis? Yes, the patient has been on warfarin since a CABG 11 years ago.

❏ *Has the patient had a CABG?* Yes, 11 years ago

❏ *If a vessel is blocked or diseased, is it an artery or vein?* vein *Is it native or a graft?* graft

❏ *If a grafted vessel is blocked, is the grafted vessel autologous, biological nonautologous, or nonbiological?* The graft used the left saphenous vein, so it is autologous.

► At this point, Tanisha is not sure of how many codes she will need. She knows that she needs to search the Index and cross-reference any instructional notes in the Tabular List before she knows what her final codes will be.

CODING PRACTICE

Exercise 14.2   **Abstracting for Circulatory System Conditions**

Instructions: Read the mini-medical-record of each patient's encounter and answer the abstracting questions. Write the answer on the line provided. Do not assign any codes.

---

1. INPATIENT HOSPITAL   Gender: F   Age: 42

Reason for admission: admitted from emergency department with subendocardial infarction

Assessment: nontransmural myocardial infarction

Plan: This is her first event so we will treat it with medication and diet.

a. What is a subendocardial infarction? _____

_____

b. What is a nontransmural infarction? _____

_____

c. What is the Main Term?_____

_____

---

2. OFFICE   Gender: F   Age: 68

Reason for encounter: Patient has been taking her BP at home and is concerned about readings that have been increasing over the past 3 months. She claims to be taking the diuretic and beta blocker as directed. Lab results show slightly low potassium.

(continued)

---

2. (continued)

Assessment: hypertensive cardiomegaly

Plan: Add spironolactone to the medication regime.

a. What is the cause of the patient's cardiomegaly?

_____

b. Should you code for low potassium? _____

_____

c. What is the Main Term? _____

---

3. INPATIENT HOSPITAL   Gender: M   Age: 68

Reason for admission: mitral porcine valvoplasty

Assessment: mitral valve regurgitation due to prolapse

a. Where is the mitral valve located? _____

_____

b. In your own words, explain what procedure was done.

_____

c. In your own words, explain why the procedure was done.

_____

(continued)

CODING PRACTICE *(continued)*

4. INPATIENT HOSPITAL   Gender: F   Age: 71

Reason for admission: Admitted from emergency department with angina. Patient has history of MI 2 years ago, as well as history of TIAs, although the TIAs did not leave any residual deficits.

Assessment: STEMI involving 90% occlusion of the right coronary artery

Procedure: CABG

a. Should you code for angina? _____

   Why or why not? _____

b. What is TIA? _____

c. What is STEMI? _____

d. What is the site of the STEMI? _____

   _____

e. Should you code for the old MI? _____

   _____

f. In your own words, describe the procedure that was done. _____

   _____

5. OFFICE   Gender: M   Age: 65

Chief complaint: increased edema and SOB since last visit

Assessment: HTN and decompensated CHF, A-fib

Plan: We will start by adjusting the diuretic, then evaluate the need for other adjustments based on response after 4 weeks. Continue long term warfarin and clopidrogel (*an antiplatelet medication*).

a. Define the abbreviations in this scenario. _____

   _____

b. Which condition are the edema and SOB most related to? _____

c. What is the causal relationship between HTN and CHF? _____

d. Which condition is the first listed diagnosis?

   _____ Why? _____

e. What type of medication is warfarin? _____

   _____

f. What type of medication is clopidrogel? _____

   _____

6. INPATIENT HOSPITAL   Gender: M   Age: 57

Reason for admission: transferred from another hospital where patient was admitted for cerebral infarct 20 hours ago and received tPA (tissue plasminogen activator), but now it is evident that a mechanical or surgical embolectomy is needed

Assessment: cerebral infarction d/t embolus in right middle cerebral artery, cerebral atherosclerosis, HTN, history of tobacco use

Procedure: surgical embolectomy

a. What is the common term for cerebral infarction?

   _____

b. What is the cause of the cerebral infarction?

   _____

c. What is an embolus? _____

   _____

d. Is the affected artery **cerebral** (*located within the brain*) or **precerebral** (*outside of the brain*)? _____

   _____

e. What other medical conditions exist? _____

   _____

f. What lifestyle habit is documented?

   _____

g. In your own words, describe the procedure that was performed. _____

   _____

ASSIGNING CODES FOR CIRCULATORY SYSTEM CONDITIONS

Diseases of the circulatory system frequently occur with multiple comorbidities from within the cardiovascular system and/or from other systems. The choice of codes is dependent on the precise wording physicians use in the documentation. The coding of hypertension, a common circulatory system condition, is an example of how documentation affects code choices. Hypertension may occur by itself, in conjunction with chronic kidney disease, heart disease, both kidney and heart disease, or many other conditions. Refer to the following examples to better understand how to interpret physician documentation when assigning codes.

> ### SUCCESS STEP
>
> ICD-10-CM does not have a separate Hypertension Table as ICD-9-CM did. Locate the Main Term **Hypertension** in the Index, then locate the appropriate subterm(s) for the condition being coded. In addition, ICD-10-CM does not distinguish between essential, benign, and malignant hypertension as ICD-9-CM did.

Hypertension

Physicians diagnose hypertension when patients have elevated blood pressure over an extended period of time. Assign a code for hypertension only when the physician has documented for this condition. Do not assign a code for hypertension simply because a patient has an incidental (*random*) high blood pressure reading (■ FIGURE 14-7).

When the diagnosis of hypertension is documented, search for the Main Term **Hypertension** in the Index. Assign the default code, **I10 Essential (primary) hypertension**, for hypertension described with the following terms:

- accelerated
- benign
- essential
- idiopathic
- malignant
- systemic

Refer to the Index entry in the ICD-10-CM manual, which identifies these terms as nonessential modifiers by the use of

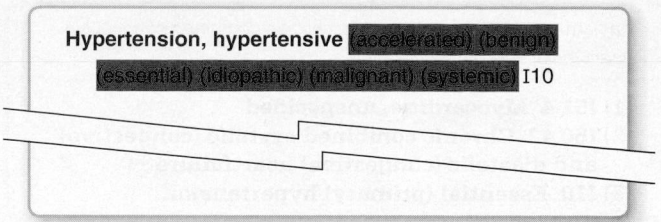

Figure 14-8 ■ Index Entry for Main Term Hypertension with Nonessential Modifiers

parentheses (■ FIGURE 14-8). Subterms identify codes for use when hypertension occurs with or due to another condition, which is discussed later in this chapter.

In the Tabular List, an instructional note, **Excludes1**, reminds coders that hypertension complicating pregnancy, childbirth, and the puerperium (*postpartum period*) is not coded here. Another instructional note, **Excludes2**, directs coders to look elsewhere for hypertension involving vessels of the brain and eye.

Hypertension and Chronic Kidney Disease

ICD-10-CM presumes a causal relationship between hypertension and **chronic kidney disease (CKD)** because hypertension is known to cause CKD and CKD is known to cause hypertension.

OGCR I.C.9.a provides guidelines on coding these conditions when they occur together. Assign codes as follows (■ FIGURE 14-9):

1. Assign a code from category **I12 Hypertensive chronic kidney disease** based on the stage of CKD documented. Refer to category **I12** in the ICD-10-CM manual to review the available codes and locate the instructional notes.

2. Assign a code from category **N18 Chronic kidney disease** as an additional code to identify the stage of CKD, as stated in the instructional note (OGCR I.C.9.a.2).

Hypertension and Heart Disease

Although hypertension is a major cause of heart failure, ICD-10-CM does *not* presume a causal relationship between hypertension and heart disease. A causal relationship must be stated or implied in order to assign a code for *hypertensive* heart disease. A causal relationship is stated definitively by documentation such as *heart disease due to hypertension* or *hypertension with heart involvement*. A causal relationship is implied by documentation such as *hypertensive heart disease*.

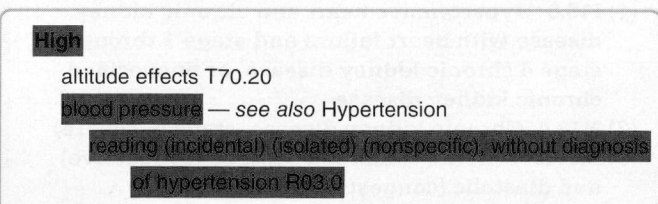

Figure 14-7 ■ Index Entry for Incidental High Blood Pressure Reading

> Patient is seen for stage 4 CKD and HTN.
>
> (1) **I12.9 Hypertensive chronic kidney disease with stage 1 through stage 4 chronic kidney disease, or unspecified chronic kidney disease**
> (2) **N18.4 Chronic kidney disease, stage 4 (severe)**

Figure 14-9 ■ Example of Assigning Codes for Hypertension and Chronic Kidney Disease

Patient is seen for myocarditis, chronic combined congestive heart failure, and hypertension.

(1) I51.4 **Myocarditis, unspecified**
(2) I50.42 **Chronic combined systolic (congestive) and diastolic (congestive) heartfailure**
(3) I10 **Essential (primary) hypertension**

Figure 14-10 ■ Example of Assigning Codes for Hypertension and Heart Disease When a Causal Relationship Is NOT Documented

SUCCESS STEP

Hypertensive heart disease is the leading cause of illness and death due to hypertension.

No Causal Relationship

When no causal relationship is documented, assign separate codes for the heart condition and hypertension. Do not assign a code for *hypertensive* heart disease (■ FIGURE 14-10).

Causal Relationship Stated or Implied

When a causal relationship exists between heart failure and hypertension, assign codes as follows:

1. Assign a code from category **I11 Hypertensive heart disease**. This category includes any condition in **I51.4** to **I51.9** that is due to hypertension (■ FIGURE 14-11).

2. Also assign a code from category **I50 Heart failure** to identify the type of heart failure as left ventricular, systolic, diastolic, combined, or unspecified. Sequence the code for hypertensive heart disease first and the code for heart failure second (■ FIGURE 14-12).

I51.4 **Myocarditis, unspecified**
　　Chronic (interstitial) myocarditis
　　Myocardial fibrosis
　　Myocarditis NOS
　　Excludes1: acute or subacute myocarditis (I40.-)
I51.5 **Myocardial degeneration**
　　Fatty degeneration of heart or myocardium
　　Myocardial disease
　　Senile degeneration of heart or myocardium
I51.7 **Cardiomegaly**
　　Cardiac dilatation
　　Cardiac hypertrophy
　　Ventricular dilatation
I51.8 **Other ill-defined heart diseases**
　　I51.81 **Takotsubo syndrome**
　　　　Reversible left ventricular dysfunction following
　　　　　sudden emotional stress
　　　　Stress induced cardiomyopathy
　　　　Takotsubo cardiomyopathy
　　　　Transient left ventricular apical ballooning syndrome
　　I51.89 **Other ill-defined heart diseases**
　　　　Carditis (acute)(chronic)
　　　　Pancarditis (acute)(chronic)
I51.9 **Heart disease, unspecified**

Figure 14-11 ■ Tabular List Entry for I51.4 to I51.9

Patient is seen for hypertensive myocarditis with chronic combined congestive heart failure.

(1) I11.0 **Hypertensive heart disease with heart failure**
(2) I50.42 **Chronic combined systolic (congestive) and diastolic (congestive) heart failure**

Figure 14-12 ■ Example of Assigning Codes for Heart Disease and Hypertension When a Causal Relationship IS Documented

SUCCESS STEP

To locate CHF in the Index, search for the Main Term **Failure**, and the subterm **heart**.

Hypertensive Kidney Disease and Hypertensive Heart Disease

The documentation may state that both hypertensive kidney disease and *hypertensive* heart disease exist. The causal relationship between hypertension and heart disease must be stated or implied, but a causal relationship between hypertension and CKD should be assumed. Assign codes as follows (■ FIGURE 14-13):

1. Assign a code from category **I13 Hypertensive heart and chronic kidney disease**.

2. Also assign a code from category **I50** when heart failure is present.

3. Assign a code from category **N18** to identify the stage of CKD.

Hypertension and Other Conditions

Whenever hypertension exists with another condition, searching Main Terms for both conditions helps ensure that nothing is omitted. Carefully review all available subterms under **Hypertension** to locate any applicable code for the comorbidity. Also locate the Index Main Term entry for the comorbid condition and search for a subterm of hypertension. Refer to OGCR I.C.9.a for additional guidelines on coding hypertension with cerebrovascular disease and retinopathy, as well as secondary, transient, controlled, and uncontrolled hypertension.

Guided Example of Assigning Codes for Circulatory System Conditions

To practice skills for assigning codes for the circulatory system, continue with the example from earlier in the chapter about

Patient is seen for hypertensive myocarditis with chronic combined CHF and stage 4 CKD.

(1) I13.0 **Hypertensive heart and chronic kidney disease with heart failure and stage 1 through stage 4 chronic kidney disease, or unspecified chronic kidney disease**
(2) N18.4 **Chronic kidney disease, stage 4 (severe)**
(3) I50.42 **Chronic combined systolic (congestive) and diastolic (congestive) heart failure**

Figure 14-13 ■ Example of Assigning Codes for Hypertensive Heart Disease and Hypertensive Chronic Kidney Disease

patient Gordon Rothe, who was admitted to Branton Medical Center due to unstable angina.

Follow along in your ICD-10-CM manual as Tanisha assigns codes. Check off each step after you complete it.

▶ First, Tanisha confirms the information she abstracted from the medical record:

❑ Unstable angina

❑ ASHD with occlusion in grafted vein

❑ Lipid-rich plaque

❑ Anticoagulant use for 11 years

❑ Tobacco use

▶ Tanisha searches the Index for the Main Term **Angina**.

❑ She locates the subterm **unstable I20.0**.

▶ Tanisha verifies code **I20.0** in the Tabular List.

❑ She reads the code title for **I20.0, Unstable angina** and confirms that this accurately describes the medical record documentation.

▶ Tanisha checks for instructional notes in the Tabular List.

❑ Tamara cross-references the beginning of category **I20** and reads the **Excludes1** note that states **atherosclerosis of coronary artery bypass graft(s) and coronary artery of transplanted heart with angina pectoris (I25.7-)**.

❑ The note tells her that **I20.0** cannot be used with a code from **I25.7-** because **Excludes1** means the codes are mutually exclusive.

❑ She decides to research the rest of her codes before deciding whether she should include **I20.0**.

▶ Next, Tanisha searches the Index for the Main Term **Atherosclerosis** (■ FIGURE 14-14, page 224).

❑ She locates the instructional note to cross-reference the Main Term **Arteriosclerosis**.

❑ She follows the indented subterms for **coronary (artery), bypass graft, autologous vein, with, angina pectoris, unstable I25.710**.

❑ She identifies that she will have a combination code for ASHD and unstable angina.

SUCCESS STEP

Arteriosclerosis (*hardening of an artery*) is usually caused by atherosclerosis (*hardening of a vessel due to plaque*), so ICD-10-CM indexes both conditions to the Main Term **Arteriosclerosis**. When you remember this, you can go directly to **Arteriosclerosis** in the Index, then locate the needed subterm, rather than searching **Atherosclerosis** first.

▶ Tanisha verifies code **I25.710** in the Tabular List.

❑ She locates the code title **Atherosclerosis of autologous vein coronary artery bypass graft(s) with unstable angina pectoris** and confirms that all components of the code description are consistent with the documentation.

❑ She also refers to OGCR I.C.9.b, which states:

▪ ICD-10-CM has combination codes for atherosclerotic heart disease with angina pectoris. When using one of these combination codes it is not necessary to use an additional code for angina pectoris. A causal relationship can be assumed in a patient with both atherosclerosis and angina pectoris, unless the documentation indicates the angina is due to something other than the atherosclerosis.

❑ She determines that because this is a combination code, she should *not* also assign **I20.0, Unstable angina**.

▶ Tanisha cross-references the beginning of the subcategory **I25.7** and reads the instructional notes.

❑ She determines that the **Excludes1** notes do not apply because they refer to other forms of ASHD.

❑ She reads that note that states **Use additional code, if applicable, to identify coronary atherosclerosis due to lipid rich plaque (I25.83)**.

❑ She confirms that the medical record documents lipid-rich plaque.

❑ She verifies code **I25.83, Coronary atherosclerosis due to lipid rich plaque**.

❑ She reads the instructional note under code **I25.83** that states **Code first coronary atherosclerosis (I25.1-, I25.7-, I25.81-)**.

❑ The note confirms that **I25.710** should be sequenced first and **I25.83** should be sequenced as an additional code.

❑ Tanisha cross-references the beginning of category **I25** and reads the instructional notes.

❑ She notices the instruction that states **Use additional code to identify: tobacco use (Z72.0)**. She verifies that tobacco use is documented in the medical record and verifies the code in the tabular list.

❑ She locates the code **Z72.0 Tobacco use**.

❑ Next, Tanisha cross-references the instructional notes for code **I25.710**. She cross-references the beginning of the block **I20-I25** and reads the instructional note that applies to all codes in the block. She determines the note does not apply because it pertains to hypertension, which is not documented in the medical record.

❑ She cross-references the beginning of **Chapter 9 (I00-I99)** for instructional notes that apply to all codes in the chapter. She determines that there are no instructional notes.

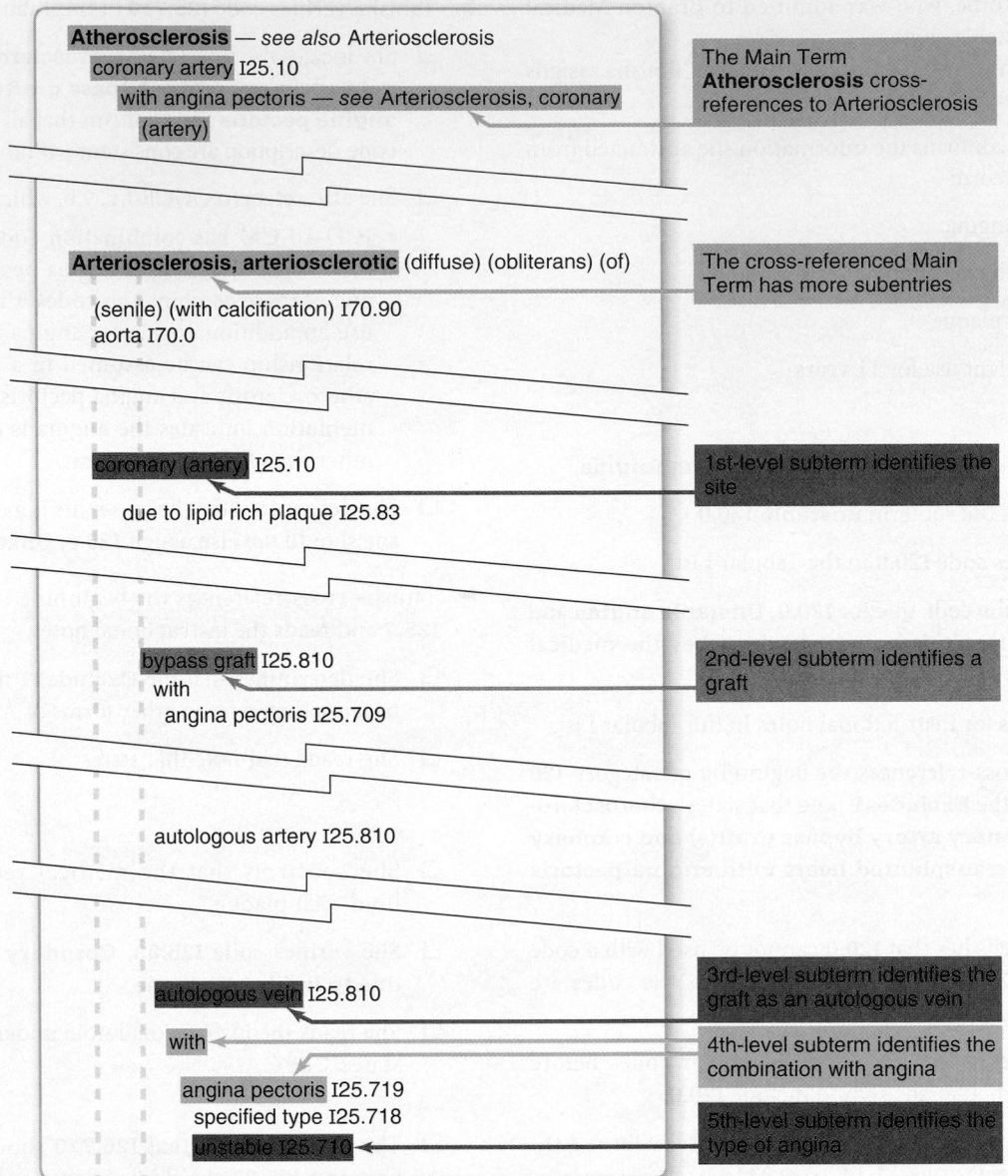

Figure 14-14 ■ Index Entry for Arteriosclerosis of a Grafted Autologous Vein with Unstable Angina

▶ Tanisha reviews the codes she has assigned so far:

❑ **I25.710 Atherosclerosis of autologous vein coronary artery bypass graft(s) with unstable angina pectoris**

❑ **I25.83 Coronary atherosclerosis due to lipid rich plaque**

❑ **Z72.0 Tobacco use**

▶ Tanisha cross-references the medical record to ensure she did not miss any details. She reads the documentation that states *patient has been on warfarin since a CABG of the left anterior descending coronary artery (LAD) 11 years ago.*

❑ She knows from experience that warfarin is an anticoagulant and that she should assign a code for it.

❑ She locates the Index Main Term **Long term drug use** with the subterm **anti-coagulant Z79.01**.

❑ She verifies **Z79.01** in the Tabular List and locates the title **Long term (current) use of anticoagulants**.

▶ Tanisha reviews the codes for this case:

❑ **I25.710 Atherosclerosis of autologous vein coronary artery bypass graft(s) with unstable angina pectoris**

❑ **I25.83 Coronary atherosclerosis due to lipid rich plaque**

❑ **Z72.0 Tobacco use**

❑ **Z79.01 Long term (current) use of anticoagulants**

▶ Next, Tanisha will review the sequencing of the codes.

CODING PRACTICE

Exercise 14.3   Assigning Codes for Circulatory System Conditions

Instructions: Read the mini-medical-record of each patient's encounter, review the information abstracted in Exercise 14.2 for questions 1 to 3. For questions 4 and 5, do the abstracting on your own. Assign ICD-10-CM diagnosis codes using the Index and Tabular List. Write the code(s) on the line provided.

1. INPATIENT HOSPITAL   Gender: F   Age: 42

Reason for admission: admitted from emergency department with subendocardial infarction

Assessment: nontransmural myocardial infarction

Plan: this is her first event so we will treat it with medication and diet

1 ICD-10-CM Code _____

2. OFFICE   Gender: F   Age: 68

Reason for encounter: Patient has been taking her BP at home and is concerned about readings that have been increasing over the past 3 months. She claims to be taking the diuretic and beta blocker as directed. Lab results show slightly low potassium.

Assessment: hypertensive cardiomegaly

Plan: Add spironolactone to the medication regime.

1 ICD-10-CM Code _____

3. INPATIENT HOSPITAL   Gender: M   Age: 68

Reason for admission: mitral porcine valvoplasty

Assessment: mitral valve regurgitation

Tip: Remember to follow the cross-references in the Index.

1 ICD-10-CM Code _____

4. EMERGENCY DEPT   Gender: M   Age: 53

Chief complaint: tachycardia

Assessment: ventricular flutter

Plan: CPR, external electric shock

Tip: You did not practice abstracting this case earlier, so see how you do on your own.

1 ICD-10-CM Code _____

5. OFFICE   Gender: F   Age: 38

Chief complaint: referred by primary care physician for pain in right leg due to varicose veins that have not improved with compression stockings

Assessment: varicose veins right calf

Plan: ultrasound to evaluate for thrombus or valve problems. Consider for sclerotherapy.

Tip: You did not practice abstracting this case earlier, so see how you do on your own.

1 ICD-10-CM Code _____

ARRANGING CODES FOR CIRCULATORY SYSTEM CONDITIONS

The circumstances of admission, OGCR, and instructional notes in the Tabular List always determine the selection of the principal or first-listed diagnosis and the sequencing of codes. In some cases sequencing is fairly straightforward and in other cases it can be challenging to sort through multiple sets of instructions. This holds true for patients who have AMI and especially for patients who have had multiple MIs. Refer to the following examples to better understand how to sequence codes for MI.

SUCCESS STEP

To locate MI in the Index, use the Main Term **Infarct** and the subterm **myocardium**.

Myocardial Infarction and Coronary Artery Disease

When a patient with CAD is admitted for an AMI, sequence codes as follows (OGCR I.C.9.b):

1. Sequence the AMI first.
2. Sequence the CAD as an additional code (■ FIGURE 14-15, page 226).

SUCCESS STEP

To locate CAD in the Index, search for the Main Term **Disease**, the first-level subterm **heart**, and the second-level subterm **ischemic**. As an alternative, you can also use the Main Term **Ischemia**.

Patient was admitted for inferior wall STEMI and also has atherosclerotic heart disease.

(1) **I21.19 ST elevation (STEMI) myocardial infarction involving other coronary artery of inferior wall**
(2) **I25.10 Atherosclerotic heart disease of native coronary artery without angina pectoris**

Figure 14-15 ■ Example of Sequencing AMI and ASHD

Acute and Subsequent Myocardial Infarction

ICD-10-CM classifies an MI as acute or current for four weeks after the event. Patients may have two or more MI events within the four-week timeframe. When this occurs, assign the first MI a code from category **I21.- ST elevation (STEMI) and non-ST elevation (NSTEMI) myocardial infarction** and assign the second event a code for a subsequent AMI from category **I22.- Subsequent ST elevation (STEMI) and non-ST elevation (NSTEMI) myocardial infarction**. Sequencing is determined by the AMI that is *chiefly responsible* for the encounter, as shown in the following examples (OGCR I.C.9.e). Refer to the examples that follow to better understand sequencing rules.

SUCCESS STEP

During the course of an admission, STEMI may evolve to NSTEMI and NSTEMI may evolve to STEMI. In both cases, assign the STEMI code (OGCR I.C.9.e.1)).

Sequencing in an Admission for AMI Followed by a Subsequent MI

When a patient is admitted for an AMI and has a second AMI during the stay, sequence the codes as follows:

1. Assign a code from category **I21.-** for the original AMI and sequence this condition first because it is the condition chiefly responsible for the admission and services provided.
2. Assign a code from category **I22.-** for subsequent AMI to the second event and sequence it second, as shown in ■ FIGURE 14-16.

SUCCESS STEP

Read the instructional notes at the beginning of categories **I21, I22,** and **I23** for definitions and sequencing guidance on MI.

Patient was admitted for STEMI of the anterolateral wall. Two days later, the patient had a separate NSTEMI.

(1) **I21.09 ST elevation (STEMI) myocardial infarction involving other coronary artery of anterior wall**
(2) **I22.2 Subsequent non-ST elevation (NSTEMI) myocardial infarction**

Figure 14-16 ■ Example of Sequencing in an Admission for AMI Followed by a Subsequent MI

Patient was admitted for a STEMI involving the inferior wall. Three weeks ago, the patient had a transmural MI to the inferoposterior wall.

(1) **I22.1 Subsequent ST elevation (STEMI) myocardial infarction of inferior wall**
(2) **I21.11 ST elevation (STEMI) myocardial infarction involving right coronary artery**

Figure 14-17 ■ Example of Sequencing in an Admission for a Subsequent AMI

Sequencing in an Admission for a Subsequent MI

When a nonhospitalized patient is admitted for a second AMI within four weeks of a previous AMI, assign and sequence codes as follows (■ FIGURE 14-17):

1. Assign a code from category **I22.-** for subsequent MI to the second event. Sequence the subsequent event as the principal diagnosis because it is the reason for the admission and services provided.
2. Assign a code from category **I21.-** for acute MI to the first event. Sequence this code second because it was not the reason for admission.

SUCCESS STEP

After four weeks, an MI is no longer considered acute and is defined as an old MI.

Sequencing a Current AMI and an Old MI

When more than four weeks elapse between MI events, the first MI is classified as an old or healed MI and only the new AMI is coded as acute. When a nonhospitalized patient is admitted for a second AMI that occurs more than four weeks after a previous AMI, assign and sequence codes as follows (■ FIGURE 14-18):

1. Assign a code for a current AMI from category **I21.-** for the new AMI. Sequence the new event as the principal diagnosis because it is the reason for the admission and services provided.
2. Assign the code **I25.2 Old myocardial infarction** to the first event. Sequence this condition as an additional code because it was not the reason for admission.

Guided Example of Arranging Codes for Circulatory System Conditions

To practice skills for sequencing codes for the circulatory system, continue with the example from earlier in the chapter

Patient was admitted for AMI involving the LAD coronary artery. Three months ago, the patient had a MI to the anterior wall.

(1) **I21.02 ST elevation (STEMI) myocardial infarction involving left anterior descending coronary artery**
(2) **I25.2 Old myocardial infarction**

Figure 14-18 ■ Example of Sequencing a Current AMI and an Old MI

about patient Gordon Rothe, who was admitted to Branton Medical Center due to unstable angina.

Follow along in your ICD-10-CM manual as Tanisha sequences the codes. Check off each step after you complete it.

▶ Tanisha reviews the codes she identified for this case:

❏ **I25.710 Atherosclerosis of autologous vein coronary artery bypass graft(s) with unstable angina pectoris**

❏ **I25.83 Coronary atherosclerosis due to lipid rich plaque**

❏ **Z72.0 Tobacco use**

❏ **Z79.01 Long term (current) use of anticoagulants**

▶ Tanisha determines the principal diagnosis.

❏ She reviews the medical record for the reason for admission, which is documented as unstable angina.

❏ She reviews the reason that balloon angioplasty was performed, which is documented as atherosclerosis of grafted vessel.

❏ She confirms that **I25.710, Atherosclerosis of autologous vein coronary artery bypass graft(s) with unstable angina pectoris** meets the definition of principal diagnosis, which is "that condition established after study to be chiefly responsible for occasioning the admission of the patient to the hospital for care" (OGCR II).

❏ She double-checks the instructional note under code **I25.710** in the Tabular List that directs her to use **I25.83, Coronary atherosclerosis due to lipid rich plaque** as

an *additional* code, meaning **I25.83** should *not* be the principal diagnosis.

❏ She double-checks the instructional note under code **I25.83** in the Tabular List that directs her to *Code first* a code from **I25.7-**, meaning that **I25.7.-** should be sequenced *before* **I25.83**.

❏ She also refers to OGCR I.C.9.b, which states:

▪ If a patient with coronary artery disease is admitted due to an acute myocardial infarction (AMI), the AMI should be sequenced before the coronary artery disease.

❏ She determines that the guideline does not affect the sequencing because the patient did not have an AMI.

❏ Therefore, she is confident that **I25.710** is the principal diagnosis and **I25.83** is sequenced second.

❏ She sequences **Z72.0, Tobacco use** third because it was specified in an instructional note.

❏ She sequences **Z79.01, Long term (current) use of anticoagulants** as the final code.

▶ Tanisha finalizes the codes and the sequencing for this case:

(1) **I25.710 Atherosclerosis of autologous vein coronary artery bypass graft(s) with unstable angina pectoris**

(2) **I25.83 Coronary atherosclerosis due to lipid rich plaque**

(3) **Z72.0 Tobacco use**

(4) **Z79.01 Long term (current) use of anticoagulants**

CODING PRACTICE

Exercise 14.4   Arranging Codes for Circulatory System Conditions

Instructions: Read the mini-medical-record of each patient's encounter, review the information abstracted in Exercise 14.2 for questions 1 to 3. For questions 4 and 5, do the abstracting on your own. Assign ICD-10-CM diagnosis codes using the Index and Tabular List, and sequence them correctly.

1. INPATIENT HOSPITAL   Gender: F   Age: 71

Reason for admission: Admitted from emergency department with angina. Patient has history of MI 2 years ago, as well as history of TIAs, although the TIAs did not leave any residual deficits

Assessment: STEMI involving 90% occlusion of the right coronary artery

Procedure: CABG

(continued)

1. (continued)

Tip: Assign a Z code for history of TIA.

3 ICD-10-CM Codes _____

_____

2. OFFICE   Gender: M   Age: 65

Chief complaint: increased edema and SOB since last visit

Assessment: HTN and decompensated CHF, A-fib

Plan: We will start by adjusting the diuretic, then evaluate the need for other adjustments based on response after 4 weeks. Continue long term warfarin and clopidrogel (an antiplatelet medication).

(continued)

CODING PRACTICE (continued)

2. (continued)

Tip: Remember to assign Z codes for the long-term use of the medications.

5 ICD-10-CM Codes _____

_____

3. INPATIENT HOSPITAL   Gender: M   Age: 57

Reason for admission: *transferred from another hospital where patient was admitted for cerebral infarct 20 hours ago and received tPA (tissue plasminogen activator), but now it is evident that a mechanical or surgical embolectomy is needed*

Assessment: *cerebral infarction d/t embolus in right middle cerebral artery, cerebral atherosclerosis, HTN, history of tobacco use*

Procedure: *surgical embolectomy*

Tip: Remember to read the instructional notes at the beginning of the category and the beginning of the block to identify what you need Z codes for.

5 ICD-10-CM Codes _____

_____

4. OFFICE   Gender: F   Age: 55

Reason for encounter: *management of CHF and A-fib*

Assessment: *A-fib, chronic diastolic CHF*

Plan: *Refer to wound clinic for a stage 1 venous stasis ulcer on left thigh*

Tip: You did not practice abstracting this case earlier, so see how you do on your own.

   Use your resources if you need assistance in defining any terms or conditions.

4 ICD-10-CM Codes _____

_____

5. INPATIENT HOSPITAL   Gender: M   Age: 45

Reason for admission: *Admitted from emergency department with angina, SOB, tachycardia, hemoptysis. Undergoing treatment for DVT*

Assessment: *pulmonary embolism, chronic DVT of left femoral vein*

Tip: You did not practice abstracting this case earlier, so see how you do on your own.

2 ICD-10-CM Codes _____

_____

CHAPTER SUMMARY

In this chapter you learned that:

- The function of the circulatory system, also called the cardiovascular (CV) system, is to distribute blood throughout the body.
- ICD-10-CM Chapter 9, Diseases of the Circulatory System (I00-I99), contains 11 blocks or subchapters that are divided by the type of disease.
- Coders need to pay close attention to detail when abstracting for the CV system because they assign codes that are very specific to anatomic sites, nature of the disease, and comorbidities.
- Diseases of the circulatory system frequently occur with multiple comorbidities from within the cardiovascular system and/or from

other systems; consequently, the choice of codes is dependent on the precise wording physicians use in the documentation.
- Sequencing of codes for multiples MIs depends on the circumstances of admission.
- ICD-10-CM provides Official Guidelines for Coding and Reporting (OGCR) for the circulatory system in OGCR section I.C.9 and provides detailed discussion regarding hypertension, atherosclerotic coronary artery disease and angina, cerebrovascular accident and disease, and acute myocardial infarction.

CONCEPT QUIZ

Take a moment to look back at the circulatory system and solidify your skills. Try to answer the questions from memory first, then refer back to the discussion in the chapter if you need a little extra help.

Completion

Instructions: Write the term that answers each question based on the information you learned in this chapter. Choose from the list below.

Some choices may be used more than once and some choices may not be used at all.

angioplasty	endarterectomy
arrhythmia	endocarditis
atherosclerosis	Holter monitor
bypass graft	ischemia
cardiac catheterization	months
cerebrovascular accident (CVA)	NSTEMI
congestive heart failure (CHF)	STEMI
days	stenosis
deep vein thrombosis (DVT)	weeks
electrocardiography	4
embolectomy	6
embolus	8

1. Another term for arteriosclerotic heart disease (ASHD) is _____.

2. The medical term for stroke is _____.

3. A thrombus that has broken loose from its point of origin and circulates through the bloodstream is a/an

   _____.

4. The inability of the heart to maintain circulation, often resulting in water retention and edema, is _____.

5. The formation of a thrombus within a deep vein, usually in the leg or pelvis, is _____.

6. Taking a vessel from another part of the body to create a new route around a blockage in a blood vessel is a/an

   _____.

7. A myocardial infarction is classified as current or acute for _____ weeks.

8. A myocardial infarction that completely occludes a vessel is called _____.

9. Removal of the diseased or damaged inner lining of an artery is a/an _____.

10. A portable EKG worn by the patient for an extended period of hours or days to measure heart activity in a variety of situations is a/an _____.

Multiple Choice

Instructions: Circle the letter of the best answer to each question based on the information you learned in this chapter.

1. Which of the following diagnostic statements states or implies a causal relationship?
   A. Chronic kidney disease and congestive heart failure
   B. Hypertensive heart disease
   C. Hypertension and heart disease
   D. STEMI and HTN

2. To locate acute myocardial infarction in the Index, you should search under the Main Term
   A. heart.
   B. acute.
   C. myocardial.
   D. infarction.

3. OGCR instructs coders to presume a causal relationship between hypertension and
   A. chronic kidney disease.
   B. acute myocardial infarction.
   C. congestive heart failure.
   D. chronic heart disease.

4. Assign a Z code for any of the following when they are present EXCEPT
   A. history of myocardial infarction.
   B. status post CABG.
   C. history of tobacco use.
   D. long-term use of anticoagulants.

5. To locate congestive heart failure in the Index, you should search under the Main Term
   A. congestive.
   B. heart.
   C. failure.
   D. myocardial.

6. Which of the following is NOT a key criterion for abstracting circulatory system disorders?
   A. Is the condition acquired or congenital?
   B. What is the patient's alcohol use?
   C. Has the patient had more than one AMI in the past four weeks?
   D. Which conditions are documented as being related to the CV condition?

7. When a patient has a second MI within four weeks of another MI, assign a code from category _____ to the FIRST MI.
   A. I21.- ST elevation (STEMI) and non-ST elevation (NSTEMI) myocardial infarction
   B. I22.- Subsequent ST elevation (STEMI) and non-ST elevation (NSTEMI) myocardial infarction
   C. I23 Certain current complications following ST elevation (STEMI) and non-ST elevation (NSTEMI) myocardial infarction
   D. I25.2 Old myocardial infarction

8. When a patient has a second MI within four weeks of another MI, assign a code from category _____ to the SECOND MI.
   A. I21.- ST elevation (STEMI) and non-ST elevation (NSTEMI) myocardial infarction
   B. I22.- Subsequent ST elevation (STEMI) and non-ST elevation (NSTEMI) myocardial infarction
   C. I23 Certain current complications following ST elevation (STEMI) and non-ST elevation (NSTEMI) myocardial infarction
   D. I25.2 Old myocardial infarction

9. _____ circulation carries blood from the aorta to the tissues of the heart.
   A. Coronary
   B. Endocardial
   C. Pulmonary
   D. Systemic

10. Mitral, tricuspid, aortic, and pulmonary are
    A. coronary arteries.
    B. chambers of the heart.
    C. valves of the heart.
    D. types of myocardial infarction.

(continued from page 231)

19. ST elevation myocardial infarction involving the anterior wall: ICD-10-CM Code(s) _____

20. Alcoholic cardiomyopathy with alcohol abuse: ICD-10-CM Code(s) _____

21. Myocardial infarction (STEMI) of left anterior descending coronary artery with old myocardial infarction involving left main coronary artery: ICD-10-CM Code(s) _____

22. Second-degree atrioventricular block, type I: ICD-10-CM Code(s) _____

23. Stuttering following a cerebral infarction, nontraumatic: ICD-10-CM Code(s) _____

24. Premature atrial beats: ICD-10-CM Code(s) _____

25. Chronic venous hypertension, both legs with inflammation: ICD-10-CM Code(s) _____

Diseases of the Blood and Blood-Forming Organs and Certain Disorders Involving the Immune Mechanism (D50-D89)

Chapter 15

Learning Objectives

After completing this chapter, you should have the skills to:

15.1 Spell and define the key words, medical terms, and abbreviations related to diseases of the blood and blood-forming organs.

15.2 Discuss the structure, function, and common conditions of the blood and blood-forming organs.

15.3 Identify the main characteristics of coding for diseases of the blood and blood-forming organs.

15.4 Abstract diagnostic information from the medical record for coding diseases of the blood and blood-forming organs.

15.5 Assign codes for diseases of the blood and blood-forming organs.

15.6 Arrange multiple diagnosis codes for diseases of the blood and blood-forming organs.

15.7 Code malignancies of the blood and blood-forming organs.

15.8 Discuss the Official Guidelines for Coding and Reporting related to diseases of the blood and blood-forming organs.

Chapter Outline

- **Blood Refresher**
- **Coding Overview of the Blood**
- **Abstracting for Conditions of the Blood**
- **Assigning Codes for Conditions of the Blood**
- **Arranging Codes for Conditions of the Blood**
- **Coding Malignancies of the Blood**

Key Terms and Abbreviations

anemia	formed element	leukocyte	thrombocyte
aplastic anemia	hemic system	nutritional anemia	vasoocclusive crisis
blood	hemoglobin (Hb)	plasma	white blood cell disorder
bone marrow	hemolytic anemia	relapse	
erythrocyte	hemostasis	remission	

In addition to the key terms listed here, students should know the terms defined within tables in this chapter.

For updates and corrections, visit our student resource site at

www.pearsonhighered.com/healthprofessionsresources

INTRODUCTION

You need to determine if your vehicle runs best on regular grade, premium, or super premium fuel because each has different components. The blood in the human body is comprised of several distinct components and, sometimes, they become out of balance and require medical attention.

A hematologist specializes in diagnosing and treating conditions of the blood and blood-forming organs. Hematologists may specialize in oncology and treat malignancies of the blood. Primary care physicians treat uncomplicated conditions of the blood and refer complex cases to a hematologist.

BLOOD REFRESHER

The function of the **blood**, also called the **hemic system**, is to transport and pass nutrients, oxygen, carbon dioxide, water, proteins, and hormones to cells and to transport waste products to excretory organs. Blood consists of **plasma** (*clear fluid*) and **formed elements**, or blood cells. There are three types of blood cells, which are created in the **bone marrow** (*connective tissue in the cavities of bones*): **erythrocytes** (*red blood cells, RBCs*), **leukocytes** (*white blood cells, WBCs*), and **thrombocytes** (*platelets*) (■ FIGURE 15-1). Blood cells are named based on their appearance and ability to accept **stain** during lab testing (■ FIGURE 15-2). **Hemoglobin** (Hb) is the oxygen-carrying component of erythrocytes. The spleen destroys old erythrocytes, filters microorganisms from the blood, and serves as a reservoir for blood.

SUCCESS STEP

The spleen functions as part of both the hemic and digestive systems.

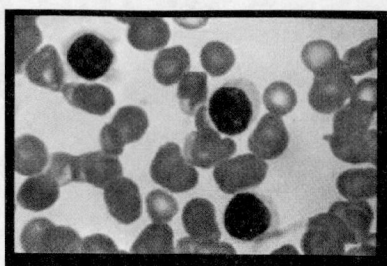

Figure 15-2 ■ Microscopic Image of a Stained Blood Cell. *Source:* © *National Institutes of Health.*

In Figure 15-1, each component of blood is labeled with its name, which is based on the medical terminology root. Refer to ■ TABLE 15-1 for a refresher on how to build medical terms related to the blood and lymphatic systems.

CODING CAUTION

Be alert for medical terms that are spelled similarly and have different meanings.

-emia (*blood condition*) and **-penia** (*lack of*)

hemostasis (*stoppage of bleeding*) and **homeostasis** (*the maintenance of a stable internal physical state*)

Conditions of the Blood

Diseases and disorders of the blood include anemias, hemostasis disorders, and white blood cell disorders. Coders use medical resources, such as a reference book on diseases, to understand conditions of the blood, diagnostic methods, and common treatments.

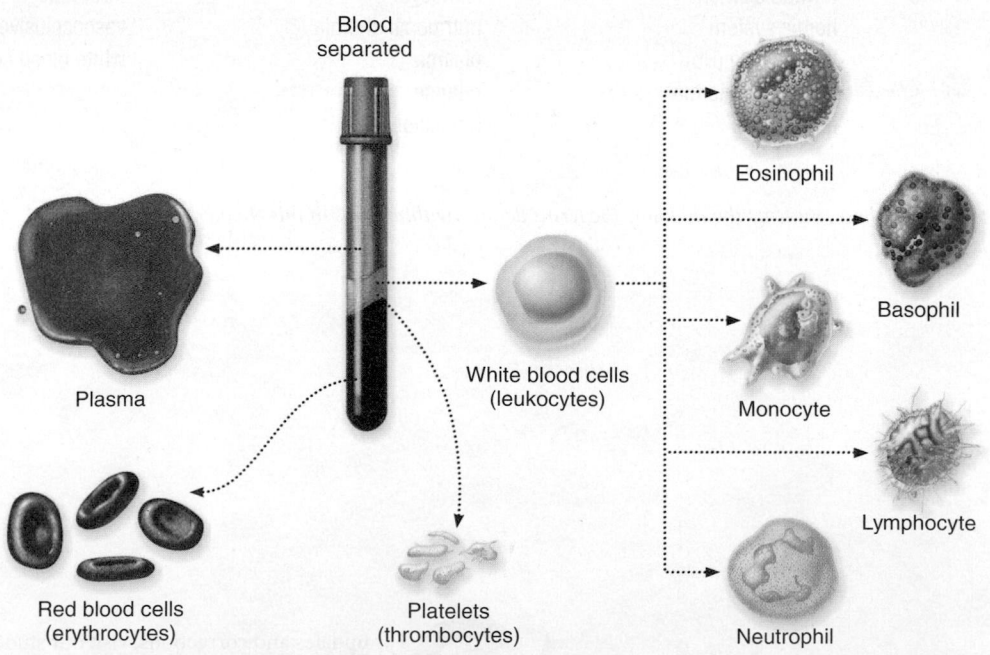

Figure 15-1 ■ Formed Elements of the Blood (Hemic System)

Table 15-1 ■ **EXAMPLE OF CONSTRUCTING MEDICAL TERMS FOR THE HEMIC SYSTEM**

Combining Form	Suffix	Complete Medical Term
hem/e, hemat/o (*blood*)		**hemato + poiesis** (*formation of blood*)
		an + emia (*lack of blood condition*)
erythr/o- (*red*)	**-emia** (*blood condition*)	**erythro + cyte** (*red blood cell*)
	-penia (*lack of*)	**erythro + cyto + penia** (*lack of red blood cells*)
	-cyte (*cell*)	**erythro + poiesis** (*formation of red blood cells*)
	-phil (*attraction*)	
leuk/o (*white*)	**-poiesis** (*formation*)	**leuko + cyte** (*white blood cell*)
		leuko + penia (*lack of white blood cells*)
		leuk + emia (*condition of white blood cells*)

Anemia is a blood disorder characterized by a reduction in the number of red blood cells, which results in less oxygen reaching the tissues. Although there are over 400 different types of anemia, they are classified into the following three groups, based on common etiology (*cause*):

- nutritional anemia—anemia due to malabsorption or poor dietary intake of iron, folate, and/or vitamin B_{12}

- hemolytic anemia—anemia due to excessive loss of erythrocytes

- aplastic anemia—anemia due to loss of red bone marrow

Anemia can result as a complication of other diseases and treatments, including chronic kidney disease (CKD), malignant neoplasms, and antineoplastic therapy such as chemotherapy, radiotherapy, and immunotherapy.

Hemostasis disorders include a range of medical problems that lead to poor clotting and continuous bleeding. Causes include platelet dysfunction, vitamin K deficiency, and clotting factor deficiencies.

White blood cell disorders diminish the body's immune response and increase the risk of infection.

Common blood conditions are summarized in ■ TABLE 15-2. Physicians diagnose blood disorders using blood tests,

Table 15-2 ■ **COMMON BLOOD CONDITIONS**

Condition	Description
Folic acid deficiency anemia	Anemia due to a lack of **folic acid**
Hemophilia	A genetic disorder in which blood takes too long to clot
Hypogammaglobulinemia	A deficiency of gamma globulins (protein fraction) and antibodies in the blood
Iron deficiency anemia	Anemia due to insufficient iron to manufacture hemoglobin
Neutropenia	A decrease in neutrophils
Pancytopenia	An abnormal reduction in the number of all (medical prefix *pan-*) types of blood cells: red, white, and platelets
Pernicious anemia	Anemia due to insufficient absorption of vitamin B_{12}, which is necessary for erythrocyte production
Polycythemia	An abnormal increase in the number of circulating red blood cells
Purpura	Small hemorrhages in the skin
Sarcoidosis	Formation of nodules in the lymph nodes, lungs, bone, and skin
Sickle cell anemia	A genetic disorder in which red blood cells take on a sickle (curved) shape and lead to hemolytic anemia; also called sickle cell disease (SCD)
Thalessemia	A genetic disorder that results in defective formation of hemoglobin
Thrombophilia	A tendency to create blood clots (thrombi)
Von Willebrand disease	A genetic disorder marked by bleeding of the mucosa

microscopic examination of blood cells, and bone marrow biopsy. Treatments include correction of nutritional deficiencies and other lifestyle changes, medication to correct the symptom or underlying problem, and transfusion of whole blood or a particular component of the blood.

Remember to keep standard reference books handy to learn more about conditions affecting the blood and blood-forming organs.

CODING PRACTICE

Exercise 15.1   Refresher on the Blood

Instructions: Use your medical terminology skills and resources to define the following conditions related to the blood and blood-forming organs, then assign the diagnosis code. Follow these steps:

- Use slash marks "/" to break down each term into its root(s) and suffix.

- Define the meaning of the word based on the meaning of each word part.
- Assign the default ICD-10-CM diagnosis code for the condition using the Index and Tabular List.

Example: leukemia leuk/emia   Meaning: *disorder of white blood cells*   ICD-10-CM Code: *C95.90*

1. hemophilia   Meaning _____   ICD-10-CM Code _____
2. neutropenia   Meaning _____   ICD-10-CM Code _____
3. thrombocytopenia   Meaning _____   ICD-10-CM Code _____
4. leukocytosis   Meaning _____   ICD-10-CM Code _____
5. eosinophilia   Meaning _____   ICD-10-CM Code _____
6. hemoglobinemia   Meaning _____   ICD-10-CM Code _____
7. panhematopenia   Meaning _____   ICD-10-CM Code _____
8. hemolymphangioma   Meaning _____   ICD-10-CM Code _____
9. erythroblastophthisis   Meaning _____   ICD-10-CM Code _____
10. leukoerythroblastosis Meaning _____   ICD-10-CM Code _____

CODING OVERVIEW OF THE BLOOD

ICD-10-CM Chapter 3, Diseases of the Blood and Blood-Forming Organs and Certain Disorders Involving the Immune Mechanism (D50-D89), contains seven blocks or subchapters that are divided by type of condition. This chapter begins at D50, in the middle, rather than at the beginning, of a letter division. Review the block names and code ranges listed at the beginning of Chapter 3 in the ICD-10-CM manual to become familiar with the content and organization.

ICD-10-CM Chapter 3 is comparable to ICD-9-CM Chapter 4 (280-289) but also includes codes that were in ICD-9-CM Chapter 3, Endocrine, Nutritional and Metabolic Disorders, as well as some codes from ICD-9-CM Chapter 1, Infectious and Parasitic Diseases.

Many categories have been expanded to increase specificity. For example, ICD-9-CM had one code for thalassemia, whereas ICD-10-CM has seven codes for specific types of thalassemia.

This ICD-10-CM chapter includes anemia due to nutritional deficiencies, hemolytic anemia, aplastic anemia, coagulation disorders, and disorders of blood-forming organs. It does not include infectious diseases, most diseases of the lymphatic system, or disorders of the circulatory system, all of which are classified in other ICD-10-CM chapters.

ICD-10-CM does not provide Official Guidelines for Coding and Reporting (OGCR) for this chapter. OGCR I.C.2.c.1) and 2) in the ICD-10-CM Chapter 2, Neoplasms, discuss the coding of anemia associated with malignancy, chemotherapy, radiotherapy, and immunotherapy. The Tabular List contains frequent instructional notes to use an additional code for associated conditions and to code first underlying diseases.

ABSTRACTING FOR THE BLOOD

Many of the conditions in this ICD-10-CM chapter can have multiple underlying causes and multiple manifestations. Therefore, coders should thoroughly abstract the symptoms, manifestations, and underlying causes documented in the medical record.

Some of these situations use combination codes, some require multiple coding, and others do not need to be coded because they are integral to the condition. For example, approximately 75 ICD-10-CM codes classify the different types

Table 15-3 ■ KEY CRITERIA FOR ABSTRACTING CONDITIONS OF THE BLOOD

- ❏ What is the condition?
- ❏ What part of the hemic system does the condition involve?
- ❏ Does the condition have an underlying cause?
- ❏ Is the condition acquired or congenital?
- ❏ If anemia exists, is it due to a neoplasm or chronic disease?
- ❏ If sickle cell disease exists, what is the specific type?
- ❏ If sickle cell disease exists, is the patient in crisis?
- ❏ If sickle cell disease exists, does the patient have a fever?
- ❏ What symptoms are integral to the condition?
- ❏ What manifestations require an additional code?
- ❏ Is the condition drug induced?

of anemia. Closely related anemias are classified to the same code. Refer to ■ Table 15-3 for guidance on how to abstract conditions of the blood and blood-forming organs, then work through the detailed example that follows. Remember that the abstracting questions are a guide and that not every question applies to, or can be answered for, every case.

Guided Example of Abstracting for Conditions of the Blood

Refer to the following example throughout this chapter to learn skills for abstracting, assigning, and sequencing codes for disorders of the blood and blood-forming organs. Scott Hood, CPC, is a fictitious coder who guides you through the coding process.

> Date: 05/11/yy   Location: Branton Medical Center Emergency Department   Provider: Robyn Akin, MD
>
> Patient: Douglas Ketron   Gender: M   Age: 10 months
>
> Reason for encounter: fever, cough, SOB, bilateral dactylitis (*painful and swollen hands and/or feet*)
>
> Assessment: vasoocclusive crisis and acute chest syndrome due to HbSS sickle cell disease (SCD)
>
> Plan: administer oxygen and IV antibiotics, then admit as inpatient

Follow along as Scott Hood, CPC, abstracts the diagnosis. Check off each step after you complete it.

▶ Scott reads through the entire record, paying special attention to the reason for the encounter and the final assessment. Scott reviews all the medical terms in the documentation to be sure he understands the case.

    ❏ He knows from his experience at East Side Hematology that vasoocclusive crisis is a form of **sickle cell crisis** in

which the patient experiences severe pain due to infarctions and that the pain may occur in nearly any location (■ Figure 15-3, page 238).

    ❏ He is also aware that acute chest syndrome (ACS) is a group of symptoms, often due to a bacterial infection or lung infarction, seen in patients with SCD and can bring on a vasoocclusive crisis.

    ❏ He notes the presenting symptoms of *fever, cough, SOB, and bilateral dactylitis*

▶ Scott refers to the Key Criteria for Abstracting Conditions of the Blood (Table 15-3).

    ❏ *What is the condition?* vasoocclusive crisis and acute chest syndrome

    ❏ *What part of the hemic system does the condition involve?* circulation

    ❏ *Does the condition have an underlying cause?* sickle cell disease

    ❏ *Is the condition acquired or congenital?* Sickle cell is congenital.

    ❏ *If anemia exists, is it due to a neoplasm or chronic disease?* Not applicable.

    ❏ *If sickle cell disease exists, what is the specific type?* HbSS

    ❏ *If sickle cell disease exists, is the patient in crisis?* Yes, vasoocclusive crisis.

    ❏ *If sickle cell disease exists, does the patient have a fever?* Yes.

    ❏ *What symptoms are integral to the condition?* fever, cough, SOB are symptoms of ACS. Dactylitis is a manifestation of SCD.

    ❏ *What manifestations require an additional code?* fever

    ❏ *Is the condition drug induced?* No.

SUCCESS STEP

At the time of initial abstracting, it may not be clear that a separate code for fever is required, but it will become clear later when assigning codes in the Tabular List. That is the reason the abstracting questions specifically ask about fever with sickle cell crisis.

▶ Scott double-checks the medical record to be certain that he has identified all of the symptoms, conditions, and manifestations.

▶ At this point, Scott has abstracted the information he needs, but he is still unsure of how many codes he will need for this case. He knows that he will need to research the Index and Tabular List to learn what combination codes are available for this case.

Hemoglobin S and Red Blood Cell Sickling

Sickle cell anemia is caused by an inherited autosomal recessive defect in Hb synthesis. Sickle cell hemoglobin (HbS) differs from normal hemoglobin only in the substitution of the amino acid valine for glutamine in both beta chains of the hemoglobin molecule.

When HbS is oxygenated, it has the same globular shape as normal hemoglobin. However, when HbS loses its oxygen, it becomes insoluble in intracellular fluid and crystallizes into rodlike structures. Clusters of rods form polymers (long chains) that bend the erythrocyte into the characteristic crescent shape of the sickle cell.

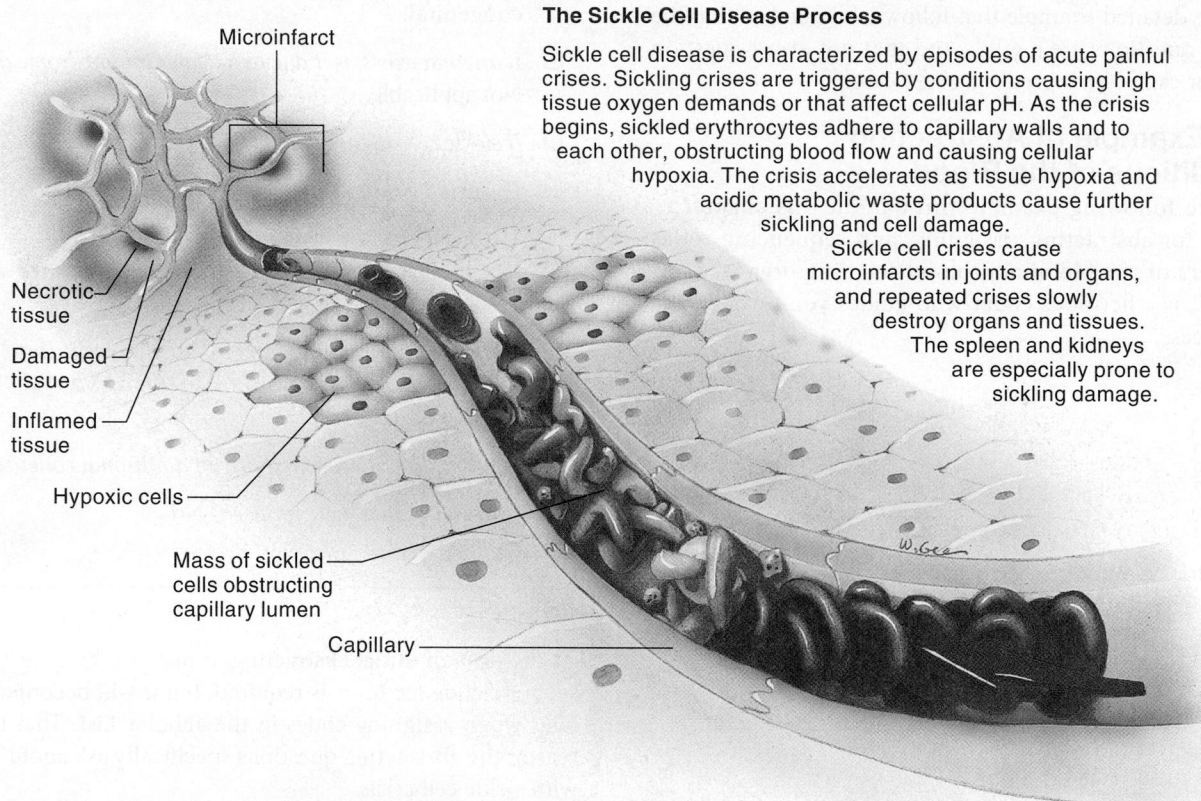

Incorrect amino acids

β chains

Hemoglobin S molecule

α chains

Polymerized deoxyhemoglobin S

Oxyhemoglobin S

Oxygenated erythrocyte

O₂

Deoxyhemoglobin S

Deoxygenated erythrocyte

Sickled erythrocyte

The Sickle Cell Disease Process

Sickle cell disease is characterized by episodes of acute painful crises. Sickling crises are triggered by conditions causing high tissue oxygen demands or that affect cellular pH. As the crisis begins, sickled erythrocytes adhere to capillary walls and to each other, obstructing blood flow and causing cellular hypoxia. The crisis accelerates as tissue hypoxia and acidic metabolic waste products cause further sickling and cell damage.

Sickle cell crises cause microinfarcts in joints and organs, and repeated crises slowly destroy organs and tissues. The spleen and kidneys are especially prone to sickling damage.

Microinfarct

Necrotic tissue

Damaged tissue

Inflamed tissue

Hypoxic cells

Mass of sickled cells obstructing capillary lumen

Capillary

Figure 15-3 ■ How Sickle Cell Disease Affects the Patient. *Source: Pearson Education/PH College.*

CODING PRACTICE

Exercise 15.2   **Abstracting for Conditions of the Blood**

Instructions: Read the mini-medical-record of each patient's encounter and answer the abstracting questions. Write the answer on the line provided. Do not assign any codes.

1. OFFICE   Gender: M   Age: 81

Chief complaint: referred by family physician for reduction in lymphocyte count which appeared on lab results from annual physical

Assessment: lymphocytopenia

Plan: further testing to determine underlying cause

a. What is the reason for referral? _____

_____

b. What is the diagnosis? _____

_____

c. Should you code the abnormal lab results?
_____ Why or why not? _____

_____

2. OFFICE   Gender: F   Age: 35

Reason for encounter: numbness in extremities, nausea and vomiting

Assessment: pernicious anemia

Plan: vitamin B-12 injections, refer to hematologist

a. What are the symptoms and signs? _____

_____

b. What is the diagnosis? _____

_____

c. Are the symptoms and signs integral to the diagnosis? _____

_____

d. Should you code for the symptoms? _____

3. OFFICE   Gender: M   Age: 52

Reason for encounter: referred by family physician for pain and swelling in LUQ

Assessment: splenomegaly due to splenitis

Plan: schedule splenectomy ASAP

(continued)

3. (continued)

a. What are the symptoms? _____

_____

b. What is splenomegaly? _____

_____

c. What is splenitis? _____

_____

d. What is a splenectomy? _____

_____

e. Where is the spleen located? _____

_____

f. What condition should you code for? _____

_____

4. INPATIENT HOSPITAL   Gender: F   Age: 59

Reason for admission: weakness, fatigue, confusion

Assessment: anemia due to chemotherapy for metastatic colon cancer

a. What are the symptoms? _____

_____

b. Are the symptoms integral to anemia? _____

_____

c. What is the cause of the anemia? _____

_____

d. What is the primary cancer site? _____

_____

e. What is metastatic cancer? _____

_____

f. What condition should be sequenced first?

_____

g. What condition should be sequenced second?

_____

h. What condition should be sequenced third?

_____

i. What adverse effect has occurred? _____

_____

(continued)

CODING PRACTICE (continued)

5. INPATIENT HOSPITAL Gender: M Age: 61

Reason for admission: tachycardia, headaches, fatigue

Assessment: anemia due to stage 3 chronic kidney disease

Plan: erythropoiesis stimulating agents (ESAs), supplemental iron

a. What are the symptoms? _____

_____

b. What is the diagnosis? _____

_____

c. Are the symptoms integral to the diagnosis?

_____

d. What is the underlying condition? _____

_____

e. Which condition is the principal diagnosis?

_____

f. What is the additional diagnosis? _____

_____

6. INPATIENT HOSPITAL Gender: F Age: 50

Reason for encounter: follow up on glucose tolerance test (GTT) and complete chemistry analysis

Assessment: hyperglycemia due to pre-diabetes, lab results also indicate iron (Fe)-deficiency anemia

Plan: manage pre-diabetes with 1,500 calorie diabetic diet, Rx Fe supplements

a. What is hyperglycemia? _____

_____

b. Should both hyperglylcemia and prediabetes be coded? _____

Why or why not? _____

_____

c. Should anemia be coded? _____

Why or why not? _____

d. What type of anemia is present? _____

_____

e. What should be the first-listed diagnosis?

_____

f. What is the additional diagnosis? _____

_____

ASSIGNING CODES FOR CONDITIONS OF THE BLOOD

When an ICD-10-CM chapter does not have any OGCR, as is the case with diseases of the blood and blood-forming organs, coders apply the general OGCR (I.A, I.B, II, and III) and follow instructional notes in the Tabular List. When coders thoroughly abstract information, they are poised to assign codes correctly.

Most types of anemia are indexed under the Main Term **Anemia**, followed by subterms that identify the specific type. Because the Index contains over 350 subterms for **Anemia**, remember to search them carefully to locate the most specific code. Refer to ■ FIGURE 15-4 for a sample Index entry showing how to locate aplastic anemia due to drugs.

SUCCESS STEP

Anemia of newborns and anemia related to pregnancy are not classified in this chapter. ICD-10-CM has separate chapters for conditions of the newborn and pregnancy-related conditions. To locate the codes for anemia of the newborn, search the Main Term **Anemia** and subterm **newborn**. To locate codes for anemia in pregnancy, search the Main Term, **Pregnancy** and subterm **complicated by anemia**.

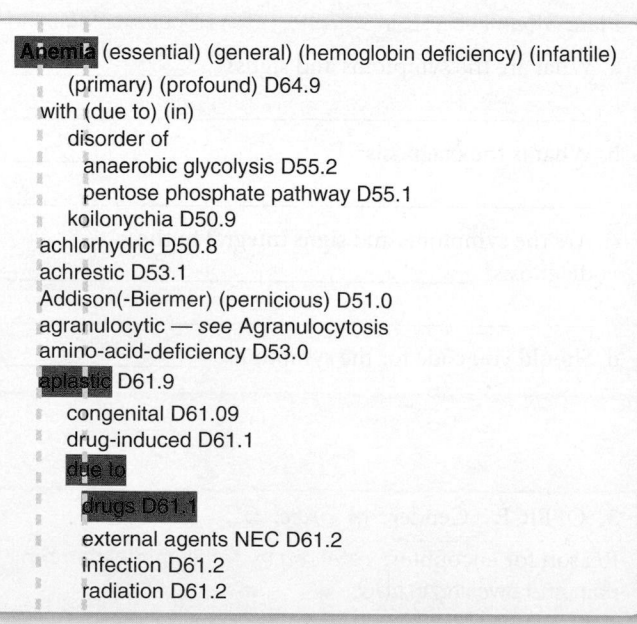

Anemia (essential) (general) (hemoglobin deficiency) (infantile) (primary) (profound) D64.9
  with (due to) (in)
    disorder of
      anaerobic glycolysis D55.2
      pentose phosphate pathway D55.1
    koilonychia D50.9
  achlorhydric D50.8
  achrestic D53.1
  Addison(-Biermer) (pernicious) D51.0
  agranulocytic — see Agranulocytosis
  amino-acid-deficiency D53.0
  aplastic D61.9
    congenital D61.09
    drug-induced D61.1
    due to
      drugs D61.1
      external agents NEC D61.2
      infection D61.2
      radiation D61.2

Figure 15-4 ■ Index Entry for Aplastic Anemia Due to Drugs

Table 15-4 ■ ANEMIA CODES FOR CANCER PATIENTS

Cause of Anemia	Code Assignment
Anemia due to the cancer itself	D63.0 Anemia in neoplastic disease
Aplastic anemia due to chemotherapy	D61.1 Drug-induced aplastic anemia
Other anemia due to chemotherapy	D64.81 Anemia due to antineoplastic chemotherapy

Anemia is often associated with cancer and may be caused by the disease itself or by adjunct therapy such as chemotherapy, radiotherapy, or immunotherapy. Review the documentation carefully to clearly identify the cause. Chemotherapy may cause anemia or aplastic anemia, which is a result of bone marrow not producing erythrocytes, and each has separate codes (■ TABLE 15-4). Information about multiple coding for anemia in cancer patients is discussed later in this chapter.

Anemia may be caused by other drugs, in addition to chemotherapy. Drugs such as nonsteriodal anti-inflammatory drugs (NSAIDs) can cause bleeding, which in turn causes anemia. Drugs that suppress the immune system can cause anemia because the hematopoietic function of the bone marrow is suppressed. Other drugs, such as certain antibiotics, **antihypertensives**, and **antiarrythmics**, can occasionally destroy erythrocytes prematurely, causing hemolytic anemia. When anemia is drug-induced, the Tabular List instructs coders to assign an external cause code for the substance. Use the Table of Drugs and Chemicals to locate the substance and intent.

Anemia may also be caused by CKD, in which case an additional code to identify the stage of kidney disease is required.

> ### SUCCESS STEP
> Refer to OGCR I.C.19.e to review the definitions of each intent column in the Table of Drugs and Poisonings.

Guided Example of Assigning Codes for Conditions of the Blood

To practice skills for assigning codes for disorders of the blood and blood-forming organs, continue with the example from earlier in the chapter about patient Douglas Ketron, age 10 months, who was seen in Branton Medical Center Emergency Department with HbSS sickle cell disease, vasoocclusive crisis, and acute chest syndrome.

Follow along in your ICD-10-CM manual as Scott Hood, CPC, assigns codes. Check off each step after you complete it.

▶ First, Scott confirms the diagnosis in the medical record: HbSS sickle cell with vasoocclusive crisis and acute chest syndrome; and the symptoms and manifestations: fever, cough, SOB, and bilateral dactylitis.

❑ He does not know how many codes he will need, so he begins by coding the main condition, HbSS sickle cell disease.

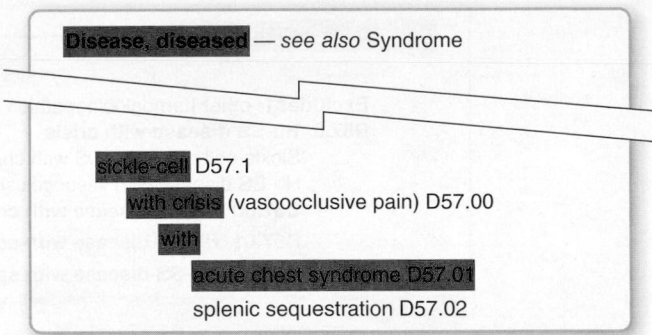

Figure 15-5 ■ Index Entry Showing a Combination Code for Sickle Cell Disease with Crisis and Acute Chest Syndrome

▶ Scott searches the Index for the Main Term **Disease**.

❑ He locates the subterm **sickle-cell** (■ FIGURE 15-5).

❑ He reviews the second-level subterms and notices that there are subterms for several types of SCD, but not HbSS.

❑ He determines that he will need to use either the default entry under **sickle-cell** or the entry for **specified NEC**, but he will not know for sure until he gets to the Tabular List.

❑ Scott reviews the subterms under **sickle-cell** and locates a third-level subterm **with crisis (vasoocclusive pain)**.

❑ He locates an additional fourth-level subterm **with** that provides a combination code for **acute chest syndrome D57.01**.

▶ Scott verifies code **D57.01** in the Tabular List.

❑ He verifies the code title **D57.01, Hb-SS disease with acute chest syndrome**, and confirms that this accurately describes the diagnosis.

❑ He notes that the Tabular List specifies the **D57.0-** category includes HbSS, so he is in the right place and does not need to locate the code for **Other specified sickle cell, NEC** that he had considered in the Index.

❑ He also verifies that this is a combination code for SCD, vasoocclusive crisis, and acute chest syndrome, so he does not need to assign additional codes for vasoocclusive crisis or ACS.

▶ Scott checks for instructional notes in the Tabular List.

❑ He cross-references the beginning of category **D57** and reads the instructional note that states **Use additional code for any associated fever (R50.81)** (■ FIGURE 15-6, page 242).

❑ Before looking up the code for fever, Scott completes the verification of **D57.01**. He cross-references the beginning of the block **Hemolytic anemias (D55-D59)** and verifies that there are no instructional notes.

❑ He then cross-references the beginning of **Chapter 3 (D50-D89)** and verifies that there are no instructional notes.

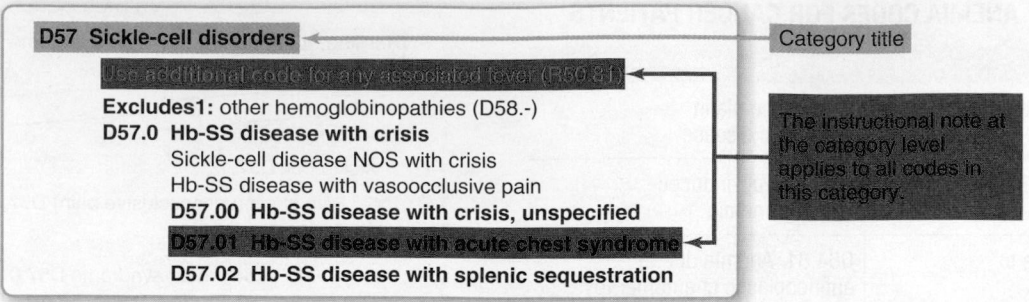

Figure 15-6 ■ Instructional Note at the Category Level in the Tabular List to Use Additional Code

▶ Now Scott verifies the code for fever contained in the first instructional note, **R50.81**.

❑ He verifies the code title **R50.81, Fever presenting with conditions classified elsewhere**, and confirms that this accurately describes the fever.

❑ He recognizes that the code is from ICD-10-CM Chapter 18, Symptoms, Signs and Abnormal Clinical and Laboratory Findings, Not Elsewhere Classified (R00-R99). He normally would hesitate to assign a code for a sign with a confirmed diagnosis that includes the three main conditions. However, because the instructional note directs him to assign a code for fever, if present, he knows he should assign it. He knows that fever is a sign of infection and that infection is a life-threatening event for a patient with SCD.

▶ Scott is unsure whether he needs to assign a code for bilateral dactylitis, so he researches this condition in the Index and Tabular List.

❑ He locates the Index Main Term **Dactylitis**.

❑ The subterms **sickle cell** then **HbSS** lead him to **D57.00**.

❑ He instantly recognizes that **D57.00** is from the same category as his previous code, **D57.01**.

❑ He verifies **D57.00** in the Tabular List and reads the code title **Hb-SS disease with crisis, unspecified**.

❑ This confirms his thinking that dactylitis is a manifestation of SCD crisis. Because he has already identified **D57.01**, which is a *more specific code* for SCD crisis, he does not also assign **D57.00**. **D57.00** is a code with unspecified manifestations, so it adds no further information (OGCR I.A.9.b).

▶ Scott reviews the codes he has assigned for this case:

❑ **R50.81 Fever presenting with conditions classified elsewhere**

❑ **D57.01 Hb-SS disease with acute chest syndrome**

▶ Next, Scott needs to confirm the sequencing.

CODING PRACTICE

Exercise 15.3 Assigning Codes for Conditions of the Blood

Instructions: Read the mini-medical-record of each patient's encounter, review the information abstracted in Exercise 15.2, and assign ICD-10-CM diagnosis codes using the Index and Tabular List. Write the code(s) on the line provided.

1. OFFICE   Gender: M   **Age:** 81

Chief complaint: *referred by family physician for reduction in lymphocyte count which appeared on lab results from annual physical*

Assessment: *lymphocytopenia*

Plan: *further testing to determine underlying cause*

Tip: The name of the condition is the Main Term.

1 ICD-10-CM Code _____

2. OFFICE   Gender: F   **Age:** 35

Reason for encounter: *numbness in extremities, nausea and vomiting*

Assessment: *pernicious anemia*

Plan: *vitamin B-12 injections, refer to hematologist*

Tip: Look for the Main Term anemia, then look for the subterm that identifies the type of anemia.

1 ICD-10-CM Code _____

3. OFFICE   Gender: M   **Age:** 52

Reason for encounter: *referred by family physician for pain and swelling in LUQ*

Assessment: *splenomegaly due to splenitis*

Plan: *schedule splenectomy ASAP*

1 ICD-10-CM Code _____

ARRANGING CODES FOR CONDITIONS OF THE BLOOD

Sequencing of codes in this ICD-10-CM chapter is based on the circumstances of admission and the instructional notes in the Tabular List. When anemia is due to an underlying condition, the Tabular List instructs coders to code the underlying condition first. When anemia has certain manifestations, the Tabular List instructs coders to assign an additional code for the manifestation. OGCR for the neoplasm chapter provides additional guidance for sequencing anemia codes for cancer patients.

Admission for Anemia Due to Neoplastic Disease

Patients with a malignancy and anemia may be admitted to treat the neoplasm or to treat the anemia. Assign and sequence codes in the same way for both situations. Assign and sequence codes as follows (OGCR I.C.2.c.1)):

1. Assign a code for the neoplasm.
2. Assign code **D63.0 Anemia in neoplastic disease** for the anemia.

Depending on the conventions used by a particular publisher, the Tabular List entry for **D63.0 Anemia in neoplastic disease** may be highlighted or appear in an italic typeface, indicating that it is a manifestation code and should not be sequenced as the first-listed or principal diagnosis (OGCR I.A.13) (■ FIGURE 15-7).

> ## CODING CAUTION
>
> Sequencing guidelines for anemia in neoplastic disease are different in ICD-10-CM than in ICD-9-CM. In ICD-10-CM, always sequence the anemia *after* the neoplasm code, even when the reason for the encounter is treatment of the anemia.

Admission for Anemia Due to Chemotherapy or Immunotherapy

When the admission or encounter is for management of an anemia associated with an adverse effect of chemotherapy or immunotherapy and the *only* treatment is for the anemia, assign and sequence codes as follows (OGCR I.C.2.c.2)):

1. Assign a code for the anemia.
2. Assign a code for the neoplasm.
3. Assign a code for the adverse effect from the Table of Drugs and Chemicals.

> ## SUCCESS STEP
>
> Although code **D64.81 Anemia due to antineoplastic chemotherapy** may seem to be a combination code that includes the external cause, it is not. You must assign an external cause code (**T45.1X5-**) from the Table of Drugs and Chemicals when using this code (OGCR I.C.2.c.2)).

Admission for Anemia Due to Radiotherapy

When the admission or encounter is for management of an anemia associated with an adverse effect of radiotherapy, assign and sequence codes as follows (OGCR I.C.2.c.2)):

1. Assign a code for the anemia.
2. Assign a code for the neoplasm.
3. Assign an external cause code for the complication, **Y84.2 Radiological procedure and radiotherapy as the cause of abnormal reaction of the patient, or of later complication, without mention of misadventure at the time of the procedure.**

> ## CODING CAUTION
>
> Notice that when the admission or encounter is for management of an anemia associated with an adverse effect of radiotherapy, anemia is sequenced first. This sequencing is different than when anemia is due to the neoplasm itself.

Admission for Adjunct Therapy

When the admission or encounter is for the purpose of administering adjunct therapy and the patient develops anemia *during* the encounter, assign and sequence codes as follows (OGCR I.C.2.e.3)):

1. First, assign the appropriate **Z** code for the therapy encounter:
   a. **Z51.11 Encounter for antineoplastic chemotherapy**
   b. **Z51.12 Encounter for antineoplastic immunotherapy**
   c. **Z51.0 Antineoplastic radiation therapy**
2. Assign a second code from the Table of Drugs and Chemicals for the adverse effect when the encounter is for chemotherapy or immunotherapy.
3. Assign a code for the anemia (See Table 15-4).
4. Assign a code for the neoplasm.
5. If the encounter was for radiotherapy, assign code **Y84.2.**

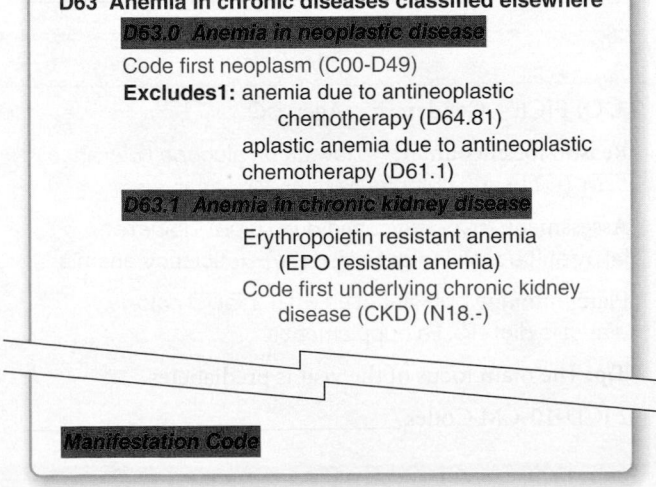

D63 Anemia in chronic diseases classified elsewhere
  D63.0 Anemia in neoplastic disease
  Code first neoplasm (C00-D49)
  Excludes1: anemia due to antineoplastic
        chemotherapy (D64.81)
      aplastic anemia due to antineoplastic
        chemotherapy (D61.1)
  D63.1 Anemia in chronic kidney disease
      Erythropoietin resistant anemia
        (EPO resistant anemia)
      Code first underlying chronic kidney
        disease (CKD) (N18.-)

Manifestation Code

Figure 15-7 ■ Tabular List Convention for a Manifestation Code

Guided Example of Arranging Codes for Conditions of the Blood

To practice skills for sequencing codes for disorders of the blood and blood-forming organs, continue with the example from earlier in the chapter about patient Douglas Ketron, age 10 months, who was seen in Branton Medical Center Emergency Department with HbSS sickle cell disease, vasoocclusive crisis, and acute chest syndrome.

Follow along in your ICD-10-CM manual as Scott Hood, CPC, sequences the codes. Check off each step after you complete it.

▶ First, Scott confirms the diagnosis codes he believes should be assigned:

❑ **R50.81 Fever presenting with conditions classified elsewhere**

❑ **D57.01 Hb-SS disease with acute chest syndrome**

▶ Scott needs to cross-reference back to the Tabular List to read the sequencing instructions.

❑ Scott reads the instructional note that appears in the Tabular List under code **R50.81**. The note states **Code first underlying condition when associated fever is present, such as with: sickle cell disease (D57.-)** (■ FIGURE 15-8).

▪ This instruction tells him that SCD should be sequenced first.

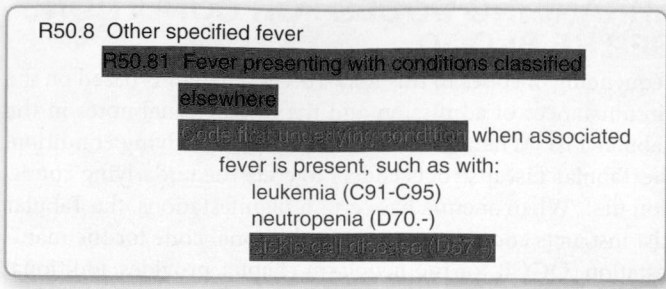

R50.8 Other specified fever

R50.81 Fever presenting with conditions classified elsewhere

Code first underlying condition when associated fever is present, such as with:
leukemia (C91-C95)
neutropenia (D70.-)
sickle cell disease (D57)

Figure 15-8 ■ Instructional Note in the Tabular List to Code First

❑ Scott double-checks the Tabular List entry for code **D57.01**.

▪ He is reminded of the instructional note at the beginning of category **D57**, which states **Use additional code for any associated fever (R50.81)**.

▪ This note confirms that the code for the fever should be sequenced as an additional, or second, code after the code for SCD.

▶ Scott finalizes the codes and sequencing for this case:

(1) **D57.01 Hb-SS disease with acute chest syndrome**

(2) **R50.81 Fever presenting with conditions classified elsewhere**

CODING PRACTICE

Exercise 15.4   Arranging Codes for Conditions of the Blood

Instructions: Read the mini-medical-record of each patient's encounter, review the information abstracted in Exercise 15.2, assign ICD-10-CM diagnosis codes using the Index and Tabular List, and sequence them correctly.

1. INPATIENT HOSPITAL   Gender: F   Age: 59

Reason for admission: weakness, fatigue, confusion

Assessment: new anemia due to chemotherapy for metastatic colon cancer

Tip: Read the instructional notes in the Tabular List and refer to OGCR I.C.2c.2) to identify all codes needed and the sequencing.

4 ICD-10-CM Codes _____

_____

2. INPATIENT HOSPITAL   Gender: M   Age: 61

Reason for admission: tachycardia, headaches, fatigue

Assessment: anemia due to stage 3 chronic kidney disease

Plan: erythropoiesis stimulating agents (ESAs), supplemental iron

Tip: Read the instructional notes in the Tabular List for sequencing guidance.

2 ICD-10-CM Codes _____

3. OFFICE   Gender: F   Age: 50

Reason for encounter: follow up on glucose tolerance test (GTT) and complete chemistry analysis

Assessment: hyperglycemia due to pre-diabetes, lab results also indicate iron (Fe)-deficiency anemia

Plan: manage pre-diabetes with 1,500 calorie diabetic diet, Rx Fe supplements

Tip: The main focus of the visit is prediabetes.

2 ICD-10-CM Codes _____

CODING MALIGNANCIES OF THE BLOOD

Malignancies of the blood and blood-forming organs do not appear in ICD-10-CM Chapter 3, Diseases of the Blood and Blood-Forming Organs and Certain Disorders Involving the Immune Mechanism (D50-D89). Codes for malignancies of the blood and blood-forming organs appear in block C81 to C96 within the neoplasm chapter.

Neoplasms, which are solid tumors, do not form in the blood, so there is no entry for blood in the Table of Neoplasms. However, hematological malignancies do affect blood, bone marrow, and lymph nodes. Leukemia and myeloma, which begin in the bone marrow, and lymphoma, which begins in the lymphatic system, are the most common types of blood cancer. The blood is also one of the primary vehicles for metastasis of malignant neoplasms in any organ because it circulates through all organs and body tissues.

Lymphomas, leukemias, and myelomas are named based on the type of cell affected and whether the disease begins in mature or immature cells, so coders must be attentive to the exact name of the malignancy. Examples include the following:

- anaplastic large cell lymphoma
- ALK-negative or acute myeloid leukemia with 11q23-abnormality
- multiple myeloma

Acute myeloid leukemia (AML) and chronic lymphocytic leukemia (CML) are the most common leukemias, according to the Leukemia and Lymphoma Society, and increase significantly in adults over age 55. Leukemia is the most common type of cancer in children, accounting for over 27% of childhood cancer. Acute lymphoblastic leukemia (ALL) accounts for 65% of acute leukemias in children, according to the Children's Cancer Research Fund.

To locate codes, search the Index for the Main Term that describes the condition, such as **Lymphoma**, **Leukemia**, or **Myeloma**. Then search for subterms that describe the type and location. Do not search the Table of Neoplasms unless the Index directs you to do so.

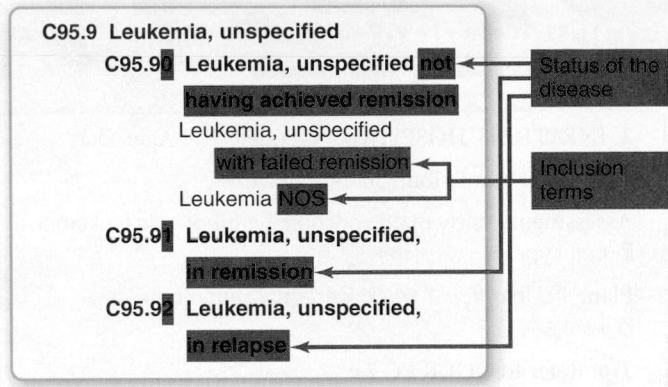

Figure 15-9 ■ Tabular List Entry for Leukemia Showing Separate Codes for the Status of the Disease

Each type of leukemia has three separate codes based on the status of the disease, as follows (OGCR I.C.2.n):

- not having achieved **remission** (*blood counts return to normal and bone marrow samples show no sign of disease*), final digit of **0**
- in remission, final digit of **1**
- in **relapse** (*the return of the disease after remission*), final digit of **2**

When the medical record does not specifically document the status of the disease, assign a code for **not having achieved remission** because the Tabular List classifies **leukemia NOS** under the codes for **leukemia, not having achieved remission** (■ FIGURE 15-9). Also assign a code for **not having achieved remission** when leukemia is documented as failed remission.

CODING CAUTION

Remember to distinguish between remission and a personal history of the disease. Personal history defines a condition that no longer exists and is not receiving treatment but has the potential for recurrence and therefore may require continued monitoring (OGCR I.C.21.c.4)). If the documentation is unclear whether the patient is in remission, query the provider (OGCR I.C.2.n).

CODING PRACTICE

Exercise 15.5 Coding Malignancies of the Blood

Instructions: Read the mini-medical-record of each patient's encounter, then abstract, assign, and sequence ICD-10-CM diagnosis codes using the Index and Tabular List. Write the code(s) on the line provided.

1. INPATIENT HOSPITAL Gender: M Age: 78

Reason for admission: induction chemotherapy

Assessment: acute myeloid leukemia M7

Tip: Acute myeloid leukemia has eight subtypes. The goal of induction chemotherapy is to achieve remission.

2 ICD-10-CM Codes _____

(*continued*)

CODING PRACTICE (continued)

2. INPATIENT HOSPITAL   Gender: F   **Age:** 65

Reason for admission: chemotherapy

Assessment: early stage chronic lymphocytic leukemia, B-cell type

Plan: FU in office 1 week. Repeat treatment 3 weeks.

Tip: Refer to OGCR I.C.2.e.

2 ICD-10-CM Codes _____

3. OFFICE   Gender: M   **Age:** 9

Reason for encounter: monitoring of acute lymphoblastic leukemia (ALL)

Assessment: ALL, in remission

Plan: RTO 3 months

1 ICD-10-CM Code _____

4. OFFICE   Gender: F   **Age:** 22

Reason for encounter: follow up biopsy of lump in neck

Assessment: classical Hodgkin's lymphoma with mixed cellularity

Plan: radiation therapy to neck

1 ICD-10-CM Code _____

5. OFFICE   Gender: F   **Age:** 36

Reason for encounter: radiation therapy

Assessment: non-Hodgkin's follicular lymphoma, grade 2, stage 3, in neck, abdomen, and pelvic nodes

Plan: treatment 5x/week for 6 weeks

Tip: Remember to distinguish between grade (how aggressive it is) and stage (how far it has spread).

2 ICD-10-CM Codes _____

CHAPTER SUMMARY

In this chapter you learned that:

- The function of the blood, also called the hemic system, is to transport and pass nutrients, oxygen, carbon dioxide, water, proteins, and hormones to cells and to transport waste products to excretory organs.

- ICD-10-CM Chapter 3, Diseases of the Blood and Blood-Forming Organs and Certain Disorders Involving the Immune Mechanism (D50-D89), contains seven blocks or subchapters that are divided by type of condition.

- Many of the conditions in this ICD-10-CM chapter can have multiple underlying causes and multiple manifestations, so coders should thoroughly abstract the symptoms, manifestations, and underlying causes documented in the medical record.

- When an ICD-10-CM chapter does not have any OGCR, as is the case with diseases of the blood and blood-forming organs,

coders apply the general OGCR (I.A, I.B, II, and III) and follow instructional notes in the Tabular List.

- Sequencing of codes in this ICD-10-CM chapter is based on the circumstances of admission and the instructional notes in the Tabular List.

- Neoplasms, which are solid tumors, do not form in the blood, but leukemia and myeloma, which begin in the bone marrow, and lymphoma, which begins in the lymphatic system, are the most common types of blood cancer.

- ICD-10-CM does not provide Official Guidelines for Coding and Reporting (OGCR) for this chapter, but the Tabular List contains frequent instructional notes to use an additional code for associated conditions and to code first underlying diseases.

CONCEPT QUIZ

Take a moment to look back at diseases of the blood and blood-forming organs and solidify your skills. Try to answer the questions from memory first, then refer back to the chapter if you need a little extra help.

Completion

Instructions: Write the term that answers each question based on the information you learned in this chapter. Choose from the list below. Some choices may be used more than once and some choices may not be used at all.

aplastic

bone marrow

erythrocytes

formed elements

hemic

hemoglobin

hemolytic

leukocytes

nutritional

plasma

polycythemia

sarcoidosis

sickle cell disease

spleen

thrombocytes

thrombophilia

1. Hb, an abbreviation for _____, is the oxygen-carrying component of erythrocytes.

2. Blood cells are created in the _____.

3. _____ anemia is due to excessive loss of erythrocytes.

4. _____ are white blood cells.

5. The blood is referred to as the _____ system.

6. _____ is the formation of nodules in the lymph nodes, lungs, bone, and skin.

7. Erythrocytes, leukocytes, and thrombocytes are blood cells, or the _____ of the blood.

8. The spleen destroys old _____ and filters the blood.

9. _____ is an abnormal increase in the number of circulating red blood cells.

10. HbSS is a type of _____.

Multiple Choice

Instructions: Circle the letter of the best answer to each question based on the information you learned in this chapter.

1. Which of the following disorders is NOT classified in ICD-10-CM Chapter 3, Diseases of the Blood and Blood-Forming Organs?
   A. Aplastic anemia
   B. Congestive heart failure
   C. Coagulation disorders
   D. Hemophilia

2. Which medical term means "formation of blood"?
   A. Hematapoiesis
   B. Hematologist
   C. Hemoglobin
   D. Hemophilia

3. Code D63.0, Anemia in neoplastic disease, describes what type of anemia?
   A. Aplastic anemia due to chemotherapy
   B. Anemia due to radiotherapy
   C. Anemia due to the cancer itself
   D. Anemia due to antineoplastic chemotherapy

4. _____ disorders include a range of medical problems that lead to poor clotting and continuous bleeding.
   A. Hemostasis
   B. Hemoglobin
   C. Anemia
   D. Purpura

5. When an ICD-10-CM chapter does not have OGCR, how does the coder know how to assign and sequence codes?
   A. Use common sense.
   B. Assign the default code listed in the Index.
   C. Ask the supervisor.
   D. Follow instructional notes in the Tabular List.

6. When anemia is due to an underlying condition, the Tabular List instructs coders to code which condition first?
   A. Anemia
   B. The underlying condition
   C. Either condition may be sequenced first.
   D. Sequencing is determined by the circumstances of admission.

7. When anemia is drug induced, the Tabular List instructs coders to assign an external cause code for
   A. the neoplasm.
   B. the injury.
   C. the substance.
   D. the anemia.

8. All of the following are key criteria for abstracting conditions of the blood EXCEPT
   A. What part of the hemic system does the condition involve?
   B. Is heart failure involved?
   C. Is the condition drug induced?
   D. Is the condition acquired or congenital?

9. All of the following are options when coding leukemia EXCEPT
   A. whether leukemia is in remission.
   B. whether leukemia has metastasized.
   C. whether leukemia has relapsed.
   D. whether leukemia has not achieved remission.

10. When the admission or encounter is for management of an anemia associated with an adverse effect of radiotherapy, the first sequenced code is
    A. anemia.
    B. neoplasm.
    C. an external cause code.
    D. Z code for the therapy encounter.

CODING CHALLENGE

Instructions: Read the mini-medical-record of each patient's encounter, then abstract, assign, and sequence ICD-10-CM diagnosis codes using the Index and Tabular List. Write the code(s) on the line provided.

1. OFFICE Gender: M Age: 61

Reason for encounter: bruising and petechiae, SOB, rapid heart rate, pelvic pain

Assessment: aplastic anemia due to chemotherapy for prostate cancer with metastasis to the pelvic bones

Plan: Admitted and started on immunosuppressant drugs, received blood transfusion and pain management. Referral to interventional radiologist to deliver targeted ablation (RFA) to bone metastasis. Pain management at weaker opioid level, RTO weekly for CBC

Tip: Refer to OGCR I.C.2.c.2) for sequencing rules.

4 ICD-10-CM Codes _____

_____

2. INPATIENT HOSPITAL Gender: M Age: 47

Reason for admission: severe anemia

Assessment: anemia due to lung cancer in right lower lobe with metastasis to the bone.

Plan: He received blood transfusions and was discharged home.

Tip: Refer to OGCR I.C.2.c.1) for sequencing rules.

3 ICD-10-CM Codes _____

_____

3. OFFICE Gender: F Age: 12

Reason for encounter: management and monitoring of thrombophilia

Assessment: congenital antithrombin III deficiency

Plan: INR protocol, anticoagulation medication

1 ICD-10-CM Code _____

4. INPATIENT HOSPITAL Gender: F Age: 53

Chief complaint: Patient states she ran out of the anticoagulant warfarin 5 days ago and now "feels funny."

Assessment: lupus anticoagulant syndrome, systemic lupus erythematosus

Plan: restart warfarin, FU in office

Tip: Remember to assign an external cause code for the medication.

3 ICD-10-CM Codes _____

_____

5. INPATIENT HOSPITAL Gender: M Age: 74

Reason for admission: bruising, petechiae, hemorrhages, nosebleeds, bleeding gums, extreme fatigue

Assessment: leukemia, anemia, and thrombocytopenia

Plan: Pt received platelet transfusion. Schedule chemotherapy, Rx anemia support medications

Tip: Pancytopenia is a deficiency of WBCs, RBCs, and platelets.

1 ICD-10-CM Code _____

6. OFFICE Gender: F Age: 32

Reason for encounter: FU on lab results from daily renal dialysis showing Hb in urine

Assessment: hemoglobinuria due to dialysis, end-stage renal failure

Plan: erythropoietin protocol, place on kidney replacement list, investigate possibility of family kidney donor. FU for test results in five days

Tip: Remember to assign an external cause code for complication from dialysis.

3 ICD-10-CM Codes _____

_____

7. INPATIENT HOSPITAL Gender: M Age: 64

Reason for admission: Fever, oral cavity lesions. CBC shows absolute neutrophil count (ANC) is below 500/microliter

Assessment: neutropenia with fever

Plan: At discharge patient provided guidelines to avoid infections, including use of saline mouth rinses. Antibiotic and/or antifungal meds as directed. RTO weekly for CBC.

Tip: Remember to read the instructional notes in the Tabular List.

2 ICD-10-CM Codes _____

8. INPATIENT HOSPITAL Gender: F Age: 28

Reason for Admission: Palpitations, rapid heartbeat, long bone pain, enlarged, painful spleen. Admit patient for transfusion, IV therapy, pain management, and splenectomy.

Assessment: Sickle cell crisis with splenic sequestration

Plan: RTO in one week for CBC and post operative check

1 ICD-10-CM Code _____

9. INPATIENT HOSPITAL Gender: F Age: 45

Reason for Admission: bone marrow transplant

Assessment: secondary myelofibrosis due to right breast cancer

Tip: Remember that "due to" means secondary.

2 ICD-10-CM Codes _____

10. INPATIENT HOSPITAL Gender: M Age: 36

Chief complaint: unexplained loss of weight, fever, weakness, night sweats, itching, tingling in legs, SOB, elevated red cell count

Assessment: Leukocytosis with polycythemia vera

Plan: FU with clinic one week

2 ICD-10-CM Codes _____

KEEP ON CODING

As a coder, you can never have too much experience. Apply everything you have learned in this chapter to code the following diagnostic statements. Use the OGCR and instructional notes in the Tabular List to help determine how many codes are required.

Instructions: Read the diagnostic statement, then use the Index and Tabular List to assign and sequence ICD-10-CM diagnosis codes. Write the code(s) on the line provided.

1. Sideropenic dysphagia: ICD-10-CM Code(s) _____

2. Alpha thalassemia: ICD-10-CM Code(s) _____

3. Sickle cell disease without crisis: ICD-10-CM Code(s) _____

4. Hereditary factor IX deficiency: ICD-10-CM Code(s) _____

5. Bandemia: ICD-10-CM Code(s) _____

6. Cyst of the spleen: ICD-10-CM Code(s) _____

7. Diffuse large B-cell lymphoma, of axilla: ICD-10-CM Code(s) _____

8. Megaloblastic anemia: ICD-10-CM Code(s) _____

9. Pancytopenia due to chemotherapy for metastatic pancreatic cancer: ICD-10-CM Code(s) _____

10. Encounter for chemotherapy for acute monocytic leukemia: ICD-10-CM Code(s) _____

11. Sarcoid arthropathy: ICD-10-CM Code(s) _____

(continued)

(continued from page 249)

12. Postprocedural hematoma of the spleen following gastric surgery: ICD-10-CM Code(s) _____

13. Cyclic neutropenia: ICD-10-CM Code(s) _____

14. Histiocytic sarcoma: ICD-10-CM Code(s) _____

15. Pyruvate kinase (PK) deficiency anemia: ICD-10-CM Code(s) _____

16. Hemolytic-uremic syndrome: ICD-10-CM Code(s) _____

17. Infantile pseudoleukemia: ICD-10-CM Code(s) _____

18. Heparin-induced thrombocytopenia: ICD-10-CM Code(s) _____

19. Leukopenia: ICD-10-CM Code(s) _____

20. Di George syndrome: ICD-10-CM Code(s) _____

21. Essential cryoglobulinemia: ICD-10-CM Code(s) _____

22. Protein deficiency anemia: ICD-10-CM Code(s) _____

23. Evans syndrome: ICD-10-CM Code(s) _____

24. Acquired pure red cell aplasia: ICD-10-CM Code(s) _____

25. Polycythemia due to stress: ICD-10-CM Code(s) _____

Diseases of the Respiratory System (J00-J99)

Chapter 16

Learning Objectives

After completing this chapter, you should have the skills to:

16.1 Spell and define the key words, medical terms, and abbreviations related to the respiratory system.

16.2 Discuss the structure, function, and common conditions of the respiratory system.

16.3 Identify the main characteristics of coding for respiratory system conditions.

16.4 Abstract diagnostic information from the medical record for coding diseases of the respiratory system.

16.5 Assign codes for diseases of the respiratory system.

16.6 Arrange multiple diagnosis codes for diseases of the respiratory system.

16.7 Code neoplasms of the respiratory system.

16.8 Discuss the Official Guidelines for Coding and Reporting related to the respiratory system.

Chapter Outline

- **Respiratory System Refresher**
- **Coding Overview of the Respiratory System**
- **Abstracting for Respiratory System Conditions**
- **Assigning Codes for Respiratory System Conditions**
- **Arranging Codes for Respiratory System Conditions**
- **Coding Neoplasms of the Respiratory System**

Key Terms and Abbreviations

acute exacerbation
acute rhinitis
aerosol therapy
airway obstruction
allergic rhinitis
alveolus
atopic
bronchodilator
bronchogenic
bronchus
bronchial tree
bronchiole

chronic bronchitis
chronic obstructive pulmonary disease (COPD)
culture and sensitivity
emphysema
endotracheal intubation
exchange
extrinsic
hospital-acquired condition (HAC)
hypercapnia
hypoxemia

laryngitis
larynx
lobe
lower respiratory tract
lung
intrinsic
nonatopic
pharyngitis
pharynx
productive cough
pulmonary function test
respiratory system

sinusitis
status asthmaticus
thoracentesis
trachea
tracheal cartilage
tracheostomy tube
upper respiratory tract
ventilation-perfusion scan
ventilator-associated pneumonia (VAP)
ventilator

In addition to the key terms listed here, students should know the terms defined within tables in this chapter.

For updates and corrections, visit our student resource site at

www.pearsonhighered.com/healthprofessionsresources

INTRODUCTION

As you travel to a higher elevation than what you're accustomed to, breathing becomes more difficult. This is not because there is less oxygen in the air but because a decrease in air pressure causes us to inhale less air with each breath.

A pulmonologist specializes in diagnosing and treating conditions of the lungs and lower respiratory system. An otolaryngologist specializes in diagnosing and treating conditions of the upper respiratory system. Primary care physicians treat uncomplicated conditions of the respiratory system and refer more complicated cases to specialists.

RESPIRATORY SYSTEM REFRESHER

The function of the **respiratory system** is to obtain oxygen (O_2) from the air and deliver it to the lungs and blood for distribution to tissue cells and to remove the gaseous waste product carbon dioxide (CO_2) from the blood and lungs and expel it. This process is called **exchange**. The respiratory system also makes it possible to cough, sneeze, and talk.

The respiratory system is divided into the **upper respiratory tract**, which consists of the nose, **pharynx** (*throat*), and **larynx** (*voice box*); and the **lower respiratory tract**,

which consists of the **trachea** (*windpipe*), bronchi, and **lungs** (■ Figure 16-1). As air enters the nasal cavity or oral cavity, it is warmed and moistened, then passes through the pharynx, larynx, and trachea. The trachea divides into two **bronchi** (*bronchial tubes*) that lead to the two lungs. Rings of **tracheal cartilage** keep the trachea and bronchi open. In the **bronchial tree**, the bronchi subdivide into smaller and smaller branches, with the smallest being the **bronchioles**, which do not contain rings of cartilage. Bronchioles end in small air sacs in the lungs, **alveoli**.

The lungs consist of spongy tissue with interlacing networks of bronchioles, alveoli, alveolar sacs, blood vessels, and capillaries. The lungs are divided into **lobes** (*segments*). The right lung has three lobes: the superior, middle, and inferior. The left lung has two lobes: the superior and inferior. The lungs receive deoxygenated blood from the heart through the pulmonary artery, reoxygenate it, and send it back to the heart through the pulmonary vein so the heart can pump the blood out to the rest of the body.

In Figure 16-1, each structure in the respiratory system is labeled with its name as well as its medical terminology root/combining form, where applicable. Refer to ■ Table 16-1 for a

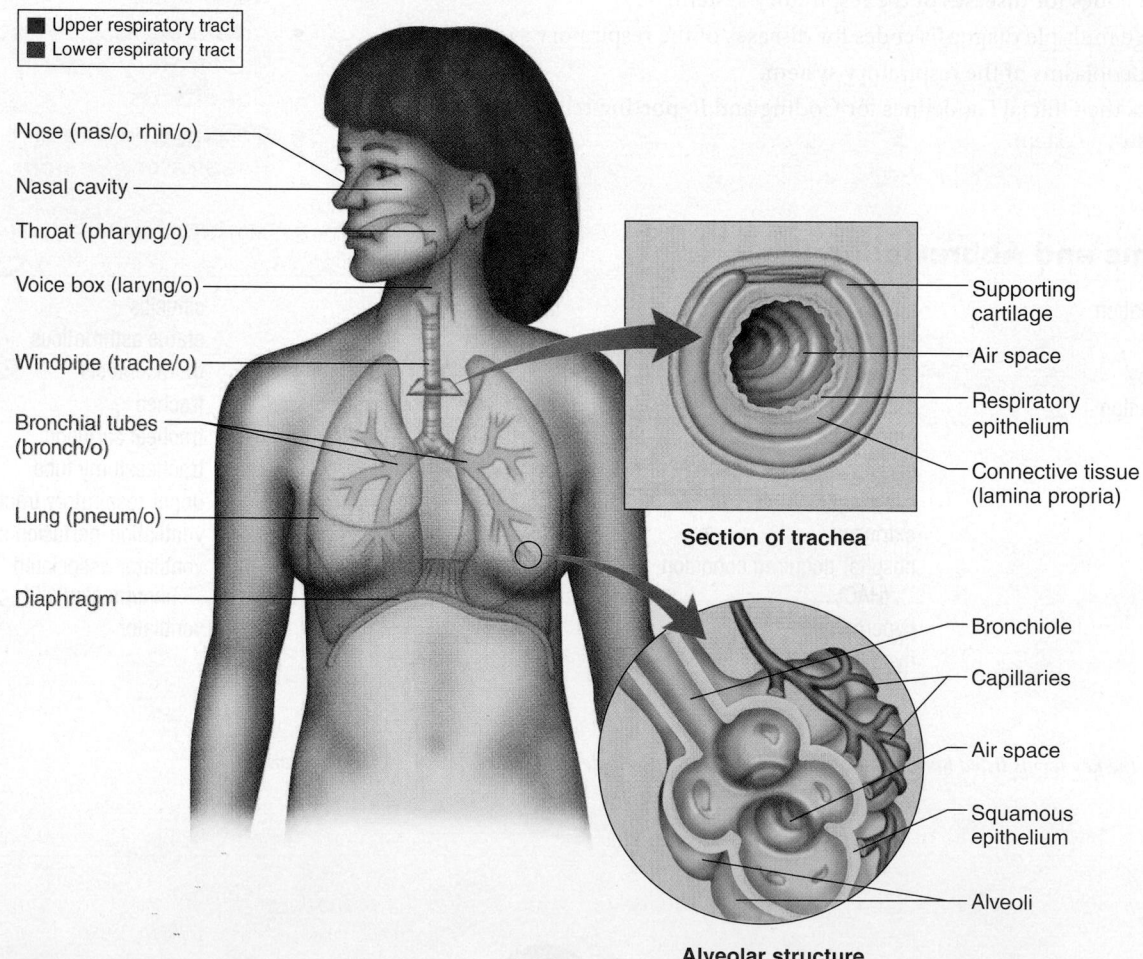

Figure 16-1 ■ The Respiratory System

Table 16-1 ■ **EXAMPLE OF CONSTRUCTING MEDICAL TERMS FOR THE RESPIRATORY SYSTEM**

Prefix/Combining Form	Suffix	Complete Medical Term
dys- (*abnormal, painful*)	-scope (*instrument to view the inside*) -ectasis (*dilation*)	dys + phonia (*difficulty speaking*) dys + pnea (*difficulty breathing*)
bronch/o (*bronchus*)	-pnea (*breathing*) -phonia (*voice*)	broncho + scope (*instrument to view the bronchus*) bronchi + ectasis (*dilated bronchus*)

refresher on how to build medical terms related to the respiratory system.

SUCCESS STEP

Remember to form the plural of most medical terms, you need to drop the last one or two letters and substitute new letters. For example, one bronch**us** becomes two bronch**i**.

CODING CAUTION

Be alert for medical terms that are spelled similarly and have different meanings.

bron<u>ch</u>itis (*inflammation of the bronchus*) and **bron<u>chiol</u>itis** (*inflammation of the bronchiole*)

py<u>o</u>thorax (*pus in the chest*) and **pneu<u>mo</u>thorax** (*air in the chest*)

emph<u>ys</u>ema (*abnormal accumulation of air in body tissue*) and **emp<u>y</u>ema** (*pus in a body cavity*)

Conditions of the Respiratory System

Respiratory conditions are divided based on whether they affect the upper or lower respiratory tract. Conditions affecting the upper respiratory tract, frequently caused by viruses, include **acute rhinitis** (*common cold*), **allergic rhinitis** (*hay fever*), **sinusitis** (*sinus infection*), **pharyngitis** (*sore throat*), and **laryngitis** (*irritated vocal cords*). Conditions affecting the lower respiratory tract include obstructive diseases (narrowing of the air passages), infection and inflammatory diseases (viral and bacterial infections), and mechanical damage (nontraumatic structural damage to the lung). Refer to ■ TABLE 16-2 for a summary of respiratory system conditions.

Coders should have an understanding of asthma, COPD, and ventilator-associated pneumonia because they pose special coding challenges. These are discussed next, followed by an overview of diagnostic and treatment methods.

Asthma

Asthma is a chronic lung disease that affects the bronchi and is characterized by inflammation and narrowing of the airway. A common symptom is wheezing due to **bronchospasms**. Asthma may be **extrinsic** or **atopic** (*due to allergens*), or **intrinsic** or **nonatopic** (*not due to allergens*). According to the American College of Allergy, Asthma, and Immunology (ACAAI), approximately 34.1 million people in the United States are diagnosed with asthma, resulting in 500,000 hospitalizations and over 10 million office visits per year.

Physicians diagnose asthma based on the frequency and type of symptoms, forced expiratory volume (FEV), and peak expiratory flow (PEF), which are measurements of lung function. Based on this information, patients' asthma is rated as intermittent or persistent and is classified into one of four severity levels:

1. Mild intermittent
2. Mild persistent
3. Moderate persistent
4. Severe persistent

An **acute exacerbation**, commonly called an asthma attack, is a sudden increase in the intensity or type of symptoms, such as shortness of breath, wheezing, and chest tightness. **Status asthmaticus** is an acute exacerbation that does not respond to the standard medical treatments of bronchodilators and **steroids**.

Chronic Obstructive Pulmonary Disease

Chronic obstructive pulmonary disease (COPD), one of the most common lung diseases, is the combination of **chronic bronchitis** and **emphysema** as comorbidities. An airway **obstruction** is a reduction in the amount of air inhaled during each breath, most commonly caused by a reduction in the diameter of the bronchioles due to inflammation.

According to the Centers for Disease Control and Prevention, approximately 13% of nursing home residents have COPD and over 6% of noninstitutionalized adults suffer from either chronic bronchitis or emphysema. COPD accounts for over 17 million physician office visits per year.

Physicians diagnose chronic bronchitis when patients present with a **productive cough** (*cough with sputum*) on most days for three months in two consecutive years. The most common cause is long-term inhalation of irritants. Emphysema is an enlargement and rupture of alveolar sacs at the end of the bronchioles, causing an abnormal accumulation of air in the tissue.

Table 16-2 ■ CONDITIONS OF THE RESPIRATORY SYSTEM

Condition	Definition
Acute respiratory distress syndrome (ARDS)	Acute respiratory failure that results in widespread injury to the endothelium in the lung, caused by sepsis, massive blood transfusion, **aspiration** of gastric contents, or pneumonia
Acute respiratory failure (ARF)	Insufficient oxygen passing from the lungs to the blood, due to hypercapnia (*high carbon dioxide level*), hypoxemia (*low oxygen level*), or both
Asthma	A chronic lung disease that affects the bronchi and is characterized by inflammation of the airway, a reversible obstruction, and reshaping of the airway
Atelectasis	Collapse of a lung, preventing the exchange of oxygen and carbon dioxide
Chronic bronchitis	Inflammation of the bronchi with a productive cough for three months in two consecutive years
Chronic obstructive pulmonary disease (COPD)	The combination of chronic bronchitis and emphysema as comorbidities
Emphysema	An enlargement and rupture of alveolar sacs at the end of the bronchioles, causing an abnormal accumulation of air in the tissue
Influenza	An acute respiratory infection with sudden onset caused by a virus and characterized by fever, chills, headache, muscle aches, cough, and sore throat
Laryngitis	Inflammation of the larynx, resulting in hoarseness
Lobar pneumonia	Bacterial pneumonia that primarily affects one lobe of the lung
Lobular pneumonia	Pneumonia that primarily affects the bronchi and lobules (*clusters of alveoli that surround each bronchial branch*); also called bronchopneumonia
Pharyngitis	Inflammation of the throat
Pleurisy	Inflammation of the lining of the lungs and thoracic cavity with oozing of fluid or fibrinous material into the pleural cavity
Pneumoconiosis	Abnormal condition of the lung caused by inhalation of dust particles, such as coal dust (anthracosis), asbestos (asbestosis), iron dust (siderosis), or quartz (silicosis)
Pneumonia	Inflammatory condition of the lung in which the alveoli and air spaces fill with fluid; caused by bacterial, virus, fungi, or chemical irritants (■ Figure 16-2)
Pneumothorax	A collection of air between the chest wall and lungs, which may cause the lung to collapse
Pulmonary edema	An abnormal accumulation of fluid in the lungs, especially the alveoli, resulting in dyspnea
Tonsillitis	Inflammation of the tonsils

The damage it causes is irreversible, unlike asthma, in which the obstruction is reversible.

Ventilator-Associated Pneumonia

Ventilator-associated pneumonia (VAP) is pneumonia that develops 48 hours or more after mechanical ventilation is initiated. Mechanical ventilation is the administration of oxygen using an endotracheal tube or **tracheostomy tube** (*a surgical opening in the neck leading to the trachea*). Intubation allows microorganisms from oral and gastric secretions to invade the tissues of the lower respiratory tract and lung. VAP is more serious than other types of pneumonia because patients who acquire it are in poorer health than the average person. In addition, the types of germs present in a hospital are often more dangerous and more resistant to treatment than those found in the community at large.

SUCCESS STEP

VAP is an example of a **hospital-acquired condition** (HAC), a serious condition that develops after admission. Medicare does not pay hospitals for the costs incurred to care for HACs and hospitals cannot bill patients for them.

Diagnosis and Treatment of Respiratory Conditions

Diseases of the respiratory system are diagnosed with a wide variety of techniques, including the following:

- arterial blood gasses to determine O_2 and CO_2 concentrations
- biopsy
- chest X-ray

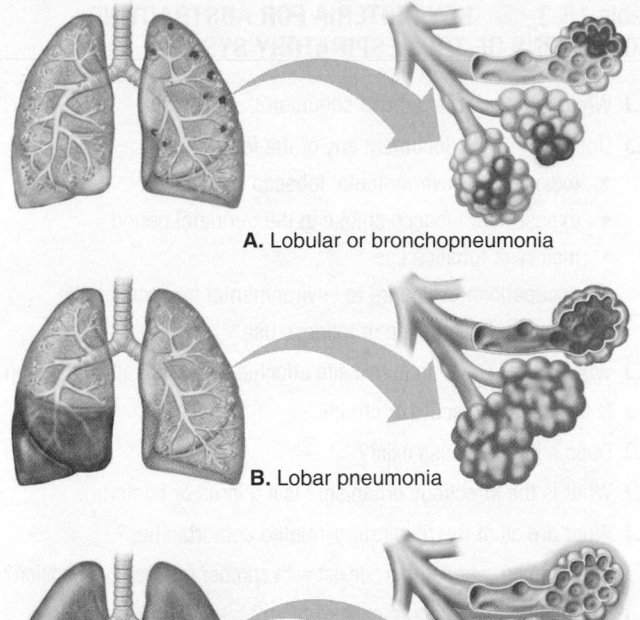

A. Lobular or bronchopneumonia

B. Lobar pneumonia

C. Interstitial pneumonia

Figure 16-2 ■ **(A)** Lobular or Bronchopneumonia with Localized Pattern **(B)** Lobar Pneumonia with a Diffuse Pattern within a Lung Lobe **(C)** Interstitial Pneumonia Is Typically Diffuse and Bilateral

- computed tomography scan
- **culture and sensitivity**—a lab test of secretions, such as sputum, to observe bacterial growth and determine antibiotic effectiveness
- endoscopy (laryngoscopy, bronchoscopy)
- **pulmonary function tests**—diagnostic tests that measure air flow in and out of the lungs, lung volumes, and gas exchange between the lungs and blood
- ultrasound scanning
- **ventilation-perfusion scan**—a nuclear medicine test useful in identifying pulmonary emboli by showing whether blood is flowing to all parts of the lung

Respiratory diseases are treated by medications, surgery, and respiratory therapy, including the following:

- **aerosol therapy**—medication suspended in a mist that is inhaled
- **bronchodilator**—a medication that relaxes muscle spasms in bronchial tubes
- **endotracheal intubation**—placement of a tube through the mouth and glottis into the trachea to create a viable airway
- **pulmonectomy or lobectomy**
- **thoracentesis**—surgical puncture of the chest wall to remove fluids
- tracheostomy

CODING PRACTICE

Exercise 16.1 **Respiratory System Refresher**

Instructions: Use your medical terminology skills and resources to define the following conditions related to the respiratory system, then assign the diagnosis code. Follow these steps:

- Use slash marks "/" to break down each term into its root(s) and suffix.

- Define the meaning of the word, based on the meaning of each word part.
- Assign the default ICD-10-CM diagnosis code for the condition using the Index and Tabular List.

Example: tonsillitis tonsil/itis   Meaning: *inflammation of the tonsils*   ICD-10-CM Code: *J03.90*

1. pneumatocele	Meaning _____	ICD-10-CM Code _____
2. bronchiolitis	Meaning _____	ICD-10-CM Code _____
3. pneumohemothorax	Meaning _____	ICD-10-CM Code _____
4. rhinorrhea	Meaning _____	ICD-10-CM Code _____
5. nasopharyngitis	Meaning _____	ICD-10-CM Code _____
6. bronchoalveolitis	Meaning _____	ICD-10-CM Code _____
7. laryngoplegia	Meaning _____	ICD-10-CM Code _____
8. pyothorax	Meaning _____	ICD-10-CM Code _____
9. tracheostenosis	Meaning _____	ICD-10-CM Code _____
10. hydropneumothorax	Meaning _____	ICD-10-CM Code _____

CODING OVERVIEW OF THE RESPIRATORY SYSTEM

ICD-10-CM Chapter 10, Diseases of the Respiratory System (J00-J99), contains 11 blocks or subchapters that are divided by type of disorder and anatomic site. Review the block names and code ranges listed at the beginning of Chapter 10 in the ICD-10-CM manual to become familiar with the content and organization.

ICD-10-CM Chapter 10 compares to ICD-9-CM Chapter 8 (460-519). ICD-10-CM includes more codes than ICD-9-CM did to report manifestations, infectious organisms, and comorbidities. It also introduces new terminology for certain conditions, such as asthma.

This chapter includes infections of the upper and lower respiratory tracts, acute and chronic obstructive diseases, lung diseases due to external agents, and respiratory failure. It does not include infectious diseases, toxic effects of smoke, symptoms and signs, perinatal conditions, or obstetric-related conditions. These conditions are classified in other ICD-10-CM chapters.

ICD-10-CM provides Official Guidelines for Coding and Reporting (OGCR) for the respiratory system in OGCR section I.C.10. OGCR provides a detailed discussion of chronic obstructive pulmonary disease and asthma, acute respiratory failure, influenza, and ventilator associated pneumonia.

An instructional note at the beginning of the ICD-10-CM Chapter 10 in the Tabular List directs coders when they should use an additional code to identify circumstances and lifestyle habits related to tobacco use and tobacco smoke exposure. An additional instructional note directs coders how to assign codes when more than one site in the respiratory system is affected. Instructional notes appear throughout the Tabular List directing coders when additional codes are required for certain categories.

ABSTRACTING FOR RESPIRATORY SYSTEM CONDITIONS

Abstracting diagnoses for the respiratory system requires knowledge of the disease processes because multiple comorbidities are common. Coders need to distinguish between diseases to ensure they abstract all of the required details. In addition to identifying the conditions, coders must also identify the infectious organism and lifestyle habits related to tobacco. ■ TABLE 16-3 lists important questions to ask when abstracting respiratory system conditions.

Guided Example of Abstracting for Respiratory System Conditions

Refer to the following example throughout this chapter to practice skills for abstracting, assigning, and sequencing respiratory system codes. Leanne Riehl, CCS, is a fictional coder who guides you through the coding process.

Table 16-3 ■ KEY CRITERIA FOR ABSTRACTING CONDITIONS OF THE RESPIRATORY SYSTEM

❑ What is the specific type of condition?

❑ Does the record document any of the following:

- exposure to environmental tobacco smoke
- exposure to tobacco smoke in the perinatal period
- history of tobacco use
- occupational exposure to environmental tobacco smoke
- tobacco dependence or tobacco use

❑ What is the lowest anatomic site affected by a respiratory infection?

❑ Is the condition acute or chronic?

❑ Does a lung abscess exist?

❑ What is the infectious organism? Is it a virus or bacteria?

❑ What are all of the respiratory-related comorbidities?

❑ Does influenza or asthma coexist with another respiratory condition?

❑ Is the condition in acute exacerbation?

❑ If asthma is documented, what is the level of severity?

❑ Is asthma in acute exacerbation or status asthmaticus?

❑ Is the condition the result of an external cause or procedural complication?

❑ If influenza is documented, what manifestations exist?

❑ Is the condition recurrent?

❑ Does the patient use supplemental oxygen or a **ventilator** (*a machine that assists in breathing*)?

Date: 6/16/yy   Location: Branton Medical Center

Provider: Gilbert Stagg, MD

Patient: Jared Hershman   Gender: M   Age: 73

Reason for admission: dehydration, started IV fluids

Assessment: Patient who previously smoked cigarettes for 50 years (nicotine dependence) was placed on ventilator due to COPD exacerbation. Patient acquired ventilator associated pneumonia (VAP) due to *Pseudomonas*. Hospital stay was prolonged due to the VAP.

Plan: discharged home after 10 days, continue antibiotics, start supplemental O_2

Follow along as Leanne Riehl, CCS, abstracts the diagnosis. Check off each step after you complete it.

▶ Leanne reads through the entire record, paying special attention to the reason for the encounter and the final assessment.

❑ She sees that there are quite a few things going on with this patient, so she needs to break it down step by step. She refers to the Key Criteria for Abstracting Conditions of the Respiratory System (Table 16-3). Because there are several coexisting conditions, she must review all the abstracting questions for each condition.

- ❏ *What is the specific type of condition?* The reason for the admission is dehydration. She notes that this condition was treated with IV fluids.

- ❏ *What are all of the respiratory-related comorbidities?* After he was admitted, the patient experienced an acute exacerbation of the COPD. Patient also developed VAP.

- ❏ *Does the patient use supplemental oxygen or a ventilator?* Yes, patient was placed on ventilator.

- ❏ *What is the infectious organism?* Pseudomonas. *Is it a virus or bacteria?* Bacteria

- ❏ *Is the condition the result of an external cause or procedural complication?* Yes, the pneumonia is ventilator associated.

- ❏ *Does the record document any current or past tobacco use?* Previously smoked cigarettes for 50 years (nicotine dependence).

▶ Leanne reviews all the information she has gathered about this case.

- ❏ The patient was admitted for dehydration.

- ❏ He has COPD.

- ❏ He experienced an acute exacerbation of COPD.

- ❏ He has a history of cigarette smoking.

- ❏ He acquired VAP due to *Pseudomonas.*

▶ At this time, Leanne does not know which of these conditions may need to be coded, nor how many codes she will end up with. She will learn about this when she moves on to assigning codes.

CODING PRACTICE

Exercise 16.2   Abstracting for Respiratory System Conditions

Instructions: Read the mini-medical-record of each patient's encounter and answer the abstracting questions. Write the answer on the line provided. Do not assign any codes.

1. OFFICE   Gender: M   Age: 31

Reason for encounter: patient with previously diagnosed extrinsic asthma presents with increased symptoms of coughing, wheezing, and SOB

Assessment: Symptoms are due to acute exacerbation of mild intermittent asthma.

Plan: oral steroids and quick relief bronchodilator inhaler

a. What condition was previously diagnosed?

_____

b. What are the presenting symptoms? _____

_____

c. What is the cause of the symptoms? _____

_____

d. Which symptoms should you code? _____

_____

e. What is the severity of the patient's asthma? _____

_____

2. OFFICE   Gender: F   Age: 69

Reason for encounter: productive cough and fever, patient is concerned that she may need medication for COPD which she has not needed for several years

Assessment: viral pneumonia unrelated to patient's history of COPD

Plan: Rx cough medicine with expectorant, take aspirin for fever, drink plenty of fluids to prevent dehydration

(continued)

2. (continued)

a. What are the patient's symptoms? _____

_____

b. Why was the patient concerned about the symptoms?

_____

c. What condition did the physician diagnose?

_____

d. What is the difference between viral pneumonia and bacterial pneumonia? _____

e. Is the pneumonia related to the past COPD?

_____

f. Should you code the symptoms? _____

Why or why not? _____

g. Should you code the COPD? _____

Why or why not? _____

Tip: If you are unsure about this, refer to OGCR IV.J.

h. Should you code the pneumonia? _____

Why or why not? _____

3. INPATIENT HOSPITAL   Gender: M   Age: 72

Reason for encounter: management of chronic obstructive pulmonary disease, recent self-administered spirometry results have been declining, increased SOB

Assessment: COPD with chronic bronchitis and emphysema

Plan: nebulizer treatment to administer bronchodilators

a. What chronic disease was previously diagnosed?

_____

b. What symptoms does the patient report at this encounter? _____

(continued)

CODING PRACTICE (continued)

3. (continued)

c. Do these symptoms lead to a new diagnosis?

_____

d. Should you code the symptoms? _____

Why or why not? _____

e. Should you code the COPD? _____

Why or why not? _____

f. Should you code chronic bronchitis and/or emphysema? _____

Why or why not? _____

---

4. INPATIENT HOSPITAL Gender: M Age: 80

Reason for admission: *patient with congestive heart failure admitted from physician's office after presenting with low fever, chills, cough. CHF increases patient risk for complications.*

Assessment: *lobular pneumonia and acute bronchitis, both due to Mycoplasma pneumoniae*

a. What are the symptoms? _____

b. Should the symptoms be coded? _____

Why or why not? _____

c. What is the role of CHF in this case? _____

_____

d. What two conditions were diagnosed? _____

_____

e. Is the bronchitis acute or chronic? _____

_____

f. What is the infectious organism? _____

_____

g. Does the patient have COPD? _____

h. What is the principal diagnosis? _____

_____

Tip: Refer to OGCR II.B.

i. What is the second diagnosis? _____

_____

j. What is the third diagnosis? _____

_____

k. What ongoing medical treatment does the patient use? _____

---

5. INPATIENT HOSPITAL Gender: F Age: 76

Reason for admission: *acute bronchitis*

(*continued*)

---

5. (continued)

Assessment: *COPD with acute bronchitis exacerbation and chronic bronchitis*

Plan: *begin oxygen therapy, patient must cease cigarette smoking as it continues to impact her respiratory conditions, counseled her regarding treatment options for tobacco dependence*

a. What is the reason for admission? _____

_____

b. What other conditions are documented? _____

_____

c. What is the relationship between COPD and the acute bronchitis? _____

_____

d. Should the acute bronchitis be coded? _____

Why or why not? _____

e. Should chronic bronchitis be coded? _____

Why or why not? _____

f. What lifestyle habit should be coded? _____

_____

Tip: You will learn the sequencing when you begin assigning the codes in Exercise 16.4.

---

6. INPATIENT HOSPITAL Gender: F Age: 78

Reason for admission: *asbestosis which is thought to be due to exposure to asbestos particles brought home by her late husband who worked in the fireproofing industry for many years and died of mesothelioma*

Assessment: *asbestosis, clubbing of fingers due to the asbestosis, mild persistent asthma*

Plan: O_2, *thoracentesis, medication, respiratory therapy*

a. What is the reason for admission? _____

_____

b. What is clubbing of the fingers due to? _____

_____

c. Should clubbing of the fingers be coded? _____

_____

Why or why not? _____

d. What other diagnosis exists? _____

_____

e. What is the severity of the asthma? _____

_____

f. Should asthma be coded? _____

Why or why not? _____

g. What is the principal diagnosis? _____

_____

ASSIGNING CODES FOR RESPIRATORY SYSTEM CONDITIONS

Coders must be attentive to the details of the case, instructional notes in the Tabular List, and the OGCR to accurately assign codes for respiratory system conditions. They should become familiar with chapter-wide coding considerations as well as information specifically for asthma, COPD, and influenza.

Chapter-Wide Coding

ICD-10-CM Chapter 10, Diseases of the Respiratory System (J00–J99), begins with two instructional notes that apply to all codes in the chapter. One instruction pertains to assigning additional codes for lifestyle habits; the other instruction describes how to code when multiple sites within the respiratory system are affected. Coders should also assign status **Z** codes when needed.

Lifestyle Habits

ICD-10-CM Chapter 10 provides an instructional note at the beginning of the chapter that instructs coders to use an additional code, when applicable, to identify various situations related to tobacco use, dependence, and exposure to tobacco smoke (■ FIGURE 16-3). Exposure may include environmental tobacco smoke, occupational exposure to tobacco smoke, and exposure to tobacco smoke during the perinatal period (before birth through the first 28 days after birth).

SUCCESS STEP

ICD-9-CM provided a chapter-wide note to assign an additional code to identify the infectious organism. Because ICD-10-CM has many combination codes that describe the condition and the organism, this chapter-wide note was eliminated. However, you still see a similar note in certain categories that do not provide a combination code.

Multiple Sites Affected

Respiratory conditions may affect more than one site within the respiratory system, such as the tonsils and adenoids, trachea and bronchi, or bronchi and lung. When the site is not specifically indexed, assign a code for the lowest anatomical site. This requires coders to follow conventions in the Index carefully and to have knowledge of respiratory system anatomy.

For example, consider a patient seen for tracheobronchitis, an inflammation (-itis) of the trachea (trache/o) and

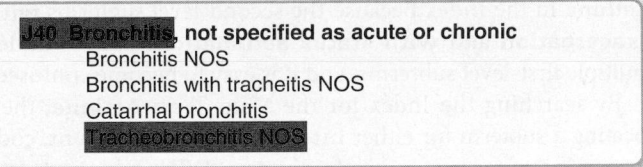

Figure 16-4 ■ Tabular List Entry for Bronchitis with Tracheobronchitis as an Inclusion Term

bronchi (bronch/o). The Index entry for the Main Term **Tracheobronchitis** cross-references coders to the Main Term **Bronchitis** because the bronchi are located lower than the trachea. The Index entry for the Main Term **Bronchitis** directs coders to **J40** (■ FIGURE 16-4). In the Tabular List, **Tracheobronchitis** appears as an inclusion term under the code **J40 Bronchitis, not specified as acute or chronic.**

Z Codes

Certain treatments for respiratory conditions require status **Z** codes. The most common are the existence of a tracheostomy, an encounter for tracheostomy care, long-term use of oxygen, and/or ventilator assistance in breathing. If there are complications from any of these devices, code the complication and do not assign a **Z** code.

Locate codes for tracheostomy status and tracheostomy care under the Main Term **Tracheostomy** in the Index. Locate the **Z** codes for oxygen and ventilator use under the Main Term **Dependence** in the Index (■ FIGURE 16-5).

Assigning Codes for Asthma

Assigning codes for asthma has new requirements in ICD-10-CM. To assign codes for asthma, coders need to identify how the physician has documented the severity of the patient's condition. Be attentive when navigating the Main Term for

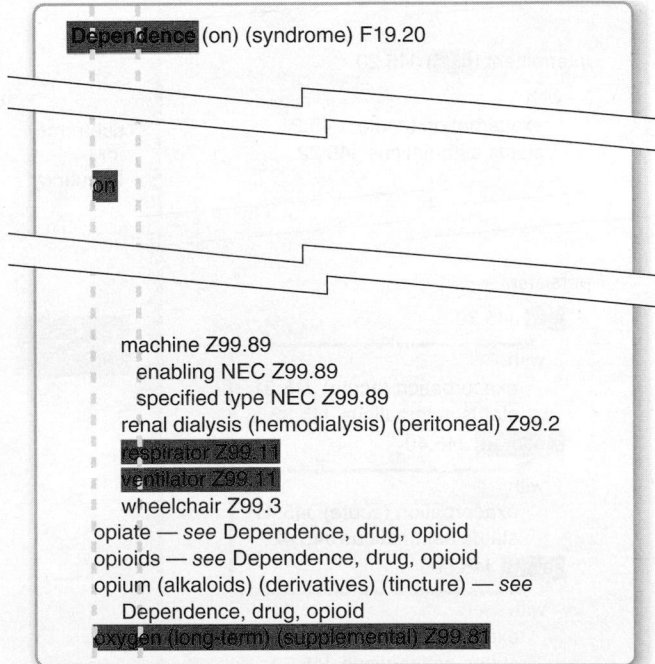

Figure 16-5 ■ Index Entries for Dependence on Ventilator or Oxygen

---

Use additional code, where applicable, to identify:
        exposure to environmental tobacco smoke (Z77.22)
        exposure to tobacco smoke in the perinatal period (P96.81)
        history of tobacco use (Z87.891)
        occupational exposure to environmental tobacco smoke
            (Z57.31)
        tobacco dependence (F17.-)
        tobacco use (Z72.0)

Figure 16-3 ■ Tabular List Instructional Notes That Apply to All Codes in Chapter 10

Asthma in the Index because the second-level subterms **with exacerbation** and **with status asthmaticus** appear under multiple first-level subterms, and it is easy to become confused.

By searching the Index for the Main Term **Asthma**, then locating a subterm for either **intermittent** or **persistent**, coders can locate most of the codes they need. The subterm **intermittent** contains only one level of severity, **mild**, then provides choices for **with exacerbation** or **with status asthmaticus**. The subterm **persistent** provides additional subterms for **mild**, **moderate**, or **severe**, then provides choices under each for **with exacerbation** or **with status asthmaticus** (■ FIGURE 16-6).

CODING CAUTION

In ICD-9-CM asthma codes were divided based on whether asthma was extrinsic or intrinsic. In ICD-10-CM, these terms lead you to default codes for unspecified asthma. Instead, you need to locate asthma based on the severity level as mild intermittent, moderate intermittent, moderate persistent, and severe persistent.

Assigning Codes for COPD and Asthma

The codes in categories **J44 Other chronic obstructive pulmonary disease** and **J45 Asthma** distinguish between uncomplicated cases and those in acute exacerbation. An acute exacerbation is a worsening of a chronic condition. An acute exacerbation is not the same as an infection superimposed on a chronic condition, although an exacerbation may be triggered by an infection.

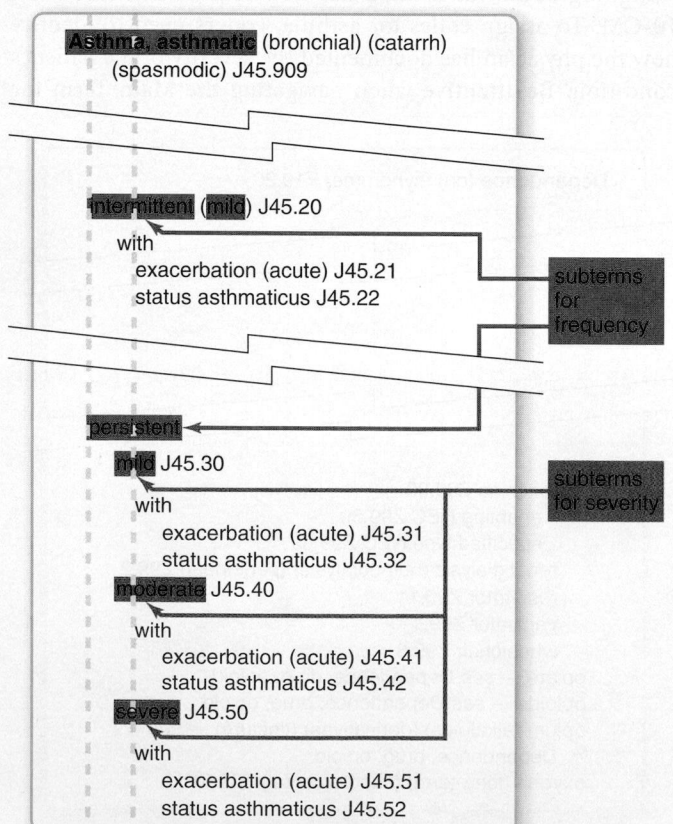

Figure 16-6 ■ Example of the Index Entry for Asthma

Patient with COPD is ▓▓▓▓▓▓▓▓▓▓▓▓▓▓▓▓▓▓ with status asthmaticus.

(1) **J45.52 Severe persistent asthma with status asthmaticus**
(2) **J44.0 Chronic obstructive pulmonary disease**

Figure 16-7 ■ Example of Assigning Codes for COPD and Asthma

When asthma occurs with COPD, the Index leads to the entry **Asthma, with chronic obstructive pulmonary disease J44.9**, which appears to be a combination code. However, the Tabular List instructs coders to assign an additional code for the type of asthma. The same holds true for chronic obstructive bronchitis with asthma. Sequencing depends on the circumstances of admission. (OGCR I.C.10.a.1)) (■ FIGURE 16-7).

Assigning Codes for Influenza

When assigning codes for influenza, coders must identify the type of influenza and the manifestations. Influenza codes are divided based on whether the disease is identified as **novel influenza A virus**, other virus, or the virus is unidentified. Novel influenza A, which includes avian influenza and H1N1, has a specific subcategory in the Tabular List (■ FIGURE 16-8). Coders should assign codes from subcategory **J09.X** and **J10** only when the virus is confirmed as one of those listed in the inclusion notes. Confirmation requires a definitive diagnostic statement from the physician but does not require a positive laboratory test. However, if the provider documents *suspected or possible or probable* avian influenza, do not assign a code from **J09.- Influenza due to certain identified influenza viruses**. Instead, assign a code from category **J11.- Influenza due to unspecified influenza virus** (OGCR I.C.10.c).

CODING CAUTION

OGCR I.C.10.c, which prohibits coding unconfirmed cases of avian or H1N1 influenza, is an exception to the hospital inpatient guideline OGCR II.H, which says to code uncertain conditions as though they exist. Remember that when there is a difference between a general coding guideline and a chapter-specific guideline, you should follow the chapter-specific guideline.

For all types of influenza, assign a combination code that describes the manifestation(s). The choices include the following:

- pneumonia
- other respiratory
- gastrointestinal
- encephalopathy
- myocarditis
- otitis media
- other

Instructional notes in the Tabular List also instruct coders to assign additional codes for lung abscess, **pleural effusion**,

4th J09 Influenza due to certain identified influenza viruses
　　Excludes1:　seasonal influenza due to other identified influenza virus (J10.-)
　　　　　　　　seasonal influenza due to unidentified influenza virus (J11.-)

　　5th J09.X Influenza due to identified novel influenza A virus
　　　　　　Avian influenza
　　　　　　Bird influenza
　　　　　　Influenza A/H5N1
　　　　　　Influenza of other animal origin, not bird or swine
　　　　　　Swine influenza virus (viruses that normally cause infections in pigs)

Figure 16-8 ■ Tabular List Inclusion and Exclusion Notes for Influenza Due to Certain Identified Influenza Viruses

perforated **tympanic membrane**, sinusitis, the type of pneumonia, and any additional manifestations.

Guided Example of Assigning Codes for Respiratory System Conditions

To practice skills for sequencing codes for the respiratory system, continue with the example from earlier in the chapter about patient Jared Hershman, who was admitted to Branton Medical Center due to dehydration.

Follow along in your ICD-10-CM manual as Leanne Riehl, CCS, assigns codes. Check off each step after you complete it.

▶ First, Leanne reviews all the information she abstracted about the patient. She will tackle each condition, one at a time.

❑ The patient was admitted for dehydration.

❑ He has COPD.

❑ He experienced an acute exacerbation of COPD.

❑ He has a history of cigarette smoking.

❑ He acquired VAP due to *Pseudomonas*.

▶ Leanne searches the Index for the Main Term **Dehydration**.

❑ She identifies the default code **E86.0**.

❑ She reviews the three subterms and verifies that none of them are documented.

▶ Leanne verifies code **E86.0** in the Tabular List.

❑ She reads the code title for **E86.0, Dehydration** and confirms that this accurately describes the documentation.

▶ Leanne checks for instructional notes in the Tabular List.

❑ She cross-references the beginning of category **E86**, reads the **Excludes1** notes, and verifies that they do not apply to this case.

❑ She then cross-references the beginning of the block **E70-E88** and the beginning of the chapter, reads the **Excludes1** notes, and verifies that they do not apply to this case.

❑ Leanne finalizes the code **E86.0, Dehydration**.

▶ Leanne proceeds to assign a code for COPD.

❑ She searches the Index for the Main Term **Disease** and subterm **lung**.

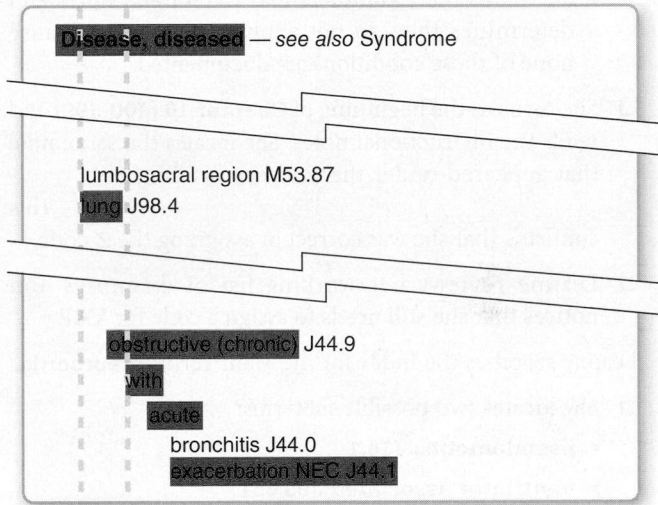

Figure 16-9 ■ Index Entry for Chronic Obstructive Pulmonary Disease with Acute Exacerbation

❑ She locates a second-level subterm **obstructive**.

❑ She locates additional subterm levels **with**, **acute**, and **exacerbation** (■ FIGURE 16-9).

❑ Now she knows she will have a combination code for COPD and the acute exacerbation. She identifies the code **J44.1**.

▶ Leanne verifies code **J44.1** in the Tabular List.

❑ She reads the code title for **J44.1, Chronic obstructive pulmonary disease with acute exacerbation** and confirms that this accurately describes the documentation.

❑ She double-checks to be sure that additional characters are not required.

▶ Leanne checks for instructional notes in the Tabular List.

❑ She reads the **Excludes2** note under code **J44.1** and determines that it does not apply to this case because the patient does not have acute bronchitis.

❑ She cross-references the beginning of category **J44** and reads the instructional notes.

　■ She determines that the **Excludes1** note does not apply to this case because none of these conditions are documented.

- She determines that the note **Code also type of asthma, if applicable (J45.-)** does not apply because asthma is not documented.

❑ She reads the **Use additional code** notes and determines that **history of tobacco use (Z87.891)** applies to this case because the patient smoked cigarettes for 50 years. This answers her question as to whether she should code the past nicotine dependence. She verifies this code in the Tabular List. **Z87.891, Personal history of nicotine dependence**.

❑ Leanne continues with cross-referencing and turns the page to the beginning of the block **Chronic lower respiratory diseases (J40-J47)**.

- She reads the **Excludes1** and **Excludes2** notes and determines they do not apply to this case because none of these conditions are documented.

❑ She turns to the beginning of **Chapter 10 (J00-J99)** and reads the instructional notes. She locates the same note that appeared under the category heading, **Use additional code for history of tobacco use (Z87.891)**. This confirms that she was correct in assigning the **Z** code.

❑ Leanne reviews her working list of diagnoses and notices that she still needs to assign a code for VAP.

▶ Leanne searches the Index for the Main Term **Pneumonia**.

❑ She locates two possible subterms:

- **pseudomonas J15.1**

- **ventilator associated J95.851**

❑ To determine whether she needs both of the codes or only one, she knows she needs to verify the codes in the Tabular List.

❑ She verifies the title for code **J15.1, Pneumonia due to Pseudomonas**, which is classified under the category **J15, Bacterial pneumonia, not elsewhere classified**.

❑ She verifies the title for code **J95.851, Ventilator associated pneumonia**, which is classified under the category **J95, Intraoperative and postprocedural complications and disorders of respiratory system, not elsewhere classified**.

❑ Leanne refers to OGCR I.C.10.d, which provides guidelines on coding VAP.

- OGCR I.C.10.d.1) states that code should be used only when the provider has documented VAP. She

double-checks the medical record to be certain it is documented.

- The guideline also states that she should assign an additional code to identify the infectious organism.

- The guideline also states that a code from **J12** to **J18** should NOT be assigned to identify the type of pneumonia.

❑ Leanne now understands that **J15.1** is for pneumonia due to *Pseudomonas* that patients acquire in the normal course of events and that **J95.851** is specifically for VAP.

❑ She returns to the Tabular List for code **J95.851** and reads the instructional note **Use additional code to identify the organism, if known (B95.-, B96.-, B97.-)**. This note is consistent with OGCR I.C.10.d, which she consulted. These codes are located in **Chapter 1, Certain Infectious and Parasitic Diseases (A00-B99)** and are used to identify infectious organisms in diseases classified in other ICD-10-CM chapters.

❑ She cross-references the block heading **J95** and sees that it is the same as the category. She sees no further instructional notes.

▶ Leanne cross-references the codes **B95.-**, **B96.-**, and **B97.-** to locate the code for *Pseudomonas*, **B96.5**, which has the title **Pseudomonas (aeruginosa) (mallei) (pseudomallei) as the cause of diseases classified elsewhere**.

❑ She notices that the terms **(aeruginosa) (mallei) (pseudomallei)** are nonessential modifiers because they are enclosed in parentheses. They describe various species of *Pseudomonas* and do not need to be present in the documentation in order to use the code.

▶ Leanne reviews the codes she has assigned for this case.

❑ **J95.851 Ventilator associated pneumonia**

❑ **Z87.891 Personal history of nicotine dependence**

❑ **J44.1 Chronic obstructive pulmonary disease with acute exacerbation**

❑ **E86.0 Dehydration**

❑ **B96.5 Pseudomonas (aeruginosa) (mallei) (pseudomallei) as the cause of diseases classified elsewhere**

▶ Next, Leanne must determine how to sequence the codes.

CODING PRACTICE

Exercise 16.3 Assigning Codes for Respiratory System Conditions

Instructions: Read the mini-medical-record of each patient's encounter, review the information abstracted in Exercise 16.2, and assign ICD-10-CM diagnosis codes using the Index and Tabular List. Write the code(s) on the line provided.

1. OFFICE   Gender: M   Age: 31

Reason for encounter: *patient with previously diagnosed extrinsic asthma presents with increased symptoms of coughing, wheezing, and SOB*

Assessment: *Symptoms are due to acute exacerbation of mild intermittent asthma.*

(*continued*)

1. (continued)

Plan: oral steroids and quick relief bronchodilator inhaler

Tip: Assign a code for the severity, not extrinsic vs. intrinsic.

1 ICD-10-CM Code _____

2. OFFICE   Gender: F   Age: 69

Reason for encounter: productive cough and fever, patient is concerned that she may need medication for COPD which she has not needed for several years

Assessment: viral pneumonia unrelated to patient's past history of COPD

Plan: Rx cough medicine with expectorant, take aspirin for fever, drink plenty of fluids to prevent dehydration

1 ICD-10-CM Code _____

3. INPATIENT HOSPITAL   Gender: M   Age: 72

Reason for encounter: management of chronic obstructive pulmonary disease, recent self-administered spirometry results have been declining, increased SOB

Assessment: COPD with chronic bronchitis and emphysema

Plan: nebulizer treatment to administer bronchodilators

Tip: Compare the codes for COPD, COPD with bronchitis, and COPD with emphysema.

1 ICD-10-CM Code _____

ARRANGING CODES FOR RESPIRATORY SYSTEM CONDITIONS

OGCR provides specific instructions regarding sequencing codes for ventilator associated pneumonia and acute respiratory failure (ARF).

Arranging Codes for Ventilator-Associated Pneumonia

VAP is pneumonia that patients acquire as a result of being on a ventilator (■ FIGURE 16-10). The relationship between ventilator use and the pneumonia must be documented by the physician. VAP is a complication of care and is classified separately from other types of pneumonia by ICD-10-CM. OGCR I.C.10.d provides instructions for how to assign codes for VAP, as follows:

1. Confirm that the provider has documented the relationship between the ventilator use and the pneumonia.
2. Assign code **J95.851 Ventilator associated pneumonia**.
3. Assign an additional code from **B95.-, B96.-,** or **B97.-** to identify the infectious organism.
4. Do not assign a code from categories **J12** to **J18** to identify the type of pneumonia.

Patients may be admitted with one type of pneumonia, then be put on a ventilator and also develop VAP. When this happens, assign and sequence codes as follows:

1. Assign a code from categories **J12** to **J18** to identify the pneumonia the patient had at admission. Sequence this as the principal diagnosis.

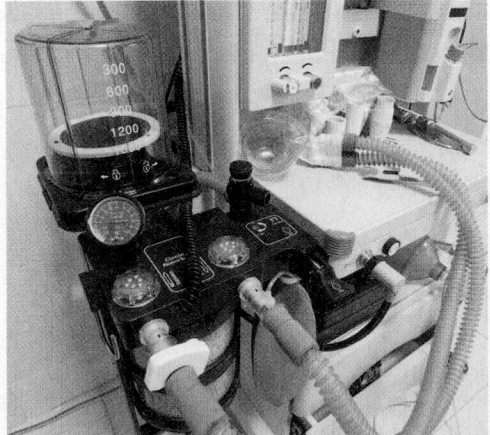
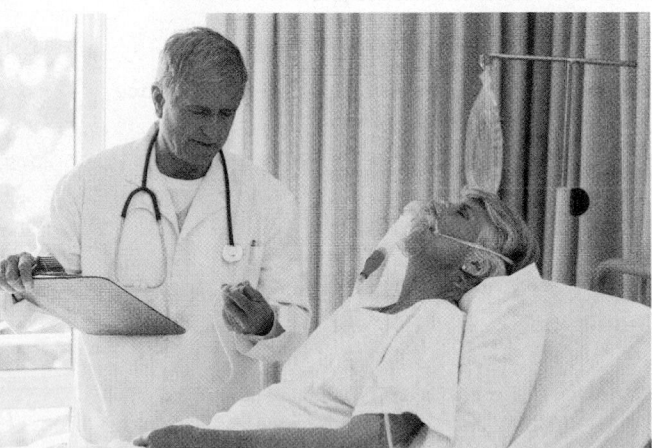

Figure 16-10 ■ Ventilators assist patients with breathing, but can also create an opportunity for pneumonia. *Sources: Paul Vinten/Shutterstock.com (left) and wavebreakmedia ltd/Shutterstock (right).*

2. Assign code **J95.851 Ventilator associated pneumonia** for VAP.

3. Assign an additional code from **B95.-, B96.-,** or **B97.-** to identify the infectious organism.

When patients are on a ventilator and do not have VAP or other ventilator-associated complications, assign code **Z99.11 Dependence on respirator [ventilator] status**.

SUCCESS STEP

To locate VAP in the Index, search for the Main Term **Pneumonia** and the subterm **ventilator associated**.

Arranging Codes for Acute Respiratory Failure

Acute respiratory failure (ARF) may be sequenced as either the principal diagnosis or a secondary diagnosis. OGCR I.C.10.b. provides the following guidance:

- When ARF meets the definition of a principal diagnosis, coders should sequence it first, unless another chapter-specific guideline, such as obstetrics, poisoning, HIV, or newborn, provides sequencing direction that takes priority.

- When ARF does not meet the criteria for the principal diagnosis, or arises after admission, coders should sequence it as an additional diagnosis.

- When ARF and another acute condition, such as myocardial infarction, cerebrovascular accident, or aspiration pneumonia, coexist, the circumstances of admission should determine the principal diagnosis.

Guided Example of Arranging Codes for Respiratory System Conditions

To practice skills for sequencing codes for the respiratory system, continue with the example from earlier in the chapter about patient Jared Hershman, who was admitted to Branton Medical Center due to dehydration.

Follow along in your ICD-10-CM manual as Leanne Riehl, CCS, sequences the codes. Check off each step after you complete it.

▶ Leanne confirms codes she has assigned.

❑ **J95.851 Ventilator associated pneumonia**

❑ **Z87.891 Personal history of nicotine dependence**

❑ **J44.1 Chronic obstructive pulmonary disease with acute exacerbation**

❑ **E86.0 Dehydration**

❑ **B96.5 Pseudomonas (aeruginosa) (mallei) (pseudo-mallei) as the cause of diseases classified elsewhere**

▶ First, she must determine the principal diagnosis, which the Uniform Hospital Data Discharge Set (UHDDS) defines as "that condition established after study to be chiefly responsible for occasioning the admission of the patient to the hospital for care" (OGCR II).

❑ Leanne checks the medical record and confirms that dehydration was the reason for admission. The COPD exacerbation and VAP developed after admission. Although these conditions were responsible for additional services and prolonged the length of stay, they do not meet the criteria for the reason for admission. She sequences **E86.0, Dehydration** as the principal diagnosis.

❑ Leanne determines that **J44.1, Chronic obstructive pulmonary disease with acute exacerbation** should be the second code because it was the reason the patient was placed on a ventilator.

❑ She sequences **J95.851, Ventilator associated pneumonia** as the third code and **B96.5, Pseudomonas** as the fourth code. The instructional notes and OGCR indicate that the organism is sequenced in addition to or after the code for VAP.

❑ The final code is **Z87.891, Personal history of nicotine dependence** because it is required by instructional notes and provides supplementary information.

▶ Leanne finalizes the code assignment and sequencing for this case:

1. **E86.0 Dehydration**

2. **J44.1 Chronic obstructive pulmonary disease with acute exacerbation**

3. **J95.851 Ventilator associated pneumonia**

4. **B96.5 Pseudomonas (aeruginosa) (mallei) (pseudo-mallei) as the cause of diseases classified elsewhere**

5. **Z87.891 Personal history of nicotine dependence**

CODING PRACTICE

Exercise 16.4 Arranging Codes for Respiratory System Conditions

Instructions: Read the mini-medical-record of each patient's encounter, review the information abstracted in Exercise 16.2, assign ICD-10-CM diagnosis codes using the Index and Tabular List, and sequence them correctly.

1. INPATIENT HOSPITAL Gender: M Age: *80*

Reason for admission: *patient with congestive heart failure admitted from physician's office after presenting with low fever, chills, cough. CHF increases patient risk for complications.*

(continued)

1. (continued)

Assessment: *lobular pneumonia and acute bronchitis, both due to Mycoplasma pneumoniae*

Tip: Be sure to distinguish between lobar pneumonia and lobular pneumonia. Remember to assign a **Z** code for the supplemental oxygen use.

4 ICD-10-CM Codes _____

_____

2. INPATIENT HOSPITAL   Gender: F   **Age:** 76

Reason for admission: *COPD with exacerbation*

Assessment: *COPD with acute bronchitis exacerbation and chronic bronchitis*

Plan: *antibiotics for the infection, begin oxygen therapy, patient must cease cigarette smoking as it continues to impact her respiratory conditions, counseled her regarding treatment options for tobacco dependence*
(continued)

2. (continued)

Tip: Read the instructional notes in the Tabular List for sequencing instructions.

3 ICD-10-CM Codes _____

_____

3. INPATIENT HOSPITAL   Gender: F   **Age:** 78

Reason for admission: *asbestosis which is thought to be due to exposure to asbestos particles brought home by her late husband who worked in the fireproofing industry for many years and died of mesothelioma*

Assessment: *asbestosis, clubbing of fingers due to the asbestosis, mild persistent asthma*

Plan: *O_2, thoracentesis, medication, respiratory therapy*

3 ICD-10-CM Codes _____

_____

CODING NEOPLASMS OF THE RESPIRATORY SYSTEM

Neoplasms of the respiratory system do not appear in ICD-10-CM Chapter 10, Diseases of the Respiratory System (J00–J99). Codes for neoplasms of the respiratory system appear in the block C30 to C39 within the neoplasm chapter.

The most common site for cancer in the respiratory system is the lung. Lung cancer, rare in people under age 45, is the deadliest type of cancer for both men and women, causing more deaths each year than breast, colon, and prostate cancers combined. Most lung cancer is **bronchogenic**, beginning in the cells that line the bronchi. Cigarette smoking is the leading cause of lung cancer; risk increases with how long people have smoked and the number of cigarettes smoked per day (■ FIGURE 16-11). However, lung cancer occurs in people who have never smoked.

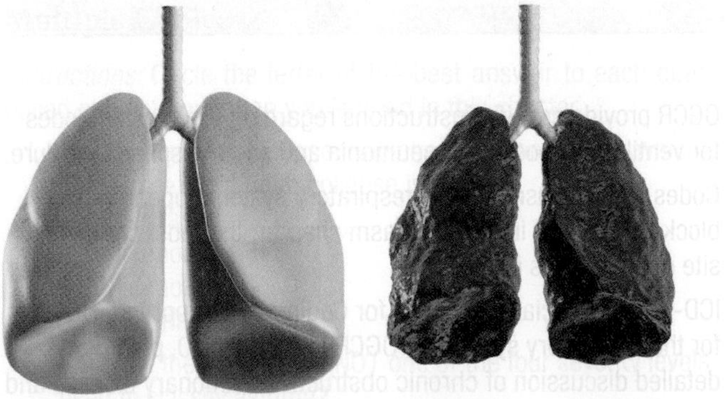

Figure 16-11 ■   Comparison of a Healthy Lung and the Lung of a Smoker. *Source: Sebastian Kaulitzki/Shutterstock.*

According to the American Cancer Society (ACS), an estimated 3,000 nonsmoking adults die each year from lung cancer related to breathing secondhand smoke. Mesothelioma is lung cancer that is usually caused by exposure to asbestos dust.

Primary lung cancer is divided into non-small-cell lung cancer (NSCLC), the most common type; small-cell lung cancer (SCLC), which is aggressive and metastasizes quickly; and mixed small cell/large cell, which includes both NSCLC and SCLC. Lung cancer commonly spreads to the liver, adrenal glands, bone, and brain. According to ACS, five-year survival rates depend on the type of lung cancer and stage when discovered but are lower (16%) compared to other cancers because it is usually not detected until metastasis has occurred. However, NSCLC found in Stage 1 and removed with surgery has a five-year survival rate of 60% to 70%.

The lung is also a common site of metastasis from other types of cancer, the most common being bladder, breast, colon, and kidney cancer. If only a small area of the lung is infiltrated and the original tumor has been cured, then surgery to remove the diseased portion of the lung can be beneficial. However, this is rare, and metastasis in the lung usually indicates that the original cancer has spread widely throughout the body and has a poor prognosis.

Although most types of lung cancer are classified in the Table of Neoplasms, coders should always search the Index first for the specific type of malignancy. Mesothelioma is classified in the Index, not the Table of Neoplasms. Codes are divided based on the site within the lung where the tumor is found and also contain laterality.

CODING CHALLENGE

Instructions: Read the mini-medical-record of each patient's encounter, then abstract, assign, and sequence ICD-10-CM diagnosis codes using the Index and Tabular List. Write the code(s) on the line provided.

1. OFFICE Gender: F Age: 1

Reason for encounter: productive cough, SOB, fever

Assessment: Chest X-ray and sputum culture positive for acute bronchitis due to *Streptococcus pneumonia*. Child exposed to cigarette smoke prenatally and currently because her mother smoked during pregnancy and still does.

Plan: OTC expectorant, acetaminophen to reduce fever, FU one week or sooner if necessary.

Tip: Assign one code for the bronchitis and two codes for smoke exposure.

3 ICD-10-CM Codes _____

_____

2. OFFICE Gender: F Age: 9

Reason for encounter: coughing, wheezing, SOB, and chest tightness during and 10 to 15 minutes after exercising during gym at school

Assessment: acute exacerbation of mild persistent asthma, intrinsic

Plan: Rx bronchodilator, use prior to exercise. FU office visit in one month.

Tip: Remember to code the severity of the asthma.

1 ICD-10-CM Code _____

3. INPATIENT HOSPITAL Gender: M Age: 82

Reason for admission: pneumonococcal pneumonia

Assessment: COPD with acute exacerbation required ventilation

Plan: discharged to skilled nursing facility with oxygen

2 ICD-10-CM Codes _____

_____

4. OFFICE Gender: F Age: 84

Reason for encounter: cracked tracheostomy tube

Assessment: Patient also has sarcoidosis with lung involvement.

Plan: replaced tracheostomy tube

(continued)

4. (continued)

Tip: A cracked tracheostomy tube is a mechanical complication of a tracheostomy.

2 ICD-10-CM Codes _____

5. INPATIENT HOSPITAL Gender: M Age: 33

Reason for encounter: ethmoidectomy and nasal reconstruction

Assessment: ethmoidal polyps and hypertrophy of nasal turbinates due to deviated nasal septum

Plan: excised polyps and repaired deviated nasal septum

3 ICD-10-CM Codes _____

_____

6. INPATIENT HOSPITAL Gender: F Age: 23

Reason for encounter: acute sinus pain, toothache, headache

Assessment: acute recurrent sinusitis, right maxillary sinus

Plan: Schedule CT scan of sinuses, analgesic, antihistamine, and antibiotic therapy. FU office visit 10 days.

1 ICD-10-CM Code _____

7. INPATIENT HOSPITAL Gender: M Age: 89

Reason for admission: admitted from emergency department due to acute respiratory failure

Assessment: ARF is due to aspiration pneumonia due to gastric secretions, lung abscess, diabetes type 2 with gastroparesis

Plan: Discharged to a skilled nursing facility.

4 ICD-10-CM Codes _____

_____

8. INPATIENT HOSPITAL Gender: M Age: 72

Reason for admission: gram-negative pneumonia

Assessment: Patient's left-sided congestive heart failure and pulmonary edema were managed in addition to the pneumonia. Patient also has chronic back pain with an unknown etiology but it was not a factor during this admission.

Plan: FU with pulmonary clinic and cardiologist in one week

2 ICD-10-CM Codes _____

9. INPATIENT HOSPITAL   Gender: M   **Age:** 36

Reason for admission: difficulty breathing

Assessment: spontaneous pneumothorax secondary to a ruptured bulla

Plan: X-ray confirmed reexpansion of lung, pulmonary clinic FU 1 week

2 ICD-10-CM Codes _____

10. INPATIENT HOSPITAL   Gender: F   **Age:** 6

Reason for encounter: **T&A**

Assessment: chronic tonsillitis with adenoiditis

Plan: FU in office 1 week

1 ICD-10-CM Code _____

KEEP ON CODING

Instructions: Read the diagnostic statement, then use the Index and Tabular List to assign and sequence ICD-10-CM diagnosis codes. Write the code(s) on the line provided.

1. Acute pharyngitis: ICD-10-CM Code(s) _____

2. Atelectasis: ICD-10-CM Code(s) _____

3. Chylous effusion of the pleura: ICD-10-CM Code(s) _____

4. Allergic rhinitis due to pollen: ICD-10-CM Code(s) _____

5. Malignant neoplasm of the ethmoid sinus, right: ICD-10-CM Code(s) _____

6. Stenosis of the larynx: ICD-10-CM Code(s) _____

7. Chlamydial pneumonia: ICD-10-CM Code(s) _____

8. Acute streptococcal tonsillitis: ICD-10-CM Code(s) _____

9. Avian flu: ICD-10-CM Code(s) _____

10. Acute bronchiolitis due to respiratory syncytial virus: ICD-10-CM Code(s) _____

11. Chronic tonsillitis: ICD-10-CM Code(s) _____

12. Exercised induced bronchospasm: ICD-10-CM Code(s) _____

13. Postprocedural respiratory failure: ICD-10-CM Code(s) _____

14. Hernia of the mediastinum: ICD-10-CM Code(s) _____

15. Mixed simple and mucopurulent chronic bronchitis: ICD-10-CM Code(s) _____

16. COPD (chronic obstructive pulmonary disease) with acute exacerbation: ICD-10-CM Code(s) _____

17. Carcinoma of the trachea: ICD-10-CM Code(s) _____

18. Acute respiratory failure with hypoxia: ICD-10-CM Code(s) _____

19. Maltworker's lung: ICD-10-CM Code(s) _____

20. Personal history of carcinoma of the lung: ICD-10-CM Code(s) _____

21. Vocal cord paralysis, bilateral: ICD-10-CM Code(s) _____

22. Tracheoesophageal fistula following tracheostomy: ICD-10-CM Code(s) _____

23. Ulcer of the left bronchus: ICD-10-CM Code(s) _____

24. Exercise induced bronchospasm: ICD-10-CM Code(s) _____

25. Pharyngeal abscess: ICD-10-CM Code(s) _____

Chapter 17

Diseases of the Nervous System and Sense Organs (G00-G99)

Chapter Outline

- **Nervous System Refresher**
- **Coding Overview of the Nervous System**
- **Abstracting for Nervous System Conditions**
- **Assigning Codes for Nervous System Conditions**
- **Arranging Codes for Nervous System Conditions**
- **Coding Neoplasms of the Nervous System**

Learning Objectives

After completing this chapter, you should have the skills to:

17.1 Spell and define the key words, medical terms, and abbreviations related to the nervous system and sense organs.

17.2 Discuss the structure, function, and common conditions of the nervous system and sense organs.

17.3 Identify the main characteristics of coding for conditions of the nervous system and sense organs.

17.4 Abstract information from the medical record required for coding conditions of the nervous system and sense organs.

17.5 Assign codes for conditions of the nervous system and sense organs.

17.6 Arrange multiple diagnosis codes for conditions of the nervous system and sense organs.

17.7 Code neoplasms of the nervous system and sense organs.

17.8 Discuss the Official Guidelines for Coding and Reporting related to the nervous system and sense organs.

Key Terms and Abbreviations

absence seizure	focal	nervous system	quadriplegia
Alzheimer disease (AD)	generalized	neurons	reflex sympathetic dystrophy
atonic	grand mal	olfactory	(RSD)
aura	gustatory	Parkinson disease (PD)	refractory
brain	hemiplegia	parkinsonian	secondary parkinsonism
central nervous system (CNS)	homeostasis	parkinsonism	simple partial
clonic	idiopathic	partial	spinal cord
complex partial	intractable	peripheral nervous system	status epilepticus
dementia	late onset	(PNS)	status migrainosus
distributed	localized	petit mal	tonic
dominance	monoplegia	pharmacoresistant	tonic-clonic
early onset	myoclonic	psychomotor	vasodilation

In addition to the key terms listed here, students should know the terms defined within tables in this chapter.

For updates and corrections, visit our student resource site at

www.pearsonhighered.com/healthprofessionsresources

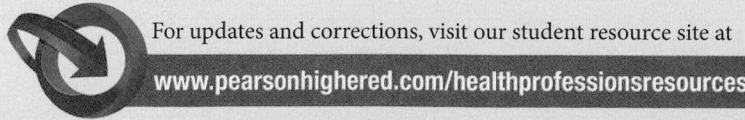

INTRODUCTION

Electrical problems can be one of the most troublesome to solve. A defect in the electrical system located in one part of a car can create a problem in a completely different area. The human nervous system is the electrical system in our bodies, sending and receiving messages that enable us to perform all functions.

A neurologist specializes in diagnosing and treating conditions of the nervous system. Neurosurgeons specialize in performing surgical procedures on the nervous system. Primary care physicians treat uncomplicated conditions of the nervous system and refer more complex cases to a specialist.

NERVOUS SYSTEM REFRESHER

The function of the nervous system is to direct the body's response to internal and external stimuli and coordinate the activities of other organ systems. It works with the endocrine system to maintain homeostasis (*maintenance of a stable internal physical state*). The nervous system consists of the central nervous system (CNS) and peripheral nervous system (PNS). The CNS acts as the control center for the nervous system by processing information and providing short-term control over other organ systems. The CNS consists of the brain and spinal cord. The brain governs perception of the senses, emotions, consciousness, memory, and voluntary movements (■ FIGURE 17-1). The spinal cord relays information to and from the brain. The PNS consists of the 12 nerves that radiate out from the brain and the 31 pairs of nerves that radiate from the spinal cord to all other areas of the body (■ FIGURE 17-2). The PNS links the CNS with other systems and the sense organs.

In Figures 17-1 and 17-2, each structure in the nervous system is labeled with its name as well as its medical terminology root/combining form where applicable. As you learn about conditions and procedures that affect the nervous system,

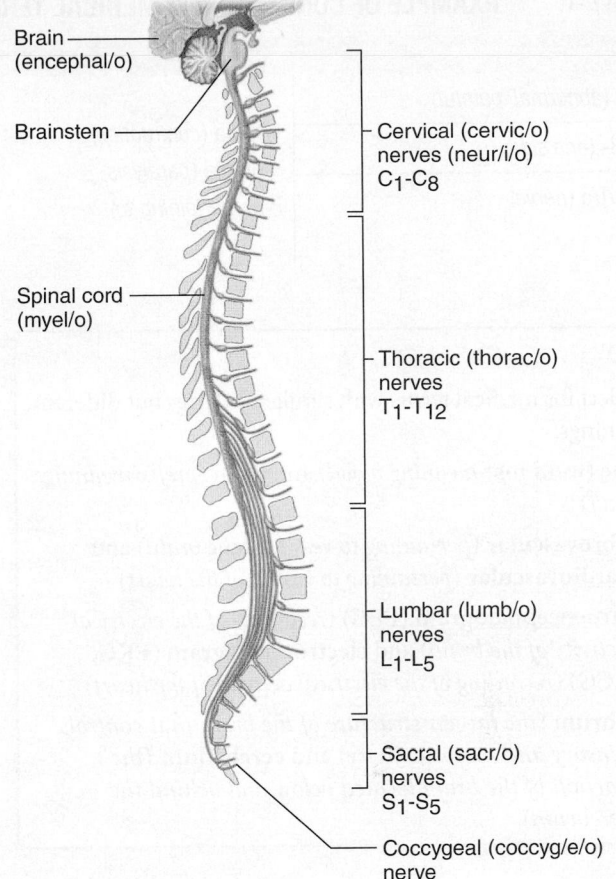

Figure 17-2   ■   The Spinal Cord and Spinal Nerves

remember to apply medical terminology skills to use word roots, prefixes, and suffixes you already know to define new terms related to the nervous system. Refer to ■ TABLE 17-1 (page 272) for a refresher on how to build medical terms related to the nervous system.

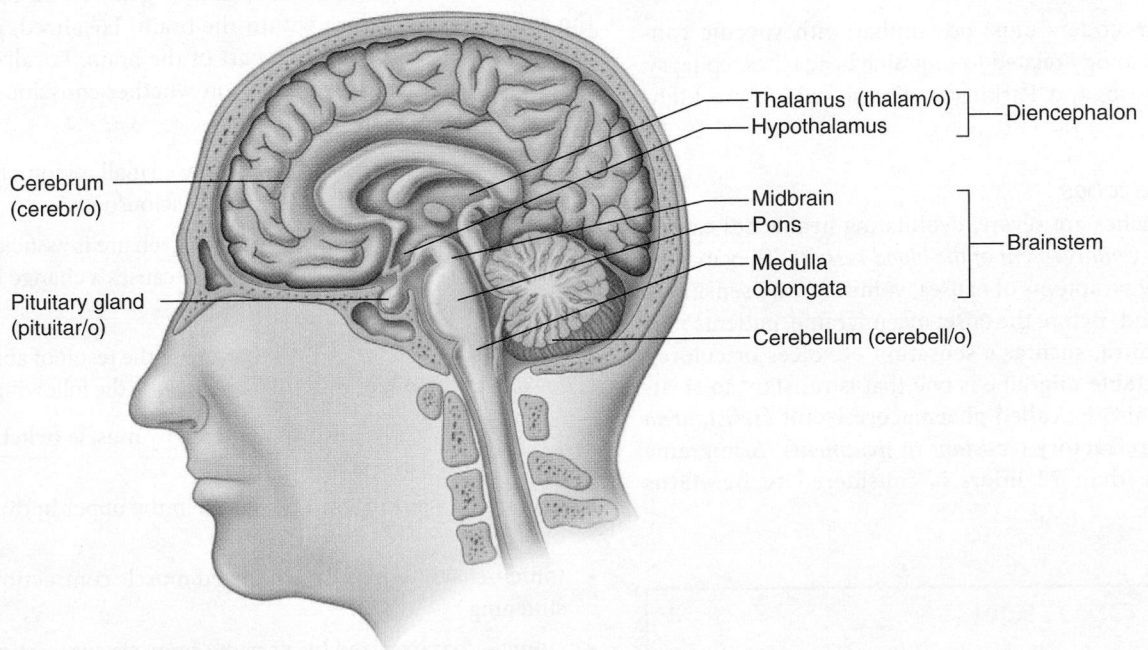

Figure 17-1   ■   The Brain

Table 17-1 ■ EXAMPLE OF CONSTRUCTING MEDICAL TERMS FOR THE NERVOUS SYSTEM

Prefix/Combining Form	Suffix	Complete Medical Term
dys- (abnormal, painful)	-tonia (contraction) -plegia (paralysis) -al (pertaining to)	dys + tonia (abnormal contraction)
hemi- (one side)		hemi + plegia (paralysis on one side of the body)
neur/i/o (nerve)		neuro + plegia (paralysis of a nerve) neur + al (pertaining to nerves)

CODING CAUTION

Be alert for medical terms with similar spellings but different meanings:

heme (*word root meaning blood*) and **hemi** (*prefix meaning half*)

cerebrovascular (*pertaining to vessels of the brain*) and **cardiovascular** (*pertaining to vessels of the heart*)

electroencephalogram (EEG) (*recording of the electrical activity of the brain*) and **electrocardiogram (EKG, ECG)** (*recording of the electrical activity of the heart*)

cerebrum (*the largest structure of the brain that controls sensory and motor activity*) and **cerebellum** (*the portion of the brain located below and behind the cerebrum*)

Conditions of the Nervous System

Diseases and disorders of the nervous system include headaches, infectious diseases, CNS disorders, and seizure disorders. Coders use medical resources, such as a reference book on diseases, to understand conditions of the nervous system, diagnostic methods, and common treatments. Refer to ■ TABLE 17-2 for a summary of diseases affecting the nervous system.

In particular, coders must be familiar with specific concepts and terminology related to migraine headaches, epilepsy, Alzheimer disease, and Parkinson disease, which are highlighted next.

Migraine Headaches

Migraine headaches are severe, debilitating headaches caused by **vasodilation** (*enlargement of the blood vessels*). They may be accompanied by symptoms of nausea, vomiting, and sensitivity to light and sound. Before the onset of a migraine, patients may experience an **aura**, such as a sensation of voices or colored light. An **intractable** migraine is one that is resistant to treatment and may also be called **pharmacoresistant** (*resistant to medication*) or **refractory** (*resistant to treatment*). A migraine that lasts more than 72 hours is considered to be **status migrainosus**.

CODING CAUTION

Do not assume that any severe headache is a migraine.

Epilepsy

Epilepsy is a brain disorder in which **neurons** (*clusters of nerve cells*) signal abnormally, causing seizures and/or unconsciousness. Epilepsy may be due to a medical condition or an injury or may be **idiopathic** (*of unknown cause*). Known causes include the following:

- alcoholism
- birth trauma
- depressed skull fracture
- penetrating wound
- infections of the brain
- dementia
- stroke or transient ischemic attack (TIA)
- other traumatic brain injury
- brain tumor

CODING CAUTION

Do not assume that all seizure activity is epilepsy. Seizures may also be caused by high fevers, psychological disorders, or other medical conditions such as narcolepsy, **Tourette syndrome**, or cardiac arrhythmia.

Seizures are classified as **localized** or **generalized** based on the source of the seizure within the brain. Localized, **partial**, or **focal** seizures occur in one part of the brain. Localized seizures are further classified based on whether consciousness is affected, as follows:

- A **simple partial** seizure affects only a small region of the brain and does not cause loss of consciousness.
- A **complex partial**, or **psychomotor**, seizure is associated with both sides of the cerebrum and causes a change in or loss of consciousness.

Generalized or **distributed** seizures are the result of abnormal activity on both sides of the brain and include the following types:

- **absence** or **petit mal**—characterized by muscle twitching or jerking for several seconds
- **myoclonic**—jerking and twitching in the upper body, arms, or legs
- **tonic**—characterized by prolonged muscle contractions or stiffening
- **clonic**—characterized by a series of muscle contractions and relaxations on both sides of the body

Table 17-2 ■ COMMON DISEASES OF THE NERVOUS SYSTEM

Condition	Definition
Alzheimer disease	A progressive degenerative brain disease
Amyotrophic lateral sclerosis (ALS) or Lou Gehrig disease	A chronic, terminal neurological disease characterized by a progressive loss of motor neurons and muscle atrophy
Bell palsy	Inflammation of the seventh (VII) cranial nerve, the facial nerve
Cerebral palsy	A functional disorder of the brain manifested by motor impairment
Chronic pain syndrome (CPS)	A collection of pain conditions lasting more than six months and unresponsive to treatment
Cluster headache	Unilateral pain in the eye or temple
Complex regional pain syndrome	A chronic pain syndrome in which an extremity experiences intense burning pain and changes in skin texture and temperature; also called **reflex sympathetic dystrophy (RSD)**
Degenerative neural disease	A class of diseases marked by degeneration of nerves and brain tissue, resulting in abnormalities in muscle and sensory functions
Dementia	A loss of brain function that affects memory, thinking, language, judgment, and behavior
Dystonia	Erratic jerky movements due to improperly functioning muscle tension
Encephalitis	A viral inflammation of the brain and meninges
Epilepsy	A brain disorder in which neurons signal abnormally, causing seizures and/or unconsciousness
Huntington chorea	An inherited progressive, degenerative disease involving loss of muscle control and personality changes
Hydrocephalus	Excess cerebrospinal fluid trapped in the brain
Meningitis	A contagious, acute inflammation of the pia mater and the arachnoid mater in the brain
Migraine headache	A severe, debilitating headache caused by vasodilation
Multiple sclerosis	A chronic, progressive disorder of the CNS characterized by muscle impairment due to patches of hardened tissue in the brain or spinal cord
Narcolepsy	A condition characterized by brief sudden attacks of deep sleep
Parkinson disease	A degenerative disease that affects muscle control and coordination
Spina bifida	A congenital neural tube defect in which vertebrae do not fuse

- **tonic-clonic** or **grand mal**—characterized by a sudden loss of consciousness and falling to the floor; affects the entire brain

- **atonic**—characterized by a brief loss of muscle tone

Epilepsy is classified as to whether it is intractable. According to the Centers for Disease Control and Prevention, approximately 70% of epilepsy is responsive to medication and 30% is intractable. **Status epilepticus** is an epileptic seizure that lasts more than 30 minutes or is a near-constant state of seizures and is a medical emergency.

Alzheimer Disease

Alzheimer disease (AD) is a progressive degenerative brain disease that doubles in prevalence with every five years of age. **Early onset** AD is diagnosed before age 65 and accounts for approximately 10% of all AD cases, according to the Centers for Disease Control and Prevention. **Late onset** AD is diagnosed after age 65 and affects 30% to 40% of people over age 85. AD is the most common cause of **dementia** (*a progressive loss of brain function that affects memory, thinking, language, judgment, and behavior*), which is classified in ICD-10-CM Chapter 5, Mental and Behavioral Disorders.

Parkinson Disease

Parkinson disease (PD) is a degenerative disease that affects muscle control and coordination, usually occurring in midlife. Symptoms include tremor, rigid muscles, and loss of normal reflexes. Dementia may be caused by PD or it may occur independently of PD. When dementia is diagnosed first, followed at a later time with an additional diagnosis of Parkinson disease, the combined condition is referred to as **parkinson*ian*** dementia or dementia with **parkinson*ism*** and assumes the existence of Lewy body disease. When PD is diagnosed first, followed at a later time with an additional diagnosis of dementia, the combined condition is referred to as Parkin*son* disease with dementia, and the existence of Lewy body disease is not assumed. **Secondary parkinsonism** is Parkinson-type abnormal movements that are caused by medication or another condition.

CODING PRACTICE

Exercise 17.1 Nervous System Refresher

Instructions: Use your medical terminology skills and resources to define the following conditions related to the nervous system, then assign the default diagnosis code.

Follow these steps:

- Use slash marks "/" to break down each term into its root(s) and suffix.
- Define the meaning of the word based on the meaning of each word part.
- Assign the default ICD-10-CM diagnosis code for the condition using the Index and Tabular List.

Example: neuropathy neuro/pathy   Meaning: *abnormal condition of a nerve*   ICD-10-CM Code: *G62.9*

1. neuroma (benign)   Meaning _____   ICD-10-CM Code _____
2. neuromyelitis   Meaning _____   ICD-10-CM Code _____
3. encephalomyeloradiculitis Meaning _____   ICD-10-CM Code _____
4. causalgia   Meaning _____   ICD-10-CM Code _____
5. neuromyotonia   Meaning _____   ICD-10-CM Code _____
6. myelinolysis   Meaning _____   ICD-10-CM Code _____
7. hemichorea   Meaning _____   ICD-10-CM Code _____
8. meningoencephalopathy   Meaning _____   ICD-10-CM Code _____
9. myasthenia   Meaning _____   ICD-10-CM Code _____
10. hemiplegia   Meaning _____   ICD-10-CM Code _____

CODING OVERVIEW OF THE NERVOUS SYSTEM

ICD-10-CM Chapter 6, Diseases of the Nervous System and Sense Organs (G00-G99), contains 11 blocks or subchapters that are divided by the type of structure affected. Review the block names and code ranges listed at the beginning of Chapter 6 in the ICD-10-CM manual to become familiar with the content and organization.

ICD-10-CM Chapter 6 is comparable to ICD-9-CM Chapter 6 (320-389). Some codes from other chapters in ICD-9-CM have been moved to the nervous system chapter in ICD-10-CM. For example, ICD-10-CM category G45, Transient cerebral ischemic attacks, includes codes from ICD-9-CM Chapter 7, Diseases of the Circulatory System. Categories for Alzheimer disease (G30), migraine headaches (G43), secondary parkinsonism (G21), and dystonia (G24) are examples of categories in which codes have been significantly expanded in ICD-10-CM. Instructional notes have been expanded in ICD-10-CM, directing coders to use an external cause code, code first the underlying disease, and code first the underlying neoplasm.

This chapter includes disorders of the central and peripheral nervous systems as well as paralytic syndromes. It also includes the **gustatory** (*taste*) and **olfactory** (*smell*) sense organs. The eye and the ear, which were both part of Chapter 6 in ICD-9-CM, each has its own chapter in ICD-10-CM. This chapter does not include congenital disorders or injuries, which are classified in other ICD-10-CM chapters. This chapter also does not include cerebrovascular disease, which is classified with the circulatory system in block I60-I69. However, it does include transient ischemic attacks and related syndromes that were classified with the circulatory system in ICD-9-CM.

ICD-10-CM provides Official Guidelines for Coding and Reporting (OGCR) for the nervous system and sense organs in OGCR section I.C.6. OGCR provide detailed discussion of coding for pain, including general coding information, postoperative pain, chronic pain, neoplasm-related pain, and chronic pain syndrome. OGCR also discuss the definitions of dominant and nondominant side when coding hemiplegia. OGCR I.C.19.g.2) discusses pain due to devices, implants, and grafts. OGCR I.C.5.a discusses pain disorders related to psychological factors.

ABSTRACTING FOR CONDITIONS OF THE NERVOUS SYSTEM

When abstracting, coders analyze the medical record to highlight the key facts of the case and to identify details that will be important when assigning and sequencing codes. As coders gain experience in assigning and sequencing codes, they are able to abstract more quickly and more accurately. Review the questions in ■ TABLE 17-3 to learn key questions to ask when analyzing cases related to the nervous system. Remember that the abstracting questions are a guide and that not every question applies to, or can be answered for, every case. Because of the variety of conditions addressed under the nervous system, coders need general criteria for abstracting conditions of the nervous system overall (Table 17-3), as well as specific criteria to abstract pain (■ TABLE 17-4), headaches (■ TABLE 17-5), epilepsy (■ TABLE 17-6), and PD (■ TABLE 17-7).

Table 17-3 ■ KEY CRITERIA FOR ABSTRACTING CONDITIONS OF THE NERVOUS SYSTEM

- ❑ What is the condition?
- ❑ What is the subtype of the condition?
- ❑ What is the anatomic site?
- ❑ What is the underlying disease, if any?
- ❑ What is external cause, if any?
- ❑ What is the infectious organism, if any?
- ❑ What laterality is documented?
- ❑ Is paralysis documented?

Table 17-4 ■ KEY CRITERIA FOR ABSTRACTING PAIN

- ❑ What is the site of the pain?
- ❑ What is the underlying cause of the pain?
- ❑ Is the pain due to a device, implant, graft, or trauma?
- ❑ Is the pain postoperative?
- ❑ Is it related to a specific postoperative complication?
- ❑ Is the pain related to a neoplasm?
- ❑ Is pain management the reason for the encounter?
- ❑ Is treatment of the underlying condition the reason for the encounter?
- ❑ Is the pain documented as chronic?
- ❑ Is chronic pain syndrome documented?
- ❑ Is complex regional pain syndrome documented?
- ❑ What psychological factors are associated with the pain?

Table 17-5 ■ KEY CRITERIA FOR ABSTRACTING HEADACHES

- ❑ What specific type of headache is documented?
- ❑ Is it documented as intractable?
- ❑ Is the headache documented as episodic or chronic?
- ❑ Does it affect the entire head or only one side?
- ❑ Is the headache accompanied with aura?
- ❑ Is status migrainosus or duration of 72 hours or more documented?
- ❑ Is the headache associated with another condition such as trauma, menstruation, cerebral infarction, or drug use?

Table 17-6 ■ KEY CRITERIA FOR ABSTRACTING EPILEPSY

- ❑ Is the seizure documented as epilepsy?
- ❑ Is it localized or generalized?
- ❑ Is it documented as intractable?
- ❑ Is status epilepticus or duration of 30 minutes or more documented?
- ❑ Are partial seizures documented as simple or complex?

Table 17-7 ■ KEY CRITERIA FOR ABSTRACTING PARKINSON DISEASE

- ❑ Is parkinsonism primary or secondary?
- ❑ Is dementia documented?
- ❑ Is dementia documented as parkinsonian dementia or Parkinson disease with dementia?
- ❑ Is secondary parkinsonism documented?
- ❑ What is the cause?

SUCCESS STEP

Several conditions have been expanded in ICD-10-CM compared to what they were in ICD-9-CM, requiring additional abstracting. The most notable of these are epilepsy, migraines, AD, secondary parkinsonism, dystonia, and myasthenia gravis. Coders who have mastered ICD-9-CM should review these categories in ICD-10-CM carefully to learn the differences and new elements required.

SUCCESS STEP

Physicians do not need to use the exact word *intractable* to allow coders to abstract a migraine or epilepsy as intractable. Acceptable terms that mean intractable are *pharmacoresistant*, *pharmacologically resistant*, *treatment resistant*, *refractory*, and *poorly controlled*.

Guided Example of Abstracting for Nervous System Conditions

Refer to the following example throughout this chapter to practice skills for abstracting, assigning, and sequencing nervous system codes. Angelia Harkey, CPC, is a fictitious coder who guides you through the coding process.

Date: 7/11/yy   Location: Branton Medical Center

Provider: Lorene Garman, MD

Patient: Catalina Piatt   Gender: F   Age: 57

Reason for encounter: patient was admitted from the emergency department where she presented with left sided hemiparesis

Assessment: Imaging studies were negative for CVA, symptoms mitigated within 24 hours leading to a diagnosis of TIA. Patient received Duradrin (*a vasoconstrictor combination medication*) for classical migraine which responded to treatment. She received routine insulin for type 1 diabetes.

Plan: She was discharged to home with no residual weakness. FU in office 1 week.

Follow along as Angelia Harkey, CPC, abstracts the diagnosis. Check off each step after you complete it.

▶ Angelia reads through the entire record, paying special attention to the reason for the encounter and the final assessment.

❑ She notes that the presenting symptoms, left sided hemiparesis, were temporary and that imaging studies were negative for CVA, which she knows is a cerebrovascular accident, or a stroke.

❑ She reviews Key Criteria for Abstracting Conditions of the Nervous System (Table 17-3).

❑ *What is the condition?* She notes there is a definitive diagnosis of TIA, which is a transient ischemic attack. A TIA is a brief episode of ischemia that has temporary symptoms but causes no permanent damage.

❑ *What is the subtype of the condition?* None was listed.

❑ *What is the anatomic site?* A TIA by definition occurs in the brain.

❑ *What is the underlying disease, if any?* None.

❑ *What is the external cause, if any?* None.

❑ *What is the infectious organism, if any?* None.

❑ *What laterality is documented?* Temporary left-sided hemiparesis.

❑ *Is paralysis documented?* Temporary weakness is documented, but no paralysis.

❑ Because the left-sided hemiparesis was temporary and the underlying cause was diagnosed as TIA, she knows she should not code for the presenting symptom.

❑ She identifies that two additional conditions were treated during the admission: classical migraine and type 1 diabetes.

▶ At this time, Angelia has a good idea that she will have three diagnoses, but she will not know for certain until she completes the next step of assigning codes.

CODING PRACTICE

Exercise 17.2 Abstracting Diagnoses for the Nervous System

Instructions: Read the mini-medical-record of each patient's encounter and answer the abstracting questions. Write the answer on the line provided. Do not assign any codes.

1. OUTPATIENT HOSPITAL Gender: F Age: 31

Reason for encounter: patient comes in today for a migraine which started 2 days ago with aura

Assessment: pharmacoresistant migraine

Plan: Administered injection of sumatriptan and discussed potential side effects and how to manage. Rx oral sumatriptan. Patient to call nurse tomorrow to discuss progress.

a. What condition is documented? _____
_____

b. Is it documented as intractable? _____
_____

c. Is it documented as affecting only one side?
_____

d. Is the migraine accompanied with aura?
_____

e. Is status migrainosus or duration of 72 hours or more documented? _____

f. Is the headache associated with another condition: trauma, menstruation, cerebral infarction, or drug use? _____

2. OUTPATIENT HOSPITAL Gender: M Age: 9

Reason for encounter: video EEG (*video to monitor brain activity in real time*) as part of ongoing epilepsy evaluation

Assessment: benign childhood epilepsy with EEG spikes, poorly controlled at this time

Plan: we are going to start with Rx gabapentin monotherapy (*single-drug therapy*) and reevaluate in 4 weeks, consult with nutritionist re: diet modifications

a. What condition is documented? _____
_____

b. What is the type of epilepsy? _____
_____

c. Is it documented as intractable? _____
_____

d. Is status epilepticus or duration of 30 minutes or more documented? _____

3. OFFICE Gender: M Age: 51

Reason for encounter: management of PD, patient reports increased tremor activity and difficulty walking since last visit

Assessment: PD has progressed

Plan: adjusted medications, referred to physical therapy

(continued)

CODING PRACTICE (continued)

3. (continued)

a. What symptoms are reported? _____

_____

b. What condition is documented? _____

_____

c. Should you code the symptoms? _____

Why or why not? _____

d. Is the condition primary or secondary?

_____

e. Is dementia documented? _____

_____

---

4. INPATIENT HOSPITAL   Gender: F   Age: 33

Reason for admission: *implant neurostimulator (a device placed under the skin that stimulates the spinal cord by tiny electrical impulses) for pain control*

Assessment: *chronic lumbar pain due to displaced disc at L3-L4 which resulted from a back injury two years ago*

Plan: *FU 2 weeks*

a. What is the reason for admission? _____

_____

b. What is the site of the pain? _____

_____

c. What is the underlying cause of the pain?

_____

d. Is the pain due to a device, implant, graft, or trauma? _____

e. Is pain management the reason for the encounter? _____

f. Is treatment of the underlying condition the reason for the encounter? _____

g. Is the pain documented as chronic? _____

h. Is chronic pain syndrome documented?

_____

---

5. INPATIENT HOSPITAL   Gender: M   Age: 86

Reason for encounter: *admitted from nursing facility due to generalized weakness*

(continued)

---

5. (continued)

Assessment: *weakness is due to hyponatremia, patient presents an elopement risk due to late onset AD, dementia with hallucinations, and wandering*

Plan: *discharged to nursing facility*

a. What symptom is documented? _____

_____

b. What is the cause of the symptom? _____

c. What type of AD is documented? _____

_____

d. What is an elopement risk? _____

e. Is the dementia accompanied with behavioral disturbances? _____

f. What is the principal diagnosis? _____

_____

g. What additional diagnosis(es) should be coded? _____ Why? _____

---

6. INPATIENT HOSPITAL   Gender: F   Age: 42

Reason for admission: *admitted from emergency department where patient presented with migraine of 4 days' duration which has not responded to the usual medication*

Assessment: *persistent migraine with cerebrovascular infarction, cerebral stenosis of right cerebellar artery, hypertension*

a. What specific type of migraine is documented?

_____

b. Is it documented as intractable? _____

_____

c. Is the migraine accompanied with aura?

_____

d. Is status migrainosus or duration of 72 hours or more documented? _____

e. What other conditions are documented?

_____

f. What is the location of the cerebral stenosis?

_____

g. What is the principal diagnosis? _____

_____

ASSIGNING CODES FOR CONDITIONS OF THE NERVOUS SYSTEM

OGCR contain specific guidelines for assigning codes for hemiplegia and monoplegia and pain.

Assigning Codes for Hemiplegia and Monoplegia

According to the instructional note at the beginning of categories **G81**, **G82**, and **G83**, codes for **hemiplegia** (*paralysis of one side of the body*), **quadriplegia** (*paralysis of all limbs*), and **monoplegia** (*paralysis of one limb*) from this ICD-10-CM chapter should be assigned when the paralysis is reported without further specification or is stated to be old or long-standing but of unspecified cause. Also use these categories in multiple coding to identify these conditions resulting from any cause. When these conditions result from cerebrovascular disease, assign codes from category **I69 Sequelae of cerebrovascular disease**.

Codes for hemiplegia and monoplegia require coders to assign a fifth character to identify a combination of laterality and dominance. Dominance refers to the side of the body an individual favors, such as being left-handed or right-handed (■ FIGURE 17-3).

For *right-handed* persons, assign the fifth character as follows:

- **1** identifies that the right side (dominant) of a right-handed person is affected.
- **4** identifies that the left side (nondominant) of a right-handed person is affected.

For *left-handed* persons, assign the fifth character as follows:

- **2** identifies that the left side (dominant) of a left-handed person is affected (■ FIGURE 17-4).
- **3** identifies that the right side (nondominant) of a left-handed person is affected.

Assign the fifth character **0** when laterality is not documented.

When laterality is documented, but dominance is not, OGCR I.C.6.a instructs coders to code the right side as

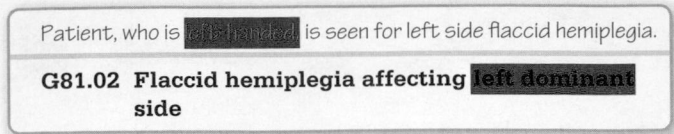

Figure 17-4 ■ Example of Hemiplegia Affecting Left Dominant Side

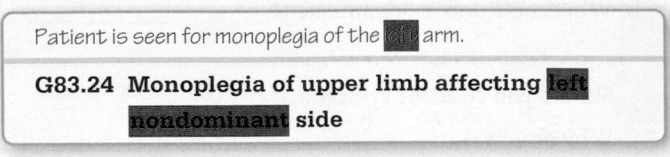

Figure 17-5 ■ Example of Monoplegia with Unspecified Dominance

dominant and the left side as nondominant (■ FIGURE 17-5). For ambidextrous patients, the default is to code the affected side as dominant.

Assigning Codes for Pain

OGCR I.C.6.b provides detailed guidance for assigning and sequencing codes from category **G89 Pain, not elsewhere classified**. Use this category *only* when pain is specified as acute or chronic, postthoracotomy, postprocedural, or neoplasm related. These codes may be used with codes from other categories and other chapters, including site-specific pain codes from ICD-10-CM Chapter 18, Symptoms, Signs and Abnormal Clinical and Laboratory Findings, when they provide additional information about the condition, such as whether the pain is acute or chronic.

SUCCESS STEP

You should code pain as acute or chronic based on the physician's documentation. There is no specific time frame that defines acute or chronic.

Coders must determine whether the underlying cause of the pain is known. If it is, assign codes from category **G89** *only* when the purpose of the encounter is to provide pain management (■ FIGURE 17-6), but not when the purpose of the encounter is to treat the underlying condition (■ FIGURE 17-7) (OGCR I.C.6.b.1 (a) and (b)).

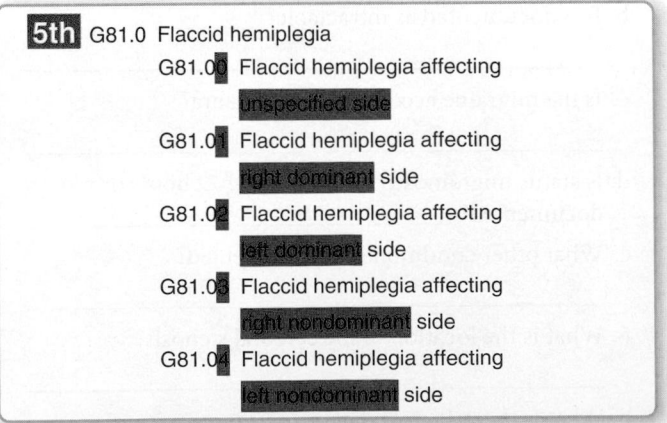

Figure 17-3 ■ Tabular List Entry Showing Dominance and Nondominance

Patient with a displaced C4-C5 disk due to trauma and associated severe chronic neck pain presents for a steroid injection in the spinal canal to relieve pain.

(1) **G89.21 Chronic pain due to trauma**
(2) **M50.22 Other cervical disc displacement, mid-cervical region**

Figure 17-6 ■ Example of an Encounter to Treat Pain

Patient with low-back pain due to a wedge compression fracture of lumbar vertebra L4 is seen ▓▓▓▓▓▓▓▓▓▓▓ *(a procedure to stabilize the vertebral segments).*

S32.040A   Wedge compression fracture of fourth lumbar vertebra, initial encounter for closed fracture

Figure 17-7 ■ Example of an Encounter to Treat the Underlying Condition

ICD-10-CM provides a specific code and specific OGCR for neoplasm related pain (OGCR I.C.6.b.5)). Assign code **G89.3 Neoplasm related pain (acute) (chronic)** when pain is documented as either acute or chronic for any of the following:

- neoplasm related
- cancer associated
- due to malignancy
- tumor associated

Also assign a code(s) for the neoplasm and/or metastases.

Refer to OGCR I.C.6.b.3) for instructions on coding postoperative pain.

CODING CAUTION

Be careful to distinguish codes for chronic pain (**G89.2-**), chronic pain syndrome (**G89.4**), and complex regional pain syndrome (CRPS) (**G90.5-**) based on the physician's documentation.

Guided Example of Assigning Codes for Nervous System Conditions

To practice assigning codes for diseases of the nervous system, continue with the example from earlier in the chapter about patient Catalina Piatt, who was admitted to Branton Medical Center due to left-sided hemiparesis.

Follow along in your ICD-10-CM manual as Angelia Harkey, CPC, assigns codes. Check off each step after you complete it.

▶ First, Angelia reviews the conditions she identified during abstracting:

❑ TIA

❑ classical migraine

❑ type 1 diabetes

▶ Angelia is most concerned about assigning a code for the migraine, so she begins with this diagnosis. She searches the Index for the Main Term **Migraine**.

❑ She locates the subterm **classical** and reads the cross-referencing note in the Index, *see* **Migraine, with aura**.

❑ Staying under the Main Term **Migraine**, she locates the subterm **with aura** (■ FIGURE 17-8).

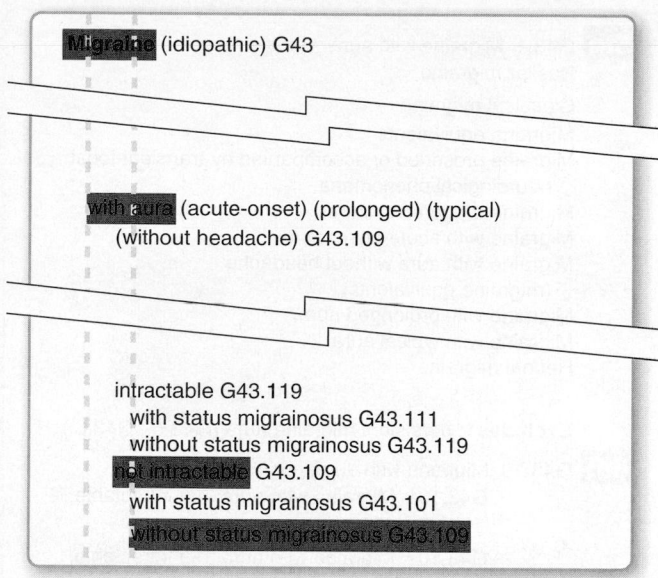

Migraine (idiopathic) G43

with aura (acute-onset) (prolonged) (typical) (without headache) G43.109

intractable G43.119
  with status migrainosus G43.111
  without status migrainosus G43.119
not intractable G43.109
  with status migrainosus G43.101
  without status migrainosus G43.109

Figure 17-8 ■ Index Entry for Migraine

❑ She notices that there are indented third-level subterms for **intractable, not intractable**, and **persistent**.

❑ She double-checks the medical record and notes that the physician documented *classical migraine which responded to treatment*. Because intractable means "not responsive to treatment," she determines that she should select a code for not intractable. Although the physician did not use the exact statement "not intractable," she is confident of the meaning of the term and proceeds.

❑ Under the entry for **not intractable**, she reads two additional indented subterms for **with** or **without status migrainosus**.

❑ She again double-checks the documentation and confirms that status migrainosus is not documented, so she selects the entry for **without status migrainosus, G43.109**.

❑ Angelia verifies code **G43.109** in the Tabular List (■ Figure 17-9, page 280).

❑ She reads the code title **G43.109, Migraine with aura, not intractable, without status migrainosus** and is concerned because the documentation did not state that the migraine was accompanied with aura.

❑ She reads the inclusion terms under the category heading **G43.1, Migraine with aura** and sees the term **Classical migraine**. The inclusion term confirms that this is the correct category to classify a classical migraine.

▶ Angelia checks for instructional notes in the Tabular List.

❑ Angelia cross-references the beginning of subcategory **G43.1, Migraine with aura** and reads the instructional notes. The note **Code also any associated seizure** does not apply because no seizure was documented.

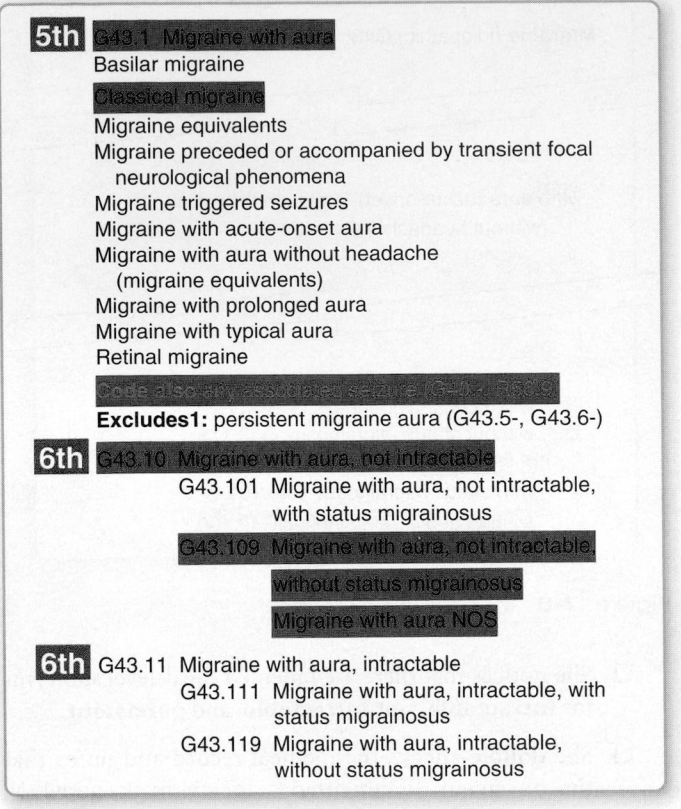

Figure 17-9 ■ Tabular List Entry for G43.1 Migraine with aura

❑ She cross-references the beginning of category **G43, Migraine** and reads the **NOTE** that defines intractable. She confirms that this case is not intractable.

❑ Angelia cross-references the beginning of the block **G40-G47 Episodic and paroxysmal disorders** and verifies that there are no instructional notes that apply to all codes in the block.

❑ She cross-references the beginning of **Chapter 6 (G00-G99)** and reviews the **Excludes2** note. She determines that it does not apply to this case because the patient does not have any of the conditions listed.

❑ Angelia finalizes the code assignment for the migraine, **G43.109, Migraine with aura, not intractable, without status migrainosus**.

▶ Next, Angelia assigns a code for the TIA. She searches the Index for the Main Term **Transient**.

❑ She reads the nonessential modifier (meaning homeless) and determines this is not the correct Main Term to use.

❑ She searches the Index for the Main Term **Attack**.

❑ She locates the subterm **transient ischemic (TIA) G45.9** and determines that this is an appropriate entry.

▶ Angelia verifies code **G45.9** in the Tabular List.

❑ She reads the code title **G45.9, Transient cerebral ischemic attack, unspecified**, and confirms that this describes the documentation.

❑ She confirms that this is the accurate code by reading the inclusion term **TIA** listed under code **G45.9**.

❑ She quickly rechecks the beginning of the category, block, and chapter for instructional notes and finds no notes that apply to this case.

❑ Angelia finalizes the code assignment **G45.9, Transient cerebral ischemic attack, unspecified**.

▶ Angelia checks her abstracting notes and identifies that she needs to assign a code for type 1 diabetes because it was treated during this admission.

❑ She searches the Index for the Main Term **Diabetes** and the subterm **type 1 E10.9**. No additional complications are documented, so none of the second-level subterms apply.

❑ She turns to the Tabular List to verify the code **E10.9, Type 1 diabetes mellitus without complications**.

❑ She cross-references the beginning of the category **E10**, the block **E08-E13**, and the chapter to identify that there are no further instructional notes that apply.

▶ Angelia reviews the codes for this case:

❑ **E10.9 Type 1 diabetes mellitus without complications**

❑ **G45.9 Transient cerebral ischemic attack, unspecified**

❑ **G43.109 Migraine with aura, not intractable, without status migrainosus**

▶ Next, Angelia must determine how to sequence the codes.

CODING PRACTICE

Exercise 17.3 Assigning Codes for Conditions of the Nervous System

Instructions: Read the mini-medical-record of each patient's encounter, review the information abstracted in Exercise 17.2, and assign ICD-10-CM diagnosis codes using the Index and Tabular List. Write the code(s) on the line provided.

1. OFFICE   Gender: F   Age: 31

Reason for encounter: *patient comes in today for a migraine which started 2 days ago with aura*

Assessment: *pharmacoresistant migraine*

(continued)

1. (continued)

Plan: *Administered injection of sumatriptan (a medication used to treat migraines) and discussed potential side effects and how to manage. Rx oral sumatriptan. Patient to call nurse tomorrow to discuss progress.*

Tip: Be sure to review the meaning of intractable.

1 ICD-10-CM Code _____

2. (continued)

Plan: *we are going to start with Rx gabapentin monotherapy (single-drug therapy) and reevaluate in 4 weeks, consult with nutritionist re: diet modifications*

Tip: Read and follow the cross-referencing instruction in the Index.

1 ICD-10-CM Code _____

2. OUTPATIENT HOSPITAL Gender: M Age: 9

Reason for encounter: *video EEG as part of ongoing epilepsy evaluation*

Assessment: *benign childhood epilepsy with EEG spikes, poorly controlled at this time*

(continued)

3. OFFICE Gender: M Age: 51

Reason for encounter: *management of PD, patient reports increased tremor activity and difficulty walking since last visit*

Assessment: *PD has progressed*

Plan: *adjusted medications, referred to physical therapy*

1 ICD-10-CM Code _____

ARRANGING CODES FOR CONDITIONS OF THE NERVOUS SYSTEM

Sequencing codes that include codes for pain is determined by the circumstances of the encounter. When the purpose of the encounter is to manage the pain, sequence the code for pain first. When the purpose of the encounter is to treat the underlying condition, sequence the code for the condition first. Follow the same procedure when coding neoplasm-related pain. Refer to the examples in ■ FIGURE 17-10 and ■ FIGURE 17-11 to learn more about sequencing codes for neoplasm-related pain.

Guided Example of Arranging Codes for Nervous System Conditions

To practice skills for sequencing codes for diseases of the nervous system, continue with the example from earlier in the chapter about patient Catalina Piatt, who was admitted to Branton Medical Center due to left-sided hemiparesis.

Follow along in your ICD-10-CM manual as Angelia Harkey, CPC, sequences the codes. Check off each step after you complete it.

▶ Angelia reviews the codes she assigned for this case:

❑ **E10.9 Type 1 diabetes mellitus without complications**

❑ **G45.9 Transient cerebral ischemic attack, unspecified**

❑ **G43.109 Migraine with aura, not intractable, without status migrainosus**

▶ First, Angelia needs to determine the principal diagnosis.

❑ She refers back to the medical record and confirms that the reason established after study for the admission and the services provided is TIA.

❑ She sequences **G45.9, Transient cerebral ischemic attack, unspecified** first, as the principal diagnosis.

❑ She refers to the OGCR I.C.4 and 6 to determine whether any sequencing guidelines apply for the migraine and diabetes but finds none.

❑ She refers to OGCR Section III, Reporting Additional Diagnoses, and verifies that because the migraine and

Patient is admitted ▮▮▮▮▮▮▮▮▮▮▮▮ related to metastatic pancreatic cancer.

(1) **G89.3 Neoplasm related pain** (acute) (chronic)
(2) **C25.9 Malignant neoplasm of pancreas, unspecified**
(3) **C79.9 Secondary malignant neoplasm of unspecified site**

Figure 17-10 ■ Example of an Encounter to Treat Neoplasm-Related Pain

Patient is admitted ▮▮▮▮▮▮▮▮▮▮▮▮ for lung cancer and also reports severe neoplasm-related pain.

(1) **C34.12 Malignant neoplasm of upper lobe, left bronchus or lung**
(2) **G89.3 Neoplasm related pain** (acute) (chronic)

Figure 17-11 ■ Example of an Encounter to Treat the Neoplasm, with Pain as an Additional Diagnosis

CONCEPT QUIZ

Take a moment to look back at the nervous system and sense organs and solidify your skills. Try to answer the questions from memory first, then refer back to the discussion in the chapter if you need a little extra help.

Completion

Instructions: Write the term that answers each question based on the information you learned in this chapter. Choose from the list below. Some choices may be used more than once and some choices may not be used at all.

30	epilepsy
60	hydrocephalus
72	laterality
brain	meningitis
CNS	PNS
dominance	spina bifida
electrocardiogram	spinal cord
electroencephalogram	status epilepticus
encephalitis	status migrainosus

1. The _____ acts as the control center for the nervous system by processing information and providing short-term control over other organ systems.

2. _____ is a viral inflammation of the brain and meninges.

3. _____ is a brain disorder in which neurons signal abnormally, causing seizures and/or unconsciousness.

4. The _____ is a common site of metastases from cancers in other organs.

5. The _____ consists of the 12 nerves that radiate out from the brain and the 31 pairs of nerves that radiate from the spinal cord to all other areas of the body.

6. When a condition is _____, it is resistant to treatment.

7. _____ refers to the side of the body an individual favors, such as being left-handed or right-handed.

8. _____ is a recording of the electrical activity of the brain.

9. _____ is a congenital neural tube defect in which vertebrae do not fuse.

10. Status epilepticus is an epileptic seizure lasting more than _____ minutes.

Multiple Choice

Instructions: Circle the letter of the best answer to each question based on the information you learned in this chapter.

1. The maintenance of a stable internal physical state of the body is
   A. hemostasis.
   B. equilibrium.
   C. homeostasis.
   D. intractable.

2. Which of the following terms does NOT mean resistant to treatment?
   A. Poorly controlled
   B. Pharmacoresistant
   C. Refractory
   D. Status migrainosus

3. _____ seizures are the result of abnormal activity on both sides of the brain.
   A. Simple partial
   B. Psychomotor
   C. Status epilepticus
   D. Generalized

4. Parkinson disease that is followed by a diagnosis of dementia at a later time is
   A. Parkinson disease with dementia.
   B. parkinsonian dementia.
   C. Lewy body disease.
   D. secondary parkinsonism.

5. Which of the following is NOT a key criterion for abstracting headaches?
   A. Is it documented as intractable?
   B. Does it affect the entire head or only one side?
   C. Is a duration of 30 minutes or more documented?
   D. Is it accompanied with aura?

6. Hemiplegia of the right arm in a left-handed person should be coded as
   A. right dominant.
   B. left dominant.
   C. right nondominant.
   D. left nondominant.

7. Codes from category G89 Pain, not elsewhere classified should NOT be assigned when
   A. pain is documented as acute.
   B. the underlying condition is the reason for the encounter.
   C. pain is related to neoplasm.
   D. pain is documented as chronic.

8. Classical migraine is the same as
   A. migraine with aura.
   B. intractable migraine.
   C. cluster headache.
   D. status migrainosus.

9. Which of the following IS a key criterion for abstracting pain?
   A. Is it due to a device, implant, graft, or trauma?
   B. Is it documented as intractable?
   C. Is paralysis documented?
   D. Is a duration of 72 hours or more documented?

10. Which of the following is the most common neoplasm of the nervous system?
    A. Primary malignant neoplasm
    B. Metastasis to the brain
    C. Benign neoplasm of the brain
    D. Benign neoplasm of the PNS

CODING CHALLENGE

Instructions: Read the mini-medical-record of each patient's encounter, then abstract, assign, and sequence ICD-10-CM diagnosis codes using the Index and Tabular List. Write the code(s) on the line provided.

1. OUTPATIENT HOSPITAL   Gender: M   Age: 36

Reason for encounter: Patient presents to the infusion center for treatment of meningitis

Assessment: *Staphylococcal* meningitis

Plan: FU in 3 days and 1 week after antibiotic infusions are complete

Tip: Read the instructional notes in the Tabular List.

2 ICD-10-CM Codes _____

2. INPATIENT HOSPITAL   Gender: M   Age: 60

Reason for admission: acute respiratory distress

Assessment: myasthenia gravis crisis, chronic inflammatory demyelinating polyneuropathy (CIDP) (*an inflammatory disorder of PNS due to abnormal immune activity*)

Plan: Rx cholinesterase inhibitor and immunosuppressant drugs. FU 1 week

2 ICD-10-CM Codes _____

3. OFFICE   Gender: F   Age: 13

Reason for encounter: increase in number and intensity of myoclonic seizures.

Assessment: poorly controlled juvenile myoclonic epilepsy (JME)

Plan: valporoic acide dosage changes

Tip: Read the cross-reference instruction in the Index.

1 ICD-10-CM Code _____

4. OFFICE   Gender: M   Age: 18

Reason for encounter: EEG

Assessment: focal seizures

Plan: Rx Dilantin

Tip: Read the cross-reference instruction in the Index.

1 ICD-10-CM Code _____

5. OFFICE   Gender: M   Age: 44

Reason for encounter: Continuing lower back pain with radiating pain in left hip. Patient has had surgical repair of several ruptured discs and is overweight and sedentary.

Assessment: chronic pain syndrome

Plan: acetaminophen, consult with dietician for weight loss plan, 12 session physical therapy followed by regular exercise, RTO in 4 weeks

2 ICD-10-CM Codes _____

6. INPATIENT HOSPITAL   Gender: F   Age: 12

Reason for admission: recurring headaches, problems with balance, poor coordination, gait disturbances

Assessment: normal-pressure hydrocephalus

Plan: placement of ventriculoperitoneal shunt (*a tube that drains fluid from the brain into the peritoneal cavity*)

1 ICD-10-CM Code _____

7. OFFICE   Gender: M   Age: 55

Reason for encounter: sleep study

Assessment: obstructive sleep apnea, nutritional obesity with BMI 33.0

Plan: Rx **continuous positive airway pressure (CPAP) device**, refer to dietician for weight loss

3 ICD-10-CM Codes _____

_____

8. OFFICE   Gender: F   Age: 68

Reason for encounter: carpal tunnel release, right hand, endoscopic

Assessment: carpal tunnel syndrome and diabetes type 2 with polyneuropathy

Plan: FU 3 weeks

2 ICD-10-CM Codes _____

(*continued*)

(continued from page 285)

---

9. OFFICE Gender: F Age: 58

Reason for encounter: pain in the calf muscle, muscle weakness and cramping in thighs and upper arms

Assessment: alcohol dependence with alcoholic myopathy

Plan: referral to alcohol counseling and nutritionist, RTO 1 week

2 ICD-10-CM Codes _____

---

10. OFFICE Gender: F Age: 43

Reason for encounter: physical therapy

Assessment: long-standing left-sided hemiplegia due to encephalitis 20 years ago

Plan: return 1 week

Tip: Refer to OGCR I.C.6.a for coding of hemiplegia. Remember that 20 years ago means that the hemiplegia is a sequela of encephalitis.

2 ICD-10-CM Codes _____

KEEP ON CODING

Instructions: Read the diagnostic statement, then use the Index and Tabular List to assign and sequence ICD-10-CM diagnosis codes. Write the code(s) on the line provided.

1. Pneumococcal meningitis: ICD-10-CM Code(s) _____

2. Metastatic carcinoma of the thalamus from primary cancer of the right breast: ICD-10-CM Code(s) _____

3. Accidental puncture of the meninges during a nervous system operative procedure: ICD-10-CM Code(s) _____

4. Alper disease: ICD-10-CM Code(s) _____

5. Migraine with an aura: ICD-10-CM Code(s) _____

6. Restless legs syndrome: ICD-10-CM Code(s) _____

7. Vascular parkinsonism: ICD-10-CM Code(s) _____

8. Amyotrophic lateral sclerosis: ICD-10-CM Code(s) _____

9. Blepharospasm: ICD-10-CM Code(s) _____

10. Epilepsy due to syphilis: ICD-10-CM Code(s) _____

11. Menstrual migraine, intractable without status migrainosus: ICD-10-CM Code(s) _____

12. Narcolepsy with cataplexy: ICD-10-CM Code(s) _____

13. Huntington chorea: ICD-10-CM Code(s) _____

14. Headache due to lumbar puncture: ICD-10-CM Code(s) _____

15. Ataxic cerebral palsy: ICD-10-CM Code(s) _____

16. Guillian-Barré syndrome: ICD-10-CM Code(s) _____

17. Myasthenia gravis without exacerbation: ICD-10-CM Code(s) _____

18. Intractable epilepsy with status epilepticus: ICD-10-CM Code(s) _____

19. Primary central sleep apnea: ICD-10-CM Code(s) _____

20. Spasmotic torticollis: ICD-10-CM Code(s) _____

21. Postpolio myelitic syndrome: ICD-10-CM Code(s) _____

22. Tropical spastic paraplegia: ICD-10-CM Code(s) _____

23. Medulloblastoma: ICD-10-CM Code(s) _____

24. Alzheimer disease: ICD-10-CM Code(s) _____

25. Episodic tension-type headache: ICD-10-CM Code(s) _____

Mental, Behavioral, and Neurodevelopmental Disorders (F01-F99)

Chapter 18

Learning Objectives

After completing this chapter, you should have the skills to:

18.1 Spell and define the key words, medical terms, and abbreviations related to mental, behavioral, and neurodevelopmental disorders.

18.2 Discuss the common types of mental, behavioral, and neurodevelopmental disorders.

18.3 Identify the main characteristics of coding for mental, behavioral, and neurodevelopmental disorders.

18.4 Abstract diagnostic information from the medical record for coding mental, behavioral, and neurodevelopmental disorders.

18.5 Assign codes for mental, behavioral, and neurodevelopmental disorders.

18.6 Arrange multiple codes for mental, behavioral, and neurodevelopmental disorders.

18.7 Discuss the Official Guidelines for Coding and Reporting related to mental, behavioral, and neurodevelopmental disorders.

Chapter Outline

- **Psychiatry Refresher**
- **Coding Overview of Psychiatry**
- **Abstracting Diagnoses for Psychiatry**
- **Assigning Diagnosis Codes for Psychiatry**
- **Arranging Diagnosis Codes for Psychiatry**

Key Terms and Abbreviations

abuse (substance)
addiction
behavioral disorder
behavioral disturbance
blood alcohol concentration (BAC)
blood alcohol content
blood alcohol level (BAL)

delirium
delusion
dependence (substance)
hallucination
in remission
intellectual disability
intoxication

Lewy body disease
mental disorder
neurodevelopmental disorder
paranoia
perceptual disturbance
psychoactive substance

psychotherapy
schizophrenia
schizothymia
tolerate
use (substance)
vascular dementia

In addition to the key terms listed here, students should know the terms defined within tables in this chapter.

 For updates and corrections, visit our student resource site at

www.pearsonhighered.com/healthprofessionsresources

INTRODUCTION

According to the National Highway Traffic Safety Administration (NHTSA), on any given day there are 1,400 injuries and 29 deaths due to drunk driving. Substance abuse is just one of many topics in the ICD-10-CM chapter on mental, behavioral, and neurodevelopmental disorders, but it occupies a significant portion of the codes.

A psychiatrist specializes in diagnosing and treating mental, behavioral, and neurodevelopmental disorders and also prescribes medications to treat those disorders. Other providers who may also treat mental, behavioral, and neurodevelopmental disorders are clinical psychologists, social workers, and therapists. However, these nonphysician providers cannot prescribe medication. Primary care physicians screen for mental, behavioral, and neurodevelopmental disorders and usually refer patients who need treatment to one of these specialists. For the sake of brevity, this chapter refers to mental, behavioral, and neurodevelopmental disorders as psychiatry.

As you read this chapter, open up your medical terminology book and keep a medical dictionary handy to refresh your memory of any unfamiliar terms. Many psychiatric conditions are part of your daily vocabulary, so a reference book will help you understand the medical meaning of these terms.

PSYCHIATRY REFRESHER

Mental, behavioral, and neurodevelopmental disorders are real, not imagined, disorders that have diagnostic criteria and are proven to respond to treatment. **Mental disorders** are psychological or physical conditions that disrupt an individual's personality, mind, and emotions in such a way that they affect the ability to function and interact with others. **Behavioral disorders** are manifestations of mental disturbances that result in extreme or disruptive conduct, such as rage, withdrawal, or substance abuse. **Neurodevelopmental disorders** are conditions that result from impaired development of the nervous system during infancy or childhood. Although mental, behavioral, and neurodevelopmental disorders are not fully understood by scientists, they are believed to be caused by a combination of psychological, environmental, biological, and social factors (■ FIGURE 18-1).

As you learn about conditions and procedures related to mental, behavioral, and neurodevelopmental disorders, remember to apply medical terminology skills to use word roots, prefixes, and suffixes you already know to define new terms. Refer to ■ TABLE 18-1 for a refresher on how to build medical terms related to mental, behavioral, and neurodevelopmental disorders.

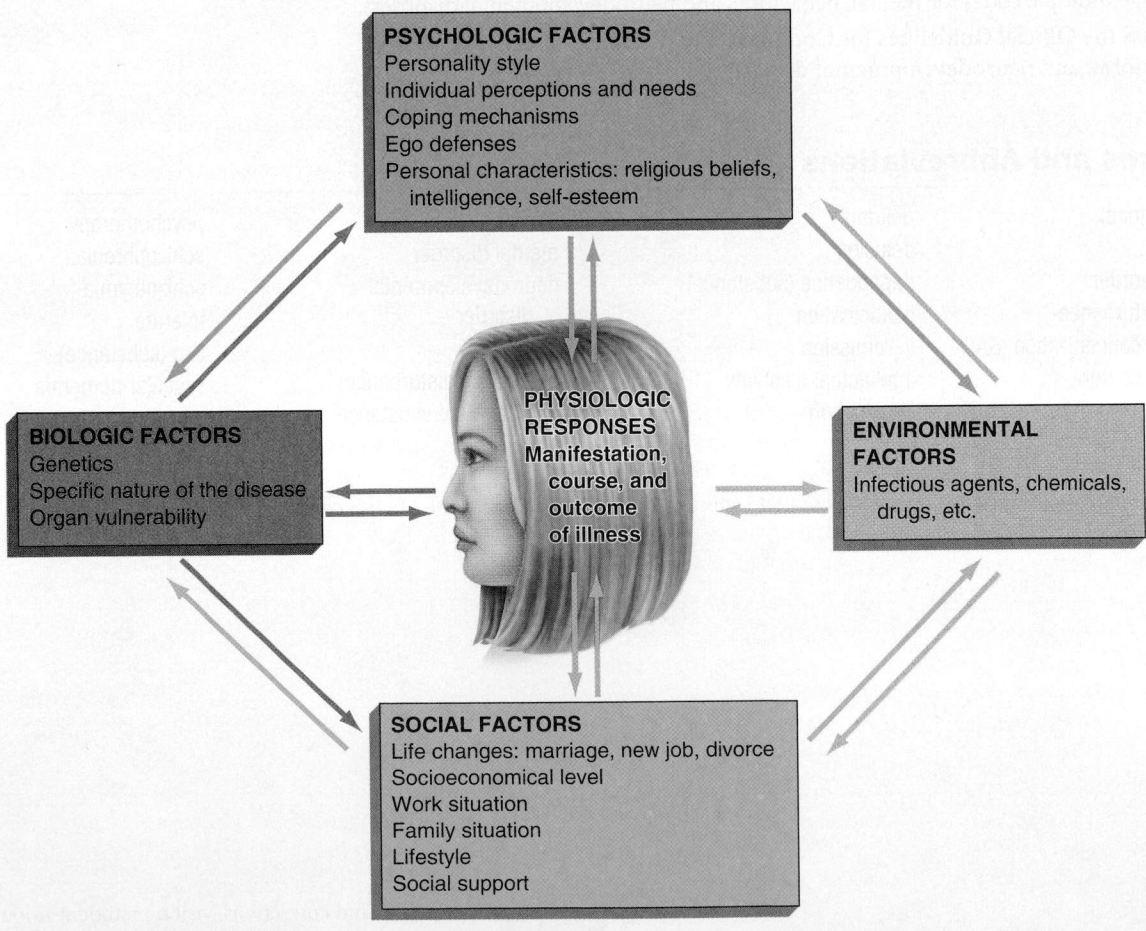

Figure 18-1 ■ Factors Contributing to Mental Health and Mental Illness

Table 18-1 ■ **EXAMPLE OF CONSTRUCTING MEDICAL TERMS FOR PSYCHIATRIC DISORDERS**

Prefix/Combining Form	Suffix	Complete Medical Term
dys- (*abnormal, painful*) para- (*beside*)	-thymia (*condition of the mind or emotion*) -phrenia (*condition of the mind*) -asthenia (*lack of strength*)	dys + thymia (*abnormal condition of the mind*) schizo + thymia (*condition of a split mind*)
schiz/o (*split*)		schizo + phrenia (*condition of a split mind*) para + phrenia (*condition beside the mind*)
psych/o (*mind*)		psycho + genic (*originating in the mind*) psycho + asthenia (*lack of strength in the mind*)

Medical terms may seem confusing because the literal meaning of the word parts may not fully describe how the word is used, particularly in the area of mental, behavioral, and neurodevelopmental disorders. For example, **para-** means *beside* or *beyond* and **-noia** means *mind*. The literal meaning of **paranoia** is beside or beyond the mind, but the word is used to mean a mental condition of delusions of persecution. The suffixes **-thymia** and **-phrenia** both mean *mind*, but **schizothymia** (*tendency toward being severely introverted*) is a different and less serious condition than **schizophrenia** (*a condition characterized by the inability to distinguish between thoughts and reality*). Coders understand that they use medical terminology skills to gain a basic understanding; they also need to know how a term is actually used within the context of the medical field.

CODING CAUTION

Be alert for medical terms that sound similar but are spelled differently and have different meanings.

thym/o (*thymus gland*) and **-thymia** (*condition of the mind*)

dysthymia (*depression*) and **dysrhythmia** (*abnormal heartbeat*)

Psychiatric Conditions

The National Institutes of Health (NIH) estimates that nearly 25% of adults experience a mental health disorder each year, and 6% of adults and 10% of children live with a serious mental disorder. Mental, behavioral, and neurodevelopmental disorders are classified into broad types (■ TABLE 18-2, page 290). Psychiatrists (*medical doctors, MDs, who diagnose and treat mental disorders*) and psychologists (*nonphysicians with advanced training, such as a masters degree or PhD, in psychology*) use written tests, observation, and interviews to diagnose mental, behavioral, and neurodevelopmental disorders. Psychiatrists prescribe medication and provide **electroconvulsive therapy** to treat mental disorders. Both psychiatrists and psychologists use **psychotherapy** to treat patients. Psychotherapy employs nonphysical techniques, such as talking, interpreting, listening, rewarding, and role playing, to treat disorders.

In particular, coders must be familiar with the terminology related to psychoactive substance use and dementia in order to code accurately.

Psychoactive Substance Disorders

Psychoactive substances have the ability to alter behavior, impair judgment, or create medical problems. Inappropriate use of such products can create legal, social, employment, family, and medical problems. Psychoactive substance disorders may involve legal substances, such as tobacco, alcohol, and, in some states, cannabis; illegal substances, such as heroin, cocaine, or cannabis; or prescribed medications, such as pain relievers or tranquilizers, that are used inappropriately. Substances may be taken orally, inhaled through breathing or smoking, injected into veins, or snorted (placed on mucosa of the mouth or nose). They are classified by their effect on the mind and body (■ TABLE 18-3, page 290).

Usage patterns of substances are described as use, abuse, dependence, or in remission, as follows:

- **use**—consuming the substance in moderate amounts that do not create significant legal, social, employment, family, or medical problems.
- **abuse**—using the substance in quantity or frequency that creates legal, employment, social, or family problems, or places the individual at physical risk, without causing physical dependence.
- **dependence**—compulsive reliance on the substance to the extent that it is physically or psychologically difficult to stop despite the significant problems it creates; also called **addiction**.
- **in remission**—a history of past drug or alcohol dependence documented by the physician.

Intoxication occurs when more of the substance is consumed than a person can physically **tolerate** (*absorb*), resulting in behavioral or physical abnormalities. The level of potential alcohol **impairment** is estimated based on a person's **blood alcohol level (BAL)**, which measures the amount of alcohol present in the blood. BAL is computed as the number of milligrams (mg) of alcohol per 100 milliliters (mL) of blood. BAL may be expressed as a ratio, a percentage, or a number. For example, a BAL of *80 mg per 100 mL* is the same as a BAL of *0.08%*, which may also be written without the percent sign as *.08*. To convert a percentage, such as *0.08%*, to a ratio, simply add a *0* to the end of the percentage and drop the leading decimal point to arrive at *80 mg per 100 mL*.

Table 18-2 ■ COMMON MENTAL, BEHAVIORAL, AND NEURODEVELOPMENTAL DISORDERS

Type of Disorder	Definition	Examples
Adjustment	Abnormal difficulty in responding to life changes	Adjustment disorder with anxiety, adjustment disorder with depressed mood
Anxiety	Abnormal anxiety that interferes with normal activities	Panic disorder, social phobia, obsessive-compulsive, posttraumatic stress disorder (PTSD)
Cognitive	Failure to develop or deterioration of mental comprehension	Autism, dementia, intellectual disability
Dissociative	Disruption in consciousness, memory, identity, or perception	Multiple personality amnesia
Eating	Serious disturbance in eating behavior	Anorexia nervosa, bulimia nervosa
Impulse-control	Extreme difficulty in controlling impulses, despite the negative consequences	Intermittent explosive disorder, **kleptomania**, **pyromania**, pathological gambling
Mood (affective)	Instability of mood	Major depression, mania, bipolar disorder
Personality	Persistent inflexible patterns of behavior that affect interpersonal relationships	Cluster A: Paranoid and schizoid Cluster B: Antisocial, borderline, histrionic, and narcissistic Cluster C: Avoidant, dependent, obsessive-compulsive
Psychotic	Delusions (*false beliefs that hinder the ability to function*) and hallucinations (*false visual, auditory, olfactory, or* **tactile** *perceptions*)	Schizophrenia (catatonic type, disorganized type, paranoid type, undifferentiated type, residual type); delusional disorder; brief psychotic disorder
Sexual	Repetitive and prolonged sexual activity and sexual dysfunction that interferes with normal relationships or daily activities	Gender identity disorder, pedophilia, voyeurism
Sleeping	Abnormal sleep problems	Insomnia, sleepwalking
Somatoform	Physical symptoms that are not explained by medical conditions	Hypochondriasis, body dysmorphoric disorder (BDD), pain disorder
Substance	Drug and alcohol use, abuse, and addiction	Alcoholism, tobacco dependence, illicit drug use

Table 18-3 ■ COMMONLY ABUSED SUBSTANCES

Classification	Effect	Examples
Alcohol (ethanol)	Reduces tension, promotes relaxation	Beer, wine, liquor (scotch, gin, vodka, rum)
Barbituate (sedative)	Reduces tension, promotes relaxation	Phenobarbital, tuinal, secobarbital, "downers"
Hallucinogen	Promotes relaxation, changes mood, thoughts, and behavior	Cannabis (marijuana), hashish, LSD, PCP
Narcotic (opiate)	Reduces physical pain and anxiety	Opium, cocaine, heroin, morphine, codeine, meperidine (Demerol), fentanyl, hydrocodone (Vicodin), oxycodone (OxyContin)
Nicotine	Stimulant, increases feelings of confidence and elevates mood	Cigarettes, cigars, pipes, smokeless tobacco, chewing tobacco
Stimulant	Increases feelings of confidence, alertness, and well-being	Amphetamine, "meth" (methamphetamine), dextroamphetamine (Dexedrine), speed, crank
Tranquilizer	Reduces anxiety, induces sleep	Diazepam (Valium), lorazepam (Ativan), alprazolam (Xanax)

Dementia

Dementia is a progressive loss of brain function that affects memory, thinking, language, judgment, and behavior. A leading cause is Lewy body disease in which patients have abnormal protein structures in certain areas of the brain. Vascular dementia is caused by many small strokes. Dementia may be a manifestation of substance abuse disorders or other nervous systems diseases such as Parkinson disease, multiple sclerosis, and Alzheimer disease. Most dementia is accompanied by behavioral disturbances such as aggression, wandering, depression, delusion or hallucinations, sleep disturbances, or poor eating habits.

CODING PRACTICE

Exercise 18.1 **Psychiatry Refresher**

Instructions: Use your medical terminology skills and resources to define the following conditions related to mental, behavioral, and neurodevelopmental disorders, then assign the diagnosis code.

Follow these steps:

- Use slash marks "/" to break down each term into its root(s) and suffix.
- Define the meaning of the word, based on the meaning of each word part.
- Assign the default ICD-10-CM diagnosis code for the condition using the Index and Tabular List.

Example: arachnophobia arachno/phobia   Meaning: *fear of spiders*   ICD-10-CM Code: *F40.210*

1. agoraphobia   Meaning _____   ICD-10-CM Code _____
2. psychasthenia   Meaning _____   ICD-10-CM Code _____
3. trichotillomania   Meaning _____   ICD-10-CM Code _____
4. hypomania   Meaning _____   ICD-10-CM Code _____
5. pedophilia   Meaning _____   ICD-10-CM Code _____
6. hematophobia   Meaning _____   ICD-10-CM Code _____
7. dysmorphophobia   Meaning _____   ICD-10-CM Code _____
8. somnambulism   Meaning _____   ICD-10-CM Code _____
9. paraphilia   Meaning _____   ICD-10-CM Code _____
10. pseudocyesis   Meaning _____   ICD-10-CM Code _____

CODING OVERVIEW OF PSYCHIATRY

ICD-10-CM Chapter 5, Mental, Behavioral, and Neurodevelopmental Disorders (F01-F99), contains 11 blocks or subchapters that are divided by the type of disorder. Review the block names and code ranges listed at the beginning of Chapter 5 in the ICD-10-CM manual to become familiar with the content and organization.

ICD-10-CM Chapter 5 is comparable to ICD-9-CM Chapter 4 (290-319). Categories for mental, behavioral, and neurodevelopmental disorders due to psychoactive substance use, F10 through F19, are expanded and more detailed in ICD-10-CM. Codes differentiate between abuse, dependence, and unspecified use and also identify complications, such as delusions, hallucinations, or sleep disturbances. Categories for intellectual disabilities, F70 through F79, provide instructional notes to code first any associated physical or developmental disorder.

This chapter includes mental, behavioral, and neurodevelopmental disorders with physiological causes; personality, mood, and schizophrenic disorders; substance disorders; intellectual disabilities; and developmental disorders. It does not include symptoms and signs, neurological disorders, or congenital conditions.

ICD-10-CM provides Official Guidelines for Coding and Reporting (OGCR) for mental, behavioral, and neurodevelopmental disorders in OGCR section I.C.5. The OGCR provide detailed discussion of pain disorders related to psychological factors and mental, behavioral, and neurodevelopmental disorders due to substance abuse. Additional guidelines related to pain appear in OGCR I.C.6.b.

The American Psychiatric Association (APA) uses the *Diagnostic and Statistical Manual of Mental Disorders* (DSM) to diagnose and classify mental disorders. In addition to codes, the manual also lists known causes of disorders, statistics regarding gender, age at onset, prognosis, and research concerning optimal approaches. DSM-5 was released in 2013. Because the DSM numbering system parallels the one that was used in ICD-9-CM, it does not correspond to the ICD-10-CM numbering system and requires that users convert or crosswalk DSM-5 codes to ICD-10-CM. DSM is not a HIPAA-approved code set and cannot be used for insurance billing.

ABSTRACTING DIAGNOSES FOR PSYCHIATRY

Many mental, behavioral, and neurodevelopmental disorders have multiple subtypes, so coders must be particularly attentive to the documented wording of the condition. For example, a substance disorder may be stated as use, abuse, or dependence, each of which has a specific meaning and different codes. Some disorders, such as dementia, may have underlying physiological conditions that must be identified and abstracted as well. Diseases and conditions classified in other ICD-10-CM body system chapters, such as digestive, circulatory, and nervous systems, contain frequent instructional notes to assign an additional code for use, abuse, or dependence on alcohol or nicotine.

The table that follows provides general criteria for abstracting mental, behavioral, and neurodevelopmental disorders (■ TABLE 18-4). Remember that the abstracting questions are a guide and that not every question applies to, or can be answered for, every case. For example, not every disorder is described based on whether it is in remission. Coders should be alert to the fact that some conditions do have this criterion, so they should always double-check the documentation to see if such information is present. Additional tables provide specific criteria for abstracting mood disorders (■ TABLE 18-5) and substance disorders (■ TABLE 18-6).

Guided Example of Abstracting Diagnoses for Psychiatry

Refer to the following example throughout this chapter to learn about abstracting, assigning, and sequencing mental,

Table 18-4 ■ KEY CRITERIA FOR ABSTRACTING GENERAL PSYCHIATRIC DISORDERS

❏ What is the disorder?

❏ What is the specific subtype of disorder?

❏ Is the disorder due to an underlying physiological condition?

❏ Does the patient report symptoms that have no medical cause?

❏ What is the severity?

❏ Is the condition in remission?

Table 18-5 ■ KEY CRITERIA FOR ABSTRACTING MOOD DISORDERS

❏ What is the disorder?

❏ Does it have psychotic features?

❏ Is the condition current or in remission?

❏ Is the current or most recent episode manic, depressed, or mixed?

❏ Is the severity mild, moderate, or severe?

❏ Is remission partial or full?

Table 18-6 ■ KEY CRITERIA FOR ABSTRACTING PSYCHOACTIVE SUBSTANCE DISORDERS

❏ What is the specific substance?

❏ What is the class of substance (opioid, sedative, stimulant, hallucinogen, inhalant)?

❏ Is the disorder one of use, abuse, or dependence?

❏ Does the provider clearly document the relationship between the mental or behavioral disorder and the substance use?

❏ What is the blood alcohol level?

❏ Is intoxication present?

❏ Is withdrawal present?

❏ Is delirium (*state of confusion, restlessness, and incoherence*) or perceptual disturbance (*misinterpretation of surroundings or events*) present?

❏ Are any associated hallucinations, delusions, or other psychotic conditions present?

❏ Is the condition in remission?

behavioral, and neurodevelopmental disorder codes. Ladonna Shuck, CPC, is a fictitious coder who will guide you through the coding process.

Date: 8/11/yy   Location: Valley Hospital

Provider: Brett Camden, MD

Patient: Cody Locust   Gender: M   Age: 58

Reason for admission: admitted from the emergency department with coma

Assessment: Alcoholic liver failure with coma for 4 hours, alcohol dependent abuse for 15 years with intoxication at admission, BAL .23%. Early onset Alzheimer dementia with behavioral disturbance was managed as well.

Plan: discharge to rehab program

Follow along as Ladonna Shuck, CPC, abstracts the diagnosis. Check off each step after you complete it.

▶ Ladonna reads through the entire record, paying special attention to the reason for the encounter and the final assessment. She notes that the patient was admitted with a coma that lasted for four hours and was later diagnosed with alcoholic liver disease.

▶ Ladonna refers to the Key Criteria for Abstracting Psychoactive Substance Disorders (Table 18-6).

  ❏ *What is the specific substance?* alcohol

  ❏ *Is the disorder one of use, abuse, or dependence?* dependence

  ❏ *Does the provider clearly document the relationship between the mental or behavioral disorder and the substance use?* Yes, alcoholic liver failure

❑ *What is the blood alcohol level?* BAL .23%

❑ *Is intoxication present?* Yes, with intoxication at admission

❑ *Is withdrawal present?* No.

❑ *Is delirium or perceptual disturbance present?* No.

❑ *Are any associated hallucinations, delusions, or other psychotic conditions present?* Early onset Alzheimer dementia with behavioral disturbance

❑ *Is the condition in remission?* No.

▶ At this time, Ladonna does not know which of these conditions may need to be coded nor how many codes she will end up with. She will learn about this when she moves on to assigning codes.

CODING PRACTICE

Exercise 18.2 Abstracting Diagnoses for Psychiatry

Instructions: Read the mini-medical-record of each patient's encounter and answer the abstracting questions. Write the answer on the line provided. Do not assign any codes.

1. OFFICE Gender: F Age: 9

Reason for encounter: *referred by pediatrician for hyperactivity, short attention span, and irritability*

Assessment: *after testing, symptoms are due to attention deficit hyperactive disorder, predominately hyperactive type*

Plan: *Start medication and behavior therapy*

a. What symptoms are reported? _____

b. What is the disorder? _____

c. What is the specific subtype of the disorder?

_____

d. What symptoms should you report? _____
   Why? _____

2. INPATIENT HOSPITAL Gender: M Age: 31

Reason for encounter: *extreme delusions of paranoia*

Assessment: *dependent continual user of coke, psychosis with delusions due to dependence and long-term use of cocaine*

Plan: *Rx to help manage delusions, transfer to rehab*

a. What is the specific substance? _____

b. Is the disorder one of use, abuse, or dependence?

_____

c. Does the provider clearly document the relationship between the mental or behavioral disorder and the substance use? _____

_____

d. Is withdrawal present? _____

(continued)

2. (continued)

e. Is delirium or perceptual disturbance present?

_____

f. Are any associated hallucinations, delusions, or other psychotic conditions present? _____

_____

3. OFFICE Gender: F Age: 21

Reason for encounter: *ongoing medical management (evaluation and renewal of prescription) of schizophrenia*

Assessment: *paranoid schizophrenia*

Plan: *medication is managing the condition well and patient is interested in getting a job. Referred to a supported employment service (a program that assists in locating community-based employment)*

a. What is the reason for the encounter? _____

_____

b. What condition does the medication treat? _____

_____

c. What is the specific subtype of disorder? _____

_____

d. Is the disorder due to an underlying physiological condition? _____

4. OFFICE Gender: M Age: 10

Reason for encounter: *I have been seeing this child for autism, but today his mother is concerned about continuing "fussing and worry about his private parts" that has been going on for quite awhile and his "desire to be like his sister."*

Assessment: *gender identity disorder*

Plan: *adjusted medications for current autism.*

(continued)

CODING PRACTICE *(continued)*

4. (continued)

a. What concerns did the mother express? _____

_____

b. What is the disorder? _____

c. What other conditions were managed? _____

d. What condition is the main reason for the
   encounter? _____

---

5. INPATIENT HOSPITAL   Gender: M   Age: 48

Reason for encounter: *admitted from emergency
department for alcohol-induced gastritis with
hemorrhaging and intoxication with BAL of .09%*

Assessment: *patient has long-term alcohol use with
dependence, prior cocaine abuser but states he no
longer uses*

Plan: *patient agreed to counseling after discharge*

a. What is the medical condition? _____

_____

b. What substance is the cause? _____

c. Does the provider clearly document the relationship
   between the mental or behavioral disorder and the
   substance use? _____

_____

d. Is the disorder one of use, abuse, or dependence?

_____

e. Is intoxication present? _____

f. What is the blood alcohol level? _____

   How do you write this number as a ratio?

   _____ mg per 100 mL

(continued)

---

5. (continued)

g. Is delirium or perceptual disturbance present?

_____

h. What substance abuse is in remission? _____

_____

---

6. INPATIENT HOSPITAL   Gender: M   Age: 56

Reason for encounter: *severe depression due to bipolar
disorder*

Assessment: *patient is also being treated for liver
cirrhosis with ascites due to chronic continuous
alcoholism*

Plan: *patient has stable living situation so we are
going to discharge him to a partial hospitalization
program (a treatment program that participants attend
during the day and return home at night)*

a. What is the mood disorder? _____

b. Is the current or most recent episode manic, depressed,
   or mixed? _____

c. Does it have psychotic features? _____

d. Is the severity mild, moderate, or severe? _____

_____

e. What physical condition exists? _____

f. What substance disorder is documented? _____

_____

g. Is the disorder one of use, abuse, or dependence?

_____

h. Are any associated hallucinations, delusions, or other
   psychotic conditions present? _____

_____

i. What condition was chiefly responsible for the
   admission and services? _____

ASSIGNING DIAGNOSIS CODES FOR PSYCHIATRY

Three types of conditions in this ICD-10-CM chapter present
challenges in assigning codes because of the level of detail that
must be reported: bipolar disorder, schizophrenic disorders,
and substance disorders.

Assigning Codes for Bipolar Disorder

Bipolar disorder has numerous variations based on the episode,
severity, and psychotic disturbances that may accompany it.

Follow these steps to assign codes for bipolar disorder
(■ FIGURES 18-2 and 18-3):

1. Locate the Main Term **Disorder** in the Index.

2. Locate the subterm **bipolar (I)**.

   ■ For bipolar II disorder, locate the subterm
     bipolar II, which follows the subterm entry for
     bipolar (I).

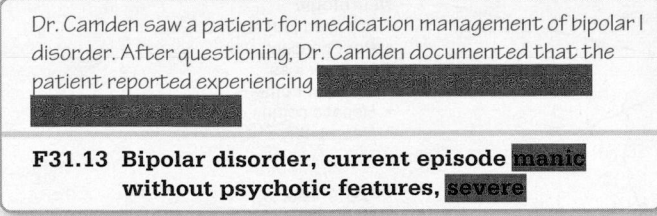

Dr. Camden saw a patient for medication management of bipolar I disorder. After questioning, Dr. Camden documented that the patient reported experiencing ▓▓▓▓▓▓▓▓▓▓ ▓▓▓▓▓▓▓▓▓▓

F31.13 Bipolar disorder, current episode manic without psychotic features, severe

Figure 18-2 ■ Example of Assigning Codes for Bipolar Disorder

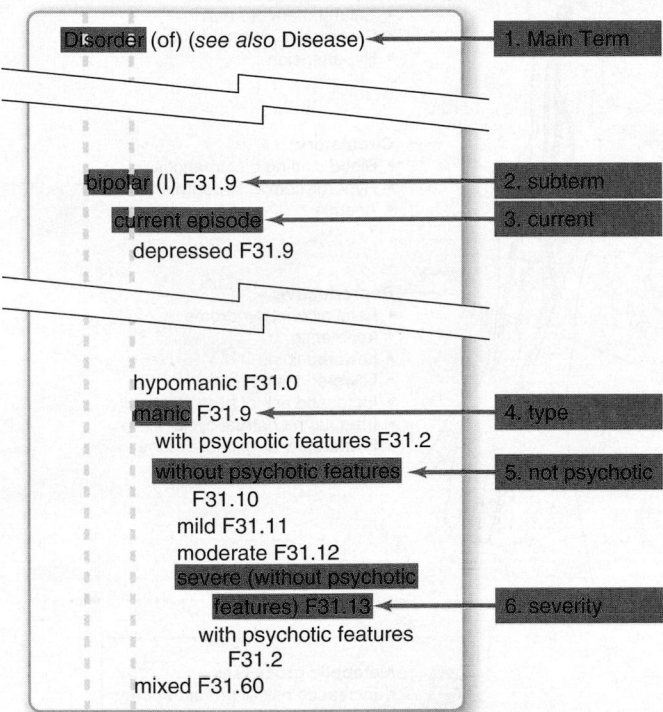

Figure 18-3 ■ Index Entry for the Bipolar Disorder

3. Determine whether the disorder is documented as **current** or **in remission** and locate the corresponding second-level subterm.

4. For current bipolar disorder, identify whether the current episode is **depressed**, **hypomanic**, **manic**, or **mixed** and locate the corresponding third-level subterm.

5. Identify whether the disorder is **with psychotic features** or **without psychotic features** and locate the corresponding fourth-level subterm.

6. For cases **without psychotic features**, select the fifth-level subterm that describes the severity as **mild**, **moderate**, or **severe**. Verify the code in the Tabular List.

7. For bipolar **in remission**, locate the corresponding second-level subterm, then identify whether the remission is **full** or **partial**. Under the corresponding third-level subterm, select the additional subterm that describes the severity. Verify the code in the Tabular List.

Assigning Codes for Schizophrenic Spectrum Disorders

Schizophrenic spectrum disorders (SSDs) include several different disorders, each with different characteristics and diagnostic criteria. Coders must be careful to identify the specific terminology documented in order to assign the correct code. Refer to ■ TABLE 18-7 for a summary of SSDs and associated codes.

Table 18-7 ■ **ASSIGNING CODES FOR SCHIZOPHRENIC SPECTRUM DISORDERS**

Condition	Description	Code(s)
Schizoaffective disorder	Characterized by an extended period in which schizophrenia is accompanied by major depressive, manic, or mixed episodes	F25.-
Schizoid of childhood (Asperger syndrome)	Severe and sustained impairment in social interactions and restricted, repetitive patterns of behaviors, interests, and activities	F84.5
Schizoid personality disorder, schizothymia	Persistent withdrawal from social relationships and lack of emotional responsiveness in most situations	F60.1
Schizophrenia	Inability to distinguish between thoughts and reality, think logically, and have normal emotional and social relationships	F20.0 through F20.5
Schizophreniform disorder	Identical to schizophrenia except that the total duration is greater than one month but less than six months; impaired social or occupational functioning may not be apparent	F20.81
Schizotypal personality disorder	Trouble with relationships and disturbances in thought patterns, appearance, and behavior	F21

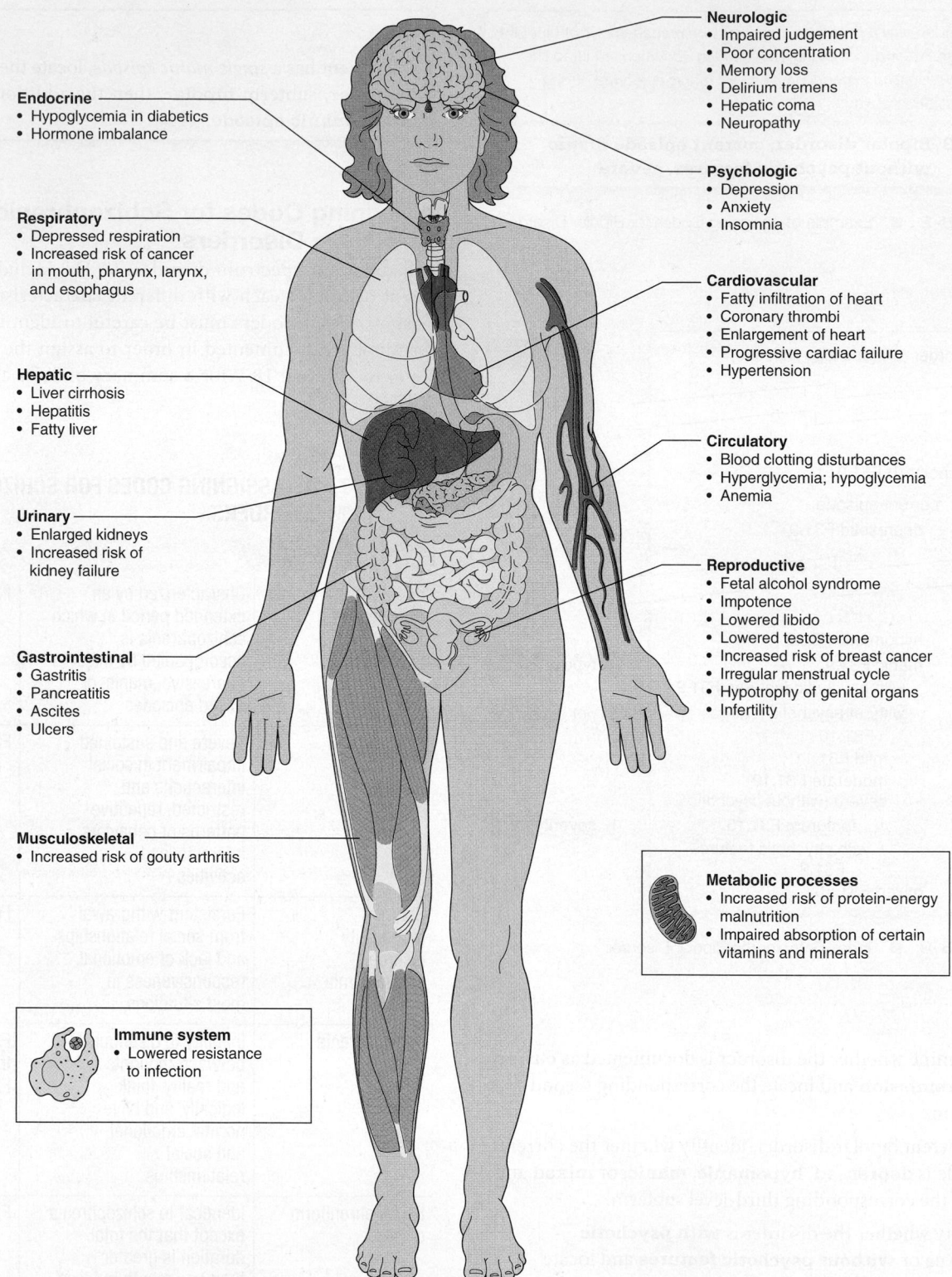

Endocrine
• Hypoglycemia in diabetics
• Hormone imbalance

Respiratory
• Depressed respiration
• Increased risk of cancer in mouth, pharynx, larynx, and esophagus

Hepatic
• Liver cirrhosis
• Hepatitis
• Fatty liver

Urinary
• Enlarged kidneys
• Increased risk of kidney failure

Gastrointestinal
• Gastritis
• Pancreatitis
• Ascites
• Ulcers

Musculoskeletal
• Increased risk of gouty arthritis

Immune system
• Lowered resistance to infection

Neurologic
• Impaired judgement
• Poor concentration
• Memory loss
• Delirium tremens
• Hepatic coma
• Neuropathy

Psychologic
• Depression
• Anxiety
• Insomnia

Cardiovascular
• Fatty infiltration of heart
• Coronary thrombi
• Enlargement of heart
• Progressive cardiac failure
• Hypertension

Circulatory
• Blood clotting disturbances
• Hyperglycemia; hypoglycemia
• Anemia

Reproductive
• Fetal alcohol syndrome
• Impotence
• Lowered libido
• Lowered testosterone
• Increased risk of breast cancer
• Irregular menstrual cycle
• Hypotrophy of genital organs
• Infertility

Metabolic processes
• Increased risk of protein-energy malnutrition
• Impaired absorption of certain vitamins and minerals

Figure 18-4 ■ The Multisystem Effects of Alcohol Use, Abuse, and Dependence

Assigning Codes for Psychoactive Substance Disorders

When mental, behavioral, and neurodevelopmental disorders are documented as being caused by or associated with psychoactive substance use, coders need to review their abstracting results carefully in order to assign accurate codes (Table 18-6).

Assign codes for substance disorders *only* when the *relationship* between the mental or behavioral disorder and the substance use is clearly documented (OGCR I.C.5.b.1)). To better understand the effect of substance abuse on the rest of the body, refer to ■ FIGURE 18-4.

SUCCESS STEP

Alcoholism is indexed under the Main Term **Dependence** and the subterm **alcohol**.

Most codes related to substance disorders contain six characters that identify several pieces of specific information. To assign codes accurately, follow these steps:

1. Determine whether the condition is **use**, **abuse**, or **dependence**. Use this word as the Main Term in the Index.
   - When the documentation mentions both use and abuse, assign a code for abuse. When it mentions both abuse and dependence, assign a code for dependence (OGCR I.C.5.b.2)).
2. Locate the subterm **drug** if the substance is other than alcohol.
   - When the substance is alcohol, go directly to the subterm **alcohol**.
3. Locate a second-level subterm for the specific substance or class of substance.
   - **Cannabis**, **cocaine**, and **nicotine** are separate subterms.
   - **Nicotine** has additional subterms for **chewing tobacco** and **cigarettes**.
   - Other substances are classified under subterms for the class of substance: **hallucinogen**, **inhalant**, **opioid**, **sedative**, **stimulant**, or **psychoactive substance NEC** (Table 18-3).
4. Review the entries under the third-level subterm **with** to locate a combination code for the substance and any manifestations.
5. When the condition is stated as in remission, select the subterm **in remission**.
6. Verify the code in the Tabular List, being certain that all aspects of code title correctly describe the documented diagnosis.

SUCCESS STEP

ICD-10-CM codes do not identify continuous or episodic substance use as ICD-9-CM did.

Guided Example of Assigning Diagnosis Codes for Psychiatry

To learn more about assigning codes for mental, behavioral, and neurodevelopmental disorders, continue with the example from earlier in the chapter about patient Cody Locust, who was admitted to Valley Hospital with a coma.

Follow along in your ICD-10-CM manual as Ladonna Shuck, CPC, assigns codes. Check off each step after you complete it.

▶ First, Ladonna confirms the conditions she abstracted:

❑ *coma that lasted for four hours*

❑ *alcoholic liver disease*

❑ *alcohol dependence of 15 years*

❑ *alcohol intoxication with BAL of .23%*

❑ *dementia with behavioral disturbance due to Alzheimer*

▶ Ladonna reads the medical record again to determine the main reason for the admission and the services provided, as determined after tests and studies were done.

❑ Although the patient was admitted with a coma, the physician linked the coma to alcoholic liver disease.

❑ Ladonna decides to begin assigning codes with alcoholic liver disease. Depending on what she finds for that condition, she will determine whether she needs to go back and also assign a code for the coma.

▶ Ladonna searches the Index for the Main Term **Disease**.

❑ She searches for a subterm for alcoholic, but does not find one. So she then searches for the subterm that describes the anatomic site, **liver**.

❑ Under **liver**, she locates a second-level subterm **alcoholic**.

❑ Under **alcoholic**, she locates a third-level subterm **failure**.

❑ Under **failure**, she locates a fourth-level subterm **with coma K70.41**.

❑ This code appears to be a combination code that includes both alcoholic liver failure and the coma.

▶ Ladonna verifies code **K70.41** in the Tabular List.

❑ She reads the code title for **K70.41, Alcoholic hepatic failure with coma**. She knows that hepatic means liver and confirms that this accurately describes the diagnosis.

▶ Ladonna checks for instructional notes in the Tabular List.

❑ She cross-references the beginning of category **K70** and reads the instructional note, **Use additional code to identify: alcohol abuse and dependence (F10.-)**.

❑ She cross-references the beginning of the block **Diseases of liver (K70-K77)** and reads the **Excludes1** and **Excludes2** notes. She determines that they do not apply to her because they do not include any of the conditions she abstracted.

❑ She cross-references the beginning of **Chapter 11 (K00-K94)** and reads the **Excludes1** and **Excludes2** notes. She determines that they do not apply to her because they do not include any of the conditions she abstracted.

❑ She has finished verifying the code **K70.41, Alcoholic hepatic failure with coma**.

▶ Next, Ladonna assigns a code for alcohol dependence.

❑ She searches the Index for the Main Term **Dependence** (■ FIGURE 18-5, page 298).

❑ She locates a subterm for **alcohol**.

- [ ] She notes that publisher-specific conventions, such as highlighting of the code title, indicates that this is a manifestation code and should be sequenced after the etiology code.

- [ ] She cross-references the instructional notes under the heading for category **F02, Dementia in other diseases classified elsewhere**.

- [ ] She reads the **Excludes1** note and determines that the conditions do not describe this case, so this note does not apply.

- [ ] She reads the note **Code first the underlying physiological condition, such as:** and locates the entry for **Alzheimer's (G30.-)**. This instruction confirms the sequencing order. The code for Alzheimer's should be sequenced before the code for dementia because it is the etiology.

- [ ] She reads the instructional note at the beginning of the block **Mental disorders due to known physiological**

conditions **(F01-F09)** that describes the purpose of this category, but the note does not change the code assigned.

- [ ] She cross-references the beginning of **Chapter 5 (F01-F99)** for instructional notes, but does not find any that relate to this case.

- [ ] She has finished verifying the code **F02, Dementia in other diseases classified elsewhere**.

▶ Ladonna reviews the codes she has assigned for this case.

- [ ] **K70.41 Alcoholic hepatic failure with coma**

- [ ] **F10.229 Alcohol dependence with intoxication, unspecified**

- [ ] **Y90.7 Blood alcohol level, 220-239 mg/100ml**

- [ ] **G30.0 Late onset Alzheimer's**

- [ ] **F02.81 Dementia in diseases classified elsewhere, with behavioral disturbance**

▶ Next, Ladonna must determine how to sequence the codes.

CODING PRACTICE

Exercise 18.3   Assigning Codes for Psychiatry

Instructions: Read the mini-medical-record of each patient's encounter, review the information abstracted in Exercise 18.2, and assign ICD-10-CM diagnosis codes using the Index and Tabular List. Write the code(s) on the line provided.

---

1. OFFICE   Gender: F   Age: 9

Reason for encounter: *referred by pediatrician for hyperactivity, short attention span, and irritability*

Assessment: *after testing, symptoms are due to attention deficit hyperactive disorder, predominately hyperactive type*

Plan: *start medication and behavior therapy*

1 ICD-10-CM Code _____

---

2. INPATIENT HOSPITAL   Gender: M   Age: 31

Reason for encounter: *extreme delusions of paranoia*

Assessment: *dependent continual user of coke, psychosis with delusions due to dependence and long-term use of cocaine*

Plan: *Rx to help manage delusions, transfer to rehab*

1 ICD-10-CM Code _____

---

3. OFFICE   Gender: F   Age: 21

Reason for encounter: *ongoing medical management of schizophrenia*

Assessment: *paranoid schizophrenia*

Plan: *Medication is managing the condition well. Renewed Rx. Patient is interested in getting a job. Referred to a supported employment service*

Tip: The first code is a Z code to issue a repeat prescription.

2 ICD-10-CM Codes _____

ARRANGING DIAGNOSIS CODES FOR PSYCHIATRY

Sequencing of codes for mental, behavioral, and neurodevelopmental disorders is determined by instructional notes in the Tabular List. When mental disorders are associated with underlying physical conditions, the Tabular List provides an instructional note, **Code first the underlying physiological condition**. Coders must read the documentation carefully to

identify when the physician documents a relationship between a mental disorder and a physiological condition.

Arranging Codes for Pain

ICD-10-CM provides codes to use when pain is documented as exclusively or partially psychological. The guidelines for coding pain are summarized next.

When pain is exclusively psychological with no identifiable medical condition and no documentation of acute or chronic pain, assign **F45.41 Pain disorder exclusively related to psychological factors.**

When pain is exclusively psychological and there is also documentation of acute or chronic pain, assign only code **F45.41** (OGCR I.C.5.a).

When the documentation reports pain with related psychological factors, assign and sequence codes as follows:

1. Assign the appropriate code from category **G89.- Pain, not elsewhere classified.**

2. Assign code **F45.42 Pain disorder with related psychological factors.**

Arranging Codes for Intellectual Disabilities

An instructional note in ICD-10-CM for intellectual disabilities (F70 through F79) directs coders to **Code first any associated physical or developmental disorders.** According to the *Diagnostic and Statistical Manual of Mental Disorders* (DSM-V), the following criteria must be met for a diagnosis of intellectual disabilities:

- an IQ below 70
- significant limitations in two or more areas of adaptive behavior
- evidence that the limitations became apparent before the age of 18

Refer to ■ FIGURE 18-8 to learn more about sequencing codes for intellectual disabilities.

SUCCESS STEP

Following the lead of mental health advocates, in 2013 the Social Security Administration adopted the term **intellectual disabilities** to replace the outdated and stigmatized term *mental retardation.*

Guided Example of Arranging Diagnosis Codes for Psychiatry

To learn more about sequencing codes for mental, behavioral, and neurodevelopmental disorders, continue with the example from earlier in the chapter about patient Cody Locust, who was admitted to Valley Hospital with a coma.

Patient with moderate intellectual disabilities is seen for neurological endemic cretinism. Patient also has associated overactive disorder and difficulty with verbal expression. Patient is dependent on assistance with personal care.

(1) **E00.0 Congenital iodine-deficiency syndrome, neurological type**
(2) **F80.1 Expressive language disorder**
(3) **F84.8 Other pervasive developmental disorders**
(4) **Z74.1 Need for assistance with personal care**
(5) **F70 Mild intellectual disabilities**

Figure 18-8 ■ Example of Sequencing Codes for Intellectual Disabilities

Follow along in your ICD-10-CM manual as Ladonna Shuck, CPC, sequences the codes. Check off each step after you complete it.

▶ First, Ladonna confirms the codes she assigned for this case.

❑ **K70.41 Alcoholic hepatic failure with coma**

❑ **F10.229 Alcohol dependence with intoxication, unspecified**

❑ **Y90.7 Blood alcohol level, 220-239 mg/100 ml**

❑ **G30.0 Late onset Alzheimer's**

❑ **F02.81 Dementia in diseases classified elsewhere, with behavioral disturbance**

▶ Ladonna takes a moment to read the medical record to review the details of the case.

❑ She confirms that the principal diagnosis is **K70.41, Alcoholic hepatic failure with coma** because it meets the definition of principal diagnosis defined by the Uniform Hospital Data Discharge Set (UHDDS) (OGCR II).

❑ She determines that the second code should be **F10.229, Alcohol dependence with intoxication, unspecified** because it further describes the principal diagnosis.

❑ Although the code for BAL relates to code **F10.229,** she decides to sequence it as the last code because it is a supplemental code.

❑ She determines that the third code should be **G30.0, Late onset Alzheimer's** because the documentation states that the condition was managed during the admission but does not qualify as the principal diagnosis.

❑ She sequences **F02.81, Dementia in diseases classified elsewhere, with behavioral disturbance** as the fourth code because it is a manifestation code for Alzheimer's and must be sequenced after **G30.0.** During the process of assigning codes, she found four instructional codes directing her to sequence the dementia code after the Alzheimer's code:

- the *[slanted brackets]* convention in the Index
- the instructional note in the Tabular List under category **G30** to **Use additional code** to identify the dementia
- a publisher's convention for the code **F02.81** in the Tabular List that identified it as a manifestation
- the instructional note in the Tabular List under category **F02** to **Code first the underlying condition,** Alzheimer's

❑ She sequences the final code as **Y90.7, Blood alcohol level, 220-239 mg/100 ml** because it is a supplemental code that provides added information but is not a diagnosis code on its own.

CODING CAUTION

When the Tabular List provides the instructional note to **Code first the underlying condition**, it does not mean that Alzheimer's should always be the principal diagnosis. The note describes the relationship between Alzheimer's (the etiology) and dementia (the manifestation) (OGCR I.A.13). The principal diagnosis is determined based on the criteria in OGCR II.

▶ Ladonna finalizes the codes and sequencing for this case:

(1) **K70.41 Alcoholic hepatic failure with coma**

(2) **F10.229 Alcohol dependence with intoxication, unspecified**

(3) **G30.0 Late onset Alzheimer's**

(4) **F02.81 Dementia in diseases classified elsewhere, with behavioral disturbance**

(5) **Y90.7 Blood alcohol level, 220–239 mg/100 ml**

CODING PRACTICE

Exercise 18.4 Arranging Diagnosis Codes for Psychiatry

Instructions: Read the mini-medical-record of each patient's encounter, review the information abstracted in Exercise 18.2, assign ICD-10-CM diagnosis codes using the Index and Tabular List, and sequence them correctly.

---

1. OFFICE   Gender: M   Age: 10

Reason for encounter: *I have been seeing this child for autism, but today his mother is concerned about continuing "fussing and worry about his private parts" that has been going on for quite awhile and his "desire to be like his sister."*

Assessment: *gender identity disorder*

Plan: *adjusted medications for current autism*

2 ICD-10-CM Codes _____

---

2. INPATIENT HOSPITAL   Gender: M   Age: 48

Reason for encounter: *admitted from emergency department for alcohol-induced gastritis with hemorrhaging and intoxication with BAL of .09*

Assessment: *patient has long-term alcohol use with dependence, prior cocaine abuser but states he no longer uses*

(continued)

---

2. (continued)

Plan: *patient agreed to counseling after discharge*

Tip: Follow instructional notes in the Tabular List to help determine sequencing.

4 ICD-10-CM Codes _____

_____

---

3. INPATIENT HOSPITAL   Gender: M   Age: 56

Reason for encounter: *severe depression due to bipolar disorder*

Assessment: *patient is also being treated for liver cirrhosis with ascites due to chronic continuous alcoholism*

Plan: *patient has stable living situation so we are going to discharge him to a partial hospitalization program*

3 ICD-10-CM Codes _____

_____

CHAPTER SUMMARY

In this chapter you learned that:

- Mental, behavioral, and neurodevelopmental disorders are real, not imagined, disorders that have diagnostic criteria and are proven to respond to treatment.

- ICD-10-CM Chapter 5, Mental, Behavioral, and Neurodevelopmental Disorders (F01-F99), contains 11 blocks or subchapters that are divided by the type of disorder.

- Many mental, behavioral, and neurodevelopmental disorders have multiple subtypes, so coders must be particularly attentive to the documented wording of the condition.

- Three types of conditions in this ICD-10-CM chapter present challenges in assigning codes because of the level of detail that must be reported: bipolar disorder, schizophrenic disorders, and substance disorders.

- When mental disorders are associated with underlying physical conditions, the Tabular List provides an instructional note to code the underlying physiological condition first.

- ICD-10-CM Official Guidelines for Coding and Reporting (OGCR) section I.C.5 provides detailed discussion of pain disorders related to psychological factors and mental, behavioral, and neurodevelopmental disorders due to substance abuse.

CONCEPT QUIZ

Take a moment to look back at mental, behavioral, and neurodevelopmental disorders and solidify your skills. Try to answer the questions from memory, first, then look back at the discussion in this chapter if you need a little extra help.

Completion

Instructions: Write the term that answers each question based on the information you learned in this chapter. Choose from the list below. Some choices may be used more than once and some choices may not be used at all.

abuse	intoxication
barbiturate	mood
cognitive	narcotic
dependence	personality
dissociative	psychotic
hallucinogen	sexual
impulse-control	use
in remission	

1. Dementia is an example of a/an _____ disorder.
2. Voyeurism is an example of a/an _____ disorder.
3. Kleptomania is an example of a/an _____ disorder.
4. Bipolar is an example of a/an _____ disorder.
5. Phenobarbital is an example of the _____ class of drugs.
6. Fentanyl is an example of the _____ class of drugs.
7. LSD is an example of the _____ class of drugs.
8. _____ occurs when more of a substance is consumed than a person can physically tolerate, resulting in behavioral or physical abnormalities.
9. Past history of a substance disorder is _____.
10. _____ of a substance is consuming it in moderate amounts that do not create significant legal, social, employment, family, or medical problems.

Multiple Choice

Instructions: Circle the letter of the best answer to each question based on the information you learned in this chapter.

1. Psychotic disorders consist of
   A. depression and mania.
   B. delusions and hallucinations.
   C. impulse and control behaviors.
   D. obsessive and compulsive behaviors.

2. Physical symptoms that are not explained by medical conditions are
   A. affective disorders.
   B. dissociative disorders.
   C. adjustment disorders.
   D. somatoform disorders.

3. Which of the following substances is a narcotic?
   A. Secobarbital
   B. PCP
   C. Heroin
   D. Amphetamine

4. Which of the following is NOT a behavioral disturbance of dementia?
   A. Memory loss
   B. Aggression
   C. Wandering
   D. Depression

5. Which of the following is NOT a key criterion for abstracting psychoactive substance disorders?
   A. What is the class of substance?
   B. Is use episodic or continuous?
   C. Is withdrawal present?
   D. Is delirium or perceptual disturbance present?

6. A BAL of 0.08% may also be expressed as
   A. 0.8 mg per 100 mL.
   B. 8 mg per 100 mL.
   C. 80 mg per 100 mL.
   D. 800 mg per 100 mL.

7. When substance abuse and dependence are both documented, how should the condition be coded?
   A. Assign a code for abuse only.
   B. Assign a code for dependence only.
   C. Assign two codes, one for abuse and one for dependence.
   D. Assign a combination code for abuse with dependence.

(continued)

(continued from page 303)

8. Which of the following is coded under category F20 Schizophrenia?
   A. Paranoid schizophrenia
   B. Schizoaffective disorder
   C. Schizothymia
   D. Schizophreniform disorder

9. How should alcoholic liver disease with coma be coded?
   A. Assign the code for coma followed by the code for alcoholic liver disease.
   B. Assign the code for alcoholic liver disease followed by the code for coma.
   C. Assign a combination code for coma due to alcoholic liver disease.
   D. Assign a combination code for alcoholic liver disease with coma.

10. An instructional note in ICD-10-CM for intellectual disabilities (F70 through F79) directs coders to
   A. code first any associated physical or developmental disorders.
   B. use additional code for any associated physical or developmental disorders.
   C. assign combination codes for the intellectual disability and any associated physical or developmental disorders.
   D. not code any associated physical or developmental disorders.

CODING CHALLENGE

Instructions: Read the mini-medical-record of each patient's encounter, then abstract, assign, and sequence ICD-10-CM diagnosis codes using the Index and Tabular List. Write the code(s) on the line provided.

1. OFFICE   Gender: M   Age: 19

Reason for encounter: *pattern of exacerbation of asthma attacks on the weekends*

Assessment: *psychogenic moderate persistent asthma*

Plan: *allergy studies are scheduled in addition to follow-up with a family systems therapist to address the psychogenic component*

Tip: Read the instructional notes in the Tabular List to determine the codes and sequencing.

2 ICD-10-CM Codes _____

2. OFFICE   Gender: F Age: 20

Reason for encounter: *veteran experiencing flashbacks accompanied by nightmares, angry outbursts, hypervigilance, and anxiousness*

Assessment: *chronic posttraumatic stress disorder*

Plan: *trauma-focused cognitive-behavioral treatments (TFCBT) 12 weeks*

1 ICD-10-CM Code _____

3. OFFICE   Gender: M   Age: 52

Reason for encounter: *review results of brain MRI, ordered after he complained at a previous visit of episodes of sleepwalking*

Assessment: *MRI shows brain metastasis from pancreatic cancer; patient has secondary diabetes d/t pancreatic cancer and is on long-term insulin*

Plan: *refer to neurologist for further workup on sleep walking*

Tip: Review OGCR I.C.2.a and b for sequencing of neoplasm codes. Review OGCR I.C.4.a.6) regarding secondary diabetes.

5 ICD-10-CM Codes _____

_____

4. OFFICE   Gender: M   Age: 26

Reason for encounter: *Patient reports feeling extremely irritable, having cold sweats, and headaches. He went cold turkey for 4 days to try and get off heroin.*

Assessment: *symptoms are due to drug withdrawal with heroin dependence*

Plan: *the patient met with a drug counselor to discuss a more appropriate way to address his addiction, started patient on methadone (opiate substitute) treatment*

Tip: Review OGCR I.C.21.c.10) regarding the use of a Z code for the drug counseling.

1 ICD-10-CM Code _____

5. INPATIENT HOSPITAL Gender: F Age: 36

Reason for encounter: severe depression, has considered suicide

Assessment: depression and suicide ideation due to persistent anxiety regarding being unemployed for the past year

Plan: psychotherapy with no-suicide contract, antidepressant medication, refer to unemployment support group

3 ICD-10-CM Codes _____

_____

6. OFFICE Gender: M Age: 43

Reason for encounter: depressed mood (3-week duration), excessive sleep, fatigue

Assessment: depressive episode due to bipolar disorder which is in partial remission

Plan: dosage change of present mood stabilizer, psychotherapy

1 ICD-10-CM Code _____

7. OFFICE Gender: F Age: 22

Reason for encounter: excessive sadness, crying, sleeping, lethargy, feeling emotionally numb. Gave birth 3 weeks ago

Assessment: postpartum depression

Plan: interpersonal relationship counseling, Rx SSRI (selective serotonin reuptake inhibitor) antidepressant meds, obtain part time mother's helper

1 ICD-10-CM Code _____

8. OFFICE Gender: F Age: 10

Reason for encounter: struggling in school with reading and spelling

Assessment: developmental dyslexia, spelling disorder

Plan: special ed schooling, teach compensating and coping skills

2 ICD-10-CM Codes _____

9. INPATIENT HOSPITAL Gender: F Age: 16

Reason for admission: admitted from psychiatrist's office for multiple personality disorder

Assessment: Multiple personality disorder and mild intellectual disability. Patient presents with learning deficiencies (IQ 65) and with physical disability of anemia due to poor nutrition.

Plan: psychotherapy weekly, transfer patient into special education program at school, home visit by social services to address nutritional issues

Tip: Assign codes for the personality disorder, the cognitive disorder, and the physical disability.

3 ICD-10-CM Codes _____

_____

10. OFFICE Gender: F Age: 25

Reason for encounter: chewing tobacco since age 13 and wants to quit

Assessment: counseling to address dependence on tobacco

Plan: RTO 1 week

Tip: Read the instructional note in the Tabular List that indicates sequencing.

2 ICD-10-CM Codes _____

KEEP ON CODING

Instructions: Read the diagnostic statement, then use the Index and Tabular List to assign and sequence ICD-10-CM diagnosis codes. Write the code(s) on the line provided.

1. Acute brain syndrome: ICD-10-CM Code(s) _____

2. Catatonic schizophrenia: ICD-10-CM Code(s) _____

3. Thumb sucking: ICD-10-CM Code(s) _____

4. Bulimia nervosa: ICD-10-CM Code(s) _____

5. Fear of flying: ICD-10-CM Code(s) _____

(continued)

(continued from page 305)

6. Nicotine dependence with withdrawal: ICD-10-CM Code(s) _____

7. Alcohol abuse with alcohol-induced sleep disorder: ICD-10-CM Code(s) _____

8. Bipolar II disorder: ICD-10-CM Code(s) _____

9. Adjustment disorder with anxiety: ICD-10-CM Code(s) _____

10. Primary hypersomnia: ICD-10-CM Code(s) _____

11. Voyeurism: ICD-10-CM Code(s) _____

12. Autistic disorder: ICD-10-CM Code(s) _____

13. Intellectual disability with IQ level 19: ICD-10-CM Code(s) _____

14. Psychogenic encopresis: ICD-10-CM Code(s) _____

15. Trichotillomania: ICD-10-CM Code(s) _____

16. Abuse of antacids: ICD-10-CM Code(s) _____

17. Dissociative stupor: ICD-10-CM Code(s) _____

18. Sleepwalking: ICD-10-CM Code(s) _____

19. Selective mutism: ICD-10-CM Code(s) _____

20. Psychogenic torticollis: ICD-10-CM Code(s) _____

21. Dysthymic disorder: ICD-10-CM Code(s) _____

22. Hypochondria: ICD-10-CM Code(s) _____

23. Clumsy child syndrome: ICD-10-CM Code(s) _____

24. Premature ejaculation: ICD-10-CM Code(s) _____

25. Cocaine dependence with withdrawal: ICD-10-CM Code(s) _____

Diseases of the Eye and Adnexa (H00-H59)

Chapter 19

Learning Objectives

After completing this chapter, you should have the skills to:

19.1 Spell and define the key words, medical terms, and abbreviations related to diseases of the eye and ocular adnexa.

19.2 Discuss the structure, function, and common conditions of the eye and ocular adnexa.

19.3 Identify the main characteristics of coding for diseases of the eye and ocular adnexa.

19.4 Abstract diagnostic information from the medical record for conditions of the eye and ocular adnexa.

19.5 Assign codes for diseases of the eye and ocular adnexa.

19.6 Arrange multiple diagnosis codes for diseases of the eye and ocular adnexa.

19.7 Code neoplasms of the eye and ocular adnexa.

19.8 Discuss the Official Guidelines for Coding and Reporting related to diseases of the eye and ocular adnexa.

Chapter Outline

- **Eye Refresher**
- **Coding Overview of the Eye**
- **Abstracting for Eye Conditions**
- **Assigning Codes for Eye Conditions**
- **Arranging Codes for Eye Conditions**
- **Coding Neoplasms of the Eye**

Key Terms and Abbreviations

adnexa	cornea	orbital cavity	sclera
choroid	lens	pupil	vitreous body
cone	ocular globe	retina	
conjunctiva	optic nerve	rod	

In addition to the key terms listed here, students should know the terms defined within tables in this chapter.

For updates and corrections, visit our student resource site at
www.pearsonhighered.com/healthprofessionsresources

INTRODUCTION

A camera, particularly a traditional film camera, collects and focuses light in a manner very similar to the human eye. In this chapter you will learn more about how the eye and ocular adnexa works, why sometimes they do not work as they should, and how physicians treat these conditions.

An ophthalmologist is a physician (MD) who specializes in diagnosing and treating diseases of the eye. Ophthalmologists may specialize in a specific part of the eye, such as the cornea or the retina. An optometrist is a doctor of optometry (OD) who specializes in examining the eyes and prescribing corrective lenses. Optometrists screen patients for certain eye diseases, such as glaucoma, and refer patients to an ophthalmologist if there are any concerns.

EYE REFRESHER

The eye and ocular **adnexa** (*associated anatomic structures*) make vision possible by receiving light from the external world and converting it into impulses that are transmitted to the brain through the **optic nerve**, which is cranial nerve II. The **ocular globe** refers to the eyeball itself. The eyeball consists of three layers: the **sclera** (*tough, white outer layer*), the **choroid** (*opaque middle layer that supplies blood to the eye*), and the **retina** (*the innermost layer that contains sensory receptor cells*). The **orbital cavity** is the bony structure around the eye, commonly known as the eye socket. The adnexa are the surrounding ocular muscles, eyelids, and **conjunctiva** (*membrane that lines the eyelids*) (■ FIGURE 19-1).

Light rays pass through the **cornea** (*the clear hard portion of the sclera that protects the lens*), **pupil** (*the black central part of*

eye that constricts and dilates in response to light), **lens** (*the clear part of the front of the eye that focuses light rays on the retina*), and **vitreous body** (*the transparent jelly that fills the eyeball and is surrounded by a membrane*) to focus on the retina. **Rods and cones** (*light-sensitive receptor cells*) in the retina are stimulated and transmit sensory impulses to the brain, which interprets the impulses as a visual image.

In Figure 19-1, each structure in the eye is labeled with its name as well as its medical terminology root/combining form where applicable. Refer to ■ TABLE 19-1 for a refresher on how to build medical terms related to the eye and ocular adnexa.

Conditions of the Eye

Refer to ■ TABLE 19-2 for a summary of diseases affecting the eye and ocular adnexa.

CODING CAUTION

Be alert for medical words that sound and are spelled similarly but have different meanings.

uvea (*the middle layer of eye consisting of the iris, ciliary body, and choroid*) and **uvula** (*a pendant fleshy lobe, most commonly referred to as the one in the back of the mouth*)

keratitis (*inflammation of the cornea*) and **keratin** (*horny tissues found in the epidermis, hair, and nails*)

choroid (*the middle layer of the eye*) and **colloid** (*gelatin-like or mucous substance found in tissues*)

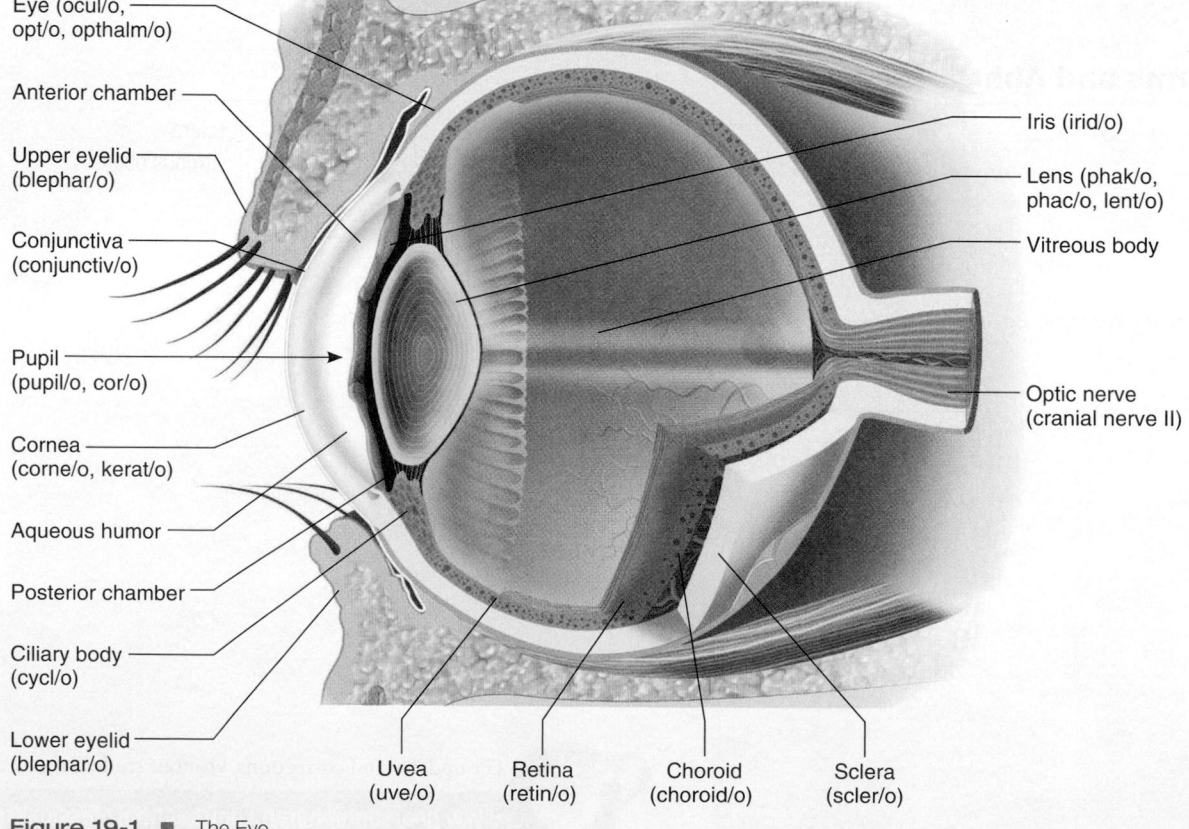

Eye (ocul/o, opt/o, opthalm/o)
Anterior chamber
Upper eyelid (blephar/o)
Conjunctiva (conjunctiv/o)
Pupil (pupil/o, cor/o)
Cornea (corne/o, kerat/o)
Aqueous humor
Posterior chamber
Ciliary body (cycl/o)
Lower eyelid (blephar/o)

Iris (irid/o)
Lens (phak/o, phac/o, lent/o)
Vitreous body
Optic nerve (cranial nerve II)

Uvea (uve/o)   Retina (retin/o)   Choroid (choroid/o)   Sclera (scler/o)

Figure 19-1 ■ The Eye

Table 19-1 ■ **EXAMPLE OF CONSTRUCTING MEDICAL TERMS FOR THE EYE AND OCULAR ADNEXA**

Combining Form	Suffix	Complete Medical Term
retin/o (*retina*)	**-itis** (*inflammation*) **-ptosis** (*drooping*) **-pathy** (*abnormal condition*)	**retin + itis** (*inflammation of the retina*) **retino + pathy** (*abnormal condition of the retina*)
blephar/o (*eyelid*)		**blephar + itis** (*inflammation of the eyelid*) **blephar + optosis** (*drooping eyelid*)
choroid/o (*vascular coat of the eye*)		**choroid + itis** (*inflammation of the vascular coat of the eye*)

Table 19-2 ■ **COMMON DISEASES OF THE EYE AND OCULAR ADNEXA**

Condition	Definition
Blepharitis	An inflammation and infection of hair follicles and glands at the margins of the eyelids due to virus, bacteria, allergic response, or exposure to irritants
Cataract	A cloudiness of the lens that usually develops slowly over time due to aging
Chalazion	A small hard cyst on the eyelid caused by blockage of a gland on the eyelid
Conjunctivitis	A viral or bacterial inflammation and infection of the conjunctiva
Diabetic retinopathy	The abnormal expansion of blood vessels and hemorrhaging in the vessels of the retina, caused by diabetes
Glaucoma	An increased fluid pressure within the eye that damages the optic nerve and can cause blindness
Hordeolum	A bacterial inflammation of a sebaceous gland on the edge or lining of the eyelid; also called a stye
Keratitis	An inflammation and ulceration of the surface of the cornea
Macular degeneration	The gradual loss of central vision due to aging, with no cure (■ FIGURE 19-2 and ■ FIGURE 19-3)
Retinal detachment	The separation of the retina from the choroid layer of the eye

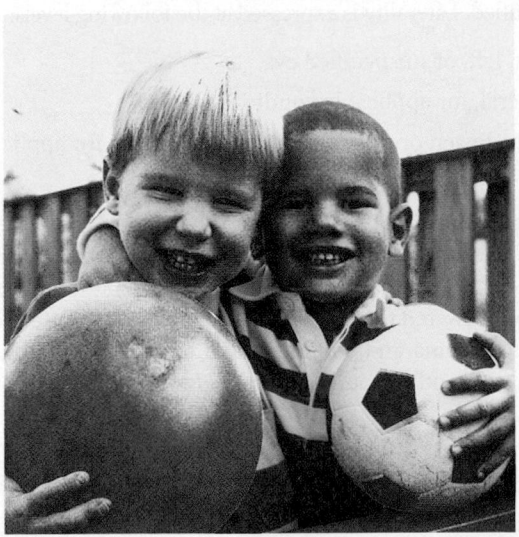

Figure 19-2 ■ Image Seen by a Person with Normal Vision. *Source: National Eye Institute, National Institutes of Health.*

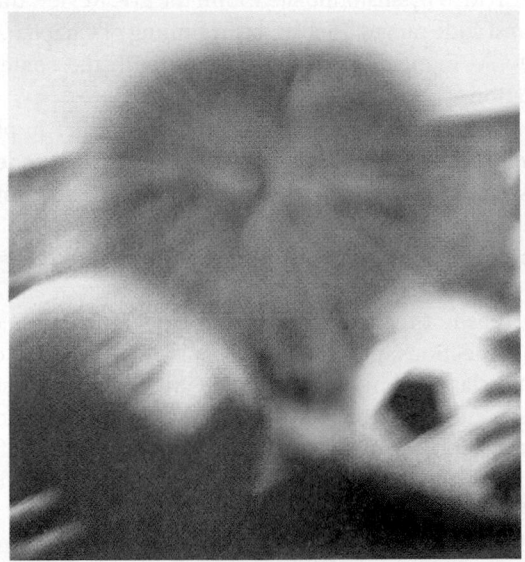

Figure 19-3 ■ Image Seen by a Person with Macular Degeneration and Related Loss of Central Vision. *Source: National Eye Institute, National Institutes of Health.*

CODING PRACTICE

Exercise 19.1   Eye Refresher

Instructions: Use your medical terminology skills and resources to define the following conditions related to the eye and ocular adnexa, then assign the default diagnosis code.

Follow these steps:

- Use slash marks "/" to break down each term into its root(s) and suffix.
- Define the meaning of the word, based on the meaning of each word part.
- Assign the default ICD-10-CM diagnosis code for the condition, including laterality, using the Index and Tabular List.

Example: conjunctivitis (right eye, acute)   Meaning: *inflammation of the lining of the eye*   ICD-10-CM Code: *H10.31*
conjunctiv/itis

1. photokeratitis (right eye)	Meaning _____	ICD-10-CM Code _____
2. retinoblastoma (left eye)	Meaning _____	ICD-10-CM Code _____
3. lagophthalmos	Meaning _____	ICD-10-CM Code _____
4. blepharoptosis (bilateral)	Meaning _____	ICD-10-CM Code _____
5. dacryoadenitis (right eye)	Meaning _____	ICD-10-CM Code _____
6. keratomalacia (bilateral)	Meaning _____	ICD-10-CM Code _____
7. retinoschisis (left eye)	Meaning _____	ICD-10-CM Code _____
8. amblyopia (bilateral)	Meaning _____	ICD-10-CM Code _____
9. iridocyclitis	Meaning _____	ICD-10-CM Code _____
10. aphakia (right eye)	Meaning _____	ICD-10-CM Code _____

CODING OVERVIEW OF THE EYE

ICD-10-CM Chapter 7, Diseases of the Eye and Adnexa (H00-H59), is a new chapter that did not exist in ICD-9-CM. In ICD-9-CM, the eye and ocular adnexa were included in Chapter 6 (360-379) for the nervous system and special senses. This is one of two chapters in which codes begin with the letter H; codes for the ear and mastoid process occupy codes H60 through H95. This chapter contains 12 blocks or subchapters that are divided by anatomic site within the eye. Review the block names and code ranges listed at the beginning of Chapter 7 in the ICD-10-CM manual to become familiar with the content and organization.

ICD-10-CM uses the term *age-related cataract* in place of *senile cataract*, which was used in ICD-9-CM. Most codes have been expanded to include greater specificity of anatomic site and laterality.

This chapter includes disorders affecting each structure within the eye, glaucoma, and visual disturbances and blindness. It does not include injuries to the eye, congenital conditions, or infectious, parasitic, or syphilis-related eye disorders, which are classified in other ICD-10-CM chapters. It also does not include diabetic or many other endocrine eye disorders, which are reported with combination codes in ICD-10-CM Chapter 4, Endocrine, Nutritional, and Metabolic Diseases (E00-E89).

ICD-10-CM provides Official Guidelines for Coding and Reporting (OGCR) in OGCR section I.C.7 regarding assigning codes for the stages of glaucoma. Instructional notes in the Tabular List guide the coder when additional codes are required. An instructional note at the beginning of the chapter directs coders to use an external cause code following the code for the eye condition when an external cause is involved in creating the eye condition. This note applies to all codes in ICD-10-CM Chapter 7.

ABSTRACTING FOR EYE CONDITIONS

The main concerns when abstracting eye conditions are identifying laterality and the presence of underlying conditions, particularly diabetes. The majority of eye conditions require that the laterality be identified. Laterality is expressed at the following levels:

- right, left, or unspecified eye
- bilateral, for applicable conditions
- upper, lower, or unspecified lid of each eye, for applicable conditions

Refer to ■ TABLE 19-3 for guidance on how to abstract conditions of the eye and ocular adnexa. Remember that the abstracting questions are a guide and that not every question applies to, or can be answered for, every case. For example, some conditions, such as glaucoma and conjunctivitis, are designated as acute or chronic, while other conditions, such as cataract(s) are not.

Abstracting Diabetic Eye Conditions

Retinopathy and cataract(s) are common diabetic manifestations. Even though diabetic eye conditions are not classified to ICD-10-CM Chapter 7, coders must know how to abstract them. Laterality is not a requirement for diabetic manifestations. Refer to ■ TABLE 19-4 to learn key criteria for abstracting ophthalmic manifestations of diabetes.

Table 19-3 ■ KEY CRITERIA FOR ABSTRACTING CONDITIONS OF THE EYE AND OCULAR ADNEXA

- ❑ What is the condition?
- ❑ What is the subtype of the condition?
- ❑ Is a more specific subtype documented?
- ❑ What is the stage (certain types of glaucoma)?
- ❑ Is laterality right, left, bilateral, or unspecified?
- ❑ For conditions affecting the eyelid, is the upper or lower lid involved?
- ❑ Is the condition acute or chronic?
- ❑ Is the eye condition secondary to diabetes or a condition from another body system?
- ❑ Do any additional eye conditions exist?
- ❑ Is the condition due to an external cause?

Table 19-4 ■ KEY CRITERIA FOR ABSTRACTING OPHTHALMIC MANIFESTATIONS OF DIABETES

- ❑ Is the diabetes type 1 or type 2?
- ❑ Is the eye condition documented as related to diabetes?
- ❑ Is the condition retinopathy, cataract(s), or other?
- ❑ What is the laterality?

For retinopathy:
- ❑ Is retinopathy proliferative or nonproliferative?
- ❑ Is nonproliferative retinopathy mild, moderate, or severe?
- ❑ Is retinopathy accompanied by macular edema?

Guided Example of Abstracting for Eye Conditions

Refer to the following example throughout this chapter to learn about abstracting, assigning, and sequencing eye and ocular adnexa codes. Megan Scheidler, CCS-P, is a fictitious coder who guides you through the coding process.

Date: 9/1/yy   Location: Branton Eye Care

Provider: Margo Bittinger, MD

Patient: Jaclyn Vandeventer   Gender: F   Age: 71

Reason for encounter: referred by optometrist after abnormal findings on a routine vision exam

Assessment: right normal tension glaucoma, mild stage (*damage to the optic nerve despite normal pressure in the eye*), age related nuclear (*centrally located*) cataracts bilaterally that are interfering with vision

Plan: drops and medication for glaucoma, we will see how that does, then see if surgery is needed, we will wait on cataract removal until the glaucoma is controlled

Follow along as Megan Scheidler, CCS-P, abstracts the diagnosis. Check off each step after you complete it.

▶ Megan reads through the entire record, paying special attention to the reason for the encounter and the final assessment.

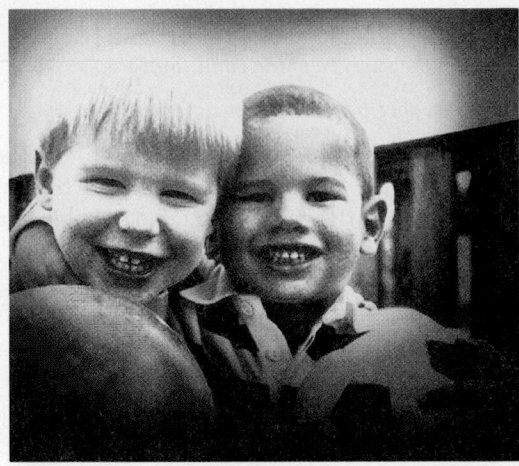

Figure 19-4 ■ Image Seen by a Person with Glaucoma and Related Tunnel Vision. *Source: National Eye Institute, National Institutes of Health.*

- ❑ She notes that the patient was seen at a clinic by an optometrist who identified some concerns that required the attention of an ophthalmologist.

▶ Megan refers to Key Criteria for Abstracting Conditions of the Eye and Ocular Adnexa (Table 19-3) and begins with glaucoma.

- ❑ *What is the condition?* glaucoma (■ Figure 19-4).
- ❑ *What is the subtype of the condition?* normal tension glaucoma
- ❑ *Is laterality right, left, bilateral, or unspecified?* right eye
- ❑ *What is the stage?* mild
- ❑ *Is the condition acute or chronic?* She notes that acute or chronic does not apply to glaucoma.
- ❑ *Is the eye condition secondary to diabetes or a condition from another body system?* No.
- ❑ *Do any additional eye conditions exist?* Yes, cataracts are documented.
- ❑ *Is the condition due to an external cause?* No.

▶ Next, Megan abstracts for cataracts (■ Figure 19-5).

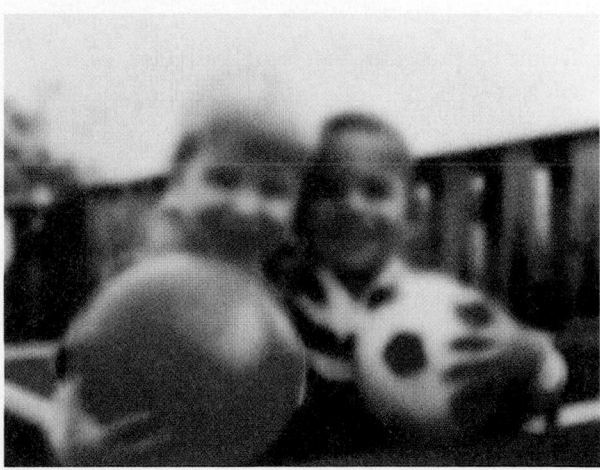

Figure 19-5 ■ Blurry Image Seen by a Person with Cataracts. *Source: National Eye Institute, National Institutes of Health.*

❑ *What is the condition?* cataracts

❑ *What is the subtype of the condition?* age related

❑ *Is a more specific subtype documented?* nuclear

❑ *Is laterality right, left, bilateral, or unspecified?* The laterality is both eyes. She notes that although the glaucoma affects only the right eye, the cataracts are bilateral.

❑ *Is the condition acute or chronic?* Acute or chronic is not applicable to cataracts.

❑ *Is the eye condition secondary to diabetes or a condition from another body system?* No.

❑ *Do any additional eye conditions exist?* No.

❑ *Is the condition due to an external cause?* No.

▶ At this time, Megan thinks she will need a code for glaucoma and a code for cataracts, but she will not know for certain until she moves on to assigning codes.

CODING PRACTICE

Exercise 19.2   **Abstracting for Eye Conditions**

Instructions: Read the mini-medical-record of each patient's encounter and answer the abstracting questions. Write the answer on the line provided. Do not assign any codes.

---

1. OFFICE   Gender: M   **Age:** 76

Reason for encounter: phacoemulsification of cataract and intraocular lens (IOL) implant

Assessment: age related nuclear cataract, left eye

Plan: FU in office, 2 days

a. Define the procedures that are the reason for the encounter. _____

b. What is the condition? _____

c. What is the subtype of the condition? _____
_____

d. What is the laterality? _____

---

2. OFFICE   Gender: F   **Age:** 84

Reason for encounter: monthly retinal injections

Assessment: wet macular degeneration, in both eyes

Plan: return, 1 month

a. Define the procedure that is the reason for the encounter. _____

b. What is the condition? _____

c. What is the subtype of the condition? _____
_____

d. What is the laterality? _____

---

3. OFFICE   Gender: F   **Age:** 69

Reason for encounter: crusty eyelids

Assessment: nonulcerative blepharitis on both upper lids

(continued)

---

3. (continued)

Plan: keep clean, Rx topical antibiotic

a. What is the condition? _____

b. What is the subtype of the condition? _____
_____

c. What is the laterality? _____

d. Is the upper or lower lid involved on the right side?
_____

   On the left side? _____

---

4. OFFICE   Gender: M   **Age:** 61

Reason for encounter: routine eye exam as part of diabetic monitoring

Assessment: moderate diabetic nonproliferative retinopathy with no macular edema

Plan: be diligent about keeping sugar and BP well controlled, to slow progression of condition

a. What is the reason for the encounter? _____
_____

b. Are there abnormal findings? _____

c. What eye condition is diagnosed? _____

e. Is it proliferative or nonproliferative? _____

e. Is it mild, moderate, or severe? _____

f. Is it accompanied by macular edema? _____
_____

g. What is the underlying condition? _____
_____

h. What is the type? _____

(continued)

5. OFFICE Gender: F Age: 53

Reason for encounter: blurred vision, eye pain, floaters in both eyes

Assessment: bilateral anterior uveitis due to juvenile rheumatoid arthritis, associated cataract with neovascularization in left eye also noted

Plan: eye drops, dark glasses

a. What is the condition? _____

b. What is the laterality? _____

c. What additional eye condition exists? _____

_____

d. What is the subtype of the additional condition? _____

e. What is the laterality of the additional condition? _____

f. Is the eye condition secondary to a condition from another body system? _____

_____

g. What is the underlying condition? _____

_____

h. What is the subtype? _____

6. OFFIEC Gender: F Age: 54

Reason for encounter: difficulty seeing, gritty feeling in eyes, ocular hyperemia (*bloodshot eye*)

Assessment: bilateral grade 2 corneal and conjunctival deposits, likely due to stage 5 renal failure, patient has been on dialysis for about 18 months

Plan: schedule cornea scraping to remove deposits

a. What are the symptoms and signs? _____

_____

b. What two eye conditions are diagnosed? _____

_____

c. What is the laterality? _____

d. Are the symptoms integral to the condition(s)? _____

_____

e. What is the underlying condition? _____

What stage? _____

f. How is the underlying condition being treated? _____

_____

ASSIGNING CODES FOR EYE CONDITIONS

Coders need to be attentive when assigning codes that involve laterality. The fifth or sixth character of the code identifies laterality. Always verify the character for laterality in the Tabular List. Although *often* the right side is **1**, the left side is **2**, and bilateral is **3**, this is not *always* the case. In some categories, laterality designations use characters other than **1**, **2**, or **3**. Some codes that have laterality do not provide an option for bilateral because the condition is commonly unilateral.

When a condition affects both eyes, but no code is provided for bilateral, assign two codes: one for the right eye and a second one for the left eye (OGCR I.B.13). For example, disorders of the eyelid have codes for right and left laterality as well as upper and lower but do not usually have codes for bilateral. (■ FIGURE 19-6).

Patient is seen for senile entropion *(turning inward)* of both upper eyelids.

| H02.031 | Senile entropion of right upper eyelid |
| H02.034 | Senile entropion of left upper eyelid |

Figure 19-6 ■ Example of Assigning Codes for a Bilateral Condition When No Code Option for Bilaterality Exists

When coding glaucoma, assign a seventh character to identify the stage of glaucoma as **unspecified, mild, moderate, severe, or indeterminate**. Assign as many codes as necessary from category **H40 Glaucoma** to fully describe the type of glaucoma, the affected eye, and the stage (OGCR I.C.7.a).

Assigning Codes for Diabetic Eye Conditions

Codes for diabetic ophthalmic manifestations are not indexed under the Main Term for the eye condition, such as retinopathy. They are indexed under the Main Term **Diabetes**, then a subterm for the type of diabetes, then a second-level subterm for the specific manifestation, such as retinopathy or cataract(s). In the Tabular List, diabetes is classified in block **E08-E13**. Each three-digit category describes a different form of diabetes. Each category has a specific subcategory for ophthalmic manifestations, which are identified with the fourth character of **3** (■ FIGURE 19-7, page 314).

The fifth and sixth characters describe the type of ophthalmic condition. Refer to ■ FIGURE 19-8 (page 314) to learn more about locating codes for diabetic eye manifestations.

Guided Example of Assigning Codes for Eye Conditions

To learn more about assigning codes for diseases of the eye and ocular adnexa, continue with the example from earlier in the

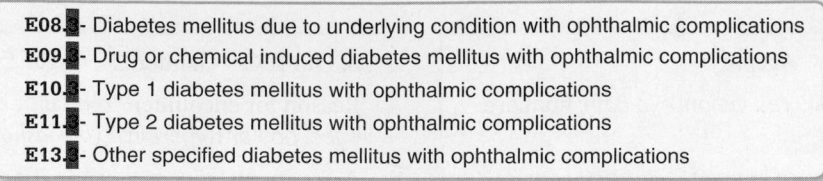

E08.**3**- Diabetes mellitus due to underlying condition with ophthalmic complications
E09.**3**- Drug or chemical induced diabetes mellitus with ophthalmic complications
E10.**3**- Type 1 diabetes mellitus with ophthalmic complications
E11.**3**- Type 2 diabetes mellitus with ophthalmic complications
E13.**3**- Other specified diabetes mellitus with ophthalmic complications

Figure 19-7 ■ Tabular List Subcategories for Diabetes with Ophthalmic Manifestations

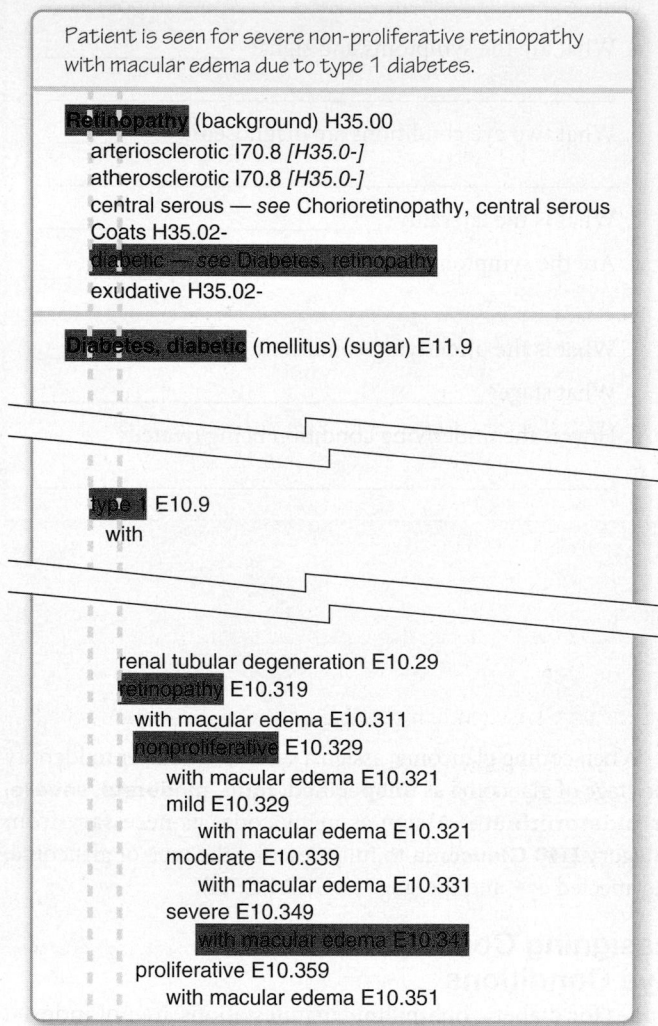

Patient is seen for severe non-proliferative retinopathy with macular edema due to type 1 diabetes.

Retinopathy (background) H35.00
   arteriosclerotic I70.8 *[H35.0-]*
   atherosclerotic I70.8 *[H35.0-]*
   central serous — *see* Chorioretinopathy, central serous
   Coats H35.02-
   diabetic — *see* Diabetes, retinopathy
   exudative H35.02-

Diabetes, diabetic (mellitus) (sugar) E11.9

   type 1 E10.9
     with

     renal tubular degeneration E10.29
     retinopathy E10.319
      with macular edema E10.311
      nonproliferative E10.329
       with macular edema E10.321
       mild E10.329
        with macular edema E10.321
       moderate E10.339
        with macular edema E10.331
       severe E10.349
        with macular edema E10.341
      proliferative E10.359
       with macular edema E10.351

Figure 19-8 ■ Example of Index Entry for Diabetic Retinopathy

chapter about patient Jaclyn Vandeventer, who was seen at Branton Eye Care due to glaucoma and cataracts.

Follow along in your ICD-10-CM manual as Megan Scheidler, CCS-P, assigns codes. Check off each step after you complete it.

▶ First, Megan confirms the conditions she abstracted.

  ❑ right normal tension glaucoma, mild stage

  ❑ bilateral age-related nuclear cataracts

▶ Megan searches the Index for the Main Term **Glaucoma** (■ FIGURE 19-9).

  ❑ She locates the subterm **low tension.**

❑ She reads the cross-reference instruction that states —*see* **Glaucoma, open angle, low-tension.**

❑ She locates the subterm **open angle, low-tension H40.12-.**

▶ Megan verifies code **H40.12-** in the Tabular List (■ FIGURE 19-10).

❑ She reads the code title for **H40.12, Low-tension glaucoma** and confirms that this accurately describes the diagnosis.

❑ She observes the symbol **6th**, indicating that a sixth digit is required for laterality.

❑ She reviews the choices for laterality and selects **H40.121, Low-tension glaucoma, right eye.**

❑ She notices the **7th** symbol and reads the instructional note under the subcategory **H40.12** to assign a seventh character to identify the stage.

❑ She checks the medical record to verify the stage as mild and selects **H40.1211, Low-tension glaucoma, right eye, mild stage.**

▶ Megan checks for instructional notes in the Tabular List.

❑ She cross-references the beginning of category **H40** and verifies that the only instructional note is an **Excludes1** note that does not apply to the low-tension glaucoma.

❑ She cross-references the beginning of the block **H40-H42** and verifies that there are no instructional notes.

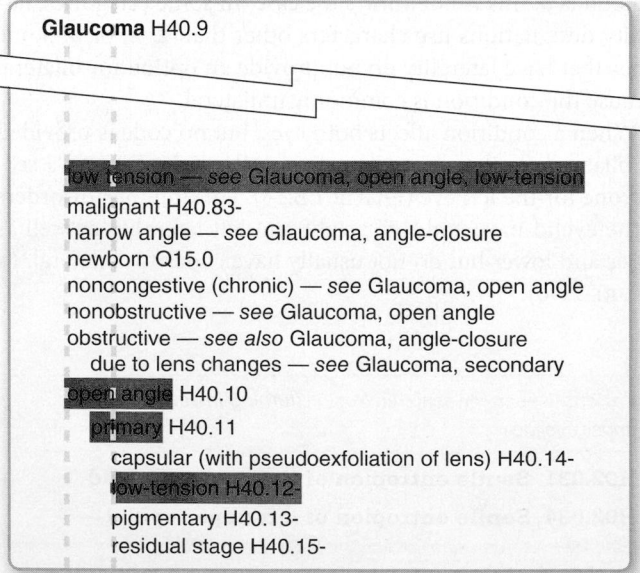

Glaucoma H40.9

   low tension — *see* Glaucoma, open angle, low-tension
   malignant H40.83-
   narrow angle — *see* Glaucoma, angle-closure
   newborn Q15.0
   noncongestive (chronic) — *see* Glaucoma, open angle
   nonobstructive — *see* Glaucoma, open angle
   obstructive — *see also* Glaucoma, angle-closure
     due to lens changes — *see* Glaucoma, secondary
   open angle H40.10
     primary H40.11
      capsular (with pseudoexfoliation of lens) H40.14-
      low-tension H40.12-
      pigmentary H40.13-
      residual stage H40.15-

Figure 19-9 ■ Index Entry for Glaucoma

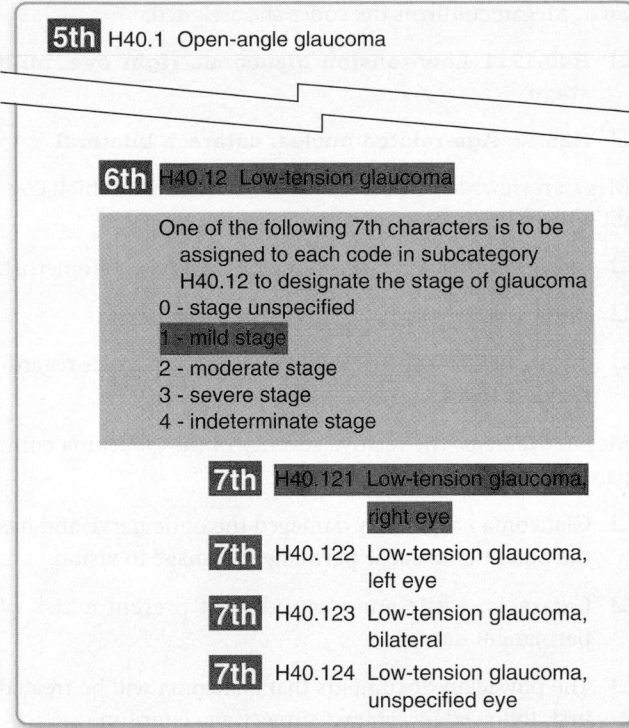

5th H40.1 Open-angle glaucoma

6th H40.12 Low-tension glaucoma

One of the following 7th characters is to be
assigned to each code in subcategory
H40.12 to designate the stage of glaucoma
0 - stage unspecified
1 - mild stage
2 - moderate stage
3 - severe stage
4 - indeterminate stage

7th H40.121 Low-tension glaucoma,
right eye

7th H40.122 Low-tension glaucoma,
left eye

7th H40.123 Low-tension glaucoma,
bilateral

7th H40.124 Low-tension glaucoma,
unspecified eye

Figure 19-10 ■ Tabular List Entry for Low-Tension Glaucoma

❑ She cross-references the beginning of **Chapter 7
(H00-H89)** and reviews the instructional note. She
determines that it does not apply to this case because
the patient's glaucoma is not related to an external cause.

▶ Megan searches the Index for the Main Term **Cataract**.

❑ She locates the subterm **age-related**.

❑ She reads the cross-reference instruction that states
—*see* **Cataract, senile**.

❑ She locates the subterm **senile**.

❑ She locates the second-level subterm **nuclear H25.1**.

▶ Megan verifies code **H25.1** in the Tabular List.

❑ She reads the code title for **H25.1, Age-related nuclear
cataract** and confirms that this accurately describes the
diagnosis.

❑ She observes the symbol **5th**, indicating that a fifth
digit is required for laterality.

❑ She reviews the choices for laterality and selects **H25.13,
Age-related nuclear cataract, bilateral**.

▶ Megan checks for instructional notes in the Tabular List.

❑ She cross-references the beginning of category **H25** and
verifies that the only instructional note is an **Excludes1**
note that does not apply to the low-tension glaucoma.

❑ She cross-references the beginning of the block **H25-H28**
and verifies that there are no instructional notes.

❑ She previously checked the beginning of **Chapter 7
(H00-H89)** and knows that the note does not apply
because the cataract is not related to an external cause.

▶ Megan reviews the codes she has assigned for this case.

❑ **H40.1211 Low-tension glaucoma, right eye, mild
stage**

❑ **H25.13 Age-related nuclear cataract, bilateral**

▶ Next, Megan must determine how to sequence the codes.

CODING PRACTICE

Exercise 19.3 Assigning Codes for Eye Conditions

Instructions: Read the mini-medical-record of each patient's encounter, review the information abstracted in Exercise 19.2, and assign ICD-10-CM diagnosis codes using the Index and Tabular List. Write the code(s) on the line provided.

---

1. OFFICE Gender: M Age: 76

Reason for encounter: phacoemulsification of cataract and intraocular lens (IOL) implant

Assessment: age related nuclear cataract, left eye

Plan: FU in office, 2 days

Tip: Follow cross-referencing instructions in the Index.

1 ICD-10-CM Code _____

---

2. OFFICE Gender: F Age: 84

Reason for encounter: monthly retinal injections

Assessment: wet macular degeneration, in both eyes

Plan: return, 1 month

1 ICD-10-CM Code _____

---

3. OFFICE Gender: F Age: 69

Reason for encounter: crusty eyelids

Assessment: nonulcerative blepharitis on both upper lids

Plan: keep clean, Rx topical antibiotic

Tip: Either code can be sequenced first.

2 ICD-10-CM Codes _____

ARRANGING CODES FOR EYE CONDITIONS

ICD-10-CM does not provide any unique instructions for sequencing codes related to diseases of the eye. Coders follow the general OGCR for selecting the principal or first-listed diagnosis. They also follow instructional notes within the Tabular List. The most common situations when coders will see instructional notes in this ICD-10-CM chapter are the following:

- When the eye condition is secondary to another condition, sequence the underlying condition first.

- When the condition is due to a drug, sequence a code for the drug first. Use the Table of Drugs and Chemicals to identify the drug.

- When another associated condition is documented, such as hypertension or glaucoma, assign codes for both conditions and sequence them according to the circumstances of the encounter.

- When the eye condition results from an adverse effect to a drug, sequence the eye condition first and the drug second. Use the Table of Drugs and Chemicals to identify the drug and intent.

Guided Example of Arranging Codes for Eye Conditions

To learn more about sequencing codes for diseases of the eye and ocular adnexa, continue with the example from earlier in the chapter about patient Jaclyn Vandeventer, who was seen at Branton Eye Care due to glaucoma and cataracts.

Follow along in your ICD-10-CM manual as Megan Scheidler, CCS-P, sequences the codes. Check off each step after you complete it.

▶ First, Megan confirms the codes she assigned.

❑ **H40.1211 Low-tension glaucoma, right eye, mild stage**

❑ **H25.13 Age-related nuclear cataract, bilateral**

▶ Megan reviews the medical record to determine which condition was the main reason for the visit.

❑ The encounter was due to a referral from the optometrist.

❑ Both conditions were evaluated during the visit.

❑ The Tabular List provides no instructional notes regarding sequencing.

▶ Megan evaluates the relative severity of the glaucoma compared to cataracts.

❑ Glaucoma has already damaged the optic nerve and has the potential to cause permanent damage to vision.

❑ Cataracts, while annoying, do not present a risk of permanent damage.

❑ The physician documents that glaucoma will be treated first, followed by cataract surgery at a later time.

❑ Based on these considerations, Megan sequences the glaucoma first.

▶ Megan finalizes the codes and sequencing for this case:

1. **H40.1211 Low-tension glaucoma, right eye, mild stage**

2. **H25.13 Age-related nuclear cataract, bilateral**

CODING PRACTICE

Exercise 19.4   Arranging Codes for Eye Conditions

Instructions: Read the mini-medical-record of each patient's encounter, review the information abstracted in Exercise 19.2, assign ICD-10-CM diagnosis codes using the Index and Tabular List, and sequence them correctly.

---

1. OFFICE   Gender: M   Age: 61

Reason for encounter: *routine eye exam as part of diabetic monitoring*

Assessment: *moderate diabetic nonproliferative retinopathy with no macular edema*

Plan: *be diligent about keeping sugar and BP well controlled, to slow progression of condition*

Tip: Assign a Z code for the reason for the encounter. Follow sequencing instructions in the Tabular List.

2 ICD-10-CM Codes _____

---

2. OFFICE   Gender: F   Age: 53

Reason for encounter: *blurred vision, eye pain, floaters in both eyes*

Assessment: *chronic bilateral anterior uveitis due to juvenile rheumatoid arthritis, associated cataract with neovascularization in left eye also noted*

Plan: *eye drops, dark glasses*

Tip: Follow cross-referencing instructions in the Index.

3 ICD-10-CM Codes _____

_____

(continued)

3. OFFICE   Gender: F   Age: 54

Reason for encounter: *difficulty seeing, gritty feeling in eyes, ocular hyperemia (bloodshot eyes)*

Assessment: *bilateral grade 2 corneal and conjunctival deposits, likely due to stage 5 renal failure, patient has been on dialysis for about 18 months*

(continued)

3. (continued)

Plan: *schedule cornea scraping to remove deposits*

Tip: Instructional notes in the Tabular List guide you to the additional codes and sequencing.

4 ICD-10-CM Codes _____

_____

CODING NEOPLASMS OF THE EYE

Neoplasms of the eye and ocular adnexa do not appear in ICD-10-CM Chapter 7, Diseases of the Eye and Adnexa (H00-H59). Codes for neoplasms of the eye and ocular adnexa appear in category **C69 Malignant Neoplasm of eye and adnexa** within the neoplasm chapter.

Among adults, the most common primary malignant neoplasm in the eye is intraocular melanoma, followed by intraocular lymphoma, although both are relatively rare. In children, the most common eye cancer is retinoblastoma (*cancer arising from cells in the retina*).

Metastatic neoplasms are more common than primary neoplasms of the eye. The most common cancers that spread to the eye are breast and lung cancers. Most often, these cancers spread to the uvea. Metastatic breast cancer usually appears

in the eye several years after breast cancer treatment has been completed. Metastatic lung cancer to the eye is often the first sign that lung cancer exists. Patients may be surprised to learn that a vision problem is a manifestation of breast or lung cancer.

Cancers of the orbit and ocular adnexa develop from tissues such as muscle, nerve, and skin around the eyeball and are classified as neoplasms of the type of tissue they arise in. For example, cancers of the eyelid are usually skin cancers and cancers of the eye muscles are usually rhabdomyosarcoma.

When eye cancer needs specific treatment, physicians use targeted radiation therapy to the eye or eye injections of chemotherapeutic drugs. Unfortunately, by the time cancer has metastasized to the eye, patients often have more serious problems to address, and the eye metastasis may not be a high treatment priority.

CODING PRACTICE

Exercise 19.5 Coding Neoplasms of the Eye

Instructions: Read the mini-medical-record of each patient's encounter, then abstract, assign, and sequence ICD-10-CM diagnosis codes using the Index and Tabular List. Write the code(s) on the line provided.

1. OFFICE   Gender: M   Age: 8

Reason for encounter: *mother is concerned about a white spot in her son's right eye and says he seems to be cross-eyed*

Assessment: *retinoblastoma*

Plan: *schedule a consultation with ophthalmologic oncologist, pediatric oncologist, and radiation oncologist to determine treatment options*

1 ICD-10-CM Code _____

2. OFFICE   Gender: F   Age: 58

Reason for encounter: *patient is concerned because she can see a dark spot on the left iris and has been having headaches*

(continued)

2. (continued)

Assessment: *melanocytoma with secondary glaucoma*

Plan: *this is benign and does not require treatment at this time, but we need to monitor the glaucoma*

2 ICD-10-CM Codes _____

3. OFFICE   Gender: F   Age: 49

Reason for encounter: *blurry vision*

Assessment: *metastatic cancer to choroid in both eyes, history of right breast cancer 5 years ago which is no longer under treatment, status post right mastectomy*

Plan: *targeted radiotherapy, referred back to her oncologist for detection of other possible metastases*

3 ICD-10-CM Codes _____

_____

(continued)

CODING PRACTICE (continued)

4. OFFICE Gender: F Age: 56

Reason for encounter: removal of lesion from right upper eyelid

Assessment: basal cell carcinoma

1 ICD-10-CM Code _____

5. OFFICE Gender: F Age: 54

Reason for encounter: review biopsy and consultation results for salmon colored patch on right conjunctiva

Assessment: malignant conjunctival lymphoma mucosa associated lymphoid tissue (MALT)

Plan: refer to oncologist for evaluation for possible systemic lymphoma, then determine course of treatment

1 ICD-10-CM Code _____

CHAPTER SUMMARY

In this chapter you learned that:

- The eye and ocular adnexa make vision possible by receiving light from the external world and converting it into impulses that are transmitted to the brain through the optic nerve.

- The majority of conditions in this chapter require that the laterality be identified.

- When a condition affects both eyes but there is no option for bilateral, assign two codes, one for the right eye and a second one for the left eye.

- ICD-10-CM does not provide any unique instructions for arranging codes related to diseases of the eye, so coders follow the general OGCR for selecting the principal or first-listed diagnosis.

- Metastatic neoplasms are more common than primary neoplasms of the eye, with the most common being metastatic breast and lung cancers.

- ICD-10-CM provides Official Guidelines for Coding and Reporting (OGCR) for coding the stages of glaucoma in OGCR I.C.7.

CONCEPT QUIZ

Take a moment to look back at the eye and ocular adnexa and solidify your skills. Try to answer the questions from memory first, then look back at the discussion in this chapter if you need a little extra help.

Completion

Instructions: Write the term that answers each question based on the information you learned in this chapter. Choose from the list below. Some choices may be used more than once and some choices may not be used at all.

adnexa	keratitis
cataract	macular degeneration
chalazion	ocular globe
conjunctivitis	optic nerve
diabetic retinopathy	orbital cavity
glaucoma	uvea
hordeolum	uvula
keratin	vitreous body

1. The ocular muscles, eyelids, and conjunctiva make up the
   _____.

2. A(an) _____ is a small hard cyst on the eyelid caused by blockage of a gland on the eyelid.

3. The transparent jelly that fills the eyeball and is surrounded by a membrane is the _____
   _____.

4. The condition of _____
   may be proliferative or nonproliferative.

5. The middle layer of eye consisting of the iris, ciliary body, and choroid is the _____.

6. The gradual loss of central vision due to aging with no cure is
   _____.

7. A(an) _____
   is a bacterial inflammation of a sebaceous gland on the edge or lining of the eyelid.

8. The eye socket is also called the _____
   _____.

9. _____ is a viral or bacterial inflammation and infection of the lining of the eyelid.

10. _____ is an inflammation and ulceration of the surface of the cornea.

Multiple Choice

Instructions: Circle the letter of the best answer to each question based on the information you learned in this chapter.

1. What is the separation of the retina from the choroid layer of the eye?
   A. Choroiditis
   B. Macular degeneration
   C. Diabetic retinopathy
   D. Retinal detachment

2. What type of codes are included in ICD-10-CM Chapter 7?
   A. Syphilis-related eye disorders
   B. Injuries to the eye
   C. Visual disturbances and blindness
   D. Diabetic eye disorders

3. Which of the following is NOT a key criterion for abstracting conditions of the eye and ocular adnexa?
   A. Is the condition malignant or benign?
   B. Is laterality right, left, bilateral, or unspecified?
   C. Is the condition acute or chronic?
   D. Is the condition due to an external cause?

4. Which character(s) of a code indicates laterality?
   A. First
   B. Second or third
   C. Fifth or sixth
   D. Seventh

5. When a condition affects both eyes but there is no option for bilateral, the coder should assign
   A. A code for unspecified eye.
   B. One code for the right eye and a second code for the left eye.
   C. A code for the dominant eye.
   D. Does not apply because all eye codes have an option for bilateral.

6. What Main Term are the codes for diabetic retinopathy indexed under?
   A. Diabetes
   B. Retinopathy
   C. Either Diabetes or Retinopathy
   D. Manifestation, diabetic

7. What subterm should be used to locate age-related cataracts in the Index?
   A. Age
   B. Old
   C. Nuclear
   D. Senile

8. When the eye condition is due to an external cause, which should be sequenced first?
   A. The place of occurrence
   B. The laterality
   C. The eye condition
   D. The external cause

9. What is nuclear cataract?
   A. Located in the center of the eye
   B. The result of exposure to radiation
   C. Beginning to become apparent
   D. Caused by diabetes

10. What is the most common neoplasm that affects the eye?
    A. Intraocular melanoma
    B. Retinoblastoma
    C. Metastasis
    D. Rhabdomyosarcoma

CODING CHALLENGE

Instructions: Read the mini-medical-record of each patient's encounter, then abstract, assign, and sequence ICD-10-CM diagnosis codes using the Index and Tabular List. Write the code(s) on the line provided.

1. OFFICE   Gender: F   Age: 28

Reason for encounter: routine vision examination

Assessment: latent nystagmus, right eye

Plan: prescription contact lenses

Tip: Assign one code for the eye exam and a second code for the finding.

2 ICD-10-CM Codes _____

2. OFFICE   Gender: M   Age: 48

Reason for encounter: light flashes for 2 months, dense shadow/curtain progressing toward central vision this morning

(continued)

2. (continued)

Assessment: detachment of retina with one break, right eye

Plan: scleral buckle surgery

1 ICD-10-CM Code _____

3. OFFICE   Gender: F   Age: 42

Reason for encounter: pain and redness in R eye

Assessment: R eye marginal corneal ulcer due to dry eye syndrome which is bilateral, so we will keep watch on the other eye as well

Plan: pain medication, tear substitute drops, discontinue contact use, RTO tomorrow

2 ICD-10-CM Codes _____

(continued)

(continued from page 319)

4. OFFICE Gender: M Age: 57

Reason for encounter: noticing mild impairment of vision, redness of eyes, foreign body sensation in eyes

Assessment: recurrent pterygium, bilateral

Plan: artificial tears, anti-inflammatory drops, RTO one month

1 ICD-10-CM Code _____

---

5. OFFICE Gender: F Age: 2

Reason for encounter: scheduled cataract removal

Assessment: subcapsular posterior juvenile cataract, cerebrotendinous xanthomatosis (*a metabolic disorder related to fat storage*)

Plan: RTO tomorrow, genetic counseling for family, referral to pediatric endocrinologist for FU

2 ICD-10-CM Codes _____

---

6. OFFICE Gender: M Age: 66

Reason for encounter: sudden painless loss of vision

Assessment: occlusion of left central retinal artery. Pt has hypertension and CAD which place her at risk for embolism

Plan: aspirin and Plavix, ocular-digital massage, admit for angiogram to evaluate carotid circulation

3 ICD-10-CM Codes _____

_____

---

7. OFFICE Gender: M Age: 9

Reason for encounter: Child referred to clinic by school teacher. Child unable to distinguish the color red from green.

(*continued*)

---

7. (continued)

Assessment: acquired color blindness

Plan: teach coping skills to distinguish colors

1 ICD-10-CM Code _____

---

8. OFFICE Gender: F Age: 31

Reason for encounter: cloudy blurred vision

Assessment: idiopathic corneal edema

Plan: hypertonic eye drops and ointment

1 ICD-10-CM Code _____

---

9. OFFICE Gender: F Age: 68

Reason for encounter: swelling of lower right eyelid, tenderness, increased tearing

Assessment: chalazion on right lower eyelid

Plan: topical antibiotic eye drops for initial infection. RTO 2 months to inject with a corticosteroid if chalazion has not disappeared

1 ICD-10-CM Code _____

---

10. OFFICE Gender: F Age: 16

Reason for encounter: pink eye, ocular itching, tearing, photophobia, watery discharge, painful socialized swelling on lid

Assessment: bilateral chronic conjunctivitis due to allergies and a stye on the edge of the right upper lid

Plan: cold compresses, NSAIDs, mast cell stabilizers, antihistamine, RTO 1 week

2 ICD-10-CM Codes _____

KEEP ON CODING

Instructions: Read the diagnostic statement, then use the Index and Tabular List to assign and sequence ICD-10-CM diagnosis codes. Write the code(s) on the line provided.

1. Abscess of both upper eyelids: ICD-10-CM Code(s) _____

2. Acute atopic conjunctivitis, both eyes: ICD-10-CM Code(s) _____

3. Kayser-Fleischer ring, left eye: ICD-10-CM Code(s) _____

4. Stable keratoconus, right eye: ICD-10-CM Code(s) _____

5. Anterior subcapsular polar age-related cataract, both eyes: ICD-10-CM Code(s) _____

6. Retinopathy of prematurity, stage 1, right eye: ICD-10-CM Code(s) _____

7. Low-tension glaucoma: ICD-10-CM Code(s) _____

8. Malignant melanoma of choroid, right eye: ICD-10-CM Code(s) _____

9. Optic nerve hypoplasia, left eye: ICD-10-CM Code(s) _____

10. Vertical strabismus, right eye: ICD-10-CM Code(s) _____

11. Sebaceous cyst of right lower eyelid: ICD-10-CM Code(s) _____

12. Low vision, both eyes: ICD-10-CM Code(s) _____

13. Cystoid macular edema post cataract surgery, left eye: ICD-10-CM Code(s) _____

14. Convergence insufficiency: ICD-10-CM Code(s) _____

15. Epiphora due to excessive discharge of tears, bilateral: ICD-10-CM Code(s) _____

16. Progressive external ophthalmoplegia, right eye: ICD-10-CM Code(s) _____

17. Horseshoe tear of retina without detachment, left eye: ICD-10-CM Code(s) _____

18. Harada disease, both eyes: ICD-10-CM Code(s) _____

19. Cortical age-related cataract, right eye: ICD-10-CM Code(s) _____

20. Staphyloma posticum: ICD-10-CM Code(s) _____

21. Pseudotumor of the left orbit: ICD-10-CM Code(s) _____

22. Ptosis of both eyelids: ICD-10-CM Code(s) _____

23. Diplopia: ICD-10-CM Code(s) _____

24. Ghost vessels in the cornea of the left eye: ICD-10-CM Code(s) _____

25. Postprocedural blebitis, stage 2: ICD-10-CM Code(s) _____

Chapter 20

Diseases of the Ear and Mastoid Process (H60-H95)

Chapter Outline

- **Ear Refresher**
- **Coding Overview of the Ear**
- **Abstracting for Ear Conditions**
- **Assigning Codes for Ear Conditions**
- **Arranging Codes for Ear Conditions**

Learning Objectives

After completing this chapter, you should have the skills to:

20.1 Spell and define the key words, medical terms, and abbreviations related to the ear and mastoid process.

20.2 Discuss the structure, function, and common conditions of the ear and mastoid process.

20.3 Identify the main characteristics of diagnosis coding for the ear and mastoid process.

20.4 Abstract diagnostic information from the medical record for conditions of the ear and mastoid process.

20.5 Assign codes for diseases of the ear and mastoid process.

20.6 Arrange multiple diagnosis codes for diseases of the ear and mastoid process.

20.7 Code neoplasms of the ear and mastoid process.

20.8 Discuss the Official Guidelines for Coding and Reporting related to diseases of the ear and mastoid process.

Key Terms and Abbreviations

auditory canal	incus	otitis media (OM)	tympanic membrane
auricle	inner ear	oval window	tympanic membrane perforation (TMP)
cerumen	labyrinth	pinna	
cochlea	malleus	purulent otitis media	tympanum
eardrum	mastoid process	saccule	utricle
equilibrium	middle ear	semicircular canal	vestibulocochlear nerve
external ear	ossicles	stapes	

In addition to the key terms listed here, students should know the terms defined within tables in this chapter.

INTRODUCTION

Many of our memories relate to sounds—a trickling brook, a thundering waterfall, or a chirping bird. If you are more of a city person, your memories may be the clacking of a train, the honking of traffic, or the music of a show. Whatever sounds are imbedded in your memory, you have your ears to thank.

An otolaryngologist is a physician who specializes in diagnosing and treating conditions of the ear, nose, and throat (ENT). Primary care physicians treat uncomplicated conditions of the ear, nose, and throat. They refer patients with more complex conditions to otolaryngologists.

Keep your medical reference resources handy as you study this chapter. The ear contains some of the smallest structures in the human body, and it is important to understand the function of each. Experienced coders keep the information they need at their fingertips.

EAR REFRESHER

The ear makes hearing possible by collecting sound waves from the external world and converting them into impulses that are transmitted to the brain through the **vestibulocochlear nerve**, cranial nerve VIII. The ear also maintains **equilibrium**, the sense of balance. The **mastoid process** is the portion of the temporal bone of the skull that juts forward behind the ear.

The ear is divided into three sections: the **external ear**, **middle ear**, and **inner ear** (■ FIGURE 20-1). The external ear consists of the **auricle** or **pinna**, the visible part of the ear, which collects sound waves; the **auditory canal**, which funnels the sound waves; and the **tympanic membrane**, also called the **tympanum** or **eardrum**, which separates the external ear from the middle ear. Glands in the auditory canal produce **cerumen** (*ear wax*) that protects and lubricates the ear.

The middle ear is a small air-filled cavity in the temporal bone that contains the **ossicles**, three small bones that are critical to the hearing process. The ossicles amplify vibrations in the middle ear and transmit them to the inner ear, from the **malleus** (*hammer*) to the **incus** (*anvil*) to the **stapes** (*stirrup*). The stapes is attached to the **oval window**, a thin membrane that covers the opening to the inner ear and passes vibrations to the cochlea.

SUCCESS STEP

The stapes is the smallest named bone in the human body. Without it, you would be unable to hear.

The inner ear, or **labyrinth**, is a fluid-filled cavity in the temporal bone that contains the **cochlea**, a snail-shaped organ that makes hearing possible, and the sensors for equilibrium, which are the **semicircular canals**, **utricle**, and **saccule**.

In Figure 20-1, each structure in the ear and mastoid process is labeled with its name as well as its medical terminology root/combining form where applicable. Refer to ■ TABLE 20-1 (page 324) for a refresher on how to build medical terms related to the ear and mastoid process.

CODING CAUTION

Be alert for medical word roots that sound and are spelled similarly but have different meanings.

ot/o (*ear*) and **opt/o** (*vision, eye*)

mastoid/o (*the combining form for the mastoid process, which is "breast shaped"*) and **mast/o** (*the combining form for the breast*)

tinnitus (*ringing in the ears*) and **tinea** (*a skin fungus*)

serous (*a clear fluid*) and **serious** (*important or somber*)

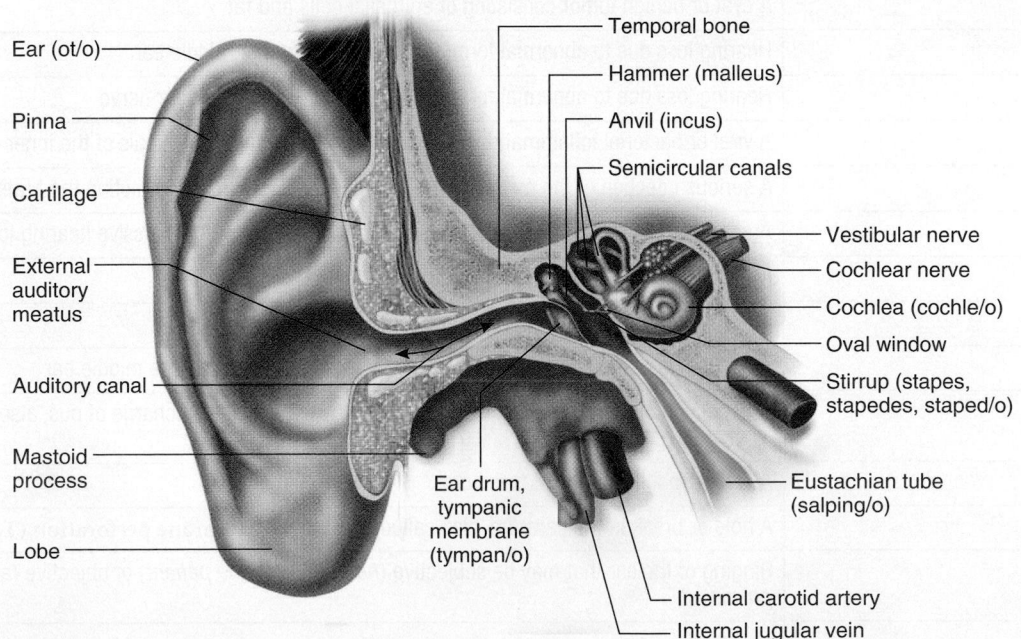

Ear (ot/o)
Pinna
Cartilage
External auditory meatus
Auditory canal
Mastoid process
Lobe
Ear drum, tympanic membrane (tympan/o)
Temporal bone
Hammer (malleus)
Anvil (incus)
Semicircular canals
Vestibular nerve
Cochlear nerve
Cochlea (cochle/o)
Oval window
Stirrup (stapes, stapedes, staped/o)
Eustachian tube (salping/o)
Internal carotid artery
Internal jugular vein

Figure 20-1 ■ The Ear and Mastoid Process

Table 20-1 ■ **EXAMPLE OF CONSTRUCTING MEDICAL TERMS FOR THE EAR AND MASTOID PROCESS**

Combining Form	Suffix	Complete Medical Term
ot/o (*ear*)		ot + itis (*inflammation of the ear*) oto + plasty (*surgical repair of the ear*)
myring/o (*eardrum*) tympan/o (*eardrum, tympanic membrane*)	-itis (*inflammation*) -plasty (*surgical repair*) -tomy (*make an incision into*)	myring + itis (*inflammation of the eardrum*) myringo + tomy (*making an incision in the eardrum*) tympano + plasty (*surgical repair of the tympanic membrane*)
staped/o (*stapes bone*)		stapedo + tomy (*make an incision in the stapes bone*)
mastoid/o (*mastoid process bone, breast shaped*)		mastoid + itis (*inflammation of the mastoid process bone*)

Conditions of the Ear

Coders must be familiar with the most common conditions of the ear: hearing loss, or deafness, and **otitis media** (OM) (*infection of the middle ear*). Approximately 17% of American adults report some degree of hearing loss, and 47% of adults age 75 or older have a hearing impairment, according to the National Institute on Deafness and Other Communication Disorders (NIDCD).

Three of every four children experience OM by the time they are three years old, according to NIDCD. Ear infections are the second most common reason for trips to the pediatrician, after wellness visits; almost half of all antibiotic prescriptions written for children are for ear infections. Untreated OM can lead to complications, such as mastoiditis, hearing loss, perforation of the tympanum, meningitis, facial nerve paralysis, and Ménière disease. Refer to ■ TABLE 20-2 for a summary of diseases affecting the ear and mastoid process.

Neoplasms of the Ear

Neoplasms of the ear are rare. Basal cell carcinoma and malignant melanoma may occur on the skin of the external

Table 20-2 ■ **COMMON DISEASES OF THE EAR AND MASTOID PROCESS**

Condition	Definition
Ceruminoma	Excessive accumulation of ear wax, also called impacted cerumen
Cholesteatoma	A cyst or benign tumor consisting of epithelial cells and fat
Hearing loss—conductive	Hearing loss due to abnormal formation of the external or middle ear
Hearing loss—sensorineural	Hearing loss due to abnormal formation of the cochlea or cochlear nerve
Labrynthitis	A viral or bacterial inflammation or infection of the semicircular canals of the inner ear
Mastoiditis	A serious infection of the mastoid process that carries the risk of infecting the brain
Ménière disease	An abnormality of the fluid of the inner ear that can lead to a progressive hearing loss
Otitis externa	An inflammation of the external ear (pinna)
Otitis media (OM)—nonsuppurative	An inflammation of the middle ear that does not produce pus
Otitis media (OM)—serous	A subtype of nonsuppurative otitis media involving clear fluid in the middle ear
Otitis media (OM)—suppurative	An infection of the middle ear, usually bacterial, involving the discharge of pus, also called **purulent otitis media**
Otosclerosis	A loss of mobility of the stapes bone
Ruptured tympanic membrane	A hole or break in the eardrum, also called **tympanic membrane perforation (TMP)**
Tinnitus	Ringing of the ear that may be subjective (*heard only by the patient*) or objective (*audible to the physician*)
Vertigo	A sensation of motion or dizziness

ear; these are classified under malignant neoplasms of the skin. Squamous cell carcinoma may occur in the ear canal; adenoid cystic carcinoma may occur in the ear glands. Acoustic neuroma, also called vestibular schwannoma, is a benign tumor of the vestibular cochlear nerve, which connects the ear to the brain. It grows slowly, and people with this condition usually do not show symptoms until after age 30.

This section provides a general reference to help understand the most common diagnoses of the ear and mastoid process. Refer to medical resources to learn more about conditions affecting the ear and mastoid process.

CODING PRACTICE

Exercise 20.1 Ear Refresher

Instructions: Use your medical terminology skills and resources to define the following conditions related to the ear and mastoid process, then assign the default diagnosis code.

Follow these steps:

- Use slash marks "/" to break down each term into its root(s) and suffix.
- Define the meaning of the word, based on the meaning of each word part.
- Assign the default ICD-10-CM diagnosis code and laterality for the condition using the Index and Tabular List.

Example: otitis (right) ot/itis   Meaning: *inflammation of the right ear*   ICD-10-CM Code: *H66.91*

1. labyrinthitis (bilateral)   Meaning _____   ICD-10-CM Code _____
2. otosclerosis (right)   Meaning _____   ICD-10-CM Code _____
3. cholesteatoma (left)   Meaning _____   ICD-10-CM Code _____
4. mastoiditis   Meaning _____   ICD-10-CM Code _____
5. presbycusis (bilateral)   Meaning _____   ICD-10-CM Code _____
6. otolith (left)   Meaning _____   ICD-10-CM Code _____
7. otorrhagia (left)   Meaning _____   ICD-10-CM Code _____
8. otorrhea   Meaning _____   ICD-10-CM Code _____
9. mastoidalgia (right)   Meaning _____   ICD-10-CM Code _____
10. tympanosclerosis (bilateral)   Meaning _____   ICD-10-CM Code _____

CODING OVERVIEW OF THE EAR

ICD-10-CM Chapter 8, Diseases of the Ear and Mastoid Process (H60-H95), is a new chapter that did not exist in ICD-9-CM. In ICD-9-CM, the ear and mastoid process were included in Chapter 6 (380-389) for the nervous system and special senses. This is the second of two ICD-10-CM chapters in which codes begin with the letter H; codes for the eye and adnexa occupy codes H00 through H59. This chapter contains five blocks or subchapters that are divided by external, middle, and internal ear. Review the block names and code ranges listed at the beginning of Chapter 8 in the ICD-10-CM manual to become familiar with the content and organization.

ICD-10-CM has expanded numerous codes in this chapter compared to ICD-9-CM. Additional codes identify laterality and greater anatomic specificity. Some categories have been reorganized. Instructional notes to code first the underlying condition have been added throughout the chapter.

This chapter includes disorders affecting the external, middle, and inner ear, as well as the mastoid process. It does not include injuries to the ear, which are classified in ICD-10-CM Chapter 19.

ICD-10-CM does not provide any Official Guidelines for Coding and Reporting (OGCR) specific to this chapter. General OGCR in sections I.A, I.B, II, III, and IV direct the coder. Instructional notes in the Tabular List guide coders when additional codes are required. An instructional note at the beginning of the chapter directs coders to use an external cause code following the code for the ear condition when an external cause created the ear condition. This note applies to all codes in ICD-10-CM Chapter 8.

ABSTRACTING FOR EAR CONDITIONS

The primary concerns in abstracting for diagnoses of the ear and mastoid process are laterality, external causes, and tobacco use or exposure. In addition, coders should be aware of the many variations of OM in order to abstract all the needed details.

Abstracting Laterality

The majority of ear conditions require that the laterality be identified. Laterality is expressed at the following levels:

- right, left, or unspecified ear
- bilateral, for applicable conditions

Table 20-3 ■ **KEY CRITERIA FOR ABSTRACTING CONDITIONS OF THE EAR AND MASTOID PROCESS**

- ❑ What is the condition?
- ❑ What is the subtype of the condition?
- ❑ Is a more specific subtype documented?
- ❑ What part of the ear is affected?
- ❑ What is the laterality?
- ❑ What other conditions coexist?
- ❑ Is there an underlying disease?
- ❑ Is the condition due to a drug or external cause?
- ❑ Is there documentation of current or past use of tobacco or exposure to tobacco smoke?

Table 20-4 ■ **KEY CRITERIA FOR ABSTRACTING OTITIS MEDIA**

- ❑ What is the subtype of otitis media?
- ❑ Is it suppurative/purulent, nonsuppurative/serous, or another subtype?
- ❑ Is it acute, acute recurrent, or chronic?
- ❑ What is the laterality?
- ❑ Is there associated rupture of the tympanic membrane?
- ❑ What is the type or extent of rupture?
- ❑ What is the laterality of the rupture?
- ❑ Is it a manifestation of another disease?
- ❑ Is there documentation of current or past use of tobacco or exposure to tobacco smoke?

When a patient has more than one ear condition, the laterality for *each* condition must be identified separately. For example, a patient may have *bilateral* OM but *unilateral* TMP in the right or left ear only.

Refer to ■ TABLE 20-3 for guidance on how to abstract conditions of the ear and mastoid process. Remember that abstracting questions are a guide and that not every question applies to, or can be answered for, every case. For example, tinnitus does not have subtype conditions.

Abstracting for Otitis Media

Otitis media requires that coders abstract the basic information required for all ear conditions, plus additional details unique to OM. Coders need to abstract the specific subtype of OM. The two most common are suppurative and serous. Serous is one form of nonsuppurative OM, but coders may occasionally encounter other nonsuppurative types, such as **mucoid**, **allergic**, **secretory**, and **seromucinous**.

CODING CAUTION

Do not assume that all conditions named *otitis* are otitis media. You need to distinguish between otitis *media*, inflammation of the middle ear, and otitis *externa*, inflammation of the external ear. These are separate conditions with different codes.

OM is classified as acute, acute recurrent, and chronic. Although there are no universal definitions of these stages, a common practice is to classify recurrent acute otitis media as chronic when it persists for longer than three months and is accompanied by changes in the lining of the middle ear. Coders abstract this information based on how physicians describe the condition in the documentation. When in doubt, query the physician for clarification. Refer to ■ TABLE 20-4 for guidance on how to abstract for otitis media, then work through the detailed example that follows.

Guided Example of Abstracting for the Ear

Refer to the following example throughout this chapter to learn about abstracting, assigning, and sequencing codes for the ear

and mastoid process. Gabrielle Javiera, CPC, is a fictitious coder who guides you through the coding process.

Date: 10/21/yy   Location: Ear, Nose, and Throat Specialists

Provider: Shauna Rotz, MD

Patient: Estela Nuno   Gender: F   Age: 4

Reason for encounter: ear pain, fever

Assessment: bilateral acute serous otitis media with total rupture of tympanic membrane of the right ear, no one in the household smokes

Plan: antibiotics, **fat-plug tympanoplasty**

Follow along as Gabrielle Javiera, CPC, abstracts the diagnosis. Check off each step after you complete it.

▶ Gabrielle reads through the entire record, with special attention to the reason for the encounter and the final assessment. She refers to the Key Criteria for Abstracting Otitis Media (Table 20-4).

- ❑ She notes the presenting symptoms: *ear pain, fever*
- ❑ *What is the condition?* otitis media
- ❑ *What is the subtype of the condition?* acute serous
- ❑ *Is it suppurative/purulent, nonsuppurative/serous, or another subtype?* serous, which is a type of nonsuppurative OM
- ❑ *What is the laterality?* bilateral
- ❑ *Is it acute, acute recurrent, or chronic?* acute
- ❑ *Is there associated rupture of the tympanic membrane?* Yes.
- ❑ *What is the type or extent of rupture?* total

❑ *What is the laterality of the rupture?* She notes that laterality of the rupture is right, although the otitis media is bilateral.

❑ *Is it a manifestation of another disease?* No.

❑ *Is there documentation of current or past use of tobacco or exposure to tobacco smoke?* no one in the household smokes

❑ Now that she has identified the conditions, she reviews the symptoms again. She determines that ear pain and fever are integral to otitis media and should not be coded (■ FIGURE 20-2).

❑ She reviews the planned treatments and concludes that they are consistent with the condition she abstracted.

▶ At this time, Gabrielle does not know how many codes she will need. She will learn about this when she moves on to assigning codes.

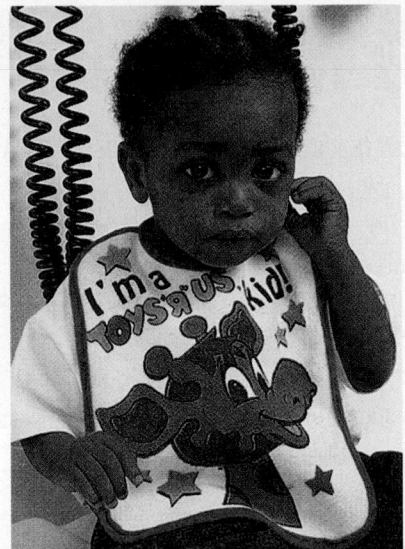

Figure 20-2 ■ Common signs of otitis media are fussiness and pulling at the ear.
Source: Pearson Education.

CODING PRACTICE

Exercise 20.2   **Abstracting for Ear Conditions**

Instructions: Read the mini-medical-record of each patient's encounter and answer the abstracting questions. Write the answer on the line provided. Do not assign any codes.

1. OUTPATIENT HOSPITAL   Gender: M   Age: 7

Reason for encounter: bilateral tympanoplasty

Assessment: bilateral chronic serous otitis media

Plan: FU in office, 2 weeks

a. What is tympanoplasty? _____

b. What is the condition? _____

c. Is it suppurative or nonsuppurative? _____

_____

d. What is the laterality? _____

e. Is the condition acute or chronic? _____

_____

2. OFFICE   Gender: F   Age: 23

Chief complaint: severe nausea, vomiting, sweating, vertigo

Assessment: symptoms are due to Meniere's disease, left ear

Plan: diazepam (*a sedative*) for vertigo, it may get better on its own or it may not, will consider surgery if necessary, but we want to follow it for awhile

(continued)

2. (continued)

a. What are the symptoms? _____

b. Will you code the symptoms? _____

Why or why not? _____

c. What condition is diagnosed? _____

d. What is the laterality? _____

3. OFFICE   Gender: F   Age: 32

Chief complaint: ringing and buzzing in right ear, difficulty hearing in right ear

Assessment: objective tinnitus

Plan: We will try electrical stimulation treatments and see how the condition responds before considering surgery.

a. What are the symptoms? _____

b. Will you code the symptoms? _____

Why or why not? _____

c. What condition is diagnosed? _____

_____

What does *objective* mean? _____

d. What is the laterality? _____

(continued)

CODING PRACTICE (continued)

4. OUTPATIENT SURGERY   Gender: M   Age: 58

Reason for encounter: bilateral stapedotomy (*making an incision in the stapes bone*) and placement of prosthesis

Assessment: bilateral conductive hearing loss due to bilateral nonobliterative otosclerosis of the stapes at the oval window

Plan: FU in office, 2 weeks

a. What is stapedotomy? _____

b. What type of hearing loss is documented? _____
_____

c. What is the laterality of the hearing loss? _____
_____

d. What is otosclerosis? _____

e. What is the type of otosclerosis? _____

f. What bone is affected by the otosclerosis? _____
_____

g. What is the laterality of the otosclerosis? _____
_____

5. OFFICE   Gender: F   Age: 12

Reason for encounter: left earache, fever, head congestion

Assessment: acute recurrent suppurative otitis media and acute recurrent sinusitis, mother is a heavy cigarette smoker

Plan: antibiotics for OM, decongestant, and fluids

a. What are the symptoms? _____

b. What condition is the first condition diagnosed?
_____

c. Is it suppurative or nonsuppurative? _____
_____

d. Is it acute or chronic? _____

e. Is it recurrent? _____

(continued)

5. (continued)

f. Which symptoms relate to the first condition?
_____

g. What is the laterality of the first condition? _____

h. What condition is the second condition
   diagnosed? _____

i. Is it acute or chronic? _____

j. Is it recurrent? _____

k. Which symptoms relate to the second condition?
_____

l. Which condition should you sequence first?
_____

   Why? _____

m. Is tobacco use or exposure documented? _____

6. OFFICE   Gender: M   Age: 19

Reason for encounter: dizziness, nausea, low back pain, headache on right side

Assessment: dizziness, nausea, and headache due to labyrinthitis, right

Plan: refer to physical therapy for balance and for LBP

a. What are the symptoms? _____

b. What is labyrinthitis? _____

c. What is the laterality? _____

d. Which symptoms relate to the labyrinthitis?
_____

e. What symptom does not relate to labyrinthitis?
_____

   Should it be coded? _____

   Why or why not? _____

ASSIGNING CODES FOR EAR CONDITIONS

The Index provides cross-referencing instructions that redirect coders to alternative Main Terms for many ear conditions. When a condition cannot be located under a Main Term, remember to refer to any alternative Main Terms provided in the cross-reference notes. This is especially helpful when assigning codes for hearing loss and OM.

Assigning Codes for Hearing Loss

Coders may use the Main Term **Deafness** for any condition described as hearing loss or deafness. Hearing loss is indexed under the Main Term **Loss** and the subterm **hearing**. Five second-level subterms direct coders to the same code, **H90.5 Unspecified sensorineural hearing loss**. A cross-reference note states *see also* **Deafness**. The Main Term **Deafness** provides over 40 subterms, which direct coders to specific codes, including the ones listed

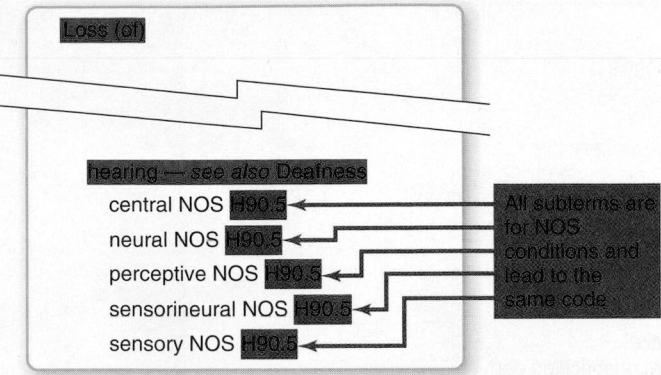

Figure 20-3 ■ Index Entry for Hearing Loss with a Cross-Reference to Deafness

under the Main Term **Loss, hearing**. Therefore, it is most efficient for coders to go directly to **Deafness** when assigning codes for hearing loss or deafness (■ FIGURE 20-3).

Assigning Codes for Otitis Media

The Index entry **Otitis, media** contains numerous cross-references between second-level subterms, which may seem confusing. Nearly all types of OM can be located under the two second-level subterms **nonsuppurative** and **suppurative**. Third- and fourth-level subterms further identify the specific subtype of OM.

SUCCESS STEP

To make navigating the Index for OM easier, highlight the subterm entries for **nonsuppurative** and **suppurative**.

Guided Example of Assigning Codes for Ear Conditions

To learn more about assigning codes for the ear and mastoid process, continue with the example from earlier in the chapter about a patient who was seen due to ear pain and fever.

Follow along in your ICD-10-CM manual and check off each step after you complete it.

▶ First, Gabrielle confirms the diagnoses.

❑ bilateral acute serous otitis media

❑ total rupture of tympanic membrane of the right ear

▶ Gabrielle searches the Index for the Main Term **Otitis** (■ FIGURE 20-4).

❑ She locates the subterm **media**.

❑ She knows that serous otitis media is a type of nonsuppurative otitis media, so she locates the second-level subterm, **nonsuppurative**.

❑ She locates the third-level subterm **acute**.

❑ She locates the fourth-level subterm **serous H65.0-**.

▶ Gabrielle verifies **H65.0-** in the Tabular List (■ FIGURE 20-5, page 330).

❑ She reads the subcategory title for **H65.0, Acute serous otitis media** and confirms that this accurately describes the condition.

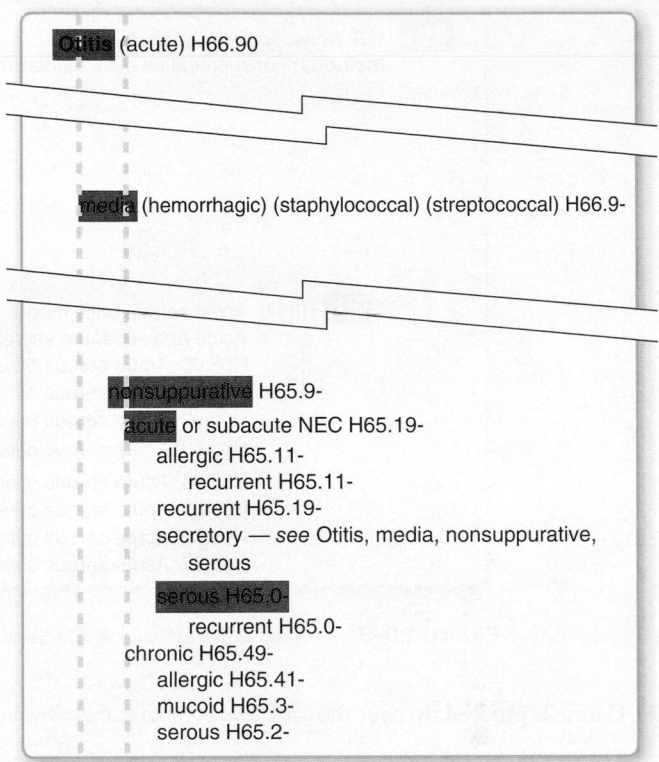

Figure 20-4 ■ Index Entry for Nonsuppurative Otitis Media

❑ She identifies the symbol **5th** in front of the subcategory number, telling her that a fifth digit is required to identify the laterality.

❑ She notices that there eight codes in this category: four for acute serous otitis media and four for acute serous otitis media, *recurrent*.

❑ She verifies that the documentation does not state recurrent, so she selects the code **H65.03, Acute serous otitis media, bilateral**.

▶ Gabrielle checks for instructional notes in the Tabular List.

❑ She cross-references the beginning of subcategory **H65.0** and verifies that there are no instructional notes.

❑ She cross-references the beginning of category **H65** and identifies several instructional notes. The first note states **Use additional code for any associated perforated tympanic membrane (H72.-)**. This tells her that she will need a separate code for the TMP.

❑ She reads the other instructional notes that direct her to use an additional code for various circumstances of tobacco use and exposure. She double-checks the medical record and determines that none of these circumstances are documented.

❑ She cross-references the beginning of the block **H65-H75** and verifies that there are no instructional notes.

❑ She cross-references the beginning of **Chapter 8 (H60-H95)** and reviews the instructional note. She determines that it does not apply to this case because the condition is not due to an external cause.

4th H65 Nonsuppurative otitis media
Includes: nonsuppurative otitis media with myringitis
Use additional code for any associated perforated tympanic membrane (H72.-)
Use additional code to identify:
exposure to environmental tobacco smoke (Z77.22)
exposure to tobacco smoke in the perinatal period (P96.81)
history of tobacco use (Z87.891)
occupational exposure to environmental tobacco smoke (Z57.31)
tobacco dependence (F17.-)
tobacco use (Z72.0)
5th H65.0 Acute serous otitis media
Acute and subacute secretory otitis
H65.00 Acute serous otitis media, unspecified ear
H65.01 Acute serous otitis media, right ear
H65.02 Acute serous otitis media, left ear
H65.03 Acute serous otitis media, bilateral
H65.04 Acute serous otitis media, recurrent, right ear
H65.05 Acute serous otitis media, recurrent, left ear
H65.06 Acute serous otitis media, recurrent, bilateral
H65.07 Acute serous otitis media, recurrent, unspecified ear

Figure 20-5 ■ Tabular List Entry for Acute Serous Otitis Media

▶ Gabrielle proceeds to code the *ruptured tympanic membrane*.

❑ She cross-references the Tabular List entry for **H72.-** that is listed in the instructional note.

❑ She notices there are a lot of codes under category **H72**.

❑ She reviews the subcategory headings until she locates subcategory **H72.82, Total perforation of tympanic membrane**.

❑ She identifies the symbol **6th** in front of the subcategory number, telling her that a sixth digit is required to identify the laterality.

❑ She double-checks the medical record to confirm that laterality for the TMP is *right*.

❑ She reviews the available code options and selects the code **H72.821, Total perforation of tympanic membrane, right ear**.

▶ Gabrielle checks for instructional notes in the Tabular List.

❑ She cross-references the beginning of category **H72** and identifies the instructional note that states **Code first any associated otitis media**.

❑ She already checked the instructional notes for the block and chapter, so she does not check them again because she knows they do not apply to this case.

▶ Gabrielle reviews the codes she has assigned for this case.

❑ **H72.821 Total perforation of tympanic membrane, right ear**

❑ **H65.03 Acute serous otitis media, bilateral**

▶ Next, Gabrielle must decide how to sequence the codes.

CODING PRACTICE

Exercise 20.3 Assigning Codes for Ear Conditions

Instructions: Read the mini-medical-record of each patient's encounter, review the information abstracted in Exercise 20.2, and assign ICD-10-CM diagnosis codes using the Index and Tabular List. Write the code(s) on the line provided.

1. OUTPATIENT SURGERY Gender: M Age: 7

Reason for encounter: bilateral tympanoplasty

Assessment: bilateral chronic serous otitis media

Plan: FU in office, 2 weeks

1 ICD-10-CM Code _____

2. OFFICE Gender: F Age: 23

Chief complaint: severe nausea, vomiting, sweating, vertigo

Assessment: symptoms are due to Meniere's disease, left ear

Plan: diazepam for vertigo, it may get better on its own or it may not, will consider surgery if necessary, but we want to follow it for awhile

1 ICD-10-CM Code _____

(continued)

3. OFFICE   Gender: F   Age: 32

Chief complaint: ringing and buzzing in right ear, difficulty hearing in right ear

Assessment: objective tinnitus

(continued)

---

3. (continued)

Plan: We will try electrical stimulation treatments and see how the condition responds before considering surgery.

1 ICD-10-CM Code _____

ARRANGING CODES FOR EAR CONDITIONS

ICD-10-CM does not provide any unique instructions for sequencing codes related to diseases of the ear. Coders follow the general OGCR for selecting the principal or first-listed diagnosis. They also follow instructional notes within the Tabular List. The most common situations in which coders will see instructional notes in this ICD-10-CM chapter are the following:

- When the ear condition is secondary to another condition, sequence the underlying condition first.

- When the ear condition results from an adverse effect of a drug, sequence the condition first and the drug second. Use the Table of Drugs and Chemicals to identify the drug and intent.

- When OM is accompanied by a perforated tympanic membrane, sequence the OM first and the perforated membrane second.

- When the ear condition is due to an external cause, sequence the ear condition first, followed by the external cause code.

- Sequence codes describing tobacco use or exposure as secondary codes.

Guided Example of Arranging Codes for Ear Conditions

To learn more about sequencing codes for the ear and mastoid process, continue with the example from earlier in the chapter about a patient who was seen due to ear pain and fever.

Follow along in your ICD-10-CM manual and check off each step after you complete it.

▶ First, Gabrielle confirms the codes she assigned.

❏ **H72.821 Total perforation of tympanic membrane, right ear**

❏ **H65.03 Acute serous otitis media, bilateral**

▶ Gabrielle reviews the instructional notes in the Tabular List to determine how to sequence the codes.

❏ The instructional note for code **H72.821** directs her to **Code first any associated otitis media.** This tells her that the code for otitis media, **H65.03**, should be sequenced first.

❏ The instructional note for code **H65.03** directs her to **Use additional code for any associated perforated tympanic membrane.** This confirms that the code for TMP, **H72.821**, should be sequenced second.

▶ Gabrielle finalizes the codes and sequencing for this case:

1. **H65.03 Acute serous otitis media, bilateral**
2. **H72.821 Total perforation of tympanic membrane, right ear**

CODING PRACTICE

Exercise 20.4   Arranging Codes for Ear Conditions

Instructions: Read the mini-medical-record of each patient's encounter, review the information abstracted in Exercise 20.2, assign ICD-10-CM diagnosis codes using the Index and Tabular List, and sequence them correctly.

---

1. OUTPATIENT SURGERY   Gender: M   Age: 58

Reason for encounter: bilateral stapedotomy and placement of prosthesis

Assessment: bilateral conductive hearing loss due to bilateral nonobliterative otosclerosis of the stapes at the oval window

Plan: FU in office, 2 weeks

Tip: Nonobliterative means nonblocking. Sequence the underlying condition first because it is the reason for the procedure.

2 ICD-10-CM Codes _____

(continued)

CODING PRACTICE *(continued)*

---

2. OFFICE   Gender: F   **Age:** 12

Reason for encounter: *left earache, fever, head congestion*

Assessment: *acute recurrent suppurative otitis media and acute recurrent sinusitis, mother is a heavy cigarette smoker in the home*

Plan: *antibiotics for OM, decongestant, and fluids*

3 ICD-10-CM Codes _____

_____

---

3. OFFICE   Gender: M   **Age:** 19

Reason for encounter: *dizziness, nausea, low back pain, headache on right side*

Assessment: *dizziness, nausea, and headache due to labyrinthitis, right*

Plan: *refer to physical therapy for balance and for LBP*

2 ICD-10-CM Codes _____

CHAPTER SUMMARY

In this chapter you learned that:

- The ear makes hearing possible by collecting sound waves from the external world and converting them into impulses that are transmitted to the brain through the vestibulocochlear nerve, cranial nerve VIII.

- ICD-10-CM Chapter 8, Diseases of the Ear and Mastoid Process (H60-H95), is a new chapter that did not exist in ICD-9-CM.

- The primary concerns in abstracting for diagnoses of the ear and mastoid process are laterality, external causes, tobacco use or exposure, and the many variations of otitis media.

- The Index provides cross-references that redirect coders to alternative Main Terms for many ear conditions.

- ICD-10-CM does not provide any unique instructions for sequencing codes related to diseases of the ear.

- ICD-10-CM provides no Official Guidelines for Coding and Reporting (OGCR) for Chapter 8.

CONCEPT QUIZ

Take a moment to look back at the ear and mastoid process and solidify your skills. Try to answer the questions from memory first, then look back at the discussion in this chapter if you need a little extra help.

Completion

Instructions: Write the term that answers each question based on the information you learned in this chapter. Choose from the list below. Some choices may be used more than once and some choices may not be used at all.

ceruminoma	labyrinthitis	recurrent
cholesteatoma	mastoid	sensorineural
chronic	Ménière	serous
conductive	disease	suppurative
external	middle	tinnitus
inner	nonsuppurative	vertigo

1. The tympanic membrane is part of the _____ ear.

2. _____ is excessive accumulation of ear wax.

3. _____ hearing loss is due to abnormal formation of the cochlea or cochlear nerve.

4. Otitis media is an infection of the _____ ear.

5. The ossicles are part of the _____ ear.

6. _____ OM involves the discharge of pus.

7. The cochlea is part of the _____ ear.

8. _____ is a viral or bacterial inflammation or infection of the semicircular canals of the inner ear.

9. _____ is a sensation of motion or dizziness.

10. A common practice is to classify recurrent acute otitis media as _____ when it persists for longer than three months and is accompanied by changes in the lining of the middle ear.

Multiple Choice

Instructions: Circle the letter of the best answer to each question based on the information you learned in this chapter.

1. How should laterality be abstracted when a patient has more than one ear condition?
   A. The laterality for each condition must be the same.
   B. The laterality for each condition must be different.
   C. The laterality for each condition must be bilateral.
   D. The laterality for each condition must be identified separately.

2. Laterality for the ear designates all of the following EXCEPT
   A. right.
   B. left.
   C. bilateral.
   D. inner.

3. What situation does an instructional note at the beginning of Chapter 8 directs coders to assign an additional code for?
   A. External cause
   B. Alcohol use
   C. Tobacco use
   D. Exposure to loud music

4. Which is NOT a subtype of otitis media?
   A. Suppurative
   B. Serous
   C. Sensorineural
   D. Allergic

5. Untreated OM can lead to all of the following EXCEPT
   A. strep throat.
   B. meningitis.
   C. mastoiditis.
   D. facial nerve paralysis.

6. What is the focus of OGCR for Chapter 8?
   A. Otitis media
   B. Laterality
   C. Hearing loss
   D. There are no OGCR for Chapter 8.

7. Serous OM is the most common type of _____ OM.
   A. suppurative
   B. nonsuppurative
   C. chronic
   D. allergic

8. What Main Term does the Index entry for Loss, hearing cross-reference coders to?
   A. Sensorineural
   B. Conductive
   C. Deafness
   D. Hearing

9. What second-level subterms are nearly all types of OM indexed under?
   A. Nonsuppurative and suppurative
   B. Acute and chronic
   C. Otitis and media
   D. Serous and recurrent

10. How should acute serous OM with TMP be coded?
   A. Assign a combination code for both OM and TMP.
   B. Assign a code for OM first, with TMP as an additional code.
   C. Assign a code for TMP first, with OM as an additional code.
   D. Assign a code for OM and do not code TMP.

CODING CHALLENGE

Instructions: Read the mini-medical-record of each patient's encounter, then abstract, assign, and sequence ICD-10-CM diagnosis codes using the Index and Tabular List. Write the code(s) on the line provided.

1. OFFICE   Gender: M   Age: 6

Reason for encounter: Earache in left ear and fever

Assessment: acute bullous myringitis, left ear

Plan: antipyrine and benzocaine ear drops for pain, amoxillin, RTO 1 week

1 ICD-10-CM Code _____

2. OFFICE   Gender: F   Age: 41

Reason for encounter: sudden loss of hearing after taking tobramycin as prescribed for an infection

Assessment: ototoxic bilateral sensorineural hearing loss

Plan: hearing workup for hearing aids

Tip: Follow any cross-reference notes you find in the Index. Remember to code for the drug using the Table of Drugs and Chemicals.

2 ICD-10-CM Codes _____

3. OFFICE   Gender: M   Age: 21

Reason for encounter: right ear pain and otorrhagia

Assessment: polyp of right middle ear and associated cholesteatoma in middle ear

Plan: removed cholesteatoma, Rx antibiotics, RTO 3 weeks

2 ICD-10-CM Codes _____

4. OFFICE   Gender: M   Age: 11

Reason for encounter: frequent ear aches

Assessment: chronic serous otitis media (CSOM), bilateral, with attic rupture of left eardrum

Plan: Rx antibiotics

1 ICD-10-CM Code _____

(continued)

(continued from page 333)

5. OFFICE Gender: M Age: 58

Reason for encounter: patient had upper respiratory infection (URI) followed by feeling of fullness, popping ears, intermittent sharp ear pain and mild disequilibrium

Assessment: acute Eustachian salpingitis, left ear, URI

Plan: 10 day course of amoxillin, nasal decongestant limited to short term and only 3-4 times daily

2 ICD-10-CM Codes _____

8. OFFICE Gender: F Age: 22

Reason for encounter: pain, swelling, discharge, and itchiness of outer ear

Assessment: malignant bilateral otitis externa due to pseudomonas aeruginosa, diabetes type 1

Plan: schedule for surgical debridement of necrotic tissue, antipseudomonal antibiotic course of 4–6 weeks, RTO in one week

3 ICD-10-CM Codes _____

_____

6. OFFICE Gender: F Age: 16

Reason for encounter: ear pain, recurrent URIs

Assessment: acute and subacute allergic serous otitis media, bilateral, recurrent; the patient smokes cigarettes and both parents smoke at home

Plan: ear drops to control pain, refer patient and parents to stop smoking clinic

2 ICD-10-CM Codes _____

9. OFFICE Gender: F Age: 9

Reason for encounter: yellow discharge, redness, and some swelling on left ear lobe after getting her ears pierced

Assessment: abscess of external ear

Plan: instruct patient on cleaning area with saline, warm salt water compresses to be performed 4x daily, RTO in 2 days if infection has not mitigated

Tip: Code for the condition only. Do not assign external cause codes.

1 ICD-10-CM Codes _____

7. OFFICE Gender: M Age: 17

Reason for encounter: mild hearing impairment, R ear; has been using q-tips to clean ears

Assessment: impacted cerumen, right ear

Plan: removed cerumen with curette, call if any further problems

1 ICD-10-CM Code _____

10. OFFICE Gender: M Age: 4

Reason for encounter: admitted for intravenous antibiotics and mastoidectomy d/t fever, mastoid swelling, deep ear pain at physician's office

Assessment: left subperiosteal mastoiditis

Plan: oral antibiotic, RTO in 1 week

1 ICD-10-CM Code _____

KEEP ON CODING

Instructions: Read the diagnostic statement, then use the Index and Tabular List to assign and sequence ICD-10-CM diagnosis codes. Write the code(s) on the line provided.

1. Diffuse cholesteatosis, right ear: ICD-10-CM Code(s) _____

2. Noise-induced hearing loss of bilateral inner ears: ICD-10-CM Code(s) _____

3. Mucosal cyst of postmastoidectomy cavity, both ears: ICD-10-CM Code(s) _____

4. Swimmer's ear, left: ICD-10-CM Code(s) _____

5. Exostosis, right external ear canal: ICD-10-CM Code(s) _____

6. Postauricular fistula, both ears: ICD-10-CM Code(s) _____

7. Aural vertigo: ICD-10-CM Code(s) _____

8. Conductive deafness: ICD-10-CM Code(s) _____

9. Cochlear otosclerosis, right ear: ICD-10-CM Code(s) _____

10. Partial loss of ear ossicles, left ear: ICD-10-CM Code(s) _____

11. Acute petrositis, both ears: ICD-10-CM Code(s) _____

12. Postoperative stenosis of right external ear canal: ICD-10-CM Code(s) _____

13. Otorrhea, left ear: ICD-10-CM Code(s) _____

14. Basal cell carcinoma of pinna of right ear: ICD-10-CM Code(s) _____

15. Chronic allergic otitis media: ICD-10-CM Code(s) _____

16. Hyperacusis, right ear: ICD-10-CM Code(s) _____

17. Adhesive otitis, left middle ear: ICD-10-CM Code(s) _____

18. Patulous Eustachian tube, both ears: ICD-10-CM Code(s) _____

19. Acute reactive otitis externa, left ear: ICD-10-CM Code(s) _____

20. Acute myringitis, bilateral: ICD-10-CM Code(s) _____

21. Labyrinthine hydrops: ICD-10-CM Code(s) _____

22. Perforation of tympanic membrane, left: ICD-10-CM Code(s) _____

23. Transient ischemic deafness, left: ICD-10-CM Code(s) _____

24. Otitic barotrauma, both ears: ICD-10-CM Code(s) _____

25. Hematoma of pinna, right ear: ICD-10-CM Code(s) _____

Chapter 21

Certain Infectious and Parasitic Diseases (A00-B99)

Chapter Outline

- **Infectious Disease Refresher**
- **Coding Overview of Infectious Diseases**
- **Abstracting for Infectious Diseases**
- **Assigning Codes for Infectious Diseases**
- **Arranging Codes for Infectious Diseases**

Learning Objectives

After completing this chapter, you should have the skills to:

21.1 Spell and define the key words, medical terms, and abbreviations related to infectious and parasitic diseases.

21.2 Discuss the nature of infectious and parasitic diseases.

21.3 Identify the main characteristics of coding for infectious and parasitic diseases.

21.4 Abstract diagnostic information from the medical record for coding infectious and parasitic diseases.

21.5 Assign codes for infectious and parasitic diseases.

21.6 Arrange multiple codes for infectious and parasitic diseases.

21.7 Discuss the Official Guidelines for Coding and Reporting related to infectious and parasitic diseases.

Key Terms and Abbreviations

acquired immunodeficiency syndrome (AIDS)
asymptomatic
bacteria
Candida
Escherichia coli (*E. coli*)

fungus
Giardia
helminth
herpes
human immunodeficiency virus (HIV)
inconclusive HIV

indeterminate HIV
localized
multiple organ dysfunction
opportunistic infection
pandemic
parasite
protozoa

Pseudomonas aeruginosa (*P. aeruginosa*)
serology
smallpox
systemic
varicella
virus

In addition to the key terms listed here, students should know the terms defined within tables in this chapter.

For updates and corrections, visit our student resource site at

www.pearsonhighered.com/healthprofessionsresources

INTRODUCTION

When you travel out of the United States or Canada, you will most likely be required to get some vaccinations. These "travel shots" help protect you from contracting an infectious disease and, as importantly, prevent you from spreading it to others. Most such infectious diseases are classified in ICD-10-CM Chapter 1.

An infectious disease physician specializes in diagnosing and treating infectious diseases. Primary care physicians treat common infectious diseases but refer patients with more complex conditions to an infectious disease specialist.

Coding infectious diseases requires working with the scientific names of microorganisms. Rely on your medical resources so you have the information you need at your fingertips.

INFECTIOUS DISEASE REFRESHER

Infectious and parasitic diseases are not a body system; they are a class of diseases that affect the entire body, called **systemic** diseases. This is in contrast to **localized** infections, which primarily affect a single organ or body system, such as pneumonia or pharyngitis. Infectious organisms (germs) live in the environment, in the air, on the skin, and inside the body. When the body's immune defenses are weaker than the organism, the organism multiplies to the extent that it causes illness. Infectious organisms are classified by scientists based on the type of cell, shape, and behavior (■ FIGURE 21-1). There are four main types of infectious organisms, as follows:

- **bacteria**—one-celled germs that multiply quickly and may release toxins that create illness. Examples are *Escherichia coli* (*E.coli*) and *Pseudomonas aeruginosa* (*P. aeruginosa*).

- **viruses**—capsules that contain genetic material and use the body's own cells to multiply. Examples are **varicella** (*chicken pox*) and **herpes** (*shingles*).

- **protozoa**—one-celled beings, more complex than bacteria, that use other living things as a source of food and a place to live. Examples are *Trichomonas vaginalis* (the cause of trichomoniases, a sexually transmitted disease) and *Giardia* (*the cause of giardiasis, an intestinal tract infection*).

- **fungi**—primitive vegetables that reproduce through spores. Examples include *Candida* (*yeast*) and *Trichophyton rubrum* (the cause of athlete's foot).

The type of infectious organism also determines how physicians treat it. For example, antibiotics treat many bacterial infections but are useless against viruses.

Parasites, also called **helminths**, are plants or animals that live in or on another living organism, or host, and often cause damage to the host. Examples are tapeworm and head lice.

Medical terms related to infectious diseases are built on the word root for the causal organism, which is often named after its shape. As you learn about infectious and parasitic diseases, remember to use medical terminology skills to distinguish between word roots for organisms, nouns that describe conditions, and adjectives that mean *pertaining to*. When the

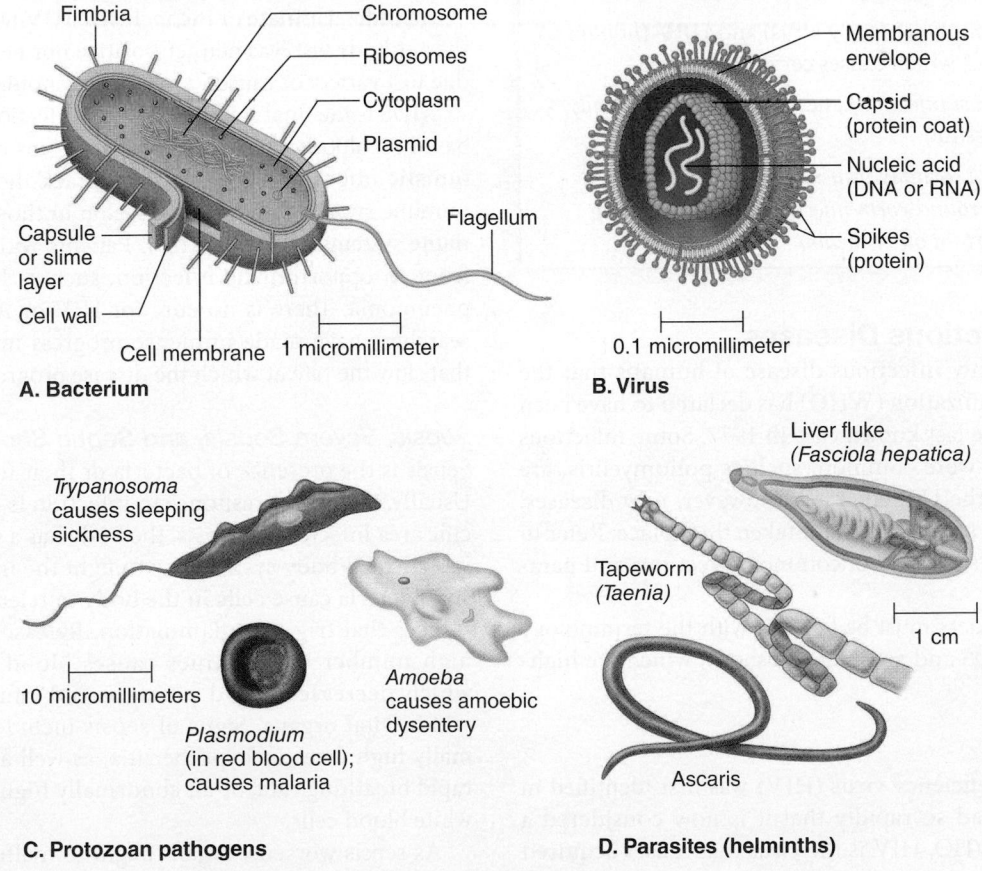

Figure 21-1 ■ Pathogens Causing Infectious and Parasitic Diseases

Table 21-1 ■ EXAMPLE OF CONSTRUCTING MEDICAL TERMS FOR INFECTIOUS AND PARASITIC DISEASES

Combining Form	Suffix	Complete Medical Term
cocc/o (*sphere*) strept/o (*twisted*) staphyl/o (*cluster*) tubercul/o (*knob or bump*) chlamyd/o (*envelope or cloak*)	-osis (*condition of*) -iasis (*condition of*) -us (*structure*)	**strepto + cocc + us** (*condition of an organism shaped like a twisted sphere*) **staphylo + cocc + us** (*condition of an organism shaped like a cluster of spheres*) **tubercul + osis** (*condition of an organism shaped like a knob*) **chlamydi + osis** (*condition of an organism shaped like a cloak*)
	-al (*pertaining to*) -ic (*pertaining to*) -in (*pertaining to*)	**strepto + cocc + al** (*pertaining to the* Streptococcus *organism.* Example: streptococcal sore throat) **staphylo + cocc + al** (*pertaining to the* Staphylococcus *organism.* Example: staphylococcal pneumonia) **chlamydi + al** (*pertaining to the* Chlamydia *organism.* Example: chlamydial cystitis) **tubercul + in** (*pertaining to a* Tuberculosis *organism.* Example: tuberculin test)

organism causes a condition, a suffix is added to create a noun or adjective. Refer to ■ TABLE 21-1 for a refresher on how to build medical terms related to infectious and parasitic diseases.

CODING CAUTION

Be alert for medical word roots that are spelled similarly but have different meanings.

HIV (*human immunodeficiency virus*) and **HPV** (*human papilloma virus*, which causes cervical cancer)

candidiasis (*a yeast infection*) and **chlamydia** (*a sexually transmitted disease*)

trichomoniasis (*a sexually transmitted disease*) and **trichinosis** (*a roundworm infection caused by eating raw pork or certain other meats*)

Common Infectious Diseases

Smallpox is the only infectious disease of humans that the World Health Organization (WHO) has declared to have been eradicated, with the last known case in 1977. Some infectious diseases that once were common, such as poliomyelitis, are now quite rare in the United States. However, new diseases, such as HIV and Lyme disease, have taken their place. Refer to ■ TABLE 21-2 for a summary of common infectious and parasitic diseases.

In particular, coders must be familiar with the terminology related to HIV/AIDS and sepsis/septic shock, which are highlighted next.

HIV and AIDS

Human **immunodeficiency virus** (HIV) was first identified in 1983 and has spread so rapidly that it is now considered a pandemic by the WHO. HIV is the virus that causes **acquired immunodeficiency syndrome** (AIDS). It is transmitted through unsafe sex, contaminated needles, blood products, breast milk, and perinatal means (the birth process). Screening of blood products for HIV has nearly eliminated the transmission of HIV through blood transfusions in developed countries.

HIV invades T4 lymphocytes and eventually paralyzes the body's immune system. People can be infected with the HIV virus and be **asymptomatic** (*have no symptoms*) for many years. During this time **serology** (*blood tests*) will be positive for the virus.

An **indeterminate** or inconclusive HIV test result means that the antibody test was neither positive nor negative. This may be due to a variety of causes, and the test should be repeated.

AIDS is the final stage of the HIV infection and is diagnosed based on blood cell counts. The symptoms of AIDS are **opportunistic infections**, diseases that attack those with weakened immune systems but do not develop in those with healthy immune systems (■ TABLE 21-3). Patients with AIDS usually die from an opportunistic infection, such as Kaposi sarcoma or pneumonia. There is no cure for HIV or AIDS, although researchers have made immense progress in developing drugs that slow the rate at which the disease progresses.

Sepsis, Severe Sepsis, and Septic Shock

Sepsis is the presence of bacteria or their toxins in the blood. Usually, the body's response to infection is limited to the specific area infected. In sepsis, the body has a systemic response, in which all body systems try to fight the infection. The invasive bacteria cause cells in the body to release cytokines, substances that trigger inflammation. Release of an abnormally high number of cytokines causes blood vessels to dilate, which decreases blood pressure and causes blood to clot within vital organs. Signs of sepsis include either an abnormally high fever or hypothermia, as well as rapid heart rate, rapid breathing rate, or an abnormally high or low number of white blood cells.

As sepsis worsens, organs begin to malfunction and blood pressure may decrease. Septic shock is diagnosed when blood

Table 21-2 ■ **COMMON INFECTIOUS AND PARASITIC DISEASES**

Condition	Definition
Acquired immunodeficiency syndrome (AIDS)	A disease caused by the HIV virus that weakens and paralyzes the immune system
Hepatitis	A viral inflammation of the liver
Herpes zoster	A painful, blistering skin rash due to the varicella-zoster virus that causes chickenpox; also called shingles
Human immunodeficiency virus (HIV)	A virus that infects and destroys helper T cells of the immune system and causes AIDS
Human papilloma virus (HPV)	A virus that causes cervical cancer
Leprosy	A chronic bacterial disease characterized by the formation of nodules on the surface of the body
Malaria	An acute or chronic disease caused by parasites and characterized by high fevers, shaking chills, flu-like symptoms, and anemia
Methicillin-susceptible *Staphylococcus aureus* (MSSA) infection	A type of staph infection that responds to commonly used antibiotics
Methicillin-resistant *Staphylococcus aureus* (MRSA) infection	A type of staph infection that does not respond to commonly used antibiotics
Mononucleosis	A viral infection causing fever, sore throat, and swollen lymph glands
Multiple drug-resistant organism (MDRO)	A bacteria that survives exposure to many different antibiotics
Nosocomial	Any hospital-acquired infection
Sepsis	A severe, life-threatening, system-wide reaction to infection caused by disease-causing organisms, especially bacteria, in the blood or tissues
Septic shock	Life-threatening low blood pressure due to sepsis
Septicemia	A systemic disease associated with the presence and persistence of bacteria, viruses, fungi, or other organisms or toxins in the blood
Severe sepsis	Acute or multiple organ dysfunction (MOD) due to sepsis
Syphilis	A sexually transmitted disease (STD) caused by bacteria that produces chancres, rashes, and systemic lesions
Systemic inflammatory response syndrome (SIRS)	An acute, system-wide inflammatory reaction with at least two manifestations: fever, tachycardia, tachypnea, leukocytosis, and/or leukopenia
Tuberculosis (TB)	A contagious bacterial infection that involves the lungs but may spread to other organs

pressure remains low despite intensive treatment. Severe sepsis is organ malfunction, which results from a blockage of blood flow to vital organs due to blood clots.

Infants, the elderly, and those with weakened immune systems are most likely to get sepsis. Physicians treat sepsis with antibiotics to kill the bacteria, fluids to maintain adequate blood pressure, and mechanical ventilation to aid breathing. Sepsis progresses rapidly, causing death in one-third of those who get it, according to the Centers for Disease Control and Prevention (CDC).

CODING CAUTION

Medicare does not reimburse inpatient hospitals for costs associated with a hospital-acquired condition (HAC) (*a preventable condition acquired during a hospital stay*).

Inpatient hospitals must report whether conditions are present on admission (POA). Because sepsis and septicemia are common HACs, it is important to correctly identify the POA status. OGCR Appendix I provides detailed guidelines on POA reporting.

Table 21-3 ■ **CONDITIONS COMMON TO AIDS**

Type of Complication	Conditions
Malignancies	Kaposi sarcoma (*malignant neoplasm of the connective tissue*) lymphoma
Infections	Candidiasis
	Herpes simplex
	Herpes zoster (shingles)
	Pneumonia (*Pneumocystis carinii* pneumonia [PCP])
	Toxoplasmosis
	Tuberculosis
Gastrointestinal symptoms	Diarrhea
	Lack of appetite
	Nausea and vomiting
Neurological symptoms	Confusion and memory loss
	Headaches and visual changes

CODING PRACTICE

Exercise 21.1 Infectious Disease Refresher

Instructions: Use your medical terminology skills and resources to define the following conditions related to infectious and parasitic diseases, then assign the default diagnosis code.

Follow these steps:
- Identify the infectious organism.
- Define the meaning of the condition.
- Assign the diagnosis code for the condition using the Index and Tabular List.

Example: chlamydial cervicitis   Organism: *Chlamydia*   Meaning: *inflammation of the cervix due to Chlamydia*   ICD-10-CM Code: *A56.09*

1. candidiasis bronchitis   Organism _____   Meaning _____   ICD-10-CM Code _____

2. syphilitic endocarditis   Organism _____   Meaning _____   ICD-10-CM Code _____

3. herpetic eyelid   Organism _____   Meaning _____   ICD-10-CM Code _____

4. typhoid meningitis   Organism _____   Meaning _____   ICD-10-CM Code _____

5. amebiasis cutaneous   Organism _____   Meaning _____   ICD-10-CM Code _____

6. parasitic stomatitis   Organism _____   Meaning _____   ICD-10-CM Code _____

7. Rickettsialpox (pox is a disease manifested through eruptions or pustules)   Organism _____   Meaning _____   ICD-10-CM Code _____

8. trichomoniasis prostate   Organism _____   Meaning _____   ICD-10-CM Code _____

9. tubercular anus   Organism _____   Meaning _____   ICD-10-CM Code _____

10. gonococcal pharyngitis   Organism _____   Meaning _____   ICD-10-CM Code _____

CODING OVERVIEW OF INFECTIOUS DISEASES

ICD-10-CM Chapter 1, Certain Infectious and Parasitic Diseases (A00-B99), contains 22 blocks or subchapters that are divided by the type of infection. Review the block names and code ranges listed at the beginning of Chapter 1 in the ICD-10-CM manual to become familiar with the content and organization. Two letters of the alphabet, A or B, are used as the first letter of codes.

Chapter 1 is comparable to ICD-9-CM Chapter 1 (001-139) and has been reorganized in some areas compared to ICD-9-CM. Certain diseases, such as malaria, leprosy, hepatitis, and mononucleosis, contain expanded or redefined codes. Codes for bacterial and viral infectious agents have been expanded for increased specificity.

This chapter includes parasitic infestations and systemic infections due to viruses, bacteria, protozoa, and fungi. It also includes the named organisms that cause localized infections. This chapter does not include localized infections, which are classified in the body system chapter. Localized infections may be assigned a combination code that identifies the condition and the causal organism, or they may require one code for the condition and a second code from Chapter 1 to identify the causal organism. Instructional notes in the Tabular List, under the code for the localized infection, identify when to assign an additional code for the infectious organism. This chapter also does not include obstetric- or newborn-related conditions, which are classified in ICD-10-CM Chapters 15 and 16, respectively.

ICD-10-CM provides Official Guidelines for Coding and Reporting (OGCR) infectious and parasitic diseases in OGCR section I.C.1. OGCR provide a detailed discussion of assigning and sequencing codes for HIV, sepsis, and septic shock. An instructional note at the beginning of Chapter 1 in the Tabular List instructs coders to assign an additional code when an infection is drug resistant. This instruction applies to all codes in Chapter 1.

SUCCESS STEP

Experienced coders will notice that this chapter has been reorganized and expanded compared to Chapter 1 in ICD-9-CM. However, as long as you follow standard coding practices for using the Index, you should have little problem locating new or changed codes.

ABSTRACTING FOR INFECTIOUS DISEASES

Coders always need to identify the scientific name of the infectious organism and subtype, as well as associated complications or manifestations. Additional details are needed when abstracting HIV/AIDS and sepsis. Refer to ■ TABLE 21-4 for guidance on

Table 21-4 ■ KEY CRITERIA FOR ABSTRACTING INFECTIOUS AND PARASITIC DISEASES

❑ What is the named organism responsible for the patient's condition?

❑ What type of organism is it (bacteria, virus, etc.)?

❑ What is the subtype of the condition?

❑ Is a more specific subtype documented?

❑ Does the patient have a condition that is due to *Streptococcus, Staphylococcus,* or *Enterococcus*?

❑ Is the infection systemic or localized (organ specific)?

❑ Is the organism the cause of a condition that exists in a specific body system?

❑ Does the documentation state that the infection is resistant to antibiotics?

Table 21-5 ■ KEY CRITERIA FOR ABSTRACTING HIV AND AIDS

❑ Does the physician clearly document a confirmed diagnosis of HIV positive?

❑ Does the patient have symptoms or complications?

❑ Is the patient being seen (or admitted) for an HIV-related condition?

❑ Is the patient being seen (or admitted) for a condition *un*related to HIV?

❑ Has the patient been previously diagnosed with an HIV-related illness?

❑ Is the purpose of the encounter HIV testing?

❑ Did the patient receive HIV counseling?

❑ Is HIV serology inconclusive?

how to abstract infectious and parasitic diseases. Remember that the abstracting questions are a guide and that not every question applies to, or can be answered for, every case. For example, the hepatitis virus has subtypes A, B, or C, but not every organism does. Also remember to abstract for symptoms and determine whether they are integral to the confirmed diagnoses.

Abstracting HIV and AIDS

When abstracting cases involving HIV and AIDS, coders must determine whether physician documentation confirms an HIV infection. In addition, coders must determine whether HIV is asymptomatic or if it manifests itself in AIDS-related conditions. For any encounter with an HIV or AIDS patient, coders must also determine if the reason for the encounter is related to HIV or AIDS or if it is unrelated, such as an accident that causes a fracture. Refer to ■ TABLE 21-5 for guidance in abstracting HIV and AIDS cases, then refer to the example that follows (■ FIGURE 21-2).

Abstracting Sepsis, Severe Sepsis, and Septic Shock

When abstracting sepsis, severe sepsis, and septic shock, coders must have a clear understanding of the definitions of these conditions. For example, patients with sepsis and associated acute organ dysfunction are classified as having severe sepsis even if the documentation does not contain the precise word *severe*

(OGCR I.C.1.d.1)(a)). When the documentation is unclear regarding the status of the patient, query the physician for clarification. Coders also abstract the underlying systemic infection, such as *Pseudomonas aeruginosa* or *Escherichia coli*. Refer to ■ TABLE 21-6 for guidance in abstracting these cases, then work through the detailed example that follows.

Table 21-6 ■ KEY CRITERIA FOR ABSTRACTING SEPSIS AND SEPTIC SHOCK

❑ What is the systemic infection underlying the sepsis?

❑ Is a more specific subtype documented?

❑ Is sepsis documented as severe?

❑ Is an *associated* acute organ dysfunction documented?

❑ Is septic shock documented?

❑ Was the severe sepsis present on admission or did it develop after admission?

❑ Does a localized (organ-specific) infection exist in addition to sepsis?

❑ Is the sepsis the complication of a procedure that was performed?

❑ Is the sepsis associated with a wound?

❑ Is the sepsis associated with a noninfectious condition (such as trauma)?

Patient with known AIDS is admitted for AIDS-related pneumocystis carinii pneumonia (PCP).

Does the physician clearly document a confirmed diagnosis of HIV positive? **Yes, a diagnosis of AIDS presumes HIV positive.**
Does the patient have symptoms or complications? **Yes, pneumonia.**
Is the patient being seen (or admitted) for an HIV-related condition? **Yes, PCP.**
Is the patient being seen (or admitted) for a condition unrelated to HIV? **No.**
Has the patient been previously diagnosed with an HIV-related illness? **Yes, patient is known to have AIDS at the time of admission.**
Is the purpose of the encounter HIV testing? **No.**
Did the patient receive HIV counseling? **No.**
Is HIV serology inconclusive? **No.**

Figure 21-2 ■ Example of Abstracting HIV/AIDS

Guided Example of Abstracting for Infectious Diseases

Refer to the following example throughout this chapter to practice skills for abstracting, assigning, and sequencing infectious and parasitic disease codes. Susanna Vannote, CPC, is a fictitious coder who guides you through the coding process.

Date: 02/11/yy   Location: Branton Medical Center

Provider: James Cruickshank, MD

Patient: Faye Gillis   Gender: F   Age: 81

Reason for admission: admitted to ICU from the emergency department due to acute respiratory failure

Assessment: Gram-negative (E. coli) sepsis with organ failure (POA)

Plan: discharged to skilled nursing facility

Follow along as Susanna Vannote, CPC, abstracts the diagnosis. Check off each step after you complete it.

▶ Susanna reads through the entire record, paying special attention to the reason for the encounter and the final assessment. She refers to the Key Criteria for Abstracting Sepsis and Septic Shock (Table 21-6).

❑ *What is the systemic infection underlying the sepsis?* E. coli

❑ *Is sepsis documented as severe?* No.

❑ *Is an associated acute organ dysfunction documented?* Yes, respiratory

❑ *Is septic shock documented?* No.

❑ *Was the severe sepsis present on admission or did it develop after admission?* Sepsis was present on admission.

❑ *Does a localized (organ-specific) infection exist in addition to sepsis?* No.

❑ *Is the sepsis the complication of a procedure that was performed?* No.

❑ *Is the sepsis associated with a wound?* No.

❑ *Is the sepsis associated with a noninfectious condition (such as trauma)?* No.

▶ At this time, Susanna does not know which of these conditions may need to be coded, nor how many codes she will end up with. She will learn about this when she moves on to assigning codes.

CODING PRACTICE

Exercise 21.2 Abstracting for Infectious Diseases

Instructions: Read the mini-medical-record of each patient's encounter and answer the abstracting questions. Write the answer on the line provided. Do not assign any codes.

---

1. OFFICE   Gender: M   Age: 18

Chief complaint: general lack of energy, fatigue, loss of appetite, fever, and chills

Assessment: suspected Epstein-Barr mononucleosis, which was confirmed by a blood test

Plan: drink fluids, get rest, acetaminophen or ibuprofen for pain and fever, recovery can take several weeks, call if abdominal pain, difficulty breathing, severe weakness, or persistent high fever

a. What are the symptoms? _____

_____

b. Is the condition uncertain or confirmed? _____

_____

c. What is the named organism? _____

_____

d. Should the symptoms be coded? _____
   Why or why not? _____

---

2. OFFICE   Gender: F   Age: 46

Reason for encounter: annual work related PPD (*purified protein derivative*) tuberculin test

Assessment: PPD positive for TB, X-ray of lung positive for nodules in lung

Plan: order sputum culture, begin pharmacotherapy

a. What is the named organism responsible for the patient's condition? _____

_____

b. Does the documentation state that the infection is resistant to antibiotics? _____

_____

c. What anatomic site is involved? _____

_____

---

3. INPATIENT HOSPITAL   Gender: F   Age: 70

Reason for admission: called in for a consult on *Staphylococcus aureus* pneumonia

Assessment: culture result shows MSSA

Plan: IV teicoplanin (*an antibiotic*) was successful and patient was discharged with instructions to help prevent recurrence

(*continued*)

3. (continued)

a. What is the named organism responsible for the patient's condition? _____

_____

b. Does the patient have a condition that is due to *Streptococcus, Staphylococcus,* or *Enterococcus*?

_____

c. Does the documentation state that the infection is resistant to antibiotics? _____

_____

5. (continued)

c. Is sepsis documented as severe? _____

_____

d. Is an associated acute organ dysfunction documented? _____

_____

e. Is the sepsis the complication of a procedure or a wound? _____

_____

4. OFFICE   Gender: M   Age: 27

Reason for encounter: *genital chancre (a firm, nonitchy skin ulcer)*

Assessment: *primary syphilis*

Plan: *antibiotics*

a. What is the named organism responsible for the patient's condition? _____

_____

b. What is the subtype of the condition? _____

_____

c. Does the patient have a condition that is due to *Streptococcus, Staphylococcus,* or *Enterococcus*?

_____

d. Does the documentation state that the infection is resistant to antibiotics? _____

_____

6. OFFICE   Gender: M   Age: 26

Reason for encounter: *lesions on the skin of this HIV positive patient*

Assessment: *Kaposi's sarcoma of the skin*

Plan: *refer to oncologist to evaluate extent of the cancer and determine treatment plan*

a. Does the physician clearly document a confirmed diagnosis of HIV positive? _____

b. Does the patient have symptoms or complications?

_____

c. Is the patient being seen (or admitted) for an HIV-related condition? _____

_____

7. EMERGENCY DEPARTMENT   Gender: M   Age: 26

Reason for encounter: *toe pain after a horse stepped on his foot*

Assessment: *fractured distal phalanx of great toe on the right foot, AIDS patient with Kaposi sarcoma of the lymph nodes which was not treated at this encounter*

Plan: *reduced fracture and applied cast, crutches, FU office 2 weeks*

a. What is the reason for the encounter? _____

_____

b. What bone was fractured? _____

_____

c. What is the laterality? _____

_____

5. INPATIENT HOSPITAL   Gender: F   Age: 35

Reason for admission: *admitted from emergency department due to septicemia*

Assessment: *Staphylococcus aureus septicemia, cause unknown, responsive to antibiotics*

Plan: *after O$_2$ and IV fluids and antibiotics, patient was discharged home in good condition*

a. What is the systemic infection underlying the sepsis?

_____

b. Does the documentation state that the infection is resistant to antibiotics? _____

_____

(continued)

(continued)

CODING PRACTICE *(continued)*

7. (continued)

d. What is the episode of care? _____

_____

e. Does the physician clearly document a confirmed diagnosis of HIV positive? _____

_____

f. Does the patient have symptoms or complications? _____

g. Is the patient being seen (or admitted) for an HIV-related condition? _____

_____

8. OFFICE   Gender: F   Age: 31

Reason for encounter: follow up on HIV test results

Assessment: positive for HIV, asymptomatic, counseled patient on managing the infection

Plan: refer to HIV support group

a. Did the physician clearly document a confirmed diagnosis of HIV positive? _____

_____

b. Does the patient have symptoms or complications?

_____

c. Is the purpose of the encounter HIV testing?

_____

d. Did the patient receive HIV counseling? _____

_____

9. OFFICE   Gender: M   Age: 45

Reason for encounter: HIV positive patient with no related conditions presents with dysuria, weakness, and fever

Assessment: urosepsis (UTI) d/t E. coli (non-Shiga toxin-producing)

Plan: antibiotics

(continued)

9. (continued)

a. What are the symptoms? _____

_____

b. What condition is diagnosed? _____

c. What is the infectious organism? _____

What is the subtype? _____

_____

d. Does the documentation state that the infection is resistant to antibiotics? _____

_____

e. Does the physician clearly document a confirmed diagnosis of HIV positive? _____

_____

f. Is the urosepsis documented as HIV related?

_____

g. What condition is the reason for the encounter?

_____

10. INPATIENT HOSPITAL   Gender: F   Age: 77

Reason for admission: admitted from SNF 1 day post-hospital-discharge with 102 F fever, dyspnea, heart rate 100 per minute, low BP

Assessment: severe sepsis d/t nosocomial MRSA and associated heart failure, septic shock

Plan: deceased

a. What is the systemic infection underlying the sepsis? _____

_____

b. Does the documentation state that the infection is resistant to antibiotics? _____

_____

c. Is sepsis documented as severe? _____

d. Is septic shock present? _____
Why or why not? _____

_____

e. Is an associated acute organ dysfunction documented? _____

_____

ASSIGNING CODES FOR INFECTIOUS DISEASES

OGCR provide many detailed guidelines for coding infectious organisms; HIV and AIDS; and sepsis, severe sepsis, and septic shock. Although coders do not need to memorize every guideline, they should memorize the *fact* that OGCR exist for these conditions and refer to OGCR every time they code these conditions.

Assigning Codes for Infectious Organisms

Guidelines describe how to code infectious organisms that are the cause of localized infections and organisms that are resistant to drugs.

Infectious Organisms in Diseases Classified Elsewhere

As discussed earlier in this chapter, localized infections are classified in body system chapters. In some cases, a combination code describes the condition and the infectious organism. In other cases, the body system chapter provides a code for the condition with an instructional note to assign an additional code for the causal agent. Assign a code from one of the following categories:

- **B95 Streptococcus, Staphylococcus, and Enterococcus as the cause of diseases classified to other chapters**
- **B96 Other bacterial agents as the cause of diseases classified to other chapters**
- **B97 Viral agents as the cause of diseases classified to other chapters**

These are causal agent codes and should be assigned only as a secondary code, in conjunction with a principal or first-listed diagnosis code for the localized infection (OGCR I.C.1.b). When an infectious organism causes a systemic infection, assign a code from elsewhere in ICD-10-CM Chapter 1 based on guidance from the Index and OGCR.

SUCCESS STEP

E. coli is classified by its strain. O157 is a strain that produces potentially harmful Shiga toxins. Shiga toxins can also be produced by other strains of *E. coli*. Review the code selections under category **B96.2** to identify codes for the various strains of *E. coli*.

Drug-Resistant Organisms

When an organism is stated as resistant to antibiotics or other drugs, report the resistance with a combination code that identifies the organism and its resistance, if one is available. *Staphylococcus aureus* is classified as either susceptible (responsive) to methicillin, described as methicillin-susceptible *Staphylococcus aureus* (MSSA), or resistant to methicillin, described as methicillin-resistant *Staphylococcus aureus* (MRSA). Combination codes for both MSSA and MRSA are located in the Index under the Main Term **MSSA** and **MRSA**, respectively, and also under the Main Term **Staphylococcus**.

> Patient is treated for *Klebsiella pneumoniae* pneumonia which is ▇▇▇▇▇▇▇▇▇▇▇▇▇▇▇▇▇▇▇▇
>
> (1) **J15.0 Pneumonia due to Klebsiella pneumoniae**
> (2) **Z16.24 Resistance to** ▇▇▇▇▇▇▇▇▇▇

Figure 21-3 ■   Example of Coding Multiple Drug-Resistant Organisms

Read the documentation carefully to identify the correct type of *Staphylococcus aureus*.

When a combination code is not available, report the resistance with two codes: (1) the infection code and (2) a code from category **Z16 Resistance to antimicrobial drugs** (OGCR I.C.1.c). Locate the code for resistance in the Index under the Main Term **Resistance** and subterms **organism, to, drug**, with a final subterm for the class of drug. When an organism is resistance to multiple drugs, select the subterm **multiple drugs (MDRO)** (■ FIGURE 21-3).

Assigning Codes for HIV and AIDS

ICD-10-CM provides detailed guidelines for assigning codes related to HIV and AIDS. Coders must be careful to use the terminology for HIV and AIDS correctly and precisely, as discussed earlier in this chapter. The codes for a patient with HIV or AIDS change as the disease progresses (■ FIGURE 21-4, page 346).

Asymptomatic HIV

Assign code **Z21 Asymptomatic human immunodeficiency virus [HIV] infection status** when the documentation describes the following circumstances (OGCR I.C.1.a.2)(d)):

- HIV positive
- known HIV
- HIV test positive
- asymptomatic HIV

To locate the code, search the Index for the Main Term **HIV** and the subterm **positive, seropositive** (■ FIGURE 21-5, page 346). Do not assign code **Z21** when the test results are documented as inconclusive or when terms AIDS or HIV *disease* are documented. These situations are discussed next.

AIDS

Assign code **B20 Human immunodeficiency virus [HIV] disease** in the following documented circumstances:

- documentation uses the terms AIDS or HIV *disease*
- the patient is treated for any HIV-related illness
- the patient is described as having any condition resulting from HIV-positive status
- the patient has been previously diagnosed with AIDS (OGCR I.C.1.a.2)(f))

To locate the code, search the Index for the Main Term **HIV** and use the default code (Figure 21-5), or search for the Main Term **AIDS** and use the default code (■ FIGURE 21-6, page 346).

Guided Example of Assigning Infectious Disease Codes

To practice skills for assigning codes for infectious and parasitic diseases, continue with the example from earlier in the chapter about patient Faye Gillis, who was admitted to Branton Medical Center due to acute respiratory failure.

Follow along in your ICD-10-CM manual as Susanna Vannote, CPC, assigns codes. Check off each step after you complete it.

▶ First, Susanna confirms the diagnoses.

  ❑ *Gram-negative (E. coli) sepsis*

  ❑ *acute respiratory failure*

▶ Susanna searches the Index for the Main Term **Sepsis** (■ FIGURE 21-9).

  ❑ She locates the subterm for the type of sepsis, **Escherichia coli A41.51**.

  ❑ As Susanna continues to review all the subterms under **Sepsis**, she notes an additional subterm that may apply.

    ▪ Immediately under **Sepsis**, she sees the subterm, **with, acute organ dysfunction R65.2**.

▶ Susanna feels confused with so many choices. She remembers that the OGCR contain several guidelines regarding sepsis, so turns to OGCR I.C.1 near the front of her ICD-10-CM manual for more information.

  ❑ OGCR I.C.1.d.1)(a) states **For a diagnosis of sepsis, assign the appropriate code for the underlying systemic infection**.

    ▪ This tells her she needs a code for *Gram-negative sepsis* because it is the underlying systemic infection.

  ❑ OGCR I.C.1.d.1)(a)(iii) states **If a patient has sepsis and associated acute organ dysfunction or multiple organ dysfunction (MOD), follow the instructions for coding severe sepsis**.

    ▪ This tells her that **acute organ dysfunction** follows the same guidelines as **severe sepsis**, even though the word *severe* was not specifically documented.

  ❑ OGCR I.C.1.d.1)(b) states **The coding of severe sepsis requires a minimum of 2 codes: first a code for**

the underlying systemic infection, followed by a code from subcategory **R65.2**.

    ▪ This confirms that she needs a code for *Gram-negative sepsis*.

    ▪ This tells her that she also needs a code from subcategory **R65.2**.

▶ Susanna verifies subcategory **R65.2, Severe sepsis** in the Tabular List.

  ❑ She observes that there are many instructional notes under the subcategory title.

  ❑ She identifies the symbol [5th] in front of the subcategory title, which tells her that a fifth character is required to complete the code.

  ❑ She locates the fifth-character codes below the instructional notes and determines that code **R65.20, Severe sepsis without septic shock** describes this case because septic shock was not documented.

▶ Susanna reviews the instructional notes in the Tabular List for **R65.20** (■ FIGURE 21-10).

  ❑ She cross-references the notes at the beginning of subcategory **R65.2**.

[5th] R65.2 Severe sepsis
Infection with associated acute organ dysfunction
Sepsis with acute organ dysfunction
Sepsis with multiple organ dysfunction
Systemic inflammatory response syndrome due to infectious process with acute organ dysfunction
Code first underlying infection, such as:
    Infection following a procedure (T81.4)
    Infections following infusion, transfusion and therapeutic injection (T80.2)
    Puerperal sepsis (O85)
    Sepsis following complete or unspecified spontaneous abortion (O03.87)
    Sepsis following ectopic and molar pregnancy (O08.82)
    Sepsis following incomplete spontaneous abortion (O03.37)
    Sepsis following (induced) termination of pregnancy (O04.87)
    Sepsis NOS A41.9
Use additional code to identify specific acute organ dysfunction, such as:
    acute kidney failure (N17.-)
    acute respiratory failure (J96.0-)
    critical illness myopathy (G72.81)
    critical illness polyneuropathy (G62.81)
    disseminated intravascular coagulopathy [DIC] (D65)
    encephalopathy (metabolic) (septic) (G93.41)
    hepatic failure (K72.0-)
  R65.20 Severe sepsis without septic shock
    Severe sepsis NOS
  R65.21 Severe sepsis with septic shock

Figure 21-10 ■ Tabular List Entry for Severe Sepsis

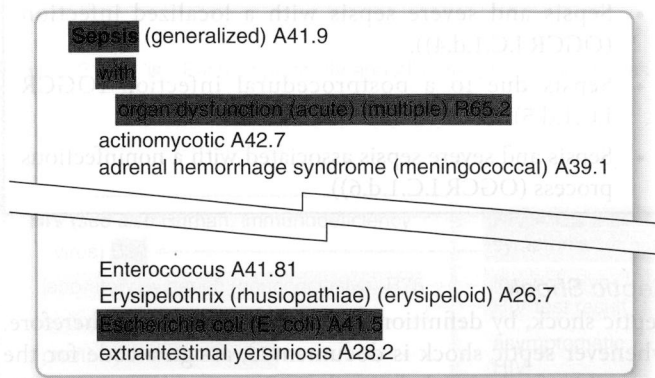

Sepsis (generalized) A41.9
  with
    organ dysfunction (acute) (multiple) R65.2
  actinomycotic A42.7
  adrenal hemorrhage syndrome (meningococcal) A39.1

  Enterococcus A41.81
  Erysipelothrix (rhusiopathiae) (erysipeloid) A26.7
  Escherichia coli (E. coli) A41.5
  extraintestinal yersiniosis A28.2

Figure 21-9 ■ Index Entry for Sepsis

❑ The inclusion notes state **Sepsis with acute organ dysfunction**. This accurately describes the case.

❑ She reviews the note **Code first underlying infection, such as:**.

❑ None of the conditions listed include the code she assigned for Gram-negative sepsis. However, she recalls that OGCR I.C.1.d.1)(b) already gave her sequencing instructions, which she will review later.

❑ She reviews the note **Use additional code to identify specific acute organ dysfunction, such as:**.

❑ She determines that this note applies because the patient had acute respiratory failure, which is listed in the instruction as **acute respiratory failure (J96.0-)**. She will finish verifying the instructional notes for **R65.20** then will assign and verify code for acute respiratory failure.

❑ She cross-references the beginning of the category **R65** and verifies that there are no instructional notes that apply to all codes in the category.

❑ She cross-references the beginning of the block **R50-R69** and verifies that there are no instructional notes that apply to all codes in the block.

❑ She cross-references the beginning of **Chapter 18 (R00-R99)** and reviews the instructional notes. These notes apply to assigning codes for symptoms and signs when a more specific diagnosis cannot be established. She determines that she should assign **R65.20** from this chapter, although a more specific diagnosis code is available, because the OGCR specifically direct her to assign a code from category **R65.2**.

▶ Next, Susanna wants to assign a code for acute respiratory failure. She locates the cross-referenced subcategory **J96.0, Acute respiratory failure** in the Tabular List.

❑ She identifies the symbol 5th in front of the subcategory title, which tells her that a fifth character is required to complete the code.

❑ She reviews the fifth-digit options and determines that the code that best describes the case is **J96.00, Acute**

respiratory failure, unspecified whether with hypoxia or hypercapnia** because neither hypoxia or hypercapnia were documented.

❑ Susanna cross-references the beginning of the category **J96**, the beginning of the block **J96-J99,** and the beginning of **Chapter 10 (J00-J99)** for additional instructional notes and finds none that apply to this case.

▶ Susanna checks her notes and realizes she still needs to verify the code she located in the Index for the underlying infection, **Sepsis, Escherichia coli A41.51**.

❑ She locates the subcategory **A41.5** in the Tabular List, which has the title **Sepsis due to other Gram-negative organisms**. She notices that it requires a fifth character.

❑ She reads the codes listed, which identify various strains of Gram-negative sepsis, and selects code **A41.51, Sepsis due to Escherichia coli [E. coli]**.

❑ She confirms that this accurately describes the documented organism.

❑ She cross-references the instructional notes at the beginning of category **A41, Other sepsis**. She determines that the conditions listed do not apply to this case.

❑ She cross-references the beginning of the block **A30-A49** and verifies that there are no instructional notes for this block.

❑ She cross-references the beginning of **Chapter 1 (A00-B99)** and reviews the instructional note that applies to all codes in this chapter. She determines that it does not apply to this case because the infection is not due to an external cause.

▶ Susanna reviews the codes she has assigned for this case.

❑ **R65.20 Severe sepsis without septic shock**

❑ **J96.00 Acute respiratory failure, unspecified whether with hypoxia or hypercapnia**

❑ **A41.51 Sepsis due to Escherichia coli [E. coli]**

▶ Next, Susanna must determine how to sequence the codes.

CODING PRACTICE

Exercise 21.3   Assigning Codes for Infectious Diseases

Instructions: Read the mini-medical-record of each patient's encounter, review the information abstracted in Exercise 21.2, and assign ICD-10-CM diagnosis codes using the Index and Tabular List. Write the code(s) on the line provided.

1. OFFICE   Gender: M   Age: 18

Chief complaint: *general lack of energy, fatigue, loss of appetite, fever, and chills*

Assessment: *suspected Epstein-Barr mononucleosis, which was confirmed by a blood test*

(continued)

CODING PRACTICE *(continued)*

1. (continued)

Plan: drink fluids, get rest, acetaminophen or ibuprofen for pain and fever, recovery can take several weeks, call if abdominal pain, difficulty breathing, severe weakness, or persistent high fever

1 ICD-10-CM Code _____

2. OFFICE   Gender: F   **Age:** 46

Reason for encounter: annual work related PPD tuberculin test

Assessment: PPD positive for TB, X-ray of lung positive for nodules in lung

Plan: order sputum culture, begin pharmacotherapy

1 ICD-10-CM Code _____

3. OFFICE   Gender: F   **Age:** 31

Reason for encounter: follow up on HIV test results

Assessment: positive for HIV, asymptomatic, counseled patient on managing the infection

Plan: refer to HIV support group

(continued)

3. (continued)

Tip: Refer to OGCR I.C.1.a.2)(d). The second code is for HIV counseling.

2 ICD-10-CM Codes _____

4. OFFICE   Gender: M   **Age:** 27

Reason for encounter: genital chancre

Assessment: primary syphilis

Plan: antibiotics

1 ICD-10-CM Code _____

5. INPATIENT HOSPITAL   Gender: F   **Age:** 35

Reason for encounter: admitted from emergency department due to septicemia

Assessment: *Staphylococcus aureus* septicemia, cause unknown, responsive to antibiotics

Plan: after O_2 and IV fluids and antibiotics, patient was discharged home in good condition

Tip: Refer to OGCR I.C.1.d.1)(a).

1 ICD-10-CM Code _____

ARRANGING CODES FOR INFECTIOUS DISEASES

Codes from this ICD-10-CM chapter are sequenced first when the systemic infection qualifies as the principal or first-listed diagnosis. Manifestations or conditions associated with the infection are sequenced after the systemic infection code. This order is indicated in the Tabular List through the use of the instructional notes **Code first** for the systemic infection and **Use additional code** for the associated condition (■ FIGURE 21-11).

CODING CAUTION

Do not confuse the guidelines for sequencing of codes for causal organisms with the sequencing guidelines for etiology and manifestation. When an etiology/manifestation relationship exists, sequencing is specifically designated in ICD-10-CM through the use of conventions, such as brackets in the Index and highlighting in the Tabular List. These conventions direct coders to sequence the etiology first and the manifestation second.

The exception to this guideline is when a localized infection is described with a code from a body system chapter but

the causal organism is *not* identified with a combination code. Assign the localized infection from the body system chapter as the first code. Assign a secondary code from the block **Bacterial and viral infectious agents (B95-B97)**, which contains codes to identify the infectious agent in diseases classified elsewhere. This order is indicated in the Tabular List through the use of the instructional notes **Code first** for the primary disease and **Use additional code** for the infectious organism (■ FIGURE 21-12).

OGCR provide specific guidelines for sequencing codes related to HIV/AIDS and sepsis/severe sepsis/septic shock. These are discussed next.

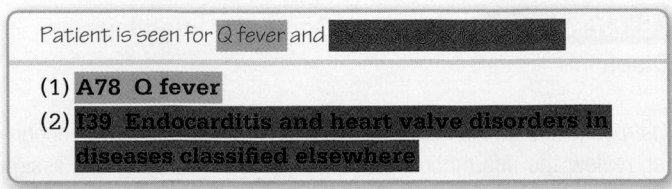

Patient is seen for Q fever and ▓▓▓▓▓▓▓▓▓▓

(1) A78 Q fever
(2) I39 Endocarditis and heart valve disorders in diseases classified elsewhere

Figure 21-11 ■ Example of Body System Disease Associated with an Infection

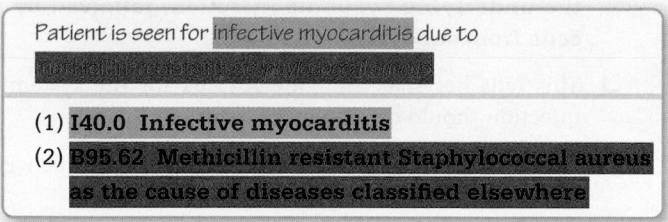

Figure 21-12 ■ Example of Sequencing for a Body System Disease Due to an Infectious Organism

Arranging Codes for HIV and AIDS

Sequencing of codes for HIV and AIDS depends on the circumstances of admission. Review the documentation and abstracting notes carefully to determine whether the patient was seen or admitted for treatment related directly to HIV or if the reason for the encounter was an unrelated condition, such as a traumatic injury.

Admission for HIV

When a patient is admitted for an HIV-related condition, assign and sequence codes as follows (OGCR I.C.1.a.2)(a)) (see Figure 21-8):

1. Assign code **B20 Human immunodeficiency virus [HIV] disease**.

2. Assign code(s) for all reported HIV-related condition(s).

Admission for a Condition Not Related to HIV

When a patient with HIV disease is admitted for an unrelated condition, assign and sequence codes as follows (OGCR I.C.1.a.2) (b)) (■ FIGURE 21-13):

1. Assign code(s) for the unrelated condition(s).

2. Assign code **B20 Human immunodeficiency virus [HIV] disease**.

3. Assign code(s) for all reported HIV-related condition(s).

Arranging Codes for Severe Sepsis and Septic Shock

Sequencing of codes for severe sepsis and septic shock is dependent on the circumstances of admission and when the condition develops.

Severe Sepsis

OGCR provide specific sequencing guidelines based on whether severe sepsis is the reason for admission or develops after admission.

Severe Sepsis Present at Admission. When severe sepsis meets the requirements of principal diagnosis, assign and sequence codes as follows (OGCR I.C.1.d.1)(b) and OGCR I.C.1.d.3)):

1. Assign a code for the underlying systemic infection or assign **A41.9 Sepsis, unspecified** if the infection is not specified.

2. Assign either **R65.20 Severe sepsis without septic shock** or **R65.21 Severe sepsis with septic shock**, as appropriate.

3. Assign code(s) for acute organ dysfunction.

Severe Sepsis That Develops after Admission. When severe sepsis develops after admission, assign and sequence codes as follows:

1. Assign code(s) for the condition(s) that meet the requirements of principal diagnosis.

2. Assign a code for the underlying systemic infection or assign **A41.9 Sepsis, unspecified** if the infection is not specified.

3. Assign either **R65.20 Severe sepsis without septic shock** or **R65.21 Severe sepsis with septic shock**, as appropriate.

4. Assign code(s) for acute organ dysfunction.

Septic Shock

OGCR provide specific sequencing guidelines based on whether septic shock is the reason for admission or develops after admission.

Septic Shock Present at Admission. When septic shock meets the requirements of principal diagnosis, assign and sequence codes as follows (OGCR I.C.1.d.2)):

1. Assign a code for the underlying systemic infection or assign **A41.9 Sepsis, unspecified** if the infection is not specified.

2. Assign code **R65.21 Severe sepsis with septic shock**.

3. Assign code(s) for acute organ dysfunction, when applicable.

Septic Shock That Develops after Admission. When septic shock develops after admission, assign and sequence codes as follows (OGCR I.C.1.d.3)) (■ FIGURE 21-14):

1. Assign code(s) for the condition(s) that meet the requirements of principal diagnosis.

2. Assign a code for the underlying systemic infection or assign **A41.9 Sepsis, unspecified** if the infection is not specified.

3. Assign code **R65.21 Severe sepsis with septic shock**.

4. Assign code(s) for acute organ dysfunction, when applicable.

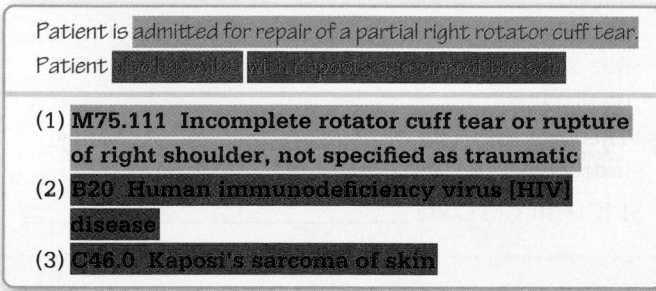

Figure 21-13 ■ Example of Sequencing for an AIDS Patient Admitted with a Nonrelated Condition

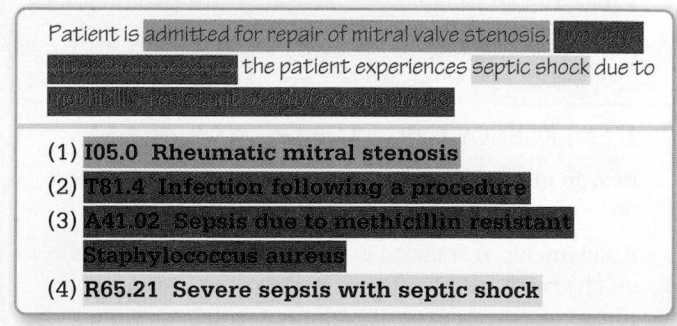

Figure 21-14 ■ Example of Sequencing for a Patient Who Develops Septic Shock Following a Procedure

Guided Example of Arranging Infectious Disease Codes

To practice skills for sequencing codes for infectious and parasitic diseases, continue with the example from earlier in the chapter about patient Faye Gillis, who was admitted to Branton Medical Center due to acute respiratory failure.

Follow along in your ICD-10-CM manual as Susanna Vannote, CPC, sequences the codes. Check off each step after you complete it.

▶ First, Susanna confirms codes she has assigned.

❑ **R65.20 Severe sepsis without septic shock**

❑ **J96.00 Acute respiratory failure, unspecified whether with hypoxia or hypercapnia**

❑ **A41.51 Sepsis due to Escherichia coli [E. coli]**

▶ Susanna refers back to the OGCR and instructional notes she read earlier.

❑ OGCR I.C.1.d.1)(b) states **The coding of severe sepsis requires a minimum of 2 codes: first a code for**

the underlying systemic infection, followed by a code from subcategory R65.2.

❑ This tells her that the code **A41.51** for the systemic infection should be sequenced before **R65.20**.

❑ She is still unsure whether **R65.20** should be sequenced before or after **J96.00**.

❑ She refers back to the instructional note under subcategory **R65.2** that states **Use additional code to identify specific acute organ dysfunction, such as: acute respiratory failure (J96.0-).**

❑ This tells her that **J96.00** should be sequenced after **R65.20** because it says that **J96.00-** is an additional code.

▶ Susanna finalizes the codes and sequencing for this case:

1. **A41.51 Sepsis due to Escherichia coli [E. coli]**
2. **R65.20 Severe sepsis without septic shock**
3. **J96.00 Acute respiratory failure, unspecified whether with hypoxia or hypercapnia**

CODING PRACTICE

Exercise 21.4 Arranging Codes for Infectious Diseases

Instructions: Read the mini-medical-record of each patient's encounter, review the information abstracted in Exercise 21.2, assign ICD-10-CM diagnosis codes using the Index and Tabular List, and sequence them correctly.

---

1. OFFICE   Gender: M   Age: 26

Reason for encounter: lesions on the skin of this HIV positive patient

Assessment: Kaposi sarcoma of the skin

Plan: refer to oncologist to evaluate extent of the cancer and determine treatment plan

Tip: Refer to OGCR I.C.1.a.2)(a) for sequencing instructions.

2 ICD-10-CM Codes _____

---

2. EMERGENCY DEPT   Gender: M   Age: 26

Reason for encounter: toe pain after a horse stepped on his foot

Assessment: fractured distal phalanx of great toe on the right foot, AIDS patient with Kaposi sarcoma of the lymph nodes which was not treated at this encounter

(continued)

---

2. (continued)

Plan: reduced fracture and applied cast, crutches, FU office 2 weeks

Tip: Refer to OGCR I.C.1.a.2)(b) and (f) for coding and sequencing instructions. Also, remember to assign an external cause code.

4 ICD-10-CM Codes _____

_____

---

3. INPATIENT HOSPITAL   Gender: F   Age: 70

Reason for encounter: called in for a consult on *Staphylococcus aureus* pneumonia

Assessment: culture result shows MSSA

Plan: IV teicoplanin was successful and patient was discharged with instructions to help prevent recurrence

Tip: Refer to OGCR I.C.1.c for coding and sequencing instructions.

1 ICD-10-CM Code _____

(continued)

4. OFFICE Gender: M Age: 45

Reason for encounter: HIV positive patient with no related conditions presents with dysuria, weakness, and fever

Assessment: urosepsis (UTI) d/t E. coli (non-Shiga toxin-producing)

Plan: antibiotics

Tip: Urosepsis is not sepsis or septicemia. Refer to OGCR I.C.1.a.2)(d) and I.C.1.b.

3 ICD-10-CM Codes _____

_____

5. INPATIENT HOSPITAL Gender: F Age: 77

Reason for admission: admitted from SNF 1 day post-hospital-discharge with 102 F fever, dyspnea, heart rate 100 per minute, low BP

Assessment: severe sepsis d/t nosocomial MRSA aureus and has associated heart failure

Plan: deceased

Tip: Refer to OGCR I.C.1.d.1) and 2).

3 ICD-10-CM Codes _____

_____

CHAPTER SUMMARY

In this chapter you learned that:

- Infectious and parasitic diseases are not a body system; they are systemic diseases that affect the entire body.

- ICD-10-CM Chapter 1, Certain Infectious and Parasitic Diseases (A00-B99), contains 22 blocks or subchapters that are divided by the type of infection.

- Coders always need to identify the scientific name of the infectious organism and subtype, as well as associated complications or manifestations.

- Although coders do not need to memorize every guideline, they should memorize the *fact* that OGCR exist for HIV and AIDS and

sepsis, severe sepsis, and septic shock; they should refer to OGCR every time they code these conditions.

- Codes from this ICD-10-CM chapter are sequenced first when the systemic infection qualifies as the principal or first-listed diagnosis, followed by codes for associated conditions.

- OGCR I.C.1 provides detailed discussion of assigning and sequencing codes for HIV, sepsis, and septic shock.

CONCEPT QUIZ

Take a moment to look back through infectious and parasitic diseases and solidify your skills. Try to answer the questions from memory first, then look back at the discussion in this chapter if you need a little extra help.

Completion

Instructions: Write the term that answers each question based on the information you learned in this chapter. Choose from the list below. Some choices may be used more than once and some choices may not be used at all.

asymptomatic	parasites
bacteria	septic shock
herpes zoster	severe sepsis
HIV	smallpox
HPV	trichinosis
inconclusive	tuberculosis
leprosy	viruses
opportunistic	

1. _____ is a virus that causes cervical cancer.

2. _____ is a roundworm infestation caused by eating raw pork.

3. _____ is a chronic bacterial disease characterized by the formation of nodules on the surface of the body.

4. _____ is organ malfunction due to sepsis.

5. _____ is a virus that causes AIDS.

6. A disease that attacks people with weakened immune systems but does not develop in those with healthy immune systems is a(an) _____ infection.

7. _____ is a painful, blistering skin rash due to the varicella-zoster virus that causes chickenpox.

8. HIV serology that is neither positive or negative is

_____.

9. *Escherichia coli* is an example of _____.

10. _____ is diagnosed when blood pressure remains low despite intensive treatment.

(continued)

(continued from page 353)

Multiple Choice

Instructions: Circle the letter of the best answer to each question based on the information you learned in this chapter.

1. Which of the following are examples of protozoa?
   A. *Trichomonas vaginalis* and *Giardia*
   B. Varicella and herpes
   C. HIV and AIDS
   D. *Escherichia coli* and *Pseudomonas aeruginosa*

2. Pneumonia and pharyngitis are examples of
   A. systemic diseases.
   B. infectious agents.
   C. localized infections.
   D. bacteria.

3. What characteristic do word roots for causal organisms often describe?
   A. Frequency
   B. Shape
   C. Toxicity
   D. Immunity

4. What is the relationship between AIDS and HIV?
   A. AIDS is the cause of HIV.
   B. AIDS is asymptomatic HIV.
   C. AIDS is an opportunistic infection.
   D. AIDS is the final stage of HIV.

5. Which of the following is a key criterion for abstracting HIV/AIDS?
   A. Is HIV acute or chronic?
   B. Is HIV serology inconclusive?
   C. Is HIV shock documented?
   D. Is it considered curable?

6. What code should be assigned for a patient who is HIV positive with no symptoms?
   A. B20, HIV disease
   B. R75, Inconclusive laboratory evidence of HIV
   C. Z0.6, Exposure to HIV
   D. Z21, Asymptomatic HIV

7. How should *E. coli* sepsis with organ failure be coded?
   A. Sepsis
   B. Severe sepsis
   C. Septic shock
   D. Two unrelated infections

8. When a patient is treated for any HIV-related illness, assign code
   A. B20, HIV disease.
   B. B97.35, HIV 2 as the cause of diseases classified elsewhere.
   C. Z0.6, Exposure to HIV.
   D. Z71.7, HIV counseling.

9. When septic shock develops after admission, what should the principal diagnosis code be?
   A. The condition that is responsible for the admission and the services provided
   B. A code for the systemic infection
   C. R65.21, Severe sepsis with septic shock
   D. A41.9, Sepsis, unspecified

10. A patient with AIDS and associated Kaposi sarcoma is admitted for repair of a torn rotator cuff. What condition is the principal diagnosis?
    A. HIV disease
    B. Kaposi sarcoma
    C. HIV as the cause of diseases classified elsewhere
    D. Rotator cuff tear

CODING CHALLENGE

Instructions: Read the mini-medical-record of each patient's encounter, then abstract, assign, and sequence ICD-10-CM diagnosis codes using the Index and Tabular List. Write the code(s) on the line provided.

1. OFFICE   Gender: F   Age: 52

Reason for encounter: bloody diarrhea, patient states she is worried she might have cancer

Assessment: Symptoms started a few days after eating hamburgers at a cookout. Hemorrhagic colitis (*inflammation and bleeding of the colon*) due to E. coli.

Plan: call back if it does not improve within 1 week

Tip: Follow the cross-references in the Index.

1 ICD-10-CM Code _____

2. OFFICE   Gender: M   Age: 44

Reason for encounter: blisters and scabs on face and left side of body, unexplained pain

Assessment: disseminated herpes zoster

Plan: Rx pain management medication, Calamine lotion applied topically to blisters and rash, RTO 1 week.

1 ICD-10-CM Code _____

3. OFFICE   Gender: M   Age: 23

Reason for encounter: HIV testing (screening) after unprotected sex with an infected partner *(continued)*

3. (continued)

Assessment: *exposure to HIV*

Plan: *FU in 1 week for results*

Tip: You need two Z codes, one for the reason for the encounter and a second for the exposure.

2 ICD-10-CM Codes _____

4. INPATIENT HOSPITAL   Gender: F   Age: 43

Reason for encounter: *antiviral therapy*

Assessment: *chronic hepatitis due to hepatitis B*

Plan: *RTO as protocol for antiviral therapy stipulates, FU liver function tests at next office visit*

1 ICD-10-CM Code _____

5. INPATIENT HOSPITAL   Gender: F   Age: 22

Reason for admission: *diarrhea and vomiting, fever*

Assessment: *gastroenteritis d/t salmonella food poisoning*

Plan: *Rx antibiotics. RTO 1 week following discharge*

1 ICD-10-CM Code _____

6. INPATIENT HOSPITAL   Gender: M   Age: 84

Reason for encounter: *redness on neck is spreading*

Assessment: *cellulitis due to group F streptococcus infection of tracheostomy tube*

Plan: *Discharge to skilled nursing facility. Rx oral antibiotics and antibiotic cream.*

3 ICD-10-CM Codes _____

_____

7. INPATIENT HOSPITAL   Gender: F   Age: 58

Reason for encounter: *recent trip to Sumatra without malaria prophylaxis, 4 day history of fever, sudden onset (SO) left upper quadrant (LUQ) pain and tenderness*

Assessment: *plasmodium vivax malaria with splenic rupture*

(*continued*)

7. (continued)

Plan: *post ICU discharge: 14 day course of chloroquine to be taken with food, RTO in 1 week*

Tip: Plasmodium vivax is the type of malaria.

1 ICD-10-CM Code _____

8. OFFICE   Gender: M   Age: 7

Reason for encounter: *itchy scalp and rash on the child's neck. Parent suspects that they have identified nits in the patient's hair.*

Assessment: *head lice infestation*

Plan: *Advise head lice shampoo (Rid, Nix).*

Tip: Read and follow the cross-reference in the Index.

1 ICD-10-CM Code _____

9. OFFICE   Gender: M   Age: 29

Reason for encounter: *numbness (temperature sensations), multiple pale, diffuse cutaneous lesions*

Assessment: *BL leprosy (borderline lepromatous leprosy)*

Plan: *multidrug therapy (Dapsone, rifampin, and clofazimine) regime initiated, RTO in 3 months*

1 ICD-10-CM Code _____

10. INPATIENT HOSPITAL   Gender: M   Age: 30

Reason for encounter: *admitted from emergency department due to septic shock*

Assessment: *sepsis is due to an infected tooth that patient has had for six months*

Plan: *Rx antibiotic, FU with dentist for extraction when patient is organism free.*

Tip: Because the infectious organism is not identified, you need to assign a default NOS code for sepsis. Refer also to OGCR I.C.1.d.1) and 2).

3 ICD-10-CM Codes _____

_____

KEEP ON CODING

Instructions: Read the diagnostic statement, then use the Index and Tabular List to assign and sequence ICD-10-CM diagnosis codes. Write the code(s) on the line provided.

1. *Salmonella* pyelonephritis: ICD-10-CM Code(s) _____

2. Glanders: ICD-10-CM Code(s) _____

3. Infant botulism: ICD-10-CM Code(s) _____

4. Gonococcal orchitis: ICD-10-CM Code(s) _____

5. Fatal familial insomnia: ICD-10-CM Code(s) _____

6. Postmeasles otitis media: ICD-10-CM Code(s) _____

7. Thrush: ICD-10-CM Code(s) _____

8. Meningococcal meningitis: ICD-10-CM Code(s) _____

9. Acute military tuberculosis: ICD-10-CM Code(s) _____

10. Monkeypox: ICD-10-CM Code(s) _____

11. Cat scratch fever: ICD-10-CM Code(s) _____

12. Postherpetic trigeminal neuralgia: ICD-10-CM Code(s) _____

13. Eczema herpeticum: ICD-10-CM Code(s) _____

14. Viral pericarditis, coxsackie: ICD-10-CM Code(s) _____

15. Toxoplasma myositis: ICD-10-CM Code(s) _____

16. *Rhodesiense* trypanosomiasis: ICD-10-CM Code(s) _____

17. Whooping cough due to *Bordetella pertussis* with pneumonia: ICD-10-CM Code(s) _____

18. Acute hepatitis E: ICD-10-CM Code(s) _____

19. Sepsis due to *Escherichia coli*: ICD-10-CM Code(s) _____

20. Jungle yellow fever: ICD-10-CM Code(s) _____

21. African histoplasmosis: ICD-10-CM Code(s) _____

22. Sequelae of leprosy: ICD-10-CM Code(s) _____

23. Rabies: ICD-10-CM Code(s) _____

24. Chlamydial conjunctivitis: ICD-10-CM Code(s) _____

25. West Nile fever: ICD-10-CM Code(s) _____

Diseases of the Genitourinary System (N00–N99)

Chapter 22

Learning Objectives

After completing this chapter, you should have the skills to:

22.1 Spell and define the key words, medical terms, and abbreviations related to the urinary system and male and female reproductive systems.

22.2 Discuss the structure, function, and common conditions of the urinary system and male and female reproductive systems.

22.3 Identify the main characteristics of coding for diseases of the urinary system and male and female reproductive systems.

22.4 Abstract diagnostic information from the medical record for conditions of the urinary system and male and female reproductive systems.

22.5 Assign codes for diseases of the urinary system and male and female reproductive systems.

22.6 Arrange multiple diagnosis codes for diseases of the urinary system and male and female reproductive systems.

22.7 Code neoplasms of the urinary system and male and female reproductive systems.

22.8 Discuss the Official Guidelines for Coding and Reporting related to diseases of the genitourinary system.

Chapter Outline

- **Genitourinary System Refresher**
- **Coding Overview of the Genitourinary System**
- **Abstracting for Genitourinary System Conditions**
- **Assigning Codes for Genitourinary System Conditions**
- **Arranging Codes for Genitourinary System Conditions**
- **Coding Neoplasms of the Genitourinary System**

Key Terms and Abbreviations

Bartholin's gland
blood creatinine
benign prostatic hyperplasia (BPH)
benign prostatic hypertrophy (BPH)
bulbo-urethral gland
clitoris
dialysis
dialysis-related amyloidosis (DRA)
ductal
electrolyte

fallopian tube
genitourinary (GU) system
glomerular filtration rate (GFR)
glomerulus
hematuria
hemodialysis (HD)
impotence
kidney
labia major
labia minor
lobular

lower urinary tract symptom (LUTS)
nephron
ovary
penis
peritoneal dialysis (PD)
peritoneal membrane
polycystic kidney disease
polynephritis
prostate
prostate-specific antigen (PSA)

reflux nephropathy
renal pelvis
reproductive duct
testis
ureter
urethra
urinary bladder
urinary tract infection (UTI)
uterus
vagina

In addition to the key terms listed here, students should know the terms defined within tables in this chapter.

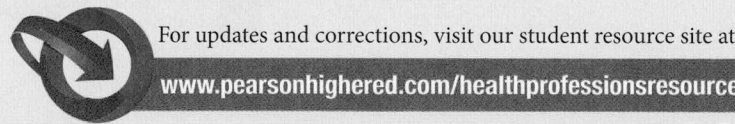

For updates and corrections, visit our student resource site at
www.pearsonhighered.com/healthprofessionsresources

INTRODUCTION

All travelers have their own strategies for managing restroom needs, but everyone driving on an interstate highway looks forward to the next Rest Area. The genitourinary system consists of three systems: urinary, male reproductive, and female reproductive; each is discussed separately within this chapter.

A urologist specializes in diagnosing and treating conditions of the urinary tract and male reproductive organs, and a nephrologist specializes in diagnosing and treating conditions of the kidney. A gynecologist specializes in diagnosing and treating conditions of the female reproductive organs. Primary care physicians treat common conditions affecting the genitourinary system and refer more complex cases to a specialist.

GENITOURINARY SYSTEM REFRESHER

The **genitourinary (GU) system** includes the urinary system and the male and female genital, or reproductive, systems. The function of the urinary system is to filter, store, and remove waste products from the blood and maintain homeostasis. The function of the genital system is sexual reproduction. The urinary and reproductive systems are grouped together in the coding manual because they arise from the same embryonic tissue, use common structures, and are in close physical proximity. Each major section of this chapter is divided into subsections on the urinary, male reproductive, and female reproductive systems.

Urinary System Refresher

The urinary system consists of two kidneys, two ureters, the urinary bladder, and the urethra (■ FIGURE 22-1). The **kidneys** produce urine and regulate the level of **electrolytes** and body fluid (■ FIGURE 22-2). The **nephrons** are the functioning

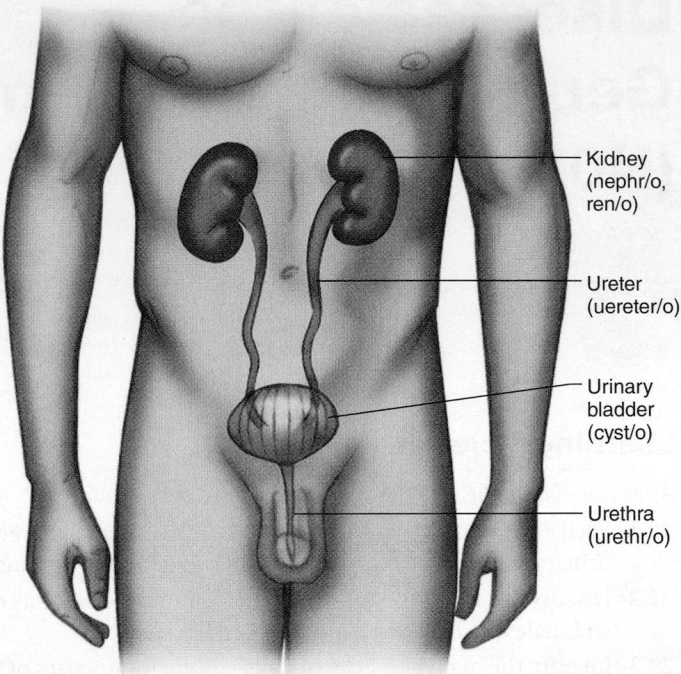

Figure 22-1 ■ The Urinary System

part of each kidney and filter waste from the blood, beginning with the **glomerulus**, a cluster of capillaries that separates the urinary space from the blood. The **renal pelvis** of each kidney collects urine, which then passes through the **ureter** (*a tube that drains each kidney*) to the **urinary bladder**, a muscular sac that holds urine until it is expelled through the **urethra** (*the tube that carries urine out of the body*).

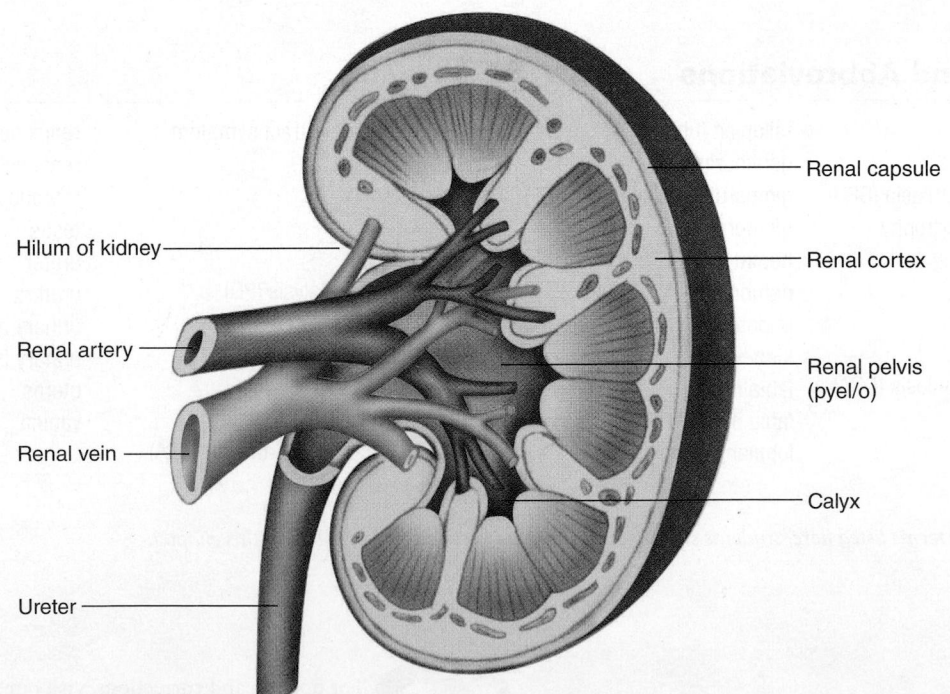

Figure 22-2 ■ The Kidney

■ Reproductive system

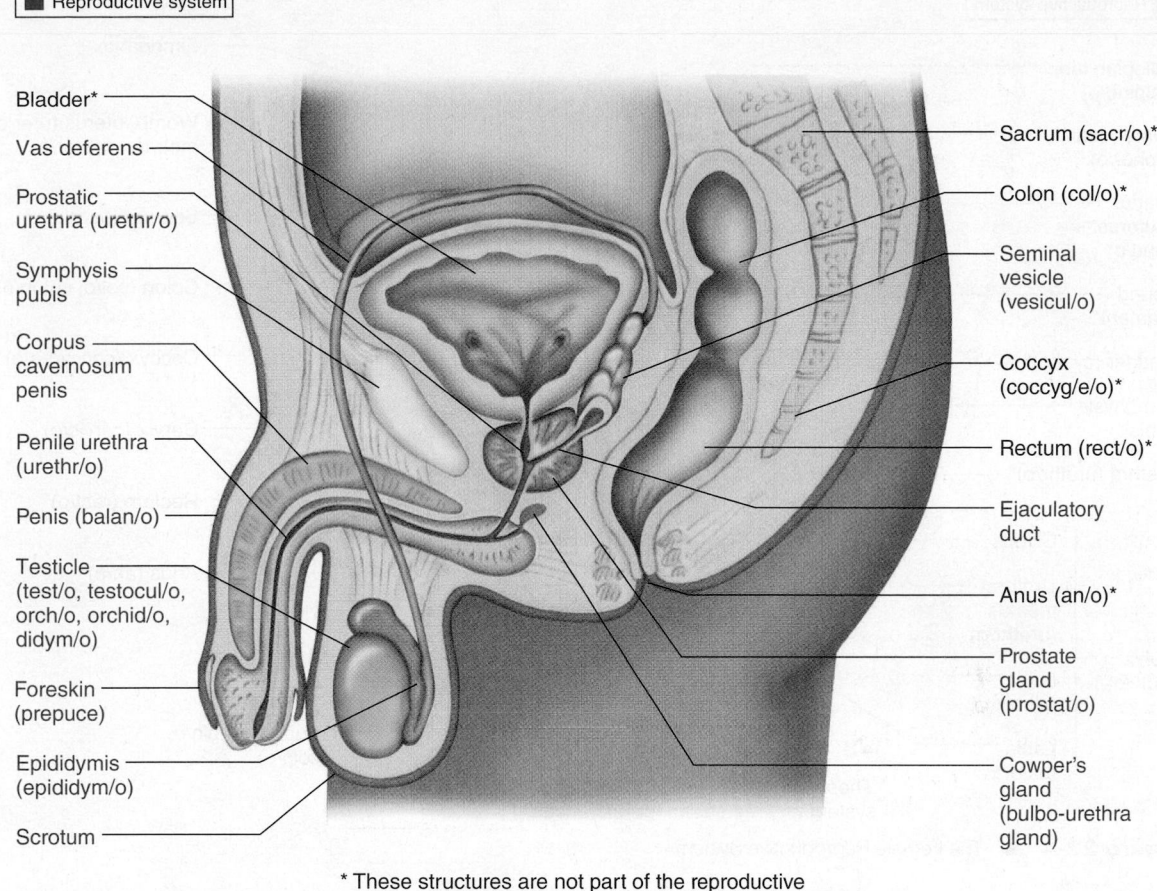

Bladder*

Vas deferens

Prostatic
urethra (urethr/o)

Symphysis
pubis

Corpus
cavernosum
penis

Penile urethra
(urethr/o)

Penis (balan/o)

Testicle
(test/o, testocul/o,
orch/o, orchid/o,
didym/o)

Foreskin
(prepuce)

Epididymis
(epididym/o)

Scrotum

Sacrum (sacr/o)*

Colon (col/o)*

Seminal
vesicle
(vesicul/o)

Coccyx
(coccyg/e/o)*

Rectum (rect/o)*

Ejaculatory
duct

Anus (an/o)*

Prostate
gland
(prostat/o)

Cowper's
gland
(bulbo-urethra
gland)

* These structures are not part of the reproductive
system and are shown for reference.

Figure 22-3 ■ The Male Reproductive System

Male Reproductive System Refresher

The male reproductive system consists of the external genital organ, internal genital organs, and associated glands (■ Figure 22-3). The **penis**, the external male sex organ, is a conduit for the urethra, which carries urine and semen out of the body. The male urethra is approximately eight inches long. Internal genital organs are the **testes** and the **reproductive ducts**. Associated glands are the **prostate** and **bulbo-urethral glands**. The testes also function as part of the endocrine system.

Female Reproductive System Refresher

The female reproductive system also consists of external and internal genital organs (■ Figure 22-4, page 360). The external genital organs are the **labia major** and **labia minor** (*folds of flesh that surround and protect the opening to the vagina and urethra*), **Bartholin's gland** (*a gland that secretes mucus*), and the **clitoris** (*a small sensitive protrusion*). The internal genital organs consist of two **ovaries**, which produce eggs; two **fallopian tubes**, which transport eggs for fertilization and implantation in the uterus; the **uterus**, which is the womb for development of the fetus; and the **vagina**, which is

the birth canal. The female urethra, which is one to two inches long and exits the body in front of the vagina, does not function in reproduction. The female breasts are also part of the reproductive system. The ovaries also function as part of the endocrine system.

In the previous figures, each structure in the genitourinary system is labeled with its name as well as its medical terminology root/combining form, where applicable. Refer to ■ Table 22-1 (page 360) for a refresher on how to build medical terms related to the genitourinary system.

CODING CAUTION

Be alert for medical word terms that are spelled similarly but have different meanings.

prostat/o (*prostate*) and **proct/o** (*anus and rectum*)

salpingitis of the **fallopian** tube (*part of the female reproductive system*) and salpingitis of the **Eustachian tube** (*located between the ear and the nasopharynx*)

ureter (*the two tubes that drain the kidneys into the bladder*) and **urethra** (*a single tube that carries urine from the bladder to the outside of the body*)

colp/o (*vagina*) and **col/o** or **colon/o** (*colon or large intestine*)

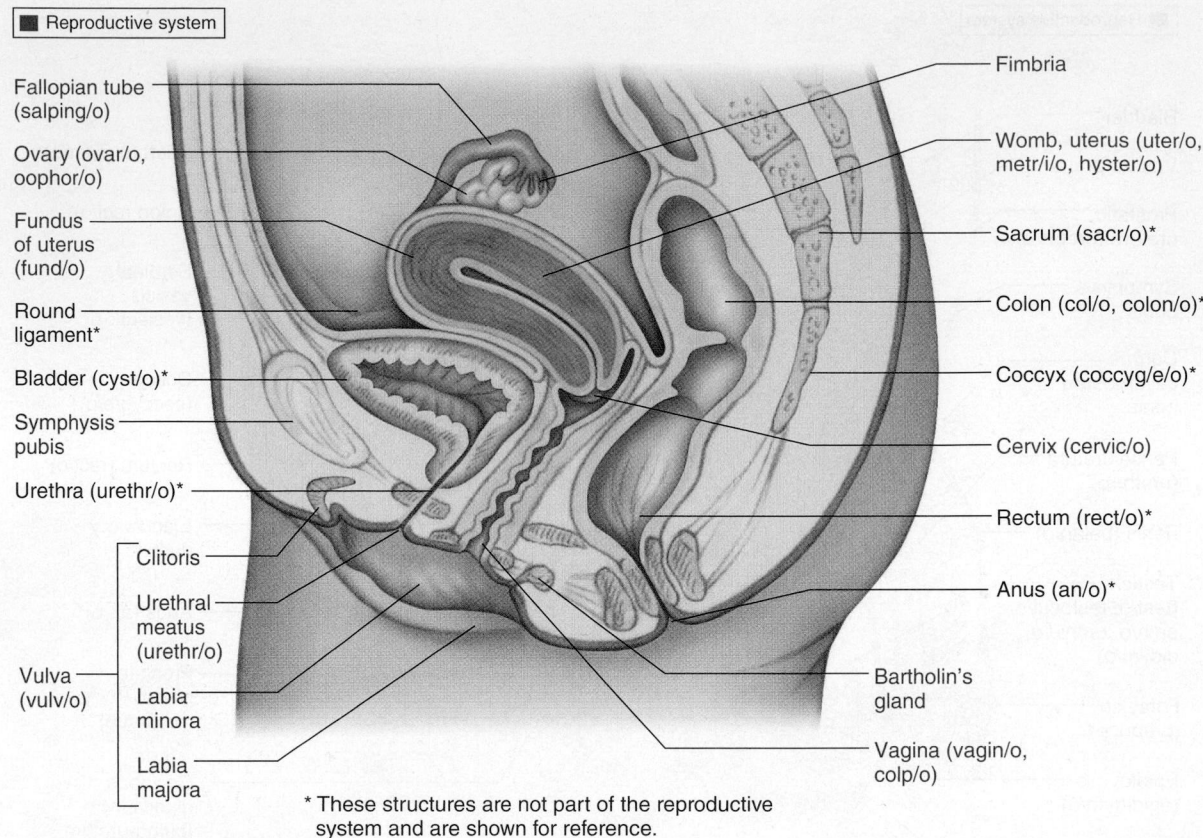

Figure 22-4 ■ The Female Reproductive System

Conditions of the Urinary System

Urologic and kidney conditions are among the most common reasons for doctor visits and hospital admissions. Over 13% of women have a urinary tract infection each year; more than 10% of the population over age 20 has chronic kidney disease, according to the National Institutes of Health (NIH).

Diseases and disorders of the urinary system include infections and inflammations of nearly any anatomic site, glomerular diseases that attack the kidneys' filtering ability, kidney failure, and obstructions. Coders use medical resources, such as reference books on diseases, to understand conditions of the genitourinary system, diagnostic methods, and common treatments. Refer to ■ TABLE 22-2 for a summary of diseases affecting the urinary system.

In particular, coders must be familiar with the terminology related to chronic kidney disease.

Chronic Kidney Disease

Chronic kidney disease (CKD), also called chronic renal failure, is the slow loss of kidney function over a period of months or years. People are able to live long periods of time with decreased kidney function; symptoms of the disease may not appear until

Table 22-1 ■ EXAMPLE OF CONSTRUCTING MEDICAL TERMS FOR GENITOURINARY SYSTEM

Combining Form	Suffix	Complete Medical Term
nephr/o- (*kidney*) **hemat/o** (*blood*) **cyst/o-** (*bladder*)	**-uria** (*condition of urine*) **-ptosis** (*to droop*) **-lithiasis** (*condition of stones*) **-itis** (*inflammation*) **-ectomy** (*surgical excision*)	**nephro + ptosis** (*drooping of the kidney*) **cyst + ptosis** (*drooping of the bladder*) **hemat + uria** (*blood in urine*) **nephro + lithiasis** (*kidney stones*) **cysto + lithiasis** (*bladder stones*)
prostat/o (*prostate*)		**prostat + itis** (*inflammation of the prostate*) **prostat + ectomy** (*surgical removal of the prostate*)
end/o (*within*) **metr/i** (*uterus*) **hyster/o** (*uterus*)		**endo + metr + itis** (*inflammation of the lining of the uterus*) **hyster + ectomy** (*surgical removal of the uterus*)

Table 22-2 ■ **COMMON DISEASES OF THE URINARY SYSTEM**

Condition	Definition
Acute kidney failure	The rapid loss of kidney function over a period of days or weeks
Acute tubular necrosis	Damage to the renal tubules due to reduced blood flow or toxins in the urine
Calculi	Stones that may accumulate in the kidneys, bladder, or ureters
Chronic kidney disease (CKD)	The slow loss of kidney function over a period of months or years
Cystitis	Bacterial infection of the urinary bladder; also called **urinary tract infection (UTI)**
Diabetic nephropathy	Accumulated damage to the glomerulus capillaries due to chronic high blood glucose
Glomerulonephritis	Inflammation of the glomerulus of the kidney, allowing protein and blood into the urine
Hydronephrosis	Distention of the renal pelvis due to excessive urine collection in the kidney, often due to ureteral obstruction (■ Figure 22-5)
Incontinence	The inability to control bladder muscles
Nephritic syndrome	A collection of disorders affecting the kidneys, characterized by nonpurulent inflammatory glomerular disorders that allow proteins and red blood cells to pass into the urine, resulting in proteinuria and **hematuria** (*blood in the urine*)
Nephroptosis	Downward placement of the kidney from its normal location
Nephrotic syndrome	A collection of disorders affecting the kidneys, characterized by proteinuria but not hematuria
Pyelonephritis	Acute or chronic infection of the renal medulla and upper urinary tract as a result of untreated cystitis, also called **polynephritis**
Uremia	Toxic blood condition due to the inability of the kidneys to remove nitrogenous substances from the blood

as little as 10% of kidney function remains. However, the loss of kidney function results in the build up of toxins in the body, which can have serious effects on most body functions, especially red blood cell production, blood pressure control, vitamin D absorption, and bone health (■ FIGURE 22-6, page 362).

Diabetes and high blood pressure account for two-thirds of the cases of CKD, according to the National Kidney Foundation.

Other conditions that cause CKD include **polycystic kidney disease**, glomerulonephritis, medications, autoimmune disorders such as lupus erythematosus and scleroderma, kidney stones, recurrent UTIs, and **reflux nephropathy**.

Kidney health is monitored through a wide range of blood tests that are included as part of most routine physical examinations. Persistent protein in the urine is an early sign of possible

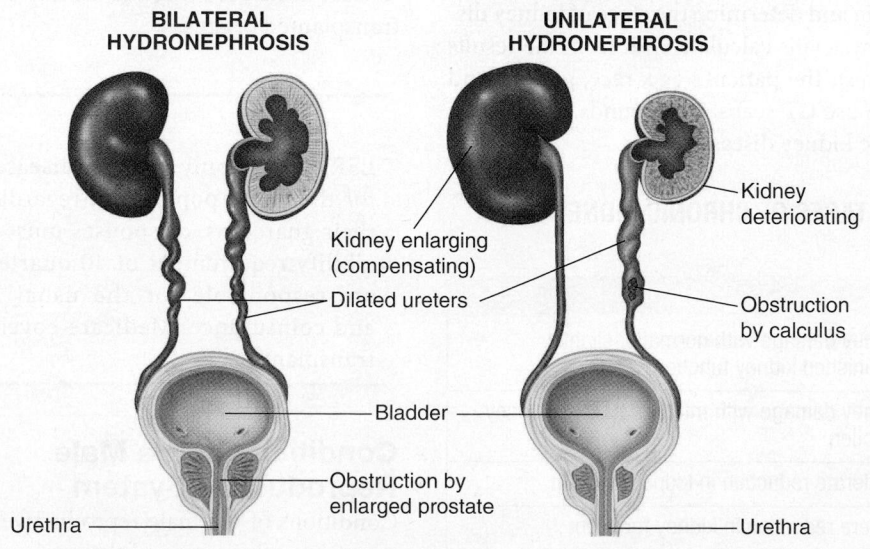

BILATERAL HYDRONEPHROSIS

UNILATERAL HYDRONEPHROSIS

Kidney enlarging (compensating)
Dilated ureters
Bladder
Obstruction by enlarged prostate
Urethra

Kidney deteriorating
Obstruction by calculus
Urethra

Figure 22-5 ■ Hydronephrosis: Bilateral and Unilateral

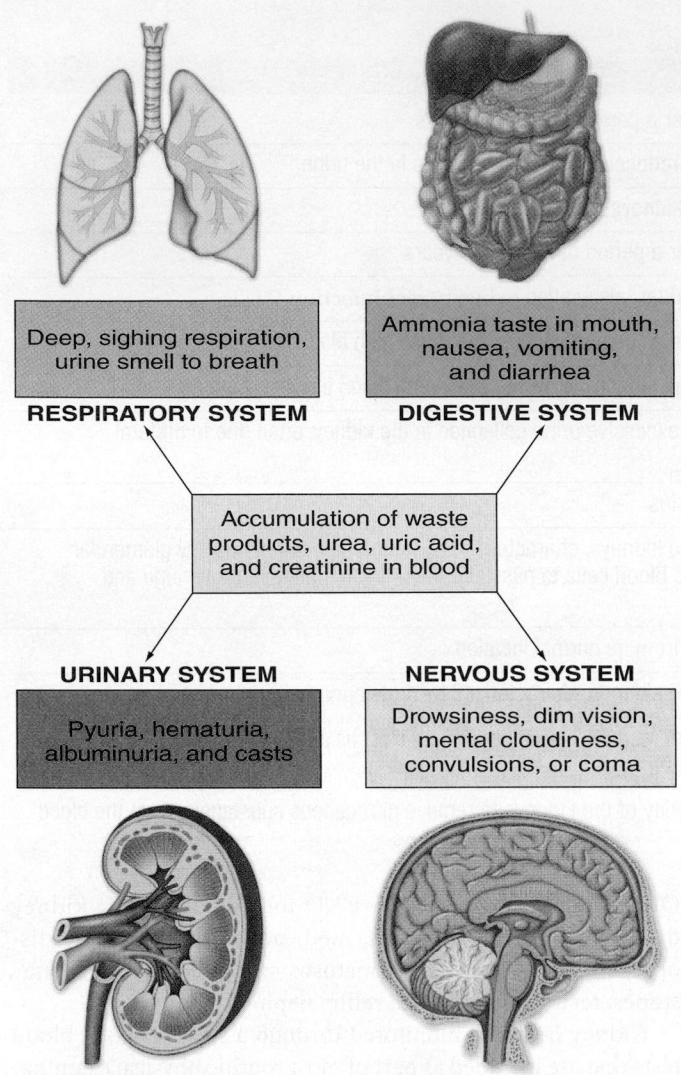

RESPIRATORY SYSTEM

Deep, sighing respiration, urine smell to breath

DIGESTIVE SYSTEM

Ammonia taste in mouth, nausea, vomiting, and diarrhea

Accumulation of waste products, urea, uric acid, and creatinine in blood

URINARY SYSTEM

Pyuria, hematuria, albuminuria, and casts

NERVOUS SYSTEM

Drowsiness, dim vision, mental cloudiness, convulsions, or coma

Figure 22-6 ■ Manifestations of Chronic Kidney Disease

CKD. **Glomerular filtration rate (GFR)** is the preferred way to measure kidney function and determine the stage of kidney disease (■ TABLE 22-3). Physicians calculate GFR from the results of a **blood creatinine** test, the patient's age, race, gender, and other factors. They also use CT scans, ultrasounds, and kidney biopsies to help evaluate kidney disease.

Table 22-3 ■ THE STAGES OF CHRONIC KIDNEY DISEASE

Stage	GFR	Description
1	130-90	Kidney damage with normal or slightly diminished kidney function
2	90-60	Kidney damage with mild reduction in kidney function
3	60-30	Moderate reduction in kidney function
4	30-15	Severe reduction in kidney function
5	15-0	Kidney failure; end-stage renal disease (ESRD)

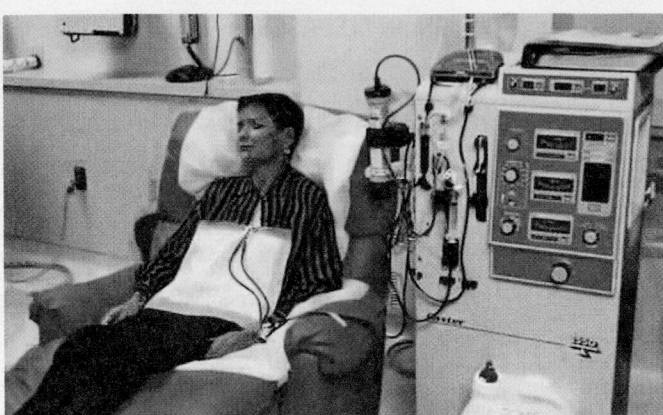

Figure 22-7 ■ A Patient Undergoing Hemodialysis. *Source: Michal Heron/Pearson Education.*

CKD is not curable, but its progress can be slowed through diet, lifestyle, and medication. When CKD reaches stage 5, the kidneys cease to function, and patients must receive **dialysis** or a kidney transplant in order to survive.

Dialysis is a treatment that filters the blood to remove waste, excess salt, and water. Over a half-million Americans are on dialysis, according to NIH. In **hemodialysis (HD)** the blood is processed through a machine (■ FIGURE 22-7). In **peritoneal dialysis (PD)**, the peritoneal membrane (*the lining of the abdomen*) is used to filter the blood. Although 99% of dialysis is performed at centralized dialysis centers, according to Home Dialysis Central, it can be done at home with proper training and support. Medicare, which covers dialysis services for ESRD, requires that all patients be offered all dialysis options. Dialysis brings on its own complications as well, including infections and hemorrhaging through the dialysis port access site, electrolyte abnormalities, anemia, cardiac dysfunction, and **dialysis-related amyloidosis (DRA)** (*deposits of the starchy substance amyloid in the joints*) in long-term dialysis patients. Kidney transplants are an option to treat ESRD, making the kidney one of the most frequently transplanted organs.

SUCCESS STEP

ESRD is the only specific disease that Medicare covers for the entire population, regardless of age. Individuals, their guardians, or spouses must meet the Medicare eligibility requirement of 40 quarters of employment and are responsible for the usual Medicare deductibles and coinsurance. Medicare covers dialysis services and transplants.

Conditions of the Male Reproductive System

Conditions of the male reproductive system relate to both the structure and function of the organs. Components may be misshaped or out of place. When portions of the system malfunction, fertility and reproduction are affected. ■ TABLE 22-4

Table 22-4 ■ COMMON DISEASES OF THE MALE REPRODUCTIVE SYSTEM

Condition	Definition
Enlarged prostate (EP)	The abnormal growth of epithelial cells of the prostate, causing compression or obstruction of the urethra; also called *benign prostatic hypertrophy* or *hyperplasia* (BPH)
Erectile dysfunction (ED)	The chronic inability to achieve or maintain a penile erection until ejaculation; also called *impotence*
Hydrocele	A fluid-filled sack in the scrotum caused by abnormal fetal development, injury, hernia, or blockages
Male factor infertility	A problem in the male genital system that diminishes reproduction, such as inability to ejaculate, lack of sperm production, or lack of live sperm
Prostatic intraepithelial neoplasia (PIN)	Neoplastic changes in the epithelial cells of the prostate ducts showing some features of cancer, but not invasive; a potential precursor of carcinoma or adenocarcinoma
Spermatocele	Benign cystic swelling of sperm in the ducts of of the epididymis

summarizes conditions of the male reproductive system covered in ICD-10-CM Chapter 14. Sexually transmitted diseases are classified in ICD-10-CM Chapter 1, Certain Infections and Parasitic Diseases (A00-B99).

Conditions of the Female Reproductive System

Conditions of the female reproductive system are related to organ position, fertility, and reproduction; they include disorders of the breast in addition to the reproductive organs located in the pelvic region (■ TABLE 22-5). Sexually transmitted diseases are classified in ICD-10-CM Chapter 1, Certain Infections and Parasitic Diseases (A00-B99).

Table 22-5 ■ COMMON DISEASES OF THE FEMALE REPRODUCTIVE SYSTEM

Condition	Definition
Cervical dysplasia	Abnormal changes in the cells on the surface of the cervix that may lead to cancer if not treated
Cervical intraepithelial neoplasia (CIN)	Cervical dysplasia seen on a cervical biopsy, classified as mild dysplasia (CIN I), moderate to marked dysplasia (CIN II), and severe dysplasia to cancer in situ (CIN III)
Endometriosis	The growth of endometrial tissue in any area other than the uterus
Female factor infertility	A problem in the female genital system that diminishes reproduction, such as scarring or obstruction of the fallopian tubes or abnormal interaction between sperm and the mucous membrane in the cervix
Fibrocystic breast disease	Lumps of benign fibrous tissue in the breast
Genital prolapse	Downward displacement of the uterus or vagina to an abnormal position
Pelvic inflammatory disease (PID)	Inflammation of the female reproductive tract above the cervix
Squamous intraepithelial lesion (SIL)	Cervical dysplasia seen on a **PAP** test, graded as low grade (LSIL), high grade (HSIL), and possibly cancerous or malignant
Vulvovaginitis	Inflammation of the vulva and vagina due to yeast, bacteria, viruses, parasites, or skin care products

This section provides a general reference to help understand the most common diagnoses of the genitourinary system but does not list everything you need to know. Use medical terminology skills discussed earlier in this chapter to learn the meaning of unfamiliar words. Remember to keep standard reference books handy in case you get stuck.

CODING PRACTICE

Exercise 22.1   Genitourinary System Refresher

Instructions: Use your medical terminology skills and resources to define the following conditions related to the genitourinary system, then assign the default diagnosis code. Follow these steps:

- Use slash marks "/" to break down each term into its root(s) and suffix.
- Define the meaning of the word, based on the meaning of each word part.
- Assign the default ICD-10-CM diagnosis code for the condition using the Index and Tabular List.

(continued)

CODING PRACTICE (continued)

Example: cystitis cyst/itis   Meaning: _inflammation of the bladder_   ICD-10-CM Code: _N30.90_

1. amenorrhea   Meaning _____   ICD-10-CM Code _____

2. cystolithiasis   Meaning _____   ICD-10-CM Code _____

3. dyspareunia   Meaning _____   ICD-10-CM Code _____

4. hydrocele   Meaning _____   ICD-10-CM Code _____

5. cystoptosis   Meaning _____   ICD-10-CM Code _____

6. nephralgia   Meaning _____   ICD-10-CM Code _____

7. urethrorrhagia   Meaning _____   ICD-10-CM Code _____

8. nephrosis   Meaning _____   ICD-10-CM Code _____

9. ureterocele   Meaning _____   ICD-10-CM Code _____

10. pyelonephrosis   Meaning _____   ICD-10-CM Code _____

CODING OVERVIEW OF THE GENITOURINARY SYSTEM

ICD-10-CM Chapter 14, Diseases of the Genitourinary System (N00-N99), contains 11 blocks or subchapters that are divided by anatomic site. Review the block names and code ranges listed at the beginning of Chapter 14 in the ICD-10-CM manual to become familiar with the content and organization.

ICD-10-CM Chapter 14 corresponds to ICD-9-CM Chapter 10 (580-629). Many codes have been added, deleted, expanded, combined, or moved. Codes for stress incontinence, nonspecific urethritis, and other ovarian hyperfunction have been moved to this chapter from other chapters in ICD-9-CM. Codes for vesicoureteral reflux, hematuria, salpingitis, and oophoritis are expanded and restructured in ICD-10-CM.

This chapter includes conditions of the male and female urinary system, the male reproductive system, the female breast, and disorders of the female genital tract. It does not include disorders related to pregnancy, which are classified in Chapter 15, Pregnancy, Childbirth and the Puerperium (O00-O9A). It also does not include injuries or congenital conditions of the genitourinary system.

ICD-10-CM provides Official Guidelines for Coding and Reporting (OGCR) diseases of the genitourinary system in OGCR section I.C.14. OGCR provides detailed discussion of chronic kidney disease. Additional OGCR related to hypertensive chronic kidney disease appear in OGCR I.C.9.a.2) and 3).

ABSTRACTING FOR GENITOURINARY SYSTEM CONDITIONS

Disorders in this chapter have a wide range of abstracting criteria because there is a wide range of organs and types of disorders. Most conditions can be adequately abstracted by being attentive to the specific type and subtype of condition. Certain conditions require additional specific criteria, such as CKD and BPH. Refer to the following tables for guidance on how to abstract conditions of the urinary system (■ TABLE 22-6),

male reproductive system (■ TABLE 22-7), and female reproductive system (■ TABLE 22-8), then work through the detailed example that follows. Remember that the abstracting

Table 22-6 ■ KEY CRITERIA FOR ABSTRACTING CONDITIONS OF THE URINARY SYSTEM

❑ What is the condition?

❑ What is the subtype or anatomic site?

❑ Does laterality apply?

❑ Is the condition acute or chronic?

❑ Is an obstruction documented?

❑ What is the infectious organism?

❑ Is there a history of recurrent UTIs?

❑ What stage is the chronic kidney disease?

❑ Does the patient receive dialysis?

❑ Is the patient on a transplant waiting list or the recipient of a transplant?

❑ Do any additional conditions coexist?

Table 22-7 ■ KEY CRITERIA FOR ABSTRACTING CONDITIONS OF THE MALE REPRODUCTIVE SYSTEM

❑ Verify the patient's gender.

❑ What is the condition?

❑ What is the subtype or anatomic site?

❑ Does laterality apply?

❑ Is the condition acute or chronic?

❑ Is an obstruction documented?

❑ What is the infectious organism?

❑ What symptoms are associated with prostatic hypertrophy?

❑ Do any additional conditions coexist?

Table 22-8 ■ KEY CRITERIA FOR ABSTRACTING CONDITIONS OF THE FEMALE REPRODUCTIVE SYSTEM

❑ Verify the patient's gender.

❑ What is the condition?

❑ What is the subtype or anatomic site?

❑ Does laterality apply?

❑ Is the condition acute or chronic?

❑ What is the infectious organism?

❑ Do any additional conditions coexist?

Date: 02/21/yy   Location: Branton Professional Group   Provider: Ann Colyer, MD

Patient: Ronald Coffield   Gender: M   Age: 53

Reason for encounter: ESRD patient presents with ongoing complaints of extreme joint pain

Assessment: joint pain is due to dialysis-related amyloidosis (DRA), ESRD, HD, on kidney transplant waiting list

Plan: begin medication regimen despite side effects, and consider surgical intervention

---

questions are a guide and that not every question applies to, or can be answered for, every case. For example, laterality applies to many, but not all, disorders of the breast, but not to most disorders of the kidneys, ureters, ovaries, or fallopian tubes, all of which are paired organs. Also remember to abstract for symptoms and determine if they are integral to the confirmed diagnoses.

CODING CAUTION

Checking patients' gender helps prevent coding errors, such as picking up a code for the wrong gender, and also helps identify potential keying errors. Never assume a patient's gender based on the name because many common names are androgynous, such as Terry, Taylor, Lynn, or Pat. In addition, if ethnic names are unfamiliar, it is impossible to "guess." Examples are Shing, which is Chinese (male); Iffat, which is Muslim (female); or Gwandoya, which is African (male).

Guided Example of Abstracting for Urinary System Conditions

Refer to the following example throughout this chapter to learn skills for abstracting, assigning, and sequencing urinary system codes. Chrystal Crago, CCA, is a fictitious coder who guides you through the coding process.

Follow along as Chrystal Crago, CCA, abstracts the diagnosis. Check off each step after you complete it.

▶ Chrystal reads through the entire record, paying special attention to the reason for the encounter and the final assessment. She refers to the Key Criteria for Abstracting Conditions of the Urinary System (Table 22-6).

❑ *What is the condition?* ongoing complaints of extreme joint pain for an ESRD patient.

❑ *Which system does this case relate to: urinary, male reproductive, or female reproductive?* Urinary.

❑ *What are the presenting symptom(s)?* ongoing extreme joint pain

❑ *What is the condition?* amyloidosis

❑ *What is the subtype?* ESRD dialysis-related (DRA)

❑ *What stage is the chronic kidney disease?* By definition, ESRD is stage 5.

❑ *Does the patient receive dialysis?* Yes, HD is documented.

❑ *Is the patient on a transplant waiting list or the recipient of a transplant?* Yes.

▶ At this time, Chrystal does not how many codes she will end up with. She will learn about this when she moves on to assigning codes.

CODING PRACTICE

Exercise 22.2   Abstracting for Genitourinary System Conditions

Instructions: Read the mini-medical-record of each patient's encounter and answer the abstracting questions. Write the answer on the line provided. Do not assign any codes.

---

1. OFFICE   Gender: F   Age: 42

Reason for encounter: surgery for endometriosis

Assessment: endometriosis of the uterus

Plan: FU in office 2 weeks

a. Which system does this case relate to: urinary, male reproductive, or female reproductive?

_____

(continued)

CODING PRACTICE (continued)

1. (continued)

b. What is the condition? _____

_____

c. What is the subtype or anatomic site? _____

_____

d. Is an infectious organism named? _____

_____

2. OFFICE   Gender: F   Age: 46

Reason for encounter: painful lumps in both breasts

Assessment: fibrocystic breast changes

Plan: OTC acetaminophen, heat and ice as needed to relieve local pain

Tip: Physicians use the term *changes* rather than the more traditional *disease* to avoid alarming patients.

a. Which system does this case relate to: urinary, male reproductive, or female reproductive?

_____

b. What is the condition? _____

_____

c. What is the anatomic site? _____

_____

d. Does laterality apply? _____

_____

e. Is an obstruction documented? _____

_____

f. Do any additional conditions coexist? _____

_____

3. OFFICE   Gender: M   Age: 61

Reason for encounter: occasional excruciating low back pain

Assessment: renal and ureteral calculi

Plan: medical expulsive therapy (MET) (*treatment with drugs to expel the calculi*) with tamsulosin (*an alpha blocker*)

a. Which system does this case relate to: urinary, male reproductive, or female reproductive?

_____

b. What are the symptoms? _____

_____

3. (continued)

c. What is the condition? _____

_____

d. Does the condition account for the symptom?

_____

e. What is the anatomic site? _____

_____

f. Does laterality apply? _____

_____

g. Is an obstruction documented? _____

_____

4. OFFICE   Gender: M   Age: 81

Reason for encounter: FU on EP with obstruction and urinary retention

Assessment: little improvement seen despite multiple medication adjustments

Plan: schedule transurethral resection of the prostate (TURP)

a. Which system does this case relate to: urinary, male reproductive, or female reproductive?

_____

b. What is the condition? _____

_____

c. Is an obstruction documented? _____

_____

d. What symptoms are associated with prostatic hypertrophy? _____

_____

5. OFFICE   Gender: F   Age: 37

Reason for encounter: vaginal discharge, burning, redness in perineal area

Assessment: lab results show bacterial vaginitis due to staphylococcus, which is treatable

Plan: antibiotics

a. Which system does this case relate to: urinary, male reproductive, or female reproductive?

_____

b. What are the symptoms? _____

(continued)

5. (continued)

c. What is the condition? _____

d. What is the subtype of the condition? _____
_____

e. What is the infectious organism? _____
_____

f. Is the organism resistant to antibiotic treatment?
_____

---

6. INPATIENT HOSPITAL   Gender: F   Age: 83

Reason for admission: nursing facility (NF) patient brought to emergency department with suspected UTI because of signs of confusion and lack of cooperation; history of UTI over the past 2 years

(continued)

---

6. (continued)

Assessment: UTI due to E. coli, (non-Shiga toxin-producing)

Plan: administered IV antibiotics, discharged after 2 days to NF with Rx

a. Which system does this case relate to: urinary, male reproductive, or female reproductive?
_____

b. What is the condition? _____

c. Is an obstruction documented? _____

d. What is the infectious organism? _____

   What is the subtype? _____

e. Is there a history of recurrent UTIs? _____
_____

ASSIGNING CODES FOR GENITOURINARY SYSTEM CONDITIONS

Two similar urinary system conditions, nephritic syndrome and nephrotic syndrome, demonstrate the importance of checking cross-referencing instructions in the Index in order to assign the most specific code available.

Assigning Codes for Nephritic Syndrome and Nephrotic Syndrome

An analysis of word roots and suffixes leads to similar descriptions of nephritis (*inflammation of the kidney*) and nephrosis (*abnormal condition of the kidney*), but, clinically, they are distinct conditions with distinct diagnostic criteria (Table 22-2).

Nephritic syndrome is a collection of disorders affecting the kidneys, characterized by nonpurulent inflammatory glomerular disorders that allow proteins and red blood cells to pass into the urine, resulting in proteinuria and hematuria. The Index entry for the Main Term **Syndrome** and the subterm **nephritic** provides a cross-referencing instruction, *see also* **Nephritis**. It provides additional subterms for **acute**, **chronic**, and **rapidly**

progressive (■ FIGURE 22-8). The subterm **with edema** provides a cross-reference *see* **Nephrosis** because edema is characteristic of nephrosis.

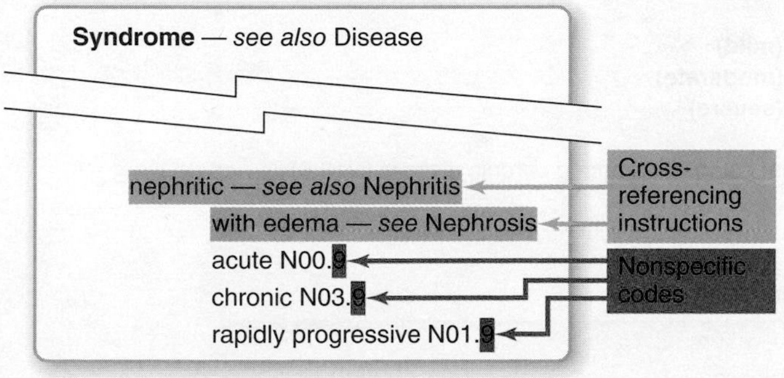

Coders may feel confused whether they should assign one of the codes listed under **Syndrome, nephritic**, or whether they must follow the cross-reference. Remember the following tips:

- When the condition is *not specified any further* in the documentation, assign the code that follows the appropriate subterm.
- When documentation *provides more details than appear in the Index entry*, follow the cross-referenced Main Term to search for a more specific code.

SUCCESS STEP

Whenever you are in doubt if you have the correct code, follow the cross-reference. It only takes a moment and either confirms your initial choice or leads you to a more specific code. Either way, cross-referencing gives you confidence in your coding skills.

Nephrotic syndrome is a collection of disorders affecting the kidneys, characterized by proteinuria and edema but *not* hematuria. The Index entry for the Main Term **Syndrome** and the subterm **nephrotic** provides a cross-referencing instruction, *see also* **Nephrosis**. It provides additional subterms for certain subtypes of the condition.

Refer to ■ FIGURE 22-9 (page 368) to learn more about when to follow the cross-referencing instructions in the Index.

When coders search only under **Syndrome, nephritic, acute**, they identify the code **N00.9 Acute nephritic syndrome with unspecified morphologic changes** (■ FIGURE 22-10, page 368). When they follow the cross-reference to

Syndrome — *see also* Disease

nephritic — *see also* Nephritis
with edema — *see* Nephrosis
acute N00.9
chronic N03.9
rapidly progressive N01.9

Cross-referencing instructions

Nonspecific codes

Figure 22-8 ■ Index Entry for Nephritic Syndrome

A mother presents with her 6 year old daughter who has blood in her urine. Urinalysis testing shows albuminuria, hematuria, and proteinuria. A kidney biopsy is also done and after results come back, the physician diagnoses her with acute nephritic syndrome with mesangial proliferative glomerulonephritis.

Index: **Nephritis, acute, diffuse, mesangial proliferative glomerulonephritis**
Tabular List: **N00.3 Acute nephritic syndrome with diffuse mesangial proliferative glomerulonephritis**

Figure 22-9 ■ Example of Assigning Codes for Nephritic Syndrome

Nephritis, then follow the subterms that describe the specific subtype, they identify code **N00.3 Acute nephritic syndrome with diffuse mesangial proliferative glomerulonephritis** (Figure 22-10). Because **N00.3** is a specific code, it is the correct code for this example.

Guided Example of Assigning Codes for Urinary System Conditions

To practice skills for assigning codes for diseases of the urinary system, continue with the example from earlier in the chapter about patient Ronald Coffield, who was seen at Branton Professional Group for ESRD and joint pain.

Follow along in your ICD-10-CM manual as Chrystal Crago, CCA, assigns codes. Check off each step after you complete it.

▶ First, Chrystal confirms the information she abstracted:

❑ ESRD

❑ HD

❑ DRA

❑ on transplant waiting list

▶ Chrystal begins with ESRD and searches the Index for the Main Term **Disease**.

❑ She locates the subterm **renal**.

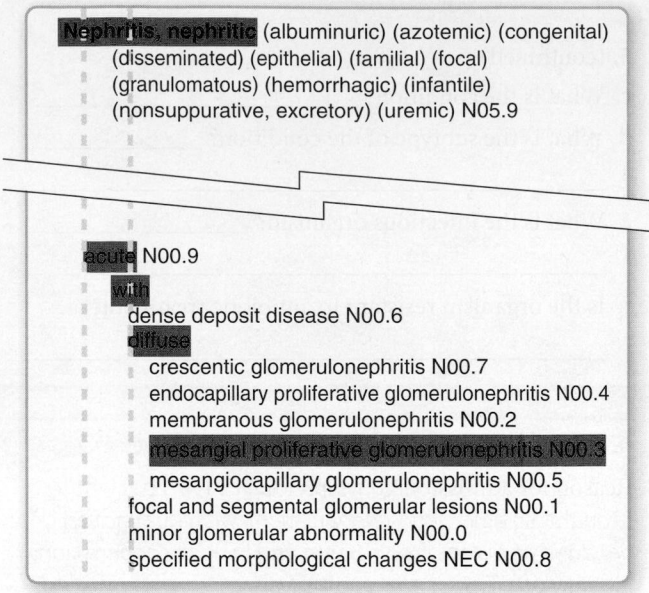

Figure 22-10 ■ Index Entry for the Main Term Nephritis

❑ She locates the second-level subterm **end stage (failure) N18.6**.

❑ She notes an additional level subterm **due to hypertension**, but concludes it does not describe this case because the patient's ESRD is not documented as due to hypertension.

▶ Chrystal verifies code **N18.6** in the Tabular List (■ **Figure 22-11**).

❑ She reads the code title for **N18.6, End stage renal disease** and confirms that this accurately describes the diagnosis.

❑ She reads the inclusion note under the code title that states **Chronic kidney disease requiring chronic dialysis**.

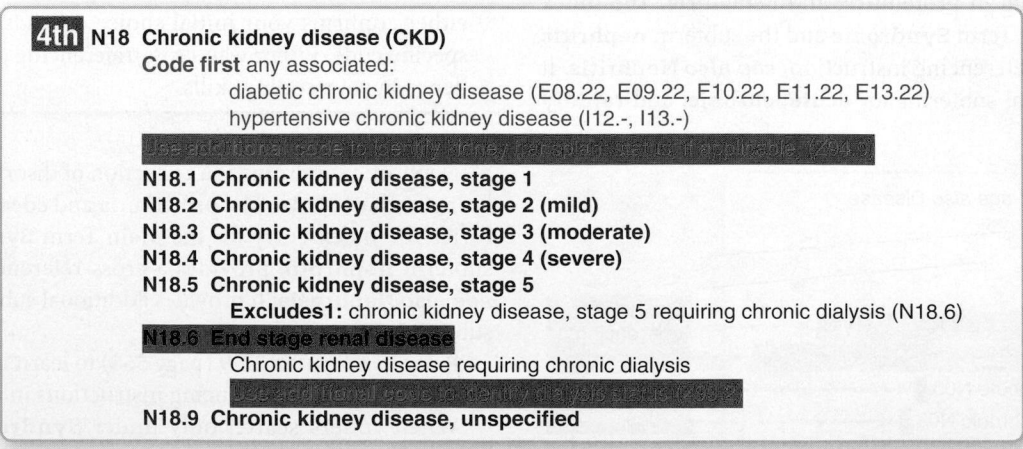

Figure 22-11 ■ Tabular List Entry for Chronic Kidney Disease

❑ She reads the instructional note under the code title that states **Use additional code to identify dialysis status (Z99.2)**.

❑ This tells her to assign a code for dialysis and that it should be a secondary code.

▶ Chrystal checks for other instructional notes in the Tabular List.

❑ She cross-references the beginning of category **N18** and reads the instructional notes.

❑ This patient does not have diabetes or hypertension, so the first two notes do not apply.

❑ The third note that states **Use additional code to identify kidney transplant status, if applicable, (Z94.0)** also does not apply because the patient has not yet received a transplant.

❑ She cross-references the beginning of the block **(N17-N19)** and reviews the **Excludes2** notes. None of them apply because they do not describe ESRD.

❑ She cross-references the beginning of **Chapter 14 (N00-N99)** and reviews the **Excludes2** notes. None of them apply.

▶ Chrystal moves on to HD and searches the Index for the Main Term **Dialysis**.

❑ She locates the subterm **renal Z99.2**.

❑ This code is the same as the one cross-referenced by the Tabular List under code **N18.6**.

❑ She reviews the rest of the subterms and does not see any others that apply.

▶ Chrystal verifies code **Z99.2** in the Tabular List.

❑ She reads the code title for **Z99.2, Dependence on renal dialysis** and confirms that this accurately describes the diagnosis.

❑ She reads the inclusion items under the code title and learns that this code describes both hemodialysis and peritoneal dialysis.

❑ She reads the **Excludes1** notes, which do not apply.

▶ Chrystal checks for instructional notes in the Tabular List.

❑ She cross-references the beginning of category **Z99.2** and verifies that there are no instructional notes.

❑ She cross-references the beginning of the block **Z77-Z99** and reads the instructional note. It does not apply because there was no follow-up examination.

❑ She cross-references the beginning of **Chapter 21 (Z00-Z99)** and reviews the instructional notes, which describe the general use and purpose of Z codes. Nothing she reads changes the code assigned.

▶ Next, Chrystal works on DRA dialysis-related amyloidosis and searches the Index for the Main Term **Amyloidosis**.

❑ She locates the subterm **hemodialysis-associated E85.3**.

❑ She reviews the rest of the subterms and does not see any others that apply.

▶ Chrystal verifies code **E85.3** in the Tabular List.

❑ She reads the code title for **E85.3, Secondary systemic amyloidosis** and confirms that this accurately describes the diagnosis.

❑ She reads the inclusion item under the code title and confirms that this code describes **Hemodialysis-associated amyloidosis**.

▶ Chrystal checks for instructional notes in the Tabular List.

❑ She cross-references the beginning of category **E85** and verifies that the **Excludes1** note regarding Alzheimer's disease does not apply.

❑ She cross-references the beginning of the block **E70-E88** and verifies that the **Excludes1** notes do not apply.

❑ She cross-references the beginning of **Chapter 14 (E00-E89)** and determines that the notes do not apply to this case because the patient does not have any of the conditions listed.

▶ Chrystal finishes with on kidney transplant waiting list and searches the Index for the Main Term **Waiting**.

❑ She locates the subterm **for organ transplant Z76.82**.

▶ Chrystal verifies code **Z76.82** in the Tabular List.

❑ She reads the code title for **Z76.82, Awaiting organ transplant status** and confirms that this accurately describes the diagnosis. She searches for, but does not find, a code specifically for kidney transplant waiting list.

▶ Chrystal checks for instructional notes in the Tabular List.

❑ She cross-references the beginning of category **Z76** and verifies that there are no instructional notes.

❑ She cross-references the beginning of the block **Z69-Z76** and verifies that there are no instructional notes.

❑ She previously cross-referenced the beginning of **Chapter 21 (Z00-Z99)** and remembers that there are not chapter-wide instructional notes that apply to this case.

▶ Chrystal reviews the codes she has assigned for this case.

❑ **N18.6 End stage renal disease**

❑ **Z99.2 Dependence on renal dialysis**

❑ **E85.3 Secondary systemic amyloidosis**

❑ **Z76.82 Awaiting organ transplant status**

▶ Next, Chrystal must determine how to sequence the codes.

CODING PRACTICE

Exercise 22.3 Assigning Codes for
Genitourinary System Conditions

Instructions: Read the mini-medical-record of each patient's encounter, review the information abstracted in Exercise 22.2, and assign ICD-10-CM diagnosis codes using the Index and Tabular List. Write the code(s) on the line provided.

---

1. OFFICE   Gender: F   **Age:** 42

Reason for encounter: *surgery for endometriosis*

Assessment: *endometriosis of the uterus*

Plan: *FU in office 2 weeks*

1 ICD-10-CM Code _____

---

2. OFFICE   Gender: F   **Age:** 46

Reason for encounter: *painful lumps in both breasts*

Assessment: *fibrocystic breast changes*

Plan: *OTC acetaminophen, heat and ice as needed to relieve local pain*

Tip: Physicians use the term *changes* rather than the more traditional *disease* to avoid alarming patients.

2 ICD-10-CM Codes _____

---

3. OFFICE   Gender: M   **Age:** 61

Reason for encounter: *occasional excruciating low back pain*

Assessment: *ureteral calculi*

Plan: *medical expulsive therapy (MET) with tamsulosin*

Tip: The presence of calculi accounts for the low-back pain.

1 ICD-10-CM Code _____

ARRANGING CODES FOR GENITOURINARY SYSTEM CONDITIONS

Coders should be attentive to instructional notes in the Tabular List regarding how to sequence codes for genitourinary conditions due to infections and codes for enlarged prostate (EP) and associated symptoms.

Arranging Codes for Genitourinary Conditions Due to Infections

Because many disorders of the genitourinary system are infections, the Tabular List provides frequent instructional notes directing coders to assign an additional code to identify the infectious organism or underlying condition. Sequence the genitourinary condition first and the infectious organism second (■ Figure 22-12).

Arranging Codes for Enlarged Prostate

An enlarged prostate (EP), or benign prostatic hypertrophy (BPH), is the abnormal growth of epithelial cells of the prostate, causing compression or obstruction of the urethra. The condition is common among men over 50 years old and may be accompanied by a variety of **lower urinary tract symptoms (LUTS)** (*symptoms relating to urine storage and voiding disturbances*). ICD-10-CM provides

separate codes for EP based on whether LUTS exist. When EP is accompanied with LUTS, coders must assign codes for LUTS and sequence them after the code for the EP (■ Figure 22-13).

CODING CAUTION

Do not confuse the abbreviation EP, which is an enlarged prostate, with the abbreviation ED, which is erectile dysfunction.

Refer to ■ Figure 22-14 to learn more about assigning and sequencing codes for EP with LUTS. The code for EP must be sequenced first, followed by the two symptoms. The order of the symptoms does not matter, unless the physician indicates that one is of greater importance.

Guided Example of Arranging Codes for Urinary System Conditions

To practice skills for sequencing codes for diseases of the urinary system, continue with the example from earlier in the chapter about patient Ronald Coffield, who was seen at Branton Professional Group for ESRD and joint pain.

Follow along in your ICD-10-CM manual as Chrystal Crago, CCA, sequences the codes. Check off each step after you complete it.

▶ First, Chrystal confirms the codes she assigned.

❑ **N18.6 End stage renal disease**

❑ **Z99.2 Dependence on renal dialysis**

❑ **E85.3 Secondary systemic amyloidosis**

❑ **Z76.82 Awaiting organ transplant status**

> *Patient is seen for acute vaginitis due to* Candida.
>
> (1) **N76.0 Acute vaginitis**
> (2) **B37.3 Candidiasis of vulva and vagina**

Figure 22-12 ■ Example of Arranging Codes for a Genitourinary Condition Due to an Infectious Organism

4th **N40   Enlarged prostate (EP)**
   Includes: adenofibromatous hypertrophy of prostate
            benign hypertrophy of the prostate
            benign prostatic hyperplasia
            benign prostatic hypertrophy (BPH)
            nodular prostate
            polyp of prostate
   Excludes1: benign neoplasms of prostate (adenoma,
            benign) (fibroadenoma) (fibroma)
            (myoma) (D29.1)
   Excludes2: malignant neoplasm of prostate (C61)
   **N40.0   Enlarged prostate without lower urinary
            tract symptoms (LUTS)**
            Enlarged prostate NOS
   **N40.1   Enlarged prostate with lower urinary tract
            symptoms (LUTS)**

            ▓▓▓▓▓▓▓▓▓▓▓▓▓▓▓▓▓▓▓▓▓▓▓
            ▓▓▓▓▓▓▓▓▓▓▓▓▓

            incomplete bladder emptying (R39.14)
            nocturia (R35.1)
            straining on urination (R39.16)
            urinary frequency (R35.0)
            urinary hesitancy (R39.11)
            urinary incontinence (N39.4-)
            urinary obstruction (N13.8)
            urinary retention (R33.8)
            urinary urgency (R39.15)
            weak urinary stream (R39.12)

Figure 22-13 ■ Tabular List Entry for Enlarged Prostate

▶ Chrystal must determine the first-listed diagnosis because this was an outpatient office visit.

❑ She reviews OGCR IV.G, which states the following:

   ▪ **List first the ICD-10-CM code for the diagnosis, condition, problem, or other reason for encounter/visit shown in the medical record to be chiefly responsible for the services provided. List additional codes that describe any coexisting conditions.**

❑ She reviews the medical record and determines that the diagnosis that best meets this definition is DRA. The

---

Patient is seen due to complaints of a weak urine stream and straining to urinate. The physician determines these symptoms are due to an enlarged prostate.

(1) **N40.1   Enlarged prostate with lower urinary tract symptoms (LUTS)**
(2) **R39.16   Straining to void**
(3) **R39.12   Poor urinary stream**

Figure 22-14 ■ Example of Arranging Codes for Enlarged Prostate with Lower Urinary Tract Symptoms

patient's ongoing complaints of severe joint pain were the main reason for the visit and the services.

❑ She assigns DRA as the first-listed diagnosis.

   ▪ Although the DRA is secondary to the ESRD, she did not see any instructional notes that directed her to sequence ESRD first.

▶ Chrystal determines that ESRD should be the second sequenced diagnosis because it is responsible for the DRA. It takes priority over the **Z** codes, which describe the status of the patient but not specific conditions.

▶ Chrystal sequences HD status as the third code because it is required by the instructional note under code **N18.6**. The instructional note also indicates that HD should be sequenced secondary to ESRD.

▶ Chrystal sequences the code for awaiting organ transplant as the final code.

▶ Chrystal reviews the medical record one final time to assure that she has captured all the details and that the final codes are consistent with the medical record.

▶ Chrystal finalizes the codes and sequencing for this case:

(1) **E85.3   Secondary systemic amyloidosis**
(2) **N18.6   End stage renal disease**
(3) **Z99.2   Dependence on renal dialysis**
(4) **Z76.82   Awaiting organ transplant status**

CODING PRACTICE

Exercise 22.4   **Arranging Codes for Genitourinary System Conditions**

Instructions: Read the mini-medical-record of each patient's encounter, review the information abstracted in Exercise 22.2, assign ICD-10-CM diagnosis codes using the Index and Tabular List, and sequence them correctly.

1. OFFICE   Gender: M   Age: 81

Reason for encounter: FU on EP with obstruction and urinary retention

Assessment: little improvement seen despite multiple medication adjustments

Plan: schedule transurethral resection of the prostate (TURP)

Tip: Follow instructional notes in the Tabular List for additional codes and sequencing.

3 ICD-10-CM Codes _____

_____

(*continued*)

CODING PRACTICE (continued)

2. OFFICE Gender: F Age: 37

Reason for encounter: *vaginal discharge, burning, redness in perineal area*

Assessment: *lab results show bacterial vaginitis due to staphylococcus, which is treatable*

Plan: *antibiotics*

Tip: The type of *Staphylococcus* is not specified.

2 ICD-10-CM Codes _____

3. INPATIENT HOSPITAL Gender: F Age: 83

Reason for admission: *nursing facility (NF) patient brought to emergency department with suspected UTI because of signs of confusion and lack of cooperation; history of UTI over the past 2 years*

Assessment: *UTI due to E. coli (non-Shiga toxin-producing)*

Plan: *administered IV antibiotics, discharged after 2 days to NF with Rx*

Tip: In the elderly, confusion and lack of cooperation may be the only symptoms of UTI.

3 ICD-10-CM Codes _____

_____

CODING NEOPLASMS OF THE GENITOURINARY SYSTEM

Neoplasms of the genitourinary system do not appear in ICD-10-CM Chapter 14, Diseases of the Genitourinary System (N00–N99). Codes for neoplasms of the genitourinary system appear in the following blocks within the neoplasm chapter:

- **C50 Malignant neoplasm of breast**

- **C51-C58 Malignant neoplasm of female genital organs**

- **C60-C63 Malignant neoplasms of male genital organs**

- **C64-C68 Malignant neoplasm of urinary tract**

The most common cancer of the urinary system is bladder cancer, which is the sixth most common cancer in the United States, according to NIH. Most bladder cancer is transitional cell carcinoma, which starts from the cells lining the bladder. The tumors are classified based on the way they grow. Papillary tumors have a wart-like appearance and are attached to a stalk. Nonpapillary tumors are less common but more invasive, with a poorer outcome. Smoking is a major risk factor for bladder cancer. Other risk factors are a family history of bladder cancer, advanced age, Caucasian race, and male gender.

The most common sites for cancer in the reproductive system are the prostate in males and the breast and ovaries in females, according to NIH.

Prostate cancer is the most common cancer in men and third most common cause of death from cancer in men of all ages. It is the most common cause of death from cancer in men over age 75. Prostate cancer is rarely found in men younger than 40. The **prostate-specific antigen (PSA)** blood test is performed to screen for prostate cancer, enabling physicians to detect prostate cancer before it causes symptoms. At an early stage, prostate cancer is very treatable through surgery and radiation.

Breast cancer is the most common cancer in women, affecting one in eight women at some point during their lifetime. Most occurrences of breast cancer are **ductal**, starting in the milk ducts. **Lobular** breast cancer starts in the lobules that produce milk. Screening mammograms are proven to be effective at identifying breast cancer in early stages. Treatment of breast cancer in the early stages, through surgery and radiation, has a high success rate.

Ovarian cancer is the fifth most common cancer among women, according to NIH. It causes more deaths than any other type of female genital cancer, largely because its symptoms of bloating, pain, and the feeling of fullness are often attributed to other causes. Ovarian cancer usually is not diagnosed until after it has metastasized, making it difficult to treat.

Genetic testing for mutations in the genes *BRCA1* and *BRCA2* can be helpful in identifying women who are at greater risk of breast or ovarian cancer and men who are at greater risk of breast cancer, prostate cancer, and several other cancers.

CODING PRACTICE

Exercise 22.5   Coding Neoplasms of the Genitourinary System

Instructions: Read the mini-medical-record of each patient's encounter, then abstract, assign, and sequence ICD-10-CM diagnosis codes using the Index and Tabular List. Write the code(s) on the line provided.

1. OFFICE   Gender: M   Age: 62

Reason for encounter: review results of needle biopsy which was performed due to elevated PSA

Assessment: stage 1 adenocarcinoma of the prostate which affects less than 5% of the prostate

Plan: brachytherapy (*placing radioactive seeds inside the prostate gland*)

1 ICD-10-CM Code _____

2. OUTPATIENT HOSPITAL   Gender: M   Age: 64

Reason for encounter: radiation therapy

Assessment: transitional cell carcinoma bladder cancer with overlapping lesions of the orifice and metastasis to the prostate

Plan: daily treatments for 3 more weeks

3 ICD-10-CM Codes _____

_____

3. OFFICE   Gender: F   Age: 60

Reason for encounter: painful and frequent urination, blood in urine

Assessment: radiation cystitis as a result of external beam radiotherapy for metastatic ovarian cancer

Tip: The fourth code is an external cause code for a complication of radiotherapy.

4 ICD-10-CM Codes _____

_____

4. OFFICE   Gender: F   Age: 44

Reason for encounter: FU on imaging for pain and hematuria

Assessment: angiomyolipoma, right kidney

Plan: embolization to reduce risk of hemorrhage and shrink the tumor

1 ICD-10-CM Code _____

5. OUTPATIENT HOSPITAL   Gender: F   Age: 58

Reason for encounter: lumpectomy

Assessment: ductal cancer in situ (DCIS) of the left breast, upper inner quadrant

1 ICD-10-CM Code _____

CHAPTER SUMMARY

In this chapter you learned that:

- The genitourinary (GU) system includes the urinary system and male and female genital, or reproductive, systems. The function of the urinary system is to filter, store, and remove waste products from the blood and maintain homeostasis. The function of the genital system is sexual reproduction.

- ICD-10-CM Chapter 14, Diseases of the Genitourinary System (N00-N99), contains 11 blocks or subchapters that are divided by anatomic site.

- Disorders in this chapter have a wide range of abstracting criteria because there is a wide range of organs and types of disorders.

- Two similar genitourinary conditions, nephritic syndrome and nephrotic syndrome, demonstrate the importance of checking cross-referencing instructions in the Index in order to assign the most specific code available.

- Coders should be attentive to instructional notes in the Tabular List regarding how to sequence codes for genitourinary conditions due to infections and codes for enlarged prostate (EP) and associated symptoms.

- The most common sites for cancer in the genital system are the prostate in males and the breast and ovaries in females, according to NIH.

- ICD-10-CM Official Guidelines for Coding and Reporting (OGCR) I.C.14 provides detailed discussion of chronic kidney disease.

CONCEPT QUIZ

Take a moment to look back through diseases of the genitourinary system and solidify your skills. Try to answer the questions from memory first, then look back at the discussion in this chapter if you need a little extra help.

Completion

Instructions: Write the term that answers each question based on the information you learned in this chapter. Choose from the list below. Some choices may be used more than once and some choices may not be used at all.

calculi

cervical dysplasia

cervical intraepithelial
   neoplasia

CKD

diabetic nephropathy

dialysis

ED

endometriosis

EP

ESRD

glomerulonephritis

glomerulus

nephritic

nephron

nephroptosis

nephrotic

renal pelvis

transplant

ureter

urethra

1. Urine passes from the renal pelvis through the _____ to the urinary bladder.

2. _____ syndrome is a collection of disorders affecting the kidneys, characterized by nonpurulent inflammatory glomerular disorders that allow proteins and red blood cells to pass into the urine, resulting in proteinuria and hematuria.

3. The _____ is a cluster of capillaries in the kidney that separates the urinary space from the blood.

4. _____ is accumulated damage to the glomerulus capillaries due to chronic high blood glucose.

5. BPH is also called _____.

6. Diseases of the _____ attack the kidneys' filtering ability.

7. _____ is abnormal changes in the cells on the surface of the cervix that may lead to cancer if not treated.

8. _____ is stage 5 chronic kidney disease.

9. Stones that may accumulate in the kidneys, bladder, or ureters are called _____.

10. _____ is a treatment that filters the blood to remove waste, excess salt, and water.

Multiple Choice

Instructions: Circle the letter of the best answer to each question based on the information you learned in this chapter.

1. In what stage of CKD do the kidneys cease to function, requiring that patients receive dialysis or a kidney transplant to survive?
   A. 1
   B. 3
   C. 4
   D. 5

2. Long-term dialysis patients may accumulate deposits of the starchy substance amyloid in the joints called
   A. dialysis-related amyloidosis.
   B. end-stage renal disease.
   C. nephritic syndrome.
   D. nephrolithiasis.

3. What is the only specific disease that Medicare covers for the entire population, regardless of age?
   A. BPH
   B. ED
   C. CKD
   D. ESRD

4. Which of the following is NOT included in ICD-10-CM Chapter 14?
   A. Conditions of the urinary system
   B. Conditions of the female breast
   C. Conditions of the kidney related to pregnancy
   D. Conditions of the male reproductive system

5. What condition does OGCR I.C.14 discuss in detail?
   A. Hypertensive kidney disease
   B. Chronic kidney disease
   C. Nephritic and nephrotic syndrome
   D. Enlarged prostate

6. What feature can assist coders when documentation provides more details than appear in the Index entry?
   A. Nonessential modifiers
   B. Fifth digits
   C. Cross-referenced Main Terms
   D. Z codes

7. What code should be assigned when an ESRD patient is receiving dialysis?
   A. N18.5, Chronic kidney disease, stage 5
   B. Z99.2, Dependence on renal dialysis
   C. I12.0, Hypertensive chronic kidney disease with end stage renal disease
   D. Z76.82, Awaiting organ transplant status

8. What codes should be sequenced after code N40.1 Enlarged prostate with lower urinary tract symptoms (LUTS)?
   A. Associated symptoms
   B. With or without obstruction
   C. Infectious organism
   D. Acute or chronic

9. Which type of cancer is often not diagnosed until after it has metastasized, making it more difficult to treat?
   A. Prostate
   B. Ovarian
   C. Breast
   D. Bladder

10. What condition does the PSA blood test screen for?
   A. Cervical cancer
   B. Enlarged prostate
   C. Prostate cancer
   D. Pyelonephritis

CODING CHALLENGE

Instructions: Read the mini-medical-record of each patient's encounter, then abstract, assign, and arrange ICD-10-CM diagnosis codes using the Index and Tabular List. Write the code(s) on the line provided.

Urinary System

1. INPATIENT HOSPITAL   Gender: M   Age: 46

Reason for encounter: oliguria, drowsy and lethargic, edema

Assessment: acute renal failure with tubular necrosis and hypertension

Plan: fluid restriction, diuretics, restrict mineral intake, dialysis if serum potassium remains high

Tip: Only chronic renal failure is assumed to be related to hypertension.

2 ICD-10-CM Codes _____

2. INPATIENT HOSPITAL   Gender: M   Age: 37

Reason for encounter: bloody urine, edema of feet, ankles, and legs, uncontrolled high BP, upper abdominal pain, general malaise

Assessment: glomerulonephrosis due to secondary DM which is a result of alcohol dependent chronic pancreatitis, 2 years on insulin

Plan: adjust BP meds, diuretics, angiotension-converting enzyme inhibitors

4 ICD-10-CM Codes _____

_____

3. OFFICE   Gender: F   Age: 56

Reason for encounter: renal dialysis

Assessment: stage V CKD due to autosomal recessive polycystic kidney disease

Plan: return in 2 days

Tip: Patients typically receive dialysis three times per week.

3 ICD-10-CM Codes _____

_____

Male Reproductive System

4. OFFICE   Gender: M   Age: 63

Reason for encounter: painful urination

Assessment: acute enterococcal prostatitis

Plan: IV antibacterial gram positive therapy

2 ICD-10-CM Codes _____

5. OFFICE   Gender: M   Age: 16

Reason for encounter: red and painful foreskin and penis with foul smelling discharge, uncircumcised

Assessment: balanitis due to E. coli

Plan: Rx antibiotics, hygiene instructions

2 ICD-10-CM Codes _____

Female Reproductive System

6. OFFICE   Gender: F   Age: 38

Reason for encounter: urinary incontinence (UI), difficulty with sexual encounters, feeling of pelvic heaviness

Assessment: cystocele and uterine prolapse, grade 3

Plan: schedule surgical rectocele and cystocele repair in 3 wk

Tip: Follow the cross-references in the Index.

1 ICD-10-CM Code _____

7. OFFICE   Gender: F   Age: 20

Reason for encounter: severe pelvic pain and cramps on the first day or two of her monthly period

Assessment: no specific problems except an incidental finding of **retroverted** uterus which I do not believe is the cause of the menstrual pain

Plan: patient advised to begin a daily walking program, ibuprofen or other NSAIDs to be taken 1-2 days prior to her period

2 ICD-10-CM Codes _____

(continued)

(continued from page 375)

---

8. OFFICE   Gender: F   Age: 22

Reason for encounter: FU on routine pap smear showing CIN II (unvaccinated for HPV)

Assessment: CIN II

Plan: schedule for Colposcopy in 2 weeks

Tip: If you are unsure whether the CIN is mild, moderate, or severe, review the inclusion notes in the Tabular List for the possible codes.

1 ICD-10-CM Code _____

---

9. OFFICE   Gender: F   Age: 81

Reason for encounter: urge incontinence, bladder droops to the vaginal opening

Assessment: urge incontinence due to grade 2 cystocele on the right side

(continued)

---

9. (continued)

Plan: Kegel exercises, pessary, RTO in 2 months to schedule surgery if no relief

1 ICD-10-CM Code _____

---

10. OUTPATIENT HOSPITAL   Gender: F   Age: 41

Reason for encounter: screening mammogram

Assessment: suspicious mass, right breast, and bilateral microcalcifications

Plan: schedule biopsy next week

3 ICD-10-CM Codes _____

_____

KEEP ON CODING

Instructions: Read the diagnostic statement, then use the Index and Tabular List to assign and sequence ICD-10-CM diagnosis codes. Write the code(s) on the line provided.

Urinary System

1. Hydroureter: ICD-10-CM Code(s) _____

2. Cystostomy malfunction: ICD-10-CM Code(s) _____

3. Carcinoma of the left kidney pelvis: ICD-10-CM Code(s) _____

4. Dysuria: ICD-10-CM Code(s) _____

5. Urethrocele: ICD-10-CM Code(s) _____

6. Interstitial nephritis: ICD-10-CM Code(s) _____

7. Trigonitis: ICD-10-CM Code(s) _____

8. End-stage renal disease currently receiving dialysis: ICD-10-CM Code(s) _____

9. Terminal atrophy of the kidney: ICD-10-CM Code(s) _____

10. Hypermobility of urethra with urinary stress incontinence: ICD-10-CM Code(s) _____

11. Urinary bladder stone: ICD-10-CM Code(s) _____

12. Ureteritis cystica: ICD-10-CM Code(s) _____

Male Reproductive System

13. Enlarged prostate with nighttime urination: ICD-10-CM Code(s) _____

14. Oligospermia: ICD-10-CM Code(s) _____

15. Priapism due to trauma: ICD-10-CM Code(s) _____

16. Infected hydrocele due to *E. coli:* ICD-10-CM Code(s) _____

17. Cyst of tunica albuginea testes: ICD-10-CM Code(s) _____

18. Erectile dysfunction due to type 2 diabetes: ICD-10-CM Code(s) _____

19. Gynecomastia: ICD-10-CM Code(s) _____

Female Reproductive System

20. Torsion of fallopian tube: ICD-10-CM Code(s) _____

21. Decubitus ulcer of cervix: ICD-10-CM Code(s) _____

22. Secondary amenorrhea: ICD-10-CM Code(s) _____

23. Anteversion of uterus: ICD-10-CM Code(s) _____

24. Endometriosis of the intestines: ICD-10-CM Code(s) _____

25. Bartholin's gland cyst: ICD-10-CM Code(s) _____

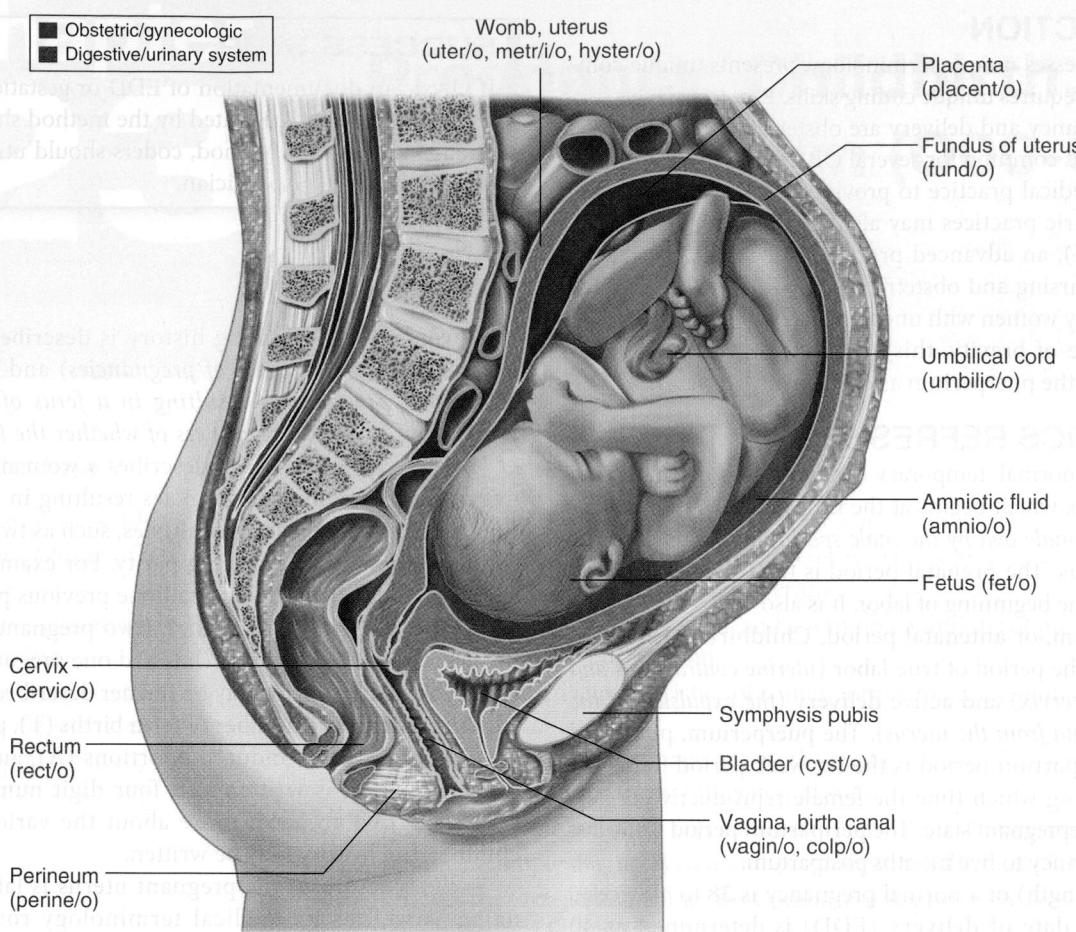

- ■ Obstetric/gynecologic
- ■ Digestive/urinary system

Womb, uterus
(uter/o, metr/i/o, hyster/o)

Placenta
(placent/o)

Fundus of uterus
(fund/o)

Umbilical cord
(umbilic/o)

Amniotic fluid
(amnio/o)

Fetus (fet/o)

Cervix
(cervic/o)

Rectum
(rect/o)

Perineum
(perine/o)

Symphysis pubis

Bladder (cyst/o)

Vagina, birth canal
(vagin/o, colp/o)

Figure 23-2 ■ Pregnant Uterus in a Full-Term Pregnancy

CODING CAUTION

Be alert for medical word terms that are spelled similarly but have different meanings.

anti- (*against*) and **ante-** (*before*)

dystocia (*difficult labor*) and **dyspnea** (*difficulty breathing*)

mastalgia (*breast pain*) and **mastitis** (*inflammation of the breast*)

In particular, coders must be familiar with the terminology related to each aspect of pregnancy, childbirth, and the puerperium.

Conditions of Pregnancy

According to the American Pregnancy Association (APA), there are over 4 million live births and another 2 million pregnancy losses every year in the United States. Approximately 20% of pregnant women experience one or more pregnancy complications.

Table 23-1 ■ **EXAMPLE OF CONSTRUCTING MEDICAL TERMS FOR OBSTETRICS**

Prefix	Root/Combining Form	Complete Medical Term
pre- (*before*) **ante-** (*before*)		**pre + natal** (*before birth*)
		ante + natal (*before birth*)
		pre + partum (*before birth*)
	natal (*birth*)	**ante + partum** (*before birth*)
peri- (*surrounding*)	**partum** (*birth*)	**peri + natal** (*surrounding birth*)
		peri + partum (*surrounding birth*)
post- (*after*)		**post + natal** (*after birth*)
		post + partum (*after birth*)

A normal pregnancy is defined as follows:

- no preexisting conditions
- no new conditions that develop during pregnancy
- single gestation
- mother will be over age 16 and under age 35 at EDD

Disorders of the pregnancy may be due to preexisting conditions of the mother, conditions that arise during pregnancy, or conditions of the fetus or amniotic cavity. Coders use medical resources, such as reference books on diseases, to understand conditions of pregnancy, childbirth, and the puerperium, diagnostic methods, and common treatments. Refer to ■ Table 23-2 for a summary of conditions affecting pregnancy.

Conditions Due to Pregnancy Compared to Preexisting Conditions

Some conditions, such as Rh incompatibility and preeclampsia, occur only during pregnancy. Other conditions, such as diabetes and hypertension, may affect people at any time during life but also have a pregnancy-related variation. When a condition has been diagnosed before a woman becomes pregnant, it is a preexisting condition. When the condition is first diagnosed during pregnancy, it is a **gestational condition**.

Characteristics of a gestational condition, such as gestational diabetes or gestational hypertension, include the following:

- The gestational disease has the same symptoms and signs as its nongestational counterpart.
- The condition is not present prior to pregnancy.
- The condition usually begins after the twentieth week of pregnancy.
- The condition returns to normal when the pregnancy is over.

When diabetes or hypertension is present, coders must review the documentation carefully to determine whether it is gestational or preexisting in order to assign the correct codes.

Multiple Gestation

Multiple gestation is a pregnancy with more than one fetus, as in twins, triplets, or sextuplets, and carries greater risk for complications than **singletons** (*pregnancies with one fetus*). The rate of twin births increased over 76% from 1980 to 2009, according to the Centers for Disease Control and Prevention, and leveled off in subsequent years. The increase in multiple gestation pregnancies is due to delayed childbearing and expanding use of reproductive technology.

Coders need to be familiar with the terminology used to describe multiple gestation because it affects code assignment. Physicians describe multiple gestation pregnancies based on the number of **amnions** or **amniotic sacs**, **chorions**, and **placentas**. This is important because it directly affects the mortality risk of the fetuses. The amniotic sac is a membrane that surrounds the embryo. The chorion is an outer membrane that surrounds the amnion. The space inside the chorion and the amnion is called the amniotic cavity and is filled with amniotic fluid. The amniotic cavity prevents the embryo from drying out and protects it against vibration and shocks. The placenta is the organ that allows for the exchange of oxygen, nutrients, and waste between the fetus and the mother. It attaches to the chorion and consists of chorionic material from the fetus and uterine material from the mother.

When multiple embryos each develop from separate **zygotes** (*fertilized eggs*), as happens with fraternal twins, each embryo always has its own amnion and chorion, making the pregnancy **dichorionic-diamniotic (DiDi)**.

Table 23-2 ■ COMMON CONDITIONS OF PREGNANCY

Condition	Definition
Chromosomal abnormality	Any of a wide range of disorders in which a fetus has an abnormal number of chromosomes or a structural abnormality in one or more chromosomes
Eclampsia	Convulsions occurring during pregnancy or the puerperium associated with preeclampsia
Gestational diabetes	Diabetes that develops during pregnancy in a woman who did not previously have diabetes
Gestational hypertension	Development of hypertension after 20 weeks of gestation in a woman who previously was not diagnosed with hypertension; also called **pregnancy-induced hypertension (PIH)**
HELLP syndrome	Severe preeclampsia with **H**emolysis, **E**levated **L**iver enzymes, and **L**ow **P**latelet count
In vitro fertilization (IVF)	Fertilization of an ova in a laboratory dish, followed by introduction into the uterus
Preeclampsia	A metabolic disorder of pregnancy that develops after the 20th week and involves gestational hypertension and proteinuria
Preexisting diabetes	Diabetes diagnosed in a woman before she becomes pregnant
Preexisting hypertension	Hypertension diagnosed in a woman before she becomes pregnant
Rhesus (Rh) incompatibility	A condition in which mother is Rh negative and develops antibodies against a fetus that is Rh positive

Monochorionic-Monoamniotic (MoMo) **Monochorionic-Diamniotic (MoDi)** **Dichorionic-Diamniotic (DiDi)**

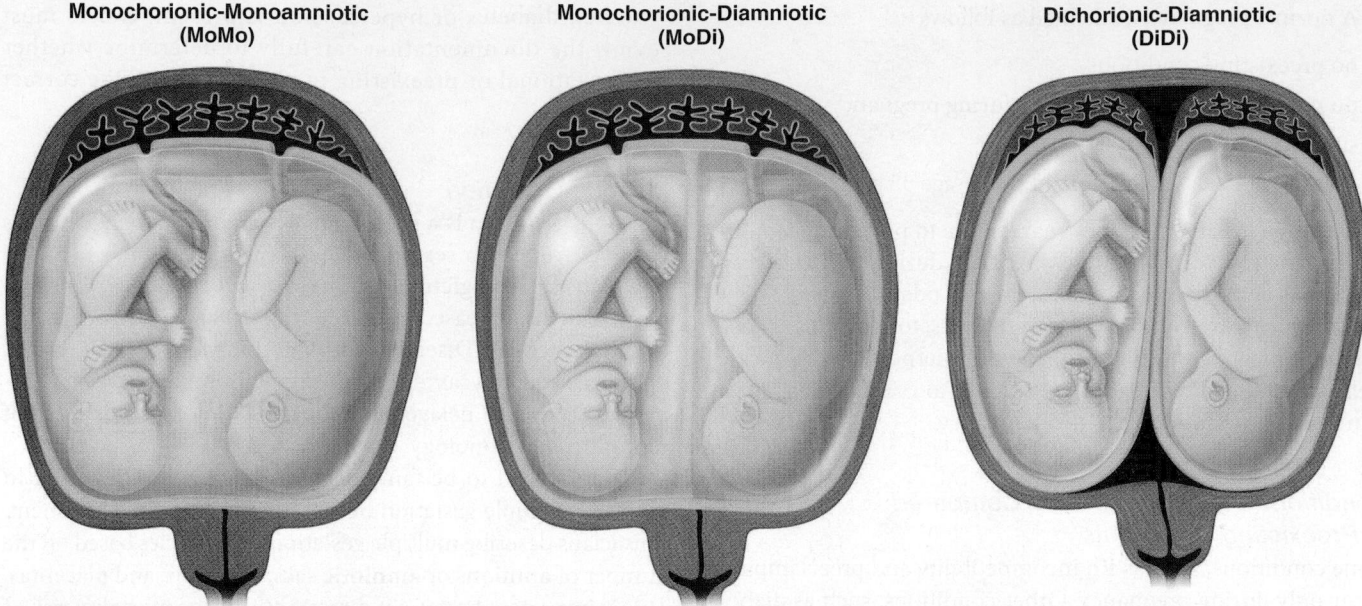

Figure 23-3 ■ Twin Configurations of the Chorion and Amnion

Table 23-3 ■ CONFIGURATIONS OF CHORION, AMNION, AND PLACENTA OF TWINS

Description	Number of Chorions	Number of Amnions	Number of Placentas	Division of Zygote
Monochorionic-monoamniotic (MoMo)	1	1	1	8–13 days after fertilization
Monochorionic-diamniotic (MoDi)	1	2	1	3–8 days after fertilization
Dichorionic-diamniotic (DiDi)	2	2	2	Less than 3–4 days after fertilization

Identical twins are created when a zygote divides to create two or more identical embryos. Normally, identical embryos are DiDi, with each embryo enclosed in its own amnion and chorion and having its own placenta. However, it is possible for more than one embryo to share a chorion or an amniotic sac. When the chorion is shared, the placenta is also shared. The sharing of the chorion and amnion is determined by how soon after fertilization the egg divides. Refer to ■ TABLE 23-3 to learn the possible combinations of twins and ■ FIGURE 23-3 to visualize the differences. Monochorionic (*sharing the chorion*) twins are at risk for more complications than DiDi twins; monoamniotic (*sharing the same amnion*) twins have the greatest risk of mortality.

Conditions of Childbirth

A normal delivery is defined as follows:

- single liveborn infant
- full-term pregnancy
- vaginal delivery with cephalic presentation
- no induction, manipulation, or instrumentation
- no complications

Any labor and delivery that does not meet these criteria is complicated. Complications can occur during any phase of labor and delivery (■ FIGURE 23-4) and multiple complications may

A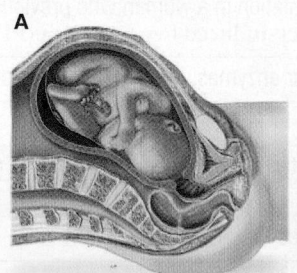

DILATION STAGE:
Uterine contractions dilate cervix

B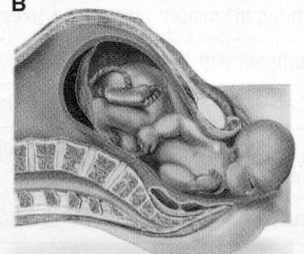

EXPULSION STAGE:
Birth of baby or expulsion

C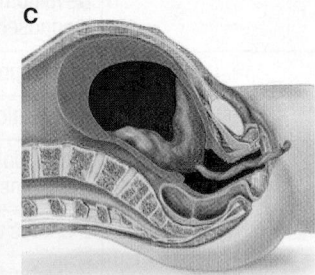

PLACENTAL STAGE:
Delivery of placenta

Figure 23-4 ■ Three Stages of Labor and Delivery

Table 23-4 ■ **COMMON CONDITIONS OF CHILDBIRTH**

Condition	Definition
Assisted delivery	A delivery of the fetus using mechanical assistance, such as forceps or vacuum extractor; pharmacologic assistance, such as drugs to induce labor; or medical assistance, such as manual rotation of the fetal position
Cephalopelvic disproportion (CPD)	A cause of obstructed labor due to a mismatch between the size of the fetal head and the mother's pelvic brim; also called fetopelvic disproportion
Cesarean delivery	Delivery of the fetus by making a surgical incision into the abdominal wall and uterus; also called abdominal delivery
Forceps delivery	Extraction of a fetus from the birth canal by grasping the head with forceps (tongs)
Malposition of fetus	Any presentation of the fetus other than occipitoanterior (OA) (*the back of the baby's head is slightly off center in the pelvis with the back of the head toward the mother's left thigh*)
Normal spontaneous vaginal birth (NSVB)	Vaginal delivery without mechanical, pharmacologic, or medical assistance
Nuchal cord	The condition of the umbilical cord becoming wrapped around the neck of the fetus
Obstructed labor	Labor in which the fetus cannot progress into the birth canal, despite adequate uterine contractions, due to a physical blockage
Pelvic girdle pain (PGP)	Pain at the back of the pelvis
Placenta previa	A condition in which the placenta partially or fully covers the cervix, posing a risk that it may separate from the wall of the uterus during labor (■ FIGURE 23-5)
Placental infarction	A scarring of the placenta due to inadequate blood supply
Premature rupture of membranes (PROM)	The rupture of the amniotic sac and chorion before the onset of labor. May also be called prelabor rupture of membranes.
Unstable lie	Repeated changes in the fetal position during or after the 36th week of pregnancy
Vaginal birth after cesarean (VBAC)	Delivery through the vagina after having a cesarean delivery in a previous pregnancy
Vaginal birth	Delivery of the fetus from the uterus through the cervix to the vagina (birth canal)

affect one mother. Refer to ■ TABLE 23-4 for a summary of conditions affecting labor and delivery.

Conditions of the Puerperium

Postpartum and puerperal conditions arise after delivery and are due to the postpregnancy state. Because some conditions, such as depression, can be preexisting, look for the physician's documentation that describes a condition as puerperal. Refer to ■ TABLE 23-5 for a summary of conditions affecting the puerperium.

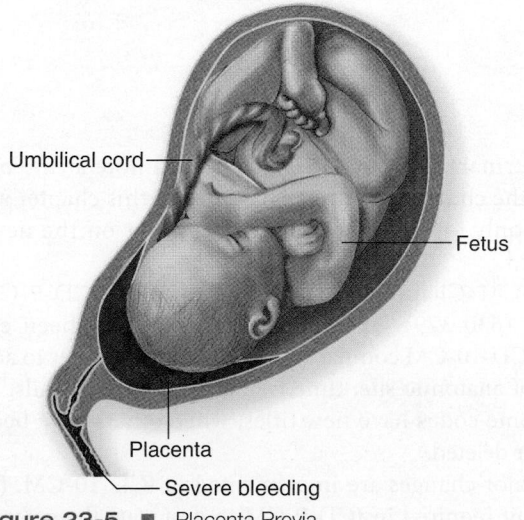

Umbilical cord

Fetus

Placenta

Severe bleeding

Figure 23-5 ■ Placenta Previa

Table 23-5 ■ **COMMON CONDITIONS OF THE PUERPERIUM**

Condition	Definition
Postpartum depression	Moderate to severe depression after giving birth
Postpartum hemorrhage (PPH)	Excessive bleeding following delivery
Postpartum psychosis	Sudden dramatic onset of psychotic symptoms after giving birth, often occurring in patients with bipolar disorder
Postpartum wound infection	Bacterial infection of a cesarean delivery wound
Puerperal mastitis	Inflammation or infection of the mammary gland in the breast during the postpartum period

CODING PRACTICE

Exercise 23.1 **Obstetrics Refresher**

Instructions: Use your medical terminology skills and resources to define the conditions, then assign the diagnosis code.

Follow these steps:

- Use slash marks "/" to break down the underlined term into its root(s) and suffix.
- Define the meaning of the word, based on the meaning of each word part.
- Assign the default diagnosis code for the condition using the Index and Tabular List.

Example: Pregnancy, complicated by, endometritis endo/metr/itis

Meaning: *inflammation of the lining of the uterus*

ICD-10-CM Code: *086.12*

1. Pregnancy, complicated by, <u>hyperemesis</u>

Meaning _____

ICD-10-CM Code _____

2. Pregnancy, complicated by, <u>antepartum hemorrhage</u>, second trimester

Meaning _____

ICD-10-CM Code _____

3. Pregnancy, complicated by, <u>amnionitis</u>, first trimester

Meaning _____

ICD-10-CM Code _____

4. Pregnancy, complicated by, <u>isoimmunization</u> Rh, second trimester

Meaning _____

ICD-10-CM Code _____

5. Pregnancy, complicated by, <u>oligohydramnios</u>, second trimester

Meaning _____

ICD-10-CM Code _____

6. Pregnancy, complicated by, <u>salpingo-oophoritis</u>, first trimester

Meaning _____

ICD-10-CM Code _____

7. Pregnancy, <u>intraperitoneal</u>

Meaning _____

ICD-10-CM Code _____

8. Pregnancy, supervision of, high risk, older mother, <u>primigravida</u>, second trimester

Meaning _____

ICD-10-CM Code _____

9. Delivery, complicated by, <u>cervical dystocia</u>, third trimester

Meaning _____

ICD-10-CM Code _____

10. Delivery, complicated by, <u>abruptio placentae</u>, third trimester

Meaning _____

ICD-10-CM Code _____

CODING OVERVIEW OF OBSTETRICS

ICD-10-CM Chapter 15, Pregnancy, Childbirth, and the Puerperium (O00-O9A), contains nine blocks or subchapters that are divided by the phase of pregnancy and the type of condition. Review the block names and code ranges listed at the beginning of Chapter 15 in the ICD-10-CM manual to become familiar with the content and organization.

This chapter includes pregnancy with abortive outcome, complications of pregnancy, delivery and complications of delivery, and disorders arising during the postpartum period. It does not include reproductive or fertility disorders, which are classified in ICD-10-CM Chapter 14, Diseases of the Genitourinary System. An instructional note at the beginning of the chapter requires that codes in this chapter are to be used only on the mother's record, never on the newborn's record.

ICD-10-CM Chapter 15 corresponds with ICD-9-CM Chapter 11 (630-379). Numerous categories have been expanded in ICD-10-CM compared to ICD-9-CM in order to add specificity of anatomic site, time frames, and other details. In addition, some codes have new titles, while others have been combined or deleted.

Three major changes are implemented in ICD-10-CM. (1) The fifth digit required in ICD-9-CM to designate the episode of care has been eliminated. Instead, conditions are classified based on the trimester in which the condition occurs. (2) An instructional note at the beginning of the chapter directs coders to assign an additional code from category **Z3A** to identify the weeks of gestation. (3) Some codes require a seventh-character to identify which fetus in a multiple gestation is affected. Examples of how to assign trimester, week, and fetus identifiers are provided later in this chapter.

ICD-10-CM provides Official Guidelines for Coding and Reporting (OGCR) pregnancy, childbirth, and the puerperium in OGCR section I.C.15. OGCR provide detailed discussion of general rules for obstetric cases, selection of OB principal or first-listed diagnosis, preexisting conditions, and several specific conditions, including hypertension, diabetes, HIV, alcohol and tobacco use, normal delivery, postpartum, and abortions. OGCR regarding the use of Z codes related to pregnancy, childbirth, and the puerperium appear in OGCR I.C.21.c.11).

ABSTRACTING DIAGNOSES FOR OBSTETRICS

Because multiple complications are common during pregnancy, childbirth, and the puerperium, coders must be attentive to which complication is the reason for the encounter or admission.

Abstracting Conditions of Pregnancy

It is important to identify all the conditions affecting a pregnant woman, but coders also must identify the main reason for the specific encounter or admission, as this will determine the first-listed or principal diagnosis. Refer to ■ TABLE 23-6 for guidance on how to abstract conditions of pregnancy. In particular, coders must be attentive to distinguish between preexisting conditions and pregnancy-related conditions. They should also be familiar with the criteria for abstracting multiple gestations.

Table 23-6 ■ **KEY CRITERIA FOR ABSTRACTING CONDITIONS OF PREGNANCY**

- ❑ Will the patient be under age 16 or age 35 and older at EDD?
- ❑ How many fetuses are there?
- ❑ What trimester is the pregnancy?
- ❑ How many weeks of gestation are completed?
- ❑ How many pregnancies has the patient had, including the current one?
- ❑ How many births has the patient had?
- ❑ What preexisting medical conditions exist?
- ❑ What complications exist?
- ❑ What is the current gestational age?
- ❑ For multiple gestations, how many chorions and amniotic sacs are present?
- ❑ For multiple gestations, which fetus is affected by the complication?
- ❑ What is the main reason for the encounter or the primary complication treated?

Abstracting Preexisting Conditions and Conditions Due to Pregnancy

Pregnant women may have a medical condition that must be treated in addition to caring for the pregnancy itself. Coders must determine, based on the documentation, if the condition is preexisting (*existed prior to the pregnancy*) or if it developed as a direct result of the pregnancy. Although the symptoms, manifestations, and complications are similar for preexisting and pregnancy-related variations of a disease, different codes are often required (OGCR I.C.15.c.). Two common conditions that fall into this category are diabetes and hypertension.

Prexisting and Gestational Diabetes. Preexisting diabetes should be clearly documented in the medical record and identified as type 1 or type 2. Coders should also identify any additional manifestations of diabetes and whether a type 2 diabetic is on long-term use of insulin. Preexisting diabetes that is treated during pregnancy is *not* gestational diabetes. Gestational diabetes mellitus (GDM) is first diagnosed during pregnancy, usually during the second or third trimester, and usually resolves after delivery. GDM should be identified as diet-controlled or insulin-controlled. For a refresher on abstracting diabetes, refer to OGCR I.C.4.a and Chapter 10 of this text.

CODING CAUTION

A patient cannot have *both* preexisting diabetes and gestational diabetes. You need to identify the condition as one or the other. If the documentation is not clear, query the physician.

Preexisting and Gestational Hypertension. Preexisting hypertension should also be clearly documented in the medical record. The type of hypertension and whether the condition involves the heart and/or kidney should also be identified. When a patient with preexisting hypertension develops preeclampsia, this combination should be noted. Gestational hypertension is first diagnosed during pregnancy and usually resolves after delivery. Coders must carefully review the documentation for gestational hypertension to determine whether it exists with significant proteinuria, which constitutes preeclampsia. Preeclampsia should be further identified as mild, moderate, severe, or HELLP syndrome. Finally, coders should note when symptoms of edema and proteinuria are documented *without* hypertension.

Abstracting Multiple Gestations

Multiple gestation is a complication of pregnancy that places both the mother and the fetuses at higher risk of developing problems. Coders must identify the number of amnions and chorions in all multiple gestation pregnancies. If the physician has documented that the number of placenta or amniotic sacs cannot be determined, this should also be noted.

Physicians identify each fetus in a multiple gestation by number, such as fetus 1, fetus 2, or fetus 3. When a fetus is affected by a prenatal or delivery complication, or the mother is affected by a condition of a fetus, coders must identify which fetus is affected (■ FIGURE 23-6, page 386).

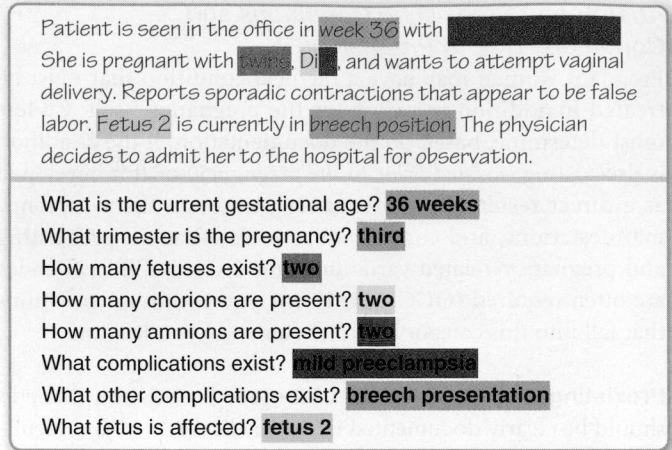

Patient is seen in the office in week 36 with ▓▓▓▓▓▓▓▓. She is pregnant with ▓▓▓▓, Di▓, and wants to attempt vaginal delivery. Reports sporadic contractions that appear to be false labor. Fetus 2 is currently in breech position. The physician decides to admit her to the hospital for observation.

What is the current gestational age? **36 weeks**
What trimester is the pregnancy? **third**
How many fetuses exist? **two**
How many chorions are present? **two**
How many amnions are present? **two**
What complications exist? **mild preeclampsia**
What other complications exist? **breech presentation**
What fetus is affected? **fetus 2**

Figure 23-6 ■ Example of Abstracting for Multiple Gestation

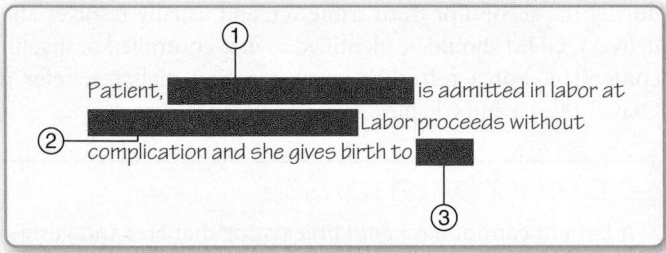

Figure 23-7 ■ Example of a Delivery with Three Complications

Abstracting Conditions of Childbirth

Any delivery that varies from the definition of a normal delivery is complicated and requires that coders identify all the complications that occurred. First, identify the main circumstance or complication of the delivery. Then, identify any additional complications. When a cesarean delivery is performed, identify the main circumstance or complication that establishes the need for the cesarean delivery.

Keep in mind that certain circumstances always qualify as complications, even though they may not seem to be a specific "problem." Circumstantial complications include the following (■ Figure 23-7):

- age at EDD under 16 or age 35 and older
- multiple gestation
- previous cesarean delivery
- delivery before 37 completed weeks of gestation

Refer to ■ Table 23-7 for guidance in abstracting conditions related to labor, delivery, and childbirth.

Abstracting Conditions of the Puerperium

Some conditions, such as depression or psychosis, may be preexisting, so coders need to distinguish between conditions that originate in the postpartum period and those that are preexisting. Refer to ■ Table 23-8 for guidance in abstracting conditions related to the puerperium.

Table 23-7 ■ KEY CRITERIA FOR ABSTRACTING CONDITIONS OF CHILDBIRTH

- ❏ What is the reason for the admission?
- ❏ In what week of pregnancy did delivery occur?
- ❏ Is the delivery vaginal or cesarean?
- ❏ What is the reason a cesarean delivery was performed?
- ❏ Has the mother had a previous cesarean delivery?
- ❏ Was there a malposition of the fetus or obstructed labor?
- ❏ What other complications are present?
- ❏ How many fetuses were delivered? Were there any stillbirths?

Table 23-8 ■ KEY CRITERIA FOR ABSTRACTING CONDITIONS OF THE PUERPERIUM

- ❏ Is the encounter less than six weeks after delivery?
- ❏ What complication or condition is treated during the encounter?
- ❏ Is the condition preexisting or does it originate during the postpartum/puerperal period?

Abstracting from Obstetric Records

Obstetric records contain unique information and abbreviations not found in other medical records. Refer to ■ Figure 23-8 to learn how to interpret the mini-medical-record used for obstetric cases in this text.

Guided Example of Abstracting Diagnoses for Obstetrics

Refer to the following example throughout this chapter to practice skills for abstracting, assigning, and sequencing pregnancy, childbirth, and the puerperium codes. Daphne Wittman, CCS-P, is a fictitious coder who guides you through the coding process.

Date of discharge: 3/1/yy   Location: Branton Medical Center   Provider: Kay Pinkney, MD

Patient: Glenna Ferrier   Gender: F   Age: 26

Gravida: 2   Para: 2   EDD: 3/6/yy

EGA: 39+1

Reason for admission: full term labor

Assessment: Attempted vaginal delivery. Labor started off well then slowed. I was concerned that prolonged labor would place the scar from the previous cesarean delivery at risk. In addition, the stress affected the fetal heart rate causing tachycardia so I proceeded with a cesarean delivery.

Delivery: 2/28/yy, cesarean delivery, TBLC, 1 girl, transferred to NICU for monitoring and management of heart rate

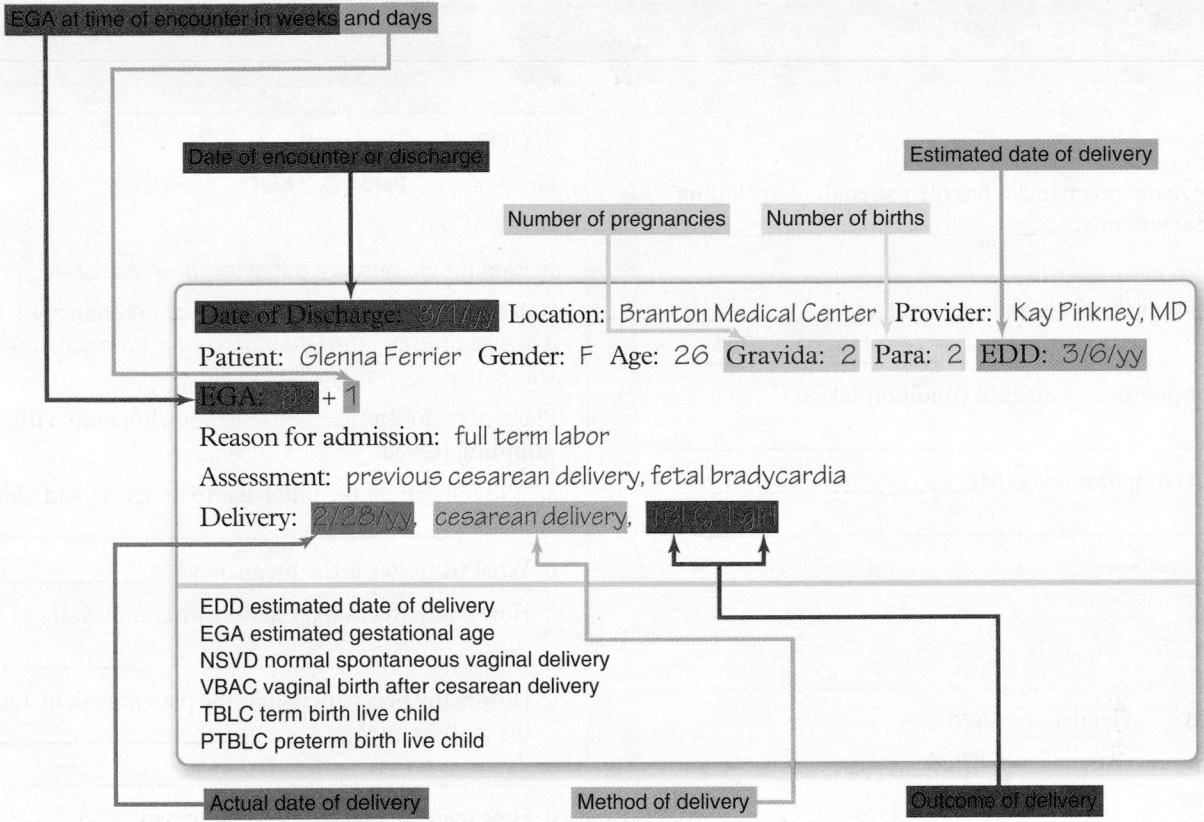

Figure 23-8 ■ Key to Interpreting the Obstetrics Mini-Medical-Record

Follow along as Daphne Wittman, CCS-P, abstracts the diagnosis. Check off each step after you complete it.

▶ Daphne reads through the entire record, paying special attention to the reason for the admission and the final delivery data. She refers to Key Criteria for Abstracting Conditions of Childbirth (Table 23-7).

❑ *What is the reason for the admission?* full term labor

❑ *In what week of pregnancy did delivery occur?* 39+1

❑ *Is the delivery vaginal or cesarean?* cesarean

❑ *What is the reason a cesarean delivery was performed?* previous cesarean delivery

❑ *Has the mother had a previous cesarean delivery?* Yes

❑ *How many fetuses were delivered?* 1 female

❑ *Were there any stillbirths?* No, TBLC

❑ *What other complications are present?* fetal tachycardia

▶ At this time, Daphne does not know how many codes she will end up with. She will learn about this when she moves on to assigning codes.

CODING PRACTICE

Exercise 23.2 **Abstracting Diagnoses for Obstetrics**

Instructions: Read the mini-medical-record of each patient's encounter and answer the abstracting questions. Write the answer on the line provided. Do not assign any codes.

1. OFFICE Gender: F Age: 33

Gravida: 3 Para: 2 EDD: 6/30/yy

EGA: 26+2

Reason for encounter: vaginal bleeding

(continued)

1. (continued)

Assessment: placenta previa, hemorrhage

Plan: bed confinement, RTO 2 weeks, cesarean delivery may be required

a. Will the patient be under age 16 or age 35 and older at EDD? _____

b. What trimester is the pregnancy? _____

How many weeks of gestation are completed?

_____

(continued)

CODING PRACTICE (continued)

1. (continued)

c. How many pregnancies has the patient had, including the current one? _____
_____

d. How many births has the patient had? _____
_____

e. What preexisting medical conditions exist?
_____

f. What complications exist? _____
_____

2. OFFICE   Gender: F Age: 24

Gravida: 1   Para: O   EDD: 3/23/yy

EGA: 40+2

Reason for encounter: prenatal visit

Assessment: unstable lie

Plan: cesarean delivery today at 1500

a. Will the patient be under age 16 or age 35 and older at EDD? _____

b. What trimester is the pregnancy? _____
How many weeks of gestation are completed?
_____

c. How many pregnancies has the patient had, including the current one? _____
_____

d. How many births has the patient had? _____
_____

e. What preexisting medical conditions exist?
_____

f. What is the current gestational age? _____
_____

g. What complications exist? _____
_____

h. Did the patient deliver at this encounter?
_____

i. What is the main reason for the encounter or the primary complication treated? _____
_____

3. OFFICE   Gender: F Age: 35

Gravida: 1   Para: O   EDD: 10/19/yy

EGA: 10+4

Reason for encounter: establish prenatal care

Assessment: discussed the risks of pregnancy at this age, need for BP and DM monitoring, no problems at this time

Plan: schedule amniocentesis and **chorionic villi sampling (CVS)**

a. Will the patient be under age 16 or age 35 and older at EDD? _____

b. What trimester is the pregnancy? _____
How many weeks of gestation are completed?
_____

c. How many pregnancies has the patient had, including the current one? _____
_____

d. How many births has the patient had? _____

e. What preexisting medical conditions exist? _____

f. What is the current gestational age? _____
_____

g. What complications exist? _____
_____

h. What is the main reason for the encounter or the primary complication treated? _____
_____

4. OFFICE   Gender: F   Age: 26

Gravida: 3   Para: 2   EDD: 7/6/yy   EGA: 24+6

Reason for encounter: prenatal visit, FU on gestational DM diagnosed at last visit

Assessment: GTT shows that the diabetes is being adequately controlled through diet

Plan: continue with nutritional plan and good eating habits

a. Will the patient be under age 16 or age 35 and older at EDD? _____

b. What trimester is the pregnancy? _____
How many weeks of gestation are completed?
_____

(continued)

4. (continued)

c. How many pregnancies has the patient had, including the current one? _____

_____

d. How many births has the patient had? _____

_____

e. What preexisting medical conditions exist?

_____

f. What is the current gestational age? _____

_____

g. What complications exist? _____

_____

h. What is the main reason for the encounter or the primary complication treated? _____

_____

---

5. OFFICE   Gender: F   Age: 25

Gravida: 2   Para: 1   EDD: 6/15/yy

EGA: 28+3

Reason for encounter: routine prenatal visit

Assessment: Rhesus incompatibility

Plan: Rho(D) immune globulin treatment on Monday

a. Will the patient be under age 16 or age 35 and older at EDD? _____

b. What trimester is the pregnancy? _____

How many weeks of gestation are completed?

_____

c. How many pregnancies has the patient had, including the current one? _____

_____

d. How many births has the patient had? _____

_____

e. What preexisting medical conditions exist?

_____

f. What is the current gestational age? _____

_____

g. What complications exist? _____

_____

h. What is the main reason for the encounter or the primary complication treated? _____

_____

---

6. INPATIENT HOSPITAL   Gender: F   Age: 18

Gravida: 1   Para: 0   EDD: 4/6/yy   EGA: 37+5

Reason for admission: full term labor

Assessment: placental infarction

Delivery: 3/22/yy, NSVD, stillborn, 1 girl

a. What is the reason for the admission? _____

_____

b. In what week of pregnancy did delivery occur?

_____

c. Is the delivery vaginal or cesarean? _____

_____

d. Has the mother had a previous cesarean delivery?

_____

e. Was there a malposition of the fetus or obstructed labor? _____

f. What other complications are present? _____

_____

g. How many fetuses were delivered? _____

Were there any stillbirths? _____

_____

---

7. OFFICE   Gender: F   Age: 30

Gravida: 2   Para: 1   EDD: 10/5/yy

EGA: 12+0

Reason for encounter: prenatal care, pernicious anemia

Assessment: blood work has improved, but still not where it should be

Plan: B12 injection

a. Will the patient be under age 16 or age 35 and older at EDD? _____

b. What trimester is the pregnancy? _____

How many weeks of gestation are completed?

_____

c. How many pregnancies has the patient had, including the current one? _____

_____

d. How many births has the patient had? _____

_____

e. What preexisting medical conditions exist? _____

_____

(continued)

CODING PRACTICE *(continued)*

7. *(continued)*

f. What is the current gestational age? _____

_____

g. What complications exist? _____

_____

h. What is the main reason for the encounter or the primary complication treated? _____

---

8. INPATIENT HOSPITAL   Gender: F   Age: 32

Gravida: 2   Para: 2   EDD: 5/18/yy

EGA: 32+2

Reason for admission: *premature rupture of membranes*

Assessment: *severe pre-eclampsia requires cesarean delivery*

Delivery: *3/22/yy, classical cesarean, PTBLC, 1 girl*

a. What is the reason for the admission? _____

_____

b. In what week of pregnancy did delivery occur?

_____

c. Is the delivery vaginal or cesarean? _____

_____

d. What is the reason a cesarean delivery was performed?

_____

e. Was there a malposition of the fetus or obstructed labor? _____

_____

f. What other complications are present? _____

_____

g. How many fetuses were delivered? _____

Were there any stillbirths? _____

_____

---

9. OFFICE   Gender: F   Age: 15

Birthday: 7/15   Gravida: 1   Para: 0

EDD: 6/1/yy   EGA: 30+4

Reason for encounter: *prenatal care, twins, MoDi*

Assessment: *dipstick shows new isolated gestational proteinuria*

Plan: *at risk for preeclampsia, RTO 4 days for repeat test.*

(continued)

---

9. *(continued)*

a. Will the patient be under age 16 or age 35 and older at EDD? _____

b. What trimester is the pregnancy? _____

How many weeks of gestation are completed?

_____

c. How many pregnancies has the patient had, including the current one? _____

_____

d. How many births has the patient had? _____

_____

e. What preexisting medical conditions exist?

_____

f. What is the current gestational age? _____

_____

g. For multiple gestations, how many chorions are present? _____ How many amniotic sacs are present?

_____

h. What complications exist? _____

_____

---

10. INPATIENT HOSPITAL   Gender: F   Age: 22

Gravida: 2   Para: 2   EDD: 3/16/yy

EGA: 41+3

Reason for admission: *post term labor*

Assessment: *obstructed labor due to CPD, severe obesity mother, BMI 41*

Delivery: *3/23/yy, cesarean delivery, TBLC, 1 boy*

a. What is the reason for the admission?

_____

b. In what week of pregnancy did delivery occur?

_____

c. Is the delivery vaginal or cesarean? _____

_____

d. Was there a malposition of the fetus or obstructed labor? _____

e. What other complications are present? _____

_____

f. What is the reason a cesarean delivery was performed?

_____

g. How many fetuses were delivered? _____

Were there any stillbirths? _____

ASSIGNING DIAGNOSIS CODES FOR OBSTETRICS

Coders should acquaint themselves with the organization of obstetrical terms in the Index and must be attentive to distinguish between codes that apply to the mother and those that apply to the infant. In addition, they should also be familiar with how to assign codes to identify the term, the pregnancy, the trimester, and the fetus. Different rules also apply for assigning codes to prenatal visits for normal and high-risk pregnancies.

Locating Obstetrical Main Terms in the Index

The Index groups codes for pregnancy under the Main Term **Pregnancy**. The first-level subterm **complicated by** occupies most of the entry and provides second- and third-level subterms for conditions that complicate pregnancy, such as **abscess** or **placenta previa**. Other first-level subterms describe the type of pregnancy, such as **normal**, **ectopic**, or **multiple gestation**.

The Index groups codes for labor and delivery under the Main Term **Delivery**. The first-level subterms **cesarean for** and **complicated by** occupy most of the entry and provide second- and third-level subterms for conditions that complicate labor and delivery, such as **cord, around neck, with compression** or **obstruction**. A limited number of other first-level subterms describe the type of delivery, such as **normal** or **forceps**.

> ### SUCCESS STEP
> Take a few minutes to review the Index entries for **Pregnancy** and **Delivery** in your ICD-10-CM manual. Highlight the beginning and end of the subterm **complicated by**.

As with any condition, most obstetrical conditions have multiple coding paths. For example, some complications of labor and delivery are also located under the Main Term **Pregnancy, complicated by**. Some conditions are also indexed under the Main Term for the name of the condition, with a subterm for pregnancy, such as **Diabetes, gestational** or **Rh, incompatibility**.

Assigning Codes for the Mother's Condition

When assigning codes for conditions related to pregnancy and childbirth, coders must recognize that although both the mother and the newborn may be affected by the same condition, they assign separate codes for each. Codes in ICD-10-CM Chapter 15 are used *only* on the mother's bill (OGCR I.C.15.a.2)). This is easy to remember because the mother's codes begin with the letter **O**.

When delivery occurs and the newborn receives medical care or occupies a bed, the baby has a separate medical record, separate bills, and separate codes. Codes for the infant begin with **P** and are assigned from ICD-10-CM Chapter 16, Certain Conditions Originating in the Perinatal Period (P00-P96). Coding for the infant is discussed in Chapter 24 of this text.

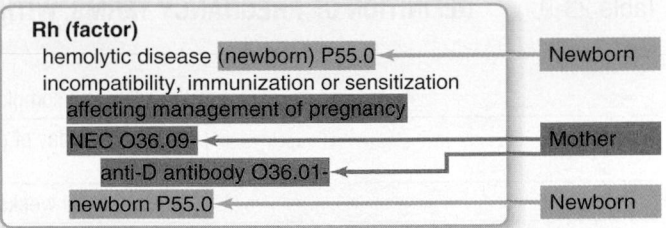

Figure 23-9 ■ Index Entry for Rh Factor, with Separate Codes for Mother and Newborn

> ### CODING CAUTION
> Codes beginning with **P** should NEVER be assigned to the mother (OGCR I.C.16.a.1)).

Careful use of the Index is required in order to identify the Main Term and subterms that distinguish between the mother and the infant. A Main Term for the condition will have separate subterms for the mother and the infant. Select the subterm that corresponds to the record being coded. For example, when a mother is treated for Rh incompatibility, the code will be different than the one used when the infant is treated for the same condition (■ FIGURE 23-9).

Assigning Codes to Identify the Term of Pregnancy

Preterm labor and delivery, as well as postterm pregnancy, constitute complications and require a code. Term lengths are defined by the gestational age at the time of the encounter (■ TABLE 23-9, page 392). Codes are indexed under the Main Term **Pregnancy**, the subterm **complicated by**, and a second-level subterm for **preterm** or **postmaturity**. Alternatively, search for the Main Term **Preterm**, **Postterm**, or **Prolonged**, then locate the appropriate subterm for **pregnancy, labor, or delivery**.

> ### SUCCESS STEP
> Be careful to distinguish between the letter **O** (oh) that begins each code, and the number **0** (zero) that occupies other positions. When making handwritten notes, use a cursive O (with a loop at the top) for the letter; write the number zero with a slash through it: Ø. By clearly distinguishing handwritten notes, you make it easier to key them in correctly. On the keyboard, use the alphabetic keys for the letter and the numeric keypad or the top row of numbers for zero. If you mix up these two similar characters, the computer in your workplace may not accept your code or, worse, the insurance company may reject your claim as unprocessable (incapable of being processed) due to an invalid code.

Assigning Codes to Identify the Trimester and Weeks

Many obstetrics codes require coders to identify the trimester and weeks of gestation. The timeframe for each trimester is defined in an instructional note at the beginning of the

Table 23-9 ■ **DEFINITION OF PREGNANCY TERMS, WITH CODES**

Term	Weeks of Gestation	Code
Preterm pregnancy, delivery, or labor	Less than 37 completed weeks of gestation	O60.1-, O60.2-
Full-term pregnancy	37 weeks, 1 day of gestation to 40 weeks, 7 days of gestation	No code
Postterm pregnancy	40 completed weeks to 42 completed weeks of gestation	O48.0
Prolonged pregnancy	More than 42 completed weeks of gestation	O48.1

chapter. Trimesters are identified in the Tabular List with the fourth, fifth, or sixth character, depending on the length of the code. The symbol **4th**, **5th**, or **6th** in front of the subcategory entry in the Tabular List indicates that an additional character is needed. The codes for each trimester are listed immediately below the subcategory heading (■ FIGURE 23-10). Conditions that only occur in one trimester, or to which the concept of trimesters does not apply, do not have a character to identify the trimester (OGCR 15.a3), 4), and 5)). For example, codes for **ectopic** (*located away from the normal site*) pregnancy do not require a trimester designation.

Assign a code from category **Z3A Weeks of gestation** to identify the number of weeks of gestation completed in the pregnancy. Locate the code in the Index under the Main Term **Pregnancy** and subterm **weeks**. Category **Z3A** appears after category **Z36** in the Tabular List.

SUCCESS STEP

Experienced coders will notice that identifying the trimester is a new concept in ICD-10-CM. The trimester designation replaces the ICD-9-CM fifth digit for episode of care, which no longer applies.

CODING CAUTION

Report codes from **Z3A** for the *completed* weeks of pregnancy. Do not count partial weeks.

Assigning Codes to Identify the Fetus

When maternal conditions affect the fetus or fetal conditions create maternal complications, assign a seventh character to identify which fetus is involved (OGCR 15.a.6)) based on physician documentation. The applicable codes are clearly designated

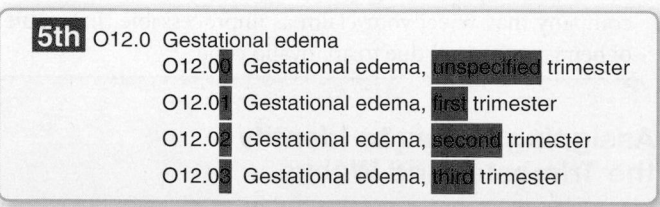

Figure 23-10 ■ Tabular List Entry for Gestational Edema, Requiring a Trimester Designation

in the Tabular List by the symbol **7th**. Seventh-character options are listed in a box at the category or subcategory level (■ FIGURE 23-11 and ■ FIGURE 23-12). Assign the seventh character of **0** in the following situations:

- for singletons

- when it is not possible for the physician to determine which fetus is affected

- when documentation does not identify the affected fetus and the coder cannot obtain clarification from the physician

SUCCESS STEP

Common sense may suggest that when there is only one fetus, you would assign the seventh character of **1**. However, the instructional note directs you to assign the seventh character **0** for a singleton. The character **1** identifies *fetus number one* in a multiple gestation pregnancy.

Assigning Codes for Prenatal Visits

ICD-10-CM provides codes for routine outpatient prenatal visits, which are classified as **Supervision of pregnancy**. Different rules apply for a normal pregnancy than for high-risk patients.

For routine outpatient visits with no complications present, assign a code from category **Z34 Encounter for supervision of normal pregnancy** as the only diagnosis code. Codes are divided based on whether it is the first pregnancy and also by trimester. If any complication from Chapter 15 (O00-O99) exists, the pregnancy is not classified as normal and coders should not assign a code from **Z34**. Locate the code in the Index by searching for the Main Term **Pregnancy**, the subterm **supervision of**, then the second-level subterm **normal**. Select the third-level subterm that identifies the pregnancy as the **first** or **specified NEC** (meaning *not the first*). Verify the code in the Tabular List in order to assign the correct character for the trimester.

For all other routine outpatient visits, assign a code from category **O09 Supervision of high-risk pregnancy** as the first listed code. Assign additional codes from ICD-10-CM Chapter 15, or other chapters as needed, to describe any complications. Women who are very young—under age 16 at EDD—or older—age 35 and older at EDD—are classified as high-risk pregnancies and should be assigned a corresponding code from

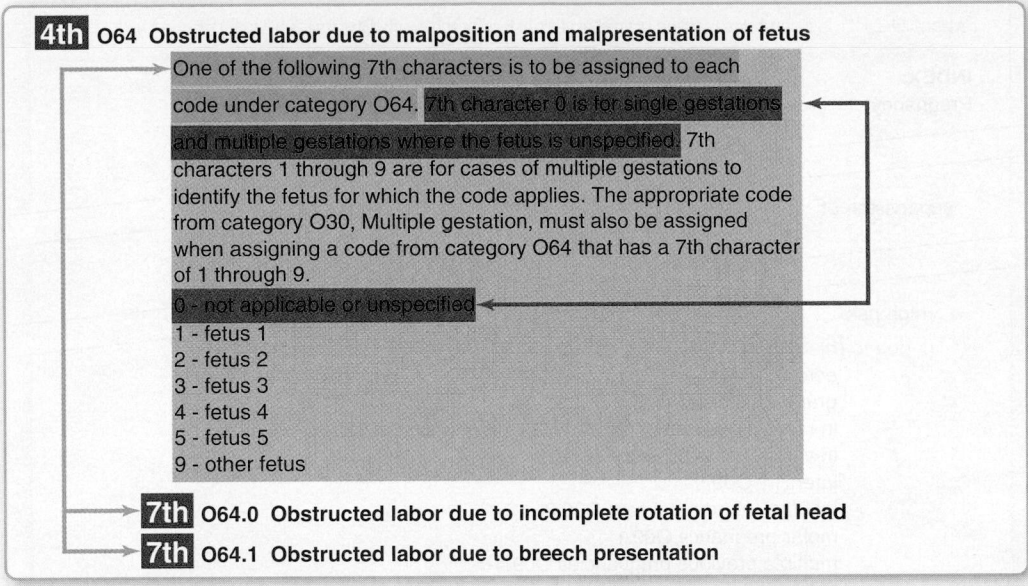

Figure 23-11 ■ Tabular List Entry for Seventh Character Identification of Fetus

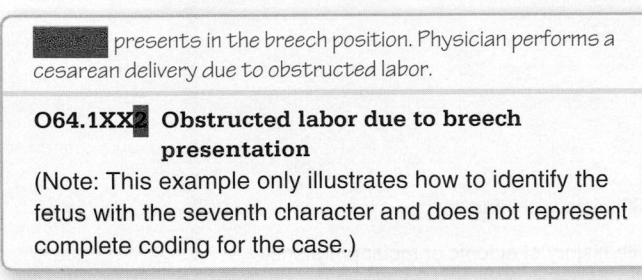

Figure 23-12 ■ Example of Assigning a Seventh Character to Identify the Fetus

category **O09**. Locate the code in the Index by searching for the Main Term **Pregnancy**, the subterm **supervision of**, then the second-level subterm **high risk**. Select the third-level subterm that describes the reason the pregnancy is high risk. Verify the code in the Tabular List in order to assign the correct character for the trimester (■ FIGURE 23-13, page 394).

SUCCESS STEP

Assign a code from category **Z32** for an encounter for pregnancy testing, childbirth instruction, and childcare instruction. Search under the Main Term **Encounter** and the subterms **pregnancy**, then **test**, then **result** or the subterm **instruction**.

Guided Example of Assigning Obstetrics Diagnosis Codes

To practice skills for assigning codes for pregnancy, childbirth, and the puerperium, continue with the example from earlier in the chapter about patient Glenna Ferrier, who was admitted to Branton Medical Center for full-term labor.

Follow along in your ICD-10-CM manual as Daphne Wittman, CCS-P, assigns codes. Check off each step after you complete it.

▶ First, Daphne confirms the circumstances and outcome of delivery:

❑ full term delivery

❑ vaginal delivery was attempted

❑ cesarean delivery performed due to previous cesarean delivery

❑ single live female infant

❑ fetal tachycardia

❑ 39 weeks of gestation

▶ Daphne begins with fetal tachycardia. She searches the Index for the Main Term **Tachycardia**.

❑ She locates a subterm for neonatal, which refers to the newborn infant, but she does not see a subterm that relates the tachycardia as a complication of delivery.

❑ She decides to go a different direction and searches the Index for the Main Term **Delivery**.

❑ She locates the subterm **complicated by**.

❑ She locates a second-level subterm for **fetal heart rate, O76**.

▶ Daphne verifies code **O76** in the Tabular List. (■ FIGURE 23-14, page 395).

❑ She reads the code title **O76 Abnormality in fetal heart rate and rhythm complicating labor and delivery**.

❑ She reads the inclusion notes under the code and sees the entry **Fetal tachycardia complicating labor and delivery**. This entry confirms that this is the correct code.

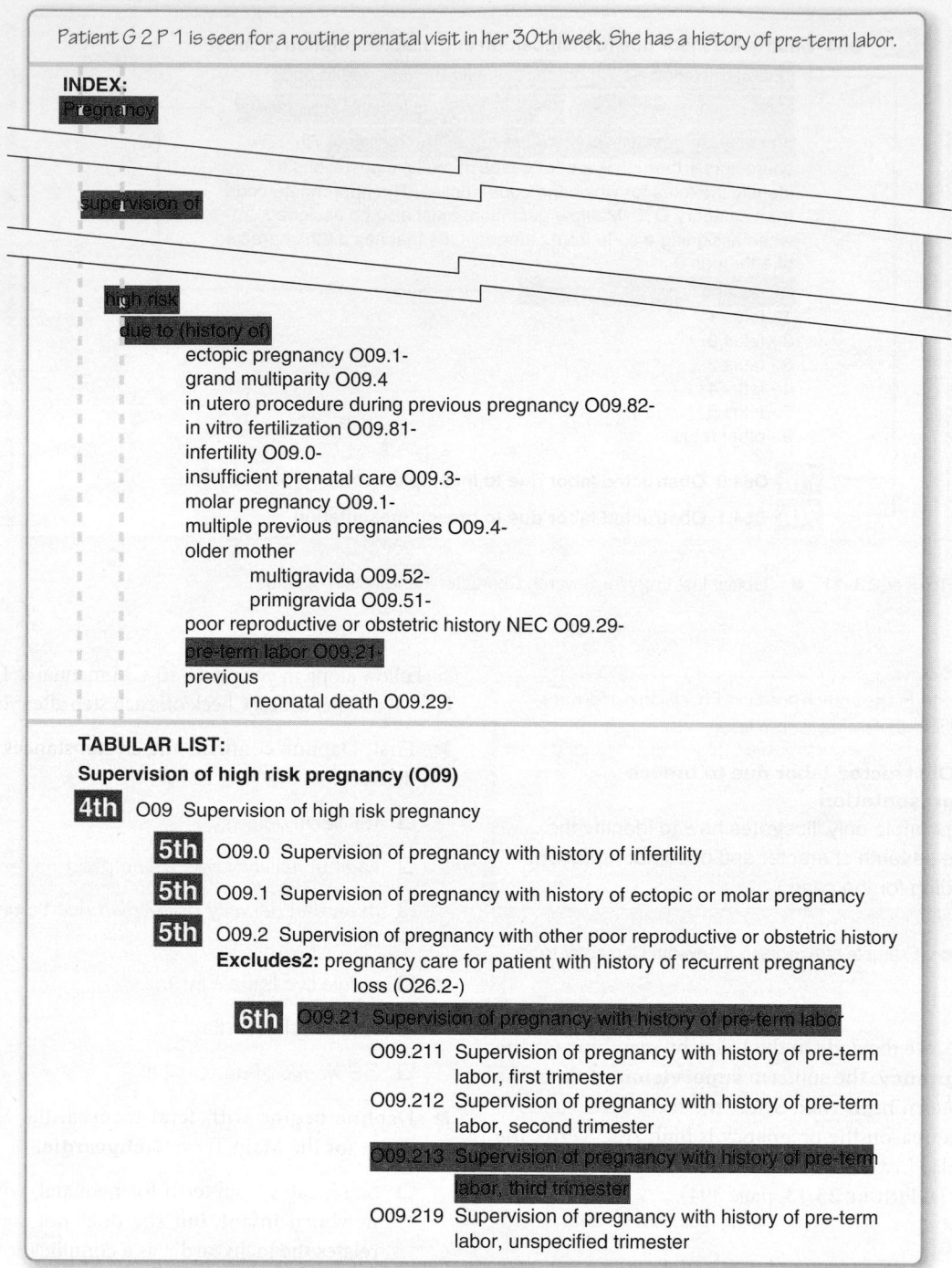

Patient G 2 P 1 is seen for a routine prenatal visit in her 30th week. She has a history of pre-term labor.

INDEX:

Pregnancy

   supervision of

      high risk

         due to (history of)

            ectopic pregnancy O09.1-

            grand multiparity O09.4

            in utero procedure during previous pregnancy O09.82-

            in vitro fertilization O09.81-

            infertility O09.0-

            insufficient prenatal care O09.3-

            molar pregnancy O09.1-

            multiple previous pregnancies O09.4-

            older mother

                multigravida O09.52-

                primigravida O09.51-

            poor reproductive or obstetric history NEC O09.29-

            pre-term labor O09.21-

            previous

                neonatal death O09.29-

TABULAR LIST:

Supervision of high risk pregnancy (O09)

4th O09 Supervision of high risk pregnancy

   5th O09.0 Supervision of pregnancy with history of infertility

   5th O09.1 Supervision of pregnancy with history of ectopic or molar pregnancy

   5th O09.2 Supervision of pregnancy with other poor reproductive or obstetric history
       Excludes2: pregnancy care for patient with history of recurrent pregnancy
          loss (O26.2-)

      6th O09.21 Supervision of pregnancy with history of pre-term labor

         O09.211 Supervision of pregnancy with history of pre-term labor, first trimester

         O09.212 Supervision of pregnancy with history of pre-term labor, second trimester

         O09.213 Supervision of pregnancy with history of pre-term labor, third trimester

         O09.219 Supervision of pregnancy with history of pre-term labor, unspecified trimester

Figure 23-13 ■ Example of Selecting the First-Listed Diagnosis for Supervision of a High-Risk Pregnancy

▶ Daphne checks for instructional notes in the Tabular List.

   ❑ Code **O76** is also a category, so there are no further instructional notes to cross-references at the category level.

   ❑ She cross-references the beginning of the block **O60-O77** and verifies that there are no instructional notes.

   ❑ She cross-references the beginning of **Chapter 15 (O00-O9A)** and reviews the instructional notes, which provide general information about using codes in this chapter. There are no notes that relate to the condition she is coding.

▶ Daphne decides to code the reason for the cesarean delivery next, which is the fact that the patient had a previous cesarean delivery. She searches the Index for the Main Term **Delivery**.

   ❑ She locates the subterm **cesarean for**.

   ❑ She locates a second-level subterm for **previous cesarean delivery O34.21**.

▶ Daphne verifies code **O34.21** in the Tabular List.

   ❑ She reads the code title **O34.21 Maternal care for scar from previous cesarean delivery**.

O76 Abnormality in fetal heart rate and rhythm complicating labor and delivery

> Depressed fetal heart rate tones complicating labor and delivery
> Fetal bradycardia complicating labor and delivery
> Fetal heart rate decelerations complicating labor and delivery
> Fetal heart rate irregularity complicating labor and delivery
> Fetal heart rate abnormal variability complicating labor and delivery
> Fetal tachycardia complicating labor and delivery
> Non-reassuring fetal heart rate or rhythm complicating labor and delivery
> **Excludes1:** fetal stress NOS (O77.9)
> > labor and delivery complicated by electrocardiographic evidence of fetal stress (O77.8)
> > labor and delivery complicated by ultrasonic evidence of fetal stress (O77.8)
> **Excludes2:** fetal metabolic acidemia (O68)
> > other fetal stress (O77.0-O77.1)

Figure 23-14 ■ Tabular List Entry for Fetal Tachycardia

▶ Daphne checks for instructional notes in the Tabular List.

❑ She cross-references the beginning of the category **O34 Maternal care for abnormality of pelvic organs** and reads the instructional notes (■ Figure 23-15).

   ▪ The **Includes** note describes the general purpose of this category.

   ▪ The second note states **Code first any associated obstructed labor (O65.5).**

   ▪ She double-checks the medical record and confirms that obstructed labor is not documented; therefore this note does not apply.

CODING CAUTION

Notice that Daphne did not *automatically* assign a code for obstructed labor when she read the instructional note. The expression "Code first *any*" means "Code obstructed labor, *if it is documented*." Because obstruction is not documented, she did not assign a code for it.

▪ The third note states **Use additional code for specific condition.**

▪ The specific condition is fetal tachycardia, which she has already coded. This note will also provide direction when it is time to sequence the codes.

❑ She cross-references the beginning of the block **O30-O48** and verifies that there are no instructional notes.

❑ She is already familiar with the instructional notes at the beginning of **Chapter 15 (O00-O9A)** and remembers that there are no notes that relate to the condition she is coding.

▶ Daphne recalls that for every encounter in which a birth occurs, OGCR require coders to assign a **Z** code for outcome of the delivery (OGCR I.C.15.b.5)).

❑ She searches the Index for the Main Term **Outcome of delivery**.

❑ She locates the subterm **single**.

❑ She reviews the second-level subterms under **single** and locates **liveborn Z37.0**.

▶ Daphne verifies the code **Z37.0** in the Tabular List.

❑ She verifies the code title **Z37.0 Single live birth** and confirms that this correctly describes the outcome.

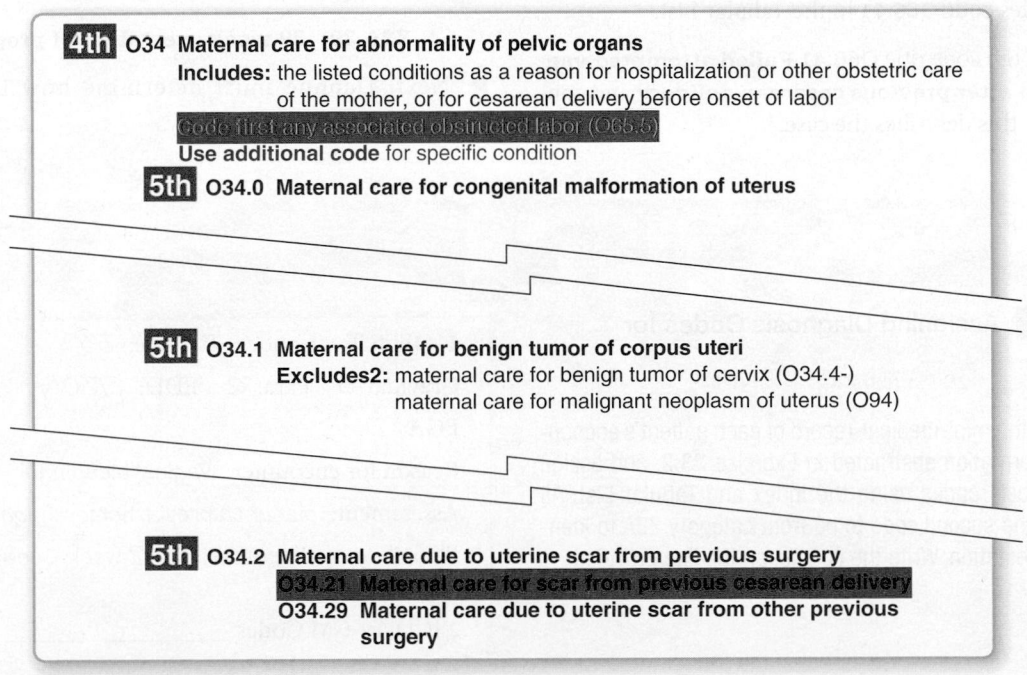

4th O34 Maternal care for abnormality of pelvic organs
Includes: the listed conditions as a reason for hospitalization or other obstetric care of the mother, or for cesarean delivery before onset of labor
Code first any associated obstructed labor (O65.5)
Use additional code for specific condition
5th O34.0 Maternal care for congenital malformation of uterus

5th O34.1 Maternal care for benign tumor of corpus uteri
Excludes2: maternal care for benign tumor of cervix (O34.4-)
maternal care for malignant neoplasm of uterus (O94)

5th O34.2 Maternal care due to uterine scar from previous surgery
O34.21 Maternal care for scar from previous cesarean delivery
O34.29 Maternal care due to uterine scar from other previous surgery

Figure 23-15 ■ Tabular List Entry Showing Instructional Notes for Code O34.21

❏ She cross-references the **NOTE:** under the category heading **Z37**, which states **This category is intended for use as an additional code to identify the outcome of delivery on the mother's record. It is not for use on the newborn record.**

❏ This note confirms that she has the correct code for the mother's record.

SUCCESS STEP

Highlight the **NOTE:** at **Z37** in your coding manual and write the word "Mother" in the margin. These tips will remind you to distinguish the codes in category **Z37**, which are used on the *mother's* record, from similar codes in category **Z38**, which are used on the *newborn's* record.

❏ Daphne quickly checks the beginning of the category **Z30-Z39** for instructional notes and finds none.

❏ She also checks the beginning of **Chapter 21 (Z00-Z99)** and reviews the instructional notes.

▶ Daphne reviews the medical record to be certain she has captured all the elements that need to be coded for this patient.

❏ She reads that a vaginal delivery was attempted first and this complicated the delivery. She determines that she needs to assign a code for a failed attempt at vaginal delivery after a previous cesarean delivery.

▶ Daphne searches the Index for the Main Term **Delivery** and the subterm **complicated by.**

❏ She locates a second-level subterm **failed.**

❏ She locates a third-level subterm **attempted vaginal birth after previous cesarean delivery O66.41.**

▶ Daphne verifies code **O66.41** in the Tabular List.

❏ She reads the code title **O66.41 Failed attempted vaginal birth after previous cesarean delivery** and confirms that this describes the case.

❏ She reads the instructional note under the code that states **Code first rupture of uterus, if applicable (O71.0-, O71.1).** She determines that the note does not apply because a uterine rupture is not documented.

❏ She has already cross-referenced the beginning of the block **O60-O77** and **Chapter 15 (O00-O9A)** for instructional notes and remembers that there are no instructions that apply to this case.

▶ Finally, Daphne assigns a code for the weeks of gestation of the pregnancy.

❏ She checks the medical record and verifies that 39 weeks of gestation were completed.

❏ She searches the Index for the Main Term **Pregnancy.**

❏ She locates the subterm **weeks.**

❏ She reviews the second-level subterms under **weeks** and locates the subterm **39** with the code **Z3A.39.**

▶ Daphne verifies the code **Z3A.39** in the Tabular List.

❏ She verifies the code title **Z3A.39 39 weeks gestation of pregnancy**, and confirms that this correctly describes the outcome.

▶ Daphne reviews the codes she has assigned for this case.

❏ **Z37.0   Single live birth**

❏ **O34.21   Maternal care for scar from previous cesarean delivery**

❏ **O76   Abnormality in fetal heart rate and rhythm complicating labor and delivery**

❏ **O66.41   Failed attempted vaginal birth after previous cesarean delivery**

❏ **Z3A.39   39 weeks gestation of pregnancy**

▶ Next, Daphne must determine how to sequence the codes.

CODING PRACTICE

Exercise 23.3   Assigning Diagnosis Codes for Obstetrics

Instructions: Read the mini-medical-record of each patient's encounter, review the information abstracted in Exercise 23.2, and assign ICD-10-CM diagnosis codes using the Index and Tabular List. All exercises require the second code to be from category Z3A to identify the weeks of gestation. Write the code(s) on the line provided.

---

1. OFFICE   Gender: F   Age: 33

Gravida: 3   Para: 2   EDD: 6/30/yy

EGA: 26+2

Reason for encounter: vaginal bleeding

Assessment: placenta previa, hemorrhage

Plan: bed confinement, RTO 2 weeks, cesarean delivery may be required

2 ICD-10-CM Codes _____

(continued)

2. OFFICE Gender: F Age: 24

Gravida: 1 Para: 0 EDD: 3/23/yy

EGA: 40+2

Reason for encounter: prenatal visit

Assessment: unstable lie

Plan: cesarean delivery today at 1500

2 ICD-10-CM Codes _____

3. OFFICE Gender: F Age: 35

Gravida: 1 Para: 0 EDD: 10/19/yy

EGA: 10+4

Reason for encounter: establish prenatal care

Assessment: discussed the risks of pregnancy at this age, need for BP and DM monitoring, no problems at this time

Plan: schedule amniocentesis and **chorionic villi sampling (CVS)**

Tip: Primigravida means first pregnancy.

2 ICD-10-CM Codes _____

4. OFFICE Gender: F Age: 26

Gravida: 3 Para: 2 EDD: 7/6/yy EGA: 24+6

Reason for encounter: FU on gestational DM diagnosed at last visit

Assessment: GTT shows that the diabetes is being adequately controlled through diet

Plan: continue with nutritional plan and good eating habits

2 ICD-10-CM Codes _____

5. OFFICE Gender: F Age: 25

Gravida: 2 Para: 1 EDD: 6/15/yy

EGA: 28+3

Reason for encounter: routine prenatal visit

Assessment: Rhesus incompatibility

Plan: Rho(D) immune globulin treatment on Monday

Tip: Select the code for the condition as it affects the mother, not the infant. Refer to OGCR I.C.15.b.2) for sequencing information.

3 ICD-10-CM Codes _____

_____

ARRANGING DIAGNOSIS CODES FOR OBSTETRICS

Coders must be attentive to selecting the principal diagnosis when a delivery occurs and to sequencing codes from Chapter 15 with codes from body system chapters. As in all coding, the principal or first-listed diagnosis is determined by the reason for the admission or encounter, OGCR, and instructional notes in the Tabular List. Table 23-10 summarizes key coding and sequencing rules for obstetrics.

Arranging Codes for When a Delivery Occurs

When a delivery occurs, a minimum of two codes are required—one for the delivery diagnosis and one for the outcome of delivery (■ TABLE 23-10). The principal diagnosis should be one of the following (OGCR I.C.15.b.4)):

- the code for normal delivery, **O80** (■ TABLE 23-11, page 398)
- the main complication of labor and delivery
- the main reason a cesarean delivery was required
- the reason for admission if unrelated to any of the above

Search the Main Term **Delivery** and subterm **complicated by** to locate the codes for complications.

The additional code is a code from category **Z37.-**, which describes the outcome of delivery in terms of the number of live infants and/or the number of stillbirths (OGCR I.C.15.b.5)). Search for the Main Term **Outcome of Delivery** for the **Z37.-** code (■ FIGURE 23-16, page 398).

SUCCESS STEP

Assign a code from **Z37.-** only during the admission in which delivery occurs. Do not assign it for subsequent admissions, even if they are for complications of delivery or for postpartum office visits. **Z37.-** is NEVER the principal or first-listed code.

Table 23-10 ■ SUMMARY OF CODE SEQUENCING FOR OBSTETRICS

Type of Encounter	Index Main Term & Subterms
Routine prenatal visit	1. Pregnancy, supervision 2. Pregnancy, weeks of gestation (**Z3A.-**)
Complications of pregnancy	1. Pregnancy, complicated by
Normal delivery	1. Delivery, normal (**O80**) 2. Outcome of delivery, single live birth (**Z37.0**)
Delivery with complications	1. Delivery, complicated by 2. Outcome of delivery (**Z37.-**)
Cesarean delivery	1. Delivery, cesarean 2. Outcome of delivery (**Z37.-**)
Birth encounter for the newborn	1. Newborn + appropriate subterm: born in hospital/born outside of hospital/twin/triplet/quadruplet/multiple born (**Z38.-**) 2. Newborn, affected by

> Patient gives birth to a baby boy who makes a cephalic presentation. Aside from requesting an epidural and having an episiotomy, the patient has no problems.
>
> (1) Index: **Delivery, normal**
>   Tabular List: **O80   Encounter for full-term uncomplicated delivery**
> (2) Index: **Outcome of delivery, single, liveborn**
>   Tabular List: **Z37.0   Single live birth**

Figure 23-16 ■ Example of Sequencing Codes for a Delivery

Table 23-11 ■ DEFINITION OF A NORMAL DELIVERY, ICD-10-CM CODE O80

Includes	Excludes
Minimal or no assistance	Fetal manipulation
Episiotomy	Rotation version
Spontaneous	Instrumentation/forceps
Cephalic presentation	Induced labor
Vaginal	Noncephalic presentation
Full-term	Cesarean delivery
Single gestation	Preterm delivery
Live-born infant	Postterm delivery
Resolved antepartum conditions	Prolonged delivery
No other complications	Multiple gestation
	Stillbirth
	Any complication

Arranging Chapter 15 Codes with Codes from Other Chapters

Many complications require a code from Chapter 15 to identify the obstetric complication and an additional code from a body system chapter to describe the details of the condition. Always sequence the Chapter 15 code first (OGCR 15.a.1)). Follow this guideline regardless of whether the condition is preexisting, as in diabetes, or is specific for the postpartum period, as in postpartum thrombophlebitis (■ FIGURE 23-17). Refer to the Tabular List for instructional notes to assign additional codes (■ FIGURE 23-18).

SUCCESS STEP

The terms *thrombophlebitis* and *phlebothrombosis* are interchangeable in ICD-10-CM. Notice that both terms contain two roots, **phleb-** (*vein*) and **thromb-** (*clot*).

Guided Example of Arranging Obstetrics Diagnosis Codes

To practice skills for sequencing codes for pregnancy, childbirth, and the puerperium, continue with the example from earlier in the chapter about patient Glenna Ferrier, who was admitted to Branton Medical Center for full-term labor.

> Patient is seen for postpartum deep venous phlebothrombosis in the tibial vein of the left leg.
>
> (1) Index: **Phlebothrombosis, puerperal, - see Thrombophlebitis, puerperal; Thrombophlebitis, puerperal, deep**
>   Tabular List: **O87.1 Deep phlebothrombosis in the puerperium**
> (2) Tabular List: **Use additional code to identify the deep vein thrombosis (I82.4-, I85.5-, I82.62-, I82.72-)**
>   **I82.442 Acute embolism and thrombosis of left tibial vein**

Figure 23-17 ■ Example of Sequencing Obstetric Complications with Codes from a Body System Chapter

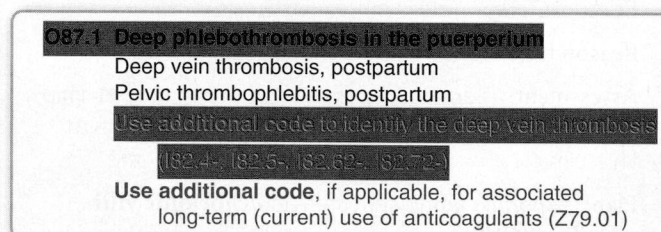

Use additional code, if applicable, for associated long-term (current) use of anticoagulants (Z79.01)

Figure 23-18 ■ Tabular List Entry for an Obstetric Complication Requiring Additional Codes from a Body System Chapter

Follow along in your ICD-10-CM manual as Daphne Wittman, CCS-P, sequences the codes. Check off each step after you complete it.

▶ First, Daphne reviews the codes she has assigned for this case:

❑ **Z37.0   Single live birth**

❑ **O34.21   Maternal care for scar from previous cesarean delivery**

❑ **O76   Abnormality in fetal heart rate and rhythm complicating labor and delivery**

❑ **O66.41   Failed attempted vaginal birth after previous cesarean delivery**

❑ **Z3A.39   39 weeks gestation of pregnancy**

▶ To better determine the sequencing rules Daphne reads OGCR I.C.15.b.4, which states the following:

❑ "In cases of cesarean delivery, the selection of the principal diagnosis should be the condition established after study that was responsible for the patient's admission. If the patient was admitted with a condition that resulted in the performance of a cesarean procedure, that condition should be selected as the principal diagnosis."

❑ Daphne reviews the medical record and the codes she assigned. The main reason a cesarean delivery was performed was because of the scar from the previous cesarean delivery.

❏ Therefore, the principal diagnosis is **O34.21 Maternal care for scar from previous cesarean delivery**.

❏ The second code should be the next most important complication, which is the fetal tachycardia.

❏ The third code is failed vaginal delivery.

❏ The fourth code is the outcome of delivery.

❏ The final code is the weeks of gestation.

▶ Daphne finalizes the codes and sequencing for this case:

(1) **O34.21 Maternal care for scar from previous cesarean delivery**

(2) **O76 Abnormality in fetal heart rate and rhythm complicating labor and delivery**

(3) **O66.41 Failed attempted vaginal birth after previous cesarean delivery**

(4) **Z37.0 Single live birth**

(5) **Z3A.39 39 weeks gestation of pregnancy**

CODING PRACTICE

Exercise 23.4 Arranging Diagnosis Codes for Obstetrics

Instructions: Read the mini-medical-record of each patient's encounter, review the information abstracted in Exercise 23.2, assign ICD-10-CM diagnosis codes using the Index and Tabular List, and sequence them correctly.

---

1. INPATIENT HOSPITAL Gender: F Age: 18

Gravida: 1 Para: 0 EDD: 4/6/yy EGA: 37+5

Reason for admission: *full term labor*

Assessment: *placental infarction*

Delivery: *3/22/yy, NSVD, stillborn, 1 girl*

Tip: Assign a code for the placental infarction, a code for the fetal death, a code for outcome of delivery, and a code for the weeks of gestation.

4 ICD-10-CM Codes _____

_____

---

2. OFFICE Gender: F Age: 30

Gravida: 2 Para: 1 EDD: 10/5/yy

EGA: 12+0

Reason for encounter: *prenatal care, pernicious anemia*

Assessment: *blood work has improved, but still not where it should be*

Plan: *B12 injection*

Tip: Read the instructional notes in the Tabular List. Assign a code for the weeks of gestation.

3 ICD-10-CM Codes _____

_____

---

3. INPATIENT HOSPITAL Gender: F Age: 32

Gravida: 2 Para: 2 EDD: 5/18/yy

EGA: 32+2

Reason for admission: *premature rupture of membranes*

Assessment: *severe pre-eclampsia requires cesarean delivery*

Delivery: *3/22/yy, classical cesarean, PTBLC, 1 girl*

Tip: Assign a code for the reason for the cesarean delivery, a code for PROM, a code for the outcome of delivery, and a code for the weeks of gestation.

4 ICD-10-CM Codes _____

_____

---

4. OFFICE Gender: F Age: 15

Birthday: 7/15 Gravida: 1 Para: 0

EDD: 6/1/yy EGA: 30+4

Reason for encounter: *prenatal care, twins, MoDi*

Assessment: *dipstick shows new isolated gestational proteinuria*

Plan: *at risk for preeclampsia, RTO 4 days for repeat test*

Tip: Assign a code for the diagnosis, a code for the mother's age, a code for the twin pregnancy, and a code for the weeks of gestation.

4 ICD-10-CM Codes _____

_____

(continued)

CODING PRACTICE *(continued)*

5. INPATIENT HOSPITAL Gender: F Age: 22

Gravida: 2 Para: 2 EDD: 3/16/yy

EGA: 41+3

Reason for admission: *post term labor*

Assessment: *obstructed labor due to CPD, severe obesity mother, BMI 41*

Delivery: *3/23/yy, cesarean delivery, TBLC, 1 boy*

(continued)

5. (continued)

Tip: Assign a delivery code for the obstruction, a code for postterm pregnancy, and a delivery code for the obesity complication, then follow instructional notes in the Tabular List. Also assign a code for the weeks of gestation.

7 ICD-10-CM Codes _____

_____

_____

CHAPTER SUMMARY

In this chapter you learned that:

- Pregnancy is a normal, temporary condition that occurs within the female body, which begins at the time of conception and ends with the birth of the fetus.

- ICD-10-CM Chapter 15, Pregnancy, Childbirth, and the Puerperium (**O00-O9A**), contains nine blocks or subchapters that are divided by the phase of pregnancy and the type of condition.

- Because multiple complications are common during pregnancy, childbirth, and the puerperium, coders must be attentive to which complication is the reason for the encounter or admission.

- Coders should acquaint themselves with the organization of obstetrical terms in the Index and must be attentive to distinguish between codes that apply to the mother and those that apply to the infant.

- Coders must be attentive to selecting the principal diagnosis when a delivery occurs and to sequencing codes from Chapter 15 with codes from body system chapters.

- ICD-10-CM provides Official Guidelines for Coding and Reporting (OGCR) in section I.C.15 that cover the general rules for obstetric cases, selection of OB principal or first-listed diagnosis, preexisting conditions, and several specific conditions, including hypertension, diabetes, HIV, alcohol and tobacco use, normal delivery, postpartum, and abortions.

CONCEPT QUIZ

Take a moment to look back at pregnancy, childbirth, and the puerperium and solidify your skills. Try to answer the questions from memory first, then look back at the discussion in this chapter if you need a little extra help.

Completion

Instructions: Write the term that answers each question based on the information you learned in this chapter. Choose from the list below. Some choices may be used more than once and some choices may not be used at all.

cephalic	gestational hypertension
conception	gravida
DiDi	HELLP syndrome
DiMo	last menstrual period
fetopelvic	MoDi
first trimester	MoMo

nuchal cord	prenatal
occipitoanterior	PROM
para	puerperium
parturition	Rhesus incompatibility
peripartum	second trimester
placenta previa	third trimester
preeclampsia	

1. The _____ period is the last month of pregnancy to five months postpartum.

2. The period of true labor is also called

   _____.

3. The estimated date of delivery is determined as 40 weeks from the _____.

4. The period from 28 weeks, 0 days until delivery is the

   _____.

5. _____ is the condition of the umbilical cord becoming wrapped around the neck of the fetus.

6. _____ is a condition in which a mother is Rh negative and develops antibodies against a fetus that is Rh positive.

7. _____ is a metabolic disorder of pregnancy that develops after the twentieth week and involves gestational hypertension and proteinuria.

8. Twin fetuses with one chorion and two amnions are _____.

9. Cephalopelvic disproportion is also called _____.

10. _____ is the rupture of the amniotic sac and chorion before the onset of labor.

Multiple Choice

Instructions: Circle the letter of the best answer to each question based on the information you learned in this chapter.

1. Which of the following terms does NOT refer to the time period from conception to the beginning of labor?
   A. Prenatal
   B. Peripartum
   C. Antepartum
   D. Antenatal

2. A woman currently pregnant, who has had one previous pregnancy and gave birth to twins, is described as
   A. gravida 1 para 2.
   B. gravida 2 para 1.
   C. gravida 2 para 2.
   D. grand multipara.

3. A normal pregnancy includes all of the following EXCEPT
   A. no preexisting conditions.
   B. no new conditions that develop during pregnancy.
   C. single gestation.
   D. gestational diabetes.

4. What is the length of a full-term pregnancy?
   A. More than 37 completed weeks of gestation
   B. 37 weeks, 0 days of gestation to 39 weeks, 6 days of gestation
   C. 40 completed weeks to 42 completed weeks of gestation
   D. More than 42 completed weeks of gestation

5. GDM is
   A. preexisting diabetes that is treated during pregnancy.
   B. preexisting hypertension that is treated during pregnancy.
   C. diabetes that is first diagnosed during pregnancy.
   D. hypertension that is first diagnosed during pregnancy.

6. Which of the following is a normal delivery?
   A. Induction of labor with vaginal delivery
   B. Vaginal delivery with cephalic presentation
   C. Vaginal delivery of twins
   D. Vaginal delivery at 36 weeks of gestation

7. When is a multiple gestation pregnancy coded as high risk?
   A. Only when the physician documents it as high risk
   B. Only when a cesarean delivery is required
   C. When there are more than two fetuses
   D. Always

8. Excessive bleeding following delivery is
   A. postpartum hemorrhage.
   B. puerperal mastitis.
   C. placenta previa.
   D. preeclampsia.

9. The seventh character of 1 identifies
   A. the first trimester.
   B. a single gestation pregnancy.
   C. fetus one in a multiple gestation pregnancy.
   D. gravida 1.

10. How many complications are documented in this case: Patient, age 15 years, 10 months, is admitted in labor at 36 weeks, 3 days gestation. Labor proceeds without complication and she gives birth to twins.
    A. None
    B. One
    C. Two
    D. Three

CODING CHALLENGE

Instructions: Read the mini-medical-record of each patient's encounter, then abstract, assign, and sequence ICD-10-CM diagnosis codes using the Index and Tabular List. Write the code(s) on the line provided.

1. EMERGENCY DEPT   Gender: F   Age: 24

Gravida: 2   Para: 1   EDD: 9/27/yy   EGA: 14+2

Reason for encounter: hurt her shoulder while lifting bags of gravel she was spreading on a walking path in the yard of her single family home, leisure status

(continued)

1. (continued)

Assessment: sprained right shoulder, does not affect pregnancy

Plan: ice and sling, FU 1 week

Tip: Remember to assign external cause codes for activity, place of occurrence, and status.

5 ICD-10-CM Codes _____
_____

(continued)

(continued from page 401)

2. OFFICE Gender: F Age: 19

Gravida: 1 Para: 0 EDD: 8/16/yy EGA: 19+6

Reason for encounter: prenatal care

Assessment: HIV positive

Plan: anti-HIV drugs beginning in second trimester, newborn to be treated within 8 hrs and for 6 months

Tip: Refer to OGCR I.C.15.f.

3 ICD-10-CM Codes _____

_____

3. OFFICE Gender: F Age: 35

Gravida: 2 Para: 0 EDD: 10/25/yy

EGA: 10+0

Reason for encounter: patient presents for prenatal care after successful IVF

Assessment: previous miscarriage

Plan: schedule pre-natal visits

Tip: Assign a separate code for each risk factor.

4 ICD-10-CM Codes _____

_____

4. INPATIENT HOSPITAL Gender: F Age: 28

Gravida: 2 Para: 2 EDD: 4/5/yy EGA: 39+1

Reason for admission: labor

Assessment: cord entanglement and compression of fetus 1

Delivery: 3/28/yy, vaginal delivery converted to cesarean delivery, TBLC, 1 girl, 1 boy

Tip: By definition, twins of the opposite sex are DiDi.

4 ICD-10-CM Codes _____

_____

5. INPATIENT HOSPITAL Gender: F Age: 31

Gravida: 2 Para: 2 Date of delivery: 3/8/yy

Reason for encounter: admitted from physician office with fever of 103 degrees F and purulent discharge from operative wound

Assessment: infected cesarean delivery wound, staphylococcus

Plan: antibiotics, FU 2 weeks

2 ICD-10-CM Codes _____

6. INPATIENT HOSPITAL Gender: F Age: 23

Gravida: 1 Para: 1 EDD: 3/27/yy EGA: 39+4

Reason for admission: full term labor

Assessment: obstructed labor due to prolapsed arm presentation, successfully converted to cephalic, with first degree perineal laceration

Delivery: 3/28/yy, NSVD, TBLC, 1 girl

4 ICD-10-CM Codes _____

_____

7. INPATIENT HOSPITAL Gender: F Age: 31

Gravida: 3 Para: 2 EDD: 10/11/yy

EGA: 12+5

Reason for admission: observation for signs of labor or other complications after failed legal abortion due to fetal chromosome abnormality

Assessment: no labor or other complications were noted

Plan: RTO FU in 2 days, supportive and genetic counseling

Tip: Assign codes for the attempted abortion and the underlying reason for the attempt. See OGCR 15.b.3).

3 ICD-10-CM Codes _____

_____

8. OFFICE Gender: F Age: 34

Gravida: 2 Para: 2 Date of Delivery: 3/15/yy

Reason for encounter: postpartum care

Assessment: abscess of right breast

Plan: Rx antibiotic, RTO 2 weeks

1 ICD-10-CM Code _____

9. OFFICE Gender: F Age: 30

Gravida: 1 Para: 0 EDD: 10/18/yy

EGA: 11+3

Reason for encounter: prenatal visit

Assessment: long standing essential hypertension

Plan: antihypertensive therapy, monitor for pre-eclampsia

2 ICD-10-CM Codes _____

10. INPATIENT HOSPITAL Gender: F Age: 21

Gravida: 2 Para: 2 EDD: 5/31/yy

EGA: 31+4

Reason for admission: premature rupture of membranes

Assessment: labor started 30 hours post admission

Delivery: 3/28/yy, VBAC, TBLC, 1 girl

4 ICD-10-CM Codes _____

_____

KEEP ON CODING

Instructions: Read the diagnostic statement, then use the Index and Tabular List to assign and sequence ICD-10-CM diagnosis codes. Write the code(s) on the line provided.

1. Tubal pregnancy: ICD-10-CM Code(s) _____

2. Supervision of elderly primigravida, 35-week pregnancy: ICD-10-CM Code(s) _____

3. Threatened abortion: ICD-10-CM Code(s) _____

4. Complication of childbirth due to bariatric surgery status, 36 weeks: ICD-10-CM Code(s) _____

5. Excessive weight gain during first 12 weeks of pregnancy: ICD-10-CM Code(s) _____

6. Pregnancy with preexisting diabetes mellitus, type 1, in puerperium: ICD-10-CM Code(s) _____

7. Pregnancy complicated by breech presentation, 39 weeks' gestation: ICD-10-CM Code(s) _____

8. Galactorrhea: ICD-10-CM Code(s) _____

9. Postpartum thyroiditis: ICD-10-CM Code(s) _____

10. Aspiration pneumonia due to anesthesia during 27th week of pregnancy (26 weeks completed): ICD-10-CM Code(s) _____

11. Acute lymphoblastic leukemia complicating the pregnancy in 31st week (30 weeks completed): ICD-10-CM Code(s) _____

12. Acute renal failure after an incomplete spontaneous abortion: ICD-10-CM Code(s) _____

13. Herpes gestationis, 10 weeks pregnant: ICD-10-CM Code(s) _____

14. Fetal anemia: ICD-10-CM Code(s) _____

15. Failed induction of labor by oxytocin, 40 weeks: ICD-10-CM Code(s) _____

16. Triplet pregnancy delivered at 38 weeks of gestation by cesarean delivery, all liveborn: ICD-10-CM Code(s) _____

17. Preterm labor without delivery, 33 weeks of pregnancy: ICD-10-CM Code(s) _____

18. Alcohol abuse complicating pregnancy at 37 weeks: ICD-10-CM Code(s) _____

19. Failed induction of labor by oxytocin, 42 weeks: ICD-10-CM Code(s) _____

20. Puerperal abscess of nipple: ICD-10-CM Code(s) _____

21. Abnormal glucose level complicating pregnancy, 22 weeks: ICD-10-CM Code(s) _____

22. Hemorrhoids complicating pregnancy at 26 weeks: ICD-10-CM Code(s) _____

23. Maternal care for incompetent cervix, 25 weeks: ICD-10-CM Code(s) _____

24. Kidney infection, in 13th week of pregnancy (12 weeks completed): ICD-10-CM Code(s) _____

25. Physical abuse complicating pregnancy in the 8th week (7 weeks completed): ICD-10-CM Code(s) _____

Chapter 24

Certain Conditions Originating in the Perinatal Period (P00-P96)

Chapter Outline

- **Perinatal Refresher**
- **Coding Overview Perinatal Conditions**
- **Abstracting for Perinatal Conditions**
- **Assigning Codes for Perinatal Conditions**
- **Arranging Codes for Perinatal Conditions**

Learning Objectives

After completing this chapter, you should have the skills to:

24.1 Spell and define the key words, medical terms, and abbreviations related to conditions originating in the perinatal period.

24.2 Discuss common conditions originating in the perinatal period.

24.3 Identify the main characteristics of coding for conditions originating in the perinatal period.

24.4 Abstract diagnostic information from the medical record for coding conditions originating in the perinatal period.

24.5 Assign codes for conditions originating in the perinatal period.

24.6 Arrange multiple diagnosis codes for conditions originating in the perinatal period.

24.7 Discuss the Official Guidelines for Coding and Reporting related to conditions originating in the perinatal period.

Key Terms and Abbreviations

chromosomal abnormality
deformation
erythroblastosis fetalis
malformation

neonatal mortality
neonate
newborn
newborn birth status

newborn clinically significant condition
perinatal condition

perinatal period
transitory

In addition to the key terms listed here, students should know the terms defined within tables in this chapter.

For updates and corrections, visit our student resource site at

www.pearsonhighered.com/healthprofessionsresources

INTRODUCTION

Newborn babies win over everyone's heart but, unfortunately, some experience medical conditions during the first few weeks of life. This chapter introduces you to some of those conditions.

A pediatrician is a physician who specializes in diagnosing and treating conditions of children, including perinatal conditions. A neonatologist is a pediatric subspecialist who diagnoses and treats complex conditions of newborns. Other medical specialties also have subspecialists in pediatrics and neonatology. For example, a neonatal cardiologist specializes in diagnosing and treating heart conditions of newborns.

PERINATAL REFRESHER

The **perinatal period** begins before birth and continues through the 28th day following birth. An infant is referred to as a **neonate** or **newborn** during the first 28 days of life (■ FIGURE 24-1). After day 28 they are classified as infants or children. **Perinatal conditions** are those that develop before birth or in the first 28 days after birth, but exclude physical **malformations** (*permanent abnormal shape of an organ or body region, resulting from arrested, delayed, or abnormal development of the embryo*), **deformations** (*a change in the size or shape of a normal structure due to physical forces*), and **chromosomal abnormalities** (*the abnormal number or structure of chromosomes*). Perinatal conditions are often **transitory** (*temporary*), but may be long term or permanent as well.

Refer to ■ TABLE 24-1 for a refresher on how to build medical terms related to conditions originating in the perinatal period.

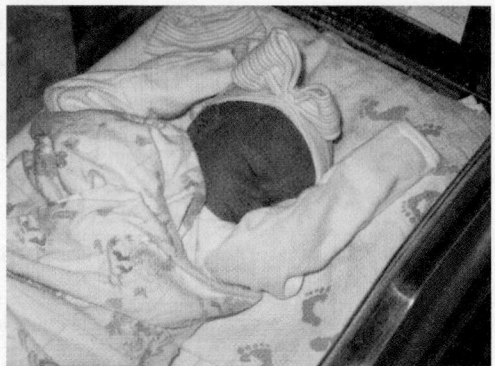

Figure 24-1 ■ A neonate or newborn is 1 to 28 days old. *Source: Bronwen Glowacki/Pearson Education.*

after the perinatal period, but because they originated during the perinatal period they are still considered perinatal conditions and are assigned codes from this ICD-10-CM chapter (■ FIGURE 24-2).

Some perinatal conditions, such as retinopathy, apnea, or tachycardia, use similar medical terms as conditions that affect adults. The condition is identified as perinatal by the use of a descriptive term, such as prematurity or newborn, in conjunction with the name of the condition. For example, retinopathy of prematurity, newborn apnea, or newborn tachycardia are perinatal conditions, whereas retinopathy, apnea, and tachycardia can originate at any age. Other perinatal conditions only occur in newborns, such as amnionitis or meconium aspiration syndrome. Refer to ■ TABLE 24-2 (page 406) for a summary of conditions originating in the perinatal period.

CODING CAUTION

Be alert for medical word roots that are spelled similarly and have different meanings.

omphal/o (*umbilicus or navel*) and **oophor/o** (*ovary*)

amni/o (*amniotic sac*), **ammon/o** (*ammonium*), and **amin/o** (*amino acid*)

Conditions Originating in the Perinatal Period

Perinatal conditions are defined by the fact that they *originated* during the perinatal period, regardless of when they are diagnosed or treated. Some conditions may not be diagnosed until

> Patient, age 15, is seen for Erb's palsy (*paralysis of the upper arm*), which resulted from damage during birth.
>
> Patient, age 60, is seen for blindness in the left eye, which he has had since birth, as a result of retinopathy of prematurity (ROP).
>
> Patient, age 35, is diagnosed with carcinoma of the vagina, due to exposure to diethylstilbestrol (DES) which her mother took during pregnancy.

Figure 24-2 ■ Examples of Perinatal Conditions Affecting Patients Later in Life

Table 24-1 ■ EXAMPLE OF CONSTRUCTING MEDICAL TERMS FOR CONDITIONS ORIGINATING IN THE PERINATAL PERIOD

Prefix	Root/Suffix	Complete Medical Term
dys- (*abnormal, painful*)		**dys + pnea** (*difficulty breathing*)
		dys + rhythmia (*abnormal heart beat*)
	-pnea (*breathing*)	
tachy- (*rapid*)	**-cardi/o** (*heart, heart rate*)	**tachy + pnea** (*rapid breathing*)
	-rhythm/o (*rhythm, beat*)	**tachy + cardia** (*rapid heart rate*)
brady- (*slow*)		**brady + pnea** (*slow breathing*)
		brady + cardia (*slow heart rate*)

Table 24-2 ■ **COMMON CONDITIONS ORIGINATING IN THE PERINATAL PERIOD**

Condition	Definition
Amnionitis	Infection or inflammation of the amniotic sac
Apgar score	An evaluation of a newborn's physical condition, performed 1 and 5 minutes after birth, to determine any immediate need for extra medical or emergency care (named after the physician who designed it, Dr. Virginia Apgar)
Appropriate for gestational age (AGA)	A fetus or newborn infant whose size is within the normal range for his or her gestational age
Birth trauma	Any physical injury to the infant during delivery
Breast engorgement	The temporary enlargement of breasts on female or male newborns, due to high levels of maternal hormones in the infant's blood
Drug withdrawal syndrome	A collection of symptoms of drug withdrawal in an infant who was exposed to narcotics in the uterus; also called neonatal abstinence syndrome (NAS)
Exceptionally large newborn	Birth weight more than 4,500 grams (9 pounds, 15 ounces)
Extremely low birth weight (ELBW)	Birth weight of less than 1,000 grams (2 pounds, 3 ounces)
Failure to thrive (FTT)	Inadequate physical growth marked by child's weight for age below the fifth percentile of the standard growth chart
Hemolytic disease of the newborn (HDN)	A blood disorder that occurs when the blood types of a mother and baby are incompatible, also called erythroblastosis fetalis
High birth weight (HBW)	Birth weight greater than 4,000 grams (8 pounds, 13 ounces)
Hyperbilirubinemia	High concentrations of bilirubin in the blood, which causes the infant's skin and sclera to turn yellow
Infant of diabetic mother (IDM)	An infant born to a woman who is diabetic
Intrauterine growth restriction (IUGR)	Poor growth of a baby while in the mother's womb during pregnancy. Specifically, it means the developing baby weighs less than 90% of other babies at the same gestational age.
Intraventricular hemorrhage (IVH)	Bleeding in the brain in very low birth weight premature babies, which usually resolves within a few days
Jaundice	A condition due to high bilirubin that causes the skin and parts of the eyes to turn a yellow color
Large for gestational age (LGA)	A fetus or newborn infant who is larger in size than normal for the baby's sex and gestational age, most commonly defined as a weight, length, or head circumference above the 90th percentile at gestational age
Low birth weight (LBW)	Birth weight less than 2,500 grams (5 pounds, 8 ounces)
Meconium aspiration syndrome (MAS)	Condition in which the newborn breathes a mixture of meconium and amniotic fluid into the lungs prior to or during delivery
Meconium peritonitis	Infection of the peritoneal cavity due to perforation of the bowel and leakage of meconium
Newborn ABO incompatibility	An infant with blood type A or B affected by comingling of type O blood from mother with blood type O
Newborn apnea	A condition in which the infant stops breathing
Newborn Rh incompatibility	Rh-positive infant affected by comingling of blood with an Rh-negative mother
Normal birth weight	Birth weight of 2,500 to 4,000 grams (5 pounds, 8 ounces to 8 pounds, 13 ounces)
Omphalitis	Infection of the umbilical stump in a newborn, usually presenting as superficial cellulitis
Respiratory distress syndrome (RDS)	A condition in which the alveolar sacs collapse due to lack of surfactant
Retinopathy of prematurity (ROP)	The abnormal growth of blood vessels in the eye that can lead to vision loss
Small for gestational age (SGA)	A fetus or newborn infant who is smaller in size than normal for the baby's sex and gestational age, most commonly defined as a weight, length, or head circumference below the 10th percentile for the gestational age
Transient tachypnea of the newborn (TTN)	Short-term condition (less than 24 hours) of rapid breathing due to retained lung fluid that occurs shortly after birth in full-term or near-term newborns
Very low birth weight (VLBW)	Birth weight of less than 1,500 grams (3 pounds, 4 ounces)

In particular, coders must be aware of conditions related to neonatal birth weight.

Birth Weight

Newborn birth weight is a major indicator of newborn health and nutritional status. Both low birth weight (LBW), under 2,500 grams, and high birth weight (HBW), over 4,000 grams, are associated with health problems. Birth weight is directly tied to the estimated gestational age (EGA) at birth. The earlier infants are born, before 37 weeks' gestation, the less they weigh. The longer a pregnancy continues, beyond 40 weeks, the more newborns weigh. Newborns of any EGA can be lighter or heavier in weight or smaller or larger in size compared to other infants of the same EGA. This condition is referred to by a variety of names such as small for gestational age, light for date, light for age, large for age, and similar.

> ### SUCCESS STEP
>
> Newborn birth weight is reported in grams using the metric system. A weight of 2,500 grams is equal to 5 pounds, 8 ounces.

LBW is a leading cause of **neonatal mortality** (*death before 29 days of age*). Although it is largely preventable in a developed country such as the United States, over 8% of infants each year are born with LBW, according to the Maternal and Child Health Bureau of the Department of Health and Human Resources, and more than 6 of every 1,000 children die before 1 year of age. LBW is associated with failure to thrive, dehydration, and feeding disorders, as well as many chronic conditions of the digestive, pulmonary, and cardiovascular systems. Premature infants

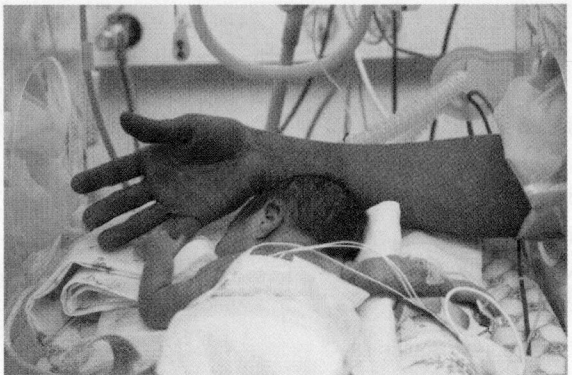

Figure 24-3 ■ Premature babies must weigh 1,800 grams before being released from an incubator. *Source: Fanfo/Fotolia.*

are weighed daily in the **neonatal intensive care unit (NICU)** and generally must weigh at least 1,800 grams (4 pounds) before being removed from the **incubator** (■ FIGURE 24-3). Each hospital sets its own weight standards for discharge, but the infant must be out of the incubator and steadily gaining weight before discharge.

High birth weight is associated with diabetes and certain childhood cancers and tumors, such as leukemia and **astrocytomas**, and possibly even adult cancers, such as breast, prostate, endometrial, and colon cancer, according to the journal *Cancer Epidemiology, Biomarkers & Prevention*.

This section provides a general reference to help understand the most common conditions originating in the perinatal period but does not list everything you need to know. Use medical terminology skills discussed earlier in this chapter to learn the meaning of unfamiliar words. Remember to keep standard reference books handy in case you get stuck.

CODING PRACTICE

Exercise 24.1   Perinatal Refresher

Instructions: Use your medical terminology skills and resources to define the following conditions related to conditions originating in the perinatal period, then assign the default diagnosis code.

Follow these steps:

- Use slash marks "/" to break down each underlined term into its root(s) and suffix.
- Define the meaning of the underlined term, based on the meaning of each word part.
- Assign the default ICD-10-CM diagnosis code for the condition using the Index and Tabular List. Locate the Main Term Newborn, then locate the subterms in the order shown.

Example: newborn <u>apnea</u> a/pnea   Meaning: <u>*lack of breathing*</u>   ICD-10-CM Code: <u>*P28.3*</u>

1. Newborn, affected by, heart
   rate, <u>tachycardia</u>   Meaning _____   ICD-10-CM Code _____

2. Newborn, affected by,
   <u>intrauterine</u> blood loss   Meaning _____   ICD-10-CM Code _____

3. Newborn, <u>hyperbilirubinemia</u>   Meaning _____   ICD-10-CM Code _____

4. Newborn, affected by,
   <u>maternal</u> <u>polyhydramnios</u>   Meaning _____   ICD-10-CM Code _____

5. Newborn, infective <u>mastitis</u>   Meaning _____   ICD-10-CM Code _____

(continued)

6. Newborn, <u>omphalitis</u>   Meaning _____   ICD-10-CM Code _____

7. Newborn, affected by, <u>hypoxic ischemic encephalopathy</u>   Meaning _____   ICD-10-CM Code _____

8. Newborn, affected by, <u>chorioamnionitis</u>   Meaning _____   ICD-10-CM Code _____

9. Newborn, <u>hyponatremia</u>   Meaning _____   ICD-10-CM Code _____

10. <u>erythroblastosis fetalis</u>   Meaning _____   ICD-10-CM Code _____

CODING OVERVIEW OF PERINATAL CONDITIONS

ICD-10-CM Chapter 16, Certain Conditions Originating in the Perinatal Period (P00-P96), contains 12 blocks or subchapters that are divided by anatomical site. Review the block names and code ranges listed at the beginning of Chapter 16 in the ICD-10-CM manual to become familiar with the content and organization.

This chapter includes newborn conditions that originate before birth or during the first 28 days of life and result from maternal conditions that are both related and unrelated to pregnancy, birth trauma, and underdevelopment during gestation. They also include respiratory, cardiovascular, metabolic, digestive, and hematological disorders. This chapter does not include fetal conditions that affect the mother or congenital abnormalities, both of which are classified in separate chapters. An instructional note at the beginning of the chapter requires that codes in this chapter are to be used *only* on the newborn's record, never on the mother's record.

ICD-10-CM Chapter 16 corresponds with ICD-9-CM Chapter 15 (760-779). Numerous categories have been expanded in ICD-10-CM compared to ICD-9-CM in order to add specificity to the diagnosis. Some codes have new titles, while others have been combined or deleted. ICD-10-CM defines all codes using the term *newborn* and omits the term *fetus*, which ICD-9-CM used in many code titles. Codes for the birth weight and gestational age of preterm infants have been redefined. Codes for birth trauma have greater specificity.

The sequencing of chapters in ICD-10-CM is different than in ICD-9-CM. In ICD-10-CM, this chapter, Certain Conditions Originating in the Perinatal Period (P00-P96), appears immediately after the obstetrics chapter, Pregnancy, Childbirth, and the Puerperium (**O00-O9A**), and is followed by Chapter 17, Congenital Malformations, Deformations and Chromosomal Abnormalities (Q00-Q99).

ICD-10-CM provides Official Guidelines for Coding and Reporting (OGCR) for conditions originating in the perinatal period in OGCR section I.C.16. OGCR provide detailed discussion of selecting the principal and additional diagnoses and how to report codes from this chapter with those from other chapters. OGCR also discuss specific coding for prematurity, low birth weight, bacterial sepsis of the newborn, and stillbirth. Additional guidelines related to assigning Z codes for newborns and infants appear in OGCR I.C.21.c.12).

ABSTRACTING FOR PERINATAL CONDITIONS

Coders must take note whether a hospitalization of a newborn includes the birth itself or whether the admission takes place after the birth episode. Abstract all **newborn clinically significant conditions**, defined as any newborn condition that meets the following criteria (OGCR I.C.16.a.6)):

- requires clinical evaluation
- requires therapeutic treatment
- requires diagnostic procedures
- extends length of hospital stay (LOS)
- increases nursing care or monitoring
- presents implications for future healthcare needs

The final criterion, conditions that present implications for future healthcare needs, is unique to newborns. When the provider documents newborn conditions that are not treated, but may have implications for future needs, coders should abstract and code this information. This type of information is *not* coded for adults.

Abstracting the birth encounter (■ Table 24-3) requires different criteria than abstracting encounters after birth

Table 24-3 ■ KEY CRITERIA FOR ABSTRACTING BIRTH ENCOUNTERS

- ❏ Was the infant born in this hospital during this admission?
- ❏ Was the infant born outside the hospital, then hospitalized?
- ❏ Was the delivery vaginal or cesarean?
- ❏ What is the birth weight?
- ❏ What is the estimated gestational age at time of delivery?
- ❏ Are any conditions documented as due to prematurity?
- ❏ Did the infant suffer any birth trauma?
- ❏ What conditions of the newborn required evaluation, treatment, extended LOS, increased care, or present implications for future healthcare needs?
- ❏ Was the newborn observed for any suspected conditions not found?
- ❏ What maternal conditions affected the infant?

Table 24-4 ■ KEY CRITERIA FOR ABSTRACTING ENCOUNTERS AFTER THE BIRTH EPISODE

❑ What is the age of the patient?

❑ What is the reason for the encounter?

❑ What condition is documented?

❑ What is the subtype of the condition?

❑ What complications and comorbidities exist?

❑ Is the condition documented as originating in the perinatal period?

Date of discharge: 4/21/yy   Location: Valley Hospital (VH)   Provider: Joann Gwinn, MD

Patient: Derek Leverette   Gender: M

DOB: 4/18/yy

Birth Weight: 1990g   EGA: 34+1   Method: cesarean

Location: VH

Assessment: cesarean performed due to maternal preeclampsia. Infant presented with transient tachypnea (TTN) due to prematurity and was admitted to NICU. O_2 and CPAP therapy were provided which restored breathing to normal within 48 hours. Patient was discharged with no symptoms.

Plan: FU in office, 2 weeks

(■ TABLE 24-4). Remember that the abstracting questions are a guide and that not every question applies to, or can be answered for, every case. For example, not all newborns are affected by a maternal condition. Also remember to abstract for symptoms and determine if they are integral to the confirmed diagnoses. After reviewing the abstracting criteria, work through the guided example that follows.

Abstracting from Newborn Records

Newborn records contain unique information and abbreviations not found in other medical records. Refer to ■ FIGURE 24-4 to learn how to interpret the mini-medical-record used for newborn cases in this text.

Guided Example of Abstracting for Perinatal Conditions

Refer to the following example throughout this chapter to practice skills for abstracting, assigning, and sequencing codes for conditions originating in the perinatal period. Aaron Randell, CCS, is a fictitious coder who guides you through the process.

Follow along as Aaron Randell, CCS, abstracts the diagnosis. Check off each step after you complete it.

▶ Aaron reads through the entire record, paying special attention to the birth data and the final assessment.

❑ He notes that this record is for the birth encounter so he refers to the Key Criteria for Abstracting Birth Encounters (Table 24-3).

❑ *Was the infant born in this hospital during this admission?* Yes.

❑ *Was the delivery vaginal or cesarean?* cesarean

❑ *What is the birth weight?* 1990 grams

❑ *What is the gestational age at time of delivery?* 34 weeks, 1 day

❑ *Are any conditions documented as due to prematurity?* transient tachypnea

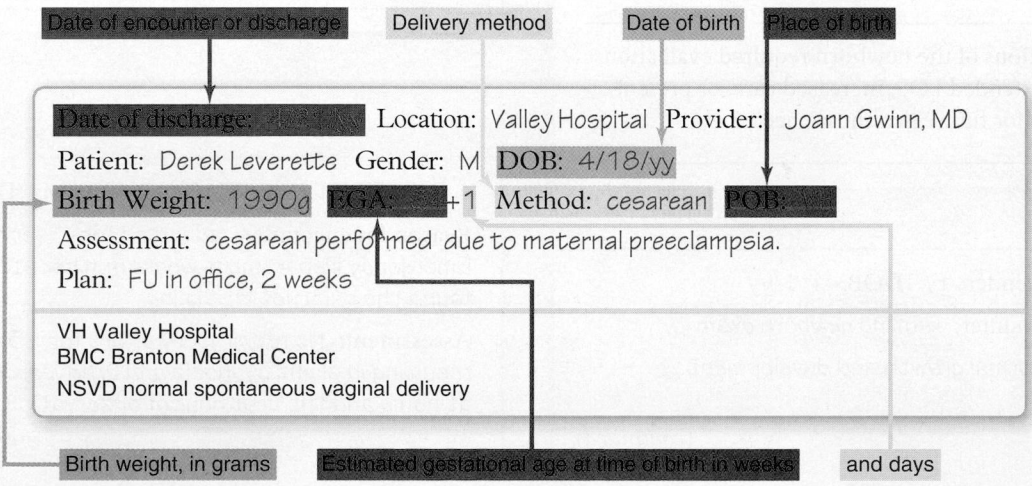

Figure 24-4 ■ Key to Interpreting the Newborn Mini-Medical-Record

❑ *Did the infant suffer any birth trauma?* No.

❑ *What conditions of the newborn required evaluation, treatment, extended LOS, increased care, or present implications for future healthcare needs?* transient tachypnea

❑ *Was the newborn observed for any suspected conditions not found?* No.

❑ *What maternal conditions affected the infant?* None. The mother had preeclampsia, but documentation does not state that it affected the infant.

▶ At this time, Aaron does not know how many codes he will end up with. He will learn about this when he moves on to assigning codes.

CODING PRACTICE

Exercise 24.2 Abstracting for Perinatal Conditions

Instructions: Read the mini-medical-record of each patient's encounter and answer the abstracting questions. Write the answer on the line provided. Do not assign any codes.

---

1. INPATIENT HOSPITAL   Gender: F   DOB: 4/22/yy

Birth Weight: 3521g   EGA: 38+2   Type: NSVD

POB: Hospital

Assessment: APGARS 6, 8

Plan: Discharged 1 day after birth. FU in office, 2 weeks

a. Was the infant born in this hospital during this admission? _____

b. Was the delivery vaginal or cesarean? _____
_____

c. What is the birth weight? _____

d. What is the estimated gestational age at time of delivery? _____

e. Are any conditions documented as due to prematurity?
_____

f. Did the infant suffer any birth trauma? _____
_____

g. What conditions of the newborn required evaluation, treatment, extended LOS, increased care, or present implications for future healthcare needs?
_____

---

2. OFFICE   Gender: F   DOB: 4/1/yy

Reason for encounter: routine newborn exam

Assessment: normal growth and development for age

(continued)

---

2. (continued)

Plan: RTO 1 month

a. What is the age of the patient? _____

b. What is the reason for the encounter? _____
_____

c. Were any abnormal conditions found? _____
_____

---

3. OFFICE   Gender: F   DOB: 4/10/yy

Reason for encounter: neonatal checkup, 13 days old

Assessment: neonatal diabetes

Plan: Start on sulfonylurea therapy and see how she does. Insulin may not be required. RTO 2 weeks.

a. What is the age of the patient? _____

b. What is the reason for the encounter? _____
_____

c. Were any abnormal conditions found? _____
_____

---

4. INPATIENT HOSPITAL   Gender: M   DOB: 4/5/yy

Reason for encounter: admitted for observation from Emergency Department where mother stated she found the baby not breathing

Assessment: No respiratory effort for 15 seconds, resulting in slight cyanosis and bradycardia times one at home and the first hour of observation. After 6

(continued)

4. (continued)

hours of observation determined to be d/t central sleep apnea

Plan: Discharged 18 days after birth. Use sleep apnea monitor and alarm

a. What is the age of the patient? _____

b. What is the reason for the encounter? _____

_____

c. What condition is documented? _____

d. What is the subtype of the condition? _____

_____

e. What complications and comorbidities exist?

_____

f. Is the condition documented as originating in the perinatal period? _____

5. INPATIENT HOSPITAL   Gender: M   DOB: 4/20/yy

Birth Weight: 3200g   EGA: 39+6

Type: forceps delivery   POB: Hospital

Assessment: admitted to NICU for observation due to fetal bradycardia during labor

Plan: d/c in excellent condition, RTO 2 weeks

a. Was the infant born in this hospital during this admission? _____

b. Was the delivery vaginal or cesarean? _____

_____

c. What is the birth weight? _____

d. What is the estimated gestational age at time of delivery? _____

e. Are any conditions documented as due to prematurity? _____

f. Did the infant suffer any birth trauma? _____

_____

g. What conditions of the newborn required evaluation, treatment, extended LOS, increased care, or present implications for future healthcare needs?

_____

h. What maternal conditions affected the infant?

_____

6. INPATIENT HOSPITAL   Gender: F   DOB: 4/21/yy

Birth Weight: 3756g   EGA: 43+3   Type: NSVD

Location: born in car on way to hospital, then admitted, mother reports discolored amniotic fluid

Assessment: meconium aspiration d/t late delivery with dyspnea and tachypnea, orotracheal intubation x 1 day, O_2 x 2 days, Rx antibiotics prophylactically

Plan: d/c in good condition, RTO 2 weeks

a. Was the infant born in this hospital during this admission? _____

b. Was the infant born outside the hospital then hospitalized? _____

c. Was the delivery vaginal or cesarean? _____

_____

d. What is the birth weight? _____

e. What is the estimated gestational age at time of delivery? _____

f. Are any conditions documented as due to prematurity?

_____

g. Did the infant suffer any birth trauma? _____

_____

h. What maternal conditions affected the infant?

_____

i. What conditions of the newborn required evaluation, treatment, extended LOS, increased care, or present implications for future healthcare needs? _____

_____

j. What is the subtype of the condition? _____

_____

7. INPATIENT HOSPITAL   Gender: F   DOB: 4/12/yy

Birth Weight: 2016g   EGA: 35+5

Type: NSVD   POB: Hospital

Reason for admission: infant was readmitted 2 days post-discharge from physician office d/t hyperbilirubinemia of prematurity

Assessment: jaundice d/t preterm delivery, resolved with phototherapy

Plan: Discharged 12 days after birth. FU in office 2 days

(continued)

CODING PRACTICE (continued)

7. (continued)

a. Was the infant born in this hospital during this admission? _____

b. Was the delivery vaginal or cesarean? _____
_____

c. What is the birth weight? _____

d. What is the estimated gestational age at time of delivery? _____

e. Are any conditions documented as due to prematurity? _____

f. Did the infant suffer any birth trauma? _____
_____

g. What conditions of the newborn required evaluation, treatment, extended LOS, increased care, or present implications for future healthcare needs? _____
_____

8. INPATIENT HOSPITAL   Gender: F   DOB: 4/2/yy

Birth Weight: 1923g   **EGA:** 37+2   **Type:** cesarean

POB: Hospital

Reason for admission: transferred from Valley Hospital on 4/3/yy for supervision of weight gain

Assessment: SGA and fetal growth restriction due to maternal preeclampsia and smoking during pregnancy

a. Was the infant born in this hospital during this admission? _____

b. Was the delivery vaginal or cesarean? _____
_____

c. What is the birth weight? _____

d. What is the estimated gestational age at time of delivery? _____

e. Are any conditions documented as due to prematurity? _____

f. Did the infant suffer any birth trauma? _____
_____

g. What maternal conditions affected the infant? _____
_____

h. What conditions of the newborn required evaluation, treatment, extended LOS, increased care, or present implications for future healthcare needs? _____

9. OFFICE   Gender: M   DOB: 4/2/yy

Reason for encounter: foul smelling urine

Assessment: UTI d/t E. coli

Plan: admit to hospital for IV antibiotics

a. What is the age of the patient? _____

b. What is the reason for the encounter? _____
_____

c. What condition is documented? _____

d. What is the subtype of the condition? _____
_____

e. What complications and comorbidities exist? _____

f. Is the condition documented as originating in the perinatal period? _____

10. OFFICE   Gender: F   DOB: 4/20/yy

Reason for encounter: first newborn check at 4 days old, baby was born at home with CNM in attendance

Assessment: Breast engorgement d/t maternal hormones which will resolve on its own. No problems with jaundice.

Plan: RTO 2 weeks

a. What is the age of the patient? _____

b. What is the reason for the encounter? _____
_____

c. What condition is documented? _____

d. What is the subtype of the condition? _____
_____

e. What complications and comorbidities exist? _____

f. Is the condition documented as originating in the perinatal period? _____

ASSIGNING CODES FOR PERINATAL CONDITIONS

To assign codes for newborns, coders must learn how to assign codes for birth status and for specific medical conditions. ICD-10-CM also provides separate codes for newborn medical examinations.

Assigning Codes for Newborn Birth Status

The **newborn birth status** code identifies the location of the birth, the delivery method, and the number of multiples. Assign this code to each mother only once and only when the hospital stay includes the birth episode. The exception is when an infant is born outside the hospital then hospitalized; in that instance, a birth status code should also be assigned. When a discharge includes the birth episode, assign a code from category **Z38.- Liveborn infants according to place of birth and type of delivery**. When a newborn is transferred from another hospital, the hospital where the infant was born reports a code from **Z38.-**. A birth status code should *not* be reported by the receiving hospital (OGCR I.C.16.a.2)).

Locate the newborn birth status code for singletons in the Index under the Main Term **Newborn**, subterm **born** (■ FIGURE 24-5). For multiple births, locate the Main Term **Newborn**, then the subterm for **twin**, **triplet**, **quadruplet**, or **quintuplet**. Each of these subterms has additional subterms for **born in hospital** and **by cesarean**. Always verify the code in the Tabular List.

Do not confuse category **Z38**, which is for use on the newborn record, with category **Z37 Outcome of delivery**, which is for use on the mother's record. Even though both categories appear to report similar information, they exist for different purposes. An instructional note at the beginning of each category in the Tabular List clearly defines the respective use and intended purpose.

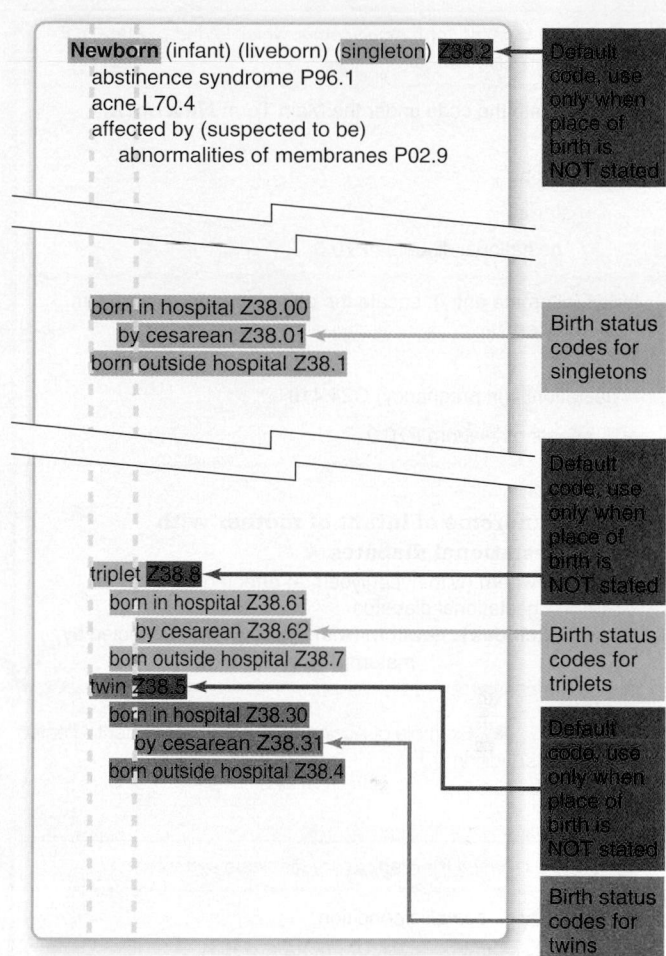

Figure 24-5 ■ Index Entries for Newborn Birth Status Codes

> ## SUCCESS STEP
>
> Highlight, flag, or draw an icon in your coding manual to remind yourself that **Z37.-** is for the mother and **Z38.-** is for the newborn. Mixing up these two code categories is a common mistake of new coders.

Assigning Codes for Conditions

Most codes for medical conditions of the newborn are indexed under the Main Term **Newborn**. The subterm **affected by** means to report the code *only* when the newborn is specifically affected by a condition. For example, when an infant is delivered with forceps assistance, assign a code only if the delivery method *affected* the infant. Do not automatically assign a code for forceps delivery to report the *fact* that forceps were used.

The subterm **maternal** describes the effect on the newborn of a condition the mother had during pregnancy, labor, or delivery. For example, when a newborn is affected by the mother's gestational diabetes (GDM), assign a code for **Newborn, affected by, maternal diabetes**. Be aware of the following distinctions among maternal and newborn codes:

- Do NOT assign code **O24.419 Gestational diabetes** to the newborn.

- Assign code **P70.0 Syndrome of infant of mother with gestational diabetes** (■ FIGURE 24-6, page 414) when the newborn is affected by maternal GDM.

- When the mother has GDM but the newborn is *not* affected by it, do not assign code **P70.0**.

When a code cannot be located under the Main Term **Newborn**, search under the name of the condition itself. Many conditions have a subterm specifically for the **newborn**, so be certain to review the subterms carefully to locate the appropriate entry (■ FIGURE 24-7, page 414). The subterm **transitory** under a newborn condition means that the condition was temporary, as many newborn conditions are.

When a condition that originated during the perinatal period is diagnosed or treated later in life, assign a perinatal code to identify the perinatal origin (OGCR I.C.16.a.4)) (■ FIGURE 24-8, page 414).

Some conditions of newborns either can be due to the birth process or be a community-acquired disease. When the documentation does not specify the cause of the condition, the default is to code it as perinatal and to assign a code from ICD-10-CM Chapter 16. When the condition is documented as community acquired, do not assign a code from Chapter 16 (OGCR I.C.16.a.5)).

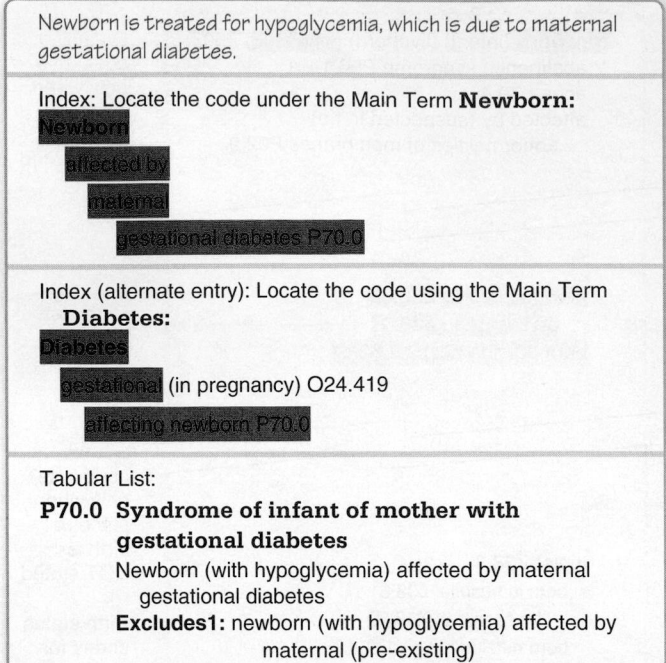

Newborn is treated for hypoglycemia, which is due to maternal gestational diabetes.

Index: Locate the code under the Main Term **Newborn:**

Newborn
affected by
maternal
gestational diabetes P70.0

Index (alternate entry): Locate the code using the Main Term **Diabetes:**

Diabetes
gestational (in pregnancy) O24.419
affecting newborn P70.0

Tabular List:

P70.0 Syndrome of infant of mother with gestational diabetes
Newborn (with hypoglycemia) affected by maternal gestational diabetes
Excludes1: newborn (with hypoglycemia) affected by maternal (pre-existing)

Figure 24-6 ■ Example of Assigning Codes for an Infant Affected by a Maternal Condition

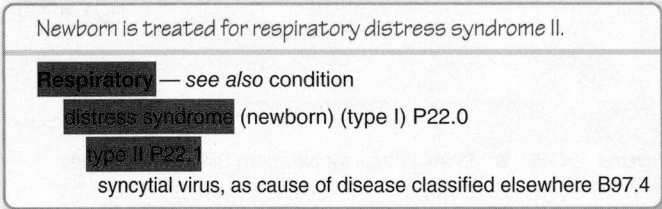

Newborn is treated for respiratory distress syndrome II.

Respiratory — *see also* condition
distress syndrome (newborn) (type I) P22.0
type II P22.1
syncytial virus, as cause of disease classified elsewhere B97.4

Figure 24-7 ■ Example of Locating a Newborn Code under the Main Term for the Condition

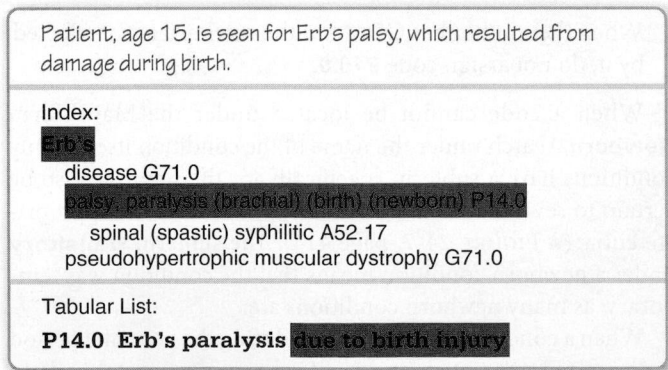

Patient, age 15, is seen for Erb's palsy, which resulted from damage during birth.

Index:
Erb's
disease G71.0
palsy, paralysis (brachial) (birth) (newborn) P14.0
spinal (spastic) syphilitic A52.17
pseudohypertrophic muscular dystrophy G71.0

Tabular List:
P14.0 Erb's paralysis due to birth injury

Figure 24-8 ■ Example of Assigning a Code for a Perinatal Condition Later in Life

Assigning Codes for Neonatal Examinations

Routine neonatal examinations are reported with **Z** codes, just as other routine physical examinations are. Search under the Main Term **Newborn** and the subterm **examination** to locate the codes in the Index. Codes are divided based on the age of

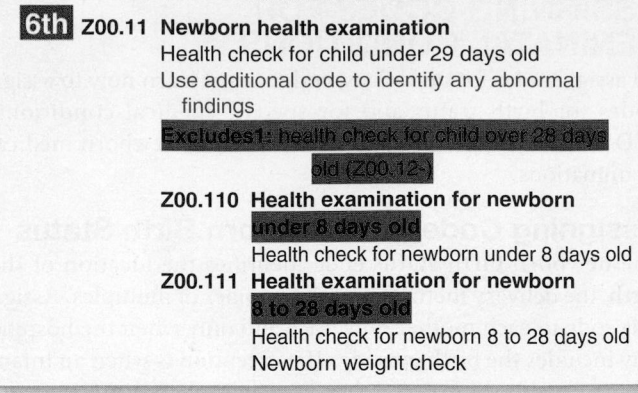

6th **Z00.11 Newborn health examination**
Health check for child under 29 days old
Use additional code to identify any abnormal findings
Excludes1: health check for child over 28 days old (Z00.12-)

Z00.110 Health examination for newborn under 8 days old
Health check for newborn under 8 days old

Z00.111 Health examination for newborn 8 to 28 days old
Health check for newborn 8 to 28 days old
Newborn weight check

Figure 24-9 ■ Tabular List Entry for Newborn Health Examination

---

SUCCESS STEP

Routine examinations for infants over 28 days in age should be assigned a code from **Z00.12- Encounter for routine child health examination**.

---

the newborn (■ FIGURE 24-9). An instructional note in the Tabular List directs coders to assign additional codes to identify any abnormal findings or conditions.

Guided Example of Assigning Perinatal Codes

To practice skills for assigning codes for conditions originating in the perinatal period, continue with the example from earlier in the chapter about patient Derek Leverette, who was born at Valley Hospital.

Follow along in your ICD-10-CM manual as Aaron Randell, CCS, assigns codes. Check off each step after you complete it.

▶ First, Aaron confirms the information he abstracted.

❑ This is a birth encounter of a preterm birth.

❑ The newborn was treated for TTN.

▶ Aaron knows that because this is a birth encounter, he must assign a code for the birth status of the infant.

▶ Aaron searches the Index for the Main Term **Newborn**.

❑ He locates the subterm **born in hospital**.

❑ He locates the second-level subterm **by cesarean Z38.01**

▶ Aaron verifies code **Z38.01** in the Tabular List.

❑ He reads the code title for **Z38.01, Single liveborn infant, delivered by cesarean**, and confirms that this accurately describes the birth.

▶ Aaron checks for instructional notes in the Tabular List.

❑ He cross-references the beginning of category **Z38** and reads the instructional note that tells him that this is the correct code for a newborn and it should never be assigned to the mother (■ FIGURE 24-10).

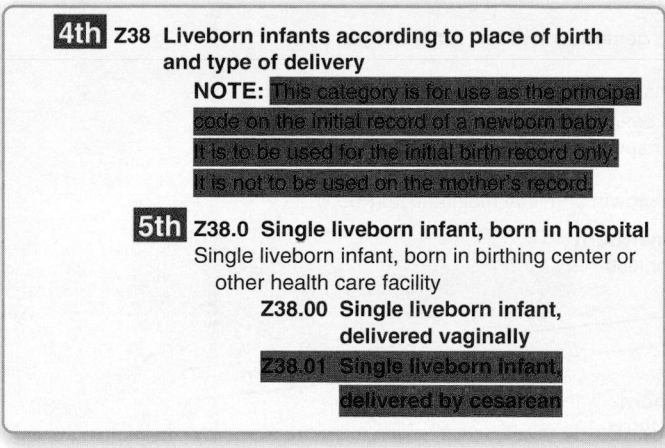

Figure 24-10 ■ Tabular List Instructional Note for Category Z38

❏ He cross-references the beginning of block **Z30-Z39** and verifies that there are no instructional notes.

❏ He cross-references the beginning of **Chapter 21 (Z00-Z99)** and reviews the instructional notes, which provide a general description about the use of Z codes. He determines there is no information that applies specifically to this code.

▶ Next, Aaron decides to assign a code for TTN.

▶ Aaron searches the Index for the Main Term **Tachypnea**.

❏ He locates the subterm **newborn P22.1**.

▶ Aaron verifies code **P22.1** in the Tabular List.

❏ He reads the code title for **P22.1, Transient tachypnea of newborn**, and confirms that this accurately describes the diagnosis.

▶ Aaron checks for instructional notes in the Tabular List.

❏ He cross-references the beginning of category **P22** and reads the **Excludes1** note. He determines that it does not apply because neither of the conditions excluded are documented for this patient.

❏ He cross-references the beginning of the block **P19-P29** and verifies that there are no instructional notes.

❏ He cross-references the beginning of **Chapter 16 (P00-P99)** and reads the instructional notes. They confirm that codes in this chapter should be used on the newborn's record.

▶ The next code Aaron decides to assign is for the preterm birth.

▶ Aaron searches the Index for the Main Term **Preterm** (■ Figure 24-11).

❏ He locates a subterm **delivery O60.10**.

❏ He reviews the remaining subterm and also locates subterm **newborn P07.30**.

❏ He notices that the codes are from different chapters because they begin with different letters. He decides to check the Tabular List for each code.

❏ He verifies the code title for **O60.10, Preterm labor with preterm delivery, unspecified trimester**.

❏ When he cross-references the beginning of the chapter, he learns that this code is from **Chapter 15 Pregnancy, Childbirth and the Puerperium (O00-O9A)**.

❏ He reads the instructional note in capital letters under the chapter title that states **CODES FROM THIS CHAPTER ARE FOR USE ONLY ON MATERNAL RECORDS, NEVER ON NEWBORN RECORDS**.

❏ This instruction tells him that he should NOT use **O60.10** because he is coding for the newborn, not the mother.

❏ Aaron returns to the Index to review the entries for the Main Term **Preterm** and subterm **newborn**.

❏ He locates a second-level subterm **gestational age**.

❏ He locates the third-level subterm **34 completed weeks (34 weeks, 0 days through 34 weeks, 6 days) P07.37**. He believes this code describes the preterm newborn of gestational age 34 weeks, which is documented in the medical record.

▶ Aaron verifies code **P07.37** in the Tabular List.

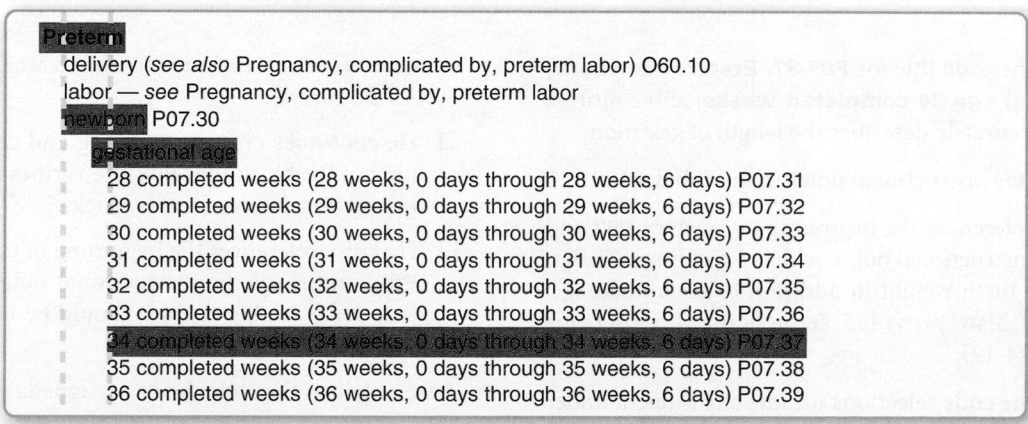

Figure 24-11 ■ Index Entry for Preterm

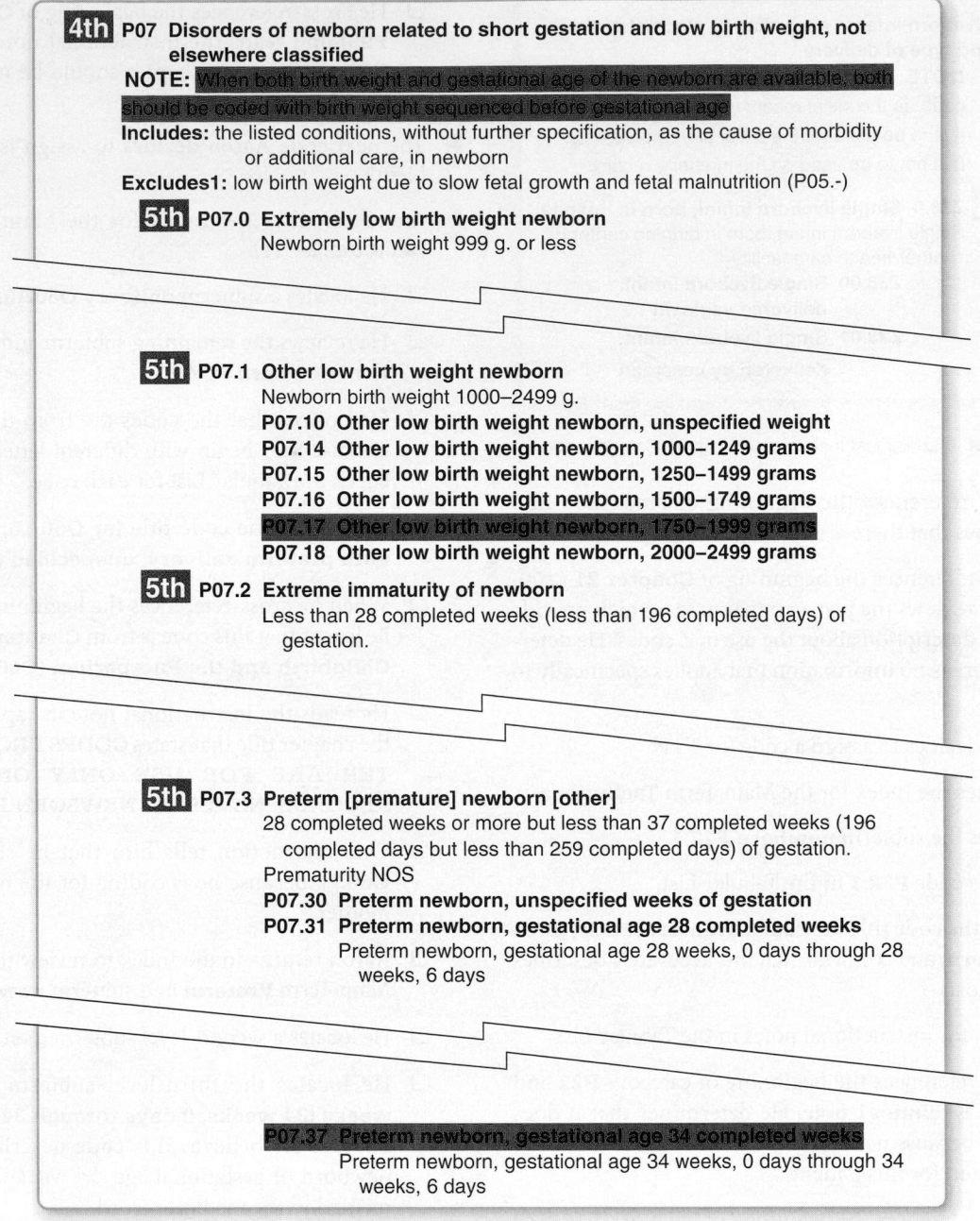

4th P07 Disorders of newborn related to short gestation and low birth weight, not elsewhere classified
NOTE: When both birth weight and gestational age of the newborn are available, both should be coded with birth weight sequenced before gestational age
Includes: the listed conditions, without further specification, as the cause of morbidity or additional care, in newborn
Excludes1: low birth weight due to slow fetal growth and fetal malnutrition (P05.-)

5th P07.0 Extremely low birth weight newborn
Newborn birth weight 999 g. or less

5th P07.1 Other low birth weight newborn
Newborn birth weight 1000–2499 g.
P07.10 Other low birth weight newborn, unspecified weight
P07.14 Other low birth weight newborn, 1000–1249 grams
P07.15 Other low birth weight newborn, 1250–1499 grams
P07.16 Other low birth weight newborn, 1500–1749 grams
P07.17 Other low birth weight newborn, 1750–1999 grams
P07.18 Other low birth weight newborn, 2000–2499 grams

5th P07.2 Extreme immaturity of newborn
Less than 28 completed weeks (less than 196 completed days) of gestation.

5th P07.3 Preterm [premature] newborn [other]
28 completed weeks or more but less than 37 completed weeks (196 completed days but less than 259 completed days) of gestation.
Prematurity NOS
P07.30 Preterm newborn, unspecified weeks of gestation
P07.31 Preterm newborn, gestational age 28 completed weeks
Preterm newborn, gestational age 28 weeks, 0 days through 28 weeks, 6 days

P07.37 Preterm newborn, gestational age 34 completed weeks
Preterm newborn, gestational age 34 weeks, 0 days through 34 weeks, 6 days

Figure 24-12 ■ Tabular List Instructional Notes for Category P07

❑ He reads the code title for **P07.37, Preterm newborn, gestational age 34 completed weeks**, and confirms that this accurately describes the length of gestation.

▶ Aaron checks for instructional notes in the Tabular List.

❑ He cross-references the beginning of category **P07** and reads the instructional notes, which direct him to assign a code for birth weight in addition to gestational age. The note also provides sequencing instructions (■ Figure 24-12).

❑ He reads the code selections for low birth weight under subcategories **P07.0** and **P07.1**. He locates the code **P07.17, Other low birth weight newborn, 1750-1999**

grams, which includes the birth weight of this baby, *1790 grams*.

❑ He continues cross-referencing and checks the beginning of the block **P05-P08**. He verifies that there are no instructional notes for this block.

❑ He cross-references the beginning of **Chapter 16 (P00-P99)** and reads the instructional notes. They confirm that codes in this chapter should be used on the newborn's record.

▶ Aaron reviews the codes he has assigned for this case.

❑ **P07.37 Preterm newborn, gestational age completed weeks**

❏ **P07.17**   **Other low birth weight newborn, 1750-1999 grams**

❏ **P22.1**   **Transient tachypnea of newborn**

❏ **Z38.01**   **Single liveborn infant, delivered by cesarean**

▶ Next, Aaron must determine how to sequence the codes.

CODING PRACTICE

Exercise 24.3   Assigning Codes for Perinatal Conditions

Instructions: Read the mini-medical-record of each patient's encounter, review the information abstracted in Exercise 24.2, and assign ICD-10-CM diagnosis codes using the Index and Tabular List. Write the code(s) on the line provided.

1. INPATIENT HOSPITAL   Gender: F   DOB: 4/22/yy

Birth Weight: 3521g   EGA: 38+2   Type: NSVD

POB: Hospital

Assessment: APGARS 6, 8

Plan: Discharged 1 day after birth. FU in office, 2 weeks

Tip: Apgar scores of 6 (one minute after delivery) and 8 (five minutes after delivery) are considered normal.

1 ICD-10-CM Code _____

2. OFFICE   Gender: F   DOB: 4/1/yy

Reason for encounter: routine newborn exam

Assessment: normal growth and development for age

Plan: RTO 1 month

1 ICD-10-CM Code _____

3. OFFICE   Gender: F   DOB: 4/10/yy

Reason for encounter: neonatal check up, 13 days old

Assessment: neonatal diabetes

Plan: Start on sulfonylurea therapy and see how she does. Insulin may not be required. RTO 2 weeks.

(continued)

3. (continued)

Tip: A checkup is the same as an examination.

2 ICD-10-CM Codes _____

4. INPATIENT HOSPITAL   Gender: M   DOB: 4/5/yy

Reason for encounter: admitted for observation from Emergency Department where mother stated she found the baby not breathing

Assessment: No respiratory effort for 15 seconds, resulting in slight cyanosis and bradycardia times one at home and the first hour of observation. After 6 hours of observation determined to be d/t central sleep apnea.

Plan: Discharged 18 days after birth. Use sleep apnea monitor and alarm at home.

1 ICD-10-CM Code _____

5. INPATIENT HOSPITAL   Gender: M   DOB: 4/20/yy

Birth Weight: 3200g   EGA: 39+6

Type: forceps delivery   POB: Hospital

Assessment: admitted to NICU for observation due to fetal bradycardia during labor

Plan: d/c in excellent condition, RTO 2 weeks

Tip: Forceps are used only in a vaginal delivery.

2 ICD-10-CM Codes _____

ARRANGING CODES FOR PERINATAL CONDITIONS

Significant perinatal sequencing guidelines relate to selecting the principal diagnosis for the birth episode, assigning codes for the weight and EGA of preterm infants, and sequencing codes for bacterial newborn sepsis.

Selecting the Principal Diagnosis for Birth Encounters

The previous section of this chapter discussed assigning a code from category **Z38** to identify the birth status on a newborn's record. This code is assigned only for hospital admissions that include the delivery or occur immediately after a birth outside the hospital. Sequence codes as follows:

1. **Z38.**- is *always* sequenced as the principal diagnosis on a newborn's record (OGCR I.C.16.a.2)). This is true regardless of any other conditions or complications that accompany the birth.

2. Sequence additional codes for any conditions that require treatment, further workup, prolong length of stay, or require resource utilization (OGCR I.C.16.c.1)). Conditions that require current treatment or workup should be sequenced based on their significance according to the provider.

3. Finally, sequence conditions documented as having implications for future healthcare needs (OGCR I.C.16.c.2)).

CODING CAUTION

Conditions not treated but documented as having implications for future healthcare needs should be coded *only* for newborns, never for adults.

Arranging Codes for Birth Weight and Estimated Gestational Age

A preterm infant may have difficulties due to short gestation or low birth weight. A postterm infant may be at risk for diabetes or other conditions. Assign codes that identify the birth weight and the EGA of the infant when these factors are documented to affect the infant's health status. Also assign codes for any specified conditions. For admissions that include the birth encounter, sequence the codes as follows (OGCR I.C.16.d and e):

1. **Z38.**- Birth status of infant, if the admission includes the birth episode

2. **P07.0**- or **P07.1**- Birth weight (Search the Index for the Main Term **Low**, subterm **birth weight.**)

3. **P07.2**- or **P07.3**- Weeks of gestation (Search the Index for the Main Term **Preterm**, subterm **newborn**, second-level subterm **gestational age.**)

4. Other specified conditions

For admissions that do not include the birth encounter, select the principal diagnosis based on the standard criteria in OGCR II.

SUCCESS STEP

Birth weight should always be sequenced *before* EGA, but weight is not the principal diagnosis.

A full-term or preterm infant may be small for its age due to slow fetal growth or malnutrition. Assign a code from **P05.- Disorders of newborn related to slow fetal growth and fetal malnutrition** in these situations.

A postterm infant may be at risk due to being large for its age. Assign a code from **P08 Disorders of newborn related to long gestation and high birth weight** in these situations.

CODING CAUTION

When you assign a code from **P05**, do *not* assign codes from **P07** for birth weight and EGA.

Arranging Codes for Bacterial Newborn Sepsis

Coding bacterial sepsis of a newborn is similar to coding any patient with sepsis, as discussed in Chapter 21 of this text and ICD-10-CM Chapter 1, Certain Infectious and Parasitic Diseases (A00-B49). One difference is that perinatal sepsis may be congenital or community acquired. When the source is not documented, the default is congenital and a newborn sepsis code should be assigned (OGCR I.C.16.f). Category **P36 Bacterial sepsis of newborn** provides combination codes that include the most common causal organisms (■ FIGURE 24-13). If the appropriate causal organism is not included in the **P36.**- code, then assign an additional code from category **B96**. Assign and sequence codes as follows:

1. Assign a code from **P36.- Bacterial sepsis of newborn**.

2. If the causal organism is *not* provided in a combination code, assign a code from **B96 Other bacterial agents as the cause of diseases classified elsewhere**.

3. When severe sepsis or septic shock is documented, assign a code from **R65.2- Severe sepsis**.

4. Assign codes for associated acute organ dysfunction(s).

Guided Example of Arranging Perinatal Codes

To practice skills for sequencing codes for diseases of the conditions originating in the perinatal period, continue with the example from earlier in the chapter about patient Derek Leverette, who was born at Valley Hospital.

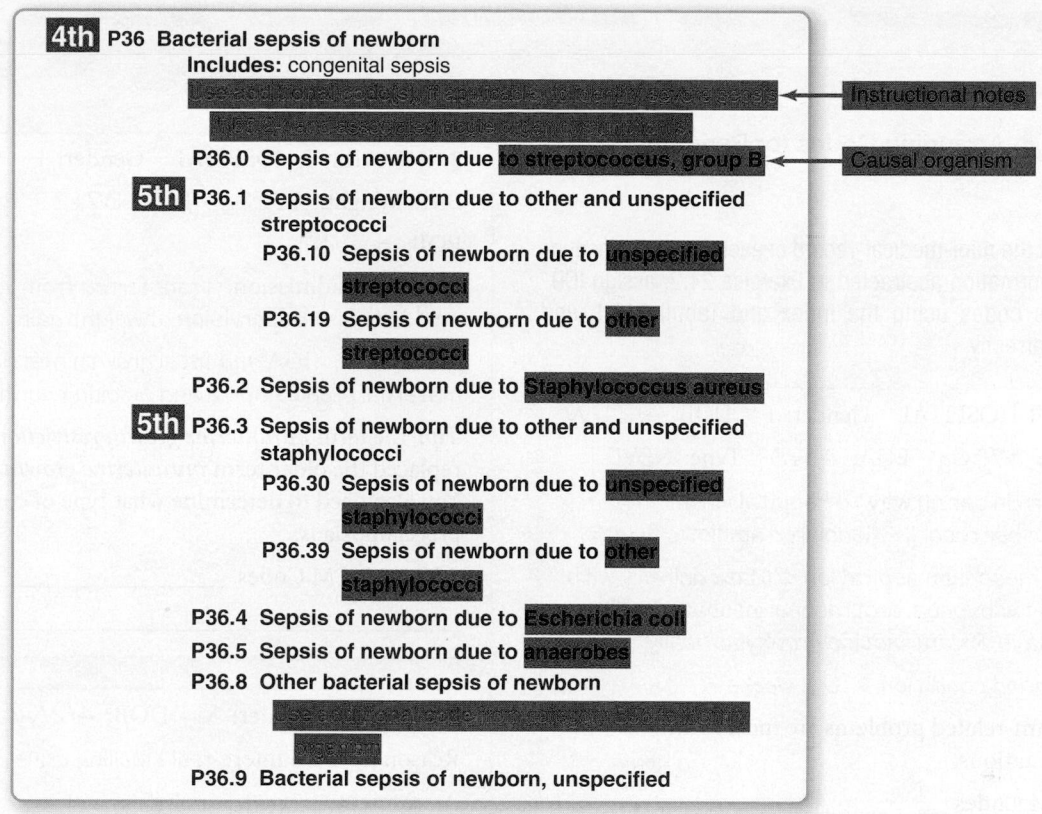

Figure 24-13 ■ Tabular List Entry for Category P36 Bacterial Sepsis of Newborn

Follow along in your ICD-10-CM manual as Aaron Randell, CCS, sequences the codes. Check off each step after you complete it.

▶ First, Aaron reviews the codes he assigned.

❑ **P07.37 Preterm newborn, gestational age 34 completed weeks**

❑ **P07.17 Other low birth weight newborn, 1750-1999 grams**

❑ **P22.1 Transient tachypnea of newborn**

❑ **Z38.01 Single liveborn infant, delivered by cesarean**

▶ Aaron refers to OGCR I.C.16.a.2), Principal Diagnosis for the Birth Record.

❑ The OGCR states that a code from **Z38** should be the principal diagnosis for the birth episode. This enables Aaron to determine that the first code should be **Z38.01**.

▶ Aaron refers to OGCR I.C.16.d, Prematurity and Fetal Growth Retardation.

❑ This OGCR states that codes should be assigned based on the documented birth weight and gestational age. It also states that the code for birth weight should be sequenced before the code for gestational age. He also recalls that he read an instructional note under category **P07** with the same information.

❑ Based on this information, Aaron determines that **P07.17** should be the second code and **P07.37** should be the third code.

❑ This leaves **P22.1** as the final code. Aaron checks the notes he wrote earlier to be certain that there are no instructional notes that affect the sequencing of this code.

▶ Aaron finalizes the codes and sequencing for this case:

1. **Z38.01 Single liveborn infant, delivered by cesarean**

2. **P07.17 Other low birth weight newborn, 1750-1999 grams**

3. **P07.37 Preterm newborn, gestational age 34 completed weeks**

4. **P22.1 Transient tachypnea of newborn**

CODING PRACTICE

Exercise 24.4 Arranging Codes for Perinatal Conditions

Instructions: Read the mini-medical-record of each patient's encounter, review the information abstracted in Exercise 24.2, assign ICD-10-CM diagnosis codes using the Index and Tabular List, and sequence them correctly.

1. INPATIENT HOSPITAL Gender: F DOB: 4/21/yy

Birth Weight: 3756g EGA: 43+3 Type: NSVD

Location: born in car on way to hospital, then admitted, mother reports discolored amniotic fluid

Assessment: meconium aspiration d/t late delivery with dyspnea and tachypnea, orotracheal intubation x 1 day, O₂ x 2 days, Rx antibiotics prophylactically

Plan: d/c in good condition, RTO 2 weeks

Tip: Meconium-related problems are most common with prolonged gestations.

3 ICD-10-CM Codes _____

_____

2. INPATIENT HOSPITAL Gender: F DOB: 4/12/yy

Birth Weight: 2016g EGA: 35+5 Type: NSVD

POB: Hospital

Reason for admission: infant was readmitted 2 days post-discharge from physician office d/t hyperbilirubinemia of prematurity

Assessment: jaundice d/t preterm delivery, resolved with phototherapy

Plan: Discharged 12 days after birth. FU in office 2 days

3 ICD-10-CM Codes _____

_____

3. INPATIENT HOSPITAL Gender: F DOB: 4/2/yy

Birth Weight: 1923g EGA: 37+2 Type: cesarean

POB: Hospital

Reason for admission: transferred from Valley Hospital on 4/3/yy for supervision of weight gain

Assessment: SGA and fetal growth restriction due to maternal preeclampsia and smoking during pregnancy

Tip: The term *intrauterine growth restriction* has largely replaced the older term *intrauterine growth retardation.* You also need to determine what type of condition preeclampsia is.

4 ICD-10-CM Codes _____

_____

4. OFFICE Gender: M DOB: 4/2/yy

Reason for encounter: foul smelling urine

Assessment: UTI d/t E. coli (NSTEC)

Plan: admit to hospital for IV antibiotics

2 ICD-10-CM Codes _____

5. OFFICE Gender: F DOB: 4/20/yy

Reason for encounter: first newborn check at 4 days old, baby was born at home with CNM in attendance

Assessment: Breast engorgement d/t maternal hormones which will resolve on its own. No problems with jaundice.

Plan: RTO 2 weeks

2 ICD-10-CM Codes _____

CHAPTER SUMMARY

In this chapter you learned that:

- The perinatal period begins before birth and continues through the 28th day following birth.
- ICD-10-CM Chapter 16, Certain Conditions Originating in the Perinatal Period (P00-P96), contains 12 blocks or subchapters that are divided by anatomical site.
- Coders must take note whether a hospitalization of a newborn includes the birth itself or whether the admission takes place after the birth episode.
- To assign codes for newborns, coders must learn how to assign codes for birth status, for specific medical conditions, and for newborn examinations.

- Significant sequencing guidelines relate to selecting the principal diagnosis for the birth episode, assigning codes for the weight and EGA of preterm infants, and sequencing codes for bacterial newborn sepsis.

- ICD-10-CM provides Official Guidelines for Coding and Reporting (OGCR) in OGCR I.C.16 regarding selecting the principal and additional diagnoses, and how to report codes from this chapter with those from other chapters, prematurity, low birth weight, bacterial sepsis of the newborn, and stillbirth.

CONCEPT QUIZ

Take a moment to look back at conditions originating in the perinatal period and solidify your skills. Try to answer the questions from memory first, then look back at the discussion in this chapter if you need a little extra help.

Completion

Instructions: Write the term that answers each question based on the information you learned in this chapter. Choose from the list below. Some choices may be used more than once and some choices may not be used at all.

1,000	Erb's palsy
1,500	LBW
2,000	LGA
2,500	MAS
4,000	meconium peritonitis
amin/o	neonate
ammon/o	omphalitis
amni/o	perinatal
amnionitis	transitory
birth trauma	VLBW

1. A newborn with a birth weight of 2,200 grams is classified as

   _____.

2. Normal birth weight is defined as _____ to
   _____ grams.

3. _____ is a condition in which the newborn breathes a mixture of meconium and amniotic fluid into the lungs prior to or during delivery.

4. A fetus or newborn infant who is larger in size than normal for the baby's sex and gestational age is classified as

   _____.

5. _____ is any physical injury to the infant during delivery.

6. Infection of the umbilical stump in a newborn is called

   _____.

7. A _____ perinatal condition is temporary.

8. An infant is referred to as a _____ during the first 28 days of life.

9. The combining form for amniotic sac is

   _____.

10. _____ grams equals 5 pounds, 8 ounces.

Multiple Choice

Instructions: Circle the letter of the best answer to each question based on the information you learned in this chapter.

1. Which type of condition is NOT classified in ICD-10-CM Chapter 16 (P00-P99)?
   A. Birth trauma
   B. Conditions that result from maternal conditions
   C. Congenital abnormalities
   D. Conditions that result from underdevelopment during gestation

2. Which of the criteria for clinically significant conditions is used ONLY for newborns?
   A. A condition that requires clinical evaluation
   B. A condition that increases nursing care or monitoring
   C. A condition that extends length of hospital stay
   D. A condition that presents implications for future healthcare needs

3. A full-term infant is born in the hospital with normal vaginal delivery and no complications. What code should be assigned to the newborn's birth record?
   A. **O80** Encounter for full-term uncomplicated delivery
   B. **Z34.03** Encounter for supervision of normal first pregnancy, third trimester
   C. **Z37.0** Single live birth
   D. **Z38.00** Single liveborn infant, delivered vaginally

4. Perinatal conditions are defined by the fact that they
   A. were diagnosed during the first 28 days.
   B. originated before birth or during the first 28 days.
   C. were treated during the first 28 days.
   D. result from a condition of the mother.

5. Which of the following conditions is NOT a perinatal condition?
   A. Gestational diabetes
   B. Retinopathy of prematurity
   C. Meconium aspiration syndrome
   D. Neonatal diabetes

6. The permanent abnormal shape of an organ or body region, resulting from arrested, delayed, or abnormal development of the embryo, is
   A. a deformation.
   B. a malformation.
   C. a chromosomal abnormality.
   D. Erb's palsy.

7. Perinatal codes can be used in all the following situations EXCEPT
   A. a 15-year-old with a permanent condition that originated at birth.
   B. a newborn condition that lasts only a few days.
   C. a fetal condition that affects the mother.
   D. a maternal condition that affects the newborn.

(continued)

(continued from page 421)

8. A birth status code from Z38 should be reported when
   A. a hospital receives a newborn from another hospital.
   B. the hospital stay includes the birth episode.
   C. a fetus is stillborn.
   D. a newborn is readmitted within 28 days of birth.

9. OGCR for Chapter 16 discuss all of the following EXCEPT
   A. selecting the principal diagnosis.
   B. low birth weight.
   C. bacterial sepsis of the newborn.
   D. neonatal diabetes.

10. A birth status code from Z38 describes the newborn's
    A. weight.
    B. gender.
    C. delivery method.
    D. gestational age.

CODING CHALLENGE

Instructions: Read the mini-medical-record of each patient's encounter, then abstract, assign, and sequence ICD-10-CM diagnosis codes using the Index and Tabular List. Write the code(s) on the line provided.

---

1. INPATIENT HOSPITAL Gender: F DOB: 4/27/yy

Birth Weight: 4555g EGA: 40+4 Type: cesarean

POB: Hospital

Assessment: LGA, watch for diabetes, otherwise healthy

Plan: Discharged 1 day after birth. FU office 2 weeks

2 ICD-10-CM Codes _____

---

2. INPATIENT HOSPITAL Gender: M DOB: 4/28/yy

Birth Weight: 3010g EGA: 42+0 Type: NSVD

POB: Hospital

Assessment: post term, otherwise healthy

Plan: Discharged 1 day after birth. FU office 2 weeks

2 ICD-10-CM Codes _____

---

3. INPATIENT HOSPITAL Gender: F DOB: 4/22/yy

Birth Weight: 1293g EGA: 30+3 Type: cesarean

POB: Hospital

Reason for admission: transferred from Valley Hospital on DOB due to heroin baby

Assessment: drug withdrawal syndrome complicated by prematurity with underdeveloped lungs

Plan: Discharged 7 days after birth. Weaned off heroin. RTO 3 days post discharge.

Tip: Follow the sequencing rules for poisonings.

4 ICD-10-CM Codes _____

_____

---

4. INPATIENT HOSPITAL Gender: F DOB: 4/20/yy

Birth Weight: 3621g EGA: 39+1 Type: cesarean

POB: Hospital

Assessment: hypoglycemia due to GDM, respiratory distress

Plan: Discharged 9 days after birth. FU weekly for first month

4 ICD-10-CM Codes _____

_____

---

5. INPATIENT HOSPITAL Gender: F DOB: 4/22/yy

Birth Weight: 3489g EGA: 38+0 Type: NSVD

POB: Hospital

Assessment: fractured clavicle during delivery d/t prolapsed arm presentation

Plan: pin long sleeved garment to the clothes to immobilize arm if discomfort observed, lift child with care, RTO 1 week

Tip: Discharged 7 days after birth. A prolapsed arm is a malpresentation.

3 ICD-10-CM Codes _____

_____

---

6. INPATIENT HOSPITAL Gender: M DOB: 4/15/yy

Reason for encounter: redness, mild bleeding, and swelling of umbilical stump

Assessment: omphalitis with hemorrhage

Plan: begin 2 week regime of antimicrobial therapy, RTO in one day for reevaluation of condition

1 ICD-10-CM Code _____

7. INPATIENT HOSPITAL   Gender: M   DOB: 3/29/yy

Birth Weight: 762g   EGA: 28   Type: NSVD

POB: Hospital

Assessment: This infant is the first born of triplets with cardiomyopathy. The second sibling was liveborn with respiratory distress syndrome and jaundice. Fetus 3 stillborn

Plan: Discharged 31 days after birth. RTO 3 days post discharge.

Tip: Each infant has its own record. Code only for the infant who is named on this record.

4 ICD-10-CM Codes _____

_____

8. INPATIENT HOSPITAL   Gender: M   DOB: 4/22/yy

Birth Weight: 3256g   EGA: 40+2   Type: NSVD

POB: Hospital

Assessment: injury to brachial plexus and cannot move arm

Plan: Discharged 7 days after birth. Refer to physical therapist for three months. Reevaluate for reconstructive surgery if no improvement in three months.

2 ICD-10-CM Codes _____

9. INPATIENT HOSPITAL   Gender: M   DOB: 4/12/yy

Reason for admission: admitted on 4/15/yy, 2 days post discharge, with acute respiratory failure d/t severe sepsis

Assessment: severe sepsis d/t staphylococcus aureus caused by amnionitis, ARF

Plan: Antibiotic therapy, careful post discharge monitoring, aggressive fluid restoration. RTO 1 week

Tip: Refer to OGCR I.C.16.f.

4 ICD-10-CM Codes _____

_____

10. INPATIENT HOSPITAL   Gender: M   DOB: 4/25/yy

Birth Weight: 3185g   EGA: 38+3   Type: NSVD

POB: Hospital

Reason for admission: transferred from Valley Hospital 6 hours after birth d/t hemolytic disease

Assessment: transfusion required for hemolytic disease due to ABO isoimmunization

Plan: Discharged 4 days after admission. FU 1 week

1 ICD-10-CM Code _____

KEEP ON CODING

Instructions: Read the diagnostic statement, then use the Index and Tabular List to assign and sequence ICD-10-CM diagnosis codes. Write the code(s) on the line provided.

1. Transient neonatal myasthenia gravis: ICD-10-CM Code(s) _____

2. Subdural hematoma due to birth injury: ICD-10-CM Code(s) _____

3. Newborn small for date, 1,150 grams: ICD-10-CM Code(s) _____

4. Newborn melena: ICD-10-CM Code(s) _____

5. Congenital pneumonia due to pseudomonas: ICD-10-CM Code(s) _____

6. Postterm newborn, 43 weeks' gestation: ICD-10-CM Code(s) _____

7. Overfeeding of newborn: ICD-10-CM Code(s) _____

8. Neonatal jaundice due to polycythemia: ICD-10-CM Code(s) _____

9. Neonatal craniotabes: ICD-10-CM Code(s) _____

10. Atelectasis of newborn: ICD-10-CM Code(s) _____

11. Transitory ileus of newborn: ICD-10-CM Code(s) _____

(continued)

(continued from page 423)

12. Neonatal aspiration of blood: ICD-10-CM Code(s) _____

13. Phrenic nerve paralysis due to birth injury: ICD-10-CM Code(s) _____

14. Newborn infant of a diabetic mother: ICD-10-CM Code(s) _____

15. Preterm newborn, 28 completed weeks: ICD-10-CM Code(s) _____

16. Noninfective neonatal diarrhea: ICD-10-CM Code(s) _____

17. Newborn affected by mother's type 1 diabetes during pregnancy: ICD-10-CM Code(s) _____

18. Neonatal goiter: ICD-10-CM Code(s) _____

19. Anemia of prematurity: ICD-10-CM Code(s) _____

20. Congenital hydrocele: ICD-10-CM Code(s) _____

21. Rh isoimmunization of newborn: ICD-10-CM Code(s) _____

22. Neonatal coma: ICD-10-CM Code(s) _____

23. Cardiac arrest of newborn: ICD-10-CM Code(s) _____

24. Massive umbilical hemorrhage of newborn: ICD-10-CM Code(s) _____

25. Transitory neonatal neutropenia: ICD-10-CM Code(s) _____

Congenital Malformations, Deformations, and Chromosomal Abnormalities (Q00-Q99)

Chapter 25

Learning Objectives

After completing this chapter, you should have the skills to:

25.1 Spell and define the key words, medical terms, and abbreviations related to congenital malformations, deformations, and chromosomal abnormalities.

25.2 Discuss common congenital malformations, deformations, and chromosomal abnormalities.

25.3 Identify the main characteristics of coding for congenital malformations, deformations, and chromosomal abnormalities.

25.4 Abstract diagnostic information from the medical record for coding congenital malformations, deformations, and chromosomal abnormalities.

25.5 Assign diagnosis codes for congenital malformations, deformations, and chromosomal abnormalities.

25.6 Arrange multiple diagnosis codes for congenital malformations, deformations, and chromosomal abnormalities.

25.7 Discuss the Official Guidelines for Coding and Reporting related to congenital malformations, deformations, and chromosomal abnormalities.

Chapter Outline

- **Congenital Abnormalities Refresher**
- **Coding Overview of Congenital Abnormalities**
- **Abstracting for Congenital Abnormalities**
- **Assigning Codes for Congenital Abnormalities**
- **Arranging Codes for Congenital Abnormalities**

Key Terms and Abbreviations

abnormal development
anomaly
arrested development
congenital abnormality
delayed development

In addition to the key terms listed here, students should know the terms defined within tables in this chapter.

CODING PRACTICE (continued)

Example: microgastria micro/gastr/ia   Meaning: _condition of a very small stomach_   ICD-10-CM Code: _Q40.2_

1. ichthyosis   Meaning _____   ICD-10-CM Code _____
2. left renal <u>agenesis</u>   Meaning _____   ICD-10-CM Code _____
3. frontal <u>encephalocele</u>   Meaning _____   ICD-10-CM Code _____
4. macrotia   Meaning _____   ICD-10-CM Code _____
5. vaginal <u>atresia</u>   Meaning _____   ICD-10-CM Code _____
6. cryptorchism   Meaning _____   ICD-10-CM Code _____
7. polydactyl   Meaning _____   ICD-10-CM Code _____
8. <u>polycystic</u> kidney disease   Meaning _____   ICD-10-CM Code _____
9. <u>bicornate</u> uterus   Meaning _____   ICD-10-CM Code _____
10. pseudohermaphroditism   Meaning _____   ICD-10-CM Code _____

CODING OVERVIEW OF CONGENITAL ABNORMALITIES

ICD-10-CM Chapter 17, Congenital Malformations, Deformations, and Chromosomal Abnormalities (Q00-Q99), contains 11 blocks or subchapters that are divided by organ system. Review the block names and code ranges listed at the beginning of Chapter 17 in the ICD-10-CM manual to become familiar with the content and organization.

This ICD-10-CM chapter compares to ICD-9-CM Chapter 14 (740-759) and appears in a different sequence within the coding manual than it did in ICD-9-CM. Numerous conditions contain more codes for greater specificity and laterality than in ICD-9-CM. Codes for cleft palate are divided by anatomic site rather than bilateral or unilateral and complete or incomplete. Codes for reduction defects of the upper and lower limbs are significantly restructured. Codes for chromosomal abnormalities have been expanded to identify the specific genetic abnormality.

This chapter includes congenital physical and chromosomal abnormalities. It does not include acquired variations of conditions that may be either congenital or acquired, which are classified in the corresponding body system chapter. It also does not include conditions originating during the birth process, which are classified in ICD-10-CM Chapter 16, Certain Conditions Originating in the Perinatal Period (P00-P96).

ICD-10-CM provides Official Guidelines for Coding and Reporting (OGCR) for congenital malformations, deformations, and chromosomal abnormalities in OGCR section I.C.17. OGCR provide discussion of sequencing codes from this chapter, multiple coding, and use of these codes throughout the patient lifespan. An instructional note at the beginning of Chapter 17 in the Tabular List states that codes from this chapter should not be used on records of mothers or unborn fetuses.

ABSTRACTING FOR CONGENITAL ABNORMALITIES

Coders must identify whether a condition is congenital and what manifestations exist. In addition, coders should follow abstracting guidelines for the body system(s) affected.

Many conditions may be either congenital or acquired. Therefore, the coder must identify the documentation regarding when the condition originated. Chromosomal abnormalities and other conditions that are, by definition, congenital, do not require explicit documentation regarding the congenital nature.

Coders should review all manifestations of the congenital condition and identify those that are integral to the condition and those that are not. When a specific code exists for a condition, coders should report only the manifestations that are related but _not integral_ to the condition. When congenital conditions do not have a unique code, assign a nonspecific code and report all manifestations.

Age is not a factor when reporting congenital conditions. Unless a congenital defect can be repaired, congenital conditions exist throughout a patient's life and may be reported at any time.

Refer to ■ TABLE 25-3 for guidance on how to abstract conditions related to congenital malformations, deformations, and chromosomal abnormalities, then work through the detailed example that follows. Remember that the abstracting questions are a guide and that not every question applies to, or can be answered for, every case. Also remember to consult key criteria for abstracting specific body system conditions. For example, to code for a congenital condition in a newborn, follow the key criteria listed here, as well as key criteria for abstracting birth encounters.

Table 25-3 ■ **KEY CRITERIA FOR ABSTRACTING CONDITIONS RELATED TO CONGENITAL ABNORMALITIES**

❏ What is the specific condition?
❏ What is the subtype?
❏ Is the condition clearly congenital?
❏ What manifestations are present?
❏ What manifestations are integral to the condition?
❏ What complications or comorbidities exist?
❏ Which condition or manifestation is the main reason for the encounter?

Guided Example of Abstracting Congenital Abnormalities

Refer to the following example throughout this chapter to practice skills for abstracting, assigning, and sequencing codes related to congenital malformations, deformations, and chromosomal abnormalities. Geneva Deckard, CPC, is a fictitious coder who guides you through the coding process.

Date: 5/21/yy   Location: Branton Medical Center

Provider: Matthew Bunker, MD

Patient: Lucia Ovalle   Gender: F   Age: 9 months

Reason for encounter: cyanosis, tachypnea, difficulty feeding, failure to thrive

Assessment: blood work and imaging studies reveal tetralogy of Fallot (TOF); congenital atrial septal defect (ASD) is also present and can be corrected at the same time as TOF surgery, if parents consent

Plan: corrective surgery

Follow along as Geneva Deckard, CPC, abstracts the diagnosis. Check off each step after you complete it.

▶ Geneva reads through the entire record, paying special attention to the reason for the encounter and the final assessment. She refers to the Key Criteria for Abstracting Conditions Related to Congenital Abnormalities (Table 25-3).

❑ *What is the specific condition?* tetralogy of Fallot

❑ *What is the subtype?* Not applicable.

❑ *Is the condition clearly congenital?* Yes, the condition is congenital by definition.

❑ *What manifestations are present?* cyanosis, tachypnea, difficulty feeding, failure to thrive

❑ *What manifestations are integral to the condition?* All manifestations listed are common with TOF.

❑ *What complications or comorbidities exist?* congenital atrial septal defect

❑ *Which condition or manifestation is the main reason for the encounter?* tetralogy of Fallot

▶ At this time, Geneva does not know which of these conditions may need to be coded, nor how many codes she will end up with. She will learn about this when she moves on to assigning codes.

CODING PRACTICE

Exercise 25.2 Abstracting for Congenital Abnormalities

Instructions: Read the mini-medical-record of each patient's encounter and answer the abstracting questions. Write the answer on the line provided. Do not assign any codes.

1. INPATIENT HOSPITAL   Gender: M   Age: 32

Reason for admission: mitral valve replacement

Assessment: mitral valve prolapse d/t congenital Marfan syndrome

Plan: valve replacement was successful, FU office 2 weeks

a. What is the specific condition? _____

b. What is the subtype? _____

c. Is the condition clearly congenital? _____

_____

d. What manifestations are present? _____

e. What manifestations are integral to the condition? _____

f. What complications or comorbidities exist?

_____

g. Which condition or manifestation is the main reason for the encounter? _____

2. INPATIENT HOSPITAL   Gender: M   Age: 23 days

Reason for admission: removal of a renal cyst

Assessment: congenital renal cyst, congenital hydronephrosis

Plan: RTO 2 weeks

a. What is the specific condition? _____

b. What is the subtype? _____

c. Is the condition clearly congenital? _____

_____

d. What manifestations are present? _____

_____

e. What manifestations are integral to the condition?

_____

f. What complications or comorbidities exist?

_____

g. Which condition or manifestation is the main reason for the encounter? _____

(continued)

CODING PRACTICE (continued)

3. OFFICE Gender: F Age: 16

Reason for encounter: referred by family physician for gynecological consult on amenorrhea

Assessment: ultrasound reveals missing uterus, which has not been surgically removed

a. What is the specific condition? _____

b. What is the subtype? _____

c. Is the condition clearly congenital? _____

_____

d. What manifestations are present? _____

e. What manifestations are integral to the condition? _____

f. What complications or comorbidities exist?

_____

g. Which condition or manifestation is the main reason for the encounter? _____

4. OFFICE Gender: F Age: 30 days

Reason for encounter: FU on endoscopy after referral from pediatrician because infant is constantly spitting up

Assessment: congenital Schatzki esophageal ring

Plan: we attempted to dilate the ring and will evaluate for surgery if that is unsuccessful

a. What is the specific condition? _____

b. What is the subtype? _____

c. Is the condition clearly congenital? _____

_____

d. What manifestations are present? _____

e. What manifestations are integral to the condition? _____

f. What complications or comorbidities exist?

_____

g. Which condition or manifestation is the main reason for the encounter? _____

5. OUTPATIENT HOSPITAL Gender: F Age: 1 year

Reason for encounter: surgical correction of polydactyly

Assessment: accessory thumb of right hand

Plan: FU office 1 week

(continued)

5. (continued)

a. What is the specific condition? _____

b. What is the subtype? _____

c. Is the condition clearly congenital? _____

_____

d. What manifestations are present? _____

e. What manifestations are integral to the condition? _____

f. What complications or comorbidities exist?

_____

g. Which condition or manifestation is the main reason for the encounter? _____

6. OFFICE Gender: F Age: 23 days

Reason for encounter: management of Down syndrome and FU on genetic testing

Assessment: Down syndrome, nonmosaic type, hypotonia, obstructive sleep apnea d/t Down-related hypertrophy of tonsils and adenoids, ASD, also Down related

Plan: FU with cardiologist and neurologist

a. What is the specific condition? _____

b. What is the subtype? _____

c. Is the condition clearly congenital? _____

_____

d. What manifestations are present? _____

e. What manifestations are integral to the condition? _____

f. Which conditions are related, but not integral, to Down syndrome? _____

g. Which condition or manifestation is the main reason for the encounter? _____

7. INPATIENT HOSPITAL Gender: M Age: 6 days

Birth Weight: 2169g EGA: 38+4 Type: NSVD

POB: Hospital

Assessment: SGA, the blood test FISH (fluorescent in situ hybridization) is positive for Prader-Willi syndrome. Hypotonia and abnormally small testes (**hypoplasia**) which cannot be detected within the scrotal sac, secondary to Prader-Willi.

(continued)

7. (continued)

Plan: follow feeding plan, evaluate for supplemental growth hormone in 1 month

a. What is the specific condition? _____

b. What is the subtype? _____

c. Is the condition clearly congenital? _____

_____

d. What manifestations are present? _____

_____

e. What manifestations are integral to the condition? _____

_____

f. What complications or comorbidities exist? _____

_____

g. Which condition or manifestation is the main reason for the encounter? _____

8. OFFICE   Gender: M   Age: 30 days

Reason for encounter: routine examination

Assessment: infant was born with microgastria and now has failure to thrive

Plan: refer to nutritionist for feeding guidance, WU for vitamin, mineral, and hormone deficiencies

a. What is the specific condition? _____

b. What is the subtype? _____

c. Is the condition clearly congenital? _____

_____

d. What manifestations are present? _____

e. What manifestations are integral to the condition? _____

f. What complications or comorbidities exist? _____

_____

g. Which condition or manifestation is the main reason for the encounter? _____

9. INPATIENT HOSPITAL   Gender: M   Age: 10 days

Birth Weight: 3216g   **EGA:** 38+2   **Type:** cesarean

POB: Hospital

Assessment: Meckel diverticulum and congenital pyloric stenosis with vomiting

Plan: Evaluate effectiveness of pyloric balloon dilation that was performed. If unsuccessful, consider surgery to correct stenosis. Surgery is not needed for Meckel unless bleeding occurs.

a. What is the specific condition? _____

b. What is the subtype? _____

c. Is the condition clearly congenital? _____

_____

d. What manifestations are present? _____

e. What manifestations are integral to the condition? _____

_____

f. What complications or comorbidities exist? _____

_____

g. Which condition or manifestation is the main reason for the encounter? _____

10. OFFICE   Gender: F   Age: 3 months

Reason for encounter: referred by pediatrician due to heart murmur

Assessment: patent foramen ovale and congenital VSD

Plan: treat VSD medically, postpone surgery if symptoms increase, no treatment needed for patent foramen ovale at this time, RTO 3 months

a. What is the specific condition? _____

b. What is the subtype? _____

c. Is the condition clearly congenital? _____

_____

d. What manifestations are present? _____

e. What manifestations are integral to the condition? _____

_____

f. What complications or comorbidities exist? _____

_____

g. Which condition or manifestation is the main reason for the encounter? _____

ASSIGNING CODES FOR CONGENITAL ABNORMALITIES

ICD-10-CM distinguishes between conditions that can be either congenital in origin or acquired. For some conditions, the default code in the Index is for congenital origin, with the acquired version appearing as a subterm. For other conditions, the default code is for the acquired version, with the congenital origin appearing as a subterm. Coders can determine which variation is identified by the default code in the Index by reading the nonessential modifiers that appear in parentheses after the Main Term. When either of these terms, congenital or acquired, appears as a nonessential modifier, the other term usually appears as a subterm. Refer to ■ FIGURE 25-1 for the Main Term **Deformity** to compare the difference between the subterm **bone**, for which the default is **(acquired)**, and the subterm **brain**, for which the default code is **(congenital)**. Notice that the code for the congenital variation is from ICD-10-CM Chapter 17 and begins with **Q**, while the code for the acquired version does not begin with **Q** but, rather, the letter from the corresponding body system chapter.

SUCCESS STEP

When the documentation does not specify either congenital or acquired, assign the default code. Remember that the nonessential modifier in parentheses does *not* have to be present in the documentation in order to assign the code.

Some conditions are congenital by definition and do not have an acquired form. When this is the case, the Index does not provide an alternative subterm for acquired and all code options begin with **Q** (■ FIGURE 25-2). Subterms describe variations of the congenital condition.

When a congenital abnormality has been corrected, assign a personal history code to identify the history of the condition (OGCR I.C.17). Search under the Main Term **History**, subterm **personal**, and the second-level subterm for the name of the condition. When the specific condition does not appear as a subterm, search under the Main Term **History**, subterm **personal**, the second-level subterm **congenital malformation**, and a third-level subterm for the body system involved (■ FIGURE 25-3).

> **Hypospadias** Q54.9
> balanic Q54.0
> coronal Q54.0
> glandular Q54.0
> penile Q54.1
> penoscrotal Q54.2
> perineal Q54.3
> specified NEC Q54.8

Figure 25-2 ■ Index Main Term for a Condition That Is Only Congenital in Origin

Guided Example of Assigning Congenital Abnormalities Codes

To practice skills for assigning codes for congenital malformations, deformations, and chromosomal abnormalities, continue with the example from earlier in the chapter about patient Lucia Ovalle, who was diagnosed at Branton Medical Center with tetralogy of Fallot and atrial septal defect.

Follow along in your ICD-10-CM manual as Geneva Deckard, CPC, assigns codes. Check off each step after you complete it.

▶ First, Geneva confirms the conditions she abstracted:

❏ tetralogy of Fallot

❏ congenital atrial septal defect

▶ Geneva searches the Index for the Main Term **Tetralogy**.

❏ She locates the entry **Tetralogy of Fallot Q21.3**.

❏ There are no subterms.

▶ Geneva verifies code **Q21.3** in the Tabular List.

❏ She reads the code title for **Q21.3, Tetralogy of Fallot**, and confirms that this accurately describes the diagnosis.

▶ Geneva checks for instructional notes in the Tabular List.

❏ She cross-references the beginning of category **Q21** and reads the **Excludes1** instructional note that directs her to *not* use this code if the cardiac septal defect is *acquired*.

❏ She determines that this note does not apply because her patient's condition is congenital.

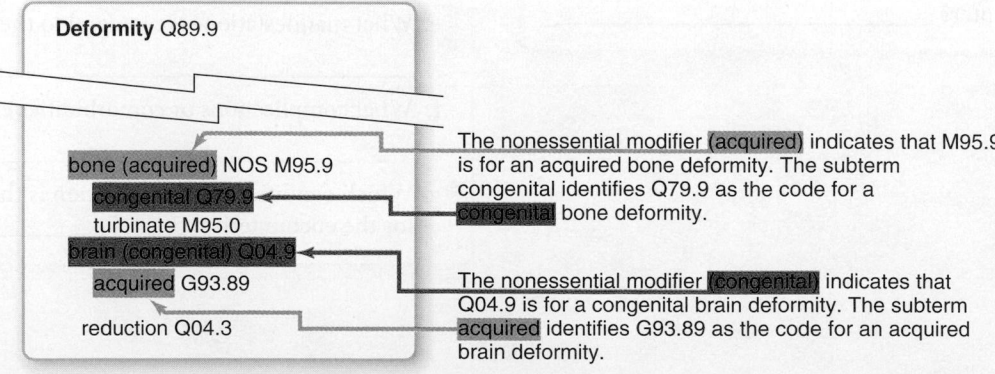

Figure 25-1 ■ Index Entry Showing Acquired and Congenital as Nonessential Modifiers and Subterms

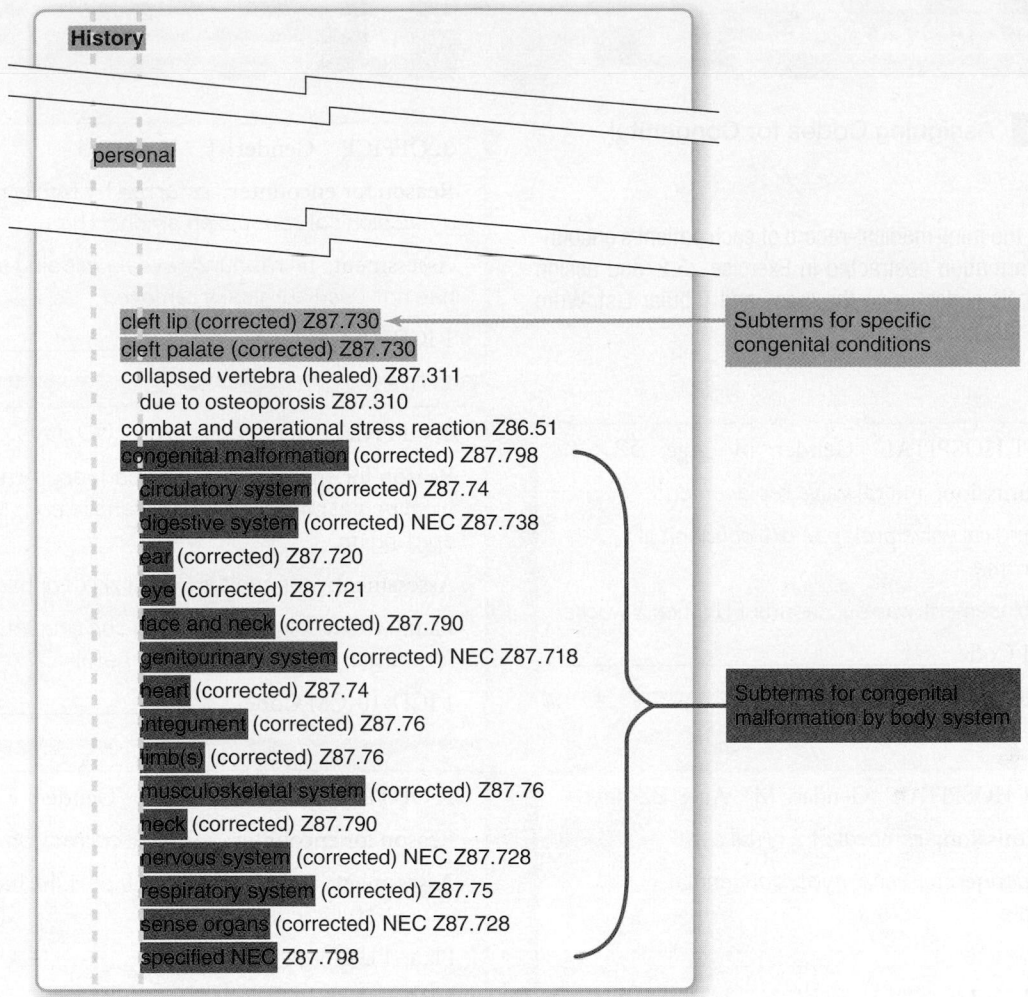

History

personal

cleft lip (corrected) Z87.730 ◄───────── Subterms for specific
cleft palate (corrected) Z87.730   congenital conditions
collapsed vertebra (healed) Z87.311
  due to osteoporosis Z87.310
combat and operational stress reaction Z86.51
congenital malformation (corrected) Z87.798
  circulatory system (corrected) Z87.74
  digestive system (corrected) NEC Z87.738
  ear (corrected) Z87.720
  eye (corrected) Z87.721
  face and neck (corrected) Z87.790
  genitourinary system (corrected) NEC Z87.718
  heart (corrected) Z87.74
  integument (corrected) Z87.76   Subterms for congenital
  limb(s) (corrected) Z87.76   malformation by body system
  musculoskeletal system (corrected) Z87.76
  neck (corrected) Z87.790
  nervous system (corrected) NEC Z87.728
  respiratory system (corrected) Z87.75
  sense organs (corrected) NEC Z87.728
  specified NEC Z87.798

Figure 25-3 ■ Index Entry for Personal History of Congenital Conditions

❏ She cross-references the beginning of the block **Q20-Q28** and verifies that there are no instructional notes.

❏ She cross-references the beginning of **Chapter 17 (Q00-Q99)** and reviews the instructional notes. She determines that the **NOTE:** does not apply to this case because the patient is not a mother or a fetus. She determines that the **Excludes1** note does not apply because the condition is not an inborn error of metabolism.

▶ Next, Geneva works on the code for *congenital atrial septal defect*.

▶ Geneva searches the Index for the Main Term **Defect**.

❏ She locates the subterm **septal (heart) NOS**.

❏ She reads the subterms and notices that there is not a subterm for congenital. However, there is a separate subterm for **acquired**, which she knows she does *not* want.

❏ She locates the second-level subterm **atrial Q21.1** and notices that it is a Q code from ICD-10-CM Chapter 17 on congenital abnormalities.

❏ The third-level subterms under **atrial** relate to myocardial infarction, which does not apply to this patient.

▶ Geneva verifies the code **Q21.1** in the Tabular List.

❏ She reads the code title for **Q21.1, Atrial septal defect**, and confirms that this accurately describes the diagnosis.

▶ Geneva checks for instructional notes in the Tabular List.

❏ She notices that this code is in the same category that code **Q21.3, Tetralogy of Fallot**, was.

❏ She believes that she remembers what the instructional notes stated for the category, block, and chapter, but does a quick double check to be certain.

▶ Geneva reviews the codes she has assigned for this case.

❏ **Q21.1   Atrial septal defect**

❏ **Q21.3   Tetralogy of Fallot**

▶ Next, Geneva must determine how to sequence the codes.

CODING PRACTICE

Exercise 25.3 Assigning Codes for Congenital Abnormalities

Instructions: Read the mini-medical-record of each patient's encounter, review the information abstracted in Exercise 25.2, and assign ICD-10-CM diagnosis codes using the Index and Tabular List. Write the code(s) on the line provided.

1. INPATIENT HOSPITAL   Gender: M   Age: 32

Reason for admission: mitral valve replacement

Assessment: mitral valve prolapse d/t congenital Marfan syndrome

Plan: valve replacement was successful, FU office 2 weeks

1 ICD-10-CM Code _____

2. INPATIENT HOSPITAL   Gender: M   Age: 23 days

Reason for admission: removal of a renal cyst

Assessment: congenital renal cyst, congenital hydronephrosis

Plan: RTO 2 weeks

2 ICD-10-CM Codes _____

3. OFFICE   Gender: F   Age: 16

Reason for encounter: referred by family physician for gynecological consult on amenorrhea

Assessment: ultrasound reveals missing uterus, which has not been surgically removed

1 ICD-10-CM Code _____

4. OFFICE   Gender: F   Age: 30 days

Reason for encounter: FU on endoscopy after referral from pediatrician because infant is constantly spitting up

Assessment: congenital Schatzki esophageal ring

Plan: we attempted to dilate the ring and will evaluate for surgery if that is unsuccessful

1 ICD-10-CM Code _____

5. OUTPATIENT HOSPITAL   Gender: F   Age: 1 year

Reason for encounter: surgical correction of polydactyly

Assessment: accessory thumb of right hand successfully removed

Plan: FU office 1 week

1 ICD-10-CM Code _____

ARRANGING CODES FOR CONGENITAL ABNORMALITIES

Codes for congenital abnormalities may be either a principal/first-listed diagnosis or a secondary diagnosis, based on the circumstances of the encounter and the definition of principal diagnosis in OGCR II (OGCR I.C.17). When a patient has multiple congenital abnormalities, which is not unusual, sequence the codes based on the circumstances of the encounter. Although this chapter does not have many instructional notes in the Tabular List, remember to always look for them and follow their direction for multiple coding and sequencing.

When coding for Down syndrome (**Q90.-**), an instructional note in the Tabular List states **Use additional code(s) to identify any associated physical conditions and the degree of intellectual disabilities (F70-F79)** (■ FIGURE 25-4).

SUCCESS STEP

When congenital abnormalities are diagnosed as part of the birth episode, assign a code from category **Z38.-** to describe the birth status of the infant. Always sequence the **Z38** code first, followed by codes for congenital or any other conditions.

SUCCESS STEP

Nonmosaic Down syndrome occurs when there is an extra copy of chromosome 21 in every cell of the body. It accounts for the majority of Down cases.

Guided Example of Arranging Congenital Abnormalities Codes

To practice skills for sequencing codes for congenital malformations, deformations, and chromosomal abnormalities, continue

Patient who has moderate mental retardation is seen for nonmosaicism Down syndrome. Patient also has associated hypothyroidism and celiac disease.

(1) **Q90.0 Trisomy 21, nonmosaicism (meiotic nondisjunction)**
(2) **F71 Moderate intellectual disabilities**
(3) **E03.9 Hypothyroidism, unspecified**
(4) **K90.0 Celiac disease**

Figure 25-4 ■ Example of Arranging Codes for Down Syndrome

with the example from earlier in the chapter about patient Lucia Ovalle, who was diagnosed at Branton Medical Center with tetralogy of Fallot and atrial septal defect.

Follow along in your ICD-10-CM manual as Geneva Deckard, CPC, sequences the codes. Check off each step after you complete it.

▶ First, Geneva confirms the codes she assigned:

❑ **Q21.1   Atrial septal defect**

❑ **Q21.3   Tetralogy of Fallot**

▶ Geneva reviews the medical record to determine which code is the principal diagnosis.

❑ The workup and studies found both conditions, and TOF is the more serious condition because it consists of four malformations. ASD is secondary to TOF.

▶ Geneva finalizes the codes and sequencing for this case:

(1) **Q21.3   Tetralogy of Fallot**

(2) **Q21.1   Atrial septal defect**

CODING PRACTICE

Exercise 25.4 **Arranging Codes for Congenital Abnormalities**

Instructions: Read the mini-medical-record of each patient's encounter, review the information abstracted in Exercise 25.2, assign ICD-10-CM diagnosis codes using the Index and Tabular List, and sequence them correctly.

---

1. OFFICE   Gender: F   Age: 23 days

Reason for encounter: management of Down syndrome and FU on genetic testing

Assessment: Down syndrome, nonmosaic type, hypotonia, obstructive sleep apnea due to Down-related hypertrophy of tonsils and adenoids, ASD, also Down related

Plan: FU with cardiologist and neurologist

Tip: Nonmosaicism is also called meiotic nondisjunction. Be careful to read any Excludes1 notes you encounter.

3 ICD-10-CM Codes _____

_____

---

2. INPATIENT HOSPITAL   Gender: M   Age: 6 days

Birth Weight: 2169g   EGA: 38+4

Type: NSVD   POB: Hospital

Assessment: SGA, the blood test FISH (fluorescent in situ hybridization) is positive for Prader-Willi syndrome. Hypotonia and abnormally small testes (**hypoplasia**) which cannot be detected within the scrotal sac, secondary to Prader-Willi

4 ICD-10-CM Codes _____

_____

---

3. OFFICE   Gender: M   Age: 30 days

Reason for encounter: routine examination

Assessment: infant was born with microgastria and now has failure to thrive

Plan: refer to nutritionist for feeding guidance, WU for vitamin, mineral, and hormone deficiencies

Tip: Be sure to check the age of the patient.

3 ICD-10-CM Codes _____

_____

---

4. INPATIENT HOSPITAL   Gender: M   Age: 10 days

Birth Weight: 3216g   EGA: 38+2

Type: cesarean   POB: Hospital

Assessment: Meckel diverticulum and congenital pyloric stenosis with vomiting

Plan: Evaluate effectiveness of pyloric balloon dilation that was performed. If unsuccessful, consider surgery to correct stenosis. Surgery is not needed for Meckel unless bleeding occurs.

3 ICD-10-CM Codes _____

_____

---

5. OFFICE   Gender: F   Age: 3 months

Reason for encounter: referred by pediatrician due to heart murmur

Assessment: patent foramen ovale and congenital VSD

Plan: treat VSD medically, postpone surgery if symptoms increase, no treatment needed for patent foramen ovale at this time, RTO 3 months

2 ICD-10-CM Codes _____

CHAPTER SUMMARY

In this chapter you learned that:

- Congenital abnormalities are specific types of perinatal conditions, which include physical malformations, deformations, and chromosomal abnormalities.
- ICD-10-CM Chapter 17, Congenital Malformations, Deformations, and Chromosomal Abnormalities (Q00-Q99), contains 11 blocks or subchapters that are divided by organ system.
- Coders must identify whether a condition is congenital and what manifestations exist.
- Coders can determine whether a condition identified by the default code in the Index is the congenital variation or the

acquired variation by reading the nonessential modifiers that appear in parentheses after the Main Term.
- Codes for congenital abnormalities may be either a principal/ first-listed diagnosis or a secondary diagnosis, based on the circumstances of the encounter.
- ICD-10-CM provides Official Guidelines for Coding and Reporting (OGCR) in OGCR section I.C.17, which discuss sequencing codes from this chapter, multiple coding, and use of these codes throughout the patient lifespan.

CONCEPT QUIZ

Take a moment to look back at congenital malformations, deformations, and chromosomal abnormalities and solidify your skills. Try to answer the questions from memory first, then look back at the discussion in this chapter if you need a little extra help.

Completion

Instructions: Write the term that answers each question based on the information you learned in this chapter. Choose from the list below. Some choices may be used more than once and some choices may not be used at all.

adults	Marfan syndrome
aortic coarctation	mothers
chromosomal abnormality	newborns
cleft palate	patent foramen ovale
deformity	Prader-Willi syndrome
Down syndrome	spina bifida
hydrocephalus	transposition of the great vessels
hydronephrosis	
hypospadias	Turner syndrome
malformation	

1. Down syndrome is an example of a _____.
2. Dislocation of the hip is an example of a
   _____.
3. _____ is a notch or division of the roof of the mouth.
4. _____ is the excessive collection of urine in the kidneys.
5. _____ is a congenital heart defect in which the aorta and pulmonary artery are switched, preventing pulmonary circulation.

6. An instructional note at the beginning of Chapter 17 in the Tabular List states that codes from this chapter should not be used on records of _____.
7. _____ is a congenital condition in which the opening of the urethra is on the underside of the penile shaft.
8. _____ is a genetic disorder of connective tissue characterized by elongated bones and ocular and circulatory defects.
9. _____ is a genetic condition in which a person has 47 chromosomes instead of the usual 46.
10. _____ is a chromosomal defect in females in which they are missing all or part of one X chromosome.

Multiple Choice

Instructions: Circle the letter of the best answer to each question based on the information you learned in this chapter.

1. Which condition is NOT part of tetralogy of Fallot?
   A. Pulmonary stenosis
   B. Atrial septal defect
   C. Overriding aorta
   D. Hypertrophy of the right ventricle

2. Prader-Willi syndrome is characterized by all of the following EXCEPT
   A. circulatory defects.
   B. short stature.
   C. muscle weakness.
   D. nonfunctioning gonads.

3. Chapter 17 (Q00-Q99) classifies
   A. acquired conditions.
   B. perinatal conditions.
   C. chromosomal abnormalities.
   D. conditions of unborn fetuses.

4. Which of the following is NOT a factor when reporting congenital conditions?
   A. Age of the patient being treated
   B. Manifestations
   C. Congenital nature of condition
   D. Comorbidities

5. Which of the following is NOT a common manifestation of tetralogy of Fallot?
   A. Blue skin
   B. Rapid breathing
   C. Rapid heart rate
   D. Difficulty feeding

6. The correct code for a congenital bone deformity is
   A. M95.9.
   B. Q79.9.
   C. Q04.9.
   D. M95.0.

7. When the documentation does not specify either congenital or acquired, what should the coder do?
   A. Assign a code for congenital.
   B. Assign a code for acquired.
   C. Assign a code for NOS.
   D. Assign the default code.

8. When a congenital abnormality has been corrected, what code should you assign?
   A. Continue to code the congenital condition.
   B. Assign a code for personal history of the condition.
   C. Assign the default code.
   D. Do not assign any code.

9. When congenital abnormalities are diagnosed as part of the birth episode, the principal diagnosis should be
   A. determined according to the circumstances of admission.
   B. the most serious congenital condition.
   C. any birth trauma.
   D. the birth status of the infant.

10. A patient has an intellectual disability, Down syndrome, hypothyroidism, and celiac disease. What is the principal diagnosis?
    A. Intellectual disability
    B. Down syndrome
    C. Hypothyroidism
    D. Celiac disease

CODING CHALLENGE

Instructions: Read the mini-medical-record of each patient's encounter, then abstract, assign, and sequence ICD-10-CM diagnosis codes using the Index and Tabular List. Write the code(s) on the line provided.

1. INPATIENT HOSPITAL   Gender: M   Age: 15 days

Birth Weight: 3421g   EGA: 39+0   Type: NSVD

POB: Hospital

Assessment: unilateral cleft lip on left side, with cleft palate, hard

Plan: Detailed review of estimated repair protocol with parents. Visiting nurse to supervise feeding for 2 days. RTO 3 days.

Tip: Infant was discharged 15 days after birth.

2 ICD-10-CM Codes _____

2. INPATIENT HOSPITAL   Gender: F   Age: 50

Reason for encounter: patient was attempting to adjust her office chair when the mechanism gave and caught and crushed her finger

Assessment: finger crush injury of right hand, congenital deficiency of the development of hands and fingers, bilaterally, complicates the repair

(continued)

2. (continued)

Plan: Arm and hand loosely wrapped in splint, elevate hand above elbow. RTO in one day, schedule reconstruction after swelling has abated.

Tip: There is not a specific external cause code for this accident. Code as exposure to inanimate mechanical forces.

4 ICD-10-CM Codes _____

_____

3. INPATIENT HOSPITAL   Gender: F   Age: 2

Reason for encounter: reconstructive heart surgery

Assessment: congenital Shone's syndrome with aortic stenosis, subaortic stenosis, aortic coarctation, bicuspid aortic valve

Plan: FU in office 3 days

4 ICD-10-CM Codes _____

_____

(continued)

(continued from page 437)

4. INPATIENT HOSPITAL   Gender: M   Age: 1 day
Birth Weight: 2421g   EGA: 36+0   Type: cesarean
POB: Hospital
Reason for encounter: spina bifida suspected at second trimester screening and confirmed by ultrasound and at birth; infant was born yesterday
Assessment: spina bifida of the thoracic region
Plan: surgical repair recommended
Tip: This is an inpatient consultation with the pediatric neurologist. When coding for the physician, do not report the birth status of the infant, which is reported only on the inpatient record.
1 ICD-10-CM Code _____

5. OFFICE   Gender: M   Age: 2
Reason for encounter: Referral from neurologist
Assessment: lingual frenum extending toward the tip of tongue, which is fused to mouth floor and affects speech
Plan: refer for speech therapy
1 ICD-10-CM Code _____

6. OFFICE   Gender: M   Age: 5
Reason for encounter: referred by pediatrician for dysphagia
Assessment: congenital esophageal web with esophageal spasm and reflux esophagitis
Plan: schedule balloon dilatation and electrocauterization
3 ICD-10-CM Codes _____
_____

7. OFFICE   Gender: M   Age: 1 year
Reason for encounter: preoperative exam for cryptorchism repair tomorrow
Assessment: cleared for surgery, bilateral perineal cryptorchism
Plan: surgery tomorrow at 11:00 am
Tip: Assign a Z code for the preoperative exam.
2 ICD-10-CM Codes _____

8. OFFICE   Gender: M   Age: 1 month
Reason for encounter: fitting of knee braces, bilateral
Assessment: congenital genu recurvatum
Plan: instruct parents on daily passive physical therapy, schedule pt treatments x 12 on weekly basis
Tip: Assign a Z code for the fitting of the braces. Genu recurvatum is a minor backward curving of knee joints causing bowed legs.
2 ICD-10-CM Codes _____

9. INPATIENT HOSPITAL   Gender: M   Age: 1 day
Birth Weight: 3011g   EGA: 38+0   Type: NSVD
POB: Hospital
Assessment: penoscrotal hypospadias
Plan: Discharged 1 day after birth. We will keep an eye on the hypospadias to see if treatment is necessary or if it will correct independently, FU in office 2 days for jaundice check
2 ICD-10-CM Codes _____

10. INPATIENT HOSPITAL   Gender: F   Age: 9 days
Birth Weight: 3011g   EGA: 38+0   Type: cesarean
POB: Hospital
Reason for encounter: open heart surgery on 9-day-old infant
Assessment: transposition of great vessels
Plan: will follow in hospital until d/c
Tip: This is an inpatient procedure by the neonatal cardiothoracic surgeon. When coding for the physician, do not report the birth status of the infant, which is reported only on the inpatient record.
1 ICD-10-CM Code _____

KEEP ON CODING

Instructions: Read the diagnostic statement, then use the Index and Tabular List to assign and sequence ICD-10-CM diagnosis codes. Write the code(s) on the line provided.

1. Congenital glaucoma: ICD-10-CM Code(s) _____

2. Accessory ovary: ICD-10-CM Code(s) _____

3. Karyotype 45, X: ICD-10-CM Code(s) _____

4. Schwannomatosis: ICD-10-CM Code(s) _____

5. Lobster-claw, left hand: ICD-10-CM Code(s) _____

6. Congenital clawfoot: ICD-10-CM Code(s) _____

7. Congenital cyst of the pancreas: ICD-10-CM Code(s) _____

8. Anomaly of the aqueduct of Sylvius: ICD-10-CM Code(s) _____

9. Ectopic kidney: ICD-10-CM Code(s) _____

10. Supernumerary nipple: ICD-10-CM Code(s) _____

11. Laryngocele: ICD-10-CM Code(s) _____

12. Cleft lip, median: ICD-10-CM Code(s) _____

13. Low-set ears: ICD-10-CM Code(s) _____

14. Anencephaly: ICD-10-CM Code(s) _____

15. Arnold-Chiari syndrome with hydrocephalus: ICD-10-CM Code(s) _____

16. Plagiocephaly: ICD-10-CM Code(s) _____

17. Marfan syndrome: ICD-10-CM Code(s) _____

18. Blue sclera: ICD-10-CM Code(s) _____

19. Ebstein's anomaly: ICD-10-CM Code(s) _____

20. Atresia of the aorta: ICD-10-CM Code(s) _____

21. Short rib syndrome: ICD-10-CM Code(s) _____

22. Congenital spondylolysis: ICD-10-CM Code(s) _____

23. Strawberry nevus: ICD-10-CM Code(s) _____

24. Epidermolysis bullosa letalis: ICD-10-CM Code(s) _____

25. Congenital hiatal hernia: ICD-10-CM Code(s) _____

SECTION THREE

ICD-9-CM Coding

Section Three, ICD-9-CM Coding, introduces to you to the diagnosis and inpatient procedure coding systems used since 1979. After the implementation of ICD-10-CM/PCS, coders will still use ICD-9-CM for limited purposes, so it is considered to be a "legacy" system, and one with which coders must be familiar. You will learn the basics of ICD-9-CM coding and how to apply the three skills of an "ace" coder—Abstract, Assign, and Arrange—in this context. This section builds on skills you learned when studying ICD-10-CM and focuses on the differences between ICD-9-CM and ICD-10-CM.

PROFESSIONAL PROFILE

MEET...

Nicolas A. Joye, BS, CCS, Senior Medical Coder
M*Modal

I have been a coder for a little over a year and landed my first job, which I love, through professional networking. I work as a remote coder on cases for outpatient clinics, outpatient surgery, physical therapy, outpatient therapy, and hospital inpatients. I use multiple electronic health record and computerized coding programs. I must meet standards for the number of charts coded per hour and a daily accuracy percentage. Until I achieved 95% accuracy, which took 4–5 months, I was employed part-time and 100% of my work was audited. Remote coding requires that I be a self-starter, well organized, and disciplined to work on my own. This setup may not work for everyone.

After my coursework was complete, I took the CCA and passed. With my certificate in hand, M*Modal hired me as a remote coder in their Coding Apprentice Program (CAP). After passing the CAP program six months later, my sights were set on the CCS certification. Working only one year as a remote coder, I studied with complete focus and passed the CCS! Education and credentials will make or break you in the HIM profession. Now that all my RHIT coursework is completed, I will take the RHIT examination after my two-week internship. These certifications and degrees are essential to climbing the ladder to a challenging and financially rewarding career.

Remote coding gives me flexibility during the workday and the ability to devote more hours to the job without a long commute. Coding never gets boring, there is always something new to learn about medicine and healthcare. This makes the job something to look forward to. With the current demand for coders because of an industry shortage and the upcoming ICD-10 implementation, I feel positive about the salary potential.

I am involved with the American Health Information Management Association (AHIMA) and Arizona HIMA (AzHIMA) rather than Arizona AHIMA. I was previously involved with California HIMA. I am a member of the Student Internship Council that was created to work on streamlining the processes of internships for prospective HIM graduates. Volunteering with HIM associations is a great way to get to know people on a personal level.

Begin networking at your local and national associations while you are in school. You will meet potential employers, and as they get to know you, you may be the first one they call when there is an opening. I found my current job by putting my name out in the field through LinkedIn, internships, and other professional networking sites/groups. It is very easy to put yourself out there and give your name to anyone who seems appropriate and to fill out lots of applications. That is what I did, and when the CAP opening became available at M*Modal, my name was passed to my current boss. This led to my current job. It is all about getting your name in the right hands and, thus, the hands of a potential employer.

In addition to networking, my advice to students is to study hard and learn the material during your course of study. You will not be able to pass the certification exams without a deep knowledge of HIM. Get your certifications as soon as you can after completing a recommended test preparation guide—pace yourself over a month or so and take one chapter at a time—learn the material well; go over what you missed the week before the test as a refresher. Finally, develop your career goals early and modify them as you see fit—there are many options in the HIM field.

Table 26-1 ■ **ORGANIZATION OF THE ICD-9-CM MANUAL**

Volume	Name of Section	Purpose
Introductory Material	<ul><li>Preface</li><li>Introduction</li><li>How to Use the ICD-9-CM</li><li>ICD-9-CM Official Conventions</li><li>Additional Conventions</li><li>ICD-9-CM Official Guidelines for Coding and Reporting</li></ul>	Information and rules on how to use the manual.
Volume 2: Index	<ul><li>ICD-9-CM Index to Diseases and Injuries (Index)</li><li>ICD-9-CM Hypertension Table</li><li>ICD-9-CM Table of Neoplasms</li><li>ICD-9-CM Table of Drugs and Chemicals</li><li>ICD-9-CM Index to External Causes of Injury and Poisoning</li></ul>	Alphabetical list of diseases and injuries, reasons for encounters, and external causes. Three tables provide quick lookups, for hypertension, neoplasms, and drugs and chemicals causing injury.
Volume 1: Tabular List	<ul><li>ICD-9-CM Tabular List of Diseases</li><li>Supplementary Classification of External Causes of Injury and Poisoning (E000-E999)</li><li>Appendix A: Morphology of Neoplasms</li><li>Appendix B: Glossary of Mental Disorders (Deleted 10/1/2004)</li><li>Appendix C: Classification of Drugs by American Hospital Formulary Service</li><li>Appendix D: Classification of Industrial Accidents According to Agency</li><li>Appendix E: List of Three-Digit Categories</li></ul>	Numerical list of diseases and injuries, reasons for encounters, and external causes. Provides additional instruction on how to use, assign, and sequence codes. The appendices provide reference information not needed by coders on a daily basis.
Volume 3: Hospital Inpatient Procedures	<ul><li>Index to Hospital Inpatient Procedures</li><li>Tabular List of Hospital Inpatient Procedures</li></ul>	Medical and surgical procedures reported by hospitals on inpatient claims.

Official Guidelines for Coding and Reporting (OGCR)

The ICD-9-CM OGCR provide directions for how to code selected conditions and establish the rules for how to identify which diagnoses should be reported on a claim for any given patient. HIPAA requires that coders adhere to OGCR when assigning and sequencing ICD-9-CM diagnosis codes. The OGCR also explain the official conventions. Many OGCR in ICD-9-CM are the same as ICD-10-CM, but there are several important changes. Coders working with both code sets must become familiar with the differences.

Conventions

Conventions are specialized rules, abbreviations, formatting, and symbols that alert users to important information. These are described at the beginning of the manual. Official conventions appear in all ICD-9-CM manuals, whereas others are specific to each publisher. Most conventions in ICD-9-CM are similar to those in ICD-10-CM, but not all ICD-10-CM conventions are present in ICD-9-CM.

Official ICD-9-CM Conventions Conventions that are an official part of the ICD-9-CM code set are explained in the OGCR and appear in ■ TABLE 26-2.

> **CODING CAUTION**
>
> ICD-9-CM has only one type of **Excludes** note, rather than the two types—**Excludes1** and **Excludes2**—found in ICD-10-CM.

Publisher-Specific Conventions Publishers of the ICD-9-CM manual may use color coding and special symbols to alert users to important information. Conventions that vary among publishers are publisher-specific conventions. Read the introductory material in the specific manual being used to learn about these conventions. A key that explains the conventions often appears at the bottom of the page in the Tabular List. Conventions are commonly used to indicate the following:

- New code
- Revised code
- Additional character(s) required
- Age-specific requirement
- Gender-specific requirement

Table 26-2 ■ **ICD-9-CM CONVENTIONS**

Convention	Meaning/Use
() Parentheses	**Index and Tabular** : Identifies nonessential modifiers, which describe the default variations of a term. These words are not required to appear in the documentation in order to use the code.
: Colon	**Tabular:** Appears after an incomplete term that requires one or more modifiers following the colon to be classified to that code or category
[] Square brackets	**Index:** Indicates sequencing on etiology/manifestation codes or other paired codes. The code in square brackets [ ] should be sequenced second. **Tabular:** Indicates synonyms, alternative wording, explanatory phrases
And	**Tabular:** Means "and/or"
Boldface (Heavy type)	**Index:** Identifies Main Terms **Tabular:** Identifies code titles
Code First/Use Additional Code	**Tabular:** Provides sequencing instructions for conditions that have both an underlying etiology and multiple body system manifestations and certain other codes that have sequencing requirements
Excludes	**Tabular:** Identifies conditions that are not classified to the chapter, subchapter, category, subcategory, or specific subclassification code under which it is found
Includes	**Tabular:** Begins with the word *Includes* and further defines, clarifies, or gives examples
Italics (Slanted type)	**Tabular:** Identifies exclusion notes, manifestation codes
NEC	**Index and Tabular:** Not Elsewhere Classifiable. The medical record contains additional details about the condition, but there is not a more specific code available to use.
NOS	**Tabular:** Not Otherwise Specified. Information to assign a more specific code is not available in the medical record.
See	**Index:** Instructs the coder to reference another Main Term or condition to locate the correct code
See Also	**Index:** Instructs the coder to refer to an alternative or additional Main Term if the desired entry is not found under the original Main Term
With	**Tabular:** In a code title, means "associated with" or "due to"

Volume 2: Index

Volume 2, which appears *first* in most ICD-9-CM coding manuals, contains three sections: the Index to Diseases and Injuries, the Table of Drugs and Chemicals, and the Index to External Causes of Injury and Poisoning. Various publishers label these sections using slightly different terminology.

Index to Diseases and Injuries

Coders use the Index to Diseases and Injuries (Index) as the first step in coding. Conditions, diseases, and reasons for seeking medical care are listed alphabetically by Main Term and subterms that aid in locating the most appropriate code. After identifying preliminary codes in the Index, they are verified in Volume 1, the Tabular List. Final code selection should never be made based only on the Index.

> **SUCCESS STEP**
>
> The Table of Neoplasms in ICD-9-CM is comparable to the one in ICD-10-CM. The Table of Drugs and Chemicals is similar, but the ICD-10-CM table incorporates several changes compared to ICD-9-CM. The Hypertension Table exists only in ICD-9-CM.

Table of Drugs and Chemicals

Coders use the Table of Drugs and Chemicals when a patient has been injured by a drug, chemical, biological, or other external agent. It contains an alphabetical list of drugs and other chemical substances, cross-tabbed with a list of causes, to identify poisonings and external causes of drug-related adverse effects, such as drug-induced attempted suicide or an adverse reaction to penicillin. Differences in the Table of Drugs and Chemicals between ICD-10-CM and ICD-9-CM are as follows:

- The ICD-9-CM Table of Drugs and Chemicals has a column titled **Poisoning** not present in ICD-10-CM. A code from this column and an **E** code from one of the intent columns must be reported for all poisonings.

- The column titled **Adverse Effect** in ICD-10-CM is titled **Therapeutic Use** in ICD-9-CM.

- ICD-9-CM does not have a column for **Underdosing**.

Alphabetic Index to External Causes of Injury and Poisoning

When a condition is caused by an accident or other external event, supplemental codes describe the circumstances, such as a

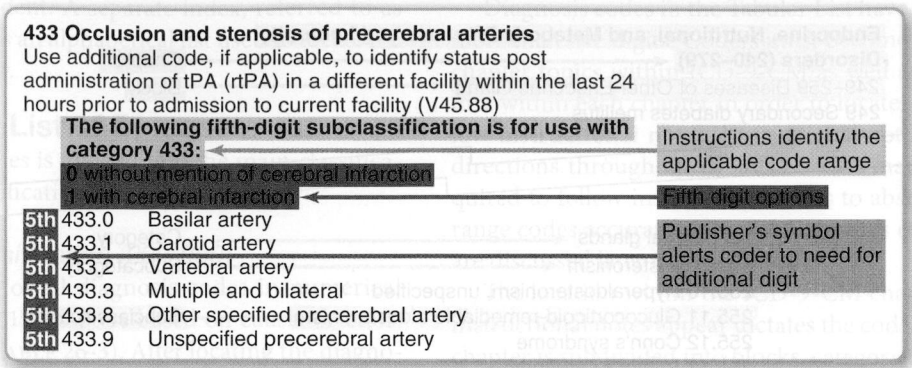

433 Occlusion and stenosis of precerebral arteries
Use additional code, if applicable, to identify status post administration of tPA (rtPA) in a different facility within the last 24 hours prior to admission to current facility (V45.88)

The following fifth-digit subclassification is for use with category 433: ◄——————————— Instructions identify the applicable code range

0 without mention of cerebral infarction
1 with cerebral infarction ◄——————————— Fifth digit options

5th 433.0   Basilar artery
5th 433.1   Carotid artery
5th 433.2   Vertebral artery
5th 433.3   Multiple and bilateral
5th 433.8   Other specified precerebral artery
5th 433.9   Unspecified precerebral artery

Publisher's symbol alerts coder to need for additional digit

Figure 26-2 ■ Tabular List Entry for Fifth-Digit Options at the Beginning of the Category.
Source: © PB Resources, Inc. Used with permission.

typically performed to treat a condition rather than to diagnose it. Assign secondary codes for additional procedures, including those for treatment or diagnosis.

Volume 3 does not have OGCR. Most of the conventions used are the same as those in Volume 1. Two unique conventions to Volume 3 are **omit code** and **[brackets]**.

- **Omit code** appears in the Index to indicate when a code should *not* be used because it is included in another, larger procedure. For example, a laparotomy is a small abdominal incision, often created when a laparoscopic procedure is performed. The Index uses the **Omit code** convention to direct coders *not* to code the laparotomy *in addition to* the laparoscopic procedure (■ FIGURE 26-3). Only the code for the laparoscopic procedure is required.

- **[Brackets]** appear in the Index to indicate that a synchronous procedure (*a procedure performed at the same time as another procedure*) should be coded along with the main procedure (■ FIGURE 26-4). The code for the synchronous procedure appears in brackets and should be sequenced second. For example, reconstruction of the bladder (**57.87**) together with the ileum appears in

Table 26-5 ■ EXAMPLE OF COMPLETE CODES FROM CATEGORY 433

Code	Description
433.00	Occlusion and stenosis of basilar artery without mention of cerebral infarction
433.01	Occlusion and stenosis of basilar artery with cerebral infarction
433.10	Occlusion and stenosis of carotid artery without mention of cerebral infarction
433.11	Occlusion and stenosis of carotid artery with cerebral infarction
433.20	Occlusion and stenosis of vertebral artery without mention of cerebral infarction
433.21	Occlusion and stenosis of vertebral artery with cerebral infarction

Table 26-6 ■ ICD-9-CM VOLUME 3 TABULAR LIST

Chapter Number	Chapter Name	Code Range
0	Procedures and Interventions, Not Elsewhere Classified	00
1	Operations on the Nervous System	01–05
2	Operations on the Endocrine System	06–07
3	Operations on the Eye	08–16
3A	Other Miscellaneous Diagnostic and Therapeutic Procedures	17
4	Operations on the Ear	18–20
5	Operations on the Nose, Mouth, and Pharynx	21–29
6	Operations on the Respiratory System	30–34
7	Operations on the Cardiovascular System	35–39
8	Operations on the Hemic and Lymphatic System	40–41
9	Operations on the Digestive System	42–54
10	Operations on the Urinary System	55–59
11	Operations on the Male Genital Organs	60–64
12	Operations on the Female Genital Organs	65–71
13	Obstetrical Procedures	72–75
14	Operations on the Musculoskeletal System	76–84
15	Operations on the Integumentary System	85–86
16	Miscellaneous Diagnostic and Therapeutic Procedures	87–99

Laparotomy NEC 54.19
  as operative approach—omit code
  exploratory (pelvic) 54.11

Figure 26-3 ■ Example of *Omit Code* Convention in Volume 3 Index

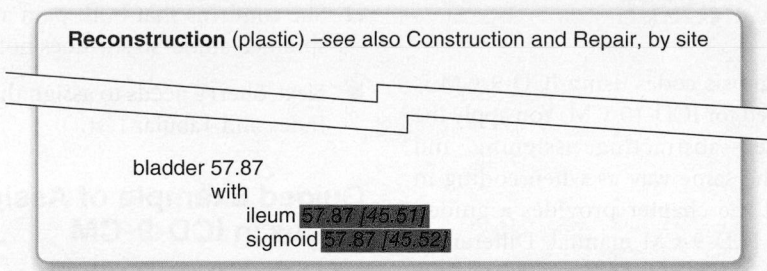

Figure 26-4 ■ Example of the Brackets Convention in Volume 3 Index

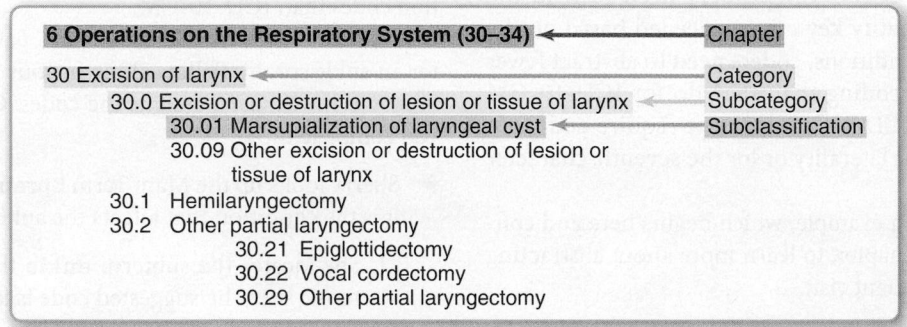

Figure 26-5 ■ Example of Chapter Organization in Volume 3. *Source: © PB Resources, Inc. Used with permission.*

the Index as **57.87 [45.51]**. Assign and sequence the codes as follows:

1. **57.87 Reconstruction of urinary bladder**

2. **45.51 Isolation of segment of small intestine**

Procedure codes in the Tabular List have either three or four digits, with a decimal point after the second digit, such as **30.21**. The Volume 3 Tabular List is organized into chapters, categories, subcategories, and subclassifications (■ FIGURE 26-5).

CODING PRACTICE

Exercise 26.1   Organization of ICD-9-CM

Instructions: Look up each code in the Tabular List using the portion of the code shown below. Identify the missing digit needed to match the description. Write the correct number in the space provided.

Example: 242.0 __1__ Toxic diffuse goiter with mention of thyrotoxic crisis or storm

1. 242.9 _____ Thyrotoxicosis without mention of goiter or other cause, and without mention of thyrotoxic crisis or storm

2. 434.1 _____ Cerebral embolism with cerebral infarction

3. 741.9 _____ Spina bifida without mention of hydrocephalus, dorsal (thoracic) region

4. 304.5 _____ Hallucinogen dependence, episodic

5. 765.0 _____ Extreme immaturity, 1,000–1,249 grams

6. 945.2 _____ Blisters, epidermal loss [second degree] of lower leg

7. 880.1 _____ Open wound of upper arm, complicated

8. E815. _____ Other motor vehicle traffic accident involving collision on the highway injuring passenger on motorcycle

9. 288.0 _____ Congenital neutropenia

10. 296.1 _____ Manic disorder, recurrent episode, in partial or unspecified remission

HOW TO CODE DIAGNOSES IN ICD-9-CM

The process of assigning diagnosis codes using ICD-9-CM is very similar to what you learned for ICD-10-CM. You apply the three skills of an "ace" coder—abstracting, assigning, and arranging codes—in much the same way as when coding in ICD-10-CM. This section of the chapter provides a guided example of coding using the ICD-9-CM manual. Differences between ICD-9-CM and ICD-10-CM are identified.

Guided Example of Abstracting for ICD-9-CM

When abstracting for ICD-9-CM, coders need to read the medical record and identify key criteria needed based on the condition. For many conditions, coders need to abstract fewer details for ICD-9-CM coding than they do for ICD-10-CM coding. For example, ICD-9-CM does not require coders to abstract information for laterality or for the seventh-character episode of care.

Refer to the following example, which begins here and continues throughout the chapter, to learn more about abstracting a diagnosis for an outpatient visit.

> Location: OFFICE   Gender: M   Age: 24
>
> Chief complaint: *Pain and swelling in right ankle. Tripped over some rocks, fell, and twisted ankle.*
>
> Assessment: *X-rays negative for fracture. Right ankle sprain, deltoid ligament*
>
> Plan: *Ice, compression wrap, crutches. Elevate foot. Keep weight off foot for 1 week. OTC acetaminophen for pain PRN. Call office if not better in 2 weeks.*

Follow along with fictional coder Sherry Whittle, CPC, as she reads the progress note from Eric Beardsley's office visit. Check off each step as you complete it.

▶ First, Sherry reviews the demographic information, and then she reads the chief complaint.

❏ She notes that *pain* is a subjective symptom experienced by the patient and *swelling* is an objective sign that Dr. Conover verified.

❏ She also notes the cause of the injury. The injury occurred when the patient *tripped over rocks, fell.*

▶ She reads the assessment, which is the physician's diagnosis.

❏ She notes that X-rays were taken to determine whether there is a fracture, which there is not.

❏ The physician diagnoses the patient with *ankle sprain, deltoid ligament.*

❏ Because she is coding using ICD-9-CM, Sherry does not need to abstract laterality.

▶ Sherry compares the signs and symptoms in the chief complaint to the diagnostic statement of a sprained ankle.

❏ She confirms that both pain and swelling are integral to a sprained ankle, so she does not need to code the symptoms.

▶ Next, Sherry needs to assign the codes using the ICD-9-CM Index and Tabular List.

Guided Example of Assigning Codes in ICD-9-CM

When assigning codes, coders first look up the Main Term in the Index, then verify the code in the Tabular List and assign the correct number of digits. In addition, more conditions require multiple coding in ICD-9-CM because it has fewer combination codes than ICD-10-CM.

Continue with the example of the patient who was treated for an ankle sprain. Follow along in your ICD-9-CM manual as Sherry Whittle, CPC, assigns the codes. Check off each step as you complete it.

▶ Sherry looks up the Main Term **Sprain** in the Index because it is the condition that affects the ankle.

❏ She locates the subterm **ankle** that identifies the anatomic site. The suggested code is **845.00**.

❏ She notices that the only additional subterm is **and foot**, which has the same code, **845.00**. She does not see a subterm for the deltoid ligament under **ankle**.

❏ Sherry looks through other first-level subterms under **Sprain** and locates **deltoid** as a separate subterm.

❏ **Deltoid** has two second-level subterms: **ankle 845.01** and **shoulder 840.8**. She chooses the entry for the ankle.

▶ Next, Sherry turns to the Index to External Causes to identify the code for falling due to tripping over rocks.

❏ In the Index to External Causes, she locates the Main Term **Fall, falling**. She notices that the subterms distinguish falls into or off of an object from falls on the same level. Under the subterm **same level**, she chooses the preposition **from**, then **slipping, stumbling, tripping E885**.

❏ In **E** codes only, the decimal point appears after the fourth character, rather than after the third, as in all other ICD-9-CM codes.

▶ Sherry has now identified two preliminary codes to verify in the Tabular List:

❏ **845.01** for the sprain of the deltoid ligament in the ankle

❏ **E885** for the external cause of tripping over rocks and falling

▶ Sherry turns to the Tabular List to verify code **845.01**.

❏ She reads the code title **Deltoid (ligament) ankle.**

❏ The code is five digits, so she knows it is a valid code.

❏ In ICD-9-CM she needs to refer to the subcategory and category titles to verify the full meaning of the code. This is different from ICD-10-CM, which provides the full code title next to each code number.

❑   The subcategory is **845.0 Ankle**.

❑   The category title is **845 Sprains and strains of ankle and foot**.

❑   The full meaning of code **845.01** is **Sprains and strains of ankle and foot, Ankle, Deltoid (ligament) ankle**.

▶ Sherry needs to check for instructional notes at the category, block, and chapter levels, just as she does when using ICD-10-CM.

❑   Category **845 Sprains and strains of ankle and foot** has no notes.

❑   She locates the block title **Sprains and Strains of Joints and Adjacent Muscles (840–848)** and reads the **Includes** and **Excludes** notes. The **Includes** note lists sprains, so this confirms that she is in the correct section.

❑   She locates the beginning of chapter **17 Injury and Poisoning (800–999)** and reads the instructional note that states **Use E code(s) to identify the cause and intent of the injury or poisoning**. This confirms that she needs to assign a code for the external cause.

▶ Next, Sherry needs to verify the external cause code. She turns to the Tabular List for External Causes to locate code **E885**.

❑   External cause codes begin with the letter E. The first two blocks in the Tabular List are **External Cause Status (E000)** and **Activity (E001-E030)**. After that, the codes move to **E800**. There are no codes numbered E031 through E799.

❑   Sherry locates **E885**, which is a category title, **Fall on same level from slipping tripping or stumbling**.

❑   She reviews the codes that appear in this category to find the one that best describes the situation. Most of the codes identify falling from scooters, roller skates, and similar devices. She notices the last code, **E885.9 Fall from other slipping tripping or stumbling**, and determines that this is the most appropriate code for tripping over rocks. There is no code that specifically describes rocks.

❑   She checks the beginning of the block **Accidental Falls (E880-E888)** and reviews the **Excludes** notes, which do not apply to this patient.

❑   Because the code **E885.9** appears in the block for accidental falls, the full description of the code is **Accidental fall from other slipping tripping or stumbling**.

▶ Next, Sherry needs to arrange the two codes she has verified in the Tabular List.

Guided Example of Arranging Codes in ICD-9-CM

When arranging codes, coders must be attentive to ICD-9-CM OGCR and instructional notes in the Tabular List. In addition, because ICD-9-CM requires more multiple coding, coders may need to arrange multiple codes more frequently when using ICD-9-CM.

The final step in diagnosis coding is to arrange, or sequence, codes in the correct order when there is more than one diagnosis code. Coders may need to assign more than one diagnosis code when patients have more than one condition that is being treated or managed during an encounter; there is an etiology/manifestation relationship; multiple coding is required; or instructional notes in the Tabular List direct the coder to additional codes needed. In addition, the OGCR discuss requirements for multiple coding related to specific diseases.

Continue with the example of the patient who was treated for an ankle sprain. Follow along in your ICD-9-CM manual as Sherry Whittle, CPC, arranges the codes. Check off each step as you complete it.

▶ To arrange the codes for this case, Sherry needs to determine whether the first-listed diagnosis should be the ankle sprain or the external cause of falling.

❑   She refers to the OGCR for external cause codes, OGCR I.C.19. In OGCR I.C.19.a.6), she reads that an **E** code can never be a principal or first-listed diagnosis.

❑   This instruction clearly directs her to sequence the code for the ankle sprain first.

▶ Sherry finalizes the ICD-9-CM codes for this case:

(1) **845.01 Sprains and strains of ankle and foot, Ankle, Deltoid (ligament) ankle**

(2) **E885.9 Accidental fall from other slipping tripping or stumbling**

CHAPTER SUMMARY

In this chapter you learned that:

• After the implementation of ICD-10-CM/PCS, ICD-9-CM continues to be used for three purposes: working with claims before the transition date; data tracking; and submitting claims for non-HIPAA transactions after the transition date.

• The ICD-9-CM manual is separated into three volumes: Volume 1 – Tabular List of Diseases; Volume 2 – Index to Diseases and Injuries; Volume 3 – Inpatient Procedures.

• ICD-9-CM provides official conventions and Official Guidelines for Coding and Reporting (OGCR), many of which are the same as those in ICD-10-CM.

• The process of assigning diagnosis codes using ICD-9-CM is very similar to that for ICD-10-CM, which requires coders to apply the three skills of an "ace" coder—abstracting, assigning, and arranging (sequencing) codes.

CONCEPT QUIZ

Take a moment to look back at ICD-9-CM coding and solidify your skills. Try to answer the questions from memory first, then refer to the discussion in this chapter if you need a little extra help.

Completion

Instructions: Write the term that answers each question based on the information you learned in this chapter. Choose from the list below. Some choices may be used more than once and some choices may not be used at all.

categories	neoplasms
conventions	one
drugs and chemicals	seven
codes	subclassifications
five	subterms
guidelines	therapeutic use
hypertension	three
inpatient procedures	underdosing

1. ICD-9-CM codes can be up to _____ characters long.

2. The ICD-9-CM manual is divided into _____ volumes.

3. Chapters in ICD-9-CM are organized into blocks, _____ _____, subcategories, and subclassifications.

4. The _____ table is present in ICD-9-CM but not in ICD-10-CM.

5. Volume 3 of ICD-9-CM provides codes for _____.

6. Physician offices do not use ICD-9-CM Volume _____.

7. ICD-9-CM Volume 2 has _____ sections.

8. _____ are specialized rules, abbreviations, formatting, and symbols that alert users to important information.

9. Main terms and _____ assist coders in locating the most appropriate code.

10. ICD-9-CM does not have a column for _____ in the Table of Drugs and Chemicals.

Multiple Choice

Instructions: Circle the letter of the best answer to each question based on the information you learned in this chapter.

1. What type of codes does ICD-9-CM contain?
   A. Diagnosis codes and outpatient procedure codes
   B. Diagnosis codes and inpatient procedure codes
   C. Inpatient procedure codes and outpatient procedure codes
   D. Diagnosis codes, inpatient procedure codes, and outpatient procedure codes

2. How many chapters does ICD-9-CM contain?
   A. 3
   B. 7
   C. 15
   D. 17

3. What is a legacy system?
   A. One that is outdated
   B. One that is used for historical purposes
   C. One that is legally mandated
   D. One that is optional

4. Which payer type is not mandated by HIPAA to adopt the ICD-10-CM/PCS code set?
   A. Workers' Compensation
   B. Private insurance
   C. Medicaid
   D. Medicare

5. Which ICD-9-CM convention identifies conditions that are not classified to the chapter, subchapter, category, subcategory, or specific subclassification code under which it is found?
   A. Square brackets [ ]
   B. NOS
   C. Excludes
   D. Includes

6. What type of conventions appears in all editions of the ICD-9-CM manual, regardless of publisher?
   A. CMS
   B. HIPAA
   C. Publisher-specific
   D. Official

7. Which of the following is a column title in the ICD-9-CM Table of Drugs and Poisonings?
   A. Adverse Effect
   B. Underdosing
   C. Therapeutic Use
   D. Self Harm

8. What section of the ICD-9-CM manual provides additional instruction on how to use, assign, and sequence codes?
   A. Tabular List
   B. Index
   C. Table of Neoplasms
   D. Official Sequencing Guidelines

9. What is the maximum number of digits possible in a Volume 3 code?
   A. 2
   B. 3
   C. 4
   D. 5

10. What does ICD-9-CM Volume 3 classify?
    A. Factors influencing health status and contact with health services
    B. External causes of injury and poisoning
    C. Outpatient hospital procedures
    D. Inpatient hospital procedures

CODING CHALLENGE

Instructions: Read the mini-medical-record of each patient's encounter, then abstract, assign, and arrange ICD-9-CM diagnosis codes using the Index and Tabular List. Write the code(s) on the line provided.

> OFFICE   Gender: M   Age: 75
>
> **Reason for encounter:** *Visit to monitor uncontrolled diabetes. C/o frequent urination.*
>
> **Assessment:** *Patient is a type 2 diabetic. Urinalysis confirms UTI. Refer to nutritionist for assistance in meal planning/preparation. Rx for antibiotic for 10 days to treat UTI.*

Part 1: Abstract

Read through the mini-medical-record. Observe the patient demographics.

1. Compare the chief complaint to the final assessment.

   a. What symptom did the patient report in the chief complaint? _____

   b. What two conditions are stated in the assessment? _____

2. Review the symptom.

   a. Is the symptom integral to one of the conditions stated in the assessment? _____

   b. Should you code for the symptom? _____

   c. Why or why not? _____

   d. What is the symptom due to? _____

Part 2: Assign

3. You can look up the conditions in any order you wish, as long as you sequence them correctly in the end based on the instructional notes you find during this exercise.

   a. Look up the Main Term **Diabetes** in the Index. What code is listed? _____

   b. Is there an instructional note in the Index? _____

   c. Verify this code in the Tabular List. Is there a symbol in front of this code indicating you need additional digits? _____

4. Select the final digit.

   a. What is the 5th digit? _____

   b. Why did you select this digit? _____

5. Check for instructional notes.

   a. Locate the beginning of this block for Diseases of Other Endocrine Glands. Read the instructional notes. Now refer back to the mini-medical-record. Do any of the notes apply? _____

   b. Review the instructional notes at the beginning of ICD-9-CM Chapter 3. Do any of the notes apply to this patient? _____

6. Look up the Main Term **Infection** in the Index, then the subterm **urinary (tract)**.

   a. What code is listed? _____

   b. Are there any second-level subterms under **urinary (tract)** that apply? _____

7. Verify this code in the Tabular List.

   a. Is there a symbol in front of this code indicating that you need additional digits? _____

   b. Are there any instructional notes below this code? _____

   c. Do they apply to this patient? _____

8. Locate the beginning of this block for Other Diseases of Urinary System. Are there any instructional notes? _____

9. Review the instructional notes at the beginning of ICD-9-CM Chapter 10. Do any of the notes apply to this patient? _____

Part 3: Arrange

10. You should have identified two codes for this case. Review your answers in the previous questions to determine the correct sequencing.

    a. Which code is sequenced first? _____

    b. Why is this code sequenced first? _____

    c. Which code is sequenced second? _____

KEEP ON CODING

Instructions: Read the diagnostic or procedural statement, then use the appropriate Index and Tabular List to assign ICD-9-CM diagnosis and procedure codes. Write the code(s) on the line provided.

Volumes 1 and 2, ICD-9-CM Diagnosis Codes

1. Acute gout: ICD-9-CM Code(s) _____

2. Rejection of transplanted liver: ICD-9-CM Code(s) _____

(continued)

(continued from page 453)

3. Diaphragm fitting: ICD-9-CM Code(s) _____

4. Struck by lightning in a public swimming pool: ICD-9-CM Code(s) _____

5. Plantar wart: ICD-9-CM Code(s) _____

6. Second-degree sunburn: ICD-9-CM Code(s) _____

7. Screening for osteoporosis: ICD-9-CM Code(s) _____

8. Toxic neutropenia: ICD-9-CM Code(s) _____

9. Concussion, was driver in motor vehicle accident, single car involved: ICD-9-CM Code(s) _____

10. Chronic adenoiditis with chronic tonsillitis: ICD-9-CM Code(s) _____

11. Autistic disorder, active: ICD-9-CM Code(s) _____

12. Family history of colon cancer: ICD-9-CM Code(s) _____

13. Epilepsy: ICD-9-CM Code(s) _____

14. Chronic gonorrhea of bladder: ICD-9-CM Code(s) _____

15. Acute PID: ICD-9-CM Code(s) _____

16. Congenital cardiospasm: ICD-9-CM Code(s) _____

17. Slipped on ice at grocery store: ICD-9-CM Code(s) _____

18. Continual alcohol dependence: ICD-9-CM Code(s) _____

Volume 3, Hospital Inpatient Procedures

19. Revision of ileostomy: ICD-9-CM Volume 3 Code(s) _____

20. Bilateral repair of inguinal hernia: ICD-9-CM Volume 3 Code(s) _____

21. Arthroscopy of knee: ICD-9-CM Volume 3 Code(s) _____

22. Removal of leg cast: ICD-9-CM Volume 3 Code(s) _____

23. Appendectomy via a laparotomy: ICD-9-CM Volume 3 Code(s) _____

24. Complete vasectomy: ICD-9-CM Volume 3 Code(s) _____

25. Arthrodesis of ankle: ICD-9-CM Volume 3 Code(s) _____

ICD-9-CM Body System Coding (000-999, V01-V99, E000-E999)

Chapter 27

Learning Objectives

After completing this chapter, you should have the skills to:

27.1 Spell and define the key words, medical terms, and abbreviations related to ICD-9-CM special topics.

27.2 Identify conditions that require different information than when coding in ICD-10-CM.

27.3 Abstract, assign, and arrange ICD-9-CM codes.

27.4 Discuss ICD-9-CM Official Guidelines for Coding and Reporting.

27.5 Describe the purpose and use of General Equivalency Mappings (GEMs).

Chapter Outline

- **ICD-9-CM Coding Guidelines**
- **Using General Equivalency Mappings**

Key Terms and Abbreviations

approximate mapping
exact mapping

General Equivalency Mappings (GEMs)

many-to-one mapping

one-to-many mapping

In addition to the key terms listed here, students should know the terms defined within tables in this chapter.

For updates and corrections, visit our student resource site at

www.pearsonhighered.com/healthprofessionsresources

INTRODUCTION

Although most drivers prefer the newer, faster road, there are times when it still is necessary to take the old road. Coders must continue to work with ICD-9-CM for claims follow-up and data analysis after the implementation of ICD-10-CM. Some coders must continue to do a limited amount of ICD-9-CM coding to prepare claims for services provided before the transition that have not yet been submitted. Depending on whether Workers' Compensation and third-party liability payers in a particular region are adopting ICD-10-CM, coders might use ICD-9-CM to prepare claims for current transactions for these non-HIPAA payers. In addition, coders doing claims follow-up must interpret ICD-9-CM codes on claims submitted before the transition. Coders also must translate how codes between the two code sets compare for data analysis purposes. In this chapter, you will learn more about ICD-9-CM Official Guidelines for Coding and Reporting (OGCR) and how they differ from ICD-10-CM. You will also learn about the General Equivalency Mappings (GEMs) used in data trending.

ICD-9-CM CODING GUIDELINES

Although the coding process for ICD-9-CM is comparable to ICD-10-CM and the general, inpatient, and outpatient Official Guidelines for Coding and Reporting (OGCR) are nearly identical, there are several conditions for which the chapter-specific OGCR or conventions are different. Some OGCR differ between the two code sets because of changes in conventions, such as the different types of **Excludes** notes, and code formatting, such as the seventh character.

This section provides an overview of how to code conditions in ICD-9-CM that have significantly different OGCR from ICD-10-CM. As you read the following information, open up your medical terminology book and keep a medical dictionary handy to refresh your memory of any unfamiliar terms. You also may find it helpful to refer to the ICD-10-CM chapters for each body system discussed.

HIV

The OGCR for HIV are nearly identical in ICD-9-CM and ICD-10-CM, but because coding this condition can be challenging, a summary of ICD-9-CM appears here. Codes for HIV and AIDS are based on the stage of the disease cycle, as summarized in ■ TABLE 27-1. In addition, assign codes for all AIDS-related illnesses. Refer to ICD-9-CM OGCR I.C.1.a for guidelines on HIV.

Anemia Associated with Malignancy

Patients with a neoplasm often experience anemia. The OGCR for sequencing were different in ICD-9-CM than they are in ICD-10-CM. In ICD-9-CM, sequencing of codes depends on whether the anemia or the neoplasm is the focus of the treatment. Refer to ICD-9-CM OGCR I.C.2.c.1) for guidelines on anemia associated with malignancy. Sequencing depends on the circumstances of admission.

When an encounter or admission is for management of the anemia, and the only treatment provided is for the anemia, sequence the codes as follows:

1. Anemia
2. Neoplasm

Table 27-1 ■ **ICD-9-CM CODING FOR STAGES OF HIV/AIDS**

Stage of Disease	ICD-9-CM Code
Exposure to HIV virus	**V01.79** Contact with or exposure to other viral diseases
HIV testing	**V73.89** Special screening examination for other specified viral diseases
Nonconclusive test results	**795.71** Nonspecific serologic evidence of human immunodeficiency virus [HIV]
Confirmed HIV (seropositive)	**V08** Asymptomatic human immunodeficiency virus [HIV] infection status
HIV counseling	**V65.44** Human immunodeficiency virus (HIV) counseling
AIDS manifestations or illnesses	**042** Human immunodeficiency virus [HIV] disease

Source: © PB Resources, Inc. Used with permission.

When an encounter or admission is for treatment of the neoplasm but anemia is also present, sequence the codes as follows:

1. Neoplasm
2. Anemia

Diabetes Mellitus

ICD-9-CM classifies diabetes mellitus (DM) differently than ICD-10-CM. In ICD-9-CM, all diabetes codes require a fifth digit to identify type I or type II and whether the diabetes is stated as being uncontrolled. Fourth characters for complications identify the body system affected, but additional codes are required to identify the specific type of complication. Refer to ICD-9-CM OGCR I.C.3 for guidelines on diabetes coding.

To code for diabetes in ICD-9-CM, locate the Main Term **Diabetes** in the Index. Select the appropriate subterm for the type of diabetes: **type I**, **type II**, or **secondary**, and a subterm for any manifestations. All diabetes codes must be verified in the Tabular List in order to assign the fifth digit and any additional codes for manifestations. Type I and type II usually lead to a code from category **250** for primary DM. In ICD-9-CM, codes for secondary DM appear in category **249** and are not divided by cause, as they are in ICD-10-CM. Acute manifestations or complications of primary diabetes are coded with subcategories (fourth digit) **.1** to **.3**. Chronic manifestations are coded with subcategories (fourth digit) **.4** through **.9**, based on body system affected (■ TABLE 27-2). For all diabetes codes, the fifth digit identifies the type of DM and whether it is stated as uncontrolled (■ TABLE 27-3).

When more than one body system is affected with complications, use a code of **250.xx** from each body system, with the fourth digit being different for each body system. (When referring to ICD-9-CM codes, use of x or xx is an informal placeholder that means that the appropriate number should be inserted to complete the code.) Be certain the fifth digit is the same for all. For each body system with manifestation(s), an additional code(s) from the body system chapter is required to specify the nature of the manifestation. The most common manifestations are listed in the instructional notes within each subcategory. Verify the manifestation code where it originally appears within the Tabular List. When a type II diabetic requires

Table 27-2 ■ **ICD-9-CM FOURTH DIGITS FOR DIABETES**

Type of Manifestation	4th Digit
No complication	0
Ketoacidosis	1
Hyperosmolarity	2
Other coma	3
Renal	4
Ophthalmic	5
Neurological	6
Peripheral circulatory	7
Other specified (hypoglycemia, hypoglycemic shock)	8
Unspecified	9

long-term insulin use, assign the additional code **V58.67** to report this information (■ FIGURE 27-1).

SUCCESS STEP

The code from category **250 Diabetes mellitus** is always sequenced before the code for the manifestation, even when the manifestation is the reason for the encounter.

Hypertension

ICD-9-CM provides the Hypertension Table to aid in coding for hypertension (■ FIGURE 27-2). The Hypertension Table appears in the Index alphabetized under the letter H. It provides

Table 27-3 ■ **ICD-9-CM FIFTH DIGITS FOR DIABETES 250.XX**

	Type I	Type II
Not stated as uncontrolled	1	0
Uncontrolled	3	2

a complete listing of all conditions associated with hypertension. The table contains four columns:

- Hypertension/hypertensive condition
- Malignant
- Benign
- Unspecified

When there are no hypertensive conditions or manifestations, select a code from the first row, **Hypertension**. When a hypertensive condition or manifestation exists, locate the row for the appropriate subterm in the first column. Then use the appropriate column—**Malignant**, **Benign**, or **Unspecified**—that corresponds to the documentation. Select the code where the row and column intersect. As with any other code, after the preliminary code has been identified in the Hypertension Table, verify the code in the Tabular List. Refer to ICD-9-CM OGCR I.C.7.a for guidelines on hypertension.

Myocardial Infarction

As a result of changes in clinical practice, the definition of a current myocardial infarction (MI) is different in ICD-9-CM than in ICD-10-CM. This is relevant when a patient has more than one MI close together. ICD-9-CM defines a current MI as one

---

> Patient is seen for Type II DM, with long-term insulin use and associated glaucoma.
>
> **250.50 Diabetes mellitus with ophthalmic manifestations, type II or unspecified type, not stated as uncontrolled**
> **365.44 Glaucoma associated with systemic disorders**
> **V58.67 Long-term (current) use of insulin**

Figure 27-1 ■ Example of ICD-9-CM Coding for Diabetes

Hypertension Table	Malignant	Benign	Unspecified
Hypertension, hypertensive (arterial) (arteriolar) (crisis) (degeneration) (disease) (essential) (fluctuating) (idiopathic) (intermittent) (labile) (low renin) (orthostatic) (paroxysmal) (primary) (systemic) (uncontrolled) (vascular)	401.0	401.1	401.9
with			
chronic kidney disease			
stage I through stage IV, or unspecified	403.00	403.10	403.90
stage V or end stage renal disease	403.01	403.11	403.91

Figure 27-2 ■ ICD-9-CM Hypertension Table

> Patient is seen for a stage III pressure ulcer of the sacrum.
>
> **707.03 Pressure ulcer, lower back**
> **707.23 Pressure ulcer, stage III**

Figure 27-8 ■ Example of ICD-9-CM Coding for Pressure Ulcers

A separate medical record is opened for all liveborn infants. The record will have a code from the range **V30-V39**, which describes the location of birth and the existence of multiple liveborn or stillborn mates. For example, **Twin, mate liveborn, V31**. Any other medical conditions of the infant are separately coded.

SUCCESS STEP

ICD-9-CM provides separate chapters and separate codes for the mother's record and the infant's record. Codes for conditions of pregnancy appear in ICD-9-CM Chapter 11 (630-679). These should never be assigned to the infant's record. Codes for perinatal conditions appear in ICD-9-CM Chapter 15 (760-779). These should never be assigned to the mother's record.

Pressure Ulcer

ICD-9-CM requires two codes to classify pressure ulcers, one for the anatomic site from subcategory **707.0 Pressure ulcer** and a second code for the stage from subcategory **707.2, Pressure ulcer stages**. ICD-10-CM requires only one code, from category **L89 Pressure ulcer**, which is a combination code for the anatomic site, laterality, and stage (■ Figure 27-8). Refer to ICD-9-CM OGCR I.C.12.a for guidelines on coding pressure ulcers.

Fractures

ICD-9-CM requires less detail for coding fractures than ICD-10-CM. ICD-9-CM does not require coding for laterality and has no characters to identify the episode of care (■ Figure 27-9). Refer to ICD-9-CM OGCR I.C.17.b.1) for guidelines on fractures.

- Assign the ICD-9-CM code for the fracture (**800-829**) while it is being actively treated.
  - ICD-10-CM provides seventh character(s) for **Initial encounter**.
- Assign ICD-9-CM **V** codes for aftercare (**V54**) when active treatment is complete and the patient is receiving routine

care during the healing phase. Refer to ICD-9-CM OGCR I.C.18.d.7) for guidelines on aftercare.
  - ICD-10-CM provides seventh character(s) for **Subsequent encounter during healing phase**.
- Assign ICD-9-CM codes for complications of surgical treatment with the appropriate complication codes.
- Assign ICD-9-CM codes for malunion (**733.81**) and nonunion (**733.82**) of a fracture with a corresponding code for the specific type of fracture.
  - ICD-10-CM provides seventh characters for **Subsequent encounter for malunion** or **nonunion**.
- Assign ICD-9-CM codes for late effects (**905**) when a late effect of the injury is treated.
  - ICD-10-CM provides seventh character(s) for **Sequela**.

Table of Drugs and Chemicals

The ICD-9-CM Table of Drugs and Chemicals differs from the one in ICD-10-CM in the following ways:

- ICD-9-CM provides a separate column with codes for Poisonings, which must be sequenced before the **E** code for the intent and substance.
- There is a column for Therapeutic Use instead of Adverse Effect.
- There is no column for Underdosing.

Refer to ICD-9-CM OGCR I.C.17.e for guidelines on coding adverse effects, poisoning, and toxic effects. Additional guidelines and definitions appear immediately before the Table of Drugs and Chemicals in the ICD-9-CM manual. The Table of Drugs and Chemicals appears at the end of the Index in most ICD-9-CM manuals (■ Figure 27-10). Use the table as follows:

1. Locate the row in the first column that contains the name of the substance; substance names are listed alphabetically on the left side of the table.
2. For poisonings only, select the preliminary code where the substance row and the **Poisoning** column intersect and sequence it first.
3. Locate the external cause column(s) that identifies the cause and intent (**Accident, Suicide Attempt, Assault, Undetermined**).
4. Locate the preliminary code where the substance row and external cause column intersect.
5. Verify all preliminary codes in the Tabular List to identify the full code.
6. When more than one substance is involved, assign separate codes for each substance.

> A patient is treated for a fracture to the base of the skull. She has closed subdural hemorrhage and was unconscious for 2 hours.
>
> **801.23 Fracture of base of the skull, closed with subarachnoid, subdural, and extradural hemorrhage, with moderate loss of consciousness**

Figure 27-9 ■ Example of ICD-9-CM Coding for Fractures

Substance	Poisoning	Accident	Therapeutic Use	Suicide Attempt	Assault	Undetermined
Antidepressants	969.00	E854.0	E939.0	E950.3	E962.0	E980.3
monoamine oxidase inhibitors (MAOI)	969.01	E854.0	E939.0	E950.3	E962.0	E980.3
specified type NEC	969.09	E854.0	E939.0	E950.3	E962.0	E980.3
SSNRI (selective serotonin and norepinephrine reuptake inhibitors)	969.02	E854.0	E939.0	E950.3	E962.0	E980.3
SSRI (selective serotonin reuptake inhibitors)	969.03	E854.0	E939.0	E950.3	E962.0	E980.3
tetracyclic	969.04	E854.0	E939.0	E950.3	E962.0	E980.3
tricyclic	969.05	E854.0	E939.0	E950.3	E962.0	E980.3
Antidiabetic agents	962.3	E858.0	E932.3	E950.4	E962.0	E980.4

Figure 27-10 ■ ICD-9-CM Table of Drugs and Chemicals

A summary of coding and sequencing rules appears in ■ Table 27-6.

V Codes

ICD-9-CM has codes for **Factors Influencing Health Status and Health Services**, known as **Z** codes in ICD-10-CM. In ICD-9-CM, the comparable codes begin with the letter **V**, so they are often referred to as **V** codes. **V** codes fall into one of three general categories: health status problems, encounter for certain services, or other health-related information relevant to the encounter. **V** codes are indexed in the alphabetical index of Volume 2. The V-code Tabular List is a supplementary classification that appears in Volume 1 after category **999**. Codes begin with the letter **V**, followed by two to four additional digits. The decimal point appears after the third character, such as **V56.31**. Refer to ICD-9-CM OGCR I.C.18 for guidelines on using **V** codes.

Among other uses, **V** codes identify encounters for preventive or administrative medical examinations (**V70 General medical examination**) and encounters that include the need for vaccinations (**V03** through **V06**). These categories differ from comparable categories in ICD-10-CM.

General Medical Examination

Coders accustomed to working in ICD-10-CM should be aware that ICD-9-CM codes for general medical examinations are *less* detailed than in ICD-10-CM. In ICD-9-CM, codes for general medical examinations report the purpose of the encounter, without reference to the findings (**V70-V82**). ICD-10-CM provides multiple codes based on whether there are any abnormal findings (**Z00-Z13**). This feature does not appear in ICD-9-CM.

ICD-9-CM classifies most administrative examinations with one code, **V70.3 Other general medical examination for administrative purposes**. ICD-10-CM provides *multiple codes* for administrative examinations, with separate codes for each type, such as camp, school, sports, or insurance. These codes appear in category **Z02 Encounter for administrative examination**.

Need for Prophylactic Vaccination

Coders accustomed to working in ICD-10-CM should be aware that ICD-9-CM codes that identify the need for vaccinations are *more detailed* than in ICD-10-CM.

ICD-9-CM provides separate codes for each vaccination that a patient needs (**V03-V06**). For example, separate codes

Table 27-6 ■ **ICD-9-CM CODING AND SEQUENCING RULES FOR POISONINGS AND ADVERSE EFFECTS**

Event	Definition	Coding and Sequencing
Poisonings	Wrong substance taken in error, overdose, accidents in the usage of drugs during medical procedures, intoxication	1. A code from the Poisoning column 2. An E code for the substance from the appropriate intent column: Accident, Suicide attempt, Assault, Undetermined 3. Code(s) to identify the medical condition that resulted
Adverse effect	Pathological reaction to therapeutic drugs taken or administered as prescribed: proper drug, proper dose	1. Code(s) to identify the medical condition that resulted 2. An E code for the substance from the Therapeutic Use column

Source: © PB Resources, Inc. Used with permission.

are provided for measles, influenza, chicken pox, and so on. ICD-10-CM provides *one code* that identifies the need for vaccination(s) as the purpose of the encounter (**Z23 Encounter for immunization**). It does not provide separate **Z** codes for

each type of vaccination. CPT codes, which also must be reported on each claim, identify the specific vaccination(s) administered.

CODING PRACTICE

Exercise 27.1 ICD-9-CM Coding Guidelines

Instructions: Read the mini-medical-record of each patient's encounter and assign ICD-9-CM diagnosis codes using the Index and Tabular List. Write the code(s) on the line provided.

---

1. OFFICE   Gender: M   Age: 62

Reason for encounter: *open sore on right heel*

Assessment: *patient has developed a foot ulcer with skin breakdown due to type II diabetes, which he has not been successful at controlling*

Plan: *Refer to wound care. Follow-up with dietician.*

2 ICD-9-CM Codes _____

---

2. INPATIENT HOSPITAL   Gender: F   Age: 26

Reason for admission: *full-term labor*

Assessment: *Attempted vaginal delivery. Labor started off well then slowed. I was concerned that prolonged labor would place the scar from the previous cesarean delivery at risk, so I proceeded with another cesarean delivery.*

(continued)

---

2. (continued)

Delivery: *cesarean delivery, live birth, 1 girl*

Tip: Assign a code for the cesarean delivery due to a previous cesarean delivery, a code for failed labor, and a code for the outcome of delivery.

3 ICD-9-CM Codes _____

---

3. OFFICE   Gender: F   Age: 31

Reason for encounter: *follow-up on HIV test results*

Assessment: *Positive for HIV, asymptomatic, counseled patient on managing the infection*

Plan: *Refer to HIV support group*

2 ICD-9-CM Codes _____

USING GENERAL EQUIVALENCY MAPPINGS

In addition to using ICD-9-CM when working with claims for services provided before the ICD-10-CM implementation date, coders may encounter ICD-9-CM data when working with reports and statistics. To compare data for services provided under ICD-9-CM with those provided under ICD-10-CM, coders and health information managers need a way to match codes between the two code sets. The **General Equivalency Mappings (GEMs)** are a set of four data files created by the Centers for Disease Control and Prevention (CDC) to be the authoritative source for comparing codes between the two code sets (■ TABLE 27-7). The files can be downloaded from the CDC or the Centers for Medicare and Medicaid Services (CMS) websites. Data managers use GEMs to program data analysis software to align codes from ICD-9-CM with those from ICD-10-CM/PCS. ICD-9-CM codes can be mapped

Table 27-7 ■ **GENERAL EQUIVALENCY MAPPING FILES**

GEM File	Purpose
ICD-9-CM Volume 1 to ICD-10-CM	Forward mapping that matches ICD-9-CM diagnosis codes with approximate ICD-10-CM codes
ICD-9-CM Volume 3 to ICD-10-PCS	Forward mapping that matches ICD-9-CM inpatient procedure codes with approximate ICD-10-PCS codes
ICD-10-CM to ICD-9-CM Volume 1	Backward mapping that matches ICD-10-CM codes with approximate ICD-9-CM diagnosis codes
ICD-10-PCS to ICD-9-CM Volume 3	Backward mapping that matches ICD-10-PCS codes with approximate ICD-9-CM inpatient procedure codes

Five-Digit Code	
250.50 ▼	Diabetes with ophthalmic manifestations, type II or unspecified type, not stated as uncontrolled
Add Date	10/1/1986
General Equivalence Mappings (GEMs)	This mapping has been designated as *approximate*. Choose one of the following codes: E11.311 Type 2 diabetes mellitus with unspecified diabetic retinopathy with macular edema E11.319 Type 2 diabetes mellitus with unspecified diabetic retinopathy without macular edema E11.36 Type 2 diabetes mellitus with diabetic cataract E11.39 Type 2 diabetes mellitus with other diabetic ophthalmic complication

Figure 27-11 ■ Example of GEMs in an Encoder. *Source: SpeedECoder. Reprinted with permission.*

"forward" to ICD-10-CM/PCS, and ICD-10-CM/PCS codes can be mapped "backward" to ICD-9-CM. Encoders (coding software programs) often include GEMs mappings (■ Figure 27-11).

GEMs are approximations, not exact matches, because there are many more codes in the ICD-10-CM and PCS code sets than in ICD-9-CM Volume 1 and Volume 3. ICD-10-CM/PCS code sets are more detailed, introduce new concepts and related codes, and eliminate outdated concepts and related codes. GEMs map four types of code matches:

- exact mapping the codes in both code sets have exactly the same definition
- approximate mapping the codes in both code sets are similar but not exactly the same
- one-to-many mapping a single code in ICD-9-CM has several possible equivalents in ICD-10-CM or vice versa
- many-to-one mapping several codes in ICD-10-CM are combined into a single equivalent code in ICD-9-CM or vice versa

Exact Mapping
Approximately one-fourth of ICD-9-CM codes have an exact match in ICD-10-CM, meaning that the codes in both manuals describe exactly the same condition.

- **ICD-9-CM: 416.0 Primary pulmonary hypertension**
  - **ICD-10-CM: I27.0 Primary pulmonary hypertension**
- **ICD-9-CM: 535.01 Acute gastritis, with hemorrhage**
  - **ICD-10-CM: K29.01 Acute gastritis with bleeding**

Only a few ICD-10-CM codes have an exact backward map to ICD-9-CM.

Approximate Mapping
Roughly half of ICD-9-CM codes have an approximate match in ICD-10-CM, meaning that the ICD-10-CM code is similar to, but not an exact duplicate of, the ICD-9-CM code.

- **ICD-9-CM: 157.4 Malignant neoplasm of islets of Langerhans**
  - **ICD-10-CM: C25.4 Malignant neoplasm of endocrine pancreas**

One-to-Many Mapping
Most remaining ICD-9-CM codes have one-to-many forward mappings, meaning there are several ICD-10-CM codes for conditions that are described by only one code in ICD-9-CM.

- **ICD-9-CM: 424.1 Aortic valve disorders**
  - **ICD-10-CM:**
    I35.0 Nonrheumatic aortic (valve) stenosis
    I35.1 Nonrheumatic aortic (valve) insufficiency
    I35.2 Nonrheumatic aortic (valve) stenosis with insufficiency
    I35.8 Other nonrheumatic aortic valve disorders
    I35.9 Nonrheumatic aortic valve disorder, unspecified

Working in reverse, some ICD-10-CM codes are mapped backward to multiple ICD-9-CM codes. This is often because of the increased use of combination codes in ICD-10-CM.

- **ICD-10-CM: E10.331 Type 1 diabetes mellitus with moderate nonproliferative diabetic retinopathy with macular edema**
  - **ICD-9-CM:**
    250.51 Diabetes with ophthalmic manifestations, type I [juvenile type], not stated as uncontrolled
    362.05 Moderate nonproliferative diabetic retinopathy
    362.07 Diabetic macular edema

Many-to-One Forward Mapping
Some ICD-9-CM codes have a many-to-one forward mapping, meaning there is only one ICD-10-CM code that correlates with several ICD-9-CM codes. In general, codes that have a one-to-many forward mapping also have many-to-one backward mapping.

- **ICD-9-CM:**
  401.0 Malignant essential hypertension
  401.1 Benign essential hypertension
  401.9 Unspecified essential hypertension
- **ICD-10-CM: I10 Essential (primary) hypertension**

A few ICD-9-CM codes have no match at all in ICD-10-CM.

Misuse of GEMs

Using GEMs to find code matches is an inexact process and should be used only for research and trending purposes, not for actually assigning codes to patient encounters for billing purposes. GEMs are intended to be used with large volumes of data that need to be compared or analyzed over a time span that includes dates both before and after ICD-10-CM/PCS implementation.

GEMs are not a substitute for learning how to use all the code sets appropriately. GEMs are not intended to be used by coders to assign codes for specific patient encounters. Doing so would be misuse of data and potentially fraudulent coding practices. **It is not possible to determine which code is the single best translation for a specific encounter without reference to the patient's medical record and without following the proper coding process of researching a code in the Index then verifying it in the Tabular List.**

CODING PRACTICE

Exercise 27.2 Using General Equivalency Mappings

Instructions: Write the definition of each of the following terms.

1. Exact mapping _____
   _____

2. One-to-many mapping _____
   _____

3. Approximate mapping _____
   _____

4. Backward mapping _____
   _____

5. Forward mapping _____
   _____

CHAPTER SUMMARY

In this chapter you learned that:

- The coding process for ICD-9-CM is comparable to ICD-10-CM, and the general, inpatient, and outpatient OGCR are nearly identical. There are several conditions for which the chapter-specific OGCR or conventions are different: HIV, anemia associated with malignancy, diabetes, hypertension, myocardial infarction, asthma, obstetrics, pressure ulcers, fractures, poisoning and adverse effects, and **v** codes.

- The General Equivalency Mappings (GEMs) are a set of four data files created by the Centers for Disease Control and Prevention

(CDC) to be the authoritative source for comparing codes between ICD-9-CM, ICD-10-CM, and ICD-10-PCS.

- GEMs are intended to be used with large volumes of data that need to be compared or analyzed over a time span that includes dates before and after the implementation.

- GEMs are *not* intended to be used by coders to assign codes for specific patient encounters.

CONCEPT QUIZ

Take a moment to look back at ICD-9-CM coding and solidify your skills. Try to answer the questions from memory first, then refer to the discussion in this chapter if you need a little extra help.

Completion

Instructions: Write the term that answers each question based on the information you learned in this chapter. Choose from the list below. Some choices may be used more than once and some choices may not be used at all.

accidental poisoning	aftercare
adverse reaction	anemia
after	before

backward	hypertension
controlled	many to one
episode of care	normal delivery
forward	uncontrolled
history (of)	vaginal delivery

1. A(n) _____ is a pathological reaction to therapeutic drugs taken or administered as prescribed: proper drug, proper dose.

2. _____ mapping matches ICD-10-PCS codes with approximate ICD-9-CM inpatient procedure codes.

3. _____ mapping matches ICD-9-CM diagnosis codes with approximate ICD-10-CM codes.

4. Diabetes mellitus is always sequenced _____ the code for the manifestation.

5. _____ is a term used for an encounter for full-term uncomplicated delivery.

6. Codes in category V54 are used to report _____.

7. _____ mapping maps several codes in ICD-10-CM into a single equivalent code in ICD-9-CM or vice versa.

8. When coding DM, the fifth digit identifies the type of DM and whether or not the DM is _____.

9. When coding an MI, the fifth digit identifies the _____.

10. _____ associated with malignancy is sequenced depending on the circumstances of admission.

Multiple Choice

Instructions: Circle the letter of the best answer to each question based on the information you learned in this chapter.

1. Which of the following encounters is appropriate for an ICD-9-CM V code?
   A. A patient seen for symptoms of a cold
   B. A patient seen to have her hearing aid adjusted
   C. A patient seen for a broken leg
   D. A patient seen for diagnosis of Alzheimer disease

2. What type of mapping is used when the codes in both code sets, ICD-9-CM and ICD-10-CM, are similar but not exactly the same?
   A. Exact mapping
   B. Approximate mapping
   C. One-to-many mapping
   D. Many-to-one mapping

3. What type of mapping is the following? ICD-9-CM: 416.0 Primary pulmonary hypertension and ICD-10-CM: I27.0 Primary pulmonary
   A. Exact mapping
   B. Approximate mapping
   C. One-to-many mapping
   D. Many-to-one mapping

4. What is the E code alphabetic index called?
   A. Alphabetic Index
   B. Tabular Index
   C. Index to External Causes of Injury
   D. Neoplasm Table

5. What does the fourth digit represent when coding an acute MI?
   A. The underlying cause of the MI
   B. The level of damage to the heart
   C. Where the infarction occurred
   D. The length of the MI

6. How should codes for primary and secondary neoplasms be sequenced?
   A. According to stage of the tumor or cancer
   B. Primary site first and secondary site second
   C. By severity
   D. Depending on the reason for the encounter

7. What does the the fifth-digit of 2 indicate in an obstetrics code?
   A. The delivery did not occur during the current episode of care; the patient has an antepartum condition or complication.
   B. The delivery occurred during the current episode of care, and the physician also documented a postpartum condition (after delivery).
   C. The delivery did not occur during the current episode of care; the patient has a postpartum condition or complication.
   D. The delivery occurred during the episode of care being coded.

8. What type of ICD-10-CM codes are ICD-9-CM V codes comparable to?
   A. F codes
   B. Z codes
   C. V codes
   D. E codes

9. What ICD-9-CM code should always be assigned to patients previously diagnosed with any HIV-related illness?
   A. V08
   B. V69.8
   C. 042
   D. 795.71

10. How should codes for multiple fractures be sequenced?
   A. From the head down
   B. From the foot up
   C. According to the severity
   D. According to size

CODING CHALLENGE

Instructions: Read the mini-medical-record of each patient's encounter, then abstract, assign, and arrange ICD-9-CM diagnosis codes using the Index and Tabular List. Write the code(s) on the line provided.

---

1. OUTPATIENT HOSPITAL Gender: F Age: 67

Reason for encounter: chemotherapy

Assessment: Female with carcinoma of the left upper-outer quadrant of the breast. Here for first chemotherapy.

Plan: Continue chemotherapy sessions.

2 ICD-9-CM Codes _____

(continued)

(continued from page 467)

19. 27-year-old primigravida married female, 12 weeks' gestation, with hyperemesis gravidarum and dehydration:
ICD-9-CM Code(s) _____

20. Postpartum varicose veins of legs: ICD-9-CM Code(s) _____

21. Ulcerated internal hemorrhoids: ICD-9-CM code(s) _____

22. Third visit for sprained left ankle, sustained while stepping off the sidewalk: ICD-9-CM code(s) _____

23. Contracture of right foot due to poliomyelitis: ICD-9-CM code(s) _____

24. Fungal meningitis: ICD-9-CM code(s) _____

25. Vesicoureteral reflux with bilateral reflux nephropathy: ICD-9-CM Code(s) _____

SECTION FOUR

CPT/HCPCS Procedure Coding

Section Four, CPT/HCPCS Procedure Coding, discusses the procedure coding systems used by physicians, nonphysician providers, and outpatient facilities to bill for services. Providers establish a fee for each procedure code, which is the basis of reimbursement calculations. Diagnosis codes provide the medical justification for the reason the services are needed. Although CPT and HCPCS are completely different coding systems from ICD-10-CM and ICD-9-CM, you are still able to apply the three skills of an "ace" coder: abstract, assign, and arrange.

PROFESSIONAL PROFILE

MEET...

Lori Dafoe, CPC
Compliance Analyst, The Doctors Clinic

I love the diversity of coding. On any given day, I could be working on a coding issue, helping a physician with documentation, working with an insurance carrier to ensure proper payment based on our contract, or helping to develop a training plan for ICD-10-CM. Sometimes it seems like coding changes come around faster than we can get the education out to providers!

I was working as a medical secretary in the 1990s and started working extended hours in the evenings and on Saturday, doing special projects for the business office manager. Eventually, I got involved in coding and earned my CPC certification in 2000. I currently split my time between Coding and Compliance Analyst and Business Office Supervisor. I support and provide coding and compliance training to physicians, clinical personnel, and billing staff. My responsibility is to establish effective communication with physicians and clinical staff on coding issues and provide auditing services to ensure accurate and ethical coding of claims.

Part of a coder's job is to provide feedback to physicians regarding correct coding. For example, I recently had a provider submit a charge for a simple closure (CPT code 12001) with excision of a genital lesion (CPT code 11420). Because simple closure is always included in the excision of a lesion, I reviewed the documentation to provide feedback to the physician. I found that that physician did not actually excise a lesion, but performed a biopsy of two separate lesions of the vulva, which should be coded with CPT codes 56605 and 56606.

Coders must educate physicians while still respecting their role and authority. We are here to work together, and coders can learn a lot from our providers. In addition to my findings, I always provide the regulations for the physician to review along with his or her documentation. If they disagree with the findings, I ask that they pinpoint areas they feel document the service according to the regulations. That gives me a better understanding of the procedure and their thought process behind the code selection. It also helps me provide additional education or offers insight that may support the original code selection and cause me to revise my audit findings.

When communicating with physicians, I must be short, concise, and to the point. When providing education in writing, I like to use bullet points outlining the most important items. When meeting with a physician in person, I review the essential elements first. That way, if time runs short or the physician gets called away, I've been able to deliver the most significant information.

Certification is required for the position I currently hold with my company. I believe it is extremely important to my career. I am currently the president of our local AAPC chapter and served as both secretary and education officer in the past. I am also on the Advisory Committee for the medical assisting program at a local college, which involves attending quarterly meetings and contributing to program updates.

My advice to students is "Don't get discouraged!" Medical billing and coding is a complex field and it takes time to learn everything.

Chapter 28

Introduction to CPT Coding

Chapter Outline

- **Overview of CPT Coding**
- **Organization of the CPT Manual**
- **Abstracting Procedures for CPT Coding**
- **Assigning CPT Codes**
- **Arranging CPT Codes**
- **CPT Coding and Reimbursement**

Learning Objectives

After completing this chapter, you should have the skills to:

28.1 Spell and define the key words, medical terms, and abbreviations related to CPT coding.

28.2 Discuss the history and purpose of CPT coding.

28.3 Identify the organization of the CPT manual, including CPT guidelines and conventions.

28.4 Explain how to abstract procedural information from the medical record.

28.5 Demonstrate how to assign CPT codes.

28.6 Discuss the principles of arranging (sequencing) CPT codes.

28.7 Explain the relationship between accurate CPT coding and reimbursement.

Key Terms and Abbreviations

837P
add-on code
ambulatory payment classification (APC)
bundling edit
category (CPT)
Category I
Category II
Category III
common descriptor

conversion factor
Current Procedural Terminology (CPT)
edit
geographic practice cost index (GPCI)
guidelines (CPT)
indented code description
instructional note (CPT)
Medicare Physician Fee Schedule (MPFS)

Medicare Physician Fee Schedule Database (MPFSDB)
modifier (CPT)
modifying term
outpatient prospective payment system (OPPS)
parent code
prepayment edit
relative value unit (RVU)
resequenced code

resource-based relative value scale (RBRVS)
section (CPT)
semicolon (CPT)
special instructions (CPT)
standalone code
subcategory (CPT)
subheading (CPT)
subsection (CPT)
unlisted procedure

In addition to the key terms listed here, students should know the terms defined within tables in this chapter.

For updates and corrections, visit our student resource site at

www.pearsonhighered.com/healthprofessionsresources

INTRODUCTION

When you go shopping, each item is marked with an item number that identifies it. Similarly, procedure codes identify the procedures and services that physicians provide to patients. Procedure coding is the act of assigning a code to a patient's procedure or service. Physician procedure codes have been standardized since 1966, which has made coding more efficient and more accurate. Accuracy in procedure coding is essential because incorrect or inadequate coding may lead to denial or delay of insurance claims. Each coding system, such as ICD-10-CM and CPT, is different, so it is important to learn what information applies to all code sets and what information is unique to each. CPT uses some of the same terms as ICD-10-CM/PCS but defines them differently, so coders must understand the meanings within the context of each code set. In this chapter you will learn the history, purpose, and terminology of CPT coding; the organization of the CPT manual; how to abstract, assign, and arrange (sequence) CPT codes; and the relationship between CPT codes and reimbursement.

OVERVIEW OF CPT CODING

Current Procedural Terminology (CPT), Fourth Edition (also referred to as CPT-4), is a listing of five-character alphanumeric codes and descriptions that report outpatient medical services and procedures. CPT codes are five digits with no decimal point, such as 99215. Certain categories of CPT codes contain a letter as the last character, such as 0500F. The Health Insurance Portability and Accountability Act (HIPAA) mandates the use of CPT for all covered entities that handle electronic claims related to outpatient healthcare services. As a result, CPT is the standard for communication among healthcare providers, regulators, and payers.

The History of CPT Coding

Before the mid-1960s, most patients paid out of pocket for their services. When they had health insurance, they submitted their own claims to insurance companies and were reimbursed directly. There were no standard medical billing forms or procedure codes. Reimbursement was cost-based, meaning that the insurance companies paid whatever fees providers charged.

With the passage of Medicare and Medicaid in 1965, the healthcare industry recognized the need to standardize the description of services provided. The Health Care Financing Administration (HCFA), now known as the Centers for Medicare and Medicaid Services (CMS), assigned the task of developing codes to the American Medical Association (AMA). The AMA developed and published the first edition of CPT in 1966, the year that the Medicare and Medicaid programs were implemented, and has been responsible for CPT codes ever since. The first edition of CPT primarily contained surgical procedures, with limited sections on medicine, radiology, and laboratory. Codes were four digits in length.

The CPT was updated several times during the 1970s until the fourth edition—still in use today— was adopted in 1977. At that time, a process was established to update the code set on a regular basis.

In 1983, the federal government adopted CPT as part of its Healthcare Common Procedure Coding System (HCPCS) and later required it to be used to report services billed to Medicare Part B and Medicaid. CPT codes are also called Level I HCPCS codes. The passage of HIPAA in 1996 required that uniform standards for electronic transactions be established. Effective October 16, 2003, CPT was designated a mandated procedure code set for covered entities for physician services and most other types of outpatient claims, including hospital outpatient procedures.

Today, the CPT manual covers all procedures approved by the Food and Drug Administration (FDA). The CPT lists over 8,800 procedural codes. CPT is updated every year, with changes taking effect January 1. Code changes are published by the AMA in conjunction with CMS. CPT updates are made to clarify code descriptions and incorporate new technologies and equipment. Use the edition of the CPT that was in effect on the date of service.

SUCCESS STEP

The transition date for CPT manuals is January 1. For patients seen on December 31, use the CPT manual for the old year. For patients seen on January 1 and after, use the CPT manual for the new year. Remember that the transition date for CPT differs from the transition date for the ICD-10-CM diagnosis coding manual, which is October 1.

The Purpose of CPT Coding

Procedure codes identify billable services provided to patients. Physicians report CPT procedure codes on insurance claims—the CMS-1500 and its electronic equivalent, the 837P—to identify the services provided and the cost of those services (■ FIGURE 28-1). Physicians are paid for CPT codes, but diagnosis codes are required to explain the reason(s) for the encounter and/or the reason services were provided. Coders must be certain to abstract and assign at least one ICD-9-CM or ICD-10-CM diagnosis code for each procedure or service billed. The same diagnosis code can be used for more than one service, but coders cannot report a service that is not supported by a diagnosis (■ FIGURE 28-2). Any service that lacks a corresponding diagnosis code will not be paid by the insurance company.

It can be challenging to find the most appropriate and accurate code for each patient encounter. For example, patient encounters for what is commonly referred to as an "office visit" may be reported with any of 30-plus codes, depending on a number of circumstances. However, only one code is correct in any given situation, so coders must become familiar with the nuances among codes that might seem to be similar. Likewise, more than 50 codes describe sutures for a wound. The correct code is based on the location, length, and depth of the wound. Coders need to be familiar with all of the criteria for coding services offered by their office to be certain they select the accurate code.

It is improper to code for a more complex service than what was actually provided in the hope of receiving higher

HEALTH INSURANCE CLAIM FORM

APPROVED BY NATIONAL UNIFORM CLAIM COMMITTEE (NUCC) 02/12

| | PICA | | | | | | | PICA | |

CARRIER

1. MEDICARE (Medicare#) **MEDICAID** (Medicaid#) **TRICARE** (ID#/DoD#) **CHAMPVA** (Member ID#) **GROUP HEALTH PLAN** [X] (ID#) **FECA BLK LUNG** (ID#) **OTHER** (ID#)

1a. INSURED'S I.D. NUMBER (For Program in Item 1)
7856321

2. PATIENT'S NAME (Last Name, First Name, Middle Initial)
DOE JOHN A

3. PATIENT'S BIRTH DATE MM 05 DD 15 YY 1980 **SEX** M [X] F

4. INSURED'S NAME (Last Name, First Name, Middle Initial)
DOE JANE M

5. PATIENT'S ADDRESS (No., Street)

6. PATIENT RELATIONSHIP TO INSURED Self [ ] Spouse [X] Child [ ] Other [ ]

7. INSURED'S ADDRESS (No., Street)
123 WASHINGTON STREET

CITY | **STATE**

8. RESERVED FOR NUCC USE

CITY BRANTON | **STATE** ST

ZIP CODE | **TELEPHONE (Include Area Code)** ( )

ZIP CODE 11111 | **TELEPHONE (Include Area Code)** ( )

9. OTHER INSURED'S NAME (Last Name, First Name, Middle Initial)

10. IS PATIENT'S CONDITION RELATED TO:

11. INSURED'S POLICY GROUP OR FECA NUMBER

a. OTHER INSURED'S POLICY OR GROUP NUMBER

a. EMPLOYMENT? (Current or Previous) YES [ ] NO [X]

a. INSURED'S DATE OF BIRTH MM DD YY **SEX** M [ ] F [ ]

b. RESERVED FOR NUCC USE

b. AUTO ACCIDENT? YES [ ] NO [X] **PLACE (State)**

b. OTHER CLAIM ID (Designated by NUCC)

c. RESERVED FOR NUCC USE

c. OTHER ACCIDENT? YES [ ] NO [X]

c. INSURANCE PLAN NAME OR PROGRAM NAME

d. INSURANCE PLAN NAME OR PROGRAM NAME

10d. CLAIM CODES (Designated by NUCC)

d. IS THERE ANOTHER HEALTH BENEFIT PLAN? YES [ ] NO [X] *If yes*, complete items 9, 9a, and 9d.

READ BACK OF FORM BEFORE COMPLETING & SIGNING THIS FORM.
12. PATIENT'S OR AUTHORIZED PERSON'S SIGNATURE I authorize the release of any medical or other information necessary to process this claim. I also request payment of government benefits either to myself or to the party who accepts assignment below.

SIGNED SOF DATE

13. INSURED'S OR AUTHORIZED PERSON'S SIGNATURE I authorize payment of medical benefits to the undersigned physician or supplier for services described below.

SIGNED SOF

PATIENT AND INSURED INFORMATION

14. DATE OF CURRENT ILLNESS, INJURY, or PREGNANCY (LMP) MM DD YY QUAL.

15. OTHER DATE QUAL. MM DD YY

16. DATES PATIENT UNABLE TO WORK IN CURRENT OCCUPATION FROM MM DD YY TO MM DD YY

17. NAME OF REFERRING PROVIDER OR OTHER SOURCE
17a.
17b. NPI

18. HOSPITALIZATION DATES RELATED TO CURRENT SERVICES FROM MM DD YY TO MM DD YY

19. ADDITIONAL CLAIM INFORMATION (Designated by NUCC)

20. OUTSIDE LAB? YES [ ] NO [ ] **$ CHARGES**

21. DIAGNOSIS OR NATURE OF ILLNESS OR INJURY Relate A-L to service line below (24E) **ICD Ind.** 0

A. I10 B. I48.91 C. J30.9 D.
E. F. G. H.
I. J. K. L.

22. RESUBMISSION CODE ORIGINAL REF. NO.

23. PRIOR AUTHORIZATION NUMBER

24. A. DATE(S) OF SERVICE						B. PLACE OF SERVICE	C. EMG	D. PROCEDURES, SERVICES, OR SUPPLIES (Explain Unusual Circumstances)		E. DIAGNOSIS POINTER	F. $ CHARGES		G. DAYS OR UNITS	H. EPSDT Family Plan	I. ID. QUAL.	J. RENDERING PROVIDER ID. #
From MM	DD	YY	To MM	DD	YY			CPT/HCPCS	MODIFIER							
01	15	YY	01	15	YY	11		99205		ABC	205	00	01		NPI	1234567890
01	15	YY	01	15	YY	11		95052		C	50	37	10		NPI	1234567890
01	15	YY	01	15	YY	11		93000		B	18	25	01		NPI	1234567890
															NPI	
															NPI	
															NPI	

PHYSICIAN OR SUPPLIER INFORMATION

25. FEDERAL TAX I.D. NUMBER 111222333 **SSN** [ ] **EIN** [X]

26. PATIENT'S ACCOUNT NO. 5831

27. ACCEPT ASSIGNMENT? (For govt. claims, see back) [X] YES [ ] NO

28. TOTAL CHARGE $ 273 62

29. AMOUNT PAID $

30. Rsvd for NUCC Use

31. SIGNATURE OF PHYSICIAN OR SUPPLIER INCLUDING DEGREES OR CREDENTIALS (I certify that the statements on the reverse apply to this bill and are made a part thereof.)
Kristin Conover, MD 1/15/20YY
SIGNED DATE

32. SERVICE FACILITY LOCATION INFORMATION
a. NPI b.

33. BILLING PROVIDER INFO & PH # (555) 555 1111
BRANTON FAMILY PRACTICE
999 MAIN STREET
BRANTON ST 00000
a. 9998887776 b.

NUCC Instruction Manual available at: www.nucc.org **PLEASE PRINT OR TYPE** APPROVED OMB-0938-1197 FORM 1500 (02-12)

Figure 28-1 ■ Example of a Completed CMS-1500 Form.

> A new patient presented in the office to establish primary care. Performed a comprehensive history, a comprehensive focused examination, and medical decision making of high complexity. Patient has a 10-year history of hypertension and 5-year history of atrial fibrillation both of which she has been taking medication for. Also complains of unknown allergies. Performed an EKG and 10 allergy patch tests. Diagnosis: hypertension, atrial fibrillation, allergic rhinitis
>
> | | |
> |---|---|
> | I10 | **Essential (primary) hypertension** |
> | I48.91 | **Unspecified atrial fibrillation** |
> | J30.9 | **Allergic rhinitis, unspecified** |
> | 99205 | **Office or other outpatient visit for the evaluation and management of a new patient, which requires these 3 key components...** |
> | 95052 | **x 10 Photo patch test(s) (specify number of tests)** |
> | 93000 | **Electrocardiogram, routine ECG with at least 12 leads; with interpretation and report** |

Figure 28-2 ■ Example of Matching Diagnosis Codes to Procedure Codes. *Source:* © PB Resources, Inc. Used with permission.

reimbursement. Doing so is considered fraud and carries severe penalties, including fines and possible imprisonment.

Coders must also be attentive to entering codes correctly into the computer or onto the CMS-1500 billing form. A typographic error in a code number can result in a rejected insurance claim, which must be corrected and rebilled, thus delaying the payment the office receives.

Medical Terminology Used in CPT Coding

Medical terms related to procedure coding use the same word roots and combining forms as those used in diagnosis coding, but the suffixes describe procedures rather than diagnoses. Coders must be able to distinguish between medical terms that describe diagnoses and those that describe procedures. They also must understand the meaning of suffixes that describe procedures so they can accurately identify the procedure performed. ■ TABLE 28-1 lists commonly used suffixes that describe procedures. Refer to ■ TABLE 28-2 (page 474) for a refresher on how to build medical terms for diagnoses and procedures related to the same anatomic site.

ORGANIZATION OF THE CPT MANUAL

Coders need to be familiar with the organization of the CPT manual so that they can find needed information quickly. Not only do you need to understand where needed information is located, you also need to identify and interpret coding guidelines, instructional notes, and conventions. The AMA publishes several editions of the CPT, and other publishers sometimes print the CPT manual with enhanced reference information. The codes and guidelines are the same in all editions, but some organize the features differently and might include enhanced features such as diagrams, color coding, and reference information. Each CPT manual shows the year on the front cover. Always use the manual that corresponds with the calendar year of the date of service, regardless of when the billing is done. The content and labeling of specific topics can change from year to year when the manual is updated. For this reason, it is important to become familiar with the specific edition of the manual

Table 28-1 ■ MEDICAL TERM SUFFIXES THAT DESCRIBE PROCEDURES

Suffix	Meaning	Example
-centesis	Surgical puncture (*withdrawal of fluid*)	Arthrocentesis (*performing surgical puncture to withdraw fluid from a joint*)
-clasis	Breaking down, fracture	Osteoclasis (*surgical fracture or refracture of a bone*)
-desis	Binding or stabilization	Arthrodesis (*stabilizing or binding together a joint*)
-ectomy	Cutting out all or part of	Arthrectomy (*cutting out part of a joint*)
-graphy	Making a recording or picture/image	Radiography (*making a picture using radiation waves*)
-lysis	Loosening or destroying (*to free from adhesion*)	Arthrolysis (*surgically loosening adhesions in a joint*)
-metry	Taking a measurement, measuring	Oximetry (*measuring oxygen [in the blood]*)
-pexy	Fixating, positioning, attaching	Cystopexy (*fixation of the bladder [to the abdominal wall]*)
-plasty	Surgical repair	Arthroplasty (*repairing a joint*)
-rrhaphy	Surgically suture or repair	Cystorrhaphy (*surgical suturing of the bladder*)
-scopy	Viewing	Arthroscopy (*viewing a joint*)
-section	Cutting apart, slicing	Small-bowel resection (*cutting apart/slicing out some or all of the small intestine*)
-stasis	Stopping or controlling	Hemostasis (*stopping bleeding*)
-stomy	Creating a new opening or mouth	Colostomy (*surgical creation of an opening into the colon*)
-therapy	Treatment	Radiotherapy (*treatment using radiation waves*)
-tomy	Cutting into, opening, making an incision	Arthrotomy (*making an incision into a joint*)
-tripsy	Crushing or destroying	Lithotripsy (*crushing or destroying stones/calculi*)

Source: © PB Resources, Inc. Used with permission.

Appendices

The CPT manual has 15 appendices that provide reference information. Several appendices summarize codes designated with special symbols throughout the CPT manual. Other appendices provide technical information used in offices that perform specialized procedures, such as nerve conduction studies, cardiac catheterization, or genetic testing. Appendices A, B, and C are used most often by coders. Look through the other appendices in the CPT manual so you become familiar with the available information.

Appendix A: Modifiers

Appendix A presents a complete description of all modifiers applicable to the current year codes. **Modifiers** are two-digit alphanumeric suffixes appended to CPT codes to further describe circumstances. Most publishers print an abbreviated list of commonly used modifiers inside the front cover, but you should develop the habit of referring to Appendix A until you are familiar with the details of how a specific modifier is to be used. Use of modifiers is introduced later in the chapter.

Appendix B: Summary of Additions, Deletions, and Revisions

Appendix B lists all the changes in the current year's manual. It is useful at the beginning of the year when the new CPT codes are released. You can quickly cross-reference the CPT codes on encounter forms to Appendix B to determine how the codes commonly used in your office might be affected by the annual revision.

Appendix C: Clinical Examples

Appendix C provides examples of E/M code scenarios for many medical specialties. These should not be used for coding but for learning and understanding how various patient encounters might be coded. The most commonly used E/M codes each have at least one example.

Index

Coders should always begin to locate a code by using the CPT Index. After identifying potential codes in the Index, users should verify them in the Tabular List. Never select the final code based only on the Index, even when only one code appears. Follow along in the Index of your CPT manual as the features are discussed next.

The Index lists procedures and services in the CPT manual alphabetically by Main Term and modifying terms that aid in locating the most appropriate code or range of codes (■ FIGURE 28-4).

Modifying terms, or subterms, are descriptive words in the Index that appear indented under the Main Term to further describe the service or procedure. When modifying terms appear, it is important to review the entire list of options before selecting the most specific term.

CODING CAUTION

Do not confuse the CPT expressions *modifying term* and *modifier*. Modifying terms are Index entries that add further detail to the Main Term. Modifiers are two-character suffixes that are appended to Category I codes to further explain the service provided.

The first level of modifying terms is aligned on the same margin as the Main Term but is set in smaller, nonboldfaced type. The second and third levels of modifying terms each are indented several spaces beyond the previous level. They further describe the Main Term in reference to anatomic site (e.g., **Endoscopy**, **Anus**); extent (e.g., **Excision**, **Clavicle**, **Partial**); procedure (e.g., **Electrocardiography**, **24-Hour Monitoring**); or similar descriptors.

When the Main Term or modifying term is too long to fit on one line, a carry-over line is used. Carry-over lines are indented the same number of spaces as the beginning of the line. It is important to read carefully to distinguish between carry-over lines and modifying terms.

Main Terms and modifying terms contain instructional notes, such as *see* or *see also*, which direct the user to synonyms for the code. For example, the entry **Pneumonotomy—see Incision, Lung** instructs the user to look under the Main Term **Incision** and the modifying term **Lung** to locate the codes for removal of the lung. In Figure 28-4, the instructional note **See Arthroscopy; Thoroscopy** directs the user to other useful Main Terms.

Code number(s) next to a Main Term indicate the most likely applicable codes. Numbers may be single codes, a range of codes, or a nonsequential list (■ TABLE 28-5).

Table 28-5 ■ DESIGNATION OF CODES AND CODE RANGES IN THE CPT INDEX

Symbol	Purpose	Example
None	Single code	Polyp 46615
Hyphen (-)	Range of codes All codes beginning with the first code number and ending with the last code number should be reviewed.	Bone Graft, Harvesting 20900–20902
Comma (,)	Nonsequential codes The specific codes listed should be reviewed, but the intervening code number(s) are not applicable or do not exist.	Biopsy, Urethra 52204, 52250, 52354, 53200

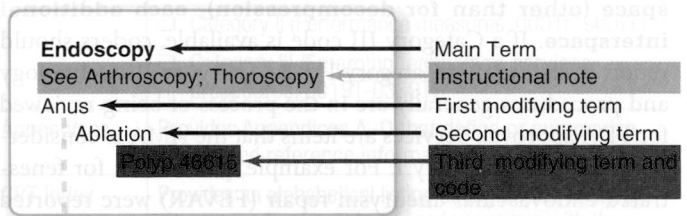

Figure 28-4 ■ Example of CPT Index Organization.

CODING PRACTICE

Exercise 28.1 Overview of CPT Coding/Organization of the CPT Manual

Instructions: Use your medical terminology skills and resources to define the following symptoms, signs, and abnormal findings, then assign the CPT code.

Follow these steps:

- Use slash marks "/" to break down each term into its root(s) and suffix.
- Define the meaning of the word, based on the meaning of each word part.
- If code(s) are listed next to the Main Term, write down the code. If no code is listed next to the Main Term, write down the first-level modifying term and the CPT code(s) listed for it.

Example: appendectomy append/ectomy   Meaning *cutting out the appendix*   First-level modifying term/code *Appendix Excision 44950, 44955, 44960*

1. ventriculography   Meaning _____   First-level modifying term/code(s) _____
2. acetabuloplasty   Meaning _____   First-level modifying term/code(s) _____
3. ureterotomy   Meaning _____   First-level modifying term/code(s) _____
4. ileostomy   Meaning _____   First-level modifying term/code(s) _____
5. pneumonolysis   Meaning _____   First-level modifying term/code(s) _____
6. urethropexy   Meaning _____   First-level modifying term/code(s) _____
7. pericardiocentesis   Meaning _____   First-level modifying term/code(s) _____
8. lymphadenectomy   Meaning _____   First-level modifying term/code(s) _____
9. laryngoscopy   Meaning _____   First-level modifying term/code(s) _____
10. neurorrhaphy   Meaning _____   First-level modifying term/code(s) _____

ABSTRACTING PROCEDURES FOR CPT CODING

Coding procedures in CPT requires the three skills of an "ace" coder—abstracting, assigning, and arranging codes. Because the CPT manual has a unique organization and unique conventions, coders must learn how using these skills differs for CPT compared with other code sets. This section of the chapter provides a guided example of coding using the CPT manual.

When abstracting for CPT, coders need to read the medical record and identify key criteria based on the services provided. Abstract only services provided during the encounter being coded. Do not code services that were previously provided or that may be planned for the future. Abstracting procedures from the patient's medical record involves three steps:

1. Identify the primary service or procedure.
2. Identify secondary services or procedures.
3. Identify the quantity of each procedure.

Identify the Primary Service or Procedure

Physicians often indicate procedure codes on the encounter form by placing a check mark next to or circling the CPT code that best describes the service provided. CPT codes may be data entered from the encounter forms directly into the practice management/billing system. However, medical offices must still audit and verify codes against the medical record on a regular basis to ensure that the documentation supports the services billed.

First, look for the chief complaint or reason for the visit, which usually provides an indication of the services that may be provided. Identify the primary procedure or the main service provided during the encounter. It is common for the E/M to be the only service provided. An E/M code includes the ongoing evaluation and management of a patient's care—specifically, taking the patient's history, conducting a physical examination, and performing the medical decision making required to create a plan of care.

When the physician orders a test to be performed at a later time, do not code for the test as part of the current encounter. Ordering the test or procedure is part of the medical decision-making component of the E/M service. Likewise, when the physician reviews test results during the encounter, do not code for the test, which was performed at a different time. The physician's review of the test results and discussion with the patient is included in the E/M code for the encounter. However, when a test is performed as part of the encounter, such as an in-office urinalysis or X-ray, code for the test in addition to the E/M service.

Identify Secondary Services or Procedures

Next, identify whether any secondary procedures were provided. Secondary procedures are any additional services documented in the medical record in addition to the primary procedure. They are abstracted and coded in the same way as the primary procedure.

At the time of abstracting, coders do not necessarily know whether an additional service or procedure can be coded because it often depends on how the specific code is defined. For example, when a surgeon removes the uterus, cervix, and fallopian tubes you may be unsure how many CPT codes are required. By identifying all the structures removed when abstracting, you are prepared. When assigning codes, you learn that only one code is required to report the removal of all three structures (**58150 Total abdominal hysterectomy (corpus and cervix), with or without removal of tube(s), with or without removal of ovary(s))**.

Identify the Quantity of Each Procedure

All services must be billed with the quantity provided. Although coders may or may not be responsible for preparing the claim, they are responsible for identifying the quantity for each code because quantity is reported differently for different codes. For many procedures the quantity is one.

For services that can be repeated multiple times during one operative session, such as removal of lesions, the quantity reported with the code varies based on the code definition. You must first identify the type and number of lesions removed, as documented in the medical record, then convert the number to agree with the quantity included in the code description. For example, code **11200** for the removal of skin tags is defined as including up to 15 lesions. Any quantity of lesions from 1 to 15 is reported with a quantity of **1** unit on the 837P electronic claim or Item 24G of the CMS-1500 form.

For services based on time, identify the number of minutes spent providing the service, then convert them to the unit of time required by the code description. For example, code **97035** for therapeutic ultrasound is reported in 15-minute increments. When 30 minutes of treatment are provided, report a quantity of **2** units on the 837P electronic claim or CMS-1500 form.

Refer to ■ TABLE 28-6 for general guidance on how to abstract procedures and services. These criteria apply to most services and procedures. More detailed abstracting criteria are presented for each body system throughout the CPT section of this text. Abstracting questions are a guide and not every question applies to, or can be answered for, every case. For example, complications do not occur with every patient.

Guided Example of Abstracting Procedures

Refer to the following example throughout this chapter to practice skills for abstracting, assigning, and arranging CPT codes.

OFFICE   Gender: M   Age: 32

Preprocedure diagnosis: lesion on the back

Procedure: Prepared the area, administered local anesthesia, and excised one lesion from the back using a scalpel. Total excised area 0.7 cm. The site was closed with simple sutures.

Postprocedure diagnosis: benign lesion on the back

Pathology report: benign lesion 0.7 cm including margins

Table 28-6 ■ **KEY CRITERIA FOR ABSTRACTING PROCEDURES (GENERAL GUIDELINES)**

❑ What service(s) were provided or procedure(s) performed at the current encounter by a physician or other qualified healthcare professional?

❑ What is the main service or procedure?

❑ What additional services or procedures were performed?

❑ What is the patient's age and gender?

For each service or procedure:

❑ What method, instrumentation, or approach was used?

❑ What anatomic site(s) were treated?

❑ What quantity was provided or time spent?

❑ What complications or unusual circumstances were encountered?

❑ Was more than one provider involved?

❑ What is the final diagnosis?

Source: © PB Resources, Inc. Used with permission.

Follow along as the fictitious coder, Sherry Whittle, CPC, abstracts the procedure. Check off each step after you complete it.

▶ Sherry reads through the entire record, paying special attention to the reason for the encounter and the final assessment. Sherry refers to Table 28-6 Key Criteria for Abstracting Procedures. (General Guidelines) (*Questions from the Key Criteria table appear in italics.* Verbiage taken directly from the medical record appears in this special font. Any other comments or observations appear in a normal font.)

❑ *What service(s) were provided or procedure(s) performed at the current encounter?* Removal of a lesion

❑ *What is the main service or procedure?* Removal of a lesion

❑ *What additional services or procedures were performed?* None

❑ *What is the patient's age and gender?* Male, 32

❑ *What method, instrumentation, or approach was used?* local anesthesia, scalpel

❑ *What anatomic site(s) were treated?* back

❑ *What quantity was provided or time spent?* one lesion, 0.7 cm

❑ *What complications or unusual circumstances were encountered?* None

❑ *Was more than one provider involved?* No

❑ *What is the final diagnosis?* Benign lesion on the back

CODING PRACTICE

Exercise 28.2   Abstracting Procedures for
CPT Coding

Instructions: Read the mini-medical-record of each patient's encounter and answer the abstracting questions. Write the answer on the line provided. Do not assign any codes.

> INPATIENT HOSPITAL   Gender: F   Age: 48
>
> Preprocedure diagnosis: metastatic breast cancer
>
> Procedure: left axillary lymphadenectomy, complete, using the open approach
>
> Postprocedure diagnosis: left breast cancer with metastasis to lymph nodes
>
> Plan: Begin radiation therapy in 3 weeks.

1. What service(s) were provided or procedure(s) performed during the current encounter? _____

2. Describe the procedure performed in your own words.
   _____

3. What is the patient's age and gender? _____

4. Are the patient's age and gender appropriate for the procedure?
   _____

5. What method, instrumentation, or approach was used?
   _____

6. What anatomic site(s) were treated? _____
   Where is this site(s) located? _____

7. What quantity was provided? _____
   What is the extent of the service (superficial or complete)?
   _____

8. What service should not be coded for this encounter?
   _____ Why? _____

9. What is the final diagnosis? _____

10. What is the principal diagnosis (the main reason the procedure was performed)? _____

ASSIGNING CPT CODES

Assigning CPT codes requires coders to research the procedure in the Index, then verify the code(s) in the Tabular List. Each of these processes includes several steps, which are discussed next. Never assign a code based on the Index alone, and do not turn to the Tabular List without first using the Index.

Research the Procedure in the Index

Use the Index to locate the preliminary code(s). This involves determining the Main Term, modifying terms, and codes or code ranges. Using the Index involves three steps.

1. Identify the Main Term.
2. Review the modifying terms and instructional notes.
3. Identify the preliminary code(s).

Identify the Main Term

The CPT Index is organized by Main Terms, the word(s) you look up in the Index to find the code(s). Each Main Term can stand alone or be followed by one to three modifying terms that provide added specificity. The CPT Index classifies Main Terms in four ways. Coders may use any of these methods to locate a code in the Index. If one method does not provide adequate information, then another method may be used. The four types of entries for Main Terms are:

- **Procedure or service name**
  - Examples: **Endoscopy, Incision, Cast**
- **Organ or anatomic site**
  - Examples: **Tibia, Colon, Lung**

- **Condition**
  - Examples: **Abscess, Clot, Fracture**
- **Synonym, eponym, or abbreviation**
  - Synonym examples: **Ocular Implant, Orbital Implant**
  - Eponym examples: **Nissen procedure, Fowler-Stephens procedure**
  - Abbreviation examples: **EKG, CD4**

The Main Term is always boldfaced, and each word begins with a capital letter. Some Main Terms are broad, with several pages of modifying terms, such as **Excision**, whereas others are quite specific, with only a single code, such as **Color Vision Examination**.

> ### SUCCESS STEP
>
> In the CPT Index, Main Terms include organs and anatomic sites, whereas in ICD-10-CM, anatomic site is not an option in the Index. Because there are many choices of how to locate a Main Term, a good guideline is to search in this order: eponym or abbreviation; procedure or service name; organ or anatomic site; disease or condition; synonym.

Review the Modifying Terms and Instructional Notes

After locating the Main Term, review the modifying terms and instructional notes. Modifying terms are entries under the Main Term that identify additional details regarding the anatomic site or procedure. Main Terms can have several levels of modifying terms. Each modifying term is a cumulative definition that

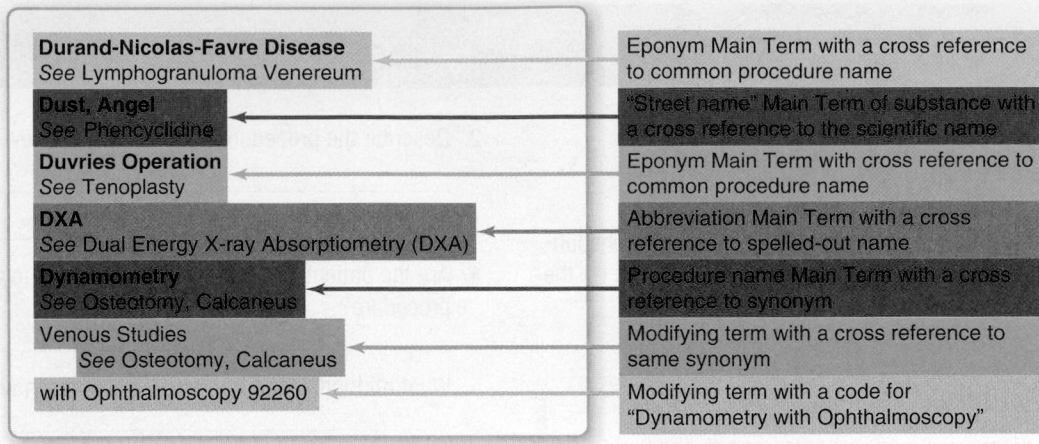

Figure 28-5 ■ Cross Reference Instructional Notes in CPT Index. *Source:* © PB Resources, Inc. Used with permission.

includes the terms at the previous levels. For example, in Figure 28-4 the meaning of the fourth-level modifying term **Polyp** is *Endoscopy of the anus with the ablation of a polyp.*

Instructional notes inform you of other Main Terms to look up if you cannot find what you need under the current term. They also tell you when to look up a synonym or other variation of the term. For example, when you look up an abbreviation or eponym in the CPT Index, it might redirect you to another entry, such as the fully spelled-out term or the generic name for the procedure. This feature assists coders in finding the appropriate Main Term more quickly (■ FIGURE 28-5).

Identify the Preliminary Code(s)

When the appropriate modifying terms are located, the preliminary code(s) is printed immediately to the right. It is helpful to jot down the preliminary codes before verifying in the Tabular List, being careful not to transpose any digits. Never use the Index to select the final code. Even when only one code appears, it must be verified in the Tabular List to be certain the code selection is accurate and to read any instructional notes.

CODING CAUTION

Be aware of how the CPT Index differs from the ICD-10-CM Index. In the ICD-10-CM Index, each Main Term or subterm provides only one possible code. In the CPT Index, a Main Term or modifying term often provides several possible codes to consider. You must read the code descriptions and instructional notes in the Tabular List to select the final code.

Verify the Code in the Tabular List

All codes must be verified in the Tabular List to ensure that the description accurately represents the service provided. Coders also need to read the guidelines, special instructions, and instructional notes printed in the Tabular List. Verifying the code in the Tabular List involves the following steps.

1. Locate the preliminary code(s) in the Tabular List.
2. Interpret Tabular List conventions.
3. Select the code with the highest level of specificity.

4. Review the code for appropriate edits, such as bundling, add-on codes, and quantity.
5. Append modifiers, if necessary.
6. Assign the code.

Locate the Preliminary Code(s) in the Tabular List

Look for the preliminary code number in the Tabular List, where codes are arranged in numerical order. The Tabular List contains six sections, each of which is divided into subsections, subheadings, categories, and subcategories based on anatomy, procedure, condition, or descriptor. Be aware that because of the expanding nature of the code set, some codes are not in strict numerical order. These are resequenced codes and are highlighted with the symbol # for easy identification.

The CPT Index does not always list every possible code for a procedure. Sometimes it will list one or two codes from a series, and the coder must review surrounding codes to locate the one needed.

CODING CAUTION

The resequenced code number appears in numerical order with an instruction that identifies the code range where the description appears. However, this cross-referenced code range can be rather broad, encompassing several code numbers. Sometimes the coder must browse multiple columns of code descriptions to locate the resequenced code.

Interpret Tabular List Conventions

Before coders verify and finalize the code, they first need to interpret the conventions presented with the code. The CPT code number appears on the left side of the column, with its description to the right. Tabular List conventions include formatting, punctuation, verbal instructions, and symbols. Conventions may appear on the same line with the code, above it, below it, or at the beginning of a subcategory, category, subheading, subsection, or section. Look carefully for any information that may be relevant to the preliminary code selection because this additional information can direct you to use a different code

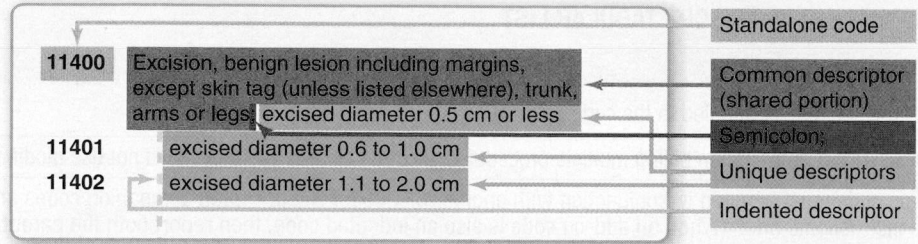

Figure 28-6 ■ Example of the Semicolon Convention. *Source:* © PB Resources, Inc. Used with permission.

or an additional code. The Tabular List conventions of the semicolon, verbal instructions, and symbols are discussed next.

Semicolon. In the Tabular List, an important convention is the use of the **semicolon** (;) and indented code descriptions. To conserve space and avoid having to repeat common terminology, some of the procedure descriptors in the Tabular List are not printed in their entirety, but rather refer back to a common portion of the procedure descriptor listed in a preceding entry. The **standalone code** or **parent code** is the one whose description is left-justified and begins with a capital letter. The shared portion of the code before the semicolon is the **common descriptor**, which is shared with indented codes. The portion after the semicolon is the unique descriptor that applies to only one code number. The **indented code description** is indented three spaces and begins with a lowercase letter. This description is the unique descriptor for that code number. The unique descriptor must be combined with the shared descriptor from the standalone code to obtain a full description of the code. Within a series of indented codes, coders *must* refer back to the preceding standalone code to determine the common descriptor of the indented code(s). Indented codes describe variations of the standalone code, such as an alternative anatomic site, alternative procedure, or extent of services.

■ FIGURE 28-6 illustrates this formatting convention. The standalone code is **11400**. The words before the semicolon— **Excision, benign lesion including margins, except skin tag (unless listed elsewhere), trunk, arms or legs;**—are the common part of the description. This common descriptor should be considered part of each of the following indented codes in that series. For example, the full procedure descriptor represented by code **11401** is:

> **11401 Excision, benign lesion including margins, except skin tag (unless listed elsewhere), trunk, arms or legs; excised diameter 0.6 to 1.0 cm**

An indented code should not be billed together with the parent code unless both services were provided. These are considered two distinct procedures or services. The common descriptor is simply a space-saving convention in the printed book.

Narrative Instructions. The CPT manual provides several types of narrative instructions that guide coders:

- **Guidelines** are instructions that appear at the beginning of each of the six sections and apply to all codes in that section. Guidelines also list commonly used modifiers and provide subsection information.

- **Special instructions** are directions within each section describing specific rules and definitions for use of codes within a particular category or subcategory. Read and interpret the special instructions before assigning a code, even if it means going back to the top of the page or a previous page to find them.

- **Instructional notes** appear in parentheses after a code description. They direct the user to alternative codes for closely related procedures or to codes that must or must not be used together (■ FIGURE 28-7).

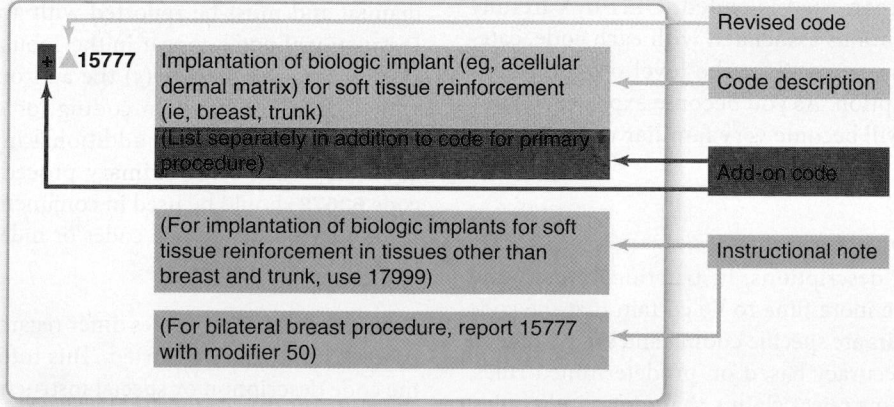

Figure 28-7 ■ Example of CPT Tabular List Conventions. *Source:* © PB Resources, Inc. Used with permission.

Table 28-7 ■ **SYMBOLS USED IN THE CPT TABULAR LIST**

Symbol	Meaning
⟲	Moderate sedation is bundled in the code description.
⊘	Modifier –51 exempt. When billing multiple procedures, a code with this symbol should not use modifier -51.
✚	Add-on code must be used in conjunction with another CPT code. The accepted companion codes are frequently provided in an instructional note. (When an add-on code is also an indented code, then report both the parent code and indented code.)
⁄	FDA approval pending. FDA approval of the vaccine described is expected to come during the current year.
( )	Parentheses enclose synonyms, eponyms, or supplementary descriptors. These terms do not have to appear in a physician's statement of condition to use the code.
•	New code in this edition of the CPT manual.
▲	Revised code. The code number is the same, but the descriptor has been updated for the current edition of the CPT manual. The descriptor should be reviewed to determine whether it is still appropriate.
►◄	Contains new or revised text. Alerts users to the fact that guidelines or instructions have been updated in the current edition of the CPT manual and should be reviewed.
#	Resequenced code. Some codes do not appear in strict numerical sequence within a section of the Tabular List. Rather than deleting and renumbering codes, which was done before 2010, resequencing allows existing codes to be relocated to an appropriate place within the CPT subsection, based on the code concept, regardless of the numerical order. This symbol is used in front of the resequenced code to help locate it.

Symbols. Symbols in the Tabular List alert the user to certain circumstances that can affect the use or interpretation of codes. A key appears at the bottom of each page. Coders should become familiar with these meanings (■ TABLE 28-7).

Select the Code with the Highest Level of Specificity

There is no universal rule that describes how many codes need to be reviewed to identify the one with the highest specificity. Sometimes, the best code is the first one listed; other times, there can be a dozen or more codes to review and additional ones to cross-reference. There also is no universal rule that governs how precise the description of the correct code will be. For example, many codes for the integumentary system include the size of the lesion or area treated, but the size is usually a range, such as a diameter of 1.1 to 2.0 cm or total area greater than 100 sq cm. If a lesion is *exactly* 1.5 cm, or the area is 110 sq cm, there is *not* a more specific code or modifier to describe the exact size. The medical record often contains more detail than what is coded. Only by carefully interpreting the conventions associated with each code, category, and section can one confirm the level of detail contained in a code description. As you become experienced in a particular office, you will become very familiar with the most frequently used codes.

Review the Code for Appropriate Edits

Carefully review code descriptions, instructional notes, and special instructions one more time to be certain that the code selected is accurate. Edits are specific coding and billing criteria that are checked for accuracy based on predetermined rules. Payers' computer systems reject claims that violate edit rules. Bundling, add-on codes, and quantity definitions are edits that should be reviewed.

Bundling Edits. Pay special attention to **bundling edits**, which are frequently triggered by the words **includes** and **not separately reportable**. These phrases indicate that multiple services are included in a single code. The words **report separately** or **use in conjunction with** indicate that additional codes should be used.

For example, the special instructions for codes **33510-33516 Coronary artery bypass, vein only** include both bundling and multiple coding situations.

- Instructions regarding bundling state: **Procurement of the saphenous vein graft is included in the description of the work for 33510-33516 and should not be reported as a separate service or co-surgery**.

- Instructions regarding multiple coding state that an additional code is needed in some situations: **to report harvesting of an upper extremity vein, use 35500 in addition to the bypass procedure.**

Add-On Codes. Add-on codes are marked with a **+** in the CPT manual and must be reported with an additional procedure. Instructional notes appear in the Tabular List below an add-on and identify which code(s) the add-on codes should be used with. For example, when coding for discectomy of multiple disks, the code for each additional interspace is reported in addition to a specific primary procedure code. CPT add-on code **63078** should be used in conjunction with **60377**. Add-on codes may be standalone codes or indented codes, as **63078** is (■ FIGURE 28-8).

Quantity Edits. CPT codes differ regarding how the quantity of procedures is to be reported. This information is provided in the code description or special instructions. For example:

- To report removal of skin tags, a single code, **11200**, describes **up to and including 15 lesions.** Although the code is

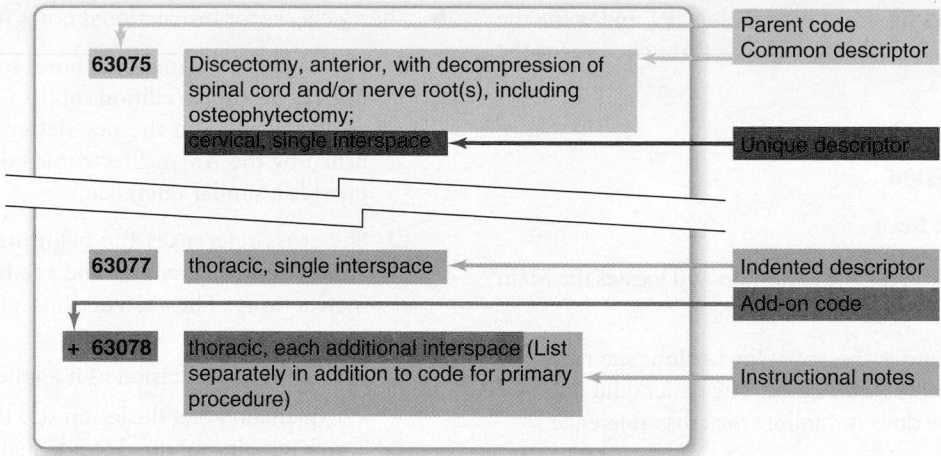

Figure 28-8 ■ Example of CPT Indented and Add-on Codes. *Source:* © PB Resources, Inc. Used with permission.

reported with a quantity of **1** in Item 24G of the CMS-1500 form, it describes any quantity from 1 to 15 lesions.

- To report shaving of epidermal or dermal lesions (**11300-11313**), each code describes a single lesion; multiple lesions of the same size and body area are reported by designating the number of lesions in Item 24G on the CMS-1500 form.

- To report end-stage renal disease services, use a single code for the entire month (**90960-90961**); the special instructions describe the scope of services included.

Codes that include a time-based element also vary in how quantity is reported. For example, codes for certain physical therapy treatments (**97032-97039**) describe 15 minutes of treatment with a quantity of **1** in the appropriate electronic field for the 837P or in Item 24G on the CMS-1500 form. Thirty minutes of treatment is reported with a quantity of **2** in the appropriate electronic field for the 837P or in Item 24G of the CMS-1500 form.

Append Modifiers, If Necessary

Modifiers are two-digit suffixes used with CPT codes to report a service or procedure that has been modified by some specific circumstance without altering or modifying the basic definition or CPT code. The proper use of modifiers can speed up claims processing and increase reimbursement. Improper use of CPT modifiers may result in claim delays or denials.

Modifiers are used for a variety of reasons:

- To report only the professional component of a procedure or service

- To report a service mandated by a third-party payer

- To indicate that a procedure was performed bilaterally

- To report multiple procedures performed during the same session by the same provider

- To report a portion of a service or procedure that was reduced or eliminated at the physician's discretion

- To report a portion of the surgical package provided by someone other than the primary surgeon.

- To report assistant surgeon services

Use of modifiers may be described in the instructional notes, special instructions, or guidelines. Modifiers may be necessary when the code(s) reported are affected by Medicare reimbursement rules. The experience of the coder is an important factor when determining whether the situation calls for any modifiers. A complete list of modifiers, with their full definitions, appears in Appendix A of the CPT manual.

Assign the Code

As a final check, with coding manual instructions fresh in your mind, refer back to the original documentation and verify that all conditions of the code agree with the medical record. If a discrepancy arises, work through the process again from the beginning. Write down the final code where indicated on your worksheet or documentation. Be certain to proofread the number as you wrote or keyed it to catch transcription errors that are easy to make. Repeat this process for any additional codes required by the medical record.

Selecting a procedure code might seem like a long and tedious process at first. As you become familiar with the services and codes used by your facility, coding becomes faster and easier, but accuracy and attention to detail are always important. Taking time and care to correctly learn the fundamentals helps create long-term success in your coding role.

Guided Example of Assigning CPT Codes

To practice skills for assigning CPT codes, continue with the example from earlier in the chapter about a patient who was seen for removal of a lesion. Follow along in your CPT manual as fictional coder Sherry Whittle, CPC, assigns codes. Check off each step after you complete it.

► First, Sherry confirms the procedure performed: *Excision, benign lesion 0.7 cm including margins.*

▶ Sherry knows that she must search the CPT Index for the Main Term for the procedure. She has three choices for the Main Term:

❑ Procedure: **Excision**

❑ Condition: **Lesion**

❑ Anatomic site: **Skin**

▶ She decides to search for the condition and locates the Main Term **Lesion**.

❑ Immediately under the entry for **Lesion**, she reads the instructional note *See* **Tumor**. The patient did not have a tumor, so she does not follow the cross-reference.

❑ She understands that a lesion on the back is located on the skin. She locates the first-level modifying term, **Skin**.

❑ She locates the second-level modifying term for the procedure, **Excision**.

❑ Under Excision, she has a choice of **Benign** or **Malignant**, so she chooses **Benign** because it is consistent with the postprocedure diagnosis.

❑ She writes down the code range listed **11400-11401**. She knows she needs to reference both of these codes in the Tabular List to determine the correct code.

▶ Sherry turns to code **11400** in the Tabular List.

❑ First, she checks the title of the category, **Excision—Benign Lesions**, which seems to correctly match the medical record.

❑ She reads the code title, **11400 Excision, benign lesion including margins, except skin tag (unless listed elsewhere), trunk, arms or legs; excised diameter 0.5 cm or less.**

❑ She also reviews code **11401**, which is an indented code description that states **excised diameter 0.6 to 1.0 cm.**

❑ She confirms the excised diameter of the lesion in the medical record, which is *0.7 cm including margin.* The size 0.7 cm is between 0.6 and 1.0 cm, so **11401** seems to identify the correct size of lesion.

❑ She confirms that the anatomic site in the parent code, **11400**, includes the back. The site of **trunk** stated in the code includes the back, as stated in the medical record.

❑ She confirms that the type of lesion in the parent code, **benign lesion**, agrees with the medical record.

❑ She combines the common portion of the parent code **11400** that comes before the semicolon with the unique description of code **11401** for a complete code description of **Excision, benign lesion including margins, except skin tag (unless listed elsewhere), trunk, arms or legs; excised diameter 0.6 to 1.0 cm.**

▶ Sherry checks for instructional notes in the Tabular List.

❑ She looks for instructional notes following the code and finds none. (Some editions of the CPT manual provide a cross-reference to the newsletter *CPT Assistant*, published by the AMA. Electronic coding programs often provide a similar reference.)

❑ She cross-references the beginning of category **Excision—Benign Lesions** and reads through the special instructions. The instructions provide the following information:

■ Definition of excision as it applies to lesions

■ Explanation that the lesion size includes the most narrow margins required to adequately excise the lesion.

■ Clarification that the code for excision includes a simple closure (single-layer closure with sutures or staples)

■ Instructions on how to code intermediate or complex closures, if required

❑ She refers back to the beginning of the subsection, **Integumentary System**, and the heading, **Skin, Subcutaneous, and Accessory Structures**, which appear before code **10030**. She finds no further instructions. She is already familiar with the **Surgery Guidelines** at the beginning of the section that include the **CPT Surgical Package Definition**. These guidelines confirm that local anesthesia is part of the surgical package and should not be coded separately.

▶ Sherry reviews the CPT code she has assigned for this case.

❑ **11401 Excision, benign lesion including margins, except skin tag (unless listed elsewhere), trunk, arms or legs; excised diameter 0.6 to 1.0 cm.**

▶ If more than one CPT code were required, she would need to determine how to sequence the codes.

▶ Sherry also assigns the ICD-10-CM diagnosis code for the lesion:

❑ **L98.9 Disorder of the skin and subcutaneous tissue, unspecified** (ICD-10-CM Index: **Lesion, skin, unspecified**)

You may have noticed in the Guided Example that the CPT Index lists only two codes under the Main Term for the condition **Lesion, Skin, Excision, Benign**: codes **11400** and **11401**. These codes describe lesions on the trunk, arm, or legs that are 1.0 cm or smaller in diameter. When the lesion diameter is *larger* than 1.0 cm or on a site *other* than the trunk, arm, or legs, neither of these codes is correct. Coders must review the other indented code descriptions through code **11471** in the Tabular List to locate the appropriate code. However, if you locate the Main Term for the type of procedure, **Excision**, and then the modifying terms **Lesion, Skin, Benign**, more codes are provided in the Index. This quirk of the CPT Index occurs frequently. When in doubt, it is a good idea to try using more than one Main Term in the Index.

CODING PRACTICE

Exercise 28.3 Assigning CPT Procedure Codes

Instructions: Refer to the mini-medical-record below that you abstracted in Exercise 28.2. Answer the questions to assign the CPT code. Write your answers on the lines provided.

> INPATIENT HOSPITAL Gender: F Age: 48
>
> Preprocedure diagnosis: *metastatic breast cancer*
>
> Procedure: *left axillary lymphadenectomy, complete, using the open approach*
>
> Postprocedure diagnosis: *left breast cancer with metastasis to lymph nodes*
>
> Plan: *Begin radiation therapy in 3 weeks.*

1. What is the Main Term for the procedure performed? _____

2. Look up the Main Term in the CPT Index. What first-level modifying term should you select? _____

3. What code(s) are listed next to the first-level modifying term? _____

4. Locate the codes in the Tabular List. Which code is a standalone code? _____

5. Which code is an indented code? _____

6. Which code best describes the procedure performed? _____

7. Write out the full description of the code. _____

8. What is the name of the category in which this code appears? _____

9. What is the name of the subheading in which this code appears? _____

10. Look at the code following the one you selected for this case. What does the **+** in front of the code indicate? _____

ARRANGING CPT PROCEDURE CODES

When more than one CPT code is required, secondary procedures are coded in the same way as primary procedures. CPT codes are prioritized from highest cost to lowest cost on the 837P electronic claim or CMS-1500 form. This is because many insurance companies pay the first procedure in full but discount additional procedures performed at the same time. In general, the E/M code is identified first because the E/M code is not subject to a price reduction when multiple procedures are performed. Other services and procedures, including those subject to payment reductions, are listed after the E/M code.

CPT CODING AND REIMBURSEMENT

CPT coding has significant impact on reimbursement because fees are attached to CPT codes. Accurate coding and accurate data entry are essential to ensuring accurate reimbursement. Improper coding can result both in lower reimbursement than the provider is entitled to and in overpayment that puts the provider at risk of refunds and fines. To code accurately, coders must link procedures to diagnoses and adhere to reimbursement edits. Coders should also understand how physicians and outpatient hospitals are reimbursed.

Diagnosis–Procedure Linking

Coders must ensure that each CPT code reported is linked, or cross-referenced, to one or more diagnosis codes that identify the medical reason each service was provided. Any CPT code not linked with an appropriate diagnosis code will not be paid by the carrier. If the coder identifies a service that does not have documentation of a diagnosis that supports the need for the service, the provider should be queried. To query a provider involves sending the physician a message that asks for the reason the service was provided and requests the physician to amend the documentation to reflect the diagnosis.

Payers, including Medicare, maintain extensive databases of which diagnoses are considered to establish the medical necessity for each CPT code.

CODING CAUTION

Coders should not manipulate codes in a manner that reports diagnoses not documented to receive reimbursement. Documentation should not be manipulated or altered to reflect diagnoses that do not actually exist. Both practices are improper and fraudulent.

On the CMS-1500 form, diagnosis codes are entered in Item 21. Date(s) of service, CPT codes, charges, and related information are entered on lines 1 through 6 of Item 24. In column 24E, enter the letter from Item 21 (A through L) that corresponds to the diagnosis that supports each service. Each service must be linked to one or more diagnosis codes. A diagnosis code can be linked to as many services as appropriate.

Reimbursement Edits

Reimbursement edits are rules regarding codes that may or may not be billed together or have special billing requirements. The purpose is to prevent overpayment associated with incorrect

Table 28-8 ■ **REIMBURSEMENT EDIT CHECKS**

Name	Description	Example
National coverage determination (NCD)	Identifies the extent to which Medicare will cover specific services, procedures, or technologies on a national basis	Bariatric Surgery for Treatment of Morbid Obesity (100.1) Specifies the types of bariatric surgery that are approved for coverage. Specifies a list of comorbidities (*simultaneous diagnoses*), one of which must be present in addition to obesity for bariatric surgery to be approved.
National Correct Coding Initiative (NCCI)	Identifies code pairs that should not be reported together because they could not be performed during the same patient encounter because they are mutually exclusive based on anatomic, time, or gender considerations or because one code is a component of the other code	**41251 Repair of laceration 2.5 cm or less; posterior one-third of tongue** cannot be reported at the same times as code **12001 Simple repair of superficial wounds of scalp, neck, axillae, external genitalia, trunk and/or extremities (including hands and feet); 2.5 cm or less**. This would be a misuse of code **12001**. **12001** can be billed with modifier **-25**, **-57**, or **-59** when supported by documentation.
Medically unlikely edits (MUEs)	Identifies the maximum units of service that a provider would report under most circumstances for a single beneficiary on a single date of service	**21920 Biopsy, soft tissue of back or flank; superficial** Medically unlikely edit (MUE): three units per patient per day per line. Some MUEs can be bypassed if the code is reported on a separate line with a modifier for separate anatomic sites, global surgery package, or modifiers **-27**, **-59**, or **-91** and documentation supports it.
Local coverage determination (LCD)	Identifies a decision by a Medicare Administrative Contractor (MAC) whether to cover a particular service or item as reasonable and necessary for providers in its region	Removal of Skin Lesion (Non-Melanoma): Medicare allows coverage and payment for only those services that are considered to be medically reasonable and necessary. The LCD indicates that the MAC will consider the removal of benign skin lesions as medically necessary, and not cosmetic, if a condition from a list of approved diagnoses is present and clearly documented in the medical record. It also provides a list of applicable CPT codes.

Source: © PB Resources, Inc. Used with permission.

coding. Rules vary by payer and by region of the country. Medicare issues the largest number of reimbursement rules, summarized in ■ TABLE 28-8. Most Medicare edits also are applicable to Medicaid. Private payers either follow Medicare edits or publish their own. Medicare publishes most of its criteria for coverage and coding edits on its website, **www.cms.gov**. Medicare Administrative Contractors (MACs) also maintain websites for each region of the country and each contractor uses its website to publish local rules.

Reimbursement edits are automated **prepayment edits**, which means that claims are electronically scanned for compliance with the rules before the payer accepts them into the claims processing system. Depending on the specific rule and codes billed, in some cases providers can append a modifier to the code in question that will allow it to be accepted.

Medicare national coverage determination (NCD) and local coverage determination (LCD) policies that provide direction regarding specific diagnosis codes will be updated for ICD-10-CM. New reference numbers will be assigned to ICD-10-CM policies to distinguish them from ICD-9-CM policies. Most encoder software contains built-in reference information (■ FIGURE 28-9) or edit checks that screen for these rules so the error can be corrected before the provider submits the claim. Electronic claims clearinghouses, which route claims from the provider to the payers, also may scrub the claims for certain edit checks. If providers repeatedly submit claims that violate the edit checks, they may be investigated by payers for compliance.

CODING CAUTION

Some medically unlikely edits (MUEs) are confidential and shared only with Medicare Administrative Contractors (MACs). Providers learn by trial and error which MUEs impact them the most.

Physician Fees

Medicare uses a **resource-based relative value scale** (RBRVS) to establish physician reimbursement rates, which are published in the **Medicare Physician Fee Schedule (MPFS)**. The MPFS lists the Medicare rates for a specific provider for each CPT code and is updated annually. A **relative value unit** (RVU) identifies the amount of work and expense involved in providing a particular service. Medicare establishes three types of RVU components for each CPT code—physician work, practice expense, and malpractice—that are added together to produce the total RVU. An RVU of 1.0 reflects an average amount of work and expense. RVUs higher than 1.0 reflect a greater than average amount of work and expense, whereas RVUs less than 1.0 reflect a lower than average amount of work and expense.

The RBRVS also factors in a **geographic practice cost index** (GPCI) for each RVU component that reflects the differences in the cost of doing business in different regions of the country and different ZIP codes. To establish fees, Medicare multiples the total RBRVS value for a CPT code by the annual **conversion factor**. For example, a conversion factor of $35 means that

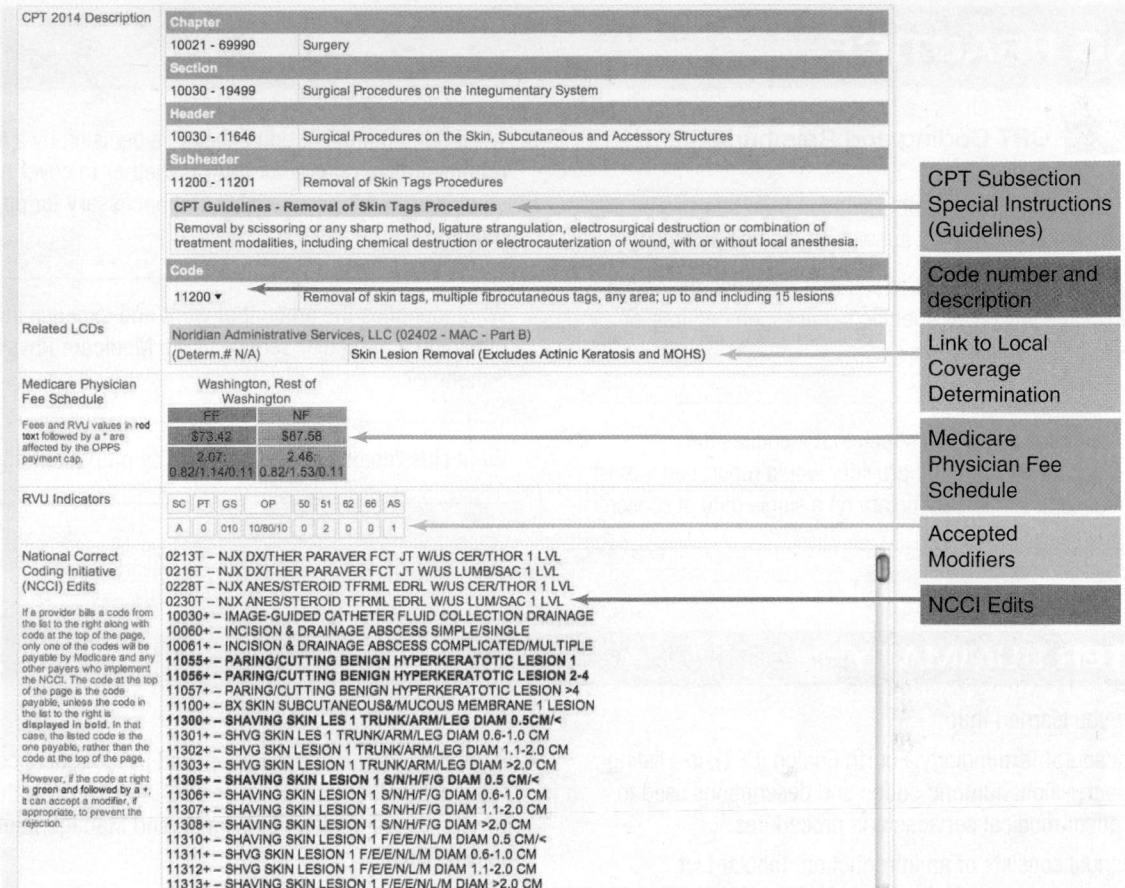

Figure 28-9 ■ Example of Reimbursement Edits in an Encoder. *Source:* http://www.speedecoder.com/app/search/detail.php?code=11200&d=CPT/. Used with permission.

an RBRVS value of 1.0 is worth $35 on the MPFS. A code with an RBRVS value of 0.5 would be worth $17.50. A code with an RBRVS value of 2.0 would be worth $70. A code with an RBRVS value of 10.0 would be worth $3,500. When Medicare adjusts prices each year, it publishes a new conversion factor that is applied to all CPT codes.

When reporting CPT codes for billing, the codes should be sequenced on the 837P electronic claim or CMS-1500 in descending order of price, which is based on the RVUs. The code with the highest price should be sequenced first, the second highest price second, and so on. When multiple services and procedures are reported for a patient on the same date of service, Medicare and many other payers pay the first CPT code at 100% and then pay subsequent CPT codes at a lower percentage. This is done because there is an efficiency of scale when multiple procedures are done concurrently. It generally takes less time and work than if each procedure were performed at separate times.

Medicare publishes RBRVS information on its website. Many encoder software programs make RBRVS information available to the user. Private payers may adopt Medicare RVUs and RBRVS, modify them, or establish their own.

The **Medicare Physician Fee Schedule Database (MPFSDB)** is the source of all information related to CPT code reimbursement for Medicare. It contains not only the fees, as the MPFS does, but also the RVUs, GPCI, CF, global surgery days (*the number of follow-up days included in a surgical procedure*), accepted modifiers, and other relevant information. A searchable version of the MPFSDB is available on the CMS website.

Physicians provide services in many settings: the medical office, an ambulatory surgery center, outpatient hospital departments such as radiology or cardiac catheterization lab, and inpatient hospitals. Although the services are provided in a location other than the medical office, physicians are still responsible for coding and billing the services they provide in those settings. Services provided at locations other than the medical office often have two billing components: the facility fee and the professional fee. The facility fee covers the cost of the building, equipment, technician, and other staff, as applicable. The professional fee covers the cost of the physician's time. The facility, such as the hospital or ambulatory surgery center, bills the facility fee, and the physician bills the professional fee.

Outpatient Hospital Reimbursement

Medicare pays outpatient hospitals using a classification called the **Ambulatory Payment Classification (APC)**. APCs are groups of CPT codes that describe similar procedures. All procedures in an APC are paid at the same rate. This system of outpatient hospital reimbursement is called the **Outpatient Prospective Payment System (OPPS)**. Private payers may adopt Medicare APCs, modify them, establish their own, or pay based on individual CPT codes.

CODING PRACTICE

Exercise 28.4 CPT Coding and Reimbursement

Instructions: Provide the term and abbreviation from this section that answers each question. Write your answer on the line provided.

1. What is the reimbursement edit check that identifies the extent to which Medicare will cover specific services, procedures, or technologies on a national basis?

2. What is the reimbursement edit check that identifies the maximum units of service that a provider would report under most circumstances for a single beneficiary on a single date of service?

3. What reimbursement edit check is a decision by a Medicare Administrative Contractor (MAC) whether to cover a particular service or item as reasonable and necessary for providers in its region?

4. What identifies the amount of work and expense involved in providing a particular service in the Medicare Physician Fee Schedule?

5. What classification system is used by outpatient hospitals?

CHAPTER SUMMARY

In this chapter you learned that:

- Current Procedural Terminology, Fourth Edition (CPT), is a listing of five-character alphanumeric codes and descriptions used to report outpatient medical services and procedures.

- The CPT manual consists of an Introduction, Tabular List, Appendices, and an Index. Coders need to know where needed information is located and how to identify and interpret coding guidelines, instructional notes, and conventions.

- When abstracting for CPT, coders need to read the medical record and identify key criteria based on the services provided.

- Assigning CPT codes requires coders to research the procedure in the Index, identify the preliminary code(s), then verify the code(s) in the Tabular List.

- In general, CPT codes are prioritized from highest cost to lowest cost on the electronic claim or CMS-1500 form, although some payers request that the Evaluation and Management (E/M) code be listed first.

- CPT coding has significant impact on reimbursement because fees are attached to CPT codes. To code accurately, coders must match procedures to diagnoses, code for the appropriate level of service, adhere to reimbursement edits, and understand how physicians and outpatient hospitals are reimbursed.

CONCEPT QUIZ

Take a moment to look back at this introduction to CPT coding and solidify your skills. Try to answer the questions from memory first, then refer to the discussion in this chapter and the Glossary at the end of this book if you need a little extra help.

Completion

Instructions: Write the term that answers each question based on the information you learned in this chapter. Choose from the following list. Some choices may be used more than once and some choices may not be used at all.

Add-on codes	edits
APC	instructional notes
Category I	modifiers
Category II	modifying terms
Category III	OPPS
common descriptor	parent code

prepayment edit   subcategory
semicolon

1. _____ codes comprise the bulk of CPT and describe widely used services and procedures approved by the FDA.

2. A _____ is a two-digit alphanumeric suffix appended to a CPT code to provide further description of the circumstances of an encounter.

3. _____ are Index entries that are indented under the Main Term and add further detail about the service or procedure.

4. _____ inform the coder of other Main Terms to look up, such as synonyms or other variations of the term.

5. _____ codes are optional, consist of four numbers followed by the letter F, and are used to collect and track data performance measurement.

6. Conventions may appear on the same line with the code, above it, below it, or at the beginning of a _____.

7. A standalone or parent code's common descriptor is shared with an indented code descriptor by the use of a

   _____.

8. _____ codes are temporary codes used for data collection and for tracking the use of emerging technology, services, and procedures.

9. Specific coding and billing criteria that are checked for accuracy based on predetermined rules are called

   _____.

10. Codes that are marked with a + in the CPT manual and must be reported with an additional procedure code are called

    _____.

Multiple Choice

Instructions: Circle the letter of the best answer to each question based on the information you learned in this chapter.

1. What is the term for sending the physician a message that asks for the reason the service was provided and requests the physician to amend the documentation to reflect the diagnosis?
   A. Memo
   B. Inquiry
   C. Query
   D. Instant message

2. What are the edits in which claims are electronically scanned for rules before a payer accepts them Into the claims processing system?
   A. Precertification
   B. Prepayment
   C. Preview
   D. Preordered

3. In what order should CPT codes be sequenced on a claim?
   A. Ascending code number
   B. Descending code number
   C. Ascending fee
   D. Descending fee

4. What type of fee covers the cost of the physician's time?
   A. Professional fee
   B. Technical fee
   C. Facility fee
   D. Referral fee

5. What is the Medicare classification system used by outpatient hospitals?
   A. Ambulatory Payment Classification (APC)
   B. Geographic Practice Cost Index (GPCI)
   C. Relative value unit (RVU)
   D. Local coverage determination (LCD)

6. Which edit identifies code pairs that should not be coded together?
   A. National coverage determination (NCD)
   B. National Correct Coding Initiative (NCCI)
   C. Medically unlikely edits (MUEs)
   D. Quick reference edits (QREs)

7. What type of fee covers the cost of the building, equipment, and other staff?
   A. Surgery suite fee
   B. OR fee
   C. Facility fee
   D. Hospital fee

8. What element establishes the medical necessity of each CPT code?
   A. Modifiers
   B. Add-on codes
   C. Procedure codes
   D. Diagnosis codes

9. What are the instructions that appear at the beginning of each CPT section?
   A. Guidelines
   B. Conventions
   C. Practices
   D. Edits

10. Which component of an E/M service includes ordering a test or procedure?
    A. History
    B. Medical decision making
    C. Examination
    D. Chief complaint

CODING CHALLENGE

Instructions: Read the mini-medical-record, then answer the questions that follow to abstract, assign, and arrange ICD-10-CM diagnosis codes and CPT procedure codes.

> OUTPATIENT HOSPITAL   Gender: F   Age: 54
>
> Reason for encounter: hematuria; patient is on insulin for type 1 diabetes
>
> Procedure: cystourethroscopy revealed 2.7-cm mass in bladder neck; mass resected using snare technique
>
> Postoperative diagnosis: pathology confirmed bladder neck mass as an adenomatoid tumor
>
> Plan: Follow-up ultrasound in 6 weeks.

(continued)

(continued from page 489)

Part 1: Abstract

1. Read through the mini-medical-record. First, abstract for the diagnosis. Compare the chief complaint to the final assessment.

   a. What symptoms did the patient report in the chief complaint? _____

   b. What condition is stated in the assessment? _____

2. Review the symptom(s).

   a. What is the meaning of the term for the symptoms? _____

   b. Should you code for the symptom? _____
   Why or why not? _____

3. Review the mini-medical-record for any other conditions.

   a. Is another condition documented? _____
   If so, list the condition. _____

   b. Should the condition be coded? _____
   Why or why not? _____

4. Next, abstract for the procedure.

   a. Break down the term into its two roots and suffix.
   _____/_____/_____

   b. What does this term mean? _____

   c. What instrument was used during this procedure? _____

   d. Through what route was the instrument inserted to reach its final objective? _____

5. Were any other procedures performed during this operative session?_____
   If so, name the additional procedure(s). _____

Part 2: Assign

6. First, assign the diagnosis codes. You can look up the conditions in any order you wish, as long as you sequence them correctly in the end based on any instructional notes and Official Guidelines for Coding and Reporting.

   a. Look up the Main Term **Tumor** in the Index of your ICD-10-CM manual, then the subterm **adenomatoid**. Are there special instructions? _____ If so, what do the special instructions tell you to do? _____

   b. Where do you locate **Neoplasm, benign, by site** in the ICD-10-CM manual? _____

   c. What first-level subterm and second-level subterm should you locate? _____

   d. What code is listed? _____

   e. Verify this code in the Tabular List. What is the final code? _____

7. Assign and verify the diagnosis code for diabetes. What is the correct code? _____
   _____

8. Now assign the procedure code. In the CPT manual, look up the Main Term **Excision** then the first-level modifying term **Bladder**.

   a. Is there an additional modifying term that should be referenced under Bladder? _____ If so, what is the term? _____

   b. What code or code range is listed? _____

9. Verify the code in the CPT Tabular List.

   a. Under what CPT section and subsection is this code located? Section _____
   subsection _____

   b. What is the code description? _____
   _____

   c. Does this code description accurately identify the procedure performed during this encounter? _____
   Why or why not?_____

   d. Is there an instructional note listed under this narrative? _____ If yes, what does the instructional note say?
   _____
   _____

   e. When you cross-reference code 52234, does it accurately describe the procedure? _____ Why or why not?
   _____
   _____

   f. Which code within the range 52234-52240 best describes the procedure performed? _____ Why?
   _____
   _____

   g. CPT codes can be indexed under several different Main Terms. Provide at least one additional Index path that can be used to locate this code. Main Term _____.
   Modifying terms _____
   _____

Part 3: Arrange

10. You identified two ICD-10-CM codes and one CPT for this case. Review your answers in the previous questions to determine the correct sequencing.

    a. Which diagnosis code is sequenced first? _____ Why?
    _____

    b. Which diagnosis code is sequenced first? _____ Why?
    _____

    c. What is the final procedure code? _____

    d. Is the procedure code supported by the first-listed diagnosis? _____ Why? _____
    _____

KEEP ON CODING

Instructions: Read the procedural statement, then use the Index and Tabular List to assign CPT procedure codes. Write the code(s) on the line provided.

1. Endoscopic placement of bronchial stent, left: CPT Code(s) _____

2. Dacryocystotomy, left: CPT Code(s) _____

3. Intermediate (layered) repair of open wound to fascia, 7.2 cm, right thigh: CPT Code(s) _____

4. Computerized tomography without contrast, head: CPT Code(s) _____

5. Swallowing function study with images: CPT Code(s) _____

6. Bone marrow biopsy from pelvic bone: CPT Code(s): _____

7. Rhinoscopy with biopsy of left sinus: CPT Code(s): _____

8. Ultrasound-guided biopsy of endomyocardial mass: CPT Code(s) _____

9. Transurethral prostatectomy: CPT Code(s) _____

10. Carpal tunnel release: CPT Code(s) _____

11. Diagnostic lumbar puncture: CPT Code(s) _____

12. Spirometry and evaluation: CPT Code(s) _____

13. Cardiac echography, spectral and color flow, 2D: CPT Code(s) _____

14. Endoscopic removal of foreign body from small intestine: CPT Code(s) _____

15. Excision of coccygeal pressure ulcer: CPT Code(s) _____

16. Endoscopic ablation of colon polyp: CPT Code(s) _____

17. Cast arm below elbow for hairline fracture, right ulna: CPT Code(s) _____

18. Cystotomy with repair of ureterocele: CPT Code(s) _____

19. Screening, computer-aided mammography: CPT Code(s) _____

20. MRI, diagnostic, right hip joint: CPT Code(s) _____

21. Ultrasound of fetus: CPT Code(s) _____

22. Nasogastric feeding tube placement with fluoroscopic guidance: CPT Code(s) _____

23. Laparoscopic splenectomy: CPT Code(s) _____

24. Vascular flow study of liver: CPT Code(s) _____

25. Aortic serialographic arteriography, abdominal: CPT Code(s) _____

Chapter 29

Introduction to HCPCS Coding (A0000-V5999)

Chapter Outline

- **Overview of HCPCS Codes**
- **Organization of the HCPCS manual**
- **Abstracting for HCPCS Codes and Modifiers**
- **Assigning HCPCS Codes**

Learning Objectives

After completing this chapter, you should have the skills to:

29.1 Spell and define the key words, medical terms, and abbreviations related to HCPCS coding.

29.2 Identify the main characteristics of HCPCS coding.

29.3 Describe the organization of the HCPCS manual.

29.4 Abstract information from the medical record for HCPCS codes and modifiers.

29.5 Assign codes using the HCPCS Index and Tabular List.

Key Terms and Abbreviations

enteral nutrition	HCPCS Table of Drugs	Level II (HCPCS)	parenteral nutrition
HCPCS Index	HCPCS Tabular List	millicurie	permanent national code
HCPCS modifier	Level I (HCPCS)	miscellaneous code	temporary national code

In addition to the key terms listed here, students should know the terms defined within tables in this chapter.

For updates and corrections, visit our student resource site at

www.pearsonhighered.com/healthprofessionsresources

INTRODUCTION

Item numbering systems differ among manufacturers, but a retailer must find ways to accommodate the various systems. Likewise, coders must adapt to multiple code sets. Procedure coding was formalized in the late 1960s and 1970s after the creation of Medicare and Medicaid. Medicare gave rise to rapid growth within the healthcare industry, and by the 1980s major updating and streamlining were needed. This led to the creation of a new coding system, the Healthcare Common Procedure Coding System (HCPCS), to classify and report services and supplies not included in the Current Procedural Terminology (CPT). This chapter introduces the HCPCS system, the organization of the HCPCS coding manual, and instructions on abstracting and assigning HCPCS codes and modifiers.

OVERVIEW OF HCPCS CODES

The **Healthcare Common Procedure Coding System (HCPCS)** was developed by the Center for Medicare and Medicaid Services (CMS) in conjunction with the American Medical Association (AMA) and was released in 1983. HCPCS has two divisions, or levels, of codes:

Level I—Current Procedural Terminology, Fourth Edition (CPT) codes

Level II—National Healthcare Common Procedure Coding System codes

Although CPT codes have been used since 1966, in 1983 they were updated and incorporated into the overall HCPCS system. However, they remain the property of the AMA. CPT codes are Level I codes within the HCPCS system. Most people refer to them as CPT codes, but you will sometimes encounter references to Level I codes when reading rules and regulations from Medicare or other payers.

Level II codes were a new code set in 1983 to classify services not included in CPT, as well as physician and nonphysician services, medical supplies, equipment, and medications. Level II codes are commonly referred to as HCPCS codes (pronounced "hick-picks"). They are owned by CMS, with the exception of codes for dental services, which are copyrighted by the American Dental Association. Examples of services, supplies, and items reported with HCPCS codes include ambulance services, medical and surgical supplies, drugs, nutrition therapy, durable medical equipment, orthotic and prosthetic procedures, and hearing and vision services.

Initially, providers were required to use HCPCS codes only for Medicare and Medicaid patients. However, many other payers found HCPCS codes to be useful and began to require that providers use them. As of 2003, HCPCS Level II became a mandated code set under the Health Insurance Portability and Accountability Act (HIPAA). CMS is responsible for maintaining Level II HCPCS codes, including yearly revisions, additions, and deletions. Updates occur quarterly throughout the year, and the full code set is published annually in January.

HCPCS codes are reported in Item 24D on the CMS-1500 form or in the comparable field on the 837P electronic claim.

Categories of HCPCS Codes

HCPCS codes have three categories:

1. Permanent national codes
2. Temporary national codes
3. Miscellaneous codes

Permanent National Codes

Permanent national codes are those that all U.S. providers and insurances can use for billing and statistical purposes. CMS created a HCPCS workgroup, which determines whether to add, revise, or delete HCPCS codes. The workgroup is responsible for maintaining the permanent codes.

Temporary National Codes

The HCPCS workgroup also creates **temporary national codes** for services and supplies that do not have a permanent code. The workgroup creates these codes in response to Medicare's needs, but any provider and insurance can use temporary codes. The workgroup can add temporary codes before the annual HCPCS code set update on January 1. Temporary codes remain temporary indefinitely until the workgroup decides to replace them with permanent codes. When the workgroup replaces a temporary code with a permanent one, it deletes the temporary code from the code set and provides a cross-reference to the new permanent code.

Miscellaneous Codes

Miscellaneous codes allow providers to immediately bill insurances for a service or item as soon as the FDA approves its use, even though there is no permanent or temporary code that describes it. Examples of miscellaneous or not otherwise specified codes include the following:

- **A9999 Miscellaneous DME supply or accessory, not otherwise specified**
- **J9999 Not otherwise classified, antineoplastic drugs**
- **V5274 Assistive listening device, not otherwise specified**

Medicare and other payers manually review claims with miscellaneous codes, so providers must submit supporting documentation to payers explaining why the patient needs the item or service. Before reporting a miscellaneous code, check with individual payers to ensure that there is not another permanent or temporary code to describe the service.

ORGANIZATION OF THE HCPCS MANUAL

There are approximately 3,000 HCPCS codes. Each is made up of a letter followed by four numbers (**A0000–V9999**). Each letter represents a group of similar services, supplies, drugs, and equipment. For example, HCPCS codes beginning with the letter **J** represent drugs, and codes beginning with the letter **D** represent dental services. The American Dental Association (ADA) created and owns the copyright to dental codes, called Current Dental Terminology (CDT) codes. These codes do not appear in the HCPCS manual and must be purchased from the

CODING PRACTICE

Instructions: For each description of services, supplies, equipment, or drugs, write down the Main Term to look for in the HCPCS Index. Locate the appropriate subterm, then list the code(s) that appear next to the subterm.

EXAMPLE: A physician provides an ankle splint to a patient. Main Term: *Splint* HCPCS Code(s): *L4392-L4398, S8451*

1. A physician orders a raised toilet seat for a patient to use at home, which the DME supplier provides. Main Term: _____ HCPCS Code(s): _____

2. A psychologist conducts a patient assessment for mental health services at an outpatient mental health facility. Main Term: _____ HCPCS Code(s): _____

3. The physician changes a lead in a patient's pacemaker, which is a transvenous VDD single pass. Main Term: _____ HCPCS Code(s) _____

4. A primary care physician (PCP) gives a patient an enteral fiber additive to assist the patient in having regular bowel movements. Main Term: _____ HCPCS Code(s): _____

5. A physician assistant administers the hepatitis B vaccine to a patient. Main Term: _____ HCPCS Code(s): _____

ABSTRACTING FOR HCPCS CODES AND MODIFIERS

The three skills of an "ace" coder—abstracting, assigning, and arranging codes—apply to HCPCS coding. As with many areas of coding, the most challenging part of working with HCPCS codes is knowing when they are needed. It takes some experience and familiarity with HCPCS codes and Medicare regulations to learn all the situations in which a HCPCS code is required. In addition, not all payers use HCPCS codes to the same extent, so it is necessary to learn and organize the requirements for the payers and services provided in your workplace.

This section provides general guidelines for abstracting HCPCS codes and modifiers. Refer to ■ TABLE 29-2 for general abstracting criteria for HCPCS codes. An answer of *yes* to any of the abstracting questions indicates a potential need for one or more HCPCS codes. Look up the supply item or service in the HCPCS Index or look up the drug in the HCPCS Table of Drugs.

For help identifying when HCPCS modifiers are needed, refer to ■ TABLE 29-3. When the answer to a question is *yes*, review the modifiers listed in the right-hand column. Look up the description of each modifier suggested in the HCPCS modifier list and determine which, if any, apply to the patient. Also refer to payer policies for guidance. Table 29-3 does not cover all modifiers or all situations, but it will help you get started. As with HCPCS codes, it takes a while to become familiar with all the HCPCS modifiers. In the workplace, you will learn which modifiers are used most often by your provider. Practice management system (PMS) software and encoders can be preprogrammed to alert to the potential need for modifiers.

Table 29-2 ■ KEY CRITERIA FOR ABSTRACTING HCPCS CODES

❑ Is the patient covered by Medicare or Medicaid?

❑ Does the patient's payer require/accept HCPCS codes?

❑ Did the patient receive durable medical equipment (DME), such as wheelchairs, crutches, hospital beds, or related accessories?

❑ Did the patient receive supplies to help treat or manage any of the following conditions:
  - urinary incontinence
  - ostomies
  - respiratory problems
  - end-stage renal disease (ESRD)/dialysis
  - need for parenteral and enteral nutrition

❑ Was radiopharmaceutical contrast administered (such as for a nuclear medicine scan)?

❑ Did the patient receive medication or drugs administered by a healthcare provider, including:
  - injections
  - chemotherapy drugs for cancer treatment
  - immunosuppressive drugs for treatment of patients whose immune systems are compromised (including patients with AIDS)
  - inhaled solutions

❑ Did the patient receive services or supplies related to orthotics or prosthetics?

❑ Did the patient receive preventive care services such as an immunization, mammogram, or colorectal cancer screening?

Source: © PB Resources, Inc. Used with permission.

Table 29-3 ■ **KEY CRITERIA FOR ABSTRACTING HCPCS MODIFIERS**

Criteria	Modifier(s)
❏ Did the patient receive a service on a paired organ or site?	LT, RT
❏ Did the patient receive a service that treated the eyelids, fingers, toes, or coronary arteries?	E1-E4, F1-FA, T1-TA, LC, LD, LM, RC, RI
❏ Was chiropractic manipulation provided?	AT
❏ Were one or more wounds dressed?	A1-A9
❏ Did the patient units of service exceed those in the medically unlikely edits (MUEs)?	GD
❏ Was a waiver of liability/Advanced Beneficiary Notice (ABN) issued or required due to the possibility of a Medicare denial for lack of medical necessity?	GA, GL, GK, GU, GZ, KB
❏ Was only the technical component of a service provided by a facility?	TC
❏ Did a dialysis patient receive dialysis-related services or non-dialysis-related services?	AX, AY, CB, CD-CF, ED-EM, G1-G6, JE, V5-V7
❏ Were psychotherapy or substance abuse services provided?	H9-HZ
❏ Did a nonphysician provider deliver the service?	AE-AJ, AS, GF, QY, SB, SD
❏ Was the service provided by a substitute or locum tenens provider?	Q5-Q6
❏ Were anesthesia services provided?	AA-AD, G8-G9, P1-P6, QX-QZ
❏ Was a screening mammogram or colonoscopy converted to a diagnostic test or done on the same day as a diagnostic version of the procedure?	GG, GH, PT
❏ Was a supply item or piece or part of equipment replaced?	FB, FC, KC, KN, KM, MS, RA, RB
❏ Did the physician admit the patient to a hospital or nursing facility during the encounter?	AI

Source: © PB Resources, Inc. Used with permission.

CODING PRACTICE

Exercise 29.2   Abstracting for HCPCS Codes and Modifiers

Instructions: Identify the appropriate modifier for each of the following situations. Refer to Table 29-3 Key Criteria for Abstracting HCPCS Modifiers to locate potential modifiers. Then look up the modifiers listed in the HCPCS manual and select the correct one. Assign the modifier only. Do not assign codes.

1. A patient received an opiate substitute as part of an opioid addiction treatment program. Modifier: _____

2. A woman delivered a 6 pound, 5 ounce infant with the assistance of a nurse-midwife. Modifier: _____

3. Dressings were changed for two wounds. Modifier: _____

4. A chalazion was removed from the right upper eyelid. Modifier: _____

5. A patient's portable respiratory suction pump malfunctioned and was replaced by the supply company. Modifier: _____

ASSIGNING HCPCS CODES

Assigning HCPCS codes requires coders to use the HCPCS Index and verify codes in the HCPCS Tabular List. This section provides details and examples of assigning codes for the most common services and supplies: transportation services, medical supplies, radiopharmaceuticals, enteral and parenteral nutrition, durable medical equipment, professional services, drugs administered by clinicians, and orthotics.

Coding for Transportation Services Including Ambulance (A0021-A0999)

HCPCS codes are used for both nonemergency and emergency transportation services. Such services use specially equipped vehicles to transport ill or injured patients. Modes of transportation include the following:

- Ambulance van
- Air ambulance, fixed wing (airplane) or rotary wing (helicopter)
- Wheelchair van
- Taxi
- Bus
- Automobile

Ambulance providers are either freestanding or institution-based services. Freestanding services include independently owned and operated ambulance services, volunteer fire and or ambulance companies, and local government-run firehouse-based ambulances. Institution-based ambulance providers are owned or operated by a hospital, critical access hospital (CAH), skilled nursing facility (SNF), comprehensive outpatient rehabilitation facility (CORF), home health agency (HHA), or hospice provider.

The company or facility that owns and provides ambulance or nonemergency transportation service is the entity that codes and bills for the service. The hospital or provider that receives a patient *does not* bill for the transportation service.

SUCCESS STEP

Employment with an ambulance service can be a potential entry-level job for coders. You have the opportunity to gain experience and confidence working with a high volume of claims that have similar but specific coding requirements.

Ambulances offer two levels of service to patients: basic life support (BLS) and advanced life support (ALS). BLS includes services from a certified emergency medical technician (EMT). ALS includes services from a certified EMT-Intermediate or an EMT-Paramedic. At least two people, including one EMT, must be in the ambulance.

Ambulance providers use HCPCS codes to bill payers for transportation services for transporting patients to the hospital, SNF, or other destination. They also use HCPCS modifier(s) with the transportation code. Ambulance services are paid a base rate for the level of service provided, a mileage rate, and fees for supplies or extra personnel. Refer to ■ TABLE 29-4 for guidance in abstracting information to code for transportation services.

Ambulance services appear under the Main Term **Ambulance** in the HCPCS Index. Coding for ambulance services involves the following steps (■ FIGURE 29-2):

1. Assign a HCPCS code for the type of transportation service provided, with the quantity of **1** (codes **A0225, A0427-A0434**).

2. If the ambulance is an institution-based provider, append one of the following modifiers to describe the type of arrangement.

   - **QM**—Ambulance service provided under arrangement by a provider of services

   - **QN**—Ambulance service furnished directly by a provider of services

Table 29-4 ■ KEY CRITERIA FOR ABSTRACTING AMBULANCE SERVICES

- ❑ Is the ambulance service freestanding or institution-based?
- ❑ What type of vehicle was used to transport the patient: ground (ambulance), air fixed wing (airplane), or air rotary wing (helicopter)?
- ❑ What type of services did the patient need: nonemergency, emergency, ALS, BLS, specialty care transport (SCT), or neonatal care?
- ❑ How many miles did the ambulance have to travel from its origin to its destination?
- ❑ Were extra personnel involved?
- ❑ What supplies were used?

Source: © PB Resources, Inc. Used with permission.

Branton Ambulance Service (freestanding supplier)
Patient was transported by ambulance from home to Branton Medical Center, after she collapsed on the kitchen floor.
Service provided: BLS, 12 miles.

A0429-RH Ambulance service, basic life support, emergency transport (BLS-emergency); origin-home (R); destination-hospital (H)
A0380 Basic life support mileage x 12

Figure 29-2 ■ Example of HCPCS Coding for Ambulance Services

3. Refer to the list of location codes (**D** through **X**) at the beginning of section **A** in the HCPCS manual. Using these codes, create a two-letter modifier than identifies the origin and destination.

   - The first letter of the modifier identifies the origin (where the patient was picked up).

   - The second letter of the modifier identifies the destination (where the patient was taken to).

4. Append the origin/destination modifier to the ambulance service code. Sequence this as the *second* modifier for institution-based providers.

5. Assign a code for the miles travelled (**A0380, A0390, A0425, A0435, A0436**), with a quantity that identifies the number of miles.

6. Assign a code for waiting time (**A0420**), if applicable, with a quantity based on the time increments shown before code **A0420** in the HCPCS Tabular List.

7. Assign codes for supplies used and any extra attendants, beyond two.

To code for nonemergency transport, follow these steps:

1. Assign a code for the mode of nonemergency transportation (**A0090-A0210**) with a quantity of **1**.

2. Assign a code for miles driven (**A0021-A0080**) with a quantity that identifies the number of miles driven.

Coding for Medical Supplies (A4026-A9300, A9900-A9999)

Healthcare providers and medical supply companies code and bill payers for supplies provided to patients. Providers can purchase supplies directly from supply companies, dispense the supply to a patient, and then bill the patient's insurance. The supply company also can provide the supply directly to the patient and then bill the patient's insurance.

Each payer, including Medicare, has unique coding, billing, and reimbursement guidelines for supplies, depending on the type of supply, the patient's diagnosis, and the circumstances involved. Some payers do not pay separately for specific supplies that they consider to be a normal part of providing a service. Instead, the payer issues one payment for the service that includes the supply costs.

To locate codes in the HCPCS Index, locate the Main Term for the supply item, such as **Catheter** or **Dressing**, or a Main Term for the condition, such as **Ostomy**.

Coding for Radiopharmaceutical Drugs (A9500-A9700)

Radiopharmaceutical drugs, also called contrasts or tracers, are used in nuclear medicine procedures. They are radioactive drugs that emit radiation, which shows on a scan and helps physicians and clinicians to determine an organ's structure and function (■ FIGURE 29-3). Radiopharmaceuticals also are used to treat diseases such as bone cancer. The tracer or contrast medium is billed by the radiologist, in addition to the CPT code for the procedure (■ FIGURE 29-4).

Medicare and other payers have specific guidelines regarding which radiopharmaceuticals providers are permitted to code and bill in addition to the radiology service. They also have guidelines for radiopharmaceuticals that should not be separately reported because they are included with payment for the CPT code. Always check individual payer guidelines to ensure that you report the correct codes.

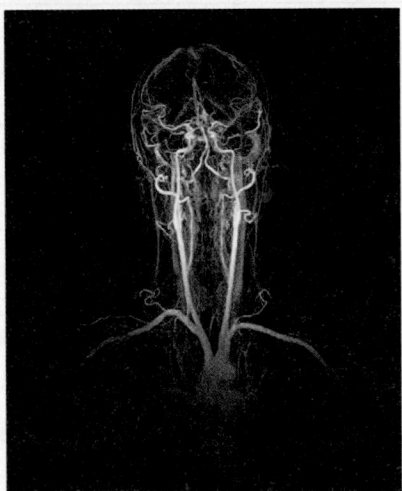

Figure 29-3 ■ Magnetic Resonance Angiography (MRA) of Arteries in the Head and Neck That Can Be Seen Using a Tracer. *Photo credit:* bendao/Shutterstock.com.

A physician performed a positron emission tomography (PET) perfusion scan with a tracer for a patient at rest. 60 millicuries of the radiopharmaceutical Rubidium Rb-82 was used in the study.

78491   **Myocardial imaging, positron emission tomography (PET), perfusion; single study at rest or stress**

A9555   **Rubidium Rb-82, diagnostic, per study dose, up to 60 millicuries x 1**

Figure 29-4 ■ Example of Coding for a Radiology Service and a Radiopharmaceutical Drug

To locate radiopharmaceutical drugs in the HCPCS Index, use the Main Term **Radiopharmaceutical**, then locate the name of the substance. You can also look up the name of the substance as the Main Term or use the Table of Drugs. The unit of measurement for radiopharmaceutical drugs is the millicurie. Report the quantity based on the dosage measurement identified in the code description. For code **A9555**, the quantity of **1** identifies 0–60 millicuries; the quantity of **2** identifies 61–120 millicuries, and so on. All radiopharmaceutical codes should be verified in the Tabular List.

Coding for Enteral and Parenteral Therapy (B4000–B9999)

HCPCS **B** codes represent supplies, equipment, and nutritional products for parenteral and enteral nutrition. Enteral nutrition therapy, also called tube feeding, is providing nutrients to patients through a tube in one of the following sites:

- nose using a nasogastric (NG) tube
- stomach using a gastrostomy (G) tube
- small intestine using a jejunostomy (J) tube

Parenteral nutrition therapy is providing nutrients intravenously because the body is unable to take in nutrients orally or by other methods. Patients who need enteral or parenteral therapy suffer from disorders or effects of surgery that prohibit them from taking food by mouth, such as swallowing disorders, neuromuscular diseases, trauma, or reconstructive procedures to treat head, neck, and bowel diseases, such as colon cancer. Patients may experience various types of infections or other complications from receiving enteral and parenteral nutrition.

Medicare and other payers may reimburse for these items when they are not part of an inpatient hospital stay, but payment depends on the place of service, the patient's diagnosis, and whether the condition is short term or long term, among other criteria.

To locate codes in the HCPCS Index, look up the Main Term for the supply item, such as **Tube**, or look up the Main Term **Parenteral nutrition** or **Enteral nutrition**, then locate the appropriate subterm. Always verify codes in the Tabular List.

Coding for Durable Medical Equipment (E0100–E8002)

HCPCS **E** codes represent DME, which includes crutches, wheelchairs, commodes, canes, walkers, hospital beds, oxygen and related respiratory equipment, pacemakers and related monitoring equipment, patient lifts and other safety equipment, fracture and traction equipment, and artificial kidney machines.

To locate codes in the HCPCS Index, look up the Main Term for the DME item, such as **Wheelchair** or **Oxygen**, then locate the appropriate subterm. Always verify codes in the Tabular List.

SUCCESS STEP

Patients must meet specific criteria of medical necessity to qualify for DME coverage by Medicare. CMS provides Certificate of Medical Necessity forms that must be completed by the DME supplier and physician to document the medical need for certain supplies and equipment (■ FIGURE 29-5, pages 500–501). Forms can be downloaded from **www.cms.gov**. Look on the *Medicare* tab for a link to *CMS Forms*.

DEPARTMENT OF HEALTH AND HUMAN SERVICES
CENTERS FOR MEDICARE & MEDICAID SERVICES

Form Approved
OMB No. 0938-0534

CERTIFICATE OF MEDICAL NECESSITY
CMS-484 — OXYGEN

DME 484.03

SECTION A	Certification Type/Date: INITIAL ___/___/___ REVISED ___/___/___ RECERTIFICATION___/___/___

PATIENT NAME, ADDRESS, TELEPHONE and HIC NUMBER

(___) ____-_____ HICN _____

SUPPLIER NAME, ADDRESS, TELEPHONE and NSC or applicable NPI NUMBER/LEGACY NUMBER

(___) ____-_____ NSC or NPI #_____

PLACE OF SERVICE_____	HCPCS CODE	PT DOB ___/___/___ Sex ____ (M/F)

NAME and ADDRESS of FACILITY
if applicable (see reverse)

_____
_____
_____
_____

PHYSICIAN NAME, ADDRESS, TELEPHONE and applicable NPI NUMBER or UPIN

(___) ____-_____ UPIN or NPI #_____

SECTION B	Information in This Section May Not Be Completed by the Supplier of the Items/Supplies.

EST. LENGTH OF NEED (# OF MONTHS): _____ 1–99 *(99=LIFETIME)*   DIAGNOSIS CODES (ICD-9): _____ _____ _____ _____

ANSWERS	ANSWER QUESTIONS 1–9. (Circle Y for Yes, N for No, or D for Does Not Apply, unless otherwise noted.)
a)_____mm Hg b)_____ % c)___/___/___	1. Enter the result of most recent test taken on or before the certification date listed in Section A. Enter (a) arterial blood gas PO2 and/or (b) oxygen saturation test; (c) date of test.
1 2 3	2. Was the test in Question 1 performed (1) with the patient in a chronic stable state as an outpatient, (2) within two days prior to discharge from an inpatient facility to home, or (3) under other circumstances?
1 2 3	3. Circle the one number for the condition of the test in Question 1: (1) At Rest; (2) During Exercise; (3) During Sleep
Y N D	4. If you are ordering portable oxygen, is the patient mobile within the home? If you are not ordering portable oxygen, circle D.
_____LPM	5. Enter the highest oxygen flow rate ordered for this patient in liters per minute. If less than 1 LPM, enter a "X".
a)_____mm Hg b)_____ % c)___/___/___	6. If greater than 4 LPM is prescribed, enter results of most recent test taken on 4 LPM. This may be an (a) arterial blood gas PO2 and/or (b) oxygen saturation test with patient in a chronic stable state. Enter date of test (c).
	ANSWER QUESTIONS 7-9 **ONLY** IF PO2 = 56–59 OR OXYGEN SATURATION = 89 IN QUESTION 1
Y N	7. Does the patient have dependent edema due to congestive heart failure?
Y N	8. Does the patient have cor pulmonale or pulmonary hypertension documented by P pulmonale on an EKG or by an echocardiogram, gated blood pool scan or direct pulmonary artery pressure measurement?
Y N	9. Does the patient have a hematocrit greater than 56%?

NAME OF PERSON ANSWERING SECTION B QUESTIONS, IF OTHER THAN PHYSICIAN (Please Print):
NAME: _____ TITLE: _____ EMPLOYER: _____

SECTION C	Narrative Description of Equipment and Cost

(1) Narrative description of all items, accessories and options ordered; (2) Supplier's charge and (3) Medicare Fee Schedule Allowance for each item, accessory and option. (See instructions on back.)

SECTION D	Physician Attestation and Signature/Date

I certify that I am the treating physician identified in Section A of this form. I have received Sections A, B and C of the Certificate of Medical Necessity (including charges for items ordered). Any statement on my letterhead attached hereto, has been reviewed and signed by me. I certify that the medical necessity information in Section B is true, accurate and complete, to the best of my knowledge, and I understand that any falsification, omission, or concealment of material fact in that section may subject me to civil or criminal liability.

PHYSICIAN'S SIGNATURE _____ DATE ___/___/___
Signature and Date Stamps Are Not Acceptable.

Form CMS-484 (09/05)

Figure 29-5 ■ Medicare Certificate of Medical Necessity for Oxygen

INSTRUCTIONS FOR COMPLETING THE CERTIFICATE
OF MEDICAL NECESSITY FOR OXYGEN (CMS-484)

SECTION A: **(May be completed by the supplier)**

CERTIFICATION TYPE/DATE: If this is an initial certification for this patient, indicate this by placing date (MM/DD/YY) needed initially in the space marked "INITIAL." If this is a revised certification (to be completed when the physician changes the order, based on the patient's changing clinical needs), indicate the initial date needed in the space marked "INITIAL," and indicate the recertification date in the space marked "REVISED." If this is a recertification, indicate the initial date needed in the space marked "INITIAL," and indicate the recertification date in the space marked "RECERTIFICATION." Whether submitting a REVISED or a RECERTIFIED CMN, be sure to always furnish the INITIAL date as well as the REVISED or RECERTIFICATION date.

PATIENT INFORMATION: Indicate the patient's name, permanent legal address, telephone number and his/her health insurance claim number (HICN) as it appears on his/her Medicare card and on the claim form.

SUPPLIER INFORMATION: Indicate the name of your company (supplier name), address and telephone number along with the Medicare Supplier Number assigned to you by the National Supplier Clearinghouse (NSC) or applicable National Provider Identifier (NPI). If using the NPI Number, indicate this by using the qualifier XX followed by the 10-digit number. If using a legacy number, e.g. NSC number, use the qualifier 1C followed by the 10-digit number. (For example. 1Cxxxxxxxxx)

PLACE OF SERVICE: Indicate the place in which the item is being used, i.e., patient's home is 12, skilled nursing facility (SNF) is 31, End Stage Renal Disease (ESRD) facility is 65, etc. Refer to the DMERC supplier manual for a complete list.

FACILITY NAME: If the place of service is a facility, indicate the name and complete address of the facility.

HCPCS CODES: List all HCPCS procedure codes for items ordered. Procedure codes that do not require certification should not be listed on the CMN.

PATIENT DOB, HEIGHT, WEIGHT AND SEX: Indicate patient's date of birth (MM/DD/YY) and sex (male or female); height in inches and weight in pounds, if requested.

PHYSICIAN NAME, ADDRESS: Indicate the PHYSICIAN'S name and complete mailing address.

PHYSICIAN INFORMATION: Accurately indicate the treating physician's Unique Physician Identification Number (UPIN) or applicable National Provider Identifier (NPI). If using the NPI Number, indicate this by using the qualifier XX followed by the 10-digit number. If using UPIN number, use the qualifier 1G followed by the 6-digit number. (For example. 1Gxxxxxx)

PHYSICIAN'S TELEPHONE NO: Indicate the telephone number where the physician can be contacted (preferably where records would be accessible pertaining to this patient) if more information is needed.

SECTION B: **(May not be completed by the supplier. While this section may be completed by a non-physician clinician, or a Physician employee, it must be reviewed, and the CMN signed (in Section D) by the treating practitioner.)**

EST. LENGTH OF NEED: Indicate the estimated length of need (the length of time the physician expects the patient to require use of the ordered item) by filling in the appropriate number of months. If the patient will require the item for the duration of his/her life, then enter "99".

DIAGNOSIS CODES: In the first space, list the ICD9 code that represents the primary reason for ordering this item. List any additional ICD9 codes that would further describe the medical need for the item (up to 4 codes).

QUESTION SECTION: This section is used to gather clinical information to help Medicare determine the medical necessity for the item(s) being ordered. Answer each question which applies to the items ordered, circling "Y" for yes, "N" for no, or "D" for does not apply.

NAME OF PERSON ANSWERING SECTION B QUESTIONS: If a clinical professional other than the treating physician (e.g., home health nurse, physical therapist, dietician) or a physician employee answers the questions of Section B, he/she must print his/her name, give his/her professional title and the name of his/her employer where indicated. If the physician is answering the questions, this space may be left blank.

SECTION C: **(To be completed by the supplier)**

NARRATIVE DESCRIPTION OF EQUIPMENT & COST: Supplier gives (1) a narrative description of the item(s) ordered, as well as all options, accessories, supplies and drugs; (2) the supplier's charge for each item(s), options, accessories, supplies and drugs; and (3) the Medicare fee schedule allowance for each item(s), options, accessories, supplies and drugs, if applicable.

SECTION D: **(To be completed by the physician)**

PHYSICIAN ATTESTATION: The physician's signature certifies (1) the CMN which he/she is reviewing includes Sections A, B, C and D; (2) the answers in Section B are correct; and (3) the self-identifying information in Section A is correct.

PHYSICIAN SIGNATURE AND DATE: After completion and/or review by the physician of Sections A, B and C, the physician's must sign and date the CMN in Section D, verifying the Attestation appearing in this Section. The physician's signature also certifies the items ordered are medically necessary for this patient.

According to the Paperwork Reduction Act of 1995, no persons are required to respond to a collection of information unless it displays a valid OMB control number. The valid OMB control number for this information collection is 0938-0534. The time required to complete this information collection is estimated to average 12 minutes per response, including the time to review instructions, search existing resources, gather the data needed, and complete and review the information collection. If you have any comments concerning the accuracy of the time estimate or suggestions for improving this form, please write to: CMS, Attn: PRA Reports Clearance Officer, 7500 Security Blvd. Baltimore, Maryland 21244.

DO NOT SUBMIT CLAIMS TO THIS ADDRESS. Please see http://www.medicare.gov/ for information on claim filing.

Form CMS-484 (09/05) INSTRUCTIONS

Figure 29-5 ■ (Continued)

Coding for Procedural/Professional Services (G0008-G9360)

HCPCS **G** codes are temporary national codes used to identify professional services and procedures that would otherwise be coded using CPT or for which no CPT code exists. Many of these codes were created for tracking by Medicare and Medicaid because they are usually more specific than CPT codes and identify services that are reimbursed in a unique way.

When a patient has Medicare or Medicaid, report the HCPCS code. CMS has specific regulations for reimbursing screening exams, including the patient's age, such as age 50 or older, and the frequency of exams, such as every 4 years (■ FIGURE 29-6).

When the patient has insurance *other than* Medicare or Medicaid, report the CPT code unless the payer requires the HCPCS code. Always check individual payer coding guidelines to be sure whether they require the HCPCS code or the CPT code (■ FIGURE 29-7).

A Medicare patient is seen for a screening colonoscopy.

G0104 Colorectal cancer screening; flexible sigmoidoscopy

Figure 29-6 ■ Example of Coding for a Colonoscopy for a Medicare Patient

---

A patient with private insurance is seen for a screening colonoscopy.

45330 Sigmoidoscopy, flexible, diagnostic; with or without collection of specimen(s) by brushing or washing (separate procedure)

Figure 29-7 ■ Example of Coding for a Colonoscopy for a Private Insurance Patient

---

SUCCESS STEP

Medical billing software can be programmed to identify whether each insurance company requires a HCPCS or CPT code. To activate this feature, the coding department must identify services that have both CPT and HCPCS codes, then give the computer technician a list of which payers require which code. Then, the billing staff member can enter only the CPT code, and the computer will substitute the HCPCS code for the required payers.

Coding for Drugs (J0000-J9999)

HCPCS **J** codes include drugs that the patient does not self-administer. They include injections, chemotherapy drugs for cancer treatment, immunosuppressive drugs for treatment of patients whose immune systems are compromised (including patients with AIDS), and inhaled solutions. Clinicians administer these drugs and monitor patients to ensure that there are no contraindications or side effects.

HCPCS also provides codes for drugs in sections **A**, **C**, **G**, **K**, **Q**, and **S**. In addition, there are HCPCS codes that represent supplies used to administer drugs, such as syringes or an IV medication bag. HCPCS codes for drugs and related supplies do not include the actual service that the clinician performs to administer the drug. CPT codes identify these services.

To locate codes for drugs in the HCPCS Index, locate the Main Term for the name of the drug. You can also locate most drugs in the Table of Drugs (■ FIGURE 29-8). The Table of Drugs provides four columns. Various publishers may use different titles for the columns, but they are similar to the following:

- **Column 1, Drug Name:** Alphabetical list of drugs by generic and brand names. Drugs that are manufactured in more than one concentration have a separate entry for each.
- **Column 2, Dose:** Identifies the quantity or dose identified by the code.
- **Column 3, Route:** The method of administration of the substance (■ TABLE 29-5).
- **Column 4, Code:** The HCPCS code that must be verified in the Tabular List.

Drug	Dosage	Route	Code
Akineton, see Biperiden			
Alatrofloxacin mesylate, injection	100 mg	IV	J0200
Albuterol	0.5 mg	INH	J7620
Albuterol, concentrated form	1 mg	INH	J7610, J7611
Albuterol, unit dose form	1 mg	INH	J7609, J7613
Aldesleukin	per single use vial	IM, IV	J9015
Aldomet, see Methyldopate HCl			
Alefacept	0.5 mg	IM, IV	J0215
Alemtuzumab	10 mg	IV	J9010
Alferon N	250.000 IU	IM	J9215
Alglucerase	per 10 units	IV	J0205
Alglucosidase alfa	10 mg	IV	J0220, J0221

Figure 29-8 ■ HCPCS Table of Drugs

Table 29-5 ■ ROUTES OF DRUG ADMINISTRATION

Abbreviation	Meaning
IA	Intra-arterial administration
IV	Intravenous administration
IM	Intramuscular administration
IT	Intrathecal (into fluid around the spinal cord)
SC	Subcutaneous administration
INH	Administration by inhaled solution
VAR	Various routes of administration (joints, cavities, tissues, topical applications, other parenteral administrations)
OTH	Other routes of administration (suppositories, catheter injections)
ORAL	Administered orally

To use the Table of Drugs, locate the drug name in the left-hand column, then identify the dose in the second and the route in the third columns. The fourth column provides the suggested code. Whether you locate codes using the Index or the Table of Drugs, always verify them in the Tabular List.

Report the quantity of a drug the patient received as a multiple of the dose listed in the second column. For example, the dose for **J9010 Alemtuzumab** is 10 mg, as shown on the Table

of Drugs and in the Tabular List. If 20 mg is administered intravenously, report a quantity of **2** for code **J9010** on the claim (20/10 = 2).

CODING CAUTION

The HCPCS Table of Drugs is different than the ICD-10-CM Table of Drugs and Chemicals. The HCPCS Table of Drugs is used to report drugs prescribed by and administered by healthcare providers. The ICD-10-CM Table of Drugs and Chemicals is used to report injuries caused by substances and due to an adverse reaction or improper use.

Orthotics (L0112-L9900)

HCPCS **L** codes represent orthotics, devices that help a patient to regain normal functioning, and prosthetics, devices that replace a body part lost to disease or trauma. Patients with orthotics and prosthetics can include those who have been diagnosed with upper or lower musculoskeletal injuries or conditions, patients with amputated limbs, and patients with spinal deformities. Examples of these devices are collars, rib braces and belts, rib aprons with straps to immobilize and support the rib cage, orthotic devices that limit the rotation of the hip, and gelatin or silicone breast implants.

To locate codes for orthotics in the HCPCS Index, locate the Main Term for the name of the item, such as **Collar** or **Boot**, or the more general term **Orthotics**. Then locate the subterm for the specific type of device. Always verify the code in the Tabular List.

CODING PRACTICE

Exercise 29.3 Assigning HCPCS Codes

Instructions: Read the mini-medical-record of each patient's encounter and assign the correct HCPCS code(s). Write the answer on the line provided.

1. INPATIENT HOSPITAL Gender: F Age: 58

Reason for encounter: anxiety disorder

Procedure: administered Librium, 100 mg

1 HCPCS Code _____

2. OFFICE Gender: F Age: 85

Assessment: diabetic polyneuropathy, callus formation

Procedure: fitted patient with a pair of custom-molded shoes

Plan: Office will schedule follow-up appointment when shoes arrive.

1 HCPCS Code _____ Quantity _____

3. OUTPATIENT HOSPITAL Gender: M Age: 65

Reason for encounter: history of malignant neoplasm of the lower GI tract 4 years ago places patient at high risk of colorectal cancer

Procedure: colorectal cancer screening

Findings: Normal

1 HCPCS Code _____

4. DME SUPPLIER Gender: M Age: 41

Reason for encounter: limited mobility due to morbid obesity, weight 400 pounds, BMI = 57 kg/m^2

Equipment: power wheelchair, group 2 heavy duty, sling/solid seat/back

1 HCPCS Code _____

(continued)

CODING PRACTICE (continued)

5. OFFICE Gender: F Age: 21

Reason for encounter: *neck pain following automobile accident 1 week ago*

Equipment: *provided patient with a cervical, flexible, nonadjustable foam collar*

Plan: *return to office 1 week*

1 HCPCS Code _____

CHAPTER SUMMARY

In this chapter you learned that:

• HCPCS codes are Level II codes of the Healthcare Common Procedure Coding System used to report services not included in CPT and for physician and nonphysician services, medical supplies, equipment, and medications.

• The HCPCS manual consists of an Index, Tabular List, Table of Drugs, and modifiers.

• The three skills of an "ace" coder—abstracting, assigning, and arranging codes—apply to HCPCS coding.

• Specific methods are required to assign modifiers and codes for transportation services, medical supplies, radiopharmaceuticals, enteral and parental nutrition, durable medical equipment, professional services, drugs administered by clinicians, and orthotics.

CONCEPT QUIZ

Take a moment to look back at HCPCS coding and solidify your skills. Try to answer the questions from memory first, then, refer to the discussion in this chapter and the Glossary at the end of this book if you need a little extra help.

Completion

Instructions: Write the term that answers each question based on the information you learned in this chapter. Choose from the list below. Some choices may be used more than once and some choices may not be used at all.

AMA	facility
CMS	guidelines
contrast medium	HCPCS
CPT	Index
dental	Medicare
diagnosis	orthotics
DME	therapy
enteral nutrition	

1. B codes represent supplies and products for _____.

2. D codes represent _____ supplies and products.

3. Each payer has unique coding, billing, and reimbursement _____ for supplies.

4. L codes represent _____ supplies and services.

5. _____ has specific regulations for reimbursing screening exams, including the patient's age and the frequency of exams.

6. _____ is billed by the radiologist, in addition to the CPT code for the procedure.

7. When the patient has insurance *other than* Medicare or Medicaid, report the _____ code unless the insurance requires the _____ code.

8. E codes represent supplies and products known as _____.

9. _____ codes represent the supplies used to administer drugs.

10. _____ codes represent the services to administer drugs.

Multiple Choice

Instructions: Circle the letter of the best answer to each question based on the information you learned in this chapter.

1. The _____ of a HCPCS code represents a group of similar services, supplies, drugs, and equipment.
   A. category
   B. letter
   C. classification
   D. Index

2. What does DME stand for?
   A. Diagnostic medical evaluation
   B. Durable medicine equipment
   C. Diagnostic modern equipment
   D. Durable medical equipment

3. What modifier is used to notify Medicare that the units of service exceed those in the medically unlikely edits (MUEs)?
   A. GA
   B. GB
   C. GL
   D. GZ

4. What do G codes identify?
   A. Hearing services
   B. Drugs other than chemotherapy
   C. Medical and surgical supplies
   D. Temporary national codes used to identify professional services

5. What abbreviation identifies that a drug is administered directly into the patient's vein?
   A. IV
   B. IT
   C. IA
   D. IM

6. Which of the following factors is not relevant when coding for an ambulance service?
   A. The type of service the patient needs
   B. The number of personnel that were needed
   C. The type of insurance reimbursing the services
   D. The type of vehicle used to transport the patient

7. What is the format of HCPCS modifiers?
   A. Alphanumeric or two letters
   B. Two numbers
   C. Two letters ranging from AA to ZZ
   D. One number and one letter

8. Where in the HCPCS code set are drugs listed in alphabetical order?
   A. Table of Drugs
   B. List of Modifiers
   C. Index
   D. Table of Brand Drugs

9. Who administers the drugs reported by J codes?
   A. The patient
   B. A healthcare professional
   C. A friend or family member
   D. All of the above

10. What does the acronym HCPCS stand for?
    A. Hospital Care Procedural Coding System
    B. Hospital Common Procedural Coding System
    C. Healthcare Common Procedure Coding System
    D. Healthcare Common Periodic Coding System

CODING CHALLENGE

Instructions: Read the mini-medical-record of each patient's encounter, then abstract, assign, and arrange ICD-10-CM diagnosis codes and HCPCS procedure codes using the appropriate Index and Tabular List. Write the code(s) on the line provided.

---

1. EMERGENCY DEPT   Gender: F   Age: 57

Reason for encounter: vomiting, nausea, and cramps

Assessment: enteritis due to *Escherichia coli*

Service provided: Ordered ampicillin sodium and sulbactam sodium IV injections 1.5 g every 6 hours. Patient received the drug for 18 hours and then was released.

Tip: Code for the supplies only.

1 ICD-10-CM Code _____

1 HCPCS Code _____

---

2. EMERGENCY DEPT   Gender: F   Age: 50

Reason for encounter: badly infected second-degree burn on her scalp that occurred in the bathroom of her home with a curling iron

Assessment: Patient has not properly cared for the wound. Treated the wound and applied an alginate dressing, 10 square inches.

(continued)

---

2. (continued)

Service Provided: Based on the wound's appearance and fluid oozing from it, I gave the patient two additional dressings to change once a week for two weeks and discharged home.

Tip: Code for the supplies only, not the service.

4 ICD-10-CM Codes _____

_____

1 HCPCS Code _____

---

3. OFFICE   Gender: M   Age: 62

Reason for encounter: visit to adjust a colostomy bag

Procedure: fitted a drainable, rubber colostomy with a faceplate and drain, and a protective solid skin barrier, size 4 inches square

1 ICD-10-CM Code _____

2 HCPCS Codes _____

(continued)

(continued from page 505)

4. OFFICE Gender: M Age: 55

Reason for encounter: review of patient's diet

Assessment: Patient currently utilizes an enteral feeding supply kit due to malnutrition from neck cancer. Patient needs additional fiber in his diet.

Service: provided patient with a fiber additive for the enteral formula

2 ICD-10-CM Codes _____

1 HCPCS Code _____

5. DME SUPPLIER Gender: F Age: 82

Patient diagnosis: Alzheimer dementia with behavioral disturbances. Patient is at risk of falling out of bed at night.

Equipment provided: hospital bed with a mattress and variable-height side rails

Tip: Code for the equipment.

2 ICD-10-CM Codes _____

1 HCPCS Code _____

6. DME SUPPLIER/HOME Gender: M Age: 68

Reason for encounter: Patient is paraplegic, needs to have his electric wheelchair motor repaired. DME repair technician makes a service call to the patient's home.

Service provided: Wheelchair motor repair, 60 minutes due to multiple nonroutine problems. Motor was running properly upon completion.

Tip: Refer to the amount of time that service was provided to calculate the units of service as stated in the code description.

1 ICD-10-CM Code _____

1 HCPCS Code _____ Quantity _____

7. OFFICE Gender: M Age: 12

Reason for encounter: congenital scoliosis

Supplies provided: cervical-thoracic-lumbar-sacral orthotic (CTLSO) (Milwaukee) brace

1 ICD-10-CM Code _____

1 HCPCS Code _____

8. SENIOR DAY CARE CENTER Gender: F Age: 100

Reason for encounter: senility

Service provided: Respite care, nursing, 1100–1600. Daughter is the regular caretaker.

Tip: Refer to the amount of time the service was provided to calculate the units of service as stated in the code description.

1 ICD-10-CM Code _____

1 HCPCS Code _____ Quantity _____

9. OFFICE Gender: M Age: 82

Reason for encounter: difficulty hearing in right ear

Assessment: hearing assessment shows conductive hearing loss in right ear

1 ICD-10-CM Code _____

1 HCPCS Code _____

10. TRANSPORT SERVICE Gender: M Age: 72

Reason for encounter: open fracture of the neck of right femur, type I, routine healing

Service provided: nonemergency transport in a wheelchair van from hospital to rehabilitation center

Distance traveled: 3 miles

1 ICD-10-CM Code _____

2 HCPCS Codes _____

Quantity _____

KEEP ON CODING

Instructions: Read the diagnostic or procedural statement, then use the appropriate Index and Tabular List to assign HCPCS codes. Write the code(s) on the line provided.

1. Injection of mitomycin, 5 mg: HCPCS Code(s) _____

2. Insulin infusion pump: HCPCS Code(s) _____

3. IV injection of Taxol, 60 mg: HCPCS Code(s) _____

4. Foley catheter, two-way, silicone: HCPCS Code(s) _____

5. Nasogastric tube, without stylet: HCPCS Code(s) _____

6. CPAP device: HCPCS Code(s) _____

7. Alcohol wipes, one box: HCPCS Code(s) _____

8. Pair of crutches, adjustable, wood: HCPCS Code(s) _____

9. Prostate screening, rectal exam: HCPCS Code(s) _____

10. Gel mattress: HCPCS Code(s) _____

11. Helicopter transport, rotary wing, per mile: HCPCS Code(s) _____

12. Pediatric gait trainer, upright support: HCPCS Code(s) _____

13. Administration, influenza virus vaccine: HCPCS Code(s) _____

14. Lightweight wheelchair, high strength, detachable arms desk, swing-away detachable elevating leg: HCPCS Code(s) _____

15. Clubfoot wedge: HCPCS Code(s) _____

16. 100 units of Pitocin IV: HCPCS Code(s) _____

17. Hearing aid assessment: HCPCS Code(s) _____

18. Nasal cannula: HCPCS Code(s) _____

19. 12-Volt battery and battery charger: HCPCS Code(s) _____

20. Basic life support ambulance services, nonemergency, 7 miles, from scene of accident to hospital: HCPCS Code(s) _____

21. Custom plastic artificial eye: HCPCS Code(s) _____

22. Contraceptive, cervical cap: HCPCS Code(s) _____

23. Orthotic device, Legg-Perthes, Scottish Rite type: HCPCS Code(s) _____

24. Standard metal bed pan: HCPCS Code(s) _____

25. Emergency ambulance transport with ALS-1 support from patient's home to helicopter pad, 21 miles: HCPCS Code(s) _____

Chapter 30

CPT Modifiers

Chapter Outline

- **Overview of CPT Modifiers**
- **Abstracting for CPT Modifiers**
- **Assigning Codes Using CPT Modifiers**
- **Arranging Codes With CPT Modifiers**

Learning Objectives

After completing this chapter, you should have the skills to:

30.1 Spell and define the key words, medical terms, and abbreviations related to CPT modifiers.

30.2 Identify the main characteristics of coding with CPT modifiers.

30.3 Abstract procedural information from the medical record for applying CPT modifiers.

30.4 Assign codes using CPT modifiers.

30.5 Arrange codes using CPT modifiers.

30.6 Discuss the CPT coding guidelines related to CPT modifiers.

Key Terms and Abbreviations

Appendix A
laterality

professional component
technical component

In addition to the key terms listed here, students should know the terms defined within tables in this chapter.

INTRODUCTION

When an item in a store is part of a special offer, the storekeeper posts a special sign to bring attention to it and may even tag and ring it up with a special code. Nothing in life is exactly the same 100% of the time, and sometimes we need a way to flag an exception to the rule so that others notice it. CPT modifiers do just that. By adding modifiers to CPT codes when needed, we may eliminate the need to write a detailed letter to the insurance company to explain how a service differs from what is usually provided. This chapter introduces you to CPT modifiers and their uses. It also helps you build skills to identify when modifiers are needed and how to apply them.

OVERVIEW OF CPT MODIFIERS

CPT modifiers are two-digit suffixes entered at the end of a CPT code to identify how the service provided varies from the usual code description. Some modifiers affect payment because they identify how a service was reduced or increased from the code description. Other modifiers are informational only and do not affect payment, such as those that identify **laterality**, the side of the body affected.

CPT provides 37 modifiers, 3 of which are used only by hospital outpatient and ambulatory surgery centers. In addition to these, approximately 50 HCPCS modifiers are listed in the CPT manual for use with CPT codes. HCPCS modifiers not listed in the CPT manual also can be used with CPT codes. They can be located in the HCPCS coding manual. HCPCS modifiers are two-character alphanumeric suffixes.

You do not need to use modifiers on every CPT code. They are used most frequently with surgical codes and, sometimes, with evaluation and management (E/M) codes. **Appendix A** of the CPT manual provides a full definition of all modifiers. Locate and refer to Appendix A frequently as you become familiar with modifiers. A list of modifiers with shortened descriptions appears inside the front cover of most CPT manuals.

CPT modifiers consist of two numbers that are placed immediately following a CPT code number. When writing a code, it is common to place a hyphen in front of the modifier to separate it from the code number or to clarify that a modifier is being referenced (■ FIGURE 30-1). The hyphen is not used when entering the modifier on a CMS-1500 form or into billing software (■ FIGURE 30-2). The CMS-1500 form and the 837P electronic claim format allow up to four modifiers to be reported with a code.

As is the case in many areas of coding, the specific requirements regarding modifier usage vary by payer. The Medicare Physician Fee Schedule Database (MPFSDB) provides

As established patient was evaluated for acute abdomen (*severe abdominal pain*). After a comprehensive examination and medical decision making of high complexity, the physician recommended surgery the following day.

99215-57 Office or other outpatient visit for an established patient (level 5)
Modifier 57 Decision for Surgery: An evaluation and management service that resulted in the initial decision to perform the surgery may be identified by adding modifier 57 to the appropriate level of E/M service.

Figure 30-1 ■ Example of Using CPT Modifiers. *Source:* © PB Resources, Inc. Used with permission.

information about certain modifiers, the codes they can be used with, and the impact on reimbursement. Medicare requires certain modifiers that other payers do not, and private payers may have requirements that do not apply to Medicare. Requirements for modifier usage can vary by the region of the country, even for a specific payer, as well as the data from the MPFSDB. As you enter the workplace, you will want to learn about modifier requirements in your area and for the specific payers billed most frequently by your facility. Medical billing software programs often can be programmed with the coding and billing requirements of individual payers. This customization provides reminder prompts to users or enters modifiers automatically, when appropriate.

CPT and HCPCS are the only codes that use modifiers. ICD-10-CM diagnosis codes and ICD-10-PCS inpatient procedure codes do not have modifiers. Modifiers are discussed before you learn the details of CPT coding because modifiers are used with codes throughout the CPT manual. An introduction to modifiers is presented in this chapter. Examples of applying modifiers in specific situations are provided in all CPT coding chapters in the sections about assigning and arranging codes.

SUCCESS STEP

Understanding modifiers when you have not yet learned how to use CPT codes can feel overwhelming. Remember that this chapter is the beginning, and you will have many opportunities to work with modifiers as you learn CPT coding. It takes time and experience to become comfortable with modifiers.

24. A. DATE(S) OF SERVICE From			To			B. PLACE OF SERVICE	C. EMG	D. PROCEDURES, SERVICES, OR SUPPLIES (Explain Unusual Circumstances) CPT/HCPCS	MODIFIER	E. DIAGNOSIS POINTER	F. $ CHARGES	G. DAYS OR UNITS	H. EPSDT Family Plan	I. ID. QUAL.	J. RENDERING PROVIDER ID. #
MM	DD	YY	MM	DD	YY										
01	05	YY				11		99125	57	AC	200 00	01		NPI	99 9999999

Figure 30-2 ■ How to Enter Modifiers on the CMS-1500 Form, Item 24D

CODING PRACTICE

Exercise 30.1 Overview of CPT Modifiers

Instructions: Write the answers to the following questions on the lines provided.

1. What is the purpose of modifiers? _____

_____

2. Which code sets use modifiers? _____

3. What is the correct way to write code 99215 with modifier -57?

_____

4. Where in the CPT manual can you find detailed information about modifiers? _____

5. What type of CPT codes most frequently require modifiers?

_____

ABSTRACTING FOR CPT MODIFIERS

Coders need to abstract information for modifiers from the patient's medical record, in addition to abstracting for diagnoses and procedures. For help identifying when CPT modifiers are needed, refer to ■ TABLE 30-1. When the answer to a question is *yes*, review the modifiers listed in the right-hand column. When you move on to assigning modifiers and codes, you will look up the description of each modifier suggested and determine which, if any, apply to the patient. Also refer to payer policies for

guidance. The fact that several modifiers are listed next to a question does not mean you can use any of them. Only specific modifiers are correct in any particular circumstance. For some patients, none of the modifiers might be needed. Table 30-1 is a tool to help you identify when a modifier *might* be needed and to help narrow down the modifiers that *might* apply. This table does not cover all modifiers or all situations but will help you get started. Throughout this text, additional criteria for abstracting modifiers are discussed relevant to the various sections of the CPT manual.

Table 30-1 ■ KEY CRITERIA FOR ABSTRACTING CPT MODIFIERS

Criteria	Modifier(s)
Was a service provided that was more extensive than usual?	-22, -23, -47, -59
Was a service reduced or discontinued?	-52, -53
Was the service mandated (required) by a third party?	-32
Was the service bilateral (performed on both members/sides of a paired organ or site)?	-50
Was more than one surgeon involved in performing a surgical procedure?	-62, -66, -80, -81, -82
Was the service provided during the global period of a surgical procedure? Was the previous procedure performed by the physician now seeing the patient? Is the current service unrelated to the previous surgery?	-24, -25, -54, -55, -56, -79
Did the physician provide only the professional component of a service that has both technical and professional components?	-26
Was the service performed in a hospital outpatient or ambulatory surgery center?	-73, -74
Was an E/M service provided on the same day or day before a surgical procedure?	-25, -57
Was the procedure repeated or a staged or unrelated procedure performed?	-58, -76, -77, -78, -79
Were surgeons other than the one who performed the surgery involved in the preoperative or postoperative care?	-54, -55, -56

Source: © PB Resources, Inc. Used with permission.

CODING PRACTICE

Exercise 30.2 Abstracting for CPT Modifiers

Instructions: Refer to Table 30-1 Key Criteria for Abstracting CPT Modifiers to answer the following questions. Identify the group of

modifiers that should be considered for each of the following situations based on the Key Criteria questions. Write the answer on the line provided. You do not need to select the final modifier.

Example: A colonoscopy was discontinued due to a drop in the patient's blood pressure. *-52, -53*

1. Monthly drug testing was ordered by the court as a condition of probation. _____

2. A patient had an emergency cholecystectomy while on vacation and was followed by her own physician for postoperative care.
_____

3. A thoracic surgeon and a neurosurgeon performed a discectomy (*excision of an intervertebral disc*). _____

4. An E/M service was provided the day before surgery.
_____

5. An appendectomy required an hour longer than usual to complete due to extensive abdominal adhesions.

ASSIGNING CODES USING CPT MODIFIERS

This section discusses the different purposes of modifiers for different types of services. As you learn how to code procedures for each body system, you will learn more about using modifiers for specific patient cases. An encoder or a practice management system often provides links to reference information or edit checks that identify which modifiers can be used with a particular CPT code (■ FIGURE 30-3). The MPFSDB also identifies the modifiers accepted for each CPT code. Some modifiers are used for multiple purposes, including those for anatomic sites. Others are limited to use with certain types of services, including Evaluation and Management (E/M), surgery, anesthesia, laboratory services,

radiology, and hospital outpatient ambulatory surgery centers. Each of these uses of CPT is discussed next. A few of the most common HCPCS modifiers also are discussed.

General CPT Modifiers

Some modifiers apply to most or all classes of CPT codes (■ TABLE 30-2, page 512). Whenever a service is mandated or required by a third-party payer, court, or other authority, modifier **-32 Mandated Services** alerts the payer.

When more than four modifiers are required on a single CPT code, they must be entered into a separate comments field (CMS-1500 Item 19), so modifier **-99 Multiple Modifiers** alerts the payer to look in that field for the modifiers.

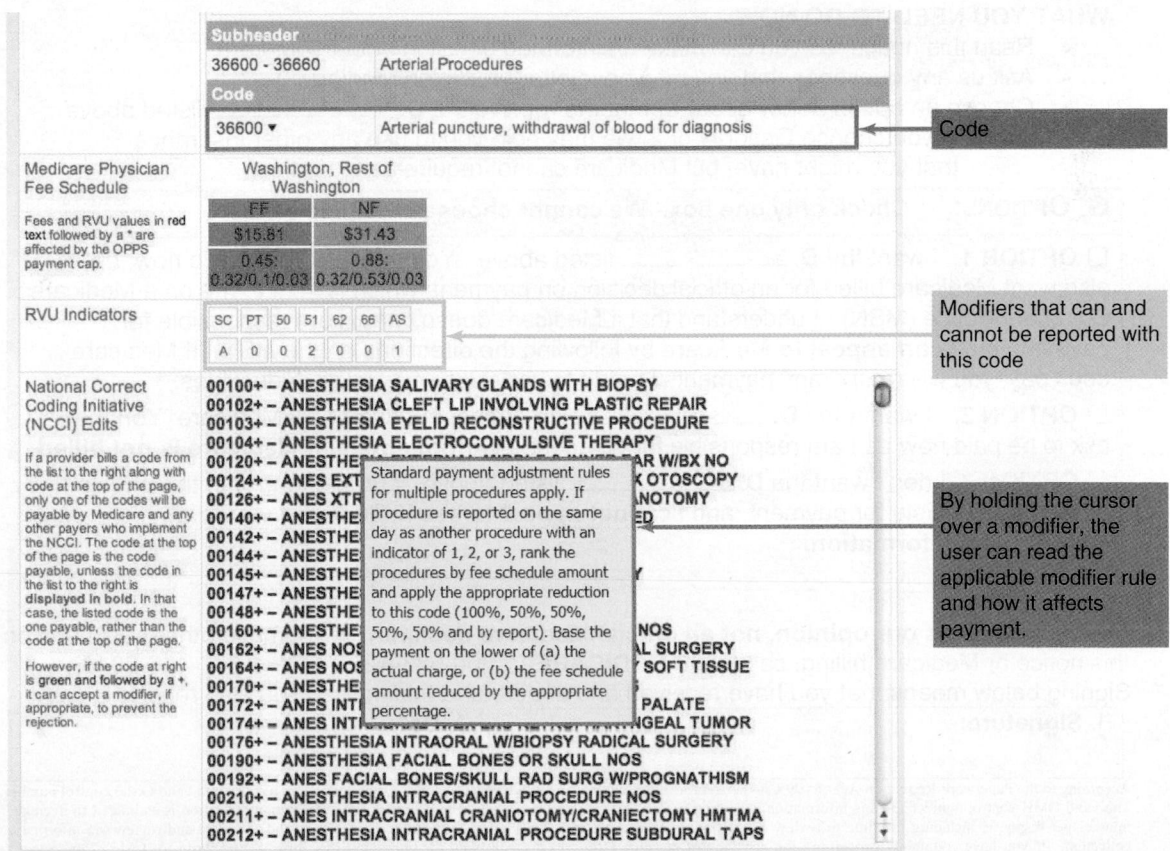

Figure 30-3 ■ Example of Modifier Rules in an Encoder. *Source: http://www.speedecoder.com/app/search/detail. php?code=36600&d=CPT. © SpeedeCoder. Reprinted with Permission.*

Table 30-2 ■ **GENERAL MODIFIERS**

Modifier	Short Description
-32	Mandated services
-99	Multiple modifiers
-GA	Waiver of liability statement on file (Medicare)
-GZ	Item or service expected to be denied as not reasonable and necessary (Medicare)

Medicare requires that patients be notified in writing when a covered service might be denied because of a lack of medical necessity. Providers must have patients sign an Advance Beneficiary Notice (ABN) acknowledging the reason for the potential denial, which makes the patient financially responsible to pay for the service (■ FIGURE 30-4). Modifier **-GA** informs Medicare that the ABN has been signed and allows the provider to bill the patient if Medicare does not pay for the service. If the service is expected to be denied and the ABN was

A. Notifier:

B. Patient Name: **C. Identification Number:**

Advance Beneficiary Notice of Noncoverage (ABN)

<u>NOTE:</u> If Medicare doesn't pay for **D.** _____ below, you may have to pay.

Medicare does not pay for everything, even some care that you or your health care provider have good reason to think you need. We expect Medicare may not pay for the **D.** _____ below.

D.	E. Reason Medicare May Not Pay:	F. Estimated Cost

WHAT YOU NEED TO DO NOW:

- Read this notice, so you can make an informed decision about your care.
- Ask us any questions that you may have after you finish reading.
- Choose an option below about whether to receive the **D.** _____ listed above.
  Note: If you choose Option 1 or 2, we may help you to use any other insurance that you might have, but Medicare cannot require us to do this.

G. OPTIONS: Check only one box. We cannot choose a box for you.
☐ **OPTION 1.** I want the **D.** _____ listed above. You may ask to be paid now, but I also want Medicare billed for an official decision on payment, which is sent to me on a Medicare Summary Notice (MSN). I understand that if Medicare doesn't pay, I am responsible for payment, but **I can appeal to Medicare** by following the directions on the MSN. If Medicare does pay, you will refund any payments I made to you, less co-pays or deductibles.
☐ **OPTION 2.** I want the **D.** _____ listed above, but do not bill Medicare. You may ask to be paid now as I am responsible for payment. **I cannot appeal if Medicare is not billed**.
☐ **OPTION 3.** I don't want the **D.** _____ listed above. I understand with this choice I am **not** responsible for payment, and **I cannot appeal to see if Medicare would pay**.

H. Additional Information:

This notice gives our opinion, not an official Medicare decision. If you have other questions on this notice or Medicare billing, call **1-800-MEDICARE** (1-800-633-4227/**TTY:** 1-877-486-2048).

Signing below means that you have received and understand this notice. You also receive a copy.

I. Signature:	J. Date:

According to the Paperwork Reduction Act of 1995, no persons are required to respond to a collection of information unless it displays a valid OMB control number. The valid OMB control number for this information collection is 0938-0566. The time required to complete this information collection is estimated to average 7 minutes per response, including the time to review instructions, search existing data resources, gather the data needed, and complete and review the information collection. If you have comments concerning the accuracy of the time estimate or suggestions for improving this form, please write to: CMS, 7500 Security Boulevard, Attn: PRA Reports Clearance Officer, Baltimore, Maryland 21244-1850.

Form CMS-R-131 (03/11)   Form Approved OMB No. 0938-0566

Figure 30-4 ■ Medicare Advance Beneficiary Notice

not signed, report modifier **-GZ**. In this case, the provider is responsible for the cost and the provider cannot bill the patient for the denied service.

Anatomic Site Modifiers

Anatomic site modifiers allow providers to specify the anatomic site more specifically than is described in a CPT code by itself. CPT codes do not specify laterality for procedures that can be performed on paired sites (■ FIGURE 30-5). Therefore, modifiers are used to distinguish laterality as follows (■ TABLE 30-3):

- All sites (right, left, or bilateral)
- Eyelids
- Fingers
- Toes
- Coronary arteries

Some CPT codes identify whether a procedure is performed on one side of the body or bilaterally. Other CPT codes do not. Laterality can be reported with modifiers **-RT Right side** or **-LT Left side**. Bilateral procedures not specified as such in the code description are reported using modifier **-50 Bilateral**. Some payers require that bilateral procedures be billed using two CPT codes: one with **-RT** and one with **-LT**. Medical billing software often can be preprogrammed with the requirements of each payer regarding how bilateral procedures should be reported. For Medicare claims, refer to the MPFS to determine whether CPT modifier **-50** is accepted with a particular procedure code.

Evaluation and Management Modifiers

Evaluation and Management (E/M) codes, which describe physician encounters such as office visits or physician hospital visits, require a modifier under certain circumstances (■ TABLE 30-4, page 514):

- A surgeon sees a patient during the postoperative period for a reason unrelated to the procedure.
- A physician provides an E/M service that should be paid separately from another service on the same day.
- The E/M service was required by a payer or legal authority (■ FIGURE 30-6, page 514).
- The E/M service resulted in a decision to perform surgery within 24 hours.
- The E/M service is the initial care provided by the admitting physician.

A patient had a chalazion removed from the right upper eyelid.

67800-E3
67800 Excision of chalazion; single
Modifier E3 Upper right eyelid

Figure 30-5 ■ Example of an Anatomic Modifier

Table 30-3 ■ **ANATOMIC SITE MODIFIERS**

Modifier	Description
All sites	
-50	Bilateral procedure
-LT	Left side (used to identify procedures performed on the left side of the body)
-RT	Right side (used to identify procedures performed on the right side of the body)
Eyelids	
-E1	Upper left eyelid
-E2	Lower left eyelid
-E3	Upper right eyelid
-E4	Lower right eyelid
Fingers	
-FA	Left hand, thumb
-F1	Left hand, second digit
-F2	Left hand, third digit
-F3	Left hand, fourth digit
-F4	Left hand, fifth digit
-F5	Right hand, thumb
-F6	Right hand, second digit
-F7	Right hand, third digit
-F8	Right hand, fourth digit
-F9	Right hand, fifth digit
Toes	
-TA	Left foot, great toe
-T1	Left foot, second digit
-T2	Left foot, third digit
-T3	Left foot, fourth digit
-T4	Left foot, fifth digit
-T5	Right foot, great toe
-T6	Right foot, second digit
-T7	Right foot, third digit
-T8	Right foot, fourth digit
-T9	Right foot, fifth digit
Coronary arteries	
-LC	Left circumflex coronary artery
-LD	Left anterior descending coronary artery
-LM	Left main coronary artery
-RC	Right coronary artery
-RI	Ramus intermedius coronary artery

Table 30-4 ■ EVALUATION AND MANAGEMENT MODIFIERS

Modifier	Short Description
-24	Unrelated evaluation and management service by the same physician or other qualified health care professional during a postoperative period
-25	Significant, separately identifiable evaluation and management service by the same physician or other qualified health care professional on the same day of the procedure or other service
-32	Mandated services
-57	Decision for surgery
-AI	Principal physician of record (Medicare)

Surgical/Procedural Modifiers

Modifiers are used on codes for medical and surgical procedures when the procedure is altered in a way that could affect its reimbursement. According to CPT guidelines, all surgical codes include specific services performed before, during, and after the procedure that are bundled into the CPT surgical package or global period. When all of these services are not provided by the same physician, a modifier is required. Surgical and procedural codes require modifiers in the following situations (■ TABLE 30-5):

- The procedure is more extensive or less extensive than described by the CPT code.
- The surgeon, not the anesthesiologist, administers general anesthesia.
- More than one surgeon is involved in the procedure.
- Preoperative or postoperative care is provided by a different surgeon than the one who performed the procedure.
- Multiple procedures are performed during the same operative session.

An insurance company requires a patient to be evaluated by a consulting physician for a second surgical opinion on back surgery. The consultant performs a comprehensive history, a comprehensive examination, and medical decision making of high complexity and concurs with the opinion of the first physician.

99245-32
99245 Office consultation for a new or established patient, which requires these 3 key components: a comprehensive history; a comprehensive examination; and medical decision making of high complexity
Modifier 32 Mandated services: Services related to mandated consultation and/or related services (e.g., third party payer, governmental, legislative or regulatory requirement) may be identified by adding modifier 32 to the basic procedure.

Figure 30-6 ■ Example of the Mandated Services Modifier.
Source: © PB Resources, Inc. Used with permission.

Table 30-5 ■ SURGICAL/PROCEDURAL MODIFIERS

Modifier	Short Description
-22	Increased procedural services
-32	Mandated services
-33	Preventive service
-47	Anesthesia by surgeon
-51	Multiple procedures
-52	Reduced services
-53	Discontinued procedure
-54	Surgical care only
-55	Postoperative management only
-56	Preoperative management only
-58	Staged or related procedure or service by the same physician or other qualified health care professional during the postoperative period
-59	Distinct procedural service
-62	Two surgeons
-63	Procedure performed on infants less than 4 kg
-66	Surgical team
-76	Repeat procedure or service by same physician or other qualified health care professional
-77	Repeat procedure by another physician or other qualified health care professional
-78	Unplanned return to the operating/procedure room by the same physician or other qualified health care professional following initial procedure for a related procedure during the postoperative period
-79	Unrelated procedure or service by the same physician or other qualified health care professional during the postoperative period
-80	Assistant surgeon
-81	Minimum assistant surgeon
-82	Assistant surgeon (when qualified resident surgeon not available)
-99	Multiple modifiers
-BL	Special acquisition of blood and blood products
-CA	Procedure payable only in the inpatient setting when performed emergently on an outpatient who expires prior to admission

- The procedure is staged, or planned to be completed over the course of several operative sessions.
- The procedure is repeated or an unplanned revision to the procedure is required (■ FIGURE 30-7).
- The surgeon who performed the procedure sees the patient for another procedure, unrelated to the first procedure, during the postoperative period.

During the postoperative period of a malignant lesion removal, the patient returned for a re-excision of the same lesion because frozen section pathology showed the margins of excision were inadequate for complete tumor removal. The final excised diameter was 3.9 cm.

11624-58
11624 Excision, malignant lesion including margins, scalp, neck, hands, feet, genitalia; excised diameter 3.1 to 4.0 cm
Modifier 58 Staged or related procedure or service by the same physician or other qualified health care professional during the postoperative period: It may be necessary to indicate that the performance of a procedure or service during the postoperative period was: (a) planned or anticipated (staged); (b) more extensive than the original procedure; or (c) for therapy following a surgical procedure. This circumstance may be reported by adding modifier 58 to the staged or related procedure.

Figure 30-7 ■ Example of Modifier for a Staged or Related Procedure. *Source: © PB Resources, Inc. Used with permission.*

Anesthesia Modifiers

General anesthesia (*using drugs to render a patient completely unaware and unable to feel pain*) is normally administered by an anesthesiologist. Anesthesiologist services are coded and billed by the anesthesiologist's office, separate from those for the surgeon. Anesthesia modifiers are used in the following situations (■ TABLE 30-6):

- All anesthesia codes require a modifier that identifies the physical status of the patient prior to surgery (■ FIGURE 30-8).

- General anesthesia was used in a procedure for which it is normally not used.

- The procedure was discontinued either before or after anesthesia was administered (outpatient hospital/ ambulatory surgery centers).

- HCPCS modifiers are used with Medicare patients to identify the type of anesthesia provider.

Radiology Modifiers

Modifiers are used on radiology codes when the service is reduced, discontinued, or repeated (■ TABLE 30-7, page 516). Radiology codes sometimes comprise two components: the technical component, which covers the cost of staffing and equipment, and the professional component, which covers the cost of a radiologist supervising the technician and interpreting the results. When the technical and professional components are provided by two different entities or individuals, modifiers are applied to identify the component of the service provided by each (■ FIGURES 30-9 and 30-10, page 516).

Laboratory Modifiers

Modifiers are used on laboratory codes when the service is reduced, discontinued, or repeated (■ TABLE 30-8, page 516).

Table 30-6 ■ **ANESTHESIA MODIFIERS**

Modifier	Short Description
-P1	A normal healthy patient
-P2	A patient with mild systemic disease
-P3	A patient with severe systemic disease
-P4	A patient with severe systemic disease that is a constant threat to life
-P5	A moribund patient who is not expected to survive without the operation
-P6	A declared brain-dead patient whose organs are being removed for donor purposes
-23	Unusual anesthesia
-52	Reduced services
-53	Discontinued procedure
-59	Distinct procedural service
-73	Discontinued outpatient hospital/ambulatory surgery center (ASC) procedure prior to the administration of anesthesia
-74	Discontinued out-patient hospital/ambulatory surgery center (ASC) procedure after administration of anesthesia
-76	Repeat procedure or service by same physician or other qualified health care professional
-77	Repeat procedure by another physician or other qualified health care professional
-78	Unplanned return to the operating/procedure room by the same physician or other qualified health care professional following initial procedure for a related procedure during the postoperative period
-79	Unrelated procedure or service by the same physician or other qualified health care professional during the postoperative period
-99	Multiple modifiers
-AA	Anesthesia services performed personally by anesthesiologist
-QX	CRNA service with medical direction by a physician
-QY	Medical direction of one certified registered nurse anesthetist (CRNA) by an anesthesiologist
-QZ	CRNA service without medical direction by a physician

Anesthesia services were provided for a ventral hernia on a patient with controlled hypertension.

00752-P2
00752 Anesthesia for hernia repairs in upper abdomen; lumbar and ventral (incisional) hernias and/or wound dehiscence
Modifier P2 Patient with mild systemic disease

Figure 30-8 ■ Example of an Anesthesia Physical Status Modifier

Table 30-7 ■ RADIOLOGY MODIFIERS

Modifier	Short Description
-26	Professional component
-32	Mandated services
-52	Reduced services
-53	Discontinued procedure
-59	Distinct procedural service
-76	Repeat procedure or service by same physician or other qualified health care professional
-77	Repeat procedure by another physician or other qualified health care professional
-78	Unplanned return to the operating/procedure room by the same physician or other qualified health care professional following initial procedure for a related procedure during the postoperative period
-79	Unrelated procedure or service by the same physician or other qualified health care professional during the postoperative period
-80	Assistant surgeon
-81	Minimum assistant surgeon
-82	Assistant surgeon (when qualified resident surgeon not available)
-99	Multiple modifiers
-GG	Performance and payment of a screening mammogram and diagnostic mammogram on the same patient, same day
-GH	Diagnostic mammogram converted from screening mammogram on same day
-TC	Technical component

When physicians send laboratory tests to an outside laboratory for processing, the laboratory can bill the patient's insurance for the test or they can bill the physician's office and allow the physician to bill the patient's insurance for the amount paid to the laboratory. This practice is a convenience to the laboratory because it saves paperwork. It is usually easy for the physician's office because it will be billing the patient's insurance for other services, including specimen collection. When the physician

73222 Magnetic resonance (e.g., proton) imaging, any joint of upper extremity; with contrast material(s)	
Total Fee	$301.74
Professional component (-26)	$62.43
Technical component (-TC)	$239.31

Figure 30-9 ■ Example of Professional and Technical Component Fees

A radiologist supervised and interpreted a transvaginal ultrasound.

76830-26
76830 Ultrasound, transvaginal
Modifier 26 Professional component: Certain procedures are a combination of a physician or other qualified health care professional component and a technical component. When the physician or other qualified health care professional component is reported separately, the service may be identified by adding modifier 26 to the usual procedure number.

Figure 30-10 ■ Example of Professional Component Modifier

Table 30-8 ■ LABORATORY MODIFIERS

Modifier	Short Description
-32	Mandated services
-52	Reduced services
-53	Discontinued procedure
-59	Distinct procedural service
-79	Unrelated procedure or service by the same physician or other qualified health care professional during the postoperative period
-90	Reference (outside) laboratory
-91	Repeat clinical diagnostic laboratory test
-92	Alternative laboratory platform testing
-99	Multiple modifiers
-QW	CLIA waived test

bills on behalf of the laboratory, the physician applies modifier -90 to the code for the laboratory test (■ FIGURE 30-11). The physician must bill the insurance company the same amount as the laboratory charged the physician. Medicare does not allow

A physician collected the specimen for a renal function panel, which he sent to a reference laboratory for analysis. The physician billed the patient's insurance company on behalf of the lab.

36415 Collection of venous blood by venipuncture
99000 Handling and/or conveyance of specimen for transfer from the office to a laboratory
80069-90
80069 Renal function panel
Modifier 90 Reference (outside) laboratory: When laboratory procedures are performed by a party other than the treating or reporting physician or other qualified health care professional, the procedure may be identified by adding modifier 90 to the usual procedure number.

Figure 30-11 ■ Example of Modifier for a Reference Laboratory. *Source: © PB Resources, Inc. Used with permission.*

this practice and it has become less common among private payers than it once was.

Hospital Outpatient/Ambulatory Surgery Center Modifiers

A specific subset of modifiers, including three unique ones, apply to hospital outpatient and ambulatory surgery centers (■ Table 30-9). The unique modifiers are **-27 Multiple Outpatient Hospital E/M Encounters on the Same Date** and modifiers **-73** and **-74**, which pertain to discontinued procedures. The other modifiers approved for use by these facilities are the same ones used by other facilities.

Table 30-9 ■ HOSPITAL OUTPATIENT/AMBULATORY SURGERY CENTER MODIFIERS

Modifier	Short Description
-25	Significant, separately identifiable evaluation and management service by the same physician or other qualified health care professional on the same day of the procedure or other service
-27	Multiple outpatient hospital E/M encounters on the same date
-50	Bilateral procedure
-52	Reduced services
-58	Staged or related procedure or service by the same physician or other qualified health care professional during the postoperative period
-59	Distinct procedural service
-73	Discontinued outpatient hospital/ambulatory surgery center (ASC) procedure prior to the administration of anesthesia
-74	Discontinued outpatient hospital/ambulatory surgery center (ASC) procedure after administration of anesthesia
-76	Repeat procedure or service by same physician or other qualified health care professional
-77	Repeat procedure by another physician or other qualified health care professional
-78	Unplanned return to the operating/procedure room by the same physician or other qualified health care professional following initial procedure for a related procedure during the postoperative period
-79	Unrelated procedure or service by the same physician or other qualified health care professional during the postoperative period
-91	Repeat clinical diagnostic laboratory test

CODING PRACTICE

Exercise 30.3   Assigning Codes Using CPT Modifiers

Instructions: Identify the specific modifier that should be used in each of the following situations. Refer to all the tables in this chapter, as needed.

Example: An X-ray of the patient's left knee was taken. *-LT*

1. A splint was applied to the patient's right middle finger. _____

2. A patient had an emergency cholecystectomy while on vacation out of town. When she returned home, a local physician provided postoperative care. _____

3. A thoracic surgeon and a neurosurgeon performed a discectomy. _____

4. An E/M service that resulted in the decision to perform surgery was provided the day before surgery. _____

5. A surgery required an hour longer than usual to complete due to extensive abdominal adhesions. _____

6. An anesthesiologist provided anesthesia services for a patient with a mild systemic disease. _____

7. A radiologist provided the professional components of supervising and interpreting a computerized tomography (CT) scan of the head. _____

8. A clinical diagnostic laboratory test had to be repeated for the same patient on the same day. _____

9. Multiple surgical procedures were performed during the same operative session. _____

10. A bilateral procedure was performed. _____

ARRANGING CODES WITH CPT MODIFIERS

There are several considerations when arranging codes using CPT modifiers. The order in which codes are arranged sometimes determines which codes receive modifiers.

The use of modifiers and the sequence of codes can impact payment. For example, when multiple surgical procedures are performed during the same operative session, the most costly procedure is sequenced first. Depending on the description of the CPT code, the secondary procedures sometimes need modifier **-51 Multiple Procedures** and are paid at a percentage of their usual rate. The discounted payment reflects the fact that less setup time is required for the secondary procedure(s) when performed during the same session as another procedure.

When a code requires more than one modifier, the order in which modifiers are applied can affect whether the claim is processed. Modifiers that affect price or payment generally are sequenced before modifiers that are used for informational

purposes. For example, a modifier such as **-26 Professional Component** affects payment because the physician does not perform all the components of code. It should be sequenced before anatomic modifiers that identify **-RT Right side** or **-LT Left side**, which are information only (■ Figure 30-12).

> A radiologist supervised and interpreted an MRI of the right shoulder.
>
> **73222-26-RT**
> **73222 Magnetic resonance (e.g., proton) imaging, any joint of upper extremity; with contrast material(s)**
> **Modifier 26 Professional component** (affects payment)
> **Modifier RT Right side** (informational)

Figure 30-12 ■ Example of Sequencing Multiple Modifiers.
Source: © PB Resources, Inc. Used with permission.

CHAPTER SUMMARY

In this chapter you learned that:

- CPT modifiers are two-digit suffixes entered at the end of a CPT code to identify how the service provided varies from the usual code description.

- As is the case in many areas of coding, the specific requirements regarding modifier usage vary by payer.

- Coders need to abstract information for modifiers from the patient's medical record, in addition to abstracting for diagnoses and procedures.

- Some modifiers are used for multiple purposes, including those for anatomic site. Others are limited to use with certain types of services, including Evaluation and Management (E/M), surgery, anesthesia, laboratory services, radiology, and hospital outpatient ambulatory surgery centers.

- The order in which codes are arranged sometimes determines which codes receive modifiers.

CONCEPT QUIZ

Take a moment to look back at CPT modifiers and solidify your skills. Try to answer the questions from memory first, then refer to the discussion in this chapter and the Glossary at the end of this book if you need a little extra help.

Completion

Instructions: Write the term that answers each question based on the information you learned in this chapter. Choose from the list below. Some choices may be used more than once and some choices may not be used at all.

-23	anesthesia
-25	surgeon
-26	payer
-27	primary care physician
-32	professional
-50	reduced service
-62	skin lesions
-63	technical
-80	toes
-81	unusual anesthesia
-82	

1. Modifier _____ is reported by the assistant surgeon.

2. Modifier _____ is used to indicate that the procedure was performed on both sides of the body.

3. When multiple modifiers are used, certain modifiers, such as _____, must be the first modifier applied to the code.

4. _____ is reported using modifier -23.

5. Modifier _____ alerts the payer that a procedure was performed on an infant weighing less than 4 kg.

6. Modifiers are used to distinguish laterality for _____.

7. Modifier _____ is used when an E/M service is required by a payer.

8. All _____ codes require a modifier that identifies the physical status of the patient prior to surgery.

9. The _____ component modifier of a radiology code is used to cover the cost of staffing and equipment.

10. Modifier _____ applies uniquely to hospital outpatient and ambulatory surgery centers.

Multiple Choice

Instructions: Circle the letter of the best answer to each question based on the information you learned in this chapter.

1. Which of the following is a modifier?
   A. -LT
   B. -MT
   C. -NT
   D. -OT

2. Which of the following is a body site that does not require a modifier to indicate the side of the body?
   A. Kidney transplant
   B. Repair of a skin laceration
   C. Lung biopsy
   D. Reduction of hip fracture

3. What modifier is used when a physician manages a patient's postoperative care only?
   A. -53
   B. -54
   C. -55
   D. -56

4. What modifier is used for interpretation of a test result?
   A. Radiology service
   B. Global service
   C. Professional component
   D. Technical component

5. What is the format of CPT modifiers?
   A. Two numbers
   B. Two letters
   C. One letter and one number
   D. One letter and one symbol

6. What modifier is used when a physician performs multiple procedures at the same operative session, such as repair of a wound on the left temporal area and removal of a cyst on the right temporal area?
   A. -50
   B. -51
   C. -LT
   D. -RT

7. Which of the following services is not included in the CPT surgical package?
   A. A surgical second opinion
   B. Evaluation 24 hours before surgery
   C. The surgical procedure
   D. Normal postoperative follow-up visits

8. What is the physical status modifier for a moribund patient undergoing anesthesia?
   A. -P3
   B. -P4
   C. -P5
   D. -P6

9. What modifier is used when an obstetrician administers a regional anesthesia block prior to an emergency cesarean delivery?
   A. -22
   B. -23
   C. -47
   D. -51

10. What modifier is used for a procedure with two co-surgeons?
    A. -62
    B. -58
    C. -51
    D. -66

CODING CHALLENGE

Instructions: Read the mini-medical-record of each patient's encounter, then identify the modifier that should be applied. Refer to the tables provided in this chapter. Write the modifier number and name on the line provided. Do not assign any codes.

Example: <u>*-22 Unusual anesthesia services*</u>

---

1. INPATIENT HOSPITAL   Gender: M   Age: 57

Preoperative assessment: Abdominal hemorrhage, 1 day postoperative from open cholecystectomy

Procedure: return to operating room for exploration of abdomen and ligation of vessels to achieve hemostasis

1 Modifier _____

---

2. OUTPATIENT HOSPITAL   Gender: M   Age: 6

Preoperative assessment: Patient had first stage of a hypospadias repair one month ago. Returns today for the second-stage repair.

Procedure: urethroplasty with free skin graft obtained from a site other than genitalia.

1 Modifier _____

---

3. OUTPATIENT SURGERY   Gender: M   Age: 17

Preoperative diagnosis: bulge in groin area for a few months

Procedure: bilateral inguinal herniorrhaphy with mesh

Postoperative diagnosis: reducible, bilateral inguinal hernias

1 Modifier _____

(continued)

(continued from page 519)

4. INPATIENT HOSPITAL   Gender: F   Age: 26

Reason for encounter: patient pulled out central line

Procedure: central line reinserted by the same cardiologist

1 Modifier _____

5. OFFICE   Gender: M   Age: 25

Reason for encounter: follow up on test results after evaluation of proximal muscle weakness, easy bruising, weight gain

Assessment: endogenous Cushing syndrome due to pituitary adenoma, evaluated for surgery

Plan: surgery scheduled to remove tumor tomorrow

1 Modifier _____

6. OUTPATIENT HOSPITAL   Gender: F   Age: 61

Reason for encounter: carpal tunnel decompression

Preoperative diagnosis: numbness, tingling, and pain in the right arm, hand, and fingers due to pinched nerve

Procedure: Carpal tunnel decompression. Regional nerve block administered by surgeon with decompression of right carpal tunnel nerve.

Postoperative diagnosis: carpal tunnel syndrome

2 Modifiers _____

7. INPATIENT HOSPITAL   Gender: F   Age: 13

Preoperative diagnosis: knee dislocated during tackle football game

Procedure: closed reduction of dislocation of right knee

Postoperative diagnosis: Dislocation of right knee

1 Modifier _____

8. EMERGENCY DEPT.   Gender: M   Age: 45

Reason for encounter: possible tibial fracture sustained when the ATV he was riding tipped over

Procedure: supervised and interpreted X-ray of lower leg that shows a transverse fracture of shaft of the right tibia

Diagnosis: transverse fracture, right tibia

2 Modifiers _____

9. OUTPATIENT SURGERY   Gender: M   Age: 48

Procedure: Cystourethroscopy with bladder biopsy. Twenty minutes into the procedure, the patient developed some arrhythmia and the surgery was stopped.

1 Modifier _____

10. OFFICE   Gender: F   Age: 25

Reason for encounter: follow-up care of fracture

Assessment: Fracture of L distal femur while skiing in Colorado. The physician in Colorado performed a closed treatment of the fracture with manipulation. Patient now sees me, as a local physician, for postoperative care.

2 Modifiers _____

Evaluation and Management Services (99201-99499)

Chapter 31

Learning Objectives

After completing this chapter, you should have the skills to:

31.1 Spell and define the key words, medical terms, and abbreviations related to evaluation and management services.

31.2 Identify the main characteristics of coding for evaluation and management services.

31.3 Discuss the CPT coding guidelines related to evaluation and management services.

31.4 Abstract information from the medical record for coding evaluation and management services.

31.5 Assign codes for evaluation and management services.

31.6 Discuss advanced coding for evaluation and management services.

Chapter Outline

- **Overview of Evaluation and Management Services**
- **Guidelines for Evaluation and Management Services**
- **Abstracting Evaluation and Management Services**
- **Assigning Codes for Evaluation and Management Services**
- **Advanced Coding for Evaluation and Management Services**

Key Terms and Abbreviations

chief complaint (CC)
concurrent care
consultation
consulting physician
content of service requirements
documentation guideline (DG)

established patient (EP)
Evaluation and Management (E/M)
facility fee
history of present illness (HPI)
initial encounter (CPT)
key component (KC)

level of service
new patient (NP)
nursing facility (NF)
past, family, and social history (PFSH)
patient type

place of service (POS)
referring physician
review of systems (ROS)
setting
subsequent encounter (CPT)
transfer of care

In addition to the key terms listed here, students should know the terms defined within tables in this chapter and the definitions of all evaluation and management categories.

INTRODUCTION

You might schedule service for a household appliance—such as a washing machine, furnace, or stove—for any number of reasons. Perhaps you experience a sudden breakdown, finally get around to having a long-standing issue fixed, or schedule preventive maintenance in the hopes of avoiding a major repair.

There are also many reasons that patients seek medical care, such as to receive preventive care, check out a new symptom or health problem, manage chronic conditions, monitor hospital care, receive emergency and critical care, or request a consultative service or second opinion. Physicians also provide case management, oversight, and coordination of care services when the patient is not present. CPT provides a special section of codes—Evaluation and Management (E/M) Services—to describe a wide variety of physician encounters.

OVERVIEW OF EVALUATION AND MANAGEMENT SERVICES

Patients meet with physicians for many different reasons. Encounters can take place in a wide variety of settings—clinics, hospitals, emergency departments, skilled nursing facilities, assisted living facilities, and even the patient's home. Physicians interview patients, perform physical examinations, and review medical data to determine the treatment plan. **Evaluation and Management (E/M)** codes describe patient encounters with a physician for the evaluation and management of a health problem. Each setting or purpose has a separate category of codes and a specific set of criteria for selecting the correct code.

E/M codes are numbered **99201** through **99499**. Although the codes begin with the numbers 99, they are located out of numerical sequence in the CPT manual. The E/M section appears first in the CPT coding manual for convenience because these are the most commonly used group of CPT codes and are used by all specialties.

During the evaluation portion of the visit, the physician does the following:

- Asks the patient questions (subjective assessment) regarding the chief complaint or reason for the encounter

- Discusses with the patient the background of the problem, symptoms or other systems affected, and past medical history, family medical history, and social (lifestyle) history

- Performs a physical examination (objective assessment) related to the patient's health and presenting problem(s)

During the management portion of the encounter, providers formulate a treatment plan—also called medical decision making—which requires them to do the following:

- Review test results or other records that are relevant to the presenting problem.
- Order further diagnostic testing.
- Refer the patient to other providers for specialized evaluation.
- Prescribe therapeutic treatments and medication.
- Schedule follow-up appointments to monitor progress.

Together, these components are referred to as the chief complaint or presenting problem, history, examination, and medical decision making.

Physicians and nonphysician practitioners (NPPs) provide E/M services. Nonphysician practitioners can be a physician assistant (PA), nurse practitioner (NP), clinical nurse specialist (CNS), or certified nurse midwife (CNM). These providers are licensed medical professionals who have less training than a physician but can diagnose patients and bill independently. The details of nonphysician practitioners' scope of practice vary by state, training, and licensure. Some nonphysician practitioners, such as physician assistants, must practice under a physician's supervision, but nurse practitioners practice independently in most states. Nonphysician practitioners also may prescribe medication in most states. They provide a cost-effective means of delivering professional, personalized care for routine medical needs.

Normally, the provider marks the E/M code on the encounter form or enters it into the electronic health record (EHR) (■ FIGURE 31-1). Coders need to ensure that documentation in the medical record is consistent with the codes marked by the provider. Offices should audit claims on a regular basis to verify that every detail of the E/M code is clearly documented. EHR systems can prompt the physician to document the various criteria required for E/M coding, then suggest the most appropriate code based on the physician's input.

Often, evaluation and management is the only service provided, but it also can be provided at the same time as other procedures, such as a laboratory test that is performed in the office, an electrocardiogram (EKG or ECG), or X-ray.

> ### SUCCESS STEP
> E/M codes used by ophthalmologists appear in the Ophthalmology subsection of the Medicine section, codes **92002** to **92014**.

E/M coding possesses some differences from the rest of CPT coding because E/M codes are assigned based on unique criteria. These criteria have specific definitions within the CPT guidelines that coders must adhere to. The criteria are:

- **Setting** – where the service is provided, such as office/outpatient, hospital, emergency department, or nursing facility; also called place of service
- **Patient type** – whether the patient is new or established
- **Level of service** – the complexity or length of service provided based on the nature of the presenting problem, the history, the examination, and the medical decision making.

The E/M section is organized by the setting in which the service is provided. The divisions of the E/M section are called categories and subcategories, rather than subsections and subheadings, as is the case in most other CPT sections. A category, the first level of division in the E/M section, identifies the setting, or place of service. Most categories are divided into subcategories based on patient type (new or established), age, or frequency. Each subcategory is divided into codes based on the level of service. Take a moment to review the table of contents

New Patient		Arthrocentesis/Aspiration/Injection			Labora
Problem Focused	99201				Amylase
Expanded Problem, Focused	99202	Small Joint		20600	B12
Detailed	99203	Interm Joint		20605	CBC &
Comprehensive	99204	Major Joint		20610	Comp N
Comprehensive/High Complex	99205	Other Invasive/Noninvasive			Chlamy
Well Exam Infant (up to 12 mos.)	99381	Audiometry		92552	Cholest
Well Exam 1–4 yrs.	99382	Cast Application			Digoxin
Well Exam 5–11 yrs.	99383	Location	Long	Short	Electrol
Well Exam 12–17 yrs.	99384	Catheterization		51701	Ferritin
Well Exam 18–39 yrs.	99385	Circumcision		54150	Folate
Well Exam 40–64 yrs.	99386	Colposcopy		57452	GC Scre
		Colposcopy w/Biopsy		57454	Glucose
		Cryosurgery Premalignant Lesion			Glucose
		Location (s):			Glycosy
Established Patient		Cryosurgery Warts			HCT
Post–Op Follow Up Visit	99024	Location (s):			HDL
Minimum	99211	Curettement Lesion			Hep BSA
Problem Focused	99212	Single		11055	Hepatit
Expanded Problem Focused	99213	2–4		11056	HGB
Detailed	99214	>4		11057	HIV
Comprehensive/High Complex	99215	Diaphragm Fitting		57170	Iron & T
Well Exam Infant (up to 12 mos.)	99391	Ear Irrigation		69210	Kidney
Well exam 1–4 yrs.	99392	ECG		93000	Lead
Well exam 5–11 yrs.	99393	Endometrial Biopsy		58100	Liver Pro
Well exam 12–17 yrs.	99394	Exc. Lesion Malignant			Mono T
Well exam 18–39 yrs.	99395	Benign			Pap Sm
Well exam 40–64 yrs.	99396	Location			Pregnan
Obstetrics		Exc. Skin Tags (1–15)		11200	Obstetr
Total OB Care	59400	Each Additional 10		11201	Pro Tim
Injections		Fracture Treatment			PSA
Administration Sub. / IM	90772	Loc			PPR
Drug		w/Reduc		w/o Reduc	Sed. Ra
Dosage		I & D Abscess Single/Simple		10060	Stool Cu

Figure 31-1 ■ Encounter Form Showing E/M Codes

for the E/M section that appears on page 1, before the E/M guidelines, in the CPT manual.

This chapter provides an overview of beginning E/M coding by discussing the guidelines and the organization of the E/M section, followed by abstracting and assigning the most common categories of E/M codes. This chapter also provides an introduction to advanced E/M coding needed for working in various medical specialties.

GUIDELINES FOR EVALUATION AND MANAGEMENT SERVICES

Four sources of guidelines must be considered when determining the level of E/M service provided:

- E/M Section Guidelines
- Category Special Instructions

- 1995 Documentation Guidelines for Evaluation and Management Services
- 1997 Documentation Guidelines for Evaluation and Management Services

The purpose of each set of guidelines is discussed next.

E/M Section Guidelines

The CPT guidelines appear at the beginning of the E/M section and provide information that applies to all codes in the section. The guidelines are several pages in length and explain the overall organization of the E/M section, define commonly used terms, and provide instructions for selecting a level of E/M service. In most editions of the CPT manual, these pages are shaded for easy identification.

1. The medical record should be complete and legible.
2. The documentation of each patient encounter should include:
   - reason for the encounter and relevant history, physical examination findings, and prior diagnostic test results;
   - assessment, clinical impression, or diagnosis;
   - plan for care; and
   - date and legible identity of the observer.
3. If not documented, the rationale for ordering diagnostic and other ancillary services should be easily inferred.
4. Past and present diagnoses should be accessible to the treating and/or consulting physician.
5. Appropriate health risk factors should be identified.
6. The patient's progress, response to and changes in treatment, and revision of diagnosis should be documented.
7. The CPT and [ICD-9/10-CM] codes reported on the health insurance claim form or billing statement should be supported by the documentation in the medical record.

Figure 31-2 ■ Principles of Medical Record Documentation. *Source: 1995 Documentation Guidelines for Evaluation and Management Services.*

SUCCESS STEP

Not only are the E/M guidelines mandatory instructions that must be followed, they provide valuable insight into the meaning of terminology in the E/M section. Read these guidelines as part of your assignment of reading this chapter of the text. Refer to them frequently as you work with E/M codes.

Category Special Instructions

Each of the 21 categories of E/M services begins with special instructions that apply to all codes within the category. Special instructions provide the following types of information:

- Explain the purpose of the category
- Describe the circumstances and settings for which codes in the category are to be used
- Define terms applicable to codes in the category
- Identify services that are and are not bundled with the codes in the category
- Redirect the coder to other categories that may be more appropriate

Many subcategories also provide instructions for that subset of codes. Coders must read the category and subcategory special instructions before selecting a code.

1995 Documentation Guidelines for Evaluation and Management Services

E/M codes were added to CPT in 1992 to replace "office visit" codes that were poorly defined. Rather than basing codes solely on the amount of time spent by providers during an encounter, E/M codes attempted to define the complexity of the visit. However, providers interpreted the CPT guidelines inconsistently, which resulted in confusion. To help provide clearer direction, the Centers for Medicare and Medicaid Services (CMS) and the American Medical Association (AMA) developed **documentation guidelines (DGs)** for the E/M services, titled *1995 Documentation Guidelines for Evaluation and Management Services* (1995 DG).

The document outlines general principles of medical documentation (■ FIGURE 31-2) and guidelines for documenting the history, examination, and medical decision making components of E/M services. It also discusses how to document an encounter dominated by counseling or coordination of care. The 1995 DG list the recognized body areas and organ systems addressed during an examination but do not clearly define the criteria for reporting the extent of the examination. 1995 DG are still used today.

1997 Documentation Guidelines for Evaluation and Management Services

After the 1995 DG were implemented, many providers desired more definition regarding how to document the physical examination. To provide clarity, CMS and the AMA developed additional guidelines, titled *1997 Documentation Guidelines for Evaluation and Management Services* (1997 DG). The 1997 DG are still in use today.

The 1997 DG further specify the requirements for a comprehensive multisystem examination, as well as single-organ system examinations frequently performed by specialists. For each type of examination, the 1997 DG provide a bulleted list of elements to be evaluated. The number of elements included in the examination determines the level of complexity of the examination: problem focused, expanded problem focused, detailed, or comprehensive.

Physicians may use either the 1995 or 1997 DG as documentation criteria for any E/M encounter. They can use 1995 DG for one patient and 1997 DG for another patient. But they cannot pick and choose from both sets of guidelines for the same encounter. In general, specialists prefer the 1997 guidelines because they delineate single-organ system examinations.

SUCCESS STEP

The 1995 DG and 1997 DG can be downloaded from the MedLearn section of the CMS website at **www.cms.gov**.

CODING PRACTICE

Exercise 31.1   Overview and Guidelines for Evaluation and Management Services

Instructions: Answer the following questions based on the information in the Overview and Guidelines sections of this chapter. Write your answer on the lines provided.

1. Where in the CPT manual are Evaluation and Management (E/M) codes located?

2. What are the three criteria that define E/M codes?

3. What guidelines describe the circumstances and settings for which codes in the category are to be used?

4. Name three examples of nonphysician practitioners.

5. What guidelines provide a bulleted list of elements to be evaluated in an examination?

ABSTRACTING EVALUATION AND MANAGEMENT SERVICES

All the information used to classify E/M services—the setting in which service was provided, the type of patient and/or frequency of the encounter, and the criteria used to determine the level of service—must be abstracted before codes can be assigned.

■ FIGURE 31-3 (page 526) provides a flow chart/decision tree for abstracting and assigning E/M codes. Refer to columns 1, 2, and 3 as you read the following material on abstracting the E/M setting and patient type.

- Column 1: Select the general setting of service as outpatient, inpatient, without direct patient contact, or other.
- Column 2: Select the type of service (E/M category) within the setting.
- Column 3: Select the subcategory of service within the type.

Abstracting the Setting

The first piece of information to abstract for E/M codes is the setting in which service was provided. The following information discusses the office, outpatient hospital, and inpatient hospital settings in detail, then provides an overview of other E/M settings. Office and inpatient settings include many types of E/M services. Therefore, several categories are provided for both of these settings, and coders must accurately select the correct one. The E/M section provides 21 categories of codes. Refer to ■ TABLE 31-1 for a general guide in abstracting the setting or category of service.

Office-Based Evaluation and Management Services

An office or other outpatient setting is a nonresidential medical facility to which patients come for several minutes or several hours at one time. Patients are outpatients until they are formally admitted to an inpatient facility. Medical offices, clinics, urgent care clinics, outpatient hospitals, and ambulatory surgery centers qualify as office or outpatient settings. CPT provides several E/M categories for office-based and outpatient services.

Table 31-1 ■ KEY CRITERIA FOR ABSTRACTING THE E/M SETTING (CATEGORY)

- ❑ In what setting was the service provided: office or other outpatient, inpatient hospital, or another setting (specify)?
- ❑ Did the service require minimal or no direct patient contact?
- ❑ Is the patient a neonate or child?
- ❑ What type of service was provided: management of a health problem, preventive care, consultation only, or other?
- ❑ If outpatient, is the patient new or established?
- ❑ If inpatient, is the encounter for the admission, continuing care, or discharge?

Source: © PB Resources, Inc. Used with permission.

In addition to encounters for the evaluation or treatment of a health problem, other E/M categories identify preventive care services, consultations, disability evaluations, and life insurance examinations provided in an office setting. The categories for office-based services do not appear next to each other within the E/M section. A description of the most commonly used outpatient E/M categories follows.

Office or Other Outpatient Services (99201-99215). Office or Other Outpatient Services (99201-99215) is the first category that appears in the E/M section, but *not all* office and outpatient services are coded here. The category **99201-99215** identifies services to diagnose or treat health problems and symptoms. The subcategory divisions are based on patient type (new or established). Within each patient type, codes are divided based on the level of service.

Office or Other Outpatient Consultations (99241-99245). A **consultation** is an evaluation of a patient requested by another physician to obtain a professional opinion on a specific problem. The provider who requests the consultation is the **referring physician**. The **consulting physician**, also called the consultant, is the one who receives the request. The consultant can recommend treatment or determine whether to accept the patient for ongoing

E/M Flow Chart

Use this chart to help locate the correct range of codes. Then, refer to the CPT® Tabular List to select and verify codes.
DO NOT code from this chart. Always read CPT code descriptions and category instructions to verify final code.

1. Identify Setting	2. Identify Category/Type of Service	3. Identify Sub-category of Service	4. Verify Code Range	5. Identify Criteria / Key Components (KC)
Office/Outpatient	Office/Outpatient (with presenting problem)	☐ New Patient	99201–99205	3 KC: H/E/MDM
		☐ Established Patient	99211–99215	2 KC: H/E/MDM
	Preventive Medicine	☐ New Patient	99381–99387	Age
		☐ Established Patient	99391–99397	Age
		☐ Individual Counseling/Risk Factor	99401–99404	Time
		☐ Individual, Behavior Change Interventions	99406–99409	Time
		☐ Group Counseling/Risk Factor	99411–99412	Time
		☐ Health Risk Assessment/Other	99420–99429	NA
	Consultation/Office	☐ Office/Outpatient (Non-Medicare)	99241–99245	3 KC: H/E/MDM
	Newborn Care	☐ Not in hospital or birthing center	99461	Setting
	Other Office/Outpatient	☐ Life/Disability Exam	99450	NA
		☐ Work Related/Medical Disability	99455–456	Treating or non-treating
		☐ Post-operative follow-up (bundled)	99024 (located in Medicine section)	
		☐ Anticoagulant Mgmt (Non-Medicare)	99363–99364	Initial/Subsequent
Hospital	Emergency Dept.	☐ Any Patient New/Established	99281–99285	3 KC: H/E/MDM
		☐ EMS direction by MD	99288	NA
	Hospital Observation (for formally admitted)	☐ Initial (New or Estab.)	99218–99220	3 KC: H/E/MDM
		☐ Subsequent (New or Estab.)	99224–99226	2 KC: H/E/MDM
		☐ Observation Discharge	99217	NA
		☐ Same Day Admit/Discharge	99234–99236	3 KC: H/E/MDM
	Hospital Inpatient (admitted)	☐ Initial Hosp Care/Admission	99221–99223	3 KC: H/E/MDM
		☐ Subsequent Hosp Care	99231–99233	2 KC: H/E/MDM
		☐ Hospital Discharge	99238–99239	Time
		☐ Same Day Admit/Discharge	99234–99236	3 KC: H/E/MDM
	Consultation/Inpatient	☐ Initial (New or Estab.)	99251–99255	3 KC: H/E/MDM
	Critical Care (CC) (life threatening condition)	☐ 6 yr and older/Adult	99291–99292	Time
	Intensive Care	☐ Neonatal/Pediatric Critical Care	99468–99482	Age/Status/Service
		☐ Neonatal/Pediatric Intensive Care	99477–99480	Age/Status/Service
		☐ Pediatric CC Transport (<=24 mo.)	99466–99486	Time/Service
	Newborn Care	☐ Normal Newborn	99460–99463	Setting
		☐ Intensive Care	99298–99300	Weight
		☐ Delivery Attendance/Resuscitation	99464–99465	Type of service
Without Direct Patient Contact	Non Face-to-Face Services (Telephone/Internet)	☐ Telephone Services	99441–99443	Time
		☐ Online Medical Evaluation	99444	NA
		☐ Interprofessional Telephone/Internet	99446–99449	Time
	Care Plan Oversight	☐ Domiciliary, Rest Home	99339–99340	Time
		☐ Home Health Agency Patient	99374–99375	Time
		☐ Hospice Patient	99377–99378	Time
		☐ Nursing Facility Patient	99379–99380	Time
	Case Management	☐ Team Conferences	99366–99368	Face to Face/Not
		☐ Transitional Care Management	99495–99496	Complexity/Time frame
	Standby-Physician		99360	Time
	Prolonged Service	☐ No Direct Face to Face Contact	99358–99359	Time
Other Settings	Nursing Facility	☐ Initial (New or Established)	99304–99306	3 KC: H/E/MDM
		☐ Subsequent (New or Established)	99307–99310	2 KC: H/E/MDM
		☐ Discharge	99315–99316	Time
		☐ Annual Assessment	99318	3 KC: H/E/MDM
	Domiciliary/Rest Home	☐ New Patient	99324–99328	3 KC: H/E/MDM
		☐ Established Patient	99334–99337	2 KC: H/E/MDM
	Home Service	☐ New Patient	99341–99345	3 KC: H/E/MDM
		☐ Established Patient	99347–99350	2 KC: H/E/MDM
	Chronic Care Management	☐ Complex Chronic Care Coordination	99487–99489	Time
Any Setting	Prolonged Service	☐ With Direct Face to Face Contact	99354–99357	Time/Report required
	Unlisted service	☐ Other/Unlisted E/M	99499	Report required

6. Evaluate Key Components
(Also refer to the Key Components Tool)

H = History   E = Exam   MDM = Medical Decision Making

For any code using H/E/MDM criteria, use the chart below to select the appropriate level of each criteria.

History	Exam	MDM
☐ Prob Focused	☐ Prob Focused	☐ Straightforward
☐ Exp Prob Focused	☐ Exp Prob Focused	☐ Low complexity
☐ Detailed	☐ Detailed	☐ Mod complexity
☐ Comprehensive	☐ Comprehensive	☐ High complexity

See CPT manual for definition of each of these levels.
2 KC = At least 2 H/E/MDM levels must meet or exceed definition
3 KC = All 3 H/E/MDM levels must meet or exceed definition

7. Evaluate Time Factor Override
Time is a factor in determining an H/E/MDM code ONLY when counseling and coordination of care occupy more than 50% of the face-to-face time.

Face to Face Time	Counseling/Coord Care Time	Couns/Coord More than 50%?
		☐ Yes ☐ No

See CPT code definition for typical time per level of care.

8. Determine if a Modifier is needed
- ☐ -24 Unrelated E/M service by same physician during post-operative period (unrelated to original procedure)
- ☐ -25 Significant, separately identifiable E/M service by same physician on the day (within 24 hr) of a (minor) procedure
- ☐ -32 Mandated services (by 3rd party)
- ☐ -57 Decision for surgery (major) made at time of visit
- ☐ -AI Admitting physician (Medicare inpatients)

See CPT manual Appendix A for full description of modifiers.

9. Determine if Special Circumstances Apply
Services provided:
- ☐ 99050 Outside of normal office hours
- ☐ 99051 During regularly scheduled eve, wkend, or holiday hrs
- ☐ 99053 10pm–8am at 24-hour facility
- ☐ 99056 Patient requests services outside of office
- ☐ 99058 Emergency basis, in office
- ☐ 99060 Emergency basis, out of office

INSTRUCTIONS
1. Identify the general setting in which service was provided.
2. Identify the type of service within the setting rows.
3. Select the subcategory of service within the category rows.
4. Reference the code range provided in the Tabular List.
5. Identify the criteria used to define the level of service and, when applicable, the # of Key Components needed.
6. Summarize the levels of the 3 KC, where applicable. Also refer to the Key Components Evaluation Tool for help.
7. Evaluate if the time factor qualifies to override the 3 KC.
8. Determine if a modifier is needed.
9. Determine if special circumstances apply.

Figure 31-3 ■ E/M Flow Chart. *Source: © PB Resources, Inc. Used with permission.*

management of one or more problems. The consulting physician reports the consultation visit using the appropriate code from **Office or Other Outpatient Consultations (99241-99245)** to identify the level of service. The request for a consultation must be documented in the patient's medical records kept both by the referring physician and the consulting physician. The consultant's findings or opinion must be reported back to the referring physician and also be documented in the patient's medical record(s).

Outpatient consultations include not only those provided in the office, outpatient department, or other ambulatory facility but also those provided to hospital observation patients and those at home, in the emergency department, or in a domiciliary or rest home.

A **transfer of care** occurs when the consulting physician assumes management of a patient's care for one or more problems or conditions. From that point forward, the physician is no longer in a consulting role and reports ongoing services with the appropriate code(s) from **Office or Other Outpatient Services (99201-99215)**. Concurrent care occurs when more than one physician treats a patient at the same time for different conditions or different aspects of the same condition. There is no code or modifier used for concurrent care.

Office or Other Outpatient Consultations (99241-99245) is a subcategory under **Consultations**. Codes are defined based on the level of care provided.

Since 2010, Medicare has not paid for consultation codes. When consultation services are provided for Medicare patients in the office or outpatient setting, report codes for **Office or Other Outpatient Services (99201-99215)** based on the type of patient and level of service provided.

Preventive Medicine Services (99381-99429). Preventive medicine services are general comprehensive checkups performed to maintain health, identify risk factors, and provide appropriate counseling, rather than to manage acute or chronic conditions. Preventive medicine subcategory divisions are based on patient type—new or established. Within each patient type, codes are divided based on the age of the patient.

Laboratory, radiology, and other screening tests can be ordered or administered during a preventive medicine visit. Vaccinations or immunizations can also be given. These services are reported with separate CPT codes, in addition to the E/M code. However, if the only service provided is a screening test or vaccination, report only that service and not an E/M code.

When a new problem is identified, or an existing problem is managed, that requires a substantial workup or evaluation, a code from **Office or Other Outpatient Services (99201-99215)** is reported for the additional work, in addition to the preventive medicine code. Apply modifier **-25** to the second code to identify that two separate E/M services were provided on the same day.

When both a preventive medicine code and a code from **Office or Other Outpatient Services (99201-99215)** are reported on the same day, be sure to assign two ICD-10-CM diagnosis codes. An ICD-10-CM code from **Z00.- Encounter for general examination without complaint, suspected or reported diagnosis** supports the preventive medicine service. (If coding from ICD-9-CM, the comparable category is **V70 General medical examination**.) A code for the condition or problem also must be assigned to support the office or other outpatient services code (■ FIGURE 31-4).

The Preventive Medicine Services category also includes subcategories for counseling and assessments:

- Individual counseling for risk factor reduction (**99401-99404**)
- Individual behavior change treatments related to smoking and alcohol abuse (**99406-99409**)
- Group counseling for risk factor reduction (**99411-99412**)
- Health risk assessment instrument (**99420**)

Other Office and Outpatient Services. Other E/M services provided in the office or outpatient setting are life and disability insurance examinations, postoperative follow-up visits, anticoagulant management, and critical care.

An established patient, age 58, comes in for his annual checkup. The patient complains of recent episodes of right leg numbness, tingling, and muscle weakness. The physician performed an evaluation and management service consisting of a detailed history, a comprehensive neurological examination, and medical decision making of high complexity.

Z00.01 Encounter for general adult medical examination with abnormal findings

99396 Periodic comprehensive preventive medicine reevaluation... established patient; 40–64 years

M54.1 Radiculopathy

99215-25 Office or other outpatient visit for the evaluation and management of an established patient (level 5) -25 Significant, Separately Identifiable Evaluation and Management Service by the Same Physician or Other Qualified Health Care Professional on the Same Day of the Procedure or Other Service

Figure 31-4 ■ Example of Coding Preventive Care and Problem Oriented E/M on Same Day.
Source: © PB Resources, Inc. Used with permission.

Life and Disability Insurance Examinations (99450-99456). Physicians sometimes provide an evaluation service to establish baseline health measurements for patients before a life insurance or disability insurance policy is issued. They also perform periodic examinations of patients who are disabled and covered by either workers' compensation or a medical disability policy. The purpose of the examination is to provide information; no active treatment is provided during the encounter. Three codes are available in the category **Special Evaluation and Management Services (99450-99456)** to report these examinations.

Postoperative Follow-up (99024). Most postoperative follow-up visits are bundled, or included, with the CPT code for the procedure performed as part of the global surgery package. However, sometimes payers require that the encounters be reported. Code **99024 Postoperative follow-up visit, normally included in the surgical package** is used for this purpose. The code carries a charge of $0.00. **99024** does not appear in the E/M section. It appears in the Medicine section, which is the last section in the CPT manual.

Anticoagulant Management (99363-99364). Anticoagulant management is provided for patients on warfarin, commonly known as a blood thinner. Patients must have blood samples drawn frequently for the laboratory test international normalized ratio (INR). The INR helps monitor the concentrations of warfarin in the blood to ensure therapeutic levels. Codes **99363** and **99364** report the physician's services to monitor lab results and make necessary adjustments to the patient's treatment regimen over a 90-day period. These services are provided for patients in the office or outpatient setting, including a domiciliary, rest home, or home. The codes for anticoagulant management appear in the **Case Management** category in the E/M section.

Medicare and some private payers require codes **99211** and **85610 (Prothrombin time)** instead of **99363** and **99364**.

Prolonged Services (99354-99360). The amount of time that physicians spend with patients or coordinating their care varies widely. Most E/M codes are defined based on the level of service provided and include a general estimate of time typically spent by physicians. The actual time spent with or in relationship to a specific patient can vary widely from the estimate and, most of the time, physicians cannot charge higher fees when the estimated time is exceeded. When the amount of time actually spent exceeds more than 30 minutes above and beyond the estimate included in the code, physicians can report the extra time with a code from the category **Prolonged Services (99354-99360).** Prolonged services less than 30 minutes beyond the usual cannot be reported separately.

For example, code **99205** includes a typical face-to-face time of 60 minutes. When the provider spends 75 minutes with the patient, there is no additional payment due for the additional time. However, when the provider spends 91 minutes or longer face to face, then it may be possible to bill for prolonged services and receive additional payment.

Prolonged service codes are add-on codes and can be used with any E/M code in any setting. This category is divided based on whether the prolonged service is direct (face to face with the patient). Codes are defined based on the amount of *excess* time. Direct patient contact codes are further defined based on whether the service was outpatient or inpatient. Refer to the category special instructions for a chart that provides an example of how to report various amounts of time (■ FIGURE 31-5). A report that describes the nature of the prolonged services should be submitted with the claim.

Critical Care Services (Age 6 to Adult) (99291, 99292). Critical care services can be provided in any setting that has the appropriate equipment and supplies. Critical care services are discussed in detail in the section "Inpatient Hospital Evaluation and Management Services" later in the chapter because they are most commonly provided in the inpatient setting. However, the same codes are reported for critical care services, regardless of the setting.

SUCCESS STEP

Especially when first learning about E/M services, it is difficult to memorize and organize all the details. The guidelines and special instructions are there to help you, so do not become frustrated or impatient about reading them.

A 13-year-old new patient is brought in by her mother due to recent symptoms of increased thirst, frequent urination, extreme hunger, and weight loss. The physician performs a comprehensive history, comprehensive examination, and medical decision making of high complexity. The physician diagnoses type 1 diabetes and spends 50 minutes discussing the disease and treatment options with the mother and daughter. A total of 95 minutes (1:35) is spent with the patient.

99205 New patient office visit (level 5)... Typically, 60 minutes are spent face-to-face with the patient and/or family.
(95 minutes – 60 minutes = 35 minutes of prolonged service)
99354 Prolonged service in the office or other outpatient setting requiring direct patient contact beyond the usual service; first hour

Figure 31-5 ■ Example of Coding for Prolonged Services

Outpatient Hospital Evaluation and Management Services

Two types of services occur in a hospital facility but are reported as outpatient services because the patient has not been admitted as an inpatient. These areas are emergency department services and hospital observation services.

Emergency Department Services (99281-99288). An emergency department (ED) is an organized, hospital-based facility that is open 24 hours per day and provides unscheduled services to patients requiring immediate medical attention, such as injury, trauma, or sudden onset of potentially life-threatening symptoms and signs. Urgent care clinics are not emergency departments, even though they may be open 24 hours per day, because they do not provide care for injuries or conditions that threaten life or limb. ED codes are divided based on the level of service provided. Patients treated in the ED are outpatients. They can be discharged, transferred, placed on observation status, or admitted as an inpatient.

When physicians treat patients in the ED then admit them, the ED services are combined with the initial inpatient services provided on the same day. Only one code, from the category **Initial Hospital Care (99221-99223)**, is reported.

Hospital Observation Services (99217-99226). Patients placed on observation status have not been formally admitted to the hospital as inpatients because they do not meet the necessary criteria for hospital admission. However, the physician wants to monitor certain symptoms or complaints that make it unsafe for a patient to be sent home. Some hospitals provide a designated observation unit and others assign observation patients to beds on inpatient units or in the emergency department. Observation status may occur for a few hours or for multiple days, until the physician decides either to admit the patient or discharge them from observation status.

Observation is an outpatient service because patients have not been formally admitted to the hospital, although they occupy hospital beds. The category **Hospital Observation Services (99217-99226)** is divided into subcategories based on patient status (initial or subsequent care) and further divided into codes based on the level of service. Separate codes are provided for **Observation Care Discharge Services (99217)** and for observation patients admitted and discharged on the same date of service (**99234-99236**).

Inpatient Hospital Evaluation and Management Services

The category **Hospital Inpatient Services (99221-99239)** classifies inpatient admission, continuing follow-up visits while an inpatient, and discharges. Visits with consulting physicians and critical care services appear in other categories. The categories for inpatient services do not appear next to each other within the E/M section. A description of the most commonly used inpatient E/M categories follows.

Hospital Inpatient Services (99221-99239). A hospital inpatient is a patient who has been formally admitted to a hospital. Beginning in 2014, Medicare requires that the patient stay span two midnights to qualify for inpatient reimbursement. The requirements of other payers vary. Codes are divided by the type of encounter—initial or subsequent. This category does not distinguish between new and established patients. Apply HCPCS modifier **-AI Principal physician of record** to the code for **Initial hospital care (99221-99223)** when the physician admits a patient during the encounter. The modifier distinguishes the admission encounter from initial inpatient visits by consulting physicians.

Partial Hospitalization Programs. A partial hospitalization program (PHP) is a mental health program, usually provided by a hospital. It consists of an intensive ambulatory treatment service of less than 24-hour daily care, but one that most patients attend daily. Patients do not stay overnight in the hospital unless they are already an inpatient. PHPs can provide a transition from inpatient to outpatient care, shorten an inpatient stay, or eliminate the need for an inpatient admission. CPT does not provide a specific E/M category for PHPs. Although PHP patients may be outpatients if they have not been formally admitted, E/M services provided for patients in a PHP setting are always coded as **Hospital Inpatient Services (99221-99239)**.

Inpatient Consultations (99251-99255). Inpatient consultations follow the same definitions as those for outpatient consultations. Codes in this category are reported for consultations provided to hospital inpatients, residents of nursing facilities, or patients in a PHP. Consulting physicians should report a consultation code only once per admission. Any follow-up or subsequent services provided during the same admission are reported with codes for **Subsequent Hospital Care (99231-99233)** or **Subsequent Nursing Facility Care (99307-99310)**.

Medicare has not paid for consultation codes since 2010. When consultation services are provided for Medicare patients in the inpatient setting, report codes for **Hospital Inpatient Services (99221-99239)** based on the type of patient and level of service provided.

Critical Care Services (Age 6 to Adult) (99291-99292). Critical care is medical treatment provided for an illness or injury that impairs one or more vital organ systems and presents a high probability of imminent or life-threatening deterioration. It involves close, constant attention by a team of specially trained healthcare providers. Critical care often takes place in an intensive care unit or ED but does not have to occur in those locations to use the critical care codes. Critical care services can also be provided in an outpatient setting, such as the emergency department or clinic. Critical care codes report the time spent providing services. Special instructions for this category in the CPT manual specify the services that are included in critical care time and should not be billed in addition to the critical care codes (■ TABLE 31-2, page 530). Any service performed not included in this list should be reported separately.

All time must be one-on-one direct care by the physician but does not have to be continuous. Report the total amount of time spent during the day. When less than 30 minutes is spent

Table 31-2 ■ SERVICES BUNDLED INTO CRITICAL CARE TIME

❑ Interpretation of cardiac output measurements (93561, 93562)

❑ Chest X-rays (71010, 71015, 71020)

❑ Pulse oximetry (94760, 94761, 94762)

❑ Blood gases (94760-94762)

❑ Information data stored in computers (e.g., ECGs, blood pressures, hematologic data [99090])

❑ Gastric intubation (43752, 43753)

❑ Temporary transcutaneous pacing (92953)

❑ Ventilatory management (94002-94004, 94660, 94662)

❑ Vascular access procedures (36000, 36410, 36415, 36591, 36600)

delivering critical care, report the appropriate E/M code, not a critical care code. Count the time spent evaluating, managing, and providing critical care services to a critically ill or injured person. The time to be billed for critical care must be spent at the immediate bedside or elsewhere on the floor as long as the physician is available to the patient. No other patients can be cared for during the time reported for critical care of a specific patient. If the physician departs to care for another patient, the clock stops, then restarts when the physician resumes critical care for the first patient.

To report the time spent on a given date, report code **99291** once for the first 30 to 74 minutes of critical care time. Then, report one unit of code **99292** for *each additional 30 minutes* of care on a given date (■ FIGURE 31-6). The special instructions for codes **99291** and **99292** provide a box that shows how to report various increments of time.

These codes are used for children age 6 and older and adults. Critical care for children younger than 6 years old is reported with neonatal and pediatric intensive care codes. Study the special instructions for reporting the critical care codes carefully to ensure that all services are properly reported.

Newborns. CPT provides specially designated codes for several newborn services, including normal newborn care, intensive care, and delivery attendance or resuscitation. Neonatal critical care is reported with critical care codes.

Normal Newborn Care Services (99460-99463).
Inpatient care for normal newborns is reported with codes **99460** to

99463. Codes are divided by setting—hospital/birthing center and other—and by initial care, subsequent care, and same-day admission and discharge. Discharges occurring after the admission date are reported with the codes for inpatient discharges, **99238** and **99239**.

Delivery/Birthing Room Attendance and Resuscitation Services (99464-99465).
When the physician performing a delivery requests another physician to be present during delivery and assist with stabilization of the newborn, report code **99464**. When a physician provides resuscitation or ventilation services to a newborn, report code **99465**. Read the instructional notes with these codes to identify codes that can and cannot be reported together.

Neonatal Intensive Care and Critical Care, and Pediatric Critical Care (99466-99486).
Neonatal and pediatric critical care codes are used for children younger than 6 years old. The same definition of critical care services for adults applies to neonates and children. However, codes for **Neonatal and Pediatric Critical Care Services (99466-99476, 99481-99482)** report all services provided per day, rather than being time based, as the adult codes are. Codes are divided based on the age of the child and whether the service is initial or subsequent. The special instructions for this category identify the services that are bundled into the critical care codes. Other services should be reported separately.

Intensive care services (**99477-99480**) are provided for newborns and children who are not critically ill but require intensive observation and frequent interventions. Infant and neonates weighing less than 5,000 grams, or about 4½ pounds, often require extended cardiac and respiratory monitoring, frequent vital sign monitoring, heat maintenance, enteral and/or parenteral nutritional adjustments, laboratory and oxygen monitoring, and constant observation by the healthcare team. Review the detailed special instructions that appear in this category to ensure proper coding.

Services Without Direct Patient Contact

A number of E/M services require minimal or no direct contact between the provider and the patient. Brief descriptions of these services include the following.

- **Non-Face-to-Face Services (99441-99443)** report telephone and Internet services that involve telephone contact with the patient but not in-person face-to-face

---

A physician provided 2.5 hours of critical care time on March 15 to a patient in acute respiratory distress.

99291 Critical care, evaluation and management of the critically ill or critically injured patient; first 30–74 minutes

99292 x 3 Critical care, evaluation and management of the critically ill or critically injured patient; each additional 30 minutes

Figure 31-6 ■ Example of Reporting Critical Care Time

contact. Read the special instructions provided in the CPT manual for each of these services. This category includes the following three types of service:

- **Telephone services** initiated by and provided to an established patient, not relating to a service within the past 7 days or next 24 hours (**99441-99443**)

- **Online medical evaluation** initiated by and provided to an established patient, not relating to a service within the past 7 days or next 24 hours (**99444**)

- **Interprofessional telephone/Internet consultations** not requiring face-to-face contact between the patient and consultant (**99446-99449**).

Read the detailed special instructions provided for all three types of services in this category to understand when these codes are appropriate to use.

- **Care Plan Oversight Services (99374-99380)** are reported by the primary supervising provider for patients under the care of home health, hospice, or nursing facilities. The work involves coordinating complex and multidisciplinary services and regular monitoring and updating of care plans. Services also include communication with a patient's family member or caregiver. Codes are divided by setting and time.

- **Case Management Services (99363-99368)** involve coordinating, managing access to, initiating, and supervising a range of healthcare services needed by the patient. Codes identify medical team conferences involving at least three health professionals from three disciplines, each of whom provide direct care to the patient. One person from each discipline may report a case management code. Patients may attend some team conferences, so codes are divided based on whether the patient is present. (The **Case Management Services** category in the CPT manual also includes codes for **Anticoagulant Management (99363-99364)**, which were discussed earlier with office and outpatient services.)

- **Transitional Care Management (TCM) Services (99495-99496)** are provided for assisting complex patients in making a transition from an inpatient setting to the patient's community setting, whether it is the patient's private residence or an assisted living or rest home type of facility. TCM consists of one face-to-face encounter with the patient, as well as a broad range of non-face-to-face services. Codes are divided based on complexity and when the face-to-face patient visit occurs. Read the special instructions carefully to understand how to report codes in this category.

- **Prolonged Service Without Direct Patient Contact (99358, 99359)** codes are reported for service above and beyond the normal E/M time, not involving direct patient contact. Codes are based on the total amount of time spent per day. Refer to the category special instructions for a chart that provides an example of how to report various amounts of time. A report that describes the nature of the prolonged services should be submitted with the claim.

Other Settings of Evaluation and Management Services

Other settings in which E/M services are provided include the following.

- **Nursing Facility Services (99304-99318)** codes are reported for E/M services provided in a **nursing facility** (NF), formerly known as a skilled nursing facility (SNF), intermediate care facility (ICF), or long-term care facility (LTCF). These are residential facilities that provide professional medical and nursing care. Codes are divided by type of encounter (initial or subsequent encounter) and the level of service provided by the physician during an E/M encounter. This category does not distinguish between new and established patients.

- **Domiciliary, Rest Home, Custodial (99324-99337; 99339-99340)** codes are reported for E/M services provided in custodial care settings such as a domiciliary, rest home, or assisted living facility. These facilities provide limited assistance with activities of daily living (ADLs) but do not provide professional medical or nursing care. Codes are divided by patient type (new or established) and the level of service provided by the physician during an E/M encounter.

- **Home Services (99341-99350)** codes are reported for E/M services provided in the patient's private residence. Codes are divided by patient type (new or established) and the level of service provided.

- **Complex Chronic Care Coordination Evaluation and Management Services (99487-99489)** codes are reported for patient-centered management and support services provided to an individual who resides at home or in a domiciliary, rest home, or assisted living facility. These services address the coordination of care by multiple disciplines and community service agencies. The codes are reported by the provider who oversees the management of services for all medical conditions, psychosocial needs, and activities of daily living. Codes are divided based on time spent during a calendar month. Be sure to read the detailed special instructions for this category in the CPT manual.

- **Other Evaluation and Management Services (99499)** codes are reported only when no other E/M code adequately describes the service provided. This is a code for an unlisted procedure and should be accompanied by a detailed report that describes the services provided.

CODING CAUTION

When billing E/M services on the CMS-1500 form or 837P electronic claim, each CPT code must be associated with a two-digit place of service (POS) identifier, entered in Item 24B. The POS identifier must be consistent with the setting of the E/M code for the claim to be processed. For example, you cannot submit a claim for E/M code **99221** (initial hospital services) with POS 11 Office. POS codes are listed in the front of most CPT manuals.

CODING PRACTICE

Exercise 31.2 Abstracting the Setting

Instructions: Name the E/M setting for each of the following scenarios. Choose from:

A. Office or other outpatient

B. Inpatient

C. Services without direct patient contact

D. Other settings

1. _____ After being seen in the emergency department, a patient is admitted to the hospital.

2. _____ A mother brings her child to an urgent care clinic.

3. _____ A physician assists with a delivery in a hospital birthing room.

4. _____ A physician provides care plan oversight services for a patient in a nursing facility.

5. _____ A patient is seen in the emergency department after an automobile accident.

6. _____ A physician provides evaluation and management services to a patient in an assisted living facility.

7. _____ A patient residing at home received physician services for complex chronic care coordination.

8. _____ A patient complaining of chest pain is kept overnight in the hospital for observation.

9. _____ A patient attends a partial hospitalization program 12 hours a day and returns home at night.

10. _____ A patient preparing to move home after a three-week stay in a rehabilitation center receives transitional care management services.

Abstracting the Patient Type

Four E/M categories divide codes based on patient type or status, which means whether the patient is new or established:

- Office or Other Outpatient Services
- Preventive Medicine Services
- Domiciliary, Rest Home, or Custodial Care Services
- Home Services

CPT provides specific definitions for new and established patients. An **established patient (EP)** is one who has received professional services from the same physician, or another physician in the group of the same specialty and subspecialty, within the previous three years (■ TABLE 31-3). All other patients are **new patients (NPs)**, who have not previously received services from a particular physician or group of physicians in the same specialty or subspecialty. Because each specialty and subspecialty has differing assessments and examinations, and because new patients require a more extensive workup than established patients, new patient E/M services are reported with separate CPT codes than established patients.

To understand the definition of an established patient, you must understand the meaning of a medical group, a medical specialty, and a subspecialty.

- A medical group is a business organization, such as a corporation or partnership, in which physicians share certain resources, such as space and staff. Revenue may be shared or may be allocated to individual physicians.

- A medical specialty is an area of study within medicine pertaining to a specific body system (cardiology), class of procedures (thoracic surgery), or patient characteristics (pediatrics).

- A subspecialty is a narrower aspect of a specialty that requires additional training, such as interventional cardiology, congenital cardiac surgery, or adolescent medicine. Not all physicians have a subspecialty.

When patients are seen by the same physician within the past three years, they are established patients. If the physician has moved from one practice to another, the patient is still established with that physician if seen within three years.

When patients cannot see the same physician as before, they may accept an appointment with another physician in the same group. If the new physician is of the same specialty and subspecialty as the previous physician, then the patient is still established, as long as it has been three years or less.

However, if the specialty is different from the previous physician, the patient is new for CPT coding purposes. If the specialty is the same as that of the previous physician but the subspecialty is different, the patient is new for CPT coding

Table 31-3 ■ KEY CRITERIA FOR ABSTRACTING ESTABLISHED PATIENT TYPE

❑ Has the patient seen the same physician within the past three years? (*If No, then the next three questions must be answered Yes to qualify as an established patient.*)

❑ Did the patient see a physician of the exact same specialty as a previous physician in the same group?

❑ If previous physician was a subspecialist, did the patient see a physician of the exact same subspecialty as the previous physician in the same group?

❑ Does the visit with the same specialist or subspecialist occur within three years of the previous visit?

Source: © PB Resources, Inc. Used with permission.

purposes. The "Evaluation and Management (E/M) Services Guidelines" section in the CPT manual provides a decision tree to assist in distinguishing new and established patients.

Some E/M categories do not distinguish between new and established patient types because other criteria are more important in defining the services provided. Patient age is used to divide categories for preventive care and certain services provided to newborns and children. Frequency, such as initial care, subsequent care, or discharge, is used for certain inpatient services. Coders must be attentive to the CPT special instructions for each category of E/M service to fully understand the basis on which categories and subcategories are defined.

CODING CAUTION

The E/M categories Inpatient Hospital Services, Hospital Observation Services, and Nursing Facility Services divide codes based on whether the encounter is initial or subsequent. **Initial encounter** refers to the first encounter by the admitting physician during the current admission. **Subsequent encounter** refers to the second or later encounter by the admitting provider during the current admission and to all encounters by other than the admitting physician. CPT definitions for initial and subsequent encounters differ from those used by ICD-10-CM.

CODING PRACTICE

Exercise 31.3   Abstracting Patient Type

Instructions: Identify whether each patient is new or established. Circle the correct answer.

1. A child is seen by a pediatric cardiologist, to whom he was referred by his regular pediatrician at the same clinic. New Established

2. A patient returns to Branton Family Practice to see her internal medicine physician, whom she last saw two years ago. New Established

3. A mother brings her newborn daughter to the same pediatrician who has cared for the older siblings for three years. New Established

4. A patient is evaluated by a thoracic surgeon prior to undergoing a coronary artery bypass graft, recommended by a cardiologist at the same clinic. New Established

5. A patient comes to Branton Family Practice for the first time to see her primary care physician, whom she last saw one year ago at another clinic. New Established

6. A patient sees a gastroenterologist for the first time at the same clinic where he goes twice a year because his previous gastroenterologist retired. New Established

7. A patient sees a general surgeon for evaluation for a hernia repair. The same surgeon repaired another hernia four years ago. New Established

8. A woman who just learned, as the result of a home pregnancy test, that she might be pregnant sees her obstetrician, who delivered her first child two years ago. New Established

9. A patient sees his regular dermatologist for evaluation and treatment of a new skin rash that he has never experienced before. New Established

10. A patient who has been out of the country for three years returns to the clinic to see the same physician who cared for her before she went abroad. She brings with her the medical records that cover the time she was away. New Established

Abstracting the Level of Service

Eight E/M categories define the level, or complexity, of service provided based on a set of three **key components (KCs)**. (■ TABLE 31-4). The key components are the history, the examination, and the medical decision making, each of which can be performed at varying levels of complexity. The combinations of the three key components define three to five levels of service within each category. Criteria that include the three key components also include three contributory factors and time. Levels of service cannot be interchanged or substituted across E/M categories. For example, the criteria for the five levels of service for a new patient office visit cannot be interchanged with the criteria for the five levels of service for an established patient office visit because the key components are combined in different ways.

Table 31-4 ■ **E/M CATEGORIES THAT USE KEY COMPONENTS**

❑ Consultation Services

❑ Domiciliary, Rest Home (e.g., Boarding Home), or Custodial Care Services

❑ Emergency Department Services

❑ Home Services

❑ Hospital Inpatient Services

❑ Hospital Observation Services

❑ Nursing Facility Services

❑ Office or Other Outpatient Services

Key components also are referred to as **content of service requirements** because they define the work done during the encounter, in contrast to codes based on time, patient age, or other elements.

Three Key Components

The three key components are the extent of the patient's history gathered by the physician, the extent of the physical examination, and the complexity of medical decision making. Each key component is divided into four levels, each of which describes the complexity of the service provided (■ TABLE 31-5).

History. History refers to the discussion between the patient and physician regarding several areas that could provide information regarding the patient's medical situation. The history is subjective because it is based on what the patient tells the physician. It includes the **chief complaint (CC)**, a **history of present illness (HPI)**, a **review of systems (ROS)**, and the patient's **past, family, and social history (PFSH)**. Each of these elements (except for the CC) also is assigned a level of complexity based on the amount of information gathered.

Examination. The physical examination is objective because it is based on the physician's examination of the patient. The type of examination is determined by the patient's chief complaint and the amount of information the physician needs to collect to make a diagnosis and formulate a treatment plan. The physician can perform a general multisystem examination or an organ-specific examination. The examination can include up to 7 defined body areas and 12 organ systems.

A general multisystem examination or a single organ system examination may be performed by any physician, regardless of specialty. The type (general multisystem or single organ system) and content of the examination are selected by the examining physician and are based on clinical judgment, the patient's history, and the nature of the presenting problem(s). The 1997 DG present a bulleted list of elements in each body system that potentially can be examined for the general multisystem

Table 31-5 ■ SUMMARY OF KEY COMPONENTS AND CONTRIBUTORY FACTORS

Three Key Components	
History levels: • Problem focused • Expanded problem focused • Detailed • Comprehensive	Subjective information that the patient provides, including four elements: 1. Chief complaint (CC) 2. History of present illness (HPI) 3. Review of systems (ROS) 4. Past, family, and/or social history (PFSH)
Examination levels: • Problem focused • Expanded problem focused • Detailed • Comprehensive	Objective information that the physician identifies during the examination of specific body areas and/or organ systems
Medical decision making levels: • Straightforward • Low • Moderate • High	The physician renders a diagnosis and makes recommendations for treatment. Medical decision making includes reviewing and analyzing three elements: • Number of possible diagnoses and/or number of management options • Amount and/or complexity of medical records, diagnostic tests, and/or other information • Risk of significant complications, morbidity and/or mortality, and comorbidities
Three Contributory Factors	
Counseling	The physician provides counseling to a patient and/or family members regarding the patient's diagnosis, treatment, and follow-up.
Coordination of care	The physician coordinates the patient's care with other healthcare providers or agencies.
Nature of presenting problem	A symptom, complaint, condition, illness, disease, sign, finding, or injury that represents the reason for the patient's encounter.
Time	
Intraservice (face-to-face) time	Face-to-face time the physician spends with the patient for office or other outpatient services, and unit/floor time for hospital and other inpatient services.

examination. The number of body areas and/or organ systems examined, and the total number of bulleted items examined, determine the level of the examination.

The 1997 DG also define 11 single-organ examinations and provide a bulleted list of elements that potentially can be examined in each organ system. The number of bulleted items actually examined and documented determines the level of the examination. These criteria may vary among organ systems.

Medical Decision Making. Medical decision making refers to the complexity of establishing a diagnosis and/or selecting a management option as measured by:

- the number of possible diagnoses and/or the number of management options that must be considered;

- the amount and/or complexity of medical records, diagnostic tests, or other information that must be obtained, reviewed, and analyzed; and

- the risk of significant complications, morbidity, or mortality, as well as comorbidities associated with the patient's presenting problem(s), the diagnostic procedure(s), and the possible management options.

The number of elements required in each of these areas determines the level of complexity of the medical decision making for a specific encounter (■ FIGURE 31-7).

Contributory Factors. In addition to the key components, E/M services have three contributory factors that are important, but not all are required at every encounter. These are counseling, coordination of care, and the nature of the presenting problem.

Counseling is the time spent with the patient and family discussing management options. Coordination of care is the time spent arranging for referrals to other provider or facilities for tests and treatments. The nature of the presenting problem is the disease, condition, or other reason for the encounter. Every encounter has a presenting problem, but not every encounter requires counseling and coordination of care. All services provided during an encounter must be medically necessary based on the nature of the presenting problem.

Table 31-6 ■ KEY CRITERIA FOR ABSTRACTING THE LEVEL OF SERVICE

❑ What are the criteria for determining the level of service: 2/3 key components, 3/3 key components, time, or other (specify)? (*You first must identify the preliminary E/M category to answer this question.*)

- What level of history was taken by the provider?
- What level of examination was performed?
- What was the complexity of medical decision making?
- How much time was spent in counseling and coordination of care?

❑ What is the age of the patient?

❑ How much time was spent providing the service?

Source: © PB Resources, Inc. Used with permission.

Time. Most E/M codes based on the three key components also provide the typical amount of time spent face to face with the patient and/or family for that level of service. Normally, codes are selected based on the levels of the three key components, not the time spent. When the actual time spent exceeds the typical time stated in the E/M code, a higher-level code cannot be selected, with one exception.

When the time spent in counseling and coordination of care exceeds 50% of total face-to-face time spent during the encounter, then time is the controlling factor to qualify for a particular level of E/M service. In this situation, a higher level of E/M code can be assigned, even if the three key components are not met. To do this, the nature of the counseling and coordination of care, and the time spent, must be thoroughly documented. The total face-to-face time must also be documented so the coder can determine whether the counseling and coordination of care comprised more than 50% of the total time.

Other Level of Service Criteria

E/M categories that do not use the three key components to establish the level of service define code levels in other ways, such as the amount of time spent by the physician or the patient's age. Coders must read the code descriptions and category special instructions to learn the criteria used to define code levels. Refer to ■ TABLE 31-6 for a guide in abstracting the level of service.

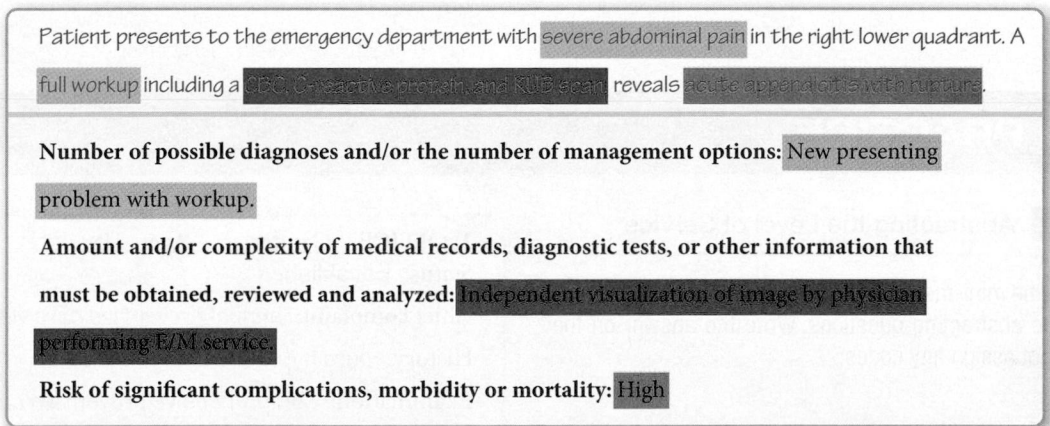

Patient presents to the emergency department with severe abdominal pain in the right lower quadrant. A full workup including a CBC, C-reactive protein and KUB scan reveals acute appendicitis with rupture.

Number of possible diagnoses and/or the number of management options: New presenting problem with workup.

Amount and/or complexity of medical records, diagnostic tests, or other information that must be obtained, reviewed and analyzed: Independent visualization of image by physician performing E/M service.

Risk of significant complications, morbidity or mortality: High

Figure 31-7 ■ Example of High Complexity of Medical Decision Making

When time is a criterion for selecting codes, the code descriptions provide the range of time applicable for each code, not an exact length of time. Depending on the code, time ranges can be expressed in minutes, hours, or even days. When a time range is provided, such as 31–60 minutes, no further coding or modifiers are required to define the specific number of minutes, such as 47 minutes.

When age is a criterion for selecting codes, the code descriptions provide an age range applicable for each code, not one code for each age. Age may be expressed in days, months, or years.

Other criteria that are sometimes used for final code selection are the setting, whether the patient is present, the specific services provided, and other details unique to a particular group of codes. Coders must read the code descriptions and identify the differences between similar codes to determine the exact criteria needed.

This provides a general overview of the criteria for E/M coding. Additional details can be found in the E/M section guidelines in the CPT manual and professional reference resources.

Guided Example of Abstracting E/M Services

Refer to the following example throughout this chapter to practice skills for abstracting and assigning E/M codes.

> OFFICE   Gender: F   Age: 32   Status: Established
>
> Chief complaint: sinus pressure, sore throat, cough
>
> History: Detailed. Extended HPI, extended ROS, pertinent PFSH. Patient was last seen by me 6 months ago for annual preventive exam.
>
> Examination: Expanded problem-focused general multisystem exam
>
> Medical decision making: Moderate complexity. New presenting problem, without workup. Sinus infection. Rx antibiotics.

Follow along as Scott Hood, CPC, abstracts the procedure. Check off each step after you complete it.

▶ Scott reads through the entire record, paying special attention to the chief complaint: sinus pressure, sore throat, cough.

▶ Scott refers to the Key Criteria for Abstracting the E/M Setting (Category) (Table 31-1).

❑ *In what setting was the service provided: office or outpatient, inpatient hospital, or another setting?* Office

❑ *What type of service was provided: management of a health problem, preventive care, consultation only, or other?* Health problem: sinus pressure, sore throat, cough

❑ *If outpatient, is the patient new or established?* Established

▶ Scott refers to Key Criteria for Abstracting Established Patient Type (Table 31-3) to confirm the patient type.

❑ *Has the patient seen the same physician within the past three years?* Yes. Patient was last seen by me 6 months ago for annual preventive exam. The patient is established because she has been seen by the same physician within the past three years.

▶ Scott refers to Key Criteria for Abstracting the Level of Service (Table 31-6) to determine the level of service.

❑ *What are the criteria for determining the level of service for code selection: 3 key components, time, or other?* 3 key components

❑ *What level of history was taken by the provider?* Detailed

❑ *What level of examination was performed?* Expanded problem-focused general multisystem exam

❑ *What was the complexity of medical decision making?* Moderate complexity

❑ *How much time was spent in counseling and coordination of care?* This information was not documented.

❑ *What is the age of the patient?* 32. Age is not a factor for this type of E/M service.

❑ *How much time was spent providing the service?* This information was not documented.

▶ Scott has abstracted the information needed. Next he needs to assign the E/M code.

CODING PRACTICE

Exercise 31.4   Abstracting the Level of Service

Instructions: Read the mini-medical-record of each patient's encounter and answer the abstracting questions. Write the answer on the line provided. Do not assign any codes.

> 1. OFFICE   Gender: F   Age: 48
> Status: Established
>
> Chief complaint: annual preventive care visit
>
> History: pure hypercholesterolemia
>
> Examination: comprehensive preventive care exam
>
> *(continued)*

1. (continued)

Medical decision making: *Cholesterol seems to be well controlled. No new problems.*

a. In what setting was the service provided: office or outpatient, inpatient hospital, or another setting (specify)? _____

b. What type of service was provided: management of a health problem, preventive care, consultation only, or other? _____

c. Is the patient new or established? _____

d. What code range is applicable for this type of encounter? _____

   What is the title of the subcategory? _____

e. What new problems were identified or managed? _____

f. What criteria are used to determine the level of service? _____

g. What patient information meets these criteria?

2. INPATIENT HOSPITAL   Gender: M   Age: 25

Chief complaint: *patient admitted by me for hematuria, severe pain in lower pelvic region*

History: *Detailed. Extended HPI, extended ROS, pertinent PFSH*

Examination: *comprehensive GU exam*

Medical decision making: *moderate complexity*

a. In what setting was the service provided: office or outpatient, inpatient hospital, or another setting? _____

b. What type of service was provided: management of a health problem, preventive care, consultation only, or other? _____

c. Is the encounter initial or subsequent? _____

d. What code range is applicable for this type of encounter? _____

   What is the title of the subcategory? _____

e. What criteria are used to determine the level of service? _____

f. What level of history was taken by the provider? _____

g. What level of examination was performed? _____

h. What was the complexity of medical decision making? _____

i. How much time was spent in counseling and coordination of care? _____

3. OFFICE   Gender: M   Age: 48   Status: New

Chief complaint: *patient was referred to me (endocrinologist) by his primary care physician for diabetes management. Refer to dietician.*

History: *comprehensive; diabetes is secondary to chronic pancreatitis*

Examination: *comprehensive general multisystem examination*

Medical decision making: *High complexity. Spent 25 minutes of this 60-minute encounter counseling patient on diet management and other lifestyle changes needed to prevent serious diabetic complications.*

a. In what setting was the service provided: office or outpatient, inpatient hospital, or another setting? _____

b. What type of service was provided: management of a health problem, preventive care, consultation only, or other? _____

c. Is the patient new or established? _____

d. What code range is applicable for this type of encounter? _____
   What is the title of the subcategory? _____

e. What criteria are used to determine the level of service? _____

f. What level of history was taken by the provider? _____

g. What level of examination was performed? _____

h. What was the complexity of medical decision making? _____

i. How much time was spent in counseling and coordination of care? _____

j. How much face to face time was spent with the patient? _____

4. OFFICE   Gender: F   Age: 61   Status: Established

Chief complaint: *cough and congestion*

History: *Expanded problem focused. Brief HPI, extended ROS, pertinent past history.*

Examination: *detailed respiratory exam*

Medical decision making: *Moderate complexity. Chest X-ray negative for pneumonia. Rx antibiotics for acute bronchitis.*

(*continued*)

the key component levels in the medical record do not exactly match those described in the code. When codes require 2/3 components, then one component can be lower than the one listed in the code, but two must meet or exceed the code. When codes require 3/3 components, then all three components must meet or exceed the levels listed in the code description.

- When a key component level in the medical record is *lower* than the one listed in the code, you must use the lower-level code.

- When a key component level in the medical record is *higher* than the one listed in the code, you cannot use the higher code unless the required number of criteria (2/3 or 3/3) match.

The Key Component Tool in ■ FIGURE 31-10 helps you match the medical record to the CPT codes for office and inpatient hospital services. Use the tool as follows:

1. In the top left-hand box labeled Patient Summary, circle the level of each criteria in your patient case. Circle OP (outpatient) or IP (inpatient). If outpatient, circle New or Established. If inpatient, circle Initial or Subsequent.

2. Locate the corresponding grids for office services (blue) on the top half of the page or inpatient services (red) on the bottom half of the page.

3. Locate the grid for a new patient/initial service (green) or established patient/subsequent service (purple) in the appropriate quadrant.

4. Compare the boxes circled on the patient summary grid with those on the grid in the appropriate quadrant of the tool. Be mindful of whether you must match 3/3 (new patient) or 2/3 (established patient) components.

5. Select the code and verify it in the Tabular List.

Also evaluate the contributory factors—counseling, coordination of care, and the nature of the presenting problem. For outpatient services, compare the total face-to-face time with the typical time stated in the code description for which you matched the key components. For inpatient services, compare the time spent on the unit or floor with the typical time stated in the code description for which you matched the key components. When the time spent in counseling and coordination of care exceeds 50% of the face-to-face or unit/floor time, you can select the code that matches the amount of face-to-face time spent (■ FIGURE 31-11, page 542).

SUCCESS STEP

Some editions of the CPT manual provide *Evaluation and Management Tables* in the Introduction section. The tables summarize the key components required for the major categories of E/M services and provide a handy reference after you become familiar with E/M coding.

Determine Whether Modifiers Are Needed

Five modifiers are used on E/M codes to alert payers that an E/M service is payable because of unique circumstances, although normally it would not be payable. Three of these circumstances relate to surgery. Recall that the global surgical package includes

a related E/M service on the day of, or day before, a surgical procedure. It also includes related E/M services during the postoperative period of 10 or 90 days for surgical follow-up. Under normal circumstances, an E/M service reported immediately before a procedure within the postoperative period would be denied by the payer. However, there are circumstances when patients receive E/M services unrelated to the surgical procedure and the physician should be paid. Each of these situations can be explained by using the appropriate modifier.

Modifier -24

The description of modifier **-24** is **Unrelated E/M service by same physician or other qualified health care professional during post-operative period (unrelated to original procedure)**. This modifier identifies that an E/M service *unrelated* to a surgical procedure was provided during a postoperative period by the *same provider* who performed the procedure. Add modifier **-24** to the E/M code and be sure to assign a diagnosis code that identifies the reason for the encounter (■ FIGURE 31-12, page 542). When the E/M service is provided by a different physician than the one who performed the surgery, a modifier is not necessary because that physician is not being paid for postoperative care.

CODING CAUTION

E/M modifiers are subject to the same concept of the *same provider* as is used to distinguish new and established patients. Same provider means the provider who performed the original service, or another physician in the same group practice who has the exact same specialty and subspecialty as the physician who performed the original service. When this is the case, the second provider should use modifiers **-24** and **-25** in the same way as if the patient had seen the original provider.

Modifier -25

The description of modifier **-25** is **Significant, separately identifiable evaluation and management service by the same physician or other qualified health care professional on the same day of the procedure or other service**. A preoperative E/M service is part of the surgical package for all major procedures and most minor procedures. When another E/M service is provided on the same day, by the same physician, for a reason unrelated to the procedure, add modifier **-25** to the E/M code. This alerts the payer that the E/M service is not part of the surgical package and should be paid. Also assign a diagnosis code to identify the reason for the E/M service and link it to the E/M code on the CMS-1500 form or the 837P electronic claim.

Modifier -57

The description of modifier **-57** is **Decision for surgery**. The E/M encounter in which the decision for surgery is made is payable separate from the surgical package. The global surgical package includes one preoperative encounter *after the decision for surgery is made* and the day of or the day before the procedure. When the decision for surgery is made within a day of performing the procedure, add modifier **-57** to the E/M code

KEY COMPONENTS TOOL

PATIENT SUMMARY:	OutPt New Estab /	InPt Initial	Subsequent
History	Problem Focused	Expanded Problem Focused	Detailed	Comprehensive
Exam	Problem Focused	Expanded Problem Focused	Detailed	Comprehensive
MDM	Straight forward	Low Complex	Moder. Complex	High Complex

Instructions: 1. Circle the patient type on the Patient Summary (Outpatient-New or Established/Inpatient-Initial or Subsequent)
2. Circle the level of each Key Component on the Pt Summary (**one** item per line).
3. Locate the corresponding Office or Inpatient chart for patient type and levels.
4. Verify that patient levels for Key Components on the Patient Summary meet <u>or exceed</u> those shown in the Office or Inpatient chart for the code selected.

Do NOT code from this tool. Always read CPT® code descriptions and category instructions before selecting final code.

Office or Outpatient (99201–99205)
New patient

99201	Required Components:		3/3
History	Problem Focused	Expanded Problem Focused	Detailed	Comprehensive
Exam	Problem Focused	Expanded Problem Focused	Detailed	Comprehensive
MDM	Straight forward	Low Complex	Moderate Complex	High Complex

99202	Required Components:		3/3
History	Problem Focused	Expanded Problem Focused	Detailed	Comprehensive
Exam	Problem Focused	Expanded Problem Focused	Detailed	Comprehensive
MDM	Straightforward	Low Complex	Moderate Complex	High Complex

99203	Required Components:		3/3
History	Problem Focused	Expanded Problem Focused	Detailed	Comprehensive
Exam	Problem Focused	Expanded Problem Focused	Detailed	Comprehensive
MDM	Straightforward	Low Complex	Moderate Complex	High Complex

99204	Required Components:		3/3
History	Problem Focused	Expanded Problem Focused	Detailed	Comprehensive
Exam	Problem Focused	Expanded Problem Focused	Detailed	Comprehensive
MDM	Straightforward	Low Complex	Moderate Complex	High Complex

99205	Required Components:		3/3
History	Problem Focused	Expanded Problem Focused	Detailed	Comprehensive
Exam	Problem Focused	Expanded Problem Focused	Detailed	Comprehensive
MDM	Straightforward	Low Complex	Moderate Complex	High Complex

Office or Outpatient (99211–99215)
Established patient

99211	Required Components:		NA
History	Minimal presenting problem may not require the presence of a physician. Typically, 5 minutes are spent performing or supervising these services.		
Exam			
MDM			

99212	Required Components:		2/3
History	Problem Focused	Expanded Problem Focused	Detailed	Comprehensive
Exam	Problem Focused	Expanded Problem Focused	Detailed	Comprehensive
MDM	Straightforward	Low Complex	Moderate Complex	High Complex

99213	Required Components:		2/3
History	Problem Focused	Expanded Problem Focused	Detailed	Comprehensive
Exam	Problem Focused	Expanded Problem Focused	Detailed	Comprehensive
MDM	Straightforward	Low Complex	Moderate Complex	High Complex

99214	Required Components:		2/3
History	Problem Focused	Expanded Problem Focused	Detailed	Comprehensive
Exam	Problem Focused	Expanded Problem Focused	Detailed	Comprehensive
MDM	Straightforward	Low Complex	Moderate Complex	High Complex

99215	Required Components:		2/3
History	Problem Focused	Expanded Problem Focused	Detailed	Comprehensive
Exam	Problem Focused	Expanded Problem Focused	Detailed	Comprehensive
MDM	Straightforward	Low Complex	Moderate Complex	High Complex

Inpatient Hospital (99221–99223)
Initial hospital care

99221	Required Components:		3/3
History	Problem Focused	Expanded Problem Focused	Detailed	Comprehensive
Exam	Problem Focused	Expanded Problem Focused	Detailed	Comprehensive
MDM	Straightforward	Low Complex	Moderate Complex	High Complex

99222	Required Components:		3/3
History	Problem Focused	Expanded Problem Focused	Detailed	Comprehensive
Exam	Problem Focused	Expanded Problem Focused	Detailed	Comprehensive
MDM	Straightforward	Low Complex	Moderate Complex	High Complex

99223	Required Components:		3/3
History	Problem Focused	Expanded Problem Focused	Detailed	Comprehensive
Exam	Problem Focused	Expanded Problem Focused	Detailed	Comprehensive
MDM	Straightforward	Low Complex	Moderate Complex	High Complex

Inpatient Hospital (99231–99233)
Subsequent hospital care

99231	Required Components:		2/3
History	Problem Focused	Expanded Problem Focused	Detailed	Comprehensive
Exam	Problem Focused	Expanded Problem Focused	Detailed	Comprehensive
MDM	Straightforward	Low Complex	Moderate Complex	High Complex

99232	Required Components:		2/3
History	Problem Focused	Expanded Problem Focused	Detailed	Comprehensive
Exam	Problem Focused	Expanded Problem Focused	Detailed	Comprehensive
MDM	Straightforward	Low Complex	Moderate Complex	High Complex

99233	Required Components:		2/3
History	Problem Focused	Expanded Problem Focused	Detailed	Comprehensive
Exam	Problem Focused	Expanded Problem Focused	Detailed	Comprehensive
MDM	Straightforward	Low Complex	Moderate Complex	High Complex

Always read CPT code descriptions and category instructions before selecting final code.

© PB Resources, Inc. CPT©American Medical Assn.

Figure 31-10 ■ Key Component Tool. *Source: © PB Resources, Inc. Used with permission.*

An established patient with type 2 diabetes is referred to an endocrinologist due to poor management of the condition. The endocrinologist performs a comprehensive history, comprehensive examination, and medical decision making of moderate complexity. He spends 45 minutes counseling the patient regarding diet and lifestyle management and reviews the potential risks if the diabetes is not brought under control. Total face to face time is 80 minutes.

99245 Office consultation for a new or established patient (level 5)
    .... Typically, 80 minutes are spent face-to-face with the patient and/or family.

The three key components qualify for code 99244 (comprehensive history; comprehensive examination; and medical decision making of moderate complexity), which has a typical face to face time of 60 minutes. Because more than half of the visit was spent in counseling and coordination of care, the code can be upgraded to 99245.

Figure 31-11 ■ Example of Coding for Time as the Controlling Factor

to inform the payer that the encounter was not a bundled preoperative visit but, rather, the initial decision for surgery. When the decision for surgery is made several days or weeks before the procedure is performed, modifier **-57** is not required. Payers can vary in how they want modifier **-57** to be used, so it is a good idea to check the policies of individual payers.

Modifier -32

The description of modifier **-32** is **Mandated services**. When an E/M service is required by a payer, court, or other third party, use modifier **-32** to alert the payer that it should be paid, when otherwise it might not. An E/M service can be mandated when a second surgical opinion or second medical evaluation is required. You may also need to submit the letter or order form from the mandating party to document who requested the service and the reason.

Modifier -AI

The description of modifier **-AI** is **Principal physician of record**. This is a HCPCS modifier required by Medicare when a

physician admits a patient to the hospital. Admitting physicians report a code from **Initial Hospital Services (99231-99233)** for the initial history and physical when they admit a patient (■ FIGURE 31-13). Consulting physicians also use these codes for an initial consultation encounter with a Medicare patient because Medicare stopped paying for inpatient consultation codes in 2010. Modifier **-AI** identifies the admitting physician and differentiates her or him from a consulting physician, who does not use a modifier.

Determine Whether Special Circumstances Apply

CPT provides codes for special circumstances for use when services are provided at unusual times (**99050-99060**) (■ FIGURE 31-14). Although the codes begin with **99**, they do not appear in the E/M section. They appear in the Medicine section at the end of the CPT Tabular List. These can be used as additional codes with E/M services, as appropriate. Medicare does not pay an additional amount for these codes, but some payers do.

Patient sees the general surgeon regarding treatment for chronic bleeding peptic ulcers. 30 days ago the same surgeon performed a laparoscopic cholecystectomy (90 day postoperative period).

K27.4 Chronic or unspecified peptic ulcer, site unspecified, with hemorrhage
99213-24 Office and other outpatient visit, established patient (level 3);
    -24 Unrelated E/M service by same physician or other qualified health care professional during post-operative period (unrelated to original procedure)

Figure 31-12 ■ Example of Modifier -24

A Medicare patient was seen in the emergency department for a fractured left hip. The same physician admitted the patient. The combined services in the ED and for the admission involved a comprehensive history, a comprehensive examination, and medical decision making of high complexity.

99223-AI Initial hospital care, per day (level 3);
    -AI Principal physician of record.

Figure 31-13 ■ Example of Coding a Hospital Admission

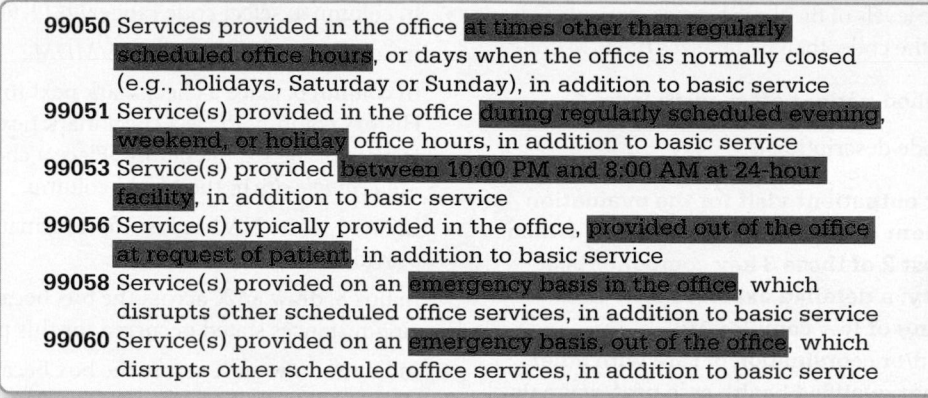

99050 Services provided in the office at times other than regularly scheduled office hours, or days when the office is normally closed (e.g., holidays, Saturday or Sunday), in addition to basic service

99051 Service(s) provided in the office during regularly scheduled evening, weekend, or holiday office hours, in addition to basic service

99053 Service(s) provided between 10:00 PM and 8:00 AM at 24-hour facility, in addition to basic service

99056 Service(s) typically provided in the office, provided out of the office at request of patient, in addition to basic service

99058 Service(s) provided on an emergency basis in the office, which disrupts other scheduled office services, in addition to basic service

99060 Service(s) provided on an emergency basis, out of the office, which disrupts other scheduled office services, in addition to basic service

Figure 31-14 ■ CPT Codes that Identify Special Circumstances

Arranging E/M Codes

Typically, an E/M code is listed first on a claim, then codes for other services are sequenced in descending price order. Some payers request that the E/M code be arranged in the appropriate place in descending price order, along with any other CPT codes being reported.

When two E/M codes are reported, as may occur during a preventive medicine visit when a problem is identified that requires a separate evaluation, report the preventive medicine code first because it is related to the reason for the encounter.

When an E/M code and a special circumstances code (**99050-99060**) are reported, sequence the E/M code first and the special circumstances code second.

Guided Example of Assigning E/M Codes

To practice skills for assigning codes for E/M services, continue with the example from earlier in the chapter about a patient who was seen for a sinus infection. Follow along in your CPT manual as Scott Hood, CPC, assigns codes. Check off each step after you complete it.

▶ First, Scott reviews the information he abstracted.

❑ An established patient was seen in the office for a sinus infection.

❑ The history was detailed.

❑ The examination was expanded problem focused.

❑ The medical decision making was of moderate complexity.

▶ Scott searches the Index for the Main Term **Evaluation and Management**.

❑ He locates the subterm **Office and Other Outpatient**.

❑ The code range is **99201-99215**.

▶ Scott turns to the Tabular List to review codes **99201** through **99215**.

❑ He reads the category title **Office or Other Outpatient Services** listed at the top of the page, before code **99201**.

❑ He reads the category special instructions and confirms that he has selected the appropriate category. He reads instructions that cross reference him to other categories

for emergency department, observation care, and inpatient care services. None of these apply because the patient was seen in the office.

❑ He reads the subcategory title, **New Patient**, which appears immediately before code **99201**.

❑ He reviews the rest of the category and locates another subcategory, **Established Patient**, which begins with code **99211**. There are no additional subcategories after this one.

❑ He believes this is the correct subcategory because the patient was an outpatient seen for a health problem and is an established patient.

▶ Scott reviews the code requirements for codes in the subcategory **Established Patient 99211-99215**.

❑ Code **99211** is a minimal visit that does not require the presence of a physician.

❑ Codes **99212** through **99215** utilize the three key components: history, examination, and medical decision making.

❑ The code descriptions confirm that the codes describe office and other outpatient visits for evaluation and management of an established patient.

❑ He reads in the code descriptions that to select a code, it must meet 2 of the 3 key components at the level stated in the code or higher.

▶ Scott compares the level of each component for the patient with those listed in the coding manual.

❑ The patient's history was detailed, which qualifies for code **99214** or lower.

❑ The patient's examination was expanded problem focused, which qualifies for code **99213** or lower.

❑ The patient's medical decision making was of moderate complexity, which qualifies for code **99214** or lower.

❑ Two of the three key components—history and medical decision making—qualify for the levels stated in code **99214**.

▶ Scott checks for any additional instructional notes under the code and finds none.

▶ Scott reconfirms the levels of the three key components to be certain they match the code, then he finalizes the E/M code.

❑ **99214 Established patient office visit, level 4.**

The full CPT code description is:

Office or other outpatient visit for the evaluation and management of an established patient, which requires at least 2 of these 3 key components: a detailed history; a detailed examination; medical decision making of low complexity. Counseling and/or coordination of care with other physicians, other qualified health care professionals, or agencies are provided consistent with the nature of the problem(s) and the patient's and/or family's needs. Usually, the presenting problem(s) are of low to moderate severity. Typically, 20 minutes are spent face-to-face with the patient and/or family.

▶ Scott also assigns an ICD-10-CM diagnosis code that supports the need for the service. The confirmed diagnosis, sinus infection, is documented. He does not assign codes for the presenting symptoms because they are integral to the confirmed diagnosis. The complete coding is:

❑ **J01.90 Acute sinusitis, unspecified**

❑ **99214 Established patient office visit, level 4**

To code this case using the tools provided in this chapter, do the following.

First, refer to Figure 31-3, E/M Flow Chart.

- In column 1, select *Office/Outpatient*.
- In column 2, select *Office/Outpatient (with presenting problem)*.
- In column 3, select *Established patient*.

- In column 4, select code range *99211-99215*.
- In column 5, select *2 KC: H/E/MDM*.
- In column 6, place a checkmark next to *Detailed* in the History column. Place a checkmark next to *Exp prob focused* in the Exam column. Place a checkmark next to *Mod complexity* in the MDM column.
- In box 7, write NA because no information on time was provided.
- In box 8, draw an X across the box because none of the circumstances stated occurred for this patient.
- In box 9, draw an X across the box because none of the circumstances stated occurred for this patient.

Next, refer to Figure 31-10, Key Component Tool, to select the code.

- In the box at the top left of the page titled Patient Summary, circle *OutPt* and *Estab*.
- In the first row, History, circle *Detailed*.
- In the second row, Exam, circle *Expanded problem focused*.
- In the third row, MDM, circle *Moder. Complex*.
- Locate the section of grids labeled *Office or Outpatient (99211-99215) Established patient*. (Notice that the colors of blue for the title and purple for the subtitle match the colors of your choices on the Patient Summary grid for outpatient [blue] and established [purple].)
- Next, locate the code grid (99214) in which at least two of the highlighted key components are equal to or lower than the components circled in the Patient Summary grid.
- Verify the code in the Tabular List.

These tools provide assistance while learning about E/M coding. As you become more familiar with E/M coding, you may find that you no longer need to use both tools.

CODING PRACTICE

Exercise 31.5 Assigning Codes for Evaluation and Management Services

Instructions: Read the mini-medical-record of each patient's encounter, review the information abstracted in Exercise 31.4, and assign CPT procedure codes using the Index and Tabular List. Write the code(s) on the line provided.

---

1. OFFICE   Gender: F   Age: 48   Status: Established

Chief complaint: annual preventive care visit

History: pure hypercholesterolemia

Examination: comprehensive preventive care exam

Medical decision making: Cholesterol seems to be well controlled. No new problems.

1 CPT Code _____

---

2. INPATIENT HOSPITAL   Gender: M   Age: 25

Chief complaint: patient admitted by me for hematuria, severe pain in lower pelvic region

History: Detailed. Extended HPI, extended ROS, pertinent PFSH

Examination: comprehensive GU exam

Medical decision making: moderate complexity

Tip: To meet 3/3 key components, all components of the encounter must be at or above the level stated in the code.

1 CPT Code _____

3. OFFICE   Gender: M   Age: 48   Status: New

Chief complaint: patient was referred to me (endocrinologist) by his primary care physician for diabetes management

History: comprehensive; diabetes is secondary to chronic pancreatitis

Examination: comprehensive general multisystem examination

Medical decision making: High complexity. Spent 25 minutes of this 60-minute encounter counseling patient on diet management and other lifestyle changes needed to prevent serious diabetic complications. Refer to dietician.

Tip: When counseling and coordination of care make up more than 50% of the encounter, the level of the code can be upgraded.

1 CPT Code _____

4. OFFICE   Gender: F   Age: 61   Status: Established

Chief complaint: cough and congestion

History: Expanded problem focused. Brief HPI, extended ROS, pertinent past history.

Examination: detailed respiratory exam

Medical decision making: Moderate complexity. Chest X-ray negative for pneumonia. Rx antibiotics for acute bronchitis.

1 CPT Code _____

5. NURSING FACILITY   Gender: F   Age: 87

Chief complaint: status post total left hip replacement

History: problem-focused history of patient whom I saw last week in this facility

Examination: expanded problem-focused MS exam

Medical decision making: Straightforward. Patient is improving.

1 CPT Code _____

6. INPATIENT HOSPITAL   Gender: M   Age: 72 (Medicare)

Chief complaint: presented to ED with complaints of chest pain, SOB

History: Comprehensive. Extended HPI, complete ROS, complete PFSH

Examination: Comprehensive CV exam

Medical decision making: High complexity. Patient experienced a myocardial infarction while being examined and I provided 1 hour, 20 minutes of critical care in addition to the other services provided. Patient was stabilized and subsequently admitted by me.

Tip: A modifier is needed.

3 CPT Codes _____

_____

ADVANCED CODING FOR EVALUATION AND MANAGEMENT SERVICES

Although this chapter has covered a great deal of information, you have only scratched the surface of E/M coding. You may be asking questions such as:

- What elements make a history *problem focused* or *expanded problem focused*?
- What elements make an examination *detailed* or *comprehensive*?
- What is the difference between medical decision making of *moderate* and *high* complexity?

All E/M codes that are based on the three key components—history, examination, and medical decision making—require additional abstracting to determine the level of each component. Physicians must document their findings for the history, examination, and medical decision making in the medical record. They cannot document a general statement such as "I conducted a problem-focused examination" or "The medical decision making was of high complexity." (Such information is provided in this chapter to assist in learning.) They must document the exact information for each sign, symptom, body area, organ system, and patient complaint. The coder or medical record auditor can read the documentation and count the exact number of elements recorded for each key component. This provides the basis for determining the levels of the key components.

CMS and the AMA defined specific criteria for each of the three key components in the 1995 DG and 1997 DG. The charts that follow provide an overview of how the key components are determined, but you are not expected to master these details now. You will learn more about this aspect of E/M coding as you progress through your coding studies. For further information, download and study the 1995 DG and 1997 DG.

Determining the Level of History

Analyzing the patient history is a detailed process because the history consists of three elements in addition to the chief complaint—HPI, ROS, and PFSH—and each of these elements consists of several factors. The HPI consists of 8 factors, the ROS can consist of up to 14 systems, and the PFSH consists of 3 major factors, each with multiple components. Thus, determining the level of history requires coders to identify as many as 25 statements in the medical record. History levels and elements are summarized in ■ TABLE 31-7 (page 546), then the content of each of the three elements are discussed. All information in each

Table 31-7 ■ **HISTORY LEVELS AND ELEMENTS**

History (3/3 required) (Chief Complaint included)	Problem Focused	Expanded Problem Focused	Detailed	Comprehensive
History of Present Illness (HPI) Location, severity, timing, modifying factors, quality, duration, context, associated signs/symptoms	Brief (1 element)	Brief (2–3 elements)	Extended (4+ elements *or* 3 chronic problems)	Extended (4+ elements *or* 3 chronic problems)
Review of Systems (ROS) Constitutional, allerg/immun, CV, ENT/M, endocrine, eyes, GI, GU, hemic/lymph, MS, neurologic, psychiatric, respiratory, skin/breast	None	Pertinent (1 system)	Extended (2–9 systems)	Complete (10+ systems)
Past, Family, and Social History (PFSH) New pt/initial hosp/consults	Pertinent (1–2 elements)	Pertinent (1–2 elements)	Pertinent (1–2 elements)	Complete (3 elements)
Established pt/subsequent hospital	Pertinent (1 element)	Pertinent (1 element)	Pertinent (1 element)	Complete (2–3 elements)

Source: Adapted with permission from Kate Gabriel-Jones, Medical Coding Evaluation and Management, Pearson Education, 2014

component must be relevant to the chief complaint. For example, a physician cannot ask a multitude of questions that are not necessary to understand the patient's chief complaint just to qualify for a higher level of history-taking.

HPI Factors

HPI consists of an interview in which the physician asks the patient questions about eight factors relating to the chief complaint. ■ Table 31-8 defines the factors and provides examples of each.

ROS Factors

The ROS continues the physician's interview with the patient. In this phase, the physician asks questions regarding how the chief complaint might impact other body systems. The ROS is not the physical examination. It consists of patients telling the physician what other signs and symptoms they are experiencing (■ Table 31-9). Refer to the 1995 DG and 1997 DG for a list of systems with examples of signs and symptoms that qualify for review.

PFSH Factors

In the PFSH, the physician asks questions about the patient's past medical history, the family medical history, and the patient's lifestyle or social history, as they pertain to the chief complaint. ■ Table 31-10 defines each of these factors.

Determining the Level of Examination

Physicians have three options for evaluating the content of the physical examination: the 1995 DG, the general multisystem examination described in the 1997 DG, and 11 single organ system examinations, also described in the 1997 DG. ■ Table 31-11 summarizes the requirements of each type of examination. Refer to the 1997 DG to read the elements required in each single organ system examination for a limited, expanded problem-focused, detailed, or comprehensive examination. You will learn about the single organ system examinations as you study CPT coding for the various medical specialties.

CODING CAUTION

All elements of the history, examination, and medical decision making must be medically necessary based on the chief complaint/presenting problem. For example, a comprehensive examination would not be medically necessary for a chief complaint of contact dermatitis. Although all the elements of a comprehensive examination may have been performed, it would be improper to code and accept payment for it, based on the diagnosis of contact dermatitis.

Table 31-8 ■ **HPI FACTORS**

HPI Factors	Physician's Question	Examples
1. Location	Where is the problem/condition located?	Left leg, stomach, elbow, head
2. Quality	Can you describe how the condition feels?	Aching, burning, radiating pain, raw, itching
3. Severity	What is the level of sensation or pain on a scale of 1 to 10, with 1 being the least severe and 10 being the most severe?	10 on a pain scale of 1 to 10
4. Duration	How long have you had the condition; when did it begin?	Started three days ago; condition has lasted two weeks
5. Timing	When does the condition occur?	Constant or comes and goes
6. Context	Does the condition appear when you are engaging in a certain activity or at a certain time of the day?	Pain occurs when lifting large objects at work; pain is worse upon awakening
7. Modifying factors	What factors improve or worsen the condition?	Pain decreases when heat is applied; pain increases when standing up
8. Associated signs and symptoms	Are there any other problems that occur along with the condition?	Numbness in toes also occurs with leg pain

Table 31-9 ■ **ROS FACTORS**

ROS Level	Number of Systems*	Description	Example
Problem-pertinent	1	The physician asks about the system directly related to the problem stated in the HPI.	The patient's CC is an earache. The ROS is positive for left ear pain. The patient denies tinnitus or a feeling of fullness in the ear. In this example, the physician reviews one system, the ear.
Extended	2 to 9	The physician asks about the system directly related to the problem stated in the HPI and also asks about additional systems.	The patient's CC is a follow-up visit after a cardiac catheterization. The patient states, "I feel great." The patient denies chest pain, syncope, palpitations, and shortness of breath. In this example, the physician reviews two systems, cardiovascular and respiratory.
Complete	10 or more	The physician asks about the system directly related to the problem stated in the HPI and also asks about additional systems.	The patient's CC is having a "fainting spell." The ROS documents related signs and symptoms of 10 body systems.

*ROS systems: constitutional, ENT/M, respiratory, GU, skin/breast, endocrine, allergic/ immunologic, eyes, CV, GI, MS, psychiatric, neurologic, hemic/lymphatic

Table 31-10 ■ **PFSH FACTORS**

PFSH Factor	Description
Past medical history (P)	The patient's past experiences with illnesses, injuries, treatments, surgeries, hospitalizations, current medications, immunizations, and allergies
Family medical history (F)	The health history of family members (parents, siblings, children), such as diseases or conditions they have or had; cause of death of deceased family members; review of hereditary medical conditions that may place the patient at risk
Social history (S)	An age-appropriate review of the patient's past and current activities, such as marital status, employment, occupation, education, sexual history, smoking, drugs, alcohol, and tobacco

Table 31-11 ■ **EXAMINATION LEVELS IN 1995 AND 1997 DOCUMENTATION GUIDELINES**

Examination	Problem Focused	Expanded Problem Focused	Detailed	Comprehensive
1995 DG physical examination	A limited exam of affected BA or OS (1 BA/OS)	A limited exam of affected BA or OS and other symptomatic or related OS (2–4 BA/OS)	An extended exam of affected BA or OS and other symptomatic or related OS (5–7 BA/OS)	A general multisystem exam or complete exam of a single OS and other symptomatic or related OS (8+ BA *or* OS, but they cannot be mixed)
1997 DG general multisystem examination	1–5 elements identified by a bullet	At least 6 elements identified by a bullet	At least 2 elements identified by a bullet from each of 6 areas/systems or at least 12 elements identified by a bullet in 2 or more areas/systems	Performance of all elements identified by a bullet in at least 9 BA/OS and documentation of at least 2 elements identified by a bullet in each of the examined systems
1997 DG single organ system examination	1–5 elements identified by a bullet	At least 6 elements identified by a bullet	At least 12 elements identified by a bullet Eye & psychiatric: At least 9 elements identified by a bullet	All elements identified by a bullet within each shaded border and at least 1 element identified by a bullet within each unshaded border

BA = body area(s); OS = organ system(s)
Bullet refers to a bulleted list of elements in the charts in the 1997 DG.
Shaded and *unshaded borders* refers to areas in the charts in the 1997 DG.

Source: Adapted with permission from Kate Gabriel-Jones, Medical Coding Evaluation and Management, Pearson Education, 2014

Table 31-12 ■ **MEDICAL DECISION MAKING LEVELS**

Medical Decision Making (2/3 required)	Straightforward	Low Complexity	Moderate Complexity	High Complexity
Number of diagnoses or management options	Established presenting problem, stable or improving	Established presenting problem, worsening	New presenting problem, without workup	New presenting problem, with workup
Amount and/or complexity of data to be reviewed	Ordering or reviewing diagnostic data	Obtaining old records or additional history from someone other than the patient	Discussion of diagnostic results with physician who performed diagnostic testing	Independent visualization of image, tracing, or scan by physician performing the E/M service
Risk of significant complications, morbidity, and/or mortality*	Minimal	Low	Moderate	High

*Refer to the Table of Risk in the 1997 DG for the criteria for minimal, low, moderate, and high risk.

Source: Adapted with permission from Kate Gabriel-Jones, Medical Coding Evaluation and Management, Pearson Education, 2014

Determining the Level of Medical Decision Making

Medical decision making consists of three elements, each of which has multiple factors. ■ TABLE 31-12 summarizes the elements and factors required for each of the four levels of medical decision making. Also refer to the 1995 DG and 1997 DG to view the Table of Risk, which specifies additional details.

As you progress through your study of coding, you will learn more about how to read a complete medical record and analyze the elements of history, examination, and medical decision making. The tables here provide you with reference information and help you understand that very specific criteria are used to evaluate the level of service provided.

Hospital Outpatient E/M Coding

The criteria for evaluating the three key components discussed in this chapter apply to individual providers, who bill for professional services. Hospitals also use E/M codes to report emergency department visits and outpatient critical care services. The hospital fee is referred to as the **facility fee**. Hospitals bill for facility resources, not professional services, so the three key components do not apply. Facility resources include nursing and support staff, supplies, medication administration, social services, and the cost of space.

Hospital emergency departments assign E/M code levels based on the resources used. Types of visits that require fewer resources are assigned to lower-level E/M codes and those using more resources are assigned to higher-level E/M codes. Each facility is directed by CMS to create its own custom crosswalk based on the types of services provided, a process called E/M "leveling." For Medicare patients, the E/M codes, and other CPT codes, are mapped to an ambulatory payment classification (APC) group based on similar clinical characteristics and costs. APC is part of Medicare's Outpatient Prospective Payment System (OPPS), under which an all-inclusive, predetermined rate is paid to outpatient hospitals for patients with similar resource consumption. APCs for outpatient services are similar in concept to Medicare

Severity-Adjusted Diagnosis Related Groups (MS-DRGs) for inpatient services.

The facility service may be mapped to a higher- or lower-level E/M code than the actual professional fee. Medicare does not require or expect a correlation between the professional E/M code and the facility E/M code for the same encounter. For example, one encounter may involve two or three physicians, each of whom bills a professional fee, but the hospital bills only one facility fee. Another example of this difference is a patient who requires limited physician care but extensive facility resources (■ FIGURE 31-15). In other situations, the facility E/M level could be lower than that reported by the physician because limited facility resources are utilized but extensive physician care is required.

A patient presents to the emergency department with vomiting due to excessive alcohol intake. The physician performs a problem focused history, a problem focused exam, and medical decision making of low complexity. The physician orders a lab test to determine the BAC, then allows the patient to sleep for several hours until he is able to be discharged safely. During this time, the nurses continually monitor the condition of the patient and assist the patient to the restroom several times due to vomiting. The patient is discharged 6 hours later.

Physician coding:
99282 Emergency department visit for the evaluation and management of a patient, which requires these 3 key components: an expanded problem focused history; an expanded problem focused examination; and medical decision making of low complexity.

Facility coding:
99283 Emergency department visit for the evaluation and management of a patient (level 3)
APC 0614 Level 3 Type A Emergency Visits

Figure 31-15 ■ Example of Professional and Facility Coding for the Same Encounter

CODING PRACTICE

Exercise 31.6 Advanced Coding for Evaluation and Management Services

Instructions: Refer to the tables in this section of the chapter to identify the following information. Write your answer on the line provided.

1. Table 31-7 History Levels and Elements: What is the level of history based on 2–3 elements of HPI, 1 system in the ROS, and 1–2 elements in a new patient PFSH?

2. Table 31-8 HPI Factors: Which HPI factor is addressed with a description of pain that started three days ago?

3. Table 31-9 ROS Factors: How many systems does an extended ROS include?

4. Table 31-10 PFSH Factors: Which PFSH factor includes a review of the patient's tobacco and alcohol use?

5. Table 31-11 Examination Levels in 1995 and 1997 Documentation Guidelines: What level of examination is described by 6 bulleted items in the 1997 DG?

6. Table 31-11 Examination Levels in 1995 and 1997 Documentation Guidelines: How many body areas or organ systems must be addressed for a detailed examination under the 1995 DG?

7. Table 31-12 Medical Decision Making Levels: What type of medical decision is required when the presenting problem is established and stable or improving?

8. Table 31-12 Medical Decision Making Levels: What type of medical decision is required when the treating physician discusses diagnostic results with the physician who performed diagnostic testing?

9. What do outpatient hospitals use as the basis for assigning E/M code levels?

10. What is the purpose of an APC?

CHAPTER SUMMARY

In this chapter you learned that:

- Physicians can provide E/M services in many settings and for a number of different purposes. Each type of encounter has a separate category of codes and a specific set of criteria for selecting the correct code.

- Four sources of guidelines must be considered when determining the level of E/M service provided: E/M Section Guidelines; Category Special Instructions; 1995 Documentation Guidelines for Evaluation and Management Services; and 1997 Documentation Guidelines for Evaluation and Management Services.

- The divisions of the E/M section are called categories and subcategories, rather than subsections and subheadings, as is the case in most other CPT sections. A category, the first level of division in the E/M section, identifies the setting of service.

- The most commonly used E/M categories for office and outpatient settings are Office or Outpatient Services, Preventive Care, Consultations, Emergency Department, and Hospital Observation.

- The most commonly used E/M categories for inpatient services are Hospital Inpatient Services, Hospital Inpatient Consultations, Critical Care Services, and Newborn, Neonatal, and Pediatric Intensive and Critical Care Services.

- An established patient is one who has received professional services from the same physician, or another physician in the group with the same specialty and subspecialty, within the previous three years. All other patients are new patients because each specialty and subspecialty has differing assessments and examinations.

- Eight E/M categories define the level, or complexity, of service provided based on a set of three key components—the history, the examination, and the medical decision making—and each key component can be performed at varying levels of complexity.

- When E/M codes require two of three key components, one component in the medical record can be lower than the one listed in the code, but two must meet or exceed the levels listed in the code description. When codes require all three components, then all three components in the medical record must meet or exceed the levels listed in the code description.

- E/M codes that are based on the three key components require additional abstracting to determine the actual level of each component. This is accomplished by following detailed instructions in the 1995 and 1997 Documentation Guidelines.

CONCEPT QUIZ

Take a moment to look back at evaluation and management services and solidify your skills. Try to answer the questions from memory first, then refer to the discussion in this chapter if you need a little extra help.

Completion

Instructions: Write the term that answers each question based on the information you learned in this chapter. Choose from the list below. Some choices may be used more than once and some choices may not be used at all.

case management	observation patient
consultation	outpatient
critical care	prolonged service
disability evaluation	preventive care
emergency department	resuscitation
home services	transfer of care
inpatient	transitional care management
intensive care	

1. _____ is an evaluation of a patient requested by another physician to obtain a professional opinion on a specific problem.

2. _____ codes also include codes for counseling and assessments.

3. The codes for anticoagulant management appear in the _____ category in the E/M section.

4. _____ codes are add-on codes and can be used with any E/M code in any setting.

5. A patient treated in the ED and discharged is a/an _____.

6. A/an _____ is a patient who has been formally admitted to a hospital spanning at least two midnights.

7. Since 2010, Medicare has not paid for _____ codes.

8. _____ and _____ codes report the time spent providing services.

9. A patient in a partial hospitalization program is considered a/an _____.

10. _____ codes are reported for services to newborns and children who are not critically ill but require close observation and frequent interventions.

Multiple Choice

Instructions: Circle the letter of the best answer to each question based on the information you learned in this chapter.

1. What criterion is used to divide categories for preventive care and certain services to newborns and children?
   A. Physician specialty
   B. Physician subspecialty
   C. Age of the patient
   D. Frequency of care

2. Which of the following divide codes based on whether the encounter is initial or subsequent?
   A. Office visits
   B. Preventive care services
   C. Outpatient hospital services
   D. Inpatient hospital services

3. What are the three key components of E/M services?
   A. Chief complaint, history, time
   B. Chief complaint, examination, medical decision making
   C. History, examination, medical decision making
   D. History, examination, time

4. An established patient is defined as one who has received professional services from the physician within how many years?
   A. One
   B. Two
   C. Three
   D. Four

5. What criterion is used for subsequent care for the low-birth-weight neonate who requires continuous monitoring?
   A. Time
   B. Age
   C. Birth weight
   D. All of the above

6. What modifier identifies the admitting physician and differentiates him from a consulting physician, who does not use a modifier?
   A. -24
   B. -25
   C. -B1
   D. -A1

7. What key component refers to the complexity of establishing a diagnosis?
   A. Chief complaint
   B. Examination
   C. History of present illness
   D. Medical decision making

8. Which contributory factor includes the time spent arranging for referrals to another provider?
   A. Counseling
   B. Coordination of care
   C. Care management
   D. Online services

9. What step should a coder take before selecting the level of service?
   A. Identify the setting
   B. Evaluate contributory factors
   C. Determine whether time is a factor
   D. Determine whether a modifier is needed

10. How many levels of medical decision making are there?
   A. Three
   B. Four
   C. Five
   D. Six

CODING CHALLENGE

Instructions: Read the mini-medical-record of each patient's encounter, then abstract, assign, and arrange ICD-10-CM diagnosis codes and CPT procedure codes using the appropriate Index and Tabular List. Write the code(s) on the line provided.

1. INPATIENT HOSPITAL   Gender: M   Age: 67 (Medicare)   Status: Initial

Chief complaint: LUQ pain and swelling, increasing over the past 3 days, indigestion. Pt is admitted.

History: Comprehensive. Pain is worse after eating; does not smoke; weekly alcohol consumption at 2–3 cases of beer x10 years.

Examination: a comprehensive GI exam; abdominal tenderness in the LUQ without masses; liver and spleen WNL

Medical decision making: moderate complexity with stool sample collected; abdominal US; IV fluids with pain control; GI consult ordered

Assessment: acute pancreatitis, alcohol induced

Tip: Refer to Medicare rules for billing this type of service.

1 ICD-10-CM Code _____

1 CPT Code _____

2. INPATIENT HOSPITAL   Gender: F   Age: 42
Status: Discharge

Reason for admission: Patient found nonresponsive. Family reports patient being on a fast.

Course of treatment: IV fluids increased to soft diet

Assessment: nondiabetic hypoglycemic coma

Plan: instructed on diet and glucometer; FU in 1 week

Time spent: 10 minutes

1 ICD-10-CM Code _____

1 CPT Code _____

3. OFFICE   Gender: F   Age: 42   Status: Established

Chief complaint: blood pressure check

History: Long-time patient with hypertension, which has been difficult to control. Patient is here for her twice weekly BP check.

Examination: Blood pressure check by the nurse. BP reading is 120/72 today.

Tip: Minimal time is spent by the nurse under supervision of the physician for a routine office visit.

1 ICD-10-CM Code _____

1 CPT Code _____

4. OFFICE   Gender: M   Age: 52   Status: New

Chief complaint: dizziness upon sudden standing, temporary visual dimming, numbness and tingling in arms and hands

History: history of present illness, ROS, and PFSH reviewed in detail

Examination: detailed constitutional exam of vital signs and general appearance; detailed CV exam

Medical decision making: BP to be checked daily and follow instructions related to lifestyle changes (i.e., improve diet and exercise); low complexity

Assessment: orthostatic hypotension

Tip: Identify the setting and the type of service.

1 ICD-10-CM Code _____

1 CPT Code _____

5. INPATIENT HOSPITAL   Gender: F   Age: 71
Status: New

Chief complaint: patient referred by Dr. Conover for consult on peripheral autonomic neuropathy

(continued)

(continued from page 551)

5. (continued)

History: *Comprehensive history. The patient also has type 2 diabetes, which has been well managed with diet and lifestyle.*

Examination: *comprehensive examination*

Medical decision making: *High complexity. Rx and tests. Return in 6 weeks. Report sent to Dr. Conover.*

Assessment: *Type 2 DM, peripheral neuropathy*

Tip: Determine whether the neuropathy is related to the diabetes. Refer to Medicare rules for billing this type of service.

1 ICD-10-CM Code _____

1 CPT Code _____

---

6. OFFICE Gender: F Age: 4 Status: Established

Reason for encounter: *routine exam of a 4-year-old*

History: *normal healthy female child; immunizations up to date; detailed history obtained*

Examination: *Detailed exam; no new findings*

Plan: *RTO in 1 year, call if any new problems*

Tip: Determine the type of service for this visit.

1 ICD-10-CM Code _____

1 CPT Code _____

---

7. EMERGENCY DEPT Gender: M Age: 24 Status: New

Chief complaint: *in pain with swollen wrist, unable to bend*

History: *patient slipped walking across an icy driveway and used his right hand to break his fall*

Examination: *expanded problem focused*

Medical decision making: *Low. X-ray of the right arm reviewed.*

Assessment: *fracture of the distal right radius*

Tip: Injury codes should be followed by external cause codes. Remember to sequence the external cause codes in the correct order.

3 ICD-10-CM Codes _____

_____

1 CPT Code _____

---

8. NURSING FACILITY Gender: F Age: 87 Status: Established

Chief complaint: *cellulitis, left leg*

History: *problem focused, cellulitis improved on IV antibiotic*

Examination: *problem-focused examination limited to left leg, less swelling*

Medical decision making: *discontinue IV antibiotic and start oral antibiotic; topical medication; DM and HTN stable*

3 ICD-10-CM Codes _____

_____

1 CPT Code _____

---

9. INPATIENT HOSPITAL Gender: M Age: 77 Status: Established

Chief Complaint: *acute renal failure*

Treatment: *reviewed lab results and renal ultrasound; discussed possible dialysis with patient and limitations due to anteroseptal MI last week; nephrologist consulted; central line discontinued*

Time spent: *critical care provided from 1700 to 1820*

1 ICD-10-CM Code _____

2 CPT Codes _____

---

10. OFFICE Gender: M Age: 59 Status: New

Chief complaint: *patient comes in today for a migraine, which started two days ago with aura*

History: *detailed; patient is referred by his PCP for neurological evaluation of pharmacoresistant migraine*

Examination: *detailed examination of multiple body areas*

Medical decision making: *low complexity; Rx for zolmitriptan and Cafergot*

Assessment: *migraine with aura*

1 ICD-10-CM Code _____

1 CPT Code _____

KEEP ON CODING

Instructions: Read the diagnostic or procedural statement, then use the appropriate Index and Tabular List to assign ICD-10-CM diagnosis codes and CPT procedure codes. Write the code(s) on the line provided.

1. Established patient office visit with a comprehensive history, comprehensive examination, and high-complexity medical decision making, resulting in a decision for major surgery the next day. CPT Code(s) _____

2. A 45-year-old male presents to the ER, where an open fracture of the left radius is diagnosed. Patient is admitted. Surgeon performs comprehensive history, comprehensive examination, and medical decision making of high complexity. Surgery is scheduled for the next day. CPT Code(s) _____

3. A new patient was seen in the physician's office for abdominal pain. The physician performs a detailed history and comprehensive examination. Medical decision making is of moderate complexity. CPT Code(s) _____

4. A patient with rectal bleeding was seen in the office of a gastroenterologist. The patient's primary care physician requested that the gastroenterologist provide advice about this case. The specialist conducted a comprehensive history and exam, and medical decision-making was high. The consultant documented his findings and communicated them via written report to the primary care physician. CPT Code(s) _____

5. An established patient seen for his monthly B12 injection. The nurse performs the service under the physician's supervision. CPT Code(s) _____

6. A new patient is seen in the physician's office for a cough, sore throat, and fever. The physician performs a problem-focused history and exam, and medical decision making was straightforward. CPT Code(s) _____

7. Consultation for newly admitted inpatient for massive, life-threatening esophageal varices hemorrhage and severe substernal pain; comprehensive history, comprehensive examination, and high-complexity medical decision making. CPT Code(s) _____

8. Established patient office visit for evaluation of a hard lump on his shoulder, status post appendectomy 10 days ago. Problem-focused history, problem-focused examination, straightforward medical decision making. CPT Code(s) _____

9. Emergency department visit for a painful sunburn with blister formation on the back. Problem-focused history; problem-focused examination; straightforward medical decision making. CPT Code(s) _____

10. Referred to office by PCP for consult for avascular necrosis of the left humeral head due to trauma. Detailed history; detailed examination; and medical decision making of low complexity. CPT Code(s) _____

11. Office visit for 18-year-old new male patient with cystic acne of the face unresponsive to over-the-counter medications. Expanded problem-focused history; expanded problem-focused examination; straightforward medical decision making. CPT Code(s) _____

12. Initial hospital visit for one-day-old with cyanosis, respiratory distress, and tachypnea. CPT Code(s) _____

13. Established patient admitted for observation following medication reaction with nausea, vomiting, and dizziness. Comprehensive history; comprehensive examination; moderate-complexity medical decision making. CPT Code(s) _____

14. First office visit of 20-year-old female for annual Pap test and discussion of contraception options. CPT Code(s) _____

15. New patient office visit for worker's compensation evaluation of acute four-extremity weakness and shortness of breath one week after exposure to toxic chemicals. Comprehensive history; comprehensive examination; medical decision making of high complexity. CPT Code(s) _____

16. Established patient seen at 6:30 p.m. after regular office hours requesting a return-to-work certificate for resolving contact dermatitis. CPT Code(s) _____

(continued)

(continued from page 553)

17. Initial hospital inpatient consultation for evaluation of patient with increased bilateral pulmonary infiltrate, hypoxemia, and sudden decrease in urine output. Comprehensive history; comprehensive examination; medical decision making of moderate complexity. CPT Code(s) _____

18. Emergency department visit for a 24-year-old who fell off a trail bike and sustained a head injury with loss of consciousness for approximately 5 minutes. Detailed history; detailed examination; medical decision making of moderate complexity. CPT Code(s)

_____

19. First office visit for removal of mole. Patient also asks physician to evaluate ingrown toenail. Expanded problem-focused history; expanded problem-focused examination; straightforward medical decision making. CPT Code(s) _____

20. First hour of critical care for a patient with acute respiratory failure from acute exacerbation of chronic obstructive emphysema. CPT Code(s) _____

21. Subsequent hospital visit for maintenance of analgesia using an IV Dilaudid infusion. Expanded problem-focused history; problem-focused examination; straightforward medical decision making. CPT Code(s) _____

22. Established patient requested to be seen at a psychiatric residential treatment center by PCP for possible purulent bacterial conjunctivitis. Problem-focused history; problem-focused examination; straightforward medical decision making. CPT Code(s)

_____

23. Office visit for an established patient with a history of bipolar disorder and migraine headaches complaining of auditory hallucinations. Comprehensive history; comprehensive examination; medical decision making of moderate complexity. CPT Code(s)

_____

24. Established patient seen by his personal nephrologist, who was called to the emergency department at midnight because patient presented with new-onset peripheral edema and increased blood pressure three months post kidney transplant. Detailed history; comprehensive examination; medical decision making of high complexity. CPT Code(s) _____

25. Critical care services in the emergency department for a patient in respiratory failure and with congestive heart failure. Ventilator management is initiated. Physician spends an hour and 50 minutes providing critical care for this patient. CPT Code(s) _____

Medicine Procedures (90281-99199, 99500-99607)

Chapter 32

Learning Objectives

After completing this chapter, you should have the skills to:

32.1 Spell and define the key words, medical terms, and abbreviations related to procedures in the Medicine section.

32.2 Identify the main characteristics of coding for procedures in the Medicine section.

32.3 Abstract procedural information from the medical record for coding services in the Medicine section.

32.4 Assign codes for procedures in the Medicine section.

32.5 Arrange codes for procedures in the Medicine section.

32.6 Code evaluation and management services for psychiatric services.

32.7 Discuss the CPT coding guidelines related to the Medicine section.

Chapter Outline

- **Medicine Procedure Basics**
- **Coding Overview of the Medicine Section**
- **Abstracting Medicine Procedures**
- **Assigning Codes for Medicine Procedures**
- **Arranging Codes for Medicine Procedures**
- **E/M Coding for Medicine**

Key Terms and Abbreviations

allergen immunotherapy	electrocardiogram (ECG or EKG)	interactive complexity	psychiatric diagnostic interview
allergenic extract	electroencephalogram (EEG)	manometry	psychotherapy
allergy testing	electromyogram (EMG)	minimally invasive (procedure)	push technique
antigen	hemodialysis	motility study	revascularization
catheter	immune globulin	noninvasive (procedure)	supervised modallty
constant attendance modality	immunization	occlusive disease	toxoid
dialysis	immunodeficiency	otorhinolaryngological	vaccine
echocardiogram (ECC)	infusion technique	peritoneal dialysis	

In addition to the key terms listed here, students should know the terms defined within tables in this chapter.

INTRODUCTION

A department store carries a wide variety of products, such as men's, women's, and children's clothing, tools, household products, kitchen products, and perhaps even furniture. This variety is in contrast to a specialized store that carries closely related products, such as only kitchen products or only children's clothing.

Similarly, the Medicine section of the CPT manual contains codes for services provided by many medical specialties but that are not suitable to the Surgery section. Any physician or qualified provider can perform procedures from the Medicine section that are within the provider's scope of practice and training.

MEDICINE PROCEDURE BASICS

Medicine procedures can be diagnostic or therapeutic, each of which can be divided into several broad types of procedures. Diagnostic procedures are performed to help analyze a patient's complaint and determine the cause of signs and symptoms. Diagnostic techniques classified in the Medicine section include an assessment or evaluation, an examination, or the use of equipment or tools to make a recording or measurement or conduct a function study.

- **Assessment/evaluation**—asking questions to arrive at a conclusion. Examples are a psychiatric diagnostic interview and a discussion of a patient's symptoms.
- **Examination**—performing a visual and physical inspection, with or without the assistance of instruments, to arrive at a conclusion. Examples are range of motion testing and any ophthalmoscopy.
- **Recording**—creating an image of a structure or process. Examples are electrocardiography and angiography.
- **Measurement**—using equipment or tools to quantify the body's response, reflex, or perception. Examples are a tonometer that measures intraocular pressure and an audiometer that measures the ear's response to sound.
- **Function study**—visualizing a physiologic function in real time to observe the processes at work. Examples are a gastric motility (*movement*) study and nerve function studies.

Although not classified in this chapter, laboratory tests, in which a fluid or tissue specimen is analyzed for certain characteristics, also are an important diagnostic tool. These codes are classified in the CPT Laboratory section (**80000-89398**). Radiographic imaging, such as X-rays, MRI, PET, fluoroscopy, and CT, is also used for diagnostic purposes. These codes are classified in the CPT Radiology section (**70000-79999**). Most physical examinations are part of the E/M code (**99201-99499**).

Therapeutic procedures treat a condition to minimize its effects, eliminate it, or cure it. Therapeutic procedures classified in the Medicine section include physical, pharmacologic, immunologic, mechanical, and mental techniques.

- **Corporeal (physical)**–applying a manual technique to the body. Examples are chiropractic manipulation or use of a hot pack.
- **Pharmacologic**–altering the body's processes via drugs or biologicals. Examples are intravenous administration of antibiotics or intravenous administration of antineoplastic drugs.
- **Immunologic/vaccine**–activating the body's defenses through administration of an immune globulin or vaccine. Examples are the hepatitis B immune globulin and the influenza vaccine.
- **Assistive device (mechanical)**–using an external device to assist or perform the body's normal function. Examples are a pacemaker and a neurostimulator.
- **Psychotherapy (mental)**–using questions, discussion, and advice to redirect mental and behavioral processes. Examples are individual, group, and family psychotherapy.

Additional therapeutic procedures appear in the CPT Surgery (**10021-69990**) and Radiology sections.

Medical Terminology

Medical terms for medical procedures combine roots for various organs or anatomic sites with prefixes and suffixes to create a term that describes a specific service or procedure. Many of the procedures in this section contain a prefix or root that identifies the organ or anatomic site that is the target of the procedure, such as heart (cardi/o), eye (opt/o), or nerve (neur/o). The prefix can describe the method or technique used, such as electrical (electro-), sound (echo-), or within a structure (intra-). The suffix describes the purpose of the procedure, such as measuring (-metry), recording an image (-graphy), or providing treatment (-therapy). Refer to ■ TABLE 32-1 for a refresher on how to build medical terms related to Medicine procedures.

Table 32-1 ■ **EXAMPLE OF CONSTRUCTING MEDICAL TERMS FOR MEDICINE PROCEDURES**

Prefix/Combining Form	Suffix	Complete Medical Term
echo- (sound)		**echo + cardio + graphy** (recording of the heart using sound waves)
		electro + cardio + graphy (recording of the heart using electrical waves)
psycho- (mind) **tympano-** (eardrum)	**-graphy** (recording) **-metry** (measurement) **-therapy** (treatment)	**psycho + metry** (measurement/testing of the mind) **tympano + metry** (measurement of the eardrum)
electro- (electrical)		**electro + convulsive + therapy** (treatment using electricity to create convulsion) **psycho + therapy** (treatment of the mind)

Source: © PB Resources, Inc. Used with permission.

CODING CAUTION

Be alert for medical words that are spelled similarly and have different meanings.

chemotherapy (*treatment using drugs*) and
  photochemotherapy (*treatment using drugs and light*)

plethysmography (*recording of the volume*) and
  polysomnography (*multiple recordings of sleep*)

SUCCESS STEP

You may recognize *gonioscopy* as a medical term because you know the suffix *–scopy* refers to a visual examination, but the root *goni/o* is probably unfamiliar. *Goni/o* means angle. Gonioscopy is the visual examination of the angle between the cornea and iris (iridocorneal angle) using a specialized tool called a gonioscope.

CODING PRACTICE

Exercise 32.1 Medicine Procedure Basics

Instructions: Use your medical terminology skills and resources to define the following procedures, then identify the applicable code or code range. Follow these steps:

- Use slash marks "/" to break down the underlined term into its root(s) and suffix.
- Define the meaning of the underlined word based on the meaning of each word part.
- Use the entire phrase to identify the code or code range shown in the CPT Index.

Example: <u>audiometry</u>, comprehensive audio/metry   Meaning *measurement of hearing*   CPT Code(s) *0212T, 92557*

1. <u>electrogastrography</u>   Meaning _____   CPT Code(s) _____

2. <u>hemofiltration</u>   Meaning _____   CPT Code(s) _____

3. <u>hydrotherapy</u>, application   Meaning _____   CPT Code(s) _____

4. <u>endomyocardial</u> biopsy   Meaning _____   CPT Code(s) _____

5. allergy tests, <u>intradermal</u>, biologicals   Meaning _____   CPT Code(s) _____

6. <u>angiography</u>, bypass graft   Meaning _____   CPT Code(s) _____

7. <u>anorectal</u> biofeedback   Meaning _____   CPT Code(s) _____

8. <u>otorhinolaryngology</u>, unlisted services and procedures   Meaning _____   CPT Code(s) _____

9. infusion therapy, <u>subcutaneous</u>   Meaning _____   CPT Code(s) _____

10. <u>ophthalmoscopy</u>   Meaning _____   CPT Code(s) _____

CODING OVERVIEW OF THE MEDICINE SECTION

The CPT section for Medicine procedures contains 34 subsections that are divided by the type of procedure. Review the subsection and category names and code ranges listed at the beginning of the Medicine section in many CPT manuals to become familiar with the content and organization. In this list, subsections and categories followed by an asterisk (*) contain special instructions that provide guidelines for using codes in that subsection or category.

The Medicine section reports **noninvasive** (*procedures performed without puncturing the skin*) and **minimally invasive** procedures (*procedures performed using only natural body openings, needles, or small incisions*) from a wide variety of medical specialties and that are not appropriate for the Surgery section. Among the procedures reported in this section are those for immunology, vaccinations, psychiatry, dialysis, gastroenterology, otorhinolaryngology, cardiovascular, pulmonology,

endocrinology, neurology, dermatology, physical medicine and rehabilitation, nutrition, and home health. The **Ophthalmology** subsection provides evaluation and management codes, in addition to other procedures. Several subsections identify procedures from complementary medicine: acupuncture, biofeedback, osteopathic, and chiropractic. Non-face-to-face services provided by nonphysician providers appear here. Moderate sedation services and qualifying circumstances for anesthesia also appear here but are discussed in the anesthesia chapter of this text.

Because the Medicine section lists codes from a wide range of medical specialties, diagnosis codes from nearly any chapter of the ICD-10-CM manual can be used to support these procedures. When tests are performed for diagnostic purposes, the CPT codes for outpatient procedures might require diagnosis code(s) for signs and symptoms if test results are not known and a definitive diagnosis has not yet been established. When test results, and the physician's interpretation of those results, are available when the record is coded, then assign the code for the diagnosis stated by the physician.

The principal diagnosis for inpatient procedures is the one determined, *after study*, to be chiefly responsible for the admission. *Study* includes many of the tests and procedures classified in the Medicine section. When a patient is admitted for testing to determine the cause of signs and symptoms, tests from this section may be performed. Keep in mind that the ordering physician must indicate the significance of the test result in determining the patient's diagnosis. Do not assign a diagnosis based solely on the test result.

CPT Medicine guidelines discuss add-on codes, separate procedures, unlisted services or procedures, special reports, and supplied materials.

Recall that add-on codes must be reported in addition to a primary service. Add-on codes do not require modifier **-51** because they are exempt from the multiple procedure concept that reduces payment for additional procedures performed at the same time. The symbol + in front of a code designates it as an add-on code. In addition, the wording of the code description includes phrases such as **each additional** or **List separately in addition to primary procedure**.

Some procedures in this section are commonly performed as an integral part of a more extensive procedure. Codes identified with the note **(separate procedure)**, for example, **92511 Nasopharyngoscopy with endoscope (separate procedure)**, should not be reported in addition to the more extensive service. Use such a code only when it is performed as a distinct, independent procedure, such as one performed during a different patient encounter, on a separate anatomic site, or not as part of another procedure. Apply modifier **-59** to alert the payer that you are reporting the code as a separate procedure.

Supplies such as procedure trays, drugs, supplies, and other materials beyond those normally included with the procedure should be reported separately. Use CPT code **99070** or a HCPCS code for the specific supply.

Because of the varied nature of procedures in the Medicine section, many subsections and categories begin with special instructions that provide additional guidelines and instructions for reporting specific procedures. Coders must read this information before assigning codes from these subsections to ensure they are properly using the codes. Frequent instructional notes in the Tabular List identify codes that may and may not be reported together, as well as cross-references to related codes.

SUCCESS STEP

As you read this chapter, also open your CPT manual and read the special instructions at the beginning of each subsection to become familiar with the guidelines.

ABSTRACTING MEDICINE PROCEDURES

Because there are so many different types of Medicine procedures, each subsection has its own abstracting rules. Some subsections require multiple sets of abstracting criteria because of

---

Table 32-2 ■ **KEY CRITERIA FOR ABSTRACTING MEDICINE PROCEDURES**

❑ What organ system or anatomic site is involved?
❑ Is the procedure diagnostic or therapeutic?
❑ What equipment and techniques are used?
❑ What is the quantity, duration, or frequency?
❑ Is the procedure part of a more extensive procedure?

Source: © PB Resources, Inc. Used with permission.

---

the wide variety of procedures included. In general, the information shown in ■ TABLE 32-2 provides a good starting point when approaching a case you are unfamiliar with. As you learn more about the specific services provided, refer to the specific abstracting tables in the discussion that follows. Finally, you will work through a detailed example for the Medicine section. Remember that the abstracting questions are a guide and that not every question applies to, or can be answered for, every case. For example, time is not a factor in every procedure.

Abstracting Immune Globulins and Immunizations

Providers of all specialties administer immunizations and immune globulins. Allergists and immunologists offer additional expertise. When the body's immune system fails or reduces in function, **immunodeficiency** results. Immunodeficiency can result from disease, an organ transplant, cancer treatment, or drug side effects. A person with immunodeficiency has a greater risk of becoming ill because his immune system cannot adequately produce antibodies to protect the body from diseases. Immunizations and immune globulins, also called immunoglobulins, assist the human body in achieving active and passive immunity (■ TABLE 32-3).

An **immunization** provides active immunity and consists of administering a vaccine (virus) or toxoid (bacteria). A **vaccine** contains antigens from a weakened strain of a virus so that the body will produce antibodies to fight it, but the person will not become ill. A **toxoid** contains bacteria that are nontoxic so that the immune system will produce antibodies, but the individual will not become ill. Later, if the person is exposed to the active virus or bacteria, then the immune system will recognize the pathogen and attack it.

Immune globulins provide passive immunity and consist of serum globulins or recombinant immune globulins. Serum globulins are proteins extracted from purified human blood plasma. Recombinant immune globulin products are created in a lab from human or animal proteins. Immune globulin protection wears off in a short period of time, typically a few months, and an individual could contract a specific disease after the effects of the immune globulin have worn off.

Protection against some conditions is available both as an immunization and as an immune globulin. Immunizations are administered as a preventive measure in patients who do not currently have, and have not been recently exposed to, a disease. Immune globulins are used when patients have already been exposed to a disease—called postexposure prophylaxis—or if their immune systems are compromised.

Table 32-3 ■ **TYPES OF IMMUNITY**

Type of Immunity	Description	Examples
Active immunity	The body's immune system produces antibodies to fight off a disease.	
Natural active immunity	A person is exposed to a disease pathogen, becomes ill, and then develops immunity toward the disease.	Chickenpox, measles, and mumps
Artificial active immunity	A person is exposed to a disease through an antigen from a vaccine or toxoid (bacteria), and then the immune system produces antibodies that attack the antigen so the person does not become ill.	Vaccines: hepatitis A, influenza virus, measles, and mumps Toxoids: diphtheria and tetanus
Passive immunity	The body's immune system receives antibodies to fight off a disease.	
Natural passive immunity	The fetus receives antibodies from the mother during gestation, which protect the baby for approximately the first six months of life.	Tetanus
Artificial passive immunity	A person receives an immune globulin that contains antibodies, which help to prevent a disease or lessen the effects of a disease to which a person has already been exposed.	Hepatitis B

■ TABLE 32-4 provides abstracting criteria for immunizations and immune globulins. Administering immunizations and immune globulins consists of two parts: the work or service of administering the injection and the actual immune globulin, vaccine, or toxoid product used, both of which are documented in the medical record. The service includes the route of administration and, for immunizations, whether counseling was provided to the family of a child. In addition, identify whether an additional E/M service was provided, such as a preventive care visit or evaluation of a health problem that created the need for the service.

Table 32-4 ■ **KEY CRITERIA FOR ABSTRACTING IMMUNIZATIONS AND IMMUNE GLOBULINS**

Immune Globulins:

❑ Is the administration method infusion or injection?

❑ Is the route subcutaneous (SQ), intramuscular (IM), intravenous (IV), or intra-arterial (IA)?

❑ How long does the infusion last?

❑ How many substances or drugs are injected?

❑ What substance(s) or drugs(s) is given?

Immunizations:

❑ What is the patient's age?

❑ Is counseling provided to the parents or family members of a child?

❑ How many vaccine components or combinations are administered?

❑ What is the route of administration of each vaccine or component?

❑ Is the vaccination provided in conjunction with a preventive medicine or other service?

❑ Is an immunization given for H1N1 influenza?

Source: © PB Resources, Inc. Used with permission.

Abstracting Psychiatry

Psychiatry services include diagnostic services, psychotherapy, and other services provided to an individual, family, or group. Psychiatry services are provided most often by a psychiatrist (MD), psychologist (PsyD), psychiatric mental health nurse practitioner (NP), clinical nurse specialist (CNS), or clinical social worker (CSW). Only psychiatrists and nurse practitioners can prescribe medication.

During a **psychiatric diagnostic interview**, or psychiatric exam, the provider assesses a patient's mental status by reviewing the patient's medical history, asking the patient a series of questions, and communicating with family members and other providers involved in the patient's care to determine the patient's diagnosis. The diagnostic interview is typically the first meeting with a patient to diagnose the patient and establish a plan for further treatment options. The interview may also be interactive, especially when treating children. The provider uses play equipment, such as dolls, to communicate with a patient who cannot or will not communicate verbally.

Psychotherapy involves the provider communicating face-to-face with the patient to determine the cause(s) of a specific condition and develop ways to effectively cope with it. Psychotherapy can be provided at the same time as medication management or medical evaluation and management services. The physician must document the components of an E/M service—history, exam, medical decision making—in addition to documentation of psychotherapy.

Psychotherapy can also be provided for families and in groups:

• **Family psychotherapy**—Family members meet with the clinician to discuss the patient's condition and how to help the patient. The patient may be present.

• **Group psychotherapy**—A group of patients with the same disorder meet with the clinician to share information to help

Table 32-5 ■ KEY CRITERIA FOR ABSTRACTING PSYCHIATRY

- ❑ What is the duration of psychotherapy services?
- ❑ Are services provided in a group or family setting?
- ❑ Is pharmacologic management provided?
- ❑ Is the service provided for crisis?
- ❑ Is interactive complexity required?
- ❑ Is testing or other services provided?
- ❑ Are separate E/M services provided?

Source: © PB Resources, Inc. Used with permission.

one another change their behaviors. An example is group psychotherapy for patients who suffer from anxiety disorders to help them to learn techniques to deal with their anxiety.

- **Multiple-family group psychotherapy**—A group of families who share the same problems meets to discuss the issues they are having. An example is a group made up of parents with children with behavioral problems. The clinician and families discuss ways to improve the children's behavior and learn effective parenting skills.

Other treatments that can be provided include electroconvulsive therapy (ECT) and hypnotherapy.

Physicians use ECT, also called shock treatment, to treat conditions such as depression when medications and psychotherapy fail. ECT involves placing the patient under anesthesia and attaching electrodes to his head. The electrodes deliver shocks to the brain and cause the patient to seize for a short time. ECT remains a controversial method of treating patients, as many clinicians feel that it causes brain damage or does not improve patients' conditions.

Hypnotherapy involves hypnotizing the patient to change specific behaviors, such as to stop smoking, lose weight, or cope with anxiety.

■ TABLE 32-5 provides abstracting criteria for psychiatry services. Psychotherapy services require coders to identify the length of time spent providing the service.

Psychiatry services have a component of **interactive complexity** when communication is challenging because of the involvement of third parties in addition to the patient, such as a parent, language interpreter, social agency, or law enforcement. Interactive complexity also includes maladaptive communication—high anxiety, repeated questions, disagreement, unhelpful caregiver emotions or behavior, mandated reporting, and use of play equipment or other physical devices to aid in communication.

Psychotherapy for crisis is an urgent assessment for a highly complex or life-threatening problem. Service includes a history of a crisis state, a mental status examination, and a final disposition or outcome. Treatment includes mobilization of resources to stabilize the crisis situation, psychotherapy, and other interventions to minimize the potential for psychological damage.

Abstracting Dialysis and ESRD Procedures

Dialysis is filtering the blood to remove impurities and toxins when the kidneys cannot perform this function. Nephrologists perform E/M and supervisory services related to dialysis.

Hemodialysis and inpatient peritoneal dialysis treatments are provided by registered nurses (RNs) specially trained in dialysis procedures and by dialysis technicians under physician supervision. Each patient's nephrologist provides a prescription for the frequency, duration, and other parameters of dialysis treatments. Physicians monitor and evaluate patients, typically one to four times per month, and adjust the dialysis prescription as needed.

Long-term dialysis, typically administered three times per week for three to four hours at a time, is provided for patients who have end-stage renal disease (ESRD). Patients need long-term dialysis to survive and receive dialysis for the rest of their lives or until they receive a kidney transplant. The only reason for long-term dialysis is ESRD, but ESRD can be caused by numerous conditions, including diabetes, primary or secondary glomerulonephritis, vasculitis, nephritis, hypertension, neoplasms, and various congenital diseases.

Short-term dialysis, typically consisting of a few treatments to several weeks of treatment, is provided for patients with acute renal failure (ARF) or certain other situations, such as a drug overdose, in which a substance needs to be removed from the blood. Patients receive short-term dialysis to recover from an acute condition but do not need it for the rest of their lives.

Both short-term and long-term dialysis patients can receive dialysis in hospitals or outpatient dialysis clinics. When properly trained, patients can administer dialysis at home, usually using **peritoneal dialysis**, a process in which the peritoneal membrane is used as the filtering agent.

Hemodialysis involves connecting a patient to dialysis equipment through a dialysis access, which consists of one of the following methods:

- inserting an intravenous (IV) catheter
- creating an arteriovenous (AV) fistula—anastomosis of an artery and vein to create a larger access route for blood
- implanting an AV graft—anastomosis of an artery and vein with a synthetic tube, called a graft, when an AV fistula does not work

Tubing is connected from the catheter, fistula, or graft to the dialysis machine. The patient's blood is circulated through an extracorporeal (*external to the body*) circuit, passed through a dialyzer fluid to filter toxins from the blood, and returned to the body, a process that takes several hours to complete.

■ TABLE 32-6 provides abstracting criteria for dialysis procedures. Coders must identify the type of service provided, the reason it was provided, the location of service, and the number of face-to-face physician encounters.

Abstracting Gastroenterology Procedures

Gastroenterologists perform gastric function studies to evaluate digestive processes. An esophageal **motility study**, also called **manometry**, evaluates muscular activity of the esophagus at rest and during swallowing to diagnose esophageal disorders involving motility or causes of heartburn.

An acid perfusion test, or Bernstein test, evaluates causes of heartburn. Physicians insert a nasogastric (NG) tube through the nose and into the esophagus. They introduce hydrochloric

Table 32-6 ■ KEY CRITERIA FOR ABSTRACTING DIALYSIS PROCEDURES

❑ What is the patient's age?

❑ Where is the service provided?

❑ Are the services ESRD related?

❑ What type of dialysis is provided: hemodialysis, peritoneal dialysis, hemofiltration, or other continuous replacement therapies?

❑ How many days of ESRD inpatient services are provided during the month?

❑ How many ESRD outpatient encounters with the physician occur during the month?

❑ Are ESRD dialysis services provided in the hospital, a clinic, or the home?

❑ Are separate evaluation and management services provided, in addition to dialysis-related evaluation and management?

❑ For inpatient dialysis, how many evaluations are required with the hemodialysis procedure?

Source: © PB Resources, Inc. Used with permission.

Table 32-7 ■ KEY CRITERIA FOR ABSTRACTING GASTROENTEROLOGY PROCEDURES

❑ What site in the gastrointestinal system is involved?

❑ What is the nature of the test?

❑ Is fluoroscopy or endoscopy used?

❑ Which components of the service are provided: professional, technical, or both?

Source: © PB Resources, Inc. Used with permission.

acid then saline solution into the esophagus to determine whether the patient experiences pain. No pain indicates a normal esophagus; pain could indicate acid reflux or another disorder, such as esophagitis.

A breath hydrogen test analyzes the patient's breath to determine normal concentrations of hydrogen and methane, followed by concentrations after introducing another substance, such as fructose (*sugar found in fruit*) or lactose (*sugar found in milk*), to determine whether the patient can adequately absorb the sugars or has an overgrowth of intestinal bacteria.

Electrogastrography uses electrodes to detect electrical activity of the stomach—gastrointestinal contractions—to diagnose stomach disorders.

■ TABLE 32-7 provides abstracting criteria for gastroenterology procedures. These are relatively straightforward to abstract because all that is needed is the nature of the test and the site involved. Identify services that involve fluoroscopy or endoscopy because these services are not coded from the Medicine section.

Abstracting Ophthalmology Services

Ophthalmology includes eye procedures such as exams, tests, and imaging. In addition to evaluation and management of eye conditions, ophthalmologists perform specialized assessments and procedures. An ophthalmologist (MD) is a physician who provides complete eye care, including medical and surgical care, and plastic surgery on the eye. An optometrist (OD) specializes in conducting eye examinations, diagnosing and treating vision disorders such as nearsightedness and farsightedness, and prescribing corrective lenses. A licensed dispensing optician (LDO) helps fit eyeglasses and contact lenses following prescriptions from ophthalmologists and optometrists. Specialized eye services include the following:

- **Gonioscopy**—Viewing the angle between the iris and cornea with a goniolens or gonioscope, a magnification lens with an attached mirror, to test for glaucoma.

- **Computerized corneal topography**—The clinician measures the shape and variations of the cornea when diseases or trauma cause it to be misshapen.

- **Tonometry**—Measuring intraocular pressure (IOP) in the eye with a tonometer to test for diseases such as glaucoma.

- **Ophthalmoscopy**—Viewing the inside of the eye with an ophthalmoscope, a viewing instrument with a lens and mirror.

- **Contact lens services**—Prescription, modification, and replacement of one or two contact lenses for the cornea or the cornea and sclera (corneoscleral).

- **Spectacle services**—Fitting and repairing various types of eyeglasses, depending on the type of eye disorder that the patient has.

SUCCESS STEP

Some specialties tend to have smaller group practices or consist of only one or two providers, such as ophthalmologists, audiologists, chiropractors, and physical therapists. Smaller practices can provide more accessible externship and employment options for new coders. They tend to work with fewer codes and often provide the opportunity to work in multiple areas of practice administration, such as patient registration, coding, billing, and insurance follow-up. This gives you a broad skill set that is an excellent foundation on which to build your career.

■ TABLE 32-8 provides abstracting criteria for ophthalmology services. Although it is always necessary to abstract a diagnosis that supports the services provided, in ophthalmology, some services are diagnosis specific, so you need to abstract the diagnosis to determine the correct CPT code. E/M services for ophthalmology appear in the Medicine section, not the

Table 32-8 ■ KEY CRITERIA FOR ABSTRACTING OPHTHALMOLOGY SERVICES

❑ Is a diagnostic and treatment program initiated? Is the patient new or established? Is the level of service intermediate or comprehensive?

❑ Is contact lens service provided?

❑ Is spectacle service provided?

❑ What ophthalmic condition(s) is treated?

❑ Is ophthalmoscopy performed?

❑ What other type(s) of ophthalmic services is provided?

❑ Is the service bilateral or unilateral?

Source: © PB Resources, Inc. Used with permission.

Evaluation and Management section. Intermediate ophthalmological services describe evaluation of a new diagnostic or management problem that requires a new treatment program. Comprehensive ophthalmological services describe a general evaluation of the complete visual system with initiation of a new treatment program. Definitions for new and established patients are the same as for other E/M services.

Identify any specialized ophthalmological services provided. Also identify the prescription and fitting of contact lenses and eyeglasses (spectacles).

Abstracting Hearing Services

In addition to physicians, speech-language pathologists and audiologists also provide some **otorhinolaryngological** (*pertaining to the ear, nose, and throat*) services. A speech-language pathologist (SLP), also called a speech therapist, assesses, diagnoses, treats, and helps to prevent disorders related to speech sounds and rhythm; understanding and producing language; cognitive communication; voice pitch and tone; swallowing; and fluency. A doctor of audiology (AuD), or audiologist, diagnoses and treats a patient's hearing and balance problems using advanced technology and procedures.

Speech, language, and swallowing difficulties can result from a variety of causes, including stroke, brain injury or deterioration, developmental delays or disorders, learning disabilities, cerebral palsy, cleft palate, voice pathology, intellectual disabilities, hearing loss, or emotional problems.

Audiologists examine patients of all ages and identify those with symptoms of hearing loss and other auditory issues, difficulties with balance, and related sensory and neural problems. Using audiometers, computers, and other testing devices, audiologists measure the volume at which a person begins to hear sounds, the ability to distinguish among sounds, and the impact of hearing loss on an individual's daily life. They also use computer equipment to evaluate and diagnose balance disorders. Audiologists interpret these results and may coordinate them with medical, educational, and psychological information to make a diagnosis and determine a course of treatment. Audiologists who diagnose and treat balance disorders often work in collaboration with physicians and physical and occupational therapists.

■ TABLE 32-9 provides abstracting criteria for hearing services. Certain diagnostic and treatment procedures are included

Table 32-9 ■ KEY CRITERIA FOR ABSTRACTING HEARING SERVICES

❑ Is an Evaluation and Management (E/M) service provided?
❑ Is the service diagnostic or therapeutic?
❑ What anatomic site(s) is evaluated or treated?
❑ What specific tests are performed?
❑ What is the purpose of any evaluation service(s) provided?
❑ How much time is spent providing the evaluation?
❑ For speech-related services, does the service evaluate speech production and language abilities or does it evaluate the effect of residual hearing abilities on speech formation?
❑ What is the purpose of any therapy provided?
❑ What devices, tools, or equipment are used?

Source: © PB Resources, Inc. Used with permission.

with evaluation and management services, such as otoscopy, anterior rhinoscopy, tuning fork test, and removal of impacted cerumen. Do not abstract these as separate procedures. Identify only services that are above and beyond an E/M service.

Coders must identify the specific site and function of the ear-nose-throat system that was evaluated or treated. Identifying any tools or equipment used also helps to determine the correct code.

Abstracting Cardiovascular Procedures

Cardiologists perform a variety of cardiovascular procedures to diagnose and treat heart disorders. Some of these procedures can be complex and involved.

Take time to review the anatomy of the heart and great vessels, also called the coronary arteries, because coronary anatomy provides the foundation for assigning the correct procedure codes (■ FIGURE 32-1). Anatomy books may use alternative names and designations of the coronary arteries. In addition, the precise anatomy and branches of the coronary arteries varies from one person to the next. For coding purposes, CPT recognizes five major coronary arteries and up to two branches of each. The **coronary arteries** are shown in boldface type and the *branches* of the coronary arteries are shown in italics.

- **Left main coronary artery (LM)**
- **Left anterior descending artery (LAD)**
  - *Diagonal* branches (D1, D2)
- **Circumflex artery (LCX)**
  - *Marginal* (M1, M2) or *obtuse marginal* (OM1, OM2) branches
- **Ramus intermedius artery** (appears only in 15% of patients; is located between the LAD and LCX)
  - No branches
- **Right coronary artery (RCA)**
  - *Posterior descending* (PDA) or *posterior intraventricular* (PIV) branches
  - *Posteroloateral* branches (PLB)

Cardiovascular procedures that appear in the Medicine section are performed to diagnose a variety of cardiac conditions, which may be treated with other Medicine section procedures or may require surgical intervention (■ TABLE 32-10). Separate abstracting criteria are provided for interventional cardiology (■ TABLE 32-11, page 564), evaluation of cardiac devices (■ TABLE 32-12, page 564), electrophysiological studies (■ TABLE 32-13, page 564), and cardiac catheterization (■ TABLE 32-14, page 565).

SUCCESS STEP

The original abbreviation of electrocardiogram is EKG, which reflects both the Greek word *kardia*, meaning heart, and the German spelling *electrokardiogram*. The more recent abbreviation ECG reflects the English spelling. Both abbreviations are correct, and some people prefer EKG because it is more easily distinguished from EEG (electroencephalogram) and ECC (echocardiogram).

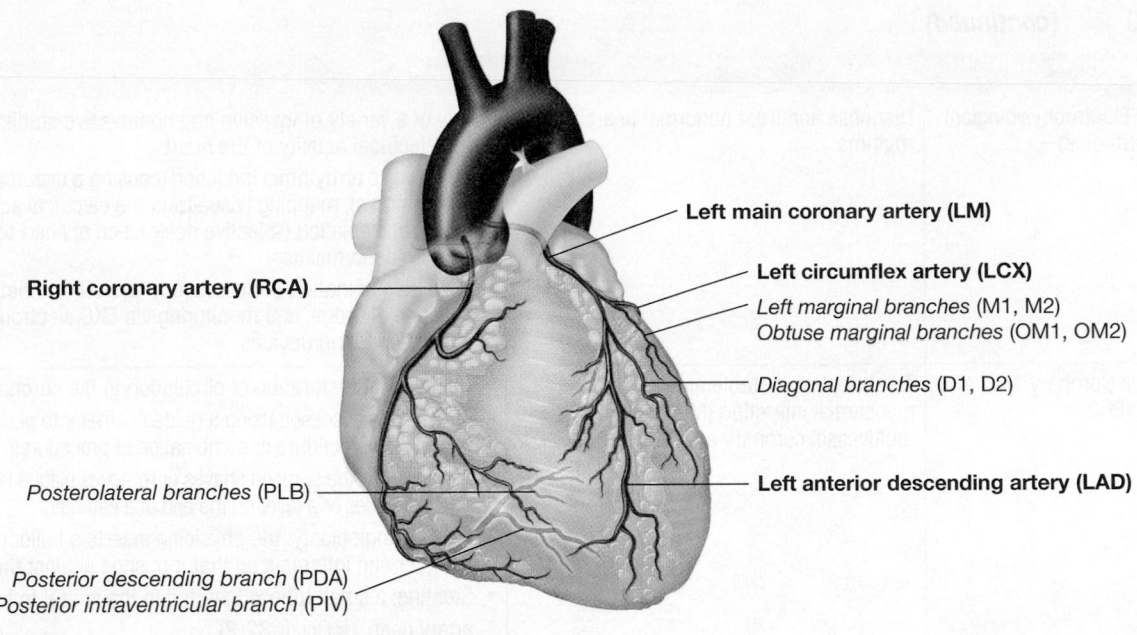

Figure 32-1 ■ Coronary Arteries Recognized by CPT

Table 32-10 ■ CARDIOVASCULAR PROCEDURES

Procedure	Purpose	Description
Angiography	Diagnose blockages; visualize vessels to guide catheter placement for diagnostic or therapeutic procedures	• Use of contrast dyes and X-rays to view the inside of vessels • Performed as part of some cardiovascular procedures
Cardiac Catheterization	View blood circulation and detect blockages affecting the heart, the coronary arteries, and the aorta	• Threading an IV catheter into the patient's vein (usually the femoral vein) to a site in the heart, aorta, or coronary arteries • A contrast dye is injected through the catheter, giving the physician a picture of the coronary vessel patency. • The image is viewed on a monitor.
Cardiopulmonary Resuscitation (CPR)	Treatment to revive a patient who has stopped breathing	Use of manual chest compressions and artificial respiration
Cardiovascular Stress Test	Monitor the heart's activity when the patient is exercising; diagnose the causes of symptoms such as chest pain	• Placement of multiple leads on the patient's chest while patient exercises on a treadmill or bicycle • The heart's response to activity is recorded on a graph, similar to EKG tracings. • Pharmacologic stress test: When a patient is unable to exercise, medication that mimics the effect of exercise on the heart is administered.
Cardioversion	Treatment of arrhythmias, such as atrial fibrillation	• Use of a low electrical current to restore normal heart rhythm • With the patient under moderate sedation, patches are placed both over the heart and to the side of the heart.
Echocardiography	View the anatomic structures of the heart	• Use of sound waves to create a moving picture of the heart • A transducer is placed on the external chest wall that sends sound waves through the chest. • The picture is more detailed than a plain X-ray image and involves no radiation exposure.
Electrocardiogram (ECG or EKG)	Monitor heart rhythm and diagnose abnormal heart rhythm	• Placement of electrode leads on the patient's chest, arms, and legs • Results are transmitted to an EKG machine that produces a graph of the electrical activity of the heart, heart rate, and any abnormal rhythm.

(continued)

Table 32-10 ■ *(continued)*

Procedure	Purpose	Description
Intracardiac Electrophysiological Studies (EP Studies)	Diagnose and treat abnormal heart rhythms	• Any of a variety of invasive and noninvasive studies to assess the electrical activity of the heart • Can involve arrhythmia induction (causing a disturbance in the heart rhythm), mapping (visualizing the electrical activity of the heart), and ablation (selective destruction of heart tissue causing abnormalities) • Uses a combination of fluoroscopy-assisted catheterization, injection of drugs, and monitoring via EKG electrodes and other monitoring devices
Percutaneous Coronary Intervention (PCI)	Treatment of unstable angina, acute myocardial infarction (MI), and multivessel coronary artery disease (CAD)	• Nonsurgical restoration of circulation to the coronary vessel • The heart is accessed using a guided catheter to perform a therapeutic procedure or combination of procedures. • Atherectomy: the surgeon shaves or removes plaque using tiny rotating blades or a laser on the end of a catheter. • Balloon angioplasty: the physician inserts a balloon through the catheter and inflates it so that it pushes against the artery wall. • Stenting: a small tube is inserted in the vessel to keep the artery open. (■ FIGURE 32-2)

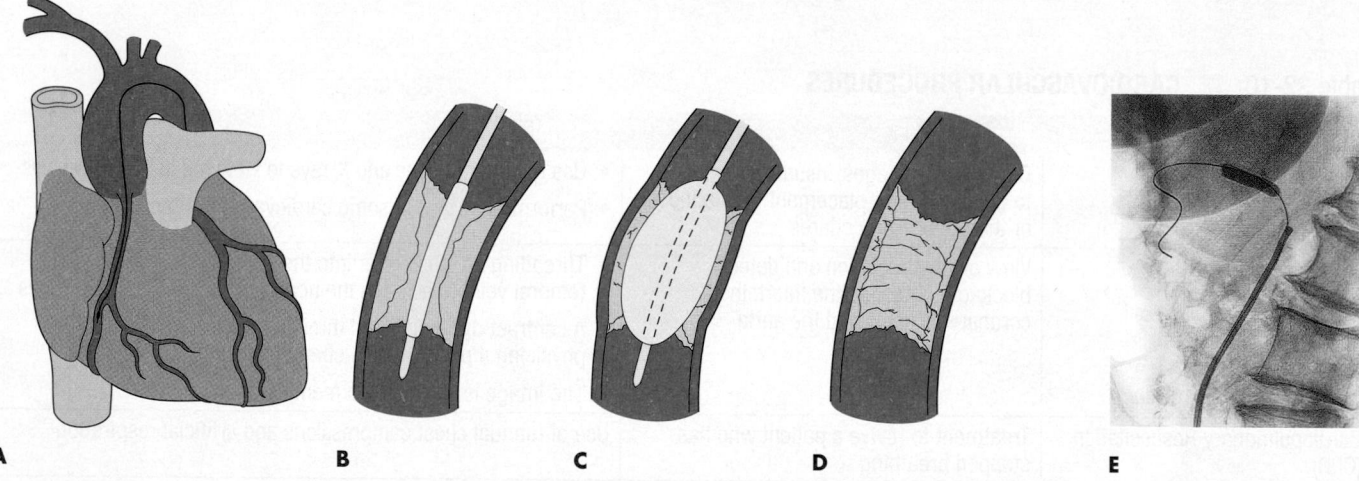

A   **B**   **C**   **D**   **E**

Figure 32-2 ■ Balloon Angioplasty Procedure. (A) The balloon catheter is threaded into the affected coronary artery. (B) The balloon is positioned across the area of obstruction. (C) The balloon is inflated. (D) Balloon is removed, leaving plaque flattened against the arterial wall. (E) X-ray angiogram of balloon catheter. *Source: Du Cane Medical Imaging Ltd./Photo Researchers, Inc.*

Table 32-11 ■ KEY CRITERIA FOR ABSTRACTING INTERVENTIONAL CARDIOVASCULAR PROCEDURES

❑ Is the procedure diagnostic or therapeutic (interventional)?
❑ How many and which coronary arteries are treated?
❑ Which branches of each coronary artery are treated?
❑ How many grafted vessels are treated?
❑ Is contrast dye used?
❑ Is a stent or balloon used?
❑ Is intravascular Doppler velocity or coronary flow measured?

Diagnostic Angiography:

❑ Is angiography performed at the same time as a coronary interventional procedure?
❑ Has the patient previously had angiography performed?
❑ Has there been a change in the patient's clinical indicators since the previous angiography?

Source: © PB Resources, Inc. Used with permission.

Table 32-12 ■ KEY CRITERIA FOR ABSTRACTING EVALUATION OF CARDIAC DEVICES

❑ What type of device is evaluated?
❑ How many leads does the device have?
❑ What type of evaluation is performed?
❑ Are programming services performed?
❑ Which components of the service are provided: professional, technical, or both?

Source: © PB Resources, Inc. Used with permission.

Table 32-13 ■ KEY CRITERIA FOR ABSTRACTING ELECTROPHYSIOLOGICAL STUDIES

❑ Which site(s) is evaluated?
❑ Is pacing performed?
❑ Is a comprehensive electrophysiologic evaluation performed?
❑ Which specific elements are evaluated?

Source: © PB Resources, Inc. Used with permission.

Table 32-14 ■ KEY CRITERIA FOR ABSTRACTING CARDIAC CATHETERIZATION

❑ Is catheterization performed for congenital heart disease?

❑ For catheterization procedures, which site(s) is catheterized: right heart, left heart, coronary arteries, bypass grafts?

❑ Is contrast dye used?

❑ Is catheterization accompanied by any of the following:

  • transeptal or transapical puncture

  • pharmacological study

  • exercise study

  • injection procedure for selective right ventricular or left atrial angiography; supravalvular aortography; pulmonary angiography

❑ Which components of the catheterization service are provided: professional, technical, or both?

❑ Is another procedure such as revascularization with a stent or balloon performed?

Source: © PB Resources, Inc. Used with permission.

Tables 32-11 through 32-14 provide abstracting criteria for a variety of cardiovascular procedures.

Abstracting Noninvasive Vascular Studies

Noninvasive vascular diagnostic studies include specialized services to study veins and arteries other than the heart and great vessels. Conventional ultrasound bounces sound waves off blood vessels and a computer creates a black and white moving image on a screen. Doppler ultrasound uses short bursts of sound to create an image that shows the speed and direction of blood flow. The image can be color coded to highlight blockages. Duplex scans combine conventional ultrasound with Doppler ultrasound. Duplex scans are useful to diagnose carotid artery occlusive disease, deep vein thrombosis, peripheral artery disease, aortoiliac occlusive disease, varicose veins, and abdominal aneurysms. ■ TABLE 32-15 provides abstracting criteria for noninvasive vascular studies.

Allergy Procedures

Allergists and immunologists most commonly perform allergy procedures. An allergy is an abnormal reaction of the human immune system. It wrongly identifies certain allergens as harmful foreign bodies and produces antibodies against them. When these antibodies are produced in excess, they release histamine and other chemicals in the body, which in turn results in an

Table 32-15 ■ KEY CRITERIA FOR ABSTRACTING NONINVASIVE VASCULAR STUDIES

❑ What body region is evaluated?

❑ Does the study involve arteries, veins, or both?

❑ What technique(s) or equipment is used?

❑ Is the study limited or complete?

❑ Is the study unilateral or bilateral?

Source: © PB Resources, Inc. Used with permission.

Table 32-16 ■ KEY CRITERIA FOR ABSTRACTING ALLERGY PROCEDURES

Allergy Testing:

❑ What method(s) of testing is used: percutaneous, intracutaneous, or inhalation?

❑ What type(s) of test is performed: allergenic extracts, venoms, biologicals, or food?

❑ How many tests of each type were performed?

Immunotherapy:

❑ Is the service injection only, provision of antigen *and* injection, or provision of antigen only?

Source: © PB Resources, Inc. Used with permission.

allergic reaction. **Allergy testing** is a skin or inhalation test to expose a patient to an allergen to determine whether it causes an allergic response. **Allergen immunotherapy** exposes a patient to allergenic extracts or insect venoms to decrease his sensitivity to the allergen, a process called desensitization.

■ TABLE 32-16 provides abstracting criteria for allergy procedures. When immunotherapy is performed, you must identify whether the medical office or the patient provided the allergen extract.

Abstracting Neurology Procedures

Neurologists specialize in conditions that affect the nervous system. They provide a wide range of tests to diagnose and treat neurological conditions.

Sleep testing is performed while the patient sleeps to assess various body functions to diagnose sleep disorders such as sleep apnea, insomnia, narcolepsy, and somnambulism. Tests include polysomnography, which includes multiple measurements of functions and activities of the heart, muscles, brain, and eyes during sleep.

Several types of tests evaluate the function and responsiveness of nerves and muscles, including evoked potentials and reflex tests, needle electromyography (EMG), nerve conduction studies, range of motion studies, and other tests.

Electroencephalography (EEG) records the electrical activity of the brain and produces a graphical report. A routine EEG usually requires 20 to 40 minutes but can be conducted for longer amounts of time. Specialized EEG monitoring can last for several days. EEG is used to diagnose seizures, epilepsy, sleep disorders, coma, encephalopathies, and brain death.

Intraoperative neurophysiology monitoring (IONM), also called surgical neurophysiology, is used during procedures that pose a risk to the nervous system. A variety of neurological modalities, such as EEG, EMG, and evoked potentials, detect changes in nerve, spinal cord, and brain activity. This provides to the surgeon real-time information that helps avoid or minimize complications such as paralysis, hearing loss, or stroke.

Central nervous system assessments evaluate the cognitive (*intellectual*) function of the central nervous system. Several types of written tests and standardized functional assessments are used, depending on the specific type of information desired, such as reasoning ability, speech, visual response, and so on.

Table 32-17 ■ KEY CRITERIA FOR ABSTRACTING NEUROLOGY PROCEDURES

❏ What site(s) is treated?

❏ What testing method(s) is used?

❏ How many studies or tests are performed?

❏ How long does a recording last, if performed?

❏ Are all services—recording, interpretation, and report—provided?

Sleep Studies:

❏ How old is the patient?

❏ What parameters are measured?

❏ Is the testing attended, unattended, or remote?

❏ Which components of the service are provided: professional, technical, or both?

Source: © PB Resources, Inc. Used with permission.

The tests produce quantitative data that is compiled and interpreted in a report written by a physician.

■ TABLE 32-17 provides abstracting criteria for neurology procedures.

CODING CAUTION

Be attentive to acronyms that are similar but identify different tests:

ECG/EKG—electrocardiogram—a recording of the electrical activity of the heart

ECC—echocardiogram—image of the heart made using sound waves

EEG—electroencephalogram—a recording of the electrical activity of the brain

EMG—electromyogram—a recording of the electrical activity of a muscle

Abstracting Infusion and Injection Procedures

Patients may need certain medications delivered under direct physician supervision, by infusion or injection, because of the nature of their condition, the type of drug needed, or other special considerations. In general, these methods deliver the medication more quickly than oral administration. The route of administration can be subcutaneous (SQ), intravenous (IV), intramuscular (IM), or intra-arterial (IA) (■ FIGURE 32-3).

Injections and infusions can be administered directly into the site or through an access port. Ports are used to avoid repeatedly penetrating the vein with a needle. An access port is a small medical appliance implanted under the skin, with a **catheter** (*small tube*) that connects to the vein. Intravenous and intra-arterial administration of drugs can be accomplished through the **infusion technique** (*a slow, steady rate of release of medication over a long period of time*) or the **push technique** (*a one-time, rapid injection of medication into the bloodstream*). When infusion is performed, a bag or bottle of solution containing the medication is hung on a stand and is connected to the site with tubing. The push technique is also called a **bolus**.

Physician services involve approval of the treatment plan and direct supervision of staff administering the procedure, usually an RN. Infusion services include the use of local anesthesia, starting the IV, accessing the indwelling catheter or port, flushing, and standard tubing, syringes, and supplies. A single drug or multiple drugs can be administered. Multiple drugs can be administered concurrently (*at the same time*) or sequentially (*one after the other*). The purpose of infusion can be any of the following:

- **Hydration**—replenishing fluid lost through dehydration, such as vomiting, diarrhea, and alcohol-related illnesses

- **Therapy**—treatment of an illness or condition, such as antibiotic administration for a serious infection

- **Prophylaxis**—preventive purposes, such as an antibiotic before surgery

- **Diagnosis**—diagnostic purposes, such as to measure the uptake or absorption of a substance

- **Chemotherapy**—antineoplastic drugs, highly complex drugs, or biologic agents for treatment of cancer or other conditions, such as cyclophosphamide for autoimmune conditions. In addition to the customary subcutaneous, intramuscular, and intravenous routes, chemotherapy can be administered via additional routes, including intra-arterial,

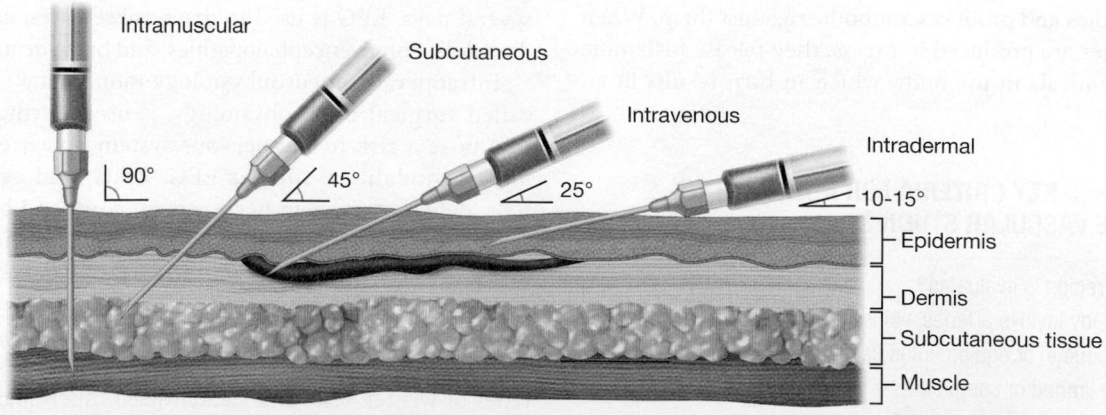

Figure 32-3 ■ Routes of Injection Administration.

Table 32-18 ■ KEY CRITERIA FOR ABSTRACTING INFUSION AND INJECTION PROCEDURES

- ❑ What is the purpose of the infusion?
- ❑ What is the route of administration?
- ❑ What administration technique is used?
- ❑ How long does the administration last?

Source: © PB Resources, Inc. Used with permission.

intralesional, intrathecal, subarachnoid, and into the pleural or peritoneal cavities.

■ TABLE 32-18 provides abstracting criteria for infusion and injection procedures.

Abstracting Physical Medicine, Osteopathic, and Chiropractic

Physical medicine and rehabilitation includes physical therapy (PT) and occupational therapy (OT) and involves evaluations, exercises, tests, and wound care management, including debridement. Services are provided for patients with any number of disorders, including physical and neurological conditions. Therapists may treat patients after a stroke or motor vehicle accident to help them to regain their physical and mental strength and abilities.

An osteopathic physician (DO), or osteopath, manually performs osteopathic manipulative treatment (OMT), which involves moving joints and muscles through various methods, such as applying pressure. This treatment can help to alleviate disorders such as migraine headaches and carpal tunnel syndrome.

A doctor of chiropractic (DC), or chiropractor, is a healthcare professional who focuses on improving patients' conditions by manipulating body areas, typically the spine, to improve the structure and function of specific sites. Chiropractors manually massage, adjust, and manipulate the spinal column to treat conditions such as low-back pain. They cannot prescribe medications in most states.

■ TABLE 32-19 provides abstracting criteria for physical medicine procedures.

CODING CAUTION

A doctor of osteopathy is a DO. A doctor of optometry is an OD. An ophthalmologist is an MD.

Table 32-19 ■ KEY CRITERIA FOR ABSTRACTING PHYSICAL MEDICINE PROCEDURES

- ❑ What site(s) is treated?
- ❑ What type of evaluation or assessment is performed (if any)?
- ❑ What modality is used?
- ❑ Is the service supervised or constant attendance?
- ❑ What is the duration of treatment for each modality?
- ❑ How many spinal or body regions were treated by a chiropractor or osteopath?

Source: © PB Resources, Inc. Used with permission.

Guided Example of Abstracting Medicine Services

Refer to the following example throughout this chapter to practice skills for abstracting, assigning, and arranging Medicine codes. Cardiovascular therapy is used as an example because it is among the more challenging services to code. Coding services in each subsection of Medicine vary based on the specific type of procedure.

OUTPATIENT HOSPITAL   Gender: M   Age: 62

Preprocedure diagnosis: ASHD with angina

Procedure: Catheterization for coronary angiography and stenting. Moderate sedation was administered. Catheterization was performed with access through the right femoral artery. Dye was injected to visualize the coronary arteries, noting significant plaque in the RCA. We proceeded to open the vessel with a stent. (Professional component provided.)

Postprocedure diagnosis: 75% blockage of RCA due to lipid-rich plaque

---

Follow along as fictitious coder Ladonna Shuck, CPC, abstracts the procedure. Check off each step after you complete it.

▶ Ladonna reads through the entire record, paying special attention to the reason for the encounter and the final assessment. She refers to the Key Criteria for Abstracting Cardiac Catheterization (Table 32-14).

- ❑ She notes the preprocedure diagnosis of ASHD and the postprocedure diagnosis of 75% blockage of RCA.

- ❑ *For catheterization procedures, which site(s) is catheterized?* coronary arteries

- ❑ *Is catheterization accompanied with any of the following?*
  - ▪ *Transseptal or transapical puncture.* No
  - ▪ *Pharmacological study.* No
  - ▪ *Exercise study.* No.
  - ▪ *Injection procedure for selective right ventricular or left atrial angiography; supravalvular aortography; pulmonary angiography.* No.

- ❑ *Is the professional component, technical component, or both components of catheterization provided?* Professional component only.

- ❑ *Is another procedure such as revascularization with a stent or balloon performed?* Yes, in the RCA.

- ❑ At this time, Ladonna does not know which services may need to be coded, nor how many codes she will end up with. She will learn about this when she moves on to assigning codes.

CODING PRACTICE

Exercise 32.2 Abstracting for Medicine Procedures

Instructions: Read the mini-medical-record of each patient's encounter and answer the abstracting questions. Write the answer on the line provided. Do not assign any codes.

1. OFFICE Gender: F Age: 67

Reason for encounter: *referred by PCP due to extreme depression since death of husband 6 months ago*

Procedure: *psychiatric diagnostic examination that included a history and review of diagnostic and laboratory studies*

Assessment: *depressive state with tremors*

a. What is the duration of psychotherapy services?

_____

b. Are services provided in a group or family setting?

_____

c. Is pharmacologic management provided?

_____

d. Is the service provided for crisis? _____

e. Is testing or other services provided?

_____

f. Are separate E/M services provided?

_____

2. INPATIENT HOSPITAL Gender: F Age: 31

Preprocedure diagnosis: *acute renal failure*

Procedure: *hemodialysis with two evaluations due to hypotensive episode after onset of treatment*

a. What is the patient's age? _____

b. Where is the service provided? _____

c. Are the services ESRD related? _____

d. What type of dialysis is provided: hemodialysis, peritoneal dialysis, hemofiltration, or other continuous replacement therapies? _____

e. Are separate evaluation and management services provided, in addition to dialysis-related evaluation and management? _____

f. For inpatient dialysis, how many evaluations are required with the hemodialysis procedure?

_____

3. HOSPITAL SLEEP LAB Gender: F Age: 31

Reason for encounter: *"I feel tired all the time."*

Assessment: *insomnia*

(continued)

3. (continued)

Procedure: *sleep study, attended by technologist, simultaneous recording of ventilation, respiratory effort, heart rate, and oxygen saturation*

Plan: *severe obstructive sleep apnea based on interpretation of sleep study. Refer to pulmonologist for further treatment.*

a. How old is the patient? _____

b. What parameters are measured? _____

c. Is the testing attended, unattended, or remote?

_____

4. OFFICE Gender: F Age: 8

Reason for encounter: *annual preventive care checkup for established patient*

Procedure: *Comprehensive periodic preventive medicine examination. Updated immunizations: IM injection TdaP (diphtheria, tetanus toxoid, acellular pertussis); oral poliovirus.*

Plan: *Counseled mother regarding potential side effects and signs to be observant for. Call office with any concerns.*

a. What is the patient's age? _____

b. How many vaccine components or combinations are administered? _____

c. What is the route of administration of each vaccine or component? _____

d. Is the vaccination provided in conjunction with a preventive medicine or other service?

_____

e. Is an immunization given for H1N1 influenza?

_____

5. OFFICE (Physical therapy) Gender: M Age: 42

Reason for encounter: *referred by PCP for therapy for low-back strain while playing golf*

Procedure: *Initial physical therapy evaluation; 15 minutes of manual electrical stimulation; 15 minutes of therapeutic exercises to increase ROM and flexibility; 15 minutes of alternating hot and cold packs*

Plan: *return 3x week for 2 weeks, per physician's order*

a. What site(s) is treated? _____

b. What type of evaluation or assessment is performed (if any)? _____

c. What modality is used? _____

(continued)

5. (continued)

d. Is the service supervised or constant attendance?

_____

e. What is the duration of treatment for each modality?

_____

6. INPATIENT HOSPITAL Gender: M Age: 72

Reason for admission: STEMI of LAD with thrombus

Procedure: Percutaneous transluminal revascularization during acute myocardial infarction using angiography. Stent and thrombectomy for acute total occlusion of LAD. Both diagonals show evidence

(continued)

6. (continued)

of chronic subtotal occlusion. Balloon angioplasty on D1 and D2 due to chronic subtotal occlusion.

a. Is the procedure diagnostic or therapeutic (interventional)? _____

b. How many and which coronary arteries are treated?

_____

c. Which branches of each coronary artery are treated?

_____

d. Is contrast dye used? _____

e. Is a stent or balloon used? _____

f. What is the extent of the occlusion in each site?

_____

ASSIGNING CODES FOR MEDICINE PROCEDURES

Because the Medicine section contains a wide range of services, coders must be certain to thoroughly read the guidelines, special instructions, and instructional notes that appear throughout the section. As you learn more about assigning Medicine section codes, follow along in your CPT manual and locate the codes and guidelines as they are discussed.

Immune Globulins and Immunizations (90281-90399, 90460-90749)

To assign CPT codes for immune globulins and immunizations, assign a code for the administration and an additional code(s) for the product(s) administered. The steps for assigning codes are discussed separately for immune globulins and immunizations. Diagnoses that support the administration of immune globulins and immunizations often are disorders from ICD-10-CM Chapter 1, **Certain Infectious and Parasitic Diseases (A00-B99)**; Chapter 18, **Symptoms, Signs, Abnormal Clinical and Laboratory Findings (R00-R99)**; Chapter 21, **Factors Influencing Health Status and Contact With Health Services (Z00-Z99)**, or the body system chapter of the affected system.

Immune Globulins

The following information outlines the steps required to assign codes for immunization administration and the product administered.

Immune Globulin Administration Immune globulin administration identifies the method and route of administration. Assign an administration code for each substance administered, as follows:

1. Search the Index for the Main Term **Immune Globulin Administration**.
2. Select the first-level modifying term **Intravenous Infusion** or **Injection** to identify the method. Identify the code(s) or code range.

3. In the Tabular List, review the codes to select the appropriate description of route and time or quantity.

In the Tabular List, infusion codes are subdivided by route (IV or SQ) and time. The parent codes for intravenous (**96365**) and subcutaneous (**96369**) identify the first hour of infusion. Add-on codes identify each additional hour and additional substances. Additional substances can be administered either sequentially or concurrently.

Injection codes are subdivided by route: subcutaneous or intramuscular (**96372**), intra-arterial (**96373**), and intravenous push (**96374**). Report additional injections using the same route (SQ/IM, IA) with an additional unit or quantity of the code. Add-on codes report additional IV push injections, divided by whether a new substance (**96375**) or the same substance (**96376**) is injected. Assign a separate administration code for each substance or dug administered.

Codes for administration contain a parenthetical instructional note that states (**specify substance or drug**). This note reminds coders to assign an additional code to identify the product.

Immune Globulin Product The immune globulin product identifies the substance administered. Assign a code for each immune globulin product, as follows:

1. Search the Index for the Main Term **Immune Globulins**.
2. Select the first-level modifying term to identify the type of substance.

ESRD patient, age 45, who receives hemodialysis service in the dialysis clinic 3 times per week, is hospitalized for 4 days. The nephrologist evaluates the patient daily while in the hospital and orders 2 hemodialysis procedures by the dialysis staff. The nephrologist also evaluates the patient 3 times as an outpatient during the month.

90935 x 2 Hemodialysis procedure with single evaluation by a physician or other qualified health care professional

90961 x 1 End-stage renal disease (ESRD) related services monthly, for patients 20 years of age and older; with 2–3 face-to-face visits by a physician or other qualified health care professional per month

Note: Also report Inpatient E/M codes (**99221–99233**) for the encounters on the two days when no hemodialysis procedure was performed.

Figure 32-6 ■ Example of Coding ESRD Services

13 times per month. They typically are evaluated by a physician one to four times per month. Codes identify the number of face-to-face physician visits during the month, not the number of clinic encounters to receive dialysis.

Clinic and home-based services are identified using codes that report a full month of physician services, when provided (**90963-90966**). When less than a full month of services is provided, codes **90951-90962** identify the number of outpatient services provided during the month.

Inpatient services are reported for each face-to-face physician encounter. When a patient from a dialysis clinic is hospitalized, inpatient dialysis services are almost always provided. Report inpatient dialysis codes for a hemodialysis procedure with physician evaluation. Report partial month outpatient dialysis services with the code that identifies the correct number of outpatient physician encounters (■ FIGURE 32-6). ■ TABLE 32-20 summarizes the division of ESRD codes by location, number of physician visits, and age.

Inpatient and outpatient services include all evaluation and management related to the dialysis procedure. E/M services not related to dialysis should be reported separately using the appropriate E/M code with modifier **-25 Significant, separately identifiable evaluation and management service**.

All patients with ESRD require a first-listed diagnosis of **N18.6 End stage renal disease** for dialysis-related services and the additional diagnosis **Z99.2 Dependence on renal dialysis**. Additional **Z** codes are available to report fitting and adjustment of a dialysis catheter (**Z49.0-**) and patient noncompliance with dialysis (**Z91.15**). In addition, physicians may identify additional diagnoses for the underlying causes of ESRD and any comorbidities.

Diagnoses for patients undergoing short-term dialysis may include acute renal failure (**N17.-**), drug overdose, and injury to the kidneys. In addition, physicians may identify additional diagnoses for the underlying causes of acute renal failure (ARF) and any comorbidities.

Gastroenterology Procedures (91010-91299)

The Gastroenterology subsection does not provide any special instructions. Frequent instructional notes appear in the Tabular List; these direct coders to codes for specific types of tests and also identify codes that can and cannot be used together. To assign codes for gastroenterology procedures, use one of the following methods to locate the Main Term in the Index.

1. Search for the Main Term **Gastric Tests**, then select the first-level modifying term, **Acid Reflux** or **Motility**, for the type of test. Identify the code(s) or code range to verify in the Tabular List.

2. Search for name or type of test as the Main Term, such as:

   - **Reflux Study**
   - **Manometric Studies**
   - **Manometry**
   - **Motility Study**

Some tests, such as manometric studies and motility studies, can be performed at a variety of anatomic sites, so

Table 32-20 ■ CODES FOR HEMODIALYSIS PHYSICIAN SERVICES

Location	Number of Physician Visits	Codes by Age Group			
		<2 Years	**2–11 Years**	**12–19 Years**	**≥20 Years**
ESRD inpatient	1 evaluation per treatment	90935	90935	90935	90935
	Repeated evaluations	90937	90937	90937	90937
ESRD clinic	1/month	90953	90956	90959	90962
	2–3/month	90952	90955	90958	90961
	≥4/month	90951	90954	90957	90960
ESRD home dialysis	Full month	90963	90964	90965	90966
ESRD clinic or home	Per day (less than a full month)	90967	90968	90969	90970
Non-ESRD	One (1) evaluation per treatment	90935-90937			

Source: © PB Resources, Inc. Used with permission. CPT codes © American Medical Association.

be certain to select the code for the correct site. Identify the code(s) or code range to verify in the Tabular List.

3. Search for the anatomic site as the Main Term, such as **Esophagus**. Locate an appropriate subterm for the procedure, such as **acid reflux, acid perfusion, balloon distention provocation study, imaging studies**. Some tests, such as manometric studies and motility studies, can be performed at a variety of anatomic sites, so be certain to select the code for the correct site.

In the Tabular List, review the codes in the relevant range and select the code that accurately describes the service provided. There are only a few add-on codes and indented codes in this subsection, so code selection tends to be straightforward. Read the instructional notes that identify codes that cannot be reported together.

Most of the procedures in the Gastroenterology subsection consist of technical and professional components, so the appropriate modifier **-26 Professional component** or **-TC Technical component** should be used as appropriate.

Diagnoses that support gastroenterology procedures most often come from ICD-10-CM Chapter 11, **Diseases of the Digestive System (K00-K95)**, or Chapter 18, **Symptoms, Signs, Abnormal Clinical and Laboratory Findings (R00-R99)**.

Ophthalmology and Hearing Services (92002-92499, 92502-92700)

Ophthalmology services include general and special ophthalmological services, as well as contact lens and spectacle services. Hearing services include a variety of evaluation and testing services.

To assign codes from these subsections, follow these steps.

1. For ophthalmological services:
   - Search the Index for the Main Term **Ophthalmology, Diagnostic**.
   - Locate the name of the specific service as the Main Term, such as **Gonioscopy** or **Contact Lens Service**.

2. For hearing services:
   - Search the Index for the Main Term **Audiologic Function Tests**, **Vestibular Function Tests**, or **Audiometry**, as appropriate.
   - To locate codes by anatomic site, locate the Main Term **Ear, Nose, and Throat**. This entry is separate from the Main Term **Ear** alone.

3. If necessary, locate the appropriate modifying term(s) that describes the specific service provided. Identify the code(s) or code range.

4. Refer to the Tabular List to select and verify the appropriate code based on the type and extent of service.

The Tabular List provides special instructions for the Ophthalmology subsection that contain detailed definitions for intermediate, comprehensive, and special ophthalmological services. Coders must be familiar with these definitions so they know the services included in each category of codes.

The subheading **General Ophthalmological Services (92001-92014)** provides codes for services that do not meet the criteria of Evaluation and Management (E/M) codes, such as yearly eye exams. The definitions of new and established patients are the same as for E/M codes, but the levels of service are different, as described in the special instructions. Do not assign an E/M code in addition to, or in place of, codes **92001** through **92014**.

Codes under the subheading **Special Ophthalmological Services (92015-92287)** describe tests that evaluate a particular part of the visual system. Assign these codes in addition to E/M codes and codes for **General Ophthalmological Services**, as appropriate.

Codes in the subheading **Contact Lens Services (92310-92326)** include the prescription, fitting, patient education, and follow-up related to contact lenses. Codes are divided by who provides the fitting and whether one eye or both eyes are treated. Report codes **92310-92313** when the fitting is provided by the same office that prescribed the lenses. Report codes **92314-92317** when the prescription is provided by one office and the fitting is performed by an independent technician. Codes **92310** and **92314** include the description **except aphakia** and are used when contact lenses are prescribed to supplement a person's natural lens. Append modifier **-52 Reduced Services** when a lens is prescribed for only one eye.

Codes that include the description **for aphakia** (*absence of a lens*) are used when the contact lens replaces a person's natural lens, as occurs with cataract removal.

The supply of the lens itself may be reported as part of the fitting service or may be reported separately using code **99070** or the appropriate HCPCS code.

Codes under the subheading **Spectacle Services (92340-92499)** include the fitting, patient education, and follow-up related to eyeglasses. Prescription of the lenses is included in code **92015 Determination of refractive state**. Codes are divided by the type of lens—monofocal, bifocal, or multifocal—and the condition: for aphakia, not for aphakia, and low-vision aids. The supply of the material is not included in the fitting service and should be reported separately using code **99070** or the appropriate HCPCS code.

Read the code descriptions to determine whether the code is unilateral or bilateral. Some services provide separate codes for one eye or both eyes, and others do not. When the code description includes the words **unilateral** or **bilateral**, select the code that describes the extent of service provided. Append the appropriate modifier, **-LT** or **-RT**, for a unilateral procedure. When the description does not specify bilateral, apply modifier **-50 Bilateral procedure**. When the procedure description states bilateral but the service was provided for only one eye, apply modifier **-52 Reduced services**.

Diagnosis codes that support the need for ophthalmological services most often come from ICD-10-CM Chapter 7, **Diseases of the Eye and Adnexa (H00-H59)**, or the section **Diabetes mellitus (E08-E13)** from Chapter 4, **Endocrine, Nutritional, and Metabolic Diseases (E00-E89)**.

Diagnosis codes that support the need for hearing services most often come from ICD-10-CM Chapter 8, **Diseases of the Ear and the Mastoid Process (H60-H95)**. Diagnosis codes for injuries to the eye and ear are in the section **Injuries to the head (S00-S09)** of ICD-10-CM Chapter 19, **Injury, Poisoning and Certain Other Consequences of External Causes**.

2. For EPS, refer to the code range listed, which includes all the codes in this subheading.

3. Refer to the Tabular List to select and verify the correct code based on the specific test provided.

In the Tabular List, read the special instructions at the beginning of this subheading. Three types of procedures are described in this subheading:

- **Arrhythmia Induction**—Recreating the arrhythmia using electrical pacing or programmed stimulation

- **Mapping**—Recording the site of origin of the tachycardia or its electrical path through the heart

- **Ablation**—Selectively destroying cardiac tissue using radiofrequency or cryo-energy

Many times, patients with arrhythmias are evaluated and treated during the same encounter. When this occurs, report the induction and ablation with one code that bundles both procedures (**93653-93655**), but report the mapping as a separate service with an add-on code (**93609** or **93613**). Read the instructional notes in the Tabular List to verify codes that can and cannot be reported together.

The bundle of His (pronounced *hiss*) recording is a test that can be performed alone or as part of an EPS. A catheter with a sensor on the end is advanced to the heart to measure the electrical activity of the bundle of His.

When more than one procedure is performed during an encounter, the second and subsequent codes from this subsection require modifier **-51 Multiple procedures**. Do not use modifier **-51** on add-on codes or codes that require modifier **-59 Distinct procedural service**.

EPS procedures are commonly supported by diagnoses for conduction disorders and cardiac arrhythmias (**I44-I49**) and signs and symptoms that may indicate the presence of these conditions. Patients might also have other cardiac conditions and a variety of comorbidities.

SUCCESS STEP

The CPT Index provides a limited number of Main Terms for specific EPS services. You may wish to write your own notes in the Index, alphabetized in the proper location. For example, write an entry under **B** to identify *Bundle of His 93600*. Write additional notes under **M**, **P**, and **R** to create Main Terms that seem logical, such as *Mapping*, *Pacing*, and *Recording*. For these entries, you can list the code range *93602-93662*.

Noninvasive Vascular Studies (93880-93998)

The subsection Noninvasive Vascular Diagnostic Studies includes specialized services to study veins and arteries other than the heart and great vessels.

To assign codes for noninvasive vascular diagnostic studies, follow these steps.

1. In the Index, locate the Main Term **Vascular Studies**.

2. Locate the first-level modifying term for the type of procedure or body site. Identify the code(s) or code range.

3. Refer to the Tabular List to select and verify the code for the body site and type of vessel treated.

In the Tabular List, codes are divided into subheadings by body site and whether the study involves an artery, vein, or both. The subsection provides special instructions that describe how the studies are performed and lists the components required for limited and complete studies of both the lower and upper extremities. In general, limited studies require measurements at one or two levels and complete studies require measurements at three or more levels. Examples of levels for the lower extremities are the high thigh, low thigh, calf, ankle, metatarsal, and toes. Examples of levels for the upper extremities are the arm, forearm, wrist, and digits.

Codes for extremity studies identify a bilateral study. When the study is unilateral, apply modifier **-52 Reduced services**.

Codes under the subheading Cerebrovascular Arterial Studies (**93880-93892**) are divided by methodology—either a duplex scan or transcranial Doppler (TCD) study. Parent codes identify a complete study; indented codes identify a limited or unilateral study. Codes in this subsection are comprised of professional and technical components, so apply modifiers **-26** and **-TC** as appropriate.

Diagnosis codes that support noninvasive vascular diagnostic studies frequently are found in the following sections of ICD-10-CM Chapter 10, **Diseases of the Circulatory System (I00-I99)**:

- **Cerebrovascular diseases (I60-I69)**

- **Diseases of the arteries, arterioles and capillaries (I70-I79)**

- **Disease of veins, lymphatic vessels and lymph nodes, not elsewhere classified (I80-89)**

Allergy Procedures (95004-95199)

The subsection **Allergy and Clinical Immunology** describes services to allergy testing and allergen immunotherapy. An **antigen** is any natural or artificial substance that produces an immune response. An **allergenic extract** is a concentration of components from the allergen, such as grass or pollen. Do not confuse allergen immunotherapy with the administration of immune globulins, discussed earlier in this chapter.

To locate codes for allergy and clinical immunology, follow these steps.

1. For allergy testing, search for the Main Term **Allergy Test** in the Index.

2. Locate the first- and second-level modifying terms that identify the type of test.

3. For allergen immunotherapy, search for the Main Term **Allergen Immunotherapy**.

4. Locate the first- and second-level modifying terms that identify the type of therapy provided. Identify the code(s) or code range.

5. Refer to the Tabular List to select and verify the code based on the type of test provided.

> ## CODING CAUTION
>
> Under the Main Term **Allergen Immunotherapy**, the first-level modifying term **Allergen** leads to codes for laboratory tests from the Pathology and Laboratory section, which begin with **8**. Codes for testing and treatment appear in the Medicine section and begin with **9**.

In the Tabular List, allergy testing codes are divided by the type of test performed. When the description states **specify number of tests**, report one unit of the code for each test performed. Ingestion challenge test codes are defined based on the length of time required for the test. Allergen immunotherapy is the periodic administration of antigens to increase a person's immune response to the allergen.

The antigen or allergenic extract can be provided by the physician or by the patient, purchased elsewhere. Codes **95115** and **95117** describe professional immunotherapy services when the physician does *not* provide the antigen. Codes **95120** and **95125** describe professional immunotherapy services when the physician *does* provide the antigen. The parent code (**95115** and **95120**) in each pair reports one injection. The indented code (**95117** and **95125**) in each pair reports two or more injections. It is not an add-on code and should not be reported with the respective parent code. Additional indented codes are provided specifically for stinging insect venoms.

Codes also are provided to report professional services for the supervision of preparation and provision of antigens by the physician.

The interpretation and reporting of allergy tests is included in the code and should not be reported separately using an E/M code. E/M codes can be reported when a significant, separately identifiable E/M service is provided. Apply modifier **-25** to the E/M code.

Codes for allergy procedures are most commonly supported by a diagnosis of an inflammatory condition of the affected anatomic site, such as rhinitis, sinusitis, conjunctivitis, otitis, dermatitis, and similar conditions.

Neurology Procedures (95782-96020)

Neurology services are typically provided as E/M consultations for outpatients and inpatients. In addition, diagnostic and therapeutic procedures can be reported separately. The subsection Neurology and Neuromuscular Procedures provides codes for a wide variety of tests including sleep testing, routine and special EEG tests, nerve and muscle function tests, and intraoperative neurophysiology.

To assign codes from the Neurology subsection, follow these steps.

1. In the Index, search for the name of the test or procedure as the Main Term.

2. Review the modifying term(s) to select the appropriate code range.

3. Refer to the Tabular List to select and verify the code based on the type of test.

The Tabular List provides special instructions that describe various tests and identify codes that can and cannot be reported together. Be attentive to how each code reports time or quantity of service.

Sleep testing (**95803-95811**) is performed while the patient sleeps to assess various body functions to diagnose sleep disorders such as sleep apnea, insomnia, narcolepsy, and somnambulism. Tests include polysomnography, which includes multiple measurements of functions and activities of the heart, muscles, brain, and eyes during sleep. Polysomnography codes are divided by the age of the patient and the number of sleep parameters evaluated.

Evoked potentials and reflex tests (**95925-95937**) are performed to diagnose neuromuscular diseases and are completed by measuring visual, auditory, and automatic nerve reflexes.

The Intraoperative Neurophysiology subheading provides two codes, **95940** and **95941**, both of which are add-on codes used in conjunction with other neurological tests performed during surgery. **95940** Reports continuous one-on-one intraoperative monitoring in the operating room and is reported in 15-minute increments. Code **95941** reports intraoperative monitoring from a remote or nearby location outside of the operating room and is reported in one-hour increments. Read the detailed special instructions with this subheading to use the codes correctly.

Most, but not all, procedures in this subsection contain professional and technical components, so apply modifiers **-26** and **-TC** as needed. When services described as bilateral are performed unilaterally, apply modifier **-52**.

Diagnosis codes that support Neurology subsection procedures most commonly are supported by codes from ICD-10-CM Chapter 6, **Diseases of the Nervous System and Sense Organs (G00-G99)**, or Chapter 18, **Symptoms, Signs, Abnormal Clinical and Laboratory Findings (R00-R99)**.

Infusion and Injection Procedures (96360-96549)

Infusion and injection procedures include hydration; therapeutic, prophylactic, and diagnostic injections and infusions; and chemotherapy administration. Administration of other highly complex drugs that require close supervision and monitoring for side effects is coded with the same codes used for chemotherapy administration.

To assign codes for infusion and injection procedures follow these steps.

1. In the Index, search for the Main Term **Infusion Therapy**.

2. Locate the first-level modifying term for the type: **Hydration**, **Intravenous**, or **Subcutaneous** (■ FIGURE 32-7, page 578).

3. For chemotherapy, locate the second-level modifying term **Chemotherapy** under **Intravenous**.

4. As an alternative, select a Main Term for the type of infusion, which leads directly to the appropriate code: **Chemotherapy**, **Hydration**, or **Intravenous Therapy**.

5. Regardless of the Main Term selected, identify the code range to verify in the Tabular List.

The Tabular List for this subsection provides detailed special instructions that identify the terms used to assign codes,

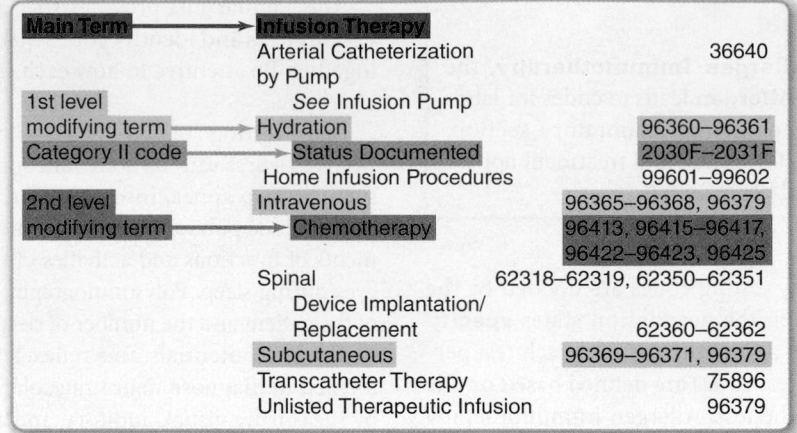

Figure 32-7 ■ CPT Index Entry for Infusion Therapy

sequencing directions, and differences between physician coding and facility coding.

When the following services are performed to facilitate the infusion or injection, they are bundled and should not be reported separately.

- Use of local anesthesia
- Starting the IV
- Access to indwelling IV, subcutaneous catheter, or port
- Flush at conclusion of infusion
- Standard tubing, syringes, and supplies

Three categories of infusion codes identify the purpose of the service:

- Hydration **96360- 96361**
- Therapeutic, prophylactic, and diagnostic services **96365-96379**
- Chemotherapy **96401-96549** (■ FIGURE 32-8)

Patient is seen for chemotherapy infusion for metastatic colon cancer. Oxaliplatin is administered through intravenous infusion for two hours followed by leucovorin for two hours. A bolus (push) of 5-fluorouracil (5-FU) is administered at the same access site.

Z51.11 Encounter for antineoplastic chemotherapy
C79.9 Secondary malignant neoplasm of unspecified site
C18.9 Malignant neoplasm of colon, unspecified
96413 x 1 Chemotherapy administration, intravenous; infusion technique, up to 1 hour
96417 x 1 Chemotherapy administration, intravenous infusion technique; each additional sequential infusion (different substance/drug), up to 1 hour
96415 x 2 Chemotherapy administration, intravenous; infusion technique, each additional hour (Note: 1 unit is the second hour of oxaliplatin infusion and 1 unit is the second hour of leucovorin infusion)
96411 Chemotherapy administration, intravenous; push technique

---

Figure 32-8 ■ Example of Coding Infusion Services

Except for hydration services, there are basic types of infusion codes: initial, concurrent, and sequential.

- **Initial infusion**—Report one code per day, unless a second, separate site is required for additional infusions. Report the second code with modifier **-59**. This is a time-based code, with an add-on code for additional time.

- **Concurrent infusion**—Report a single code for infusion of a second substance or drug infused at the same time as another substance or drug. If a third substance is administered concurrently, do not report it.

- **Sequential infusion**—Report an infusion or IV push of a new substance or drug following a primary or initial service.

Physicians report infusion therapy for nonfacility or office-based services only. Physicians report the infusion that is the main reason for the encounter, regardless of the chronological order in which infusions are provided. Facilities follow a hierarchy of sequencing priorities, which is discussed later in the chapter.

A significant, separately identifiable office or other outpatient E/M service can be reported on the same day as the infusion, when performed. Apply modifier **-25** in addition to the infusion code(s) **96360-96549**.

Thousands of diagnoses can support infusion and injection procedures. Hydration services frequently are supported with codes from ICD-10-CM Chapter 4, **Endocrine, Nutritional, and Metabolic Diseases (E00-E89)**, for volume depletion (**E86**) and disorders of fluid, electrolyte, and acid–base imbalance (**E87**). Chemotherapy services are often, but not always, supported by codes from ICD-10-CM Chapter 2, **Neoplasms (C00-D49)**.

Physical Medicine, Osteopathic, and Chiropractic (97001-97799, 98925-98929, 98940-98943)

Physical medicine and rehabilitation services include physical therapy modalities, therapeutic procedures, active wound care management, tests and measurements, and orthotic and prosthetic management. Many services can be located by searching the Index for the name of the procedure.

To assign codes for physical medicine follow these steps.

1. Search the Index for the Main Term **Physical Medicine/ Therapy/Occupational Therapy**.

2. Locate the first- and second-level modifying terms for the specific service or modality, such as **Evaluation, Physical Therapy** or **Modalities, Traction**. Some services also appear directly under a Main Term for the name of the service, such as **Traction Therapy** or **Wound, Care**.

3. Identify the code(s) or code range to verify in the Tabular List.

4. In the Tabular List, select the code and determine the quantity to be reported based on the code description.

Modalities are physical therapy treatments that use thermal (*heat*), acoustic (*sound*), luminous (*light*), mechanical, or electric energy to produce beneficial changes in biologic tissue. Codes for modalities are divided into supervised and constant attendance.

Supervised modalities do not require continuous one-on-one contact with the patient by the provider. The provider sets up the treatment then can leave the room while the modality runs. Examples are the application of hot packs or mechanical traction. Supervised modality codes (**97010-97028**) are reported with one unit of service regardless of the amount of time the modality operates.

Constant attendance modalities require constant one-on-one contact with the patient by the provider. The provider personally applies the modality and is present with the patient the entire time. Examples are ultrasound and contrast baths. Constant attendance modality codes (**97032-97039**) are time-based codes in which 15 minutes equals one unit of service, 30 minutes equals two units of service, and so on.

The subheading **Therapeutic Procedures (97110-97546)** provides codes for other types of therapy, training, and activities. Code descriptions identify those that are time-based.

Read the documentation carefully to determine the exact type of service provided. Some modalities can be applied using either supervision or constant attendance. For example, electrical stimulation can be either supervised/unattended (**97014**) or constant attendance/manual (**97032**). Whirlpool (**96365**) and paraffin baths (**97018**) are supervised, and contrast baths (**97034**) and the Hubbard tank (**97036**) are constant attendance. Mechanical traction is supervised (**97012**), and manual traction is reported with a time-based code (**97140**) from the Therapeutic Procedures subheading (■ FIGURE 32-9).

To assign codes for chiropractic or osteopathic manipulation, locate the Main Term **Chiropractic Treatment** or **Osteopathic Manipulation**, respectively. The Tabular List provides special instructions for both of these subsections. Select codes based on the number of body regions treated, which are defined in the special instructions.

SUCCESS STEP

Medicare covers chiropractic treatment only for acute injuries supported by radiographic (X-ray) evidence. Append HCPCS modifier -**AT Acute Treatment** to the code. Contact your local Medicare Administrative Contractor (MAC) for detailed guidelines on chiropractic billing.

Patient receives physical therapy treatment for a back sprain. The physical therapist applies unattended electrical stimulation for 15 minutes, then provides therapeutic exercises for 30 minutes. The session concludes with 15 minutes of manual therapy including traction.

S33.5XXA Dislocation and sprain of joints and ligaments of lumbar spine and pelvis

97110 x 2 Therapeutic procedure, 1 or more areas, each 15 minutes; therapeutic exercises to develop strength and endurance, range of motion and flexibility

97140 x 1 Manual therapy techniques (eg, mobilization/manipulation, manual lymphatic drainage, manual traction), 1 or more regions, each 15 minutes

97014 Application of a modality to 1 or more areas; electrical stimulation (unattended)

Figure 32-9 ■ Example of Coding for Physical Medicine

Diagnoses that support physical medicine services can come from many chapters of the ICD-10-CM manual because nearly every body system can be affected by conditions for which patients can be helped by physical medicine. Conditions from ICD-10-CM Chapter 19, **Injury, Poisoning and Certain Other Consequences of External Causes (S00-T88)**, also frequently require physical medicine services. Chiropractic services often require codes from specific categories such as **M99 Biomechanical lesions, not elsewhere classified** or codes for **Subluxation and dislocation of** the cervical (**S13.1-**), thoracic (**S23.1-**), or lumbar (**S33.1-**) vertebra to qualify for reimbursement.

Other Medicine Procedures

The Medicine section contains many additional subsections beyond the ones discussed here. Use the three skills of an Ace coder—Abstract, Assign, and Arrange—to approach new coding situations that you have not encountered before. The special instructions and instructional notes in the Tabular List provide the needed guidance for any given subsection or category.

Biofeedback (90901–90911)

Biofeedback teaches patients to regulate certain body functions through mental or physical exercises. Patients who experience increased heart rate, respirations, and blood pressure in response to stress can learn to control their mental processes to regulate their body functions. For example, patients who suffer from irritable bowel syndrome (IBS) or fecal incontinence (*inability to control the bowels*) can learn to relax or constrict their anal sphincters to manage their disorders. Many payers cover biofeedback training because, in the long run, biofeedback can successfully resolve many conditions. To locate codes for biofeedback, search the Index for the Main Term **Biofeedback Training**.

Pulmonary Procedures (94002-97499)

Pulmonologists treat conditions related to the function of the lungs. Pulmonary diagnostic testing and therapies includes many different diagnostic breathing tests to identify pulmonary and respiratory disorders by assessing lung functions and therapeutic services to help patients to breathe more easily. To locate codes for pulmonary procedures, search the Index for the Main Term **Pulmonology** then the first-level modifying term **Diagnostic** or **Therapeutic**. Then locate the additional modifying term(s) for the type of procedure. Alternatively, search for the Main Term for the name of the procedure.

Endocrinology (95250–95251)

The Endocrinology subsection contains two codes for ambulatory continuous glucose monitoring of interstitial tissue fluid. Some diabetic patients need this service. A continuous monitoring device is implanted under the abdominal skin to measure glucose concentrations every 5 minutes for 72 hours. The device transmits the results to a monitor worn by the patient. Report codes for these services only once a month.

To locate endocrinology codes in the Index, search for the Main Term **Glucose**, the first-level modifying term **Interstitial Fluid**, and the second-level modifying term **Continuous Monitoring**. An alternative coding path is to locate the Main Term **Monitoring** then the modifying terms **Glucose** and **Interstitial Fluid**.

Non-Face-to-Face Services (98966-98969) and Special Services (99000-99091)

The Medicine section provides subsections for non-face-to-face services provided by nonphysicians, online medical evaluation, and special services, procedures, and reports. Take a few moments to review these subsections and become familiar with the codes. To locate these codes in the Index, use the subsection or category title as the Main Term.

Guided Example of Assigning Medicine Codes

To practice skills for assigning codes for Medicine services, continue with the example from earlier in the chapter about a patient who was seen for cardiac therapy. Follow along in your CPT manual as Ladonna Shuck, CPC, assigns codes. Check off each step after you complete it.

▶ First, Ladonna confirms cardiac catheterization of the right heart followed by balloon angioplasty of the right coronary artery.

▶ Ladonna searches the Index for the Main Term **Catheterization**.

❑ She locates the modifying term **Cardiac**, which provides a cross-reference *See* **Cardiac Catheterization**. This tells her to look under a different Main Term.

❑ She locates the Main Term entry for **Cardiac Catheterization**, which provides a cross reference **See Catheterization, Cardiac**. This is confusing at first because that is where she just looked. Then she notices additional modifying terms that identify various anatomic sites.

❑ She reads all of the modifying terms until she locates **for Angiography**, which lists several modifying terms. She selects the second-level modifying term **Coronary** because the coronary arteries were catheterized. The codes listed for **Coronary** are **93454-93461, 93563, 93571**.

▶ Ladonna locates codes **93454-93461, 93563, 93571** in the Tabular List and reads the code descriptions of each. She needs to determine the differences between the parent code and the indented codes under it (■ TABLE 32-23).

❑ **93454 Catheter placement in coronary artery(s) for coronary angiography, including intraprocedural injection(s) for coronary angiography, imaging supervision and interpretation**

❑ **93455** identifies **for bypass graft angiography**, which is not documented.

❑ **93456** identifies **with right heart catheterization**, which is not documented.

❑ **93457** identifies **for bypass graft angiography** and **right heart catheterization**, which are not documented.

❑ **93458** identifies **with left heart catheterization**, which is not documented.

❑ **93459** identifies **with left heart catheterization** and **bypass graft angiography**, which are not documented.

❑ **93460** identifies **with right and left heart catheterization**, which is not documented.

❑ **93461** identifies **with right and left heart catheterization** and **bypass graft angiography**, which are not documented.

❑ **93471** is an add-on code that identifies **intravascular Doppler velocity**. She rejects this code because intravascular Doppler velocity is not documented.

▶ Ladonna concludes that code **93454** is the code that describes the procedure, but she would not have known this without reviewing all the codes listed in the Index.

Table 32-23 ■ SUMMARY OF CARDIAC CATHETERIZATION CODES (93451-93461)

	Right Heart	Left Heart	Coronary Arteries	Coronary Arteries + Bypass Graft
Right Heart	93451	93453	93456	93457
Left Heart	93453	93452	93458	93459
Coronary Arteries	93456	93457	93454	93455
Right + Left Heart	93453	93453	93460	93461

Source: © PB Resources, Inc. Used with permission. CPT codes © American Medical Association.

▶ Ladonna checks the special instructions under the category heading **Cardiac Catheterization**.

❏ She reads the description of each target site: right heart catheterization, left heart catheterization, catheter placement in coronary arteries.

❏ She also reads that cardiac catheterization codes **include contrast injection(s), imaging supervision, interpretation, and report**, as well as **all roadmapping angiography**.

❏ She does not read any instructions that indicate the codes include balloon angioplasty or stenting.

▶ Ladonna rereads the documentation and identifies that a stent was inserted in the RCA. Because the code for catheterization does not include stenting, she knows she must find another code.

▶ Ladonna locates the Main Term **Stent** in the CPT Index.

❏ She locates the first-level modifying term **for Revascularization, Intracoronary** and identifies the codes listed: **92937-92938, 92941, 92943-92944**.

❏ Just to be sure, she also checks the Main Term **Angioplasty** and the first-level modifying term **Coronary Artery** with the second-level modifying term **with stent placement**. The same codes are listed, with the addition of **92928-92929**.

▶ Ladonna turns to the Tabular List to verify the codes.

❏ When she locates code **92928** in numerical sequence, she reads an instructional note that states: **92928 is out of numerical sequence. See 92998-93000**.

❏ She locates code **92998**, then finds **92928** in the code series that follows.

▶ Now Ladonna must identify the differences among codes **92928-92929, 92937-92938, 92941**, and **92943-92944**.

❏ **92928** and **92929** identify stenting without any qualifications or criteria. She thinks **92928** might be a possibility, but needs to read the remaining codes.

❏ **92937** and **92938** identify stenting of a **bypass graft**, which is not documented.

❏ **92941** identifies stenting during a **myocardial infarction**, which is not documented.

❏ **92943** and **92944** identify stenting to correct **chronic total occlusion**. She thinks **92943** might be a possibility, but is

unsure whether 75% *occlusion* documented in the medical record qualifies as **chronic total occlusion**.

▶ Ladonna checks the special instructions under the category heading **Coronary Therapeutic Services and Procedures**.

❏ She reads that **Chronic total occlusion of a coronary vessel is present when there is no antegrade flow through the true lumen**. She further reads that **subtotal occlusion… [is] not considered chronic total occlusion**.

❏ Based on this information, she concludes that 75% *occlusion* is subtotal occlusion, not chronic total occlusion. Therefore, **92943** is not appropriate because it specifies **chronic total occlusion**.

❏ She selects code **92928 Percutaneous transcatheter placement of intracoronary stent(s), with coronary angioplasty when performed; single major coronary artery or branch**.

▶ Ladonna reads the rest of the special instructions before code **92920** and learns that angiography (**99354**) cannot always be reported with a code from **92920-92944**.

❏ She reads that **Diagnostic angiography performed at the time of a coronary interventional procedure may be separately reportable if: 1. No prior catheter-based coronary angiography study is available, and a full diagnostic study is performed, and a decision to intervene is based on the diagnostic angiography**.

❏ The situation she is coding meets this criterion because a full diagnostic study was performed and, based on the result, a decision was made to perform the angioplasty and stent placement. Therefore, she is confident that she can use both codes.

▶ Ladonna reviews the procedure codes she has assigned for this case.

❏ **92928 Percutaneous transcatheter placement of intracoronary stent(s), with coronary angioplasty when performed; single major coronary artery or branch**

❏ **93454 Catheter placement in coronary artery(s) for coronary angiography, including intraprocedural injection(s) for coronary angiography, imaging supervision and interpretation**

▶ Next, Ladonna must determine how to sequence the codes and whether any modifiers are needed.

CODING PRACTICE

Exercise 32.3   **Assigning Codes for Medicine Procedures**

Instructions: Read the mini-medical-record of each patient's encounter. Review the information abstracted in Exercise 32.2 for questions 1 through 3. For questions 4 and 5, do the abstracting on your own. Assign CPT procedure codes using the Index and Tabular List. Write the code(s) on the line provided.

(continued)

that only the technical component is provided. In cases where the facility also hires the medical staff, do not report either modifier, indicating that both components were provided.

Common services with both professional and technical components include:

- Cardiac catheterization
- Echocardiogram
- Electroencephalogram
- Nerve conduction studies
- Pulmonary function tests
- Reflux studies
- Sleep studies

Check the Medicare Physician Fee Schedule (MPFS) on the CMS website (**www.cms.gov**) to identify codes that have professional and technical components. Many encoders also provide this information (■ FIGURE 32-10). In the workplace, the billing software is usually preloaded with information about which codes have professional and technical components and which component(s) is normally provided by your company.

Modifier -59 Distinct Procedural Service

When a procedure that is normally performed as part of a larger, more extensive procedure is performed by itself, modifier **-59 Distinct procedural service** may be required to identify that the procedure performed is separate and distinct and should be paid.

Diagnostic angiography (**93454-93461**) requires modifier **-59** when performed as a separate service during the same encounter as percutaneous coronary revascularization (**92920-92944**). Special instructions before code **92920** describe when angiography can be reported with PCI. Apply modifier **-59** to the angiography code.

Coronary Artery Modifiers

When procedures are performed on the coronary arteries, apply a HCPCS modifier to identify the artery. The modifiers are:

-LM Left main coronary artery
-LD Left anterior descending coronary artery
-LC Left circumflex coronary artery
-RI Ramus intermedius coronary artery
-RC Right coronary artery

There are no modifiers for coronary artery branches.

Guided Example of Arranging Medicine Codes

To practice skills for arranging codes for Medical procedures, continue with the example from earlier in the chapter about the patient who was seen for cardiac therapy. Follow along in your CPT manual as Ladonna Chuck, CPC, arranges the codes. Check off each step after you complete it.

▶ Ladonna reviews the procedure codes she identified:

❏ **92928 Percutaneous transcatheter placement of intracoronary stent(s), with coronary angioplasty when performed; single major coronary artery or branch**

❏ **93454 Catheter placement in coronary artery(s) for coronary angiography, including intraprocedural injection(s) for coronary angiography, imaging supervision and interpretation**

▶ Ladonna knows that procedures should be ranked in order of descending cost on the claim.

❏ **93454** is the more extensive procedure, has the higher price, and should be sequenced first.

❏ **92928** is less extensive and should be sequenced second.

▶ Ladonna needs to determine whether modifiers are needed.

❏ She reads that modifier **-59 Distinct procedural service** is required on code **93454** to identify that the diagnostic angiography is separate and distinct from the stent placement.

❏ Cardiac catheterization codes consist of a technical component and a professional component. Assign modifier **-26 Professional component** to indicate that the physician provided only the professional component. Sequence this as the first modifier because it affects payment.

❏ **92928** requires HCPCS modifier **-RC Right coronary artery** to identify the location of the stent.

▶ Ladonna finalizes the procedure codes and sequencing for this case:

(1) **93454-26-59 Catheter placement in coronary artery(s) for coronary angiography, including**

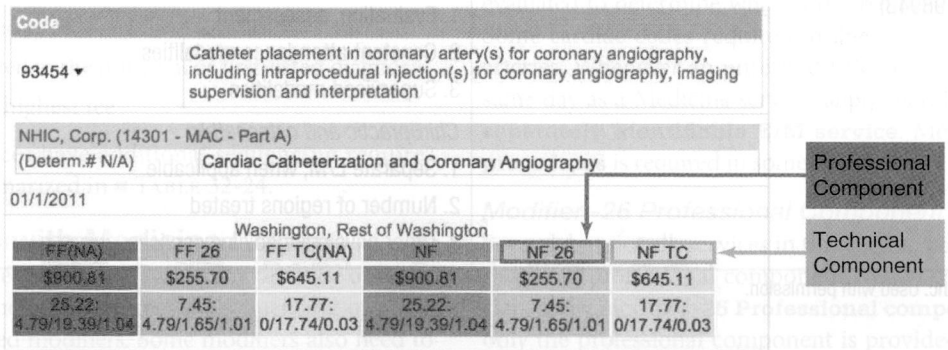

Figure 32-10 ■ Encoder Screen Showing Professional and Technical Components for CPT Code 93454. Source: Screen shot courtesy of SpeedECoder.

intraprocedural injection(s) for coronary angiography, imaging supervision and interpretation; -59 Distinct procedural service

(2) **92928-RC Percutaneous transcatheter placement of intracoronary stent(s), with coronary angioplasty when performed; single major coronary artery or branch; -RC Right coronary artery**

▶ Ladonna also assigns and sequences the ICD-10-CM diagnosis codes that support the need for the service.

(1) **I25.119 Atherosclerotic heart disease of native coronary artery with unspecified angina pectoris**

(2) **I25.83 Coronary atherosclerosis due to lipid rich plaque**

CODING PRACTICE

Exercise 32.4   Arranging Codes for Medicine Procedures

Instructions: Read the mini-medical-record of each patient's encounter. Review the information abstracted in Exercise 32.2 for questions 1 through 3. For questions 4 and 5, do the abstracting on your own. Assign CPT procedure codes using the Index and Tabular List, and arrange them correctly.

1. OFFICE   Gender: F   Age: 8

Reason for encounter: *annual preventive care checkup for established patient*

Procedure: *Comprehensive periodic preventive medicine examination. Updated immunizations: IM injection TdaP (diphtheria, tetanus toxoid, acellular pertussis); oral poliovirus.*

Plan: *Counseled mother regarding potential side effects and signs to be observant for. Call office with any concerns.*

Tip: Code for the E/M service, vaccine administration, and vaccine products.

5 CPT Codes _____

_____

2. OFFICE (Physical therapy)   Gender: M   Age: 42

Reason for encounter: *referred by PCP for therapy for low-back strain while playing golf*

Procedure: *Initial physical therapy evaluation; 15 minutes of manual electrical stimulation; 15 minutes of therapeutic exercises to increase ROM and flexibility; 15 minutes of alternating hot and cold packs*

Plan: *return 3x week for 2 weeks, per physician's order*

Tip: Indicate the quantity to be reported for each modality.

4 CPT Codes _____

_____

3. INPATIENT HOSPITAL   Gender: M   Age: 62

Reason for admission: *STEMI of LAD with thrombus*

Procedure: *Percutaneous transluminal revascularization during acute myocardial infarction using angiography. Stent and thrombectomy for acute total occlusion of LAD. Both diagonals show evidence of chronic subtotal occlusion. Balloon angioplasty on D1. Balloon angioplasty and atherectomy on D2.*

Tip: Use a modifier to identify the coronary artery. Review the section of this chapter that discusses the coronary arteries and branches. Read the CPT special instructions about coronary artery branches and the instructional notes under the code(s) in the Tabular List.

3 CPT Codes _____

4. OFFICE   Gender: F   Age: 32

Reason for encounter: *eye examination*

Procedure: *ophthalmological examination and evaluation of established patient, intermediate; prescription and fitting of contact lens, both eyes*

Assessment: *astigmatism, myopia*

Tip: You did not abstract this case in Exercise 32.2, so do the abstracting before you code it. Code for the services and for supply of the product.

3 CPT Codes _____

5. INPATIENT HOSPITAL   Gender: M   Age: 66

Preprocedure diagnosis: *single-lead pacemaker insertion for right bundle branch block*

Procedure (Cardiologist): *Periprocedural evaluation and programming of single-lead pacemaker before surgery. Reevaluation and parameter adjustment after surgery. Analysis, review, and report pre- and postprocedure.*

Plan: *FU in office 1 week*

Tip: You did not abstract this case in Exercise 32.2, so do the abstracting before you code it. Read the instructional notes to determine the quantity to report. The physician provided the professional component of service.

1 CPT Code _____

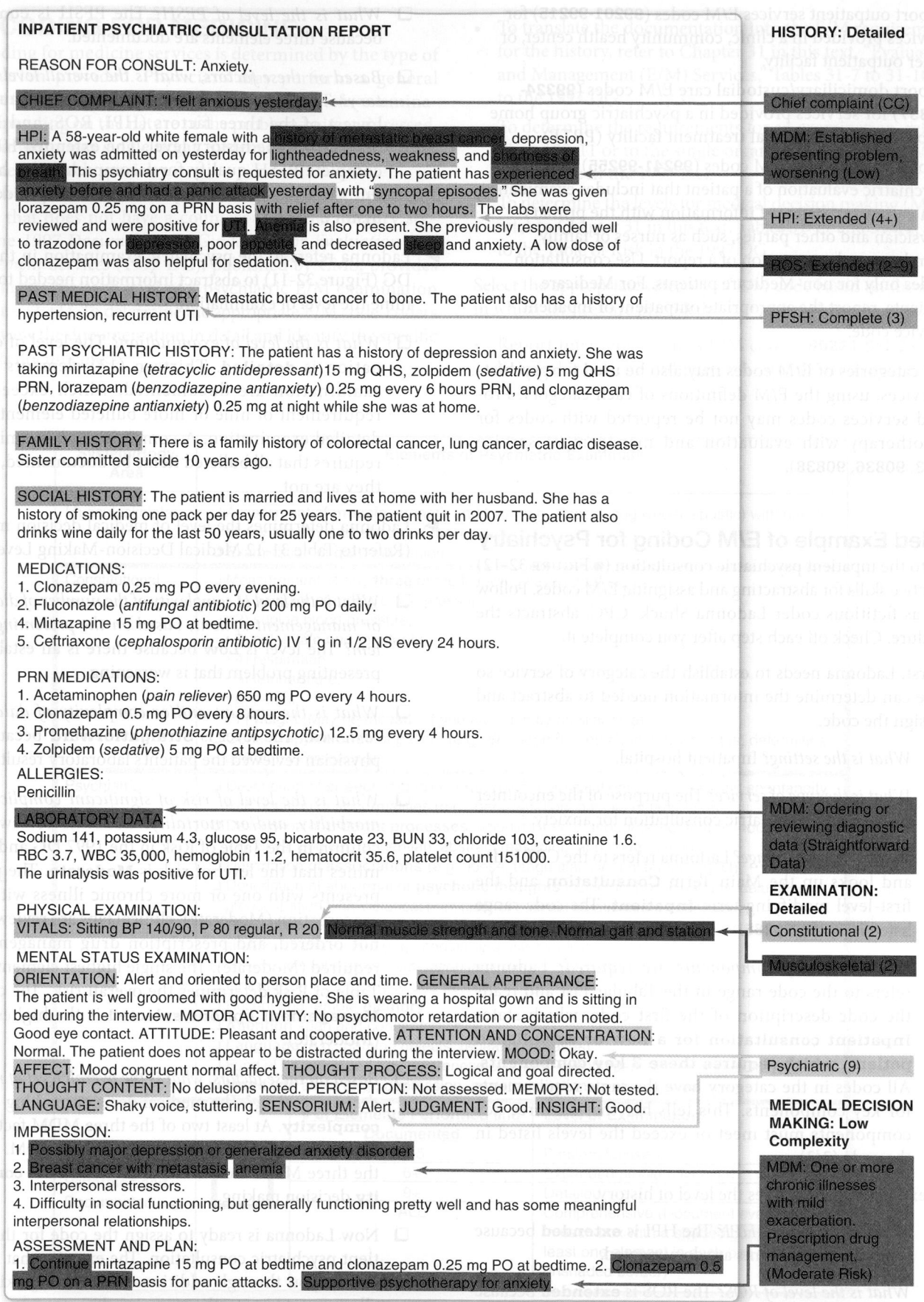

INPATIENT PSYCHIATRIC CONSULTATION REPORT

HISTORY: Detailed

REASON FOR CONSULT: Anxiety.

CHIEF COMPLAINT: "I felt anxious yesterday."

→ Chief complaint (CC)

HPI: A 58-year-old white female with a history of metastatic breast cancer, depression, anxiety was admitted on yesterday for lightheadedness, weakness, and shortness of breath. This psychiatry consult is requested for anxiety. The patient has experienced anxiety before and had a panic attack yesterday with "syncopal episodes." She was given lorazepam 0.25 mg on a PRN basis with relief after one to two hours. The labs were reviewed and were positive for UTI. Anemia is also present. She previously responded well to trazodone for depression, poor appetite, and decreased sleep and anxiety. A low dose of clonazepam was also helpful for sedation.

→ MDM: Established presenting problem, worsening (Low)

→ HPI: Extended (4+)

→ ROS: Extended (2–9)

PAST MEDICAL HISTORY: Metastatic breast cancer to bone. The patient also has a history of hypertension, recurrent UTI

→ PFSH: Complete (3)

PAST PSYCHIATRIC HISTORY: The patient has a history of depression and anxiety. She was taking mirtazapine (*tetracyclic antidepressant*)15 mg QHS, zolpidem (*sedative*) 5 mg QHS PRN, lorazepam (*benzodiazepine antianxiety*) 0.25 mg every 6 hours PRN, and clonazepam (*benzodiazepine antianxiety*) 0.25 mg at night while she was at home.

FAMILY HISTORY: There is a family history of colorectal cancer, lung cancer, cardiac disease. Sister committed suicide 10 years ago.

SOCIAL HISTORY: The patient is married and lives at home with her husband. She has a history of smoking one pack per day for 25 years. The patient quit in 2007. The patient also drinks wine daily for the last 50 years, usually one to two drinks per day.

MEDICATIONS:
1. Clonazepam 0.25 mg PO every evening.
2. Fluconazole (*antifungal antibiotic*) 200 mg PO daily.
4. Mirtazapine 15 mg PO at bedtime.
5. Ceftriaxone (*cephalosporin antibiotic*) IV 1 g in 1/2 NS every 24 hours.

PRN MEDICATIONS:
1. Acetaminophen (*pain reliever*) 650 mg PO every 4 hours.
2. Clonazepam 0.5 mg PO every 8 hours.
3. Promethazine (*phenothiazine antipsychotic*) 12.5 mg every 4 hours.
4. Zolpidem (*sedative*) 5 mg PO at bedtime.

ALLERGIES:
Penicillin

LABORATORY DATA:
Sodium 141, potassium 4.3, glucose 95, bicarbonate 23, BUN 33, chloride 103, creatinine 1.6. RBC 3.7, WBC 35,000, hemoglobin 11.2, hematocrit 35.6, platelet count 151000. The urinalysis was positive for UTI.

→ MDM: Ordering or reviewing diagnostic data (Straightforward Data)

PHYSICAL EXAMINATION:
VITALS: Sitting BP 140/90, P 80 regular, R 20. Normal muscle strength and tone. Normal gait and station

EXAMINATION: Detailed

→ Constitutional (2)

→ Musculoskeletal (2)

MENTAL STATUS EXAMINATION:
ORIENTATION: Alert and oriented to person place and time. GENERAL APPEARANCE: The patient is well groomed with good hygiene. She is wearing a hospital gown and is sitting in bed during the interview. MOTOR ACTIVITY: No psychomotor retardation or agitation noted. Good eye contact. ATTITUDE: Pleasant and cooperative. ATTENTION AND CONCENTRATION: Normal. The patient does not appear to be distracted during the interview. MOOD: Okay. AFFECT: Mood congruent normal affect. THOUGHT PROCESS: Logical and goal directed. THOUGHT CONTENT: No delusions noted. PERCEPTION: Not assessed. MEMORY: Not tested. LANGUAGE: Shaky voice, stuttering. SENSORIUM: Alert. JUDGMENT: Good. INSIGHT: Good.

→ Psychiatric (9)

MEDICAL DECISION MAKING: Low Complexity

IMPRESSION:
1. Possibly major depression or generalized anxiety disorder.
2. Breast cancer with metastasis, anemia.
3. Interpersonal stressors.
4. Difficulty in social functioning, but generally functioning pretty well and has some meaningful interpersonal relationships.

→ MDM: One or more chronic illnesses with mild exacerbation. Prescription drug management. (Moderate Risk)

ASSESSMENT AND PLAN:
1. Continue mirtazapine 15 mg PO at bedtime and clonazepam 0.25 mg PO at bedtime. 2. Clonazepam 0.5 mg PO on a PRN basis for panic attacks. 3. Supportive psychotherapy for anxiety.

KEY: HPI History of the present illness ROS Review of systems
PFSH Past, family, and social history MDM Medical decision making

Figure 32-12 ■ Psychiatric Encounter. *Source: © PB Resources, Inc. Used with permission.*

CODING PRACTICE

Exercise 32.5   E/M Coding for Medicine

Instructions: Refer to the *1997 Documentation Guidelines for Evaluation and Management Services* (available at **www.cms.gov**) or Chapter 31, "Evaluation and Management Services" (Tables 31-7 to 31-12) in this text. Answer the following questions about the Inpatient Psychiatric Consult (Figure 32-12).

1. a. Which elements of the HPI are documented? Circle all that apply. Location, Quality, Severity, Duration, Timing, Context, Modifying factors, Associated signs and symptoms

   b. How many elements are documented? _____

   c. What is the level of HPI? _____

2. a. Which systems are reviewed in the ROS? Circle all that apply. Constitutional, Allergic/immunologic, CV, Endocrine, ENT/M, Eyes, GI, GU, Hemic/lymphatic, MS, Neurologic, Psychiatric, Respiratory, Skin/breast

   b. How many systems are documented? _____

   c. What is the level of ROS? _____

3. a. Which PFSH elements are documented? Circle all that apply. Past medical, Family, Social

   b. What is the level of PFSH? _____

   c. What is the overall level of history? (The lowest history factor—HPI, ROS, or PFSH—determines the level of history.)
   _____

4. Refer to Figure 32-11 (1997 DG for Psychiatric Examination).

   a. Which bulleted items are documented for the examination? (Check off the bulleted items documented.)

   b. How many bulleted items are documented? _____

   c. What is the level of the examination? _____

5. Refer to Table 31-12 Medical Decision-Making Levels or the 1997 DG.

   a. What is the MDM level for the number of diagnoses or management options? _____

   b. What is the MDM level for the amount and/or complexity of data to be reviewed? _____

   c. Refer to the Table of Risk in the 1997 DG. Which elements of risk are documented for each risk factor?

      1. Presenting problem: _____

      2. Diagnostic procedures ordered: _____

      3. Management Options Selected: _____

   d. What is the level of risk? _____

   e. What is the overall level of MDM? (2/3 MDM factors are needed to determine the overall level.) _____

6. a. What is the setting? _____

   b. What is the type of service? _____

   c. What is the code range? _____

   d. How many key components are required? _____

   e. What is the level of history? _____

   f. What is the level of examination? _____

   g. What is the level of medical decision making?
   _____

   h. What is the correct code for the inpatient psychiatric consultation? _____

7. Abstract, assign, and arrange (sequence) the diagnosis code(s) that support the E/M code.

   ICD-10-CM Code(s) _____

CHAPTER SUMMARY

In this chapter you learned that:

- Diagnostic techniques classified in the Medicine section include an assessment or evaluation, an examination, or the use of equipment or tools to make a recording or measurement or conduct a function study.

- Therapeutic procedures classified in the Medicine section include physical, pharmacologic, immunologic, mechanical, and mental techniques.

- Medical terms for medical procedures combine roots for various organs or anatomic sites with prefixes and suffixes to create a term that describes a specific service or procedure.

- The CPT section for Medicine procedures contains 34 subsections, divided by the type of procedure, and reports noninvasive and minimally invasive procedures from a wide variety of medical specialties that are not appropriate for the Surgery section.

- Each Medicine subsection has its own abstracting rules; some subsections require multiple sets of abstracting criteria for different types of procedures.

- Coders must be certain to thoroughly read the guidelines, special instructions, and instructional notes that appear throughout the Medicine section to guide them when assigning codes.

- Arranging codes for Medicine procedures follows general CPT sequencing rules.

- To provide E/M services for Medicine procedures, physicians may perform a general multisystem examination or a single organ system examination, depending on the nature of the problem being addressed.

CONCEPT QUIZ

Take a moment to look back at the Medicine section and solidify your skills. Try to answer the questions from memory, first. Then, refer to the discussion in this chapter if you need a little extra help.

Completion

Instructions: Write the term that answers each question based on the information you learned in this chapter. Choose from the list below. Some choices may be used more than once and some choices may not be used at all.

anesthesia	immunization
antigen	mapping
arrhythmia induction	medicine
cardioversion	nephrology
chiropractor	osteopathic physician
ECT	physical therapist
EKG	plethysmography
EMG	polysomnography
EPS	psychiatry
immune globulin	

1. A(n)_____ is administered as a preventive measure in patients who do not currently have, and have not been recently exposed to, a disease.

2. A(n) _____ is any natural or artificial substance that produces an immune response.

3. _____ is used to treat arrhythmias such as atrial fibrillation.

4. _____ includes invasive diagnostic tests that assess the electrical activity in the heart.

5. A(n) _____ focuses on improving patients' conditions by manipulating body areas, typically the spine, to improve the structure and function of specific sites.

6. _____ is a recording of volume.

7. _____ is one of the few specialties in the Medicine section that does not have a counterpart in the Surgery section.

8. _____ is used to treat conditions such as depression when medications and psychotherapy fail.

9. _____ is the recording of the electrical activity of a muscle.

10. _____ is the recording the site of origin of tachycardia or its electrical path through the heart.

Multiple Choice

Instructions: Circle the letter of the best answer to each question based on the information you learned in this chapter.

1. What physician specialist provides E/M and supervisory services for dialysis?
   A. Nephrologist
   B. Neurologist
   C. Gastroenterologist
   D. Oncologist

2. What type of immunity occurs when the body's immune system receives antibodies to fight off a disease?
   A. Artificial active
   B. Artificial passive
   C. Natural active
   D. Natural passive

3. Which modifier should a physician report to identify that only the professional component of a service was provided?
   A. -59
   B. -52
   C. -PC
   D. -26

4. What test records the electrical activity of the brain?
   - A. ECC
   - B. EEG
   - C. EKG
   - D. EMG

5. What modifier identifies the left main coronary artery?
   - A. -LC
   - B. -LA
   - C. -LM
   - D. -LT

6. For what type of service does Medicare require radiographic evidence to be eligible for coverage?
   - A. Cardiac catheterization
   - B. Physical therapy
   - C. Dialysis
   - D. Chiropractic manipulation

7. What type of procedure is performed for revascularization?
   - A. PCI
   - B. ECG
   - C. TCD
   - D. EPS

8. What type of procedure enables physicians to visualize vessels to guide catheter placement for diagnostic or therapeutic cardiac procedures?
   - A. Angiography
   - B. Echocardiography
   - C. Intracardiac electrophysiological studies
   - D. Cardiac catheterization

9. What type of provider specializes in conducting eye examinations and diagnosing and treating vision disorders?
   - A. Audiologist
   - B. Ophthalmologist
   - C. Optometrist
   - D. Otolaryngologist

10. How many code(s) should be assigned when a child receives two immunizations?
    - A. Two combination codes: one for each immunization given
    - B. Three codes: one for the E/M and two for the immunizations
    - C. Three codes: one for administration and two for the products
    - D. Four codes: two for administration and two for the products

CODING CHALLENGE

Instructions: Read the mini-medical-record of each patient's encounter, then abstract, assign, and arrange ICD-10-CM and CPT codes using the Index and Tabular List. Provide the correct quantity of each CPT code with more than one unit of service. Write the codes on the lines provided.

1. OUTPATIENT HOSPITAL   Gender: F   Age: 63

Reason for encounter: intermittent chest pain

Assessment: unspecified chest pain

Procedure: left heart catheterization via femoral artery. I moved catheter to right and left coronary arteries during angiography. No blockage or defects noted.

1 ICD-10-CM Code _____

1 CPT Code _____

2. EMERGENCY DEPARTMENT   Gender: M   Age: 23

Reason for encounter: patient presents with dry mouth, dry skin, minimal output during past 24 hours

Assessment: dehydration

Procedure: IV fluids for 24 hours

Plan: no work for 24 hours, increase fluids, follow up with PCP

1 ICD-10-CM Code _____

2 CPT Codes _____

3. OUTPATIENT HOSPITAL   Gender: M   Age: 17

Reason for encounter: family history of stroke; patient needs clearance to play basketball

Procedure: transthoracic echocardiogram

2 ICD-10-CM Codes _____

1 CPT Code _____

4. OFFICE   Gender: F   Age: 72

Reason for encounter: hearing aid check

Assessment: patient has sensorineural hearing loss and wears hearing aids in both ears

Procedure: inspection and cleaning of both hearing aids, replaced batteries

1 ICD-10-CM Code _____

1 CPT Code _____

5. OFFICE   Gender: M   Age: 85

Reason for encounter: recheck of open-angle glaucoma

Procedure: comprehensive ophthalmologic examination

1 ICD-10-CM Code _____

1 CPT Code _____

(continued)

(continued from page 591)

6. OFFICE   Gender: M   Age: 48

Reason for encounter: *pain in the right hip*

Procedure: *chiropractic manipulation of the lumbar and sacroiliac spinal regions*

Plan: *Return to clinic in two days*

1 ICD-10-CM Code _____

1 CPT Code _____

7. OUTPATIENT HOSPITAL   Gender: F   Age: 36

Reason for encounter: *chemotherapy needed for cancer of left breast that has metastasized to the spinal column*

Procedure: *chemotherapy infusion administered intravenously for 90 minutes*

3 ICD-10-CM Codes _____

_____

2 CPT Codes _____

8. HOME   Gender: F   Age: 58

Reason for encounter: *Acute osteomyelitis of the left ankle. Patient is completing IV antibiotics at home.*

Procedure: *administration of antibiotic infusion for 4 hours*

(continued)

8. (continued)

Plan: *I will return tomorrow to administer another dose of antibiotic.*

1 ICD-10-CM Code _____

2 CPT Codes _____

9. OFFICE   Gender: M   Age: 13

Reason for encounter: *patient's mother requests allergy testing due to constant sneezing*

Procedure: *percutaneous tests using 10 allergen extracts, with immediate type reaction*

Plan: *Tests indicate patient is allergic to animal dander. Patient should avoid close contact with animals.*

1 ICD-10-CM Code _____

1 CPT Code _____

10. OUTPATIENT HOSPITAL   Gender: F   Age: 45

Reason for encounter: *Patient has asthma. Lately, she has been wheezing and having difficulty catching her breath.*

Procedure: *conducted vital capacity test*

Plan: *Rx for rescue inhaler, continue with steroids to manage asthma.*

1 ICD-10-CM Code _____

1 CPT Code _____

KEEP ON CODING

Instructions: Read the procedural statement, then use the Index and Tabular List to assign and sequence CPT procedure codes. Provide the correct quantity of each CPT code with more than one unit of service. Write the code(s) on the line provided.

1. IM injection for rabies human immune globulin: CPT Code(s) _____

2. Routine EKG with 12 leads: CPT Code(s) _____

3. Individual psychotherapy, 30 minutes: CPT Code(s) _____

4. Peritoneal dialysis with one evaluation by physician: CPT Code(s) _____

5. Bilateral computerized corneal topography with interpretation and report: CPT Code(s) _____

6. Color vision exam to test for color blindness: CPT Code(s) _____

7. Impedance tympanometry: CPT Code(s) _____

8. 30 minutes of acupuncture with 11 needles without electrical stimulation: CPT Code(s) _____

9. Scratch tests, 5 trees: CPT Code(s) _____

10. Optical coherence biometry diagnostic test: CPT Code(s) _____

11. EEG, awake and asleep, supervision, interpretation, and report: CPT Code(s) _____

12. Chemotherapy administration via IV infusion, push technique: CPT Code(s) _____

13. Professional service for gastroesophageal reflux test: CPT Code(s) _____

14. PUVA photochemotherapy: CPT Code(s) _____

15. Gait and stairs retraining, 40 minutes: CPT Code(s) _____

16. CPAP: CPT Code(s) _____

17. Psychoanalysis: CPT Code(s) _____

18. Chiropractic treatment, 3 areas of spine: CPT Code(s) _____

19. Colon motility study: CPT Code(s) _____

20. Spirometry: CPT Code(s) _____

21. Comprehensive eye exam, new patient: CPT Code(s) _____

22. IM injection of hepatitis B and 4-type HPV vaccines: CPT Code(s) _____

23. Complete bilateral study of extracranial arteries using a duplex scan: CPT Code(s) _____

24. Speech Stenger test: CPT Code(s) _____

25. Catheterization of right heart with measurement of oxygen saturation (professional service only): CPT Code(s) _____

Table 33-1 ■ **COMMON SURGICAL METHODS**

Method*	CPT Definition
Ablation	Separating, detaching, or destroying
Amputation	Cutting off all or a portion of a body part, such as a leg or arm
Anastomosis	Joining two structures that are not normally joined together
Biopsy	Removing skin, tissue, muscle, or bone to test for the presence of disease
Closure	Closing an open wound with stitches, staples, or other mechanism
Debridement	Cleaning out an area using various methods, such as scraping or irrigation, to remove contaminated or necrotic tissue
Decompression	Removing pressure
Destruction	Reducing to tiny fragments
Dilation/dilatation	Expanding or stretching an opening
Drainage	Removing fluids
Endoscopy	Viewing a body cavity using a long, narrow, hollow instrument that has a light and a camera
Excision	Cutting out all or part of an organ or tissue; sometimes used synonymously with resection
Exploration	Examining an organ or structure to determine a diagnosis
Fusion/arthrodesis	Joining together two or more bones, joints, or vertebrae
Graft	Attaching a piece of skin, fascia, muscle, or bone from one area of the body to another
Incision	Cutting with a sharp instrument
Incision and drainage (I&D)	Cutting into and releasing fluid
Injection	Forcing a fluid or other substance into a cavity, tissue, or vessel
Introduction/insertion	Putting something in place
Laparotomy	Cutting into the abdominal cavity
Ligation	Tying off using any substance, such as cotton, silk, or wire
Manipulation/reduction	Using force to move a bone
Reconstruction	Restoring or reforming a part of the body
Removal	Taking something out
Repair	Restoring damaged or diseased tissues to normal function
Resection	Removing all or part of a structure or organ; sometimes used synonymously with excision
Revision	Repairing or replacing work performed during a previous procedure
Suture	Closing a wound with stitches
Transplant	Replacing an organ or tissue with organ or tissue from a donor

*The procedures in this table apply to CPT coding. Definitions vary from those for ICD-10-PCS Root Operations.

Purpose

A surgical procedure can be performed for any of three purposes: screening, diagnosis, or therapy.

- A **screening procedure** is performed to determine whether an abnormality exists in a person showing no signs or symptoms of disease. A common example is a screening colonoscopy, which is recommended to be performed every 10 years to detect early signs of malignancy.

- A **diagnostic procedure**, or exploratory procedure, is performed to identify a suspected abnormality. An example

is diagnostic colonoscopy performed to detect the cause of bleeding or to collect a specimen.

- A **therapeutic procedure** is performed to treat a condition. An example is therapeutic colonoscopy performed to remove polyps or control bleeding.

The physician performs the procedure in the same way, regardless of the purpose, except that in a therapeutic procedure additional steps may be performed to treat the problem. A diagnosis code always identifies the reason the procedure was performed. CPT does not provide modifiers or supplemental

Table 33-2 ■ **SURGICAL SUFFIXES**

Suffix	Meaning	Example
-centesis	Drainage, withdrawal of fluid	Arthrocentesis—withdrawing fluid from a joint
-desiccation	Destruction	Electrodesiccation—destruction using electricity
-desis	Stabilization or fusing together	Arthrodesis—fusing joints together
-ectomy	Excision, surgical removal	Appendectomy—surgical removal of the appendix
-lysis	Destruction	Ureterolysis—destruction of the ureter
-pexy	Surgical fixation	Hysteropexy—surgical fixation of the uterus to keep it from moving
-plasty	Surgical repair	Dermatoplasty—surgical repair of skin using grafts
-rraphy	Suturing	Nephrorrhaphy—suture of a kidney wound
-scopy	Visual examination	Colonoscopy—visual examination of the colon
-stomy	Surgical creation of an opening	Tracheostomy—surgical creation of an opening in the trachea
-tomy	Incision, cutting into	Thoracotomy—cutting into the thorax or chest
-tripsy	Crushing	Lithotripsy—crushing of stones or calculi, as in kidney stones

Table 33-3 ■ **EXAMPLES OF CONSTRUCTING MEDICAL TERMS FOR SURGERY**

Combining Form	Suffix	Complete Medical Term
nephr/o (*kidney*)	**-ectomy** (*surgical removal*) **-rraphy** (*suture*) **-plasty** (*surgical repair*) **-scopy** (*visual examination*)	**nephr + ectomy** (*surgical removal of the kidney*) **nephro + rraphy** (*suture of the kidney*) **nephro + plasty** (*surgical repair of the kidney*) **nephro + scopy** (*visual examination of the kidney with an endoscope*)
gastr/o (*stomach*)		**gastr + ectomy** (*surgical removal of the stomach*) **gastro + rraphy** (*suture of the stomach*) **gastro + plasty** (*surgical repair of the stomach*) **gastro + scopy** (*visual examination of the stomach*)

Source: © PB Resources, Inc. Used with permission.

codes to identify the purpose of the procedure as screening, diagnostic, or therapeutic. For some procedures, CPT provides separate codes for screening, diagnosis, and/or treatment. Procedures that qualify as a preventive care service under the Patient Protection and Affordable Care Act (PPACA) require modifier **-33 Preventive services** if the CPT code description does not identify the procedure as a screening or preventive in nature. A screening colonoscopy is an example.

When a procedure that is begun as screening or diagnostic becomes a therapeutic procedure during the operative session, the procedure should be coded as therapeutic if a separate code is provided. Do not also assign a code for the diagnostic procedure performed at the same time using the same method.

The Surgical Facility

The **surgical facility** is the setting or location in which surgery is performed. The choice of the facility is determined by the type of procedure to be performed, patient condition and risk factors, availability, and surgeon preference. Common sites of surgery and an example of the type of procedure performed include the following:

- Office—Example: destruction of skin lesions
- Ambulatory surgery center (ASC)—Example: arthroscopic joint surgery
- Outpatient hospital procedure room—Example: screening or diagnostic colonoscopy
- Outpatient hospital operating room (OR)—Example: arthroscopic joint surgery
- Bedside in the inpatient hospital room—Example: wound debridement
- Inpatient operating room (OR)—Example: heart bypass, hip replacement

Physicians bill for providing the professional service of performing the surgical procedure. The facility bills for the use of the facility, supplies, and staff.

Facility Billing

The facility provides the operating room, the staff, and the instruments, drugs, and supplies used during the procedure. The facility charges an operating room fee that includes use of the room and staff. Other charges are itemized then consolidated into revenue codes (*four-digit accounting codes that summarize inpatient hospital cost center [department] charges*). For Medicare inpatients, the operating room costs are paid under the Medicare Severity-Adjusted Diagnosis Related Group (MS-DRG), a predetermined, all-inclusive amount for the inpatient admission based on the patient's diagnosis and procedure. Facility services provided to Medicare patients at an ambulatory surgery center are paid under the ambulatory payment classification (APC), a predetermined, all-inclusive amount for the outpatient procedure based on the patient's diagnosis and procedure. Private payers might use MS-DRGs and APCs but substitute their own reimbursement amounts, modify the Medicare systems, or create their own methodology, such as a per diem (*daily*) payment rate.

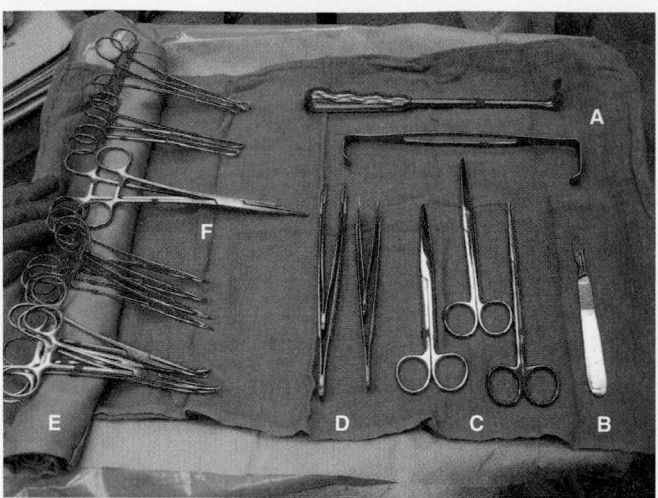

Figure 33-1 ■ Typical General Surgery Instruments: Retractors (A), Scalpel (B), Scissors (C), Forceps (D), Hemostats/Locking Forceps (E), Needle Holders (F)

SUCCESS STEP

Inpatient hospitals bill using ICD-10-PCS codes. All other facility locations are outpatient and bill using CPT codes.

Facility Staff

Except for minor procedures performed in the office or at the patient's bedside, surgery requires staff in addition to the surgeon. An anesthesia provider—either an anesthesiologist, certified registered nurse anesthetist (CRNA), or anesthesia assistant (AA)—administers most types of anesthesia other than local, topical, or a nerve block to the hand or foot. Types of anesthesia are discussed in detail in Chapter 34 of this text. Anesthesiologists typically belong to a medical group practice that contracts with the facility to provide anesthesia services. The group practice is responsible to code and bill for the services of the anesthesia providers, although this task can be outsourced to a medical billing service or the hospital billing department.

The operating room staff consists of a scrub and a circulator. The scrub is a nurse or surgical technician who adopts a sterile state (*washing hands and forearms in the prescribed manner and wearing a sterile surgical gown, gloves, mask, and hair covering*), prepares the table or tray of sterile supplies and instruments (■ FIGURE 33-1), passes instruments and supplies to the surgeon, and assists the surgeon by holding retractors or anatomic sites as requested. Some surgeons provide their own scrub so they can work with the same person all the time—someone who is familiar with their operating techniques and preferences. The circulator, required to be a registered nurse (RN) in most states, is responsible for the overall nursing care, maintains safety, transfers the patient into and out of the operating room, and assists in positioning the patient and preparing the surgical site.

Variations occur for minor procedures, which do not always require a full operating room setup or a scrub and circulator, and for more extensive procedures, which can require a team of multiple surgeons, additional operating room staff, or special equipment.

CODING PRACTICE

Exercise 33.1 Surgery Basics

Instructions: Use your medical terminology skills and resources to define the following procedures, then identify the applicable code or code range. Follow these steps.

- Use slash marks "/" to break down the underlined term into its root(s) and suffix.
- Define the meaning of the underlined word based on the meaning of each word part.
- Use the entire phrase to identify the code or code range shown in the CPT Index.

Example: <u>arthroplasty</u>, ankle arthro/plasty   Meaning *surgical repair of a joint*   CPT Code(s) *27700-27703*

1. <u>cystourethroscopy</u> with brush biopsy   Meaning _____   CPT Code(s) _____

2. posterior <u>colporrhaphy</u>   Meaning _____   CPT Code(s) _____

3. <u>ureterocalycostomy</u>   Meaning _____   CPT Code(s) _____

4. <u>tenotomy</u>, elbow   Meaning _____   CPT Code(s) _____

5. hemorrhoidopexy by stapling   Meaning _____   CPT Code(s) _____

6. diagnostic amniocentesis   Meaning _____   CPT Code(s) _____

7. partial adrenalectomy   Meaning _____   CPT Code(s) _____

8. penetrating keratoplasty   Meaning _____   CPT Code(s) _____

9. intrapleural pneumonolysis   Meaning _____   CPT Code(s) _____

10. subtalar arthrodesis   Meaning _____   CPT Code(s) _____

CODING OVERVIEW OF THE SURGERY SECTION

The CPT **Surgery (10021-69990)** section contains 19 subsections divided by body system. Each subsection is further divided into subheadings and categories by type of procedure and anatomic site. Review the subsection names and code ranges in ■ TABLE 33-4 to become familiar with the content and organization.

Surgery section guidelines appear in the CPT manual at the beginning of the Surgery section, before the list of codes. The guidelines provide general information that applies to all codes in this section, including the definition of the **CPT surgical package**, which identifies services in addition to the operative procedure included in the procedure code. These services cannot be billed separately.

The guidelines list codes for unlisted services or procedures for the subsections and subheadings within the Surgery section. When a physician performs a unique, experimental, or new procedure not represented by a CPT Category I or Category III code, assign the corresponding code for an unlisted procedure. Submit a report with the claim that describes the service provided, including the nature of, extent of, and need for the procedure, as well as the time, effort, and equipment required.

The guidelines provide information about coding for **surgical destruction**, also called lysis. Destruction is the obliteration of tissue using electrosurgery, cryosurgery, laser, or chemical treatment. It is a part of a surgical procedure and should not be coded separately unless the destruction technique substantially alters the standard management of a problem or condition.

The guidelines discuss CPT codes that carry the instructional note **(separate procedure)**. This note identifies a procedure that sometimes is performed by itself and sometimes is part of a more extensive procedure. Assign the code for the separate procedure only when it is performed alone or is not bundled into the main procedure (■ FIGURE 33-2). When it is performed with a more extensive procedure that includes the service identified as separate procedure, only assign a code for the more extensive procedure (■ FIGURE 33-3, page 600).

Special instructions that pertain to specific groups of codes appear at the beginning of subsections, subheadings, and categories throughout the Surgery section. Instructional notes providing further information on the use of specific codes appear in the Tabular List.

All surgical codes must be supported by the appropriate diagnosis codes that identify the reason(s) the procedure is performed.

Table 33-4 ■ SURGERY SUBSECTIONS

Subsection Name	Code Range
General	10021–10022
Integumentary System	10030–19499
Musculoskeletal System	20005–29999
Respiratory System	30000–32999
Cardiovascular System	33010–37799
Hemic and Lymphatic Systems	38100–38999
Mediastinum and Diaphragm	39000–39599
Digestive System	40490–49999
Urinary System	50010–53899
Male Genital System	54000–55899
Reproductive System Procedures	55920
Intersex Surgery	55970-55980
Female Genital System	56405–58999
Maternity Care and Delivery	59000–59899
Endocrine System	60000–60699
Nervous System	61000–64999
Eye and Ocular Adnexa	65091–68899
Auditory System	69000–69979
Operating Microscope	69990

The surgeon performs a bilateral pelvic lymphadenectomy on a patient with bladder cancer, to determine whether it has metastasized to the lymph nodes.

C67.9 Malignant neoplasm of bladder, unspecified
38770–50 Pelvic lymphadenectomy, including external iliac, hypogastric, and obturator nodes (separate procedure); –50 Bilateral procedure

Figure 33-2 ■ Example of Coding a Separate Procedure

The surgeon performs a complete cystectomy with a bilateral pelvic lymphadenectomy on a patient with bladder cancer with metastases to the pelvic lymph nodes.

C67.9 Malignant neoplasm of bladder, unspecified
C77.5 Secondary and unspecified malignant neoplasm of intrapelvic lymph nodes
51575 Cystectomy, complete; with bilateral pelvic lymphadenectomy, including external iliac, hypogastric, and obturator nodes

Figure 33-3 ■ Example of a Separate Procedure Included in a More Extensive Procedure

ABSTRACTING SURGERY SECTION PROCEDURES

The details of abstracting for surgery are provided for each body system in subsequent chapters of this text. Also refer to Table 28-6 Key Criteria for Abstracting Procedures (General Guidelines). The discussion that follows provides information about the nature of surgery that aids in determining which details must be abstracted.

A surgical procedure has several **integral components**, tasks that are part of the intraoperative service and are not coded or billed separately (■ TABLE 33-5). Coders must be familiar with these components and should not attempt to assign separate codes.

Three components that can be especially helpful to the coder in understanding the procedure are the patient position, surgical approach, and incision site. This information helps to identify certain details that can affect the choice of codes.

Patient Position

Patients must be arranged in a particular **position** that enables the surgeon to best access the operative site. Proper positioning of the patient helps prevent injury from loss of circulation, impaired respiration, or diminished skin integrity. The position of the patient (■ FIGURE 33-4) is not coded but can help determine whether an anterior or posterior approach is used in certain types of procedures, such as those performed on the spinal column.

Table 33-5 ■ INTEGRAL COMPONENTS OF A SURGICAL PROCEDURE

❑ Assess the patient in the preoperative area to determine readiness for surgery.
❑ Transfer the patient to the operating room.
❑ Prepare the patient for surgery, including removing hair and cleaning the surgical site.
❑ Position the patient for surgery, including elevating specific anatomic sites, such as a knee.
❑ Drape the patient (*cover the patient and surrounding area with a sterile surgical drape to separate sterile from nonsterile areas*).
❑ Administer local and, sometimes, regional anesthesia (by the surgeon).
❑ Make a surgical incision through multiple layers to access the surgical site.
❑ Explore specific areas of the patient, including further investigation of an anatomic site.
❑ Perform lysis of lesions or adhesions necessary to access the surgical site.
❑ Debride or excise necrotic or contaminated tissue and remove foreign bodies.
❑ Perform the procedure.
❑ Perform lavage/irrigation (*washing out*).
❑ Achieve hemostasis (*stoppage of bleeding*).
❑ Close the incision after surgery, including closing multiple layers of tissue.
❑ Transfer the patient to the postoperative care area.
❑ Document the procedure.

Surgical Approach

The **surgical approach** identifies how the surgeon reaches the surgical site (■ TABLE 33-6). The approach must be abstracted because CPT provides separate codes for open procedures and those performed endoscopically. CPT code descriptions assume an open approach. An endoscopic or percutaneous approach is specified in the code description.

Table 33-6 ■ TYPES OF SURGICAL APPROACH*

Name	Description	Documentation Example
Endoscopic via natural opening	An endoscope is inserted through an existing orifice (*body opening*), such as the nose, mouth, anus, vagina, or urethra.	A #21 French cystoscope was then used to visualize the entire urethra and bladder.
Endoscopic percutaneous	Several small incisions, 5–10 mm in length, are made, through which instruments and a camera, linked to an external video monitor, are inserted (■ FIGURE 33-5, page 602).	A stab incision was made within the umbilicus. The standard four trocars were inserted uneventfully.
Open	An extended incision is made through the skin, subcutaneous tissue (with division or dissection of the fascia), and muscle when necessary.	A McBurney's incision was made. A transverse right lower quadrant incision was made.
Percutaneous	A needle is used to penetrate the skin and subcutaneous tissue.	A long 20-gauge spinal needle was passed to the level of the foramen ovale. ...The needle was withdrawn.

*Note: These approaches and definitions vary from those defined with the ICD-10-PCS system.

Source: © PB Resources, Inc. Used with permission.

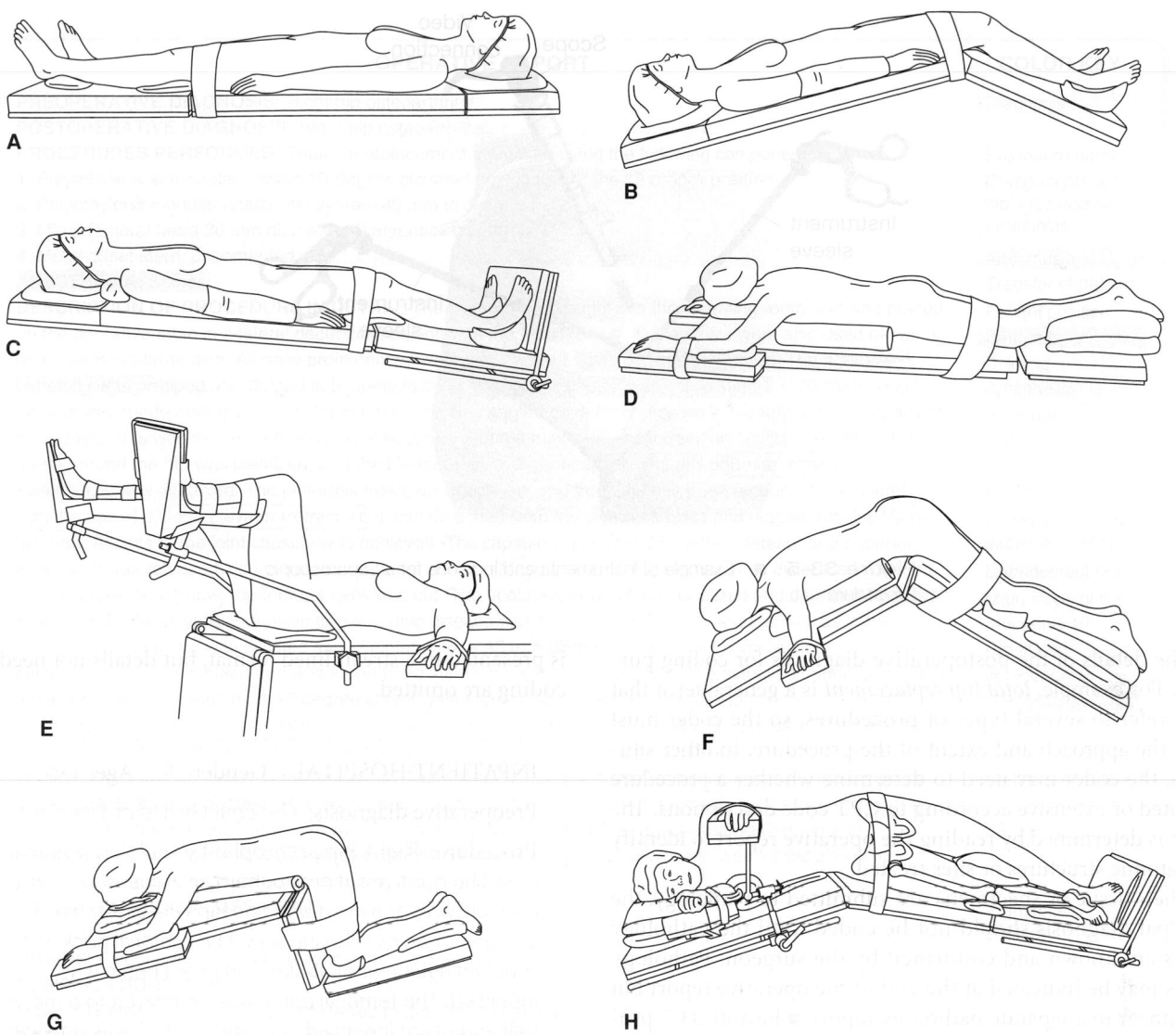

Figure 33-4 ■ Patient Positions for Surgery: Dorsal Recumbent/Supine (A), Trendelenburg (B), Reverse Trendelenburg (C), Prone (D), Lithotomy (E), Kraske/Jacknife (F), Knee–Chest (G), Lateral (H)

In operative reports, the approach is not always explicitly stated or described. For example, when a surgeon documents, *A 4-cm upper midline incision was made*, the word *open* is not used. The approach is open because an extended incision was made. Descriptions of endoscopic percutaneous procedures mention the creation of short or stab incisions, use of a trocar, and insertion of an endoscope. *Endoscopy* is a general term that often takes on the name of the anatomic site treated, such as arthroscopy, laparoscopy, colonoscopy, and so on.

Incision Site

The operative report also identifies the **incision site** (*the anatomic location at which the surgeon cuts through the skin and subcutaneous tissue*) (■ FIGURE 33-6, page 602). Although the incision site is not coded, it helps provide an understanding of the procedure and the internal structures that might be accessed.

Operative Report

At the conclusion of a procedure or operation, the physician dictates the **operative report**, which is a detailed narrative description of the procedure that includes:

- Patient name, age, and date
- Name and role of all physicians
- Preoperative and postoperative diagnoses
- Name of procedure
- Type of anesthesia
- Detailed description of the procedure, including site and length of incision, division of subcutaneous layers, visualization of anatomic structures, removal of tissue, and new tissue or tissue substitute(s) introduced
- Closure of the wound, hemostasis, and transfer to postoperative area
- Instruments, materials, and supplies used

Although the diagnosis and name of the procedure are stated at the beginning of the operative report, coders must read and analyze the entire report to confirm the details of the procedure and diagnosis necessary for coding. The terminology used by the physician may differ from the terms in the coding manuals, so it is necessary to confirm the exact nature of the procedure

2. Identify the appropriate first- and second-level modifying term(s). Examples:

   - Main Term **Arthroplasty**; first-level modifying term **Hip**; second-level modifying term **Total Replacement**.
   - Main Term **Replacement**; first-level modifying term **Hip**.
   - Main Term **Hip**; first-level modifying term **Arthroplasty**.

3. Identify the code(s) or code range. Example: **27130-27132**

4. Refer to the Tabular List to select and verify the code.
   Example: **27130 Arthroplasty, acetabular and proximal femoral prosthetic replacement (total hip arthroplasty), with or without autograft or allograft.** (Note: Code **27132** describes the conversion of a previous hip surgery to total hip arthroplasty. This example is not a conversion.)

5. Read all applicable guidelines, special instructions, and instructional notes.

6. Assign modifiers, as needed. Example: **-RT Right side**

7. Repeat this process for each procedure performed.

Surgical Care Process

To understand the use of Surgery codes and modifiers, developing a good understanding of the surgical care process is useful, beginning with a patient's first encounter with a physician regarding a problem, through the preoperative preparation, the surgical procedure, and postoperative healing and follow-up period. ■ TABLE 33-7 summarizes the major steps a patient experiences and identifies the diagnosis and procedure codes assigned by both physicians and hospitals.

Table 33-7 ■ **OVERVIEW OF THE SURGICAL CARE PROCESS: TOTAL RIGHT HIP REPLACEMENT DUE TO OSTEOARTHRITIS**

Services Provided	Physician Coding	Hospital Coding
Patient with chronic osteoarthritis of the right hip presents to PCP with complaints of increased hip pain. After evaluation and discussion, patient agrees to an evaluation by an orthopedic surgeon for possible joint replacement.	PCP codes and bills for the encounter. ICD-10-CM: **M16.11 Unilateral primary osteoarthritis, right hip** CPT*: **99213**	Not applicable
The PCP orders an updated X-ray at the request of the orthopedic surgeon. Patient presents to the radiology department at the hospital where the X-ray will be performed.	Neither the PCP nor orthopedic surgeon codes or bills for ordering the X-ray. The service is factored into the E/M service when the patient is evaluated. The radiologist who contracts with the hospital codes for the professional component of the X-ray. ICD-10-CM: **M16.11** CPT: **73510-26-RT Radiologic examination, hip, unilateral; complete, minimum of 2 views; -26 Professional component; -RT Right side**	Outpatient radiology codes for the technical component of the X-ray. ICD-10-CM: **M16.11** CPT: **73510-TC-RT**
Patient presents to the orthopedic surgeon, who evaluates the patient and determines she is a good candidate for the procedure. The patient and surgeon decide to schedule a total hip replacement procedure.	The orthopedic surgeon codes for the E/M visit for surgical evaluation. ICD-10-CM: **M16.11** CPT*: **99245 Office consultation for a new or established patient, Level 5**	Not applicable
The day before the procedure, the patient presents to the orthopedic surgeon for preoperative clearance. She also reports to the hospital outpatient laboratory for preoperative tests.	The orthopedic surgeon does not charge for the preoperative visit because it is part of the global surgical package.	The outpatient laboratory codes and enters charges for the tests into the hospital's computer. The tests will be bundled into an inpatient admission.
The patient reports to the hospital, where she is admitted. The orthopedic surgeon performs a successful procedure.	The orthopedic surgeon codes for a total right hip replacement. ICD-10-CM: **M16.11** CPT: **27130-RT Arthroplasty, acetabular and proximal femoral prosthetic replacement (total hip arthroplasty), with or without autograft or allograft; -RT Right side**	The hospital codes and enters charges for the use of the operating room and supplies. The hospital enters a charge for the technical component of the pathology evaluation. ICD-10-CM: **M16.11** CPT: **88304-TC (Technical component)**

Table 33-7 ■ *(continued)*

Services Provided	Physician Coding	Hospital Coding
	The anesthesiologist codes and bills for services provided during the procedure. ICD-10-CM: **M16.11** CPT: **01214-P1 Anesthesia for open procedures involving hip joint; total hip arthroplasty; -P1 Normal healthy patient**	
	The pathologist codes and bills for evaluation of joint material removed from the patient during surgery. ICD-10-CM: **M16.11** CPT: **88304-26 Level III - Surgical pathology, Femoral head, other than fracture; -26 Professional component**	
The patient remains in the hospital for three days following surgery. The surgeon visits the patient each day and evaluates her progress.	The orthopedic surgeon does not charge for the postoperative visits because they are part of the global surgical package, which includes a 90-day postoperative period. ICD-10-CM#: **M16.11, Z96.641 Presence of right artificial hip joint** CPT: **99024 Postoperative follow-up visit** (The code is reported once for each visit with the corresponding date. There is no charge attached to reporting the postoperative follow-up visit on the claim. The code alerts the payer that the visit occurred as part of the global surgery package.)	The hospital enters charges for daily room and board, which includes nursing care.
The patient is discharged on the fourth day following surgery.	The orthopedic surgeon does not charge for the discharge because it is part of the global surgical package. ICD-10-CM: **Z47.1 Aftercare following joint replacement surgery, Z96.641** CPT: **99024**	The hospital generates a bill for all charges accumulated during the patient's stay. ICD-10-CM: **M16.11** ICD-10-PCS*: **0SR902Z Replacement of Right Hip Joint with Metal on Polyethylene Synthetic Substitute, Open Approach**
The patient follows up with the orthopedic surgeon for postoperative evaluation 2, 4, 8, and 12 weeks after surgery.	The orthopedic surgeon does not charge or bill for the postoperative visits because they are part of the global surgical package. ICD-10-CM: **Z47.1, Z96.641** CPT: **99024** (The code is reported once for each postoperative visit with the corresponding date.)	Not applicable
The orthopedic surgeon refers the patient to physical therapy at the hospital.	The orthopedic surgeon does not charge or bill for writing orders because it is included in the surgical package.	The hospital's outpatient physical therapy department bills for the services provided during each visit, such as therapeutic exercise and gait training. ICD-10-CM: **Z47.1, Z96.641** CPT*: **97110 Therapeutic exercises** **97116 Gait training**

* The codes shown are examples. The actual code is determined based on documentation of the service performed.

Seventh characters that identify the episode of care are not used on code M16.11, so Z codes for aftercare are reported.

Source: © PB Resources, Inc. Used with permission.

Notice that several different physicians, each with a unique role, become involved at various stages of the process. Also, notice the differences between what the physician(s) codes for and what the hospital codes for. Finally, notice how the diagnosis code(s) evolves, depending on the phase of surgical care and the provider. This particular example involves a patient who is admitted as an inpatient for a total right hip replacement due to osteoarthritis. The codes provided are examples only. Actual codes could vary based on the actual situation and the documentation of services provided.

Surgical Package

The surgical package identifies a group of services that all relate to a single surgery, including preoperative, intraoperative, and postoperative services. The **global period** is the number of days during which the provider must render all services related to the surgery. Each payer establishes its own time frames for the global period for each procedure then issues one payment to cover all services performed during that time.

CPT guidelines provide a definition of the CPT surgical package. Medicare defines its own global surgical package. The policies of private payers vary.

CPT Surgical Package

The Surgery guidelines, which appear at the beginning of the Surgery section in the CPT manual, provide the CPT definition of a surgical package. ■ TABLE 33-8 identifies the elements included, or bundled, in the CPT surgical package and those that can be billed separately. The required modifier, if any, for the additional services is also shown.

Medicare Global Surgical Package

Medicare providers render services that are related to the global surgical package in any setting, including hospitals, ambulatory surgery centers (ASCs), and physicians' offices. Medicare defines services that are included in the **Medicare global surgical package**, which varies slightly from the CPT surgical package (■ TABLE 33-9).

Table 33-8 ■ **CPT SURGICAL PACKAGE**

CPT Surgical Package	Additional Services
Before the Procedure	
Subsequent to (*after*) the decision for surgery, conducting one related E/M encounter on the date immediately prior to or on the date of procedure, including history and physical	The initial encounter, and any related tests, in which the physician evaluates the patient and the decision for surgery is made (append modifier -**57** to the E/M code when the decision for surgery is made within 24 hours of the procedure)
During the Procedure	
Local anesthesia, metacarpal/metatarsal/digital block, topical anesthesia The procedure(s) performed Supplies and materials usually included with the procedure Immediate postoperative care, including dictating operative notes and talking with the family and other physicians Evaluating the patient in the postanesthesia recovery area	General anesthesia is billed by the anesthesiologist using codes from the Anesthesia section. (If general anesthesia is provided by the surgeon, append modifier -**47** to the surgical procedure code.) Supplies and materials over and above those usually included with the procedure (identify using CPT code **99070** or the appropriate HCPCS code) Surgeries for which services performed are significantly greater than usually required (identify with modifier -**22**) Surgeries for which services performed are significantly less than usually required (identify with modifier -**52**)
After the Procedure	
Writing orders Typical postoperative follow-up care based on the number of days in the follow-up period as defined by the payer (identify with code **99024**.) Care for typical complications from the procedure	Services provided by other physicians, except when the surgeon and the other physician(s) agree on the transfer of care E/M services provided by the surgeon during the postoperative period that are *unrelated* to the procedure (identify with modifier -**24**) *Unrelated* procedures performed by the same physician during the postoperative period (identify with modifier -**79**) Care of the condition for which a diagnostic procedure was performed Care for comorbid conditions Repeat procedure by the same or another physician (identify with modifier -**76** or -**77**, respectively) Unplanned return to the operating room during the postoperative period (identify with modifier -**78**)

Source: © PB Resources, Inc. Used with permission.

Table 33-9 ■ **MEDICARE GLOBAL PACKAGE**

Medicare Global Surgical Package	Additional Services
Before the Procedure	
For minor surgery: the initial encounter in which the physician evaluates the patient and the decision for surgery is made Preoperative visits	For major surgery: the initial encounter in which the physician evaluates the patient and the decision for surgery is made (append modifier **-57** to the E/M code when the decision for surgery is made within 24 hours of the procedure) Diagnostic tests and procedures, including diagnostic radiology procedures
During the Procedure	
Intraoperative services (*the procedure itself and any directly related services*) Supplies, except for those identified as exclusions by the payer Surgical tray (for most payers) (HCPCS code **A4550**)	Splints and casting supplies Supplies identified as exclusions by the payer Surgeries for which services performed are significantly greater than usually required (identify with modifier **-22**) Surgeries for which services performed are significantly less than usually required (identify with modifier **-52**)
After the Procedure	
Complications following surgery that do not require additional trips to the operating room Postoperative visits and services, such as dressing changes, removal of sutures, wires, drains, cases, splints, and tubes Postsurgical pain management	Visits unrelated to the diagnosis for which the surgical procedure is performed Treatment for the underlying condition Clearly distinct surgical procedures that are conducted during the postoperative period that are not reoperations or treatment for complications A more extensive procedure required when an original, less extensive procedure fails Treatment for postoperative complications that requires a return trip to the operating room (identify with modifier **-78**) Immunosuppressive therapy for organ transplants Critical care services unrelated to the surgery where a seriously injured or burned patient is critically ill and requires the physician's constant attendance (identify with codes **99291** and **99292**)

Source: © PB Resources, Inc. Used with permission.

Medicare assigns a global period of 0, 10, or 90 days to each procedure. A global period of 0 includes only the day of surgery. Minor procedures have a global period of 10 days *plus* the day of surgery. Major procedures have a global period of 90 days *plus* one day before surgery and the day of surgery itself. CMS publishes Medicare's number of global days for specific CPT codes in the **Medicare Physician Fee Schedule Database (MPFSDB)**, which can be accessed through the CMS website and many encoder software programs. The MPFSDB contains not only the relative value units (RVUs) and allowable fees for each CPT code, it also identifies other rules, such as the global period, the modifiers accepted, and reimbursement impact of modifiers. When multiple procedures are performed during one operative session, the global period is determined by the primary procedure. Add-on and secondary procedures do not add to the length of the global period.

Some private payers follow Medicare's global period, and others establish their own criteria. Check with individual payers to learn the length of the global period and the services included in the surgical package.

CODING CAUTION

The length of a month affects the end date of the postoperative period. For example, a 10-day postoperative period for a procedure performed on February 25 ends on March 7 in a non–leap year and on March 6 in a leap year. A 10-day postoperative period for a procedure performed on March 25 ends on April 4 because March has 31 days. A 90-day postoperative period for a procedure performed in June or July must take into account that both July and August contain 31 days. Remember to count the day *after* surgery as the first day of a 10- or 90-day period.

Surgery Modifiers

Modifiers provide payers with information about the services or procedures that vary from the standard protocol so that they will consider the claim for payment. (Refer to Table 30-1 Key Criteria for Abstracting CPT Modifiers.) A wide variety of surgical circumstances requires modifiers. After the decision for surgery is made, the most common use of modifiers is to report multiple procedures, multiple surgeons, or portions of the surgical package. A modifier for increased procedural services—those that require substantial additional work— is also available but should be used infrequently.

-57 Decision for Surgery

When an E/M encounter results in a decision for major surgery and the procedure is performed within 24 hours, the physician reports the E/M code and applies modifier **-57**. This indicates that the decision for surgery occurred within the Medicare global period, which begins the day before the procedure. Commercial payers may follow different policies. Example: **99215-57**.

-22 Increased Procedural Services

When the physician work required to provide a service is substantially greater than usual, apply modifier **-22** to the usual CPT code (■ FIGURE 33-8). This modifier should be used only in the most unusual of circumstances, such as increased intensity, time, and technical difficulty of the procedure, severity of the patient's condition, and physical and mental effort required. Medicare and some private payers require that the unusual circumstance must require at least 50% more time than usual. Some payers allow it when the procedure time is increased by 25%. Increase the charge reported for the service in proportion to the increased work when the claim is billed because payers do not automatically increase the amount paid. Medicare increases payment by 18% for this modifier. Private payers may do the same or follow a different policy.

Examples of unusual circumstances include morbid obesity, excessive hemorrhaging, extensive adhesions that block access to the surgical site, and medical emergencies, such as cardiac arrest. Documentation must describe in detail the nature of unusual circumstance, the reason additional work was required, and the time spent providing the service. In addition to the diagnosis code reported for the service itself, also report diagnosis codes that describe the nature of the unique circumstance.

The surgeon performs a laparoscopic cholecystectomy due to acute cholecystitis, but cannot access the gall bladder because of extensive adhesions in the abdominal cavity. He changes to an open approach and spends an additional 35 minutes lysing the adhesions. Once the gall bladder can be accessed, then he completes the procedure without further problems. The work on the adhesions increases the length of the procedure by 50% to 1 hour, 35 minutes.

K81.0 Acute cholecystitis
K66.0 Peritoneal adhesions
47600–22 Cholecystectomy; –22 Increased procedural services

Usual charge: $1,200.00
Charge for this patient: $1,800.00

Figure 33-8 ■ Example of Coding with Modifier -22. *Source:* © *PB Resources, Inc. Used with permission. CPT codes only © American Medical Association.*

When the reason is morbid obesity, report a diagnosis code for morbid obesity (**Z68.-**).

Modifier **-22** can be used with all CPT codes except E/M services.

SUCCESS STEP

Place a self-adhesive tab on the top edge of this page with the label *Surgery Modifiers*. Doing so will make it easy to refer back to this important information as you proceed through your coding class.

Multiple Procedures

When multiple procedures are performed during the same operative session or during the global period, modifiers **-50**, **-51**, and **-59** explain the circumstances. Coders also need to understand how to use the National Correct Coding Initiative (NCCI) to identify when multiple procedures can be billed and when they are bundled together. When repeat, staged, or unplanned procedures are performed during the postoperative period, CPT provides modifiers **-58**, **-76**, **-77**, **-78**, and **-79**.

-50 Bilateral Procedure When a procedure is performed on paired anatomic sites or organs, such as both hands or both eyes, it is a bilateral procedure. To code bilateral procedures, assign the CPT code for the unilateral procedure and append modifier **-50** (■ FIGURE 33-9). Report a quantity of **1** in Item 24G on the CMS-1500 claim form or the corresponding field on the 837P electronic claim. In general, double the charge for the service, understanding that the payer may take a discount. Medicare pays the second procedure at 50% of the standard fee. Payment policies of private payers vary.

When the code description contains the word **bilateral**, do not apply modifier **-50** because the bilateral nature of the procedure is already identified. When the code description states **unilateral or bilateral**, the same code is reported whether the procedure is done on one side or both (■ FIGURE 33-10). Do not append a modifier and do not adjust the fee. The MPFSDB identifies CPT codes for which modifier **-50** is allowed.

-51 Multiple Procedures When more than one procedure is performed during the same operative session by the same individual, report the CPT code for the first procedure, then append modifier **-51** to the second and subsequent procedures. Modifier **-51** identifies the following situations:

- Multiple, related surgical procedures performed by the same surgeon during the same operative session

- A combination of surgical procedures that may be performed through either the same or different incisions and at either the same or a different anatomic site

- A combination of medical and surgical procedures performed during the same session

Do not report modifier **-51** on E/M codes, add-on codes (designated with the symbol + in the CPT manual), or codes

The surgeon performs carpal tunnel decompression on both hands.

G56.01 Carpal tunnel syndrome, right upper limb
G56.02 Carpal tunnel syndrome, left upper limb
64721–50 Neuroplasty and/or transposition; median
nerve at carpal tunnel; –50 Bilateral
procedure

21. DIAGNOSIS OR NATURE OF ILLNESS OR INJURY Relate A-L to service line below (24E)									ICD Ind. 0		22. RESUBMISSION CODE			ORIGINAL REF. NO.	
A. G56.01			B. G56.02			C.		D.							
E.			F.			G.		H.			23. PRIOR AUTHORIZATION NUMBER				
I.			J.			K.		L.							

24. A. DATE(S) OF SERVICE						B. PLACE OF SERVICE	C. EMG	D. PROCEDURES, SERVICES, OR SUPPLIES (Explain Unusual Circumstances)		E. DIAGNOSIS POINTER	F. $ CHARGES		G. DAYS OR UNITS	H. EPSDT Family Plan	I. ID. QUAL.	J. RENDERING PROVIDER ID. #
From MM	DD	YY	To MM	DD	YY			CPT/HCPCS	MODIFIER							
01	05	YY				22		64721	50	AB	900	00	01		NPI	99 99999999

Note: If usual fee for the procedure is $450.00, then bill $900.00 for a bilateral procedure, unless the payer provides other direction. For example, CMS allows 150% of the usual price of one procedure for a bilateral procedure, which would be $675.00 here.

Figure 33-9 ■ Example of Coding a Bilateral Procedure with Modifier -50. *Source: © PB Resources, Inc. Used with permission. CPT codes only © American Medical Association.*

exempt from modifier **-51** (designated with the symbol ⊘ in the CPT manual). The MPFSDB identifies CPT codes for which modifier **-51** is allowed.

-59 Distinct Procedural Service Use modifier **-59** to identify that a procedure or service is separate and distinct from other services provided during the same session. Use this modifier only when no other modifier is appropriate. It identifies services that are not normally reported together but are appropriate in the current situation because of:

- a different operative session;
- a different anatomic site or organ system;
- a different procedure or surgery;
- a separate incision or excision;
- a separate lesion; or
- a separate injury or separate area of injury in extensive injuries.

Modifier **-59** informs the payer that although the procedure is normally bundled with another procedure, in this case it is not. More information about bundling and unbundling related to the National Correct Coding Initiative is discussed next.

National Correct Coding Initiative The **National Correct Coding Initiative (NCCI)** was implemented to promote correct coding and to control improper coding leading to inappropriate payment. NCCI identifies pairs of codes that normally cannot be reported together. NCCI code pair edits are automated **prepayment edits** for Medicare and other payers, which means that the payer's computer analyzes codes before the claim is processed and flags claims that might result in improper payment. The goal is to prevent improper payment when certain codes are submitted for services covered by Medicare Part B for the same patient, on the same date, by the same provider.

The NCCI data are presented in a table that consists of several columns. **Column 1** contains a list of all payable CPT codes.

The surgeon performs a cystectomy of both ovaries.

N83.20 Unspecified ovarian cysts
58925 Ovarian cystectomy, unilateral or bilateral

21. DIAGNOSIS OR NATURE OF ILLNESS OR INJURY Relate A-L to service line below (24E)								ICD Ind. 0		22. RESUBMISSION CODE			ORIGINAL REF. NO.	
A. N83.20			B.		C.		D.							
E.			F.		G.		H.			23. PRIOR AUTHORIZATION NUMBER				
I.			J.		K.		L.							

24. A. DATE(S) OF SERVICE						B. PLACE OF SERVICE	C. EMG	D. PROCEDURES, SERVICES, OR SUPPLIES (Explain Unusual Circumstances)		E. DIAGNOSIS POINTER	F. $ CHARGES		G. DAYS OR UNITS	H. EPSDT Family Plan	I. ID. QUAL.	J. RENDERING PROVIDER ID. #
From MM	DD	YY	To MM	DD	YY			CPT/HCPCS	MODIFIER							
01	05	YY				21		58925		A	800	00	01		NPI	99 99999999

Figure 33-10 ■ Example of Coding a Bilateral Procedure That Does Not Require Modifier -50. *Source: © PB Resources, Inc. Used with permission. CPT codes only © American Medical Association.*

Column 2 contains the code that is not payable with a particular Column 1 code unless a modifier is permitted and submitted (■ TABLE 33-10). The column labeled Modifier Indicator identifies whether the code in Column 2 can be billed with the code in Column 1.

0–Not Allowed. No modifiers associated with NCCI are allowed to be used with this code pair. There are no circumstances in which both procedures of the code pair should be paid for the same beneficiary on the same day by the same provider.

1–Allowed. The modifiers -25, -57, or -59 are allowed on the Column 2 code of the code pair when clinically appropriate, such as when one of the circumstances listed in the preceding subheading for modifier -59 exists or when an E/M service provided during the global period is not part of the global surgical package (-25, -57).

9–Not Applicable. An NCCI edit does not apply to this code pair. A previous edit was deleted.

Any code *not* listed in Column 2 can be reported with the Column 1 code without any NCCI restrictions. However, all other coding and billing rules apply, and modifiers may be necessary for other reasons.

The NCCI table contains additional columns with historical and other supplemental information. Instructions on how to use the NCCI tables are available on the CMS website (**www.cms.gov**). Many encoders and billing software programs contain the NCCI edits and provide a warning or reminder when a code pair is used that is not allowed or requires a special modifier.

Staged, Repeat, and Unplanned Procedures When staged, repeat, or unplanned procedures are performed during the postoperative period, CPT provides modifiers -58, -76, -77, -78, and -79. Multiple procedures may be performed during the postoperative period for several reasons. A modifier identifies the reason for an additional procedure and alerts the payer that it is a separate procedure that should be paid. If the appropriate modifier is not used, the payer considers the procedure to be a duplicate bill or a service included in the global surgical package and does not pay it. Coders must apply the modifiers correctly on the original claim. If a modifier is omitted that results in a denied claim, it is difficult to persuade the payer to accept the modifier retroactively.

Table 33-10 ■ EXAMPLES OF NCCI CODE PAIRS

Column 1	Column 2	Modifier Indicator
39561	96375	1
39561	96376	1
39561	99148	0
39561	99149	0
39561	99150	0
39561	99211	1
39561	99212	1

Source: Centers for Medicare and Medicaid Services

-58 Staged or related procedure or service by the same physician or other qualified health care professional during the postoperative period A series of procedures is planned to accomplish the operative objective, such as skin grafts or breast reconstruction. A procedure that is more extensive than the original is performed, such as amputation of additional gangrenous digits. A therapeutic procedure is performed following a surgical procedure, such as a mastectomy performed after a breast biopsy is positive for carcinoma. Append modifier -58 to the code for the subsequent procedure(s). The modifier alerts the payer that the staged procedure is separate and distinct, and a new postoperative period should begin. Do not report this modifier when CPT provides separate codes for each stage of the treatment.

-76 Repeat procedure or service by same physician or other qualified health care professional The provider who performed the original service needs to repeat the same procedure, such as X-rays or EKGs performed for comparative purposes over a period of time. Append modifier -76 to the code for the repeat procedure reported by the same physician. The modifier alerts the payer that this is not a duplicate billing of the same procedure, but it was performed for a specific reason.

-77 Repeat procedure or service by another physician or other qualified health care professional The same procedure as the original is repeated by a different provider than performed the original, such as when the original physician is not available, the patient chooses to see a different physician, or a physician of a different specialty repeats the procedure for a medically necessary reason. Append modifier -77 to the code for the repeat procedure reported by the second physician. The modifier alerts the payer that this is not a duplicate billing of the same procedure, but it was performed for a specific reason.

-78 Unplanned return to the operating/procedure room by the same physician or other qualified health care professional following initial procedure for a related procedure during the postoperative period A procedure to treat a complication arising from the original procedure is performed by the same surgeon who performed the original procedure, such as returning to the operating room to control postoperative hemorrhaging. Append modifier -78 to the code for the unplanned procedure. The modifier alerts the payer that the procedure should be paid, even though it occurs during the global postoperative follow-up period. When the unplanned procedure is performed by a different physician, no modifier is required because the follow-up days of the global package apply only to the original physician.

-79 Unrelated procedure or service by the same physician or other qualified health care professional during the postoperative period A procedure not related to the original procedure is performed by the same surgeon who performed the original procedure, such as an emergency appendectomy during the postoperative period of a cholecystectomy. Append modifier -79 to the code for the unrelated procedure. The modifier alerts the payer that the procedure should be paid, even though it occurs during the global postoperative follow-up period, because it is unrelated to the original procedure. When the unrelated procedure is performed by a different physician, no modifier is required because the follow-up days of the global package apply only to the original physician.

Multiple Surgeons

Most surgical procedures are performed by one surgeon, but in some situations multiple surgeons are needed. Coders must understand the various roles of surgeons so that each physician's involvement in the procedure can be coded and billed correctly. The role of each physician is identified on the operative report and is reported using a modifier. Each surgeon bills the same CPT code, then appends the modifier that identifies his or her role in the procedure. The total amount of reimbursement for the procedure is prorated among all surgeons involved, based on the role of each. The MPFSDB identifies CPT codes for which each of these modifiers is allowed and how the reimbursement is prorated. Other payers can follow Medicare's criteria or develop their own.

-66 Surgical Team A surgical team is a group of several physicians or other qualified health professionals, usually of different specialties, who work together to perform highly complex procedures, such as organ transplants. Each provider performs a specific part of the procedure for which they have been specially trained. Each surgeon reports the same CPT code with modifier -**66**. Payment is split between the two surgeons based on the work that each performed.

-62 Two Surgeons Cosurgeons are two surgeons of different specialties who work together as primary surgeons to perform separate parts of a procedure. An example is spinal surgery, in which a thoracic surgeon makes the surgical incision and creates access to the spine and a neurosurgeon performs the spinal procedure. Each surgeon reports the same CPT code with modifier -**62**. Payment is split between the two surgeons based on the work that each performed.

-80 Assistant Surgeon An assistant surgeon actively assists the primary surgeon in performing the procedure and is present for all, or a substantial portion, of the procedure. The assistant surgeon must be medically necessary. Fewer than 5% of surgical cases require an assistant surgeon. The assistant surgeon reports the same CPT code as the primary surgeon and appends modifier -**80**.

-81 Minimum Assistant Surgeon A minimum assistant surgeon assists the surgeon for a short time during the procedure.

The medical necessity of a minimum assistant surgeon must be documented, and this situation is rare.

-82 Assistant Surgeon When a Qualified Resident is Not Available A qualified resident surgeon is a licensed physician who is receiving advanced training after completing medical school. Hospitals with a teaching program often use a qualified resident surgeon when an assistant surgeon is needed. The cost of residents is incorporated into the overall reimbursement rates for the hospital. When a resident surgeon is not available, then another surgeon, who is not paid by the hospital or paid at a different rate, must fill the assistant surgeon role.

Assistant surgeons and minimum assistant surgeons report the same CPT code as the primary surgeon and append the appropriate modifier. The primary surgeon reports the CPT code with no modifier.

Portions of the Surgical Package

Surgeons' services include all care included in the global package. When the same surgeon does not provide all phases of the global package—preoperative, procedural, and postoperative— then each surgeon involved must use a modifier to identify the portion of the global package provided. The MPFSDB identifies the portion of the procedure fee paid to each physician who provides part of the surgical package, based on the role of each. Private payers establish their own payment criteria.

-56 Preoperative Management Only When a surgeon provides the preoperative visit but does not perform the procedure or provide the postoperative follow-up, report the CPT code for the surgical procedure and append modifier -**56**.

-54 Surgical Care Only When a surgeon performs the surgical procedure but does not provide preoperative and postoperative care, report the CPT code for the surgical procedure and append modifier -**54**.

-55 Postoperative Management Only When a surgeon provides the postoperative follow-up visits, but not the preoperative visit, and does not perform the procedure, report the CPT code for the surgical procedure and append modifier -**55**.

When a surgeon provides two components of the surgical package, such as providing preoperative care and performing the procedure, report the CPT code for the surgical procedure and append the modifiers for the two components provided.

CODING PRACTICE

Exercise 33.3 Assigning Surgery Codes

Instructions: Circle either *Yes* or *No* to indicate whether each of the following services is part of the CPT surgical package.

1. The initial encounter, and any related tests, in which the physician evaluates the patient and the decision for surgery is made.   Yes   No

2. Local anesthesia.   Yes   No

3. General anesthesia.   Yes   No

4. Care for typical complications from the procedure.   Yes   No

5. Care for comorbid conditions.   Yes   No

ARRANGING SURGERY CODES

Sequence multiple surgical procedures in descending order by the dollar charge or RVU. Ideally, both methods result in the same order because the price should reflect the RVU. The **Medicare Physician Fee Schedule (MPFS)** (*a listing of CPT codes and Medicare allowable fees published by the Centers for Medicare and Medicaid Services*) is based on RVUs, so price order and RVU order should be the same. Other payers may have specific instructions regarding whether price or RVU takes priority. Some payers' computer systems, including Medicare's, automatically rearrange codes to the desired order. Most payers allow the full amount of the first procedure and reduce the value of subsequent procedures that carry modifier **-51** to 50% of the allowed amount. The reduction is based on the efficiencies gained when multiple procedures are performed during the same operative session compared with being performed alone. More specific guidance on sequencing Surgery codes appears in the subsections for each body system.

SURGERY: GENERAL SUBSECTION (10021-10022)

The first and smallest subsection of the Surgery chapter is General, which includes only two codes. The codes identify fine-needle aspiration without imaging guidance (**10021**) and with imaging guidance (**10022**).

Fine-needle aspiration biopsy (FNAB, FNA, or NAB) is a procedure in which a physician inserts a fine (*thin*), hollow needle under the skin to obtain aspirate, a small sample of cells, tissue, or fluid. It can be performed on nearly any anatomic site to help determine the cause of a lump, mass, infection, or inflammation. The physician can use imaging, such as ultrasound, fluoroscopy, MRI, or CT, to visualize the needle and determine where to move it. The cells from the sample are placed on a glass slide and stained, and a pathologist views them under a microscope.

Table 33-11 ■ KEY CRITERIA FOR ABSTRACTING FINE-NEEDLE ASPIRATION

❏ Is the aspiration procedure specified as *fine-needle* aspiration?

❏ Is imaging guidance performed?

❏ Is a specimen being obtained?

Locate other codes if the answer to any of the following questions is *Yes*.

❏ Is the specimen being evaluated? (Use laboratory codes.)

❏ Does the aspirate consist of orbital contents? (Use eye codes.)

❏ Is the transendoscopic method used to obtain the aspirate from the esophagus, stomach, duodenum, or colon? (Use gastrointestinal system codes.)

❏ Is a percutaneous or core needle biopsy performed? (Use appropriate code for the anatomic site.)

Source: © PB Resources, Inc. Used with permission.

When abstracting for fine-needle aspiration, verify that the documentation identifies fine-needle aspiration and not another type of needle biopsy, such as a percutaneous core needle biopsy, which uses a larger needle and is classified by anatomic site (■ TABLE 33-11).

To assign codes for fine-needle aspiration, search the Index for the Main Term **Fine Needle Aspiration**. Locate the first-level modifying term **Diagnostic**, which refers you to the codes **10021** and **10022**. Review the other first-level modifying terms listed to be sure that none apply.

Instructional notes in parentheses direct you to assign other codes for radiologic supervision, laboratory analysis of the sample, and percutaneous needle biopsy other than fine needle. For other types of needle biopsies, search for the Main Term **Biopsy** and the first-level modifying term for the anatomic site.

CODING PRACTICE

Exercise 33.4 Surgery: General Subsection

Instructions: Code the following services using the Index and Tabular List. Write the code(s) on the line provided.

1. Fine-needle aspiration biopsy of the pancreas, with imaging guidance   1 CPT Code _____

2. Percutaneous core needle biopsy of the left breast
   1 CPT Code _____

3. Transendoscopic fine-needle biopsy of the colon
   1 CPT Code _____

4. FNAB of the thyroid   1 CPT Code _____

5. Fine-needle aspiration biopsy of the orbital contents
   1 CPT Code _____

CHAPTER SUMMARY

In this chapter you learned that:

• Surgery is the branch of medicine that treats diseases, injuries, and deformities through the use of instruments or manual techniques. A surgical procedure is a combination of a surgical method and an anatomic site.

• Surgery section guidelines appear in the CPT manual at the beginning of the Surgery section, before the list of codes. The guidelines provide general information that applies to all codes in this section, including the definition of the CPT surgical package, which identifies services in addition to the operative procedure included in the procedure code.

- A surgical procedure has several integral components—tasks that are considered part of the procedure and are not coded or billed separately.

- Medicare defines services that are included in the Medicare global surgical package, which varies slightly from the CPT surgical package.

- To assign Surgery codes, follow the standard process for assigning CPT codes. Modifiers provide payers with more information about the services so they will consider the claim for payment.

- Sequence multiple surgical procedures in descending order by the dollar charge or relative value unit (RVU).

- The first and smallest subsection of the Surgery chapter is General, which includes only two codes for fine-needle aspiration.

CONCEPT QUIZ

Take a moment to look back at the Surgery section and solidify your skills. Try to answer the questions from memory first, then refer to the discussion in this chapter if you need a little extra help.

Completion

Instructions: Write the term that answers each question based on the information you learned in this chapter. Choose from the list below. Some choices may be used more than once and some choices may not be used at all.

ablation	exploration
anastomosis	fusion
biopsy	laparotomy
decompression	ligation
dilation	reconstruction
drainage	resection
excision	suturing

1. _____ is the method used to relieve pressure.

2. _____ is cutting into the abdominal cavity.

3. _____ is joining together two or more bones, joints, or vertebrae.

4. _____ is the surgical method used to remove fluid.

5. The purpose of a(n) _____ is to remove skin, tissue, muscle, or bone to test for the presence of disease.

6. _____ may be done to examine an organ or structure to determine a diagnosis.

7. _____ is tying off using any substance, such as cotton, silk, or wire.

8. _____ describes a procedure in which all or part of a structure or organ is removed.

9. The surgical method called _____ is used to separate, detach, or destroy.

10. _____ is expanding or stretching an opening.

Multiple Choice

Instructions: Circle the letter of the best answer to each question based on the information you learned in this chapter.

1. Which service is part of the CPT surgical package?
   A. The encounter in which the decision for surgery is made
   B. Care for typical complications from the procedure
   C. General anesthesia
   D. A repeat procedure by the same physician

2. How many days is the Medicare postoperative period for minor procedures?
   A. 0
   B. 5
   C. 10
   D. 15

3. What modifier is assigned when a surgeon provides the preoperative visit but does not perform the procedure or provide postoperative follow-up?
   A. -53
   B. -54
   C. -55
   D. -56

4. What modifier identifies services that are not normally billed together but are appropriate in the current situation?
   A. -59
   B. -22
   C. -80
   D. -81

5. What type of surgery is medically necessary but can be delayed at least 24 hours?
   A. Emergency
   B. Screening
   C. Optional
   D. Elective

6. Which of the following is an integral component of a surgical procedure?
   A. Anesthesia administered by a CRNA
   B. Preoperative lab work
   C. Transferring the patient to the operating room
   D. Postoperative follow-up

7. What is the surgical approach for a procedure that begins with a McBurney's incision?
   A. Percutaneous
   B. Open
   C. Endoscopic via natural opening
   D. Endoscopic percutaneous

(continued)

(continued from page 613)

8. Where does the coder find Medicare's number of global days for specific CPT codes?
   A. Medicare Global Period Schedule
   B. Appendix A of the CPT code book
   C. Medicare Physician Fee Schedule
   D. CPT Surgical Package Schedule

9. What is the last day of a 90-day postoperative period for a procedure performed on October 3?
   A. January 1
   B. January 2
   C. January 3
   D. January 4

10. When is it appropriate to use modifier -22?
    A. Multiple procedures are performed during the same operative session
    B. Services performed are significantly greater than usually required
    C. E/M services unrelated to an operative procedure are provided by the surgeon during the postoperative period of the procedure
    D. There is an unplanned return to the operating room during the postoperative period

Anesthesia Procedures (00100-01999)

Chapter 34

Learning Objectives

After completing this chapter, you should have the skills to:

34.1 Spell and define the key words, medical terms, and abbreviations related to anesthesia.

34.2 Discuss the types of anesthesia services.

34.3 Identify the main characteristics of coding for anesthesia.

34.4 Abstract procedural information from the medical record for coding anesthesia.

34.5 Assign codes for anesthesia procedures.

34.6 Arrange codes for anesthesia procedures.

34.7 Discuss the CPT coding guidelines related to anesthesia.

Chapter Outline

- **Anesthesia Basics**
- **Coding Overview of the Anesthesia Section**
- **Abstracting Anesthesia Procedures**
- **Assigning Anesthesia Codes**
- **Arranging Anesthesia Codes**

Key Terms and Abbreviations

anesthesia
anesthesia code package
anesthesia conversion factor
anesthesia time
anesthesiologist

base unit (B)
certified registered nurse anesthetist (CRNA)
controlled hypotension
Mallampati score

modifying unit (M)
monitored anesthesia care (MAC)
patient-controlled analgesia (PCA)

physical status score
postoperative anesthesia care unit (PACU)
time unit (T)
total-body hypothermia

In addition to the key terms listed here, students should know the terms defined within tables in this chapter.

INTRODUCTION

When you take a car to the repair shop, mechanics can begin work immediately, without advance preparation to protect the vehicle. However, when people need surgery, they must be protected from pain and discomfort through the use of anesthesia. In this chapter you will learn about the specialized area of anesthesia services and how to code for them, including the unique anesthesia payment formula. Although the Anesthesia section appears before the Surgery section in the CPT manual, this text presented the introduction to the Surgery section first so that you understand the basics of surgery before tackling anesthesia services.

ANESTHESIA BASICS

Anesthesia is a medical specialty that works in conjunction with surgical specialties to manage a patient's status during a surgical procedure. The surgeon is solely responsible for performing the operative procedure; the anesthesia provider keeps the patient immobile and unaware of pain while the procedure is performed. Coders must be familiar with the types of anesthesia providers, the anesthesia patient care cycle, and the various types of anesthesia.

Anesthesia Providers

Anesthesia providers include anesthesiologists, certified registered nurse anesthetists, and anesthesiologist assistants. **Anesthesiologists** are physicians who specialize in providing perioperative care, developing anesthesia plans, and administrating anesthetics. Some anesthesiologists specialize in anesthesia for cases in pediatrics, obstetrics, cardiothoracic, neurosurgical, orthopedics, critical care, trauma, organ transplant, ambulatory, and pain management. Most procedures require only one anesthesia provider. Anesthesiologists also can be responsible for supervising other anesthesia providers, such as certified registered nurse anesthetists and anesthesiologist assistants.

A **certified registered nurse anesthetist (CRNA)** is a registered nurse with advanced education and training in the field of anesthesia. CRNAs can work alone on cases, with other CRNAs, or under the supervision of an anesthesiologist. An anesthesiologist has more education and training than a CRNA and is licensed to practice medicine. CRNAs can work in hospitals and ambulatory surgery centers, as well as surgery suites, physician offices, and pain management clinics.

An **anesthesiologist assistant (AA)** is a specialty physician assistant who assists the anesthesiologist and can also work alongside a CRNA. An anesthesia technician, certified anesthesia technician, and certified anesthesia technologist assist the anesthesiologist, AA, and CRNA. They also operate, maintain, and monitor equipment and oversee supplies.

The Centers for Medicare and Medicaid Services (CMS) requires that anesthesia services be provided by one of the following providers to qualify for reimbursement:

- anesthesiologist
- physician other than an anesthesiologist, including licensed residents and fellows
- dentist, oral surgeon, or podiatrist who is qualified to administer anesthesia under state law

- CRNA under the supervision of the operating surgeon or an anesthesiologist who is immediately available if needed, meaning that they are physically located in the same area
- AA under the supervision of an anesthesiologist who is immediately available if needed

Anesthesia providers work in a facility, such as an inpatient hospital, outpatient hospital, ambulatory surgery center (ASC), or pain clinic. In most cases, anesthesia providers are not employed by the facility. Individual providers belong to a group practice that contracts with one or more facilities to provide anesthesia services. They bill using CPT codes. Billing is done by the group practice staff or is contracted out to a billing service or a hospital's billing department. Payment is issued to the anesthesia practice.

Anesthesia Care Cycle

The patient care cycle for anesthesia services includes preoperative, intraoperative, and postoperative services.

Preoperative care includes evaluation of the patient's current health and readiness for anesthesia. The **physical status score** identifies the patient's health status at the time anesthesia begins, on a scale of 1 through 5. The **Mallampati score** rates the potential difficulty of endotracheal intubation on a scale of I through IV. Preoperative care also includes placing monitoring devices on the patient and facilitating anesthesia administration with other equipment, such as an endotracheal tube. Anesthesia administration begins when the anesthesia provider induces the patient; it includes monitoring the patient's vital signs to ensure that the patient receives the correct amount of anesthesia and has no adverse reactions.

Intraoperative anesthesia care involves monitoring and managing the patient's physiological status during a procedure and ensuring the patient's safety. If a patient experiences complications to anesthesia, then the anesthesia provider must render appropriate care to the patient, including life-saving interventions, such as cardiopulmonary resuscitation, restoration of fluids and blood, and respiratory therapy. Routine monitoring includes electrocardiography (ECG, EKG), oximetry (*measurement of the concentration of oxygen in the blood*), capnography (*measurement of the concentration of carbon dioxide in the blood*), and mass spectrometry (*measurement of the amount of gases and anesthetics the patient inhales and exhales*), as well as monitoring of temperature and blood pressure. In unusual situations, monitoring may be performed using an intra-arterial catheter (*one inserted into an artery*), a Swan-Ganz (*a catheter inserted into the pulmonary artery*), and a central venous catheter (CVC) (*one inserted into one of the large veins near the heart*).

Because of the risks inherent in anesthesia administration, physicians use the lowest level of anesthesia necessary to keep the patient comfortable and pain free. For example, regional, rather than general, anesthesia is used whenever possible because it poses less risk to the patient. For many patients even major joint procedures, such as total hip replacement, can be performed using regional anesthesia. However, the nature and extent of some procedures leave no option other than general anesthesia.

Table 34-1 ■ **EXAMPLE OF CONSTRUCTING MEDICAL TERMS FOR ANESTHESIA**

Combining Form	Prefix/Suffix	Complete Medical Term
algesi/o (*sense of pain*) **esthesi/o** (*nervous sensation*) **mnesi/o** (*memory*)	**a-/an-** (*lack of*) **-ia** (*condition*)	**an + alges + ia** (*condition of lack of pain*) **an + esthes + ia** (*condition of lack of nervous sensation*) **a + mnes + ia** (*condition of lack of memory*)

Source: © PB Resources, Inc. Used with permission.

After surgery is complete, the patient is taken to a **postoperative anesthesia care unit (PACU)** or other area to recover from the surgical procedure and effects of anesthesia. Anesthesia administration ends when the anesthesia provider turns over the care and supervision of the patient to PACU nursing staff. After the anesthesia provider and PACU staff ensure that the patient has no negative effects or complications, the patient is moved out of the PACU. Outpatients are discharged to home. Inpatients are transferred to an inpatient room, where they are monitored for one or more days until discharged by the attending physician.

Types of Anesthesia

Anesthesia is a temporary state, induced by drugs, of unconsciousness, loss of memory, lack of pain, and/or muscle relaxation. The three components of anesthesia are analgesia (*pain relief*), amnesia (*loss of memory*), and immobilization (■ TABLE 34-1). Some drugs may achieve all three components, but often a combination of drugs is used, each with a unique effect (■ TABLE 34-2). General anesthetics cause a reversible loss of consciousness, and local anesthetics cause a reversible loss of sensation in a limited region of the body while maintaining consciousness. Additional drugs, called reversal agents, are administered to reverse the effects of anesthesia when the procedure is complete.

Anesthesia providers give patients anesthesia through various methods, including intravenous injection or infusion, a face mask, an endotracheal tube, intranasal spray, or an injection directly into the anatomic site where surgery will occur. Patients receive specific types of anesthesia depending on the procedure performed, their physical condition and health history, and the potential for possible complications (■ TABLE 34-3, page 618).

Although advances in anesthesia enable providers to eliminate patients' pain during many types of surgeries, anesthesia is not without risks. Patients with comorbidities are at a greater risk for developing complications from anesthesia than are normal, healthy patients. Risks also depend on the complexity of a procedure and the type of anesthesia administered.

CODING CAUTION

Although the terms *asleep* and *awake* are often used when speaking of anesthesia, the state of unconsciousness induced by anesthesia is not sleep and does not provide the restorative benefits of natural sleep.

Monitored Anesthesia Care

Monitored anesthesia care (MAC) is a planned procedure during which the patient undergoes local anesthesia together with sedation and analgesia. MAC is the first choice in 10–30% of

Table 34-2 ■ **COMMONLY USED ANESTHETIC DRUGS**

Generic Name (Brand Name)	Drug Class
Articaine/epinephrine (Septocaine, Orabloc, Articadent, Zorcaine)	Local anesthetic
Bupivacaine (Marcaine, Sensorcaine)	Local anesthetic
Cisatracurium (Nimbex)	Neuromuscular blocking agent
Dexamethasone (Baycadron, DexPak, Zema Pak, etc.)	Corticosteroid
Fentanyl (Sublimaze)	Narcotic analgesic
Flumazenil (Romazicon)	Reversal agent
Hyoscyamine (Anaspaz, Cystospaz, etc.)	Anticholinergic/antispasmodic
Ketamine (Ketalar)	General anesthetic
Lidocaine (Anesthacaine, Xylocaine, etc.)	Topical anesthetic
Meperidine (Demerol)	Narcotic analgesic
Mepivacaine (Carbocaine, Polocaine, Scandonest)	Local or regional anesthetic
Methohexital (Brevital Sodium)	Barbiturate
Midazolam (Versed)	Benzodiazepine sedative
Naloxone (Narcan)	Reversal agent
Prilocaine (none)	Topical anesthetic
Propofol (Diprivan)	General anesthetic
Succinylcholine (Anectine, Quelicin)	Neuromuscular blocking agent

surgical procedures because it is less physically demanding and allows for faster recovery than general anesthesia. The fundamental principles of MAC are safe sedation, anxiety control, and pain control.

MAC may include varying levels of sedation as necessary. The provider of monitored anesthesia care must be prepared and qualified to convert to general anesthesia when necessary. If the patient loses consciousness and the ability to respond purposefully, the anesthesia care is a general anesthetic, irrespective of whether airway instrumentation is required.

Third-party payers reimburse for MAC services only when they are medically necessary based on the patient's condition and medical history and patient information documented in the anesthesia record.

Table 34-3 ■ **TYPES OF ANESTHESIA**

Type	Description	Examples/Uses
Topical	Numbs the surface area of a body part.	Removal of a foreign object from the eye
Local	Numbs a small area of a body part. Patient is awake and alert.	Cyst removal from the skin Tooth extraction
Moderate (conscious) sedation	Uses a mild sedative to relax the patient and pain medicine to relieve pain. Patient stays awake but may not remember the procedure afterward.	Colonoscopy or endoscopy, dental reconstructive surgery or dental prosthetics
Regional	Epidural, spinal, and peripheral nerve blocks. Blocks pain in an area of the body, such as an arm or leg. Patient feels nothing in that area of the body.	Cesarean delivery, many orthopedic procedures
General	Affects the whole body, including the brain. Patient feels nothing and has no memory of the procedure afterward.	Open-heart surgery, abdominal surgery

Special Anesthesia Techniques

Anesthesia providers occasionally use controlled hypotension and total-body hypothermia to help reduce patients' risk pertaining to certain conditions.

Controlled hypotension, also called induced hypotension or hypotensive anesthesia, is a technique that lowers the mean arterial blood pressure (MAP) by 30% during surgery, with the goal of reducing intraoperative blood loss and minimizing the risk of fluid overload. This reduces the need for blood transfusions and may also decrease the risk of fluid-related complications, such as edema and deep vein thrombosis (DVT) (*the formation of blood clots in the legs*). Hypotension is accomplished by administering vasodilators (*drugs that widen the diameter of blood vessels*). It is most often used with patients at high risk of these conditions who are undergoing orthopedic, spinal, or maxillofacial surgery.

Total-body hypothermia, also called induced hypothermia or hypothermic anesthesia, is a technique that lowers the core body temperature below 35°C (95°F) during surgery, with the goal of protecting neurons from injury or degeneration. Hypothermia is accomplished by administering antipyretics (*drugs that lower fever*) and using various physical mechanisms such as ice packs, fans, and cooling blankets and caps. It is most often used with comatose cardiac arrest survivors, head injury victims, and patients with neonatal encephalopathy.

Patient-Controlled Analgesia

Patient-controlled analgesia (PCA) is a method of pain control that patients can administer in response to the level of pain experienced. A PCA pump is an electronically controlled analgesia pump that delivers pain medication intravenously. The patient pushes a button on a hand-held device to direct the pump to deliver the medication. The provider sets a limit on the maximum amount of medication that the pump can deliver to the patient during a specific time interval. PCA pumps help postoperative and terminally ill patients with pain control.

CODING PRACTICE

Exercise 34.1 Anesthesia Basics

Instructions: Use your medical terminology skills and resources to define the following procedures, then identify the applicable code or code range. Follow these steps:

- Use slash marks "/" to break down the underlined term into its root(s) and suffix.
- Define the meaning of the underlined word based on the meaning of each word part.
- Locate the Main Term *Anesthesia* in the CPT Index, then identify the code(s) shown for the procedure in the CPT Index.

Example: Anesthesia, <u>Angiography</u>   Angio/graphy   Meaning *recording of vessels*   CPT Code *01920*

1. Anesthesia, <u>cystolithotomy</u>   Meaning _____   CPT Code _____

2. Anesthesia, <u>vitreoretinal</u> surgery   Meaning _____   CPT Code _____

3. Anesthesia, <u>tenodesis</u>   Meaning _____   CPT Code _____

4. Anesthesia, <u>abdominoperineal</u> resection   Meaning _____   CPT Code _____

5. Anesthesia, <u>urethrocystoscopy</u>   Meaning _____   CPT Code _____

6. Anesthesia, <u>retropharyngeal</u> tumor excision   Meaning _____   CPT Code _____

7. Anesthesia, <u>vulvectomy</u>   Meaning _____   CPT Code _____
8. Anesthesia, <u>lymphadenectomy</u>   Meaning _____   CPT Code _____
9. Anesthesia, <u>colporrhaphy</u>   Meaning _____   CPT Code _____
10. <u>Omphalocele</u>   Meaning _____   CPT Code _____

CODING OVERVIEW OF THE ANESTHESIA SECTION

The CPT **Anesthesia (00100-01999)** section contains 19 subsections, most of which are divided by anatomic site. The last four subsections are divided by the type of procedure: radiological, burn excisions or debridement, obstetric, and other. Review the subsection names and code ranges listed at the beginning of the Anesthesia section in the CPT manual to become familiar with the content and organization.

This chapter includes codes reported by anesthesia providers for the administration of anesthesia services. Do not report codes from this section when the surgeon administers anesthesia. Instead, append modifier **-47 Anesthesia by surgeon** to the CPT code for the procedure. Codes for moderate sedation appear in the **Moderate Sedation (99143-99150)** category of the Medicine section. Do not report a moderate sedation code when it is included in the procedure, which is indicated by the symbol ⊙ to the left of the CPT code in the Tabular List, unless the moderate sedation is administered by someone other than the primary surgeon. CPT codes that include moderate sedation also appear in CPT Appendix G.

Codes in the Anesthesia section are supported by the same diagnosis code(s) reported by the surgeon.

CPT Anesthesia section guidelines provide information regarding time reporting, supplied materials, multiple procedures, anesthesia modifiers, and qualifying circumstances. These guidelines are discussed throughout this chapter.

None of the categories in the Anesthesia section provide special instructions.

Instructional notes in the Tabular List redirect coders to other codes for specific procedures, as appropriate, and provide instructions regarding codes that may and may not be reported together.

ABSTRACTING ANESTHESIA PROCEDURES

Abstracting for anesthesia services differs from abstracting for the actual surgical procedure. First, identify the actual surgical procedure performed, then abstract the additional details needed to assign anesthesia codes and modifiers. Necessary documentation includes the preanesthesia evaluation form (■ FIGURE 34-1, page 620) and anesthesia record (■ FIGURE 34-2, page 621), both of which are completed by the anesthesia provider; the postanesthesia record completed by the anesthesia provider and the PACU team; and the operative report completed by the surgeon. In this text, key information from these reports is summarized in the mini-medical-record.

The medical record of anesthesia includes details about the patient's anesthesia administration and monitoring from the beginning of a procedure to the time the patient is recovering postoperatively. The anesthesia provider documents intraoperative anesthesia services including administration and monitoring of anesthesia, drugs administered, techniques used, fluids or blood products given, vital signs, complications, and adverse reactions. The anesthesia provider also documents postanesthesia information in the patient's medical record.

Refer to ■ TABLE 34-4 for guidance on how to abstract Anesthesia procedures. Remember that the abstracting questions are a guide and that not every question applies to, or can be answered for, every case. For example, anesthesiologists do not always supervise other anesthesia providers. The following information discusses how to abstract anesthesia time and the patient's physical status.

To abstract the surgical procedure, identify the anatomic site, type of procedure, and approach, such as open or closed. If more than one surgical procedure is performed, abstract only the primary or principal procedure. However, calculate the anesthesia time for the total duration of all procedures. Anesthesia time begins when the anesthesia provider begins to prepare the patient for the induction of anesthesia and ends when the anesthesia provider is no longer in personal attendance and the patient can be safely placed under postoperative supervision. Anesthesia time is always greater than the time it takes the surgeon to perform the procedure. The start and stop times for anesthesia are documented on the anesthesia record.

The physical status of the patient, also documented on the anesthesia record, is expressed in categories defined by the American Society of Anesthesiologists (ASA) as follows:

P1 A normal healthy patient
P2 A patient with mild systemic disease
P3 A patient with severe systemic disease
P4 A patient with severe systemic disease that is a constant threat to life
P5 A moribund patient who is not expected to survive without the operation
P6 or E (*expired*) A declared brain-dead patient whose organs are being removed for donor purposes

When abstracting the diagnoses, verify that documentation includes diagnoses to support the systemic disease and comorbidities identified by the physical status category.

PRE-ANESTHESIA EVALUATION

AGE	SEX	HEIGHT	WEIGHT	PRE-PROCEDURE VITAL SIGNS			
	☐ M ☐ F	in./cm.	lb./kg.	B/P	P	R	T

PROPOSED PROCEDURE

PREVIOUS ANESTHESIA/OPERATIONS (*If none, check here* ☐)

CURRENT MEDICATIONS (*If none, check here* ☐)

FAMILY HISTORY OF ANESTHESIA COMPLICATIONS (*If none, check here* ☐)

ALLERGIES (*If NKDA, check here* ☐)

AIRWAY/TEETH/HEAD AND NECK

HISTORY FROM
☐ PARENT/GUARDIAN ☐ POOR HISTORIAN ☐ CHART
☐ SIGNIFICANT OTHER ☐ PATIENT

SYSTEM	WNL	COMMENTS	PERTINENT STUDY RESULTS
RESPIRATORY Asthma Pneumonia Bronchitis Productive cough COPD Recent cold Dyspnea SOB Orthopnea Tuberculosis	☐	Tobacco Use: ☐ No ☐ Yes ____ Pack/Day for ____ Years	Chest X-ray Pulmonary Studies
CARDIOVASCULAR Angina MI Arrhythmia Murmur CHF MVP Exercise Tolerance Pacemaker Hypertension Rheumatic fever	☐		EKG
HEPATO/GASTROINTESTINAL Bowel obstruction Jaundice Cirrhosis N&V Hepatitis Reflux/heartburn Histal hernia Ulcers	☐	Ethanol Use: ☐ No ☐ Yes Frequency_____	
NEURO/MUSCULOSKELETAL Arthritis Paresthesia Back problems Syncope CVA/stroke Seizures DJD TIAs Headaches Weakness Loss of consciousness Neuromuscular disease Paralysis	☐		
RENAL/ENDOCRINE Diabetes Renal failure/Dialysis Thyroid disease Urinary retention Urinary tract infection Weight loss/gain	☐		
OTHER Anemia Bleeding tendencies Hemophilia Pregnancy Sickle cell trait Transfusion history			

PROBLEM LIST/DIAGNOSES	ASA PS	LAB STUDIES Hgb/HcT/CBC Electrolytes Urinalysis
	1	
	2	
PLANNED ANESTHESIA/SPECIAL MONITORS	3	Other
	4	
	5	
	E	**POST-ANESTHESIA NOTE**

PRE-ANESTHESIA MEDICATIONS ORDERED

SIGNATURE OF EVALUATOR(S)

Signed _____ Date _____ Time _____

OPTIONAL FORM 517 BACK

Figure 34-1 ■ Example of a Preanesthesia Evaluation Form. *Source: US General Services Administration (OF517).*

AUTHORIZED FOR LOCAL REPRODUCTION

MEDICAL RECORD–ANESTHESIA

PROCEDURE	ITEM	START	STOP
	Anesthesia		
	Procedure		

DATE	OR NO.	PAGE OF	SURGEON(S)

PRE–PROCEDURE
- ☐ Identified ☐ ID Band ☐ Questioning
- ☐ Chart Review ☐ Permit Signed
- ☐ NPO Since _____
- Pre-anesthetic State: ☐ Calm
- ☐ Awake ☐ Asleep
- ☐ Apprehensive ☐ Confused
- ☐ Uncooperative ☐ Unresponsive

PATIENT SAFETY
- ☐ Anes. Machine # _____ Checked
- ☐ Safety Belt On ☐ Axillary Roll
- ☐ Arm Restraints ☐ Arms Tucked
- ☐ Pressure points checked and padded
- ☐ Eye Care: ☐ Ointment ☐ Saline
- ☐ Taped ☐ Pads ☐ Goggles

MONITORS AND EQUIPMENT
- ☐ Steth ☐ Esoph ☐ Precord ☐ Other
- ☐ Non-Invasive B/P ☐ Nerve Stimulator
- ☐ Continuous EKG ☐ V Lead EKG
- ☐ Pulse Oximeter ☐ Oxygen Analyzer
- ☐ End Tidal CO_2 ☐ Resp Gas Anlyzr
- ☐ Temp _____ ☐ EEG
- ☐ Warming Blanket ☐ Fluid Warmer
- ☐ Airway Humidifier ☐
- ☐ NG/OG Tube ☐ Foley Catheter
- ☐ Art Line _____
- ☐ CVP _____
- ☐ PA Line _____
- ☐ IV(s) _____
- ☐

ANESTHETIC TECHNIQUES
- Method: ☐ General ☐ Spinal
- ☐ Epidural ☐ Caudal ☐ Brachial
- ☐ Bier Block ☐ Ankle Blk ☐ M.A.C.
- General: ☐ Pre-O_2 ☐ L.T.A.
- ☐ Rapid Sequence ☐ Cricoid Pressure
- ☐ Intravenous ☐ Inhalation
- ☐ Intramuscular ☐ Rectal
- Regional: ☐ Position _____
- ☐ Prep _____ ☐ Local _____
- ☐ Needle _____
- ☐ Drug(s) _____
- ☐ Dose _____ ☐ Attempts x _____
- ☐ Site _____ ☐ Level _____
- ☐ Catheter _____ ☐ See Remarks

AIRWAY MANAGEMENT
- ☐ Intubation ☐ Oral ☐ Nasal
- ☐ Direct Vision ☐ Magill's ☐ Blind
- ☐ Diff. see Rmks ☐ Fiber Op ☐ Stylet
- ☐ Attempts x _____ ☐ Blade _____
- ☐ Tube size _____ ☐ Endobronchial
- ☐ Regular ☐ RAE ☐ Armored ☐ Laser
- ☐ Cuffed ☐ Min. occ. pres. ☐ Air ☐NS
- ☐ Uncuffed, leaks at _____ cm H_2O
- ☐ Secured at _____ ☐ ET CO_2 Present
- ☐ Breath Sounds _____
- ☐ Circuit: ☐ Circle ☐ Non-rebreathing
- ☐ Airway: ☐ Oral ☐ Nasal ☐ Natural
- ☐ Mask Case ☐ Via Tracheostomy
- ☐ Nasal Cannula ☐ Simple O_2 Mask

RECOVERY ROOM

Time	B/P	O_2 Sat.
☐ PACU	P	R	T
☐ ICU ☐ L&D		

- ☐ Awake ☐ Spont Resp ☐ Oral Airway
- ☐ Asleep ☐ Ventilator ☐ Nasal Airway
- ☐ Stable ☐ Extubated ☐ Face Shield O_2
- ☐ Unstable ☐ Intubated ☐ T-Piece O_2

CONTROLLED DRUGS

Drug	Used	Destroyed	Returned

Provider _____ Witness _____

TIME:

AGENTS
- ☐ Hal ☐ Enf ☐ Iso (%)
- ☐ N_2O ☐ Air (L/min)
- Oxygen (L/min)
- ( )
- ( )
- ( )
- ( )
- ( )

FLUIDS

MONITORS
- Urine (ml)
- EBL (ml)
- EKG
- % O_2 Inspired (FIO_2)
- O_2 Saturation (SaO_2)
- End Tidal CO_2
- Temp: ☐ °C ☐ °F

VITAL SIGNS
- Baseline Values
- 200
- 180
- 160
- 140
- 120
- 100
- 80
- 60
- 40
- 20
- B/P
- P
- R

VENT
- Tidal Vol. (ml)
- Resp. Rate
- Peak Pres. (cm H_2O)
- PEEP (cm H_2O)

Symbols for Remarks

Position

TOTALS

SYMBOLS
- ✕ ANESTHESIA
- ⊙ OPERATION
- ∨ ∧ B/PCUFF PRESSURE
- ⊥ ARTERIAL LINE PRESSURE
- Δ MEAN ARTERIAL PRESSURE
- ● PULSE
- ○ SPONTANEOUS RESP
- ⊘ ASSISTED RESP
- ⊗ CONTROLLED RESP
- T TOURNIQUET

ANESTHESIA PROVIDER(S)

REMARKS

PATIENT'S IDENTIFICATION (For typed or written entries give: Name–last, first, middle: ID No. (SSN or other); hospital or medical facility.)

ANESTHESIA
Medical Record
OPTIONAL FORM 517 (7–95)
Prescribed by GSA/ICMR,
FPMR (41 CFR) 101–11.203(b)(10)

Figure 34-2 ■ Example of an Anesthesia Record. *Source: US General Services Administration (OF517).*

CODING PRACTICE (continued)

5. (continued)

b. What is the diagnosis(es)? _____

c. How old is the patient? _____

d. What type of anesthesia is provided (local, regional, general)? _____

e. How long was anesthesia care provided? _____

f. What is the health status of the patient? _____

g. What type of anesthesia provider is in attendance?

_____

h. Are anesthesia services provided personally by the anesthesiologist? _____

i. How many anesthesia providers did the physician supervise, if any? _____

j. Are any unusual forms of monitoring used (intra-arterial, central venous, Swan-Ganz)? _____

---

6. INPATIENT HOSPITAL   Gender: F   Age: 79

Status: P4

Start time: 1015   Stop time: 1245

Anesthesia provider: MD in personal attendance

Anesthesia type: general, with Swan-Ganz monitoring and controlled hypotension

(continued)

6. (continued)

Diagnosis: *fracture of the neck of the left scapula, hypertension, DVT*

Procedure: *open scapula repair with controlled hypotension*

a. What is the anatomic site, type of procedure, and approach for the main procedure performed?

_____

b. What is the diagnosis(es)? _____

c. How old is the patient? _____

d. What type of anesthesia is provided (local, regional, general)? _____

e. How long was anesthesia care provided? _____

f. What is the health status of the patient? _____

g. What type of anesthesia provider is in attendance?

_____

h. Are anesthesia services provided personally by the anesthesiologist? _____

i. How many anesthesia providers did the physician supervise, if any? _____

j. Is controlled hypotension used? _____

k. Are any unusual forms of monitoring used (intra-arterial, central venous, Swan-Ganz)? _____

ASSIGNING ANESTHESIA CODES

The **anesthesia code package** includes preoperative visits, administration of anesthesia, intraoperative monitoring (■ TABLE 34-5), and postoperative services. Drugs, tray supplies, and materials above and beyond those usually included with the service are reported in addition to the basic service. These are usually reported by the facility, not the anesthesia provider. Assigning codes for anesthesia services requires the following steps, which are discussed in the next sections.

1. Identify the surgical procedure.
2. Assign the Anesthesia code.

Table 34-5 ■ INTRAOPERATIVE SERVICES INCLUDED IN THE ANESTHESIA CODE PACKAGE

❏ Blood administration

❏ Fluid administration

❏ Electrocardiogram (ECG, EKG)

❏ Temperature

❏ Blood pressure

❏ Oximetry

❏ Capnography

❏ Mass spectrometry

3. Assign the physical status modifier.
4. Assign any qualifying circumstances code(s).
5. Assign any moderate sedation code(s).
6. Assign CPT and HCPCS modifiers.
7. Assign codes for any unusual monitoring services.
8. Calculate the anesthesia payment formula.

Identify the Surgical Procedure

The actual surgical procedure was identified during abstracting, but you do not need to assign a code for it. You do need to know the anatomic site, the type of procedure, and the approach to accurately assign the code for anesthesia services. Anesthesia codes are less specific than Surgery codes. CPT provides fewer than 300 Anesthesia codes but thousands of Surgery codes. Thus, a single Anesthesia code is intended to be used with a large number of Surgery codes.

SUCCESS STEP

The ASA publication *CROSSWALK: A Guide for Surgery/Anesthesia CPT Codes* links CPT Surgery codes to the appropriate Anesthesia code(s) and provides tips for code selection.

Assign the Anesthesia Code

Anesthesia providers report only one Anesthesia code per operative session, with the exception of Anesthesia add-on codes for burn excisions or debridement and obstetric services. Report an Anesthesia code for the most extensive or most complex procedure performed.

Coders also must identify the circumstances for which they should *not* assign codes from the Anesthesia section.

- Topical or local anesthesia and metacarpal/metatarsal/digital blocks are included in the CPT surgical package.

- Anesthesia administered by the surgeon, rather than an anesthesia provider, is reported with modifier **-47** appended to the Surgery section code.

- Moderate sedation is reported with Medicine section codes **99143-99150**.

Locating Anesthesia Codes

To assign codes for anesthesia services, search for the Main Term **Anesthesia** in the Index (■ Figure 34-3). Most procedures are indexed in multiple ways under the **Anesthesia** entry: by anatomic site, type of procedure, and, often, synonym. First-level modifying terms that identify the anatomic site provide a second-level modifying term for the procedure (e.g., **Anesthesia, Hip, Arthroplasty**). First-level modifying terms that identify the procedure provide a second-level modifying term for the anatomic site (e.g., **Anesthesia, Arthroplasty, Hip**). Some procedures are indexed both by the medical term and the synonym (e.g., **Anesthesia, Replacement, Hip**).

Do not use the actual procedure name as the Main Term because the Main Term for a procedure, such as **Angiography**, leads to the code for the procedure, not the related anesthesia services.

The Tabular List of the Anesthesia section provides a separate category for each anatomic region. Codes within an anatomic region are divided by the specific site and/or the general type of procedure.

Add-on Codes for Burn and Cesarean Delivery Procedures

The Anesthesia section provides three add-on codes: one for burn excisions or debridement and two for cesarean deliveries. Anesthesia for burn excision or debridement is reported based on the percentage of total body surface area (TBSA) treated. Two codes identify treatment of less than 4% of TBSA (**01951**) and 4% to 9% of TBSA (**01952**). The add-on code **01953** reports each additional 9% of TBSA, or portion thereof, beyond the first 9%.

The Obstetric category provides two add-on codes to be used with code **01967 Neuraxial labor analgesia/anesthesia for planned vaginal delivery.**

- Code **01968** identifies **Anesthesia for cesarean delivery following neuraxial labor analgesia/anesthesia.**

- Code **01969** identifies **Anesthesia for cesarean hysterectomy following neuraxial labor analgesia/anesthesia.**

Assign the Physical Status Modifier (P1-P6)

A physical status modifier must be assigned for each anesthesia patient. It is appended to the Anesthesia code for the primary or most extensive procedure performed. The CPT modifiers correspond with the ASA physical status indicators discussed earlier in this chapter. The ASA category is documented on the anesthesia record; coders do not determine the physical status based on patients' diagnoses. The modifiers also appear in the CPT guidelines at the beginning of the Anesthesia section.

Assign Any Moderate Sedation Codes (99143-99150)

Assign codes for moderate sedation when it is not bundled into the CPT code, as designated by the symbol ☉. Codes that include moderate sedation also appear in CPT Appendix G. Do not assign moderate sedation codes for services listed in the Anesthesia section (**00100-01999**). Moderate sedation can be administered by the physician performing the procedure or by a second anesthesia provider.

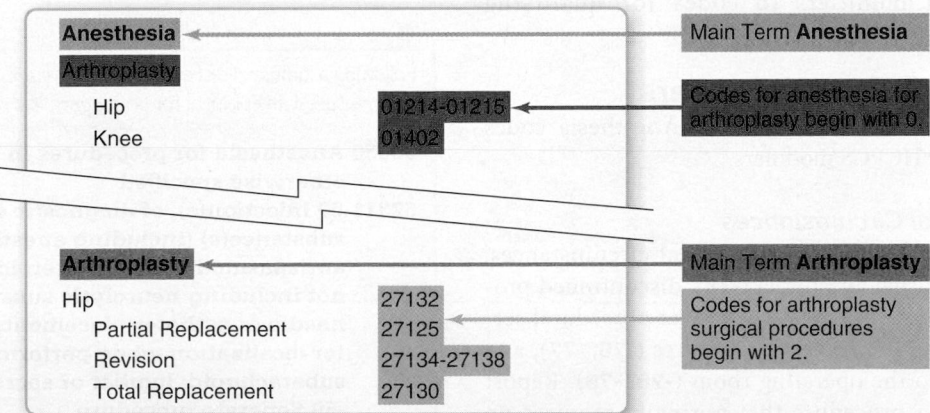

Figure 34-3 ■ CPT Index Entries for **Anesthesia–arthroplasty** and **Arthroplasty**.
Source: Annotations © PB Resources, Inc. Used with permission. CPT codes only © American Medical Association.

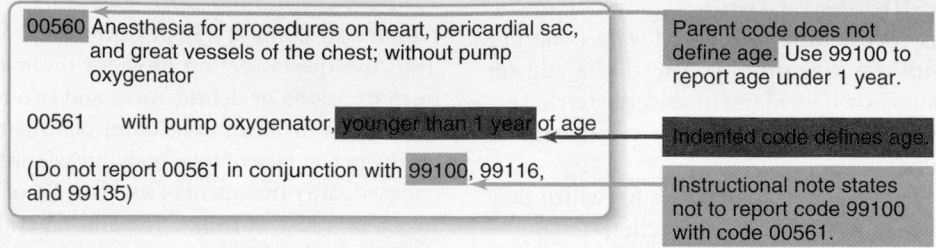

Figure 34-4 ■ Example of a Code that Includes Age

Search the Index for the Main Term **Sedation**, which has one first-level modifying term, **Moderate**. The Tabular List provides two parent codes (**99143** and **99148**), each of which has one indented code and one indented add-on code.

Codes **99143** to **99145** are reported when the physician performing the primary procedure also administers the moderate sedation. Codes **99143** and **99144** are divided by age and include up to 30 minutes of intraservice time. Code **99145** reports each additional 15 minutes of service.

Codes **99148** to **99150** are reported when a physician other than the one performing the primary procedure administers the moderate sedation. Codes **99148** and **99149** are divided by age and include up to 30 minutes of intraservice time. Code **99150** reports each additional 15 minutes of service.

Assign Any Qualifying Circumstances Codes (99100-99140)

Qualifying circumstances codes are add-on codes that identify four situations that increase the difficulty of anesthesia administration. They include codes for age younger than 1 year or older than 70 (**99100**) (■ Figure 34-4); use of total-body hypothermia (**99116**); use of controlled hypotension (**99135**); and emergency circumstances (**99140**). Do not use the code for age younger than one year when the Anesthesia code already includes the age. The codes appear in the CPT guidelines at the beginning of the Anesthesia section and can also be located under the Main Term **Anesthesia** and the first-level modifying term **Special Circumstances**. In the Tabular List, they appear in numerical order in the Medicine section.

Do not append modifiers to codes for qualifying circumstances.

Assign CPT and HCPCS Modifiers

In addition to physical status modifiers, Anesthesia codes accept both CPT and HCPCS modifiers.

Unusual Procedural Circumstances

CPT modifiers describe unusual procedural circumstances, such as those for unusual anesthesia (**-23**), discontinued procedures (**-53**), reduced services (**-52**), distinct procedural service (**-59**) (■ Figure 34-5), repeat procedures (**-76**, **-77**), and unplanned returns to the operating room (**-78**, **-79**). Report modifier **-23** when a procedure that normally requires no anesthesia or local anesthesia instead requires general anesthesia. Two modifiers used specifically by outpatient hospitals and ASCs report discontinued procedures:

-73 Discontinued outpatient hospital/ambulatory surgery center (ASC) procedure prior to the administration of anesthesia
-74 Discontinued outpatient hospital/ambulatory surgery center (ASC) procedure after administration of anesthesia

Refer to Appendix A of the CPT manual for full descriptions of these modifiers.

Monitored Anesthesia Care

When MAC is provided, report one of the following HCPCS modifiers:

-QS MAC (monitored anesthesia care, informational)
-G8 Monitored anesthesia care (MAC) for deep complex, complicated, or markedly invasive surgical procedures.
-G9 Monitored anesthesia care for patient who has history of severe cardiopulmonary condition

Anesthesia Providers and Medical Direction

Anesthesiologists may personally provide services to some patients and provide only medical direction for other patients whose direct anesthesia provider is a CRNA or anesthesiologist assistant.

When the anesthesiologist personally provides anesthesia services, assign the appropriate Anesthesia code for the procedure and append modifier **-AA Anesthesia services performed personally by anesthesiologist**.

In some states, and for some payers, CRNAs can provide anesthesia services independently, without medical direction.

Following a lumbar disk replacement procedure, the anesthesiologist administered an epidural for postoperative pain control.

00630 Anesthesia for procedures in lumbar region; not otherwise specified
62311-59 Injection(s), of diagnostic or therapeutic substance(s) (including anesthetic, antispasmodic, opioid, steroid, other solution), not including neurolytic substances, including needle or catheter placement, includes contrast for localization when performed, epidural or subarachnoid; lumbar or sacral (caudal).
-59 Separate procedure

Figure 34-5 ■ Example of Using Modifier -59 with Anesthesia Services

In this situation, assign the appropriate Anesthesia code for the procedure and append modifier **-QZ CRNA service: without medical direction by a physician**.

Medicare and some other payers, and some states, require CRNAs to work under the medical direction of an anesthesiologist. To qualify for medical direction, physicians must meet the following criteria:

- perform the preanesthesia evaluation and examination and develop the plan for anesthesia
- personally administer various procedures, when appropriate, including the induction of and emergence from anesthesia
- oversee another anesthesia provider involved in anesthesia care
- frequently monitor anesthesia care of the patient
- be physically available to provide emergency care if needed
- provide postanesthesia care

The CRNAs and the MD use different modifiers. Each CRNA bills the Anesthesia code appropriate for his or her case and appends modifier **-QX CRNA service: with medical direction by physician**. The MD bills a separate Anesthesia code for each case being supervised, using the same code as the CRNA for each case, then appends a modifier that identifies the number of cases being supervised concurrently (■ FIGURE 34-6):

> **-QY Medical direction of one CRNA by an anesthesiologist**
> **-QK Medical direction of two, three, or four concurrent anesthesia procedures involving qualified individuals**
> **-AD Medical supervision by a physician: more than four concurrent anesthesia procedures**

The payment for anesthesia services is prorated between the MD and the CRNA for each case.

CODING CAUTION

Do not use modifiers for laterality (**-50, -RT, -LT**) on Anesthesia codes, even if a paired anatomic site, such as one arm or leg, receives a regional block.

An anesthesiologist provides medical direction of three CRNAs, each providing anesthesia services for a different patient.

Patient #1: Pancreatectomy
00794 Anesthesia for intraperitoneal procedures in upper abdomen including laparoscopy; pancreatectomy, partial or total (e.g., Whipple procedure)
CRNA: **00794-QX CRNA service: with medical direction by physician**
MD: **00794-QK Medical direction of two, three, or four concurrent anesthesia procedures involving qualified individuals**

Patient #2: Ventral hernia repair
00832 Anesthesia for hernia repairs in lower abdomen; ventral and incisional hernias
CRNA: **00832-QX CRNA service: with medical direction by physician**
MD: **00832-QK Medical direction of two, three, or four concurrent anesthesia procedures involving qualified individuals**

Patient #3: Vaginal hysterectomy
00944 Anesthesia for vaginal procedures (including biopsy of labia, vagina, cervix or endometrium); vaginal hysterectomy
CRNA: **00944-QX CRNA service: with medical direction by physician**
MD: **00944-QK Medical direction of two, three, or four concurrent anesthesia procedures involving qualified individuals**

Figure 34-6 ■ Example of Coding Anesthesia Medical Direction. *Source: © PB Resources, Inc. Used with permission. CPT codes only © American Medical Association.*

Assign Code(s) for Any Unusual Monitoring Services

Assign codes for unusual monitoring services not included in the Anesthesia package when the catheter insertion is separate and distinct from the operative procedure (■ TABLE 34-6). When the catheter is inserted as part of the operative procedure, do not assign a separate code. When a Swan-Ganz catheter is

---

Table 34-6 ■ **ASSIGNING CODES FOR CATHETER MONITORING DURING ANESTHESIA**

Catheter Type	Main Term	Modifying Terms	Code(s)
Central venous (CVC) (centrally inserted)	**Central Venous Catheter Placement**	**Insertion, Central, Non-Tunneled**	**36555** Patient <5 years old **36556** Patient ≥5 years
Peripherally inserted central venous (PICC)	**Central Venous Catheter Placement**	**Insertion, Peripheral, without Port or Pump**	**36568** Patient <5 years old **36599** Patient ≥5 years
Intra-arterial (A-line)	**Catheterization**	**Arterial System**	**36625 Cutdown** **36620 Percutaneous**
Swan-Ganz	**Swan-Ganz Catheter**	**Insertion**	**93503**

Source: © PB Resources, Inc. Used with permission. CPT codes only © American Medical Association.

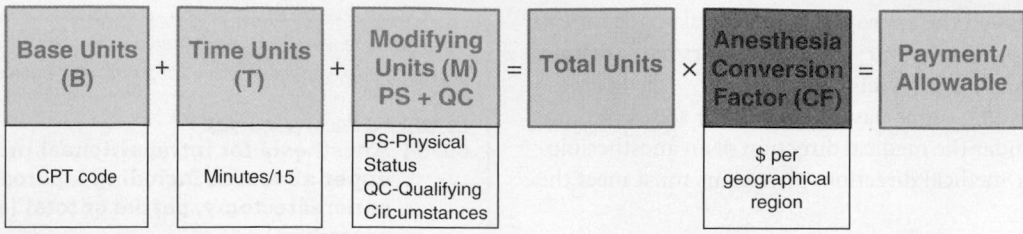

Figure 34-7 ■ Anesthesia Payment Formula. *Source: © PB Resources, Inc. Used with permission.*

inserted through an existing CVC, assign a code for insertion of the Swan-Ganz only. Do not assign a code for the CVC because it was not inserted during the current treatment.

Calculate the Anesthesia Payment Formula

Anesthesia services are reimbursed using a unique payment formula, which varies slightly between Medicare and commercial payers (■ FIGURE 34-7). Rather than basing payment on relative value units (RVUs), as is done with other CPT codes, payment for Anesthesia codes is based on unit values. The ASA assigns base unit values to anesthesia codes, qualifying circumstances codes, and physical status modifiers, updating base unit values yearly in the *Relative Value Guide* (*RVG*). The components of the anesthesia payment formula are three unit values and an anesthesia conversion factor expressed as $(B + T + M) \times CF$.

- **Base units (B)**—A number that represents the complexity of the anesthesia, the risk to the patient, and the skills needed by the anesthesia provider to render services for each CPT Anesthesia code. Use the base units for the most complex or extensive Anesthesia service provided. (Assign a minimum of five units for procedures of the head, neck, or shoulder girdle that require field avoidance and procedures performed in a position other than supine or lithotomy.)

- **Time units (T)**—The total minutes of anesthesia service provided for all procedures divided by 15.

- **Modifying units (M)**—Numbers assigned to each physical status modifier and each qualifying circumstance code to represent the added difficulty of the procedure (■ TABLE 34-7).

Table 34-7 ■ SUMMARY OF ANESTHESIA UNITS FOR MODIFYING FACTORS

Modifier	Modifying Units
-P1, -P2, -P6	0
-P3	1
-P4	2
-P5	3

Code	Modifying Units
99100	1
99116	5
99135	5
99140	2

Some payers, including Medicare, do not pay extra for modifying units.

- **Anesthesia conversion factor**—A dollar value, adjusted for geographic differences in cost, that Medicare (and other payers) assigns to one base unit of anesthesia. The anesthesia conversion factor is different than the overall conversion factor established by Medicare (and other payers) for other CPT codes.

To compute the payment or allowable amount, follow these steps (■ FIGURE 34-8).

1. Look up the numbers for the base units, time units, and modifying units (physical status and qualifying circumstances).

2. Add the number of units together to arrive at a total.

3. Multiply the total number of units by the anesthesia conversion factor.

4. The resulting number is the payment or allowable amount for the procedure.

An anesthesiologist provides anesthesia services for a pancreatectomy. The physical status is P1, a normal healthy patient. Total anesthesia time is 3 hours (180 minutes).

00794-AA Anesthesia for intraperitoneal procedures in upper abdomen including laparoscopy; pancreatectomy, partial or total (eg, Whipple procedure). -AA Anesthesia services performed personally by anesthesiologist

1. *Look up the numbers for the base units, time units, and modifying units.*
   B-Base units: 8
   T-Time units: 180/15 = 12
   M-Modifying units: 0
2. *Add the number of units together to arrive at a total.*
   Total units: 8 + 12 = 20
   CF-Anesthesia conversion factor: $22.89
3. *Multiply the total number of units times the anesthesia conversion factor.*
   Payment or allowable: 20 × $22.89 = $274.68
4. *The resulting number is the payment or allowable amount for the procedure.*
   $274.68

Figure 34-8 ■ Example of Calculating Anesthesia Payment. *Source: © PB Resources, Inc. Used with permission. CPT codes only © American Medical Association.*

When reporting Anesthesia services on a claim, report only time units in Item 24G on the CMS-1500 form or the corresponding field on the 837P electronic claim. Payers' claims processing systems automatically calculate the base units and modifying units using preloaded data. Some payers might require that actual minutes be reported instead of time units. In some areas of the country, time longer than 4 hours is calculated in 10-minute intervals.

SUCCESS STEP

Base units and conversion factors can be downloaded from the Anesthesiologists Center on the CMS website (**www.cms.gov**). Most medical billing systems automatically calculate the anesthesia payment formula based on preloaded data, even though it is not entered on the CMS-1500 form or 837P electronic claim.

Guided Example of Assigning Anesthesia Codes

To practice skills for assigning codes from the Anesthesia section, continue with the example from earlier in the chapter about a patient who was seen for a total hip replacement with regional anesthesia. Follow along in your CPT manual as Jacob Bates, CCS, assigns codes. Check off each step after you complete it.

▶ First, Jacob confirms the procedure of a total hip replacement performed under regional anesthesia.

▶ Second, Jacob assigns the code for anesthesia services.

❑ He searches the Index for the Main Term **Anesthesia**.

❑ He locates the first-level modifying term **Arthroplasty** and the second-level modifying term **Hip**.

❑ He writes down the code range listed: **01214-01215**.

❑ As a double check, he also looks under the Main Term **Anesthesia** and the first-level modifying term **Hip**. The same codes are listed: **01214-01215**.

▶ Jacob consults the Tabular List to verify codes **01214-01215** and select the appropriate code.

❑ He notices that both codes are indented codes under the parent code **01210 Anesthesia for open procedures involving hip joint**.

❑ He reads the description for **01214 Total hip arthroplasty** and compares it with code **01215 Revision of total hip arthroplasty**.

❑ Because code **01215** describes a revision of a previous hip arthroplasty, it does not apply to this case.

▶ Jacob checks for instructional notes in the Tabular List and finds none.

❑ As a double check, he scans the rest of the codes under the category **Upper Leg (Except Knee)**. The other codes for open procedures are not for a total hip arthroplasty.

The remaining codes describe closed procedures, which does not describe this case.

❑ The full description of code **01214** is **Anesthesia for open procedures involving hip joint; total hip arthroplasty**.

▶ Third, Jacob assigns the physical status modifier that is appended to the anesthesia code.

❑ He verifies the physical status modifier in the medical record, **P3 A patient with severe systemic disease**.

❑ He verifies that the description is consistent with congestive heart failure.

▶ Fourth, Jacob assigns a qualifying circumstances code because of the patient's age.

❑ **99100 Anesthesia for patient of extreme age, younger than 1 year and older than 70**

▶ Fifth, Jacob must assign a code for the intra-arterial monitoring.

❑ He locates the Main Term **Catheterization** and the first-level modifying term **Arterial system**.

❑ He reviews the second-level modifying terms and selects **Percutaneous 36620**.

❑ He verifies code **36620 Arterial catheterization or cannulation for sampling, monitoring or transfusion (separate procedure); percutaneous**.

❑ He makes note of the symbol ⊘ which identifies that this code is exempt from modifier **-51 Multiple procedures**.

▶ Sixth, Jacob assigns CPT and HCPCS modifiers.

❑ Code **01214** requires the modifier **-P3** to identify the physical status of the patient at the beginning of the procedure.

❑ Code **01214** also requires modifier **-AA Anesthesia services performed personally by anesthesiologist**.

❑ Code **99100** does not require any modifiers. Modifiers **-P3** and **-AA** are assigned to the Anesthesia service code only.

❑ Code **36620** does not require any modifiers because it is exempt from modifier **-51**. National Correct Coding Initiative (NCCI) edits do not place any restrictions on these codes being reported together.

▶ Seventh, Jacob calculates the anesthesia payment formula.

❑ The base units for this procedure are 8.

❑ The time units for 3 hours, 10 minutes are 190 minutes/15 = 13 (12.66 rounded up).

❑ The modifying unit for the physical status **P3** is 1.

❑ The modifying unit for qualifying circumstances code **99100** is 1.

❑ The total units are 8 + 13 + 1 + 1 = 23.

❑ The conversion factor for the local geographic region is $22.67.

❑ The total payment or allowable is 23 units × $22.67 = $521.41.

❑ Code **36620** will be paid in addition to the anesthesia payment.

▶ Next, Jacob must determine how to sequence the codes.

CODING PRACTICE

Exercise 34.3 Assigning Anesthesia Codes

Instructions: Each question has three parts.

Part a: Read the mini-medical-record of each patient's encounter. Review the information abstracted in Exercise 34.2 for questions 1–3. For questions 4–6, abstract the case on your own. Assign CPT codes using the Index and Tabular List, and arrange the codes in the proper sequence. Assign modifiers for physical status, type of provider, and any other applicable circumstances. Write the code(s) and modifier(s) on the line provided.
Part b: Determine the time units.
Part c: Calculate the modifying units. PS is the number of physical status units. QC is the number of qualifying circumstances units.

1. OUTPATIENT HOSPITAL   Gender: M   Age: 67
Status: P1

Start time: 0900   Stop time: 1115

Anesthesia provider: CRNA without medical direction

Anesthesia type: patient requested general anesthesia rather than conscious sedation because he was anxious about remaining awake for the procedure

Diagnosis: corneal edema that is a sequela of an automobile accident five years ago

Procedure: corneal transplant, right eye

Tip: Assign a modifier for unusual anesthesia.

a. 1 CPT Code _____

b. Anesthesia time (minutes) ____/15 = ____ Time units

c. PS ____ + QC ____ = ____ Modifying units

2. INPATIENT HOSPITAL   Gender: M   Age: 28
Status: P4

Start time: 0600   Stop time: 0930

Anesthesia provider: MD in personal attendance

Anesthesia type: general

Diagnosis: ESRD

Procedure: kidney transplant, open

a. 1 CPT Code _____

b. Anesthesia time (minutes) ____/15 = ____ Time units

c. PS ____ + QC ____ = ____ Modifying units

3. OUTPATIENT HOSPITAL   Gender: M   Age: 66
Status: P1

Start time: 1115   Stop time: 1330

Anesthesia provider: CRNA under medical direction of an anesthesiologist

Anesthesia type: spinal

Diagnosis: benign prostatic hyperplasia (BPH)

Procedure: transurethral resection of the prostate (TURP)

Tip: Code only for the CRNA.

a. 1 CPT Code _____

b. Anesthesia time (minutes) ____/15 = ____ Time units

c. PS ____ + QC ____ = ____ Modifying units

4. INPATIENT HOSPITAL   Gender: F   Age: 3 months
Status: P4

Start time: 0700   Stop time: 1245

Anesthesia provider: MD in personal attendance

Anesthesia type: general

Diagnosis: atrial septal defect

Procedure: open-heart surgery with pump oxygenator

Tip: Abstract this scenario on your own before coding.
Base units = 25

a. 1 CPT Code _____

b. B ____ + T ____ + M ____ = ____ TU × $22.89 =
   $ ____

5. INPATIENT HOSPITAL Gender: M Age: 61

Status: P5

Start time: 0345 Stop time: 0845

Anesthesia provider: MD in personal attendance

Anesthesia type: general

Diagnosis: dissecting abdominal aortic aneurysm

Procedure: emergency repair of AAA

Tip: Abstract this scenario on your own before coding. The abdominal aorta is a major abdominal blood vessel. Assign one code for the anesthesia and one code for the qualifying circumstances.

a. 2 CPT Codes _____

b. Anesthesia time (minutes) ____/15 = ____ Time units

c. PS ____ + QC ____ = ____ Modifying units

6. INPATIENT HOSPITAL Gender: F Age: 34

Status: P3

Start time: 1345 Stop time: 1700

Anesthesia provider: anesthesiologist in personal attendance

Anesthesia type: general with MAC due to morbid obesity, which significantly increased the complexity of the procedure

Diagnosis: morbid obesity, obstructive sleep apnea, hypertension

Procedure: gastric banding

Tip: Abstract this scenario on your own before coding.

a. 1 CPT Code _____

b. Anesthesia time (minutes) ____/15 = ____ Time units

c. PS ____ + QC ____ = ____ Modifying units

ARRANGING ANESTHESIA CODES

Many times anesthesia cases require only one code. Even when multiple surgical procedures are performed, only one anesthesia code—the one for the most complex procedure—is assigned. Multiple codes are required when there is a qualifying circumstance or an additional anesthesia service not included in the anesthesia package. When this occurs, sequence the codes as follows:

1. Anesthesia service (**00100-01999**) with **P** modifier

2. Additional services

3. Qualifying circumstances (**99100-99140**)

When a code requires multiple modifiers, remember to sequence the modifiers that affect payment before those that are informational only.

Guided Example of Arranging Anesthesia Codes

To practice skills for arranging codes for the Anesthesia section, continue with the example from earlier in the chapter about the patient who was seen for a total right hip arthroplasty. Follow along in your CPT manual as Jacob Bates, CCS, arranges (sequences) the codes. Check off each step after you complete it.

▶ Jacob reviews the sequencing guidelines for Anesthesia.

❑ The Anesthesia code **01214** is the primary service provided and has the highest price, so should be sequenced first. The code requires two modifiers, **-P3** and **-AA**.

Modifier **-P3** is required on Anesthesia codes and affects payment because it adds modifying units to the payment formula. **-AA** is informational only and does not affect payment, so **-P3** is sequenced first, followed by **-AA**.

❑ The modifying circumstances code **99100** has no RVU or monetary value, so it is sequenced last.

❑ Code **36620** for the arterial line monitoring is sequenced second. The MFPS assigns 1.47 RVUs to this code.

▶ Jacob finalizes the procedure codes, modifiers, and sequencing for this case:

(1) **01214-P3-AA Anesthesia for open procedures involving hip joint; total hip arthroplasty. -P3 A patient with severe systemic disease. -AA Anesthesia services performed personally by anesthesiologist**

(2) **36620 Arterial catheterization or cannulation for sampling, monitoring or transfusion (separate procedure); percutaneous**

(3) **99100 Anesthesia for patient of extreme age, younger than 1 year and older than 70**

▶ Jacob assigns and sequences the ICD-10-CM diagnosis codes that support the need for the service.

(1) **M16.11 Unilateral primary osteoarthritis, right hip**

(2) **I50.9 Heart failure, unspecified**

CODING PRACTICE

Exercise 34.4 Arranging Anesthesia Codes

Instructions: **Part a.** Read the mini-medical-record of each patient's encounter. Review the information abstracted in Exercise 34.2 for questions 1–3. For questions 4–6, abstract the case on your own. Assign CPT codes using the Index and Tabular List, and arrange the codes in the proper sequence. Assign modifiers for physical status, type of provider, and any other applicable circumstances. Write the code(s) and modifier(s), if any, on the line provided.

Part b: Calculate the time and modifying units. Using the base units provided in the *Tip* and a conversion factor of $22.89, calculate the anesthesia payment formula. Base units (B) + time units (T) + modifying units (M) = Total units (TU) × $22.89 = Anesthesia payment/allowable.

---

1. OUTPATIENT HOSPITAL   Gender: M   Age: 78
Status: P3

Start time: 1315   Stop time: 1500

Anesthesia provider: CRNA without medical direction

Anesthesia type: local with moderate sedation

Diagnosis: cardiac arrhythmia

Procedure: pacemaker insertion

Tip: Base units = 4.

a. 2 CPT Codes _____

b. B _____ + T _____ + M _____ = _____ TU × $22.89 =
   $ _____

---

2. INPATIENT HOSPITAL   Gender: M   Age: 54
Status: P4

Start time: 1415   Stop time: 1945

Anesthesia provider: CRNA under medical direction of an MD who is supervising 3 cases

Anesthesia Type: general

Diagnosis: third-degree burns are the result of a house fire that occurred last week

Procedure: burn excision and debridement of the trunk involving 20% of total body surface area. Supplemental monitoring provided using a CVC (nontunneled).

Tip: Base units = 7. Provide the quantity for the anesthesia codes. Code for the CRNA only.

a. 3 CPT Codes (CRNA) _____ × _____
   _____ × _____

b. B _____ + T _____ + M _____ = _____ TU × $22.89 =
   $ _____

---

3. INPATIENT HOSPITAL   Gender: F   Age: 79
Status: P4

Start time: 1015   Stop time: 1245

Anesthesia provider: MD in personal attendance

(continued)

---

3. (continued)

Anesthesia Type: general, with Swan-Ganz monitoring and controlled hypotension

Diagnosis: fracture of the neck of the left scapula, hypertension, DVT

Procedure: open scapula repair with controlled hypotension

Tip: Base units = 3. Sequence the code for the Swan-Ganz catheter second.

a. 4 CPT Codes _____
   _____

b. B _____ + T _____ + M _____ = _____ TU × $22.89
   = $ _____

---

4. INPATIENT HOSPITAL   Gender: F   Age: 26
Status: P1

Start time: 1215   Stop time: 1345

Anesthesia provider: MD in personal attendance

Anesthesia Type: anesthesia for cesarean delivery following neuraxial labor analgesia for planned vaginal delivery

Diagnosis: cephalopelvic disproportion and obstructed labor

Procedure: cesarean delivery after planned vaginal delivery, 1 healthy baby boy delivered

Tip: Abstract this scenario on your own before coding. Base units = 7.

a. 2 CPT Codes _____

b. B _____ + T _____ + M _____ = _____ TU × $22.89
   = $ _____

---

5. OUTPATIENT HOSPITAL   Gender: M   Age: 9
months   Status: P1

Start time: 1030   Stop time: 1300

(continued)

5. (continued)

Anesthesia provider: CRNA under medical direction of an anesthesiologist. MD provides medical direction to 5 cases.

Anesthesia Type: general

Diagnosis: undescended left testicle

Procedure: open orchiopexy

Tip: Abstract this scenario on your own before coding. Assign codes for both the CRNA and anesthesiologist (MD).

a. 2 CPT Codes (CRNA) _____

2 CPT Codes (MD) _____

b. Anesthesia time (minutes) _____/15 = _____ Time units

c. PS _____ + QC _____ = _____ Modifying units

6. DENTAL OFFICE Gender: M Age: 5

Start time: 0945 Stop time: 1030

Anesthesia provider: anesthesiologist provided sedation, monitoring, and observation while dentist performed the procedure

Anesthesia Type: moderate sedation provided in response to mother's request that child is afraid of needles and does not like to sit still

Diagnosis: advanced tooth decay

Procedure: tooth extraction

Tip: Abstract this scenario on your own before coding. This code does not require modifiers or the anesthesia payment formula.

2 CPT Codes _____

CHAPTER SUMMARY

In this chapter you learned that:

- Anesthesia is a medical specialty that works in conjunction with surgical specialties to manage the patient's status during a surgical procedure by keeping the patient immobile and unaware of pain while the procedure is performed.

- The CPT **Anesthesia (00100-01999)** section contains 19 subsections, most of which are divided by anatomic site and are used by anesthesia providers for the administration of anesthesia services.

- Abstracting for anesthesia services differs from abstracting for the actual surgical procedure because first you need to identify the actual surgical procedure performed, then you need to abstract the additional details needed to assign anesthesia codes and modifiers.

- The Anesthesia code package includes preoperative visits, administration of anesthesia, intraoperative monitoring, and postoperative services; several steps are required to assign all required codes and modifiers.

- Multiple Anesthesia codes are required when there is a qualifying circumstance or an additional anesthesia service not Included in the anesthesia package.

- CPT Anesthesia section guidelines provide information regarding time reporting, supplied materials, multiple procedures, anesthesia modifiers, and qualifying circumstances.

CONCEPT QUIZ

Take a moment to look back at anesthesia coding and solidify your skills. Try to answer the questions from memory first, then, refer to the discussion in this chapter if you need a little extra help.

Completion

Instructions: Write the term that answers each question based on the information you learned in this chapter. Choose from the list to the right. Some choices may be used more than once and some choices may not be used at all.

analgesia	controlled hypotension	moderate (conscious) sedation	patient-controlled analgesia
amnesia	immobilization	monitored anesthesia care (MAC)	provider
anesthesia	intra-arterial	oximetry	regional
capnography	mass spectrometry	patient care cycle	Swan-Ganz
central venous	medical specialty		total-body hypothermia

(continued)

(continued from page 633)

1. _____ manages a patient's status during a surgical procedure.

2. The _____ for anesthesia services includes pre-, intra-, and postoperative services.

3. The three components of anesthesia care are _____, _____, and _____.

4. _____ is a planned procedure during which the patient undergoes local anesthesia together with sedation and analgesia.

5. The technique that lowers mean arterial blood pressure to reduce intraoperative blood loss and minimize the risk of fluid overload is _____.

6. _____, _____, and _____ monitoring are considered unusual forms of anesthesia monitoring.

7. _____ uses a mild sedative to relax and pain medicine for pain while the patient stays awake but may not remember the procedure afterward.

8. A method of pain control that patients can administer in response to the level of pain they are experiencing is _____.

9. Epidural, spinal, and peripheral nerve blocks are examples of _____ anesthesia.

10. _____ is a technique that lowers the core body temperature during surgery to protect neurons from injury or degeneration.

Multiple Choice

Instructions: Circle the letter of the best answer to each question based on the information you learned in this chapter.

1. How is the drug *ketamine* classified?
   A. Neuromuscular blocking agent
   B. Reversal agent
   C. General anesthetic
   D. Narcotic analgesic

2. What is a planned procedure during which the patient undergoes local anesthesia together with sedation and analgesia?
   A. Regional block
   B. Monitored anesthesia care
   C. Patient-controlled analgesia
   D. Moderate sedation

3. What modifier reports that general anesthesia was administered by the surgeon?
   A. -47
   B. -23
   C. -AA
   D. -GS

4. What is a registered nurse with advanced education and training in the field of anesthesia?
   A. RNFA
   B. AA
   C. ARN
   D. CRNA

5. What score identifies a patient's health status on a scale of 1 through 5 at the time anesthesia is begun?
   A. Anesthesia score
   B. Physical status score
   C. Apgar score
   D. Mallampati score

6. What is the first step in assigning codes for anesthesia services?
   A. Identify the surgical procedure.
   B. Select the qualifying circumstances code(s).
   C. Calculate the anesthesia payment formula.
   D. Determine the physical status modifier.

7. What is the anesthesia payment formula?
   A. $B + T + M + CF$
   B. $B + PS + QC$
   C. $(B + T + QC) \times CF$
   D. $(B + T + M) \times CF$

8. What is a dollar value that Medicare assigns to one base unit of anesthesia?
   A. Anesthesia geographic factor
   B. Anesthesia allowable amount
   C. Anesthesia conversion factor
   D. Anesthesia payment formula

9. What type of code identifies the anesthesia provider?
   A. A qualifying circumstance code
   B. A HCPCS Level II modifier
   C. An add-on code
   D. An anesthesia status modifier

10. When is more than one anesthesia code reported?
    A. An anesthesia add-on code is required
    B. More than one anesthesiologist participates in the procedure
    C. More than one surgical procedure is performed during the same operative session
    D. Complications arise due to the anesthesia

CODING CHALLENGE

Instructions: Read the mini-medical-record of each patient's encounter, then abstract, assign, and arrange ICD-10-CM and CPT codes using the Index and Tabular List.

1. Append physical status modifiers and any applicable CPT modifiers.

2. Assign applicable qualifying circumstances codes.

3. Assign HCPCS modifiers identifying the anesthesia provider and/or MAC.

4. Report the total elapsed time in hours and minutes and the number of time units for the procedure (15 minutes = 1 time unit).

1. INPATIENT HOSPITAL   Gender: F   Age: 32
Status: P1

Start time: 0800   Stop time: 1300

Anesthesia provider: CRNA without medical direction

Anesthesia type: general

Diagnosis: Lumbar spondylolisthesis

Procedure: Posterior lumbar interbody fusion (PLIF),
L3-L4

1 ICD-10-CM Code _____

1 CPT Code _____

Time _____ hours_____ minutes. Time units _____

2. INPATIENT HOSPITAL   Gender: M   Age: 74
Status: P4

Start time: 1245   Stop time: 1900

Anesthesia provider: MD in personal attendance

Anesthesia type: General, with induced hypothermia

Diagnosis: Coronary atherosclerosis

Procedure: CABG with pump oxygenator

1 ICD-10-CM Code _____

3 CPT Code(s) _____

_____

Time _____ hours_____ minutes. Time units _____

3. INPATIENT HOSPITAL   Gender: F   Age: 42
Status: P4

Start time: 0603   Stop time: 0718

Anesthesia provider: CRNA

Anesthesia type: Spinal, general

Diagnosis: Preterm premature rupture of membranes
(PPROM), 33 weeks 2 days, primigravida, hypertensive
chronic renal disease stage 1

Procedure: Low transverse cesarean delivery following
attempted vaginal delivery

Tip: Assign codes for PPROM, supervision of pregnancy,
weeks of gestation, outcome of delivery, hypertensive
kidney disease, and the stage of chronic kidney disease.

6 ICD-10-CM Codes _____

_____

2 CPT Codes _____

Time _____ hours_____ minutes. Time units _____

4. OUTPATIENT SURGERY   Gender: M   Age: 63
Status: P2

Start time: 0915   Stop time: 1145

Anesthesia provider: anesthesiologist assistant
under direction of the anesthesiologist who is
supervising one other concurrent procedure

Anesthesia type: Conscious sedation

Diagnosis: Sinoatrial node dysfunction, mild
congestive heart failure

Procedure: Radiofrequency sinus node ablation

2 ICD-10-CM Codes _____

1 CPT Code _____

Time _____ hours_____ minutes. Time units _____

5. OFFICE   Gender: M   Age: 19   Status: P3

Start time: 0930   Stop time: 1245

Anesthesia provider: oral surgeon personally
administers the local anesthetic

Anesthesia type: Local

Diagnosis: Gingival hyperplasia, mandibular; type 1
diabetes

Procedure: Excision of lesion of gum with one
suture

2 ICD-10-CM Codes _____

1 CPT Code _____

Time _____ hours _____ minutes. Time units _____

6. OUTPATIENT SURGERY   Gender: M   Age: 71
Status: P4

Start time: 1330   Stop time: 1415

Anesthesia provider: anesthesiologist in personal
attendance

Anesthesia type: Monitored anesthesia care (MAC)

Diagnosis: Morbid obesity (BMI = 47 kg/m^2);
obstructive sleep apnea; hypertension

Procedure: Laparoscopic placement of gastric
band

4 ICD-10-CM Codes _____

_____

2 CPT Codes _____

Time _____ hours_____ minutes. Time units _____

(*continued*)

(continued from page 635)

7. INPATIENT HOSPITAL   Gender: F   Age: 66   Status: P3

Start time: 0745   Stop time: 1145

Anesthesia provider: CRNA under medical direction of an anesthesiologist

Anesthesia type: General

Diagnosis: Left breast cancer, primary

Procedure: radical mastectomy—removal of the breast, pectoral muscles, axillary lymph nodes, and associated skin and subcutaneous tissue

1 ICD-10-CM Code _____

1 CPT Code _____

Time _____ hours_____ minutes. Time units _____

8. INPATIENT HOSPITAL   Gender: M   Age: 21 days   Status: P4

Start time: 1415   Stop time: 1845

Anesthesia provider: anesthesiologist in personal attendance

Anesthesia type: General

Diagnosis: Atrial septal defect

Procedure: Open repair interarterial septal defect with pump oxygenator

1 ICD-10-CM Code _____

1 CPT Code _____

Time _____ hours_____ minutes. Time units _____

9. OUTPATIENT SURGERY   Gender: F   Age: 14   Status: P1

Start time: 1015   Stop time: 1115

Anesthesia provider: anesthesiologist in personal attendance

Anesthesia type: Monitored anesthesia care (MAC)

Diagnosis: Calcaneal bone spur, right

Procedure: Excision of calcaneal bone spur, right

1 ICD-10-CM Code _____

1 CPT Code _____

Time _____ hours_____ minutes. Time units _____

10. OUTPATIENT HOSPITAL   Gender: M   Age: 47   Status: P2

Start time: 0750   Stop time: 0855

Anesthesia provider: MD supervising 3 other concurrent procedures

Anesthesia type: Regional, peripheral block

Diagnosis: Ganglion cyst of left wrist, hypercholesterolemia

Procedure: Arthroscopic excision of lesion, left wrist

2 ICD-10-CM Codes _____

1 CPT Code _____

Time _____ hours_____ minutes. Time units _____

KEEP ON CODING

Instructions: Read the procedural statement, then use the Index and Tabular List to assign and sequence CPT procedure codes. Assign modifiers and qualifying circumstances codes as appropriate. Do not calculate the time. Write the code(s) on the line provided.

1. Otherwise healthy patient for removal of bladder calculus by incision with bladder spoon and anesthesia provided by CRNA with medical direction from physician: CPT Code(s) _____

2. Anesthesia for an otherwise healthy patient for left carpal tunnel release; anesthesia provided by CRNA without medical direction: CPT Code(s) _____

3. Anesthesia for a Coumadin patient for arthroscopic partial medial meniscectomy; anesthesia supervised by physician with five concurrent anesthesia procedures: CPT Code(s) _____

4. Anesthesia for a patient with mild hypertension has right hemilaminectomy of L1 and L2 and discectomy of L1; anesthesia personally provided by anesthesiologist: CPT Code(s) _____

5. Anesthesia for a controlled diabetic patient for right ankle arthrodesis; anesthesia provided by CRNA without physician supervision: CPT Code(s) _____

6. Anesthesia for an oncology patient for radical hysterectomy, bilateral salpingo-oophorectomy, extended pelvic lymphadenectomy; anesthesia personally provided by anesthesiologist: CPT Code(s) _____

7. Anesthesia for a mild congestive heart failure patient for arthroscopic removal of an osteochondritis dissecans of right glenohumeral joint; anesthesia provided by CRNA without physician supervision: CPT Code(s) _____

8. Anesthesia for a patient with severe carotid stenosis for left carotid endarterectomy with bovine patch angioplasty; anesthesia provided by a physician providing medical direction of three concurrent anesthesia procedures involving qualified individuals: CPT Code(s) _____

9. Anesthesia for a 78–year-old patient for craniotomy to evacuate frontal hematoma; anesthesia personally provided by anesthesiologist: CPT Code(s) _____

10. Anesthesia for an emergency patient for debridement of second-degree burn of 6% total body surface area; anesthesia provided by CRNA without direction by a physician: CPT Code(s) _____

11. Anesthesia for an oncology patient for the Whipple procedure; anesthesia provided by physician providing medical direction of three concurrent anesthesia procedures involving qualified individuals: CPT Code(s) _____

12. Anesthesia for a healthy pregnant female for vaginal delivery; supervision of two concurrent services under the anesthesiologist's direction: CPT Code(s) _____

13. Anesthesia for a patient with systemic lupus erythematous for open reduction and internal fixation of proximal femoral shaft fracture; anesthesia provided by the surgeon: CPT Code(s) _____

14. Anesthesia for a patient with severe hypertension for arthroscopic removal of bone fragment in the left elbow joint; anesthesia provided by CRNA without physician direction: CPT Code(s) _____

15. Anesthesia for a patient with 90% occlusion in the left carotid artery for balloon angioplasty and stent placement; anesthesia personally performed by the anesthesiologist: CPT Code(s) _____

16. Anesthesia for a brain-dead patient on life support for harvesting organs for donor purposes; medical direction of one concurrent anesthesia procedure by qualified individuals: CPT Code(s) _____

17. Anesthesia for a patient with 100% coronary artery blockage for CABG without pump oxygenator; anesthesia provided by CRNA without direction by a physician: CPT Code(s) _____

18. Anesthesia for an obese patient for therapeutic right L5 and L6 nerve blocks in lateral decubitus position; anesthesia provided by a physician with medical direction of one CRNA: CPT Code(s) _____

19. Anesthesia for a 21-year-old female patient with intellectual disabilities for vaginal examination and Pap test; anesthesia provided by CRNA with medical direction by physician: CPT Code(s) _____

20. Anesthesia for an emergency patient for pulmonary thromboendarterectomy with pump oxygenator, controlled hypotension and hypothermia, and cardiac arrest; anesthesia personally performed by the anesthesiologist: CPT Code(s) _____

21. Anesthesia for an oncology patient for breast reconstruction with implants and monitored anesthesia care: CPT Code(s) _____

22. Anesthesia for an otherwise healthy orthopedic patient for fusion across the sacroiliac joint; anesthesiologist performs anesthesia services: CPT Code(s) _____

23. Anesthesia for a healthy 71-year-old patient for smaller saphenous varicose vein procedure; anesthesia performed under medical direction of one CRNA by anesthesiologist: CPT Code(s) _____

24. Anesthesia for an otherwise healthy 15-year-old girl for tonsillectomy; anesthesia performed by anesthesiologist: CPT Code(s) _____

25. Anesthesia for a patient with Cushing disease due to left adrenal gland adenoma for unilateral adrenalectomy; anesthesia performed by anesthesiologist: CPT Code(s) _____

Chapter 35

Digestive System Procedures (40490-49999)

Chapter Outline

- **Digestive System Procedure Basics**
- **Coding Overview of Digestive System Procedures**
- **Abstracting Digestive System Procedures**
- **Assigning Codes for Digestive System Procedures**
- **Arranging Codes for Digestive System Procedures**
- **E/M Coding for Gastroenterology**

Learning Objectives

After completing this chapter, you should have the skills to:

35.1 Spell and define the key words, medical terms, and abbreviations related to digestive system procedures.

35.2 Discuss the types of digestive system procedures.

35.3 Identify the main characteristics of coding for the Digestive System.

35.4 Abstract procedural information from the medical record for coding digestive system procedures.

35.5 Assign codes for Digestive System procedures.

35.6 Arrange codes for Digestive System procedures

35.7 Code evaluation and management services for gastroenterology.

35.8 Discuss the CPT coding guidelines related to Digestive System.

Key Terms and Abbreviations

allotransplantation	capsule endoscopy	proximal	transnasal
anastomosis	incidental appendectomy	pull-through	transoral
by report	multiple endoscopy rule	reducible	

In addition to the key terms listed here, students should know the terms defined within tables in this chapter.

INTRODUCTION

It is exciting when a favorite store offers a BOGO sale—buy one, get one at half-price. Insurance companies require a similar discount when physicians bill for multiple procedures done at the same time. Coders indicate this circumstance with a modifier. Modifiers and multiple endoscopy payment rules are among the skills to be mastered when coding for the Digestive System.

DIGESTIVE SYSTEM PROCEDURE BASICS

Gastroenterology is a subspecialty of internal medicine that specializes in the digestive system. Gastroenterologists perform medical procedures such as endoscopies and gastric function studies, but they do not perform surgery. General surgeons perform surgery on digestive system organs and structures. Plastic surgeons perform reconstructive repairs involving the lips and mouth, such as cleft palate repair. Oral and maxillofacial surgeons (OMSs) also perform surgery on the face, mouth, and jaws.

For procedural purposes, the digestive system is divided into four parts:

- Upper gastrointestinal (GI) tract—lips through ileum
- Lower gastrointestinal (GI) tract—cecum through anus
- Accessory organs—salivary glands, liver, gallbladder, and pancreas
- Surrounding structures—abdomen, peritoneum, and omentum

Physicians use a variety of dividing points between the upper and lower GI tract, depending on the context:

- Diagnosis of bleeding—Bleeding above the duodenal junction is classified as upper GI bleeding, and bleeding below the duodenal junction is classified as lower GI bleeding.
- Endoscopic access—An upper GI endoscopy includes the mouth through the duodenum, and a lower GI endoscopy includes the cecum through the anus. The jejunum and ileum are not accessible to endoscopy procedures.
- Embryonic development—Developmentally, the GI tract is divided into three parts—the upper, from the mouth to the major duodenal papilla (*opening of the pancreatic duct into the duodenum*); middle, from the duodenal papilla to the mid-transverse colon; and lower, from the mid-transverse colon to the anus—based on the derivation from the foregut, midgut, and hindgut, respectively.

Because the digestive, or alimentary, tract consists of and connects several anatomic sites, medical terms frequently contain word roots of multiple sites, which are combined with a procedural suffix. To understand terminology, identify the suffix, then break down each word into the combining forms for each site. Refer to ■ TABLE 35-1 for a refresher on how to build medical terms related to digestive system procedures.

> **CODING CAUTION**
>
> Be alert for medical terms that are spelled similarly and have different meanings.
>
> **cholecystectomy** (*excision of the gall bladder*) and **chole<u>docho</u>cystectomy** (*excision of the common bile duct*)
>
> **laparo<u>tomy</u>** (*cutting into the abdomen*) and **laparo<u>scopy</u>** (*visual examination of the abdomen*)
>
> **an/o** (combining form for *anus*) and **an-** (prefix meaning *none*)

Procedures commonly performed on each section of the digestive system are discussed next. Refer to detailed anatomic diagrams of specific parts of the digestive system when you need to refresh your memory of the relationship of organs and sites to each other.

Procedures of the Upper GI Tract

Procedures commonly performed on the upper GI tract are summarized in ■ TABLE 35-2 (pages 640–641). In particular, coders need to understand upper GI endoscopy, anastomosis, and foreign body removal.

Upper GI Endoscopy

Endoscopy is a procedure that is performed for screening, diagnostic, and therapeutic purposes. In the upper GI tract, the endoscope access can be **transoral** (*through the oral cavity*) or **transnasal** (*through the nose*) and can access the esophagus, stomach, and duodenum. Transnasal procedures are performed

Table 35-1   ■   **EXAMPLE OF CONSTRUCTING MEDICAL TERMS FOR DIGESTIVE SYSTEM PROCEDURES**

Root/Combining Form	Suffix	Complete Medical Term
esophag/o- (*esophagus*)	**-scopy** (*visual examination*) **-ectomy** (*excision*)	**esophago + scopy** (*visual examination of the esophagus*) **gastro + scopy** (*visual examination of the stomach*) **duodeno + scopy** (*visual examination of the duodenum*) **esophago + gastro + duodeno + scopy** (*visual examination of the esophagus, stomach, and duodenum*)
gastr/o (*stomach*) **duoden/o** (*duodenum*)		**esophag + ectomy** (*excision of the esophagus*) **gastr + ectomy** (*excision of the stomach*) **duoden + ectomy** (*excision of the duodenum*)

Source: © PB Resources, Inc. Used with permission.

Table 35-2 ■ **COMMON PROCEDURES OF THE UPPER GASTROINTESTINAL TRACT**

Procedure Name	Definition	Reason Performed
Antrectomy • Distal gastrectomy	The distal (*lowest*) portion of the stomach is excised. (Open)	Gastric ulcers, neoplasms
Billroth I • Gastroduodenostomy	The pylorus is removed and the **proximal** (*toward the center of the body*) stomach is anastomosed (*connected*) directly to the duodenum in an end-to-end manner. (Open)	Reestablish gastrointestinal continuity after excision of portions of one or more organs
Billroth II • Gastrojejunostomy	The greater curvature of the stomach is connected to the first part of the jejunum in a side-to-side manner. (Open)	Reestablish gastrointestinal continuity after excision of portions of one or more organs
Cleft lip/cleft palate repair	Abnormally oriented and attached muscles are repositioned to repair the functionality of soft palate musculature. (Open)	Cleft lip or cleft palate (*incomplete formation of the lip or roof of the mouth*)
Endoscopic balloon dilation (EBD)	Through-the-scope (TTS) balloon dilators or plastic dilators are moved over a guide wire to stretch the esophagus, pyloric valve, or duodenum. (Endoscopic)	Stricture (*narrowing*) of the esophagus, pylorus, or duodenum due to a variety of conditions (e.g., gastric outlet obstruction [GOO], peptic ulcers, Crohn's disease)
Endoscopic sclerotherapy	A solution that causes inflammation and scarring is injected into a vein to close it off. (Endoscopic)	Esophageal varices
Esophagectomy • Transhiatal esophagectomy (THE) • Transthoracic esophagectomy (TTE)	All or part of the esophagus is surgically removed. (Open)	Barrett esophagus, localized esophageal cancer
Esophagogastroduodenoscopy (EGD) • Upper gastrointestinal endoscopy	The endoscope is inserted through the mouth and moved down the throat into the esophagus, stomach, and duodenum. (Endoscopic)	Esophagitis, gastritis, gastroesophageal reflux disease (GERD), esophageal stricture (*narrowing*), varices, Barrett esophagus, hiatal hernia, ulcers, cancer
Foreign body removal (FBR)	An object is retrieved from within the body. (Endoscopic or open)	Removal of an object from outside the body that has made its way into the body, usually into a hollow organ, such as the nose, ear, or throat
Gastric bypass	The stomach is divided to create a small pouch and causes food to bypass part of the small intestine. (Laparoscopic or open)	Reduce calorie absorption
Heller myotomy • Esophagomyotomy	The esophageal sphincter muscle is cut. (Laparoscopic)	Achalasia (*a disorder of the esophagus that makes it difficult for foods and liquids to pass into the stomach*)
Laparoscopically adjustable gastric banding (LABG) • Lap-band • A-band • Gastric restriction	An inflatable silicone device is placed around the top portion of the stomach to divide it into a smaller pouch and a larger pouch. (Laparoscopic or open)	Slow and reduce food consumption
Nissen fundoplication	The upper part of the stomach is wrapped around the lower esophageal sphincter (LES). (Laparoscopic or open)	Strengthen the sphincter, prevent acid reflux, repair a hiatal hernia
Paraesophageal hernia repair • Hiatal hernia repair • Hiatus hernia repair • Fundoplication	The diaphragm is repaired using sutures or mesh; part of the stomach may be wrapped around the esophagus (fundoplication). (Laparoscopic or open)	Paraesophageal hernia (part of the stomach bulges through the hiatus [*opening in the diaphragm*])
Percutaneous endoscopic gastrostomy (PEG)	A tube is passed into a patient's stomach through the abdominal wall. (Percutaneous)	Feed patients who cannot swallow due to conditions such as stroke and neurological diseases

Table 35-2 ■ (*continued*)

Procedure Name	Definition	Reason Performed
Roux-en-Y (RNY) • Gastrojejunostomy	The stomach and small bowel are joined using an end-to-side anastomosis. (Laparoscopic or open)	Reestablish gastrointestinal continuity after excision of portions of one or more organs
Sialolithotomy	Calculus is removed from the salivary gland(s). (Open)	Sialolithiasis (*calculi in the salivary gland*)
Tonsillectomy/adenoidectomy (T&A)	The tonsils and adenoids are surgically removed. (Open)	Acute tonsillitis, obstructive sleep apnea, nasal airway obstruction, peritonsillar abscess
Vagotomy • Truncal vagotomy (TV) • Selective vagotomy (SV) • Highly selective vagotomy (HSV)	A portion of the vagus nerve in the stomach is excised. (Laparoscopic or open)	Peptic ulcer disease

Source: © PB Resources, Inc. Used with permission.

with a rigid endoscope. Transoral procedures can be performed with either a rigid or flexible endoscope. Rigid endoscopes provide excellent lighting and visualization and have tips of varying angles and sizes. They enable tissue collection, surgery, and procedures such as cauterization. Flexible endoscopes are smaller in diameter and can be manipulated in tight areas but require two hands to operate. Historically, flexible endoscopes have provided inferior lighting and images, but these have improved with the development of digital endoscopes. Among procedures most commonly performed with an endoscope are:

- collection of specimens by brushing or washing
- injections
- biopsies
- removal of foreign bodies
- dilation of strictures
- removal of tumors or polyps
- electrocauterization
- hemostasis
- ultrasound examination
- cyst drainage
- resection

Endoscopes cannot access the jejunum or ileum, so physicians may opt to use capsule endoscopy to examine the small intestine. **Capsule endoscopy** is a technology in which patients swallow a video capsule the size of a large pill that contains a video microchip, light bulb, battery, and radio transmitter. As the capsule moves through the alimentary tract, it takes about 14 photographs per second and transmits them to a receiver worn by the patient. When the capsule passes through the anus, it is flushed down the toilet. The physician downloads thousands of photographs from the receiver and analyzes them to formulate a diagnosis or plan for further testing.

Anastomosis

Sometimes all or part of a digestive organ must be removed because of disease. The excision interrupts the continuous flow of GI tract, so continuity is reestablished through anastomosis. **Anastomosis** is a surgical connection between two, usually tubular, structures such as the organs in the digestive tract or blood vessels. Several techniques can be used to join the structures:

- End-to-end—the ends of both tubes are connected
- End-to-side—the end of one tube is connected to an opening in the side of another
- Side-to-side—the sides of two tubes are connected with an opening between them

The choice of technique depends on the condition, the exact sites removed, and the surgeon's preference (■ FIGURE 35-1).

In an operative note, anastomosis can be described as a **pull-through**, which means that the surgeon removes the diseased portion of organ and connects the healthy segment to the adjacent organ. The pull-through procedure was originally developed to treat Hirschsprung disease (*nerve cells normally present in the wall of the intestine do not form properly during fetal development*). Part of the colon is excised, then joined to the anus in a posterior sagittal anorectoplasty (PSARP) procedure. The pull-through became preferred over a colostomy, and the technique was eventually adapted for use in other portions of the digestive tract.

SUCCESS STEP

An anastomosis is described with the suffix -*stomy* for the creation of a new opening and word roots that identify the two body parts joined. For example, *gastro/duodeno/stomy* describes the joining of the stomach and the duodenum.

Foreign Body Removal

Foreign bodies can enter the digestive tract through the mouth. They can pass through the system without incident or become lodged. Some objects, such as a coin, normally pass through without a problem and are excreted. An object that becomes lodged can create an obstruction or perforation and poses a medical risk.

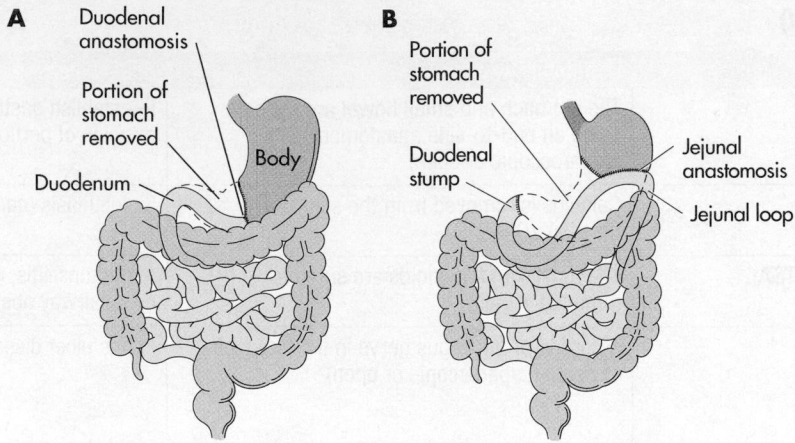

Figure 35-1 ■ Anastomoses. (A) End-to-End Gastroduodenostomy. (B) End-to-Side Gastrojejunostomy

Objects that are potentially poisonous must be removed immediately. For example, ingested batteries have potential for corrosive injury. X-rays are used to identify the type and location of foreign objects. Many can be retrieved endoscopically, but others require an open procedure to access the site.

Procedures of the Lower GI Tract

Procedures commonly performed on the lower GI tract are summarized in ■ TABLE 35-3. Endoscopy and ostomy procedures of the lower GI tract require special attention from coders.

Lower GI Endoscopy

Endoscopy of the lower GI tract is named after the sites examined: anoscopy (*endoscopy of the anus*), proctosigmoidoscopy (*endoscopy of the anus, rectum, and part of the descending colon*), sigmoidoscopy (*endoscopy of the anus, rectum, and part of the sigmoid colon*), and colonoscopy (*endoscopy of the entire colon from the rectum to the cecum and possibly the terminal ileum*). A colonoscopy is the preferred method of screening for colorectal cancer, which is recommended by the American Cancer Society and the Centers for Disease Control and Prevention (CDC)

Table 35-3 ■ COMMON PROCEDURES OF THE LOWER GASTROINTESTINAL TRACT

Procedure Name	Definition	Reason Performed
Appendectomy	Surgical removal of the appendix (Laparoscopic or open)	Appendicitis
Colectomy • Bowel resection • Total colectomy • Partial (subtotal) • Hemicolectomy • Proctocolectomy	Surgical removal of all or part of the large intestine (Laparoscopic or open)	Bleeding, bowel obstruction, Crohn's disease, colon cancer, ulcerative colitis, diverticulitis
Colonoscopy	Use of an endoscope to view the colon (*a thin, flexible tube with small video camera attached to take pictures or video*)	Ulcers, colon polyps, tumors, and areas of inflammation or bleeding; biopsy, screening for malignant neoplasm
Colostomy	Division (*cutting*) of the colon (*large intestine*), bringing the proximal end out through a stoma (*opening*) in the abdominal wall, bypassing the rectum and anus (Laparoscopic or open)	Bowel blockage (*obstruction*), bowel resection, injuries
Ileostomy • Enterostomy	Division of the ileum (*small intestine*) bringing the proximal end out to a stoma in the abdominal wall, bypassing the colon, rectum, and anus (Laparoscopic or open)	Inflammatory bowel disease, colon or rectal cancer, familial polyposis, birth defects involving the intestines, injuries
Polypectomy	Surgical removal of a polyp(s) (*abnormal growth from the mucous membrane*) (Laparoscopic or open)	Polyps
Small bowel transplant	Surgical removal of a diseased small intestine and replacement with some or all of a small intestine from a healthy person (Open)	Intestinal failure and complications related to parenteral nutrition (PN)

Source: © PB Resources, Inc. Used with permission.

every 10 years from ages 50 to 75. When abnormalities are found by a screening colonoscopy, such as polyps that are removed, it becomes a therapeutic, or surgical, procedure.

Ostomy

An ostomy is a temporary or permanent surgically created opening that connects an internal organ to the surface of the body. In the lower GI tract, ostomies are performed most commonly to reroute the contents of the ileum or colon because of rectal cancer or inflammatory bowel disease. A temporary ostomy may be performed when the intestinal tract cannot be properly prepared for surgery, as occurs when it is blocked by disease (e.g., tumors) or scar tissue, or when inflammation or an operative wound needs to heal without contamination by stool. Temporary ostomies can usually be reversed with minimal or no loss of intestinal function. A permanent ostomy may be required when disease, or its treatment, impairs normal intestinal function or when the pelvic and anal sphincter muscles that control elimination do not work properly. After the procedure, an ostomy appliance (*a bag or pouch that is adhered to the body with an adhesive*) collects bowel contents. The appliance is quite secure and is emptied or changed as needed. Whenever a portion of the small or large intestines is removed, the excision procedure must be followed by an anastomosis or ostomy.

> ### SUCCESS STEP
>
> An ostomy is described with the word root of the organ involved and the suffix -*stomy* for the creation of a new opening. For example, *ileo/stomy* describes connecting the ileum to the abdominal wall, and *colo/stomy* describes connecting the colon to the abdominal wall.

Procedures of the Accessory Digestive Organs

Commonly performed procedures on the accessory digestive organs are summarized in ■ TABLE 35-4. In particular, coders need to be familiar with procedures on the biliary tract and transplant procedures.

Biliary Tract

The biliary tract, or biliary tree, consists of the gall bladder, cystic duct, common bile duct, extrahepatic ducts, and pancreatic duct (■ FIGURE 35-2, page 644). The sphincter of Oddi is a muscular valve that joins the biliary tree to the duodenum. Any of these structures can become inflamed or obstructed, requiring surgery that may involve multiple components. A cholecystectomy can be either a laparoscopic or open procedure. It can be

---

Table 35-4 ■ COMMON PROCEDURES OF ACCESSORY DIGESTIVE ORGANS

Procedure Name	Definition	Reason performed
Autologous islet cell transplantation	The pancreas is surgically removed and the islet cells are isolated then injected into the portal vein. (Open)	Prevent or minimize the risk of diabetes after a pancreatectomy
Cholecystectomy	Surgical removal of the gall bladder (Laparoscopic or open)	Gallstones, infected or inflamed gallbladder
Common bile duct (CBD) exploration	Injection of a dye into the duct, visualization on an X-ray, removal of calculi, and introduction of a drainage bag when necessary (Laparoscopic)	Obstructive jaundice, stones in bile ducts
Endoscopic retrograde cholangiopancreatography (ERCP)	Injection of contrast medium into the bile ducts via a tube through the ampulla of Vater to visualize the entire biliary tree (*pancreatic, common bile, cystic, and hepatic ducts*)	Obstructive jaundice, stones in bile ducts, pancreatitis, biliary strictures due to cancer
Hepatectomy • Liver resection	Surgical removal of all or part of the liver (Open)	Donor for, or recipient of, liver transplantation, usually due to neoplasms of the liver or cirrhosis
Lithotripsy of gallstones	Use of high-frequency sound waves to break up gallstones (External)	Cholelithiasis, choledocholithiasis
Liver biopsy	Surgical removal of a small piece of the liver (Percutaneous, transvenous, or laparoscopic)	Determine the presence of liver disease
Liver transplant	Surgical removal of a diseased liver and replacement with some or all of a healthy liver from another person (Open)	Acute and end-stage liver failure, usually due to neoplasms of the liver or cirrhosis
Pancreatectomy	Surgical removal of all or part of the pancreas (Open)	Chronic pancreatitis, malignant neoplasm
Pancreaticoduodenectomy • Whipple procedure	Surgical removal of parts of the pancreas, duodenum, common bile duct, and, if required, portions of the stomach (Open)	Pancreatic cancer, neuroendocrine (islet cell) tumors, chronic pancreatitis, cancer of the ampulla of Vater (ampullary cancer), duodenal cancer, cancer of the distal bile duct

Source: © PB Resources, Inc. Used with permission.

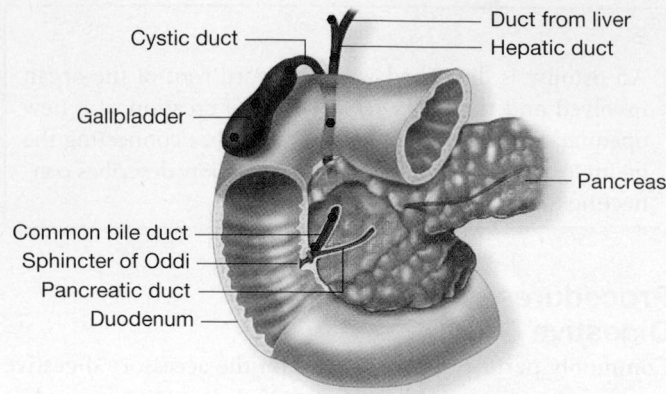

Figure 35-2 ■ Biliary Tract. (Red Dots Identify Common Sites of Calculi.)

performed alone, aided by cholangiography, with exploration and/or excision of the common bile duct, with anastomosis of the intestinal tract, and with a sphincteroplasty or sphincterotomy. Calculi can occur in the gall bladder, common bile duct, or both. When gallstones become symptomatic, they must be excised or destroyed using a method such as lithotripsy.

Transplantation

The liver and pancreas are two of the six organs that can be transplanted between individuals. Organ transplantation involves three distinct components: harvesting the donor organ, backbench work to prepare the organ, and recipient **allotransplantation** (*receiving an organ from another person*).

Liver transplantation is the replacement of a diseased liver with some or all of a healthy liver from another person. It is a viable treatment option for acute liver failure and end-stage liver disease, which can be caused by cirrhosis (*scarring of the liver*), chronic hepatitis B or C, bile duct diseases, genetic diseases, autoimmune liver diseases, primary liver cancer, alcoholic liver disease, and fatty liver disease.

Surgeons remove the diseased liver and replace it with the donor organ in the same anatomic location. The donor organ usually comes from a cadaver, but recent advances in transplant medicine now make it possible for living donors to donate a portion of their liver. Typically, the right lobe of the donor's liver is removed. The liver begins to regenerate almost immediately and continues to do so for about a year.

Although all transplants are complicated procedures, liver transplants are even more intricate because of the number of disconnections and reconnections of abdominal and hepatic tissue and blood vessels. A liver transplant typically requires 4 to 12 hours and three surgeons, two anesthesiologists, and up to four nurses.

Pancreas transplants are provided for diabetic patients, often in conjunction with a kidney transplant. The diseased pancreas is not removed during the operation. The donor pancreas is usually placed in the right lower part of the patient's abdomen. Blood vessels from the new pancreas are anastomosed to the patient's blood vessels. The donor duodenum, if retained, is anastomosed to the patient's intestine or bladder. Pancreas transplant surgery takes about 3 hours; a combination kidney/pancreas transplant requires about 6 hours.

Pancreatic islets, also called islets of Langerhans, are tiny clusters of cells scattered throughout the pancreas. Autologous (*from the same person*) islet cell transplantation is an option for patients who require a pancreatectomy because of chronic pancreatitis that cannot be managed by other treatments. The surgeon removes the pancreas from the patient, extracts and purifies islets, and infuses them into the patient's liver using a catheter. The goal is to give the body enough healthy islets to make insulin. Type 1 diabetics cannot receive autologous islet cell transplants because their beta cells (*islet cells that produce insulin*) do not function. Allotransplantation from a cadaver is an experimental procedure approved for limited use by the Food and Drug Administration (FDA) and is being tested as an option for type 1 diabetics.

SUCCESS STEP

The six organs that can be transplanted are, in descending order of frequency, kidney, liver, heart, lung, pancreas, and intestine.

Procedures of the Abdominal Structures

Procedures commonly performed on the abdominal structures that surround the digestive organs are summarized in ■ TABLE 35-5. When extensive adhesions impede access to an intended operative site, surgeons must perform adhesiolysis as part of the procedure.

Hernias can occur in several locations and are named by site (■ FIGURE 35-3). Some hernias are **reducible**, which means they can be corrected by the physician pushing the tissue back into place, whereas others require surgical repair, suturing, or insertion of a mesh prosthesis to reinforce the abdominal wall.

This section provides a general reference to help understand the most common digestive system procedures. Remember to keep standard reference books handy in case you get stuck.

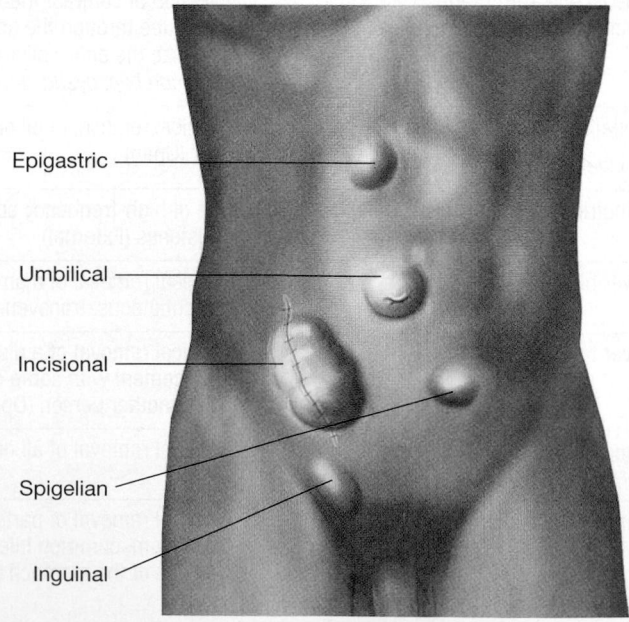

Figure 35-3 ■ Common Types of Hernias

Table 35-5 ■ **COMMON PROCEDURES WITHIN THE ABDOMINAL CAVITY**

Procedure Name	Definition	Reason Performed
Adhesiolysis	Use of scalpel or electric current to destroy or cut free adhesions (*scar tissue between organs or structures*) (Laparoscopic or open)	Abdominal adhesions
Hernia repair • Hernioplasty • Herniorrhaphy • Herniotomy	Surgical correction of a hernia through the use of manual manipulation, sutures, or mesh (External, laparoscopic, or open)	Bulging of internal organs or tissues through a defect in the wall of a body cavity
Omental flap	Removal of part of the omentum with blood vessel supply intact (Open)	Reconstruction of other anatomic sites, such as the chest wall or abdomen
Paracentesis	A surgical puncture of a body cavity to remove ascites (*excess fluid*) (Percutaneous)	Remove excess fluid caused by conditions such as infection, inflammation, cirrhosis, cancer, or injuries.

Source: © PB Resources, Inc. Used with permission.

CODING PRACTICE

Exercise 35.1 Digestive System Procedure Basics

Instructions: Use your medical terminology skills and resources to define the following procedures, then identify the applicable code or code range. Follow these steps:

- Use slash marks "/" to break down the underlined term into its root(s) and suffix.
- Define the meaning of the underlined word based on the meaning of each word part.
- Use the entire phrase to identify the code(s) or code range shown in the CPT Index.

Example: <u>appendectomy</u>, laparoscopic
append/ectomy   Meaning <u>*cutting out of the appendix*</u>   CPT Code <u>*44970*</u>

1. <u>Operculectomy</u>   Meaning _____   CPT Code _____
2. <u>Pancreatorrhaphy</u>   Meaning _____   CPT Code _____
3. <u>Sialodochoplasty</u>   Meaning _____   CPT Code _____
4. Anus, sphincter, <u>sphincterectomy</u> Meaning _____   CPT Code _____
5. <u>Proctosigmoidoscopy</u>, biopsy Meaning _____   CPT Code _____
6. <u>Cholangiopancreatography</u>, endoscopic retrograde, with papillotomy   Meaning _____   CPT Code _____
7. <u>Vermilionectomy</u>   Meaning _____   CPT Code _____
8. <u>Pyloromyotomy</u>   Meaning _____   CPT Code _____
9. <u>Enterolysis</u>   Meaning _____   CPT Code _____
10. <u>Cheiloplasty</u>   Meaning _____   CPT Code _____

CODING OVERVIEW OF DIGESTIVE SYSTEM PROCEDURES

The CPT Surgery subsection **Digestive System (40490-49999)** contains 18 subheadings divided by anatomic site. Anatomic sites are arranged by the order in which they occur in the alimentary (*digestive*) tract, beginning with the lips and ending with the anus. The last four subheadings identify sites that aid in digestion but are not part of the alimentary tract: the liver; biliary tract; pancreas; and abdomen, peritoneum, and omentum. Each subheading contains categories divided by the type of procedure, such as incision, excision, introduction, endoscopy, destruction, repair, and other procedures. The specific category titles vary by subheading based on what is applicable to a particular anatomic site. Review the subheadings, categories, and code ranges listed at the beginning of the Digestive System subsection in many CPT manuals, to become familiar with the content and organization.

This chapter includes invasive, minimally invasive, and noninvasive surgical procedures on the digestive system. Codes for diagnostic tests on the digestive system appear in the Medicine section. The medical necessity of any procedure codes always must be supported by diagnosis codes. CPT codes in the Digestive System subsection are frequently supported by diagnosis codes from ICD-10-CM **Chapter 11 Diseases of the Digestive System (K00-K95)**, as well as neoplasms, symptoms and signs, and injuries (■ TABLE 35-6). ICD-10-CM classifies injuries of the lips, mouth, and tongue with injuries of the face. Injuries of the throat are classified with injuries of the neck. These are the most commonly used codes to support procedures on the digestive system; however, diagnosis codes from any ICD-10-CM chapter are permissible.

CPT guidelines at the beginning of the Surgery section apply to Digestive System procedures. There are no special instructions at the beginning of this subsection, but there are some for subheadings and categories that provide definitions and coding information. A special instruction that appears in each endoscopy or laparoscopy category is that a surgical endoscopy or laparoscopy always includes a diagnostic endoscopy or laparoscopy. To report a diagnostic laparoscopy as a separate procedure, use code **49320**. Instructional notes appear throughout the Tabular List to alert coders to the need for modifiers, provide cross-references to codes for similar procedures on other sites, identify when additional codes might be needed for radiological services, and highlight resequenced and recently deleted codes.

ABSTRACTING DIGESTIVE SYSTEM PROCEDURES

Abstracting digestive system procedures requires paying special attention to the detailed anatomy of the digestive system and the order of the digestive organ within the GI tract, starting from either end. Knowledge of the order of the alimentary tract is necessary to determine the path of an endoscope and the farther site reached. Refer to Chapter 9 in this text for a refresher on digestive system anatomy.

In addition to familiarity with each structure, coders must be able to locate specific anatomic landmarks within the mouth, salivary glands, stomach (■ FIGURE 35-4), or colon. Coders need to read operative or procedure reports and determine the exact organ(s) and site(s) accessed, treated, excised, and/or reconnected to another site.

Refer to ■ TABLE 35-7 for guidance on how to abstract procedures on the Digestive System, then work through the detailed example that follows. Remember that the abstracting questions are a guide and that not every question applies to, or can be answered for, every case. For example, anastomosis is not performed in every procedure. Age is a factor for tonsillectomies and some hernia repairs.

Guided Example of Abstracting Digestive System Procedures

Refer to the following example throughout this chapter to practice skills for abstracting, assigning, and arranging Digestive System procedure codes.

Table 35-7 ■ **KEY CRITERIA FOR ABSTRACTING DIGESTIVE SYSTEM PROCEDURES**

❑ What is the patient's age?
❑ What site(s) is treated?
❑ What primary procedure is performed?
❑ What other procedure(s), if any, are performed?
❑ Is the treatment screening, diagnostic, or therapeutic?
❑ What is the approach?
❑ What exact sites within an organ are excised or treated?
❑ What type of anastomosis, if any, is performed?
❑ What sites are joined in the anastomosis?

Endoscopy

❑ What approach (access) is used?
❑ What is the farthest site reached?
❑ Is the purpose of the service preventive care?
❑ Does a screening or diagnostic endoscopy convert to a therapeutic procedure?
❑ Is the endoscopy a separate procedure?
❑ Was more than one treatment performed during the endoscopy?
❑ Is the patient covered by Medicare?

Table 35-6 ■ **LOCATING ICD-10-CM AND ADDITIONAL CPT CODES FOR THE DIGESTIVE SYSTEM**

Type of Code	Codes
ICD-10-CM Digestive System-Related Codes	
Digestive system conditions	K00-K95
Neoplasms	C00-C26
Symptoms and signs	R10-R19
Injuries	S09.93, S19.9, S36.-, T28.-
CPT Digestive System-Related Codes	
Medicine procedures	91010-91299
Radiologic procedures	
• Diagnostic radiology	74210-74363
• Diagnostic ultrasound	76700-76766, 76975
• Radiologic guidance	77001-77022
• Nuclear medicine, diagnostic	78201-78299
Laboratory organ/disease panels	80074-80076

Source: © PB Resources, Inc. Used with permission.

Source: © PB Resources, Inc. Used with permission.

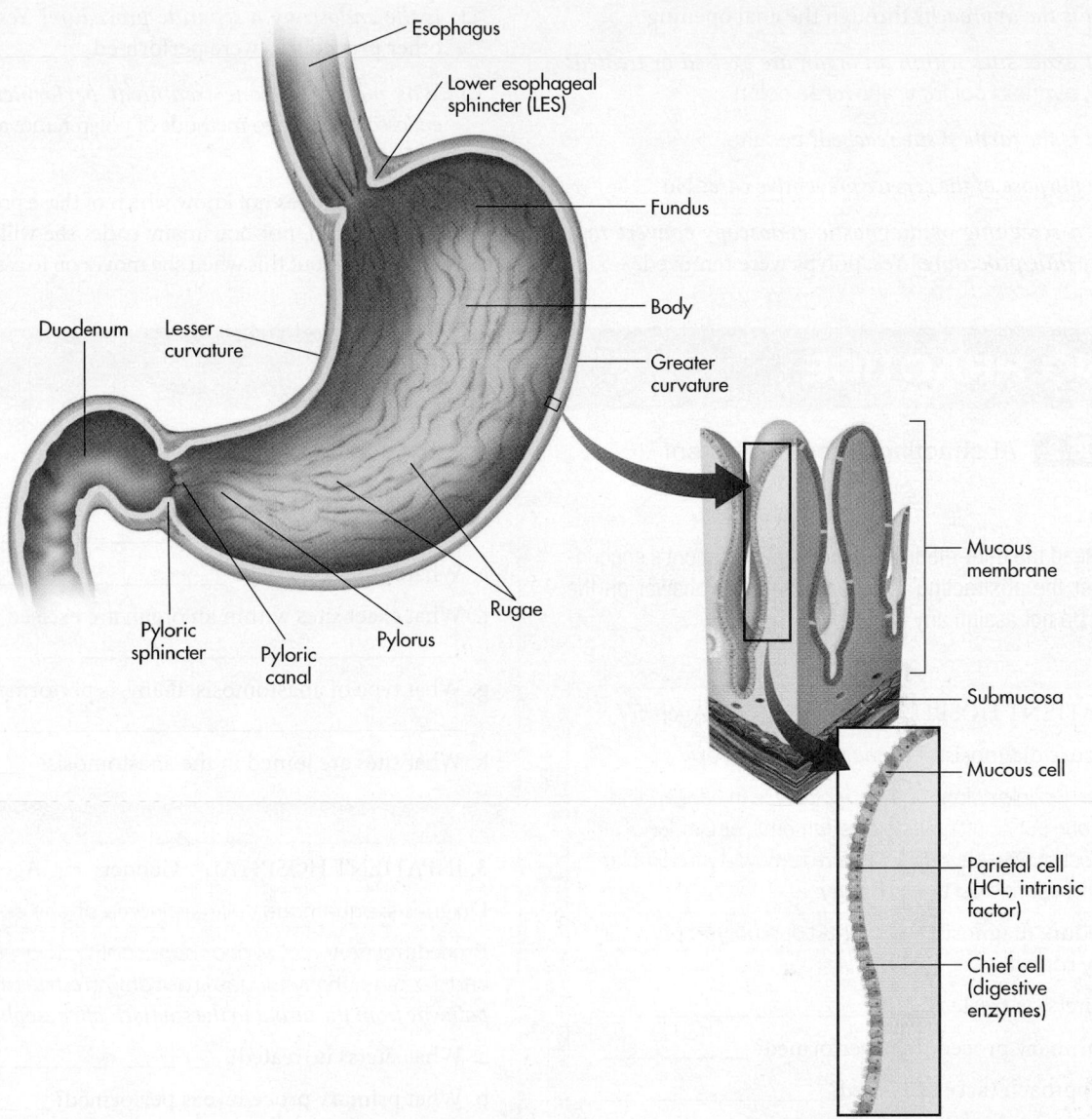

Figure 35-4 ■ Anatomic Landmarks of the Stomach

OUTPATIENT HOSPITAL   Gender: M   Age: 57

Preoperative diagnosis: hematochezia

Procedure: Colonoscopy, polypectomy, hemorrhoidectomy. Inspection of anus immediately revealed internal hemorrhoids. Colonoscopic examination identified 2 polyps in the sigmoid colon at 20 cm that were removed with hot forceps and one polyp in the transverse colon at 100 cm that was removed with a snare. Remainder of colon to cecum was unremarkable. Hemorrhoids were ligated with rubber bands. Patient tolerated procedure well and was transferred to the recovery area. Polyps were submitted to pathology.

Postoperative diagnosis: internal first-degree hemorrhoids, colonic polyps

Pathology report: benign adenomatous polyps

Follow along as fictitious coder Jill Hynes, CPC, abstracts the procedure. Check off each step after you complete it.

▶ Jill reads through the entire record, paying special attention to the reason for the encounter, the procedure performed, and the postoperative diagnosis. She refers to the Key Criteria for Abstracting Digestive System Procedures (Table 35-7).

❑ She notes the preoperative diagnosis, hematochezia (*bloody stool*).

❑ *What is the patient's age?* 57

❑ *What site is treated?* colon

❑ *What primary procedure is performed?* colonoscopy

❑ *What other procedure(s), if any, are performed?* polypectomy, hemorrhoidectomy

❑ *Is the treatment screening, diagnostic, or therapeutic?* diagnostic because of hematochezia

❑ *What is the approach?* through the anal opening

❑ *What exact sites within an organ are excised or treated?* anus, sigmoid colon, transverse colon

❑ *What is the farthest site reached?* cecum

❑ *Is the purpose of the service preventive care?* No

❑ *Does a screening or diagnostic endoscopy convert to a therapeutic procedure?* Yes, polyps were removed.

❑ *Is the endoscopy a separate procedure?* Yes, because no other procedures were performed.

❑ *Was more than one treatment performed during the endoscopy?* Yes, two methods of polyp removal: hot forceps and snare

▶ At this time, Jill does not know which of these procedures may need to be coded, nor how many codes she will end up with. She will learn about this when she moves on to assigning codes.

CODING PRACTICE

Exercise 35.2 **Abstracting Digestive System Procedures**

Instructions: Read the mini-medical-record of each patient's encounter and answer the abstracting questions. Write the answer on the line provided. Do not assign any codes.

1. OUTPATIENT HOSPITAL Gender: M Age: 57

Preprocedure diagnosis: screening colonoscopy

Procedure: flexible colonoscopy, two polyps in descending segment, one polyp in transverse segment, remainder of colon to cecum was clear. Polyps were removed with bipolar cautery and submitted to pathology

Postprocedure diagnosis: adenomatous polyps per pathology report

a. What site(s) is treated? _____

b. What primary procedure is performed? _____

c. What approach (access) is used? _____

d. What is the farthest site reached? _____

e. Is the purpose of the service preventive care? _____

f. Does a screening or diagnostic endoscopy convert to a therapeutic procedure? _____

g. Is the endoscopy a separate procedure? _____

h. Was more than one treatment performed during the endoscopy? _____

2. INPATIENT HOSPITAL Gender: F Age: 33

Diagnosis: morbid obesity, BMI = 43 kg/m^2

Procedure: laparoscopic gastric bypass and Roux-en-Y gastroenterostomy (100 cm)

a. What site(s) is treated? _____

b. What primary procedure is performed? _____

c. What other procedure(s), if any, are performed? _____

(continued)

2. (continued)

d. Is the treatment screening, diagnostic, or therapeutic? _____

e. What is the approach? _____

f. What exact sites within an organ are excised or treated? _____

g. What type of anastomosis, if any, is performed? _____

h. What sites are joined in the anastomosis? _____

3. INPATIENT HOSPITAL Gender: F Age: 48

Diagnosis: squamous cell carcinoma of the esophagus

Procedure: near-total esophagectomy, thoracotomy, end-to-side pharyngogastrostomy (*restructuring of the pathway from the throat to the stomach after esophagectomy*)

a. What site(s) is treated? _____

b. What primary procedure is performed? _____

c. What other procedure(s), if any, are performed? _____

d. Is the treatment screening, diagnostic, or therapeutic? _____

e. What is the approach? _____

f. What exact sites within an organ are excised or treated? _____

g. What type of anastomosis, if any, is performed? _____

h. What sites are joined in the anastomosis? _____

4. OUTPATIENT HOSPITAL Gender: M Age: 64

Diagnosis: initial incarcerated incisional hernia

Procedure: incarcerated incisional hernia repair with mesh

a. What site(s) is treated? _____

b. What primary procedure is performed? _____

(continued)

4. (continued)

c. What other procedure(s), if any, are performed?
_____

d. Is the treatment screening, diagnostic, or therapeutic?
_____

e. What is the approach? _____

5. (continued)

c. What is the approach? _____

d. What is the farthest site reached? _____

e. Does a screening or diagnostic endoscopy convert to a therapeutic procedure? _____

f. Was more than one treatment performed during the endoscopy? _____ If so, name the additional procedures. _____

5. OUTPATIENT HOSPITAL   Gender: M   Age: 61

Preoperative diagnosis: *melena, hematemesis*

Procedure: *EGD was initiated with flexible scope through the mouth. Identified bleeding ulcers in esophagus and duodenum, which were successfully cauterized. Features of chronic gastritis were noted. No masses or hiatal hernia. Obtained biopsy from the antrum. Biopsies submitted to pathology for H&E* (hematoxylin and eosin stain test to detect cancer) *and CLO* (Campylobacter-*like organism test for* H. pylori).

Postoperative diagnosis: *bleeding esophageal ulcer and bleeding peptic ulcer*

Pathology report: *biopsies negative for H. pylori and carcinoma*

a. What site(s) is treated? _____

b. What primary procedure is performed? _____

(continued)

6. INPATIENT HOSPITAL   Gender: M   Age: 3 months

Diagnosis: *bilateral cleft lip and nasal deformity*

Procedure: *primary repair of a bilateral cleft lip and nasal deformity; repair of soft tissue of cleft palate and closure of alveolar ridge*

a. What site(s) is treated? _____

b. What primary procedure is performed? _____

c. What other procedure(s), if any, are performed?
_____

d. Is the treatment screening, diagnostic, or therapeutic?
_____

e. What is the approach? _____

f. What exact sites within an organ are excised or treated?
_____

ASSIGNING CODES FOR DIGESTIVE SYSTEM PROCEDURES

This section reviews coding rules for several commonly performed Digestive System procedures: tonsillectomy, appendectomy, anastomosis, endoscopy, transplants, and repairs. Learning about these procedures will reinforce basic coding skills that you can use throughout the CPT manual.

Tonsillectomy

Tonsillectomy and adenoidectomy (**42820-42870**) provide several coding options based on patient age and the combination of procedures performed. Codes *do not* distinguish among the surgical method used: tonsillotome (*scalpel*), cryosurgery, laser, or electrocautery.

To assign codes, search the Index for the Main Term **Tonsillectomy**; **Tonsils** with the first-level modifying term **Excision**; or **Adenoids** with the first-level modifying term **Excision**. Review and verify the codes in the Tabular List based on the following criteria.

When a tonsillectomy and adenoidectomy are performed together, select the code based on patient age: **42820** for **younger than 12** and **42821** for **age 12 or over**.

When only a tonsillectomy is performed, select the code based on patient age: **42825** for **younger than 12** and **42826** for **age 12 or over**.

When only an adenoidectomy is performed, determine whether the procedure is primary (*the patient's first adenoidectomy*) or secondary (*the patient's second adenoidectomy performed to remove regrowth after a previous surgery*). Then select the code based on the patient's age. Codes **42830** and **42831** identify a primary adenoidectomy; codes **42835** and **42836** identify a secondary adenoidectomy.

Codes for other tonsil procedures, such as radical resection, excision of tonsil tags, and excision of the lingual tonsil, also are provided.

SUCCESS STEP

When you see the term *tonsil*, be sure to identify the anatomic site of the tissue. *Tonsil* refers to a small rounded mass of lymphoid tissue. The palatine (*pertaining to the palate*) tonsils are located at the back of the throat and are commonly referred to simply as tonsils. There are several other sites of tonsil tissue throughout the mouth and throat, and there is even tonsil tissue in the cerebellum.

Appendectomy

Although there are only six codes in the Appendix subheading, they are used frequently, and coders must understand the differences. To locate codes in the Index, search for the Main Term **Appendix** or **Appendectomy**. In the Tabular List, CPT provides one code for **Incision and drainage of appendiceal abscess, open** (**44900**), three codes for open appendectomies, and one code for a laparoscopic appendectomy (plus a code for an unlisted laparoscopic procedure).

An **incidental appendectomy** is the removal of the appendix as a preventive measure during another procedure, such as a cholecystectomy. Incidental appendectomies are usually not coded.

When an appendectomy is performed for an indicated (specific) reason, assign the code as follows. Refer to the CPT manual to observe the formatting of codes and read the full code descriptions.

- When an open appendectomy is performed and the appendix has not ruptured, assign **44950**.

- When an open appendectomy is performed for a ruptured appendix with abscess or generalized peritonitis, assign **44960**.

- When an open appendectomy is done for an indicated reason at the same time as another procedure, assign the add-on code **44955**.

- For a laparoscopic appendectomy, assign **44970**.

Anastomosis

Anastomosis is not a standalone procedure; it is performed in conjunction with a total or partial excision of an organ. When an excision is performed on the alimentary tube or a duct, either an anastomosis or an ostomy is almost always necessary.

To locate codes in the Index, search for the Main Term **Anastomosis**, a first-level modifying term for the site treated, and a second-level modifying term for the site connected to.

Refer to the Tabular List to select the correct code based on the details of the procedure. Read the code options to determine how anastomosis is to be coded:

- bundled into the code for the main procedure
- an indented code under the main code
- an add-on code
- a separate standalone code

Identify the two sites that are connected and the type of connection created, such as Roux-en-Y, end to end, end to side, and side to end. The specific type of connection is sometimes, but not always, coded.

Endoscopy

CPT differentiates between endoscopy and laparoscopy in the Digestive System subsection. Endoscopy codes describe access through the mouth, nose, or rectum. Laparoscopy codes describe percutaneous access through the abdomen. The subheadings Esophagus and Intestines provide codes for both endoscopy and laparoscopy. The subheading Anus provides endoscopy codes only. The subheadings Stomach; Appendix; Liver; and Abdomen, Peritoneum, and Omentum provide laparoscopy codes only because these sites, except for the stomach, cannot be reached endoscopically. Endoscopy of the stomach and duodenum is classified with the esophagus because the stomach and duodenum are examined in conjunction with the esophagus.

Each category for endoscopy or laparoscopy presents special instructions that define the extent of the examinations for the respective anatomic sites. The special instructions also direct that a surgical scope procedure always includes a diagnostic scope procedure. This instruction means that when an endoscopic or laparoscopic procedure begins as a screening or diagnostic procedure and is converted to a surgical procedure, only the surgical procedure should be coded.

For example, during a screening colonoscopy, the physician may remove a polyp. The polypectomy coverts the procedure from screening to surgical, but only one code—the one for the polypectomy—should be reported.

Assign endoscopy codes based on the farthest site accessed. In the upper GI system, when the esophagus, stomach, and duodenum are examined, assign a code for esophagogastroduodenoscopy only; do not also assign a code for esophagoscopy. In the lower GI system, when the entire colon is examined, assign a code for colonoscopy only; do not also assign codes for anoscopy, proctosigmoidoscopy, and sigmoidoscopy, even if procedures were done in those areas (■ FIGURE 35-5).

Multiple Endoscopy Rule

The **multiple endoscopy rule** explains how to assign endoscopy codes when more than one procedure is performed during the same session. Endoscopy codes are divided into families, each with a base code. The base code is a screening/diagnostic endoscopy for a particular region. The other codes in the family are therapeutic/surgical procedures, such as biopsy, dilation, or tumor excision. You may assign as many surgical codes from one family as necessary, but do not assign the *base* diagnostic endoscopy code together with a *surgical* endoscopy code. The Medicare Physician Fee Schedule Database (MPFSDB) identifies the codes subject to this rule and the corresponding base codes (■ TABLE 35-8). The descriptions of the base codes include the designation (**separate procedure**), which means that the base code should be reported only when it is done as a distinct procedure and not as part of a more extensive surgical procedure. Each code in the family includes the work RVU and price of the base code service, plus the additional work and price for the surgical procedure. Although more than one surgical endoscopy code from the same family can be billed, a special endoscopy payment formula excludes the price of the base service from all but the first code reported (■ FIGURE 35-6, page 652).

Upper GI Endoscopy

CPT provides endoscopy codes for esophagoscopy and esophagogastroduodenoscopy. Special instructions at the beginning of the Endoscopy category define an esophagoscopy as extending

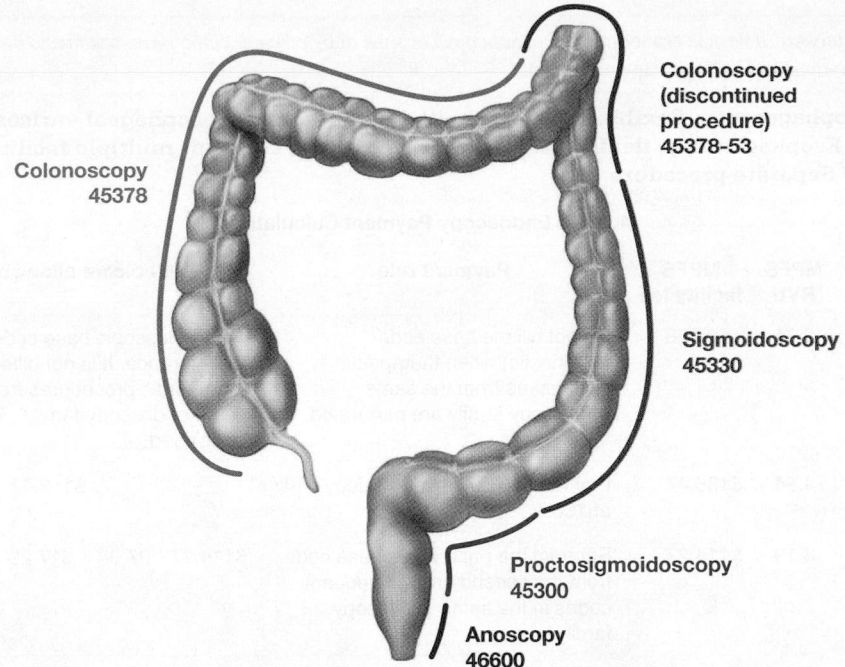

Colonoscopy
(discontinued
procedure)
45378-53

Colonoscopy
45378

Sigmoidoscopy
45330

Proctosigmoidoscopy
45300

Anoscopy
46600

Figure 35-5 ■ Lower GI Endoscopy Codes

from the upper esophageal sphincter to the gastroesophageal junction. When only the esophagus is examined, assign a code for esophagoscopy (**43191-43232**). Esophagoscopy codes are divided based on whether the endoscope is rigid (parent code **43191**) or flexible. Flexible endoscopy codes are divided based on whether the access is transnasal (parent code **43197**) or transoral (parent code **43200**). Each of these code families is subdivided based on the additional procedures performed during the examination, such as a biopsy, foreign body removal, or polyp removal.

When the stomach and duodenum are examined, assign a code for esophagogastroduodenoscopy (**43235-43259**). Do not

Table 35-8 ■ ENDOSCOPIC CODE FAMILIES FOR THE DIGESTIVE SYSTEM

Base Code	Short Description	Code Family
43191	Esophagoscopy, rigid, transoral; diagnostic	43192-43196
43197	Esophagoscopy, flexible, transnasal; diagnostic	43198
43200	Esophagoscopy, flexible, transoral; diagnostic	43201-43232
43235	Esophagogastroduodenoscopy, flexible, transoral; diagnostic	43233-43259, 43270
43260	Endoscopic retrograde cholangiopancreatography (ERCP); diagnostic	43261- 43265, 43274-43278
44360	Small intestinal endoscopy, enteroscopy beyond second portion of duodenum, not including ileum; diagnostic	44361-44373
44376	Small intestinal endoscopy, enteroscopy beyond second portion of duodenum, including ileum; diagnostic	44377-44379
44388	Colonoscopy through stoma; diagnostic	44389-44397
45300	Proctosigmoidoscopy, rigid; diagnostic	45303-45327
45330	Sigmoidoscopy, flexible; diagnostic	45331-45345
45378	Colonoscopy, flexible; diagnostic	45379-45392
46600	Anoscopy; diagnostic	46604-46615
47552	Biliary endoscopy, percutaneous via T-tube or other tract; diagnostic	47553-47556
49320	Laparoscopy, abdomen, peritoneum, and omentum; diagnostic	49321-49325

Source: © PB Resources, Inc. Used with permission. CPT codes only © American Medical Association.

Patient underwent a flexible transoral esophagoscopy because of bleeding. A biopsy was taken and band ligation of esophageal varices was performed.

43205 Esophagoscopy, flexible, transoral; with band ligation of esophageal varices facility
43202-59 Esophagoscopy, flexible, transoral; with biopsy, single or multiple facility;
    -59 Separate procedure

			Multiple Endoscopy Payment Calculation	
Code	MPFS RVU	MPFS facility fee	Payment rule	Medicare allowable
Endoscopic base code 43200	2.71	$97.08	Do not bill the base code (diagnostic) when therapeutic procedures from the same endoscopy family are performed.	The endoscopic base code is used for reference. It is not billed because therapeutic procedures from the same endoscopy family were performed.
43205	4.34	$155.47	Pay (allow) the first endoscopy at 100%	$155.47
43202	3.19	$114.27	Subtract the price of the base code from the second and subsequent codes in the same endoscopy family.	$114.27 - 97.08 = $17.29
			Total	$172.76

Figure 35-6 ■ Example of Multiple Endoscopy Payment Rule. *Source: © PB Resources, Inc. Used with permission. CPT codes only © American Medical Association.*

also assign a code for esophagoscopy because the service is included in the code for the esophagogastroduodenoscopy. Code **43235** is the parent code for this code family. Codes are divided based on the additional procedures performed during the examination. CPT provides an important instructional note at the beginning of the esophagogastroduodenoscopy code family. When the examination includes the stomach but not the duodenum, assign a code for esophagogastroduodenoscopy with modifier **-52** or **-53**. The choice of modifier depends on whether the physician intends to repeat the examination to include the duodenum.

- When the duodenum is not examined because it is not considered clinically relevant to the reason for the procedure, assign modifier **-52 Reduced services** (■ FIGURE 35-7).

- When the duodenum is not examined because an issue, such as retained gastric contents, prevents safe access to the duodenum, and the physician plans to repeat the procedure

under better conditions, assign modifier **-53 Discontinued procedure** (■ FIGURE 35-8).

- When a repeat examination is not planned, assign modifier **-52 Reduced services**.

CODING CAUTION

Many codes in the Digestive System have been resequenced. The cross-referencing instruction provided in the Tabular List does not always lead to the exact location of the resequenced code. It is worthwhile to take a few minutes to locate the new code, then write a note next to where the code number appears in numerical order. For example, the cross-reference next to code **46945** states **See 46200-46288.** Because this is a large range to search, next to **46945** write *see after code 46221* so you can immediately locate the resequenced code.

Patient underwent an endoscopic examination of the esophagus and stomach because of suspected reflux disease. The physician does not examine the duodenum because it is not clinically pertinent.

43235-52 Esophagogastroduodenoscopy, flexible, transoral; diagnostic, including collection of specimen(s) by brushing or washing, when performed (separate procedure); -52 Reduced services

Figure 35-7 ■ Example of Coding an EGD with Modifier -52

Patient underwent an esophagogastroduodenoscopy for peptic ulcers. The physician cannot move the endoscope past the gastroduodenal junction because the patient did not prepare properly and there is still food in the duodenum. The patient is instructed about the necessity of proper preparation. The procedure is rescheduled for next week.

43235-53 Esophagogastroduodenoscopy, flexible, transoral; diagnostic, including collection of specimen(s) by brushing or washing, when performed (separate procedure); -53 Discontinued procedure

Figure 35-8 ■ Example of Coding an EGD with Modifier -53

Table 35-9 ■ HCPCS LEVEL II CODES FOR COLON CANCER SCREENING

HCPCS Code	HCPCS Code Descriptor
G0104	Colon cancer screening; flexible sigmoidoscopy
G0105	Colon cancer screening; colonoscopy on individual at high risk
G0106	Colon cancer screening; barium enema as an alternative to G0104
G0107	Colon cancer screening; FOBT, 1–3 simultaneous determinations
G0120	Colon cancer screening; barium enema as an alternative to G0105
G0121	Colon cancer screening; colonoscopy for individuals not meeting criteria for high risk
G0122	Colon cancer screening; barium enema (noncovered)
G0328	Colon cancer screening; as an alternative to G0107; fecal occult blood test, immunoassay, 1–3 simultaneous determinations

Source: Centers for Medicare and Medicaid

Medicare Colonoscopy Coding

Medicare has special rules for coding screening colonoscopies. The code for a screening colonoscopy for non-Medicare patients is **45378**. Medicare requires that a HCPCS Level II code be used. **G0105** identifies a screening for an individual at high risk of developing colon cancer, which Medicare has established specific criteria for. **G0121** is used for a screening colonoscopy for a person who does not meet Medicare's high-risk criteria. Medicare also provides HCPCS Level II codes for other types of colorectal cancer screening: fecal occult blood testing, flexible sigmoidoscopy, colonoscopy, and screening barium enema (■ TABLE 35-9). Medicare provides detailed instructions regarding how these codes should be used and the diagnoses needed to support them.

When a screening colonoscopy is converted to a diagnostic or surgical endoscopy—for example, when polyps are removed—assign the HCPCS Level II modifier -**PT Colorectal cancer screening test, converted to diagnostic test or other procedure** (■ FIGURE 35-9).

Physician performs a screening colonoscopy on a patient not at high risk. During the procedure, two polyps were found and removed using hot forceps.

G0121-PT Colon cancer screening; colonoscopy for individuals not meeting criteria for high risk; -PT Colorectal cancer screening test, converted to diagnostic test or other procedure

Figure 35-9 ■ Example of Coding for a Medicare Screening Colonoscopy

Transplants

Each type or organ transplant has three groups of codes for the three main parts of the transplant process: donor organ harvesting, backbench work, and recipient transplantation. Special instructions at the beginning of each transplant category (liver, pancreas, and small intestine) describe the division and use of codes.

For liver transplants, different codes are used for a cadaver hepatectomy (**47133**) than for a living donor. Codes for a living donor hepatectomy are divided based on which segments of the liver are removed (**47140-47142**). Codes for backbench preparation and reconstruction are divided based on the extent of work performed (**47143-47174**). Recipient codes are divided based on whether the transplant is orthotopic (*the transplanted organ is placed in the same position as the original organ*) or heterotopic (*the transplanted organ is placed in a position other than that of the original organ*) (**47135-47136**).

The donor and recipient require different diagnosis codes. A living donor is assigned a **Z** code indicating the donor status. Diagnosis codes for the organ recipient identify the condition(s) that describes why the transplant is necessary, as well as any comorbid conditions.

It is common for multiple physicians to be involved in various parts of the transplantation process, so each physician reports the appropriate code(s) for the services personally provided (■ FIGURE 35-10, page 654).

Modifier rules vary among the six types of organ transplants. Carefully review the MPFSDB to determine which transplant codes accept modifier -**66 Surgical team** and which codes require modifier -**51 multiple procedures**.

Repairs

Repair involves closing an opening—such as a laceration, fistula, or ostomy—or restructuring/reconstructing an anatomic site. This is in contrast to an incision made for drainage or to create an opening and in contrast to an excision, which removes tissue. Most Digestive System subheadings provide a category for Repair. To locate Repair codes in the Index, search for the one of the following:

- the Main Term **Repair** and a first-level modifying term for the anatomic site
- the name of the procedure, which usually ends with the suffix -plasty, -rraphy, or -pexy
- the name of the anatomic site and a first-level modifying term for **Repair**

In the Tabular List, review the details of the codes to select the one that describes the details of the procedure. Repair codes may appear as a parent code with several indented codes that describe variations of the procedure (■ FIGURE 35-11, page 654).

Adhesions

When performing procedures in the abdominal cavity, surgeons frequently encounter adhesions resulting from scarring from previous surgeries or inflammation. They must loosen, excise, or destroy the adhesions to reach the surgical site. CPT

A living donor match is found for a pediatric patient with congenital biliary atresia who has been on the liver transplant list. The transplant team consists of two surgeons. Surgeon A performs a hepatectomy of the left lateral segment on the living donor. Surgeon B performs the backbench reconstruction with two venous anastomoses and two arterial anastomoses. Both surgeons transplant the liver segment into the patient recipient. The transplant is orthotopic.

Surgeon A
Living donor:
Z52.6 Liver donor
47140 Donor hepatectomy (including cold preservation), from living donor; left lateral segment only (segments II and III)

Surgeon B
Backbench reconstruction:
Q44.2 Atresia of bile ducts
47147 x 2 Backbench reconstruction of cadaver or living donor liver graft prior to allotransplantation; arterial anastomosis, each
47146-51 x 2 Backbench reconstruction of cadaver or living donor liver graft prior to allotransplantation; venous anastomosis, each; -51 Multiple procedures

Surgeon A and Surgeon B
Transplant recipient:
Q44.2 Atresia of bile ducts
47135-66 Liver allotransplantation; orthotopic, partial or whole, from cadaver or living donor, any age; -66 Surgical team

Figure 35-10 ■ Example of Coding a Liver Transplant. *Source:* © *PB Resources, Inc. Used with permission. CPT codes only* © *American Medical Association.*

guidelines state that surgical destruction is part of a surgical procedure and, usually, should not be reported separately. This includes adhesions. When adhesions are so extensive that the surgeon spends a significant amount of time destroying or removing them to enable access to the surgical site, it might be possible to append modifier **-22 Increased procedural services** to the CPT code for the procedure. Documentation must identify the amount of excess time required, describe in detail what the surgeon did, and explain why the added time was necessary. In general, modifier **-22** should be used only when the added work has increased the operative time by 50% or more.

Separate codes for adhesiolysis are reported in the unusual circumstance when lysis is performed as a separate procedure. To locate adhesiolysis codes in the Index, search for the Main Term **Adhesions** and the first-level modifying term for the anatomic site.

Surgeon performs an esophagoplasty and closes a tracheoesophageal fistula using the thoracic approach.

43312 Esophagoplasty (plastic repair or reconstruction), thoracic approach; with repair of tracheoesophageal fistula

Figure 35-11 ■ Example of Coding a Repair on the Esophagus

Guided Example of Assigning Digestive System Procedure Codes

To practice skills for assigning codes for the Digestive System, continue with the guided example from earlier in the chapter about a patient who was seen for a colonoscopy. Follow along in your CPT manual as Jill Hynes, CPC, assigns codes. Check off each step after you complete it.

▶ First, Jill confirms the procedures: *colonoscopy, polypectomy, hemorrhoidectomy.*

▶ Jill searches the Index for the Main Term **Colonoscopy**.

 ❑ She locates the first-level modifying term **Flexible**.

 ❑ She locates the second-level modifying term **Removal**, then **Polyp**.

 ❑ She identifies the codes to verify: **45384, 45385**.

▶ Jill turns to the Tabular List to review and verify codes **45384-45385**.

 ❑ She notices that **45384-45385** are indented codes, so she traces back through the Tabular List to locate the parent code, **45378**.

 ❑ She reads the common part of code **45378** that appears before the semicolon: **Colonoscopy, flexible**. This code describes the basic colonoscopy provided, which extended from the anus to the cecum. She reads the second part of the code description, **diagnostic, including collection of specimen(s) by brushing or washing, when performed (separate procedure)**, and confirms that it does not describe this procedure because a therapeutic procedure also was performed.

❏ She reads the indented description for code **45384, with removal of tumor(s), polyp(s), or other lesion(s) by hot biopsy forceps** and confirms that this accurately describes the two polyps found in the sigmoid colon.

❏ She reads the indented description for code **45385, with removal of tumor(s), polyp(s), or other lesion(s) by snare technique** and confirms that this accurately describes the polyp found in the transverse colon.

▶ Jill checks for instructional notes in the Tabular List.

❏ She looks for instructional notes after the parent code, **45378**, and the indented codes she plan to use, **45384** and **45385**, and finds none.

❏ She refers to the beginning of the category **Endoscopy**, which appears before code **45300**, and reviews the special instructions that include definitions of endoscopic procedures on the colon.

❏ She understands that even though a polypectomy occurred in the sigmoid segment of the colon, she should not report a sigmoidoscopy; she should assign codes based on the farthest extent of the procedure, which was the entire length of the colon from the rectum to the cecum.

❏ She also reads the statement **Surgical endoscopy always includes diagnostic endoscopy**. This tells her that she should not use a separate code for the diagnostic portion of the procedure in addition to the codes for the polypectomies.

❏ She checks for special instructions at the beginning of the Digestive System subsection, before code **40490**, and finds none.

❏ She reviews the Surgery section guidelines that appear before code **10021** but does not find any information specific to endoscopies.

▶ Jill returns to the codes for the polypectomies: **45384** and **45385**.

❏ Because these codes share the same parent code (**45378**), she needs to determine whether they can both be reported.

❏ She confirms that there were no instructional notes directing her to not use the codes together.

❏ She recalls the multiple endoscopy rule that permits multiple codes from the same code family to be reported together. Both of these codes belong to the code family with the base code **43578**, so she knows that she can report both codes.

▶ Jill turns her attention to the hemorrhoidectomy.

▶ Jill searches the Index for the Main Term **Hemorrhoidectomy**.

❏ She locates the first-level modifying term **Ligation**.

❏ She identifies the code range to verify: **46221, 46945-46946**.

▶ Jill turns to the Tabular List to review and verify the codes.

❏ First she locates code **46221** and notices that codes **46945-46946** appear next because they are resequenced codes. She likes being able to review and compare all three codes together.

❏ She reads the description for code **46221, Hemorrhoidectomy, internal, by rubber band ligation(s)**. This sounds like the right description but she checks the other codes to be certain.

❏ She notices that code **46945** is a parent code for **46946**, and the common descriptor is **Hemorrhoidectomy, internal, by ligation other than rubber band;**

❏ She double checks the documentation and confirms the ligation method: Hemorrhoids were ligated with rubber bands. The documentation confirms that **46221** is the correct code because the code specifies **by rubber band ligation**.

▶ Jill reviews the Tabular List for instructional notes and finds two.

❏ The first instructional note appears after code **46221: (Do not report 46221 in conjunction with 45350, 45398)**. This note does not apply because she already determined that she is not reporting code **45350** or **45398**.

❏ The second instructional note appears after code **46946: (Do not report 46221, 46945, and 46946, in conjunction with 0249T.)** This note does not apply because she is not using code **0249T**.

❏ Jill also reviews the special instructions at the beginning of the subheading **Anus**, before code **46020**. The special instructions define the codes to use for various types of hemorrhoids and confirm that she selected the correct code for ligation of internal hemorrhoids.

▶ Jill reviews the procedure codes she has assigned for this case.

❏ **46221 Hemorrhoidectomy, internal, by rubber band ligation(s)**

❏ **45384 Colonoscopy, flexible; with removal of tumor(s), polyp(s), or other lesion(s) by hot biopsy forceps**

❏ **45385 Colonoscopy, flexible; with removal of tumor(s), polyp(s), or other lesion(s) by snare technique**

▶ Next, Jill must determine what modifiers are needed and how to sequence the codes.

CODING PRACTICE

Exercise 35.3 Assigning Codes for Digestive System Procedures

Instructions: Read the mini-medical-record of each patient's encounter. Review the information abstracted in Exercise 35.2 for questions 1–3. For questions 4–6, do the abstracting on your own. Assign CPT procedure codes using the Index and Tabular List. Write the code(s) on the line provided.

1. OUTPATIENT HOSPITAL   Gender: M   Age: 57

Preprocedure diagnosis: screening colonoscopy

Procedure: flexible colonoscopy, 2 polyps in descending segment, 1 polyp in transverse segment, remainder of colon to cecum was clear. Polyps were removed with bipolar cautery and submitted to pathology

Postprocedure diagnosis: adenomatous polyps per pathology report

Tip: Apply a modifier to identify this as a preventive service.

1 CPT Code _____

2. INPATIENT HOSPITAL   Gender: F   Age: 33

Diagnosis: morbid obesity, BMI = 43

Procedure: laparoscopic gastric bypass and Roux-en-Y gastroenterostomy (100 cm)

Tip: Identify the meaning of *gastroenterostomy* to determine the Roux-en-Y sites.

1 CPT Code _____

3. INPATIENT HOSPITAL   Gender: F   Age: 48

Diagnosis: squamous cell carcinoma of the esophagus

Procedure: near-total esophagectomy, thoracotomy, end-to-side pharyngogastrostomy (*restructure of the pathway from the throat to the stomach after esophagectomy*)

1 CPT Code _____

4. EMERGENCY DEPT   Gender: M   Age: 2

Reason for encounter: Mother brings in her son, who swallowed a toy piece

Procedure: rigid esophagoscopy through the mouth, retrieved plastic toy piece, no damage or laceration apparent

Diagnosis: esophagoscopy with foreign body removal

Tip: Abstract this procedure on your own before attempting to assign codes.

1 CPT Code _____

5. EMERGENCY DEPT   Gender: F   Age: 26

Diagnosis: abscess under the tongue

Procedure: superficial sublingual incision and drainage

Tip: Abstract this procedure on your own. Do not confuse the sublingual site within the mouth with the sublingual salivary gland.

1 CPT Code _____

6. LOCATION   Gender: M   Age: 36

Preprocedure diagnosis: rectal mass

Procedure: transsacral proctotomy to excise rectal tumor

Postprocedure diagnosis: stage I carcinoma of the rectum

Tip: Abstract this procedure on your own before attempting to assign codes.

1 CPT Code _____

ARRANGING CODES FOR DIGESTIVE SYSTEM PROCEDURES

When more than one procedure is performed during an operative session, coders must be attentive to modifiers and how to arrange (sequence) codes. The order of codes sometimes determines the modifiers needed. Some modifiers can be assigned at the same time the code is assigned, and some modifiers cannot be assigned until the codes are sequenced. Certain modifiers are required even when only one procedure is performed.

In general, multiple surgical procedures are sequenced in descending order of RVU, which corresponds to the complexity and price of the procedure. RVUs are provided in the MPFSDB and in most encoders and billing software programs.

Modifiers

Modifiers that have a special application for specific Digestive System codes have been discussed throughout this chapter and examples have been provided. This section summarizes those modifiers and introduces some new ones. These are not the only modifiers that can be used with Digestive System codes. Refer to Appendix A of the CPT manual and to Chapters 29 and 31 of this text for more information about modifiers.

-33 Preventive Service

Modifier **-33** identifies certain procedures, such as a screening colonoscopy, as preventive care services under the Patient Protection and Affordable Care Act (PPACA). The United States Preventive Services Task Force (USPSTF) assigns one of five letter grades (A, B, C, D, or I) to recommend the likelihood of the net benefit of providing a preventive service. The PPACA requires that services rated as A or B be covered in full by private health plans. Copayments, coinsurances, and deductibles are not owed for these services under PPACA.

When a service on the approved list does not have a CPT code specifically described as preventive, assign modifier **-33** to indicate that the service was provided for preventive care. For example, CPT provides codes for preventive medicine E/M visits, so those codes do not need modifier **-33**. However, CPT does not provide a dedicated code for screening colonoscopies, so the code for a diagnostic colonoscopy (**45378**) must be reported. Append modifier **-33** to identify the colonoscopy as preventive in nature. The insurance company will waive the patient's copayment, coinsurance, and deductible and pay 100% of the allowed fee to the provider (■ Figure 35-12). A copayment may still apply if preventive care is not the *primary* purpose of the office visit or other services that require copayment are provided.

SUCCESS STEP

The USPSTF list of A and B services is updated annually and is available at **http://www.uspreventiveservicestaskforce .org/**. Other services eligible for modifier **-33** include certain routine immunizations recommended by the CDC and certain preventive care and screening services for children and women supported by the Health Resources and Services Administration (HRSA).

-51 Multiple Procedures

When multiple procedures are performed at the same operative session by the same provider, modifier **-51** indicates that payment should be reduced on the second and subsequent procedures because of the efficiencies gained. Procedures should be ordered in descending order by RVU, so that the most extensive procedure is paid in full and payment is reduced for the less extensive procedures. The standard Medicare rule for payment of multiple surgeries is to allow the full amount of the first procedure and allow the second through fifth procedures at 50% of the Medicare Physician Fee Schedule (MPFS) rate. Multiple procedures beyond six are priced **by report** (*based on a report submitted by the physician*). Private payers establish their own guidelines for payment of multiple procedures.

Do not append modifier **-51** to add-on codes or to codes with the symbol ⊘ (**modifier-51 exempt**). The MPFSDB and most encoders identify the codes for which this modifier is applicable.

-52 Reduced Services

The subcategory **Esophagogastroduodenoscopy** provides special instructions regarding modifier **-52** that appear before code **43235**. When the duodenum is not examined because it is not judged clinically relevant, append modifier **-52**. Likewise, if the duodenum cannot be examined for some other reason, such as retention of gastric contents, and a repeat examination is not planned, append modifier **-52**. Reduce the fee to be billed based on the extent of the service actually provided. Use of this modifier is required.

Special instructions at the beginning of the **Endoscopy** category for **Colon and Rectum** provide further direction on modifier **-52**. There are times when a therapeutic colonoscopy cannot proceed all the way to the cecum or small intestine, usually due to retained fecal matter. In this situation, append modifier **-52** to the therapeutic colonoscopy code. Submit appropriate documentation with the claim to explain the reason the procedure was reduced.

-53 Discontinued Procedure

The special instructions for the subcategory **Esophagogastroduodenoscopy** also include directions about modifier **-53**. In

---

Physician performs a routine screening colonoscopy on a patient, age 50.					
45378-33 Colonoscopy, flexible, proximal to splenic flexure; diagnostic, with or without collection of specimen(s) by brushing or washing, with or without colon decompression (separate procedure); -33 Preventive services					
Modifier -33 Payment Calculation					
Code	Modifier	Allowed fee	Patient co-insurance	Patient pays	Insurance pays
45378	33	$400.00	Waived	$0.00	$400.00
45378	None	$400.00	20%	$80.00	$320.00

Figure 35-12 ■ Example of Using Modifier -33. *Source: © PB Resources, Inc. Used with permission. CPT codes only © American Medical Association.*

the situation that the duodenum cannot be examined and a repeat examination *is planned*, append modifier -**53**.

CPT special instructions at the beginning of the **Endoscopy** category for **Colon and Rectum** provide additional guidance regarding this modifier. When a screening colonoscopy cannot proceed all the way to the cecum or small intestine, report the code for the full colonoscopy and append modifier -**53** to indicate that the procedure could not be completed. Use of this modifier is required. Reduce the fee to be billed based on the extent of the service actually provided. Submit appropriate documentation with the claim to explain the reason the procedure was discontinued.

-59 Distinct Procedural Service

Modifier -**59** is used to clarify that two procedures that might be considered to be bundled were performed on distinct sites or lesions or through distinct procedures. When the NCCI assigns the indicator 1 to a pair of surgical codes, modifier -**59** identifies that two separate services were provided. A common example of this with Digestive System procedures is when multiple therapeutic procedures from the same endoscopic code family are performed, as described under the multiple endoscopy rule discussed earlier in this chapter. Both indented codes are reported and modifier -**59** is appended to the second code of the pair.

In 2015, the Centers for Medicare and Medicaid (CMS) introduced four HCPCS modifiers to selectively identify subsets of procedures that would otherwise be reported with modifier -**59**. They are referred to as **X** modifiers and describe specific reasons that services should be considered as separate and distinct. When appropriate, use one of the following modifiers instead of modifier -**59** for Medicare patients. Check with other payers to learn how they want these modifiers applied:

- **-XE Separate Encounter**—a service that is distinct because it occurred during a separate encounter

- **-XS Separate Structure**—a service that is distinct because it was performed on a separate organ/structure

- **-XP Separate Practitioner**—a service that is distinct because it was performed by a different practitioner

- **-XU Unusual Non-Overlapping Service**—the use of a service that is distinct because it does not overlap usual components of the main service

-66 Surgical Team

Surgical teams are used for liver and pancreas transplants. Each surgeon reports modifier -**66** on the code for the recipient transplantation. Payment is prorated among the surgeons based on the role of each documented in the operative report. Surgical teams are not paid for all components of a transplant. For example, harvesting a cadaver organ or backbench preparation may not qualify for a surgical team. Intestinal transplants do not qualify for a surgical team. In some cases, a cosurgeon (modifier -**62**) or assistant surgeon (modifier -**80**) is allowed. The MPFSDB identifies the modifiers accepted for each code. Many encoders and billing software programs also provide modifier information.

-PT Colorectal Cancer Screening Test, Converted to Diagnostic Test or Other Procedure

Assign this HCPCS Level II modifier for Medicare patients when a screening colonoscopy or other colorectal cancer screening test is converted to a diagnostic or therapeutic procedure. This includes any time that a treatment is performed during the screening, including removing a polyp, cauterization, dilation, and so on.

Guided Example of Arranging Digestive System Procedure Codes

To practice skills for assigning modifiers and arranging codes for procedures of the Digestive System, continue with the example from earlier in the chapter about the patient who was seen for a colonoscopy. Follow along in your CPT manual as Jill Hynes, CPC, arranges the codes. Check off each step after you complete it.

▶ First, Jill confirms the CPT codes.

- ❑ **46221 Hemorrhoidectomy, internal, by rubber band ligation(s)**

- ❑ **45384 Colonoscopy, flexible; with removal of tumor(s), polyp(s), or other lesion(s) by hot biopsy forceps**

- ❑ **45385 Colonoscopy, flexible; with removal of tumor(s), polyp(s), or other lesion(s) by snare technique**

▶ Jill reviews the RVUs for each code. She selects the facility RVUs because the physician is performing the procedure at an outpatient hospital facility rather than at a location he personally owns and operates. The RVU schedule defines *facility RVU* as a facility owned by a third party (other than the physician). Facility RVUs are used when the physician performing the service does not own the facility where the procedure is performed. Nonfacility RVUs are used when the physician performing the service owns the location where the procedure is performed. The facility RVUs and pricing do not reimburse the physician for facility-related costs, so they are lower than nonfacility RVUs and pricing, which reimburse the physician for facility-related costs, such as those for the building, equipment, and staff. (Note: Although this is not a Medicare patient, the MPFSDB is used because many private payers use Medicare RVUs and assign their own prices. In the workplace, follow the rules of each payer.)

- ❑ Code **45385** for the polypectomy using the snare technique is the most extensive service, with a facility RVU of 8.78. She sequences this code first.

- ❑ Code **45384** for the polypectomy using hot forceps is the second most extensive service, with a facility RVU of 7.74. She sequences this code second. Although two polyps were removed, the code description identifies the entire procedure. It does not provide direction to assign multiple occurrences of the code for each polyp removed, so she reports this code only once.

21. DIAGNOSIS OR NATURE OF ILLNESS OR INJURY Relate A-L to service line below (24E)				ICD Ind. 0	22. RESUBMISSION CODE	ORIGINAL REF. NO.

A. D12.3   B. D12.5   C. K64.0   D. ____

E. ____   F. ____   G. ____   H. ____

I. ____   J. ____   K. ____   L. ____

23. PRIOR AUTHORIZATION NUMBER

24. A. DATE(S) OF SERVICE						B. PLACE OF SERVICE	C. EMG	D. PROCEDURES, SERVICES, OR SUPPLIES (Explain Unusual Circumstances)		E. DIAGNOSIS POINTER	F. $ CHARGES	G. DAYS OR UNITS	H. EPSDT Family Plan	I. ID. QUAL.	J. RENDERING PROVIDER ID. #
From MM	DD	YY	To MM	DD	YY			CPT/HCPCS	MODIFIER						
1 01	05	YY				22		45385		A	314 52	01		NPI	99 99999999
2 01	05	YY				22		45384	59	B	277 27	01		NPI	99 99999999
3 01	05	YY				22		46221	51	C	195 59	01		NPI	99 99999999

Figure 35-13 ■ CMS-1500 Form Billing for the Guided Example. *Source:* © PB Resources, Inc. Used with permission. CPT codes only © American Medical Association.

❑ Code **46221** for the hemorrhoid ligation is the least extensive service, with a facility RVU of 5.46. She sequences this code third.

▶ Jill reviews the codes to determine the need for modifiers. (Refer to Table 30-1 Key Criteria for Abstracting CPT Modifiers or Appendix A in the CPT manual.)

❑ Code **45385** does not require any modifiers because it is the primary procedure performed. She will link a diagnosis code for a polyp of the transverse colon to support this procedure.

❑ Code **45384** requires modifier -59 **Distinct procedural service** to clearly identify that the hot forceps polypectomy was a different lesion than the snare polypectomy. This will be clarified further when she links the diagnosis code for a polyp of the sigmoid colon. This procedure will be paid under the multiple endoscopy rule, not the multiple procedures rule, so modifier -51 **Multiple procedures** is not needed. (Some private payers might require modifier -51 in addition to modifier -59.)

❑ Code **46221** requires modifier -51 **Multiple procedures** because the hemorrhoidectomy was performed during the same session as the colonoscopy. The payment will be reduced to 50% of the usual fee.

▶ Jill finalizes the procedure codes, modifiers, and sequencing for this case (■ FIGURE 35-13):

(1) **45384 Colonoscopy, flexible; with removal of tumor(s), polyp(s), or other lesion(s) by hot biopsy forceps**

(2) **45385-59 Colonoscopy, flexible; with removal of tumor(s), polyp(s), or other lesion(s) by snare technique; -59 Distinct procedural service**

(3) **46221-51 Hemorrhoidectomy, internal, by rubber band ligation(s); -51 Multiple procedures**

▶ Jill also assigns and sequences the ICD-10-CM diagnosis codes that support the need for the service.

(1) **D12.3 Benign neoplasm of transverse colon**

(2) **D12.5 Benign neoplasm of sigmoid colon**

(3) **K64.0 First degree hemorrhoids**

CODING PRACTICE

Exercise 35.4 Arranging Codes for Digestive System Procedures

Instructions: Read the mini-medical-record of each patient's encounter, and review the information abstracted in Exercise 35.2 for questions 1-3. For questions 4-6, do the abstracting on your own. Assign CPT codes and modifiers using the Index and Tabular List, and arrange the codes in proper sequence. Write the code(s) on the line provided.

1. OUTPATIENT HOSPITAL   Gender: M   Age: 64

Diagnosis: initial incarcerated incisional hernia

Procedure: incarcerated incisional hernia repair with mesh

2 CPT Codes _____

2. OUTPATIENT HOSPITAL   Gender: M   Age: 61

Preoperative diagnosis: melena, hematemesis

Procedure: EGD was initiated with flexible scope through the mouth. Identified bleeding ulcers in esophagus and duodenum, which were successfully cauterized. Features of chronic gastritis were noted. No masses or hiatal hernia. Obtained biopsy from the antrum. Biopsies submitted to pathology for H&E

(continued)

CODING PRACTICE (continued)

2. (continued)

(*hematoxylin and eosin stain test to detect cancer*) and CLO (Campylobacter-*like organism test for* H. pylori).

Postoperative diagnosis: bleeding esophageal ulcer and bleeding peptic ulcer

Pathology report: biopsies negative for H. pylori and carcinoma

Tip: EGD with control of bleeding has a higher RVU than EGD with biopsy.

2 CPT Codes _____

3. INPATIENT HOSPITAL   Gender: M   Age: 3 months

Diagnosis: bilateral cleft lip with nasal deformity and cleft palate

Procedure: primary repair of a bilateral cleft lip and nasal deformity; repair of soft tissue of cleft palate and closure of alveolar ridge

Tip: Primary repair identifies a one-stage procedure.

2 CPT Codes _____

4. HOSPITAL   Gender: F   Age: 58

Preprocedure diagnosis: breast cancer with metastasis to the ileum and abdominal cavity

Procedure: Made a midline incision in the abdominal cavity. Excised tumors of 5 cm, 7 cm, 9 cm, and 12 cm in diameter from the peritoneum. Turned our attention to the ileum, from which a 75-cm segment was resected, and the healthy bowel was anastomosed in an end-to-end manner.

(continued)

4. (continued)

Tip: Abstract this procedure on your own. To locate the Main Term, use the medical term for cutting out part of the small intestine.

2 CPT Codes _____

5. INPATIENT HOSPITAL   Gender: M   Age: 57

Diagnosis: malignant ascites

Procedure: Under general anesthesia, created trocar ports in the abdomen and chest. Using the laparoscope, we inserted a tunneled intraperitoneal catheter, then inserted a subcutaneous extension from the catheter to exit from the chest.

Tip: Abstract this procedure on your own. A trocar is a sharp tool used to create openings and hold instruments used for laparoscopic surgery.

2 CPT Codes _____

6. INPATIENT HOSPITAL   Gender: M   Age: 74

Diagnosis: dysphagia following stroke

Procedure: Administered moderate sedation. Injected contrast medium. Under fluoroscopic guidance created gastrostomy, inserted feeding tube, and then converted to gastrojejunostomy tube.

Tip: Abstract this procedure on your own. The surgeon provided the image documentation and report.

2 CPT Codes _____

E/M CODING FOR GASTROENTEROLOGY

The *1997 Documentation Guidelines for Evaluation and Management Services* (1997 DG), published by CMS, do not provide guidelines for a single-system gastroenterology examination. Gastroenterologists use the multisystem examination criteria (■ FIGURE 35-14). To determine the appropriate E/M code, coders must review the documentation in detail and identify the specific elements documented.

- To translate the documentation into the E/M requirements for the history, refer back to Chapter 31, "Evaluation and Management Services (99201-99499)," Tables 31-7 to 31-10, or the 1997 DG.

- To determine the requirements for an examination, refer to Figure 35-14 or to the general multisystem examination in the 1997 DG.

- To determine the levels for medical decision making (MDM), refer to Chapter 31, Table 31-12, and to the Table of Risk in the 1997 DG.

Guided Example of E/M Coding for Gastroenterology

Refer to ■ Figure 35-15 Gastroenterology Encounter (page 663) to practice skills for abstracting and assigning E/M codes. Follow along as fictitious coder Jill Hynes, CPC, abstracts the procedure. Check off each step after you complete it.

▶ First, Jill needs to establish the category of service so she can determine the information needed to abstract and assign the code.

❑ *What is the setting?* Office.

System/Body Area	Elements of Multi-System Examination
Constitutional	❑ Measurement of any **three** of the following seven **vital** signs: • 1) sitting or standing blood pressure, • 2) supine blood pressure, • 3) pulse rate and regularity, • 4) respiration, • 5) temperature, • 6) height, • 7) weight (May be measured and recorded by ancillary staff) ❑ General **appearance** of patient (eg, development, nutrition, body habitus, deformities, attention to grooming)
Eyes	❑ Inspection of **conjunctivae** and **lids** ❑ Examination of **pupils** and **irises** (eg, reaction to light and accommodation, size and symmetry) ❑ Ophthalmoscopic examination of **optic discs** (eg, size, C/D ratio, appearance) and posterior segments (eg, vessel changes, exudates, hemorrhages
Ears, Nose, Mouth and Throat	❑ External **inspection** of ears and nose (eg, overall appearance, scars, lesions, masses) ❑ Otoscopic examination of external **auditory canals** and **tympanic membranes** ❑ Assessment of **hearing** (eg, whispered voice, finger rub, tuning fork) ❑ Inspection of **nasal mucosa, septum** and **turbinates** ❑ Inspection of **lips, teeth** and **gums** ❑ Examination of **oropharynx:** oral mucosa, salivary glands, hard and soft palates, tongue, tonsils and posterior pharynx
Neck	❑ Examination of **neck** (eg, masses, overall appearance, symmetry, tracheal position, crepitus) ❑ Examination of **thyroid** (eg, enlargement, tenderness, mass)
Respiratory	❑ Assessment of **respiratory effort** (eg, intercostal retractions, use of accessory muscles, diaphragmatic movement) ❑ **Percussion** of chest (eg, dullness, flatness, hyperresonance) ❑ **Palpation** of chest (eg, tactile fremitus) ❑ **Auscultation** of lungs (eg, breath sounds, adventitious sounds, rubs)
Cardiovascular	❑ **Palpation of heart** (eg, location, size, thrills) ❑ **Auscultation** of heart with notation of abnormal sounds and murmurs Examination of: ❑ **carotid arteries** (eg, pulse amplitude, bruits) ❑ **abdominal aorta** (eg, size, bruits) ❑ **femoral arteries** (eg, pulse amplitude, bruits) ❑ **pedal pulses** (eg, pulse amplitude) ❑ **extremities** for edema and/or varicosities
Chest (Breasts)	❑ **Inspection** of breasts (eg, symmetry, nipple discharge) ❑ **Palpation** of breasts and axillae (eg, masses or lumps, tenderness)
Gastrointestinal (Abdomen)	❑ Examination of **abdomen** with notation of presence of masses or tenderness ❑ Examination of **liver** and **spleen** ❑ Examination for presence or absence of **hernia** ❑ Examination (when indicated) of **anus, perineum** and **rectum,** including sphincter tone, presence of hemorrhoids, rectal masses ❑ Obtain **stool sample** for occult blood test when indicated
Genitourinary	**MALE:** ❑ Examination of the **scrotal contents** (eg, hydrocele, spermatocele, tenderness of cord, testicular mass) ❑ Examination of the **penis** ❑ Digital rectal examination of **prostate** gland (eg, size, symmetry, nodularity, tenderness) **FEMALE:** Pelvic examination (with or without specimen collection for smears and cultures), including ❑ Examination of **external genitalia** (eg, general appearance, hair distribution, lesions) and **vagina** (eg, general appearance, estrogen effect, discharge, lesions, pelvic support, cystocele, rectocele) ❑ Examination of **urethra** (eg, masses, tenderness, scarring) ❑ Examination of **bladder** (eg, fullness, masses, tenderness) Cervix (eg, general appearance, lesions, discharge) ❑ **Uterus** (eg, size, contour, position, mobility, tenderness, consistency, descent or support) ❑ **Adnexa**/parametria (eg, masses, tenderness, organomegaly, nodularity)

Figure 35-14 ■ 1997 DG for Multisystem Examination. *Source: Centers for Medicare and Medicaid Services,* *1997* Documentation Guidelines for Evaluation and Management Services *(with formatting adjustments).*

Lymphatic	Palpation of lymph nodes in **two or more** areas: ❑ Neck ❑ Axillae ❑ Groin ❑ Other
Musculoskeletal	❑ Examination of **gait and station** ❑ Inspection and/or palpation of **digits** and **nails** (eg, clubbing, cyanosis, inflammatory conditions, petechiae, ischemia, infections, nodes) Examination of joints, bones and muscles of **<u>one or more</u>** of the following six areas: ❑ 1) head and neck; ❑ 2) spine, ribs and pelvis; ❑ 3) right upper extremity; ❑ 4) left upper extremity; ❑ 5) right lower extremity; and ❑ 6) left lower extremity. The examination of a given area includes: • Inspection and/or palpation with notation of presence of any **misalignment,** asymmetry, crepitation, defects, tenderness, masses, effusions • Assessment of **range of motion** with notation of any pain, crepitation or contracture • Assessment of **stability** with notation of any dislocation (luxation), subluxation or laxity • Assessment of muscle **strength** and **tone** (eg, flaccid, cog wheel, spastic) with notation of any atrophy or abnormal movements
Skin	❑ **Inspection** of skin and subcutaneous tissue (eg, rashes, lesions, ulcers) ❑ **Palpation** of skin and subcutaneous tissue (eg, induration, subcutaneous nodules, tightening)
Neurologic	❑ Test **cranial nerves** with notation of any deficits ❑ Examination of **deep tendon reflexes** with notation of pathological reflexes (eg, Babinski) ❑ Examination of **sensation** (eg, by touch, pin, vibration, proprioception)
Psychiatric	❑ Description of the patient's **judgment** and **insight** *Brief assessment of mental status including:* ❑ **Orientation** to time, place and person ❑ Recent and remote **memory** ❑ **Mood** and affect (eg, depression, anxiety, agitation, hypomania, lability)

Total # Bullets Performed and Documented →	⬜	# of Elements Performed and Documented	Level of Examination
		1–5	Problem focused
		6+	Expanded problem focused
		6 organ systems/body areas @ 2 bullet points each OR: 12 elements in at least 2 organ systems/body areas	Detailed
		ALL	Comprehensive (Perform all elements identified by a bullet in **at least nine** organ systems or body areas and document **at least two elements** identified by a bullet from **each of nine** areas/systems)

Figure 35-14 ■ *(continued)*

❑ *What is the type of service?* The encounter qualifies as a consultation because the gastroenterologist's advice is requested by the referring physician and the gastroenterologist sends a report back to the referring physician at the conclusion of the encounter.

❑ *What is the code range?* Jill refers to the CPT Index and looks up the Main Term **Evaluation and Management** and the subterm **Consultation**. The code range listed is **99241-99255**.

❑ *How many key components are required?* Jill refers to the code range in the Tabular List and notices that the Consultation subheading is divided into two categories:

Office or other outpatient and **Inpatient**. She selects the **Office or other outpatient** category and reads the code description of the first code, which states **Office consultation for a new or established patient, which requires these 3 key components**. All codes in the category have the same requirements for key components. This tells her that all three key components must meet or exceed the levels listed in the code (3/3).

▶ Next, Jill identifies the level of history.

❑ *What is the level of HPI?* The HPI is **extended** because seven elements are documented.

GASTROENTEROLOGY ENCOUNTER

HISTORY: Detailed

Chief complaint (CC)

CHIEF COMPLAINT: Nausea and abdominal pain after eating.

HPI: Extended (4+)

HPI: The patient is a 33 year old white female, came to the office. She is referred to me by her internal medicine physician for evaluation for a cholecystectomy. Patient complains of pain after eating fatty food, dark colored urine, subjective chills, subjective low-grade fever, nausea and sharp stabbing pain. Symptoms started about 2 months ago. Symptoms are relieved when lying on right side and with antacids. Prior workup by internist includes abdominal ultrasound positive for cholelithiasis without CBD obstruction. Laboratory studies include elevated total bilirubin and elevated WBC.

Consultation referral

MDM Management: New presenting problem, without workup (Moderate Management Options)

MDM Data: Ordering or reviewing diagnostic data (Straightforward Data)

PAST MEDICAL HISTORY: No significant past medical problems.
PAST SURGICAL HISTORY: Diagnostic laparoscopic exam for pelvic pain/adhesions.
ALLERGIES: No known drug allergies.
CURRENT MEDICATIONS: No current medications.
SOCIAL HISTORY: Marital status: married. Patient states smoking history of 1 pack per day. Patient quit smoking 1 year ago. Admits to no history of using alcohol. States use of no illicit drugs.
FAMILY MEDICAL HISTORY: There is no significant, contributory family medical history.
OB GYN HISTORY: LMP: 4/03/YY. Gravida: 2. Para: 2. Date of last pap smear: 8/25/YY.

PFSH: Complete (3)

REVIEW OF SYSTEMS:
Cardiovascular: Denies angina, MI history, dysrhythmias, palpitations, murmur, pedal edema, orthopnea, TIAs, stroke.
Pulmonary: Denies cough, hemoptysis, wheezing, dyspnea, bronchitis, emphysema, TB exposure or treatment.
Neurological: Denies seizures and ataxia.
Skin: Denies scaling, rashes, blisters, photosensitivity.

ROS: Extended (2–9)

PHYSICAL EXAMINATION:
Appearance: Healthy appearing. Moderately overweight.
HEENT: Normocephalic. EOMs (*extraocular movements*) intact. PERRLA. Oral pharynx without lesions.
Neck: Neck mobile. Trachea is midline.
Lymphatic: No apparent cervical, supraclavicular, axillary or inguinal adenopathy.
Breast: Normal appearing breasts bilaterally, nipples everted. No nipple discharge, skin changes.
Chest: Normal breath sounds heard bilaterally without rales or rhonchi. No pleural rubs. No scars.
Cardiovascular: Regular heart rate and rhythm without murmur or gallop. No signs of edema.
Abdominal: Bowel sounds are high pitched.
Extremities: Lower extremities are normal in color, touch and temperature. No ischemic changes are noted. Range of motion is normal.
Skin: Normal color, temperature, turgor and elasticity; no significant skin lesions.

EXAMINATION: Detailed

(12 elements in at least 2 organ systems/body areas)

IMPRESSION: Abdominal pain due to acute cholecystitis.

DISCUSSION: Reviewed laparoscopic cholecystectomy procedure sheet and answered questions. The patient gave verbal and written consent for the procedure.

MEDICAL DECISION MAKING: Moderate Complexity

MDM Risk: Acute illness with systemic symptoms, Elective major surgery (open, percutaneous or endoscopic) with no identified risk factors (Moderate Risk)

PLAN: We will proceed with laparoscopic cholecystectomy with intraoperative cholangiogram. Report sent to the referring physician with my assessment and recommendation.

MEDICATIONS PRESCRIBED: None.

Consultation report

PROCEDURES SCHEDULED: Laparoscopic cholecystectomy scheduled in 2 weeks on 5/11/YY at outpatient surgery center.

KEY: HPI History of the present illness   ROS Review of systems
PFSH Past, family, and social history   MDM Medical decision making

Figure 35-15 ■ Gastroenterology Encounter. *Source: © PB Resources, Inc. Used with permission.*

❏ *What is the level of ROS?* The ROS is **extended** because four systems are documented.

❏ *What is the level of PFSH?* The PFSH is **complete** because three elements are documented.

❏ *Based on these factors, what is the overall level of history?* The level of history is **detailed** because the lowest of the three factors (HPI, ROS, and PFSH) determines the history

level. The HPI and PFSH qualify for a comprehensive history, but the ROS qualifies for only a detailed history.

▶ Jill refers to the multisystem examination in the 1997 DG (Figure 35-14) to abstract information needed to determine the level of the examination.

❏ *What is the level of examination?* The level of examination is **detailed**. Nineteen (19) elements in 4 organ systems are documented, which exceeds the requirement of 12 or more elements in 2 organ systems for a detailed examination. A comprehensive examination requires documentation of at least two elements identified by a bullet from each of nine systems, which they are not.

▶ Jill determines the level of medical decision making. (Refer to Table 31-12 Medical Decision Making Levels.)

❑ *What is the level of complexity of the number of diagnoses or management options based on the presenting problem?* The level is **moderate** because there is a new presenting problem without a workup by this provider. The workup was done by the referring provider.

❑ *What is the amount and/or complexity of data to be reviewed?* The level is **Straightforward** because diagnostic data were reviewed.

❑ *What is the level of risk of significant complications, morbidity, and/or mortality?* She reviews each column in the Table of Risk in the 1997 DG and determines that the level of risk is **Moderate** because the patient has an acute illness with systemic symptoms and elective major surgery is agreed to. The patient has no identified risk

factors. The single highest element in the Table of Risk determines the overall risk. Both of these risk elements are classified as **Moderate**.

❑ *Based on these factors, what is the overall level of medical decision making?* The medical decision making is **Moderate complexity**. At least two of the three MDM factors are required to qualify for a specific level of MDM. Two of the three MDM factors meet or exceed moderate decision making.

Now Jill is ready to assign the code for the GI encounter. The exercise that follows guides you through additional abstracting skills and allows you to assign the correct code.

CODING CAUTION

Verify that the physician signature is present in the medical record and is legible. If it is not, the physician must sign an attestation statement, which identifies the author. If the documentation for an encounter is not signed or attested to, Medicare considers the claim to be *insufficiently documented* and can deny or recoup payment.

CODING PRACTICE

Exercise 35.5 Evaluation and Management Coding for Gastroenterology

Instructions: Refer to the *1997 Documentation Guidelines for Evaluation and Management Services* (available at **www.cms.gov**) or Chapter 31, "Evaluation and Management Services (99201-99499)" (Tables 31-7 to 31-12), in this text. Answer the following questions about the Gastroenterology Encounter (Figure 35-15).

1. a. Which elements of the HPI are documented? Circle all that apply. Location, Quality, Severity, Duration, Timing, Context, Modifying factors, Associated signs and symptoms

   b. How many elements are documented? _____

   c. What is the level of HPI? _____

2. a. Which systems are reviewed in the ROS? Circle all that apply. Constitutional, Allergic/immunologic, CV, Endocrine, ENT/M, Eyes, GI, GU, Hemic/lymphatic, MS, Neurologic, Psychiatric, Respiratory, Skin/breast

   b. How many systems are documented? _____

   c. What is the level of ROS? _____

3. a. Which PFSH elements are documented? Circle all that apply. Past medical, Family, Social

   b. What is the level of PFSH? _____

   c. What is the overall level of history? (The lowest history factor—HPI, ROS, or PFSH—determines the level of history.)

   _____

4. a. Refer to Figure 35-14 (1997 DG for Multisystem Examination). Which bulleted items are documented for the examination? (Check off the items documented.)

   b. How many bulleted items are documented? _____

   c. What is the level of the examination? _____

5. Refer to Table 31-12 Medical Decision Making Levels or the 1997 DG.

   a. What is the MDM level for the number of diagnoses or management options? _____

   b. What is the MDM level for the amount and/or complexity of data to be reviewed? _____

   c. Refer to the Table of Risk in the 1997 DG. Which elements of risk are documented for each risk factor?

      1. Presenting problem: _____

      2. Diagnostic procedures ordered: _____

      3. Management options selected: _____

   d. What is the level of risk? _____

   e. What is the overall level of MDM? (2 of the 3 MDM factors are needed to determine the overall level.) _____

6. a. What is the setting? _____

   b. What type of service? _____

   c. What is the code range? _____

   d. How many key components are required? _____

   e. What is the level of history? _____

   f. What is the level of examination? _____

   g. What is the level of medical decision making? _____

   h. What is the correct code? _____

   i. Is modifier -57 required? _____ Why or why not? _____

7. Abstract, assign, and arrange (sequence) the diagnosis codes that support the E/M code.

   1 ICD-10-CM Code _____

CHAPTER SUMMARY

In this chapter you learned that:

- Because the digestive, or alimentary, tract consists of and connects several anatomic sites, medical terms frequently contain word roots of multiple sites, which are combined with a procedural suffix.

- The CPT Surgery subsection Digestive System (**40490-49999**) contains 18 subheadings divided by anatomic site. Anatomic sites are arranged by the order in which they occur in the alimentary (digestive) tract, beginning with the lips and ending with the anus.

- Abstracting digestive system procedures requires special attention to the detailed anatomy of the digestive system and the order of the digestive organs within the GI tract, starting from either end.

- Coding for tonsillectomy, appendectomy, anastomosis, endoscopy, transplants, and repairs reinforces basic coding skills that you can use throughout the CPT manual.

- The order of codes sometimes determines the modifiers needed. Some modifiers can be assigned at the same time the code is assigned, and some cannot be assigned until the codes are sequenced. Certain modifiers are required even when only one procedure is performed.

- Gastroenterologists use the multisystem examination criteria because the *1997 Documentation Guidelines for Evaluation and Management Services* do not provide guidelines for a single-system gastroenterology examination.

- The Digestive System does not have any subsection guidelines or special instructions, but some subheadings and categories provide definitions and coding information. A special instruction that appears in each endoscopy or laparoscopy category directs that a surgical endoscopy or laparoscopy always includes a diagnostic one.

CONCEPT QUIZ

Take a moment to look back at the digestive system and solidify your skills. Try to answer the questions from memory first, then refer to the discussion in this chapter if you need a little extra help.

Completion

Instructions: Write the term that answers each question based on the information you learned in this chapter. Choose from the list below. Some choices may be used more than once and some choices may not be used at all.

anastomosis

antrectomy

colostomy

endoscopic sclerotherapy

ERCP

gastric bypass

herniorrhaphy

ileostomy

lap band

lithotripsy

Nissen fundoplication

paracentesis

Roux-en-Y

transthoracic esophagectomy

vagotomy

1. During a(n) _____, the upper part of the stomach is wrapped around the lower esophageal sphincter (LES).

2. A(n) _____ may be created to relieve a bowel blockage or obstruction in the large intestine.

3. _____ is a surgical puncture of a body cavity to remove excess fluid.

4. Gastrojejunostomy is another term used to describe a(n) _____.

5. A(n) _____ may be performed to repair bulging of internal organs or tissues through a defect in the wall of a body cavity.

6. The treatment of Barrett esophagus may include a(n) _____.

7. High-frequency sound waves, or _____, are used to break up gallstones.

8. A(n) _____ is the removal of the distal portion of the stomach due to gastric ulcers.

(continued)

(continued from page 665)

9. To reestablish gastrointestinal continuity after excision of portions of one or more organs, a(n) _____ may be performed.

10. When treating peptic ulcer disease, an open or laparoscopic _____ may be performed to relieve acid secretion.

Multiple Choice

Instructions: Circle the letter of the best answer to each question based on the information you learned in this chapter.

1. What HCPCS Level II code is used for a screening colonoscopy on a Medicare patient at high risk for colorectal cancer?
   A. G0104
   B. G0105
   C. G0107
   D. G0121

2. What procedure is an examination of the rectum, sigmoid colon, and part of the descending colon?
   A. Proctosigmoidoscopy
   B. Anoscopy
   C. Sigmoidoscopy
   D. Colonoscopy

3. What is the collective name for the salivary glands, liver, gall bladder, and pancreas?
   A. Accessory organs
   B. Omentum
   C. Hepatic system
   D. Digestive tract

4. What is the special instruction that appears in each endoscopy category?
   A. Surgical endoscopy always includes diagnostic endoscopy.
   B. Refer to CPT coding guidelines, Endoscopy.
   C. Surgical endoscopy codes should not be used with surgical laparoscopy codes.
   D. Surgical endoscopy includes radiologic guidance.

5. Which of the following codes is the base code for ERCP, diagnostic?
   A. 43260
   B. 43261
   C. 43274
   D. 43277

6. What abstracting question should be answered for an endoscopic procedure on the digestive system?
   A. Does the surgeon administer general anesthesia?
   B. How long does the procedure take?
   C. Is the procedure open or closed?
   D. What is the farthest site reached?

7. How are multiple surgical procedures sequenced?
   A. In numerical order
   B. In descending order of complexity and price
   C. In the order listed by the surgeon in the operative report
   D. According to the modifier(s) used

8. What modifier should be used when the duodenum is not examined during an EGD because it is not judged clinically relevant?
   A. -51
   B. -52
   C. -53
   D. -58

9. What does pull-through refer to?
   A. A surgical approach for an open procedure
   B. A type of laparoscopic procedure
   C. An anastomosis technique
   D. An ostomy technique

10. What modifier is used when a hemorrhoidectomy is performed during the same session as a colonoscopy?
    A. -51
    B. -52
    C. -58
    D. None

CODING CHALLENGE

Instructions: Read the mini-medical-record of each patient's encounter, then abstract, assign, and arrange ICD-10-CM diagnosis codes and CPT procedure codes using the appropriate Index and Tabular List. Write the code(s) on the line provided.

---

1. OUTPATIENT HOSPITAL   Gender: F   Age: 61

Diagnosis: recurrent inguinal hernia on the right side

Procedure: right inguinal herniorrhaphy

1 ICD-10-CM Code _____

1 CPT Code _____

---

2. OFFICE   Gender: M   Age: 52

Reason for encounter: lump and tenderness in jaw

Assessment: abscess, submandibular salivary gland; heavy current tobacco use

Procedure: incision and drainage of abscess

Tip: Read the instructional note under the code for the salivary gland abscess to identify the second code.

2 ICD-10-CM Codes _____

1 CPT Code _____

3. INPATIENT HOSPITAL   Gender: M   Age: 38

Diagnosis: fecal incontinence due to nontraumatic anal sphincter tear, which has not improved

Procedure: sphincteroplasty

Tip: Read the instructional notes under the code for nontraumatic anal sphincter tear to identify the second code.

2 ICD-10-CM Codes _____

1 CPT Code _____

---

4. INPATIENT HOSPITAL   Gender: F   Age: 52

Reason for encounter: RUQ pain, T 102 degrees, vomiting

Diagnosis: ultrasound revealed acute cholecystitis with CBD calculus causing obstruction

Procedure: laparoscopic cholecystectomy

1 ICD-10-CM Code _____

1 CPT Code _____

---

5. OUTPATIENT HOSPITAL   Gender: M   Age: 47

Reason for encounter: foreign body–like sensation in his proximal esophagus after a meal

Assessment: evaluated with lateral C-spine films and soft-tissue films without any evidence of perforation. The patient then was taken to the endoscopy suite.

Procedure: EGD with removal of a foreign body from gastroesophageal junction (piece of fish bone)

1 ICD-10-CM Code _____

1 CPT Code _____

---

6. OUTPATIENT HOSPITAL   Gender: F   Age: 57

Assessment: multiple severe external hemorrhoids

Procedure: removal of external hemorrhoids

1 ICD-10-CM Code _____

1 CPT Code _____

---

7. OUTPATIENT HOSPITAL   Gender: M   Age: 67

Reason for encounter: screening colonoscopy

Procedure: colonoscopy with snare removal of two adenomatous polyps, biopsy of suspicious lesion in transverse colon to rule out malignancy

Pathology report: benign polyps, benign lesion

Tip: Refer to the OGCR for sequencing guidelines for the diagnoses codes.

3 ICD-10-CM Codes _____

_____

2 CPT Codes _____

---

8. OUTPATIENT HOSPITAL   Gender: M   Age: 9

Diagnosis: chronic hypertrophic tonsillitis and adenoiditis, chronic otitis media refractory to antibiotics, left ear

Procedure: tonsillectomy and adenoidectomy, insertion of myringotomy tube under general anesthesia

2 ICD-10-CM Codes _____

2 CPT Codes _____

---

9. INPATIENT HOSPITAL   Gender: F   Age: 49

Diagnosis: ulcerative colitis involving primarily the rectosigmoid, unresponsive to steroids

Procedure: laparoscopic total abdominal colectomy with end ileostomy; splenorrhaphy to repair accidental puncture of spleen

2 ICD-10-CM Codes _____

2 CPT Codes _____

---

10. INPATIENT HOSPITAL   Gender: M   Age: 53

Assessment: admitted to the intensive care unit with complaints of abdominal pain and unstable vital signs

Procedure: repair of perforated duodenal ulcer, gastrojejunostomy and feeding jejunostomy placement

Postoperative diagnosis: perforated duodenal ulcer

1 ICD-10-CM Code _____

3 CPT Codes _____

_____

KEEP ON CODING

Instructions: Read the procedural statement, then use the appropriate Index and Tabular List to assign CPT procedure codes. Write the code(s) on the line provided.

1. Percutaneous endoscopic colostomy: CPT Code(s) _____

2. Transnasal biopsy of esophagus: CPT Code(s) _____

3. Esophagogastroduodenoscopy with cold forceps biopsy: CPT Code(s) _____

4. Hemiglossectomy: CPT Code(s) _____

5. Laparoscopic appendectomy converted to open due to extensive intestinal adhesions, which were lysed to provide access to the appendix. Enterolysis increased the time for the procedure by 50%: CPT Code(s) _____

6. Endoscopic retrograde cholangiopancreatography with stent placement: CPT Code(s) _____

7. Orthotopic liver transplantation by a surgical team with choledochostomy, standard bench prep of donor organ: CPT Code(s)

   _____

8. Open drainage of subphrenic abscess: CPT Code(s) _____

9. Left colon resection with colorectal anastomosis; complete mobilization of the splenic flexure: CPT Code(s) _____

10. Laparoscopic cholecystectomy with needle biopsy of liver: CPT Code(s) _____

11. Repair of nasolabial fistula: CPT Code(s) _____

12. Small-bowel resection for congenital atresia, approximately 1.5 feet; jejunostomy; placement of an abdominal wound VAC, wound surface area 20 sq cm: CPT Code(s) _____

13. Parotid gland needle biopsy: CPT Code(s) _____

14. Incarcerated ventral hernia repair: CPT Code(s) _____

15. Excision of full-thickness lip lesion with local flap reconstruction: CPT Code(s) _____

16. Flexible sigmoidoscopy with removal of foreign body: CPT Code(s) _____

17. Esophagogastroduodenoscopy with esophageal variceal band ligation: CPT Code(s) _____

18. Pelvic exenteration for colorectal malignancy with proctectomy and colostomy: CPT Code(s) _____

19. Revision of ileostomy: CPT Code(s) _____

20. Endoscopic ultrasound of sigmoid colon: CPT Code(s) _____

21. Gastric lavage: CPT Code(s) _____

22. EGD with dilation of gastric outlet for obstruction and biopsy of esophagus: CPT Code(s) _____

23. Closure of gastrostomy: CPT Code(s) _____

24. Suture of bleeding gastric ulcer: CPT Code(s) _____

25. Closure of anal fistula: CPT Code(s) _____

Endocrine System Procedures (60000-60699)

Learning Objectives

After completing this chapter, you should have the skills to:

36.1 Spell and define the key words, medical terms, and abbreviations related to endocrine system procedures.

36.2 Discuss the fundamentals of Endocrine System procedures.

36.3 Identify the main characteristics of coding for the Endocrine System.

36.4 Abstract procedural information from the medical record for coding Endocrine System procedures.

36.5 Assign codes for Endocrine System procedures.

36.6 Arrange codes for Endocrine System procedures.

36.7 Code evaluation and management services for endocrinology.

36.8 Discuss the CPT coding guidelines related to the Endocrine System.

Chapter Outline

- **Endocrine System Procedure Basics**
- **Coding Overview of Endocrine System Procedures**
- **Abstracting Endocrine System Procedures**
- **Assigning Codes for Endocrine System Procedures**
- **Arranging Codes for Endocrine System Procedures**
- **E/M Coding for Endocrinology**

Key Terms and Abbreviations

cervical approach
contralateral lobectomy
dorsal approach

neck dissection
partial thyroid lobectomy
secondary thyroidectomy

subtotal thyroid lobectomy
total thyroid lobectomy
total/complete thyroidectomy

transabdominal approach
transthoracic approach

In addition to the key terms listed here, students should know the terms defined within tables in this chapter.

CODING OVERVIEW OF ENDOCRINE SYSTEM PROCEDURES

The CPT subsection **Endocrine System (60000-60699)** contains two subheadings that are divided by anatomic site. Review the subheadings, categories, and code ranges listed at the beginning of the Endocrine System subsection in the CPT manual to become familiar with the content and organization. This subsection has approximately 30 codes.

The Endocrine System subsection includes invasive and minimally invasive surgical procedures on four of the nine endocrine glands: the thyroid, parathyroid, thymus, and adrenal glands. Procedures for removal of a tumor from the carotid body (*a small cluster of chemoreceptor cells near the bifurcation [splitting in two] of the carotid artery in the neck*) also appear in this subsection. The carotid body is considered an endocrine gland because it secretes erythropoiesis hormones. Although the pancreas appears in the second subheading title, no procedures on the pancreas appear in the Tabular List. Several endocrine glands also function as part of other organ systems. Procedures on five endocrine glands appear in other Surgery subsections, as follows:

- Ovaries—Female Genital System (58600-58960)
- Pancreas—Digestive System (48000- 48999)
- Pineal gland—Nervous System (61105-61576)
- Pituitary gland —Nervous system (61546-61548)
- Testes—Male Genital System (54500-56499)

Codes for diagnostic tests on the Endocrine System appear in the Medicine section. Many endocrine conditions are managed medically, so patients may have codes only for Evaluation and Management (E/M) encounters. CPT codes in the Endocrine System subsection are frequently supported by diagnosis codes from ICD-10-CM **Chapter 4 Endocrine, Nutritional, and Metabolic Diseases (E00-E89)**, as well as neoplasms, symptoms and signs, and injuries (■ TABLE 36-3). These codes are most commonly assigned to support procedures on the endocrine system; however, diagnosis codes from any ICD-10-CM chapter are permissible.

CPT guidelines for the Surgery section apply to the Endocrine System. This subsection has no additional guidelines or special instructions. Instructional notes in the Tabular List redirect coders when different or additional codes are required. One add-on code, for parathyroid autotransplantation, appears in this section. An instructional note identifies the standalone codes it can be reported with.

ABSTRACTING ENDOCRINE SYSTEM PROCEDURES

Surgical approach always identifies the technique used, such as open, endoscopic, or external. The anatomic approach identifies the site of the incision and the direction from which the surgical site is accessed. Certain thyroidectomy and thymectomy procedures can be performed through an incision in the neck, which is a **cervical approach**, or through an incision in the chest, which is a **transthoracic approach**. An adrenalectomy can be performed through an incision in the abdomen,

Table 36-3 ■ LOCATING ICD-10-CM AND CPT CODES FOR THE ENDOCRINE SYSTEM

Type of Code	Codes
ICD-10-CM Endocrine System-Related Codes	
Endocrine system conditions	E00-E89
Neoplasms	C75, C78.89, D09.3, D35, D44
Symptoms and signs	R62, R94.7
Screening	Z13.2
CPT Endocrine System-Related Codes	
Medicine procedures	95250-95251
Radiologic procedures	
• Diagnostic ultrasound	76536
• Nuclear medicine	78012-78099
Laboratory tests	
• Organ/disease panels	80047-80050
• Chemistry	80400-80435, 81506, 84431-84445

Source: © PB Resources, Inc. Used with permission.

which is a **transabdominal approach**; the lower back, which is a lumbar approach; or the midback, which is a **dorsal approach**.

Refer to ■ TABLE 36-4 for guidance on how to abstract procedures on the Endocrine System, then work through the detailed example that follows. Remember that the abstracting questions are a guide and that not every question applies to, or can be answered for, every case. For example, some, but not all, codes are divided based on whether the purpose of an excision is to remove a malignancy.

Guided Example of Abstracting Endocrine System Procedures

Refer to the following example throughout this chapter to practice skills for abstracting, assigning, and arranging Endocrine System codes.

Table 36-4 ■ KEY CRITERIA FOR ABSTRACTING ENDOCRINE SYSTEM PROCEDURES

- ❑ What endocrine gland is treated?
- ❑ What is the surgical approach (e.g., open, endoscopic)?
- ❑ What is the anatomic approach (e.g., cervical, thoracic)?
- ❑ Is the procedure partial, subtotal, or total/complete?
- ❑ Is the procedure done to remove a malignancy?
- ❑ Were any adjacent tumors removed?
- ❑ What is the extent of lymph node excision, if any?

Source: © PB Resources, Inc. Used with permission.

INPATIENT HOSPITAL   Gender: F   Age: 35

Preoperative diagnosis: suspected carcinoma per result of fine-needle aspiration (FNA) done last week

Procedure: Thyroidectomy with radical neck dissection. With the patient in the supine position, a horizontal 10-cm incision was made just below the larynx. The skin flaps were separated and the muscle and fascia were divided, exposing the thyroid gland. Being diligent to protect the recurrent laryngeal nerve from trauma, we excised all of both thyroid lobes and the first five regions of bilateral cervical lymph nodes and the internal jugular vein (IJV), spinal accessory nerve (SAN), and sternocleidomastoid muscle (SCM). Hemostasis was achieved, the operative wound was closed, and the patient was transferred to postoperative care in stable condition. Tissue was submitted to pathology.

Postoperative diagnosis: differentiated thyroid cancer (DTC) with lymph node metastases

Pathology report: papillary thyroid cancer, metastatic cancer in lymph nodes

Follow along as fictitious coder, Tamara Brownlee, CCS-P, abstracts the procedure. Check off each step after you complete it.

▶ Tamara reads through the entire record, paying special attention to the reason for the encounter, the procedure performed, and the postoperative diagnosis. She refers to the Key Criteria for Abstracting Endocrine System Procedures (Table 36-4).

❑ She notes the preoperative diagnosis. She does not code the FNA because it was performed last week and coded at that time.

❑ *Which gland is treated?* thyroid

❑ *What is the surgical approach?* Open, as indicated by the excision.

❑ *What is the anatomic approach?* Cervical

❑ *Is the procedure partial, subtotal, or total/complete?* Total, all of both thyroid lobes.

❑ *Is the procedure done to remove a malignancy?* Yes, suspected carcinoma, confirmed by pathology.

❑ *Were any adjacent tumors removed?* No.

❑ *What was the extent of lymph node excision, if any?* Radical; first five regions of cervical lymph nodes.

▶ Tamara also reviews the general criteria for abstracting procedures (Table 28-6).

❑ *Is the name of the procedure consistent with the documented details?* Yes, a total thyroidectomy involves excision of all, or nearly all, of the thyroid. An RND involves excision of cervical lymph nodes I–V and the internal jugular vein (IJV), spinal accessory nerve (SAN), and sternocleidomastoid muscle (SCM).

❑ *What is the final diagnosis?* differentiated thyroid cancer (DTC) with lymph node metastases

At this time, Tamara does not know how many codes she will end up with. She will learn about this when she moves on to assigning codes.

CODING PRACTICE

Exercise 36.2   Abstracting Endocrine System Procedures

Instructions: Read the mini-medical-record of each patient's encounter and answer the abstracting questions. Write the answer on the line provided. Do not assign any codes.

1. OUTPATIENT HOSPITAL   Gender: F   Age: 4

Preprocedure diagnosis: abscess, thyroglossal duct

Procedure: I&D, cyst in the thyroglossal duct. Punctured the cyst with a needle, drained exudate, and applied a sterile dressing.

Postprocedure diagnosis: infected thyroglossal duct cyst

(continued)

1. (continued)

a. What endocrine gland is treated? _____

b. What is the surgical approach? _____

c. What is the anatomic approach? _____

d. What procedure is performed? _____

e. Is the procedure done to remove a malignancy?

_____

f. Were any adjacent tumors removed? _____

g. What was the extent of lymph node excision, if any?

_____

(continued)

CODING PRACTICE (continued)

2. INPATIENT HOSPITAL   Gender: F Age: 45

Preoperative diagnosis: myasthenia gravis, thymoma

Procedure: Transthoracic thymectomy. Made a length-wise incision in the chest slightly left of the midline. Explored the chest and excised the entire thymus gland. No adjacent structures were disturbed. Inspected the surgical field to ensure no residual thymic tissue. Closed surgical wound and transferred patient to the postoperative area in stable condition.

Postoperative diagnosis: thymoma, benign

a. What endocrine gland is treated? _____

b. What is the surgical approach? _____

c. What is the anatomic approach? _____

d. What procedure is performed? _____

e. Is the procedure done to remove a malignancy?

_____

f. Were any adjacent tumors removed? _____

g. What was the extent of lymph node excision, if any?

_____

3. OUTPATIENT HOSPITAL   Gender: M Age: 35

Preoperative diagnosis: adrenal adenoma, Cushing syndrome

Procedure: laparoscopic adrenalectomy, right adrenal gland

Postoperative diagnosis: benign adrenal tumor

a. What endocrine gland is treated? _____

b. What is the surgical approach? _____

c. What procedure is performed? _____

d. On which side of the body is the procedure performed?

_____

e. Is the procedure done to remove a malignancy?

_____

f. Were any adjacent tumors removed? _____

g. What was the extent of lymph node excision, if any?

_____

4. INPATIENT HOSPITAL   Gender: F Age: 38

Preoperative diagnosis: hyperthyroidism

Procedure: excision of both lobes of the thyroid gland through an incision in the neck

Postoperative diagnosis: thyroid tissue negative for malignancy   (*continued*)

4. (continued)

a. What endocrine gland is treated? _____

b. What is the surgical approach? _____

c. What is the anatomic approach? _____

d. What procedure is performed? _____

e. Is the procedure done to remove a malignancy?

_____

f. Were any adjacent tumors removed? _____

g. What was the extent of lymph node excision, if any?

_____

5. INPATIENT HOSPITAL   Gender: F Age: 47

Diagnosis: four-gland hyperparathyroidism

Procedure: transthoracic parathyroidectomy with mediastinal exploration and parathyroid autotransplantation, left forearm

a. What endocrine gland is treated? _____

b. What is the surgical approach? _____

c. What is the anatomic approach? _____

d. What is the primary procedure? _____

e. What is the secondary procedure? _____

f. Is the procedure done to remove a malignancy?

_____

g. Were any adjacent tumors removed? _____

h. What was the extent of lymph node excision, if any?

_____

i. What is the site of autotransplantation?

_____

6. OUTPATIENT HOSPITAL   Gender: F Age: 42

Diagnosis: recurrent nodular goiter

Procedure: secondary thyroidectomy, cervical, bilateral

a. What endocrine gland is treated? _____

b. What is the surgical approach? _____

c. What is the anatomic approach? _____

d. What procedure is performed? _____

e. What is the laterality? _____

f. Is the procedure done to remove a malignancy?

_____

g. Were any adjacent tumors removed? _____

h. What was the extent of lymph node excision, if any?

_____

ASSIGNING CODES FOR ENDOCRINE SYSTEM PROCEDURES

To locate codes for Endocrine System procedures in the Index, search for the Main Term that names the gland, such as **Thyroid Gland**, **Adrenal Gland**, **Parathyroid Gland**, or **Thymus Gland**, then locate the appropriate first-level modifying term and second-level modifying term that describe the procedure. Alternatively, search for the Main Term that identifies the procedure, such as **Thyroidectomy**, **Lobectomy**, **Adrenalectomy**, or **Thymectomy**, and the appropriate modifying terms.

When verifying codes in the Tabular List, be alert for indented codes and the parent codes they are paired with. Codes for thyroid lobectomy procedures are divided based on whether tissue is removed from one or both lobes and whether the excision of one lobe is partial, subtotal, or complete (■ FIGURE 36-2). When all tissue is removed from both lobes, assign a code for a total thyroidectomy (**60240-60274**).

Adrenalectomy codes are divided based on whether the procedure is open (**60640, 60645**) or laparoscopic (**60650**). A surgical laparoscopy includes a diagnostic laparoscopy, when performed. One code encompasses several variations of an adrenalectomy procedure:

- partial or complete
- exploratory with or without biopsy
- transabdominal, lumbar, or dorsal approach

Open adrenalectomy has an indented code for use when a retroperitoneal tumor is excised at the same time as the adjacent adrenal gland (**60545**).

CODING CAUTION

Although there are only 30 codes in this subsection, you must still navigate the Tabular List carefully to identify variations described by indented codes.

Guided Example of Assigning Endocrine System Procedure Codes

To practice skills for assigning codes for the Endocrine System, continue with the example from earlier in the chapter about a patient who was seen for a thyroidectomy. Follow along in your CPT manual as Tamara Brownlee, CCS-P, assigns codes. Check off each step after you complete it.

▶ First, Tamara confirms the procedure, *thyroidectomy with radical neck dissection*.

▶ Tamara searches the Index for the Main Term **Thyroidectomy**.

❑ She locates the first-level modifying term **Total**.

❑ She locates the second-level modifying term **for Malignancy** and the indented term **Radical Neck Dissection**.

❑ She identifies the code **60254**.

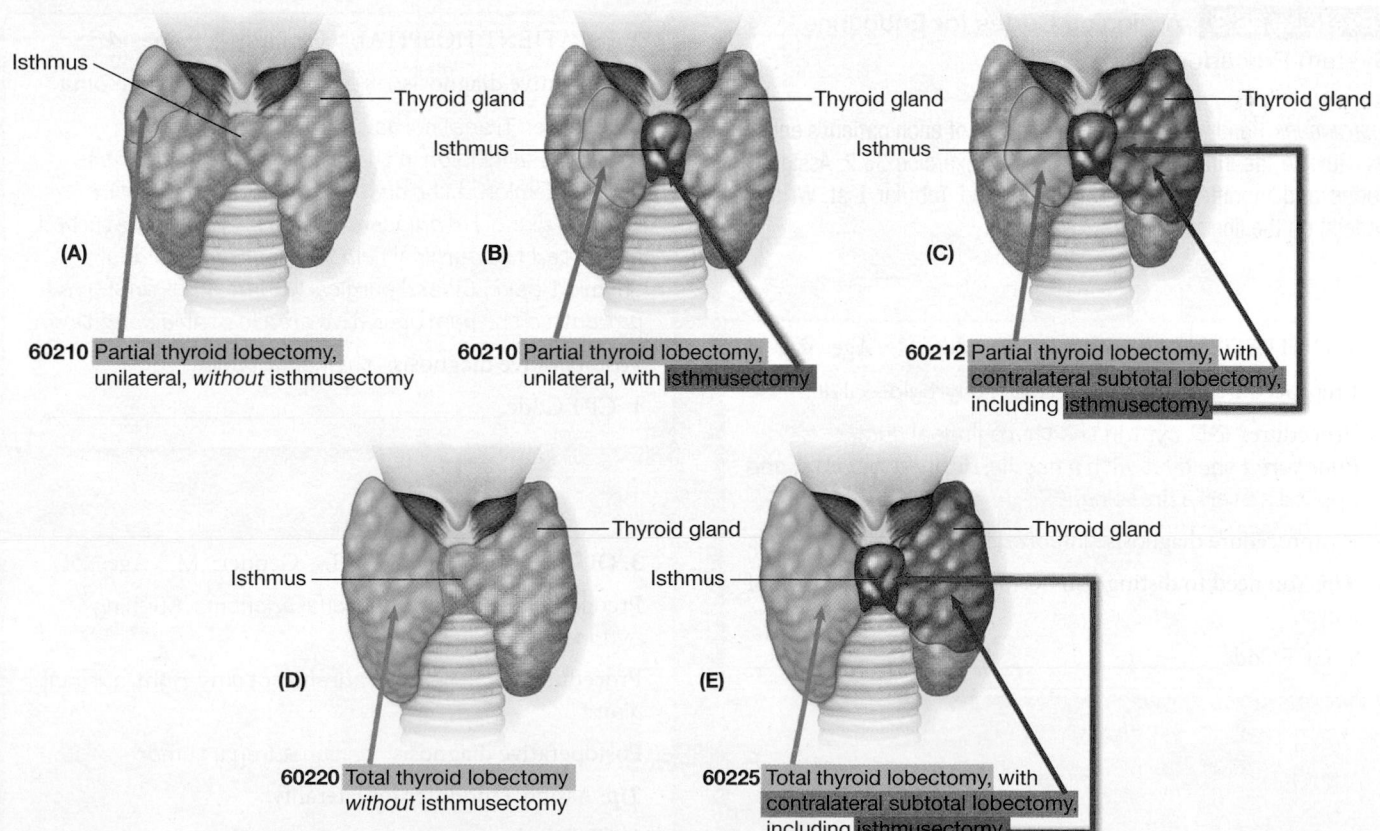

Figure 36-2 ■ Coding Thyroid Lobectomy Procedures. *Source: Annotations © PB Resources, Inc. CPT codes only © American Medical Association.*

▶ Tamara verifies code **60254** in the Tabular List.

❑ She reads the code title for **60254 with radical neck dissection** and recognizes this as an indented code because the description is indented two spaces and begins with a lowercase letter.

❑ She notices that the preceding code, **60252**, is a parent code because the description is left justified, begins with a capital letter, and contains a semicolon. The parent code description reads **Thyroidectomy, total or subtotal for malignancy; with limited neck dissection**. The portion of the description before the semicolon is the common descriptor that applies to the indented code. The only difference between the parent code and the indented code is that the parent code describes a *limited* neck dissection and the indented code describes a *radical* neck dissection.

❑ She confirms that the medical record describes a radical neck dissection and concludes that **60254** accurately describes the procedure.

❑ She combines the common descriptor from the parent code with the descriptor from the indented code to arrive at the full description for code **60254 Thyroidectomy,**

total or subtotal for malignancy; with limited neck dissection.

▶ Tamara checks for instructions in the Tabular List.

❑ She looks for instructional notes immediately before and after the code family **60252-60254** and finds none.

❑ She cross-references the beginning of the subcategory **Excision** and the category **Excision** and verifies that there are no special instructions.

❑ She cross-references the beginning of the subheading **Endocrine** and verifies that there are no special instructions.

❑ She cross-references the beginning of the **Surgery** section and reviews the guidelines. She determines that there are no further instructions or guidelines to direct the coding of this case.

▶ Tamara double-checks the medical record to determine whether there are any other procedures that she should code. Because the lymphadenectomy is included in the code for the thyroidectomy, she does not need to assign a separate code.

▶ Next, Tamara must determine whether she needs a modifier.

CODING PRACTICE

Exercise 36.3 Assigning Codes for Endocrine System Procedures

Instructions: Read the mini-medical-record of each patient's encounter. Review the information abstracted in Exercise 36.2. Assign CPT codes and modifiers using the Index and Tabular List. Write the code(s) on the line provided.

1. OUTPATIENT HOSPITAL Gender: F Age: 4

Preprocedure diagnosis: abscess, thyroglossal duct

Procedure: I&D, cyst in the thyroglossal duct. Punctured the cyst with a needle, drained exudate, and applied a sterile dressing.

Postprocedure diagnosis: infected thyroglossal duct cyst

Tip: You need to distinguish between I&D and excision of a cyst.

1 CPT Code _____

2. INPATIENT HOSPITAL Gender: F Age: 45

Preoperative diagnosis: myasthenia gravis, thymoma

Procedure: Transthoracic thymectomy. Made a length-wise incision in the chest slightly left of the midline. Explored the chest and excised the entire thymus gland. No adjacent structures were disturbed. Inspected the surgical field to ensure no residual thymic tissue. Closed surgical wound and transferred patient to the postoperative area in stable condition.

Postoperative diagnosis: thymoma, benign

1 CPT Code _____

3. OUTPATIENT HOSPITAL Gender: M Age: 35

Preoperative diagnosis: adrenal adenoma, Cushing syndrome

Procedure: laparoscopic adrenalectomy, right adrenal gland

Postoperative diagnosis: benign adrenal tumor

Tip: Assign a modifier for laterality.

1 CPT Code _____

ARRANGING CODES FOR ENDOCRINE SYSTEM PROCEDURES

Although the endocrine section is relatively short, there are several specific situations in which coders must use multiple codes and/or modifiers. These include bilateral procedures, separate procedures, modified radical neck dissection, and imaging guidance.

Bilateral Procedures

Although the thyroid gland contains two lobes, it is a single organ and is not coded as bilateral. When a single lobe is excised, assign a code for a lobectomy. When both lobes are excised at the same time, assign a code for thyroidectomy. When one lobe is removed and the next day the other lobe is removed, assign a code for a lobectomy for the first procedure and a code for secondary thyroidectomy for the second procedure. Assign modifier **-50 Bilateral procedure** to the secondary thyroidectomy when tissue is removed from both sides.

Lymph nodes are bilateral because they occur in paired chains on either side of the body. Cervical lymph nodes occur on both sides of the neck. When a thyroidectomy includes bilateral neck dissection with excision of lymph nodes, assign modifier **-50 Bilateral procedure**. Per the National Correct Coding Initiative (NCCI), Medicare does not pay additional for a bilateral lymphadenectomy performed with a thyroidectomy. However, the *CPT Assistant* newsletter, published by the American Medical Association, directs coders to apply the bilateral modifier (November 2000, volume 10, issue 11). Therefore, for private payers, use modifier **-50** for thyroidectomy with bilateral neck dissection and lymph node removal. Payment policies vary by payer.

The adrenal glands are bilateral organs because one adrenal gland exists suprarenally (*at the top of the kidneys*) on each side of the body. An instructional note in the Tabular List following code **60545** directs **For bilateral procedure, report 60540 with modifier 50**.

-59 Distinct Procedural Service

The Endocrine System subheading contains three codes with the designation **(separate procedure)** as part of the code description: **60520** and **60521** (thymectomy) and **60540** (adrenalectomy). An adrenalectomy is often performed as part of a nephrectomy and is bundled into the nephrectomy code. When the adrenal gland(s) is removed as an independent procedure, assign code **60540**.

A thymectomy is a separate procedure when performed with most thyroidectomy procedures because the two procedures require separate incisions. Append modifier **-59 Distinct procedural service** when a thymectomy is performed with a thyroidectomy (■ Figure 36-3) to indicate that it is separate from the thyroidectomy. The exception is when a transthoracic thyroidectomy (**60270**) is performed; then, the thymectomy (**60520-60522**) can be performed through the same incision. Because the thymus gland is located in the upper portion of the thorax, it can be accessed through the same incision as a transthoracic thyroidectomy, so the procedures are bundled.

Surgeon performs a total thyroidectomy and a transcervical thymectomy through a separate incision in the lower neck.

60240 Thyroidectomy, total
60520-59 Thymectomy, partial or total; transcervical approach (separate procedure); -59 separate procedure

Figure 36-3 ■ Example of Coding a Thyroidectomy with a Thymectomy. *Source: © PB Resources, Inc. Used with permission. CPT codes only © American Medical Association.*

Surgeon performs a total thyroidectomy with a bilateral modified radical neck dissection.

38724-50 Cervical lymphadenectomy (modified radical neck dissection); -50 bilateral procedure
60240-51 Thyroidectomy, total; -51 multiple procedures

Figure 36-4 ■ Example of Coding a Thyroidectomy With Modified Radical Neck Dissection. *Source: © PB Resources, Inc. Used with permission. CPT codes only © American Medical Association.*

Modified Radical Neck Dissection

CPT provides combination codes for a thyroidectomy with a limited or radical neck dissection. When a modified neck dissection is performed, report two codes: one for the thyroidectomy and one for a modified radical neck dissection (■ Figure 36-4). The modified radical neck dissection is worth 42.00 RVUs, compared with 26.36 RVUS for the thyroidectomy, so the lymph node dissection is sequenced first. Append modifier **-50** to the bilateral lymphadenectomy. Append modifier **-51** to the thyroidectomy. Although the thyroidectomy is the main reason surgery is performed, it is not sequenced by physicians as the primary procedure because the code with the highest RVU is sequenced first.

Both modifiers **-50** and **-51** can impact payment. Payers might allow up to a 50% increase in payment for bilateral procedures. At the same time, they might reduce payment for a secondary procedure by as much as 50% (■ Table 36-5).

Imaging Guidance

When imaging guidance is performed to assist with a percutaneous core needle biopsy, assign an additional code from the Radiology section. An instructional note following code **60100** identifies the appropriate Radiology codes (**76942, 77002, 77012, 77021**) based on the type of imaging required (■ Figure 36-5).

Table 36-5 ■ **IMPACT OF CODE SEQUENCING AND MODIFIERS ON REIMBURSEMENT**

CPT Code	Fee Schedule	Modifier Adjustment	Allowed Amount
38724-50	$1,504.56	150%	$2,256.84
60240-51	$944.29	50%	$472.14
Total	**$2,448.85**		**$2,728.98**

Source: © PB Resources, Inc. Used with permission. CPT codes only © American Medical Association.

Surgeon performs a percutaneous core needle biopsy of the thyroid with fluoroscopic guidance.

60100 Biopsy thyroid, percutaneous core needle
77002 Fluoroscopic guidance for needle placement (eg, biopsy, aspiration, injection, localization device)

Figure 36-5 ■ Example of Coding Thyroid Biopsy With Fluoroscopic Guidance. *Source: © PB Resources, Inc. Used with permission. CPT codes only © American Medical Association.*

Guided Example of Arranging Endocrine System Procedure Codes

Continue with the example from earlier in the chapter about the patient who was seen for a thyroidectomy. Although no sequencing is required because only one code is needed, modifiers must be reviewed. Follow along in your CPT manual as Tamara Brownlee, CCS-P, finalizes the coding. Check off each step after you complete it.

▶ First, Tamara confirms the procedure **60254 Thyroidectomy, total or subtotal for malignancy; with radical neck dissection**.

❑ She confirms that no additional procedure codes are needed.

❑ She reviews the procedure to determine the need for modifiers.

❑ She identifies that the thyroidectomy procedure does not require a bilateral modifier.

❑ She confirms that the radical neck dissection was performed on both sides and assigns modifier **-50 Bilateral procedure**.

▶ Tamara finalizes the procedure code and modifier for this case:

(1) **60254-50 Thyroidectomy, total or subtotal for malignancy; with radical neck dissection; -50 Bilateral procedure**

▶ Tamara also assigns and sequences the ICD-10-CM diagnosis codes that support the need for the procedure.

(1) **C73 Malignant neoplasm of thyroid gland**

(2) **C77.0 Secondary and unspecified malignant neoplasm of lymph nodes of head, face and neck**

CODING PRACTICE

Exercise 36.4 Arranging Codes for Endocrine System Procedures

Instructions: Read the mini-medical-record of each patient's encounter. Review the information abstracted in Exercise 36.2. Assign CPT codes and modifiers using the Index and Tabular List, and arrange the codes in the proper sequence. Write the code(s) on the line provided.

1. INPATIENT HOSPITAL   Gender: F   Age: 38

Preoperative diagnosis: hyperthyroidism

Procedure: excision of both lobes of the thyroid gland through an incision in the neck

Postoperative diagnosis: thyroid tissue negative for malignancy

1 CPT Code _____

2. INPATIENT HOSPITAL   Gender: F   Age: 47

Diagnosis: four-gland hyperparathyroidism

Procedure: transthoracic parathyroidectomy with mediastinal exploration and parathyroid autotransplantation, left forearm

2 CPT Codes _____

3. OUTPATIENT HOSPITAL   Gender: F   Age: 42

Diagnosis: recurrent nodular goiter

Procedure: secondary thyroidectomy, cervical, bilateral

Tip: Read the instructional note following this code in the Tabular List.

1 CPT Code _____

E/M CODING FOR ENDOCRINOLOGY

Neither the *1995* nor *1997 Documentation Guidelines for Evaluation and Management Services* (DG) provide a single organ system examination for the endocrine system. Endocrinologists use a multisystem E/M physical examination (■ FIGURE 36-6). Documentation guidelines for the history and medical decision making are the same for the 1995 DG and the 1997 DG. The requirements of the physical examination vary. Physicians and their coders can use either the 1995 DG or 1997 DG for any encounter. They can assign an E/M code based on whichever set of criteria is most beneficial, but they cannot be combined or intermixed for the same encounter. They do not need to use the

Body Areas (BA)	Organ Systems (OS)
❑ Head, including the face ❑ Neck ❑ Chest, including breasts and axillae ❑ Abdomen ❑ Genitalia, groin, buttocks ❑ Back, including spine Each extremity: ❑ Right arm ❑ Left arm ❑ Right leg ❑ Left leg	❑ Constitutional (e.g., vital signs, general appearance) ❑ Eyes ❑ Ears, nose, mouth, and throat ❑ Cardiovascular ❑ Respiratory ❑ Gastrointestinal ❑ Genitourinary ❑ Musculoskeletal ❑ Skin ❑ Neurologic ❑ Psychiatric ❑ Hematologic/lymphatic/immunologic
(A) Total number of body areas:	(B) Total number of organ systems:

(A) + (B)	(C)	# of ❑ Elements Performed and Documented	Level of Examination
Total # body areas + organ systems →	☐	1 body area or organ system (C)	Problem focused
		2–4 body areas and/or organ systems (C)	Expanded problem focused
		5–7 body areas and/or organ systems (C)	Detailed
		8+ body areas (A) _or_ 8+ organ systems (B), but they cannot be combined	Comprehensive

Figure 36-6 ■ 1995 DG for Multisystem Examination. *Source: © PB Resources, Inc. Used with permission. Based on Centers for Medicare and Medicaid Services, 1995 Documentation Guidelines for Evaluation and Management Services.*

same DG for all patients. To determine the appropriate E/M code using the 1995 DG, coders must review the documentation in detail and identify the specific elements documented.

- To translate the documentation into the E/M requirements for the history, refer back to Chapter 31, "Evaluation and Management Services (99201-99499)," Tables 31-7 to 31-10, or to the 1995 DG.
- To determine the requirements for an examination, refer to Figure 36-6. The 1995 DG provide general examination criteria but do not quantify the number of elements required. This chapter reviews the 1995 DG multisystem examination and follows the generally accepted quantitative guidelines for each examination level shown in the figure.
- To determine the levels for medical decision making (MDM), refer to Chapter 31, Table 31-12, and to the Table of Risk in the 1995 DG.

Guided Example of E/M Coding for Endocrinology

Refer to the endocrinology encounter (■ FIGURE 36-7) to practice skills for abstracting and assigning E/M codes. This example demonstrates use of the 1995 DG. Follow along as fictitious coder Tamara Brownlee, CCS-P, abstracts the service. Check off each step after you complete it.

▶ First, Tamara needs to establish the category of service so she can determine the information needed to abstract and assign the code.

❑ *What is the setting?* Endocrine clinic (office)

❑ *What is the type of service?* Established patient

❑ *What is the code range?* Tamara refers to the CPT Index and looks up the Main Term **Evaluation and Management**. She must determine whether the encounter should be coded as a consultation or an office visit. She reviews the definition of a consultation, which requires that one physician request the opinion of another physician with a report back on the findings. This patient is established with the endocrinology clinic and is returning for a 6-month checkup. Management of the patient's diabetes is under the ongoing care of the endocrinologist, so this is not a consultation.

❑ Tamara returns to the CPT Index and locates the subterm **Office and other outpatient**. The code range listed is **99201-99215**. Tamara refers to the code range in the Tabular List and notices that the code range is divided into two categories: **New Patient** and **Established Patient**. She selects the code range for **Established patient 99211-99215**.

❑ *How many key components are required?* Tamara refers to the code range in the Tabular List. The first code, **99211**, is described as a minimal visit that does not require the presence of a physician; it probably does not apply to this encounter because the patient met with the physician and the service was more than minimal. She

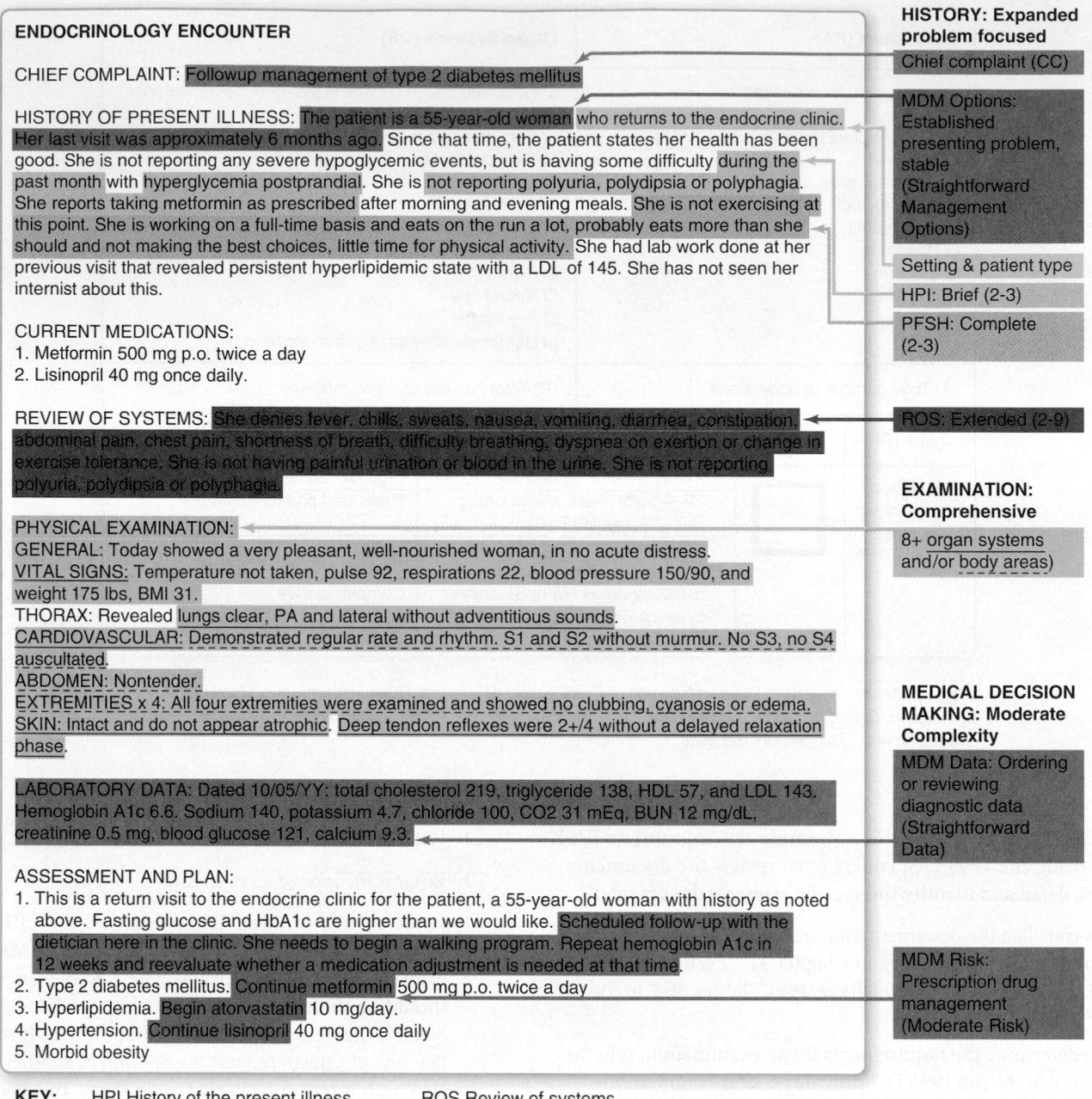

ENDOCRINOLOGY ENCOUNTER

CHIEF COMPLAINT: Followup management of type 2 diabetes mellitus

HISTORY OF PRESENT ILLNESS: The patient is a 55-year-old woman who returns to the endocrine clinic. Her last visit was approximately 6 months ago. Since that time, the patient states her health has been good. She is not reporting any severe hypoglycemic events, but is having some difficulty during the past month with hyperglycemia postprandial. She is not reporting polyuria, polydipsia or polyphagia. She reports taking metformin as prescribed after morning and evening meals. She is not exercising at this point. She is working on a full-time basis and eats on the run a lot, probably eats more than she should and not making the best choices, little time for physical activity. She had lab work done at her previous visit that revealed persistent hyperlipidemic state with a LDL of 145. She has not seen her internist about this.

CURRENT MEDICATIONS:
1. Metformin 500 mg p.o. twice a day
2. Lisinopril 40 mg once daily.

REVIEW OF SYSTEMS: She denies fever, chills, sweats, nausea, vomiting, diarrhea, constipation, abdominal pain, chest pain, shortness of breath, difficulty breathing, dyspnea on exertion or change in exercise tolerance. She is not having painful urination or blood in the urine. She is not reporting polyuria, polydipsia or polyphagia.

PHYSICAL EXAMINATION:
GENERAL: Today showed a very pleasant, well-nourished woman, in no acute distress.
VITAL SIGNS: Temperature not taken, pulse 92, respirations 22, blood pressure 150/90, and weight 175 lbs, BMI 31.
THORAX: Revealed lungs clear, PA and lateral without adventitious sounds.
CARDIOVASCULAR: Demonstrated regular rate and rhythm. S1 and S2 without murmur. No S3, no S4 auscultated.
ABDOMEN: Nontender.
EXTREMITIES x 4: All four extremities were examined and showed no clubbing, cyanosis or edema.
SKIN: Intact and do not appear atrophic. Deep tendon reflexes were 2+/4 without a delayed relaxation phase.

LABORATORY DATA: Dated 10/05/YY: total cholesterol 219, triglyceride 138, HDL 57, and LDL 143. Hemoglobin A1c 6.6. Sodium 140, potassium 4.7, chloride 100, CO2 31 mEq, BUN 12 mg/dL, creatinine 0.5 mg, blood glucose 121, calcium 9.3.

ASSESSMENT AND PLAN:
1. This is a return visit to the endocrine clinic for the patient, a 55-year-old woman with history as noted above. Fasting glucose and HbA1c are higher than we would like. Scheduled follow-up with the dietician here in the clinic. She needs to begin a walking program. Repeat hemoglobin A1c in 12 weeks and reevaluate whether a medication adjustment is needed at that time.
2. Type 2 diabetes mellitus. Continue metformin 500 mg p.o. twice a day
3. Hyperlipidemia. Begin atorvastatin 10 mg/day.
4. Hypertension. Continue lisinopril 40 mg once daily
5. Morbid obesity

HISTORY: Expanded problem focused

Chief complaint (CC)

MDM Options: Established presenting problem, stable (Straightforward Management Options)

Setting & patient type

HPI: Brief (2-3)

PFSH: Complete (2-3)

ROS: Extended (2-9)

EXAMINATION: Comprehensive

8+ organ systems and/or body areas)

MEDICAL DECISION MAKING: Moderate Complexity

MDM Data: Ordering or reviewing diagnostic data (Straightforward Data)

MDM Risk: Prescription drug management (Moderate Risk)

KEY: HPI History of the present illness   ROS Review of systems
PFSH Past, family, and social history   MDM Medical decision making

Figure 36-7 ■ Endocrinology Encounter

reads the code description of the second code, **99212**, which states **Office or other outpatient visit for the evaluation and management of an established patient, which requires at least 2 of these 3 key components**. Codes **99212-99215** have the same requirements for key components. This tells her that two out of three (2/3) key components must meet or exceed the levels listed in the code.

▶ Next, Tamara identifies the level of history.

❑ *What is the level of HPI?* The HPI is **Extended** because four elements are documented.

❑ *What is the level of ROS?* The ROS is **Extended** because two to nine systems are documented.

❑ *What is the level of PFSH?* The PFSH is **Complete** because two to three elements are documented, which qualifies as a complete PFSH for an established patient.

❑ *Based on these factors, what is the overall level of history?* The level of history is **Expanded problem-focused** because the lowest of the three factors (HPI, ROS, and PFSH) determines the history level. The ROS and PFSH qualify for a higher level of history, but the HPI qualifies for only an **Expanded problem-focused** history.

▶ Tamara refers to the multisystem examination in the 1995 DG (Figure 36-6) to abstract information needed to determine the level of the examination.

- ❏ *What is the level of examination?* The level of examination is **Comprehensive**. Ten (10) body areas and organ systems are documented, which exceeds the requirement of eight or more bulleted elements for a comprehensive examination.

▶ Tamara determines the level of medical decision making (Refer to Table 31-12).

- ❏ *What is the level of complexity of the number of diagnoses or management options, based on the presenting problem?* The level is **Straightforward** because the presenting problem is established and with only a mild exacerbation.

- ❏ *What is the amount and/or complexity of data to be reviewed?* The amount of data to be reviewed is **Straightforward** because the physician reviews several laboratory tests.

- ❏ *What is the level of risk of significant complications, morbidity, and/or mortality?* Tamara reviews each column in the Table of Risk in the 1995 DG. She identifies that the

level of risk is **Moderate** because the patient presents with one stable chronic illness (low), clinical labs are reviewed but not ordered, and prescription drug management is required (moderate). The single highest element in the Table of Risk determines the overall risk.

- ❏ *Based on these factors, what is the overall level of medical decision making?* The medical decision making is **Straightforward complexity**. At least two of the three MDM factors are required to qualify for a specific level of MDM. Two of the three MDM factors are straightforward, so this qualifies for a straightforward complexity of decision making.

Now Tamara is ready to assign the code for the endocrinology encounter. The exercise that follows guides you through additional abstracting skills and allows you to assign the correct code.

SUCCESS STEP

Physicians use their clinical judgment and the nature of the patient's presenting problem(s) to determine the depth of history needed to complete the service.

CODING PRACTICE

Exercise 36.5   Evaluation and Management Coding for Endocrinology

Instructions: Refer to the *1995 Documentation Guidelines for Evaluation and Management Services* (available at www.cms.gov) or Chapter 31, "Evaluation and Management Services (99201-99499)" (Tables 31-7 to 31-12), in this text. Answer the following questions about the outpatient endocrinology encounter (Figure 36-7).

1. a. Which elements of the HPI are documented? Circle all that apply. Location, Quality, Severity, Duration, Timing, Context, Modifying factors, Associated signs and symptoms

   b. How many elements are documented? _____

   c. What is the level of HPI? _____

2. a. Which systems are reviewed in the ROS? Circle all that apply. Constitutional, Allergic/ immunologic, CV, Endocrine, ENT/M, Eyes, GI, GU, Hemic/lymphatic, MS, Neurologic, Psychiatric, Respiratory, Skin/breast

   b. How many systems are documented? _____

   c. What is the level of ROS? _____

3. a. Which PFSH elements are documented? Circle all that apply. Past medical, Family, Social

   b. What is the level of PFSH? _____

c. What is the overall level of history? (The lowest history factor—HPI, ROS, or PFSH—determines the level of history.) _____

4. Refer to Figure 36-6 (1995 DG for Multisystem Examination).

   a. How many organ systems are documented for the examination? Circle all that apply. Constitutional (e.g., vital signs, general appearance); Eyes; ENT/M; CV; Respiratory; GI; GU; MS; Skin; Neurologic; Psychiatric; Hematologic/ lymphatic/immunologic

   b. How many body areas are documented for the examination? Circle all that apply. Head, including the face; Neck; Chest, including breasts and axillae; Abdomen; Genitalia, groin, buttocks; Back, including spine; Each extremity (×4)

   c. What is the total number of body areas and organ systems documented? _____

   d. What is the level of the examination? _____

5. Refer to Table 31-12 Medical Decision Making Levels or the 1995 DG.

   a. What is the MDM level for the number of diagnoses or management options? _____

   b. What is the MDM level for the amount and/or complexity of data to be reviewed? _____

(continued)

(continued from page 683)

2. (continued)

isthmus. Performed with modified radical dissection of cervical lymph nodes on both sides.

1 ICD-10-CM Code _____

1 CPT Code _____

---

3. OUTPATIENT HOSPITAL   Gender: M   **Age:** 33

Diagnosis: Thyroid nodule

Procedure: Percutaneous core needle biopsy. Using ultrasound guidance, positioned the core needle (*an automatic spring–powered device with a hollow inner needle*) over the nodule and extracted tissue sample. Tissue submitted to pathology for analysis.

Pathology report: Negative

1 ICD-10-CM Code _____

2 CPT Codes _____

---

4. OUTPATIENT HOSPITAL   Gender: M   **Age:** 24

Preoperative diagnosis: Difficulty swallowing due to large thyroid nodule

Procedure: Removal of colloid cyst in thyroid

Postoperative diagnosis: Malignant neoplasm of thyroid

Pathology report: Positive for malignant neoplasm of thyroid

1 ICD-10-CM Code _____

1 CPT Code _____

---

5. INPATIENT HOSPITAL   Gender: F   **Age:** 14

Diagnosis: Hashimoto disease

Procedure: Thyroidectomy. Made incision below voice box. Removed thyroid, including extension into the thorax below the sternum. Parathyroid remains intact.

1 ICD-10-CM Code _____

1 CPT Code _____

---

6. INPATIENT HOSPITAL   Gender: M   **Age:** 67

Preoperative diagnosis: small mass on both adrenal glands, suspected carcinoma

Procedure: Made transverse incision to visualize both adrenals. Carefully removed each adrenal. Kidneys showed no sign of further concern.

Postoperative diagnosis: Adrenal cortical carcinoma

Pathology report: Adrenal cortical carcinoma, 3 cm left, 5 cm right

2 ICD-10-CM Codes _____

1 CPT Code _____

---

7. OUTPATIENT HOSPITAL   Gender: M   **Age:** 15

Diagnosis: Thyroglossal duct cyst

Procedure: Made small transverse incision over area of cyst. Cyst was isolated and removed along with the tract, following it to base of tongue. Cyst was sent to lab for review.

Pathology report: Simple cyst. No malignancy noted.

1 ICD-10-CM Code _____

1 CPT Code _____

---

8. INPATIENT HOSPITAL   Gender: F   **Age:** 55

Preprocedure diagnosis: Hurthle cell tumor

Procedure: Standard neck incision is made. Performed partial left lobectomy with contralateral subtotal right lobectomy. Removed isthmus with thyroid.

1 ICD-10-CM Code _____

1 CPT Code _____

---

9. INPATIENT HOSPITAL   Gender: F   **Age:** 56

Diagnosis: Myasthenia gravis in crisis

Procedure: Sternum was separated and mediastinum was explored. Radical mediastinal dissection was performed and thymus was removed.

1 ICD-10-CM Code _____

1 CPT Code _____

10. OUTPATIENT HOSPITAL   Gender: M   Age: 66

Diagnosis: Carotid body tumor

Procedure: Horizontal incision is made in the midneck. Carotid body tumor is isolated and removed. Carotid artery is also dissected and removed.

Pathology report: Benign carotid body tumor

Tip: A carotid body is a small tissue mass of nerves and cells in the carotid artery.

1 ICD-10-CM Code _____

1 CPT Code _____

KEEP ON CODING

Instructions: Read the procedural statement, then use the appropriate Index and Tabular List to assign CPT procedure codes. Write the code(s) on the line provided.

1. Subtotal thyroidectomy for carcinoma with limited neck dissection: CPT Code(s) _____

2. Unilateral total thyroid lobectomy with contralateral subtotal lobectomy and isthmusectomy and parathyroid autotransplantation: CPT Code(s) _____

3. Excision of carotid body tumor: CPT Code(s) _____

4. Reexploration of parathyroid glands: CPT Code(s) _____

5. Laparoscopic adrenalectomy with biopsy, left side, lumbar approach: CPT Code(s) _____

6. Parathyroidectomy: CPT Code(s) _____

7. Excision of cyst in thyroglossal duct: CPT Code(s) _____

8. Aspiration of a thyroid cyst: CPT Code(s) _____

9. Bilateral thyroidectomy including substernal thyroid, cervical approach: CPT Code(s) _____

10. Partial thymectomy, sternal approach, with radical mediastinal dissection (separate procedure): CPT Code(s) _____

Chapter 37

Integumentary System Procedures (10030-19499)

Chapter Outline

- **Integumentary System Procedure Basics**
- **Coding Overview of Integumentary System Procedures**
- **Abstracting Integumentary System Procedures**
- **Assigning Codes for Integumentary System Procedures**
- **Arranging Codes for Integumentary System Procedures**
- **E/M Coding for Dermatology**

Learning Objectives

After completing this chapter, you should have the skills to:

37.1 Spell and define the key words, medical terms, and abbreviations related to integumentary system procedures.

37.2 Discuss the fundamentals of integumentary system procedures.

37.3 Identify the main characteristics of coding for the Integumentary System.

37.4 Abstract procedural information from the medical record for coding Integumentary System procedures.

37.5 Assign codes for Integumentary System procedures.

37.6 Arrange codes for Integumentary System procedures.

37.7 Code evaluation and management services for the integumentary system.

37.8 Discuss the CPT coding guidelines related to the Integumentary System.

Key Terms and Abbreviations

adjacent tissue transfer/
   rearrangement (ATT/R)
allograft
area measurement
autograft

cosmetic
flap
full-thickness skin graft (FTSG)
linear measurement
Lund-Browder classification

primary intention healing
reconstructive
secondary intention healing
single quantity
split-thickness skin graft (STSG)

tertiary intention healing
xenograft

In addition to the key terms listed here, students should know the terms defined within tables in this chapter.

For updates and corrections, visit our student resource site at

www.pearsonhighered.com/healthprofessionsresources

INTRODUCTION

When you buy beverages such as soda pop, you can choose among various sizes and packaging: single cans, liter bottles, six-packs, twelve-packs, mini cans, and so on. Each package has one price, regardless of the number of bottles or cans it contains. CPT codes often work the same way. When coding for removal of lesions in the integumentary system, the number of lesions described by a single CPT varies from 1 to 15, depending on the type of lesion and method of removal.

INTEGUMENTARY SYSTEM PROCEDURE BASICS

Dermatologists diagnose and treat disorders of the skin and also perform surgical procedures. Plastic surgeons perform both **reconstructive** (*relating to restoring normal function or appearance*) procedures and **cosmetic** (*relating to aesthetics or appearance*) procedures. Podiatrists diagnose and treat conditions of the foot, including the skin of the foot and the toenails.

Review the anatomic structure of the skin and the associated medical terms for the layers (Figure 11-1). This knowledge helps in determining the extent and complexity of many procedures. Refer to ■ TABLE 37-1 for a refresher on how to build medical terms for integumentary system procedures.

CODING CAUTION

Be alert for combining forms that are spelled similarly and have different meanings.

ungu/o (*nail*) and **lingu/o** (*tongue*)

xen/o (*stranger, foreign material*) and **xanth/o** (*yellow*) and **xer/o** (*dryness*)

hydr/o (*water*) and **hidr/o** (*sweat*)

Procedures of the Integumentary System

Procedures commonly performed on the integumentary system are summarized in ■ TABLE 37-2. Coders must understand the basic principles of measurements when working with excision procedures and wound repair. Reviewing the wound healing process is also helpful. Additional procedures to be familiar

Table 37-1 ■ EXAMPLE OF CONSTRUCTING MEDICAL TERMS FOR INTEGUMENTARY SYSTEM PROCEDURES

Root/Combining Form	Suffix	Complete Medical Term
derm/o (*stomach*)	-plasty (*surgical repair, formation*)	**dermo + plasty** (*surgical repair of the skin*)
		lipo + plasty (*surgical formation of fat*)
lip/o (*fat*) **electr/o-** (*electrical*)	-lysis (*surgical destruction, loosening*)	**dermo + lysis** (*surgical loosening of the skin*)
		lipo + lysis (*surgical destruction of fat*)
		electro + lysis (*surgical destruction using electricity*)

Source: © PB Resources, Inc. Used with permission.

with are Mohs micrographic surgery, burns, tissue transfer and skin replacement, and breast removal and reconstruction. These are discussed next.

Measurements

Working with the integumentary system requires knowledge of measurements because many procedures are classified by size. Lesions and wound repairs are described by linear measurements, tissue repairs are classified by area, and burn treatments are classified by the percentage of total body surface area (TBSA). Linear and area measurements are reported using the metric system, which consists of meters (m), centimeters (cm), and millimeters (mm). A **linear measurement** identifies the distance between two points and is used to classify the length of wound repairs and the diameter (*distance from one side to the other*) of excised lesions. An **area measurement** describes the space inside a boundary and is used to classify the amount of skin treated in a tissue repair or skin graft. Area is calculated as the length multiplied by the width of the affected tissue (L × W) and is expressed in square centimeters (sq cm) (■ FIGURE 37-1). The details of how to use measurements to assign codes are discussed later in this chapter.

Physicians are trained to use metric units in documentation, but understanding the relationship between the metric system and the English system is helpful for coders so they can spot

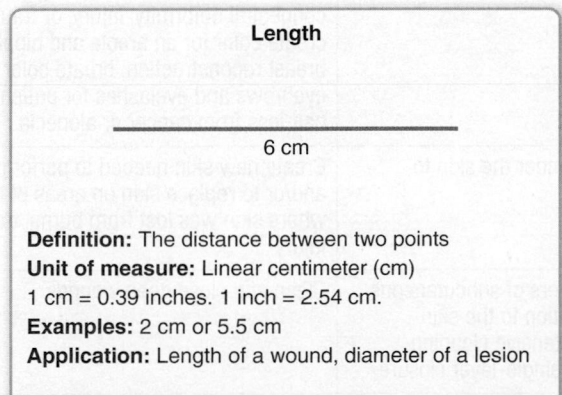

Length

6 cm

Definition: The distance between two points
Unit of measure: Linear centimeter (cm)
1 cm = 0.39 inches. 1 inch = 2.54 cm.
Examples: 2 cm or 5.5 cm
Application: Length of a wound, diameter of a lesion

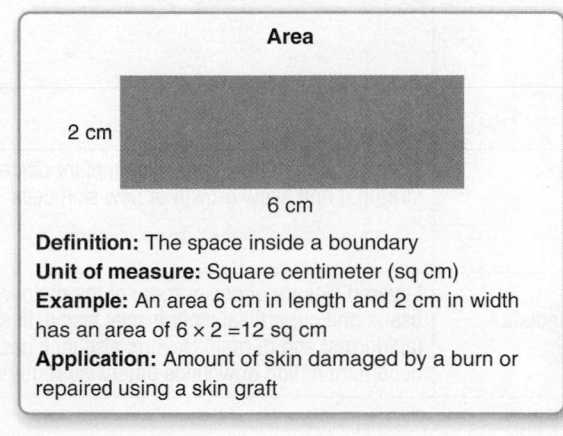

Area

2 cm

6 cm

Definition: The space inside a boundary
Unit of measure: Square centimeter (sq cm)
Example: An area 6 cm in length and 2 cm in width has an area of 6 × 2 =12 sq cm
Application: Amount of skin damaged by a burn or repaired using a skin graft

Figure 37-1 ■ Length and Area

Table 37-2 ■ **COMMON PROCEDURES OF THE INTEGUMENTARY SYSTEM**

Procedure Name	Definition	Reason Performed
Adjacent tissue transfer/rearrangement (ATT/R)	Transfer of a section of skin or flap from that immediately next to the damaged skin and that can be moved without completely detaching it	Repair or replace damaged skin
Autograft	Use of a patient's own tissue from one site to replace damaged tissue at another site	Repair or replace damaged skin
Avulsion	Forceful tearing of the nail plate	Treat onychocryptosis (*ingrown toenail*), perform a biopsy, or treat an infection
Chemosurgery	Use of a chemical agent (e.g., trichloroacetic acid, hydroxy acid, silver nitrate) to destroy tissue	Remove lesions
Cryotherapy	Use of liquid nitrogen to destroy tissue	Remove lesions
Destruction	Rendering tissue into tiny fragments	Remove lesions
Electrocauterization	Use of a hot instrument to destroy tissue	Remove lesions
Electrosurgical destruction	Use of high-frequency electric current to destroy tissue	Remove lesions
Excision	Use of scissors, scalpel, or other sharp instrument to cut out tissue	Full-thickness removal of diseased or damaged tissue
Flap transfer	Moving a section of skin and subcutaneous tissue (sometimes including muscle, fascia, and bone), with blood vessels intact, from one site to another; with anastomosis to vessels at the recipient site	Repair or replace damaged skin and vasculature
Intralesional injection	Injection of a drug, such as a corticosteroid, into a skin lesion	Treat keloids, psoriasis, hypertrophic scars, cystic acne, and eczema
Ligature	Tying off a skin tag at its base with thread, eliminating blood flow to the skin tag; it eventually dies and falls off	Remove skin tags
Mohs micrographic surgery	A multistage procedure in which a malignant lesion is excised in microscopic layers. The physician performing the procedure also performs pathological evaluation of each tissue layer. When no further malignancy is found, the site is closed.	Basal cell carcinoma, squamous cell carcinoma
Paring/cutting/curettement	Use of a scalpel, blade, or curette (*surgical instrument with a scoop or ring at then end*) to scrape away the tissue	Remove dead or infected tissue
Shaving	Use of a sharp instrument	Remove an epidermal or dermal lesion without a full-thickness excision
Skin replacement	Use of skin from the patient's own body or a donor to replace damaged skin that cannot be repaired with sutures alone	Repair or replacement of damaged skin
Skin substitute	Use of synthetic (artificial) material to replace damaged skin	Temporary repair or replacement of damaged skin while the body generates new skin tissue
Tattooing	Injection of a colored pigment into the skin	Hide a discoloration caused by disease, a congenital deformity, injury, or trauma; create color for an areola and nipple after breast reconstruction; create color for eyebrows and eyelashes for patients with hair loss from cancer or alopecia
Tissue expander	A temporary inflatable or saline implant placed under the skin to stretch it and allow growth of new skin cells	Create new skin needed to perform surgery and/or to replace skin on areas of the body where skin was lost from burns, trauma, or injury
Wound repair–intermediate	Layered closure of one or more of the deeper layers of subcutaneous tissue and superficial (nonmuscle) fascia, in addition to the skin (epidermal and dermal) closure; also includes extensive cleaning/decontamination of wounds otherwise requiring single-layer closure	Clean and close deep wounds

(continued)

Table 37-4 ■ BREAST PROCEDURES

Procedure	Description
Treatment procedures	
Mastotomy	Incision and drainage of a breast abscess
Partial mastectomy (lumpectomy, tylectomy)	Removal of only enough breast tissue to ensure that the margins of the specimen are free of malignant cells
Subcutaneous mastectomy	Excision of breast tissue but not the overlying skin, nipple, and areola, making it possible for the breast form to be reconstructed
Simple complete mastectomy	Removal of only the breast tissue, nipple, and a small portion of the overlying skin, also called simple mastectomy and total mastectomy
Modified radical mastectomy	A simple mastectomy plus removal of axillary lymph nodes but not the pectoralis major muscle
Radical mastectomy	Removal of the breast, pectoralis major and minor muscles, axillary lymph nodes, and associated skin and subcutaneous tissue
Repair and reconstruction procedures	
Mastopexy	A skin reduction with removal or reduction of underlying breast muscles to reorient the breasts into a higher position
Mammaplasty	Repair or reconstruction of the breast
Latissimus dorsi (LD) flap	Use of a latissimus dorsi muscle flap, often commonly combined with a tissue expander or implant, to reconstruct the breast
Deep inferior epigastric perforator (DIEP) flap	Use of blood vessels called deep inferior epigastric perforators (DIEPs), and the skin and connected fat, or skin only (but no muscle), from the wall of the lower belly to rebuild the breast
Transverse rectus abdominis myocutaneous (TRAM) flap	Use of the transverse rectus abdominis myocutaneous tissue to reconstruct the breast
Periprosthetic capsulectomy	Removal of a breast implant and the entire contracture capsule surrounding the breast implant

Source: © PB Resources, Inc. Used with permission.

CODING PRACTICE

Exercise 37.1 Integumentary System Procedure Basics

Instructions: Use your medical terminology skills and resources to define the following procedures, then identify the applicable code or code range. Follow these steps:

- Use slash marks "/" to break down the underlined term into its root(s) and suffix.
- Define the meaning of the underlined word, based on the meaning of each word part.
- Use the entire phrase to identify the code or code range shown in the CPT Index.

Example: mastectomy, partial mast/ectomy   Meaning *surgical removal of the breast*   CPT Code *19301-19302*

1. cryotherapy, acne   Meaning _____   CPT Code(s) _____
2. mammaplasty, reduction   Meaning _____   CPT Code(s) _____
3. ischiectomy, with pressure ulcer excision   Meaning _____   CPT Code(s) _____

(continued)

Table 37-2 ■ *(continued)*

Procedure Name	Definition	Reason Performed
Wound repair—simple	One-layer closure of epidermis, dermis, or subcutaneous tissue without significant involvement of deeper structures; includes local anesthesia and electrocauterization, when used	Close lacerations and wounds
Wound repair—complex	A layered closure that also requires scar revision, debridement, extensive undermining (*freeing the skin from the underlying tissue along lateral edge of the wound*), stents, or retention sutures (*reinforcing sutures placed around the primary suture line*)	Restructure or reinforce deep wounds

Source: © PB Resources, Inc. Used with permission.

potential errors, such as a misplaced decimal. A comparison of metric measure and English measures follows:

- 1 meter = 3.28 feet (*3 feet, 3 inches*)
- 1 centimeter (*1/100th [0.01] of a meter*) = 0.39 inches (*just less than ½ inch*)
- 1 millimeter (*1/1000th of a meter [0.001] or 1/10th [0.10] of a centimeter*) = 0.039 inches (*1/25th of an inch*)

CODING CAUTION

Metric numbers less than 1 should be written with a 0 in front of the decimal, such as 0.25, to avoid potential confusion with a similar whole number, such as 25.

Wound Healing

Wound healing is an intricate process in which the body regenerates skin cells; it can be summarized in four basic phases (■ TABLE 37-3). External assistance helps to speed the healing

Table 37-3 ■ SUMMARY OF THE PHASES OF WOUND HEALING

Phase	Name	Description	Time Frame (After Injury)
1	Hemostasis	Platelets stop bleeding.	1–60 minutes
2	Inflammation	Neutrophils, mast cells, and macrophages phagocytize (*clean up or digest cells*) wound debris to prevent infection.	6 hours to 4 days
3	Proliferation/ granulation	Fibroblasts rebuild the base of the wound and pericytes regenerate the outer layers of capillaries (angiogenesis), endothelial cells rebuild the lining (granulation), keratinocytes create new epithelial tissue (epithelialization), and the wound begins to close (contracture).	5–21 days
4	Maturation/ remodeling	Fibroblasts rebuild, reinforce, and strengthen dermal tissues.	3 weeks to 2 years

process and prevent infection. Physicians use three types of wound healing protocols based on the severity of the wound.

- **Primary intention healing** is wound closure performed with sutures, staples, or adhesive tape or glue. It is used for uncomplicated lacerations and healing after most surgeries.
- **Secondary intention healing** is an extended process in which the wound is not closed with sutures but left open to granulate (*generate new connective tissue and vasculature*). The surgeon may pack the wound with gauze or use a drainage system. Wound care is performed daily to remove wound debris and allow for granulation. It is used for tooth extraction sockets burns, severe lacerations, and pressure ulcers.
- **Tertiary intention healing** is delayed primary closure. The wound is initially cleaned, debrided, and left open for observation for several days before closure. It is used for healing after a tissue graft.

Negative-pressure wound therapy (NPWT) is a treatment in which a sealed wound dressing is connected to a vacuum pump that removes fluids, debris, and infectious materials from the wound. The process helps promote granulation and is used with secondary or tertiary intention healing protocols. The type of healing undertaken provides information on the type of procedure performed. For example, when a physician documents, The wound was left to close by secondary intention, you know that no suturing was performed.

Mohs Micrographic Surgery

Mohs micrographic surgery is an advanced technique used to excise skin cancer lesions and is considered highly successful. It is used to remove large, complex, rapidly growing, recurring, or ill-defined skin cancer and requires that 100% of the surgical margin be examined. The roots of a skin cancer may extend beyond the visible portion of the tumor. If these roots are not removed, the cancer will recur. Examination of the surgical margin helps determine whether the entire malignancy has been removed.

What makes the Mohs technique unique is that one physician functions as both surgeon and pathologist. After the affected area has been numbed, the surgeon removes the visible tumor and a margin. This margin tissue is subdivided, put on slides, and examined under a microscope by the surgeon. If there is evidence of cancer, another layer of tissue is taken from the area where the cancer was detected. This ensures that only cancerous tissue is removed during the procedure, minimizing the loss of healthy tissue. These steps are repeated until all samples are free of cancer. Most tumors require one to three stages for complete removal.

Burns

Burns are classified based on the percentage of TBSA affected. Physicians estimate the extent, depth, and percentage of burns using the **Lund-Browder classification**, a system that identifies the percentage of the total body comprised by various body areas (■ FIGURE 37-2). It is similar in concept to the Rule of Nines used in diagnosis coding but is considered more accurate because it divides the body into smaller areas and accommodates the varying proportions of the body as children grow. Using a preprinted or electronic chart, the physician shades a diagram to show the areas of the body affected by first-, second-, and third-degree burns then determines the percentage of TBSA affected using the data in the accompanying table.

Tissue Transfer and Skin Replacement

When an area of skin is damaged to the extent that it will not heal on its own, a tissue transfer, skin graft, or skin substitute might be used. In an **adjacent tissue transfer/rearrangement (ATT/R)**, part of the skin transferred remains connected to its original site to maintain the blood supply when it is attached to the new site.

Skin replacement and skin substitutes include skin grafts and other materials to repair defects and replace skin. In an **autograft**, skin is removed from one area of the body—the donor site—and transferred to the recipient site, where the wound or defect exists. Autografts consist of grafts, flaps, and skin substitutes. In a **split-thickness skin graft (STSG)** (*a skin graft consisting of the epidermis and a portion of dermis or a mucosal graft consisting of only a partial thickness of mucosa*) or **full-thickness skin graft (FTSG)** (*a skin graft consisting of the epidermis and the full depth of the dermis*), skin from the donor site is completely removed from its connecting blood supply before the physician transfers it to the recipient site. In a **flap**, the blood supply remains intact, or the physician removes the skin and blood vessels and connects them to the recipient site. Flaps can also involve subcutaneous tissue, muscle, fascia, and bone.

Skin substitutes can be an **allograft** (*skin from another person*), **xenograft** (*skin from another species, such as a pig*), or a synthetic substitute. Because these materials are foreign to the recipient's body and will not be accepted long term, they are used for temporary coverage only while the patient grows new skin and must be replaced with an autograft.

Skin replacement procedures are generally named based on the visual configuration of the tissue, such as Z-plasty, W-plasty, rotation flap, or tubed flap. Refer to a pathophysiology text or reliable Internet resource to learn more about the specific types of graft and flaps.

Breast Removal and Reconstruction Procedures

Although physiologically the breast is classified as part of the reproductive system, breast procedures are classified with the Integumentary System in CPT because they involve the skin and subcutaneous tissue. Procedures are identified based on the

Area	Age (years)					% 1°	% 2°	% 3°	% Total
	0–1	1–4	5–9	10–15	Adult				
Head	19	17	13	10	7				
Neck	2	2	2	2	2				
Ant. trunk	13	13	13	13	13				
Post. trunk	13	13	13	13	13				
R. buttock	2½	2½	2½	2½	2½				
L. buttock	2½	2½	2½	2½	2½				
Genitalia	1	1	1	1	1				
R.U. arm	4	4	4	4	4				
L.U. arm	4	4	4	4	4				
R.L. arm	3	3	3	3	3				
L.L. arm	3	3	3	3	3				
R. hand	2½	2½	2½	2½	2½				
L. hand	2½	2½	2½	2½	2½				
R. thigh	5½	6½	8½	8½	9½				
L. thigh	5½	6½	8½	8½	9½				
R. leg	5	5	5½	6	7				
L. leg	5	5	5½	6	7				
R. foot	3½	3½	3½	3½	3½				
L. foot	3½	3½	3½	3½	3½				
					Total				

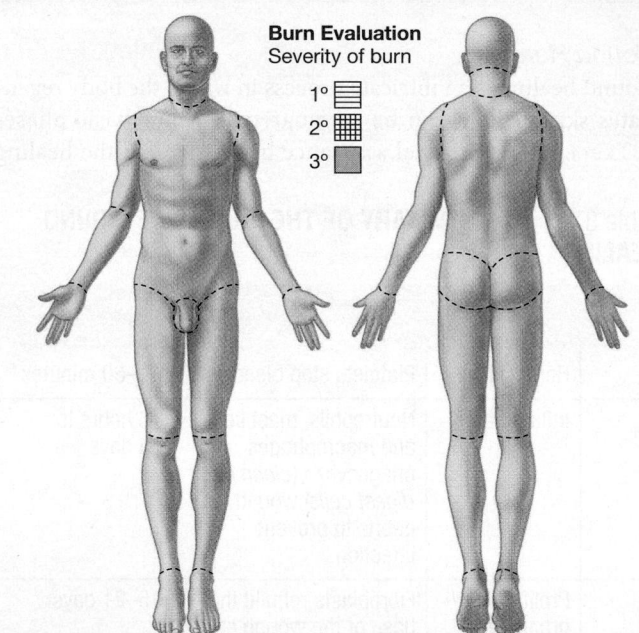

Burn Evaluation
Severity of burn

1°
2°
3°

Figure 37-2 ■ Lund-Browder Classification Chart for Burns

extent of skin, breast tissue, lymph nodes, and/or chest muscles removed. Breast reconstruction is performed using other muscles and tissue to replace the tissue removed. Procedures are named based on the technique and specific muscles used. ■ TABLE 37-4 identifies breast treatment and reconstruction procedures in progressive order, from least to most complex.

This section provides a general reference to help understand the most common integumentary system procedures. Remember to keep standard reference books handy in case you get stuck.

CODING PRACTICE *(continued)*

4. <u>rhytidectomy</u>, forehead   Meaning _____   CPT Code(s) _____
5. <u>mastopexy</u>   Meaning _____   CPT Code(s) _____
6. <u>blepharoplasty</u>   Meaning _____   CPT Code(s) _____
7. <u>hidradenitis</u>, excision   Meaning _____   CPT Code(s) _____
8. evacuation of hematoma, <u>subungual</u>   Meaning _____   CPT Code(s) _____
9. <u>escharotomy</u>, graft site   Meaning _____   CPT Code(s) _____
10. skin graft and flap, <u>fasciocutaneous</u>   Meaning _____   CPT Code(s) _____

CODING OVERVIEW OF INTEGUMENTARY SYSTEM PROCEDURES

The CPT subsection **Integumentary System (10030-19499)** contains seven subsections that are divided by anatomic site and type of procedure. Review the subheading and category names and code ranges listed in the Integumentary System table of contents, which appears at the beginning of the Integumentary System in the CPT manual, immediately after the Surgery section guidelines. Become familiar with the content and organization of this subsection. In this list, subheadings and categories followed by an asterisk (*) contain special instructions that provide guidelines for using codes in that subheading or category.

This chapter includes invasive, minimally invasive, and noninvasive surgical procedures on the skin, subcutaneous tissue, nails, and breast. Codes for diagnostic tests on the skin appear in the Medicine section. CPT codes in the Integumentary System subsection are frequently supported by diagnosis codes from ICD-10-CM **Chapter 12 Diseases of the Skin and Subcutaneous Tissue (L00-L99)** and **Chapter 14 Diseases of the Genitourinary System, Disorders of the Breast (N60-N65)**. Diagnosis codes for neoplasms, symptoms and signs, and superficial injuries (■ TABLE 37-5) also support Integumentary System procedures. ICD-10-CM codes for superficial injuries appear throughout the injury chapter **(S00-T88)** because injury codes are organized by anatomic site from head to foot, and the skin covers all sites. These are the codes most commonly used to support procedures on the integumentary system; however, diagnosis codes from any ICD-10-CM chapter are permissible.

CPT guidelines for the Surgery section apply to the Integumentary System. In addition, be alert for special instructions that provide definitions and coding guidelines at the beginning of many categories. Coding rules vary quite a bit for specific types of procedures within the Integumentary System, so the special instructions explain the relevant rules for each code category. In particular, study the special instructions for excision of benign and malignant lesions, wound repairs, and various types of flaps and grafts.

Instructional notes appear throughout the Tabular List to alert coders to the need for modifiers, provide cross-references to codes for similar procedures on other sites, identify when additional codes might be needed, and highlight resequenced and recently deleted codes.

The Integumentary System Tabular List contains many parent/indented code families and add-on codes. Indented code descriptions identify alternative anatomic sites where the parent code procedure can be performed, as well as alternative quantities, lengths, or sizes (square centimeters) of the affected area. Add-on codes identify additional quantities or sizes to be reported in addition to those of the stand-alone code.

ABSTRACTING INTEGUMENTARY SYSTEM PROCEDURES

Although the Integumentary System includes a variety of procedures, a few basic concepts apply to most procedures: site, complexity, size, method, and quantity. The details of these criteria vary for different classes of procedures, such as

Table 37-5 ■ **LOCATING ICD-10-CM AND ADDITIONAL CPT CODES FOR THE INTEGUMENTARY SYSTEM**

Type of Code	Codes
ICD-10-CM Integumentary System–related codes	
Integumentary system conditions	L00-L99, N60-N65
Neoplasms	C43-C44
Symptoms and signs	R20-R23
Injuries (superficial)	S00-T88
CPT Integumentary System–related codes	
Medicine procedures	96900-96999, 97597-97610
Radiologic procedures • Diagnostic radiology	77051-77059

Source: © PB Resources, Inc. Used with permission.

Table 37-6 ■ KEY CRITERIA FOR ABSTRACTING INTEGUMENTARY SYSTEM PROCEDURES

❑ What is the procedure?

❑ What is the anatomic site?

❑ What is the depth or complexity of the repair or treatment?

❑ What is the size (length or area) of site treated?

❑ What method is used?

❑ What is the quantity?

❑ Is a malignancy involved?

Source: © PB Resources, Inc. Used with permission.

excisions, repairs, and grafts. As discussed earlier, the size for lesion excisions is reported as diameter, wound repairs as length, and grafts as area, but size is still the basic criteria. Complexity is also reported differently. The complexity of burns is expressed as first, second, or third degree, whereas the complexity of wound repairs is expressed as wound depth and type of closure.

Refer to ■ TABLE 37-6 for guidance on how to abstract procedures on the Integumentary System, then work through the detailed example that follows. Remember that the abstracting questions are a guide and that not every question applies to, or can be answered for, every case. For example, not every procedure requires a length or area measurement.

Guided Example of Abstracting Integumentary System Procedures

Refer to the following example throughout this chapter to practice skills for abstracting, assigning, and arranging Integumentary System codes.

INPATIENT HOSPITAL   Gender: F   Age: 84

Preoperative diagnosis: Stage 4 pressure ulcer, right hip

Procedure: Excision of pressure ulcer with ischiectomy and flap closure, 30 sq cm. After administration of anesthesia, an incision was made around the ulcerated region of the ischium. The skin was cut in an elliptical fashion around the wound and the ulcerated tissue was excised down to the ischium bone; 1 cm of the ischium was excised. Purulent drainage was copiously irrigated. Defect area was 5 cm by 6 cm, needing a 30-sq cm repair. The patient's skin integrity adjacent to the ulcer was compromised, and I felt that an adjacent transfer rotational flap was contraindicated.

The abdominal tissue was intact, so a myocutaneous flap was created from the abdomen and relocated to cover the wound on the ischium. The surgical site was closed with staples and a 1/0 Jackson-Pratt drain was placed. The donor site, measuring 30 sq cm, was closed with an adjacent transfer rotational flap of 32 sq cm. Patient tolerated the procedure well and was transferred to postoperative care in stable condition. The excised tissue and bone fragments were sent to pathology.

Pathology report: Tissue consistent with decubitus ulcer. Bone fragments show evidence of osteomyelitis.

Postoperative diagnosis: Stage 4 pressure ulcer, right hip. Acute osteomyelitis of the ischium.

Follow along as fictitious coder, Joshua Grider, CPC, abstracts the procedure. Check off each step after you complete it.

▶ Joshua reads through the entire record, paying special attention to the reason for the encounter, the procedure performed, and the postoperative diagnosis. He refers to the Key Criteria for Abstracting Integumentary System Procedures (Table 37-6).

❑ He notes the diagnosis of Stage 3 pressure ulcer, right hip.

❑ *What is the anatomic site?* skin, right hip. Joshua understands that although the pressure ulcer is on the right hip, the organ system treated is the skin.

❑ *What is the primary procedure performed?* Excision of pressure ulcer

❑ *What is the depth or complexity of the repair or treatment?* Stage 4 pressure ulcer

❑ *What method is used?* excision

❑ *What is the quantity?* One

❑ *Is a malignancy involved?* No

❑ *What additional procedure is performed?* ischiectomy

❑ *What additional procedure is performed?* full-thickness myocutaneous flap closure

❑ *What is the size (area) of site treated?* 30 sq cm

▶ At this time, Joshua does not know which of these procedures may need to be coded, nor how many codes he will end up with. He will learn about this when he moves on to assigning codes.

CODING PRACTICE

Exercise 37.2 Abstracting Integumentary System Procedures

Instructions: Read the mini-medical-record of each patient's encounter and answer the abstracting questions. Write the answer on the line provided. Do not assign any codes.

---

1. OFFICE   Gender: F   Age: 39

Preprocedure diagnosis: rough scaly lesions on arms, face, and neck

Procedure: surgical curettement of 20 lesions ranging in size from 2 to 6 mm

Pathology report: premalignant actinic keratoses

Postprocedure diagnosis: premalignant actinic keratoses

a. What is the procedure? _____

b. What is the anatomic site? _____

c. What is the size of the lesions? _____

d. What method is used? _____

e. What is the quantity? _____

f. Is a malignancy involved? _____

---

2. INPATIENT HOSPITAL   Gender: M   Age: 26

Preprocedure diagnosis: multiple second-degree burns nearly covering both lower legs and feet

Procedure: removed blisters, debrided necrotic tissue, and applied dressings

Postprocedure diagnosis: leg burns, 21% TBSA second-degree

a. What is the procedure? _____

b. What is the anatomic site? _____

c. What is the depth or complexity of the repair or treatment? _____

d. What is the size (length or area) of the site treated? _____

e. What method is used? _____

---

3. INPATIENT HOSPITAL   Gender: F   Age: 35

Diagnosis: facial nerve paralysis from Bell palsy

Procedure: Harvested a fascia lata (*deep thigh*) free graft from right leg and applied to face to restore facial nerve function. Defect area 20 sq cm

a. What is the procedure? _____

b. Where is the recipient site? _____

c. Where is the donor site? _____

d. What type of donor tissue is used? _____

e. What is the size (length or area) of the site treated? _____

f. What method is used? _____

---

4. OUTPATIENT SURGERY   Gender: M   Age: 46

Preprocedure diagnosis: chronic infection and necrosis of the abdominal wall from internal dehiscence (*splitting open*) following a hernia repair 3 weeks ago

Procedure: Removed the mesh prosthesis from the hernia repair, then, using a curette, debrided 30 sq cm of subcutaneous tissue, fascia, and muscle in the abdominal wall. Applied antibiotics and packed with saline-soaked gauze for healing by secondary intention.

Postprocedure diagnosis: infection due to mesh prosthesis and internal wound dehiscence following ventral hernia repair

a. What is the primary procedure? _____

b. What is the anatomic site? _____

c. What is the depth or complexity of the repair or treatment? _____

d. What is the area of the site treated? _____

e. What method is used? _____

f. What additional procedure is performed? _____

g. What is the site of the secondary procedure? _____

---

5. OFFICE   Gender: F   Age: 37

Preprocedure diagnosis: suspicious lesions on back, arm, and hand

Procedure: Excised two lesions from the back, 1.5 and 2.1 cm including margins. One lesion from the arm, 0.5 cm including margins. One lesion from the hand, 0.4 cm including margins. All sites sutured in one layer. Tissue was submitted to pathology.

Pathology: Four specimens received, all consistent with malignant melanoma

Postprocedure diagnosis: malignant melanoma on back, arm, and hand

a. What is the procedure? _____

b. What is the anatomic site(s)? _____

c. What is the depth or complexity of the repair or treatment? _____

d. What is the size (length or area) of the site treated? _____

e. What method is used? _____

f. What is the quantity? _____

g. Is a malignancy involved? _____

6. EMERGENCY DEPT   Gender: F   Age: 16

Preprocedure diagnosis: *multiple lacerations from crash that occurred when she was driving an off-road vehicle in the woods*

Procedure: *Closed a 7.0-cm wound on the neck with a one-layer closure, a 2.5-cm wound on the face with heavy contamination requiring extensive debris removal and a simple closure, and a 10.2-cm wound on the right forearm with complex closure with debridement*   (*continued*)

6. (continued)

Postprocedure diagnosis: *lacerations*

a. What is the procedure? _____

b. What is the anatomic site? _____

c. What is the complexity of each repair? _____

d. What is the length of each wound? _____

e. What is the quantity? _____

ASSIGNING CODES FOR INTEGUMENTARY SYSTEM PROCEDURES

In addition to locating Main Terms and modifying terms for Integumentary System procedures in the Index, coders must understand how code families are organized in this subsection and how to determine the quantity applicable to the code. After reviewing these basics, essentials of coding for lesions, wound repair, mastectomy procedures, and skin grafts and flaps are highlighted.

Using the Index

To locate codes in the Integumentary System, search for the Main Term **Skin**, a first-level modifying term for the procedure, and a second-level modifying term for the details of the procedure. Do not select a Main Term for the anatomic site, such as back or arm, because these generally lead to codes about procedures on the structure itself, not on the skin covering the structure. If a Main Term for the procedure, such as **Excision**, or condition, such as **Lesion**, is selected, be sure to locate a first-level modifying term for Skin, not an anatomic site. Using the Main Term **Skin** is the most direct path to the code, and the code ranges listed in the Index are more detailed under **Skin** than under other potential Main Terms (■ FIGURE 37-3).

In addition to the Main Term **Skin**, the CPT Index provides separate Main Term entries for **Skin Graft and Flap** and **Skin Substitute Graft**, so be sure to look for these entries when coding these procedures. Procedures not performed directly on the skin are indexed under Main Terms that identify the site, such as **Nails** and **Pilonidal Cyst**.

Code Families

The Tabular List organizes many codes into code families divided by anatomic site and size, area, and/or complexity. Code families are clusters of parent codes and indented codes. The common descriptor (*the portion before the semicolon*) in the parent code applies to the indented codes and is part of the description of the indented code, even though it is not reprinted for each code number. Code families follow a specific structure within many code categories of the Integumentary System (■ FIGURE 37-4).

- The first portion of the parent code's common descriptor describes the *type of procedure* for category and is *similar* for all parent codes in the category.

- The second portion of the parent code common descriptor describes the *anatomic sites* included in the code family and applies to all codes in one family. However, this portion is *different* for each parent code in the category.

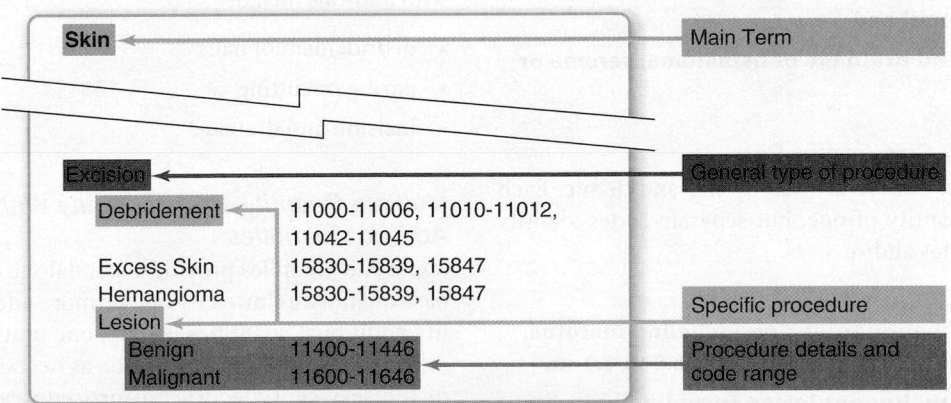

Figure 37-3 ■ CPT Index Entry for the Main Term Skin. *Source:* © *PB Resources, Inc. Used with permission. CPT codes only © American Medical Association.*

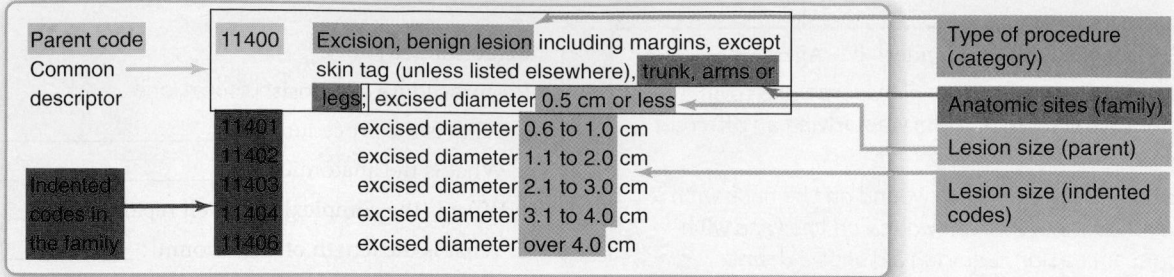

Figure 37-4 ■ Example of a Code Family in the Integumentary Subsection. *Source: Formatting © PB Resources, Inc. Used with permission. CPT codes only © American Medical Association.*

- The unique descriptor in the parent code and each indented code identifies the characteristics of the specific code, such as *size* or *quantity*. The unique descriptors tend to be *similar for all code families* within a category.

Determining Quantity

To determine the correct code in the integumentary system, coders must evaluate how the number of lesions or area of skin relates to the number of units identified in the code description. Methods of determining quantity include single quantity, single quantity by size and/or type, multiple quantiles, and add-together quantities. To understand the method used in a specific code family, read the code description and identify the unit of measure. Also read the surrounding codes for indented and add-on codes that report additional quantities and identify the type of quantities described.

Single Quantity

Single quantity refers to codes for which one unit is reported for each service performed. This is the default method for reporting CPT codes. Categories of skin procedures that use a single quantity include:

- incision and drainage (I&D)
- some nail procedures
- various other procedures

  For example:

- **11760 Repair of nail bed**
- **10140 Incision and drainage of hematoma, seroma or fluid collection**

Single Quantity By Size and/or Site

Single quantity codes can be divided by size and/or site. Each code identifies a quantity of one, but separate codes identify different anatomic sites and/or sizes.

  For example:

- **11601 Excision, malignant lesion including margins, trunk, arms, or legs; excised diameter 0.6 to 1.0 cm**
- **11621 Excision, malignant lesion including margins, scalp, neck, hands, feet, genitalia; excised diameter 0.6 to 1.0 cm**

Anatomic sites are grouped together based on the difficulty of treating the area. For example, the trunk, arms, and legs are often grouped together. Sizes or areas are reported in ranges. For example, lesions ranging in size from 0.6 to 1.0 cm are grouped together by site. Lesions of the same anatomic group and size range can be coded with multiple units. Categories of skin procedures that use a single quantity by size and site include:

- shaving of epidermal or dermal lesions
- excision of benign and malignant lesions
- destruction of malignant lesions
- some nail procedures

Details on assigning codes (with regard to coding lesions) using this type of quantity are discussed later in this chapter.

Multiple Quantity Ranges

A code family can be organized to report quantities of more than one for a particular procedure. Each code in the family reports a different quantity or range. Coders must read all the code descriptions in the code family to determine the correct range to use. For example:

- **11720 Debridement of nail(s) by any method(s); 1 to 5**
- **11721 Debridement of nail(s) by any method(s); 6 or more**

Select the code that identifies the quantity of the service performed. Categories of procedures that use a multiple quantity with add-ons include:

- debridement of nails
- paring or cutting
- incision and drainage

Multiple Quantity, Base Quantity With Add-on Quantities

Some code families provide a standalone code that identifies a base quantity followed by one or more add-on codes that identify additional quantities. Report one unit of the base code and as many units of the add-on code as necessary to report the rest of the service. Categories of procedures that use a multiple quantity with add-ons include:

- destruction of benign or premalignant lesions
- removal of skin tags
- tissue transfer and replacement

Physician removes 10 skin tags using electrosurgical destruction and 23 skin tags using chemical destruction, for a total of 33.

11200 Removal of skin tags, multiple fibrocutaneous tags, any area; up to and including 15 lesions

11201 x 2 Removal of skin tags, multiple fibrocutaneous tags, any area; each additional 10 lesions, or part thereof (List separately in addition to code for primary procedure)

Figure 37-5 ■ Example of Coding Multiple Quantities

In the example in ■ FIGURE 37-5, codes for skin tag removal include all methods, so the 33 lesions can be combined for coding purposes. Report **11200** for the first 15 lesions, leaving 18 lesions. Each unit of **11201** reports up to 10 lesions, so the first unit reports the 16th to 25th lesions; the second unit reports the 26th to 33rd lesions. Do not append modifier **–51** to code **11201** because it is an add-on code.

Add-Together Quantities

Procedures that involve measurement of length and area require that multiple measurements be added together. Sum the measurement of areas in the same anatomic grouping and of the same level of complexity. For example, the lengths of all intermediate wound repairs on the scalp, axillae, trunk, and extremities are summed to arrive at a total combined length:

- **12036 Repair, intermediate, wounds of scalp, axillae, trunk and/or extremities (excluding hands and feet); 20.1 cm to 30.0 cm**

Categories of procedures that use add-together quantities include:

- wound repair
- skin replacement surgery
- adjacent tissue transfer or rearrangement
- skin flaps
- burns, local treatment

Details about how to assign codes for these types of procedures are discussed later in this chapter.

SUCCESS STEP

Annotating your CPT coding manual can help you navigate the extensive list of parent and indented code families. In each parent code description, highlight the anatomic sites included. In each indented description, highlight the size. Highlighting only *selected* words within each description, rather than highlighting the entire description, makes it easier to identify the differences. This helps make your coding faster and more accurate.

Lesion Removal

To assign codes for lesion removal, you need to determine the following criteria:

- method of removal
- whether the lesion is benign, premalignant, or malignant

- anatomic site
- size

To locate codes in the Index, search for the Main Term **Skin**; the first-level modifying term for the method used, such as **Destruction**, **Excision**, **Shaving**, **Paring**, or **Removal**; and additional modifying terms, if necessary, for the type of lesion. The modifying term **Removal** is used for skin tags. Identify the code range and turn to the Tabular List to select and verify the code(s).

The Tabular List provides detailed special instructions at the beginning of categories for lesion removal. Take time to read and understand these definitions and instructions. To select a code in the Tabular List, follow the following steps.

1. Confirm that you have the correct category based on the method of removal, type of lesion, and benign or malignant status.

2. Review the parent codes in the code families to identify the correct anatomic group. Lesion sites are grouped into three code families: (1) trunk, arms, and legs; (2) sites on the face; (3) scalp, neck, hands, feet, and genitalia (■ FIGURE 37-6).

3. Select the code for the appropriate lesion size. Read the size options provided with the indented codes to determine the appropriate code. All sizes are given as a range. There is no additional code or modifier to identify the exact size of a specific lesion.

4. When more than one lesion of same size range in the same anatomic group is excised, report a multiple quantity for the code (■ FIGURE 37-7).

5. Assign separate codes for multiple lesions of different sizes or different anatomic groups.

A physician measures the size of the lesion before removing it. In excisions, size is determined by the diameter of the lesion itself plus the most narrow margin (*healthy tissue around the lesion*) required to adequately excise it, based on the physician's judgment (■ FIGURE 37-8). Adequate margins are necessary to prevent regrowth of the lesion and are especially important with malignant lesions. Lesion measurements are reported in centimeters.

The global surgical package concept applies to codes for lesion removal. Codes for shaving of epidermal and dermal lesions have a postoperative global period of 0 days. Codes for removal of skin tags and excision of lesions and most codes for destruction of a lesion have a 10-day postoperative global period. Destruction of cutaneous vascular proliferative lesions (**17103-17108**) has a 90-day global period. Local anesthesia and simple, nonlayered closure of the operative wound is included in the code. Do not assign additional codes for these bundled services. When a wound resulting from an excision requires an intermediate or complex closure, assign an additional code for the repair. Repair codes are discussed next.

When the physician uses electrocautery to remove the entire lesion, do not assign a code for shaving. Instead, assign a code for destruction of a lesion (**17000–17250**). Shaving does not require suture closure of the wound.

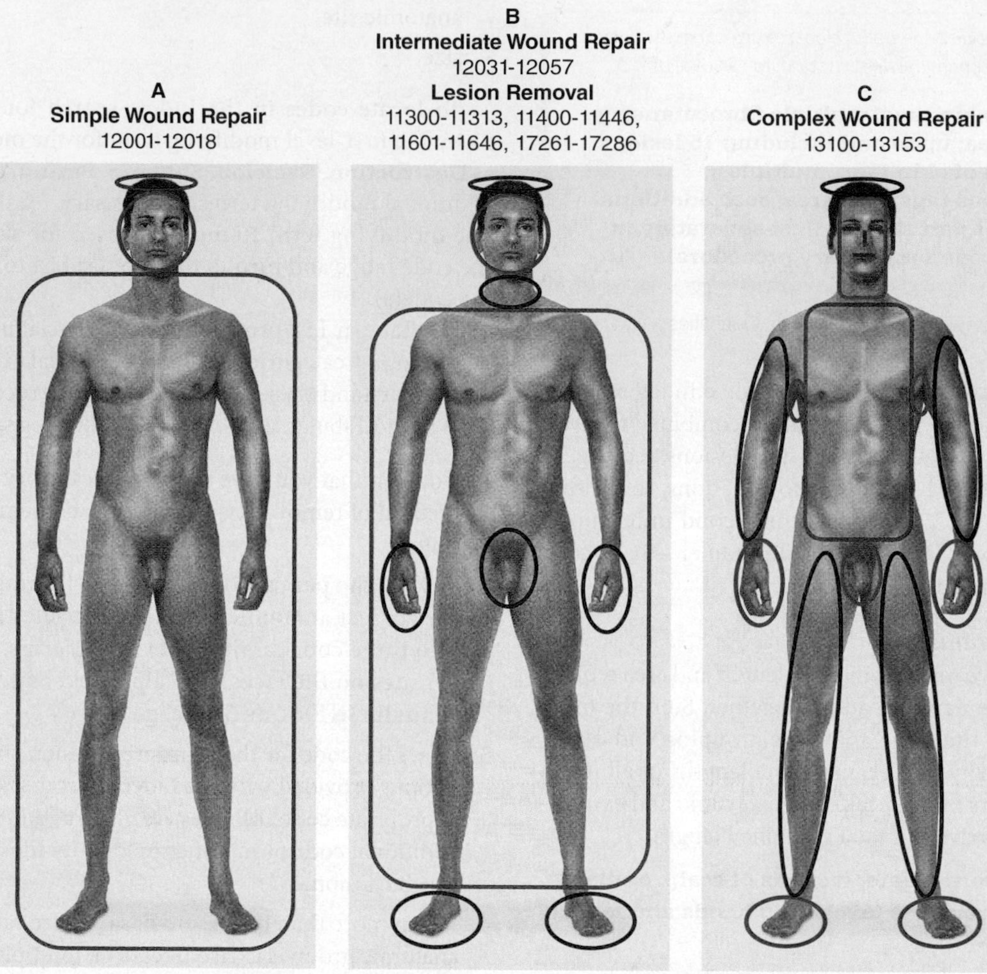

A
Simple Wound Repair
12001-12018

B
Intermediate Wound Repair
12031-12057
Lesion Removal
11300-11313, 11400-11446,
11601-11646, 17261-17286

C
Complex Wound Repair
13100-13153

Figure 37-6 ■ Code Families for Lesion Removal and Wound Repair

SUCCESS STEP

All parent codes for anatomic groupings have indented codes for similar sizes. Identify the correct anatomic code family *first*, then select the code for lesion size.

Mohs Micrographic Surgery

To assign codes for Mohs, search the Index for the Main Term **Mohs Micrographic Surgery**, then refer to the code range in the Tabular List. To select codes in the Tabular List, determine the number of blocks (*each division of the tissue*) and stages (*each phase of excision*) involved in the procedure.

The code category includes special instructions that define the process and five codes. The two parent codes (**17311**

and **17313**) are divided based on anatomic site and include up to five tissue blocks. The *first* stage of excision is described by the parent code. Each *additional* stage is reported with add-on codes (**17312** and **17314**). When more than five tissue blocks are examined, report add-on code **17315** for each additional block.

When one of the functions—surgeon or pathologist—is delegated to a physician who reports codes separately, the procedure is no longer Mohs, so the codes in this category should not be used.

Physician excises the two benign lesions, one of 0.75 cm from the right arm and one of 1.0 cm from the right leg.

11401-51 x 2 Excision, benign lesion including margins, except skin tag (unless listed elsewhere), trunk, arms or legs; excised diameter 0.6 to 1.0 cm

Figure 37-7 ■ Example of Coding Excision of a Lesion

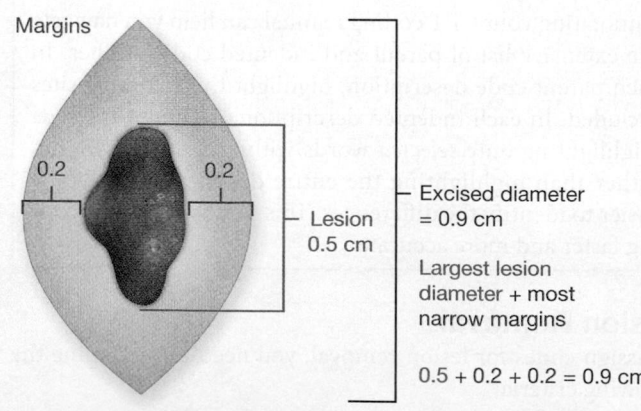

Margins

0.2   0.2

Lesion
0.5 cm

Excised diameter
= 0.9 cm

Largest lesion
diameter + most
narrow margins

0.5 + 0.2 + 0.2 = 0.9 cm

Figure 37-8 ■ How to Calculate Lesion Size

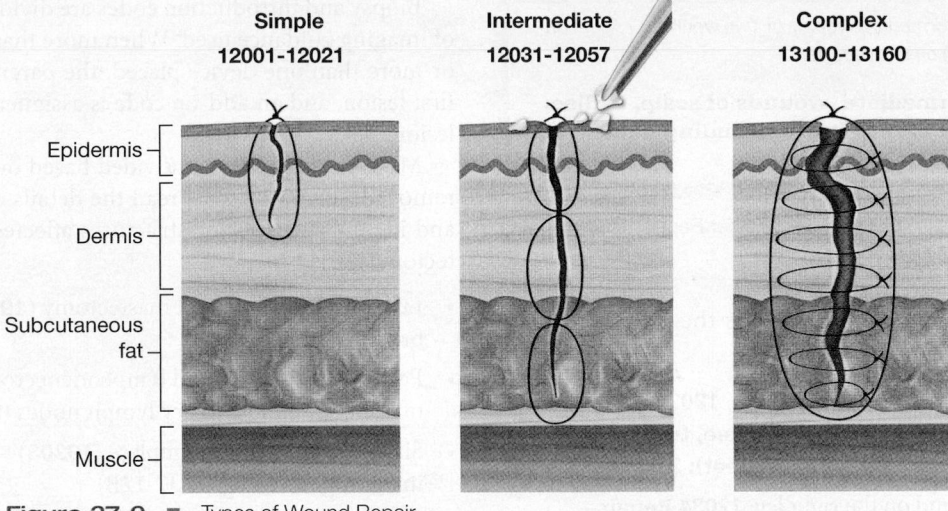

Simple
12001-12021

Intermediate
12031-12057

Complex
13100-13160

Epidermis

Dermis

Subcutaneous fat

Muscle

Figure 37-9 ■ Types of Wound Repair

Wound Repair

To assign a code for wound repair, you need to determine the following criteria:

- anatomic site
- complexity of the repair
- length

To locate codes in the Index, search for the Main Term **Wound Repair**, the first-level modifying term for the anatomic site, and a second-level modifying term for the complexity of the repair. Identify the code range and turn to the Tabular List to select and verify the code(s).

Wound repairs are classified as simple, intermediate, or complex based on the depth of the wound, the amount of debris, and the need for extensive site preparation, reconstruction, or repair (■ FIGURE 37-9). The special instructions under the **Repair (Closure)** subheading, before code **12001**, define the various types of repair, bundled services, and additional coding. Read these carefully to ensure that you assign codes accurately.

To select a code in the Tabular List, follow the following steps.

1. Confirm that you have the correct category based on the complexity of the repair.

2. Review the parent codes in the code families to identify the correct anatomic group. Select the code for the appropriate lesion length. Read the size options provided with the indented codes to determine the appropriate code. ■ FIGURE 37-10 shows metric measurements used to classify lengths

of wound repair compared to an adult's arm. All sizes in code descriptions are given as a range. There is no additional code or modifier to identify the exact size of a specific wound.

3. When more than one wound of the same complexity in the same anatomic group is excised, sum the lengths of all wounds and select the code that identifies the total combined length.

4. Assign separate codes for wound repairs of different complexities or different anatomic groups.

The anatomic sites for wound repair codes are different for each type of repair. Read the parent code of each code family within the category to determine how the sites are grouped:

- Simple repair—2 code families: (1) all sites except the face and (2) sites on the face (see Figure 37-6A)

- Intermediate repair—3 code families: (1) trunk, arms, and legs; (2) sites on the face; and (3) scalp, neck, hands, feet, and genitalia (see Figure 37-6B)

- Complex repair—4 code families: (1) trunk; (2) scalp, arms, and legs; (3) forehead, cheeks, chin, mouth, neck, axillae, genitalia, hands, and feet; and (4) eyes, nose, mouth, and ears (see Figure 37-6C)

In the example in ■ FIGURE 37-11, the two intermediate repairs occur within the same anatomic group (scalp, axillae, trunk, and/or extremities), so the lengths of the wounds are added together (7.5 + 8.0 = 15.5) to arrive at the correct code, **12035**.

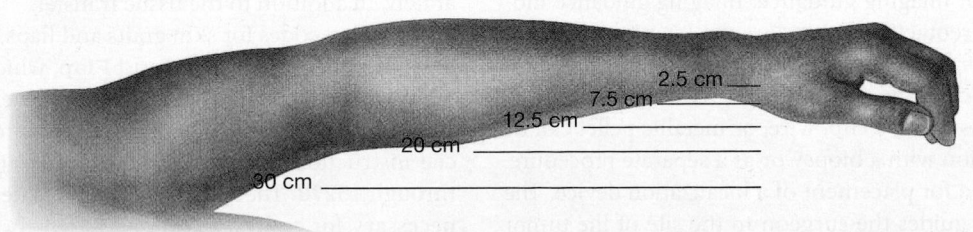

2.5 cm

7.5 cm

12.5 cm

20 cm

30 cm

Figure 37-10 ■ Approximate Lengths Relative to an Adult Arm

> Physician performs intermediate repair of two wounds: 7.5 cm on the right arm and 8 cm on the right leg.

> **12035 Repair, intermediate, wounds of scalp, axillae, trunk and/or extremities (excluding hands and feet); 12.6 cm to 20.0 cm**

Figure 37-11 ■ Example of Adding Together Repair Lengths

If either wound were coded alone as the only repair, the codes would be as follows:

- For the 7.5-cm wound on the right arm: **12032 Repair, intermediate, wounds of scalp, axillae, trunk and/or extremities (excluding hands and feet); 2.6 cm to 7.5 cm**

- For the 8.0-cm wound on the right leg: **12034 Repair, intermediate, wounds of scalp, axillae, trunk and/or extremities (excluding hands and feet); 7.6 cm to 12.5 cm**

Do not report the two codes separately when the procedures are performed at the same time because CPT special instructions state: **When multiple wounds are repaired, add together the lengths of those in the same classification (see above) and from all anatomic sites that are grouped together into the same code descriptor.**

Do not combine repairs of different complexity, such as a simple repair and an intermediate repair, and do not combine repairs of different anatomic groupings, such as an intermediate repair of the trunk and an intermediate repair of the face.

The global surgical package concept applies to codes for wound repair, which have a 10-day postoperative global period. Local anesthesia is included in the code.

Simple closure of operative wounds for excision of lesions is included in the lesion removal. When a wound resulting from an excision requires an intermediate or complex closure, assign a code for the repair in addition to the code for the lesion removal.

Breast Procedures

Breast procedures include biopsy, cyst and lesion excision, mastectomy, repair, and reconstruction. To assign codes, locate the Main Term **Breast** in the Index, then locate the first-level modifying term for the type of procedure. Second-level modifying terms identify details of the procedure and provide the code(s) or code range.

The Breast subheading in the Tabular List provides special instructions for the **Excision** and **Introduction** categories. The **Excision** instructions also provide guidelines for **Mastectomy**, even though it is a separate category.

Biopsy procedures can be percutaneous or open (incisional) and with or without imaging guidance. Imaging guidance modalities include stereotactic mammography (*specialized mammography imaging from two angles at the same time*), ultrasound (US), and magnetic resonance imaging (MRI). In addition, a localization device such as a clip, wire, or metallic pellet can be placed in conjunction with a biopsy or as a separate procedure. Imaging is also used for placement of a localization device. The localization device guides the surgeon to the site of the tumor during surgery performed at a later time.

Biopsy and introduction codes are divided based on the type of imaging guidance used. When more than one site is biopsied or more than one device placed, the parent code identifies the first lesion, and an add-on code is assigned for each additional lesion.

Mastectomy codes are divided based on the extent of tissue removed, so coders must read the details of the operative note and identify the specific structures affected. The types of mastectomy are:

- Lumpectomy or partial mastectomy (**19301**)—part of the breast

- Partial mastectomy and lymphadenectomy (**19302**)—part of the breast and axillary lymph nodes (■ FIGURE 37-12A)

- Simple mastectomy, complete (**19303**)—the entire breast, including skin (Figure 37-12B)

- Subcutaneous mastectomy (**19304**)—the breast tissue under the skin but not the skin itself (Figure 37-12C)

- Modified radical mastectomy (**19307**)—the breast, pectoralis minor (but not pectoralis major) muscle, and axillary lymph nodes (Figure 37-12D)

- Radical mastectomy (**19305**)—the breast, pectoralis major and minor muscles, and axillary lymph nodes

- Radical mastectomy (Urban-type operation) (**19306**)—the breast, pectoralis major and minor muscles, axillary lymph nodes, and internal mammary lymph nodes (Figure 37-12D)

Repair and reconstruction codes are divided based on the type of reconstructive technique and type of flap. Refer to the documentation to identify the technique used, then select the corresponding code.

Mastectomy codes are unilateral, so when the same type of procedure is performed on both breasts, assign modifier **-50 Bilateral procedure**. When a different type of mastectomy is performed on each breast, assign the appropriate code and assign the modifier **-RT** or **-LT** to identify the laterality.

Skin Replacements

CPT provides separate coding paths for various types of skin replacement procedures. To assign codes for adjacent tissue transfers, search the Index for the Main Term **Skin** and the first-level modifying term **Adjacent tissue transfer**. One code range is provided, so turn to the Tabular List to select and verify the code. Codes are divided into code families by anatomic site, then are arranged by size within the site. The size identifies the area of the defect. Adjacent tissue transfers include lesion excisions, so do not report them separately. Adjacent tissue transfers include simple repair; however, when the physician performs intermediate or complex repair, report the repair separately, in addition to the tissue transfer.

To assign codes for skin grafts and flaps, search the Index for the Main Term **Skin Graft and Flap**, which is a separate Main Term entry after **Skin**. Locate the first-level modifying term for the type of graft or flap. The Tabular List provides extensive special instructions for this category, which includes codes **15002** through **15278**. The special instructions define the terminology necessary for code selection and identify procedures that are bundled and those that are coded separately. Codes are divided

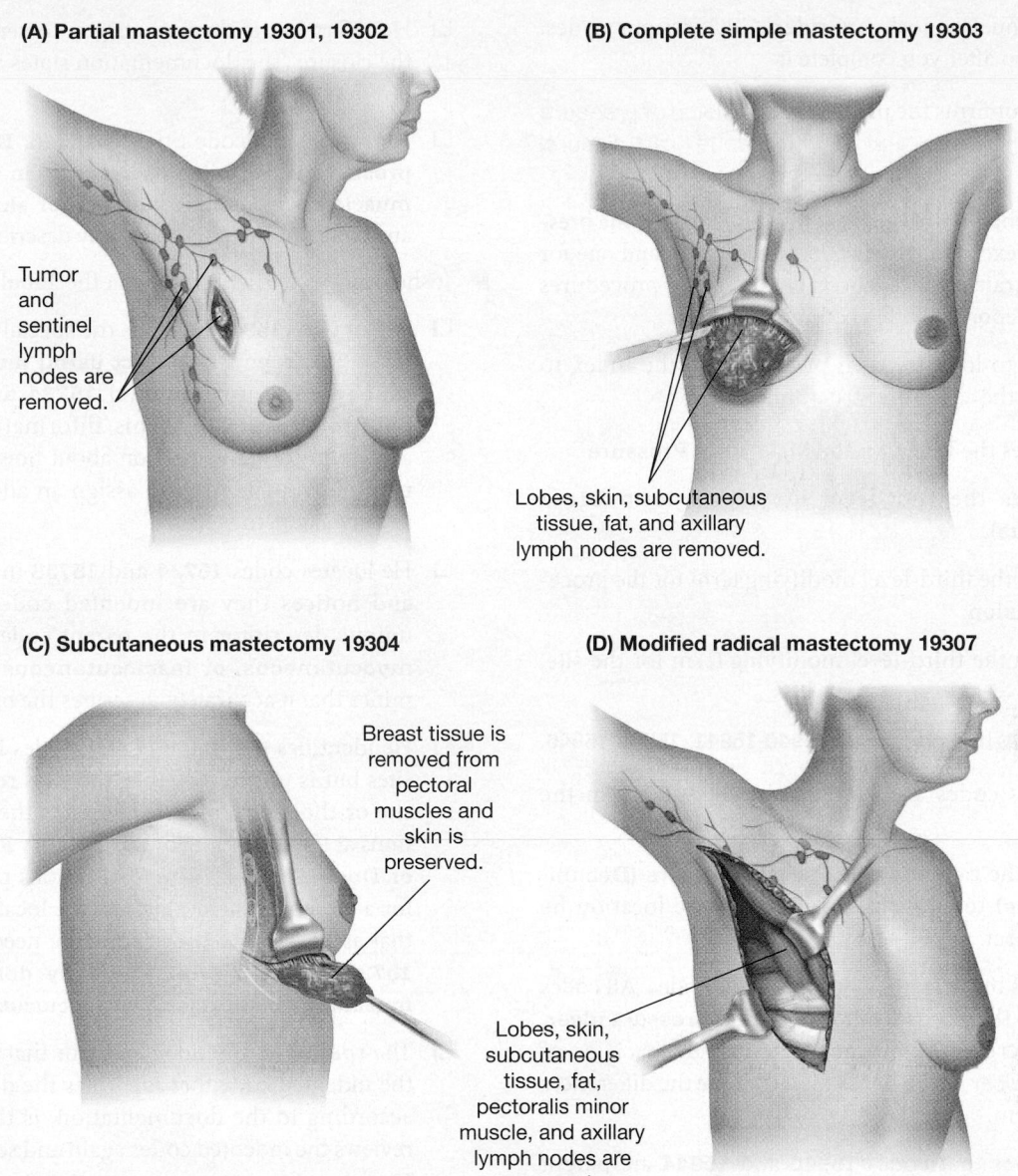

(A) Partial mastectomy 19301, 19302

Tumor and sentinel lymph nodes are removed.

(B) Complete simple mastectomy 19303

Lobes, skin, subcutaneous tissue, fat, and axillary lymph nodes are removed.

(C) Subcutaneous mastectomy 19304

Breast tissue is removed from pectoral muscles and skin is preserved.

(D) Modified radical mastectomy 19307

Lobes, skin, subcutaneous tissue, fat, pectoralis minor muscle, and axillary lymph nodes are removed.

Figure 37-12 ■ Types of Mastectomy Procedures

by the type of graft, such as epidermal, dermal, split thickness, full thickness, and tissue culture, then by anatomic site and size. Many of the code families for anatomic site provide a parent code for a specific area, such as 25 or 100 sq cm, and an add-on code for each additional unit of the same size. The parent code has a higher RVU than the add-on codes.

To assign codes for skin substitute grafts, search the Index for the Main Term **Skin Substitute Graft**, which is a separate Main Term entry after the entries for **Skin** and **Skin Graft and Flap**. Locate the first-level modifying term for the anatomic site. The Tabular List special instructions at the beginning of the category **Skin Replacement Surgery** apply to the subcategory for **Skin Substitute Grafts**. Codes are divided by anatomic site and size. Many of the code families for anatomic site provide a parent code for a specific area, such as 100 sq cm, and an add-on code for each additional unit of the same size. Coding instructions state that the areas listed in code descriptors pertain to the recipient site, not the donor site.

Codes also are provided for surgical preparation or creation of a recipient site for a graft, flap, skin replacement, or skin substitute (**15002–15005**), which involves cleaning the site and ensuring that the surface is appropriate for repair of the defect. Do not report codes **15002–15005** for surgical preparation and debridement of a wound left to heal by secondary intention, which is a wound without surgical closure that heals on its own. Instead, report wound management or debridement codes.

When the physician must repair a donor site with a skin graft or local flap, assign one code for the recipient site procedure and an additional code for the donor site repair.

Guided Example of Assigning Integumentary System Procedure Codes

To practice skills for assigning codes for the Integumentary System, continue with the example from earlier in the chapter about a patient who was seen for a pressure ulcer. Follow along in your CPT manual as Joshua Grider, CPC, assigns codes. Check off each step after you complete it.

▶ First, Joshua confirms the procedures, Excision of pressure ulcer with ischiectomy and myocutaneous graft closure, 30 sq cm.

- ❑ He is not sure if he needs three codes—one for the pressure ulcer excision, one for the ischiectomy, and one for the skin graft closure—or if one or more procedures might be reported with a combination code.

- ❑ He needs to look up each procedure in the Index to learn how the codes are structured.

▶ Joshua searches the Index for the Main Term **Pressure**.

- ❑ He locates the first-level modifying term **Ulcer (Decubitus)**.

- ❑ He locates the third-level modifying term for the procedure, **Excision**.

- ❑ He locates the third-level modifying term for the site, **Ischial**.

- ❑ He identifies the code ranges **15940-15941, 15944-15946**.

▶ Joshua locates codes **15940-15941, 15944-15946** in the Tabular List.

- ❑ He reads the category title **Pressure Ulcers (Decubitus Ulcers)** to confirm that he is in the location he would expect.

- ❑ He reviews the range of five contiguous codes. All codes begin with the words **Excision, ischial pressure ulcer**, which describes the procedure performed, excision of pressure ulcer, so he needs to determine the differences among them.

- ❑ He observes that codes **15940** and **15944** are parent codes, each with an indented code, **15941** and **15945**, respectively, that states **with ostectomy (ischiectomy)**. Code **15946** is a standalone code that also includes **with ostectomy**.

- ❑ The procedure he is coding includes with ischiectomy and 1 cm of the ischium was excised. He must read the remaining portion of the code descriptions to select the most appropriate code.

- ❑ To determine the difference between codes **15941** and **15945**, he knows that he must refer to the common descriptor in each parent code because it also applies to the indented code. He identifies that the difference between the parent codes is the nature of the wound closure. Code **15940** describes **with primary suture** and code **15945** describes **with skin flap closure**. He thinks this might be the right code, but knows he should also check code **15946**.

- ❑ The description for code **15946** states **in preparation for muscle or myocutaneous flap or skin graft closure**.

- ❑ He refers to the documentation to verify the nature of the closure. The documentation states a myocutaneous flap was created.

- ❑ He rereads the code title for **15946, Excision, ischial pressure ulcer, with ostectomy, in preparation for muscle or myocutaneous flap or skin graft closure** and confirms that this accurately describes the procedure.

▶ Joshua checks for instructions in the Tabular List.

- ❑ Under code **15946** he reads the special instructions that state: **(For repair of defect using muscle or myocutaneous flap, use code(s) 15734 and/or 15738 in addition to 15946.)** This information provides an answer to Joshua's question about how many codes are needed by telling him to assign an additional code for the myocutaneous flap.

- ❑ He locates codes **15734** and **15738** in the Tabular List and notices they are indented codes. He reads the unique descriptor in the parent code **15732 Muscle, myocutaneous, or fasciocutaneous flap;** and determines that it accurately describes the base procedure.

- ❑ He identifies that the indented codes identify alternate sites but is unsure whether the sites refer to the donor site or the recipient site. He reads the special instructions at the beginning of the category **Flaps (Skin and/or Deep Tissues)**. The instructions provide guidance for a variety of situations, and he locates the statement that applies to the code family he needs to use: **Codes 15732-15738 are described by donor site of the muscle, myocutaneous, or fasciocutaneous flap.**

- ❑ The special instructions confirm that he should select the indented code that identifies the donor site, which, according to the documentation, is the abdomen. He reviews the indented codes again and selects code **15734 Muscle, myocutaneous, or fasciocutaneous flap; abdomen**.

- ❑ He rereads the special instructions and notices a comment about repair of the donor site: **A repair of a donor site requiring a skin graft or local flaps is considered an additional separate procedure.** He checks the documentation and identifies: The donor site . . . was closed with an adjacent transfer rotational flap.

- ❑ Because the donor site was closed with a local flap, he needs to assign an additional code. Instructional notes below the special instructions provide a cross-reference: **(For adjacent tissue transfer flaps, see 14000-14302)**.

▶ Joshua needs to assign a code for the adjacent transfer rotational flap at the donor site.

- ❑ He locates codes **14000-14302** and reviews how they are organized. He identifies several pairs of parent codes and indented codes. He determines that the parent codes are divided by anatomic site and the indented codes are divided by defect size.

❏ He identifies that the common descriptor in parent code **14000** includes the trunk: **Adjacent tissue transfer or rearrangement, trunk;**. The area defined by **14000** is a **defect 10 sq cm or less** and the area defined by the indented code **14001** is a **defect 10.1 sq cm to 30.0 sq cm.**

❏ He refers to the documentation to verify the size of the defect, which is *5 cm by 6 cm, needing a 30-sq cm repair.* This information points to code **14011** because it includes the appropriate area.

❏ Joshua reads the special instructions for the category **Adjacent Tissue Transfer or Rearrangement.** He reads the last paragraph that begins with the statement **Skin graft necessary to close secondary defect is considered an additional procedure.** As he reads the rest of the paragraph, he learns that he might have incorrectly determined the size of the defect area. He had previously identified the size of the defect at the recipient site, but the special instructions state that he should determine the area of the secondary, or donor, site and that the measurement includes the size of the defect *plus* the size of the transfer necessary to repair it.

❏ He refers to the documentation again and locates the measurements of the secondary (donor) site: *The donor site, measuring 30 sq cm, was closed with an adjacent transfer rotational flap of 32 sq cm.* The secondary defect is 30 cm and the transfer necessary to repair it is 32 cm, for a total of 62 sq cm. Now he must determine how to code the new size of the repair.

❏ When he rereads code **14001**, he determines that this code is no longer appropriate because it describes a **defect 10.1 sq cm to 30.0 sq cm.** Because it does not say *each additional 30.0 sq cm*, he knows that he cannot report multiple units of this code, such as ×2 or ×3.

❏ He reviews all the codes in the category **14000-14350** to look for possible add-on codes.

❏ He locates code **14301 Adjacent tissue transfer or rearrangement, any area; defect 30.1 sq cm to 60.0 sq cm**. He recognizes that this code is used to report an ATT larger than the 30 sq cm allowed by code **14001**. However, the total secondary defect is 62 sq cm, so he still needs an additional code.

❏ He identifies the add-on code **14302 Adjacent tissue transfer or rearrangement, any area; each additional 30.0 sq cm, or part thereof** and the instructional note that follows: **(Use 14302 in conjunction with 14301)**. This instructional note directs him to report code **14302** for the **additional 30 sq cm** with code **14301**, *not* code **14002**.

❏ He reviews all the code descriptions, special instructions, and instructional notes again and is confident he has selected the appropriate codes.

▶ Joshua reviews the procedure codes he has assigned for this case.

❏ **14001 Adjacent tissue transfer or rearrangement, trunk; defect 10.1 sq cm to 30.0 sq cm**

❏ **14302 Adjacent tissue transfer or rearrangement, any area; each additional 30.0 sq cm, or part thereof (List separately in addition to code for primary procedure)**

❏ **15946 Excision, ischial pressure ulcer, with ostectomy, in preparation for muscle or myocutaneous flap or skin graft closure**

❏ **15734 Muscle, myocutaneous, or fasciocutaneous flap; trunk**

▶ Next, Joshua must determine how to sequence the codes.

CODING PRACTICE

Exercise 37.3   Assigning Codes for Integumentary System Procedures

Instructions: Read the mini-medical-record of each patient's encounter. Review the information abstracted in Exercise 37.2 for questions 1–3. For questions 4–6, abstract the case on your own. Assign CPT codes, quantities, and modifiers using the Index and Tabular List. Write the code(s) on the line provided.

1. OFFICE   Gender: F   Age: 39

Preprocedure diagnosis: *rough scaly lesions on arms, face, and neck*

Procedure: *surgical curettement of 20 lesions ranging in size from 2–6 mm*

Pathology report: *premalignant actinic keratoses*

Postprocedure diagnosis: *premalignant actinic keratoses*

1 CPT Code _____

(continued)

CODING PRACTICE (continued)

2. INPATIENT HOSPITAL Gender: M Age: 26

Preprocedure diagnosis: multiple second-degree burns nearly covering both lower legs and feet

Procedure: removed blisters, debrided necrotic tissue, and applied dressings

Postprocedure diagnosis: leg burns, 21% TBSA second-degree

1 CPT Code _____

3. INPATIENT HOSPITAL Gender: F Age: 35

Diagnosis: facial nerve paralysis from Bell palsy

Procedure: Harvested a fascia lata (*deep thigh*) free graft from right leg and applied to face to restore facial nerve function. Defect area 20 sq cm

1 CPT Code _____

4. OUTPATIENT SURGERY Gender: M Age: 4

Preprocedure diagnosis: wound, right thigh

Procedure: Applied acellular dermal replacement on the right thigh as a temporary repair. Defect was measured and consists of 1% of the patient's body area
(*continued*)

4. (continued)

Postprocedure diagnosis: wound, to heal by secondary intention, RTO 1 week

1 CPT Code _____

5. OFFICE Gender: M Age: 16

Diagnosis: acne

Procedure: Chemical exfoliation (*peeling off layers of skin*). Applied salicylic acid over the acne with a cotton-tipped swab, let rest for a few seconds to desquamate (*peel off*) the acne. Treatment was successful.

1 CPT Code _____

6. OFFICE Gender: F Age: 55

Preprocedure diagnosis: breast reconstruction following a left breast mastectomy

Procedure: Tattooed nipples on both breasts, total area of 15 sq cm

1 CPT Code _____

ARRANGING CODES FOR INTEGUMENTARY SYSTEM PROCEDURES

Multiple coding is common for Integumentary System procedures because more than one lesion removal or wound repair is often performed at the same time. Multiple procedures can be identified by reporting multiple quantities of one code, using add-on codes, using additional standalone codes, and/or appending modifier(s). Read code descriptions carefully to determine which method should be used with any specific code. Although codes are usually arranged (sequenced) based on complexity, or RVU value, the process is not as intuitive as it might be with other types of procedures.

Sequencing Excision of Lesion Codes

The complexity of Integumentary System procedures is affected both by the size of the lesion or defect and by the anatomic site. For lesions of differing sizes but the same anatomic code family, excision of the larger lesion always has a higher RVU. For lesions of the same size but different anatomic code families, excision of lesions of the trunk, arm, or legs has the lowest RVU; excision of lesions of the scalp, neck, hands, and feet has the next highest RVU; and excision of lesions of the face, ears, eyelids, mouth, lips, and mucous membrane has the highest RVU. Excision of a malignant lesion has a higher RVU than excision of a benign lesion of the same size and same anatomic site. However, when lesions are different sizes and of different anatomic code families, no general rule applies.

Use the quantity designation **x 2** when two procedures are performed and both are described by the same code.

Example: Excision of benign lesions, 0.6 cm on the arm and 0.75 cm on the leg: **11401 x 2**

Append modifier **-51 Multiple procedures** to the second and subsequent codes (■ FIGURE 37-13). The lesions of the right arm and right leg are identified by the same code, so two units of code **11401** are reported. Sequence codes in descending RVU order. Append modifier **-51** to the second and third codes.

CODING CAUTION

Add together the lengths of similar repairs or the areas of similar grafts, but *do not* add together the diameters of multiple excised lesions. Report each lesion separately.

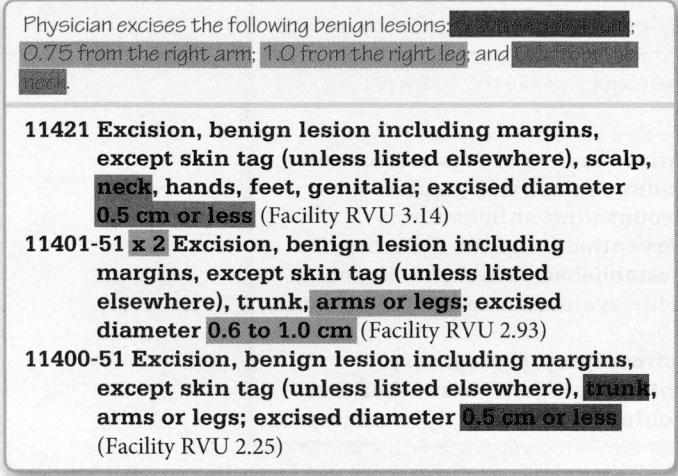

Figure 37-13 ■ Example of Sequencing Codes for Excision of Lesions. *Source:* © *PB Resources, Inc. Used with permission. CPT codes only* © *American Medical Association.*

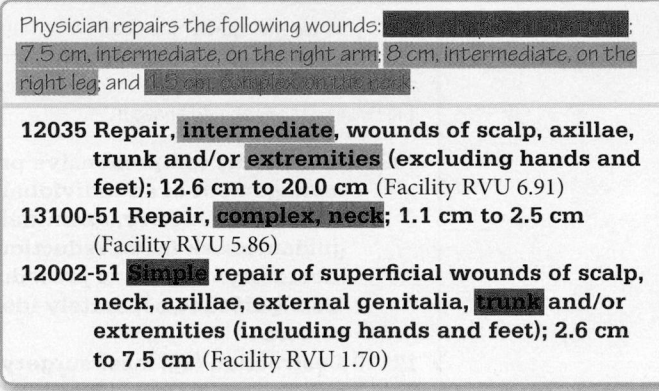

Figure 37-14 ■ Example of Sequencing Wound Repair Codes. *Source:* © *PB Resources, Inc. Used with permission. CPT codes only* © *American Medical Association.*

Sequencing Wound Repair Codes

The RVUs for repair codes are affected by the complexity of the repair, the length, and the anatomic code family. A small complex repair can have a lower RVU value than a longer simple or intermediate repair. No general rule applies, so the Medicare Physician Fee Schedule Database (MPFSDB)—or other payer's source—must be consulted to obtain RVU information.

Compare the facility RVU for the intermediate repair code **12053** for a 5.1- to 7.5-cm wound to complex repair codes for 1.1- to 2.5-cm wounds. Code **12053** for an intermediate repair of 5.1 to 7.5 cm has a *higher* RVU than code **13100** but a *lower* RVU than code **13120**:

- **12053 Repair, intermediate, wounds of face, ears, eyelids, nose, lips and/or mucous membranes; 5.1 cm to 7.5 cm** (6.20 RVU)

- **13100 Repair, complex, trunk; 1.1 cm to 2.5 cm** (5.86 RVU)

- **13120 Repair, complex, scalp, arms, and/or legs; 1.1 cm to 2.5 cm** (6.72 RVU)

After adding together wound repairs of the same anatomic code family and same complexity, sequence codes in descending RVU order. Append modifier -51 **Multiple procedures** to the second and third codes (■ FIGURE 37-14).

Using Modifiers with Integumentary System Codes

Several modifiers are commonly used when coding procedures from the Integumentary System subsection. These include modifier -25, which might be used on an E/M code in conjunction with an integumentary system procedure; several laterality and anatomic modifiers; modifier -51 for multiple procedures; modifier -58 for staged procedures; and modifier -59 to identify a separate procedure in certain circumstances. These modifiers are discussed next.

-25 Significant, separately identifiable E/M

Removal of lesions is often a relatively simple procedure and may be done when a patient is being seen for another reason, such as an annual physical. When a separately identifiable E/M service is provided at the same time as lesion removal (or any procedure), assign an E/M code in addition to the procedure. Append modifier **-25 Significant, separately identifiable evaluation and management service by the same physician or other qualified health care professional on the same day of the procedure or other service** to the E/M code only. Do not apply the modifier to the procedure code. The modifier informs the payer that the E/M is a separate service that should be paid. To use this modifier, the E/M service should be a separate and significant workup, in addition to the evaluation of the lesion (■ FIGURE 37-15).

Laterality Modifiers

Because the skin is not a bilateral organ, do not use modifiers **-50 Bilateral procedure**, **-RT Right**, and **-LT**, except on the breast.

Example: Mastotomy of the left breast with drainage of an abscess, deep: **19020-LT**

Example: Simple repair of a 2.5-cm laceration on the left cheek: **12011**

Use HCPCS Level II modifiers **FA-F9** for the fingernails, but not for the skin on the fingers; use modifiers **TA-T9** for the toenails, but not for the skin on the toes.

Example: Evacuation of a subungual hematoma on the right great toe: **11740-T5**

Example: Shaving of an epidermal lesion on the right great toe: **11300**

-51 Multiple Procedures

Use modifier **-51 Multiple procedures** when two different procedures are performed on the same date by the same provider. Append **-51** to the second procedure only.

Example: Excision of benign lesions, 0.6 cm on arm and 1.5 cm on leg: **11402, 11401-51**

A 37 year old male patient is seen for an annual physical. During the examination, the patient asks about a dark spot on the neck that "comes and goes." The physician identifies the lesion as benign seborrheic keratosis, removes it using cryotherapy, and instructs the patient that if it returns, they should shave it.

99395-25 Periodic comprehensive preventive medicine reevaluation and management of an individual including an age and gender appropriate history, examination, counseling/anticipatory guidance/risk factor reduction interventions, and the ordering of laboratory/diagnostic procedures, established patient; 18-39 years; -25 Significant, separately identifiable evaluation and management service

17110 Destruction (eg, laser surgery, electrosurgery, cryosurgery, chemosurgery, surgical curettement), of benign lesions other than skin tags or cutaneous vascular proliferative lesions; up to 14 lesions

Figure 37-15 ■ Example of Using Modifier -25 with the Integumentary System

-58 Staged Procedure

A staged procedure is one that is usually planned in advance to be performed during the postoperative period of another related procedure. The staged procedure may be planned or anticipated, be more extensive than the original procedure, or represent a therapy following the original surgical procedure. Modifier **-58 Staged or related procedure or service by the same physician or other qualified health care professional during the postoperative period** alerts the payer that the second procedure was performed as part of the overall treatment for the condition and is not part of the global surgical package.

Examples of staged procedures that may be performed on the integumentary system include the insertion of a prosthesis after a skin graft, removal of a malignancy following a biopsy, or breast reconstruction following a mastectomy (■ FIGURE 37-16).

Do not use modifier **-58** in the following circumstances. Instead, code as indicated.

- A problem related to the first procedure that requires a return to the operating room during the global period. Use modifier **-78 Unplanned Return to the Operating/ Procedure Room by the Same Physician**.

- Procedures during the global period that are *unrelated* to the original procedure. Use modifier **-79 Unrelated Procedure or Service by the Same Physician**.

- Related procedures with a global period of 0 days performed during the global period of another procedure. Report these as part of the surgical package.

- Procedures described as staged in the code descriptor, such as Mohs micrographic surgery. Report the code(s) for the procedures performed, following CPT special instructions.

- Procedures following a related procedure that has a global period of 0 days, such as some biopsies. Report the second procedure without a modifier.

-59 Distinct Procedural Service

Use modifier **-59 Distinct procedural service** to report two procedures performed at the same time but not normally performed together, such as a different site, different lesion, different incision/excision, or codes that can be reported only when performed as a separate and distinct procedure; the phrase (**separate procedure**) often appears in the code description.

Example: Radical resection of a 3-cm sarcoma from the forearm and excision of a separate, benign lesion 0.6 cm from the forearm during the same session: **25077, 11404-59**.

Some payers may require that the HCPCS modifier **-XS Separate structure** be reported instead of modifier **-59** to clarify that a second site was treated.

Guided Example of Arranging Integumentary System Procedure Codes

To practice skills for arranging codes for procedures of the Integumentary System, continue with the example from earlier in the chapter about the patient who was seen for a pressure ulcer excision. Follow along in your CPT manual as Joshua Grider, CPC, arranges the codes. Check off each step after you complete it.

▶ First, Joshua confirms the procedure, area, and anatomic sites.

   ❑ Excision of pressure ulcer with ischiectomy, myocutaneous flap closure, 30 sq cm

   ❑ Myocutaneous flap created from the abdomen, donor site 30 sq cm, closed with an adjacent transfer rotational flap of 32 sq cm

6/6/yy: Surgeon performs a quadrantectomy on the right breast of a 47 year old woman, after an incisional biopsy done on 6/1/yy was positive for carcinoma. The incisional biopsy procedure (19101) has a global period of 10 days.

19301-58-RT Mastectomy, partial (eg, lumpectomy, tylectomy, quadrantectomy, segmentectomy); -58 Staged procedure; -RT Right side

Figure 37-16 ■ Example of Using Modifier -58 with the Integumentary System

▶ Joshua reviews the procedure codes.

❑ **14001 Adjacent tissue transfer or rearrangement, trunk; defect 10.1 sq cm to 30.0 sq cm**

❑ **14302 Adjacent tissue transfer or rearrangement, any area; each additional 30.0 sq cm, or part thereof (List separately in addition to code for primary procedure)**

❑ **15946 Excision, ischial pressure ulcer, with ostectomy, in preparation for muscle or myocutaneous flap or skin graft closure**

❑ **15734 Muscle, myocutaneous, or fasciocutaneous flap; trunk**

▶ Joshua arranges the codes in descending RVU order according to the Medicare Physician Fee Schedule Database (MPFSDB). He uses the facility RVU because the procedure was performed at the hospital, not at the physician's office. The RVU order is consistent with what Joshua intuitively expected; however, this is not always the case.

❑ **15946** Facility RVU = 47.09

❑ **15734** Facility RVU = 37.90

❑ **14001** Facility RVU = 18.59

❑ **14302** Facility RVU = 6.37

▶ Joshua reviews the codes to determine the need for modifiers. (Refer to Table 30-1 Key Criteria for Abstracting CPT Modifiers or Appendix A in the CPT manual.)

❑ Code **15946** does not require a modifier because it is the primary procedure and there are no extenuating circumstances. A modifier for laterality is not required because the skin is not a bilateral organ.

❑ Code **15734** requires modifier **-51 Multiple procedures** because it was performed during the same operative session as another procedure. The payment will be reduced to 50% of the usual fee.

❑ Code **14001** requires modifier **-51 Multiple procedures** because it was performed during the same operative session as another procedure. The payment will be reduced to 50% of the usual fee.

❑ Code **14302** does not require a modifier because it is an add-on code.

▶ Joshua finalizes the procedure codes and sequencing for this case:

(1) **15946 Excision, ischial pressure ulcer, with ostectomy, in preparation for muscle or myocutaneous flap or skin graft closure**

(2) **15734-51 Muscle, myocutaneous, or fasciocutaneous flap; trunk; -51 Multiple procedures**

(3) **14001-51 Adjacent tissue transfer or rearrangement, trunk; defect 10.1 sq cm to 30.0 sq cm; -51 Multiple procedures**

(4) **14302-51 Adjacent tissue transfer or rearrangement, any area; each additional 30.0 sq cm, or part thereof (List separately in addition to code for primary procedure)**

▶ Joshua also assigns and sequences the ICD-10-CM diagnosis codes that support the need for the service.

(1) **L89.2 Pressure ulcer of right hip, stage 4**

(2) **M86.059 Other acute osteomyelitis, unspecified femur**

CODING PRACTICE

Exercise 37.4 Arranging Codes for Integumentary System Procedures

Instructions: Read the mini-medical-record of each patient's encounter. Review the information abstracted in Exercise 37.2 for questions 1–3. For questions 4–6, abstract the case on your own. Assign CPT codes, quantities, and modifiers using the Index and Tabular List, and arrange the codes in proper sequence. Write the code(s) on the line provided.

---

1. OUTPATIENT SURGERY   Gender: M   Age: 46

Preprocedure diagnosis: *chronic infection and necrosis of the abdominal wall from internal dehiscence (splitting open) following a hernia repair 3 weeks ago*

(continued)

---

1. (continued)

Procedure: *Removed the mesh prosthesis from the hernia repair, then, using a curette, debrided 30 sq cm of subcutaneous tissue, fascia, and muscle in the abdominal wall. Applied antibiotics and packed with saline-soaked gauze for healing by secondary intention.*

Postprocedure diagnosis: *infection due to mesh prosthesis and internal wound dehiscence following ventral hernia repair*

Tip: A modifier is needed because this procedure was performed during the 90-day global period for the hernia repair.

2 CPT Codes _____

(continued)

CODING PRACTICE (continued)

2. OFFICE   Gender: F   Age: 37

Preprocedure diagnosis: suspicious lesions on back, arm, and hand

Procedure: Excised two lesions from the back, 1.5 and 2.1 cm, including margins. One lesion from the arm, 0.5 cm including margins. One lesion from the hand, 0.4 cm including margins. All sites sutured in one layer. Tissue was submitted to pathology.

Pathology: Four specimens received, all consistent with malignant melanoma

Postprocedure diagnosis: malignant melanoma on back, arm, and hand

Tip: In this exercise, codes for the larger lesions earn higher RVUs. RVUs for codes of the *same size range* but different families are ranked as follows: The code family for the scalp, neck, hands, feet, and genitalia has the highest RVUs. The code family for trunk, arms, or legs has the lowest RVUs.

4 CPT Codes _____

_____

3. EMERGENCY DEPT   Gender: F   Age: 16

Preprocedure diagnosis: multiple lacerations from crash that occurred when she was driving an off-road vehicle in the woods

Procedure: Closed a 7.0-cm wound on the neck with a one-layer closure, a 2.5-cm wound on the face with heavy contamination requiring extensive debris removal and a simple closure, and a 10.2-cm wound on the right forearm with complex closure with debridement

Postprocedure diagnosis: lacerations

Tip: Add together the length of wounds in the same code family of related anatomic sites.

4 CPT Codes _____

_____

4. OFFICE   Gender: F   Age: 14

Preprocedure diagnosis: multiple lesions

Procedure: 1.0 cm with 0.5-cm margins from the cheek, 2.0 cm with 1.0-cm margins from the neck, and 3.0 cm with 0.5-cm margins from the forehead

Pathology report: benign lesions

Postprocedure diagnosis: benign lesions

2 CPT Codes _____

5. OFFICE   Gender: F Age: 23

Preprocedure diagnosis: epidermal lesions

Procedure: Injected local anesthesia and using a #15 scalpel performed shave removal of a 0.5-cm lesion from the right eyelid, a 0.6-cm lesion from the left eyelid, and a 1.0-cm lesion from the left cheek

Pathology report: 3 specimens submitted, all benign lesions

Postprocedure diagnosis: benign epidermal lesions

Tip: Identify the code family(ies), determine the number of lesions in each code family, then identify the number of lesions in the size range listed in each code.

2 CPT Codes _____

6. OFFICE   Gender: F   Age: 23

Preprocedure diagnosis: malignant lesions

Procedure: Mohs micrographic surgery. Removed lesion from right arm, prepared six tissue blocks, which under microscopic examination showed clear margins. Removed lesion from hand, prepared three tissue blocks. Margins were not clear under microscopic examination, so removed additional tissue, which was divided into two tissue blocks. Both blocks were clear under microscopic examination. All sites closed with sutures.

Postprocedure diagnosis: squamous cell carcinoma

Tip: Two procedures were performed: one that required one stage and one that required two stages. Assign a code for each procedure's first stage. Assign a code for each additional stage. Determine the number of tissue blocks examined for each code and assign a code for any excess blocks. Sequence codes by descending RVU: 17311 (18.32 RVU), 17312 (17.13 RVU), 17313 (17.13 RVU), 17314 (10.30 RVU), 17315 (2.21 RVU).

4 CPT Codes _____

_____

E/M CODING FOR DERMATOLOGY

The *1997 Documentation Guidelines for Evaluation and Management Services* (1997 DG), published by CMS, provides requirements for each level of an examination of the skin (■ FIGURE 37-17). Dermatologists are not limited to using the guidelines for a skin examination only. They can also use guidelines for a general multiorgan system examination, or any other single organ system examination, based on what is most advantageous for a specific encounter. However, physicians cannot combine elements from more than one type of examination for a given encounter. The skin examination guidelines typically provide the best results when a detailed skin examination is performed.

To determine the appropriate E/M code, coders must review the documentation in detail and identify the specific elements documented.

- To translate the documentation into the E/M requirements for the history, refer back to Chapter 31, Evaluation and Management (E/M) Services (99201-99499), Tables 31-7 to 31-10, or to the 1997 DG.

- To determine the requirements for an examination, refer to Figure 37-17 or to the single organ system examination for the skin in the 1997 DG.

- To determine the levels for medical decision making (MDM), refer to Chapter 31, Tables 31-11 and 31-12, and also to the Table of Risk in the 1997 DG.

Guided Example of E/M Coding for Integumentary System

Refer to the dermatology encounter (■ FIGURE 37-18) to practice skills for abstracting and assigning E/M codes. Follow along as fictitious coder Joshua Grider, CPC, abstracts the procedure. Check off each step after you complete it.

▶ First, Joshua needs to establish the category of service so he can determine the information needed to abstract and assign the code.

❑ *What is the setting?* Urgent care clinic, which is office or other outpatient.

❑ *What is the type of service?* Established.

❑ *What is the code range?* Joshua refers to the CPT Index and looks up the Main Term **Office or Other Outpatient Services** and the first-level modifying term **Office visit**, then the second-level modifying term **Established patient**. The code range listed is **99211-99215**.

❑ *How many key components are required?* Joshua refers to the code range in the Tabular List and reads the code description of the first full code (**99211** is a nurse-only visit), which states **Office or other outpatient visit for the evaluation and management of an established patient, which requires at least 2 of these 3 key components**. Codes **99212-99215** in the category have the same requirements for key components. This tells him that two of three key components must meet or exceed the levels listed in the code (2/3).

▶ Next, Joshua identifies the level of history.

❑ *What is the level of HPI?* The HPI is **Extended** because four or more elements are documented.

❑ *What is the level of ROS?* There is no ROS because no systems are documented.

❑ *What is the level of PFSH?* The PFSH is **Pertinent** because one element is documented.

❑ *Based on these factors, what is the overall level of history?* The level of history is **Problem focused** because the lowest of the three factors (HPI, ROS, and PFSH) determines the history level. The ROS qualifies for a problem-focused history. Although the HPI and PFSH qualify for higher levels of history, Joshua is restricted to selecting the overall history level based on the ROS, which is the lowest.

▶ Joshua refers to the Skin examination in the 1997 DG (Figure 37-17) to abstract information needed to determine the level of the examination.

❑ *What is the level of examination?* The level of examination is **Problem focused**. One bulleted element of the examination is documented, which meets the requirement of one to five bulleted elements for a problem-focused examination.

▶ Joshua determines the level of medical decision making. (Refer to Table 31-12 Medical Decision Making Levels.)

❑ *What is the level of complexity of the number of diagnoses or management options, based on the presenting problem?* The level is **Moderate** because there is a new presenting problem, without workup.

❑ *What is the amount and/or complexity of data to be reviewed?* No data are reviewed.

❑ *What is the level of risk of significant complications, morbidity, and/or mortality?* He reviews each column in the Table of Risk in the 1995 DG and determines that the level of risk is **Moderate**. The patient presents with one stable chronic illness (Low), clinical labs are reviewed but not ordered, and prescription drug management is required (Moderate). The single highest element in the Table of Risk determines the overall risk. The column **Management options selected** is the highest level (Moderate).

❑ *Based on these factors, what is the overall level of medical decision making?* The medical decision making is **Moderate complexity**. At least two of the three MDM factors are required to qualify for a specific level of MDM. Two of the three MDM factors—the nature of the presenting problem and the level of risk—meet moderate-level decision making. Although the data factor is at a lower level (none), it can be disregarded because two of the three factors meet the criteria for **Moderate complexity**.

CODING PRACTICE (continued)

5. Refer to Table 31-12 Medical Decision Making Levels or the 1997 DG.

   a. What is the MDM level for the number of diagnoses or management options? _____

   b. What is the MDM level for the amount and/or complexity of data to be reviewed? _____

   c. Refer to the Table of Risk in the 1997 DG. Which elements of risk are documented for each risk factor?

      1. Presenting problem: _____

      2. Diagnostic procedures ordered: _____

      3. Management Options Selected: _____

   d. What is the level of risk? (The highest of the three areas determines the overall level of risk.) _____

   e. What is the overall level of MDM? (2/3 MDM factors are needed to determine the overall level.) _____

6. a. What is the setting? _____

   b. What is the patient (or service) type? _____

   c. What is the code range? _____

   d. How many key components are required? _____

   e. What is the level of history? _____

   f. What is the level of examination? _____

   g. What is the level of medical decision making? _____

   h. What is the correct code? _____

7. Abstract, assign, and arrange (sequence) the diagnosis code that supports the E/M code.

   1 ICD-10-CM Code(s) _____

CHAPTER SUMMARY

In this chapter you learned that:

- Coders must understand the basic principles of measurements and wound healing when working with excision procedures and wound repair. Additional procedures to be familiar with are Mohs micrographic surgery, burns, tissue transfer and skin replacement, and breast removal and reconstruction.

- The CPT subsection **Integumentary System (10030-19499)** contains seven subsections that are divided by anatomic site and type of procedure.

- Although the Integumentary System includes a variety of procedures, a few basic concepts apply to most procedures: site, complexity, size, method, and quantity.

- To locate codes in the Integumentary System, search for the Main Term **Skin**, a first-level modifying term for the procedure, and a second-level modifying term for the details of the procedure. The

- Tabular List organizes many codes into code families divided by anatomic site and size, area, and/or complexity.

- Multiple coding is common for Integumentary System procedures because more than one lesion removal or wound repair is often performed at the same time. Read code descriptions carefully to determine whether multiple procedures require reporting of multiple quantities of one code, use of add-on codes, use of additional standalone codes, and/or modifier(s).

- The *1997 Documentation Guidelines for Evaluation and Management Services* (1997 DG), published by CMS, provides requirements for each level of an examination of the skin.

- CPT provides special instructions and instructional notes throughout the Integumentary System that define terminology and bundling rules.

CONCEPT QUIZ

Take a moment to look back at the Integumentary System and solidify your skills. Try to answer the questions from memory, first, then refer to the discussion in this chapter if you need a little extra help.

Completion

Instructions: Write the term that answers each question based on the information you learned in this chapter. Choose from the list to the right. Some choices may be used more than once and some choices may not be used at all.

abrasion	flap transfer
adjacent tissue transfer/ rearrangement	intermediate
allograft	ligature
autograft	Mohs micrographic surgery
cryotherapy	shaving
destruction	simple
excision	skin replacement
flap graft	skin substitute
	tattooing

1. _____ is performed by injecting a colored pigment into the skin.

2. _____ is moving a section of skin and subcutaneous tissue from one site to another, with blood vessels intact, and anastomosis to vessels at the recipient site.

3. _____ uses a sharp instrument to remove an epidermal or dermal lesion without a full-thickness excision.

4. _____ is a procedure that removes skin tags by tying off the skin tag at its base with thread.

5. _____ is using liquid nitrogen to remove lesions by destroying the tissue.

6. _____ involves relocating a section of skin or flap from a donor site that is immediately next to the damaged skin and can be moved without completely detaching it.

7. A(n) _____ uses a patient's own tissue from one site to replace damaged tissue at another site.

8. A(n) _____ wound repair is a one-layered closure of epidermis, dermis, or subcutaneous tissue without significant involvement of deeper structures.

9. _____ is a multistage procedure in which a malignant lesion is excised in microscopic layers and the physician performing the procedure also performs the pathological evaluation of each tissue layer.

10. A(n) _____ is the use of synthetic (artificial) material to temporarily repair or replace damaged skin.

Multiple Choice

Instructions: Circle the letter of the best answer to each question based on the information you learned in this chapter.

1. What type of measurement identifies the distance between two points and is used to classify length of wound repairs and diameter of excised lesions?
   A. Metric unit
   B. Total body surface area
   C. Area measurement
   D. Linear measurement

2. How should the excision of multiple lesions be reported?
   A. Sum the diameters of all lesions.
   B. Report the diameter of each lesion separately.
   C. Report the percentage of TBSA affected.
   D. Report only the largest lesion.

3. What tool helps physicians estimate the extent, depth, and percentage of body area affected by burns?
   A. Complexity of burns chart
   B. Total body surface area formula
   C. Lund-Browder classification
   D. Burn rate chart

4. How should Integumentary System codes be reported when specific instructions are not provided in the code description or special instructions?
   A. Single quantity
   B. Length
   C. Single quantity by size and/or type
   D. Diameter

5. Which type of procedure restores normal function or appearance as it relates to the Integumentary System?
   A. Restorative
   B. Repair
   C. Revive
   D. Reconstructive

6. What type of graft involves skin from another species, such as a pig, and is used for temporary coverage while the patient grows new skin?
   A. Free flap graft
   B. Autograft
   C. Xenograft
   D. Flap transfer graft

7. What type of measurement defines a space inside a boundary and is used to classify the amount of skin treated in a tissue repair or skin graft?
   A. Area conversion
   B. Area measurement
   C. Add-on code
   D. Intermediate unit

8. What type of procedure obtains tissue for pathologic examination and is performed independently or is unrelated or distinct from other procedures/services provided at that time?
   A. Biopsy
   B. Excision
   C. Paring/cutting
   D. Shaving

9. What type of skin graft consists of the epidermis and a portion of the dermis?
   A. Punch graft
   B. Split-thickness skin graft
   C. Pedicle flap skin graft
   D. Rotational flap skin graft

10. How should the debridement of multiple wounds be reported?
    A. Sum the length of all wounds that are at the same depth
    B. Sum the length of all wounds
    C. Sum the surface area of wounds that are at the same depth
    D. Sum the surface area of all wounds

CODING CHALLENGE

Instructions: Read the mini-medical-record of each patient's encounter, then abstract, assign, and arrange ICD-10-CM diagnosis codes and CPT procedure codes using the appropriate Index and Tabular List. Assign quantities and modifiers where needed. Write the code(s) on the line provided.

1. OUTPATIENT SURGERY   Gender: M   Age: 39

Preprocedure diagnosis: Male pattern baldness

Procedure: Hair transplant, 21 punch grafts

1 ICD-10-CM Code _____

1 CPT Code _____

2. OUTPATIENT SURGERY   Gender: M   Age: 22

Preprocedure diagnosis: Ingrown toenail, right great toe

Procedure: Wedge excision of the skin of the nail fold, right great toe

Postprocedure diagnosis: Ingrowing nail, right great toe

1 ICD-10-CM Code _____

1 CPT Code _____

3. OFFICE   Gender: M   Age: 43

Preprocedure diagnosis: Skin lesion, left forearm; two skin lesions, left shoulder region

Procedure: Punch biopsy of three lesions

Postprocedure diagnosis: Blue nevus, left forearm; blue nevus, left shoulder region ×2

Pathology report: 3 lesions consistent with blue nevi

Tip: Obtaining tissue specifically for pathologic examination is distinct and unrelated to any other procedure/services provided during this encounter.

1 ICD-10-CM Code _____

3 CPT Codes _____

_____

4. EMERGENCY DEPARTMENT   Gender: F   Age: 26

Preprocedure diagnosis: Multiple lacerations from a motor vehicle accident where she was a passenger in a car

Procedure: Layered closure of a 20.3-cm laceration of the face; one-layer closure of a 4.0-cm laceration of the neck; one-layer closure of a 5.5-cm laceration of the face; layered closure (superficial fascia) of a 15.2-cm laceration of the face

(continued)

4. (continued)

Postprocedure diagnosis: Wound repair of multiple lacerations of the face and neck

Tip: ICD-10-CM: Remember to code the External Cause and Intent of the reported injury(ies).

CPT: When multiple wounds are repaired, add together the lengths of those in the same classification and from all anatomic sites that are grouped together.

3 ICD-10-CM Codes _____

_____

3 CPT Codes _____

_____

5. OUTPATIENT SURGERY   Gender: F   Age: 57

Preprocedure diagnosis: Suspected carcinoma of the skin; two lesions on each arm and one lesion on the forehead

Procedure: Performed Mohs procedure on two lesions on each arm, first stage, 3 blocks on each lesion. Pathology confirmed. Performed Mohs procedure on one lesion on forehead; first stage, 2 blocks. Pathology confirmed.

Postprocedure diagnosis: Basal cell carcinoma of the skin of both arms and the skin of the forehead

Pathology report: Confirms basal cell carcinoma of the skin on each arm and the skin of the forehead

Tip: The surgeons treated a total of 12 blocks in first stage for both arms (2 lesions on each arm = 4 lesions × 3 blocks each = 12)

3 ICD-10-CM Codes _____

_____

3 CPT Codes _____

_____

6. INPATIENT HOSPITAL   Gender: F   Age: 46

Preprocedure diagnosis: Left breast cancer with metastasis to the regional axillary lymph nodes

Procedure: Removed the entire left breast, pectoral muscles, and left axillary lymph nodes

Postprocedure diagnosis: Invasive ductal carcinoma, left breast with metastasis to the regional axillary lymph nodes

2 ICD-10-CM Codes _____

1 CPT Code _____

7. OFFICE Gender: F Age: 41

Preprocedure diagnosis: Annual checkup, established patient

Procedure: During the examination, the patient asked to have skin tags removed. Removed 9 skin tags from the right side of the neck; removed 7 skin tags from the left side of the neck; removed 12 skin tags from the chest. Separate E/M services were not performed for the skin tags. Patient is otherwise healthy.

Tip: Remember to add the appropriate modifier to the E/M code for the additional service provided at the time of the annual checkup.

2 ICD-10-CM Code _____

3 CPT Codes _____

_____

8. INPATIENT HOSPITAL Gender: M Age: 82

Preprocedure diagnosis: Stage 4 pressure ulcer of the sacral region

Procedure: 22-sq cm excision of the pressure ulcer with partial excision of sacrum. A 24-sq cm myocutaneous flap graft was placed on the defect. An adjacent tissue transfer of 26 sq cm was performed and this defect was closed using a single-layered closure. Bone from sacrum was sent to pathology.

Postprocedure diagnosis: Stage 4 pressure ulcer; sacral region; osteomyelitis of the sacrum

Pathology report: Osteomyelitis of the sacrum

Tip: Remember to sum the size of the graft and the size of the adjacent tissue transfer for the total defect size.

2 ICD-10-CM Codes _____

3 CPT Codes _____

_____

9. INPATIENT HOSPITAL Gender: M Age: 31

Preprocedure diagnosis: Second-degree burns to both upper arms, subsequent encounter

Procedure: Debridement of blisters and skin on both upper arms measuring 180 sq cm. A skin substitute was applied.

Tip: Remember that a second-degree burn is also called a partial-thickness burn.

2 ICD-10-CM Codes _____

4 CPT Codes _____

_____

10. OUTPATIENT HOSPITAL Gender: F Age: 64

Preprocedure diagnosis: Squamous cell carcinoma, skin of right hand and left cheek

Procedure: Used laser to destroy 2 lesions of cheek: first lesion 0.2-cm excised diameter, second lesion 0.5-cm excised diameter, and 1 lesion of hand, 1.1-cm excised diameter

Postprocedure diagnosis: Squamous cell carcinoma, skin of hand; two premalignant lesions on skin of cheek

Pathology report: Confirms squamous cell carcinoma on the skin of hand; finds two lesions on skin of face are actinic keratosis (premalignant)

2 ICD-10-CM Codes _____

3 CPT Codes _____

_____

KEEP ON CODING

Instructions: Read the procedural statement, then use the appropriate Index and Tabular List to assign CPT procedure codes. Write the code(s) on the line provided.

1. Lumpectomy of breast: CPT Code(s) _____

2. Removal of lesion using Mohs procedure, left thorax; first stage, eight blocks; second stage, four blocks: CPT Code(s)

_____

3. Excision of pressure ulcer of hip, partial ostectomy of the trochanter, and a skin flap closure: CPT Code(s) _____

4. One-layer repair, 1.6-cm laceration of forehead: CPT Code(s) _____

5. Excision of pilonidal cyst, coccygeal region: CPT Code(s) _____

6. Removal of subungual hematoma by evacuation: CPT Code(s) _____

(continued)

(continued from page 715)

7. Cryotherapy to remove malignant melanomas of skin; 0.9-cm lesion on back; 1.3-cm lesion on thigh; 0.4-cm lesion on upper eyelid: CPT Code(s) _____

8. Debridement and application of dressing for second-degree burn, calf; 3% TBSA: CPT Code(s) _____

9. Application of skin substitute graft to anterior trunk (65 sq cm) and arm (33 sq cm): CPT Code(s) _____

10. Breast reduction, bilateral: CPT Code(s) _____

11. Superficial fascial repair of 2.7-cm open wound of thigh: CPT Code(s) _____

12. Intralesional injection of skin of scalp, four lesions: CPT Code(s) _____

13. Excision of umbilical hidradenitis with intermediate repair: CPT Code(s) _____

14. Needle biopsy of breast: CPT Code(s) _____

15. Excision of 2-sq cm cutaneous vascular lesion of neck using laser: CPT Code(s) _____

16. Application of split-thickness tissue-cultured skin autograft to adult trunk (85 sq cm) and legs (52 sq cm): CPT Code(s) _____

17. Layered closure of 1.2 cm of abdomen, 0.3 cm of foot, and 1.2 cm of shoulder: CPT Code(s) _____

18. Excision of malignant skin lesions including margins; 0.5 cm on scalp, 0.8 cm on neck, 1.4 cm on shoulder: CPT Code(s) _____

19. Removal of 3 epidermal lesions by shaving: 0.2 cm on one hand, 0.7 on the cheek, 1.15 cm on the other hand: CPT Code(s) _____

20. Lipectomy of abdomen, suction assisted: CPT Code(s) _____

21. Stereotactic guidance to place radioactive seeds into breast lesion: CPT Code(s) _____

22. Removal of 19 skin tags on upper back and 8 on the neck: CPT Code(s) _____

23. Paring of three corns on toes: CPT Code(s) _____

24. Incision and drainage of breast abscess: CPT Code(s) _____

25. Wound debridement and layered closure of 1.3-cm cheek wound: CPT Code(s) _____

Musculoskeletal System Procedures (20005-29999)

Learning Objectives

After completing this chapter, you should have the skills to:

38.1 Spell and define the key words, medical terms, and abbreviations related to musculoskeletal procedures.

38.2 Discuss the fundamentals of musculoskeletal procedures.

38.3 Identify the main characteristics of coding for Musculoskeletal System procedures.

38.4 Abstract procedural information from the medical record for coding the Musculoskeletal System.

38.5 Assign codes for Musculoskeletal System procedures.

38.6 Arrange codes for Musculoskeletal System procedures.

38.7 Code evaluation and management services for orthopedics.

38.8 Discuss the CPT coding guidelines related to the Musculoskeletal System.

Chapter Outline

- **Musculoskeletal System Procedure Basics**
- **Coding Overview of Musculoskeletal System Procedures**
- **Abstracting Procedures for the Musculoskeletal System**
- **Assigning Codes for Musculoskeletal System Procedures**
- **Arranging Codes for Musculoskeletal System Procedures**
- **E/M Coding for Orthopedics**

Key Terms and Abbreviations

chondroplasty	level (spinal)	reduction	transfer
external fixation	manipulation	release	uniplane fixator
hemiarthroplasty	multiplane fixator	repair	vertebral segment
internal fixation	multiple endoscopy rule	stabilization	
interspace	reconstruction	synovectomy	

In addition to the key terms listed here, students should know the terms defined within tables in this chapter.

For updates and corrections, visit our student resource site at

www.pearsonhighered.com/healthprofessionsresources

INTRODUCTION

Someone shopping in a hardware store might be bewildered by the vast array of tools and fasteners, yet each is designed for a specific purpose. The table of surgical instruments in an orthopedic operating room might look like a hardware store to some people because orthopedic surgeons use saws, drills, screwdrivers, and fasteners to perform repairs on the musculoskeletal system.

MUSCULOSKELETAL SYSTEM PROCEDURE BASICS

Several medical specialties focus on the musculoskeletal (MS) system. Orthopedic (also spelled *orthopaedic*) surgeons evaluate, treat, and perform surgery related to trauma, sports injuries, degenerative diseases, infections, tumors, and congenital disorders of the musculoskeletal system. Orthopedic surgeons can specialize in one or more specific anatomic sites, such as the knee, shoulder, back, or hip. When patients seek orthopedic surgery, it is important that they work with a surgeon who specializes in the specific site and specific problem. Any given orthopedic procedure can be performed using a variety of techniques, which can involve specific types of sutures and bone anchors aimed at promoting maximum stability and preventing reinjury. Patients need to discuss the surgeon's technique and choose the one they are most comfortable with.

Because the nerves are closely related to the function of the musculoskeletal system, neurologists may be part of the surgical team. For example, spinal surgery may be necessary when a bone deformity impacts neurological function. In general orthopedic surgeons perform procedures related to deformities or injuries to the bone and muscle. Neurosurgeons perform procedures involving the nerves, brain, and spinal cord. Podiatrists perform procedures on the foot. Oral maxillofacial surgeons (OMSs) perform procedures on the face and mouth bones, such as those performed for facial injuries, dental implants, oral cancer, and tumors and cysts of the jaws.

Orthopedic surgeons receive referrals from other medical specialties, such as primary care physicians, physiatrists (*physical medicine and rehabilitation physicians*), rheumatologists, pain medicine physicians, and athletic trainers. They may refer postsurgical patients to any of these specialists, as well as to physical therapists, psychologists, and psychiatrists.

Medical terminology related to Musculoskeletal System procedures can be challenging because of the number of bones, muscles, and connecting structures involved. (Refer to Figure 12-1 to review the anatomy of the skeletal system.) Joints are named for the two bones they connect, such as the radioulnar joint, which consists of the ends of the radius and ulna. Muscles, tendons, and ligaments often are named for the sites they connect or their shape (■ FIGURE 38-1). For example, the sternocleidomastoid muscle connects the sternum, clavicle (*cleido-*), and mastoid process. The iliofemoral tendon joins the ilium and femur. The deltoid muscle is triangular in shape, named after the Latin word *delta*, meaning triangle. The anterior and posterior cruciate ligaments form a cross-like shape and are named after the Latin terms *cruc-* or *crux*, meaning "cross." Chapter 12 of this text provides additional information on musculoskeletal system anatomy and conditions. Refer to ■ TABLE 38-1 for a refresher on how to build medical terms related to the musculoskeletal system.

> ## SUCCESS STEP
>
> Although you may not be able to specifically name every bone, muscle, tendon, and ligament, you can use your knowledge of combining forms to understand the location of unfamiliar structures.

> ## CODING CAUTION
>
> Be alert for anatomic terms that are spelled similarly and have different meanings.
>
> **metacarp/o** (*long bone of the hand that connects the carpus [wrist bones] to the phalanges [fingers]*) and **metatars/o** (*long bone of the foot that connects the tarsus [ankle bones] to the phalanges [toes]*)
>
> **ilium** (*uppermost and largest bone of the pelvis*) and **ischium** (*lower and back part of the hip bone*)
>
> **patella** (*kneecap*) and **palate** (*roof of the mouth*)

Table 38-1 ■ **EXAMPLE OF CONSTRUCTING MEDICAL TERMS FOR MUSCULOSKELETAL SYSTEM PROCEDURES**

Combining Form	Suffix	Complete Medical Term
capsul/o (*joint capsule, a thin membrane around the joint that contains synovial fluid*)		**capsulo + desis** (*surgical fusion of the joint capsule*)
		arthro + desis (*surgical fusion of the joint*)
	-desis (*surgical fusion*) **-ectomy** (*excision*) **-tomy** (*cutting into*)	**capsul + ectomy** (*surgical excision of the joint capsule*)
		arthr + ectomy (*surgical excision of the joint*)
arthr/o (*joint, the location where bones meet*)		**capsulo + tomy** (*cutting into the joint capsule*)
		arthro + tomy (*cutting into the joint*)

Source: © PB Resources, Inc. Used with permission.

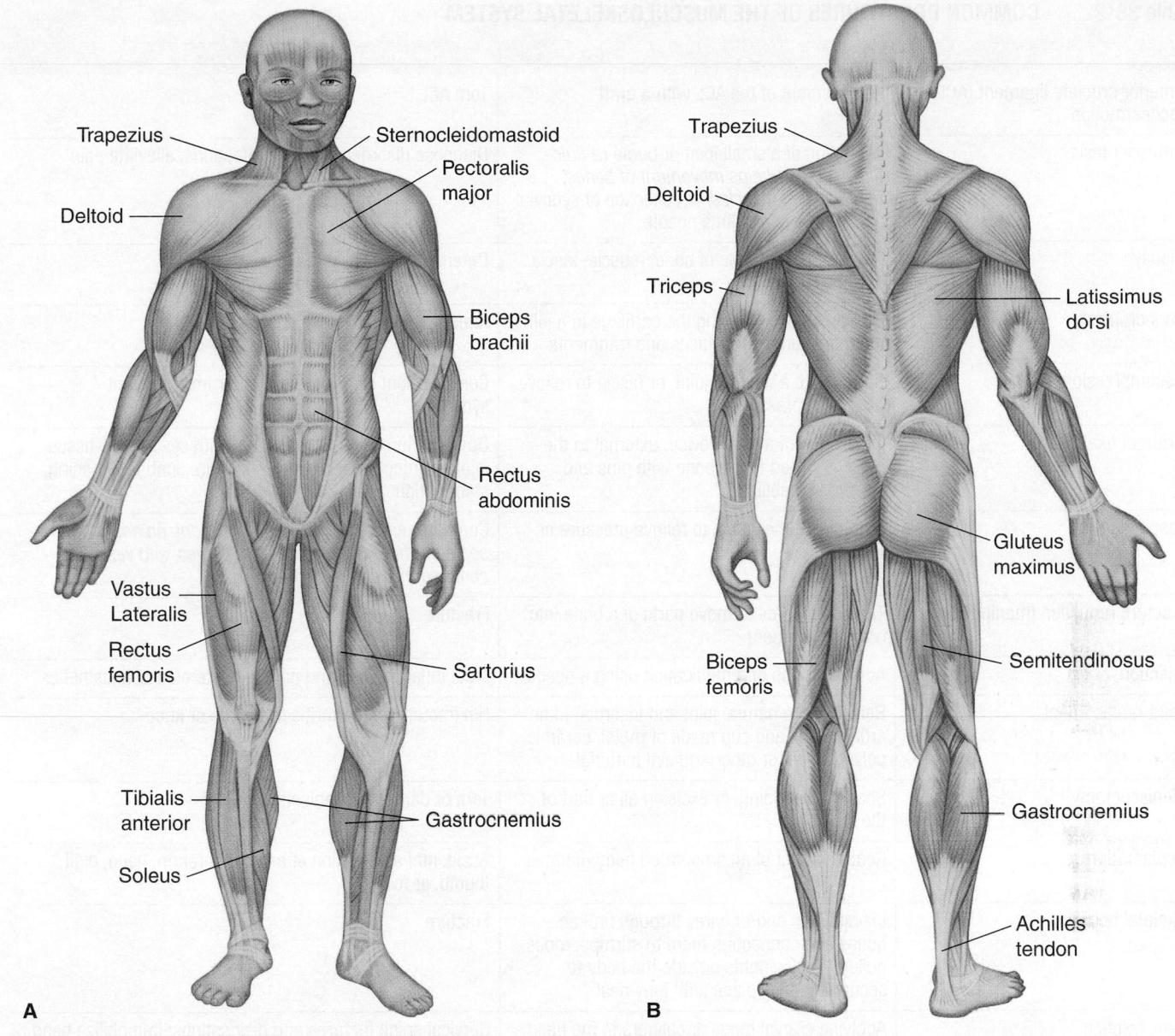

Figure 38-1 ■ The Muscular System: Anterior View (A) and Posterior View (B)

Procedures of the Musculoskeletal System

Procedures commonly performed on the Musculoskeletal System are summarized in ■ TABLE 38-2. In particular, coders need to understand arthroscopy, joint replacement, fracture treatment, and soft-tissue repair and reconstruction.

Arthroscopy

Knee arthroscopy is the most commonly performed procedure on the musculoskeletal system. Arthroscopy is also performed on other major joints, such as the shoulder, elbow, wrist, hip, and ankle. Although arthroscopy can be done as an independent procedure for diagnostic purposes, therapeutic procedures often are performed at the same time. These may include aspiration of fluid, **chondroplasty** (*reshaping of cartilage*), **synovectomy** (*surgical removal of the synovial membrane*), debridement, and a variety of repairs. Repairs can be performed using either an open or arthroscopic approach.

Joint Replacement

The most commonly replaced joints are the knee, hip, and shoulder. The most common reason for joint replacement is osteoarthritis. Pathologic hip fractures due to osteoporosis can also result in joint replacement. In a total joint replacement, also called arthroplasty, the patient's anatomy is replaced with artificial ball-and-socket components that perform the same function. The ends of the long bone(s) forming the joint are cut off and replaced with a ball on a stem that inserts into the remaining bone. In the knee the distal end of the femur and the proximal end of the tibia are replaced; in the hip the head of the femur is replaced; in the shoulder the head of the humerus is replaced. The cup or socket is also reamed out and replaced with a prosthetic component. In the knee the patella is replaced; in the hip the acetabulum is replaced; in the shoulder the glenoid is replaced.

The surgeon selects the type of prosthetic material—metal alloy, ceramic, or polyethylene—based on a number of factors,

Table 38-2 ■ COMMON PROCEDURES OF THE MUSCULOSKELETAL SYSTEM

Procedure Name	Definition	Reason Performed
Anterior cruciate ligament (ACL) reconstruction	Replacement of the ACL with a graft	Torn ACL
Arthrocentesis	Aspiration of a small joint or bursa (*a fluid-filled sac that helps movement of bones, tendons, and muscles*) or collection of synovial fluid from a joint with a needle	Diagnose disorders such as infections; alleviate pain
Biopsy	Removal of a sample of bone, muscle, fascia, or other tissue	Determine the presence of disease
Chondroplasty	Reshaping and cleaning the cartilage in a joint to remove uneven surfaces and fragments	Knee or shoulder injury
Decompression	Cutting into a muscle, joint, or fascia to relieve tension or pressure	Compartment syndrome, shoulder impingement syndrome
External fixation	Installation of a rigid device, external to the body, attached to the bone with pins and screws to stabilize it	Open fractures, closed fractures with severe soft-tissue injuries, infected nonunion of fracture, limb lengthening, stabilization
Fasciotomy	Cutting into the fascia to relieve pressure or tension	Compartment syndrome (*Compartment: an anatomic segment that involves muscles, nerves, and vessels confined by a fascia membrane*)
Fracture reduction (manipulation)	The use of force to move parts of a bone into normal alignment	Fracture
Injection	Administration of a medication using a needle	Treat inflammation and pain with steroids or anesthetics
Joint replacement	Removal of a natural joint and insertion of an artificial ball and cup made of metal, ceramic, polyethylene, or other artificial material	Hip fracture, osteoarthritis of the hip or knee
Meniscectomy	Shaving, debriding, or excising all or part of the meniscus	Torn or damaged meniscus
Replantation	Reattachment of an amputated body member	Accidental amputation of an arm, forearm, hand, digit, thumb, or foot
Skeletal traction	Placing pins and/or wires through broken bones and connecting them to stirrups, ropes, pulleys, and weights outside the body to secure bones in place until they heal	Fracture
Skull traction	Applying cranial tongs or calipers to the head and attaching them to ropes and weights on the outside, which secure the spine into place	Cervical spine factures and dislocations; immobilize head for stereotactic radiosurgery or radiation therapy
Spinal fusion	Joining together two vertebrae to stabilize them and help alleviate persistent pain	Herniated disk, stenosis, or spinal injury
Tendon repair	Sewing together the damaged or torn ends of a tendon	Torn or damaged tendon
Wound exploration	Enlargement, dissection, and examination of a wound to determine the wound depth or perform a procedure	Foreign body removal; debridement; repair of tissue, fascia, muscle, or blood vessel

Source: © PB Resources, Inc. Used with permission.

such as the patient's activity level, age, weight, and health. The same material can be used for all components or a different material used for the ball than the socket. The implant may be cemented (*attached to the bone with surgical cement*) or cement-less (*attached to the bone with a fine mesh into which the bone grows*), or a different method can be used on each component.

Joint replacement procedures have many variations. Some patients require that only one component of the joint be replaced, which is called a partial joint replacement or **hemiarthroplasty**. Prosthetic material wears down through use, just as the natural components do, and may require replacement or modification in the future. Technology related to joint replacements is constantly advancing, so new techniques and materials continue to be developed.

Patients must participate in physical therapy after a joint replacement procedure to help rebuild strength and develop stability. Most patients enjoy significant pain relief and increased mobility after joint replacement.

Fracture Treatment

Fractures comprise approximately 16% of all musculoskeletal injuries in the United States each year, accounting for 3.5 million visits to the emergency department. The most common fracture site for people younger than age 75 is the wrist, whereas the most common fracture site for people older than age 75 is the hip. Although the treatment of fractures varies based on the site, type of fracture, and patient health, it generally consists of stabilization and/or restorative treatment.

Stabilization. Stabilization involves immobilizing the fracture site to prevent further injury and allow for healing. Fractures can be stabilized using straps, splints, or a variety of casts. Sometimes stabilization is the only treatment needed. In other situations, stabilization is an initial or temporary measure taken until restorative treatment can be performed. The physician who stabilizes the fracture may provide that service only or may also provide all the follow-up care.

Restorative Treatment. Restorative treatment is surgical repair or manipulation of displaced bones. Not all fractures result in displaced bones, but when they do, the bones must be realigned. **Manipulation** or **reduction** is the realignment of bone fragments or segments. Closed reduction is performed through the direct application of force. Open reduction requires a surgical incision to expose the bone, then realign it.

After reduction, the bones are stabilized with a cast, fixation device, or traction so they heal in the proper position. **External fixation** is the use of a rigid frame, external to the body, which is attached to the bone(s) using screws and pins. It may be used temporarily until the patient is able to withstand surgery or may be the primary mode of treatment and left in place until the fracture heals. A **uniplane fixator** has a single external rod that runs parallel to a long bone and is used almost exclusively on fractures of the shaft. A **multiplane**

fixator has a ring-shaped frame that surrounds the treatment site. Wires apply tension to the frame to hold it in position. **Internal fixation** is the use of special implants, such as plates, screws, nails, rods, and/or wires, applied directly to the bone(s). The implants may be removed when the fracture has healed or may be left in permanently.

CODING CAUTION

Open and closed reductions are identified based on the surgical approach used to realign displaced bones. The terms have no bearing on whether the fracture itself is open (*piercing the skin*) or closed (*not piercing the skin*). For example, a closed displaced fracture may be treated with either open or closed reduction and either external or internal fixation.

Fracture Follow-up. Surgeons monitor patients during the postoperative follow-up period, which is usually 90 days for Medicare. They may take X-rays to ensure the bones maintain correct alignment during healing. In the event of nonunion, malunion, or infection, additional treatment may be required.

Soft-Tissue Repair and Reconstruction

Muscles, tendons, and ligaments may need to be repaired because of injury, disease, or deformity. In a **release**, the tissue is freed from surrounding adhesions so that it can move freely within the tendon sheath; for example, tenolysis of the ankle. In a **repair**, a torn or damaged tissue, such as a muscle, is sewn together; for example, suturing of a ruptured hamstring muscle. In a **transfer**, one end of a muscle or tendon is moved to a new site to replace a damaged or nonfunctional muscle or tendon; for example, transfer of the iliopsoas muscle from the lesser trochanter of the femur to the greater trochanter to compensate for weak hip abductor muscles. In **reconstruction**, the original tissue is replaced with grafted tissue to create a new structure; for example, replacement of the anterior cruciate ligament (ACL) with a graft from the patellar tendon.

This section provides a general reference to help understand the most common musculoskeletal system procedures. Remember to keep standard reference books handy in case you get stuck.

CODING PRACTICE

Exercise 38.1 Musculoskeletal System Procedure Basics

Instructions: Use your medical terminology skills and resources to define the following procedures related to the Musculoskeletal System, then identify the code(s) or code range listed in the CPT Index. Follow these steps:

- Use slash marks "/" to break down each term into its root(s) and suffix.
- Define the meaning of the word based on the meaning of each word part.
- Identify the CPT code(s) or code range listed in the CPT Index.
- Use the entire phrase to identify the code or code range shown in the CPT Index.

(continued)

CODING PRACTICE (continued)

Example: <u>arthrodesis</u>, knee arthro/desis   Meaning _fusion of a joint_   CPT Code _27580_

1. <u>tenomyotomy</u>   Meaning _____   CPT Code _____

2. <u>sesamoidectomy</u>, finger   Meaning _____   CPT Code _____

3. <u>patellectomy</u>, complete   Meaning _____   CPT Code _____

4. <u>osteoplasty</u>, ulna   Meaning _____   CPT Code _____

5. <u>tenolysis</u>, foot   Meaning _____   CPT Code _____

6. <u>orbitocraniofacial</u> reconstruction, secondary   Meaning _____   CPT Code _____

7. <u>fasciotomy</u>, palm   Meaning _____   CPT Code _____

8. <u>capsulorrhaphy</u>, posterior   Meaning _____   CPT Code _____

9. talus, <u>diaphysectomy</u>   Meaning _____   CPT Code _____

10. <u>synovectomy</u>, glenohumeral joint   Meaning _____   CPT Code _____

CODING OVERVIEW OF MUSCULOSKELETAL SYSTEM PROCEDURES

The CPT section/subsection **Musculoskeletal System (20005-29999)** contains 15 subheadings that are divided by anatomic site (■ TABLE 38-3). Within each anatomic site, codes are divided by the type of procedure, such as incision, excision, introduction, and so on. Review the subheading and category names and code ranges listed in the Musculoskeletal System subsection to become familiar with the content and organization. Some editions of the CPT manual provide a summary list of the subheadings and categories at the beginning of the Musculoskeletal System subsection, which also displays an asterisk (*) next to categories that contain special instructions.

This chapter includes invasive, minimally invasive, and noninvasive surgical procedures on the Musculoskeletal System. Codes for diagnostic tests on the Musculoskeletal System appear in the Medicine section. CPT codes in the Musculoskeletal System subsection are frequently supported by diagnosis codes from ICD-10-CM **Chapter 13 Diseases of the Musculoskeletal System and Connective Tissue (M00-M99)**, as well as neoplasms, symptoms and signs, and injuries (■ TABLE 38-4). These are the codes most commonly used to support procedures on the Musculoskeletal System; however, diagnosis codes from any ICD-10-CM chapter are permissible. CPT codes must always be linked with diagnosis codes that support the medical necessity of the procedure.

CPT guidelines for the Surgery section apply to the Musculoskeletal System.

Special instructions at the beginning of the Musculoskeletal System subsection provide definitions and coding guidelines for treatment of fractures and excision of tumors. This information applies to all codes within the Musculoskeletal System and should be studied before attempting to assign codes for these procedures. Additional special instructions appear at the beginning of many categories throughout the subsection. The **Spine (Vertebral Column)** subheading in particular provides numerous instructions regarding the use of modifiers and multiple coding.

Instructional notes appear throughout the Tabular List to alert coders to the need for modifiers, provide cross-references to codes for similar procedures on other sites, identify when additional codes for radiological services might be needed, and highlight resequenced and recently deleted codes.

Table 38-3 ■ **MUSCULOSKELETAL SYSTEM SUBHEADINGS**

Subheading	Code Range
General	20005-20999
Head	21010-21499
Neck (Soft Tissues) and Thorax	21501-21899
Back and Flank	21920-21936
Spine (Vertebral Column)	22010-22899
Abdomen	22900-22999
Shoulder	23000-23929
Humerus (Upper Arm) and Elbow	23930-24999
Forearm and Wrist	25000-25999
Hand and Fingers	26010-26989
Pelvis and Hip Joint	26990-27299
Femur (Thigh Region) and Knee Joint	27301-27599
Leg (Tibia and Fibula) and Ankle Joint	27600-27899
Foot and Toes	28001-28899
Application of Casts and Strapping	29000-29799
Endoscopy/Arthroscopy Procedures	29800-29999

Table 38-4 ■ LOCATING ICD-10-CM AND ADDITIONAL CPT CODES FOR THE MUSCULOSKELETAL SYSTEM

Type of Code	Codes
ICD-10-CM Musculoskeletal System-Related Codes	
Musculoskeletal system conditions	M00-M99
Neoplasms	C40-C41
Symptoms and signs	R25-R29
Injuries	S00-T89
CPT Musculoskeletal System-Related Codes	
Medicine procedures	96000-96004, 91001-97799, 97760-97762, 97810-97814, 89825-89829, 98940-98943
Radiologic procedures	
• Diagnostic radiology	70010-73725
• Radiologic guidance	77001-77022
• Diagnostic ultrasound	76506-76645, 76801-76857, 76881-76886
• Bone/joint studies	77071-77084
• Nuclear medicine, diagnostic	78300-78399

Source: © PB Resources, Inc. Used with permission.

Table 38-6 ■ KEY CRITERIA FOR ABSTRACTING TREATMENT OF FRACTURES AND DISLOCATIONS

❑ What bone is fractured or dislocated?

❑ What site on the bone is fractured?

❑ What is the laterality?

❑ What type of reduction is provided (open or closed)?

❑ What general type of stabilization is provided (fixation or immobilization)?

❑ What type of fixation is provided (internal or external/percutaneous)?

❑ What type of traction is provided (skeletal or skin)?

❑ Is re-reduction of the injury required?

For application of casts and strapping:

❑ What anatomic site is treated?

❑ Is the service an initial treatment?

❑ Is restorative treatment provided?

❑ Is restorative treatment provided by the same individual who applied the cast/strapping?

❑ Is the cast removed or repaired by the same individual who applied it?

Source: © PB Resources, Inc. Used with permission.

ABSTRACTING PROCEDURES FOR THE MUSCULOSKELETAL SYSTEM

Because the Musculoskeletal System is a combination of two systems, separate abstracting guidelines are provided. Abstracting for skeletal system procedures (■ TABLE 38-5) requires special attention not only to the general anatomic site, such as the tibia, but also sometimes the specific location, such as the shaft, neck, or head. Abstract information about any implants, prostheses, hardware, or cement used and left in place. Spinal procedures require identification of the procedural approach, such as open, percutaneous, or endoscopic, as well as the anatomic approach, such as anterior, posterior, or posterolateral. Abstracting for fractures and dislocations (■ TABLE 38-6) also requires that coders take note of the types of reduction, stabilization, fixation, and traction provided.

For muscular system procedures, identify the specific type of procedure, for example, an excision, repair, transfer, release, or reconstruction; the type of soft tissue treated; and the deepest layer reached (■ TABLE 38-7). Remember that the abstracting

Table 38-5 ■ KEY CRITERIA FOR ABSTRACTING SKELETAL SYSTEM PROCEDURES

❑ What is the general anatomic site?

❑ What is the specific location and/or compartment within the anatomic site?

❑ What is the laterality?

❑ What is the procedural approach (open or endoscopic)?

❑ What is the anatomic approach for spine procedures (posterior, anterior, anterolateral, or a combination)?

❑ What is the purpose of the procedure (diagnostic or therapeutic)?

❑ Is a foreign body removed?

❑ What type(s) of materials are used and/or prostheses/devices implanted?

❑ Which components of a joint are replaced (total or partial)?

Source: © PB Resources, Inc. Used with permission.

Table 38-7 ■ KEY CRITERIA FOR ABSTRACTING MUSCULAR SYSTEM PROCEDURES

❑ Is the procedure an excision, release, repair, transfer, or reconstruction or other type of procedure?

❑ Is the tissue a muscle, tendon, ligament, fascia, or other?

❑ What is the anatomic site?

❑ What is the laterality?

❑ What is the deepest layer of tissue treated?

❑ Is a foreign body removed?

❑ Is a malignancy involved?

Source: © PB Resources, Inc. Used with permission.

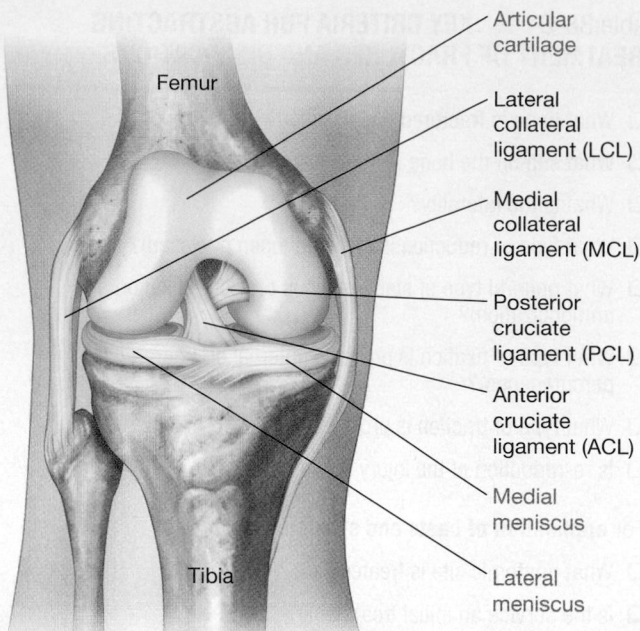

Figure 38-2 ■ Anatomy of the Knee

questions are a guide and that not every question applies to, or can be answered for, every case. For example, materials and prostheses are not used in all cases.

Guided Example of Abstracting Musculoskeletal System Procedures

Refer to the following example throughout this chapter to practice skills for abstracting, assigning, and arranging Musculoskeletal System codes. ■ FIGURE 38-2 provides a review of the anatomy of the knee.

OUTPATIENT SURGERY   Gender: M   Age: 37

Preoperative diagnosis: Current tear of medial meniscus, chondromalacia of the patella, right knee

Procedure: Right knee arthroscopy with partial medial meniscectomy and lateral meniscorrhaphy. A #11-blade stab incision was made, followed by the insertion of a trocar. An arthroscopy probe was inserted and a systematic tour of the knee compartments was performed. All menisci were probed. All articular cartilage surfaces of the tibia, femur, and patella were probed. A posterior horn tear of the medial meniscus was complex in nature. Due the tear being irreparable, it was debrided back to a stable margin using an arthroscopy meniscal biter and a #4.0 shaver. A separate peripheral tear in the lateral meniscus also was visualized in the red-red zone. This was not identified on the previous MRI and appeared amenable to repair. The edges were reduced with electrocautery and approximated, then closed with 6-0 Vicryl sutures. The chondromalacia changes were all stable

---

and did not require any chondroplasty. Patient tolerated the procedure well and was transferred to PACU in stable condition.

Postoperative diagnosis: 1) Complex posterior horn tear around medial meniscus in the white-white to white-red zone. 2) peripheral tear in the lateral meniscus in the red-red zone. 3) Chondromalacia changes of grade 2 of the patellofemoral compartment.

Postoperative plan: oral analgesics, oral anti-inflammatory medications. Ice and elevation of the limb. Weight bearing as tolerated. RTO 6–10 days for postoperative wound examination, suture removal, and referral to physical therapy.

Follow along as fictitious coder, Jacob Bates, CCS, abstracts the procedure. Check off each step after you complete it.

▶ Jacob reads through the entire record, paying special attention to the reason for the encounter, the procedure performed, and the postoperative diagnosis. He refers to the Key Criteria for Abstracting Muscular System Procedures (Table 38-7).

❑ He notes the preoperative diagnosis: Tear of medial meniscus, chondromalacia of the patella

❑ *Is the site a joint or a bone?* joint

❑ *What procedure is performed?* partial medial meniscectomy

❑ *What is the anatomic site?* knee/medial meniscus

❑ *What is the laterality?* right

❑ *What is the procedural approach (open or endoscopic)?* Endoscopic (arthroscopy)

❑ *What additional procedure was performed?* lateral meniscorrhaphy

❑ *What is the anatomic site?* knee/lateral meniscus

❑ *What is the laterality?* right

❑ *What is the procedural approach (open or endoscopic)?* Endoscopic (arthroscopy)

❑ *What is the purpose of the procedure (diagnostic or therapeutic)?* Both diagnostic (exploratory/examination) and therapeutic (debridement, suturing) services are provided, so the procedure is classified as therapeutic.

▶ At this time, Jacob does not know which of these procedures may need to be coded, nor how many codes he will end up with. He will learn about this when he moves on to assigning codes.

CODING PRACTICE

Exercise 38.2 Abstracting Procedures for the Musculoskeletal System

Instructions: Read the mini-medical-record of each patient's encounter and answer the abstracting questions. Write the answer on the line provided. Do not assign any codes.

1. OUTPATIENT SURGERY   Gender: M   Age: 33

Preprocedure diagnosis: fracture of left tibia shaft

Procedure: adjusted an external fixation system, including replacing the pins, under anesthesia

a. What is the general anatomic site? _____

b. What is the specific location and/or compartment within the anatomic site? _____

c. What is the laterality? _____

d. What is the procedural approach? _____

e. What type(s) of materials are used and/or prostheses/devices implanted? _____

2. OFFICE   Gender: M   Age: 12

Preprocedure diagnosis: fracture, left radius. Cast applied by another physician while the boy was attending summer camp.

Procedure: removal of long arm cast

a. What anatomic site is treated? _____

b. Is the service an initial treatment? _____

c. Is restorative treatment provided? _____

d. Is the cast removed or repaired by the same individual who applied it? _____

3. INPATIENT HOSPITAL   Gender: F   Age: 46

Preprocedure diagnosis: mass, abdominal wall

Procedure: Excised a tumor from the intramuscular tissue of the right anterior abdominal wall. The tumor measures 4.0 cm in diameter.

Pathology report: benign desmoid tumor

a. Is the procedure an excision, release, repair, transfer, or reconstruction or other type of procedure? _____

b. Is the tissue a muscle, tendon, ligament, fascia, or other? _____

(continued)

3. (continued)

c. What is the anatomic site? _____

d. What is the laterality? _____

e. What is the deepest layer of tissue treated? _____

f. Is a foreign body removed? _____

g. Is a malignancy involved? _____

4. INPATIENT HOSPITAL   Gender: M   Age: 65

Preprocedure diagnosis: pain in the thoracic spine due to degenerated and protruding discs

Procedure: arthrodesis on T9–T10 and T10–T11 interspace using an anterolateral approach

Postprocedure diagnosis: degeneration and protrusion, T9–T10 and T10–T11

a. What is the general anatomic site? _____

b. What is the specific location and/or compartment within the anatomic site? _____

c. What is the laterality? _____

d. What is the procedural approach (open or endoscopic)? _____

e. What is the anatomic approach (posterior, anterior, anterolateral, or a combination)? _____

f. What is the purpose of the procedure (diagnostic or therapeutic)? _____

5. EMERGENCY DEPARTMENT   Gender: M   Age: 25

Preprocedure diagnosis: Index finger and middle finger on right hand were completely amputated during automobile accident.

Procedure: reattach both fingers, including distal tip to sublimis tendon insertion

a. What is the general anatomic site? _____

b. What is the specific location within the anatomic site? _____

c. What is the laterality? _____

d. What is the procedural approach? _____

e. What type(s) of materials are used and/or prostheses/devices implanted? _____

(continued)

CODING PRACTICE (continued)

---

6. INPATIENT HOSPITAL Gender: F Age: 42

Preprocedure diagnosis: *chronic lower back pain due to degenerative disc disease*

Procedure: *Arthroplasty L4–L5 and L5-L6. Using an anterior approach excised the entire disc L4–L5 and inserted an implant. We then moved to L5-L6 where we also excised the entire disc L4–L5 and inserted an implant. Patient tolerated procedure well and was moved to PACU in stable condition.*

Postprocedure diagnosis: *intervertebral disc degeneration L4-L5, L5-L6*

a. What is the general anatomic site? _____

(continued)

---

6. (continued)

b. What is the specific location and/or compartment within the anatomic site? _____

c. What is the laterality? _____

d. What is the procedural approach (open or endoscopic)? _____

e. What is the anatomic approach (posterior, anterior, anterolateral, or a combination)? _____

f. What is the purpose of the procedure (diagnostic or therapeutic)? _____

ASSIGNING CODES FOR MUSCULOSKELETAL SYSTEM PROCEDURES

Whenever possible, search the Index for the name of the specific muscle or bone treated because these Main Terms usually provide the most detail and lead most directly to the desired code. In addition to searching for a specific site, such as **Ulna**, you can also search for a more general anatomic term, such as **Arm**. However, the results may not be as specific. Other alternatives are to search for the name of the procedure or condition. When you have difficulty locating the appropriate code, remember to search for it using an alternative Main Term. Two areas requiring special attention are using the Index to locate the appropriate anatomic site and coding for fracture care.

Indexing of Joints and Bones

The Index sometimes provides multiple Main Term entries for a joint, each with a different nuance. Therefore, coders must read beyond the first applicable Main Term entry they locate. For example, Index entries for the knee include **Knee**, **Knee Joint**, **Knee Prosthesis**, and **Kneecap**. The Main Term **Knee** classifies procedures on the tissues of the knee, such as the muscles and ligaments, whereas the entries for the Main Term **Knee Joint** classify procedures on the bony structure of the knee, including joint replacement. Arthroscopy appears only under **Knee** because arthroscopy is performed in the knee compartments, not on the bone itself. The Main Term **Knee** also provides an instructional note **See Femur; Fibula; Patella; Tibia**, so refer to these additional Main Terms if you cannot find an appropriate code. The Main Term **Knee Prosthesis** provides a cross reference to the Main Term **Prosthesis** and the first-level modifying term **Knee**. These codes classify prosthesis introduction and removal procedures. The Main Term **Kneecap** classifies procedures on the patella itself.

The Index also provides multiple Main Terms for **Hip** and **Hip Joint**, as well as **Shoulder** and **Shoulder Joint**. When locating Main Terms for the back, distinguish between the **Back** (soft tissue), **Spine** (bone), **Spinal Cord** (bundle of nerves), **Vertebra** (each bony segment of the spine), and **Intervertebral Disc** (pad of fibrocartilage between the vertebrae). Procedures on the back, spine, and vertebrae are classified under the Musculoskeletal System, whereas procedures on the spinal cord and intervertebral discs are classified under the Nervous System. Most of these Main Term entries also provide cross-references to more specific sites, so take the time to review the entries in detail and follow all cross-references, especially when you are having difficulty locating the appropriate code.

In the Tabular List, codes for the spinal column often are divided by the section of the spine—cervical, thoracic, and lumbar—with add-on code(s) for each additional vertebra, also called a **level** or **vertebral segment**. When coding for procedures on the spine, distinguish between vertebrae and intervertebral discs. In documentation, each vertebra is identified by a letter–number combination, such as C4 for the fourth cervical vertebra, L2 for the second lumbar vertebra, and so on. An intervertebral disc, or **interspace**, is the space between two vertebra and is identified by the vertebrae above and below. For example, the L2-L3 interspace is the disc situated between the second and third lumbar vertebrae. On a vertebral procedure, L2-L3 refers to *two* vertebrae (■ FIGURE 38-3), whereas on disc procedures, L2-L3 refers to *one* interspace (■ FIGURE 38-4). This distinction is important when assigning quantity and codes to spinal procedures.

Assigning Codes for Fracture Care

Assigning codes for fracture care depends on careful abstracting of who performs the service, as well as the extent of services provided. According to the National Correct Coding Initiative

Surgeon performed an osteotomy on L2, L3, and L4 using the posterolateral approach.

> **22214 Osteotomy of spine, posterior or posterolateral approach, 1 vertebral segment; lumbar**
> **22216 x 2 Osteotomy of spine, posterior or posterolateral approach, 1 vertebral segment; each additional vertebral segment**

Figure 38-3 ■ Example of Coding Procedures on Multiple Vertebrae

Surgeon replaced artificial discs at L2-L3 and L3-L4 using the anterior approach.

> **22862 Revision including replacement of total disc arthroplasty (artificial disc), anterior approach, single interspace; lumbar**
> **0165T Revision including replacement of total disc arthroplasty (artificial disc), anterior approach, each additional interspace, lumbar**

Figure 38-4 ■ Example of Coding Procedures on Multiple Discs

(NCCI), the initial encounter for fracture care with a 90-day global period usually involves an Evaluation and Management (E/M) code, a treatment code, and HCPCS codes for the materials used or the generic CPT code **99070 Supplies**. CPT provides separate codes for restorative treatment and casting. For procedures with a global period of 0 or 10 days, the initial evaluation is considered to be included in the treatment code. The exception is the application of casts and strapping, in which case an E/M code can be reported, subject to documentation and the nature of the service provided. Medicare Administrative Contractors (MACs) and private insurance companies may have additional claim edits that apply.

To locate codes for restorative fracture care, search the Index for the Main Term that identifies the bone(s) involved, such as **Tibia** or **Clavicle**, then locate the first-level modifying term **Fracture**. Additional modifying terms identify the type of treatment provided. Codes for restorative treatment include services such as open or closed treatment, with or without manipulation, and application of internal or external fixation. The subheadings for each anatomic site within the Musculoskeletal System subsection contain a category titled **Fracture and/or Dislocation**.

To locate codes for the application of casts and strapping, search the Index for the Main Term **Cast**, then locate the first-level modifying term for the type of cast. Codes are divided based on the region of the body, such as **Below knee to toes** or **Finger**, but not for each specific bone. If you cannot find the description needed as a first-level modifying term, look under the first-level modifying term **Type**, then locate the specific cast in the list of second-level modifying terms.

In the Tabular List, all codes for casting and strapping appear under the subheading **Application of Casts and Strapping 29000-29799**. Codes are divided by the upper and lower

extremities, with subdivisions for casts, splints, and straps. Special instructions appear before code **29000** and provide guidance regarding when cast application and strapping should be coded separately from the E/M code and/or restorative treatment.

- When the *same* provider applies the initial cast or strapping and also provides restorative treatment for the fracture and all follow-up care, assign a code for the restorative treatment that identifies the type of service provided. The initial cast application is included in the code for restorative care. Coding is as follows:
  - An E/M code for the type of service provided
  - A code from the category for the anatomic site that describes the type of restorative treatment provided
  - A HCPCS code or code **99070 Supplies** for the materials used
- When *different providers* perform the preoperative care, restorative treatment, and/or postoperative care, assign the code for the restorative treatment with the corresponding modifier(s) to identify the phase of care: **-54 Surgical care only, -55 Postoperative management only, -56 Preoperative management only**. Temporary cast application is not classified as preoperative care by CPT. Only the provider who performs the preoperative management codes an E/M code, which identifies the preoperative encounter at which the initial evaluation is performed and the decision for surgery is made (■ FIGURE 38-5).
- When cast application or strapping is the *only* service provided, and no other treatment is performed or anticipated, assign codes as follows (■ FIGURE 38-6):
  - An E/M code for the type of service provided
  - A code from **29000-29799** that describes the type of cast or strapping applied
  - A HCPCS code or CPT code **99070 Supplies** for the materials used
- When cast application or strapping is a *replacement* procedure during or after follow-up care, assign a code from **29000-29584** for the type of cast or strapping applied.
- When the cast is *removed* or repaired by a different individual than the one who applied it, assign a code from the category **Removal or Repair 29700-29750**.

SUCCESS STEP

Remember that when the E/M service is provided on the same day as the restorative treatment and results in a decision for surgery, apply modifier **-57 Decision for surgery** to the E/M code.

Guided Example of Assigning Musculoskeletal System Procedure Codes

To practice skills for assigning codes for the Musculoskeletal System, continue with the example from earlier in the chapter about a patient who was seen for a right knee arthroscopy.

Physician A evaluates the patient's fractured tibia, left leg, in the emergency department. He performs an expanded problem focused history, an expanded problem focused examination, and medical decision making of moderate complexity. X-rays reveal a fracture of the distal tibia. Physician A performs closed treatment with manipulation, and applies a short leg cast. The patient was on vacation at the time. When she returns home, Physician B provides the postoperative followup care, including X-rays to monitor proper healing and cast removal.

Physician A
99283-57 Emergency department visit for the evaluation and management of a patient, which requires these 3 key components: An expanded problem focused history; An expanded problem focused examination; and Medical decision making of moderate complexity. -57 Decision for surgery
27825-54-56-LT Closed treatment of fracture of weight bearing articular portion of distal tibia (eg, pilon or tibial plafond), with or without anesthesia; with skeletal traction and/or requiring manipulation; -54 Surgical care only; -56 Preoperative management only; -LT Left

Physician B
27825-55-LT Closed treatment of fracture of weight bearing articular portion of distal tibia (eg, pilon or tibial plafond), with or without anesthesia; with skeletal traction and/or requiring manipulation; -55 Postoperative management only; -LT Left

Figure 38-5 ■ Example of Coding for Fracture Care by Multiple Providers. *Source: © PB Resources, Inc. Used with permission. CPT codes only © American Medical Association.*

A patient presents to urgent care with right wrist pain. The patient reports that he fell yesterday and braced himself with his hand. The physician performs an expanded problem focused history, and examination, and medical decision making of moderate complexity. X-rays reveal no fracture. The physician diagnoses a sprain and applies a static short arm splint to stabilize the joint. No further treatment is planned.

99282-57 Emergency department visit for the evaluation and management of a patient, which requires these 3 key components: An expanded problem focused history; An expanded problem focused examination; and Medical decision making of moderate complexity. -57 Decision for surgery
29125-RT Application of short arm splint (forearm to hand); static; -RT Right

Figure 38-6 ■ Example of Coding for Application of Casts and Strapping. *Source: © PB Resources, Inc. Used with permission. CPT codes only © American Medical Association.*

Follow along in your CPT manual as Jacob Bates, CCS, assigns codes. Check off each step after you complete it.

▶ First, Jacob confirms *Right knee arthroscopy with partial medial meniscectomy and lateral meniscorrhaphy.*

▶ Jacob searches the Index for the Main Term **Knee**. Because both procedures are arthroscopic procedures on the right knee, he thinks that he will find the codes close together, so he begins with a general search on the knee and will refine it later, as needed.

❏ He locates the first-level modifying term **Arthroplasty**. Then he locates another first-level modifying term, **Arthroscopy**. He notices that different codes are listed after each entry, so he must decide which entry is preferred. He recalls that the default approach for surgical

procedures is open and then recognizes that **Arthroplasty** identifies an open procedure, whereas **Arthroscopy** identifies an endoscopic procedure. An arthroscopy was performed, so **Arthroscopy** is the Main Term he needs.

❏ He reads the second-level modifying terms **Diagnostic** and **Surgical**. The procedure performed has both diagnostic and surgical features. He recognizes that surgical procedures always include diagnostic procedures at the same site, so he selects the modifying term **Surgical**.

❏ He identifies the relevant codes **29866-29868, 29871, 29873-29877, 29879-29889**. He recognizes that numerous codes and code ranges are provided, so he will need to research the Tabular List carefully to be certain he doesn't miss anything. He also notices that, in the Index, there are no modifying terms to help distinguish between the meniscectomy and meniscorrhaphy.

▶ Jacob turns to the Tabular List to review and select the codes. He decides to begin with **29866**, the first code listed.

❑ He notices that the first three codes (**29866-29868**) are a code family that describes **osteochondral autografts**, **allografts**, and **meniscal transplantation**. Although the meniscus was treated, a transplantation was not involved. Therefore, none of these codes are correct for this case.

❑ He identifies that the next code, **29871**, is a parent code for all entries through code **29887**. The common descriptor states **Arthroscopy, knee, surgical**; He reads all the indented code descriptions to identify one that describes the procedure performed.

  ▪ Code **29877** describes **debridement/shaving of articular cartilage (chondroplasty)**. Debridement was performed, so he identifies this code as a possibility.

  ▪ Codes **29880** and **29881** describe **meniscectomy**. A medial meniscectomy was performed, so he identifies these codes as a possibility.

  ▪ Codes **29882** and **29883** describe **meniscus repair**. The lateral meniscus was sutured, so he identifies this code as a possibility.

❑ The final two codes listed in the Index, **29899** and **29899** describe the **anterior** and **posterior cruciate ligaments**, respectively. These ligaments were not treated, so these codes are not correct.

▶ Jacob reviews the five codes he identified as possibilities.

❑ Although code **29877** describes debridement and shaving, the site is articular cartilage, not the medial meniscus. He refers to the documentation and confirms that the articular cartilage was probed and evaluated and did not require any chondroplasty. Therefore, he determines that this code is not correct.

❑ Code **29880** describes **meniscectomy** and **meniscal shaving** but identifies the **medial AND lateral** ligaments. Although both the medial lateral menisci were treated, only the medial meniscus was debrided. Jacob determines that this code probably is not correct.

❑ Code **29881** describes **meniscectomy** and **meniscal shaving** and identifies the **medial OR lateral** ligaments. Because only the medial meniscus was debrided, he thinks this code could be the one he needs. However, he knows he must review all the codes to determine if there is another code that accurately describes both procedures. He reads in the code description that the code includes **debridement/shaving of articular cartilage (chondroplasty) . . . when performed**. He recognizes that the words **when performed** do not require that a chondroplasty be performed to use this code.

❑ Codes **29882** and **29883** describe **meniscus repair**. Jacob refers to the documentation and determines that no repair was performed on the medial meniscus because the damage was irreparable. That is the reason the debridement was performed. The lateral meniscus was repaired with sutures, so he thinks one of these codes could be correct.

❑ He compares the descriptions of codes. Code **29882** describes **meniscus repair** and identifies **medial OR lateral**. Because only the lateral meniscus was debrided, he determines that this code probably is correct.

❑ Code **29883** describes **meniscus repair** and identifies **medial AND lateral**. He determines this code is not correct because, although both the medial and lateral menisci were treated, only the lateral meniscus was repaired.

❑ After reviewing all codes listed in the code range and verifying the details of anatomic site and procedure with the documentation, Jacob determines that code **29881** is the correct code for partial medial meniscectomy and code **29882** is the correct code for the lateral meniscorrhaphy.

❑ He must combine the *common descriptor* portion of parent code **29871** with the *unique descriptors* of codes **29881** and **29882** to arrive at the complete code descriptions.

▶ Jacob checks for instructions in the Tabular List.

❑ He looks for instructional notes immediately before or after codes **29881** and **29882** to identify any information about whether the two codes can be used together. After careful checking, he does not find any warnings or instructions that prohibit reporting both codes.

❑ He cross-references the special instructions at the beginning of **Endoscopy/Arthroscopy** that state **Surgical endoscopy/arthroscopy always includes a diagnostic endoscopy/arthroscopy**. This confirms that the diagnostic inspection of the rest of the knee compartment and the articular cartilage surfaces is bundled with the code for the surgical procedures and should not be coded separately.

❑ He cross-references the special instructions at beginning of the subcategory **Musculoskeletal System** and verifies that there are no additional instructions that apply to this procedure.

▶ Jacob reviews the procedure code he has assigned for this case.

❑ **29881 Arthroscopy, knee, surgical; with meniscectomy (medial OR lateral, including any meniscal shaving) including debridement/shaving of articular cartilage (chondroplasty), same or separate compartment(s), when performed**

❑ **29882 Arthroscopy, knee, surgical; with meniscus repair (medial OR lateral)**

▶ Next, Jacob must determine how to sequence the codes.

cartilage (chondroplasty), same or separate compartment(s), when performed

❑ **29882 Arthroscopy, knee, surgical; with meniscus repair (medial OR lateral)**

▶ Jacob arranges the codes in descending RVU order according to the Medicare Physician Fee Schedule Database (MPFSDB). He uses the facility RVU because the procedure was performed at the outpatient surgery center, not at the physician's office.

❑ **29882** Facility RVU = 20.00

❑ **29881** Facility RVU = 15.47

▶ Jacob examines the need for modifiers. (Refer to Table 30-1 Key Criteria for Abstracting CPT Modifiers or Appendix A in the CPT manual.)

❑ Code **29882** requires two modifiers. Modifier **-RT** identifies the right knee. The National Correct Coding Initiative (NCCI) identifies **29882** as a Column 2 code when reported with code **29881**. This designation means that the lateral meniscus repair should be specifically identified as distinct from meniscectomy on the medial meniscus because it was performed to correct a separate injury at a separate site and in a different compartment of the knee. Modifier **-59 Distinct procedural service** reports this information. There are no additional modifiers that identify each different knee compartment or meniscus. The Column 2 indicator identifies that code **29882** is bundled into code **29881** when both are done on the same site. It is unusual that code **29882**, the code with the higher RVU, is bundled into code **29881**, the code with the lower RVU of the pair. Jacob sequences modifier **-59**

first because it provides information used for determining payment. Modifier **-RT** is informational only.

❑ Code **29881** requires modifiers **-RT Right** to identify the right knee. This code is unusual because it has a lower RVU value even though it is actually the more extensive procedure. Jacob appends modifier **-51 Multiple procedures** because it was performed during the same operative session as another procedure. Jacob is reminded by the encoder he uses that because arthroscopy was performed, the codes are subject to the **multiple endoscopy rule** for modifier **-51** (■ FIGURE 38-8). The multiple endoscopy rule states that when two codes from the same code family are reported, 100% is allowed on the first procedure and the allowed amount for second procedure is the *difference* in price between the second code and the endoscopic base code, which in this case is **29870** (facility RVU = 11.76). The MPFSDB identifies the endoscopic base code for each code family. (Refer to Figure 35-6 Example of Multiple Endoscopy Payment Rule.) Jacob sequences modifier **-51** first because it provides information used to calculate payment. Modifier **-RT** is informational only.

❑ He sequences code **29882** first because it has the higher RVU value, even though it requires modifier **-59**.

❑ He sequences code **29881** second because it has a lower RVU value and thus a lower payment.

▶ Jacob finalizes the procedure codes and sequencing for this case:

(1) **29882-59-RT Arthroscopy, knee, surgical; with meniscus repair (medial OR lateral); -59 Distinct procedural service; -RT Right**

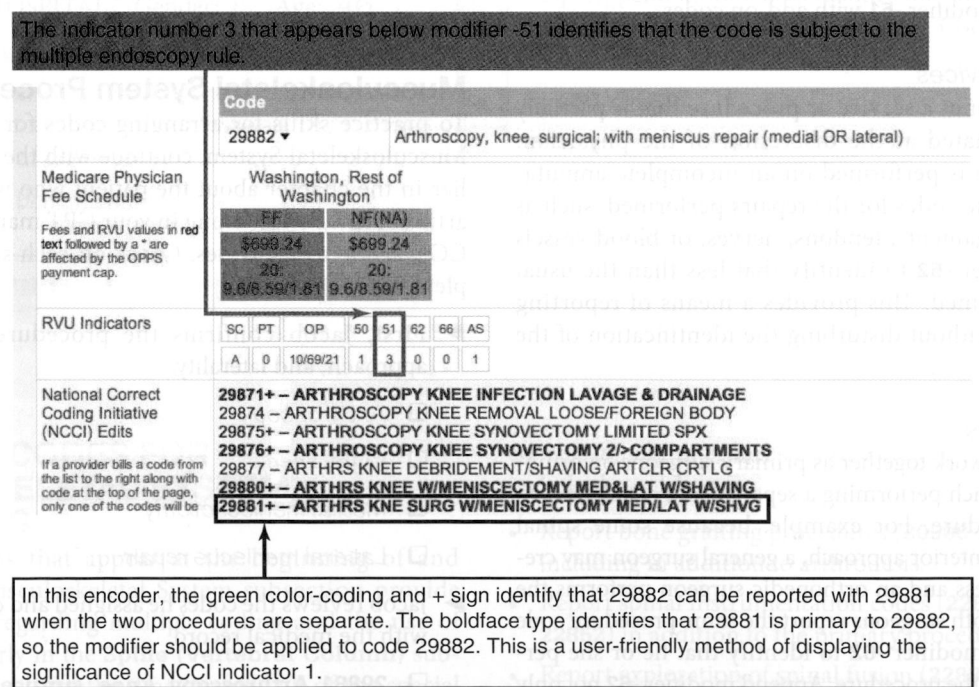

The indicator number 3 that appears below modifier -51 identifies that the code is subject to the multiple endoscopy rule.

Code	
29882 ▾	Arthroscopy, knee, surgical; with meniscus repair (medial OR lateral)

Medicare Physician Fee Schedule	Washington, Rest of Washington	
Fees and RVU values in **red** text followed by a * are affected by the OPPS payment cap.	FF	NF(NA)
	$699.24	$699.24
	20: 9.6/8.59/1.81	20: 9.6/8.59/1.81

RVU Indicators	SC	PT	OP	50	51	62	66	AS
	A	0	10/69/21	1	3	0	0	1

National Correct Coding Initiative (NCCI) Edits

If a provider bills a code from the list to the right along with code at the top of the page, only one of the codes will be

29871+ – ARTHROSCOPY KNEE INFECTION LAVAGE & DRAINAGE
29874 – ARTHROSCOPY KNEE REMOVAL LOOSE/FOREIGN BODY
29875+ – ARTHROSCOPY KNEE SYNOVECTOMY LIMITED SPX
29876+ – ARTHROSCOPY KNEE SYNOVECTOMY 2/>COMPARTMENTS
29877 – ARTHRS KNEE DEBRIDEMENT/SHAVING ARTCLR CRTLG
29880+ – ARTHRS KNEE W/MENISCECTOMY MED&LAT W/SHAVING
29881+ – ARTHRS KNE SURG W/MENISCECTOMY MED/LAT W/SHVG

In this encoder, the green color-coding and + sign identify that 29882 can be reported with 29881 when the two procedures are separate. The boldface type identifies that 29881 is primary to 29882, so the modifier should be applied to code 29882. This is a user-friendly method of displaying the significance of NCCI indicator 1.

Figure 38-8 ■ Example of Encoder Screen Showing Coding Rules for Code 29882.
Source: Copyright © SpeedeCoder. Reprinted with Permission.

(2) **29881-51-RT Arthroscopy, knee, surgical; with meniscectomy (medial OR lateral, including any meniscal shaving) including debridement/shaving of articular cartilage (chondroplasty), same or separate compartment(s), when performed; -51 Multiple procedures; -RT Right**

▶ Jacob also assigns and sequences the ICD-10-CM diagnosis codes that support the need for the service. He sequences the diagnosis code for the tear of the lateral meniscus first because the repair of the lateral meniscus is the first-listed procedure. He understands that it is acceptable to report diagnoses in a different order than they appear in the postoperative diagnosis in the operative report, based on coding and billing guidelines. A diagnosis for chondromalacia is reported, even though the condition was not directly treated,

because it is part of the diagnostic evaluation and the physician documents it as significant in the operative report.

(1) **S83.261A Peripheral tear of lateral meniscus, current injury, right knee, initial encounter**

(2) **S83.231A Complex tear of medial meniscus, current injury, right knee, initial encounter**

(3) **M94.261 Chondromalacia, right knee**

SUCCESS STEP

If you do not have an encoder available, you can search the MPFSDB to identify the modifier indicator and the NCCI database to identify the NCCI bundling rules. Both databases are available at **www.cms.gov**.

CODING PRACTICE

Exercise 38.4 Arranging Codes for Musculoskeletal System Procedures

Instructions: Read the mini-medical-record of each patient's encounter. Review the information abstracted in Exercise 38.2 for questions 1–3. For questions 4–6, abstract the case on your own. Assign CPT codes, quantities, and modifiers using the Index and Tabular List, and arrange the codes in proper sequence. Write the code(s) on the line provided.

1. INPATIENT HOSPITAL   Gender: M   Age: 65

Preprocedure diagnosis: pain in the thoracic spine due to degenerated and protruding discs

Procedure: arthrodesis on T9–T10 and T10–T11 interspace using an anterolateral approach

Postprocedure diagnosis: degeneration and protrusion, T9–T10 and T10–T11

2 CPT Codes _____

2. EMERGENCY DEPARTMENT   Gender: M   Age: 25

Preprocedure diagnosis: Index finger and middle finger on right hand were completely amputated during automobile accident.

Procedure: reattached both fingers, including distal tip to sublimis tendon insertion

Tip: Identify the quantity to be reported with the code. Assign modifiers to identify the digits treated.

1 CPT Code _____

3. INPATIENT HOSPITAL   Gender: F   Age: 42

Preprocedure diagnosis: chronic lower back pain due to degenerative disc disease

Procedure: Arthroplasty L4–L5 and L5–L6. Using an anterior approach excised the entire disc L4–L5 and inserted an implant. We then moved to L5-L6 where we also excised the entire disc L4–L5 and inserted an implant. Patient tolerated procedure well and was moved to PACU in stable condition.

Postprocedure diagnosis: intervertebral disc degeneration L4-L5, L5-L6

Tip: Read the instructional notes in the Tabular List to identity the second code.

2 CPT Codes _____

4. OUTPATIENT HOSPITAL   Gender: F   Age: 33

Preprocedure diagnosis: fractures of vertebrae L3 and L4

Procedure: percutaneous vertebroplasty, injected bone cement bilaterally into both vertebrae

Tip: Code only for the treatment, not the E/M or supplies.

2 CPT Codes _____

(continued)

5. EMERGENCY DEPARTMENT   Gender: M   Age: 22

Preprocedure diagnosis: ATV accident, open fracture of the distal clavicle and deeply embedded debris in left shoulder

Procedure: Reduced fracture and applied internal fixation device consisting of wire and screws to stabilize bone. Excised debris from subcutaneous and subfascial tissue in left shoulder.

Tip: The treatment is open because internal fixation was applied.

2 CPT Codes _____

6. OUTPATIENT HOSPITAL   Gender: F   Age: 26

Preprocedure diagnosis: right PCL avulsion

Procedure: arthroscopically aided open repair of the right posterior cruciate ligament. Used an assistant surgeon (from the same medical group).

Tip: Code for both the surgeon and the assistant surgeon, using the appropriate modifier.

2 CPT Codes _____

E/M CODING FOR ORTHOPEDICS

The *1997 Documentation Guidelines for Evaluation and Management Services* (1997 DG), published by CMS, provides requirements for each level of a musculoskeletal E/M examination (■ FIGURE 38-9). Orthopedists are not limited to using the guidelines for a musculoskeletal examination only. They can also use guidelines for a general multiorgan system examination, or any other single organ system examination, based on what is most advantageous for a specific encounter. However, physicians cannot combine elements from more than one type of examination for a given encounter. The musculoskeletal examination guidelines typically provide the best results when a detailed musculoskeletal examination is performed.

To determine the appropriate E/M code, coders must review the documentation in detail and identify the specific elements documented.

- To identify the category and type of service, identify whether the encounter is a consultation—a service requested by another physician with a report back—or an office or inpatient visit in which the orthopedist is managing the care of the problem.

- To translate the documentation into the E/M requirements for the history, refer back to Chapter 31, Evaluation and Management Services (99201-99499), Tables 31-7 to 31-10, or to the 1997 DG.

- To determine the requirements for an examination, refer to Figure 38-9 or to the single organ system examination for the musculoskeletal system in the 1997 DG.

- To determine the levels for medical decision making (MDM), refer to Chapter 31, Table 31-12, and also the Table of Risk in the 1997 DG.

Guided Example of E/M Coding for the Musculoskeletal System

Refer to the orthopedic encounter (■ FIGURE 38-10) to practice skills for abstracting and assigning E/M codes. Follow along as fictitious coder Jacob Bates, CCS, abstracts the procedure. Check off each step after you complete it.

▶ First, Jacob needs to establish the category of service so he can determine the information needed to abstract and assign the code.

❏ *What is the setting?* Office.

❏ *What is the type of service?* Established patient.

❏ *What is the code range?* Jacob refers to the CPT Index and looks up the Main Term **Evaluation and Management** and the subterm **Office and other outpatient**. The code range listed is **99201-99215**.

❏ *How many key components are required?* Jacob refers to the code range in the Tabular List and identifies that **99211-99215** identify established patient visits. All codes in the category except **99211** have the same requirements for key components. He reads the code description of the second code, which states **two out of three**. This tells him that two of three key components must meet or exceed the levels listed in the code (2/3).

▶ Next, Jacob identifies the level of history.

❏ *What is the level of HPI?* The HPI is **Extended** because four elements are documented.

❏ *What is the level of ROS?* The ROS is **Pertinent** because one system is documented.

System/Body Area	Elements of Musculoskeletal System Examination
Constitutional	❑ Measurement of any **three** of the following seven **vital** signs: • 1) sitting or standing blood pressure, • 2) supine blood pressure, • 3) pulse rate and regularity, • 4) respiration, • 5) temperature, • 6) height, • 7) weight (May be measured and recorded by ancillary staff) ❑ General **appearance** of patient (eg, development, nutrition, body habitus, deformities, attention to grooming)
Cardiovascular	❑ **Examination of peripheral vascular system by** • **observation** (eg, swelling, varicosities) • **palpation** (eg, pulses, temperature, edema, tenderness)
Lymphatic	Palpation of lymph nodes in **two or more** areas: ❑ Neck ❑ Axillae ❑ Groin ❑ Other
Musculoskeletal	❑ Examination of **gait** and **station** Examination of joints, bones and muscles of **four** of the following six areas: ❑ 1) head and neck; ❑ 2) spine, ribs and pelvis; ❑ 3) right upper extremity; ❑ 4) left upper extremity; ❑ 5) right lower extremity; and ❑ 6) left lower extremity. The examination of a given area includes: • Inspection and/or palpation with notation of presence of any **misalignment**, asymmetry, crepitation, defects, tenderness, masses, effusions • Assessment of **range of motion** with notation of any pain, crepitation or contracture • Assessment of **stability** with notation of any dislocation (luxation), subluxation or laxity • Assessment of muscle **strength** and **tone** (eg, flaccid, cog wheel, spastic) with notation of any atrophy or abnormal movements NOTE: For the **comprehensive** level of examination: all four of the **elements** identified by a bullet must be performed and documented for **each of four anatomic** areas. For the **problem focused, expanded problem focused, and detailed levels** of examination: Count each element **separately** for each body area. For example, assessing range of motion in two extremities constitutes two elements.
Skin	**Inspection and/or palpation** of skin and subcutaneous tissue (eg, scars, rashes, lesions, café-au-lait spots, ulcers) in **four** of the following six areas: ❑ 1) head and neck; ❑ 2) spine, ribs and pelvis; ❑ 3) right upper extremity; ❑ 4) left upper extremity; ❑ 5) right lower extremity; and ❑ 6) left lower extremity. NOTE: For the **comprehensive** level of examination: the examination of all **four anatomic** areas must be performed and documented. For the **problem focused, expanded problem focused, and detailed levels** of examination: Count each body area **separately**. For example, inspection and/or palpation of the skin and subcutaneous tissue of two extremities constitutes two elements.
Neurological/ Psychiatric	❑ Test **coordination** (eg, finger/nose, heel/ knee/shin, rapid alternating movements in the upper and lower extremities, evaluation of fine motor coordination in young children) ❑ Examination of **deep tendon reflexes** and/or nerve stretch test with notation of pathological reflexes (eg, Babinski) ❑ Examination of **sensation** (eg, by touch, pin, vibration, proprioception) Brief assessment of **mental status** including ❑ **Orientation** to time, place and person ❑ **Mood** and **affect** (eg, depression, anxiety, agitation)

Total # Bullets Performed and Documented →	☐	# of ❑ Elements Performed and Documented	Level of Examination
		1–5	Problem focused
		6–11	Expanded problem focused
		12	Detailed
		ALL	Comprehensive (Document **every** element in each box with a shaded border and at least **one** element in each box with an unshaded border)

Figure 38-9 ■ 1997 DG for Musculoskeletal System Examination. *Source: Centers for Medicare and Medicaid Services, 1997 Documentation Guidelines for Evaluation and Management Services (with formatting adjustments).*

ORTHOPEDIC ENCOUNTER

CHIEF COMPLAINT: Left wrist pain.

HISTORY OF PRESENT PROBLEM: The patient has a previous history of a left traumatic wrist injury, which has left him with a chronic scapholunate problem and possibly other problems in his wrist, which I have seen him for multiple times over the past five years, most recently about 18 months ago. He was doing relatively fine and tolerating the wrist soreness that he had, which varies day to day, but it has not gotten much worse until this most recent injury. He lifted a box out of the back of his car three weeks ago and it started to hurt with a sharp stabbing pain. Since then he was significantly more affected than he was before, and now he reports a dull aching pain on the ulnar side of his wrist. He presents to my office for evaluation.

CLINICAL/PHYSICAL EXAMINATION:
Musculoskeletal: An examination of the left wrist shows that the patient has point tenderness to palpation along the ulnar styloid extensor carpi ulnaris (ECU) ridge with some minor tenderness at the triangular fibrocartilage complex (TFC) region, as well as the lunotriquetral joint. There is some minor soreness, but not nearly as sore at the scapholunate (SL) ligament with dorsiflexion 30°, palmar flexion 30°, radial deviation 5° and ulnar deviation 0°. Supination/pronation grossly intact without significant signs of instability. Negative piano key sign compared to the contralateral side.
Skin: No skin breakdown or hyperhidrosis.
Neurologic: Negative signs of compressive median nerve neuropathy.
Vascular: Intact.

RADIOLOGICAL/LABORATORY EXAM: X-rays, three views of the wrist of good penetrance and quality, reveal scapholunate widening of a slack wrist with a possible ulnar styloid nonunion, with a possible occult distal radius fracture fibrous union. MRI report reviewed.

EVALUATION/TREATMENT PLAN: The MRI is consistent with edema and swelling in the ulnar styloid region, which is consistent with the injury pattern that he is claiming and where he is most sore. He has a chronic problem that needs to potentially be addressed. Sometimes with these acute on chronic problems, what was tolerated initially may no longer be tolerated by the patient, which we talked about. Our focus still should be on the initial injury which brought him in at this time. It is a three-week-old injury. Given the MRI, we probably have seen on radiographs a fibrous union between that ulnar styloid and the remaining portion of the ulna, which may have been torn or injured, especially consistent with the MRI. Therefore, I would cast him initially to get that to heal, and then reassess. All questions were answered, and we will make the treatment plans accordingly. He will followup in two weeks. We casted him.

KEY: HPI History of the present illness ROS Review of systems
PFSH Past, family, and social history MDM Medical decision making

HISTORY: Problem focused
Chief complaint (CC)
PFSH: Pertinent (1)
ROS: None (0)
MDM Management: Established presenting problem, worsening (Low Complexity Management Options)
HPI: Extended (4+)
Setting & patient type

EXAMINATION: Problem focused
(1-5 elements)

MDM Data: Independent visualization of image, tracing, or scan by physician performing the E/M service (High Complexity Data)

MEDICAL DECISION MAKING: Moderate Complexity
MDM Risk: Acute illness with systemic symptoms, Elective major surgery (open, percutaneous or endoscopic) with no identified risk factors (Moderate Risk)

Figure 38-10 ■ Orthopedic Encounter. *Source: © PB Resources, Inc. Used with permission.*

❑ *What is the level of PFSH?* The PFSH is **Pertinent** because one element is documented.

❑ *Based on these factors, what is the overall level of history?* The level of history is **Expanded problem focused** because the lowest of the three factors (HPI, ROS, and PFSH) determines the history level. The HPI qualifies for a detailed history but the ROS and PFSH qualify for an expanded problem-focused history.

▶ Jacob refers to the musculoskeletal system examination in the 1997 DG (Figure 38-9) to abstract information needed to determine the level of the examination.

❑ *What is the level of examination?* The level of examination is **Problem focused**. Three (3) elements of the examination are documented, which exceeds the requirement of one to five bulleted elements for a problem-focused examination.

▶ Jacob determines the level of medical decision making. (Refer to Table 31-12 Medical Decision Making Levels.)

❑ *What is the level of complexity of the number of diagnoses or management options, based on the presenting problem?* The level is **Low complexity** because there is an established presenting problem that is worsening as a result of a recent exacerbation.

❑ *What is the amount and/or complexity of data to be reviewed?* The level is **High complexity** because the physician providing the E/M service performed an independent visualization of the X-rays and MRI.

❑ *What is the level of risk of significant complications, morbidity, and/or mortality?* Jacob reviews each column in the Table of Risk in the 1997 DG and determines that the level of risk is **Moderate**. The patient presents with a chronic condition with mild exacerbation (Moderate),

X-rays and an MRI were ordered (Minimal), and casting was performed (Minimal). The single highest element in the Table of Risk determines the overall risk. The column **Presenting problem** is the highest level (Moderate).

❑ *Based on these factors, what is the overall level of medical decision making?* The medical decision making is **Moderate complexity**. At least two of the three MDM factors are required to qualify for a specific level of

MDM. Because the complexity of data to be reviewed is high and the risk of complications is moderate, two of the three MDM factors meet or exceed moderate decision making.

Now Jacob is ready to assign the code for the orthopedic encounter. The exercise that follows guides you through additional abstracting skills and allows you to assign the correct code.

CODING PRACTICE

Exercise 38.5   E/M Coding for Orthopedics

Instructions: Refer to the *1997 Documentation Guidelines for Evaluation and Management Services* (available at www.cms.gov) or Chapter 31 Evaluation and Management Services (Tables 31-7 to 31-12) in this text. Answer the following questions about the orthopedic encounter (Figure 38-10).

1. a. Which elements of the HPI are documented? Circle all that apply. Location, Quality, Severity, Duration, Timing, Context, Modifying factors, Associated signs and symptoms

   b. How many elements are documented? _____

   c. What is the level of HPI? _____

2. a. Which systems are reviewed in the ROS? Circle all that apply. Constitutional, Allergic/ immunologic, CV, Endocrine, ENT/M, Eyes, GI, GU, Hemic/lymphatic, MS, Neurologic, Psychiatric, Respiratory, Skin/breast

   b. How many systems are documented? _____

   c. What is the level of ROS? _____

3. a. Which PFSH elements are documented? Circle all that apply. Past medical, Family, Social

   b. What is the level of PFSH? _____

   c. What is the overall level of history? (The lowest history factor—HPI, ROS, or PFSH—determines the level of history.) _____

4. Refer to Figure 38-9 (1997 DG for Musculoskeletal System Examination).

   a. Which bulleted items are documented for the examination? (Check off the items documented.)

   b. How many bulleted items are documented? _____

   c. What is the level of the examination? _____

5. Refer to Table 31-12 Medical Decision Making Levels or the 1997 DG.

   a. What is the MDM level for the number of diagnoses or management options? _____

   b. What is the MDM level for the amount and/or complexity of data to be reviewed? _____

   c. Refer to the Table of Risk in the 1997 DG. Which elements of risk are documented for each risk factor?

      1. Presenting problem: _____

      2. Diagnostic procedures ordered: _____

      3. Management options selected: _____

   d. What is the level of risk? (The highest of the three risk factors determines the overall level of risk.) _____

   e. What is the overall level of MDM? (2/3 MDM factors are needed to determine the overall level.) _____

6. a. What is the setting? _____

   b. What is the patient (or service) type? _____

   c. What is the code range? _____

   d. How many key components are required? _____

   e. What is the level of history? _____

   f. What is the level of examination? _____

   g. What is the level of medical decision making? _____

   h. What is the correct code? _____

   i. What modifier(s) is required? _____

7. Abstract and assign the diagnosis code that supports the E/M code. There are no appropriate external cause codes.

   1 ICD-10-CM Code _____

CHAPTER SUMMARY

In this chapter you learned that:

- Any given orthopedic procedure can be performed using a variety of techniques, which can involve specific types of sutures and bone anchors aimed at promoting maximum stability and preventing reinjury.

- The CPT section/subsection **Musculoskeletal System (20005-29999)** contains 15 subheadings that are divided by anatomic site.

- Because the Musculoskeletal System is a combination of two systems, separate abstracting guidelines are provided for skeletal system, fractures and dislocations, and muscular system procedures.

- Two areas requiring special attention when assigning codes are using the Index to locate the appropriate anatomic site and coding for fracture care.

- Special instructions that appear at the beginning of and throughout the Musculoskeletal System subsection provide detailed guidance regarding multiple coding and the use of modifiers, particularly in the **Spine (Vertebral Column)** subheading.

- The *1997 Documentation Guidelines for Evaluation and Management Services* (1997 DG), published by CMS, provides requirements for each level of a musculoskeletal E/M examination, but orthopedists are not limited to using the guidelines for a musculoskeletal examination only.

- CPT provides guidelines about fracture treatment and excision of muscular system tumors at the beginning of the Musculoskeletal System subsection. Detailed special instructions and instructional notes throughout the subsection provide guidance regarding coding spinal procedures, modifiers, and multiple coding.

CONCEPT QUIZ

Take a moment to look back at the Musculoskeletal System and solidify your skills. Try to answer the questions from memory first, then refer to the discussion in this chapter if you need a little extra help.

Completion

Instructions: Write the term that answers each question based on the information you learned in this chapter. Choose from the list below. Some choices may be used more than once and some choices may not be used at all.

arthroplasty	internal fixation
biopsy	interspace
chondroplasty	manipulation
decompression	reconstruction
discectomy	replantation
external fixation	spinal fusion
fasciotomy	tenolysis
hemiarthroplasty	vertebral segment

1. _____ is another term for fracture stabilization with a rigid frame and one or more screws.

2. _____ is the use of force to move parts of a bone into normal alignment.

3. To relieve shoulder impingement a(n) _____ may be performed.

4. _____ is removing a sample of muscle to determine the presence of disease such as a muscular dystrophy.

5. In a(n) _____, two vertebrae are joined together to provide stabilization.

6. A(n) _____ may be performed when a knee injury requires reshaping and cleaning of the cartilage.

7. A partial replacement of a joint is called a(n) _____.

8. _____ is the release of a tendon.

9. A reattachment of a complete amputation of a thumb is also called a(n) _____.

10. On disc procedures, L2-L3 refers to one _____.

Multiple Choice

Instructions: Circle the letter of the best answer to each question based on the information you learned in this chapter.

1. What is the medical term for surgical excision of a joint?
   A. Arthrotomy
   B. Arthroplasty
   C. Arthrectomy
   D. Arthrodesis

2. Which type of treatment involves manipulation of displaced bones?
   A. Restorative
   B. Palliative
   C. Stabilization
   D. External fixation

3. What is the Main Term that classifies procedures on the patella?
   A. Knee
   B. Knee joint
   C. Knee bone
   D. Kneecap

4. What modifier is used when a neurosurgeon and an orthopedic surgeon each perform a portion of an anterior cervical discectomy and fusion at C5-C6?
   A. -51
   B. -54
   C. -62
   D. -80

5. What resource helps the coder to determine sequencing of CPT codes?
   A. Multiple Endoscopy Rule
   B. Medicare Physician Fee Schedule
   C. Appendix A of the CPT code book
   D. Appendix G of the CPT code book

6. During an ORIF of the femur, the patient developed tachycardia and the procedure was terminated. What modifier would the surgeon use?
   A. -33
   B. -52
   C. -53
   D. -54

7. What criteria must be abstracted to assign a code for excision of subcutaneous connective soft-tissue tumors?
   A. The approach used
   B. Location and size of the tumor

C. Type of bone involved
D. Complexity of the repair

8. When should a code for cast application be reported?
   A. When the cast is removed or repaired by a different individual than the one who applied it
   B. When different providers perform the preoperative care, restorative treatment, and/or postoperative care
   C. When the provider who applies the initial cast or strapping also provides restorative treatment for the fracture and all follow-up care
   D. When cast application or strapping is the only service provided and no other treatment is anticipated

9. What modifier is used when an arthrocentesis of the hip and ankle are performed during the same surgical episode by the same physician?
   A. -51
   B. -52
   C. -59
   D. -76

10. What resource identifies bundling rules?
    A. MPFS
    B. RVU
    C. OPPS
    D. NCCI

CODING CHALLENGE

Instructions: Read the mini-medical-record of each patient's encounter, then abstract, assign, and arrange ICD-10-CM diagnosis codes and CPT procedure codes using the appropriate Index and Tabular List. Assign quantities and modifiers where needed. Write the code(s) on the line provided.

1. OUTPATIENT SURGERY   Gender: M   Age: 12

Preprocedure diagnosis: malunion, proximal humerus fracture, right arm

Procedure: Repair of malunion of the right proximal humerus with internal fixation using a 2-hole, 16-mm pin plate

1 ICD-10-CM Code _____

1 CPT Code _____

2. OUTPATIENT SURGERY   Gender: F   Age: 56

Preprocedure diagnosis: chronic diabetic ulcer of left midfoot with muscle necrosis

Procedure: below-the-knee amputation, left leg

Postprocedure diagnosis: diabetic ulcer of plantar surface of the left midfoot with muscle necrosis

2 ICD-10-CM Codes _____

1 CPT Code _____

3. OUTPATIENT SURGERY   Gender: F   Age: 27

Preprocedure diagnosis: contractures due to excessive scarring of the tendon bed of the 4th and 5th fingers of the left hand from previous knife injury

Procedure: excision of flexor tendon of 4th and 5th fingers and implantation of synthetic rods, left hand

Postprocedure diagnosis: excessive scarring of the tendon bed of the 4th and 5th fingers of the left hand

Tip: Identify the digits using modifiers.

1 ICD-10-CM Code _____

2 CPT Codes _____

4. OUTPATIENT SURGERY   Gender: F   Age: 49

Preprocedure diagnosis: hammer toe deformity of left foot, third and fourth digits

Procedure: arthroplasty of the third and fourth digits proximal interphalangeal joint laterally of left foot

Postprocedure diagnosis: hammer toe deformity of left foot, third and fourth digits

1 ICD-10-CM Code _____

2 CPT Codes _____

(continued)

(continued from page 739)

5. EMERGENCY DEPT   Gender: M   Age: 26

Reason for encounter: worsening pain ×3 days in right lower leg extending to the foot, expanded problem-focused history, expanded problem-focused examination, low-complexity medical decision making

Procedure: short leg splint applied for stabilization

Assessment: acute right ankle sprain, possible small avulsion fracture

Plan: immobilize the ankle and make an appointment with the orthopedic surgeon in the next three days

Tip: Code only for the treatment, not the E/M or supplies.

1 ICD-10-CM Code _____

1 CPT Code _____

6. PHYSICIAN OFFICE   Gender: F   Age: 66

Reason for encounter: pathologic fracture of right radius, return to office for short arm cast change

Procedure: replaced short arm cast with a fiberglass gauntlet cast

Assessment: right radial fracture healing as expected; for cast change

Plan: return to office in two weeks

Tip: Code for the service and the supply.

1 ICD-10-CM Code _____

2 CPT Codes _____

7. INPATIENT HOSPITAL   Gender: F   Age: 50

Reason for encounter: chronic plantar fasciitis, right foot; morbidly obese at 327 lb; insulin-dependent diabetic

Procedure: open plantar fasciotomy, right foot

Assessment: failed conservative care; patient desires corrective surgery

Plan: walker boot post-op with full weight bearing, return to office in 4 days

4 ICD-10-CM Codes _____

_____

1 CPT Code _____

8. INPATIENT HOSPITAL   Gender: F   Age: 58

Preprocedure diagnosis: probable osteomyelitis

Procedure: open biopsy of left upper femur

Postprocedure diagnosis: acute and chronic osteomyelitis of the femur

Pathology report: acute and chronic osteomyelitis

Tip: Review the guidelines for anatomic modifiers.

2 ICD-10-CM Codes _____

1 CPT Code _____

9. PHYSICIAN OFFICE   Gender: M   Age: 52

Preprocedure diagnosis: subpatellar bursitis, left knee

Procedure: aspiration of fluid from bursa; excision of suspicious mole on left thigh

Postprocedure diagnosis: subpatellar bursitis, left knee; septic knee ruled out; malignant melanoma of thigh

2 ICD-10-CM Codes _____

2 CPT Codes _____

10. EMERGENCY DEPT   Gender: F   Age: 62

Reason for encounter: fall at home after stepping on a dog toy, now with pain and swelling of the left lower arm

Procedure: Closed reduction of left ulnar olecranon process

Assessment: X-ray reveals a nondisplaced fracture of the left ulnar olecranon process

Plan: referred to orthopedic surgeon for follow-up

Tip: Code for the diagnosis and the external cause. Apply seventh characters as required. Code only for the treatment, not the E/M or supplies.

3 ICD-10-CM Codes _____

_____

1 CPT Code _____

KEEP ON CODING

Instructions: Read the procedural statement, then use the appropriate Index and Tabular List to assign CPT procedure codes, quantities, and modifiers. Write the code(s) on the line provided.

1. Cemented right total hip replacement: CPT Code(s) _____

2. Kyphoplasty, T3, T4: CPT Code(s) _____

3. Endoscopic repair of rotator cuff tendon: CPT Code(s) _____

4. Arthroscopic repair of left and right medial menisci: CPT Code(s) _____

5. Arthroscopic repair of the anterior cruciate ligament, left knee: CPT Code(s) _____

6. Arthroscopic subacromial decompression: CPT Code(s) _____

7. Arthroscopic medial meniscectomy, right knee: CPT Code(s) _____

8. Removal of Stableloc external fixator from left wrist: CPT Code(s) _____

9. Left total knee replacement: CPT Code(s) _____

10. Hemiarthroplasty, femoral neck fracture: CPT Code(s) _____

11. Sternal debridement for wound infection: CPT Code(s) _____

12. Aspiration of three ganglion cysts of the wrist: CPT Code(s) _____

13. Complete amputation of second toe of left foot at the MTP joint: CPT Code(s) _____

14. ORIF right proximal humeral head: CPT Code(s) _____

15. Percutaneous drainage of right knee fluid: CPT Code(s) _____

16. Posterior interbody arthrodesis of lumbar vertebrae L1-L2: CPT Code(s) _____

17. Repair of fracture of the femoral shaft with intramedullary rod: CPT Code(s) _____

18. C4-C5, C5-C6 laminectomy for nerve root decompression: CPT Code(s) _____

19. ORIF bimalleolar fracture: CPT Code(s) _____

20. Lumbar laminectomy for decompression with foraminotomies L3-L4, L4-L5: CPT Code(s) _____

21. Open reduction internal fixation of ulnar shaft fracture with placement of long arm cast: CPT Code(s) _____

22. Radical resection of a 2.5-cm sarcoma of the scalp: CPT Code(s) _____

23. Incision and drainage with extensive debridement, left shoulder, with removal of total shoulder arthroplasty: CPT Code(s) _____

24. Removal of ulnar nail: CPT Code(s) _____

25. Open intramedullary nail fixation with locking screws of a left tibial shaft fracture: CPT Code(s) _____

Chapter 39

Cardiovascular System Procedures (33010-37799)

Chapter Outline

- **Cardiovascular System Procedure Basics**
- **Coding Overview of Cardiovascular System Procedures**
- **Abstracting Cardiovascular System Procedures**
- **Assigning Codes for Cardiovascular System Procedures**
- **Arranging Codes for Cardiovascular System Procedures**
- **E/M Coding for Cardiology**

Learning Objectives

After completing this chapter, you should have the skills to:

39.1 Spell and define the key words, medical terms, and abbreviations related to cardiovascular procedures.

39.2 Discuss the fundamentals of cardiovascular procedures.

39.3 Identify the main characteristics of coding for the Cardiovascular System.

39.4 Abstract procedural information from the medical record for coding cardiovascular procedures.

39.5 Assign codes for Cardiovascular System procedures.

39.6 Arrange codes for Cardiovascular System procedures.

39.7 Code evaluation and management services for cardiology.

39.8 Discuss the CPT coding guidelines related to the Cardiovascular System.

Key Terms and Abbreviations

bypass graft
cardiopulmonary bypass (CPB)
contralateral
ipsilateral
nonselective catheter placement
open heart surgery
selective catheter placement
vascular family

In addition to the key terms listed here, students should know the terms defined within tables in this chapter.

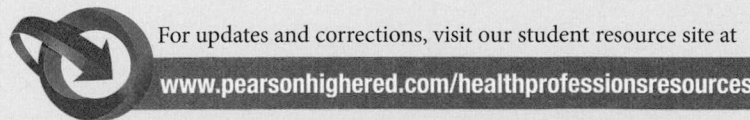

For updates and corrections, visit our student resource site at
www.pearsonhighered.com/healthprofessionsresources

INTRODUCTION

Traveling to a shopping destination may take you through a network of roads and streets. A primary destination, such as a mall, may be located next to a main highway, but to reach a small neighborhood shop you probably need to make turns onto a series of side streets. In a similar way, the cardiovascular system is a hierarchy of vessels, each leading to a more remote site than the previous one.

CARDIOVASCULAR SYSTEM PROCEDURE BASICS

Cardiology is a subspecialty of internal medicine that specializes in the cardiovascular system. Cardiologists perform medical procedures such as cardiac function tests and cardiac catheterization but do not perform surgery. Cardiothoracic surgeons perform surgery on the heart and surrounding structures, including the lung when necessary. Vascular surgeons perform surgery on the vessels. Some surgeons specialize further in areas such as heart valve surgery, neonatal cardiac surgery, and pediatric cardiac surgery. Chapter 14 of this text provides more information on cardiovascular system anatomy and conditions. Refer to ■ TABLE 39-1 for a refresher on how to build medical terms related to the cardiovascular system.

CODING CAUTION

Be alert for medical terms that are spelled similarly and have different meanings.

endarterectomy (*excision of the lining of a vessel*) and **enterectomy** (*excision of the intestine*)

arteriotomy (*incision into an artery*) and **ar<u>th</u>rotomy** (*incision into a joint*)

v<u>a</u>lvuloplasty (*surgical repair of a valve*) and **v<u>u</u>lvuloplasty** (*surgical repair of the vulva*)

Table 39-1 ■ EXAMPLE OF CONSTRUCTING MEDICAL TERMS FOR CARDIOVASCULAR PROCEDURES

Root/Combining Form	Suffix	Complete Medical Term
angi/o (*vessel*)		phlebo + tomy (*cutting into a vein*)
arteri/o (*artery*)		veni + puncture (*piercing a vein*)
	-tomy (*cutting into*) -puncture (*piercing*) -graphy (*recording*)	arterio + tomy (*cutting into an artery*)
		arterial + puncture (*piercing an artery*)
ven/o (*vein*)		angio + graphy (*recording of a vessel*)
phleb/o (*vein*)		veno + graphy (*recording of a vein*)
		arterio + graphy (*recording of an artery*)

Source: © PB Resources, Inc. Used with permission.

Procedures of the Cardiovascular System

Procedures commonly performed on the cardiovascular system are summarized in ■ TABLE 39-2. After discussing approaches to heart surgery, this section discusses procedures for pacemakers, catheterization, and congenital heart defects.

Approaches to Heart Surgery

Surgeons can operate on the heart using open-heart surgery, off-pump heart surgery, and minimally invasive heart surgery.

Open Heart Surgery Open heart surgery involves exposing the heart through a 30-cm (6 to 8 inches) incision in the chest wall that requires cutting through the sternum. For some types of surgery, the surgeon also may open the heart, but the term *open* refers to the chest, not the heart. After the heart is exposed, the patient is connected to a **cardiopulmonary** (*heart–lung*) **bypass** (CPB) machine that takes over the pumping action of the heart. A specialist oversees the CPB machine. It moves blood away from the heart, allowing the surgeon to operate on a heart that is not beating and does not have blood flowing through it. A breathing tube is placed through the throat into the lungs and is connected to a ventilator. After the procedure is completed, blood flow is restored to the heart and the patient is disconnected from the equipment. The sternum is closed with wires that remain in the body permanently. Open heart surgery is used to perform CABGs, repair or replace heart valves, treat atrial fibrillation, do heart transplants, and implant VADs and TAHs.

Off-Pump Heart Surgery Off-pump coronary artery bypass (OPCAB) surgery is also an open procedure, but a CPB machine is not used. The surgeon steadies the heart with a mechanical device and operates while blood is pumping through it. Although OPCAB is believed to reduce certain risks and complications associated with open heart surgery, it requires special training for the surgeon, and not all patients are candidates.

Minimally Invasive Heart Surgery For minimally invasive heart surgery, a surgeon makes small incisions (10–12 cm in length) in the side of the chest between the ribs. The surgeon connects a graft to diseased coronary arteries on a beating heart without any artificial support to the circulation. Because of the nature of the operation, suturing must be done under direct vision and the coronary artery to be bypassed must lie directly beneath the incision. Consequently, this procedure is only designed to bypass one or two coronary arteries. This procedure provides the most minimally invasive heart surgery alternative to limited CABG and angioplasty currently practiced.

Minimally invasive heart surgery is used to do some bypass and maze surgeries. Surgeons also used this approach to repair or replace heart valves, insert pacemakers or implantable cardioverter-defibrillators (ICDs), or harvest a vein or artery to use as a **bypass graft** (*inserting a new vessel to permanently redirect blood flow to avoid a blockage in an artery*) for CABG.

This type of procedure is also known as limited access coronary artery surgery and includes port-access coronary artery bypass (PACAB or PortCAB), which uses a heart–lung machine, and minimally invasive direct coronary artery bypass graft (MIDCAB), which does not.

Table 39-2 ■ **COMMON PROCEDURES OF THE CARDIOVASCULAR SYSTEM**

Procedure Name	Definition	Reason Performed
Arteriovenous (AV) fistula creation	Creation of a connection between an artery and vein	Hemodialysis access
Arteriovenous (AV) fistula repair	Closure of an abnormal connection between two vessels	Congenital or acquired AV fistula
Atherectomy	Threading through the veins a catheter that has a rotating shaver on its tip to cut away plaque from the artery	Atherosclerosis
Catheter ablation/ radiofrequency ablation	Use of a fluoroscopy-guided catheter to the exact site of arrhythmia in the heart to emit radiofrequency energy that destroys heart muscle cells in a very small area (about 1/5 of an inch)	Arrhythmia, supraventricular tachyarrhythmia
Coronary artery bypass grafting (CABG)	Grafting (*connecting*) a healthy artery or vein from elsewhere in the body to a blocked coronary artery	Coronary artery disease (CAD), arterial stenosis, lesions, atherosclerosis, or peripheral vascular occlusive disease
Endovascular aneurysm repair (EVAR)	Replacement of a weak section of an artery or heart wall with a patch, stent, or graft	Aneurysm
Excisional embolectomy/ thrombectomy	Incision into a vein or artery and removal of a clot	Embolus (*a moving blood clot or obstruction*) or thrombus (*a stationery blood clot*)
Fenestrated endovascular aneurysm repair (FEVAR)	Reinforcement of a weak section of the aorta with a stent that has holes customized to accommodate arterial branches	Aneurysm located at a site where a traditional stent would block one or more arteries
Heart transplant	Replacement of a diseased heart with a healthy heart from a deceased donor	End-stage heart failure
Maze surgery	Creation of new paths for the heart's electrical signals to travel through	Atrial fibrillation
Mechanical thrombectomy	A transcatheter procedure that uses a thrombolytic agent, radiological guidance, and a small blade or water jet to fragment, then suction out, a clot from an artery or vein	Thrombus
Pacemaker insertion	Placement under the skin of the chest or abdomen of a small device with wires connected to the heart chambers that transmit low-energy electrical pulses to control heart rhythm	Arrhythmia
Total artificial heart (TAH) implantation	Insertion of a device that replaces the ventricles	End-stage heart failure
Transmyocardial revascularization (TMR)	Use of lasers to make small channels through the heart muscle and into the left ventricle	Angina
Valve repair or replacement	Opening or tightening flaps on a heart valve	Valvular stenosis, regurgitation, or prolapse
Ventricular assist device (VAD) implantation	Insertion of a mechanical pump used to support heart function and blood flow	End-stage heart failure

Source: © PB Resources, Inc. Used with permission.

CODING CAUTION

Remember to distinguish between the terms *bypass graft* and *cardiopulmonary bypass*. A bypass graft refers to the *procedure* of inserting a new vessel to permanently redirect blood flow to avoid a blockage in an artery. Cardiopulmonary bypass refers to use of a *machine* to temporarily replace the function of the heart during surgery by directing the flow of blood away from the heart, through the bypass pump, and back into the body.

Pacemaker Procedures

Pacemakers and ICDs are small devices with a battery-operated pulse generator connected to leads (*wires*). Electrodes are attached to the leads, which then are attached to the heart. Physicians implant pacemakers in a skin pocket in the chest or abdomen to help control abnormal heart rhythms. They place leads directly on the epicardium (*outer layer of the heart*) through a thoracoscopy (*thoracotomy with endoscopy*) or transvenously (*through a vein*) and then into the right atrium or right ventricle (■ FIGURE 39-1). ICD electrodes are usually placed

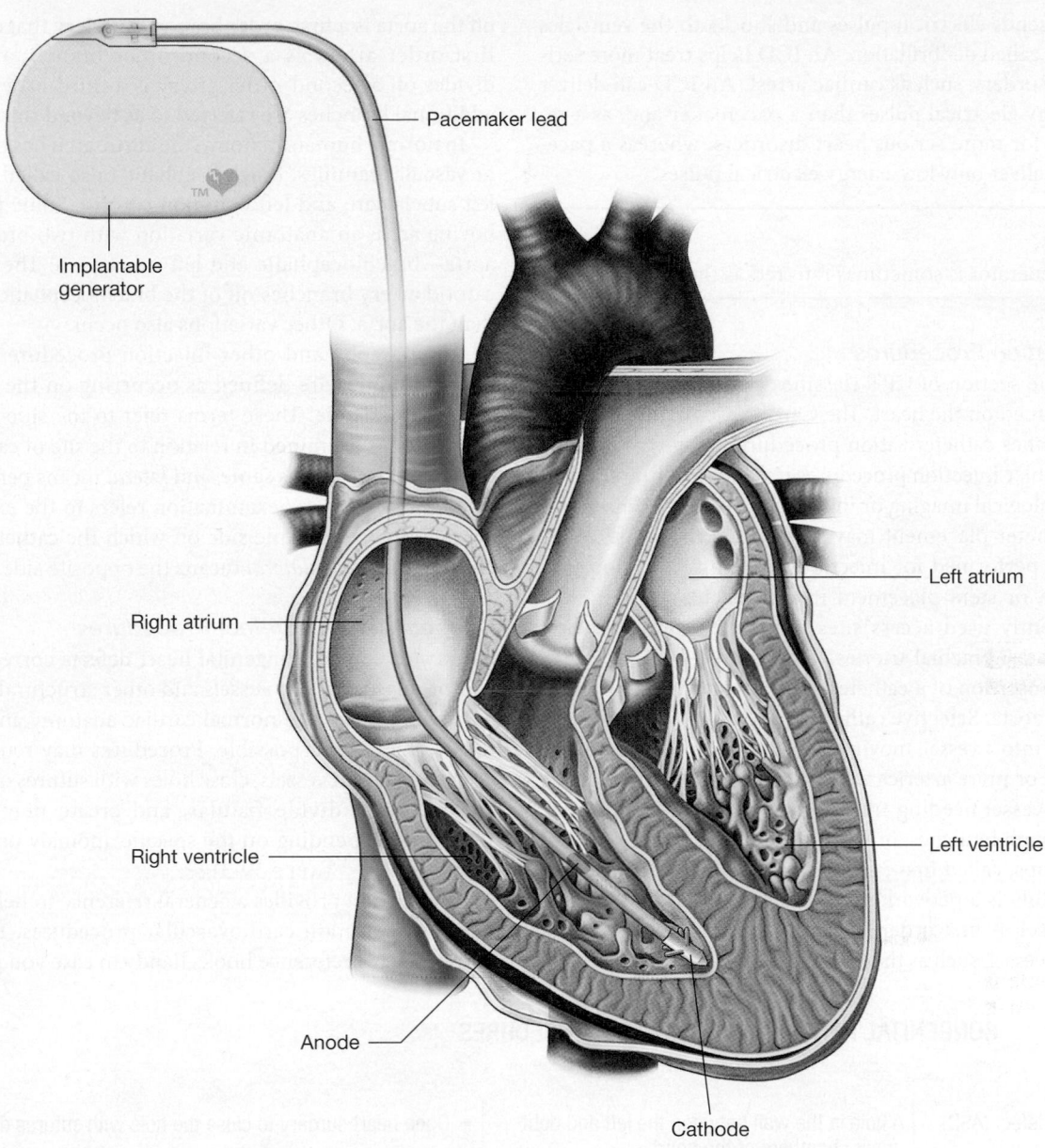

Figure 39-1 ■ Pacemaker Components

transvenously, but some can also be placed in a subcutaneous pocket with the pulse generator.

A pacemaker or ICD monitors heart rhythm and sends electrical pulses or shocks during an emergent situation to prompt the heart to beat at a normal rate. These devices are for patients with arrhythmias, disorders of heart rhythm including tachycardia and bradycardia. A pacemaker also records the heart's electrical activity and rhythm. The physician analyzes the recordings to adjust a patient's pacemaker so that it functions well.

Pacemakers have one to three wires that are each placed in different chambers of the heart.

• The wires in a single-chamber pacemaker usually carry pulses between the right ventricle and the pulse generator.

• The wires in a dual-chamber pacemaker carry pulses between the right atrium and the right ventricle and the pulse generator. The pulses help coordinate the timing of these two chambers' contractions using two leads.

• The wires in a biventricular pacemaker, also called a cardiac resynchronization therapy (CRT) device, carry pulses between an atrium and both ventricles and the generator. The pulses help coordinate electrical signaling between the two ventricles using three leads.

Pacemakers can be temporary or permanent. Temporary pacemakers are used to treat temporary heartbeat problems, such as a slow heartbeat caused by a heart attack, heart surgery, or an overdose of medicine. Temporary pacemakers also are used during emergencies until a permanent pacemaker can be implanted or until the temporary condition subsides. Permanent pacemakers are used to control long-term heart rhythm problems.

Pacemaker batteries last between 5 and 15 years, with an average of 7 years, depending on how active the pacemaker is. Physicians replace both the pulse generator and the battery before the battery starts to run down. Replacing the generator and battery is less-involved than the original surgery to implant the pacemaker. Eventually, the pacemaker's wires may also need to be replaced.

An ICD sends electrical pulses and shocks to the ventricles of the heart, called defibrillation. An ICD helps treat more serious heart disorders, such as cardiac arrest. An ICD can deliver higher-energy electrical pulses than a pacemaker and, as a result, is used for more serious heart disorders, whereas a pacemaker can deliver only low-energy electrical pulses.

SUCCESS STEP

A pulse generator is sometimes referred as the battery.

Catheterization Procedures

The Medicine section of CPT classifies catheterization procedures performed on the heart. The Cardiovascular System subsection classifies catheterization procedures performed on the vessels. Vascular injection procedures involve injecting contrast dye for radiological imaging or injecting medication into blood vessels. Catheter placement may be nonselective or selective and may be performed for injection procedures, angioplasty, atherectomy, or stent placement in the vascular system. The most frequently used access sites are the common femoral artery (CFA) and brachial arteries. **Nonselective catheter placement** is the insertion of a catheter that remains in the accessed vessel or the aorta. **Selective catheter placement** is the insertion of a catheter into a vessel, moving it to the aorta, then moving it through one or more arteries that branch off the aorta to reach the specific vessel needing treatment. Vessels connect to one another through branches, or vascular families, and are categorized in groups, called first-, second-, or third-order vessels. A **vascular family** is a network of vessels branching off the same primary vessel. A first-order branch is the first division off of the primary vessel, such as the aorta. The first artery that divides off the aorta is a first-order branch; an artery that divides off the first-order artery is a second-order branch; an artery that divides off a second-order artery is a third-order branch; any additional branches are referred to as beyond third-order.

In normal human anatomy, the aortic arch has three branches or vascular families: brachiocephalic (also called innominate), left subclavian, and left common carotid. Some people have a bovine arch, an anatomic variation with two branches off the aorta—brachiocephalic and left subclavian. The left common carotid artery branches off of the brachiocephalic artery rather than the aorta. Other variations also occur.

Angiography and other injection procedures on the head and extremities are defined as occurring on the **ipsilateral** or **contralateral** side. These terms refer to the side on which the circulation is examined in relation to the site of catheterization. The prefix *ipsi-* means same, and *lateral* means pertaining to the side, so an *ipsilateral* examination refers to the examination of circulation on the same side on which the catheterization was performed. *Contralateral* means the opposite side.

Congenital Heart Defect Procedures

Surgery to correct congenital heart defects corrects misplaced and/or misconfigured vessels and other structural anomalies in an attempt to restore normal cardiac anatomy and function to the greatest extent possible. Procedures may require that surgeons reposition vessels, close holes with sutures or a patch, create openings, divide fistulas, and create new divisions or structures, depending on the specific anomaly or combination of anomalies (■ TABLE 39-3).

This section provides a general reference to help understand the most common cardiovascular procedures. Remember to keep standard reference books handy in case you get stuck.

Table 39-3 ■ CONGENITAL HEART DEFECT REPAIR PROCEDURES

Name	Condition	Procedure(s)
Atrial septal defect (ASD) repair	A hole in the wall between the left and right upper chambers of the heart	• Open heart surgery to close the hole with sutures or a patch • Transcatheter placement of metal clamp or plug to close the hole
Coarctation of the aorta repair	Presence of a coarctation (*an abnormally narrow section*) in the aorta	• Synthetic (Gor-Tex) or autologous (subclavian artery) graft to widen the vessel • Removal of the coarctation followed by anastomosis • Creation of a bypass around the coarctation using a tube • Stent placement to widen the lumen
Hypoplastic left heart syndrome (HLHS) repair	Underdeveloped aorta and left ventricle in which the aortic and mitral valves are either too small to allow sufficient blood flow or are completely atretic (*closed*)	3-stage repair: • Creation of one blood vessel from the pulmonary artery and the aorta to carry blood to the lungs and the rest of the body (Norwood procedure) • Connect the superior vena cava directly to pulmonary arteries (Glenn shunt or hemi-Fontan procedure) • Connect the inferior vena cava directly to the pulmonary arteries (Fontan procedure)
Patent ductus arteriosus (PDA) ligation	Failure of the ductus arteriosus (*a blood vessel in the fetus that connects the aorta and the pulmonary artery*) to close after birth	• Medication • Insertion of a metal coil to block the opening • Surgery to divide and ligate the vessel

(continued)

Table 39-3 ■ *(continued)*

Name	Condition	Procedure(s)
Tetralogy of Fallot repair	Presence of four defects: • Ventricular septal defect (VSD) • Pulmonary stenosis (*obstructed outflow of blood from the right ventricle to the lungs*) • Dextroposition/overriding aorta (*blood flow from the aorta into both ventricles*) • Right ventricular hypertrophy (*thickened wall of the right ventricle*)	• Widening the pulmonary stenosis • Patching the right ventricle and pulmonary artery • Closing the VSD • Replacing the pulmonary valve • Shunting to move blood flow
Total anomalous pulmonary venous return (TAPVR) correction	The pulmonary veins bring oxygen-rich blood from the lungs back to the right side of the heart instead of the left	• Route pulmonary veins back to the left side of the heart, close any abnormal connections; ligate PDA, if present
Transposition of the great vessels repair	The placement of the aorta and pulmonary artery are switched, preventing pulmonary circulation	• Arterial switch: divide the aorta and pulmonary artery; connect pulmonary artery to right ventricle; connect aorta and coronary arteries to left ventricle
Tricuspid atresia repair	Narrowed, deformed, or absent tricuspid valve	• Medication (temporary) • Repair or replace tricuspid valve • One or a series of shunts to direct blood to the lungs
Truncus arteriosus repair	The aorta, coronary arteries, and pulmonary artery all come out of one common trunk	• Separate pulmonary arteries from the aortic trunk; patch defects; close VSD, if present
Ventricular septal defect (VSD) repair	A hole in the wall between the left and right lower chambers of the heart	• Place a patch through open heart surgery or using a guidewire

Source: © PB Resources, Inc. Used with permission.

CODING PRACTICE

Exercise 39.1   Cardiovascular System Procedure Basics

Instructions: Use your medical terminology skills and resources to define the following procedures related to the cardiovascular system, then identify the code(s) or code range listed in the CPT Index. Follow these steps:

• Use slash marks "/" to break down each term into its root(s) and suffix.

• Define the meaning of the word based on the meaning of each word part.

• Identify the CPT code(s) or code range listed in the CPT Index.

Example: <u>aortoplasty</u> aorto/plasty   Meaning *surgical repair of the aorta*   CPT Code *33417*

1. <u>pericardiocentesis</u>   Meaning _____   CPT Code _____

2. <u>thrombolysis</u>, cranial vessels   Meaning _____   CPT Code _____

3. ablation, heart <u>arrhythmogenic</u> focus   Meaning _____   CPT Code _____

4. <u>valvotomy</u>, mitral valve   Meaning _____   CPT Code _____

5. <u>septoplasty</u>   Meaning _____   CPT Code _____

6. aneurysm repair, <u>thoracoabdominal</u> aorta   Meaning _____   CPT Code _____

7. <u>thromboendarterectomy</u>, brachial artery   Meaning _____   CPT Code _____

8. <u>angioscopy</u>, noncoronary vessels   Meaning _____   CPT Code _____

9. <u>endovascular</u> repair, vena cava, repositioning   Meaning _____   CPT Code _____

10. <u>arteriovenous</u> fistula, revision, without thrombectomy   Meaning _____   CPT Code _____

CODING OVERVIEW OF CARDIOVASCULAR SYSTEM PROCEDURES

The CPT subsection **Cardiovascular System (33010-37799)** contains two subheadings: **Heart and Pericardium (33010-33999)**, which includes procedures on the conduction system, and **Arteries and Veins (34001-36556)**. Each subheading contains numerous categories divided by the anatomic site, condition, and type of procedure. Review the subheading and category names and code ranges listed in the Cardiovascular System subsection to become familiar with the content and organization. Some editions of the CPT manual provide a summary list of the subheading and categories at the beginning of the Cardiovascular System subsection and also display an asterisk (*) next to categories that contain special coding instructions.

This chapter includes invasive, minimally invasive, and noninvasive surgical procedures on the cardiovascular system. Codes for diagnostic tests on the cardiovascular system appear in the Medicine section. Procedures represented by CPT codes must be linked on a claim with diagnosis codes to support their medical necessity. CPT codes in the Cardiovascular System subsection are frequently supported by diagnosis codes from ICD-10-CM **Chapter 9 Diseases of the Circulatory System (I00-I99)**, as well as symptoms and signs and congenital malformations (■ TABLE 39-4). These are the codes most commonly used to support procedures on the cardiovascular system; however, diagnosis codes from any ICD-10-CM chapter are permissible.

CPT guidelines for the Surgery section apply to the Cardiovascular System.

Special instructions at the beginning of the subsection direct how to code for catheterization within a vascular family. CPT

Appendix L, Vascular Families, shows the designation of first-, second-, and third-order branches within vascular families for catheterization beginning at the aorta.

Detailed special instructions and a table in the category **Pacemaker or Pacing Cardioverter-Defibrillator** provide guidance on coding for related services. The "Central Venous Access Procedures Table" appears in the subcategory **Central Venous Access Procedures (36555-36598)**. Additional special instructions provide definitions and coding guidelines at the beginning of many categories.

Instructional notes appear throughout the Tabular List to alert coders to the need for modifiers, provide cross-references to codes for similar procedures on other sites, identify when additional codes for radiological services might be needed, and highlight resequenced and recently deleted codes.

ABSTRACTING CARDIOVASCULAR SYSTEM PROCEDURES

Various types of cardiovascular procedures require unique abstracting criteria. Criteria for procedures on the heart (■ TABLE 39-5) include specialized criteria for CABG and central venous access procedures. Pacemaker procedures and ICD procedures can be abstracted using similar criteria (■ TABLE 39-6). Vascular procedures include specialized criteria for catheterization and vascular injection procedures (■ TABLE 39-7). Most other cardiovascular procedures can be abstracted successfully using the general criteria for abstracting operative procedures.

Remember that the abstracting questions are a guide and that not every question applies to, or can be answered for, every

Table 39-4 ■ LOCATING ICD-10-CM AND ADDITIONAL CPT CODES FOR THE CARDIOVASCULAR SYSTEM

Type of Code	Codes
ICD-10-CM Cardiovascular System-Related Codes	
Cardiovascular system conditions	I00-I99
Congenital malformations	Q20-Q28
Symptoms and signs	R00, R01, R50-R69
CPT Cardiovascular System-Related Codes	
Medicine procedures	92920-93998
Radiologic procedures	
• Diagnostic radiology	75557-75989
• Diagnostic ultrasound	76604-76645, 76881-76886
• Radiologic guidance	77001-77022
• Nuclear medicine, diagnostic	78414-78499
Laboratory organ/disease panels	80050, 80053, 80061

Source: © PB Resources, Inc. Used with permission. CPT codes only © American Medical Association.

Table 39-5 ■ KEY CRITERIA FOR ABSTRACTING CARDIAC PROCEDURES

❑ What type of procedure is performed?
❑ What is the anatomic site?
❑ Is a device implanted or removed?
❑ Was imaging supervision and interpretation provided by the surgeon?

For CABG:

❑ How many grafted vessels are used?
❑ How many and which arteries are used for grafting?
❑ How many and which veins are used for grafting?
❑ Is a venous graft obtained endoscopically?
❑ How many distal anastomoses are performed?
❑ Is cardiopulmonary bypass used?

For central venous access procedures:

❑ What type of procedure is performed (insertion, repair, partial or complete replacement, removal)?
❑ Is the catheter inserted centrally or peripherally?
❑ Is the centrally inserted catheter tunneled or nontunneled?
❑ Is a pump or port included?
❑ What is the age of the patient?

Source: © PB Resources, Inc. Used with permission.

Table 39-6 ■ KEY CRITERIA FOR ABSTRACTING PACEMAKER AND ICD PROCEDURES

❏ What is the type of device (pacemaker, implantable [transvenous] cardioverter-defibrillator, or subcutaneous cardioverter-defibrillator)?

❏ What type of procedure is performed (initial placement, removal, replacement, upgrade, or repair)?

❏ Which components are involved (pulse generator and/or lead)?

❏ How many and which chambers are involved?

❏ What type of leads does the pulse generator have (atrial, ventricular, dual, multiple)?

❏ How many leads are removed and/or inserted transvenously? How many leads are reused?

❏ What approach is used (open [thoracotomy], endoscopic, or transvenous)?

❏ Is the device temporary or permanent?

❏ What other related services were provided (device evaluation, skin pocket relocation, defibrillator threshold testing)?

Source: © PB Resources, Inc. Used with permission.

Table 39-7 ■ KEY CRITERIA FOR ABSTRACTING VASCULAR PROCEDURES

❏ What site is treated?

❏ Is a catheter used?

❏ What type of procedure is performed?

❏ What is the surgical approach?

❏ Is a stent, filter, or other prosthesis used?

For vascular injection procedures:

❏ Is the catheterization nonselective, selective, or both?

❏ How many access sites are used?

❏ What is the point(s) of access (e.g., femoral, radial, jugular, brachial)?

❏ Does the procedure begin at the aorta?

❏ Which vascular family(ies) is accessed?

❏ What is the first-order branch?

❏ Is more than one first-order branch (family) accessed?

❏ What is the second-order branch?

❏ What is the site of the examination/injection (e.g., ipsilateral or contralateral)?

❏ What is the most distal anatomic site to where the catheter is manipulated?

❏ What imaging studies are performed?

Source: © PB Resources, Inc. Used with permission.

case. Some cases will require additional abstracting after you identify the preliminary codes and research code options in the Tabular List.

Guided Example of Abstracting Cardiovascular System Procedures

Refer to the following example throughout this chapter to practice skills for abstracting, assigning, and arranging Cardiovascular System codes.

INPATIENT HOSPITAL   Gender: M   Age: 67

Preoperative diagnosis: *chronic unstable angina, acute STEMI right inferoposterior wall*

Procedure: *Coronary artery bypass grafting (CABG) times three utilizing the left internal mammary artery (LIMA) to the left anterior descending (LAD) artery and two segments of the reversed autologous great saphenous vein graft (SVG) to the posterior descending (PDA) branch of the right coronary artery (RCA) and the obtuse marginal (OM) branch of the left main (LM) coronary artery, total cardiopulmonary bypass (CPB), cold blood potassium cardioplegia (introduction of a solution to stop the heart) for myocardial protection. The sternotomy was performed, the heart was physically stabilized, and the pericardium was entered. The PDA branch of the right coronary artery was identified, opened, and anastomosed in an end-to-side fashion to the reversed autologous SV. The OM was identified and opened and end-to-side anastomosis was performed to a second segment of the reversed autologous SV. The LIMA was clipped distally, divided, and spatulated (spread open) for anastomosis. The LAD was identified and opened. End-to-side anastomosis was performed through the LIMA. The mammary pedicle was sutured to the heart. Aortotomies were made and the veins were cut to fit these and sutured in place. Ventricular and atrial pacing wires were placed. The patient was fully warmed and weaned from CPB. Good hemostasis was noted. A single mediastinal and left pleural chest tube was placed. The sternum was closed with interrupted wire, and the linea alba, sternal fascia, and subcutaneous tissue were closed. The patient tolerated the procedure well and was transferred to PACU in stable condition.*

Postoperative diagnosis: *Acute STEMI right inferoposterior wall; atherosclerotic heart disease of RCA with 95% blockage in PDA; 85% blockage in OM; and 90% blockage in LAD, with unstable angina due to 50 years of cigarette nicotine dependence*

Follow along as fictitious coder, Tanisha Riemann, CCS-P, abstracts the procedure. Check off each step after you complete it.

▶ Tanisha reads through the entire record, paying special attention to the reason for the procedure, the procedure performed, and the postoperative diagnosis. She refers to the Key Criteria for Abstracting Cardiac Procedures (Table 39-5).

❏ She notes preoperative diagnosis. *chronic unstable angina, acute STEMI right inferoposterior wall*

❏ *What is the patient's age?* 67

❏ *What site is treated?* heart

❑ *What is the primary procedure performed?* Coronary artery bypass grafting

❑ *What is (are) the harvested vessels?* left internal mammary artery (LIMA) and two segments of the reversed autologous great saphenous vein

❑ *How many grafted vessels are used?* Coronary artery bypass grafting times three

❑ *How many distal anastomoses are performed?* Three, identified as follows: (1) The PDA branch of the right coronary artery was identified, opened, and anastomosed in an end-to-side fashion to the reversed autologous SV. (2) The OM was identified and opened

and end-to-side anastomosis was performed to a second segment of the reversed autologous SVG. (3) The LAD was identified and opened. End-to-side anastomosis was performed through the LIMA.

❑ *Is a venous graft obtained endoscopically?* No

❑ *Is cardiopulmonary bypass used?* Yes, total cardiopulmonary bypass (CPB)

▶ At this time, Tanisha does not know which of these procedures may need to be coded, nor how many codes she will end up with. She will learn about this when she moves on to assigning codes.

CODING PRACTICE

Exercise 39.2 **Abstracting Cardiovascular System Procedures**

Instructions: Read the mini-medical-record of each patient's encounter and answer the abstracting questions. Write the answer on the line provided. Do not assign any codes.

1. OUTPATIENT HOSPITAL Gender: F Age: 64

Preprocedure diagnosis: arrhythmia

Procedure: Administered conscious sedation and implanted a continuous-loop cardiac event recorder into the subcutaneous tissue of the chest

a. What type of procedure is performed? _____

b. What is the anatomic site? _____

c. Is a device implanted or removed? _____

2. OUTPATIENT HOSPITAL Gender: M Age: 79

Preprocedure diagnosis: pulmonary edema with acute pericardial effusion

Procedure: Using ultrasound guidance provided by the radiologist, advanced the needle into the pericardial space. Aspirated fluid from the pericardial sac into a syringe. Patient tolerated procedure well.

a. What type of procedure is performed? _____

b. What is the anatomic site? _____

c. Is a device implanted or removed? _____

d. Was imaging supervision and interpretation provided by the surgeon? _____

e. What is the medical term for this procedure?
_____

3. INPATIENT HOSPITAL Gender: M Age: 57

Preprocedure diagnosis: acute anterior wall MI

Procedure: CABG ×1 using radial artery bypass, aorta to LAD. Patient placed on CPB.

a. What type of procedure is performed? _____

b. What is the anatomic site? _____

c. Is a device implanted or removed? _____

d. How many grafted vessels are used? _____

e. How many and which arteries are used for grafting?
_____

f. How many and which veins are used for grafting?
_____

g. Is a venous graft obtained endoscopically?
_____

h. How many distal anastomoses are performed?
_____

i. Is cardiopulmonary bypass used? _____

4. INPATIENT HOSPITAL Gender: M Age: 63

Preprocedure diagnosis: coronary artery disease

Procedure: CABG ×4; left radial artery from the aorta to the PDA branch of the RC; LIMA from the aorta to the ramus intermedius coronary artery (RI) and then sequentially to the diagonal branch of the LAD; left saphenous vein graft to the obtuse marginal branch of the left circumflex (LCX). The assistant surgeon performed an endoscopic video-assisted harvesting of the saphenous vein.

a. What type of procedure is performed? _____

(continued)

4. (continued)

b. What is the anatomic site? _____

c. Is a device implanted or removed? _____

d. How many grafted vessels are used? _____

e. How many and which arteries are used for grafting?

_____

f. How many and which veins are used for grafting?

_____

g. Is a venous graft obtained endoscopically?

_____

h. How many distal anastomoses are performed?

_____

i. Is cardiopulmonary bypass used? _____

5. (continued)

j. Which vascular family(ies) is accessed?

_____

k. What is the first-order branch? _____

l. Is more than one first-order branch (family) accessed?

_____

m. What is the second-order branch? _____

n. What is the site of the examination/injection (e.g., ipsilateral or contralateral)? _____

o. What is the most distal anatomic site to where the catheter is manipulated? _____

p. What imaging studies are performed?

_____

5. OUTPATIENT HOSPITAL   Gender: M   Age: 47

Preprocedure diagnosis: Occlusion and stenosis of carotid artery vascular family with cerebral infarction

Procedure: Selective catheter placement with angiography and stent. Inserted catheter percutaneously in the left femoral artery and maneuvered it to the aorta, where angiography was performed on the cervicocerebral arch. Moved catheter into the left common carotid artery, proceeded to the internal carotid artery then into the left middle cerebral branch. Performed angiography of the ipsilateral common carotid circulation. Radiological supervision and interpretation done by surgeon

Postprocedure diagnosis: Occlusion and stenosis of left middle cerebral artery with cerebral infarction

a. What site is treated? _____

b. Is a catheter used? _____

c. What type of procedure is performed? _____

d. What is the surgical approach? _____

e. Is a stent, filter, or other prosthesis used?

_____

f. Is the catheterization nonselective, selective, or both?

_____

g. How many access sites are used? _____

h. What is the point(s) of access (e.g., femoral, radial, jugular, brachial)? _____

i. Does the procedure begin at the aorta?

_____

(continued)

6. INPATIENT HOSPITAL   Gender: F   Age: 68

Preprocedure diagnosis: ICD that was implanted two years ago for ventricular tachycardia

Procedure: upgrade ICD in right ventricle to dual chamber. Removed pulse generator in the subcutaneous pocket in the chest. Tested existing lead, which was found to be in good condition, so it was reused. Under fluoroscopic guidance, threaded a new lead into the right ventricle and right atrium. Inserted new pulse generator.

a. What is the type of device (pacemaker or implantable cardioverter-defibrillator)? _____

b. What type of procedure is performed (initial placement, removal, replacement, upgrade, or repair)?

_____

c. Which components are involved (pulse generator and/ or lead)? _____

d. How many and which chambers are treated?

_____

e. How many leads are removed and/or inserted transvenously? _____ How many leads are reused? _____

f. What approach is used (open [thoracotomy], endoscopic, or transvenous)? _____

g. Is the device temporary or permanent?

_____

h. What other related services were provided (device evaluation, skin pocket relocation, defibrillator threshold testing)? _____

ASSIGNING CODES FOR CARDIOVASCULAR SYSTEM PROCEDURES

The Cardiovascular System provides extensive special instructions throughout the Tabular List that clarify definitions, code assignment, and bundling rules. To aid in understanding these guidelines, this section provides a discussion and a special guided example of examining CPT guidelines and instructions. The remainder of the section discusses coding highlights for blood draws, pacemaker procedures, catheterization, congenital heart defect procedures, and CABG. Finally, the guided example introduced earlier in the chapter, about a patient who was seen for CABG, is continued.

Researching CPT Guidelines

Sometimes extensive special instructions can be challenging to understand because they occupy more space in the CPT manual than the code descriptions and may be written from the perspective of a physician rather than a coder. Every year new codes and new guidelines are added or revised, so even the experienced coder needs to analyze and comprehend new information. Remember that it may be necessary to read through the special instructions several times, refer to anatomic charts, use a medical dictionary, and compare the code descriptions to fully understand the category. Just as key criteria questions help in abstracting information for specific types of procedures, they also can help coders understand new CPT guidelines and codes (■ TABLE 39-8).

In 2014, CPT added a new category, **Fenestrated Endovascular Repair of the Visceral and Infrarenal Aorta**, with several new codes (**34839-34848**) for services previously reported with Category III temporary codes. Fenestrated endovascular aneurysm repair (FEVAR) is the reinforcement of a section of the aorta weakened by a bulge, using a customized prosthesis. Holes in the prosthesis material, positioned to align with connecting arteries, allow blood flow to be maintained and allow for stents and catheters to be placed or maneuvered through the fenestration. FEVAR provides a treatment alternative when the aneurysm is situated near arterial branches. Traditional endovascular aneurysm repair (EVAR), which uses a nonperforated

prosthesis, is usually less successful in these situations because of its inability to provide support around the arteries.

Guided Example of Researching CPT Guidelines

Use the category **Fenestrated Endovascular Repair of the Visceral and Infrarenal Aorta (34839-34848)** as an example of learning to read and understand special instructions. Read through the special instructions and follow along in your CPT manual as Tanisha Riemann, CCS-P, identifies the key points.

▶ *What is the purpose of the procedure(s)?*

❑ The fenestrated (*perforated*) endoprosthesis (*prosthesis within a vessel*) is deployed (*placed*) within the visceral aorta. Fenestrations (perforations) within the fabric allow for selective catheterization of the visceral and/or renal arteries. They also allow for an endoprosthesis such as a bare metal or covered stent to be placed at a later time to maintain flow to the visceral artery.

▶ *How are anatomic sites or regions defined?*

❑ The thoracic aorta extends from the aortic valve to the aortic segment, just above the celiac artery.

❑ The visceral aorta is the upper abdominal aorta that contains the celiac, superior mesenteric, and renal arteries.

❑ The infrarenal (*below the kidney*) aorta is the lower abdominal aorta, below the renal arteries. (This definition is not stated in the special instructions but is based on anatomy.)

▶ *How are codes divided?*

❑ Codes **34839-34844** describe repairs using endoprostheses that span from the visceral aorta to the infrarenal aorta. Code descriptions specify one, two, three, or four visceral artery origins. The prostheses in these codes *do not* extend into the common iliac arteries.

❑ Codes **34845-34848** describe repairs using endoprostheses that span from the visceral aorta through the infrarenal aorta *into the common iliac arteries*. Code descriptions specify one, two, three, or four visceral artery origins.

▶ *What services are included in the code descriptions?*

❑ Proximal abdominal aortic extension prostheses and distal extension prostheses that terminate in the aorta or the common iliac arteries

❑ Placement of unilateral or bilateral docking devices used in the infrarenal aorta

❑ Introduction of guide wires and catheters in the aorta and visceral and/or renal arteries

❑ Balloon angioplasty within the target treatment zone of the endograft, either before or after endograft deployment

❑ Fluoroscopic guidance and radiological supervision and interpretation

---

Table 39-8 ■ KEY CRITERIA FOR READING CPT GUIDELINES

❑ What is the purpose of the category and procedure(s)?

❑ How are anatomic sites or regions defined?

❑ How are the codes divided?

❑ What services are included in the code descriptions (not separately reportable)?

❑ What services can be reported separately?

❑ What standalone codes, indented codes, and add-on codes appear in the category?

❑ What instructional notes appear within the code descriptions in the Tabular List?

❑ What Main Term in the Index leads most directly to these codes?

Source: © PB Resources, Inc. Used with permission.

▶ *What services can be reported separately?*

❏ Distal extension prostheses that terminate in the internal iliac, external iliac, or common femoral arteries (e.g., **34825** and **34826**)

❏ Catheterization of the hypogastric artery(ies) and/or arterial families outside the treatment zone of the graft

❏ Exposure of the access vessels (e.g., **34812**)

❏ Extensive repair of an artery (e.g., **35226**, **35286**)

❏ Other interventional procedures such as:
  ▪ arterial embolization
  ▪ intravascular ultrasound
  ▪ balloon angioplasty
  ▪ stenting of native artery(ies) outside the endoprosthesis target zone

▶ *What standalone codes, indented codes, and add-on codes appear in the category?* To answer this question, read the code descriptions in the category. Look for CPT conventions, such as indented code descriptions and the add-on code symbol (+). This category has two standalone codes and six indented code descriptions, as follows:

❏ Standalone code **34841** reports repair of the visceral aorta.

❏ Standalone code **34845** reports repair of both the visceral aorta and infrarenal aorta.

❏ Each standalone code reports the use of one endoprosthesis.

❏ Indented code descriptions under each standalone code report the use of two, three, or four or more endoprostheses.

▶ *What instructional notes appear within the code descriptions in the Tabular List?*

❏ Several instructional notes appear at the end of the category, after code **34848**, that identify codes that should not be reported together and provide clarification and cross-references.

▶ *What Main Term in the Index leads most directly to these codes?* The special instructions do not provide this information, so you need to investigate it yourself. To identify the best Main Term, try locating codes in the Index using the methods suggested by CPT in the introduction to the Index: anatomic site, procedure name, condition, synonym, eponym, abbreviation, or acronym.

❏ Follow the basic CPT procedure of looking first under the anatomic site, which is **Aorta**. A first-level modifying term identifies **Visceral** and additional second-level modifying terms identify **Repair, Endovascular**. The code range **34839, 34841-34848**, leads to the appropriate category in the Tabular List.

❏ As an alternative approach, look up the procedure **Endovascular Repair** as the Main Term. A first-level modifying term identifies **Visceral Aorta** with second-level modifying terms that identify the various types of endografts listed in this category.

Use a process similar to this whenever you encounter complex guidelines or special instructions. Make a list or create a summary table to help visualize the information provided.

Blood Collection

The collection of a blood specimen submitted for laboratory tests is coded from the Cardiovascular System. Blood specimens can be collected from a capillary, vein, or artery, an implantable venous access device, or an established catheter (■ TABLE 39-9). To locate codes for blood collection in the Index, search for the Main Term **Collection and Processing**, then the subterm **Specimen**. Alternatively, search for the Main Term **Specimen Collection**, then the subterm **Specimen**. Then locate the source of the specimen. To locate blood collection using an arterial puncture, search for the Main Term **Puncture**, then the subterm **Artery**.

SUCCESS STEP

The CPT Index does not provide a Main Term for Blood Draw or Blood Collection. However, you can create your own reminder by writing the words *Blood Draw* under *B* in your CPT Index, then writing a cross-reference such as *See "Collection and Processing, Specimen"* or *See "Specimen Collection."* This will direct you to the correct Main Terms.

Pacemaker Procedures

To locate codes in the Index for pacemaker or ICD procedures, search for the Main Term **Pacemaker** or **Implantable Defibrillator**. Subterms identify the type of procedure performed. Subcutaneous devices are coded with temporary Category III codes.

The number of codes required varies based on the procedure. Some procedures are reported with a single code, whereas others require separate codes for each component, that is, the pulse generator and the lead(s). When verifying codes in the Tabular List, refer to the chart of pacemaker and ICD procedures that

Table 39-9 ■ **CODES FOR OBTAINING BLOOD SAMPLES**

Source of Blood Sample	Code(s)
Artery (puncture)	36600
Capillary	36416
Implantable venous access device	36591
Vein (venipuncture)	36415 (routine) 36420 (cutdown <1 year) 36400-36410 (nonroutine)
Venous catheter (established)	36592

appears before or near code **33202**. To use this chart, follow these steps:

1. In the first column, identify the type of transvenous procedure performed.

2. Select code(s) from the second (Pacemaker) or third (ICD) column that corresponds to the type of device in use.

3. Verify the code descriptions in the Tabular List.

4. Read the instructional notes following the code for variations of the procedure and bundling rules.

5. Review the special instructions for this category and ensure that all guidelines are followed.

Nonselective and Selective Catheterization

Vascular catheterization consists of inserting a catheter at a specific point and moving it through the arteries or veins to arrive at the site the physician wishes to examine or treat. Arterial catheterization most often begins at the femoral or radial artery then proceeds to the aorta, from where the desired vessel(s) are accessed. Central venous access is made through the inferior vena cava or the jugular, subclavian, or femoral veins. Peripheral venous access is made through other sites, such as the basilic or cephalic vein.

When coding for selective catheter placement, code for the most distal anatomic site reached (■ FIGURE 39-2). The

> Catheter was threaded from the aorta into the brachiocephalic artery (*first-order*), through the subclavian artery (*second-order*), and into the right vertebral artery (*third-order*).
>
> **36217 Selective catheter placement, arterial system; initial third order or more selective thoracic or brachiocephalic branch, within a vascular family**

Figure 39-2 ■ Example of Coding Selective Catheterization to a Third-Order Branch

procedure report should identify the access point and the path the catheter takes, naming each successive branch accessed (■ FIGURE 39-3). CPT **Appendix L, Vascular Families** lists vascular families and the first-, second-, and third-order branches. It is a useful reference to help identify the names of the vessels and the order they represent. ■ FIGURE 39-4 illustrates how to follow the hierarchal progression within vascular families. Begin identifying vascular families at the point where the examination begins. Do not code the movement of the catheter from the access point to the beginning point of examination. For example, when the catheter is inserted in the femoral artery and moved to the aorta, where the examination

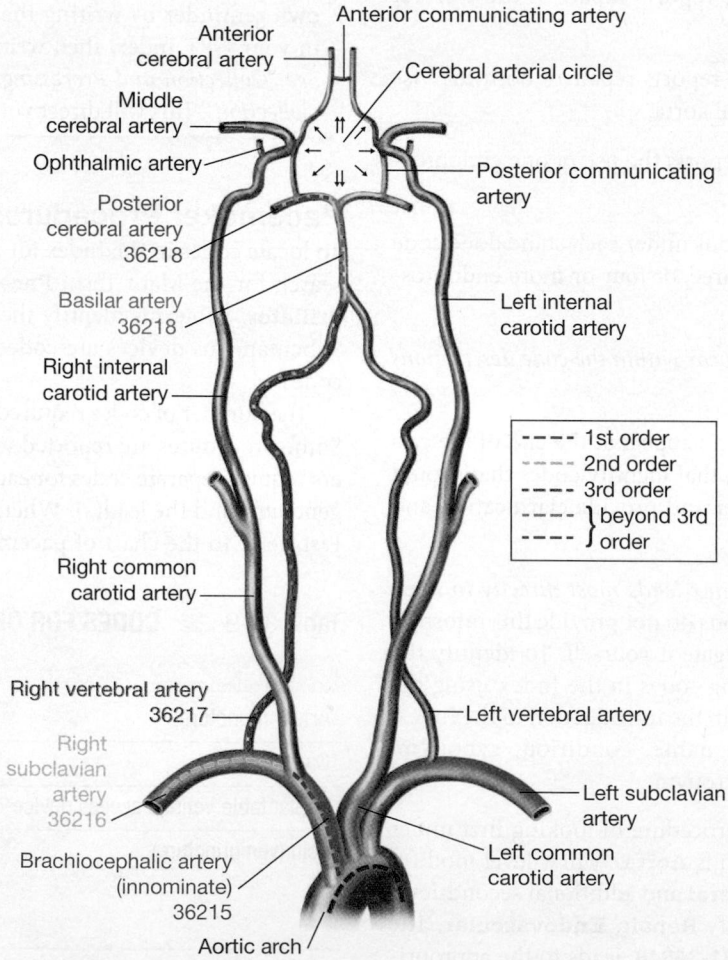

Figure 39-3 ■ Anatomy of Selective Catheterization Coding

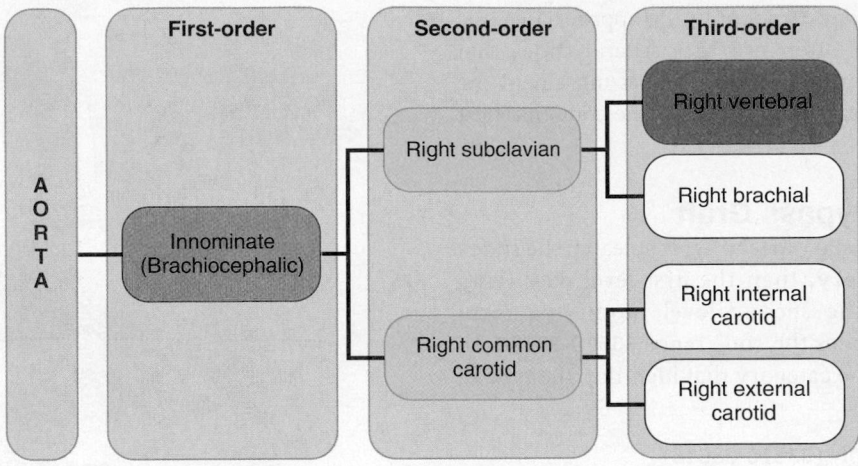

Figure 39-4 ■ Branches of a Vascular Family (Partial)

is begun, begin coding the vascular family branches at the aorta, not the femoral artery.

When the catheter is partially retracted then redirected through an additional branch of the same vascular family, assign an additional code for the most distal anatomic site reached in the additional branch (■ FIGURE 39-5).

To locate codes for vascular procedures, search the Index for the Main Term **Artery** or **Vein** and the first-level modifying term for the specific vessel. Identify the second-level modifying term for the type of procedure performed. In some cases, the first-level modifying term identifies the procedure, rather than the vessel.

The CPT Tabular List divides codes based on whether catheterization is performed in arteries or veins and whether the upper or lower body, as divided at the diaphragm, is accessed. Review code descriptions to identify separate codes for specific arteries accessed and the extent of the catheterization: first-, second-, third-order and beyond branches. Codes for angiography include catheter placement, angiography, and all associated radiological supervision and interpretation, so these services should not be reported separately. However, assign codes for additional imaging studies performed. ■ TABLE 39-10 summarizes the rules for catheterization coding.

CODING CAUTION

Be aware that many vessels are referred to by more than one name. For example, the innominate artery listed in CPT **Appendix L, Vascular Families** is the same as the brachiocephalic artery named in the Tabular List.

SUCCESS STEP

Vascular families are similar to a highway system. If you think of the aorta as analogous to an interstate highway, the first-order branch would be the first main road turned onto from an exit ramp. When you turn off of the main road onto a secondary road, it is similar to a second-order branch. Turning onto a side street is similar to a third-order branch, and so on.

Congenital Heart Defect Procedures

To locate codes for repair of a congenital heart anomaly, search the Index for the name of the condition as the Main Term. Read

---

Catheter was threaded from the aorta into the brachiocephalic artery (*first-order*), through the subclavian artery (*second-order*), and into the right vertebral artery (*third-order*). It was then retracted back to the brachiocephalic artery and threaded into the right common carotid artery (*additional second-order*).

36217 Selective catheter placement, arterial system; initial third order or more selective thoracic or brachiocephalic branch, within a vascular family

36218 Selective catheter placement, arterial system; additional second order, third order, and beyond, thoracic or brachiocephalic branch, within a vascular family (List in addition to code for initial second or third order vessel as appropriate)

Figure 39-5 ■ Example of Coding Multiple Selective Catheterizations

---

Table 39-10 ■ SUMMARY OF RULES FOR CATHETERIZATION CODING

❏ Code each access separately.

❏ Code each vascular family separately.

❏ Code additional second- or third-order catheterizations within a family.

❏ Code additional imaging studies within a family above the basic examination included in the code.

❏ Do not code both selective and nonselective catheter placement from the same access and in the same vascular family. Code only the selective catheterization.

the modifying terms, if any, to identify the appropriate code range. The Tabular List often provides several codes that describe variations of a procedure, so coders must read the details of the operative report to determine the code that best describes the operation.

Coronary Artery Bypass Graft

To locate codes for a coronary artery bypass, search the Index for the Main Term **Artery**, then the first-level modifying term **Coronary** and the second-level modifying term **Bypass**. The Index provides the code range **33510-33536**. In the Tabular List, select the category that identifies the type of graft used:

- Use of venous grafts only (**33510-33516**)
- Use of both arterial and venous grafts (**33517-33523**)
- Use of arterial grafts only (**33533-33536**)

Within each category, codes are divided based on the number of grafts performed. The number of grafts reported is identified by the number of distal anastomoses. The proximal anastomosis connects the graft to the aorta. The distal anastomosis connects the graft to a coronary artery beyond the blockage or to another graft. To report combined arterial-venous grafting, report a standalone code(s) for the arterial graft(s) and an add-on code(s) for the venous graft(s). Refer to ■ FIGURE 39-6 to better understand arterial and venous grafting.

Harvesting of the vessel to be used for grafting may or may not be reported separately, as summarized below:

- Upper extremity artery—report harvesting with code **35600** in addition to the bypass procedure
- Upper extremity vein—report harvesting with code **35500** in addition to the bypass procedure
- Femoropopliteal vein segment—report harvesting with code **35572** in addition to the bypass procedure
- Saphenous vein—harvesting is included in the description of the work for **33517-33523** and should not be reported separately
- Artery (other than upper extremity)—harvesting is included in the description of the work for **33533-33536** and should not be reported separately
- Video-assisted harvesting—report code **33508** in addition to the bypass procedure, including when the procurement is otherwise bundled (e.g., saphenous vein)

When a surgical assistant performs arterial and/or venous graft procurement, add modifier **-80** to codes **33517-33523** and **33533-33536**. Refer to the special instructions for each CABG category for more information.

SUCCESS STEP

To locate codes for a *peripheral* artery or venous bypass, search the Index for the Main Term **Artery** or **Vein**, then the first-level modifying term for name of the vessel and the second-level modifying term **Bypass Graft**.

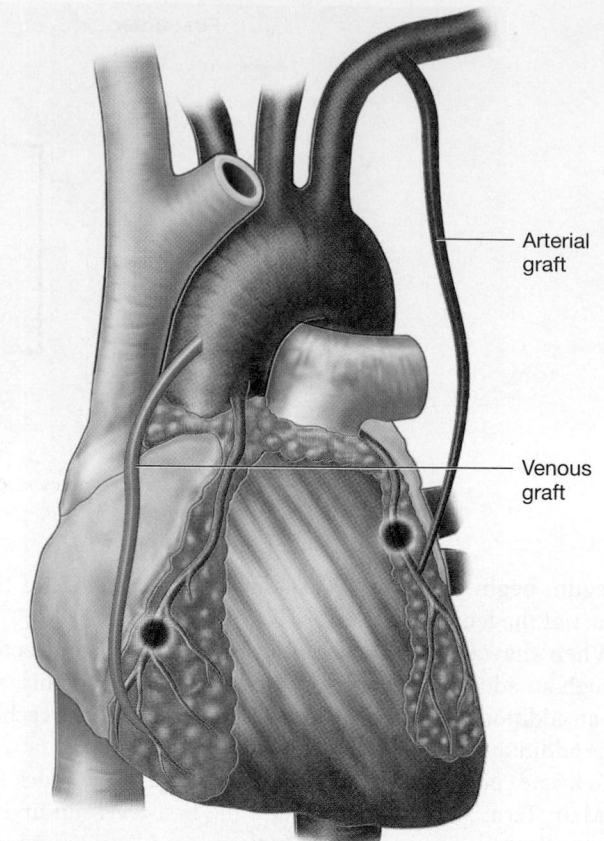

A. Venous and arterial grafts

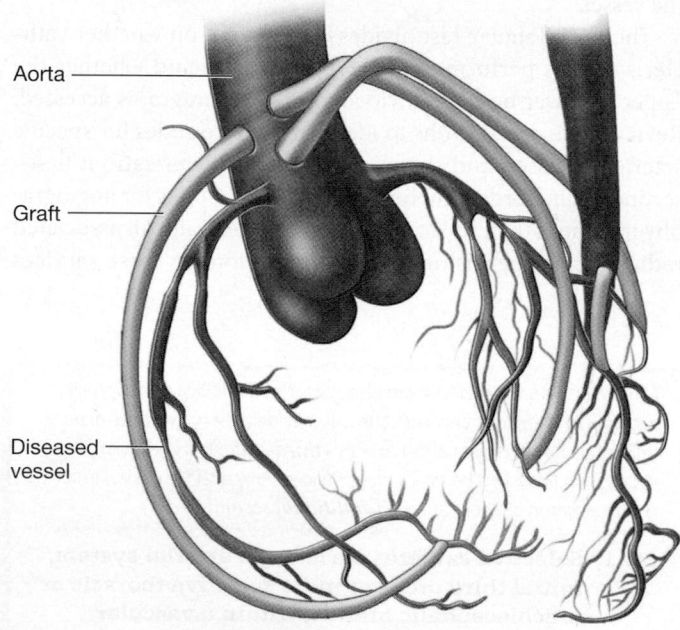

B. Graft bypassing the diseased vessel

Figure 39-6 ■ Coronary Artery Bypass Grafting

Guided Example of Assigning Cardiovascular System Procedure Codes

To practice skills for assigning codes for the Cardiovascular System, continue with the example from earlier in the chapter about a patient who was seen for CABG. Follow along in your

CPT manual as Tanisha Riemann, CCS-P, assigns codes. Check off each step after you complete it.

▶ First, Tanisha confirms the procedure *CABG ×3*.

▶ Tanisha searches the Index for the Main Term **Coronary Artery Bypass Graft (CABG)**.

❑ She locates the first-level modifying term **Arterial-Venous Graft** because both an artery (LIMA) and a vein (SV) were used. If only an artery had been used, she would select the subterm **Arterial Bypass**. If only a vein had been used, she would select the subterm **Venous Bypass**.

❑ She identifies the code range **33517-33519, 33521-33523**. (Note: The CPT Index also lists code **33531**, but no such code exists.)

▶ Tanisha turns to the Tabular List to select and verify the code(s).

❑ She notices that all the codes in the category **Combined Arterial-Venous Grafting for Coronary Bypass** are add-on codes. She is a little confused because she knows that add-on codes cannot be used alone but must be used in conjunction with a standalone code.

❑ She notices special instructions at the beginning of the category, so decides to read them to see whether she can learn more about how to code the CABG. The special instructions state that:

▪ the codes in this category **may NOT be used alone**.

▪ **two codes** must be reported: one from this category for the combined arterial-venous graft and one from code **33533-33536** for the arterial graft.

▪ **procurement of the saphenous vein graft is included** in codes **31517-33523** and **should not be reported as a separate service**.

▪ **procurement of the artery for grafting** is included in codes **33533-33536** and **should not be reported as a separate service**.

❑ Before beginning to select codes, she refers to the category **Arterial Grafting for Coronary Artery Bypass**, which contains the standalone codes **33533-33536**, to review the special instructions. The special instructions state that:

▪ the codes in this category are used **to report coronary artery bypass procedures using either arterial grafts only or a combination of arterial-venous grafts**.

▪ the codes **include the use of the internal mammary artery**, as well as several other arteries.

▪ **it is necessary to report two codes**, as stated in the previous instructions.

▪ **procurement of the artery for grafting** is included in codes from this category.

❑ Because this category provides the standalone code needed, Tanisha reads the code descriptions for the arterial graft so she can select this code first.

▪ Codes **33533-33536** are divided by the number of arterial grafts used.

▪ She refers to the documentation and confirms that the only arterial graft was the LIMA and it was used for one anastomosis. (*The LAD was identified and opened. End-to-side anastomosis was performed through the LIMA.*)

▪ She reads the code title for **33533**, **Coronary artery bypass, using arterial graft(s); single arterial graft**, and confirms that this accurately describes the principal procedure.

▶ Next, Tanisha needs to select the code for the venous grafting from the code ranges **33517-33519, 33521-33523**.

❑ Codes in this category are divided by the number of venous grafts used.

❑ The common portion of the descriptor appears in code **33517 Coronary artery bypass, using venous graft(s) and arterial graft(s)**.

❑ She refers to the documentation and confirms that the *great saphenous vein* was procured. It was used for two anastomoses (*two segments of the reversed autologous great saphenous vein graft (SVG) to the posterior descending (PDA) branch of the right coronary artery (RCA) and the obtuse marginal (OM) coronary artery*).

❑ She selects code **33518, 2 venous grafts (List separately in addition to code for primary procedure)**.

❑ She reads the instructional note under this code, which states **(Use 33518 in conjunction with 33533-33536)**, and confirms that she has followed this rule.

▶ Tanisha rechecks the special instructions in the Tabular List.

❑ She cross-references the special instructions that she read previously to be certain that she did not miss any details.

❑ She cross-references the beginning of the subheading **Heart and Pericardium** and verifies that there are no special instructions.

❑ She cross-references the beginning of the subsection **Cardiovascular System** and reviews the special instructions. She determines that these instructions apply to selective catheterization and not to CABG.

▶ Tanisha has learned through her experience coding for cardiac surgery that a Category II code can be reported as an optional code when the LIMA is used for a CABG.

❑ To locate the code, she searches the Index for the Main Term **Artery**, the first-level modifying term **Coronary**, and the second-level modifying term **Bypass**. Under **Bypass**, she locates **Internal Mammary Artery** and the Category II code **4110F**.

❑ She verifies the code description in the Category II Tabular List, which appears after code **99607**.

▶ Tanisha reviews the procedure codes she has assigned for this case.

- ❏ **33518 Coronary artery bypass, using venous graft(s) and arterial graft(s); 2 venous grafts**
- ❏ **33533 Coronary artery bypass, using arterial graft(s); single arterial graft**
- ❏ **4110F Internal mammary artery graft performed for primary, isolated coronary artery bypass graft procedure**

▶ Next, Tanisha must determine how to sequence the codes.

CODING PRACTICE

Exercise 39.3 Assigning Codes for Cardiovascular System Procedures

Instructions: Read the mini-medical-record of each patient's encounter. Review the information abstracted in Exercise 39.2 for questions 1–3. For questions 4–6, abstract the case on your own. Assign CPT codes, quantities, and modifiers using the Index and Tabular List. Write the code(s) on the line provided.

1. OUTPATIENT HOSPITAL   Gender: F   Age: 64

Preprocedure diagnosis: arrhythmia

Procedure: Administered conscious sedation and implanted a continuous loop cardiac event recorder into the subcutaneous tissue of the chest

1 CPT Code _____

2. OUTPATIENT HOSPITAL   Gender: M   Age: 79

Preprocedure diagnosis: pulmonary edema with acute pericardial effusion

Procedure: Using ultrasound guidance provided by the radiologist, advanced the needle into the pericardial space. Aspirated fluid from the pericardial sac into syringe. Patient tolerated procedure well.

1 CPT Code _____

3. INPATIENT HOSPITAL   Gender: M   Age: 57

Preprocedure diagnosis: acute anterior wall MI

Procedure: CABG ×1 using radial artery bypass, aorta to LAD. Patient placed on CPB.

Tip: Report harvesting of the radial artery in addition to the CABG.

2 CPT Codes _____

4. INPATIENT HOSPITAL   Gender: F   Age: 46

Preprocedure diagnosis: blood clot in right leg

Procedure: thrombectomy of the femoral artery using a leg incision. The vascular return is reestablished.

1 CPT Code _____

5. INPATIENT HOSPITAL   Gender: M   Age: 66

Preprocedure diagnosis: visceral and infrarenal AAA

Procedure: FEVAR repair involving endoprostheses in the visceral aorta for the celiac and renal arteries and infrarenal repair extending to the right and left iliac arteries

1 CPT Code _____

6. OUTPATIENT SURGERY   Gender: M   Age: 43

Preprocedure diagnosis: ESRD

Procedure: Created AV fistula for dialysis in left upper arm between the brachial artery and cephalic vein using an autogenous graft.

Tip: AV fistulas can be created directly by anastomosing an artery to a vein or indirectly by using an autogenous or synthetic graft.

1 CPT Code _____

ARRANGING CODES FOR CARDIOVASCULAR SYSTEM PROCEDURES

Multiple cardiac procedures are often performed together, and there is no set pattern for what is normally done because each patient's circumstances are unique. Follow the standard CPT guidelines for sequencing codes in descending RVU order. In addition, there are special considerations in coding for associated radiological services and multiple surgeons.

Radiology Services

Many services in the Cardiovascular System section involve radiological imaging, supervision, and interpretation. Read the code descriptions, special instructions, and instructional notes to identify when radiological services are bundled in the code and when they should be reported separately.

> ## CODING CAUTION
>
> When radiological services are to be reported separately, code them only if the physician for whom you are coding provided the radiological service. If you are coding for the cardiac surgeon and the radiological services are provided by a radiologist from another practice, do not assign radiology codes.

Multiple Surgeons

Cardiac surgery may involve multiple physicians, so remember to append the appropriate modifiers to identify the role of the physician for whom you are coding. When two surgeons work together as primary surgeons, each physician reports the same CPT code and appends modifier **-62 Two surgeons**. Each surgeon receives 50% of the payment. When a surgical team, usually consisting of distinct specialists, works together to perform a procedure, such as a CABG, each surgeon reports the same CPT code and appends modifier **-66 Surgical team**. Payment is split between the surgeons based on the work that each performed. When an assistant surgeon participates in a procedure with a primary surgeon, the assistant surgeon reports the same CPT code as the primary surgeon and appends modifier **-80 Assistant surgeon**. When the assistant surgeon independently performs a distinct and separately billable procedure, such as video-assisted harvesting of a vessel, then the assistant surgeon reports only the CPT code for the service performed and appends modifier **-80**.

Not all CPT codes are eligible for payment for multiple physicians. The Medicare Physician Fee Schedule Database (MPFSDB) identifies the modifiers accepted for each procedure.

Laterality

Most veins and arteries occur in pairs on opposite sides of the body. Use modifiers **-RT Right side** and **-LT Left side** to identify the laterality of vascular procedures. Do not assign laterality modifiers to procedures on the heart, heart chambers, or valves.

Coronary Arteries

HCPCS modifiers identify each of the coronary arteries:

- **-LC Left circumflex coronary artery**
- **-LD Left anterior descending coronary artery**
- **-LM Left main coronary artery**
- **-RC Right coronary artery**
- **-RI Ramus intermedius coronary artery**

Assign these modifiers when procedures are performed on the coronary arteries, including CABG.

Guided Example of Arranging Cardiovascular System Procedure Codes

To practice skills for arranging codes for procedures of the Cardiovascular System, continue with the example from earlier in the chapter about the patient who was seen for CABG. Follow along in your CPT manual as Tanisha Riemann, CCS-P, arranges the codes. Check off each step after you complete it.

▶ Tanisha reviews the procedure codes she has assigned for this case.

- ❑ **33518 Coronary artery bypass, using venous graft(s) and arterial graft(s); 2 venous grafts**

- ❑ **33533 Coronary artery bypass, using arterial graft(s); single arterial graft**

- ❑ **4110F Internal mammary artery graft performed for primary, isolated coronary artery bypass graft procedure**

▶ Tanisha recalls that the Tabular List and special instructions provide sequencing guidance for these codes.

- ❑ **33518** is an add-on code, so it cannot be sequenced first.

- ❑ The code description for **33518** states **(List separately in addition to code for primary procedure)**. Code **33533** for the arterial graft is the primary procedure.

- ❑ The instructional note after code **33518** states **(Use 33518 in conjunction with 33533-33536)**.

- ❑ Because the informational code **4110F** does not affect payment, she sequences it last.

▶ Tanisha examines the need for modifiers. (Refer to Table 30-1 Key Criteria for Abstracting CPT Modifiers or Appendix A in the CPT manual.)

- ❑ Neither of these codes requires a modifier because add-on codes do not require a modifier for a multiple or separate procedure. No other extenuating circumstances exist.

▶ Tanisha finalizes the procedure codes and sequencing for this case:

(1) **33533-LD-LC Coronary artery bypass, using arterial graft(s); single arterial graft;**

(2) **33518-RC 2 Coronary artery bypass, using venous graft(s) and arterial graft(s); 2 venous grafts;**

(3) **4110F Internal mammary artery graft performed for primary, isolated coronary artery bypass graft procedure**

▶ Tanisha also assigns and sequences the ICD-10-CM diagnosis codes that support the need for the service.

(1) **I21.11 ST elevation (STEMI) myocardial infarction involving right coronary artery**

(2) **I25.110 Atherosclerotic heart disease of native coronary artery with unstable angina pectoris**

(3) **F17.218 Nicotine dependence, cigarettes, with other nicotine-induced disorders**

CODING PRACTICE

Exercise 39.4 Arranging Codes for Cardiovascular System Procedures

Instructions: Read the mini-medical-record of each patient's encounter. Review the information abstracted in Exercise 39.2 for questions 1–3. For questions 4–6, abstract the case on your own. Assign CPT codes, quantities, and modifiers using the Index and Tabular List, and arrange the codes in the proper sequence. Write the code(s) on the lines provided.

1. INPATIENT HOSPITAL   Gender: M   Age: 63

Preprocedure diagnosis: *coronary artery disease*

Procedure: *CABG x4; left radial artery from the aorta to the PDA branch of the RC; LIMA from the aorta to the ramus intermedius coronary artery (RI) and then sequentially to the diagonal branch of the LAD; left saphenous vein graft to the obtuse marginal branch of the left circumflex (LCX). The assistant surgeon performed an endoscopic video-assisted harvesting of the saphenous vein.*

Tip: Code for the primary surgeon who performed the CABG and the assistant surgeon's graft procurement.

5 CPT Codes _____

_____

2. OUTPATIENT HOSPITAL   Gender: M   Age: 47

Preprocedure diagnosis: *Occlusion and stenosis of carotid artery vascular family with cerebral infarction*

Procedure: *Selective catheter placement with angiography and stent. Inserted catheter percutaneously in the left femoral artery and maneuvered it to the aorta, where angiography was performed on the cervicocerebral arch. Moved catheter into the left common carotid artery, proceeded to the internal carotid artery then into the left middle cerebral branch. Performed angiography of the ipsilateral common carotid circulation. Radiological supervision and interpretation done by surgeon.*

Postprocedure diagnosis: *Occlusion and stenosis of left middle cerebral artery with cerebral infarction*

Tip: The left middle cerebral vertebral artery is an intracranial branch of the left internal carotid artery

2 CPT Codes _____

3. INPATIENT HOSPITAL   Gender: F   Age: 68

Preprocedure diagnosis: *ICD that was implanted two years ago for ventricular tachycardia*

Procedure: *upgrade ICD in right ventricle to dual chamber. Removed pulse generator in the subcutaneous pocket in the chest. Tested existing lead, which was found to be in good condition, so it was reused. Under fluoroscopic guidance, threaded a new lead into the right ventricle and right atrium. Inserted new pulse generator.*

Tip: Refer to the pacemaker/ICD coding chart in the CPT manual.

2 CPT Codes _____

4. INPATIENT HOSPITAL   Gender: M   Age: 64

Preprocedure diagnosis: *arteriosclerosis*

Procedure: *Percutaneous revascularization of the right common iliac artery with transluminal angioplasty; revascularization of the ipsilateral external iliac artery with angioplasty and transluminal stent placement*

3 CPT Codes _____

5. INPATIENT HOSPITAL   Gender: F   Age: 35

Preprocedure diagnosis: *pain and swelling in both legs*

Procedure: *femoral vein valvuloplasty in both legs*

1 CPT Code _____

6. OUTPATIENT SURGERY   Gender: M   Age: 71

Preprocedure diagnosis: *heart failure*

Procedure: *Conversion of existing pacemaker system to biventricular. Removed the current pulse generator and replaced with a new pulse generator with a multiple-lead system with biventricular pacing capabilities. Inserted left ventricular pacing electrode at the same time.*

Tip: Code for the replacement of the pulse generator and insertion of the LV lead.

2 CPT Codes _____

E/M CODING FOR CARDIOLOGY

The *1997 Documentation Guidelines for Evaluation and Management Services* (1997 DG), published by CMS, provides requirements for each level of a cardiovascular E/M examination (■ FIGURE 39-7). Specialists are not limited to using only the guidelines for a cardiovascular examination. They can also use guidelines for a general multiorgan system examination or any other single organ system examination based on what is most advantageous for a specific encounter. However, physicians cannot combine elements from more than one type of examination for a given encounter. Typically, the cardiovascular examination guidelines provide the best results when a detailed examination is performed.

To determine the appropriate E/M code, coders must review the documentation in detail and identify the specific elements documented.

- To translate the documentation into the E/M requirements for the history, refer back to Chapter 31, Evaluation and Management Services (99201-99499), Tables 31-7 to 31-10, or to the 1997 DG.

- To determine the requirements for an examination, refer to Figure 39-7 or to the single organ system examination for the cardiovascular system in the 1997 DG.

- To determine the levels for medical decision making (MDM), refer to Chapter 31, Table 31-12, and also to the Table of Risk in the 1997 DG.

Guided Example of E/M Coding for Cardiology

Refer to the cardiology encounter (■ FIGURE 39-8) to practice skills for abstracting and assigning E/M codes. This Guided Example illustrates the 1997 DG for cardiovascular examination. In the workplace, coders must evaluate each encounter against the 1995 DG, the 1997 general multisystem DG, and the single organ system DG to identify the criteria that provide the optimal level of coding. Follow along as fictitious coder Tanisha Riemann, CCS-P, abstracts the procedure. Check off each step after you complete it.

▶ First, Tanisha needs to establish the category of service so she can determine the information needed to abstract and assign the code.

❑ *What is the setting?* admitted to hospital last evening

❑ *What is the type of service?* hospital inpatient services

❑ *What is the code range?* Tanisha refers to the CPT Index and looks up the Main Term **Evaluation and Management** and the subterm **Hospital**. The code range **99221-99233 is listed**.

  ▪ Tanisha refers to the code range in the Tabular List and notices that the **Hospital Inpatient Services** subsection is divided by **Initial Hospital Care** and **Subsequent Hospital Care**. She reads the special instructions for the category **Initial Hospital Care** that state, in part, **The following codes are used to report the first hospital inpatient encounter with**

the patient by the admitting physician. For initial inpatient encounters by physicians other than the admitting physician, see initial inpatient consultation codes (99251-99255) or subsequent hospital care codes (99231-99233) as appropriate.

  ▪ The special instructions tell Tanisha that because this is not the admission encounter and the physician is not documented as the admitting physician, she should not use the **Initial Hospital Care** category, despite the fact that this is the physician's first encounter with the patient.

  ▪ Although the documentation uses the term *consultation* at the end of the report, this encounter does not meet the criteria for a consultation code because there is no documentation of a request for the cardiologist's evaluation or a report back to the requesting physician. Therefore, Tanisha understands that she must code this as **Subsequent Hospital Care (99231-99233)**.

❑ *How many key components are required?* Tanisha reads the code description of the first code, which states **2 of these 3 key components**. All codes in the category have the same requirements for key components. This tells her that two of the three key components must meet or exceed the levels listed in the code (2/3).

▶ Next, Tanisha identifies the level of history.

❑ *What is the level of HPI?* The HPI is **Extended** because five elements are documented.

❑ *What is the level of ROS?* The ROS is **Extended** because five systems are documented.

❑ *What is the level of PFSH?* The PFSH is **Complete** because three elements are documented.

❑ *Based on these factors, what is the overall level of history?* The level of history is **Detailed** because the lowest of the three factors (HPI, ROS, and PFSH) determines the history level. The HPI and ROS qualify for a detailed history, and the PFSH qualifies for a detailed or comprehensive history.

▶ Tanisha refers to the cardiovascular examination in the 1997 DG (Figure 39-7) to abstract information needed to determine the level of the examination.

❑ *What is the level of examination?* The level of examination is **Expanded Problem Focused**. Eight (8) elements of the examination are documented, which exceeds the requirement of six or more bulleted elements for an expanded problem-focused examination. A detailed examination requires that 12 bulleted items be documented, which they are not.

▶ Tanisha determines the level of medical decision making. (Refer to Table 31-12 Medical Decision Making Levels.)

❑ *What is the level of complexity of the number of diagnoses or management options, based on the presenting problem?* The level is **Moderate** because there is a new presenting problem, without workup.

System/Body Area	Elements of Cardiovascular Examination
Constitutional	❏ Measurement of any <u>**three**</u> of the following seven **vital** signs: • 1) sitting or standing blood pressure, • 2) supine blood pressure, • 3) pulse rate and regularity, • 4) respiration, • 5) temperature, • 6) height, • 7) weight (May be measured and recorded by ancillary staff) ❏ General **appearance** of patient (eg, development, nutrition, body habitus, deformities, attention to grooming)
Eyes	❏ Inspection of **conjunctivae** and **lids** (eg, xanthelasma)
Ears, Nose, Mouth and Throat	❏ Inspection of **lips, teeth, gums** and **palate** ❏ Inspection of **oral mucosa** with notation of presence of **pallor** or **cyanosis**
Neck	❏ Examination of **jugular veins** (eg, distension; a, v or cannon a waves) ❏ Examination of **thyroid** (eg, enlargement, tenderness, mass)
Respiratory	❏ Assessment of **respiratory effort** (eg, intercostal retractions, use of accessory muscles, diaphragmatic movement) ❏ **Auscultation** of lungs (eg, breath sounds, adventitious sounds, rubs)
Cardiovascular	❏ **Palpation of heart** (eg, location, size, and forcefulness of the point of maximal impact; thrills; lifts; palpable S3 or S4) ❏ **Auscultation** of heart with notation of abnormal sounds and murmurs ❏ Measurement of **blood pressure in two or more extremities** when indicated (eg, aortic dissection, coarctation) Examination of: ❏ **carotid arteries** (eg, pulse amplitude, bruits) ❏ **abdominal aorta** (eg, size, bruits) ❏ **femoral arteries** (eg, pulse amplitude, bruits) ❏ **pedal pulses** (eg, pulse amplitude) ❏ **extremities** for edema and/or varicosities
Gastrointestinal (Abdomen)	❏ Examination of **abdomen** with notation of presence of masses or tenderness ❏ Examination of **liver** and **spleen** ❏ Obtain **stool sample** for occult blood from patients who are being considered for thrombolytic or anticoagulant therapy
Musculoskeletal	❏ Examination of the **back** with notation of **kyphosis** or **scoliosis** ❏ Examination of **gait** with notation of ability to undergo **exercise** testing and/or participation in exercise programs ❏ Assessment of **muscle strength** and **tone** (eg, flaccid, cog wheel, spastic) with notation of any atrophy and abnormal movements
Extremities	❏ Inspection and palpation of **digits** and **nails** (eg, clubbing, cyanosis, inflammation, petechiae, ischemia, infections, Osler's nodes)
Skin	❏ Inspection and/or palpation of **skin and subcutaneous tissue** (eg, stasis dermatitis, ulcers, scars, xanthomas)
Neurological/ Psychiatric	Brief assessment of mental status including: ❏ **Orientation** to time, place and person ❏ **Mood** and affect (eg, depression, anxiety, agitation)

Total # Bullets Performed and Documented →	☐	# of ❏ **Elements Performed and Documented**	**Level of Examination**
		1–5	Problem focused
		6–11	Expanded problem focused
		12	Detailed
		ALL	Comprehensive (Document **every** element in each box with a shaded border and at least **one** element in each box with an unshaded border)

Figure 39-7 ■ 1997 DG for Cardiovascular Examination. *Source: Centers for Medicare and Medicaid Services, 1997 Documentation Guidelines for Evaluation and Management Services (with formatting adjustments)*

CARDIOLOGY ENCOUNTER

HISTORY OF PRESENT ILLNESS: The patient is a charming and delightful 46-year-old woman admitted to this hospital last evening with palpitations and presyncope. This is my first encounter with the patient.

The patient is active and a previously healthy young woman, who has had seven years of occasional heart palpitations. Symptoms occur three to four times per year and follow no identifiable pattern. She has put thought and effort in trying to identify precipitating factors or circumstances but has been unable to do so. Symptoms can last for an hour or more and she feels as if her heart is going very rapidly. She said that has not measured her heart rate. The last two episodes, the most recent of which was yesterday, she also "felt lightheaded and dizzy." On neither occasion did she lose consciousness.

Yesterday, she had a modestly active morning taking a walk with her dogs and performing her normal routines. While working on a computer, she had a spell. Palpitations persisted for a short time thereafter as outlined in the hospital's admission note prompting her to seek evaluation at the hospital. She was in sinus rhythm on arrival and has been asymptomatic since.

No history of exogenous substance abuse, alcohol abuse, or caffeine abuse. She does have a couple of sodas and a few cups of coffee daily. She is a nonsmoker. She is a mother of one. There is no family history of congenital heart disease. She has had no history of thoracic trauma. No symptoms to suggest thyroid disease.

No known history of diabetes, hypertension, or dyslipidemia. Family history is negative for ischemic heart disease. She underwent an ACL repair 15 years ago, complicated by contact urticaria from a neoprene cast.
No regular medications prior to admission.
The only allergy is the neoprene reaction outlined above.

PHYSICAL EXAMINATION: Vital signs as charted. Pupils are reactive. Sclerae nonicteric. Mucous membranes are moist. Neck veins not distended. No bruits. Lungs are clear. Cardiac exam is regular without murmurs, gallops, or rubs. Abdomen is soft without guarding, rebound masses, or bruits. Extremities well perfused. No edema. Strong and symmetrical distal pulses.

A 12-lead EKG shows sinus rhythm with normal axis and intervals. No evidence of preexcitation.

LABORATORY STUDIES: Unremarkable. No evidence of myocardial injury. Thyroid function is pending.

Two-dimensional echocardiogram shows no evidence of clinically significant structural or functional heart disease.

IMPRESSION/PLAN: Episodic palpitations over a seven-year period. Outpatient workup would be appropriate after discharge. Event recorder should be obtained and the patient can be seen again in the office upon completion of that study. Suppressive medication (beta-blocker or Cardizem) was discussed with the patient for symptomatic improvement, though this would be unlikely to be a curative therapy. The patient expresses a preference to avoid medical therapy if possible. Caffeine avoidance was discussed.

Thank you for this consultation. We will be happy to follow her both during this hospitalization and following discharge.

HISTORY: Detailed

Chief complaint (CC)

Setting & patient type

HPI: Extended (4+)

ROS: Extended (2-9)

PFSH: Complete (3)

EXAMINATION: Expanded Problem Focused

(6-11 bulleted elements)

MEDICAL DECISION MAKING: Moderate Complexity

MDM Risk: Undiagnosed new problem with uncertain prognosis (Moderate Risk)

MDM Data: Independent visualization of image (High Data)

MDM Management: New presenting problem, with workup (Moderate Management Options)

KEY: HPI History of the present illness   ROS Review of systems
PFSH Past, family, and social history   MDM Medical decision making

Figure 39-8 ■ Cardiology Encounter

❑ *What is the amount and/or complexity of data to be reviewed?* The level is **High** because the physician provided independent visualization of the CT scan.

❑ *What is the level of risk of significant complications, morbidity, and/or mortality?* Tanisha reviews each column in the Table of Risk in the 1997 DG and determines that the level of risk is **Moderate**. The patient presents with an undiagnosed new problem with uncertain prognosis illness (Moderate), clinical labs are reviewed and an event recorder is ordered (Minimal), and prescription drugs are discussed but not implemented (Moderate). The single highest element in the Table of Risk deter-

mines the overall risk. The column **Presenting problem** is the highest level (Moderate).

❑ *Based on these factors, what is the overall level of medical decision making?* The medical decision making is **Moderate complexity**. At least two of the three MDM factors are required to qualify for a specific level of MDM. Two of the three MDM factors meet or exceed Moderate decision making.

Now Tanisha is ready to assign the code for the cardiovascular encounter. The exercise that follows guides you through additional abstracting skills and allows you to assign the correct code.

CODING PRACTICE

Exercise 39.5 E/M Coding for Cardiology

Instructions: Refer to the *1997 Documentation Guidelines for Evaluation and Management Services* (available at www.cms.gov) or Chapter 31 Evaluation and Management (E/M) Services (99201-99499) (Tables 31-7 to 31-12) in this text. Answer the following questions about the Cardiology Encounter (Figure 39-8).

1. a. Which elements of the HPI are documented? Circle all that apply. Location, Quality, Severity, Duration, Timing, Context, Modifying factors, Associated signs and symptoms

    b. How many elements are documented? _____

    c. What is the level of HPI? _____

2. a. Which systems are reviewed in the ROS? Circle all that apply. Constitutional, Allergic/ immunologic, CV, Endocrine, ENT/M, Eyes, GI, GU, Hemic/lymphatic, MS, Neurologic, Psychiatric, Respiratory, Skin/breast

    b. How many systems are documented? _____

    c. What is the level of ROS? _____

3. a. Which PFSH elements are documented? Circle all that apply. Past medical, Family, Social

    b. What is the level of PFSH? _____

    c. What is the overall level of history? (The lowest history factor—HPI, ROS, or PFSH—determines the level of history.)

    _____

4. Refer to Figure 39-7 (1997 DG for Cardiovascular Examination).

    a. Which bulleted items are documented for the examination? (Check off the items documented.)

    b. How many bulleted items are documented? _____

    c. What is the level of the examination? _____

5. Refer to Table 31-12 Medical Decision Making Levels or the 1997 DG.

    a. What is the MDM level for the number of diagnoses or management options?

    b. What is the MDM level for the amount and/or complexity of data to be reviewed?

    c. Refer to the Table of Risk in the 1997 DG. Which elements of risk are documented for each risk factor?

        1. Presenting problem: _____

        2. Diagnostic procedures ordered: _____

        3. Management options selected: _____

    d. What is the level of risk? (The highest of the three risk factors determines the overall level of risk.) _____

    e. What is the overall level of MDM? (2/3 MDM factors are needed to determine the overall level.) _____

6. a. What is the setting? _____

    b. What is the patient (or service) type? _____

    c. What is the code range? _____

    d. How many key components are required? _____

    e. What is the level of history? _____

    f. What is the level of examination? _____

    g. What is the level of medical decision making? _____

    h. What is the correct code? _____

7. Abstract and assign the diagnosis code that supports the E/M code.

    1 ICD-10-CM Code _____

CHAPTER SUMMARY

In this chapter you learned that:

- Cardiology is a subspecialty of internal medicine that specializes in the cardiovascular system. Cardiothoracic surgeons perform surgery on the heart and surrounding structures, including the lung when necessary. Vascular surgeons perform surgery on the vessels.

- Surgeons can operate on the heart using open heart surgery, off-pump heart surgery, and minimally invasive heart surgery.

- The CPT subsection **Cardiovascular System (33010-37799)** contains two subheadings: **Heart and Pericardium (33010-33999)**, which includes procedures on the conduction system,

and **Arteries and Veins (34001-36556)**. Each subheading contains numerous categories divided by the type of anatomic site, condition, and type of procedure.

- Various types of cardiovascular procedures require unique abstracting criteria, including coronary artery bypass grafts, central venous access procedures, pacemakers and implantable cardiodefibrillators, and vascular procedures.

- The Cardiovascular System provides extensive special instructions throughout the Tabular List that clarify definitions, code assignments, and bundling rules.

- Multiple cardiac procedures are often performed together, and there is no set pattern for what is normally done because each patient's circumstances are unique. Follow the standard CPT guidelines for sequencing codes in descending RVU order. In addition, there are special considerations when coding associated radiological services and multiple surgeons.

- The *1997 Documentation Guidelines for Evaluation and Management Services* (1997 DG), published by CMS, provides requirements for each level of a cardiovascular E/M examination.

- Special instructions at the beginning of the subsection direct how to code for catheterization within a vascular family. CPT **Appendix L, Vascular Families**, shows the designation of first-, second-, and third-order branches within vascular families for catheterization beginning at the aorta.

- Detailed special instructions and a table in the category **Pacemaker or Pacing Cardioverter-Defibrillator** provide guidance on coding for related services. The "Central Venous Access Procedures Table" appears in the subcategory **Central Venous Access Procedures (36555-36598)**.

CONCEPT QUIZ

Take a moment to look back at the cardiovascular system and solidify your skills. Try to answer the questions from memory first, then refer to the discussion in this chapter if you need a little extra help.

Completion

Instructions: Write the term that answers each question based on the information you learned in this chapter. Choose from the list below. Some choices may be used more than once and some choices may not be used at all.

abdominal aortic aneurysm	synthetic
arterial	tetralogy of Fallot
autologous	total artificial heart implantation
endovascular aneurysm repair	
fenestrated stent	transmyocardial revascularization
heart transplant	ventricular assist device implantation
hemodialysis	
maze surgery	ventricular septal defect
patent ductus arteriosus ligation	

1. When the ductus arteriosus fails to close after birth, a(n) _____ is performed.

2. If a traditional stent would block one or more arteries in the repair of an aneurysm, a(n) _____ can be used.

3. One treatment for atrial fibrillation that creates new paths for the heart's electrical signal is _____.

4. A(n) _____ employs the use of lasers in the treatment of angina.

5. A(n) _____ is repaired through placement of a patch through open heart surgery or using a guidewire.

6. One of the four defects found in _____ is pulmonary stenosis.

7. A patch, stent, or graft may be used to replace a weak section of an artery during a(n) _____.

8. A(n) _____ or autologous graft may be used to widen the vessel in coarctation of the aorta.

9. End-stage heart failure may require a(n) _____, in which a device replaces the ventricles.

10. An AV fistula may be used to create _____ access.

Multiple Choice

Instructions: Circle the letter of the best answer to each question based on the information you learned in this chapter.

1. What reference table appears in the Cardiovascular System subsection?
   A. The Central Venous Access Procedures Table
   B. The Coronary Artery Bypass Graft Table
   C. The Vascular Family Branches Table
   D. The EVAR/FEVAR Table

2. What term is used to describe interventional procedures?
   A. Therapeutic
   B. Operative
   C. Invasive
   D. Selective

3. What branch order is the subclavian artery when a catheter is threaded from the aorta into the brachiocephalic artery, through the subclavian artery, and into the right vertebral artery?
   A. First
   B. Second
   C. Third
   D. Additional third order

4. What is the starting point for vascular families when determining the branch order?
   A. Femoral artery
   B. Inferior vena cava
   C. Radial artery
   D. Aorta

5. What procedure is bundled in the codes for TAVR according to the CPT guidelines for cardiac valves?
   A. Diagnostic left heart catheterization
   B. Percutaneous coronary interventional procedure
   C. Angiography
   D. Cardiopulmonary bypass support

6. What service can be reported separately at the time of a PCI under certain conditions?
   A. Diagnostic angiography
   B. Selective catheterization
   C. Fluoroscopic guidance
   D. Closure of arteriotomy

(continued)

(continued from page 765)

7. What modifier is used when a surgical assistant performs graft procurement?
   A. -51
   B. -62
   C. -80
   D. -81

8. What do add-on codes for endovascular revascularization of the lower extremities indicate?
   A. Distinct lesions
   B. Different vessels
   C. Radiologic supervision and interpretation
   D. Open or percutaneous approach

9. Which graft procurement can be coded separately in addition to a bypass procedure?
   A. Greater saphenous vein
   B. Tibial vein
   c. Radial artery
   D. Femoropopliteal artery

10. What should the coder identify to determine the total number of grafts that a surgeon performs?
    A. Number of grafts harvested
    B. Percentage of blockage of the artery(ies)
    C. Distal anastomoses performed
    D. Amount of time on CPB

CODING CHALLENGE

Instructions: Read the mini-medical-record of each patient's encounter, then abstract, assign, and arrange ICD-10-CM diagnosis codes and CPT procedure codes using the appropriate Index and Tabular List. Assign quantities and modifiers where needed. Write the code(s) on the line provided.

---

1. INPATIENT HOSPITAL Gender: F Age: 47

Preprocedure diagnosis: metastatic breast cancer needing vascular access for chemotherapy

Procedure: percutaneous placement of a single-lumen Hickman catheter through the left subclavian vein with fluoroscopic guidance

Postprocedure diagnosis: metastatic breast cancer

Tip: Know the age of the patient and whether the catheter is tunneled or nontunneled to select the right code.

2 ICD-10-CM Codes _____

2 CPT Codes _____

---

2. OUTPATIENT HOSPITAL Gender: M Age: 54

Preprocedure diagnosis: left superficial femoral artery subtotal stenosis; arterial insufficiency, left lower extremity

Procedure: left lower extremity angiogram; left superficial femoral artery laser atherectomy; left superficial femoral artery percutaneous transluminal balloon angioplasty

Postprocedure diagnosis: total stenosis, left superficial femoral artery; arterial insufficiency, left lower extremity

Tip: Be sure to read the instructional guidelines for endovascular revascularization (open or percutaneous, transcatheter).

2 ICD-10-CM Codes _____

1 CPT Code _____

---

3. OUTPATIENT HOSPITAL Gender: F Age: 68

Reason for encounter: insertion of pacemaker due to tachybrady syndrome with chronic atrial fibrillation

Procedure: implantation of a single-chamber pacemaker, right ventricular lead placement under fluoroscopic guidance

Assessment: successful implantation of pacemaker, pacing and sensing appropriately

Plan: admit overnight for observation; chest X-ray to verify lead position and rule out pneumothorax

2 ICD-10-CM Code _____

1 CPT Code _____

---

4. OUTPATIENT SURGERY Gender: F Age: 45

Reason for encounter: end-stage hypertensive renal failure; on chronic hemodialysis with thrombosed dialysis access

Procedure: thrombectomy and open revision of left forearm AV fistula

Assessment: thrombosed AV fistula, awaiting kidney transplant

Plan: continue dialysis three times a week

Tip: Follow the instructions in the ICD-10-CM Tabular List to **Use additional code**.

5 ICD-10-CM Codes _____

_____

1 CPT Code _____

5. INPATIENT HOSPITAL   Gender: M   Age: 78

Reason for encounter: pacemaker battery at end of life

Procedure: pulse generator replacement, removal of a Medtronic unit and insertion of Biotronik Stratos LV with biventricular port

Assessment: previous aortic valve replacement with subsequent insertion of a dual-chamber pacemaker for underlying chronic atrial fibrillation, and now the pacemaker has shown signs of battery at the end of life

Plan: potential need for biventricular pacemaker

3 ICD-10-CM Codes _____

_____

1 CPT Code _____

6. OUTPATIENT HOSPITAL   Gender: F   Age: 17

Reason for encounter: congenital renal arteriovenous malformation; uncontrolled secondary hypertension

Procedure: angiographically guided embolization of the malformation with absolute alcohol

Assessment: renal angiogram of the right kidney revealed a large lower-pole congenital AVM amenable to embolization

Plan: embolization followed by regulation of hypertension

2 ICD-10-CM Codes _____

1 CPT Code _____

7. HOSPITAL OUTPATIENT   Gender: M   Age: 72

Preprocedure diagnosis: bilateral carotid artery occlusive disease; peripheral vascular disease

Procedure: bilateral carotid cerebral angiogram and right femoral-popliteal angiogram.

Tip: A modifier is used for both procedures.

2 ICD-10-CM Codes _____

2 CPT Codes _____

8. INPATIENT HOSPITAL   Gender: M   Age: 62

Preprocedure diagnosis: postoperative femoral-tibial bypass thrombus formation in saphenous vein graft

Procedure: return to surgery for thrombectomy

Tip: Assign a modifier to report the return to surgery.

1 ICD-10-CM Code _____

1 CPT Code _____

9. HOSPITAL INPATIENT   Gender: M   Age: 84

Reason for encounter: second-degree protein–calorie malnutrition due to end-stage kidney disease

Procedure: insertion of a tunneled femoral triple lumen catheter for TPN

Assessment: protein–calorie malnutrition, moderate

Plan: central venous access for total parenteral nutrition

2 ICD-10-CM Codes _____

1 CPT Code _____

10. HOSPITAL INPATIENT   Gender: F   Age: 68

Reason for encounter: mitral valve regurgitation

Procedure: Mitral valve replacement with a 27-mm CarboMedics mechanical valve with cardiopulmonary bypass; intraoperative transesophageal echocardiogram to assess new valve for continued regurgitation

Assessment: mitral valve regurgitation, cardiomyopathy with left ventricular failure

Plan: monitor in cardiovascular intensive care unit

3 ICD-10-CM Codes _____

_____

2 CPT Codes _____

KEEP ON CODING

Instructions: Read the procedural statement, then use the appropriate Index and Tabular List to assign CPT procedure codes, quantities, and modifiers. Write the code(s) on the line provided.

1. Aortobifemoral bypass using a bifurcated Hemashield graft: CPT Code(s) _____

2. Endovascular abdominal aortic aneurysm repair using a Gore Excluder bifurcated endoprosthesis; bilateral common iliac artery angioplasties: CPT Code(s) _____

3. Right carotid endarterectomy with patch angioplasty: CPT Code(s) _____

4. Thrombectomy, left forearm arteriovenous Gore-Tex bridge fistula: CPT Code(s) _____

(continued)

(continued from page 767)

5. Ligation (clip interruption) of patent ductus arteriosus: CPT Code(s) _____

6. Resection of right internal carotid artery aneurysm with transposition of external to internal carotid artery and patch angioplasty: CPT Code(s) _____

7. Transvenous dual-chamber ICD implantation: CPT Code(s) _____

8. Popliteal embolectomy and a fem-pop bypass with harvested saphenous vein: CPT Code(s)

_____

9. Three saphenous vein grafts in a coronary artery bypass procedure for arteriosclerosis of native arteries: CPT Code(s) _____

10. Heel stick by physician assistant: CPT Code(s) _____

11. Popliteal artery thromboendarterectomy: CPT Code(s) _____

12. Endoscopic ligation of perforator veins, subfascial: CPT Code(s) _____

13. Percutaneous internal carotid angiography and angioplasty: CPT Code(s) _____

14. Endovascular insertion of IVC filter: CPT Code(s) _____

15. Distal revascularization and internal ligation (DRIL) of the upper extremity: CPT Code(s) _____

16. Ligation and stripping of left greater saphenous vein to the level of the knee: CPT Code(s)

_____

17. Embolization of the uterine arteries for management of hemorrhage: CPT Code(s) _____

18. Coronary artery bypass graft ×3, including left internal mammary artery to the left anterior descending artery, saphenous vein graft to the first diagonal artery, and saphenous vein graft to the circumflex artery: CPT Code(s)

_____

19. Return to the operating room for control of postoperative hemorrhage following carotid endarterectomy: CPT Code(s)

_____

20. Insertion of dual-chamber rate-modulated (DDDR) permanent pacemaker with pulse generator and transvenous electrode placement: CPT Code(s) _____

21. Intravenous tPA (*tissue plasminogen activator*) for cerebral thrombolysis: CPT Code(s)

_____

22. Repair of infrarenal AAA using a 2-limb modular bifurcated prosthesis: CPT Code(s) _____

23. Replacement of a peripherally inserted central catheter (PICC) through the same access: CPT Code(s)

_____

24. Percutaneous removal of intra-aortic balloon pump (IABP): CPT Code(s) _____

25. Repair of congenital atrial septal defect, secundum, with bypass and patch: CPT Code(s)

_____

Hemic and Lymphatic Systems (38199-38999) and Mediastinum and Diaphragm Procedures (39000-39599)

Chapter 40

Learning Objectives

After completing this chapter, you should have the skills to:

40.1 Spell and define the key words, medical terms, and abbreviations related to hemic and lymphatic systems, mediastinum, and diaphragm procedures.

40.2 Discuss the fundamentals of hemic and lymphatic systems, mediastinum, and diaphragm procedures.

40.3 Identify the main characteristics of coding for the Hemic and Lymphatic Systems, Mediastinum, and Diaphragm.

40.4 Abstract procedural information from the medical record for coding hemic and lymphatic systems, mediastinum, and diaphragm procedures.

40.5 Assign codes for Hemic and Lymphatic Systems, Mediastinum, and Diaphragm procedures.

40.6 Arrange codes for Hemic and Lymphatic Systems, Mediastinum, and Diaphragm procedures.

40.7 Code evaluation and management services for the hemic and lymphatic systems, mediastinum, and diaphragm.

40.8 Discuss the CPT coding guidelines related to the Hemic and Lymphatic Systems, Mediastinum, and Diaphragm.

Chapter Outline

- **Hemic and Lymphatic Systems Procedure Basics**
- **Coding Overview of Hemic and Lymphatic Systems Procedures**
- **Abstracting Hemic and Lymphatic Systems Procedures**
- **Assigning Codes for Hemic and Lymphatic Systems Procedures**
- **Arranging Codes for Hemic and Lymphatic Systems Procedures**
- **E/M Coding for the Hemic and Lymphatic Systems**

Key Terms and Abbreviations

allogeneic	diaphragm	lymph chain	sentinel lymph node
autologous	hemic	lymph node	T-lymphocytes
bone marrow	lymph	mediastinum	

In addition to the key terms listed here, students should know the terms defined within tables in this chapter.

For updates and corrections, visit our student resource site at www.pearsonhighered.com/healthprofessionsresources

INTRODUCTION

The shelves of drugstores and health food stores are lined with products to boost your immune system and ward off illness. Such products may support the lymphatic and hemic systems, which are central to fighting many illnesses and diseases. For the sake of brevity, this chapter refers to the hemic and lymphatic systems, mediastinum, and diaphragm collectively as the hemic and lymphatic systems.

HEMIC AND LYMPHATIC SYSTEMS PROCEDURE BASICS

The **hemic** (*blood*) and lymphatic systems are studied together because blood and lymph are two of the body's main fluids, which are circulated through two separate but interconnected vessel systems. The hemic system consists of the blood, whereas the cardiovascular/circulatory system consists of the heart, great vessels, and blood vessels. Blood is circulated through arteries, veins, and capillaries by the pumping action of the heart. Chapter 15 of this text provides additional information on the anatomy and conditions of the hemic system.

The lymphatic system is part of the body's immune system, or defense against invading organisms. It transports **lymph** (*a clear fluid containing proteins, salts, organic substances, and water*) from body tissues to the blood. The lymphatic system consists of vessels or channels, nodes, ducts, and the accessory organs of the tonsils, adenoids, thymus, and spleen (■ FIGURE 40-1).

Lymph nodes are small masses of tissue that range from the size of a pinhead to about one inch in diameter and are located along the lymph vessels. Lymph nodes assist the bone marrow to produce lymphocytes, which in turn produce antibodies to defend the body against disease, bacteria, and viruses. **Lymph chains** are sequential groupings of lymph nodes in a localized area along lymph vessels, occurring in sites where the body is most vulnerable to infection. Lymph nodes and lymph chains are identified by the general anatomic area where they occur, such as cervical or pelvic, but each anatomic area is generally subdivided into several levels of nodes based on the flow of lymphatic fluid. A **sentinel lymph node** is the first node or group of nodes in a chain.

Lymph fluid drains from lymphatic capillaries in body tissue, through lymph vessels, and into the large veins of the circulatory system located in the upper chest. Lymph fluid is not pumped and does not circulate in the same way blood does. Muscles contract around the lymph vessels to move the fluid forward. Valves within the lymphatic system provide for a one-way flow created by muscular action.

The thymus contributes to the production of T-lymphocytes, which are white blood cells that protect against viruses and bacteria. The thymus decreases in size after a person reaches puberty. The thymus also performs endocrine functions.

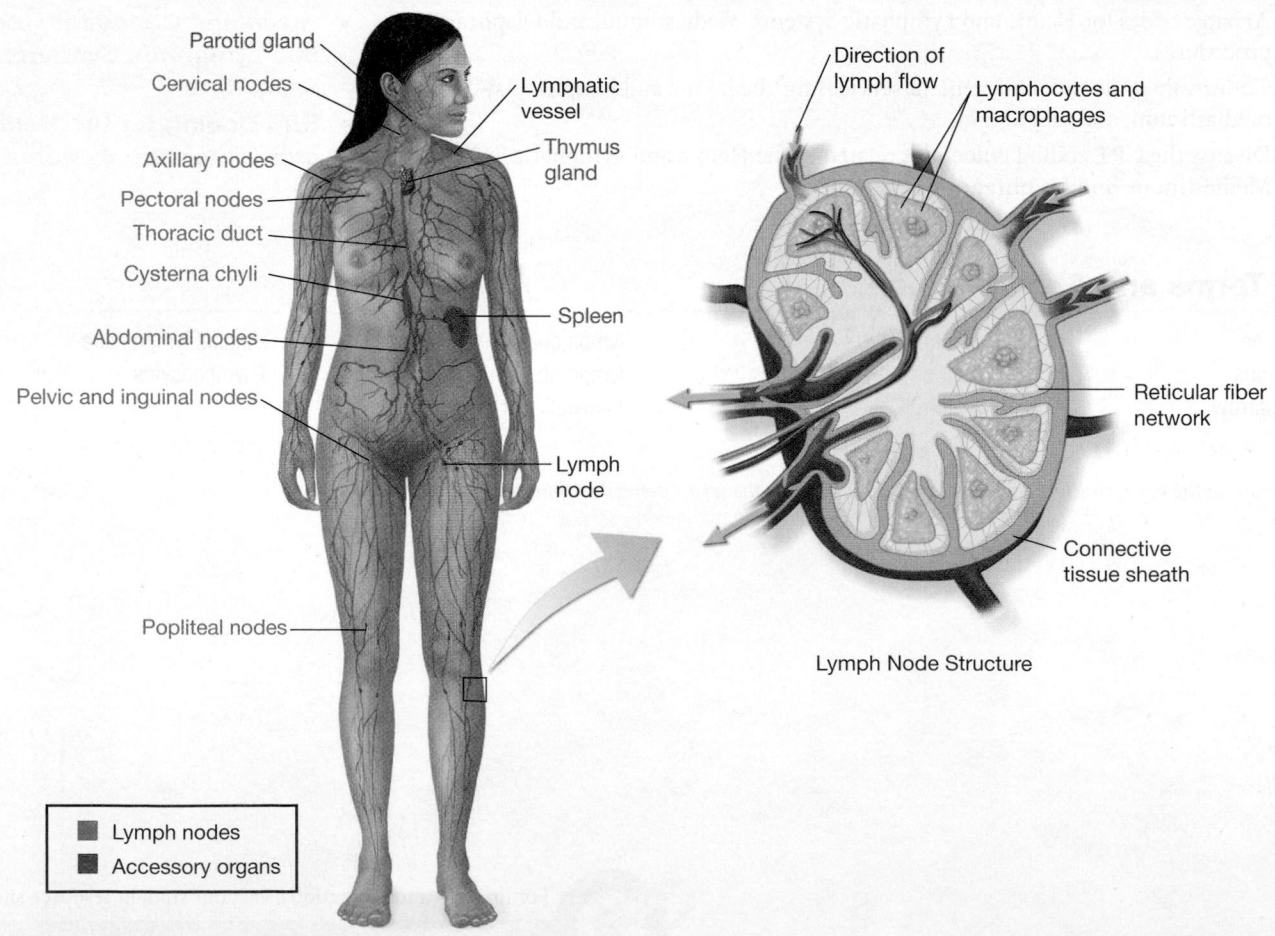

Parotid gland
Cervical nodes
Axillary nodes
Pectoral nodes
Thoracic duct
Cysterna chyli
Abdominal nodes
Pelvic and inguinal nodes
Popliteal nodes

Lymphatic vessel
Thymus gland
Spleen
Lymph node

■ Lymph nodes
■ Accessory organs

Direction of lymph flow
Lymphocytes and macrophages
Reticular fiber network
Connective tissue sheath

Lymph Node Structure

Figure 40-1 ■ The Lymphatic System

SUCCESS STEP

The lymphatic system is one of the avenues by which cancer metastasizes (*spreads*) to areas of the body distant from its origin. Surgeons often sample lymph nodes to help stage cancer (*evaluate how far cancer has spread*) and usually remove affected nodes to help diminish further spread of the malignancy.

Bone marrow is soft, spongy tissue inside bones. The body produces red blood cells (RBCs), white blood cells (WBCs), platelets, and stem cells in bone marrow. Stem cells help the body to repair damaged tissue and can grow to become other types of cells through a process called differentiation. Red bone marrow produces blood cells and platelets, and yellow marrow is made up of fat cells.

Refer to ■ FIGURE 40-2 to visualize the location of the mediastinum and diaphragm in relationship to other structures in the thoracic cavity. The **mediastinum** is located in the thorax and is surrounded by connective tissue. It separates the lungs and contains the esophagus, heart, and superior and inferior vena cava and aorta. Procedures performed on the mediastinum include removal of tumors and treatment of infections such as mediastinitis.

The **diaphragm** is a muscle shaped like half of a dome and is located between the thoracic and abdominal cavities. It contracts and flattens during inhalation and relaxes during exhalation. Procedures on the diaphragm include repairs of diaphragmatic hernias, a paralyzed phrenic nerve (*a sensory and motor nerve that conveys signals to the pleura, pericardium, and diaphragm*), and eventration (*a congenital anomaly of poor diaphragmatic muscle development*). Refer to ■ TABLE 40-1 for a

Table 40-1 ■ **EXAMPLE OF CONSTRUCTING MEDICAL TERMS FOR HEMIC AND LYMPHATIC SYSTEMS PROCEDURES**

Combining Form	Suffix	Complete Medical Term
lymph/o (*lymph fluid*) **angi/o** (*vessel*) **aden/o** (*gland*)	**-ectomy** (*excision*)	**lymph + aden + ectomy** (*surgical excision of a lymph gland*)
	-graphy (*recording*)	**lymph + angio + graphy** (*recording a lymph vessel*)
hemat/o (*blood*) **hem/e** (*blood*)	**-pheresis** (*removal*)	**hema + pheresis** (*removal of blood*)
	-poiesis (*formation*)	**hemato + poiesis** (*formation of blood*)

Source: © PB Resources, Inc. Used with permission.

refresher on how to build medical terms related to the hemic and lymphatic systems.

Procedures commonly performed on the hemic and lymphatic systems are discussed next.

CODING CAUTION

Be alert for medical word roots that are spelled similarly and have different meanings.

globin (*a byproduct of hemoglobin*) and **glob<u>ul</u>in** (*a protein molecule that comprises immunoglobulins*)

eryth<u>ro</u>cyte (*red blood cell*) and **eryth<u>em</u>a** (*redness*) and **eryth<u>rem</u>ia** (*polycythemia vera—a circulatory disorder*)

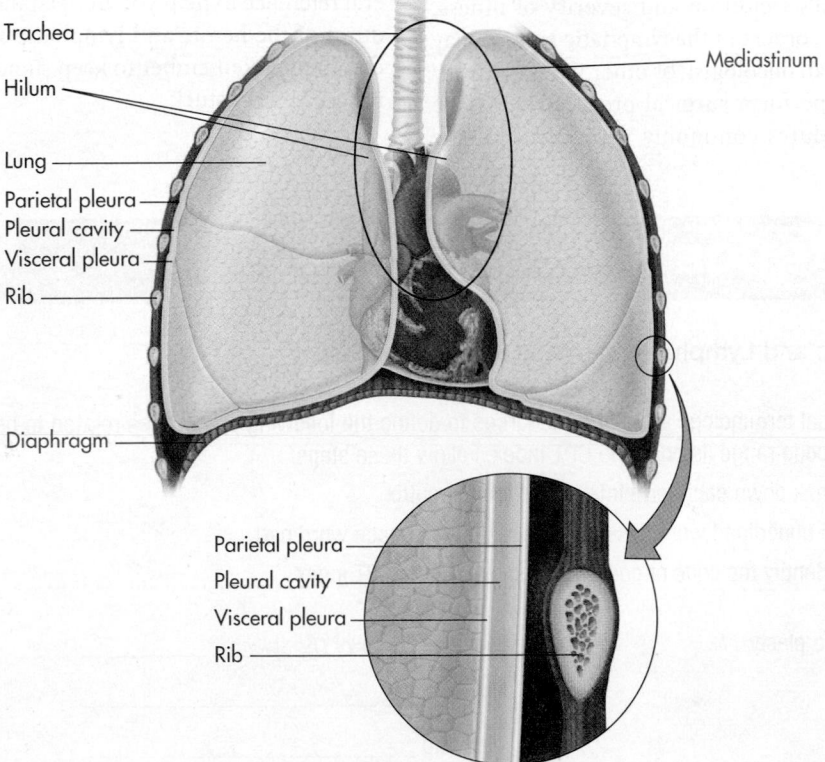

Figure 40-2 ■ The Mediastinum and Diaphragm

Table 40-2 ■ **COMMON PROCEDURES OF THE HEMIC AND LYMPHATIC SYSTEMS, MEDIASTINUM, AND DIAPHRAGM**

Procedure Name	Definition	Reason Performed
Cannulation of thoracic duct	Insertion of a tube (cannulation) into the thoracic duct to collect lymph	Diagnosis of disorders of lymph flow
Imbrication of the diaphragm	Repair of the diaphragm to resemble normal anatomy	Eventration (*a condition in which the diaphragm is relaxed and not shaped like a dome, leading to paralysis*)
Limited lymphadenectomy	Removal of lymph nodes	Staging or treatment of cancer
Lymphangiography	Radiology procedure where contrast medium is injected into the patient to visualize lymph nodes and lymph circulation	Diagnosis of diseases, such as cancer
Lymphangiotomy	Incision into a vessel of the lymphatic system	Drainage of an abscess
Mediastinotomy	Incision into the mediastinum	Drainage, exploration, or foreign body removal
Radical lymphadenectomy	Removal of lymph nodes and nearby structures	Staging or treatment of cancer
Splenectomy	Total or partial excision of the spleen	Injury, cancer, blood disorders such as idiopathic thrombocytopenic purpura (ITP) (*an autoimmune condition in which antibodies target blood platelets*)
Splenorrhaphy	Repair of ruptured spleen, with or without partial splenectomy	Injured or ruptured spleen
Transplantation	Replacement of bone marrow or hematopoietic progenitor cells (HPCs) (*stem cells in the umbilical cord and bone marrow*), including harvesting, cryopreservation, thawing, and specific cell depletion, **allogeneic** (*from a different person*) or **autologous** (*from the same person*)	Treatment of various conditions, such as cancer

Source: © PB Resources, Inc. Used with permission.

Procedures of the Hemic and Lymphatic Systems

Depending on the patient's condition and severity of illness, diagnosing and treating disorders of the lymphatic system may involve an immunologist, an oncologist, or other types of physicians. General surgeons perform surgical procedures on the lymphatic system. Procedures commonly performed on the hemic and lymphatic systems, mediastinum, and diaphragm are summarized in ■ TABLE 40-2. This section provides a general reference to help you understand the most common procedures of the hemic and lymphatic systems, mediastinum, and diaphragm. Remember to keep standard reference books handy in case you get stuck.

CODING PRACTICE

Exercise 40.1 Hemic and Lymphatic Systems Procedure Basics

Instructions: Use your medical terminology skills and resources to define the following procedures related to hemic and lymphatic systems, then identify the code(s) or code range listed in the CPT Index. Follow these steps:

- Use slash marks "/" to break down each term into its root(s) and suffix.
- Define the meaning of the underlined word based on the meaning of each word part.
- Use the entire phrase to identify the code or code range shown in the CPT Index.

Example: <u>splenoplasty</u> spleno/plasty   Meaning *repair of the spleen*   CPT Code *38115*

1. <u>splenectomy</u>, total   Meaning _____   CPT Code _____

2. <u>splenorrhaphy</u>   Meaning _____   CPT Code _____

3. <u>lymphadenectomy</u>, cervical   Meaning _____   CPT Code _____

4. <u>splenoportography</u>, injection procedure   Meaning _____   CPT Code _____

5. <u>retroperitoneal</u> transabdominal lymphadenectomy   Meaning _____   CPT Code _____

6. injection for <u>lymphangiography</u>   Meaning _____   CPT Code _____

7. <u>mediastinotomy</u>, cervical approach   Meaning _____   CPT Code _____

8. <u>lymphangiotomy</u>   Meaning _____   CPT Code _____

9. excision of axillary cystic <u>hygroma</u>   Meaning _____   CPT Code _____

10. bone marrow harvesting, <u>allogeneic</u>   Meaning _____   CPT Code _____

CODING OVERVIEW OF HEMIC AND LYMPHATIC SYSTEMS PROCEDURES

The CPT subsection **Hemic and Lymphatic Systems (38100-38999)** contains codes that represent procedures related to the spleen, bone marrow, blood, lymph nodes, and lymphatic channels (vessels). It has several subheadings: **Spleen**, **General**, **Transplantation and Post-Transplantation Cellular Infusions**, and **Lymph Nodes and Lymphatic Channels**. Each subheading contains several categories based on the type of procedure. The CPT subsection **Mediastinum and Diaphragm (39000-39599)** contains two subheadings—**Mediastinum** and **Diaphragm**—each with categories for the type of procedure.

Review the subheading and category names and code ranges listed in both of these subsections to become familiar with the content and organization. Some editions of the CPT manual provide a summary list of the subheadings and categories at the beginning of each subsection, which also displays an asterisk (*) next to categories that contain special coding instructions.

Codes for diagnostic tests on the hemic and lymphatic systems appear in the Medicine, Laboratory, and Radiology sections. The medical necessity of procedures represented by CPT codes must be justified by diagnosis codes. CPT codes in the Hemic and Lymphatic Systems subsection are frequently supported by diagnosis codes from ICD-10-CM **Chapter 1 Certain Infectious and Parasitic Diseases (A00-B99)**, as well as selected sections of the circulatory and integumentary systems chapters, neoplasms, symptoms and signs, and injuries (■ TABLE 40-3). These are the codes used most commonly to support procedures on the hemic and lymphatic systems; however, diagnosis codes from any ICD-10-CM chapter are permissible.

CPT guidelines for the Surgery section apply to the Hemic and Lymphatic Systems subsections as well as the Mediastinum and Diaphragm subsection. There are no additional guidelines at the beginning of these subsections.

Special instructions that describe how the codes should be reported appear at the beginning of the categories **Bone Marrow or Stem Cell Services/Procedures** and **Transplantation and Post-Transplantation Cellular Infusions**.

Instructional notes appear throughout the Tabular List to alert coders to the need for modifiers, provide cross-references to codes for similar procedures on other sites, identify bundled services, determine when additional codes might be needed for radiological services, and highlight resequenced and recently deleted codes.

Table 40-3 ■ LOCATING ICD-10-CM AND ADDITIONAL CPT CODES ON THE HEMIC AND LYMPHATIC SYSTEMS

Type of Code	Codes
ICD-10-CM Hemic and Lymphatic System-Related Codes	
Hematological conditions	D50-D89
Lymphatic/immune conditions	A00-B99, I88-I89, L03-L04
Neoplasms	C81-C96, D18, D46-D47
Symptoms and signs	R50-R69, R70-R79
Injuries	S35, S36
CPT Hemic and Lymphatic System-Related Codes	
Medicine procedures	90281-90749, 93880-93998
Radiologic procedures	
• Diagnostic radiology	75600-75989
• Radiologic guidance	77001-77022
• Diagnostic ultrasound	76506-76645, 76801-76857, 76881-76886
• Nuclear medicine, diagnostic	78102-78299
Laboratory organ/disease panels, tests	80047, 80050, 80074, 80075, 85002-85999, 86000-86849

Source: © PB Resources, Inc. Used with permission.

ABSTRACTING HEMIC AND LYMPHATIC SYSTEMS PROCEDURES

Familiarity with the anatomy of the lymphatic system is fundamental to abstracting because coding is based on the site and extent of treatment. Lymph nodes are identified by the anatomic region where they occur. Procedures on the lymph nodes can be performed to determine the stage of cancer metastasis; they can also be described as radical, complete, partial, or superficial depending on the specific structures treated. Codes depend on these descriptions of extent and/or on the specific sites of nodes excised. Refer to ■ TABLE 40-4 for guidance on how to abstract procedures on the hemic and lymphatic systems, then work through the detailed example that follows. Remember that the abstracting questions are a guide and that not every question applies to, or can be answered for, every case.

Table 40-4 ■ KEY CRITERIA FOR ABSTRACTING HEMIC AND LYMPHATIC SYSTEMS PROCEDURES

❑ What is the procedure?

❑ What is the anatomic site?

❑ What is the surgical approach?

❑ Is the procedure performed during the same operative session as another major procedure?

For bone marrow and stem cell transplant services:

❑ Is the harvest allogeneic or autologous?

❑ How many donors are used?

❑ What components are depleted or removed?

For lymph nodes and lymphatic channel procedures:

❑ Is the service a biopsy, limited removal for staging, or radical resection?

❑ Which specific nodes and/or chains are removed?

❑ Is the procedure bilateral (where applicable)?

Source: © PB Resources, Inc. Used with permission.

Guided Example of Abstracting Hemic and Lymphatic Systems Procedures

Refer to the following example throughout this chapter to practice skills for abstracting, assigning, and arranging Hemic and Lymphatic Systems codes. Follow along as fictitious coder Scott Hood, CPC, abstracts the procedure. Check off each step after you complete it.

OUTPATIENT HOSPITAL Gender: M Age: 32

Preoperative diagnosis: Stage 4 Hodgkin lymphoma involving multiple lymph nodes above and below the diaphragm

Procedure: Prepared hematopoietic progenitor cells (HPCs) for transplant, including thawing and washing previously frozen harvests from two allogeneic donors,

and performed specific T-cell (lymphocyte) depletion within both harvests. Proceeded with the transplantation of both harvests using sequential injections into an intravenous (IV) drip.

► Scott reads through the entire record, paying special attention to the preoperative diagnosis and the procedure performed. He refers to the Key Criteria for Abstracting Hemic and Lymphatic Systems Procedures (Table 40-4) and takes note of the added criteria for bone marrow and stem cell services.

❑ He notes preoperative diagnosis: Hodgkin lymphoma involving multiple lymph nodes

❑ *What is the patient's age?* 32

❑ *What is the procedure?* prepare hematopoietic progenitor cells (HPCs) for transplant and allogeneic transplantation.

❑ *What is the anatomic site?* hematopoietic progenitor cells

❑ *What is the surgical approach?* The approach does not apply to the preparation. The transplantation is performed using injections into an intravenous (IV) drip.

❑ *Is the procedure performed during the same operative session as another major procedure?* Two HPC procedures are performed: thawing and washing and specific T-cell (lymphocyte) depletion within harvests. In addition, the transplant is performed. No other procedures are performed.

❑ *What components are depleted or removed?* T-cell (lymphocyte) depletion

❑ *Is the harvest allogeneic or autologous?* allogeneic

❑ *How many donors are used?* two

► At this time, Scott does not know which of these procedures may need to be coded, nor how many codes he will end up with. He will learn about this when he moves on to assigning codes.

CODING PRACTICE

Exercise 40.2 Abstracting Hemic and Lymphatic Systems Procedures

Instructions: Read the mini-medical-record of each patient's encounter and answer the abstracting questions. Write the answer on the line provided. Do not assign any codes.

1. INPATIENT HOSPITAL Gender: M Age: 32

Preprocedure diagnosis: lacerated spleen sustained as a result of automobile accident

Procedure: laparoscopic splenectomy

a. What is the procedure? _____

b. What is the anatomic site? _____

c. What is the surgical approach? _____

d. Is the procedure performed during the same operative session as another major procedure? _____

2. OUTPATIENT HOSPITAL   Gender: F   Age: 45

Preprocedure diagnosis: leukemia

Procedure: bone marrow aspiration from the sternum

a. What is the procedure? _____

b. What is the anatomic site? _____

c. What is the surgical approach? _____

d. Is the procedure performed during the same operative session as another major procedure? _____

3. INPATIENT HOSPITAL   Gender: F   Age: 37

Preprocedure diagnosis: mediastinal tumor

Procedure: substernal mediastinectomy, open

Postprocedure diagnosis: benign tumor

a. What is the procedure? _____

b. What is the anatomic site? _____

c. What is the surgical approach? _____

d. Is the procedure performed during the same operative session as another major procedure? _____

4. INPATIENT HOSPITAL   Gender: F   Age: 56

Preprocedure diagnosis: metastasis of lung cancer (middle lobe)

Procedure: complete axillary lymphadenectomy, bilateral

Postprocedure diagnosis: metastasis of lung cancer (middle lobe)

a. What is the procedure? _____

b. What is the anatomic site? _____

c. What is the surgical approach? _____

d. Is the procedure performed during the same operative session as another major procedure? _____

e. Is the service a biopsy, limited removal for staging, or radical resection? _____

f. Which specific nodes and/or chains are removed?

_____

g. Is the procedure bilateral (where applicable)?

_____

5. INPATIENT HOSPITAL   Gender: M   Age: 46

Preprocedure diagnosis: CT scan shows evidence of ruptured spleen following automobile accident

Procedure: splenectomy; incised the abdomen below the left ribs and exposed the spleen. Rupture and parenchymal fragmentation was evident. Ligated and divided splenic arteries and veins. Freed the spleen from surrounding structures and ligaments. Removed the spleen in its entirety. Irrigated the surgical site, placed a drain, and performed a layered closure. Patient tolerated procedure well.

Postprocedure diagnosis: splenic rupture with parenchymal fragmentation

a. What is the procedure? _____

b. What is the anatomic site? _____

c. What is the surgical approach? _____

d. Is the procedure partial or total? _____

6. OUTPATIENT SURGERY   Gender: M   Age: 28

Preprocedure diagnosis: Acute myeloid leukemia

Procedure: thawed previously frozen HPCs harvested from a single donor, without washing, and performed RBC depletion for HPC boost, which was administered by IV

Postprocedure diagnosis: Acute myeloid leukemia

a. What is the procedure? _____

b. What is the surgical approach? _____

c. Is the procedure performed during the same operative session as another major procedure? _____

d. Is the harvest allogeneic or autologous?

_____

e. How many donors are used? _____

f. What components are depleted or removed?

_____

ASSIGNING CODES FOR HEMIC AND LYMPHATIC SYSTEM PROCEDURES

To assign codes for procedures on the hemic and lymphatic systems, mediastinum, and diaphragm, search the Index for the Main Term of the anatomic site, such as **Spleen**, **Mediastinum**, or **Diaphragm**. Locate the first-level modifying term for the type of procedure and the second-level modifying term for any additional details, as required. Verify codes in the Tabular List, paying special attention to the code descriptions and instructional notes. Additional considerations for coding bone marrow/stem cell services, transplant-related cellular infusions, and lymphadenectomies are discussed next.

Bone Marrow/Stem Cell/Transplantation Procedures

To locate codes for bone marrow or stem cell services, procedures, and cellular infusions, search the Index for the Main Term **Bone Marrow** or **Stem Cell**. Locate the first-level modifying term for the type of service or procedure provided and identify the code(s) or code range to be verified in the Tabular List. In the Tabular List, codes for these services appear under the subheading **General** in the subsection **Hemic and Lymphatic Systems**. Codes are divided into two categories.

The category **Bone Marrow or Stem Cell Services/Procedures** contains codes that describe the steps used to harvest, preserve, prepare, and purify bone marrow or stem cells, also called HPCs, for a transplant or reinfusion procedure. Special instructions at the beginning of the category state that codes in this category are reported only once per patient per day, regardless of the quantity of cells treated. The exception is codes whose descriptions contain the phrase **per donor**. When cells from more than one donor are thawed, report one code for each donor (■ FIGURE 40-3). After cells are harvested from a donor, they are frozen and stored for later use. When needed for a procedure, they are thawed and usually washed to remove the preserving solution and other impurities. Components of the harvest might be removed or reduced to create a product suitable for the transplant recipient. Separate codes report each of these services.

The category **Transplantation and Post-Transplantation Cellular Infusions** contains four codes for the actual transplantation or infusion procedure. The special instructions at the beginning of the category outline the services and activities included in the code descriptions and those that can be reported separately. Separately reportable services include management of post-transplant adverse reactions and administration of medications and/or hydration *unrelated* to the transplant. Codes in this category are divided based on whether the procedure is a transplant, post-transplant boost, or lymphocyte infusion. Transplant codes are divided based on whether the harvest is autologous or allogeneic. Allogeneic transplants are reported per donor harvest when harvests are administered sequentially.

CODING CAUTION

Medicare publishes a medically unlikely edit (MUE) of 1 for allogeneic transplantation (**38240 Hematopoietic progenitor cell (HPC); allogeneic transplantation per donor**), meaning that the code can be reported only once per day, despite the code descriptor stating **per donor**. Some private carriers follow Medicare MUEs, whereas others do not, so checking with individual carriers regarding how to report this service is helpful.

Lymphadenectomy

To locate codes for procedures on the lymphatic system, search the Index for the Main Term **Lymph Duct**, **Lymph Nodes**, **Lymph Vessels**, or **Lymphadenectomy**. The Main Term **Lymph Nodes** provides the most detailed code listing. Identify the first-level modifying term for the anatomic site and/or type of procedure. In the Tabular List, codes for procedures on the lymph nodes and lymphatic channels are divided by the type and extent of the procedure. Within each procedure category, unique codes are provided for distinct anatomic regions and sites. A lymphadenectomy can be performed as a biopsy, a cancer staging procedure, or a complete excision. When staging is performed, the surgeon first injects a radioactive dye to identify the sentinel lymph node. The injection procedure is coded in addition to the staging procedure.

A lymphatic biopsy and/or lymphadenectomy is often performed in conjunction with the partial or total excision of another organ—such as the breast, ovary(ies), prostate, or colon—because of the presence of cancer. The procedures most commonly performed with a lymphadenectomy often include code options for bundled lymphadenectomy in the CPT subsection for the primary organ. However, when a lymphadenectomy is performed in conjunction with procedures on the esophagus, trachea, thyroid, and parathyroid, the lymphadenectomy is usually reported separately. Coders must refer to the documentation, code descriptions, and instructional notes to determine when the lymphadenectomy is reported as a standalone procedure (■ FIGURE 40-4), when it is bundled with another procedure (■ FIGURE 40-5), and when it is reported separately (■ FIGURE 40-6).

Physician thawed and washed previously frozen HPC harvests from two separate donors, then performed plasma volume depletion on each.

38214 x 1 Transplant preparation of hematopoietic progenitor cells; plasma (volume) depletion
38209 x 2 Transplant preparation of hematopoietic progenitor cells; thawing of previously frozen harvest, with washing, per donor

Figure 40-3 ■ Example of Reporting Codes Per Donor.
Source: © PB Resources, Inc. Used with permission. CPT codes only © American Medical Association.

Surgeon injects a radioactive tracer to identify the sentinel node then performs a limited pelvic lymphadenectomy for staging of prostate cancer.

38562 Limited lymphadenectomy for staging (separate procedure); pelvic and para-aortic

38792-51 Injection procedure; radioactive tracer for identification of sentinel node; -51 Multiple procedures

Figure 40-4 ■ Example of Coding a Standalone Lymphadenectomy. *Source:* © PB Resources, Inc. Used with permission. CPT codes only © American Medical Association.

Surgeon performs a radical perineal prostatectomy, including a limited excision of pelvic lymph nodes, to treat prostate cancer.

55812 Prostatectomy, perineal radical; with lymph node biopsy(s) (limited pelvic lymphadenectomy)

Figure 40-5 ■ Example of Coding a Bundled Lymphadenectomy. *Source:* © PB Resources, Inc. Used with permission. CPT codes only © American Medical Association.

Surgeon performs a transthoracic thyroidectomy, including substernal thyroid, and a thoracic lymphadenectomy via thoracotomy of the low cervical and upper paratracheal nodes.

60270 Thyroidectomy, including substernal thyroid; sternal split or transthoracic approach

38746 Thoracic lymphadenectomy by thoracotomy, mediastinal and regional lymphadenectomy (List separately in addition to code for primary procedure)

Figure 40-6 ■ Example of Coding a Separate Lymphadenectomy. *Source:* © PB Resources, Inc. Used with permission. CPT codes only © American Medical Association.

Guided Example of Assigning Hemic and Lymphatic Systems Procedure Codes

To practice skills for assigning procedure codes for the hemic and lymphatic systems, continue with the example from earlier in the chapter about a patient who was seen for an HPC transplant. Follow along in your CPT manual as Scott Hood, CPC, assigns codes. Check off each step after you complete it.

▶ First, Scott confirms the procedures:

❑ thawing and washing of previously frozen harvests

❑ specific T-cell (lymphocyte) depletion

❑ transplantation of both harvests

▶ Scott searches the Index for the Main Term **Transplantation**.

❑ He locates the first-level modifying term **Stem Cells** and identifies the code range **38240-38242**.

❑ He reviews the second-level modifying terms and locates entries for **T-cell depletion 38210** and **Thawing 38208-38209**.

❑ He believes that these entries will address everything that was done during the procedure, but just to be certain he also looks up **Stem Cells** as a Main Term. He locates the first-level modifying terms for **T-cell depletion 38210**, **Thawing 38208-38209, 88241**, and **Transplantation 38240-38242**. He also notices a first-level modifying term for **Hematopoietic Progenitor Cells** that cross-references him to a Main Term entry for the same. This Main Term entry provides similar first- and second-level modifying terms with the same code ranges.

▶ Scott verifies the codes in the Tabular List. Because they are located close together, he can check all the codes in one search.

▶ He begins with thawing because that is the first procedure completed. According to the Index, he has two choices for thawing: codes **38208** and **38209**.

❑ In the Tabular List, he notices that both these codes are indented codes under the parent code **38207**. The common portion of the descriptor for code **38207** is **Transplant preparation of hematopoietic progenitor cells;**

❑ He compares the descriptions of codes and identifies that code **38208** is **thawing of previously frozen harvest, without washing, per donor** and code **38209** is the same description except **with washing**.

❑ Scott refers to the medical record and confirms that this thawing was performed with washing, so he selects code **38209**.

❑ He also identifies that the code description identifies the quantity as **per donor**. He refers to the medical record again to verify that two donors were used, which means that he will need to report the quantity as 2.

❑ He reads the full code title for code **38209** by combining the common descriptor portion of the parent code with the descriptor of the standalone code and confirms that this accurately describes the procedure: **Transplant preparation of hematopoietic progenitor cells; thawing of previously frozen harvest, with washing, per donor**.

❑ He reads the instructional note in the Tabular List after code **38208** that states **(For diagnostic thawing and expansion of frozen cells, use 88241)**. Code **88241** is reported by laboratories for processing the specimen and appears in the Index entry for the Main Term **Stem Cells** and subterm **Thawing**.

▶ Next, Scott assigns the code for specific T-cell (lymphocyte) depletion within both harvests. The Index directs him to code **38210**, which is also indented under the parent code **38207**.

❑ The unique descriptor for code **38210** is **specific cell depletion within harvest, T-cell depletion**.

❑ He refers to the medical record and confirms that the description correctly reflects the documentation.

▶ Finally, Scott must assign a code for the actual transplantation procedure. The Index directs him to the code range **38240-38242**.

❑ In the Tabular List, he notices that code **38240** is the parent code for **38241**. The common portion of the descriptor for code **38240** is **Hematopoietic progenitor cells**;

❑ He compares the unique descriptors for both and identifies that code **38240** is **allogeneic transplantation per donor** and code **38241** is **autologous transplantation**.

❑ He refers to the medical record and confirms that the transplant is from *two allogeneic donors*, so he believes that code **38240** is correct. However, the Index also listed **38242** as an option, so he reads that code before making a final decision.

❑ The description for code **38242** is **Allogeneic lymphocyte infusions**. This is not what was done, so he confirms the selection of **38240**.

❑ He also identifies that the code description for **38240** identifies the quantity as **per donor**. He refers to the medical record again to verify that *two* donors were used, which means that he will need to report the quantity as 2.

▶ Scott checks for special instructions and instructional notes in the Tabular List.

❑ He already read the instructional note following codes **38207** and **38208**, which did not apply, and does not find any notes after code **38209**.

❑ He reads several instructional notes following code **38242**. They all direct the coder to alternative codes for procedures not performed during this encounter, so they do not apply.

❑ Next, he cross-references the beginning of the category **Transplantation and Post-Transplantation Cellular Infusions** and finds extensive special instructions. He uses a highlighter to mark information that applies to this case:

   ▪ **Hematopoietic cell transplantation (HCT) refers to the infusion of hematopoietic progenitor cells (HPC) obtained from bone marrow, peripheral blood apheresis, and/or umbilical cord blood.**

   ▪ **HCT may be autologous (when the HPC donor and recipient are the same person) or allogeneic (when the HPC donor and recipient are not the same person). Code 38241 is used to report any autologous transplant while 38240 is used to report an allogeneic transplant.**

   ▪ **In some cases allogeneic transplants involve more than one donor and cells from each donor are infused sequentially whereby one unit of 38240 is reported for each donor infused.**

❑ Other information in these guidelines applies to other codes or to the bundling and reporting of services not documented for this case.

❑ He cross-references the beginning of the category **Bone Marrow or Stem Cell Services/Procedures** and finds more special instructions, which apply to all codes in this category, 38204-38232. **Each code may be reported only once per day regardless of the quantity of bone marrow/stem cells manipulated.**

❑ When Scott reviews the codes he selected from this category, he identifies that code **38209** specifically states to assign the code once **per donor**. However, code **38210** does not include the designation *per donor*, so he confirms that code **38210** should be reported **once per day**. He cross-references the beginning of the section **Hemic and Lymphatic Systems** and verifies that there are no special instructions.

▶ Scott reviews the procedure codes and quantities he has assigned for this case.

❑ **38209 x 2 Transplant preparation of hematopoietic progenitor cells; thawing of previously frozen harvest, with washing, per donor**

❑ **38210 x 1 Transplant preparation of hematopoietic progenitor cells; specific cell depletion within harvest, T-cell depletion**

❑ **38240 x 2 Hematopoietic progenitor cell (HPC); allogeneic transplantation per donor**

▶ Next, Scott must determine how to sequence the codes.

CODING PRACTICE

Exercise 40.3 Assigning Codes for Hemic and Lymphatic Systems Procedures

Instructions: Read the mini-medical-record of each patient's encounter. Review the information abstracted in Exercise 40.2 for questions 1–3. For questions 4–6, abstract the case on your own. Assign CPT codes, quantities, and modifiers using the Index and Tabular List. Write the code(s) on the line provided.

1. INPATIENT HOSPITAL   Gender: M   Age: 32

Preprocedure diagnosis: lacerated spleen sustained as a result of automobile accident

Procedure: laparoscopic splenectomy

1 CPT Code _____

---

2. OUTPATIENT HOSPITAL   Gender: F   Age: 45

Preprocedure diagnosis: leukemia

Procedure: bone marrow aspiration from the sternum

1 CPT Code _____

---

3. INPATIENT HOSPITAL   Gender: F   Age: 37

Preprocedure diagnosis: mediastinal tumor

Procedure: substernal mediastinectomy, open

Postprocedure diagnosis: benign tumor

1 CPT Code _____

---

4. OUTPATIENT HOSPITAL   Gender: F   Age: 41

Preprocedure diagnosis: leukocytosis

Procedure: bone marrow biopsy. Inserted the trocar through the skin over the iliac crest and pushed the needle into the bone marrow. Confirmed needle position was accurate, then proceeded to excise the bone marrow, which was transferred to a specimen container and sent to pathology.

1 CPT Code _____

---

5. OUTPATIENT SURGERY   Gender: M   Age: 22

Preprocedure diagnosis: tenderness and swelling in neck

Procedure: I & D of a cervical lymph node abscess, extensive

Postprocedure diagnosis: abscess, cervical lymph node

1 CPT Code _____

---

6. INPATIENT HOSPITAL   Gender: M   Age: 61

Preprocedure diagnosis: prostate cancer

Procedure: limited pelvic lymphadenectomy for staging

Pathology report: sentinel nodes are negative for metastasis

Postprocedure diagnosis: carcinoma of the prostate with no metastasis to lymph nodes

1 CPT Code _____

ARRANGING CODES FOR HEMIC AND LYMPHATIC SYSTEMS PROCEDURES

Many codes in the Hemic and Lymphatic Systems subsection can be performed at the same time as another major procedure. The instructional note **(separate procedure)** at the end of a code description reminds coders to assign the code only when the procedure is not bundled with another one or is performed at a separate site or through a separate incision. When the code description for the primary procedure includes lymph node excision, do not assign an additional code from the Hemic and Lymphatic Systems subsection.

Modifiers

In addition to modifier **-51 Multiple procedures**, modifiers for laterality and distinct procedural services are important to proper coding for the lymphatic and hemic systems.

Laterality

Most lymph nodes occur in pairs on opposite sides of the body, similar to many blood vessels. Append modifiers for laterality (**-50 Bilateral procedure**, **-RT Right side**, or **-LT Left side**) for procedures on lymph nodes that occur bilaterally, such as suprahyoid (**38700**), cervical (**38720**, **38724**), axillary (**38740**, **38745**), inguinofemoral (**38760**, **38765**), and pelvic (**38770**). Laterality does not apply to thoracic and abdominal lymphadenectomies.

Coders should assign laterality whenever a site or structure occurs bilaterally. Although CPT does not usually provide instructional notes to assign laterality, occasionally it does so when laterality might be overlooked. CPT instructional notes that direct coders to report modifier **-50** for bilateral procedures appear below the codes for inguinofemoral and pelvic lymphadenectomies. The lack of such a laterality note below suprahyoid, cervical, and axillary lymphadenectomies does not mean that laterality modifiers are unnecessary for these codes.

-59 Distinct Procedural Service

When the surgeon performs a complete lymphadenectomy on one side but a lesser procedure—such as a biopsy—on the

Surgeon performs a complete cervical lymphadenectomy on the right side and biopsy of the cervical nodes on the left side.

38720-RT Cervical lymphadenectomy (complete)
38500-59-LT Biopsy or excision of lymph node(s); open, superficial

Figure 40-7 ■ Example of Using Modifier -59 with the Lymphatic System. *Source: © PB Resources, Inc. Used with permission. CPT codes only © American Medical Association.*

contralateral side or using a separate incision, assign separate codes to each service that describes the work done. Append modifier **-59** to the less extensive service. Laterality modifiers help clarify that the procedures are classified as separate because they were performed on contralateral sites (■ FIGURE 40-7). Medicare and some other payers may request that modifier **-XS Separate structure** may be reported instead of modifier **-59**.

Guided Example of Arranging Hemic and Lymphatic Systems Procedure Codes

To practice skills for arranging codes for procedures on the hemic and lymphatic systems, continue with the example from earlier in the chapter about a patient who was seen for an HPC transplant. Follow along in your CPT manual as Scott Hood, CPC, arranges the codes. Check off each step after you complete it.

▶ First, Scott confirms the procedure codes he assigned.

❑ **38209 x 2 Transplant preparation of hematopoietic progenitor cells; thawing of previously frozen harvest, with washing, per donor**

❑ **38210 x 1 Transplant preparation of hematopoietic progenitor cells; specific cell depletion within harvest, T-cell depletion**

❑ **38240 x 2 Hematopoietic progenitor cell (HPC); allogeneic transplantation per donor**

▶ Scott arranges the codes in descending RVU order according to the Medicare Physician Fee Schedule Database (MPFSDB). He uses the facility RVU because the procedure was performed at the hospital, not at the physician's office.

❑ **38240** Facility RVU = 6.44

❑ **38210** Facility RVU = 2.27

❑ **38209** Facility RVU = 0.34

▶ Scott examines the need for modifiers. (Refer to Table 30-1 Key Criteria for Abstracting CPT Modifiers or Appendix A in the CPT manual.)

❑ Code **38240** does not require modifiers because it is the first-listed code and no unusual circumstances apply.

❑ Code **38210** requires modifier **-51 Multiple procedures** because it is an additional procedure and is not an add-on code.

❑ Code **38209** requires modifier **-51 Multiple procedures** because it is an additional procedure and is not an add-on code.

▶ Scott finalizes the procedure codes and sequencing for this case:

(1) **38240 x 2 Hematopoietic progenitor cell (HPC); allogeneic transplantation per donor**

(2) **38210-51 x 1 Transplant preparation of hematopoietic progenitor cells; specific cell depletion within harvest, T-cell depletion**

(3) **38209-51 x 2 Transplant preparation of hematopoietic progenitor cells; thawing of previously frozen harvest, with washing, per donor**

▶ Scott also assigns the ICD-10-CM diagnosis code that supports the need for the service.

(1) **C81.98 Hodgkin lymphoma, unspecified, lymph nodes of multiple sites**

CODING PRACTICE

Exercise 40.4 Arranging Codes for Hemic and Lymphatic System Procedures

Instructions: Read the mini-medical-record of each patient's encounter. Review the information abstracted in Exercise 40.2 for questions 1–3. For questions 4–6, abstract the case on your own. Assign CPT codes, quantities, and modifiers using the Index and Tabular List, and arrange the codes in proper sequence. Write the code(s) on the line provided.

1. INPATIENT HOSPITAL   Gender: F   Age: 56

Preprocedure diagnosis: metastasis of lung cancer (middle lobe)

Procedure: complete axillary lymphadenectomy, bilateral

Postprocedure diagnosis: metastasis of lung cancer (middle lobe)

1 CPT Code _____

2. INPATIENT HOSPITAL   Gender: M   Age: 46

Preprocedure diagnosis: CT scan shows evidence of ruptured spleen following automobile accident

Procedure: splenectomy; incised the abdomen below the left ribs and exposed the spleen. Rupture and parenchymal fragmentation was evident. Ligated and divided splenic arteries and veins. Freed the spleen from surrounding structures and ligaments. Removed the spleen in its entirety. Irrigated the surgical site, placed a drain, and performed a layered closure. Patient tolerated procedure well.

Postprocedure diagnosis: splenic rupture with parenchymal fragmentation

1 CPT Code _____

3. OUTPATIENT SURGERY   Gender: M   Age: 28

Preprocedure diagnosis: Acute myeloid leukemia

Procedure: thawing previously frozen HPC harvest from a single donor, without washing, and performed RBC depletion for HPC boost, which was administered by IV

Postprocedure diagnosis: Acute myeloid leukemia

Tip: An HPC boost is an additional infusion of stem cells from the original donor after the initial transplant.

3 CPT Codes _____

_____

4. INPATIENT HOSPITAL   Gender: F   Age: 55

Preprocedure diagnosis: edema of her left side, splenic mass

Procedure: partial splenectomy, abdominal lymph node biopsy

Pathology report: benign neoplasm of the spleen

Postprocedure diagnosis: benign splenic neoplasm as indicated by pathology report, sentinel node negative for malignancy

2 CPT Codes _____

5. EMERGENCY DEPT   Gender: M   Age: 25

Preprocedure diagnosis: a piece of metal is embedded in the mediastinum, creating an open wound

Procedure: laceration repair of the diaphragm, transthoracic mediastinotomy

Postprocedure diagnosis: embedded foreign object

2 CPT Codes _____

6. INPATIENT HOSPITAL   Gender: F   Age: 42

Preprocedure diagnosis: suspected metastases

Procedure: pelvic diagnostic laparoscopy followed by bilateral total pelvic lymphadenectomy also performed with laparoscope

Postprocedure diagnosis: metastasis of carcinoma of the bladder per pathology

1 CPT Code _____

E/M CODING FOR THE HEMIC AND LYMPHATIC SYSTEMS

The *1997 Documentation Guidelines for Evaluation and Management Services* (1997 DG), published by the Centers for Medicare and Medicaid Services (CMS), provides requirements for each level of a hematologic/lymphatic/immunologic E/M examination (■ FIGURE 40-8). Hematologists are not limited to using the guidelines for the hematologic/lymphatic/immunologic examination only. They can also use guidelines for a general multiorgan system examination, or any other single organ system examination, based on what is most advantageous for a specific encounter. However, physicians cannot combine elements from more than one type of examination for a given encounter. The hematologic/lymphatic/immunologic examination guidelines typically provide the best results when a detailed examination is performed.

To determine the appropriate E/M code, coders must review the documentation in detail and identify the specific elements documented.

- To translate the documentation into the E/M requirements for the history, refer back to Chapter 31, Evaluation and Management Services (99201-99499), Tables 31-7 to 31-10, or the 1997 DG.
- To determine the requirements for an examination, refer to Figure 40-8 or to the single organ system examination for hematologic/lymphatic/immunologic in the 1997 DG.
- To determine the levels for medical decision making (MDM), refer to Chapter 31, Table 31-12, and the Table of Risk in the 1997 DG.

System/Body Area	Elements of Hematologic/Lymphatic/Immunologic Examination
Constitutional	❑ Measurement of any **three** of the following seven **vital** signs: • 1) sitting or standing blood pressure, • 2) supine blood pressure, • 3) pulse rate and regularity, • 4) respiration, • 5) temperature, • 6) height, • 7) weight (May be measured and recorded by ancillary staff) ❑ General **appearance** of patient (eg, development, nutrition, body habitus, deformities, attention to grooming)
Head and Face	❑ Palpation and/or percussion of **face** with notation of presence or absence of **sinus tenderness**
Eyes	❑ Inspection of **conjunctivae** and **lids**
Ears, Nose, Mouth and Throat	❑ Otoscopic examination of external **auditory canals** and **tympanic membranes** ❑ Inspection of **nasal mucosa, septum** and **turbinates** ❑ Inspection of **teeth** and **gums** ❑ Examination of **oropharynx**: oral mucosa, salivary glands, hard and soft palates, tongue, tonsils and posterior pharynx
Neck	❑ Examination of **neck** (eg, masses, overall appearance, symmetry, tracheal position, crepitus) ❑ Examination of **thyroid** (eg, enlargement, tenderness, mass)
Respiratory	❑ Assessment of **respiratory effort** (eg, intercostal retractions, use of accessory muscles, diaphragmatic movement) ❑ **Auscultation** of lungs (eg, breath sounds, adventitious sounds, rubs)
Cardiovascular	❑ **Auscultation** of heart with notation of abnormal sounds and murmurs ❑ Examination of **peripheral vascular system** by observation (eg, swelling, varicosities) and palpation (pulses, temperature, edema, tenderness)
Gastrointestinal (Abdomen)	❑ Examination of **abdomen** with notation of presence of masses or tenderness ❑ Examination of **liver** and **spleen**
Lymphatic	❑ Palpation of **lymph nodes** in neck, axillae, groin, and/or other location
Extremities	❑ Inspection and palpation of **digits** and **nails** (eg, clubbing, cyanosis, inflammation, petechiae, ischemia, infections, nodes)
Skin	❑ Inspection and/or palpation of **skin** and **subcutaneous tissue** (eg, rashes, lesions, ulcers, ecchymoses, bruises)
Neurological/ Psychiatric	Brief assessment of mental status including: ❑ **Orientation** to time, place and person ❑ **Mood** and affect (eg, depression, anxiety, agitation)

Total # Bullets Performed and Documented →		# of ❑ Elements Performed and Documented	Level of Examination
	□	1–5	Problem focused
		6–11	Expanded problem focused
		12	Detailed
		ALL	Comprehensive (Document **every** element in each box with a shaded border and at least **one** element in each box with an unshaded border)

Figure 40-8 ■ 1997 DG for Hematologic/Lymphatic/Immunologic Examination. *Source: Centers for Medicare and Medicaid Services, 1997 Documentation Guidelines for Evaluation and Management Services (with formatting adjustments).*

Guided Example of E/M Coding for the Hemic and Lymphatic Systems

Refer to the hematology encounter (■ FIGURE 40-9) to practice skills for abstracting and assigning E/M codes. Follow along as fictitious coder Scott Hood, CPC, abstracts the procedure. Check off each step after you complete it.

▶ First, Scott needs to establish the category of service so he can determine the information needed to abstract and assign the code.

❑ *What is the setting?* Hospital inpatient

❑ *What is the type of service?* Subsequent care

HISTORY: Detailed

HEMATOLOGY ENCOUNTER

Chief complaint (CC)

CHIEF COMPLAINT: Newly diagnosed high-risk acute lymphoblastic leukemia; extensive deep vein thrombosis, right iliac vein and inferior vena cava (IVC), status post balloon angioplasty, and mechanical and pharmacologic thrombolysis following placement of a vena caval filter.

Setting & patient type

HISTORY OF PRESENT ILLNESS: The patient was transferred to this hospital the evening of 3/13/20YY from another hospital with a new diagnosis of high-risk acute lymphoblastic leukemia based on confirmation by flow cytometry of peripheral blood lymphoblasts that afternoon. History related to this illness probably dates back to last October when he had onset of swelling and discomfort in the left testicle with what he described as a residual "lump" posteriorly. The left testicle has continued to be painful off and on since. In early November, he developed pain in the posterior part of his upper right leg, which he initially thought was related to skateboarding and muscle strain. Physical therapy was prescribed and the discomfort temporarily improved. In December, he noted onset of increasing fatigue. He used to work out regularly, lifting weights, doing abdominal exercises, and playing basketball and found he did not have energy to pursue these activities. He has lost 10 pounds since December and feels his appetite has decreased. Night sweats and cough began in December, for which he was treated with a course of Augmentin. However, both of these problems have continued. He also began taking Accutane for persistent acne in December (this agent was stopped on 3/9/YY). Despite increasing fatigue and lethargy, he continues his studies at University of Denver, has a biology major (he aspires to be an ophthalmologist).

MDM Management: New presenting problem, intensive workup (High Management Options)

HPI: Extended (4-9)

ROS

on 2/9/20YY, he in the morning awakened with severe right inguinal and right lower quadrant pain. He was seen in Emergency Room where it was noted that he had an elevated WBC of 18,000. CT scan of the abdomen was obtained to rule out possible appendicitis and on that CT, a large clot in the inferior vena cava extending to the right iliac and femoral veins was found. He promptly underwent appropriate treatment in interventional radiology with the above-noted angioplasty and placement of a vena caval filter followed by mechanical and pharmacologic thrombolysis. Repeat ultrasound there on 3/10/20YY showed no evidence of deep venous thrombosis (DVT). Continuous intravenous unfractionated heparin infusion was continued. Because there was no obvious cause of this extensive thrombosis, occult malignancy was suspected. Appropriate blood studies were obtained and he underwent a PET/CT scan as part of his diagnostic evaluation. This study showed moderately increased diffuse bone marrow metabolic activity. Because the WBC continued to rise and showed a preponderance of lymphocytes, the smear was reviewed by pathologist and flow cytometry was performed on the peripheral blood. These studies became available the afternoon of 3/13/20YY, and confirmed the diagnosis of precursor-B acute lymphoblastic leukemia. The patient was transferred here that evening after stopping of the continuous infusion heparin and receiving a dose of Lovenox 60 mg subcutaneously for further diagnostic evaluation and management of the acute lymphoblastic leukemia (ALL).

MDM Data: Ordering or reviewing diagnostic data (Straightforward Data)

MEDICAL DECISION MAKING: High Complexity

MDM Risk: management options include drug therapy of therapeutic heparin maintenance that requires intensive monitoring for toxicity (High Risk)

ALLERGIES: NO KNOWN DRUG ALLERGIES. HE DOES SEEM TO REACT TO CERTAIN ADHESIVES.

CURRENT MEDICATIONS:
1. Lovenox 60 mg subcutaneously q.12h. initiated.
2. Coumadin 5 mg p.o., was administered on 3/9/20YY and 3/12/20YY.
3. Protonix 40 mg intravenous (IV) daily.
4. Vicodin p.r.n.
5. Levaquin 750 mg IV on 3/13/20YY.

IMMUNIZATIONS: Up-to-date.

PAST SURGICAL HISTORY: The treatment of the thrombosis as noted above on 3/9/20YY and 3/10/20YY.

PFSH: Complete (3)

FAMILY HISTORY: Two half-brothers, ages 26 and 28, both in good health. Parents are in good health. A maternal great-grandmother had a deep venous thrombosis (DVT) of leg in her 40s. A maternal great-uncle developed leukemia around age 50. A maternal great-grandfather had bone cancer around age 80. His paternal grandfather died of colon cancer at age 73, which he had had since age 68. Adult-onset diabetes is present in distant relatives on both sides.

SOCIAL HISTORY: The patient is a student at the University majoring in biology. He lives in a dorm there. His parents live in Breckenridge. He admits to having smoked marijuana off and on with friends and drinking beer off and on as well.

REVIEW OF SYSTEMS: He has had emesis off and on related to Vicodin and constipation since 3/9/2007, also related to pain medication. He has had acne for about two years, which he describes as mild to moderate. He denied shortness of breath, chest pain, hemoptysis, dyspnea, headaches, joint pains, rashes, except where he has had dressings applied, and extremity pain except for the right leg pain noted above.

ROS: Extended (2-9)

Figure 40-9 ■ Hematology Encounter. *Source: © PB Resources, Inc. Used with permission.*

(continued on page 784)

PHYSICAL EXAMINATION: GENERAL: Alert, cooperative, moderately ill-appearing young man.
VITAL SIGNS: At the time of admission, pulse was 89, respirations 21, blood pressure 125/65, temperature 98.6, height 5'10", weight 170 pounds, and pulse oximetry on room air 95%.
HAIR AND SKIN: Mild facial acne.
HEENT: Extraocular muscles (EOMs) intact. Pupils equal, round, and reactive to light and accommodation (PERRLA), fundi normal.
CARDIOVASCULAR: A 2/6 systolic ejection murmur (SEM), regular sinus rhythm (RSR).
LUNGS: Clear to auscultation with an occasional productive cough.
ABDOMEN: Soft with mild lower quadrant tenderness, right more so than left; liver and spleen each decreased 4 cm below their respective costal margins.
MUSCULOSKELETAL: Mild swelling of the dorsal aspect of the right foot and distal right leg. Mild tenderness over the prior catheter entrance site in the right popliteal fossa and mild tenderness over the right medial upper thigh.
GENITOURINARY: Testicle exam disclosed no firm swelling with mild nondiscrete fullness in the posterior left testicle.
NEUROLOGIC: Exam showed him to be oriented x4. Normal fundi, intact cranial nerves II through XII with downgoing toes, symmetric muscle strength, and decreased patellar deep tendon reflexes (DTRs).

LABORATORY DATA: White count 24,800 (26 neutrophils, 1 band, 7 lymphocytes, 1 monocyte, 1 myelocyte, 64 blasts), hemoglobin 14.3, hematocrit 39.8, and 323,000 platelets. Electrolytes, BUN, creatinine, phosphorus, uric acid, AST, ALT, alkaline phosphatase, and magnesium were all normal. LDH was elevated to 1925 units/L (upper normal 670), and total protein and albumin were both low at 6.1 and 3.2 g/dL respectively. Calcium was also slightly low at 8.7 mg/dL. Low molecular weight heparin test was low at 0.25 units/mL. PT was 11.9, INR 1.2, and fibrinogen 369. Urinalysis was normal.

ASSESSMENT: 1. Newly diagnosed high-risk acute lymphoblastic leukemia.
2. Deep vein thrombosis of the distal iliac and common femoral/right femoral and iliac veins, status post vena caval filter placement and mechanical and thrombolytic therapy, on continued anticoagulation.
3. Probable chronic left epididymitis.

PLAN: 1. Proceed with diagnostic bone marrow aspirate/biopsy and lumbar puncture as soon as these procedures can be safely done with regard to the anticoagulation status.
2. Prompt reassessment of the status of the deep venous thrombosis with Doppler studies.
3. Ultrasound/Doppler of the testicles.
4. Maintain therapeutic anticoagulation as soon as the diagnostic procedures for ALL can be completed.

EXAMINATION:
Expanded problem focused

(6-11 elements)

MDM Risk

KEY: HPI History of the present illness   ROS Review of systems
       PFSH Past, family, and social history   MDM Medical decision making

Figure 40-9 ■ (Continued)

▶ Scott refers to the CPT Index and looks up the Main Term **Evaluation and Management** and the subterm **Hospital**. The code range listed is **99221-99233**.

❑ *How many key components are required?* Scott refers to the code range in the Tabular List and identifies two categories: **Initial Hospital Care** and **Subsequent Hospital Care**. This encounter is not documented as the initial encounter because the patient was admitted the previous evening, so he selects the category **Subsequent Hospital Care** and reads the description of the first code, which states **requires at least 2 of these 3 key components**. All codes in the category have the same requirements for key components. This tells him that two key components must meet or exceed the levels listed in the code (2/3).

▶ Next, Scott identifies the level of history.

❑ *What is the level of HPI?* The HPI is **extended** because four or more elements are documented.

❑ *What is the level of ROS?* The ROS is **extended** because two to nine systems are documented.

❑ *What is the level of PFSH?* The PFSH is **complete** because two to three elements are documented.

❑ *Based on these factors, what is the overall level of history?* The level of history is **detailed** because all three factors (HPI, ROS, and PFSH) qualify for this level.

▶ Scott refers to the hematologic/lymphatic/immunologic examination in the 1997 DG (Figure 40-8) to abstract information needed to determine the level of the examination.

❑ *What is the level of examination?* The level of examination is **expanded problem focused**. Eight (8) elements of the examination are documented, which exceeds the requirement of 6–11 bulleted elements for an expanded problem-focused examination. A comprehensive examination requires that 12 bulleted items be documented, which they are not.

▶ Scott determines the level of medical decision making. (Refer to Table 31-12 Medical Decision-Making Levels.)

❑ *What is the level of complexity of the number of diagnoses or management options based on the presenting problem?* The level is **High** because there is a new presenting problem, with workup.

❑ *What is the amount and/or complexity of data to be reviewed?* The level is **Straightforward** because the physician reviewed a previous summary of CT/PET and ultrasound tests and reviewed laboratory results, but there was no documented indication of an independent review of images.

❏ *What is the level of risk of significant complications, morbidity, and/or mortality?* Scott reviews each column in the Table of Risk in the 1997 DG and determines that the level of risk is **High**. The patient presents with one or more chronic illnesses with mild exacerbation, progression, or side effects of treatment illness (Moderate), diagnostic procedures ordered include obtaining bone marrow aspirate from lumbar puncture (Moderate), and management options include drug therapy of therapeutic heparin maintenance, which requires intensive monitoring for toxicity (High). The single highest element in the Table of Risk determines the overall risk. The column **Management Options Selected** is the highest level (High).

❏ *Based on these factors, what is the overall level of medical decision making?* The medical decision making is **High complexity**. At least two of the three MDM factors are required to qualify for a specific level of MDM. Two of the three MDM factors —the number of diagnosis/management options and the risk of complications, morbidity, mortality—meet high-complexity decision making.

Now Scott is ready to assign the code for the hematology encounter. The exercise that follows guides you through additional abstracting skills and allows you to assign the correct code.

CODING CAUTION

CMS requires that the medical record be authenticated with either a handwritten or electronic signature. If the signature in the medical record is illegible or missing, the physician must attest to (*verify*) the signature. If the physician does not provide an attestation statement, CMS then considers the claim to be insufficiently documented and can deny payment.

CODING PRACTICE

Exercise 40.5   E/M Coding for the Hemic and Lymphatic Systems

Instructions: Refer to the *1997 Documentation Guidelines for Evaluation and Management Services* (available at www.cms.gov) or Chapter 31 Evaluation and Management Services (99201-99499) (Tables 31-7 to 31-12) in this text. Answer the following questions about the Hematology Encounter (Figure 40-9).

1. a. Which elements of the HPI are documented? Circle all that apply. Location, Quality, Severity, Duration, Timing, Context, Modifying factors, Associated signs and symptoms

   b. How many elements are documented? _____

   c. What is the level of HPI? _____

2. a. Which systems are reviewed in the ROS? Circle all that apply. Constitutional, Allergic/immunologic, CV, Endocrine, ENT/M, Eyes, GI, GU, Hemic/lymphatic, MS, Neurologic, Psychiatric, Respiratory, Skin/breast

   b. How many systems are documented? _____

   c. What is the level of ROS? _____

3. a. Which PFSH elements are documented? Circle all that apply. Past medical, Family, Social

   b. What is the level of PFSH? _____

   c. What is the overall level of history? (The lowest history factor—HPI, ROS, or PFSH—determines the level of history.) _____

4. Refer to Figure 40-8 (1997 DG for Hematologic/Lymphatic/Immunologic Examination).

   a. Which bulleted items are documented for the examination? (Check off the items documented.)

   b. How many bulleted items are documented? _____

   c. What is the level of the examination? _____

5. Refer to Table 31-12 Medical Decision-Making Levels or the 1997 DG.

   a. What is the MDM level for the number of diagnoses or management options?

   b. What is the MDM level for the amount and/or complexity of data to be reviewed?

   c. Refer to the Table of Risk in the 1997 DG. Which elements of risk are documented for each risk factor?

      1. Presenting problem: _____

      2. Diagnostic procedures ordered: _____

      3. Management options selected: _____

   d. What is the level of risk? (The highest of the three risk factors determines the overall level of risk). _____

      _____

   e. What is the overall level of MDM? (2/3 MDM factors are needed to determine the overall level.) _____

(*continued*)

CODING PRACTICE (continued)

6. a. What is the setting? _____

   b. What is the patient (or service) type? _____

   c. What is the code range? _____

   d. How many key components are required? _____

   e. What is the level of history? _____

   f. What is the level of examination? _____

   g. What is the level of medical decision making? _____

   h. What is the correct code? _____

7. Abstract, assign, and arrange (sequence) the diagnosis code(s) that supports the E/M code.

   5 ICD-10-CM Code(s) _____

   _____

CHAPTER SUMMARY

In this chapter you learned that:

- The hemic and lymphatic systems are studied together because blood and lymph are two of the body's main fluids, which are circulated through two separate but interconnected vessel systems.

- The CPT subsection **Hemic and Lymphatic Systems (38100-38999)** contains codes that represent procedures related to the bone marrow, blood, lymph nodes, and lymphatic channels (vessels) and contains three subheadings for the spleen, general, and lymph nodes and lymphatic channels. The CPT subsection **Mediastinum and Diaphragm (39000-39599)** contains two subheadings—one for the mediastinum and one for the diaphragm—each with categories for the type of procedure.

- Familiarity with the anatomy of the lymphatic system is fundamental to abstracting because coding is based on the site and extent of treatment.

- To assign codes for procedures on the hemic and lymphatic systems, mediastinum, and diaphragm, search the Index for the Main Term of the anatomic site, then locate the first-level modifying term for the type of procedure.

- The instructional note **(separate procedure)** at the end of a code description reminds coders to assign the code only when the procedure is not bundled with another one or is performed at a separate site or through a separate incision.

- The *1997 Documentation Guidelines for Evaluation and Management Services* (1997 DG), published by the Centers for Medicare and Medicaid Services (CMS), provides requirements for each level of a hematologic/lymphatic/immunologic E/M examination.

- CPT provides guidelines and instructional notes to alert coders to the need for modifiers, provide cross-references to codes for similar procedures on other sites, identify bundled services, determine when additional codes might be needed for radiological services, and highlight resequenced and recently deleted codes.

CONCEPT QUIZ

Take a moment to look back at the hemic and lymphatic systems, mediastinum, and diaphragm and solidify your skills. Try to answer the questions from memory first, then refer to the discussion in this chapter if you need a little extra help.

Completion

Instructions: Write the term that answers each question based on the information you learned in this chapter. Choose from the list below. Some choices may be used more than once and some choices may not be used at all.

cannula

cannulation

differentiation

eventration

limited lymphadenectomy

lymph nodes

lymphangiography

lymphangiotomy

mediastinotomy

radical lymphadenectomy

respiratory

splenectomy

splenorrhaphy

stem cells

transplantation

1. A/an _____ is used to treat idiopathic thrombocytopenic purpura.

2. A physician may perform a/an _____ to diagnose cancer.

3. A/An _____ is a repair of the diaphragm to resemble normal anatomy.

4. Stem cells repair damaged tissues through _____.

5. _____ is performed to replace bone marrow or HPCs.

6. A physician may insert a/an _____ to diagnose disorders of lymph flow.

7. A physician may perform a/an _____ to stage cancer.

8. The function of the _____ is to produce antibodies to defend the body.

9. A/An _____ is performed to repair a ruptured spleen.

10. A physician may perform a/an _____ to drain an abscess.

Multiple Choice

Instructions: Circle the letter of the best answer to each question based on the information you learned in this chapter.

1. How often can a code for allogeneic transplantation be reported, according to the MUE?
   A. Up to three times a day
   B. Once per donor
   C. Once per day
   D. Only one time

2. How do physicians stage cancer?
   A. Lymph node sampling
   B. Lymphangiotomy
   C. T-cell transplantation
   D. Thoracic cannulation

3. What is the name of the first node or group of nodes in a chain?
   A. Primary lymph node
   B. Sentinel node
   C. Lymph chain
   D. T-lymphocyte

4. In what procedure might specific cellular components be depleted or removed?
   A. Lymph node sampling
   B. Imbrication of the diaphragm
   C. Splenectomy
   D. Bone marrow transplantation

5. What structure separates the lungs and contains the esophagus and heart?
   A. Abdominal cavity
   B. Diaphragm
   C. Thoracic cavity
   D. Mediastinum

6. What type of transplant uses tissue or cells from a person other than the patient?
   A. Autogeneic
   B. Autologous
   C. Allogeneic
   D. Allologous

7. How many bulleted elements must be performed and documented for a physical examination to meet the criteria of a detailed hematologic/lymphatic/immunologic system E/M examination?
   A. 10
   B. 11
   C. 12
   D. 13

8. What is a group of lymph nodes in a limited area along lymph vessels where the body is most prone to infection?
   A. Lymph node
   B. Lymph chain
   C. Lymphocyte
   D. Sentinel lymph node

9. What type of cell does the thymus help produce to protect against viruses and bacteria?
   A. Red blood cells
   B. White blood cells
   C. T-lymphocytes
   D. Stem cells

10. What are hematopoietic progenitor cells?
    A. Stem cells
    B. Lymphocytes
    C. White bone marrow
    D. T-cells

CODING CHALLENGE

Instructions: Read the mini-medical-record of each patient's encounter, then abstract, assign, and arrange ICD-10-CM diagnosis codes and CPT procedure codes using the appropriate Index and Tabular List. Assign quantities and modifiers where needed. Write the code(s) on the line provided.

---

1. INPATIENT HOSPITAL   Gender: M   Age: 18

Preprocedure diagnosis: Benign neoplasm of mediastinum

Procedure: Resection of mediastinal tumor

1 ICD-10-CM Code _____

1 CPT Code _____

---

2. OUTPATIENT SURGERY   Gender: F   Age: 47

Preprocedure diagnosis: Malignant neoplasm, upper-inner quadrant left breast

Procedure: Injection for identification of sentinel node

1 ICD-10-CM Code _____

1 CPT Code _____

---

3. OUTPATIENT SURGERY   Gender: M   Age: 12

Preprocedure diagnosis: Iron-deficiency anemia

Procedure: Bone marrow aspiration

1 ICD-10-CM Code _____

1 CPT Code _____

(continued)

(continued from page 787)

4. OUTPATIENT SURGERY   Gender: F   Age: 33

Preprocedure diagnosis: Volunteer for bone marrow donation

Procedure: Bone marrow harvesting

1 ICD-10-CM Code _____

1 CPT Code _____

5. OUTPATIENT SURGERY   Gender: F   Age: 72

Preprocedure diagnosis: Postoperative bleeding following partial splenectomy

Procedure: Additional repair of the spleen

Tip: A modifier is needed.

1 ICD-10-CM Code _____

1 CPT Code _____

6. EMERGENCY DEPARTMENT   Gender: M   Age: 63

Preprocedure diagnosis: Lacerated diaphragm, initial encounter

Procedure: Repair of diaphragm with sutures

1 ICD-10-CM Code _____

1 CPT Code _____

7. OUTPATIENT SURGERY   Gender: F   Age: 22

Preprocedure diagnosis: Sarcoidosis of lymph nodes

Procedure: Endoscopy of mediastinum with lymph node biopsy

1 ICD-10-CM Code _____

1 CPT Code _____

8. OUTPATIENT SURGERY   Gender: F   Age: 27

Preprocedure diagnosis: Subsequent encounter for foreign body in median sternum

Procedure: Median sternotomy

1 ICD-10-CM Code _____

1 CPT Code _____

9. INPATIENT HOSPITAL   Gender: F   Age: 46

Preprocedure diagnosis: Acute diaphragmatic hernia

Procedure: Repair of acute traumatic diaphragmatic hernia

1 ICD-10-CM Code _____

1 CPT Code _____

10. INPATIENT HOSPITAL   Gender: F   Age: 26

Preprocedure diagnosis: Spontaneous ruptured spleen

Procedure: Repair of ruptured spleen with partial splenectomy

1 ICD-10-CM Code _____

1 CPT Code _____

KEEP ON CODING

Instructions: Read the procedural statement, then use the appropriate Index and Tabular List to assign CPT procedure codes, quantities, and modifiers. Write the code(s) on the line provided.

1. Aortic lymphadenectomy: CPT Code(s) _____

2. Needle bone marrow biopsy: CPT Code(s) _____

3. Partial splenectomy due to traumatic injury: CPT Code(s) _____

4. Repair of ruptured spleen: CPT Code(s) _____

5. Resection of benign neoplasm from mediastinum: CPT Code(s) _____

6. Mediastinoscopy: CPT Code(s) _____

7. Drainage of right axilla lymph node abscess: CPT Code(s) _____

8. Laparoscopic splenectomy: CPT Code(s) _____

9. Repair hernia of diaphragm in neonate: CPT Code(s) _____

10. Superficial needle biopsy of inguinal lymph node: CPT Code(s) _____

11. Bone marrow harvest for allogeneic transplant: CPT Code(s) _____

12. Bone marrow biopsy, sternum, using trocar: CPT Code(s) _____

13. Total splenectomy: CPT Code(s) _____

14. Suprahyoid lymphadenectomy: CPT Code(s) _____

15. Transplant of patient's own bone marrow: CPT Code(s) _____

16. Open biopsy of the deep axillary nodes: CPT Code(s) _____

17. Transplantation of allogeneic stem cells: CPT Code(s) _____

18. Incision and drainage of lymph node abscess, extensive: CPT Code(s) _____

19. Excision of cyst from mediastinum: CPT Code(s) _____

20. Surgical laparoscopy with retroperitoneal lymph node sampling, single: CPT Code(s) _____

21. Stem cell thawing, without washing: CPT Code(s) _____

22. Injection procedure for splenoportography: CPT Code(s) _____

23. Repair of chronic diaphragmatic hernia: CPT Code(s) _____

24. Transplantation of platelet depletion stem cells: CPT Code(s) _____

25. Exploration of mediastinum with mediastinotomy for drainage via cervical area: CPT Code(s) _____

Procedures commonly performed on each section of the respiratory system are discussed next. Refer to detailed anatomic diagrams of specific parts of the respiratory system when you need to refresh your memory of the relationship of organs and sites to each other.

Procedures of the Respiratory System

Procedures commonly performed on the Respiratory System are summarized in ■ TABLE 41-2. In particular, coders need to understand the types of lung procedures and the types of endoscopies.

Recall that there are two lungs with a total of five lobes; the right lung has three lobes, whereas the left lung has two lobes. Procedures on the lung are defined based on the extent of tissue removed:

- **pneumonectomy**—surgical excision of an entire lung
- **lobectomy**—surgical excision of one lobe
- **bilobectomy**—surgical excision of two lobes
- **segmentectomy** or **wedge excision**—surgical excision of tissue from part of one lobe

Endoscopy is the preferred approach for respiratory system procedures whenever possible because it is minimally invasive

and can be used to perform a wide variety of procedures. A **rigid endoscope** consists of a hard tube with a series of prisms and lenses that reflect the image. A **flexible endoscope** is a soft tube with fiber-optic bundles that transmit the image. An **operating endoscope** is equipped with irrigation and suction channels, as well as channels for inserting special instruments, such as biopsy forceps, to obtain tissue samples. Specialized endoscopes are sized and configured for various sites within the respiratory system and are named after the site they are designed to access, such as a laryngoscope—used to access the larynx; a bronchoscope—used to access the bronchi and lungs; and a thoracoscope—used to access the lung and chest cavity through the chest wall. An endoscopy can be diagnostic or therapeutic. It may be done to perform an examination, obtain a specimen or biopsy, place a stent or catheter, or perform surgical excision or repair. Fluoroscopic guidance, in which a live X-ray image of the region being accessed is viewed on a monitor, is used in some endoscopic procedures to assist the surgeon to visualize the correct placement and maneuvering of the endoscope.

This section provides a general reference to help you understand the most common respiratory system procedures. Remember to keep standard reference books handy in case you get stuck.

Table 41-2 ■ **COMMON PROCEDURES OF THE RESPIRATORY SYSTEM**

Procedure Name	Definition	Reason Performed
Caldwell-Luc procedure	Incision of the gum and bone to create an opening to the maxillary sinus	Chronic sinusitis; removal of antrochoanal (*in the maxillary sinus*) polyps, cysts, or lesions
Cricoid split	Incision of the cricoid cartilage (*ring-shaped cartilage at the larynx base*) to open the airway	Congenital or acquired subglottic (*below the glottis*) stenosis
Displacement therapy (Proetz type)	Irrigation of sinuses with a saline solution that is then suctioned out	Ethmoiditis or allergies
Ethmoidectomy	Opening of the ethmoid sinus cavity	Chronic sinusitis; removal of an obstruction
Laryngeal reinnervation by neuromuscular pedicle	Use of a neuromuscular pedicle (*a graft consisting of a nerve and a muscle*) to restore nerves	Dystonia (*a neuromuscular disorder that causes the patient to speak in a whispered or strained voice*); vocal fold paralysis
Laryngectomy	Excision of all or part of the larynx	Laryngeal cancer, trauma
Laryngoscopy (direct)	Use of a laryngoscope inserted through the mouth or nose to view the larynx and hypolarynx/subglottis (*area below the vocal cords*)	Foreign body removal; swallowing, breathing, and bleeding disorders
Laryngoscopy (indirect)	Use of a mirror to view the base of the tongue, larynx, and hypolarynx	Foreign body removal; swallowing, breathing, and bleeding disorders
Lateral rhinotomy	Creation of an incision along the nose from the inner eyebrow to the nasolabial fold (*the crease that runs from the bottom of each nostril to the corner of the mouth*)	Foreign body removal
Lavage	Irrigation of the maxillary or sphenoid sinus by puncturing the antrum or creating an ostium (*opening*)	Removal of infected mucus from chronic sinusitis, a tooth infection that spread to the sinus, or trauma that does not improve with antibiotics
Maxillectomy	Removal of all or part of the upper jaw bone	Malignant neoplasm
Pleurodesis	Use of an irritant to create inflammation within the pleural space to cause the two pleura to adhere together	Prevention of pleural effusion (*excess fluid in the pleural cavity*)
Pneumonolysis	Separation of the parietal pleura from the fascia of the chest wall	Permit the collapse of a lung; formerly used to treat tuberculosis

(continued)

Table 41-2 ■ *(continued)*

Procedure Name	Definition	Reason Performed
Rhinoplasty (primary)	Surgical repair of the nose	Congenital deformity, such as a cleft lip or cleft palate; carcinoma; aesthetics (elective or due to trauma)
Rhinoplasty (secondary)	A second rhinoplasty that may be more complex than the primary one, including grafts of cartilage, bone, or tissue to reconstruct the nose or repair the nasal septum	Unsuccessful primary rhinoplasty; trauma to the nose following the initial procedure; patient dissatisfaction with the outcome of the initial procedure
Septoplasty	Surgical repair of the nasal septum, with or without cartilage scoring (incising), contouring, or replacement with graft	Deviated, or displaced, nasal septum
Thoracentesis/pleural tap	Withdrawal of air or fluid from the pleural space using a needle or tube	Cancer, pneumonia, pneumothorax (*air or gas in the pleural space*), hemothorax (*blood in the pleural space*), or congestive heart failure
Thoracoscopy	Insertion of an endoscope through a small incision in the chest wall	Examination of the lungs, pleura, or mediastinum; biopsy; removal of fluid, cysts, or lung tissue
Thoracostomy	Creation of an opening through the chest to place a chest tube or intercostal catheter into the pleural space	Empyema (*pus in the pleural space*) or pneumothorax (*air or gas in the pleural space*)
Thoracotomy	Incision into the pleural space	Procedures on the heart and lungs, including removing neoplasms and foreign bodies and performing a biopsy
Tracheobronchoscopy	Insertion of an endoscope through an established tracheostomy incision to view the trachea and bronchi	Diagnosis of causes of tracheal stenosis
Tracheostomy	Creation of an opening in the trachea through which a breathing tube is inserted	Obstructed airway, respiratory failure
Tracheotomy	Incision through the neck into the trachea	Preoperative airway clearance; emergency treatment for the inability to breathe
Video-assisted thoracoscopic surgery (VATS)	Use of an endoscope and video camera to perform procedures traditionally performed using a thoracotomy (*incision in the chest wall*)	Management of pulmonary, mediastinal, and pleural conditions

Source: © PB Resources, Inc. Used with permission.

CODING PRACTICE

Exercise 41.1 Respiratory System Procedure Basics

Instructions: Use your medical terminology skills and resources to define the following procedures related to the Respiratory System, then identify the code(s) or code range listed in the CPT Index. Follow these steps:

• Use slash marks "/" to break down the underlined term into its root(s) and suffix.

• Define the meaning of the underlined word based on the meaning of each word part.

• Use the entire phrase to identify the code or code range shown in the CPT Index.

Example: thoraco/scopy, diagnostic, without biopsy

thora/scopy	Meaning *visual examination of the chest cavity*	CPT Code *32601*
1. septoplasty	Meaning _____	CPT Code _____
2. lateral rhinotomy	Meaning _____	CPT Code _____
3. planned tracheostomy	Meaning _____	CPT Code _____
4. maxillary sinusotomy	Meaning _____	CPT Code _____
5. arytenoidopexy	Meaning _____	CPT Code _____
6. sphenoidotomy	Meaning _____	CPT Code _____
7. thorascopic pleurodesis	Meaning _____	CPT Code _____
8. pharyngolaryngectomy	Meaning _____	CPT Code _____
9. tracheobronchoscopy	Meaning _____	CPT Code _____
10. pneumonolysis	Meaning _____	CPT Code _____

Table 41-3 ■ **RESPIRATORY SYSTEM SUBHEADINGS**

Subheading	Code Range
Nose	30000-30999
Accessory Sinuses	31000-31299
Larynx	31300-31599
Trachea and Bronchi	31600-31899
Lungs and Pleura	32035-32999

CODING OVERVIEW OF RESPIRATORY SYSTEM PROCEDURES

The CPT section/subsection **Respiratory System (30000-32999)** contains five subheadings that are divided by anatomic site (■ TABLE 41-3). Within each anatomic site, codes are divided by the type of procedure, such as incision, excision, introduction, and so on. Review the subheading and category names and code ranges listed in the Respiratory System subsection to become familiar with the content and organization. Some editions of the CPT manual provide a summary list of the subheadings and categories at the beginning of the Respiratory System subsection; these also display an asterisk (*) next to categories that contain special coding instructions.

This chapter includes invasive, minimally invasive, and noninvasive surgical procedures on the respiratory system. Codes for diagnostic tests on the respiratory system appear in the Medicine section. CPT codes in the Respiratory System subsection are frequently supported by diagnosis codes from ICD-10-CM **Chapter 10 Diseases of the Respiratory System (J00-J99)**, as well as neoplasms, symptoms and signs, and injuries (■ TABLE 41-4). These are the codes most commonly used to support procedures on the respiratory system; however, diagnosis codes from any ICD-10-CM chapter are permissible. CPT procedure codes must be linked on a claim to diagnosis codes that justify medical necessity.

CPT guidelines for the Surgery section apply to the Respiratory System. Special instructions provide definitions and coding guidelines at the beginning of many categories. The subheading **Lungs and Pleura** provides detailed special instructions about lung resections and biopsies. The categories **Stereotactic Radiation Therapy** and **Lung Transplantation** provide detailed definitions and coding instructions.

Instructional notes appear throughout the Tabular List to alert coders to the need for modifiers, provide cross-references to codes for similar procedures on other sites, identify when additional codes might be needed for radiological services, and highlight resequenced and recently deleted codes.

ABSTRACTING RESPIRATORY SYSTEM PROCEDURES

Abstracting for the respiratory system requires attention to the anatomic approach and procedure type or variation. Abstracting criteria include a special section on endoscopy procedures, in addition to questions that apply to all respiratory procedures.

Anatomic Approach

In addition to classifying procedures based on the surgical approach—open, endoscopic, or percutaneous—CPT also classifies Respiratory System procedures based on the anatomic approach. Some procedures on the nose can be performed using an **external approach** (*through the skin on the outside of the nasal structure*) or **internal approach** (*from within the nasal passage or through the mucous membrane inside the nasal passage*). For example, some excision and destruction procedures can be performed externally, by making an incision along the fold of the nose, or internally, by making an incision into the mucous membrane of the nasal passage.

Most sites within the respiratory system can be accessed through multiple routes, so the procedure description often identifies the route used. The route is described using word roots that identify the structures accessed and/or prefixes that identify the action. For example, endoscopy can be performed using a **transnasal** (*through the nose*) or **transoral** (*through the mouth*) approach or through an established tracheostomy. The frontal sinus can be accessed using a transnasal or a **transorbital** (*through an incision in the orbit of the eye*) route. When you encounter an unfamiliar term, remember to break it down into word parts; then you can usually envision the action and site being described. Also refer to a medical terminology text or a medical dictionary for clarification.

Procedure Type or Variation

Procedures are sometimes described by their type, extent, or other variation.

- Many procedures are classified by difficulty, such as simple or complex; the definition is dependent on the specific procedure performed. For example, a simple revision of a tracheostoma does not include a flap rotation, whereas a complex revision does.

Table 41-4 ■ **LOCATING ICD-10-CM AND ADDITIONAL CPT CODES FOR THE RESPIRATORY SYSTEM**

Type of Code	Codes
ICD-10-CM Respiratory System-Related Codes	
Respiratory system conditions	J00-J99
Neoplasms	C30-C39
Symptoms and signs	R00-R09, R47-R49
Injuries	S20-S29
CPT Respiratory System-Related Codes	
Medicine procedures	94002-94799
Radiologic procedures	
• Diagnostic radiology	70010-70559, 71010-71555
• Radiologic guidance	77001-77022
• Diagnostic ultrasound	76506-76642
• Nuclear medicine, diagnostic	78579-78599
Laboratory organ/disease panels	None are applicable specifically to the respiratory system.

Source: © PB Resources, Inc. Used with permission. CPT codes only © American Medical Association.

Table 41-5 ■ KEY CRITERIA FOR ABSTRACTING RESPIRATORY SYSTEM PROCEDURES

- ❑ What is the anatomic site?
- ❑ What is the procedure?
- ❑ What is the surgical approach (open, endoscopic, external)?
- ❑ What is the anatomic approach (transnasal, transthoracic, laterovertical, etc.)?
- ❑ What is the purpose or variation of the procedure?
- ❑ What is the extent of the procedure (partial, total, etc.)?
- ❑ What is the laterality?
- ❑ What additional procedures were performed during the same session?

For endoscopy:

- ❑ What type of endoscope is used?
- ❑ Is the procedure diagnostic, surgical, or both?
- ❑ What procedure(s) are performed during the endoscopy?
- ❑ Is the endoscopy a preoperative survey or scout?
- ❑ Is an endoscopic procedure converted to an open procedure?
- ❑ Is a decision made to perform an additional procedure during the same encounter based on the results of the endoscopy?
- ❑ What is the farthest anatomic site reached with the endoscope?

Source: © PB Resources, Inc. Used with permission.

- Procedures can be described by extent, such as limited or complete or partial and total, and definitions are dependent on the specific procedure. For example, a simple sinus excision involves a portion of a sinus cavity, whereas a complete excision involves the entire cavity.

- The technique or type of equipment can affect code classification. For example, a laryngoscopy can be direct, using an endoscope, or indirect, using a mirror and a light.

- Multiple procedures can be performed at the same time. For example, a bronchoscopy can have many variations depending on its purpose and other procedures performed, such as the type of biopsy or specimen collection, placement of a stent or catheter, removal of a foreign body, and so on.

Coders must be attentive to the details of each procedure and each code description. When you are reading and abstracting a medical record for a procedure that is unfamiliar, you may not always be certain of what information you will need to assign the code. Remember that you may need to cross-reference between the medical record and the coding manual several times before identifying all the information needed to assign the correct code. This is a normal part of the coding process.

Refer to ■ TABLE 41-5 for guidance on how to abstract procedures on the respiratory system, then work through the detailed example that follows. Remember that the abstracting questions are a guide and that not every question applies to, or can be answered for, every case. For example, not all procedures are described by extent, such as total or partial.

Guided Example of Abstracting Respiratory System Procedures

Refer to the following example throughout this chapter to practice skills for abstracting, assigning, and arranging Respiratory System codes.

OUTPATIENT HOSPITAL   Gender: M   Age: 58

Preoperative diagnosis: Lung mass on CT scan

Procedure: diagnostic bronchoscopy with biopsy and ultrasound. Administered conscious sedation. When patient was comfortable, advanced flexible bronchoscope into the left lower lobe of the lung, where a mass was visualized on CT. Acquired a biopsy of the nodule in that lobe. It was difficult to determine whether the mass penetrated the lung wall, so we elected to perform an endobronchial ultrasound. Signs of invasion were apparent. Three images were taken and will be reviewed by radiology. Specimen was submitted to pathology.

Postoperative diagnosis: carcinoma of the lower left lobe

Pathology report: carcinoma

Follow along as fictitious coder, Leanne Riehl, CCS, abstracts the procedure. Check off each step after you complete it.

▶ Leanne reads through the entire record, paying special attention to the reason for the encounter, the procedure performed, and the postoperative diagnosis. She refers to the Key Criteria for Abstracting Respiratory System Procedures (Table 41-5).

- ❑ She notes the preoperative diagnosis. Lung mass on CT scan

- ❑ *What is the patient's age?* 58

- ❑ *What site is treated?* lung

- ❑ *What primary procedure is performed?* diagnostic bronchoscopy with biopsy and ultrasound

- ❑ *What type of endoscope is used?* flexible bronchoscope

- ❑ *Is the procedure diagnostic, surgical, or both?* diagnostic

- ❑ *What procedure(s) are performed during the endoscopy?* biopsy, endobronchial ultrasound

- ❑ *Is the endoscopy a preoperative survey or scout?* No

- ❑ *Is an endoscopic procedure converted to an open procedure?* No

- ❑ *Is a decision made to perform an additional procedure during the same encounter based on the results of the endoscopy?* No

- ❑ *What is the farthest anatomic site reached with the endoscope?* left lower lobe of the lung

▶ At this time, Leanne does not know which of these procedures may need to be coded, nor how many codes she will end up with. She will learn about this when she moves on to assigning codes.

CODING PRACTICE

Exercise 41.2 **Abstracting Respiratory System Procedures**

Instructions: Read the mini-medical-record of each patient's encounter and answer the abstracting questions. Write the answer on the line provided. Do not assign any codes.

---

1. EMERGENCY DEPT Gender: F Age: 48

Preprocedure diagnosis: patient presents with complaints of nasal pain, edema, and purulent (pus) discharge. CT scan and lab tests reveal a nasal septum abscess

Procedure: incision and drainage (I & D) nasal septum abscess; made small incision within the nasal septum over the abscess. Suctioned purulent fluid and flushed with sterile saline. Packed the nasal cavity with gauze.

Postprocedure diagnosis: nasal septum abscess due to *Staphylococcus aureus*

a. What is the anatomic site? _____

b. What is the procedure? _____

c. What is the surgical approach (open, endoscopic, external)? _____

d. What is the purpose or variation of the procedure?

_____

---

2. EMERGENCY DEPT Gender: F Age: 4

Preprocedure diagnosis: Child is brought in by her mother who noticed her pressing her nose and picking at it. When questioned, child said a marble fell up her nose.

Procedure: Examined the nose and removed the marble with forceps. Patient was awake and alert during the procedure.

Postprocedure diagnosis: Foreign body in nose

a. What is the anatomic site? _____

b. What is the procedure? _____

c. What is the surgical approach (open, endoscopic, external)? _____

---

3. OFFICE Gender: M Age: 54

Preprocedure diagnosis: Patient states: "I can't stop coughing and always feel that there is a lump in my throat." Hoarseness is evident.

Procedure: transoral direct laryngoscopy under general anesthesia; inserted laryngoscope into the throat and visualized tumor. Excised tumor with a scalpel. Used forceps to strip the epithelium of the vocal cords. Patient tolerated procedure well. Submitted specimens to pathology.

Postprocedure diagnosis: carcinoma of the larynx per pathology report

a. What is the anatomic site? _____

b. What is the procedure? _____

c. What is the surgical approach (open, endoscopic, external)? _____

d. What is the anatomic approach (transnasal, transthoracic, laterovertical, etc.)?

e. What is the purpose or variation (direct/indirect) of the procedure? _____

f. What additional procedures were performed during the same session? _____

---

4. EMERGENCY DEPT Gender: M Age: 28

Preprocedure diagnosis: uncontrolled bilateral epistaxis

Procedure: limited cautery and packing of nasal hemorrhage. Used nasal speculum to locate site of bleeding in the right anterior nasal passage, cleaned, and applied silver nitrate stick to cauterize. Repeated on the left anterior passage. Hemostasis was achieved.

Postprocedure diagnosis: epistaxis

a. What is the anatomic site? _____

b. What is the procedure? _____

c. What is the surgical approach (open, endoscopic, external)? _____

d. What is the anatomic approach (transnasal, transthoracic, laterovertical, etc.)? _____

e. What is the purpose or variation of the procedure?

_____

f. What is the laterality? _____

5. OUTPATIENT SURGERY   Gender: M   Age: 36

Preprocedure diagnosis: mucocele frontal sinus

Procedure: left transorbital frontal sinusotomy; made an incision along the inner wall of the orbit of eye to reach the ethmoid sinus. Made an opening into the ethmoid sinus to reach the frontal sinus. Removed mucocele from the frontal sinus using curette. Performed layered closure.

a. What is the anatomic site? _____

b. What is the procedure? _____

c. What is the surgical approach (open, endoscopic, external)?_____

d. What is the anatomic approach (transnasal, transthoracic, laterovertical, etc.)? _____

e. What is the purpose or variation of the procedure? _____

f. What is the laterality? _____

g. What additional procedures were performed during the same session? _____

6. LOCATION   Gender: M   Age: 68

Preprocedure diagnosis: hemoptysis

Procedure: Conscious sedation was administered, and when the patient was comfortable we inserted flexible fiberoptic bronchoscope through nose and examined nasal passages, with no findings. Advanced into the larynx, where no abnormalities were noted. Advanced to the trachea, where no abnormalities were noted, then to the right bronchus, which was also negative.

(continued)

6. (continued)

Retracted bronchoscope, then advanced to left bronchus. Dried blood was visualized in the alveoli. We placed a fiducial marker near the apparent source and performed bronchial alveolar lavage to cleanse area and obtain specimens. Bronchoscope was withdrawn and specimens were submitted to pathology. Patient tolerated procedure well.

Postprocedure diagnosis: bronchial hemorrhage, pathology pending

a. What is the anatomic site? _____

b. What is the procedure? _____

c. What is the surgical approach (open, endoscopic, external)? _____

d. What is the anatomic approach (transnasal, transthoracic, laterovertical, etc.)? _____

e. What type of endoscope is used? _____

f. Is the procedure diagnostic, surgical, or both? _____

g. What procedure(s) are performed during the endoscopy?_____

h. What is the laterality? _____

i. Is the endoscopy a preoperative survey or scout? _____

j. Is an endoscopic procedure converted to an open procedure? _____

k. Is a decision made to perform an additional procedure at the same encounter based on the results of the endoscopy? _____

l. What is the farthest anatomic site reached with the endoscope? _____

ASSIGNING CODES FOR RESPIRATORY SYSTEM PROCEDURES

To assign codes for the Respiratory System, search the Index for the Main Term for the anatomic site, the first-level modifying term for the type of procedure, and a second-level modifying term for variations of the procedure. In the Tabular List, select the appropriate code for the anatomic approach and the variation of the procedure performed. Review instructional notes in the Tabular List carefully because they provide valuable guidance on bundling and redirect you to alternative codes for similar procedures.

The National Correct Coding Initiative (NCCI) provides extensive guidelines regarding the bundling of procedures on the respiratory system. The following sections discuss how to assign

codes for procedures on adjacent sites or systems, biopsies, and endoscopies. Other topics addressed by NCCI are control of bleeding, intubation, and chest tube procedures.

Adjacent Sites or Systems

Some procedures on the nose and mouth may be performed near the mucocutaneous (*pertaining to the skin and mucous membranes*) margins and could potentially be coded as a procedure on the respiratory system, digestive system, or integumentary system. The exact site of the procedure—such as a lesion removal or biopsy—determines the system under which the procedure is classified. Internal procedures on the mucous membrane of the nose are classified as respiratory system procedures, whereas external procedures on the skin of the nose are generally classified as integumentary system procedures. Procedures on the larynx are classified as respiratory system procedures, whereas procedures on the pharynx and mucous membranes of the oral cavity are classified as digestive system procedures.

Sometimes procedures from multiple systems are bundled into a single code. For example, CPT provides a Respiratory System code for septoplasty that includes the graft in the code descriptor. Assign only the code from the Respiratory System: **30520 Septoplasty or submucous resection, with or without cartilage scoring, contouring or replacement with graft**. Do not also assign a code from the Integumentary System subsection for the tissue transfer because the service is included in the Respiratory System code.

CODING CAUTION

When a procedure is performed near the border of two distinct sites, you may need to review codes and guidelines from both sites to determine the best code to assign. Never assign two codes, one from each site, for the same procedure.

Biopsy

When a biopsy is performed in conjunction with a more extensive nasal or sinus procedure, do not code the biopsy in addition to the more extensive procedure. Code only the more extensive procedure (■ FIGURE 41-2). The exception is when the biopsy is examined pathologically and, based on the findings, the more extensive procedure is performed (■ FIGURE 41-3).

Patient presents with an obstruction in the ethmoid sinus that was identified on a CT scan. The surgeon performs an endoscopic anterior ethmoidectomy and sends a tissue specimen to pathology upon completion of the procedure.

31254 Nasal/sinus endoscopy, surgical; with ethmoidectomy, partial (anterior)

Figure 41-2 ■ Example of Coding for a More Extensive Procedure Only. *Source: © PB Resources, Inc. Used with permission. CPT codes only © American Medical Association.*

Patient presents with several intranasal lesions that are not interfering with her breathing. The surgeon performs a biopsy of one lesion and sends it to pathology where a frozen section is performed. Pathology determines that the lesion is malignant, so the surgeon proceeds with complete removal of the initial lesion, as well as three additional similar lesions.

30117 Excision or destruction (eg, laser), intranasal lesion; internal approach
30100-51 Biopsy, intranasal; -51 Multiple procedures

Figure 41-3 ■ Example of Coding for a Biopsy and a More Extensive Procedure. *Source: © PB Resources, Inc. Used with permission. CPT codes only © American Medical Association.*

Endoscopy

Many procedures on the nose, sinuses, larynx, bronchi, and lungs are performed endoscopically. As is true in other Surgery subsections, a surgical endoscopy includes a diagnostic endoscopy, so when both are performed, report only the code for the surgical endoscopy. This is stated in special instructions at the beginning of the **Endoscopy** category for each anatomic site. In addition, special instructions under the **Endoscopy** category for **Sinus** state that a **surgical sinus endoscopy (when appropriate) includes a sinusotomy and diagnostic sinus endoscopy**. In most cases, only the surgical sinus endoscopy should be reported, not the sinusotomy or diagnostic endoscopy.

When the findings of a diagnostic endoscopy lead to the decision to perform a nonendoscopic surgical procedure during the same patient encounter, assign two codes: one for the endoscopy and one for the surgical procedure. Diagnostic endoscopy does not include using an endoscope to survey or scout the surgical field before an open procedure; the preoperative check is considered part of the surgical procedure, so the endoscopy should not be reported separately.

Endoscopy of one site includes examination of all the access sites the endoscope passes through to reach the final site. For example, a transnasal endoscopy of the sinuses includes examination of the nose. A transoral endoscopy of the lungs includes examination of the larynx, trachea, and bronchi. Report an endoscopy code only for the farthest site reached. The exception is when it is medically appropriate to perform distinct procedures using different types of endoscopes on separate sites (■ Figure 41-4).

When an endoscopic procedure cannot be completed and is converted to an open procedure, code only the open procedure, not the endoscopy.

To locate codes for endoscopy, search the Index for the Main Term for the anatomic site and the first-level modifying term **Endoscopy**. Alternatively, search the Index for the Main Term **Endoscopy** and the first-level modifying term for the anatomic site. Review the second-level modifying terms and code descriptions in the Tabular List carefully because endoscopy codes are divided based on the purpose of the procedure, such as tumor excision, biopsy, lavage, foreign body removal, and so on.

Guided Example of Assigning Respiratory System Procedure Codes

To practice skills for assigning codes for the Respiratory System, continue with the example from earlier in the chapter

Physician uses a fiberoptic laryngoscope to perform a diagnostic laryngoscopy for a laryngeal mass. She then uses a fiberoptic bronchoscope to examine a lung mass.

31622 Bronchoscopy, rigid or flexible, including fluoroscopic guidance, when performed; diagnostic, with cell washing, when performed
31575 Laryngoscopy, flexible fiberoptic; diagnostic

Figure 41-4 ■ Example of Coding Two Endoscopies. *Source: © PB Resources, Inc. Used with permission. CPT codes only © American Medical Association.*

about a patient who was seen for a bronchoscopy. Follow along in your CPT manual as Leanne Riehl, CCS, assigns codes. Check off each step after you complete it.

▶ First, Leanne confirms *diagnostic bronchoscopy with biopsy and ultrasound, left lower lobe of the lung, where a mass was visualized on CT*.

▶ Leanne searches the Index for the Main Term **Bronchoscopy**.

❑ She locates the first-level modifying term for the first procedure, **Biopsy**.

❑ She identifies the code ranges **31625-31629, 31632-31633**.

❑ She also locates the first-level modifying term for the second procedure, **Ultrasound**.

❑ She identifies the suggested code **31620**.

▶ Leanne turns to the Tabular List to review, select, and verify the code for the biopsy.

❑ She identifies that all the codes listed for the first-level modifying term **Biopsy** are indented codes under code **31622**.

▪ She knows she must refer to the common portion of code **31622** to understand the full description of the other codes: **Bronchoscopy, rigid or flexible, including fluoroscopic guidance, when performed;**. This accurately describes the basic procedure performed, *flexible bronchoscopy*.

▪ The indented codes describe additional procedures done during the bronchoscopy.

❑ She reads through the unique descriptors for the codes listed in the Index—**31625-31629, 31632-31633**—to identify possible codes for *Acquired a biopsy of the nodule in the left lobe of the lung*. She identifies three potential codes: **31625, 31628, 31632**. She compares the code descriptions to determine the differences between them.

▪ Code **31625** describes a bronchoscopy **with bronchial or endobronchial biopsy(s), single or multiple sites**.

▪ Code **31628** describes a bronchoscopy **with transbronchial lung biopsy(s), single lobe**.

▪ Code **31632** describes a bronchoscopy **with transbronchial lung biopsy(s), each additional lobe (List separately in addition to code for primary procedure)**.

▪ She identifies the differences: code **31625** identifies a bronchial or *endo*bronchial biopsy, which is a biopsy of or *within* a bronchus; code **31638** identifies a *trans*bronchial biopsy of the lung, in which the lung is accessed *through* the bronchus; and code **31632** identifies transbronchial lung biopsies in *more* than one lobe.

❑ She refers to the medical record to confirm that a biopsy was taken from a single lobe, then verifies the full code title for **31628, Bronchoscopy, rigid or flexible, including fluoroscopic guidance, when performed; with transbronchial lung biopsy(s), single lobe** and confirms that this accurately describes the procedure.

❑ She reads the instructional note that appears below the code description in the Tabular List that states (**31628 should be reported only once regardless of how many transbronchial lung biopsies are performed in a lobe**). Only one biopsy in this lobe was documented, so the note does not apply. If more than one biopsy had been performed in the lower left lobe, this note tells her that they would not be reported separately. However, if an additional biopsy had been performed in another lobe, she would report it using add-on code **31632** that she reviewed earlier.

▶ Leanne returns to the Tabular List to review, select, and verify the code for the endobronchial ultrasound.

❑ She locates code **31620** that was suggested in the Index and reads the code description: **Endobronchial ultrasound (EBUS) during bronchoscopic diagnostic or therapeutic intervention(s) (List separately in addition to code for primary procedure[s])**.

❑ The description accurately describes the procedure and no alternative codes were listed in the Index; she did not see any additional codes for EBUS when she reviewed the codes in this CPT category.

❑ She notes that this is an add-on code, as indicated by the + symbol in front of the code number.

❑ She reads the instructional note that appears below the code description in the Tabular List that states (**Use 31620 in conjunction with 31622-31646**). Code **31628** for the lung biopsy falls within the acceptable code range.

▶ Leanne checks for additional instructions in the Tabular List. She has already reviewed the instructional notes that follow the codes selected.

❑ She cross-references the beginning of the category **Endoscopy** and reads the special instructions. The instructions provide direction regarding how to code multiple anatomic sites, surgical and diagnostic bronchoscopies performed by the same physician during the same encounter, and the use of fluoroscopic guidance. None of these criteria apply to this patient case because only one site was examined and neither surgery nor fluoroscopy was performed.

❑ She cross-references the beginning of the subheading **Trachea and Bronchi** and verifies that there are no instructional notes.

❑ She cross-references the beginning of the subsection **Respiratory** and verifies that there are no instructional notes.

▶ Leanne reviews the procedure codes she has assigned for this case.

❑ **31620 Endobronchial ultrasound (EBUS) during bronchoscopic diagnostic or therapeutic intervention(s) (List separately in addition to code for primary procedure[s])**

❑ **31628 Bronchoscopy, rigid or flexible, including fluoroscopic guidance, when performed; with transbronchial lung biopsy(s), single lobe**

▶ Next, Leanne must determine how to sequence the codes.

CODING PRACTICE

Exercise 41.3 Assigning Codes for Respiratory System Procedures

Instructions: Read the mini-medical-record of each patient's encounter. Review the information abstracted in Exercise 41.2 for questions 1–3. For questions 4–6, abstract the case on your own. Assign CPT codes, quantities, and modifiers using the Index and Tabular List. Write the code(s) on the line provided.

1. EMERGENCY DEPT Gender: F Age: 48

Preprocedure diagnosis: patient presents with complaints of nasal pain, edema, and purulent (pus) discharge. CT scan and lab tests reveal a nasal septum abscess

Procedure: incision and drainage (I & D) nasal septum abscess; made small incision within the nasal septum over the abscess. Suctioned purulent fluid and flushed with sterile saline. Packed the nasal cavity with gauze.

Postprocedure diagnosis: nasal septum abscess due to *Staphylococcus aureus*

1 CPT Code _____

2. EMERGENCY DEPT Gender: F Age: 4

Preprocedure diagnosis: Child is brought in by her mother, who noticed her pressing her nose and picking at it. When questioned, child said a marble fell up her nose.

Procedure: Examined the nose and removed the marble with forceps. Patient was awake and alert during the procedure.

Postprocedure diagnosis: Foreign body in nose

1 CPT Code _____

3. OFFICE Gender: M Age: 54

Preprocedure diagnosis: Patient states: "I can't stop coughing and always feel that there is a lump in my throat." Hoarseness is evident.

Procedure: transoral direct laryngoscopy under general anesthesia; inserted laryngoscope into the throat and visualized tumor. Excised tumor with a scalpel. Used forceps to strip the epithelium of the vocal cords. Patient tolerated procedure well. Submitted specimens to pathology.

Postprocedure diagnosis: carcinoma of the larynx per pathology report

1 CPT Code _____

4. OUTPATIENT HOSPITAL Gender: F Age: 38

Preprocedure diagnosis: chronic cough and chest pain

Procedure: bronchoscopy with endobronchial biopsies of the right upper and lower lobes.

Postprocedure diagnosis: acute bronchitis per pathology report

1 CPT Code _____

5. OUTPATIENT SURGERY Gender: F Age: 2

Preprocedure diagnosis: congenital obstruction of the nasolacrimal duct

Procedure: fractured the turbinates bilaterally and then repositioned them

1 CPT Code _____

6. OUTPATIENT SURGERY Gender: M Age: 68

Preprocedure diagnosis: extensive scarring on tracheostoma

Procedure: reconstructed tracheostoma; removed scar tissue and repaired with a rotation flap

1 CPT Code _____

ARRANGING CODES FOR RESPIRATORY SYSTEM PROCEDURES

Information about bundling, multiple coding, code sequencing, and modifiers in the Respiratory System subsection appears in special instructions, instructional notes, and code descriptions. Special instructions at the beginning of several categories, especially those for endoscopy, provide direction about when multiple codes are needed and when multiple services are bundled into a single code. Extensive instructional notes throughout the subsection identify specific codes that cannot be reported together, those that should be reported together, and when additional codes might be needed.

Code descriptions identify whether the quantity for procedures on the lungs is reported as one per procedure, per lung, per lobe, or per segment or using another unit of measure. Be attentive to the occurrence of a parent code that has multiple indented codes, each with a different unit for reporting quantity.

> ## CODING CAUTION
>
> Although the variations in how quantity is reported may seem confusing at first, they are dependent on the type of procedure, so no general rule exists. Coders must give special consideration to this portion of the descriptor to be certain they are accurately reporting the quantity.

Modifiers

Because multiple procedures on the respiratory system can be performed during the same encounter, coders should review the use of modifiers **-59** and **-51** and laterality modifiers. These modifiers and examples are discussed next.

-59 Distinct Procedural Service

Append modifier **-59 Distinct procedural service** to codes for services that are usually bundled but are performed as a separate procedure at a distinct site, through a separate incision, or during a different operative session. Medicare and some private payers may require the use of a HCPCS modifier instead of modifier -59, to provide more specific information, such as

- **-XE Separate encounter**
- **-XS Separate structure**
- **-XP Separate practitioner**
- **-XU Unusual non-overlapping service**

-51 Multiple Procedures

When more than one procedure is performed during the same operative session, remember to append modifier **-51 Multiple procedures** to the second and subsequent codes. Do not append modifier **-51** to add-on codes or codes designated with the symbol ⊘ for **Modifier-51 exempt**.

Laterality

The use of modifiers to identify laterality varies for Respiratory System procedures. Because the paranasal sinuses are paired sites, assign the modifier **-LT Left side**, **-RT Right side**, or **-50 Bilateral procedure**. Most bilateral sinus procedures qualify for reimbursement at 150% of the rate for a unilateral procedure by most payers. This is indicated by an instructional note that states (**To report bilateral procedure, use . . . with modifier 50**) following several procedures (■ FIGURE 41-5).

Procedures involving the bronchi, including transbronchial procedures performed on the lung, do not accept laterality or bilateral modifiers. Transbronchial lung procedures are reported with add-on codes for each additional lobe treated, but laterality modifiers **-LT**, **-RT**, and **-50** are not reported. Because the left lung has two lobes and the right lung has three lobes, some procedures are reported separately for each lobe, but the lobe itself is not identified (■ FIGURE 41-6). When one left lobe and one right lobe are treated, do not append modifier **-50** for a bilateral procedure.

Procedures on the lungs using an approach other than transbronchial are often reported with modifiers **-RT** and **-LT** to

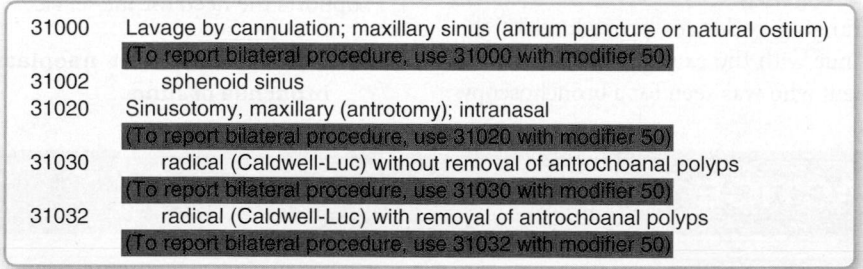

Figure 41-5 ■ Example of Tabular List Instructional Note to Report Modifier -50. *Source: © PB Resources, Inc. Used with permission. CPT codes only © American Medical Association.*

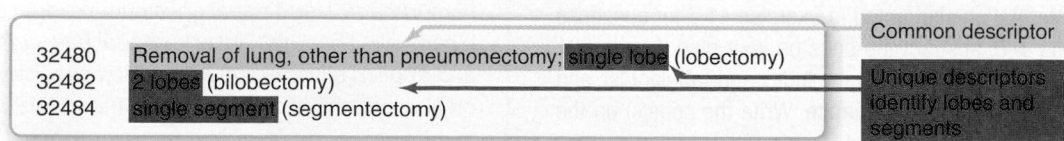

Figure 41-6 ■ Example of Tabular List Entry to Report Lung Lobes and Segments. *Source: © PB Resources, Inc. Used with permission. CPT codes only © American Medical Association.*

> Surgeon performed a thoracotomy and acquired two wedge biopsies of nodules in the left lung and one wedge biopsy of a nodule in the right lung.

32097-RT Thoracotomy, with diagnostic biopsy(ies) of lung nodule(s) or mass(es) (eg, wedge, incisional), unilateral; -RT Right side
32097-LT Thoracotomy, with diagnostic biopsy(ies) of lung nodule(s) or mass(es) (eg, wedge, incisional), unilateral; -LT Left side

Figure 41-7 ■ Example of Coding Separately for Each Lung. *Source:* © PB Resources, Inc. Used with permission. CPT codes only © American Medical Association.

identify laterality, but not modifier **-50** for bilateral procedures. Such procedures are followed by an instructional note to not report the procedure more than once per lung, which means that a separate code/modifier combination should be reported for each procedure performed (■ FIGURE 41-7).

When procedures are followed by instructional notes that specify to use modifier **-50** to report a bilateral procedure, the code can be reported once with modifier **-50** to indicate the procedure was performed on both sides.

When a procedure that is inherently bilateral is performed on only one side, append modifier **-52 Reduced services**.

SUCCESS STEP

This text provides general guidelines for reporting laterality. Various payers establish their own guidelines for how to report laterality. In the workplace you can refer to payer guidelines and the Medicare Physician Fee Schedule Database (MFSDB) for more detailed information.

Guided Example of Arranging Respiratory System Procedure Codes

To practice skills for arranging codes for procedures of the Respiratory System, continue with the example from earlier in the chapter about the patient who was seen for a bronchoscopy.

Follow along in your CPT manual as Leanne Riehl, CCS, arranges the codes. Check off each step after you complete it.

▶ First, Leanne confirms the procedure codes she assigned.

❑ **31620 Endobronchial ultrasound (EBUS) during bronchoscopic diagnostic or therapeutic intervention(s) (List separately in addition to code for primary procedure[s])**

❑ **31628 Bronchoscopy, rigid or flexible, including fluoroscopic guidance, when performed; with transbronchial lung biopsy(s), single lobe**

▶ Leanne reviews the codes where they appear in the Tabular List and reconfirms that code **31620** is an add-on code. Therefore, it should be sequenced second, after code **31628**, which is the primary procedure code.

▶ Leanne examines the need for modifiers. (Refer to Table 30-1 Key Criteria for Abstracting CPT Modifiers or Appendix A in the CPT manual.)

❑ Code **31628** does not require a modifier because there are no extenuating circumstances. Laterality modifiers are not used for transbronchial lung procedures.

❑ Code **31620** does not require a modifier for a separate procedure or multiple procedure because it is an add-on code.

▶ Leanne finalizes the procedure codes and sequencing for this case:

(1) **31628 Bronchoscopy, rigid or flexible, including fluoroscopic guidance, when performed; with transbronchial lung biopsy(s), single lobe**

(2) **31620 Endobronchial ultrasound (EBUS) during bronchoscopic diagnostic or therapeutic intervention(s) (List separately in addition to code for primary procedure[s])**

▶ Leanne also assigns the ICD-10-CM diagnosis code that supports the need for the service.

(1) **C34.32 Malignant neoplasm of lower lobe, left bronchus or lung**

CODING PRACTICE

Exercise 41.4 Arranging Codes for Respiratory System Procedures

Instructions: Read the mini-medical-record of each patient's encounter. Review the information abstracted in Exercise 41.2 for questions 1–3. For questions 4–6, abstract the case on your own. Assign CPT codes, quantities, and modifiers using the Index and Tabular List, and arrange the codes in the proper sequence. Write the code(s) on the line provided.

1. EMERGENCY DEPT   Gender: M   Age: 28

Preprocedure diagnosis: uncontrolled bilateral epistaxis

Procedure: limited cautery and packing of nasal hemorrhage. Used nasal speculum to locate site of bleeding in the right anterior nasal passage, cleaned, and applied silver nitrate stick to cauterize. Repeated on the left anterior passage. Hemostasis was achieved.

Postprocedure diagnosis: epistaxis

1 CPT Code _____

2. OUTPATIENT SURGERY Gender: M Age: 36

Preprocedure diagnosis: mucocele frontal sinus

Procedure: left transorbital frontal sinusotomy; made an incision along the inner wall of the orbit of eye to reach the ethmoid sinus. Made an opening into the ethmoid sinus to reach the frontal sinus. Removed mucocele from the frontal sinus using curette. Performed layered closure.

1 CPT Code _____

3. OUTPATIENT SURGERY Gender: M Age: 68

Preprocedure diagnosis: hemoptysis

Procedure: Conscious sedation was administered, and when the patient was comfortable we inserted a flexible fiberoptic bronchoscope through the nose and examined nasal passages with no findings. Advanced into the larynx, where no abnormalities were noted. Advanced to the trachea, where no abnormalities were noted, then to the right bronchus, which was also negative. Retracted bronchoscope, then advanced to left bronchus. Dried blood was visualized in the alveoli. We placed a fiducial marker near the site and performed bronchial alveolar lavage to cleanse area and obtain specimens. Bronchoscope was withdrawn and specimens were submitted to pathology. Patient tolerated procedure well.

Postprocedure diagnosis: bronchial hemorrhage, pathology pending

Tip: Laterality modifiers are not required.

2 CPT Codes _____

4. OFFICE Gender: M Age: 33

Preprocedure diagnosis: nasal congestion and facial pain

Procedure: performed a bilateral nasal endoscopy and excised two polyps on the right and three polyps on the left

Postprocedure diagnosis: nasal polyps

1 CPT Code _____

5. OFFICE Gender: F Age: 63

Preprocedure diagnosis: lifelong cigarette smoker, personal history of breast cancer with R breast mastectomy six years ago. Recent hemoptysis, loss of appetite, and shortness of breath

Procedure: thoracotomy with biopsy of nodules in both right and left lungs

Postprocedure diagnosis: metastatic CA to lung

Tip: Assign separate codes and modifiers for each lung.

2 CPT Codes _____

6. LOCATION Gender: F Age: 22

Preprocedure diagnosis: cystic fibrosis, double-lung transplant candidate

Procedure: Double-lung transplant including cadaver pneumonectomy, backbench preparation, and transplantation of both lungs into recipient with use of a heart–lung machine.

Tip: Assign codes for the pneumonectomy, the backbench preparation, and the transplant.

3 CPT Codes _____

_____

E/M CODING FOR PULMONOLOGY

The *1997 Documentation Guidelines for Evaluation and Management Services* (1997 DG), published by CMS, provides requirements for each level of a respiratory E/M examination (■ FIGURE 41-8). Pulmonologists are not limited to using the guidelines for a skin examination only. They can also use guidelines for a general multiorgan system examination, or any other single organ system examination, based on what is most advantageous for a specific encounter. However, physicians cannot combine elements from more than one type of examination for a given encounter. The respiratory examination guidelines typically provide the best results when a detailed respiratory examination is performed.

To determine the appropriate E/M code, coders must review the documentation in detail and identify the specific elements documented.

- To translate the documentation into the E/M requirements for the history, refer back to Chapter 31, Evaluation and Management Services (99201-99499), Tables 31-7 to 31-10, or to the 1997 DG.

- To determine the requirements for an examination, refer to Figure 41-8 or to the single organ system examination for respiratory in the 1997 DG.

- To determine the levels for medical decision making (MDM), refer to Chapter 31, Table 31-12, and to the Table of Risk in the 1997 DG.

Guided Example of E/M Coding for Pulmonology

Refer to the pulmonology encounter (■ FIGURE 41-9) to practice skills for abstracting and assigning E/M codes. Follow along as fictitious coder Leanne Riehl, CCS, abstracts the procedure. Check off each step after you complete it.

System/Body Area	Elements of Respiratory System Examination
Constitutional	❑ Measurement of any <u>three</u> of the following seven **vital** signs: • 1) sitting or standing blood pressure, • 2) supine blood pressure, • 3) pulse rate and regularity, • 4) respiration, • 5) temperature, • 6) height, • 7) weight (May be measured and recorded by ancillary staff) ❑ General **appearance** of patient (eg, development, nutrition, body habitus, deformities, attention to grooming)
Ears, Nose, Mouth and Throat	❑ Inspection of **nasal mucosa, septum** and **turbinates** ❑ Inspection of **teeth** and **gums** ❑ Examination of **oropharynx:** oral mucosa, salivary glands, hard and soft palates, tongue, tonsils and posterior pharynx
Neck	❑ Examination of **neck** (eg, masses, overall appearance, symmetry, tracheal position, crepitus) ❑ Examination of **thyroid** (eg, enlargement, tenderness, mass) ❑ Examination of **jugular veins** (eg, distention, a, v or cannon a waves)
Respiratory	❑ **Inspection** of chest with notation of symmetry and expansion ❑ Assessment of **respiratory effort** (eg, intercostal retractions, use of accessory muscles, diaphragmatic movement) ❑ **Percussion** of chest (eg, dullness, flatness, hyperresonance) ❑ **Palpation** of chest (eg, tactile fremitus) ❑ **Auscultation** of lungs (eg, breath sounds, adventitious sounds, rubs)
Cardiovascular	❑ **Auscultation** of heart with notation of abnormal sounds and murmurs ❑ Examination of peripheral vascular system by observation (eg, swelling, varicosities) and palpation (pulses, temperature, edema, tenderness)
Gastrointestinal (Abdomen)	❑ Examination of **abdomen** with notation of presence of masses or tenderness ❑ Examination of **liver** and **spleen**
Lymphatic	Palpation of lymph nodes in **two or more** areas: ❑ Neck ❑ Axillae ❑ Groin ❑ Other
Musculoskeletal	❑ Assessment of muscle **strength** and **tone** (eg, flaccid, cog wheel, spastic) with notation of any atrophy or abnormal movements ❑ Examination of **gait** and **station**
Extremities	❑ Inspection and/or palpation of **digits** and **nails** (eg, clubbing, cyanosis, inflammatory conditions, petechiae, ischemia, infections, nodes)
Skin	❑ **Inspection** of skin and subcutaneous tissue (eg, rashes, lesions, ulcers)
Neurologic/ Psychiatric	*Brief assessment of mental status including:* ❑ **Orientation** to time, place and person ❑ **Mood** and affect (eg, depression, anxiety, agitation, hypomania, lability)

Total # Bullets Performed and Documented →	☐	# of ❑ Elements Performed and Documented	Level of Examination
		1–5	Problem focused
		6–11	Expanded problem focused
		12	Detailed
		ALL	Comprehensive (Document **every** element in each box with a shaded border and at least **one** element in each box with an unshaded border)

Figure 41-8 ■ 1997 DG for Respiratory System Examination. *Source:* Centers for Medicare and Medicaid Services, *1997 Documentation Guidelines for Evaluation and Management Services* (with formatting adjustments).

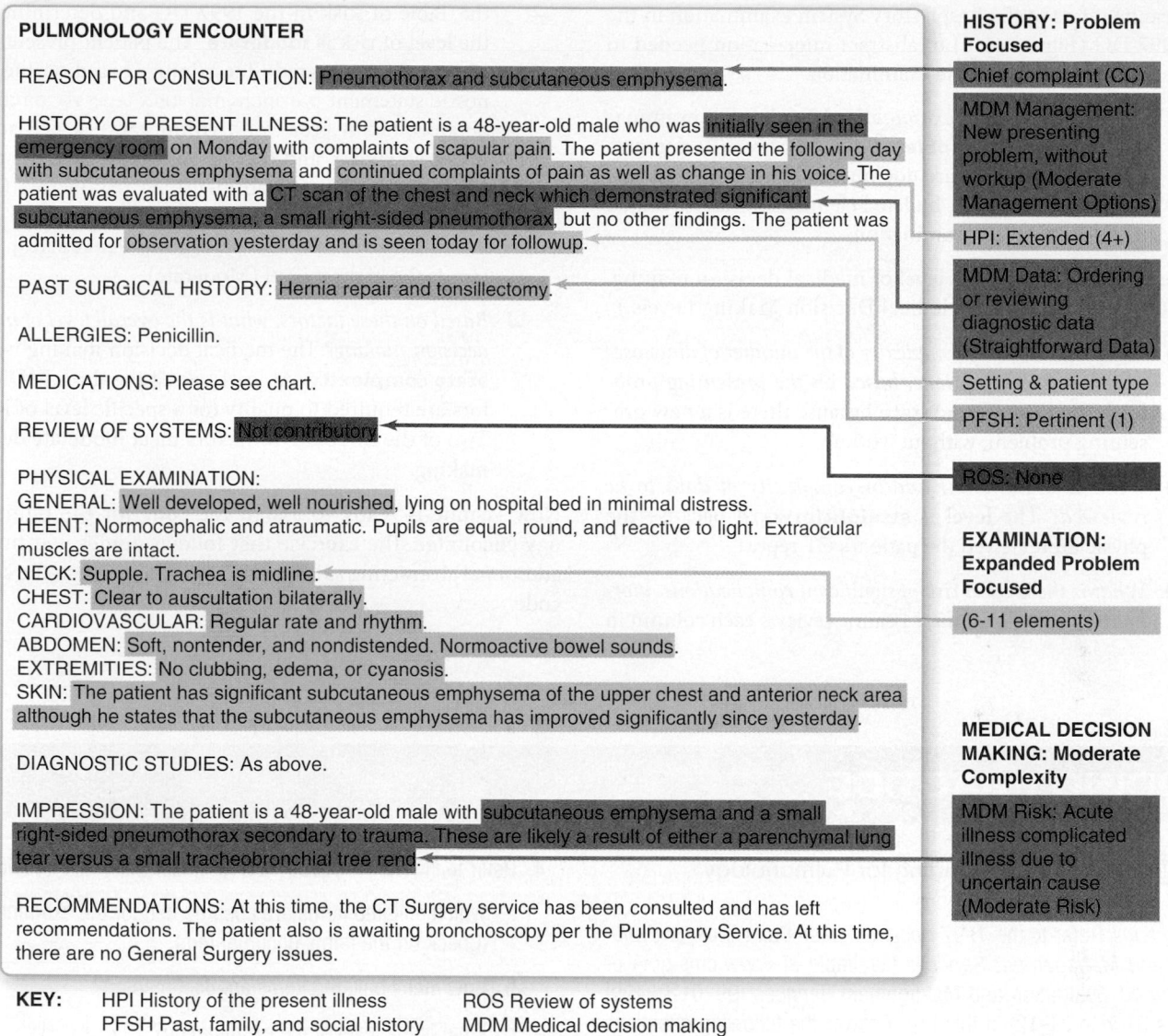

PULMONOLOGY ENCOUNTER

REASON FOR CONSULTATION: Pneumothorax and subcutaneous emphysema.

HISTORY OF PRESENT ILLNESS: The patient is a 48-year-old male who was initially seen in the emergency room on Monday with complaints of scapular pain. The patient presented the following day with subcutaneous emphysema and continued complaints of pain as well as change in his voice. The patient was evaluated with a CT scan of the chest and neck which demonstrated significant subcutaneous emphysema, a small right-sided pneumothorax, but no other findings. The patient was admitted for observation yesterday and is seen today for followup.

PAST SURGICAL HISTORY: Hernia repair and tonsillectomy.

ALLERGIES: Penicillin.

MEDICATIONS: Please see chart.

REVIEW OF SYSTEMS: Not contributory.

PHYSICAL EXAMINATION:
GENERAL: Well developed, well nourished, lying on hospital bed in minimal distress.
HEENT: Normocephalic and atraumatic. Pupils are equal, round, and reactive to light. Extraocular muscles are intact.
NECK: Supple. Trachea is midline.
CHEST: Clear to auscultation bilaterally.
CARDIOVASCULAR: Regular rate and rhythm.
ABDOMEN: Soft, nontender, and nondistended. Normoactive bowel sounds.
EXTREMITIES: No clubbing, edema, or cyanosis.
SKIN: The patient has significant subcutaneous emphysema of the upper chest and anterior neck area although he states that the subcutaneous emphysema has improved significantly since yesterday.

DIAGNOSTIC STUDIES: As above.

IMPRESSION: The patient is a 48-year-old male with subcutaneous emphysema and a small right-sided pneumothorax secondary to trauma. These are likely a result of either a parenchymal lung tear versus a small tracheobronchial tree rend.

RECOMMENDATIONS: At this time, the CT Surgery service has been consulted and has left recommendations. The patient also is awaiting bronchoscopy per the Pulmonary Service. At this time, there are no General Surgery issues.

HISTORY: Problem Focused

Chief complaint (CC)

MDM Management: New presenting problem, without workup (Moderate Management Options)

HPI: Extended (4+)

MDM Data: Ordering or reviewing diagnostic data (Straightforward Data)

Setting & patient type

PFSH: Pertinent (1)

ROS: None

EXAMINATION: Expanded Problem Focused

(6-11 elements)

MEDICAL DECISION MAKING: Moderate Complexity

MDM Risk: Acute illness complicated illness due to uncertain cause (Moderate Risk)

KEY: HPI History of the present illness   ROS Review of systems
PFSH Past, family, and social history   MDM Medical decision making

Figure 41-9 ■ Pulmonology Encounter. *Source:* © PB Resources, Inc. Used with permission.

▶ First, Leanne needs to establish the category of service so she can determine the information needed to abstract and assign the code.

❏ *What is the setting?* Hospital observation

❏ *What is the type of service?* Subsequent, because patient was admitted yesterday

❏ *What is the code range?* Leanne refers to the CPT Index and looks up the Main Term **Evaluation and Management** and the subterm **Hospital Services Observation Care.** The codes listed are 99217-99220, 99224-99226, 99234-99236.

❏ *How many key components are required?* Leanne refers to the code ranges in the Tabular List and identifies **99224-99226** as the correct category because this is subsequent observation care. She reads the code description of the first code, which states **at least 2 of these 3 key components.** All codes in the category have the

same requirements for key components. This tells her that two key components must meet or exceed the levels listed in the code (2/3).

▶ Next, Leanne identifies the level of history.

❏ *What is the level of HPI?* The HPI is **Extended** because four elements are documented.

❏ *What is the level of ROS?* No systems are documented for the ROS. The physician's statement, *not contributory,* does not describe what the physician did.

❏ *What is the level of PFSH?* The PFSH is **pertinent** because one element is documented.

❏ *Based on these factors, what is the overall level of history?* The level of history is **problem focused** because the lowest of the three factors (HPI, ROS, and PFSH) determines the history level. The HPI and PFSH qualify for a detailed history, but the ROS qualifies for only a problem-focused history.

▶ Leanne refers to the Respiratory System examination in the 1997 DG (Figure 41-8) to abstract information needed to determine the level of the examination.

❑ *What is the level of examination?* The level of examination is **expanded problem focused**. Seven (7) elements of the examination are documented, which exceeds the requirement of 6–11 bulleted elements for an expanded problem-focused examination.

▶ Leanne determines the level of medical decision making. (Refer to Table 31-12 Medical Decision Making Levels.)

❑ *What is the level of complexity of the number of diagnoses or management options, based on the presenting problem?* The level is **moderate** because there is a new presenting problem, without workup.

❑ *What is the amount and/or complexity of data to be reviewed?* The level is **straightforward** because the physician reviewed the patient's CT report.

❑ *What is the level of risk of significant complications, morbidity, and/or mortality?* Leanne reviews each column in the Table of Risk in the 1997 DG and determines that the level of risk is **moderate**. The patient presents with an acute, complicated illness/injury based on the diagnostic statement parenchymal lung tear vs. small tracheobronchial tree rent (Moderate), a CT scan is reviewed (Low), and the management option is minor elective surgery with no identified risk factors (Low). The single highest element in the Table of Risk determines the overall risk. The column **Presenting Problem** is the highest level (Moderate).

❑ *Based on these factors, what is the overall level of medical decision making?* The medical decision making is **moderate complexity**. At least two of the three MDM factors are required to qualify for a specific level of MDM. Two of the three MDM factors meet moderate decision making.

Now Leanne is ready to assign the code for the pulmonology encounter. The exercise that follows guides you through additional abstracting skills and allows you to assign the correct code.

CODING PRACTICE

Exercise 41.5 **E/M Coding for Pulmonology**

Instructions: Refer to the *1997 Documentation Guidelines for Evaluation and Management Services* (available at www.cms.gov) or Chapter 31 Evaluation and Management Services (99201-99499) (Tables 31-7 to 31-12) in this text. Answer the following questions about the Pulmonology Encounter (Figure 41-9).

1. a. Which elements of the HPI are documented? Circle all that apply. Location, Quality, Severity, Duration, Timing, Context, Modifying factors, Associated signs and symptoms

   b. How many elements are documented? _____

   c. What is the level of HPI? _____

2. a. Which systems are reviewed in the ROS? Circle all that apply. Constitutional, Allergic/ immunologic, CV, Endocrine, ENT/M, Eyes, GI, GU, Hemic/lymphatic, MS, Neurologic, Psychiatric, Respiratory, Skin/breast

   b. How many systems are documented? _____

   c. What is the level of ROS? _____

3. a. Which PFSH elements are documented? Circle all that apply. Past medical, Family, Social

   b. What is the level of PFSH? _____

   c. What is the overall level of history? (The lowest history factor—HPI, ROS, or PFSH—determines the level of history.) _____

4. Refer to Figure 41-8 (1997 DG for Respiratory Examination).

   a. Which bulleted items are documented for the examination? (Check off the items documented.)

   b. How many bulleted items are documented? _____

   c. What is the level of the examination? _____

5. Refer to Table 31-12 Medical Decision Making Levels or the 1997 DG.

   a. What is the MDM level for the number of diagnoses or management options? _____

   b. What is the MDM level for the amount and/or complexity of data to be reviewed? _____

   c. Refer to the Table of Risk in the 1997 DG. Which elements of risk are documented for each risk factor?

      1. Presenting problem: _____

      2. Diagnostic procedures ordered: _____

      3. Management options selected: _____

   d. What is the level of risk? (The highest of the three risk factors determines the overall level of risk.) _____

   e. What is the overall level of MDM? (2/3 MDM factors are needed to determine the overall level.) _____

6. a. What is the setting? _____

   b. What is the patient (or service) type? _____

6. (continued)

c. What is the code range? _____

d. How many key components are required? _____

e. What is the level of history? _____

f. What is the level of examination? _____

g. What is the level of medical decision making? _____

h. What is the correct code? _____

i. What modifier(s) is required? _____

7. Abstract, assign, and arrange (sequence) the diagnosis code(s) that support the E/M code.

ICD-10-CM Code(s) _____

CHAPTER SUMMARY

In this chapter you learned that:

- It is important to understand the anatomy of the paranasal sinuses, also called accessory sinuses, because codes are divided based on the location of the sinus.

- The CPT section/subsection **Respiratory System (30000-32999)** contains five subheadings that are divided by anatomic site.

- Abstracting for the respiratory system requires attention to the anatomic approach and procedure type or variation. Abstracting criteria include a special section on endoscopy procedures, in addition to questions that apply to all respiratory procedures.

- To assign codes for the Respiratory System, search the Index for the Main Term for the anatomic site, the first-level modifying term for the type of procedure, and a second-level modifying term for variations of the procedure. In the Tabular List, select the appropriate code for the anatomic approach and the variation of the procedure performed.

- Information about bundling, multiple coding, code sequencing, and modifiers in the Respiratory System subsection appears in special instructions, instructional notes, and code descriptions.

- The *1997 Documentation Guidelines for Evaluation and Management Services* (1997 DG), published by CMS, provides requirements for each level of a respiratory E/M examination.

- CPT provides guidelines and instructional notes throughout the Tabular List to alert coders to the need for modifiers, provide cross-references to codes for similar procedures on other sites, identify when additional codes might be needed for radiological services, and highlight resequenced and recently deleted codes.

CONCEPT QUIZ

Take a moment to look back at the Respiratory System and solidify your skills. Try to answer the questions from memory first, then refer to the discussion in this chapter if you need a little extra help.

Completion

Instructions: Write the term that answers each question based on the information you learned in this chapter. Choose from the list below. Some choices may be used more than once and some choices may not be used at all.

Caldwell-Luc procedure	pneumothorax
congenital subglottic stenosis	rhinoplasty
dystonia	septoplasty
ethmoidectomy	thoracentesis
laryngoscopy	thoracotomy
maxillectomy	tracheostomy
pleurodesis	tracheotomy
pneumonolysis	VATS

1. A malignant neoplasm of the upper jaw may require a partial _____.

2. _____ is surgical repair of the nose.

3. Laryngeal reinnervation by neuromuscular pedicle may be performed to treat _____.

4. A(n) _____ creates an opening to the maxillary sinus by incising the gum and bone.

5. A(n) _____ is a minimally invasive procedure to access the pleural cavity.

6. _____ can be performed to remove fluid from the pleural space using a needle.

7. _____ is the creation of an opening through the chest to place an intercostal catheter.

8. _____ introduces an irritant in the pleural cavity to prevent pleural effusion.

9. A(n) _____ is an incision through the neck into the windpipe.

10. An indirect _____ uses a mirror to view the base of the tongue, larynx, and the hypolarynx.

Multiple Choice

Instructions: Circle the letter of the best answer to each question based on the information you learned in this chapter.

1. What approach is used for procedures in the Incision category that relate to drainage of an abscess or hematoma from the nose?
   A. Chemical
   B. External
   C. Internal
   D. Lateral

(continued)

(continued from page 807)

2. What codes are needed when a physician performs a surgical endoscopy?
   A. One code (surgical endoscopy)
   B. One code (diagnostic endoscopy)
   C. Two codes (surgical and diagnostic endoscopy)
   D. Two codes (surgical and repair endoscopy)

3. Where are the ethmoid sinuses located?
   A. Over the eyes
   B. Under the eyes
   C. Between the eyes
   D. At the back of the nose

4. How is a sinus procedure that was done on both the right and left sides reported?
   A. Code each procedure separately
   B. Append modifiers -LT, -RT
   C. Send a copy of the procedure report with the final bill
   D. Append modifier -50

5. What codes are needed when the findings of a diagnostic endoscopy lead to the decision to perform a nonendoscopic surgical procedure during the same patient encounter?
   A. One for the surgical endoscopy only
   B. One for endoscopy and one for the surgical procedure
   C. One for the surgical procedure only
   D. One for the diagnostic endoscopy only

6. What site is examined using a laryngoscope?
   A. Hypopharynx
   B. Trachea
   C. Oral cavity
   D. Nasal passage

7. Which code can be reported with code 32506?
   A. 32501
   B. 32502
   C. 32504
   D. 32505

8. What does the abbreviation *VATS* stand for?
   A. Video access thoracoscopic surgery
   B. Video-assisted thoracoscopic surgery
   C. Video-assisted therapeutic surgery
   D. Video access thoracic surgery

9. What abstracting criterion does *laterovertical* describe?
   A. Surgical approach
   B. Anatomic approach
   C. Extent of procedure
   D. Laterality

10. Which procedure may involve collaboration between a surgeon and a radiation oncologist?
    A. Lung transplantation
    B. VATS lobectomy
    C. SRS/SBRT
    D. Ablation therapy

CODING CHALLENGE

Instructions: Read the mini-medical-record of each patient's encounter, then abstract, assign, and arrange ICD-10-CM diagnosis codes and CPT procedure codes using the appropriate Index and Tabular List. Assign quantities and modifiers where needed. Write the code(s) on the line provided.

1. OFFICE   Gender: F   Age: 2

Reason for encounter: Father noticed child place an object into her nose

Procedure: under mild sedation, a pebble was removed from her nasal passage

Assessment: toddler noted to have an object in her nostril

Plan: parents given signs and symptoms of complications to watch for and instructions to give the child acetaminophen for pain.

1 ICD-10-CM Code _____

1 CPT Code _____

2. OUTPATIENT SURGERY   Gender: F   Age: 60

Preprocedure diagnosis: bilateral pulmonary infiltrates

Procedure: fiberoptic bronchoscopy with transbronchial biopsies ×3 from various subsegments of both the right lower lobe and right middle lobe under fluoroscopic guidance

Postprocedure diagnosis: diffuse tracheobronchitis; bilateral pneumonia

Tip: Pay attention to the instructional note under Endoscopy in the tabular list.

2 ICD-10-CM Codes _____

2 CPT Codes _____

3. INPATIENT HOSPITAL   Gender: M   Age: 56

Preprocedure diagnosis: *squamous cell carcinoma of the supraglottis; two pack per day cigarette smoker*

Procedure: *total laryngectomy; bilateral modified radical neck dissection, type 1*

Postprocedure diagnosis: *squamous cell carcinoma of the supraglottis*

Tip: Follow the instruction at the diagnosis category in the Tabular List to identify the second diagnosis code.

2 ICD-10-CM Codes _____

1 CPT Code _____

---

4. OUTPATIENT SURGERY   Gender: M   Age: 38

Preprocedure diagnosis: *nasal septal deviation with bilateral inferior turbinate hypertrophy*

Procedure: *nasal septoplasty; bilateral submucous resection of the inferior turbinates*

Postprocedure diagnosis: *nasal septal deviation with bilateral inferior turbinate hypertrophy*

2 ICD-10-CM Codes _____

2 CPT Codes _____

---

5. INPATIENT HOSPITAL   Gender: F   Age: 74

Preprocedure diagnosis: *left malignant pleural effusion secondary to a left lung adenocarcinoma*

Procedure: *left video thoracoscopy, drainage of pleural effusion and talc poudrage*

Postprocedure diagnosis: *left malignant pleural effusion secondary to a left lung adenocarcinoma*

Tip: Be sure to follow the instruction in the Tabular List to sequence the diagnosis codes correctly.

2 ICD-10-CM Codes _____

1 CPT Code _____

---

6. OUTPATIENT SURGERY   Gender: M   Age: 17

Preprocedure diagnosis: *hyperhidrosis involving the soles of the feet, hands, and underarms*

Procedure: *bilateral endoscopic thoracic sympathectomy*

Postprocedure diagnosis: *hyperhidrosis involving the soles of the feet, hands, and underarms*

3 ICD-10-CM Codes _____

_____

1 CPT Code _____

---

7. OUTPATIENT HOSPITAL   Gender: F   Age: 38

Reason for encounter: *patient with multiple enlarged, soft upper pretracheal and lower paratracheal lymph nodes, suggestive of lymphoma.*

Procedure: *mediastinoscopy; mediastinal lymph node biopsy with frozen section; insertion of left subclavian MediPort device under fluoroscopy.*

Assessment: *primary mediastinal B-cell lymphoma*

Plan: *follow-up in the office with referral to oncology for discussion of chemotherapy and radiation therapy options*

Tip: A Mediport, or portacath, is inserted in a vein.

1 ICD-10-CM Code _____

3 CPT Codes _____

_____

---

8. INPATIENT HOSPITAL   Gender: F   Age: 64

Preprocedure diagnosis: *left lung mass; rule out primary lung cancer*

Procedure: *fiberoptic bronchoscopy with bronchioalveolar lavage; exploratory left thoracotomy; left lower lobe wedge resection for frozen section; left pneumonectomy.*

Postprocedure diagnosis: *squamous cell carcinoma, left lower lobe*

Tip: Read the instructional notes for Lungs and Pleura in the CPT Tabular List to help decide which codes to use.

1 ICD-10-CM Code _____

3 CPT Codes _____

_____

---

9. OUTPATIENT SURGERY   Gender: M   Age: 33

Reason for encounter: *patient is a cocaine addict, now with a large perforated septum*

Procedure: *a nasal button was inserted in the opening and fastened in place with sutures to repair the septum*

Assessment: *perforated nasal septum*

Plan: *patient is in a rehab facility and in remission of his cocaine dependence; see in office in one week*

2 ICD-10-CM Codes _____

1 CPT Code _____

(continued)

(continued from page 809)

10. INPATIENT HOSPITAL   Gender: M   Age: 46

Reason for encounter: sinus pain, facial numbness

Procedure: maxillary endoscopy with antrostomy and removal of squamous cell carcinoma (SCCA) of the right maxillary sinus

Assessment: squamous cell carcinoma of maxillary sinus

(continued)

10. (continued)

Plan: to be followed with radiotherapy and chemotherapy

1 ICD-10-CM Code _____

1 CPT Code _____

KEEP ON CODING

Instructions: Read the procedural statement, then use the appropriate Index and Tabular List to assign CPT procedure codes, quantities, and modifiers. Write the code(s) on the line provided.

1. Bilateral nasal endoscopy with total ethmoidectomy: CPT Code(s) _____

2. Direct laryngoscopy with stripping of vocal cords: CPT Code(s) _____

3. Bronchoalveolar lavage: CPT Code(s) _____

4. Flexible fiberoptic laryngoscopy performed for removal of a dime lodged in the patient's larynx: CPT Code(s) _____

5. Flexible bronchoscopy with cell washings, brushings, and biopsy: CPT Code(s) _____

6. Cadaver donor pneumonectomy: CPT Code(s) _____

7. Tracheostomy with division of thyroid isthmus: CPT Code(s) _____

8. Ultrasound-guided thoracentesis: CPT Code(s) _____

9. Percutaneous needle biopsy of the right upper lobe of the lung: CPT Code(s) _____

10. Rhinoplasty: CPT Code(s) _____

11. Cauterization of epistaxis, left nasal septum; fiberoptic nasal laryngoscopy: CPT Code(s) _____

12. Fluoroscopy-guided bronchoalveolar lavage: CPT Code(s) _____

13. Diagnostic bronchoscopy and limited left thoracotomy with partial pulmonary decortication and insertion of chest tubes ×2: CPT Code(s) _____

14. Bronchoscopy with laser destruction of a lesion of the bronchus: CPT Code(s) _____

15. Ultrasound-guided right pleurocentesis: CPT Code(s) _____

16. Tracheostomy tube change: CPT Code(s) _____

17. Endoscopic sinus surgery: CPT Code(s) _____

18. Flexible bronchoscopy with thermoplasty, right middle lobe and left upper lobe: CPT Code(s) _____

19. Backbench preparation of one cadaver donor lung: CPT Code(s) _____

20. Partial excision of the inferior turbinates: CPT Code(s) _____

21. Emergency endotracheal intubation: CPT Code(s) _____

22. VATS wedge resection of left lung, upper and lower lobes: CPT Code(s) _____

23. Revision of tracheostomy scar: CPT Code(s) _____

24. Bilateral endoscopic nasal polypectomy: CPT Code(s) _____

25. Laryngoscopy with excision of a vocal cord polyp using an operating microscope: CPT Code(s) _____

Nervous System Procedures (61000-64999)

Learning Objectives

After completing this chapter, you should have the skills to:

42.1 Spell and define the key words, medical terms, and abbreviations related to Nervous System procedures.

42.2 Discuss the types of Nervous System procedures.

42.3 Identify the main characteristics of coding for the Nervous System.

42.4 Abstract procedural information from the medical record for coding for the Nervous System.

42.5 Assign codes for Nervous System procedures.

42.6 Arrange codes for Nervous System procedures.

42.7 Code evaluation and management services for the Nervous System.

42.8 Discuss the CPT coding guidelines related to the Nervous System.

Chapter Outline

- **Nervous System Procedure Basics**
- **Coding Overview of Nervous System Procedures**
- **Abstracting Nervous System Procedures**
- **Assigning Codes for Nervous System Procedures**
- **Arranging Codes for Nervous System Procedures**
- **E/M Coding for Neurology**

Key Terms and Abbreviations

annulus fibrosus	endovascular therapy	intervertebral disc	nucleus pulposus
approach procedure (skull base)	facet	lamina	process
craniostomy	foramen	laminectomy	vertebral body
definitive procedure (skull base)	hemilaminectomy	laminotomy	

In addition to the key terms listed here, students should know the terms defined within tables in this chapter.

INTRODUCTION

When going into a store for the first time, it might take a while to learn how it is configured and how to locate what you are looking for. However, you can rely on your experience of common store layouts to help navigate the new setting. When coding for the nervous system, you might encounter unfamiliar medical terms and anatomic designations. By using your knowledge of medical terminology and the three skills of an "ace" coder—abstracting, assigning, and arranging codes—you can apply what you already know to help navigate the new and sometimes complex material in this chapter.

NERVOUS SYSTEM PROCEDURE BASICS

Neurological surgery, or neurosurgery, is a medical discipline and surgical specialty that provides care for patients in the treatment of pain or disease processes that affect the nervous system. Coders should be familiar with the organization of the nervous system, including the central nervous system (CNS) and peripheral nervous system (PNS) (■ FIGURE 42-1). The supporting structures include the meninges (*a three-layer membrane around the brain and spinal cord consisting of the dura mater, arachnoid mater, and pia mater*) (■ FIGURE 42-2), skull, skull base, and vertebral column; the vascular supply includes intracranial, extracranial, and spinal blood vessels.

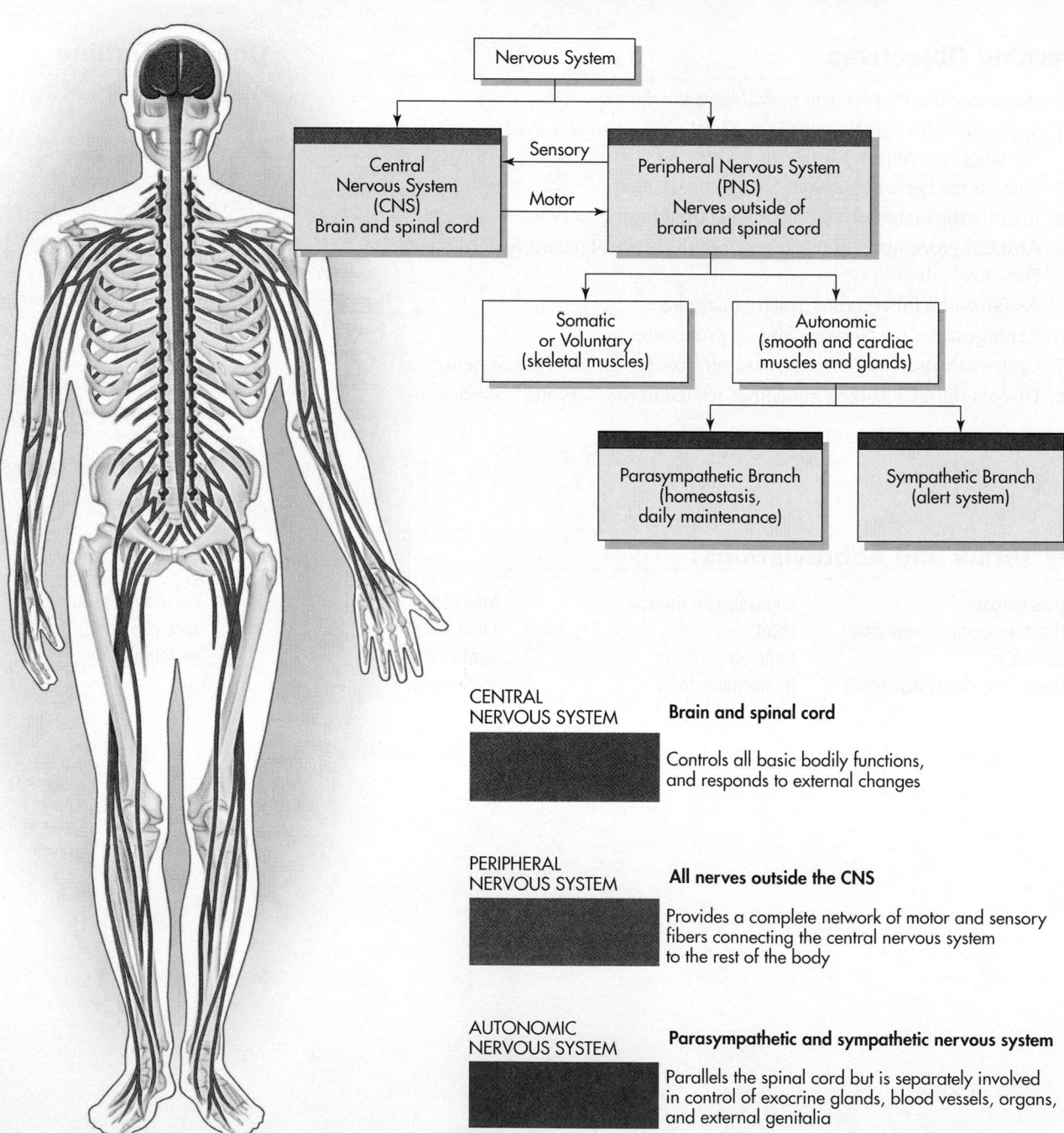

CENTRAL NERVOUS SYSTEM **Brain and spinal cord**

Controls all basic bodily functions, and responds to external changes

PERIPHERAL NERVOUS SYSTEM **All nerves outside the CNS**

Provides a complete network of motor and sensory fibers connecting the central nervous system to the rest of the body

AUTONOMIC NERVOUS SYSTEM **Parasympathetic and sympathetic nervous system**

Parallels the spinal cord but is separately involved in control of exocrine glands, blood vessels, organs, and external genitalia

Figure 42-1 ■ The Meninges of the Brain and Spinal Cord

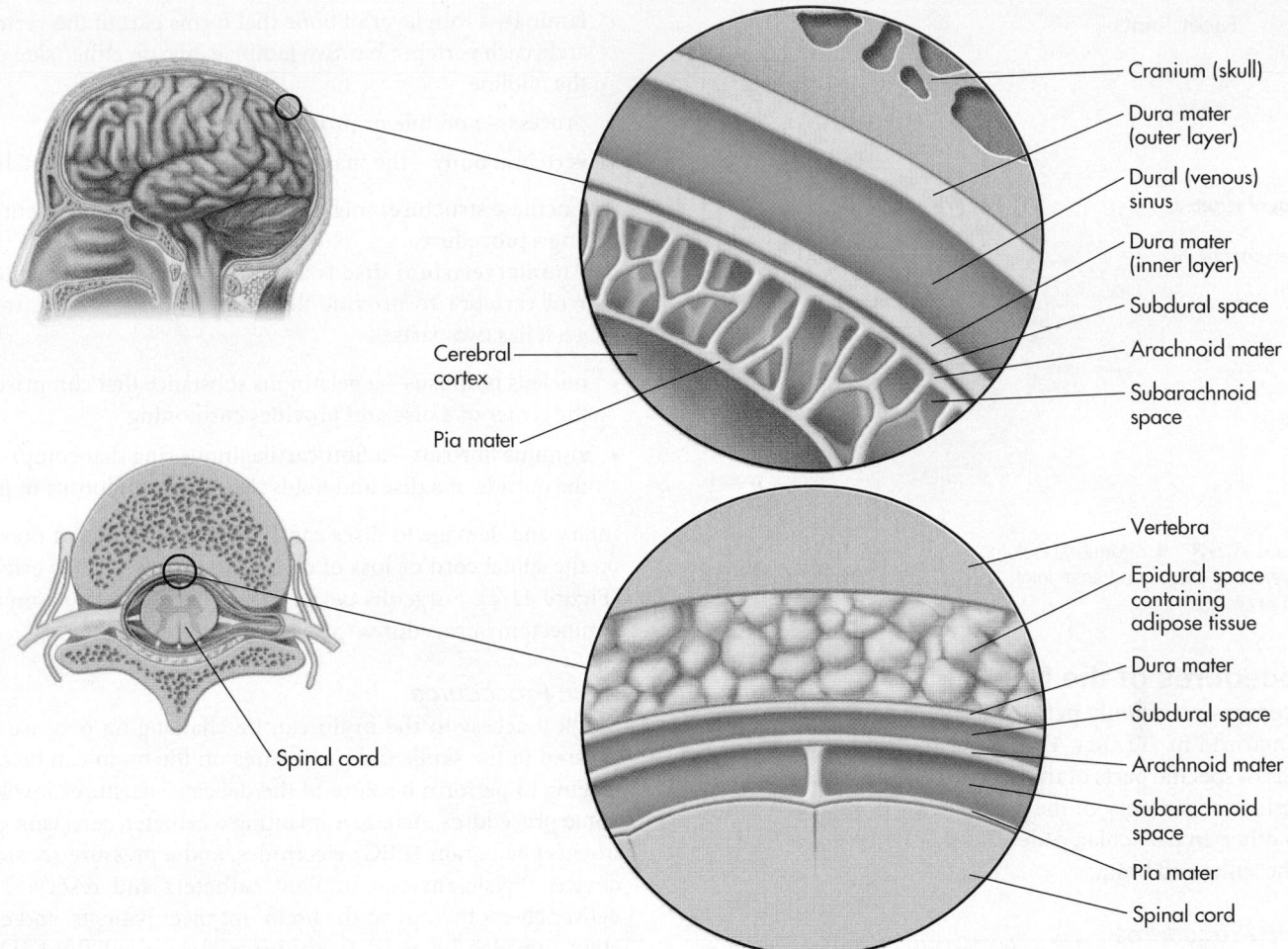

Figure 42-2 ■ Organization of the Nervous System

Operative procedures include endovascular surgery, functional and restorative surgery, stereotactic radiosurgery, and spinal fusion and instrumentation. Neurosurgeons might concentrate their practice on procedures in a particular anatomic region, such as the brain or spinal cord. Because the nervous system and musculoskeletal system are closely related, orthopedic surgeons perform some procedures involving the nervous system, such as spinal fusion. Neurosurgeons must consider possible problems that could arise during or after surgery and must work with an interdisciplinary team of otolaryngologists, ophthalmologists, plastic surgeons, and physical and occupational therapists to effectively manage patients' care.

Chapter 17 of this text provides more information on the anatomy and conditions of the nervous system. Refer to ■ TABLE 42-1 for a refresher on how to build medical terms related to the nervous system.

CODING CAUTION

Be alert for medical terms that are spelled similarly and have different meanings.

aphagia (*lack of ability to swallow*) and **apha̲sia** (*lack of ability to speak*)

ata̲xia (*lack of coordination*) and **apra̲xia** (*inability to perform motor tasks*)

Table 42-1 ■ **EXAMPLE OF CONSTRUCTING MEDICAL TERMS FOR NERVOUS SYSTEM PROCEDURES**

Combining Form	Suffix	Complete Medical Term
neur/o (*nerve*)		**neur + ectomy** (*excision of a nerve*)
		crani + ectomy (*excision of part of the skull*)
		lamin + ectomy (*excision of the lamina*)
crani/o (*skull*)	-**ectomy** (*excision*) -**tomy** (*incision into*) -**plasty** (*repair*)	**neuro + tomy** (*incision into a nerve*)
		cranio + tomy (*incision into the skull*)
		lamino + tomy (*incision into the lamina*)
lamin/o (*lamina*)		**neuro + plasty** (*repair of a nerve*)
		cranio + plasty (*repair of part of the skull*)
		lamino + plasty (*repair of the lamina*)

Source: © PB Resvources, Inc. Used with permission.

Facet Joints

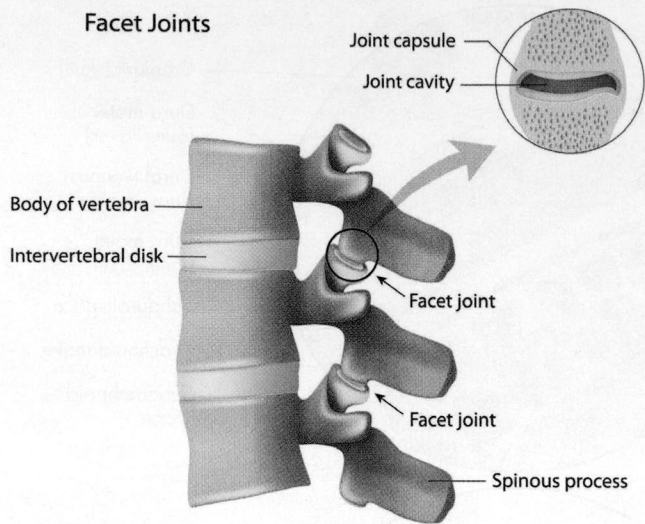

Figure 42-3 ■ Vertebral Column Showing the Vertebral Body, Intervertebral Disc, and Facet Joint. *Source: Shutterstock.com © Alila Medical Media.*

Procedures of the Nervous System

Procedures commonly performed on the Nervous System are summarized in ■ TABLE 42-2. Refer to detailed anatomic diagrams of specific parts of the nervous system when you need to refresh your memory of the relationship of organs and sites to each other. In particular, coders need to understand procedures on the spine and brain.

Spine Procedures

Spine procedures can be performed on the vertebrae (*the 26 bones of the spine*), the intervertebral discs (*the soft tissue between the vertebrae*), or the spinal cord (*the band of nerve tissue that extends from the brain to the lower back through the foramina [openings in the vertebrae]*). The prominent features of a vertebra used to describe procedures include the following:

- **facet**—a flat surface on the edge of the spinous process that forms the connection between vertebrae (■ FIGURE 42-3)

- **foramen**—an opening in the vertebra that surrounds the spinal cord (■ FIGURE 42-4)

- **lamina**—a thin layer of bone that forms part of the vertebral arch; each vertebra has two laminae, one on either side of the midline

- **process**—a nodule or projection of a bone

- **vertebral body**—the main anterior bony part of a vertebra

Any of these structures might be removed, modified, or cut into during a procedure.

An **intervertebral disc** is a plate that occurs between each pair of vertebra to provide flexibility and movement to the spine. It has two parts:

- **nucleus pulposus**—a gelatinous substance that comprises the center of a disc and provides cushioning

- **annulus fibrosus**—a fibrocartilaginous ring that comprises the outside of a disc and holds the nucleus pulposus in place

Injury and damage to discs can cause pain because of pressure on the spinal cord or loss of cushioning between the vertebrae (Figure 42-4). Surgeons perform a variety of discectomy and laminectomy procedures to help correct the situation.

Brain Procedures

Surgical access to the brain can be challenging because it is encased in the skull, and procedures on the brain can be challenging to perform because of the delicate structures involved. Some procedures include implanting a catheter, reservoir, electroencephalogram (EEG) electrodes, and a pressure recording device. Physicians can implant catheters and reservoirs to deliver chemotherapy to the brain in cancer patients, and catheters can also be used to drain cerebrospinal fluid (CSF). Implanted EEG electrodes monitor brain functions in patients with seizures and brain damage, and pressure-recording devices help physicians to detect intracranial pressure.

Aspiration procedures include removing CSF to test it for specific disorders, such as meningitis, or removing excess fluid caused by hydrocephalus or head trauma. The physician orders a CT scan or MRI first to determine the extent of CSF present and then withdraws fluid or directs it elsewhere in the body.

In a **craniostomy**, a physician drills or cuts into the skull to drain a hematoma or abscess or to remove part of the bone of

THE VERTEBRAL COLUMN

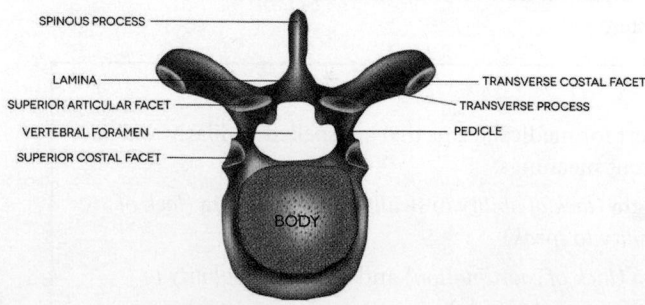

Figure 42-4 ■ A Vertebra Showing the Vertebral Body, Foramen, and Lamina. *Source:* Shutterstock.com © GRei.

Table 42-2 ■ **COMMON PROCEDURES OF THE NERVOUS SYSTEM**

Procedure Name	Definition	Reason Performed
Carpal tunnel release	Cutting of the transverse carpal ligament to release pressure on the median nerve	Carpal tunnel syndrome
Catheter procedures	Implantation, revision, or repositioning of a tunneled intrathecal or epidural catheter	Long-term medication administration; removal of an intrathecal or epidural catheter
Cerebrospinal fluid (CSF) shunt	Creation, removal, or reprogramming of a shunt and replacement or irrigation of a catheter that transports fluid from one area of the body to another (■ FIGURE 42-5)	Drainage of CSF from one area of the body into another (such as from the ventricles to the peritoneum)
Chemodenervation	Injection of a substance into a muscle group or glands to stop overactivity	Overactivity, such as muscle spasms or hyperhidrosis
Cisternal puncture	Withdrawal of CSF from the cisterna magna (*space between the pia mater and arachnoid membrane [thin layer of tissue covering the brain and spinal cord]*)	Diagnostic testing
Decompression	Excision of part of the skull or other body site	Drainage, excess pressure, such as from excess CSF
Deep brain stimulation (DBS)	Implantation of electrodes into a patient's brain to provide electrical stimulation to specific locations in the brain and reduce or eliminate involuntary movements	Parkinson disease, essential tremor (*hand tremors*), dystonia (*repeated muscle contractions*), torticollis (*rotation and tilting of neck muscles*)
Discectomy	Removal of all or part of an intervertebral disc	Herniated disc
Electrocorticography	Implantation of electrodes on the brain to record electrical impulses and identify areas to surgically remove	Epilepsy
Facetectomy	Excision of the vertebral facet	Nerve decompression, pain
Hemispherectomy	Excision of one of the two cerebral hemispheres	Epilepsy
Laminectomy	Excision of the lamina	Removal of neoplasms or abnormal intervertebral discs
Lobectomy	Excision of a lobe of the brain	Epilepsy
Nerve block	Introduction or injection of an anesthetic agent	Diagnosis of source of pain or treatment of pain
Neuroendoscopy	Use of an endoscope to visualize the CNS	Dissect adhesions, remove foreign bodies, excise tumors
Neuroplasty	Any of a variety of surgical procedures to repair or alter a nerve	Nerve decompression, adhesiolysis
Neurostimulator procedures	Implantation of electrodes under the skin; removal or revision of spinal electrodes, plates, or paddles; insertion, replacement, revision, or removal of a spinal pulse generator or receiver	Intractable pain
Reservoir/pump implantation	Implantation, replacement, or removal of subcutaneous reservoir or pump; electronic analysis of programmable implanted pump	Intrathecal or epidural drug infusion
Spinal tap or puncture	Insertion of a needle into the lumbar back to collect a sample of CSF	Diagnostic testing
Stereotactic radiosurgery	Use of narrow beams of radiation with three-dimensional guidance to target lesions in difficult-to-treat areas	Brain tumors or lesions
Subdural tap	Withdrawal of CSF through a fontanelle (*a soft spot, or gap, in an infant's skull where bones have not yet formed*)	Diagnostic testing
Tractotomy	Incision of a nerve tract (*group of nerve fibers*) in the brainstem or spinal cord	Chronic pain
Ventricular puncture	Withdrawal of CSF from the ventricles of the brain by drilling a hole in the skull	Diagnostic testing

Source: © PB Resources, Inc. Used with permission.

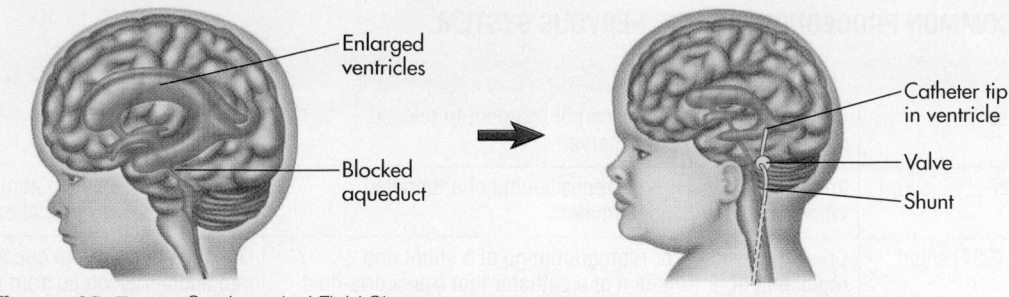

Figure 42-5 ■ Cerebrospinal Fluid Shunt

the skull to gain access to perform further surgery. The procedures are named for the equipment that a physician uses to perform them—a burr and a trephine are types of saws, and a twist drill has a drill bit that is twisted.

Endovascular therapy involves inserting microcatheters (*small catheters*) into blood vessels to treat aneurysms, lesions, and neoplasms, including intracranial tumors. Treatment includes inserting balloons and stents into blood vessels or performing embolizations. In endovascular therapy neurosurgeons work with interventional radiologists to coordinate a patient's treatment and care.

This section provides a general reference to help understand the most common nervous system procedures. Remember to keep standard reference books handy in case you get stuck.

CODING CAUTION

A *ventricle* is a cavity in a body part or organ. Both the heart and the brain have ventricles, so when the term is used, remember to identify what type of ventricle is being referenced.

CODING PRACTICE

Exercise 42.1 **Nervous System Procedure Basics**

Instructions: Use your medical terminology skills and resources to define the following procedures related to the Nervous System, then identify the code(s) or code range listed in the CPT Index. Follow these steps:

- Use slash marks "/" to break down the underlined term into its root(s) and suffix.
- Define the meaning of the underlined word based on the meaning of each word part.
- Use the entire phrase to identify the code or code range shown in the CPT Index.

Example: <u>neuroplasty</u>, cranial nerve

  neuro/plasty   Meaning *surgical repair of a nerve*   CPT Code *64716*

1. <u>discectomy</u>, cervical   Meaning _____   CPT Code _____

2. <u>corpectomy</u>   Meaning _____   CPT Code _____

3. <u>neurorrhaphy</u>, peripheral nerve, conduit   Meaning _____   CPT Code _____

4. <u>cranioplasty</u>, autograft   Meaning _____   CPT Code _____

5. <u>myelomeningocele</u>, repair   Meaning _____   CPT Code _____

6. <u>sympathectomy</u>, cervical   Meaning _____   CPT Code _____

7. <u>neurolysis</u>, internal   Meaning _____   CPT Code _____

8. <u>myelography</u>, spine, thoracic   Meaning _____   CPT Code _____

9. <u>cordotomy</u>, thoracic   Meaning _____   CPT Code _____

10. <u>hemilaminectomy</u>   Meaning _____   CPT Code _____

CODING OVERVIEW OF NERVOUS SYSTEM PROCEDURES

The CPT subsection **Nervous System (61000-64999)** contains three subheadings that are divided by anatomic site (■ TABLE 42-3). Within each anatomic site subheading, categories are divided by the type of procedure, such as injection, repair, or excision; some categories are further divided into subcategories to provide more specific information. Review the subheading and category names and code ranges listed in the Nervous System subsection to become familiar with the content and organization. Some editions of the CPT manual provide a summary list of the subheadings and categories at the beginning of the Nervous System subsection, which also displays an asterisk (*) next to categories that contain special coding instructions.

This chapter includes invasive, minimally invasive, and non-invasive surgical procedures on the nervous system. Codes for diagnostic tests on the nervous system appear in the Medicine section. Procedures represented by CPT codes must be linked on a claim to diagnosis codes that justify the medical necessity. CPT codes in the Nervous System subsection are frequently supported by diagnosis codes from ICD-10-CM **Chapter 6 Nervous System (G00-G99)**, as well as neoplasms, symptoms and signs, and injuries (■ TABLE 42-4). These are the codes most commonly used to support procedures on the nervous system; however, diagnosis codes from any ICD-10-CM chapter are permissible.

CPT guidelines for the Surgery section apply to the Nervous System.

Special instructions provide definitions and coding guidelines at the beginning of many categories, including:

- **Surgery of Skull Base**

- **Injection, Drainage, or Aspiration** located under the **Spine and Spinal Cord** subheading

- **Stereotactic Radiosurgery** and **Neurostimulators** categories, both of which occur under multiple subheadings

Remember to study these guidelines thoroughly to understand how to code accurately for these procedures. Instructional notes appear throughout the Tabular List to alert coders to the need for modifiers, provide cross-references to codes for similar procedures on other sites, identify when additional codes for radiological services might be needed, and highlight new, resequenced, and recently deleted codes.

ABSTRACTING NERVOUS SYSTEM PROCEDURES

When abstracting for nervous system procedures, coders must pay special attention to the anatomic approach used to access the surgical site because distinct codes often identify each approach. The anatomic approach identifies the direction from which the surgical site is accessed and often is described in relation to nearby anatomic structures (■ TABLE 42-5). Approach descriptions vary based on the anatomic site being accessed because the nearby anatomic structures are different. Some spine and brain procedures are accessed from two directions, such as anterior and posterior.

Table 42-3 ■ NERVOUS SYSTEM SUBHEADINGS

Subheading	Code Range
Skull, Meninges, and Brain	61000-62258
Spine and Spinal Cord	62263-63746
Extracranial Nerves, Peripheral Nerves, and Autonomic Nervous System	64400-64999

Table 42-4 ■ LOCATING ICD-10-CM AND ADDITIONAL CPT CODES FOR THE NERVOUS SYSTEM

Type of Code	Codes
ICD-10-CM Nervous System-Related Codes	
Nervous system conditions	G00-G99
Neoplasms	C7A, C7B, C69-C72
Symptoms and signs	R25-R29, R40-R49
Injuries	S00-T88
CPT Nervous System-Related Codes	
Medicine procedures	95803-96020
Radiologic procedures	
• Diagnostic radiology	70010-73725
• Radiologic guidance	77001-77022
• Diagnostic ultrasound	76506-76356, 76800
• Nuclear medicine, diagnostic	78600-78699
Laboratory/drug assays	80300-80377

Source: © PB Resources, Inc. Used with permission. CPT codes only © American Medical Association.

SUCCESS STEP

When you encounter an approach description you are unfamiliar with, look for a prefix that identifies the direction and the root that identifies the structure. A quick Internet search for the medical term can help locate images to visualize the approach.

Refer to ■ TABLE 42-6 for guidance on how to abstract procedures on the nervous system, then work through the detailed example that follows. Supplemental questions are provided to help identify the many variations of spine procedures. Remember that the abstracting questions are a guide and that not every question applies to, or can be answered for, every case. For example, laterality is reported for a laminectomy or laminotomy because two laminae are present—one on each side of the midline of a vertebra—but not for a discectomy because there is only one disc between each pair of vertebrae.

Table 42-5 ■ ANATOMIC APPROACHES FOR NERVOUS SYSTEM PROCEDURES

Approach	Definition
Anterior	From the front
Bicoronal	Through both coronal sutures (*junction of the frontal bone with the two parietal bones*) in the skull
Costovertebral	Pertaining to a rib and its adjoining vertebra
Dural	Relating to the dura mater
Epidural	From outside the dura mater
Extracranial	From outside the skull
Extradural	From outside the dura mater but within the skull
Infratentorial	Beneath the tentorium cerebelli (*fissure that divides the cerebrum and cerebellum*)
Intracranial	From within the cranium
Intradural	Within or between the membranes of the dura mater
Orbitocranial zygomatic	From the eye socket and cheek bone
Posterior	From the back
Posterolateral	From the side, toward the back
Subarachnoid	Under the arachnoid membrane
Subdural	Under the dura mater or between the dura mater and the arachnoid
Subtentorial	Same as *infratentorial*
Supratentorial	Above the tentorium cerebelli
Transcochlear	Through the cochlea
Transcondylar	Through the far lateral side of the jaw
Transcranial	Through the skull
Transorbital	Through the eye socket
Transpedicular	Through the pedicle (*base*) of a vertebra
Transpetrosal	Through a large arch extending from the temporal bone, to above and around the ear, to behind the base of the ear
Transtemporal	Through the mastoid bone

Source: © PB Resources, Inc. Used with permission.

Guided Example of Abstracting Nervous System Procedures

Refer to the following example throughout this chapter to practice skills for abstracting, assigning, and arranging Nervous System codes.

Table 42-6 ■ KEY CRITERIA FOR ABSTRACTING NERVOUS SYSTEM PROCEDURES

❑ What procedure is performed?

❑ What is the anatomic site(s)?

❑ What is the surgical approach (open, closed, percutaneous, endoscopic)?

❑ What is the anatomic approach (anterior, posterior, epidural, subdural, etc.)?

❑ Is this an initial procedure or a revision/replacement?

❑ What other procedures are performed during the same encounter?

For vertebral procedures (laminectomy, discectomy, corpectomy):

❑ Which part(s) of the vertebra is treated (vertebral body, lamina, foramen, facet, disc, etc.)?

❑ How many and which segments or interspaces are treated?

❑ What is the purpose of the procedure?

❑ Is a facetectomy performed at the same time as another vertebral procedure?

❑ What is the laterality?

Source: © PB Resources, Inc. Used with permission.

INPATIENT HOSPITAL Gender: M Age: 45

Preoperative diagnosis: spinal stenosis L3-L4 and L4-L5 visualized on imaging studies

Procedure: Bilateral laminotomy with decompression of nerve root and partial facetectomy at L3-L4, posterior approach, open with endoscopic assistance; right laminotomy with decompression of nerve root, partial facetectomy, and foraminotomy at L4-L5, posterior approach, open with endoscopic assistance; followed by arthrodesis of L3-L4-L5, posterior approach.

Follow along as fictitious coder, Angelia Harkey, CPC, abstracts the procedure. Check off each step after you complete it.

▶ Angelia reads through the entire record, paying special attention to the reason for the encounter, the procedure performed, and the postoperative diagnosis. She refers to the Key Criteria for Abstracting Nervous System Procedures (Table 42-6).

❑ She notes the preoperative diagnosis spinal stenosis.

❑ *What is the patient's age?* 45

❑ *What site is treated?* spine

❑ *How many and which segments or interspaces are treated?* two interspaces: L3-L4 and L4-L5

❑ *What is the primary procedure performed?* laminotomy

- ❑ *What other procedures are performed during the same encounter?* decompression of nerve root and partial facetectomy; decompression of nerve root, partial facetectomy, and foraminotomy; arthrodesis

- ❑ *What is the anatomic site of the **first** laminotomy?* L3-L4

- ❑ *What is the purpose of the procedure?* decompression of nerve root

- ❑ *What is the surgical approach (open, closed, percutaneous)?* open with endoscopic assistance

- ❑ *What is the anatomic approach (anterior, posterior, epidural, subdural, etc.)?* posterior

- ❑ *Is this an initial procedure or a revision/replacement?* Initial

- ❑ *Which part(s) of the vertebra is treated (vertebral body, lamina, foramen, facet, disc, etc.)?* lamina, nerve root, and facet

- ❑ *Is a facetectomy performed at the same time as another vertebral procedure?* Yes

- ❑ *What is the laterality?* Bilateral

- ❑ *What is the anatomic site of the **second** laminotomy?* L4-L5

- ❑ *What is the purpose of the procedure?* decompression of nerve root

- ❑ *What is the surgical approach (open, closed, percutaneous)?* open with endoscopic assistance

- ❑ *What is the anatomic approach (anterior, posterior, epidural, subdural, etc.)?* posterior

- ❑ *Is this an initial procedure or a revision/replacement?* Initial

- ❑ *Which part(s) of the vertebra is treated (vertebral body, lamina, foramen, facet, disc, etc.)?* lamina, nerve root, facet, foramen

- ❑ *Is a facetectomy performed at the same time as another vertebral procedure?* Yes

- ❑ *What is the laterality?* Right

- ❑ *What additional procedures are performed?* arthrodesis

- ❑ *What is the site?* L3-L4 and L4-L5

- ❑ *What is the anatomic approach?* posterior

- ❑ *Is a cage or device used?* No

▶ At this time, Angelia does not know which of these procedures may need to be coded, nor how many codes she will end up with. She will learn about this when she moves on to assigning codes.

CODING PRACTICE

Exercise 42.2   Abstracting Nervous System Procedures

Instructions: Read the mini-medical-record of each patient's encounter and answer the abstracting questions. Write the answer on the line provided. Do not assign any codes.

---

1. INPATIENT HOSPITAL   Gender: F   Age: 23

Preprocedure diagnosis: skull fracture with hemorrhage

Procedure: exploratory craniotomy with catheter placement. Created multiple burr holes supratentorially to explore for the source of bleeding; inserted a catheter to close off the hemorrhaging blood vessel.

a. What procedure is performed? _____

b. What is the anatomic site(s)? _____

c. What is the surgical approach (open, closed, percutaneous, endoscopic)? _____

d. What is the anatomic approach (anterior, posterior, epidural, subdural, etc.)? _____

e. Is this an initial procedure or a revision/replacement?

_____

f. What other procedures are performed during the same encounter? _____

---

2. INPATIENT HOSPITAL   Gender: M   Age: 18

Preprocedure diagnosis: congenital hydrocephalus with a ventricular shunt in place to divert CSF; recently developed headaches and visual disturbances

Procedure: punctured the shunt tube to aspirate the excess CSF

a. What procedure is performed? _____

b. What is the anatomic site(s)? _____

c. What is the surgical approach (open, closed, percutaneous, endoscopic)? _____

d. What is the anatomic approach (anterior, posterior, epidural, subdural, etc.)? _____

e. What other procedures are performed during the same encounter? _____

(continued)

CODING PRACTICE (continued)

3. INPATIENT HOSPITAL Gender: F Age: 87

Preprocedure diagnosis: cerebral meninges adhesions

Procedure: intracranial neuroendoscopy. Created burr hole and introduced neuroendoscope through the trocar. Dissected adhesions. We removed the trocar and connected the ventricular catheter to an external collection bag. Closed and dressed the wound. Patient tolerated procedure well.

a. What procedure is performed? _____

b. What is the anatomic site(s)? _____

c. What is the surgical approach (open, closed, percutaneous, endoscopic)? _____

d. What is the anatomic approach (anterior, posterior, epidural, subdural, etc.)? _____

e. What other procedures are performed during the same encounter? _____

4. INPATIENT HOSPITAL Gender: F Age: 30

Preprocedure diagnosis: nerve root compression of the cervical spine

Procedure: cervical neck discectomy, anterior approach C3-C4, C4-C5

a. What procedure is performed? _____

b. What is the anatomic site(s)? _____

c. What is the surgical approach (open, closed, percutaneous, endoscopic)? _____

d. What is the anatomic approach (anterior, posterior, epidural, subdural, etc.)? _____

e. Is this an initial procedure or a revision/replacement? _____

f. What other procedures are performed during the same encounter? _____

g. Which part(s) of the vertebra is treated (vertebral body, lamina, foramen, facet, disc, etc.)? _____

h. How many and which segments or interspaces are treated?

i. What is the purpose of the procedure? _____

j. Is a facetectomy performed at the same time as another vertebral procedure? _____

k. What is the laterality? _____

5. OUTPATIENT SURGERY Gender: M Age: 35

Preprocedure diagnosis: lacerations to the right thumb and index finger

Procedure: neurorrhaphy to the right thumb and index finger

a. What procedure is performed? _____

b. What is the anatomic site(s)? _____

c. What is the surgical approach (open, closed, percutaneous, endoscopic)? _____

d. What is the anatomic approach (anterior, posterior, epidural, subdural, etc.)? _____

e. Is this an initial procedure or a revision/replacement? _____

f. What is the laterality? _____

6. INPATIENT HOSPITAL Gender: F Age: 48

Preprocedure diagnosis: stenosis C4-C5, foraminal stenosis L5-S1

Procedure: right hemilaminectomy at C4-C5, posterior approach; left hemilaminectomy with foraminotomy at L5-S1, posterior approach

a. What procedure is performed? _____

b. What is the anatomic site(s)? _____

c. What is the surgical approach (open, closed, percutaneous, endoscopic)? _____

d. What is the anatomic approach (anterior, posterior, epidural, subdural, etc.)? _____

e. Is this an initial procedure or a revision/replacement? _____

f. What other procedures are performed during the same encounter? _____

g. Which part(s) of the vertebra is treated (vertebral body, lamina, foramen, facet, disc, etc.)? _____

h. How many and which segments or interspaces are treated?

i. What is the purpose of the procedure? _____

j. Is a facetectomy performed at the same time as another vertebral procedure? _____

k. What is the laterality? _____

ASSIGNING CODES FOR NERVOUS SYSTEM PROCEDURES

To assign codes for Nervous System procedures, search the Index for the Main Term for the anatomic site, such as **Skull** or **Nerve**, then locate the first-level modifying term and any second-level modifying terms for the type of procedure. If you cannot find the necessary procedure under the anatomic site, then search for the Main Term for the name of the procedure, such as **Laminectomy**. In particular, coders should pay special attention to assigning codes for basilar (*pertaining to the base*) skull procedures and laminectomies.

Assigning Codes for Basilar Skull Procedures

Procedures in the category of **Surgery of Skull Base** include removal of many different types of lesions of the skull base (■ TABLE 42-7). The surgery is difficult, involved, and time-consuming because the skull base is not easily accessible and often requires a team of specialized surgeons to perform various components of the surgery. Skull base surgery often requires more than one CPT code.

CPT provides detailed guidelines about coding skull base procedures. Codes are divided by the three parts of a skull base procedure, listed as the subcategories **Approach Procedures**, **Definitive Procedure**, and **Repair or Reconstruction Procedure**.

Approach Procedure

The **approach procedure** is performed to access or expose the lesion. It is described based on the anatomic site—the location where the physician gains access to a lesion in the skull base. Approach procedure codes (**61580-61598**) are divided as follows:

- **Anterior cranial fossa**—procedures on the anterior lobe of the brain
- **Middle cranial fossa**—procedures on the temporal lobes of the brain
- **Posterior cranial fossa**—procedures on the occipital lobes of the brain

Codes are further divided by the anatomic approach to access the specific part of the cranial fossa, such as craniofacial or infratemporal. Approach procedures can also include other procedures that the physician must perform at the same time, such as a rhinotomy (*incision into the nose*).

Definitive Procedure

The **definitive procedure** is performing the repair, biopsy, resection, or excision of a lesion. It includes primary closure of the dura, mucous membranes, and skin. CPT arranges definitive procedures (**61610-61616**) by anatomic site: the base of the anterior, middle, or posterior cranial fossa. Codes are further divided based on the approach, such as extradural or intradural. Add-on codes for definitive procedures (**61609-61612**) identify variations of transection or ligation of the carotid artery.

Repair or Reconstruction Procedure

Repair and reconstruction procedures are reported if extensive dural grafts, cranioplasty, local myocutaneous pedicle flaps (*skin flap with muscle attached*), or extensive skin grafts are required. There are only two codes for a repair/reconstruction procedure: repair by free tissue graft (**61618**) or repair by pedicle or myocutaneous flap (**61619**).

Assigning Codes for Multiple Procedures or Multiple Surgeons

To assign codes for the approach or definitive skull base procedure, search the Index for the Main Term **Skull Base Surgery**, then locate the first-level modifying term of the location, including anterior cranial fossa, middle cranial fossa, or posterior cranial fossa. Locations are further divided by second-level modifying terms that identify the type of approach, such as bicoronal or craniofacial. To assign codes for a skull base repair/reconstruction procedure, search the Index for the Main Term **Skull Base Surgery**, then locate the first-level modifying term **Dura** and the second-level modifying term **Repair of cerebrospinal fluid leak**.

To assign codes for multiple skull base procedures and/or multiple surgeons, follow these guidelines:

- When separate physicians each perform distinct parts of a skull base procedure, identified by separate CPT codes, each physician should report a code for the procedure that he or she completes (■ FIGURE 42-6).
- When multiple surgeons work together to perform a single procedure, both report the same CPT code and append the appropriate modifier to indicate their respective roles. Modifiers are discussed later in this chapter.

Table 42-7 ■ **TYPES OF SKULL BASE LESIONS**

Type of Lesion	Description
Aneurysm	Excessive blood vessel dilation, which could lead to a ruptured blood vessel or vein
Arteriovenous malformation (AVM)	Abnormal connection between arteries and veins, usually congenital
Basilar skull fracture	A linear fracture in the anterior or middle skull base or the posterior fossa
CSF fistula	An abnormal connection between the subarachnoid space around the brain and either the sinuses or the ear that allows the passage of CSF
Giant-cell bone tumor	A rare, aggressive, benign tumor, generally occurring in adults between the ages of 20 and 40 years
Neurofibroma	A benign tumor of nerve fibers and connective tissue
Orbital tumor	A benign or malignant tumor in the eye socket or tissues that surround the eyeball; sometimes originating from the surrounding paranasal sinuses, brain, or nasal cavity
Pituitary tumor	An abnormal growth in the pituitary gland that is usually benign

Source: © PB Resources, Inc. Used with permission.

Dr. A and Dr. B work together to treat a patient with a carotid aneurysm. Dr. A performs the access to the cavernous sinus using an infratemporal post-auricular approach to middle cranial fossa. Dr. B dissects and ligates the carotid aneurysm, reapproximates the scalp, and sutures the wound closed.

Dr. A—Approach procedure:

61591 Infratemporal post-auricular approach to middle cranial fossa (internal auditory meatus, petrous apex, tentorium, cavernous sinus, parasellar area, infratemporal fossa) including mastoidectomy, resection of sigmoid sinus, with or without decompression and/or mobilization of contents of auditory canal or petrous carotid artery

Dr. B—Definitive procedure:

61613 Obliteration of carotid aneurysm, arteriovenous malformation, or carotid-cavernous fistula by dissection within cavernous sinus

Figure 42-6 ■ Example of Coding Skull Base Procedures. *Source: © PB Resources, Inc. Used with permission. CPT codes only © American Medical Association.*

- When one physician performs more than one part of a skull base procedure and each part is identified by separate CPT codes, report a code for each procedure, sequencing the most complex procedure first and appending modifier **-51 Multiple procedures** to the lesser procedure(s).

Assigning Codes for Laminectomy Procedures

Laminotomy and laminectomy are spinal decompression surgeries involving the lamina, a thin bony layer that covers and protects the spinal canal and spinal cord. Laminotomy, also called a **hemilaminectomy**, is the partial removal of the lamina, whereas **laminectomy** is the complete removal of the lamina. CPT indexes *laminotomy* under the Main Term **Hemilaminectomy** and *laminectomy* under the Main Term **Laminectomy**. Each of these Main Terms leads to separate codes in the Tabular List. In noncoding the terms often are used interchangeably, so it is important to understand the work performed and to review the code descriptions thoroughly.

A laminectomy often is done in conjunction with another procedure to resolve a problem, such as disc compression or a herniated disk (■ FIGURE 42-7). Procedures such as

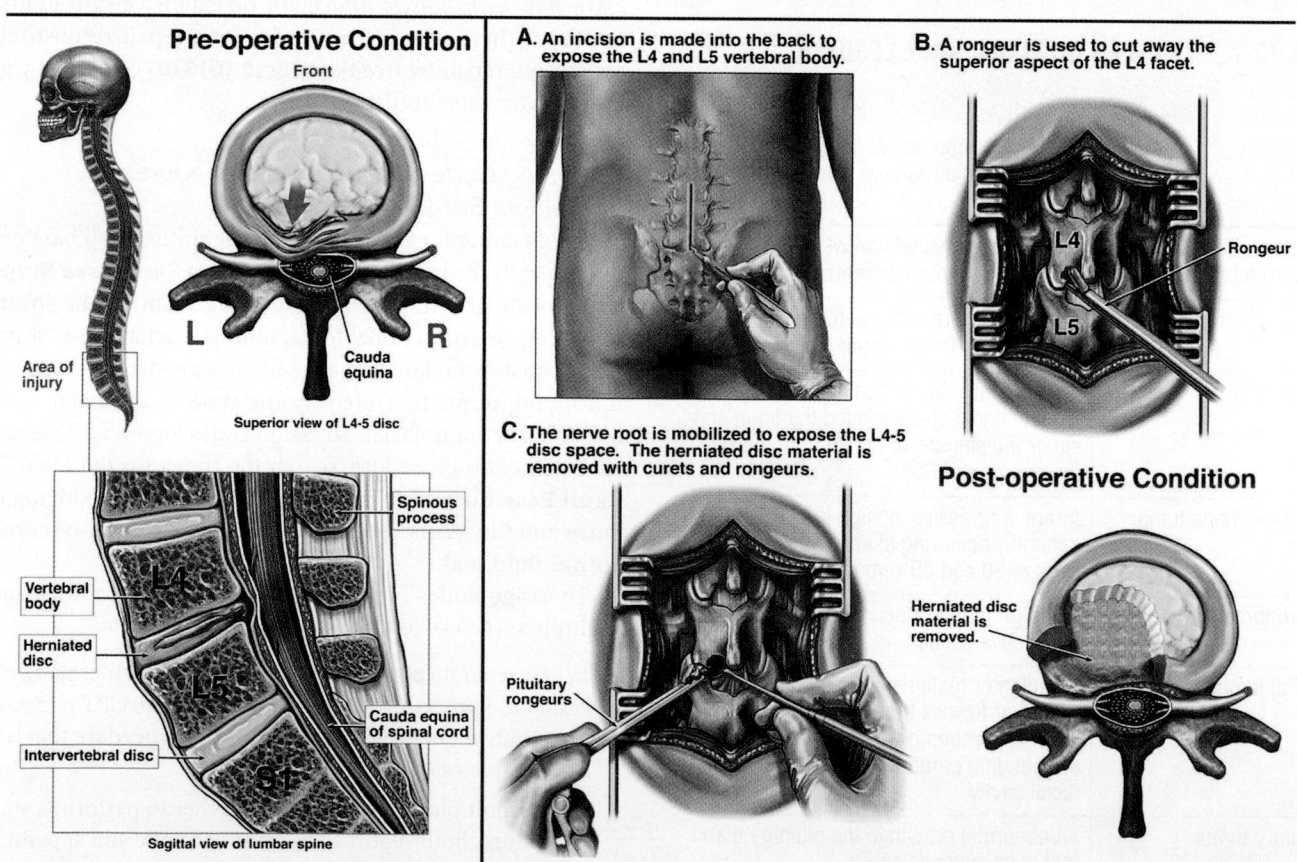

Figure 42-7 ■ Discectomy Procedure. *Source: © Nucleus Medical Art Inc./Alamy.*

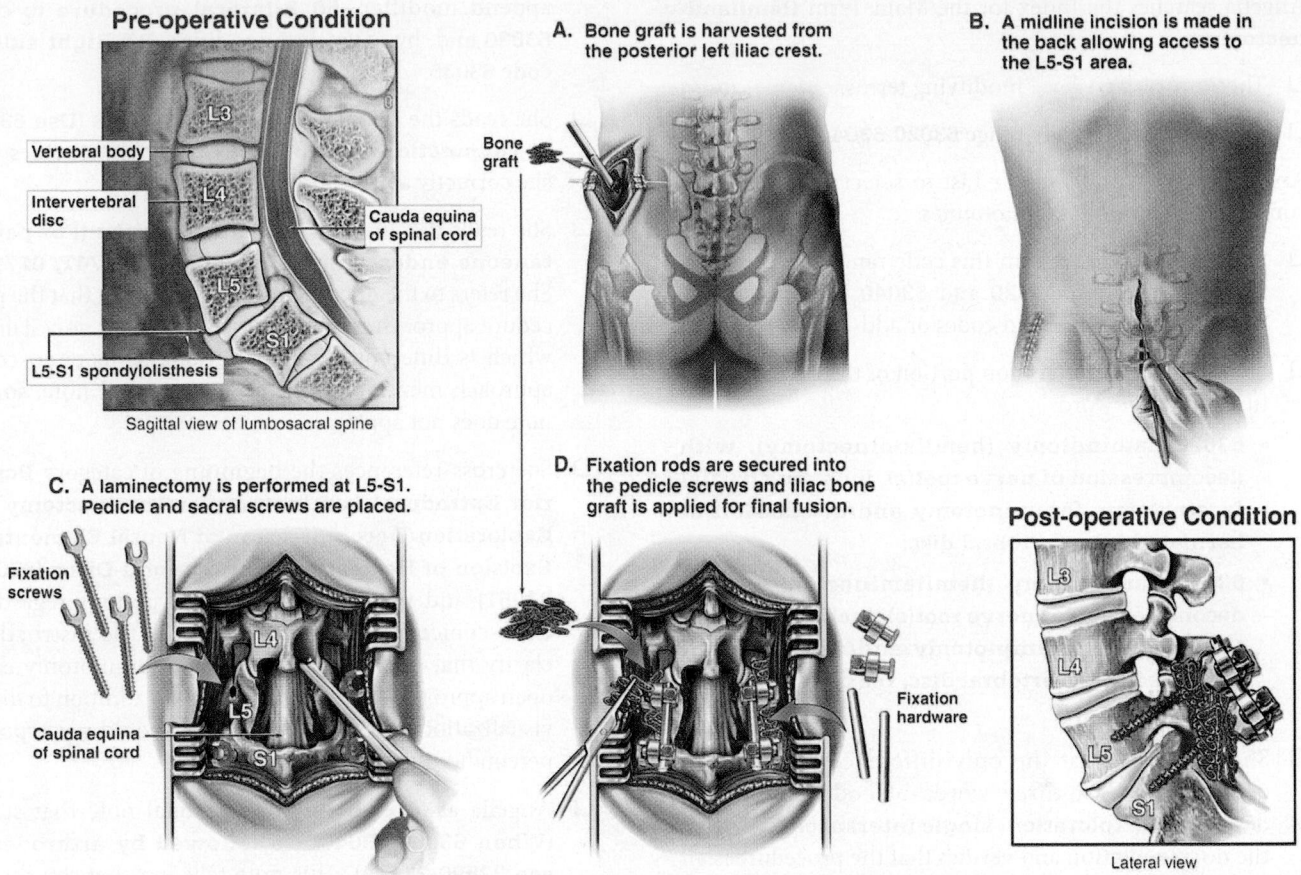

Pre-operative Condition

Vertebral body

Intervertebral disc

Cauda equina of spinal cord

L5-S1 spondylolisthesis

Sagittal view of lumbosacral spine

A. Bone graft is harvested from the posterior left iliac crest.

Bone graft

B. A midline incision is made in the back allowing access to the L5-S1 area.

C. A laminectomy is performed at L5-S1. Pedicle and sacral screws are placed.

Fixation screws

Cauda equina of spinal cord

D. Fixation rods are secured into the pedicle screws and iliac bone graft is applied for final fusion.

Fixation hardware

Post-operative Condition

Lateral view

Figure 42-8 ■ Laminectomy Procedure with Bone Graft and Fixation. *Source: © Nucleus Medical Art Inc./Alamy.*

foraminotomy, facetectomy, discectomy, and/or bone grafts are often bundled into a single code. Therefore, in both the Index and Tabular List coders must be alert for code variations. Also be alert for procedures that should be coded separately, such as arthrodesis (■ FIGURE 42-8).

To locate codes for spinal procedures, search the Index for either the anatomic site or the procedure name. When searching by anatomic site, if the desired procedure or site does not appear under Main Term **Spine**, refer to a Main Term for the appropriate part of the spine, such as **Spinal Cord**, **Intervertebral Disc**, or **Vertebra**. Using procedure names such as **Laminectomy**, **Hemilaminectomy**, or **Discectomy** as the Main Term often more directly leads to the desired code.

CODING CAUTION

Be aware that many of these entries list codes for both nervous system—beginning with the number 6—and musculoskeletal system procedures—beginning with the number 2. Review code descriptions carefully to be sure you select the correct code based on the documentation.

In the Tabular List one or more parent codes may appear with slightly different variations of a laminectomy, followed by indented codes for alternative regions of the spine. Codes for vertebral corpectomy provide separate parent codes for each spinal region with an add-on for additional segments

in the same region. To select and verify codes, follow these steps:

1. Compare the unique descriptors of the parent codes to locate the correct code family.
2. Identify the correct indented code to identify the appropriate spinal region.
3. Locate add-on codes for additional vertebra or interspaces, when applicable.
4. Read instructional notes to identify any procedures, such as arthrodesis, that might need to be coded separately.

Guided Example of Assigning Nervous System Procedure Codes

To practice skills for assigning codes for the Nervous System, continue with the example from earlier in the chapter about a patient who was seen for a laminotomy and arthrodesis. Follow along in your CPT manual as Angelia Harkey, CPC, assigns codes. Check off each step after you complete it.

▶ First, Angelia confirms the procedures:

❑ bilateral laminotomy with decompression of nerve root and partial facetectomy at L3-L4

❑ right laminotomy with decompression of nerve root, partial facetectomy, and foraminotomy at L4-L5

❑ arthrodesis of L3-L4 and L4-L5

▶ Angelia searches the Index for the Main Term **Hemilaminectomy**.

❑ There are no first-level modifying terms.

❑ She identifies the code range **63020-63044**.

▶ Angelia turns to the Tabular List to select and verify the codes needed for both laminotomies.

❑ She identifies that within this code range there are two standalone codes: **63020** and **63040**. The remaining codes are either indented codes or add-on codes.

❑ She compares the common portion of the code descriptions word for word:

  ▪ **63020 Laminotomy (hemilaminectomy), with decompression of nerve root(s), including partial facetectomy, foraminotomy and/or excision of herniated intervertebral disc;**

  ▪ **63040 Laminotomy (hemilaminectomy), with decompression of nerve root(s), including partial facetectomy, foraminotomy and/or excision of herniated intervertebral disc, reexploration, single interspace;**

❑ She identifies that the only difference between the codes is the last three words of code **63040** that describes **reexploration, single interspace**. She reads the documentation and verifies that the procedure is an initial treatment, not a reexploration.

❑ Code **63020** is the correct parent code, but Angelia needs to locate the indented code that identifies the lumbar region. Code **63030** is the indented code that shares the common descriptor of code **63020** and provides the unique descriptor **1 interspace, lumbar**.

❑ She confirms that the full description of code **63030** accurately describes the primary procedure: **Laminotomy (hemilaminectomy), with decompression of nerve root(s), including partial facetectomy, foraminotomy and/or excision of herniated intervertebral disc; 1 interspace, lumbar**.

▶ Code **63030** reports one lumbar interspace (L3-L4). Angelia must determine how to report the second interspace (L4-L5). She does not know whether she should report **63030** twice or whether there is an add-on code for additional sites.

❑ She reviews the Tabular List and locates add-on code **63035**, which also is indented under the parent code **63020**. Its unique descriptor is **each additional interspace, cervical or lumbar (List separately in addition to code for primary procedure)**.

▶ Angelia checks for instructions in the Tabular List.

❑ She reads the instructional notes following codes **63030** and **63035** in the Tabular List and locates a statement following each code: **(For bilateral procedure, report . . . with modifier 50)**. She refers to the laterality details in the documentation and understands that she should append modifier **-50 Bilateral procedure** to code **63030** and, by extension, modifier **-RT Right side** to code **63035**.

❑ She reads the instructional note that states **(Use 63035 in conjunction with 63020-63030)**. This verifies that she correctly applied the add-on code.

❑ She reads the instructional note that states **(For percutaneous endoscopic approach, see 0274T, 0275T)**. She refers to the documentation to confirm that the procedure approach is *open with endoscopic assistance*, which is different than the percutaneous endoscopic approach mentioned in the instructional note, so the note does not apply.

❑ She cross-references the beginning of category **Posterior Extradural Laminotomy or Laminectomy for Exploration/Decompression of Neural Elements or Excision of Herniated Intervertebral Discs (63001-63051)** and reads the special instructions regarding endoscopically assisted laminotomy. The instructions clarify that endoscopically assisted laminotomy is an open approach that uses endoscopy in addition to direct visualization and confirm that she should not report a percutaneous endoscopy procedure.

❑ Angelia also reads the instructional note that states **(When 63001-63048 are followed by arthrodesis, see 22590-22614)**. This note tells her that she should report an additional code for the arthrodesis procedure that was performed.

❑ She cross-references the beginning of the subheading **Spine and Spinal Cord** and verifies that there are no instructional notes that apply to this case.

▶ Angelia must assign codes for the arthrodesis, as stated in the instructional note. She refers to the code range listed in the note, **22590-22614**.

❑ She observes that the codes are divided by the region of the spine treated and include two standalone codes: one parent code with three indented codes and one add-on code.

❑ She reads the unique descriptor for code parent code **22600 Arthrodesis, posterior or posterolateral technique, single level;**

❑ She locates the indented code description for the lumbar spine, **22612 Arthrodesis, posterior or posterolateral technique, single level; lumbar (with lateral transverse technique, when performed)**. This code accurately describes the first arthrodesis procedure performed. However, because two interspaces were fixated, she needs a second code.

❑ She locates an add-on code that reports the second interspace treated: **22614 Arthrodesis, posterior or posterolateral technique, single level; each additional vertebral segment (List separately in addition to code for primary procedure).**

❏ She reads the instructional notes that appear after the codes. She also reads the special instructions for the subcategory **Posterior, Posterolateral or Lateral Transverse Process Technique**. These instructions provide definitions of vertebral segment and an interspace.

▶ Angelia reviews the procedure codes she has assigned for this case.

❏ **22612** Arthrodesis, posterior or posterolateral technique, single level; lumbar (with lateral transverse technique, when performed)

❏ **22614** Arthrodesis, posterior or posterolateral technique, single level; each additional vertebral segment

❏ **63030** Laminotomy (hemilaminectomy), with decompression of nerve root(s), including partial facetectomy, foraminotomy and/or excision of herniated intervertebral disc; 1 interspace, lumbar

❏ **63035** Laminotomy (hemilaminectomy), with decompression of nerve root(s), including partial facetectomy, foraminotomy and/or excision of herniated intervertebral disc; each additional interspace, cervical or lumbar

▶ Next, Angelia must assign modifiers and determine how to sequence the codes.

CODING PRACTICE

Exercise 42.3 Assigning Codes for Nervous System Procedures

Instructions: Read the mini-medical-record of each patient's encounter. Review the information abstracted in Exercise 42.2 for questions 1–3. For questions 4–6, abstract the case on your own. Assign CPT codes, quantities, and modifiers using the Index and Tabular List. Write the code(s) on the line provided.

1. INPATIENT HOSPITAL   Gender: F   Age: 23

Preprocedure diagnosis: skull fracture with hemorrhage

Procedure: exploratory craniotomy with catheter placement. Created multiple burr holes supratentorially to explore for the source of bleeding; inserted a catheter to close off the hemorrhaging blood vessel.

1 CPT Code _____

2. INPATIENT HOSPITAL   Gender: M   Age: 18

Preprocedure diagnosis: congenital hydrocephalus with a ventricular shunt in place to divert CSF; recently developed headaches and visual disturbances

Procedure: punctured the shunt tube to aspirate the excess CSF

Tip: The Main Term is the anatomic site where the shunt is placed.

1 CPT Code _____

3. INPATIENT HOSPITAL   Gender: F   Age: 87

Preprocedure diagnosis: cerebral meninges adhesions

Procedure: intracranial neuroendoscopy. Created burr hole and introduced neuroendoscope through the trocar. Dissected adhesions. We removed the trocar and connected the ventricular catheter to an external collection bag. Closed and dressed the wound. Patient tolerated procedure well.

1 CPT Code _____

4. EMERGENCY DEPT   Gender: M   Age: 16

Preprocedure diagnosis: injury to hand from broken glass

Procedure: sutured the right ulnar motor nerve

1 CPT Code _____

5. INPATIENT HOSPITAL   Gender: F   Age: 27

Preprocedure diagnosis: depressed skull fracture

Procedure: repair of dura to elevate skull

1 CPT Code _____

6. INPATIENT HOSPITAL   Gender: M   Age: 63

Preprocedure diagnosis: 14-mm arteriosclerotic brain aneurysm in the frontal portion of skull

Procedure: removed the aneurysm by intracranial and cervical occlusion of the carotid artery

1 CPT Code _____

ARRANGING CODES FOR NERVOUS SYSTEM PROCEDURES

Many spinal procedures are grouped into code families with separate parent codes describing the procedure at a single vertebral level in the cervical, thoracic, or lumbar region of the spine. Within some code families an add-on code reports the same procedure at each additional level, but the spinal region is not specified. Surgeons may operate on various combinations of spinal regions and vertebral levels. The National Correct Coding Initiative (NCCI) provides the following instructions for reporting procedures on multiple vertebral segments or multiple interspaces:

- When vertebral levels from different spinal regions are treated, report a parent code for each spinal region treated.
  - *Example*: When both C4 and T3 are treated, report a parent code for the cervical region and a parent code for the thoracic region.

- When multiple procedures from one code family are performed at contiguous vertebral levels, report the parent code for one level and add-on codes for any additional levels within the same family.
  - *Example*: When C3, C4, and C5 are treated, report the parent code for the cervical region and the add-on code times two.

- When the contiguous levels are in two different spinal regions, report the parent code from the first spinal region for the first level and an add-on code for the second level.
  - *Example*: When T12 and L1 are treated, report the parent code for the thoracic region and one add-on code because these segments are contiguous.

Remember that vertebrae are identified singly, such as the C4 or L2 vertebral segment. Interspaces and discs are identified by the vertebrae above and below the space, such as the C4-C5 interspace. Assign only one code for each interspace, even though it is identified using the two adjacent vertebrae.

Modifiers

Among the more commonly used modifiers for Nervous System procedures are those for multiple procedures, laterality, and multiple surgeons.

-51 Multiple Procedures

Append modifier **-51** when more than one procedure is performed during the same operative session by the same surgeon, except for add-on codes. Only one code (**61107**) in the Nervous System subsection is exempt from modifier **-51**, indicated by the symbol ⊘. Do not append modifier **-51** when two procedures are performed, each by a different surgeon.

Laterality

Report laterality for paired nerves or paired anatomic sites, including laminae. Be alert for instructional notes in the Tabular List that direct when to use modifier **-50 Bilateral procedure**. Do not report laterality for procedures on vertebrae or discs.

Multiple Surgeons

Nervous system procedures may involve multiple surgeons, including a surgical team, cosurgeons, or a primary and assistant surgeon. The operative report should identify the name and role of each surgeon. In the workplace you will be coding for a specific surgeon or for all surgeons from a specific practice, but you will not code for surgeons from other practices. When two or more surgeons perform distinct parts of one procedure with one CPT code, assign a modifier to identify the role of the specific surgeon for whom you are coding. The most commonly used modifiers in this situation are

- **-62 Two surgeons**
- **-66 Surgical team**
- **-80 Assistant surgeon**

When two surgeons each perform a different procedure, each with a different CPT code, as may occur with skull base procedures, a modifier is not necessary.

Guided Example of Arranging Nervous System Procedure Codes

To practice skills for arranging codes for procedures of the Nervous System, continue with the example from earlier in the chapter about the patient who was seen for a laminotomy and arthrodesis. Follow along in your CPT manual as Angelia Harkey, CPC, arranges the codes. Check off each step after you complete it.

▶ First, Angelia reviews the procedure codes she has assigned for this case.

❑ **22612 Arthrodesis, posterior or posterolateral technique, single level; lumbar (with lateral transverse technique, when performed)**

❑ **22614 Arthrodesis, posterior or posterolateral technique, single level; each additional vertebral segment**

❑ **63030 Laminotomy (hemilaminectomy), with decompression of nerve root(s), including partial facetectomy, foraminotomy and/or excision of herniated intervertebral disc; 1 interspace, lumbar**

❑ **63035 Laminotomy (hemilaminectomy), with decompression of nerve root(s), including partial facetectomy, foraminotomy and/or excision of herniated intervertebral disc; each additional interspace, cervical or lumbar**

▶ The laminotomy is the primary procedure, so code **63030** is sequenced first, followed by the related add-on code for the second laminotomy, **63035**.

▶ The arthrodesis procedures are secondary, so code **22612** is sequenced next, followed by the related add-on code for the second interspace **22614**.

▶ Angelia examines the need for modifiers. (Refer to Table 30-1 Key Criteria for Abstracting CPT Modifiers or Appendix A in the CPT manual.)

❑ Both of these codes require laterality modifiers. She verifies the procedures in the medical record and confirms that **63030** is a bilateral procedure, so she appends modifier **-50**.

❑ Code **63035** identifies a procedure performed on the right side, so she appends modifier **-RT**. Although the code description specifies cervical or lumbar interspace, there is no CPT modifier used to identify which spinal region is treated.

❑ Arthrodesis procedures are performed on the full interspace, so laterality modifiers are not required.

❑ Because code **22612** is a standalone code and is an additional procedure performed during the same operative session, modifier **-51 Multiple procedures** is required. Use of this modifier is discussed in the special instructions in the subheading **Arthrodesis** that appears before code **22532** in the Tabular List.

❑ Because code **22614** is an add-on code, modifier **-51** is not used.

▶ Angelia finalizes the procedure codes and sequencing for this case:

(1) **63030-50 Laminotomy (hemilaminectomy), with decompression of nerve root(s), including partial facetectomy, foraminotomy and/or excision of herniated intervertebral disc; 1 interspace, lumbar; -50 Bilateral procedure**

(2) **63035-RT Laminotomy (hemilaminectomy), with decompression of nerve root(s), including partial facetectomy, foraminotomy and/or excision of herniated intervertebral disc; each additional interspace, cervical or lumbar; -RT Right side**

(3) **22612-51 Arthrodesis, posterior or posterolateral technique, single level; lumbar (with lateral transverse technique, when performed); -51 Multiple procedures**

(4) **22532 Arthrodesis, posterior or posterolateral technique, single level; each additional vertebral segment**

▶ Angelia also assigns and sequences the ICD-10-CM diagnosis codes that support the need for the service.

(1) **M48.06 Spinal stenosis, lumbar region**

CODING PRACTICE

Exercise 42.4 Arranging Codes for Nervous System Procedures

Instructions: Read the mini-medical-record of each patient's encounter. Review the information abstracted in Exercise 42.2 for questions 1–3. For questions 4–6, abstract the case on your own. Assign CPT codes, quantities, and modifiers using the Index and Tabular List, and arrange the codes in proper sequence. Write the code(s) on the line provided.

1. INPATIENT HOSPITAL   Gender: F   Age: 30

Preprocedure diagnosis: *nerve root compression of the cervical spine*

Procedure: *cervical neck discectomy, anterior approach C3-C4, C4-C5*

2 CPT Codes _____

2. OUTPATIENT SURGERY   Gender: M   Age: 35

Preprocedure diagnosis: *lacerations to the right thumb and index finger*

Procedure: *neurorrhaphy to the right thumb and index finger*

Tip: A digital nerve is one in the finger.

2 CPT Codes _____

3. INPATIENT HOSPITAL   Gender: F   Age: 48

Preprocedure diagnosis: *stenosis C4-C5, foraminal stenosis L5-S1*

Procedure: *right hemilaminectomy at C4-C5, posterior approach; left hemilaminectomy with foraminotomy at L5-S1, posterior approach*

Tip: The two procedures are performed on different spinal regions, so assign separate parent codes.

2 CPT Codes _____

4. INPATIENT HOSPITAL   Gender: M   Age: 84

Preprocedure diagnosis: *return to the operating room because of a subdural hematoma following surgery I performed yesterday*

Procedure: *craniotomy to evacuate the hematoma; used a skull trephine craniotome to access the hematoma, then, under direct visualization, suctioned out the hematoma*

Tip: Use the Main Term **Craniotomy**. Append a modifier for the return to the operating room.

1 CPT Code _____

(continued)

CODING PRACTICE (continued)

5. INPATIENT HOSPITAL   Gender: M   Age: 68

Preprocedure diagnosis: *primary malignant neoplasm of the cranial fossa*

Procedure: Surgeon A: *resection of the posterior cranial fossa, extradural; removed entire tumor*

Surgeon B: *performed the transtemporal approach*

Tip: Code for both surgeons.

Surgeon A: 1 CPT C ode _____

Surgeon B: 1 CPT Code _____

6. OUTPATIENT SURGERY   Gender: M   Age: 28

Preprocedure diagnosis: *lumbar back pain*

Procedure: *fluoroscopic-guided destruction of paravertebral facet joint nerves bilaterally at L2 and L3 with use of a neurolytic agent*

Tip: Read the instructional notes in the Tabular List regarding the use of a modifier.

2 CPT Codes _____

E/M CODING FOR NEUROLOGY

The *1997 Documentation Guidelines for Evaluation and Management Services* (1997 DG), published by CMS, provides requirements for each level of a neurological E/M examination (■ Figure 42-9). Neurologists are not limited to using the guidelines for a neurology examination only. They can also use guidelines for a general multiorgan system examination, or any other single organ system examination, based on what is most advantageous for a specific encounter. However, physicians cannot combine elements from more than one type of examination for a given encounter. The neurological examination guidelines typically provide the best results when a detailed neurological examination is performed.

To determine the appropriate E/M code, coders must review the documentation in detail and identify the specific elements documented.

- To translate the documentation into the E/M requirements for the history, refer back to Chapter 31, Evaluation and Management Services (99201-99499), Tables 31-7 to 31-10, or the 1997 DG.

- To determine the requirements for an examination, refer to Figure 42-9 or to the single organ system examination for neurology in the 1997 DG.

- To determine the levels for medical decision making (MDM), refer to Chapter 31, Table 31-12, and the Table of Risk in the 1997 DG.

Guided Example of E/M Coding for Neurology

Refer to the neurology encounter (■ Figure 42-10) to practice skills for abstracting and assigning E/M codes. Follow along as fictitious coder Angelia Harkey, CPC, abstracts the procedure. Check off each step after you complete it.

▶ First, Angelia needs to establish the category of service so she can determine the information needed to abstract and assign the code.

❑ *What is the setting?* Physician office

❑ *What is the type of service?* This is a consultation because the patient was referred by her primary care physician (PCP) and a report of the visit is sent to the PCP.

❑ *What is the code range?* Angelia refers to the CPT Index and looks up the Main Term **Evaluation and Management** and the subterm **Consultation**. The code range listed is **99241-99255**.

❑ *How many key components are required?* Angelia refers to the code range in the Tabular List and locates the category **Office or Other Outpatient Consultations, New or Established Patient**. She reads the description of the first code, which states **requires these 3 key components**. All codes in the category have the same requirements for key components. This tells her that all three key components must meet or exceed the levels listed in the code (3/3).

▶ Next, Angelia identifies the level of history.

❑ *What is the level of HPI?* The HPI is **extended** because four elements are documented.

❑ *What is the level of ROS?* The ROS is **complete** because 10 systems were examined. Although the specific systems have not been documented, the documentation provides adequate information to support an extended ROS. However, it would best for the physician to specify the exact systems reviewed.

❑ *What is the level of PFSH?* The PFSH is **complete** because three elements are documented.

❑ *Based on these factors, what is the overall level of history?* The level of history is **comprehensive** because all three factors (HPI, ROS, and PFSH) meet the criteria for a comprehensive history.

▶ Angelia refers to the neurological examination in the 1997 DG (Figure 42-9) to abstract information needed to determine the level of the examination.

System/Body Area	Elements of Neurological Examination
Constitutional	❑ Measurement of any **three** of the following seven **vital** signs: • 1) sitting or standing blood pressure, • 2) supine blood pressure, • 3) pulse rate and regularity, • 4) respiration, • 5) temperature, • 6) height, • 7) weight (May be measured and recorded by ancillary staff) ❑ General **appearance** of patient (eg, development, nutrition, body habitus, deformities, attention to grooming)
Eyes	❑ Ophthalmoscopic examination of **optic discs** (eg, size, C/D ratio, appearance) and posterior segments (eg, vessel changes, exudates, hemorrhages
Cardiovascular	❑ Examination of **carotid arteries** (eg, pulse amplitude, bruits) ❑ **Auscultation** of heart with notation of abnormal sounds and murmurs ❑ Examination of **peripheral vascular system** by observation (eg, swelling, varicosities) and palpation (eg, pulses, temperature, edema, tenderness)
Musculoskeletal	❑ Examination of **gait** and **station** ❑ Inspection and/or palpation of **digits** and **nails** (eg, clubbing, cyanosis, inflammatory conditions, petechiae, ischemia, infections, nodes) Assessment of motor function including: ❑ Muscle strength in upper and lower extremities ❑ Muscle tone in upper and lower extremities (eg, flaccid, cog wheel, spastic) with notation of any atrophy or abnormal movements (eg, fasciculation, tardive dyskinesia)
Extremities	[See musculoskeletal]
Neurological	Evaluation of higher integrative functions including: ❑ **Orientation** to time, place and person ❑ Recent and remote **memory** ❑ **Attention span** and concentration ❑ **Language** (eg, naming objects, repeating phrases, spontaneous speech) ❑ **Fund of knowledge** (eg, awareness of current events, past history, vocabulary) Test the following cranial nerves: ❑ **2nd** cranial nerve (eg, visual acuity, visual fields, fundi) ❑ **3rd, 4th** and **6th** cranial nerves (eg, pupils, eye movements) ❑ **5th** cranial nerve (eg, facial sensation, corneal reflexes) ❑ **7th** cranial nerve (eg, facial symmetry, strength) ❑ **8th** cranial nerve (eg, hearing with tuning fork, whispered voice and/or finger rub) ❑ **9th** cranial nerve (eg, spontaneous or reflex palate movement) ❑ **11th** cranial nerve (eg, shoulder shrug strength) ❑ **12th** cranial nerve (eg, tongue protrusion) ❑ Examination of **sensation** (eg, by touch, pin, vibration, proprioception) ❑ Examination of **deep tendon reflexes** in upper and lower extremities with notation of pathological reflexes (eg, Babinski) ❑ Test **coordination** (eg, finger/nose, heel/knee/shin, rapid alternating movements in the upper and lower extremities, evaluation of fine motor coordination in young children)

Total # Bullets Performed and Documented →	☐	# of ❑ Elements Performed and Documented	Level of Examination
		1–5	Problem focused
		6–11	Expanded problem focused
		12+	Detailed
		ALL	Comprehensive (Perform **all** elements identified by a bullet; document **every** element in each box with a shaded border and at least **one** element in each box with an unshaded border.)

Figure 42-9 ■ 1997 DG for Neurological Examination. *Source: Centers for Medicare and Medicaid Services, 1997 Documentation Guidelines for Evaluation and Management Services (with formatting adjustments).*

NEUROLOGY ENCOUNTER

HISTORY:
Comprehensive

REASON FOR CONSULTATION: New-onset seizure.

Chief complaint (CC)

HISTORY OF PRESENT ILLNESS: The patient is a 3 year old female seen in my office on referral by her primary care physician because of new-onset seizure. She has a history of known febrile seizures and was placed on Keppra oral solution at 150 mg b.i.d. to help prevent febrile seizures. Although this has been a very successful treatment in terms of her febrile seizure control, she is now having occasional brief periods of pauses and staring, where she becomes unresponsive, but does not lose her postural tone. The typical spell according to father lasts anywhere from 10 to 15 seconds, mother says 3 to 4 minutes, which likely means probably somewhere in the 30- to 40-second period of time. Mom did note that an episode had happened outside of a store recently, was associated with some perioral cyanosis, but there has never been a convulsive activity noted. There have been no recent changes in her Keppra dosing and she is currently only at 20 mg/kg per day, which is overall a low dose for her.

Setting & patient type

HPI: Extended (4+)

ROS: Complete (10+)

PAST MEDICAL HISTORY: Born at 36 weeks' gestation by C-section delivery at 8 pounds 3 ounces. She does have a history of febrile seizures and what parents reported as an abdominal migraine, but on further questioning, it appears to be more of a food intolerance issue.

PAST SURGICAL HISTORY: She has undergone no surgical procedures.

FAMILY MEDICAL HISTORY: There is a strong history of epilepsy on the maternal side of family including mom with some nonconvulsive seizure during childhood and additional seizures in maternal great grandmother and a maternal great aunt. There is no other significant neurological history on the paternal side of the family.

PFSH: Complete (3)

SOCIAL HISTORY: Currently lives with both parents and two siblings. She is at home full time and does not attend day care.

REVIEW OF SYSTEMS: Clear review of 10 systems are taken and revealed no additional findings other than those mentioned in the history of present illness.

EXAMINATION:
Detailed

PHYSICAL EXAMINATION:

(12 elements in at least 2 organ systems/body areas)

Vital Signs: Weight was 15.6 kg. She was afebrile. Other vital signs were stable and within normal ranges for her age as per the medical record.

General: She was awake, alert, and oriented. She was in no acute distress, only slightly flustered when trying to place the EEG leads.

HEENT: Showed normocephalic and atraumatic head. Her conjunctivae were nonicteric and sclerae were clear. Her eye movements were conjugate in nature. Her tongue and mucous membranes were moist.

Neck: Trachea appeared to be in the midline.

Chest: Clear to auscultation bilaterally without crackles, wheezes or rhonchi.

Cardiovascular: Showed a normal sinus rhythm without murmur.

Abdomen: Showed soft, nontender, and nondistended, with good bowel sounds. There was no hepatomegaly or splenomegaly, or other masses noted on examination.

Extremities: Showed IV placement in the right upper extremity with appropriate restraints from the IV. There was no evidence of clubbing, cyanosis or edema throughout. She had no functional deformities in any of her peripheral limbs.

Neurological: From neurological standpoint, her cranial nerves were grossly intact throughout. Her strength was good in the bilateral upper and lower extremities without any distal to proximal variation. Her overall resting tone was normal. Sensory examination was grossly intact to light touch throughout the upper and lower extremities. Reflexes were 1+ in bilateral patella. Toes were downgoing bilaterally. Coordination showed accurate striking ability and good rapid alternating movements. Gait examination was deferred at this time due to EEG lead placement.

MEDICAL DECISION MAKING: Moderate Complexity

ASSESSMENT: A 3 year old female with history of febrile seizures, now with concern for spells of unclear etiology, but somewhat concerning for partial complex seizures and to a slightly lesser extent nonconvulsive generalized seizures.

MDM Risk: Uncertain diagnosis, unclear prognosis (Moderate Risk)

RECOMMENDATIONS

1. For now, we will go ahead and try to capture EEG as long as she tolerates it; however, if she would require sedation, I would defer the EEG until further adjustments to seizure medications are made and we will see her response to these medications.

MDM Data: Ordering or reviewing diagnostic data (Straightforward Data)

2. As per the above, I will increase her Keppra to 300 mg p.o. b.i.d. bringing her to a total daily dose of just under 40 mg/kg per day. If further spells are noted, we may increase upwards again to around 4.5 to 5 mL each day.

3. I do not feel like any specific imaging needs to be done at this time until we see her response to the medication and review her EEG findings. EEG, hopefully, will be able to be reviewed first thing tomorrow morning; however, I would not delay discharging the patient to wait on the EEG results. The patient has been discharged and we will contact the family as an outpatient.

MDM Management: New presenting problem, with workup (High Management Options)

4. The patient will need followup arrangement with me in 5 to 6 weeks' time, so we may recheck and see how she is doing and arrange for further followup then.

5. Report on the above has been sent to her primary care provider.

KEY: HPI History of the present illness   ROS Review of systems
         PFSH Past, family, and social history   MDM Medical decision making

Figure 42-10 ■ Neurology Encounter. *Source:* © *PB Resources, Inc. Used with permission.*

❏ *What is the level of examination?* The level of examination is **detailed**. Although 18 elements of the examination are documented, a comprehensive examination requires that all bulleted items within the shaded borders be documented, which they are not. Therefore the examination meets the requirement of 12 or more bulleted items for the detailed level.

▶ Angelia determines the level of medical decision making. (Refer to Table 31-12 Medical Decision Making Levels.)

❏ *What is the level of complexity of the number of diagnoses or management options based on the presenting problem?* The level is **moderate** because there is a new presenting problem, with workup.

❏ *What is the amount and/or complexity of data to be reviewed?* The level is **straightforward** because the physician reviewed the patient's medical record and ordered tests.

❏ *What is the level of risk of significant complications, morbidity, and/or mortality?* Angelia reviews each column in the Table of Risk in the 1997 DG and determines that the level of risk is **moderate**. The patient presents with an undiagnosed new problem with uncertain prognosis illness (Moderate), an EEG is ordered (Minimal), and prescription drug management is provided (Moderate). The single highest element in the Table of Risk determines the overall risk. The columns **Presenting Problem** and **Management Options Selected** both are the same level (Moderate).

❏ *Based on these factors, what is the overall level of medical decision making?* The medical decision making is **moderate complexity**. At least two of the three MDM factors are required to qualify for a specific level of MDM. Two of the three MDM factors meet moderate decision making.

Now Angelia is ready to assign the code for the neurology encounter. The exercise that follows guides you through additional abstracting skills and allows you to assign the correct code.

CODING PRACTICE

Exercise 42.5   Evaluation and Management Coding for Neurology

Instructions: Refer to the *1997 Documentation Guidelines for Evaluation and Management Services* (available at www.cms.gov) or Chapter 31 Evaluation and Management Services (99201-99499) (Tables 31-7 to 31-12) in this text. Answer the following questions about the Neurology Encounter (Figure 42-10).

1. a. Which elements of the HPI are documented? Circle all that apply. Location, Quality, Severity, Duration, Timing, Context, Modifying factors, Associated signs and symptoms

   b. How many elements are documented? _____

   c. What is the level of HPI? _____

2. a. Which systems are reviewed in the ROS? Circle all that apply. Constitutional, Allergic/immunologic, CV, Endocrine, ENT/M, Eyes, GI, GU, Hemic/lymphatic, MS, Neurologic, Psychiatric, Respiratory, Skin/breast

   b. How many systems are documented? _____

   c. What is the level of ROS? _____

3. a. Which PFSH elements are documented? Circle all that apply. Past medical, Family, Social

   b. What is the level of PFSH? _____

   c. What is the overall level of history? (The lowest history factor—HPI, ROS, or PFSH—determines the level of history.) _____

4. Refer to Figure 42-9 (1997 DG for Neurological Examination).

   a. Which bulleted items are documented for the examination? (Check off the items documented.)

   b. How many bulleted items are documented? _____

   c. What is the level of the examination? _____

5. Refer to Table 31-12 Medical Decision Making Levels or the 1997 DG.

   a. What is the MDM level for the number of diagnoses or management options? _____

   b. What is the MDM level for the amount and/or complexity of data to be reviewed? _____

   c. Refer to the Table of Risk in the 1997 DG. Which elements of risk are documented for each risk factor?

      1. Presenting problem: _____

      2. Diagnostic procedures ordered: _____

      3. Management options selected: _____

   d. What is the level of risk? (The highest of the three risk factors determines the overall level of risk.) _____

   e. What is the overall level of MDM? (2/3 MDM factors are needed to determine the overall level.) _____

6. a. What is the setting? _____

   b. What is the patient (or service) type? _____

(continued)

CODING PRACTICE (continued)

c. What is the code range? _____

d. How many key components are required? _____

e. What is the level of history? _____

f. What is the level of examination? _____

g. What is the level of medical decision making?

_____

h. What is the correct code? _____

i. Why can a code for a higher-level visit not be assigned?

_____

7. Abstract, assign, and arrange (sequence) the diagnosis code(s) that support the E/M code.

3 ICD-10-CM Code(s) _____

CHAPTER SUMMARY

In this chapter you learned that:

- Neurological surgery, or neurosurgery, is a medical discipline and surgical specialty that provides care for patients in the treatment of pain or disease processes that affect the nervous system.

- The CPT subsection **Nervous System (61000-64999)** contains three subheadings that are divided by anatomic site.

- When abstracting for nervous system procedures, coders must pay special attention to the anatomic approach used to access the surgical site because distinct codes often identify each approach.

- Coders should pay special attention to assigning codes for basilar skull procedures and laminectomies.

- Many spinal procedures are grouped into code families with separate parent codes describing the procedure at a single vertebral level in the cervical, thoracic, or lumbar region of the spine.

- The *1997 Documentation Guidelines for Evaluation and Management Services* (1997 DG), published by CMS, provides requirements for each level of a neurologic E/M examination.

- Special instructions at the beginning of many categories provide definitions and coding guidelines. Instructional notes appear throughout the Tabular List to alert coders to important coding rules and cross-references.

CONCEPT QUIZ

Take a moment to look back at the Nervous System and solidify your skills. Try to answer the questions from memory first, then refer to the discussion in this chapter if you need a little extra help.

Completion

Instructions: Write the term that answers each question based on the information you learned in this chapter. Choose from the list below. Some choices may be used more than once and some choices may not be used at all.

anterior

aphagia

aphasia

ataxia

chemodenervation

craniostomy

facets

hemispherectomy

laminae

nerve block

neurostimulator

posterior

posterolateral

stereotactic

subdural

1. _____ is the medical term for lack of coordination.

2. Intractable pain can be alleviated by _____ procedures such as implantation of electrodes under the skin.

3. _____ refers to in-between membranes of the dura mater.

4. An approach that is from the front is called a(n) _____ approach.

5. Brain tumors are sometimes treated with _____ radiosurgery to target lesions in difficult-to-treat areas.

6. Injection of a substance into a muscle group or glands to stop overactivity is called _____.

7. Loss of the ability to swallow is called _____.

8. Each vertebra has two _____, one on either side of the midline.

9. In a(n) _____, a physician drills or cuts into the skull.

10. A(n) _____ approach is from the side, toward the back.

Multiple Choice

Instructions: Circle the letter of the best answer to each question based on the information you learned in this chapter.

1. How does CPT arrange definitive procedures in the range of 61600-61616?
   A. Alphabetically
   B. Numerically
   C. Anatomically
   D. By complexity

2. What is the gelatinous substance that comprises the center of a disc and provides cushioning?
   A. Nucleus pulposus
   B. Annulus fibrosus
   C. Lamina
   D. Spinal cord

3. Which of the following is a treatment for epilepsy?
   A. Nerve block
   B. Epidural pump
   C. Tractotomy
   D. Hemispherectomy

4. What is the operative approach through the far lateral side of the jaw called?
   A. Transcochlear
   B. Transcondylar
   C. Transcranial
   D. Transpedicular

5. Which of the following is a surgical approach?
   A. Endoscopic
   B. Anterior
   C. Posterior
   D. Extradural

6. What procedure collects fluid through fontanelles?
   A. Ventricular puncture
   B. Subdural tap
   C. Cisternal puncture
   D. Puncture of shunt tubing or reservoir

7. In what type of procedure do neurosurgeons work with interventional radiologists to coordinate a patient's treatment and care?
   A. Musculoskeletal surgery
   B. Spinal fusion instrumentation
   C. Restorative surgery
   D. Endovascular surgery

8. Which of the following is an anatomic approach?
   A. Open
   B. Subdural
   C. Percutaneous
   D. Endoscopic

9. What part of the nervous system consists of the brain and spinal cord?
   A. Somatic
   B. Autonomic
   C. Central
   D. Peripheral

10. According to the NCCI, what should a coder do when vertebral levels from different spinal regions are treated?
    A. Report a parent code for each spinal region treated.
    B. Report the parent code for one level and add-on codes for any additional levels within the same family.
    C. Report the parent code from the first spinal region for the first level and an add-on code for the second level.
    D. Report the parent code with modifier -51, multiple procedures, appended.

CODING CHALLENGE

Instructions: Read the mini-medical-record of each patient's encounter, then abstract, assign, and arrange ICD-10-CM diagnosis codes and CPT procedure codes using the appropriate Index and Tabular List. Assign quantities and modifiers where needed. Write the code(s) on the line provided.

1. OUTPATIENT SURGERY   Gender: F   Age: 32

Preoperative diagnosis: left carpal tunnel syndrome

Procedure: release of left carpal tunnel under general anesthesia. The median nerve was freed up along the bands from the ligament. Subcutaneous tissue and skin were closed and a dressing applied.

1 ICD-10-CM Code _____

1 CPT Code _____

2. OUTPATIENT SURGERY   Gender: M   Age: 45

Preoperative diagnosis: C6 radiculopathy confirmed by EMG

Procedure: posterior cervical laminoforaminotomy. Decompressive hemilaminectomy performed, with the neural elements freely mobile. The wound was irrigated and closed with sutures.

1 ICD-10-CM Code _____

1 CPT Code _____

(continued)

(continued from page 833)

3. HOSPITAL INPATIENT Gender: F Age: 29

Preoperative diagnosis: chronic lumbar pain due to displaced disc at L3-4, which resulted from a back injury two years ago

Procedure: percutaneous neurostimulator implant. The spinal cord stimulator electrode was placed though the spinal cord stimulator needle into the epidural space and advanced under fluoroscopic guidance. Multiple electrode settings were applied with excellent stimulation.

Tip: Review OGCR I.C.6.b.1)(a) and (b)(ii) for diagnosis sequencing instructions.

2 ICD-10-CM Codes _____

1 CPT Code _____

4. OUTPATIENT HOSPITAL Gender: F Age: 34

Preoperative diagnosis: right occipital arteriovenous malformation

Procedure: CT-guided frameless stereotactic radiosurgery for the right occipital arteriovenous malformation using dynamic tracking. The patient underwent stereotactic radiosurgery to deliver 20 Gy to the AVM margin.

Plan: MRI scan in 6 months

1 ICD-10-CM Code _____

1 CPT Code _____

5. INPATIENT HOSPITAL Gender: F Age: 81

Preoperative diagnosis: acute subdural hematoma 100%, right, with herniation syndrome. This procedure is being done as a life-saving emergency procedure

Procedure: right frontotemporoparietal craniotomy, evacuation of acute subdural hematoma. A single burr hole was made at the frontoparietal junction. The subdural hematoma was evacuated and while we were closing the dura the patient went into cardiac arrest and could not be resuscitated.

Postoperative diagnosis: pronounced dead in the operating room

2 ICD-10-CM Codes _____

1 CPT Code _____

6. OFFICE Gender: F Age: 47

Preoperative diagnosis: traumatic complete amputation of the right arm at the elbow six months ago. The stump has healed well. Seen today for relief of pain. Here for a lumbar sympathetic block to manage phantom limb pain.

Procedure: lumbar sympathetic block injection at L3. After locating the L3 spinous process, anesthetic was slowly injected. Patient tolerated procedure well and was sent home in good condition.

1 ICD-10-CM Code _____

1 CPT Code _____

7. INPATIENT HOSPITAL Gender: M Age: 9

Preoperative diagnosis: malfunction of ventriculoatrial shunt with recurring headaches, problems with balance, poor coordination, gait disturbances

Procedure: endoscopic ventriculoatrial shunt irrigation. Proximal shunt was partially obstructed with debris at the lumen. Debris was removed and shunt flushed normally, with no need to replace. Wound closed and sterile dressing applied. Patient was transferred to ICU in stable condition.

1 ICD-10-CM Code _____

2 CPT Codes _____

8. OUTPATIENT SURGERY Gender: F Age: 18

Preoperative diagnosis: possible symptomatic hydrocephalus; patient has been followed in the office for 6 months complaining of headaches, now with ataxic gait.

Procedure: placement of lumbar drain for CSF drainage under regional anesthesia. Tuohy needle inserted at the L4-L5 interspace. Catheter was inserted through the needle, and 12 mL of CSF was drained. Catheter was connected to a drainage system, which we will leave in place for the next 2–3 days to continue drainage.

1 ICD-10-CM Code _____

1 CPT Code _____

9. INPATIENT HOSPITAL   Gender: M   Age: 59

Preoperative diagnosis: admitted from the ED due to laceration of superficial branch of the lateral plantar nerve and flexor digiti minimi brevis tendon, left foot. Loss of sensation across the side of the foot, with obvious open injury. Taken immediately to the OR for repair. Of note, the patient takes warfarin for prophylaxis due to atrial fib.

Procedure: A 2-cm piece of sural nerve was harvested to serve as graft to the proximal and distal ends of the lateral plantar nerve. Following this the tendon was repaired and the wound closed. Patient was admitted for overnight observation.

3 ICD-10-CM Codes _____

_____

2 CPT Codes _____

10. OUTPATIENT SURGERY   Gender: M   Age: 56

Preoperative diagnosis: recurrent intractable low back and left lower extremity pain following L4-L5 discectomy three months ago. No radiculopathy noted. MRI showed epidural fibrosis with lower spinal nerve root compression as the cause of patient's pain.

Procedure: under IV sedation using an operating microscope, I performed a left L4-L5 transforaminal neuroplasty with nerve root decompression and lysis of adhesions. Procedure was well tolerated.

Plan: discharge home and see in the office in two weeks

Tip: Code the use of the operating microscope as a separate procedure. Search the Index for the Main Term *Operating Microscope*.

2 ICD-10-CM Codes _____

2 CPT Codes _____

KEEP ON CODING

Instructions: Read the procedural statement, then use the appropriate Index and Tabular List to assign CPT procedure codes, quantities, and modifiers. Write the code(s) on the line provided.

1. Injection of lidocaine, brachial plexus: CPT Code(s) _____

2. Decompression craniectomy for treatment of intracranial hypertension: CPT Code(s) _____

3. Neuroplasty of the right ring finger using operating microscope: CPT Code(s) _____

4. Excision of neuroma of peripheral nerve of left foot: CPT Code(s) _____

5. Repair of 6-cm myelomeningocele: CPT Code(s) _____

6. Laminectomy and excision of intradural lumbar lesion: CPT Code(s) _____

7. Suture repair of posterior tibial nerve: CPT Code(s) _____

8. Sciatic neuroplasty, left leg: CPT Code(s) _____

9. Ventriculoperitoneal shunt procedure: CPT Code(s) _____

10. Suture of digital nerves to the right thumb and second finger: CPT Code(s) _____

11. Therapeutic lumbar spinal tap for drainage of fluid: CPT Code(s) _____

12. Burr holes for drainage of subdural hematoma: CPT Code(s) _____

13. Stellate ganglion block: CPT Code(s) _____

14. Removal of intrathecal infusion pump: CPT Code(s) _____

15. Lumbar laminectomy for decompression with foraminotomies L3-L4, L4-L5, L5-S1 microtechniques; repair of CSF fistula, microtechniques L5-S1, application of DuraSeal: CPT Code(s) _____

16. Endoscopy-assisted transsphenoidal exploration and radical excision of pituitary adenoma: CPT Code(s) _____

17. Left and right frontal craniotomy for placement of deep-brain stimulator electrode: CPT Code(s) _____

18. Subcutaneous ulnar nerve transposition, at elbow: CPT Code(s) _____

19. Neuroendoscopic placement of left ventriculostomy catheter via twist drill: CPT Code(s) _____

20. Percutaneous balloon angioplasty, basilar artery: CPT Code(s) _____

21. Anastomosis of the facial-phrenic nerves: CPT Code(s) _____

22. Craniotomy for evacuation of cerebral hematoma : CPT Code(s) _____

23. Stereotactic biopsy of lesion spinal cord at T3: CPT Code(s) _____

24. Bifrontal cranioplasty, 11-cm defect: CPT Code(s) _____

25. C4-C5, C5-C6 anterior cervical discectomy: CPT Code(s) _____

Chapter 43

Eye and Ocular Adnexa Procedures (65091-68899)

Chapter Outline

- **Eye Procedure Basics**
- **Coding Overview of Eye Procedures**
- **Abstracting Eye Procedures**
- **Assigning Codes for Eye Procedures**
- **Arranging Codes for Eye Procedures**
- **E/M Coding for Ophthalmology**

Learning Objectives

After completing this chapter, you should have the skills to:

43.1 Spell and define the key words, medical terms, and abbreviations related to eye and ocular adnexa procedures.

43.2 Discuss the types of eye and ocular adnexa procedures.

43.3 Identify the main characteristics of coding for the Eye and Ocular Adnexa.

43.4 Abstract procedural information from the medical record for coding the Eye and Ocular Adnexa.

43.5 Assign codes for Eye and Ocular Adnexa procedures.

43.6 Arrange codes for Eye and Ocular Adnexa procedures.

43.7 Code evaluation and management services for ophthalmology.

43.8 Discuss the CPT coding guidelines related to the Eye and Ocular Adnexa.

Key Terms and Abbreviations

intraocular lens (IOL)
intraocular pressure (IOP)
OD
operating microscope
OS
OU

In addition to the key terms listed here, students should know the terms defined within tables in this chapter.

For updates and corrections, visit our student resource site at

www.pearsonhighered.com/healthprofessionsresources

INTRODUCTION

Big gifts sometimes come in small packages. The eye is a small package but contains complex working mechanisms plus muscles, nerves, and blood vessels. Coding eye procedures requires knowledge of anatomic sites and terminology not encountered in other organ systems. In this chapter you will learn about the unique aspects of coding for procedures on the eye and ocular adnexa.

EYE PROCEDURE BASICS

Ophthalmology is the branch of medicine that studies and treats diseases of the eye. Ophthalmologists are MDs who provide medical evaluation of eye conditions and perform surgery to correct eye problems. Subspecialties of ophthalmology are cornea and external disease, glaucoma, neuro-ophthalmology, ophthalmic pathology, ophthalmic plastic surgery, pediatric ophthalmology, and vitreoretinal diseases. Cornea ophthalmologists might be referred to as specializing in the front of the eye and vitreoretinal ophthalmologists might be referred to as specializing in the back of the eye. Neurologists treat diseases of the ocular nerves and orthopedic surgeons might treat disorders of the surrounding bones, such as fracture of the ocular orbit. Optometrists conduct vision testing; opticians fit patients for corrective lenses; and ocularists fit patients with eye prostheses.

Figure 19-1 depicts the internal structures of the eye. Chapter 19 of this text provides additional information on the anatomy, diseases, and conditions of the eye. Refer to ■ TABLE 43-1 for a refresher on how to build medical terms related to the eye.

CODING CAUTION

Be alert for medical terms that are spelled similarly and have different meanings.

trichiasis (*turning inward of the eyelashes*) and **trichinosis** (a *disease caused by trichinae parasites*)

pupil (*the opening in the iris that dilates and constricts*) and **papilla** (*a small vascular protrusion of connective tissue or skin*)

retinal (*pertaining to the retina*) and **renal** (*pertaining to the kidney*)

Procedures of the Eye and Ocular Adnexa

Procedures commonly performed on the Eye and Ocular Adnexa are summarized in ■ TABLE 43-2. In particular, coders need to understand the various types of keratoplasty (*corneal repair or transplant*) (■ TABLE 43-3). Physicians transplant corneas for patients whose corneas are damaged by trauma or disease that results in corneal scarring or corneal edema that causes partial or complete blindness. The corneal endothelium pumps fluid from the cornea, resulting in clear vision. Patients with corneal edema have corneas that are unable to pump fluid, and the fluid accumulates on the cornea, causing hazy, white, cloudy, or smoky vision.

A corneal transplant, also called a cornea graft, is removal of the damaged or diseased cornea and replacement with a cadaveric cornea. Penetrating keratoplasty (PKP) is removal of the entire cornea and transplantation of a full-thickness cornea. Lamellar keratoplasty is a partial-thickness transplant involving a graft of only specific corneal layers. PKP, which involves suturing the entire cornea in place, has been the standard corneal transplant for many years. Recovery from PKP is a long process, and it can take several months to two years for a patient to fully recover visually and completely heal from the procedure.

A newer corneal transplant procedure, called Descemet's stripping endothelial keratoplasty (DSEK), is replacing PKP. It involves stripping Descemet's membrane and removing only the corneal endothelium layer, replacing it with a cadaveric endothelium. In DSEK surgery, the physician uses an air bubble, instead of sutures, to hold the new corneal cells in place. Patients experience a much shorter recovery time with improved vision relatively quickly.

This section provides a general reference to help understand the most common eye procedures. Remember to keep standard reference books handy in case you get stuck.

Table 43-1   ■   **EXAMPLE OF CONSTRUCTING MEDICAL TERMS FOR EYE PROCEDURES**

Combining Form	Suffix	Complete Medical Term
kerat/o (*cornea*)		**kerato + plasty** (*repair of the cornea*)
		irido + plasty (*repair of the iris*)
		conjunctivo + plasty (*repair of the conjunctiva*)
irid/o (*iris*)	**-plasty** (*repair*) **-ectomy** (*excision*)	**kerat + ectomy** (*excision of the cornea*)
		irid + ectomy (*excision of the iris*)
		conjunctiv + ectomy (*excision of the conjunctiva*)
conjunctiv/o (*conjunctiva*)		

Source: © PB Resources, Inc. Used with permission.

CODING PRACTICE

Exercise 43.1 Eye Procedure Basics

Instructions: Use your medical terminology skills and resources to define the following procedures related to the Eye and Ocular Adnexa, then identify the code(s) or code range listed in the CPT Index. Follow these steps:

- Use slash marks "/" to break down the underlined term into its root(s) and suffix.
- Define the meaning of the underlined word based on the meaning of each word part.
- Use the entire phrase to identify the code or code range shown in the CPT Index.
- Do not assign laterality in this exercise.

Example: retinopathy, treatment, cryotherapy

    retino/pathy   Meaning *disease of the retina*   CPT Code *67229*

1. vitrectomy, with retinal prosthesis placement   Meaning _____   CPT Code _____
2. orbitotomy, with removal of foreign body   Meaning _____   CPT Code _____
3. tarsorrhaphy   Meaning _____   CPT Code _____
4. trabeculotomy, ab externo   Meaning _____   CPT Code _____
5. keratoprosthesis   Meaning _____   CPT Code _____
6. canthoplasty   Meaning _____   CPT Code _____
7. pupillometry   Meaning _____   CPT Code _____
8. dacryoadenectomy, total   Meaning _____   CPT Code _____
9. conjunctivorhinostomy, with tube   Meaning _____   CPT Code _____
10. blepharoptosis, repair   Meaning _____   CPT Code _____

CODING OVERVIEW OF EYE PROCEDURES

The CPT section/subsection **Eye and Ocular Adnexa (65091-68899)** contains five subheadings that are divided by anatomic site (■ TABLE 43-4). Within each subheading, codes are further divided by more specific anatomic sites and the type of procedure, such as incision, excision, repair, destruction, and so on. Review the subheading and category names and code ranges listed in the Eye and Ocular Adnexa subsection to become familiar with the content and organization. Some editions of the CPT manual provide summary list of the subheading and categories at the beginning of the Eye and Ocular Adnexa subsection, which also displays an asterisk (*) next to categories that contain special coding instructions.

This CPT subsection includes invasive, minimally invasive, and noninvasive surgical procedures on the eye and ocular adnexa.

Table 43-4 ■ **EYE AND OCULAR ADNEXA SUBHEADINGS**

Subheading	Code Range
Eyeball	65091-65290
Anterior Segment	65400-66999
Posterior Segment	67005-67299
Ocular Adnexa	67311-67999
Conjunctiva	68020-68899

Codes for diagnostic tests on the eye appear in the Medicine section. CPT codes in the Eye and Ocular Adnexa subsection must be supported by diagnosis codes to justify the medical necessity of the procedure. Codes for eye procedures are frequently supported by diagnosis codes from ICD-10-CM **Chapter 7 Diseases of the Eye and Adnexa (H00-H59)**, as well as neoplasms, symptoms and signs, and injuries (■ TABLE 43-5). These are the codes used most commonly to support procedures on the eye; however, diagnosis codes from any ICD-10-CM chapter are permissible.

CPT guidelines for the Surgery section apply to the Eye and Ocular Adnexa.

Special instructions identify services that are bundled with certain codes and also identify codes that should and should not be reported together. Subcategories with special instructions include the following:

- **Anterior Segment, Cornea, Keratoplasty (65710-65757)**
- **Anterior Segment, Cornea, Other Procedures (65760-65782)**
- **Posterior Segment, Retina or Choroid, Prophylaxis (67141-67145)**
- **Posterior Segment, Retina or Choroid, Destruction (67208-67229)**
- **Ocular Adnexa, Eyelids, Excision, Destruction (67800-67850)**
- **Ocular Adnexa, Eyelids, Excision, Reconstruction (67930-67975)**

Table 43-5 ■ LOCATING ICD-10-CM AND ADDITIONAL CPT CODES FOR THE EYE

Type of Code	Codes
ICD-10-CM Eye-Related Codes	
Eye and ocular adnexa conditions	H00-H59
Neoplasms	C69, D09, D31
Symptoms and signs	Not applicable. Most eye signs and symptoms are classified in H00-H59.
Injuries	S00-S09, T26
CPT Eye-Related Codes	
Medicine procedures	92002-92499
Radiologic procedures	
• Diagnostic radiology	70010-70559
• Radiologic guidance	77001-77022
• Diagnostic ultrasound	76506-76536
Laboratory organ/disease panels	None

Source: © PB Resources, Inc. Used with permission.

Instructional notes appear throughout the Tabular List to alert coders to the need for modifiers, provide cross-references to codes for similar procedures on other sites, identify when additional codes for radiological services might be needed, and highlight resequenced and recently deleted codes.

ABSTRACTING EYE PROCEDURES

Some operative techniques used in eye procedures are rarely used to treat other body systems, such as phacoemulsification and recession. Although the eye is a small structure compared with other organs, it has numerous specific sites that affect the choice of codes, such as the pars plana, trabecular network, and extraocular muscles. The direction of extraocular muscles—vertical, lateral, or oblique—must be identified (■ FIGURE 43-2). Be aware of these unique procedures and detailed anatomy when abstracting and coding procedures on the eye. Refer to your medical resources to understand terms you may be unfamiliar with.

Laterality is always relevant for eye procedures. For procedures on the eyelid, also abstract whether the upper or lower lid is treated. In addition, identify procedures in which a graft or prosthesis—such as an IOL or implant—is used.

Some clinicians might use Latin-based abbreviations to designate the laterality of the eyes: **OD** (*oculus dexter*) for the right eye; **OS** (*oculus sinister*) for the left eye; **OU** (*oculus uterque*) for each eye or both eyes. These abbreviations are not on The Joint Commission's (TJC) required *Do Not Use List*. However, they are on TJC's supplemental list of abbreviations that they suggest institutions may wish to prohibit through internal policy. They also appear on the list *Error-Prone Abbreviations, Symbols, and Dose Designations* published by the Institute for Safe Medication Practices (ISMP).

Refer to ■ TABLE 43-6 for guidance on how to abstract procedures on the Eye and Ocular Adnexa, then work through the detailed example that follows. Take note of the specialized

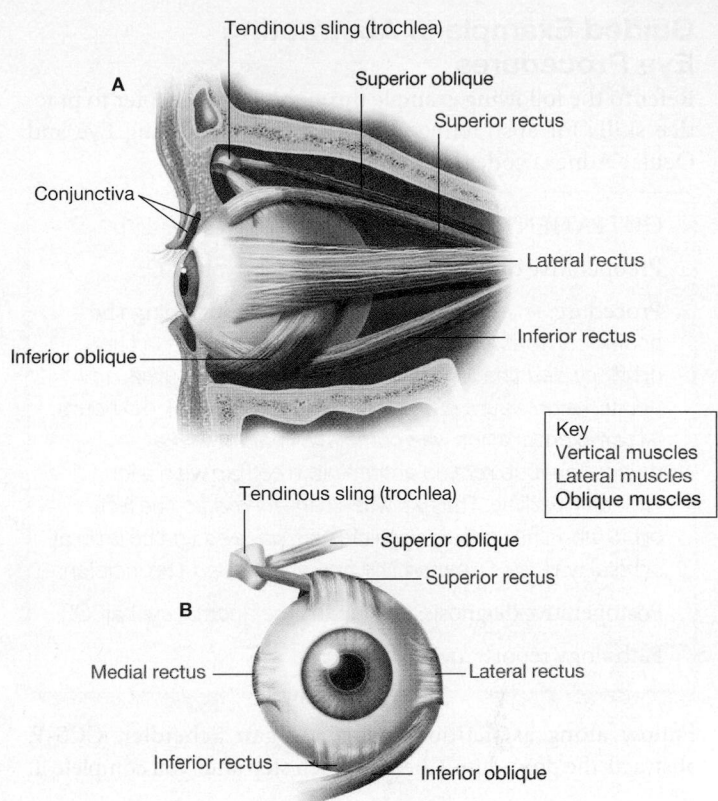

Figure 43-2 ■ Extraocular Muscles, Left Eye: Lateral View (A) and Anterior View (B)

questions for procedures on the eyelids and keratoplasty. Remember that the abstracting questions are a guide and that not every question applies to, or can be answered for, every case. For example, when a prosthesis is used, you must identify its type, but not every procedure requires a prosthesis.

Table 43-6 ■ KEY CRITERIA FOR ABSTRACTING EYE PROCEDURES

❑ What is the procedure?

❑ What part(s) of the eye is affected?

❑ What is the laterality?

❑ What is the surgical approach?

❑ What is the anatomic approach?

❑ What type of prosthesis is used?

For procedures on the eyelid(s):

❑ Is the upper or lower lid involved?

❑ Is only the skin involved, or are parts of eye and adnexa also involved?

For keratoplasty:

❑ How much of the cornea is removed (endothelium, epithelium, slice, partial thickness, full thickness)?

❑ Is the cornea reshaped?

❑ Is the patient's cornea reinserted or is a donor graft used?

❑ Is a graft secured with sutures or an air bubble?

Source: © PB Resources, Inc. Used with permission.

Guided Example of Abstracting Eye Procedures

Refer to the following example throughout this chapter to practice skills for abstracting, assigning, and arranging Eye and Ocular Adnexa codes.

OUTPATIENT SURGERY   Gender: F   Age: 51

Preoperative diagnosis: cancer of the eyeball, OS

Procedure: exenteration of the left eye, including the ocular contents and muscle; placed dry gauze in the orbit, closed the wound using absorbable sutures, and applied a pressure patch to remain in place for 48 hours. After exenteration was complete I harvested a myocutaneous rectus abdominis free flap with a long vascular pedicle. The flap was transferred to the left orbit, and the vascular pedicle was passed to the lateral orbital wall. We trimmed the flap and closed the incision.

Postoperative diagnosis: malignant melanoma, eyeball, OS

Pathology report: uveal melanoma

Follow along as fictitious coder, Megan Scheidler, CCS-P, abstracts the procedure. Check off each step after you complete it.

▶ Megan reads through the entire record, paying special attention to the reason for the encounter, the procedure performed, and the postoperative diagnosis. She refers to the Key Criteria for Abstracting Eye Procedures (Table 43-6).

❑ She notes preoperative diagnosis cancer of the eyeball, OS.

❑ *What is the patient's age?* 51

❑ *What site is treated?* left eye

❑ *What is the primary procedure performed?* exenteration

❑ *What is the laterality?* left eye

❑ *What part(s) of the eye is affected?* ocular contents and muscle

❑ *What is the surgical approach?* open

❑ *What is the anatomic approach?* not applicable

❑ *What type of prosthesis is used?* A prosthesis is not inserted at this time.

❑ *What other procedures are performed?* myocutaneous rectus abdominis free flap

▶ At this time, Megan does not know which of these procedures may need to be coded, nor how many codes she will end up with. She will learn about this when she moves on to assigning codes.

CODING PRACTICE

Exercise 43.2   **Abstracting Eye Procedures**

Instructions: Read the mini-medical-record of each patient's encounter and answer the abstracting questions. Write the answer on the line provided. Do not assign any codes.

---

1. OFFICE   Gender: F   Age: 27

Preprocedure diagnosis: Perforating laceration to the left cornea. Cannot see out of her left eye and has severe eye pain. She was hit in the eye with a softball bat during a softball game.

Procedure: repaired the corneal laceration, OS. The uveal tissue and the vascular layer beneath the sclera were intact.

Plan: steroid eye drops and antibiotics

a. What is the procedure? _____

b. What part(s) of the eye is affected? _____

c. What is the laterality? _____

d. What is the surgical approach? _____

e. What is the anatomic approach? _____

f. What type of prosthesis is used? _____

---

2. EMERGENCY DEPT   Gender: F   Age: 53

Preprocedure diagnosis: partial retinal detachment with multiple defects in the OD

Procedure: retinal repair, right eye. Applied scleral buckle using encircling procedure, with drainage of subretinal fluid

a. What is the procedure? _____

b. What part(s) of the eye is affected? _____

c. What is the laterality? _____

d. What is the surgical approach? _____

e. What is the anatomic approach? _____

f. What type of prosthesis is used? _____

3. EMERGENCY DEPT Gender: F Age: 67

Preprocedure diagnosis: spontaneous hemorrhage obscuring vision, OD

Procedure: mechanical vitrectomy; removed vitreous fluid from the eye through incisions in the pars plana

a. What is the procedure? _____

b. What part(s) of the eye is affected? _____

c. What is the laterality? _____

d. What is the surgical approach? _____

e. What is the anatomic approach? _____

f. What type of prosthesis is used? _____

4. OUTPATIENT SURGERY Gender: M Age: 72

Preprocedure diagnosis: cataract, right eye

Procedure: extracapsular cataract removal with lens implantation, right eye. Performed phacoemulsification using hydrodissection to separate the lens nucleus by injecting fluid into the capsule, then suctioned out the lens and fluid. Inserted an intraocular lens in the posterior chamber and checked for leakage.

a. What is the procedure? _____

b. What part(s) of the eye is affected? _____

c. What is the laterality? _____

d. What is the surgical approach? _____

e. What is the anatomic approach? _____

f. What type of prosthesis is used? _____

5. OFFICE Gender: M Age: 83

Preprocedure diagnosis: diabetic macular edema, right eye

Procedure: injects triamcinolone acetonide 10 mg into the Tenon's capsule (*a membrane covering the eyeball behind the conjunctiva*)

a. What is the procedure? _____

b. What part(s) of the eye is affected? _____

c. What is the laterality? _____

d. What is the surgical approach? _____

e. What is the anatomic approach? _____

f. What type of prosthesis is used? _____

6. OFFICE Gender: M Age: 5

Preprocedure diagnosis: exotropia (*eye turns outward*), left eye

Procedure: strabismus surgery, recession (*lengthening*) of left lateral rectus muscle. Placed adjustable sutures to adjust alignment postoperatively when muscles are not affected by anesthesia.

a. What is the procedure? _____

b. What part(s) of the eye is affected? _____

c. What is the laterality? _____

d. What is the surgical approach? _____

e. What is the anatomic approach? _____

f. What type of prosthesis is used? _____

ASSIGNING CODES FOR EYE PROCEDURES

To locate codes for eye procedures, search the Index for the Main Term of the anatomic site, such as **Cornea** or **Retina**, and identify the first-level modifying term for the type of procedure or condition, such as **Astigmatism** or **Removal**. This approach usually leads to the largest selection of codes. However, you may search the Index for the Main Term of the procedure, such as **Keratoplasty** or **Vitrectomy**, and identify the first-level modifying term for the variation of the procedure, which might specify the anatomic approach, such as **Anterior** or **Pars plana**.

Remember that CPT uses a variety of Main Terms to index procedures, including anatomic site, procedure name, condition, synonym, eponym, and abbreviation. If you cannot find what you are looking for using one approach, try a different one, because not all possible codes are indexed the same under all possible Main Terms. Always read the code description in the Tabular List, including any parent codes and even surrounding codes not listed in the Index. Also read the instructional notes that appear after the code and special instructions that appear at the beginning of the category to help identify the correct code.

Many eye procedures involve the use of an **operating microscope**, which is a specially designed microscope used to assist in the performance of delicate microsurgical procedures, such as operations on the eye, middle ear, or nerves. Code **69990** is an add-on code to report use of the operating microscope: **Microsurgical techniques, requiring use of operating microscope**. An instructional note at the beginning of the Eye and Ocular Adnexa subsection states **(Do not report code 69990 in addition to codes 65091-68850)**. This instruction tells you that the operating microscope is bundled into codes and should not be reported separately, even when documented.

Pay special attention to the details of blepharoplasty, cataract removal, and iridectomy.

- Identify whether a blepharoplasty procedure involves the eyelid margin, tarsus, or conjunctiva or only the skin of the eyelids. Procedures that involve the lid margin, tarsus, or conjunctiva are classified under the Eye and Ocular Adnexa (**67930-67975**)

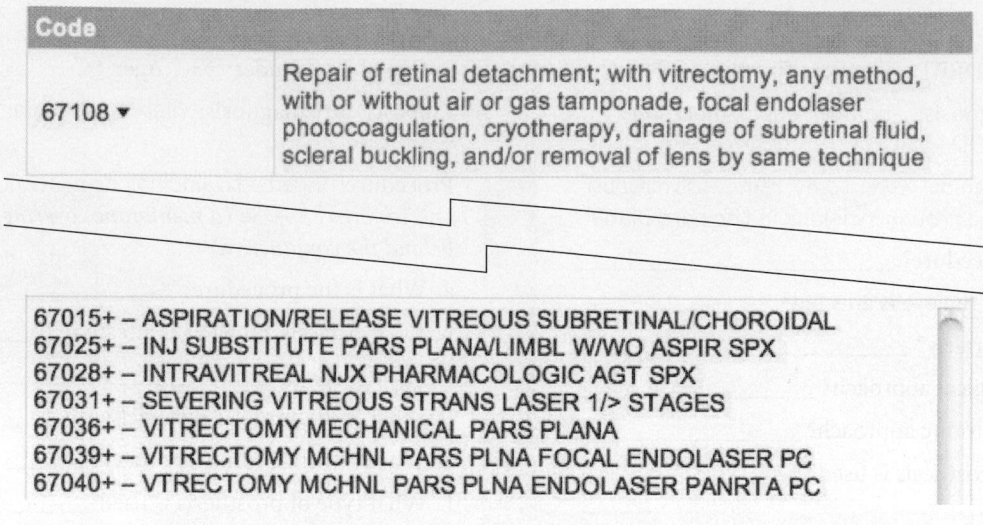

Code	
67108 ▼	Repair of retinal detachment; with vitrectomy, any method, with or without air or gas tamponade, focal endolaser photocoagulation, cryotherapy, drainage of subretinal fluid, scleral buckling, and/or removal of lens by same technique

67015+ – ASPIRATION/RELEASE VITREOUS SUBRETINAL/CHOROIDAL
67025+ – INJ SUBSTITUTE PARS PLANA/LIMBL W/WO ASPIR SPX
67028+ – INTRAVITREAL NJX PHARMACOLOGIC AGT SPX
67031+ – SEVERING VITREOUS STRANS LASER 1/> STAGES
67036+ – VITRECTOMY MECHANICAL PARS PLANA
67039+ – VITRECTOMY MCHNL PARS PLNA FOCAL ENDOLASER PC
67040+ – VTRECTOMY MCHNL PARS PLNA ENDOLASER PANRTA PC

National Correct Coding Initiative (NCCI) Edits
If a provider bills a code from [this list] along with code [above the break line], only one of the codes will be payable by Medicare and any other payers who implement the NCCI. The code [above the break line] is the code payable, unless the code in [this list] is displayed in bold. In that case, the code in [this list] is the one payable, rather than the code [above the break line]. However, if the code in [this list] is green and followed by a +, it can accept a modifier, if appropriate, to prevent the rejection.

Figure 43-3 ■ Example of Encoder Screen with NCCI Edits for Code 67108. *Source: Screen shot courtesy of SpeedECoder.*

and are usually performed by ophthalmologists. Blepharoplasty that involves only the skin of the eyelids is classified under the Integumentary System (**15820-15823**) and is usually performed by plastic surgeons.

- CPT codes describing cataract removal (**66982-66986**) are mutually exclusive of each other, so report only one code for cataract removal for the same eye on the same date of service.

- CPT codes describing repair of retinal detachment (**67101-67113**) are mutually exclusive of each other, so report only one code for retinal detachment repair for the same eye on the same date of service. Some retinal detachment repair procedures include procedures on the vitreous body, which are not separately reportable. For example, the procedure described by CPT code **67108** includes the procedures described by CPT codes **67015**, **67025, 67028, 67031, 67036, 67039,** and **67040**. The exclusions are not identified in the CPT manual but do appear in the National Correct Coding Initiative (NCCI) and, as such, are flagged by many encoders (■ FIGURE 43-3).

Guided Example of Assigning Eye Procedure Codes

To practice skills for assigning codes for the Eye and Ocular Adnexa, continue with the example from earlier in the chapter about a patient who was seen for orbital exenteration. Follow along in your CPT manual as Megan Scheidler, CCS-P, assigns codes. Check off each step after you complete it.

▶ First, Megan confirms the procedure: *exenteration of the left eye*

▶ Megan searches the Index for the Main Term **Eye**.

❑ She locates the first-level modifying term **Exenteration**.

❑ She identifies the potential codes **65110, 65112, 65114**.

▶ Megan turns to the Tabular List to review the codes.

❑ She identifies that code **65110** is a parent code with the unique descriptor **Exenteration of orbit (does not include skin graft), removal of orbital contents**.

❑ She identifies that codes **65112** and **65114** are indented codes in the same code family. She reviews the unique descriptors to determine the differences between the codes.

- Code **65110** describes removal of the orbital contents **only**.

- Code **65112** describes **therapeutic removal of bone**.

- Code **65114** describes **with muscle or myocutaneous flap**.

❑ She refers to the documentation and confirms a myocutaneous flap was part of the procedure, so code **65114** correctly describes the procedure. The descriptor also tells her that she does not need an additional code to report the myocutaneous flap.

▶ Megan checks for instructions in the Tabular List.

❑ She reads the instructional notes that follow code **65114** in the Tabular List:

- **(For skin graft to orbit (split skin), see 15120, 15121; free, full thickness, see 15260, 15261)**

- **(For eyelid repair involving more than skin, see 67930 et seq)**

❏ Although a myocutaneous graft was performed and is bundled with the procedure, a skin graft or other eyelid repair was not performed, so these notes do not apply to this case.

❏ She cross-references the beginning of the category **Removal of the Eye** and verifies that there are no special instructions.

❏ She cross-references the beginning of the subheading **Eyeball** and verifies that there are no instructional notes.

❏ She cross-references the beginning of the subsection **Eye and Ocular Adnexa** and reviews the instructional notes. She determines that they do not apply because the operating microscope was not used.

▶ Megan appends modifier **-LT Left side** to identify the laterality.

▶ Megan reviews the procedure code she has assigned for this case.

(1) **65114-LT Exenteration of orbit (does not include skin graft), removal of orbital contents; with muscle or myocutaneous flap; -LT Left side**

▶ Megan also assigns and sequences the ICD-10-CM diagnosis code that supports the need for the service.

(1) **C69.92 Malignant neoplasm of unspecified site of left eye**

▶ Next, Megan codes a follow-up procedure.

CODING PRACTICE

Exercise 43.3   Assigning Codes for Eye Procedures

Instructions: Read the mini-medical-record of each patient's encounter. Review the information abstracted in Exercise 43.2 for questions 1–3. For questions 4–6, abstract the case on your own. Assign CPT codes, quantities, and modifiers using the Index and Tabular List. Write the code(s) on the line provided.

1. OFFICE   Gender: F   Age: 27

Preprocedure diagnosis: Perforating laceration to the left cornea. Cannot see out of her left eye and has severe eye pain. She was hit in the eye with a softball bat during a softball game.

Procedure: repaired the corneal laceration, OS. The uveal tissue and the vascular layer beneath the sclera were intact.

Plan: steroid eye drops and antibiotics

1 CPT Code _____

2. EMERGENCY DEPT   Gender: F   Age: 53

Preprocedure diagnosis: partial retinal detachment with multiple defects, OD

Procedure: retinal repair, OD. Applied scleral buckle using encircling procedure, with drainage of subretinal fluid

Tip: A scleral buckle is a silicone strap applied around the eyeball.

1 CPT Code _____

3. EMERGENCY DEPT   Gender: F   Age: 67

Preprocedure diagnosis: spontaneous hemorrhage obscuring vision, OD

Procedure: mechanical vitrectomy, OD, removed vitreous fluid from the eye through incisions in the pars plana

Tip: The pars plana is a narrow area between the iris and the choroid.

1 CPT Code _____

4. OUTPATIENT SURGERY   Gender: F   Age: 17

Preprocedure diagnosis: tearing, eyelash encrustation with probable tear duct obstruction, OS

Procedure: nasolacrimal duct, OS, explored under general anesthesia. Some mild resistance was found distally and we were able to navigate through this using the probe. Patency was confirmed through the naris.

Postprocedure diagnosis: distal nasolacrimal duct stenosis with obstruction, OS

1 CPT Code _____

(continued)

CODING PRACTICE (continued)

5. OFFICE   Gender: M   Age: 27

Preprocedure diagnosis: *eye infections for the past year that have been resistant to multiple antibiotic therapies*

Procedure: *expressed conjunctival follicles in both eyes in an attempt to determine the cause*

Postprocedure diagnosis: *follicular conjunctivitis OU*

1 CPT Code _____

6. OUTPATIENT SURGERY   Gender: M   Age: 74

Preprocedure diagnosis: *open angle glaucoma, OD, uncontrolled by maximum tolerated medical therapy*

Procedure: *fistulization of sclera with trabeculectomy ab externo, OD. At the end of the procedure the anterior chamber was filled with balanced salt solution; it was noted that there was a very small amount of fluid tricking out of the scleral flap, and the pressure in the anterior chamber was considered adequate. Eye patch and eye shield were placed over the eye.*

Postprocedure diagnosis: *open angle glaucoma, OD*

1 CPT Code _____

ARRANGING CODES FOR EYE PROCEDURES

The NCCI provides direction for when separate procedures should be reported with cataract removal. When an iridectomy is performed to complete a cataract extraction, it is an integral part of the cataract procedure and is not separately reportable. Similarly, the minimal vitreous loss occurring during routine cataract extraction does not represent a vitrectomy and is not separately reportable.

When an iridectomy or vitrectomy that is separate and distinct from the cataract extraction is performed for an unrelated reason during the same patient encounter, the iridectomy and/or vitrectomy may be reported separately with an NCCI-associated modifier, such as modifier **-59 Distinct procedural**

service. The medical record must document the distinct medical necessity of each procedure.

The descriptors for CPT code **67108** (**Repair of retinal detachment...**) and **67113** (**Repair of complex retinal detachment...**) include removal of lens, if performed. CPT codes for removal of lens or cataract extraction (**66830-66984**) should not be reported separately.

A trabeculectomy is separately reportable with a cataract extraction when performed for a purpose unrelated to the cataract extraction, such as glaucoma (■ Figure 43-4). However, when a trabeculectomy is performed as a preventative service for an expected temporary increase in intraocular pressure after cataract removal, without documentation of glaucoma, it is *not* separately reportable (■ Figure 43-5).

Surgeon performs an extracapsular cataract phacoemulsification and implants a posterior IOL in the right eye. During the same operative session, he performs a bilateral trabeculectomy to treat the patient's longstanding glaucoma.

66170-50 Fistulization of sclera for glaucoma; trabeculectomy ab externo in absence of previous surgery; -50 Bilateral procedure
66984-59-RT Extracapsular cataract removal with insertion of intraocular lens prosthesis (1 stage procedure), manual or mechanical technique (eg, irrigation and aspiration or phacoemulsification);-59 Distinct procedural service; -RT Right eye
V2632-RT Posterior chamber intraocular lens

Figure 43-4 ■ Example of Multiple Coding for Cataract Removal and Trabeculectomy. *Source: © PB Resources, Inc. Used with permission. CPT codes only © American Medical Association.*

> Surgeon performs an extracapsular cataract phacoemulsification and implants a posterior IOL in the right eye. During the same operative session, he performs a right trabeculectomy as a precaution, to prevent any potential rise in IOP postoperatively.

66984-RT Extracapsular cataract removal with insertion of intraocular lens prosthesis (1 stage procedure), manual or mechanical technique (eg, irrigation and aspiration or phacoemulsification)
V2632-RT Posterior chamber intraocular lens

Figure 43-5 ■ Example of Coding for Trabeculectomy Bundled with Cataract Removal. *Source: © PB Resources, Inc. Used with permission. CPT codes only © American Medical Association.*

Guided Example of Arranging Eye Procedure Codes

To practice skills for arranging codes for procedures on the Eye and Ocular Adnexa, continue with the example from earlier in the chapter about the patient who was seen for exenteration of the eye. Follow along in your CPT manual as Megan Scheidler, CCS-P, codes for a follow-up procedure six weeks after the exenteration service. Check off each step after you complete it.

> OUTPATIENT SURGERY   Gender: F   Age: 51
>
> Preoperative diagnosis: *exenteration of the left eye, including the ocular contents and muscle*
>
> Procedure: *orbital implant, OS. Attached the prosthetic eyeball outside of the muscle cone (the gathering point of the extraocular muscles that move the eye) of the left eye.*
>
> Plan: *Refer to ocularist for ocular implant.*

▶ First, Megan performs the abstracting for the follow-up procedure and determines that this procedure involves insertion of an orbital implant, the prosthetic eyeball.

▶ Megan searches the Index for the Main Term **Orbital Implant**.

❑ She notices the cross-reference instruction under the Main Term that says **See Ocular Implant**. She knows she can disregard this instruction because an ocular implant is the glass, plastic, or acrylic cover that will be inserted by the ocularist over the orbital implant and under the eyelid.

❑ She locates the subterm **Insertion** and notes the only code **67550**.

▶ Megan turns to the Tabular List to verify code **67550**.

❑ The code description is **Orbital implant (implant outside muscle cone); insertion** and correctly describes the procedure performed.

❑ The other code in this code family, **67560**, describes **removal or revision** of the orbital implant, which was not performed.

▶ Megan appends modifier **-LT Left side** to identify the laterality.

▶ Megan refers to the global surgery schedule provided by the patient's insurance company. The exenteration procedure has a global period of 90 days. The global period means that any additional services performed during this time period are assumed to be bundled with the original procedure.

❑ Megan knows she needs a modifier to alert the payer that the orbital implant is a planned and legitimate procedure, separate from the exenteration. (Refer to Table 30-1 Key Criteria for Abstracting CPT Modifiers or Appendix A in the CPT manual.)

❑ She appends modifier **-58 Staged or related procedure or service by the same physician or other qualified health care professional during the postoperative period.**

▶ Megan finalizes the procedure codes and sequencing for this case:

(1) **67550-58-LT Orbital implant (implant outside muscle cone); insertion; -58 Staged or related procedure or service by the same physician or other qualified health care professional during the postoperative period; -LT Left side**

▶ Megan also assigns and sequences the ICD-10-CM diagnosis codes that support the need for the service. She needs a code to identify the postoperative status of the patient and a code to identify the history of the malignant neoplasm. She assigns a history code, rather than one for a current neoplasm, because the neoplasm was removed in its entirety.

(1) **Z98.89 Other specified postprocedural states**

(2) **Z85.840 Personal history of malignant neoplasm of eye**

CODING PRACTICE

Exercise 43.4 Arranging Codes for Eye Procedures

Instructions: Read the mini-medical-record of each patient's encounter. Review the information abstracted in Exercise 43.2 for questions 1–3. For questions 4–6, abstract the case on your own. Assign CPT codes, quantities, and modifiers using the Index and Tabular List, and arrange the codes in proper sequence. Write the code(s) on the line provided.

1. OUTPATIENT SURGERY Gender: M Age: 72

Preprocedure diagnosis: cataract, right eye

Procedure: extracapsular cataract removal with lens implantation, right eye. Performed phacoemulsification using hydrodissection to separate the lens nucleus by injecting fluid into the capsule, then suctioned out the lens and fluid. Inserted intraocular lens in the posterior chamber and checked for leakage.

Tip: Assign a CPT code for the procedure and a HCPCS code for the lens.

2 CPT/HCPCS Codes _____

2. OFFICE Gender: M Age: 83

Preprocedure diagnosis: diabetic macular edema, right eye

Procedure: injected triamcinolone acetonide 10 mg into the Tenon's capsule (*a membrane covering the eyeball behind the conjunctiva*)

Tip: Assign a CPT code for the procedure and a HCPCS code for the drug.

2 CPT/HCPCS Codes _____

3. OFFICE Gender: M Age: 5

Preprocedure diagnosis: exotropia (*eye turns outward*), left eye

Procedure: strabismus surgery, recession (*lengthening*) of left lateral rectus muscle. Placed adjustable sutures to adjust alignment postoperatively when muscles are not affected by anesthesia.

Tip: The left lateral rectus muscle is a horizontal muscle.

2 CPT Codes _____

4. OFFICE Gender: M Age: 59

Preprocedure diagnosis: significant pterygium, right eye

Procedure: pterygium excision with graft, right eye, with 0.2 mg mitomycin. The pterygium was excised over the conjunctiva with Westcott scissors and undermined to sclera. Hemostasis was maintained with cautery. A sponge with approximately 0.2 mg mitomycin was placed over the previous pterygium site over the sclera. This was held in place for approximately one minute. Upon conclusion of the procedure the eye was patched.

Tip: Assign a CPT code for the procedure and a HCPCS code for the drug.

2 CPT/HCPCS Codes _____

5. INPATIENT HOSPITAL Gender: F Age: 48

Preprocedure diagnosis: blind, painful right eye with conjunctival scarring

Procedure: evisceration with implant, right eye; conjunctivoplasty, right eye; frost suture for temporary tarsorrhaphy. The conjunctivoplasty began by carefully unrolling and dissecting the conjunctiva back around the muscle insertion to carefully release scar bands and to maximize the length of the conjunctiva. The technical difficulty of this procedure required substantially more time to complete. Frost suture consisting of #6-0 silk was placed, going to the tarsal plates of the upper and lower eyelids to achieve temporary eyelid closure.

Postprocedure diagnosis: blind painful eye, right eye, with conjunctival scarring; microcornea, right eye

Tip: 3 CPT Codes _____
_____

6. OFFICE Gender: M Age: 8

Preprocedure diagnosis: left orbital pseudotumor

Procedure: anterior orbitotomy with excision of lacrimal sac, left orbit. Sharp dissection through the orbicularis muscle was continued to the level of the orbital septum, where the pseudotumor was excised. The orbital portion of the lacrimal gland prolapsed through the wound. Partial excision of the lacrimal gland was performed. Pseudotumor and lacrimal tissue sent to pathology.

Pathology report: left orbital pseudotumor, normal lacrimal tissue

2 CPT Codes _____

System/Body Area	Elements of Eye Examination
Eyes	❑ Test **visual acuity** (Does not include determination of refractive error) ❑ **Gross visual field** testing by confrontation ❑ Test **ocular motility** including primary gaze alignment ❑ Inspection of bulbar and palpebral **conjunctivae** ❑ Examination of **ocular adnexae** including lids (eg, ptosis or lagophthalmos), lacrimal glands, lacrimal drainage, orbits and preauricular lymph nodes ❑ Examination of **pupils and irises** including shape, direct and consensual reaction (afferent pupil), size (eg, anisocoria) and morphology ❑ Slit lamp examination of the **corneas** including epithelium, stroma, endothelium, and tear film ❑ Slit lamp examination of the **anterior chambers** including depth, cells, and flare ❑ Slit lamp examination of the **lenses** including clarity, anterior and posterior capsule, cortex, and nucleus ❑ Measurement of **intraocular pressures** (except in children and patients with trauma or infectious disease) Ophthalmoscopic examination of: ❑ **Optic discs** including size, C/D ratio, appearance (eg, atrophy, cupping, tumor elevation) and nerve fiber layer ❑ **Posterior segments** including retina and vessels (eg, exudates and hemorrhages)
Neurological/ Psychiatric	Brief assessment of mental status including: ❑ **Orientation** to time, place and person ❑ **Mood** and affect (eg, depression, anxiety, agitation, hypomania, lability)

Total # Bullets Performed and Documented →	☐	# of ❑ **Elements Performed and Documented**	**Level of Examination**
		1–5	Problem focused
		6–8	Expanded problem focused
		9+	Detailed
		ALL	Comprehensive (Document **every** element in each box with a shaded border and at least **one** element in each box with an unshaded border)

Figure 43-6 ■ 1997 DG for Eye Examination. *Source: Centers for Medicare and Medicaid Services, 1997 Documentation Guidelines for Evaluation and Management Services (with formatting adjustments).*

E/M CODING FOR OPHTHALMOLOGY

The *1997 Documentation Guidelines for Evaluation and Management Services* (1997 DG), published by CMS, provides requirements for each level of an ophthalmologic E/M examination (■ FIGURE 43-6). Ophthalmologists are not limited to using the guidelines for an eye examination only. They can also use guidelines for a general multiorgan system examination, or any other single organ system examination, based on what is most advantageous for a specific encounter. However, physicians cannot combine elements from more than one type of examination for a given encounter. The eye examination guidelines typically provide the best results when a detailed eye examination is performed.

To determine the appropriate E/M code, coders must review the documentation in detail and identify the specific elements documented.

- To translate the documentation into the E/M requirements for the history, refer back to Chapter 31, Evaluation and Management Services (99201-99499), Tables 31-7 to 31-10, or the 1997 DG.
- To determine the requirements for an examination, refer to Figure 43-6 1997 DG for Eye Examination or to the single organ system examination for the eye in the 1997 DG.

- To determine the levels for medical decision making (MDM), refer to Chapter 31, Table 31-12, and the Table of Risk in the 1997 DG.

Guided Example of E/M Coding for Ophthalmology

Refer to the ophthalmology encounter (■ FIGURE 43-7) to practice skills for abstracting and assigning E/M codes. Follow along as fictitious coder Megan Scheidler, CCS-P, abstracts the procedure. Check off each step after you complete it.

▶ First, Megan needs to establish the category of service so she can determine the information needed to abstract and assign the code.

❑ *What is the setting?* Office

❑ *What is the type of service?* New patient

❑ *What is the code range?* Megan refers to the CPT Index and looks up the Main Term **Evaluation and Management** and the subterm **Office and other outpatient**. The code range listed is **99201-99215**.

❑ *How many key components are required?* Megan refers to the code range in the Tabular List and locates the

OPHTHALMOLOGY ENCOUNTER

Patient is an 85-year-old white female who presents to the eye clinic today for the first time because of decreased vision in the left eye over the past week.

She has a past ocular history including cataract extraction with lens implants in both eyes 10 years ago. She also has a history of glaucoma diagnosed 25 years ago and macular degeneration. She has been followed at home and is here visiting family and was brought in on an urgent basis today.

Her past medical history includes hypertension and hypercholesterolemia and hypothyroidism.

Her medications include betaxolol hydrochloride 0.5% eye drops to both eyes twice a day and pilocarpine 2% OU three times a day. She took both the drops this morning. She takes levothyroxine for hypothyroidism and felodipine for blood pressure.

She is allergic to penicillin.

She has a family history of blindness in her brother as well as glaucoma and hypertension.

Her visual acuity today at distance without correction is 20/25 in the right and count fingers at 3 feet in the left eye. Manifest refraction showed no improvement in either eye. The intraocular pressures by applanation were 8 in the right eye and 17 in the left eye. Gonioscopy showed grade 4 open angles in both eyes. Humphrey visual field testing done elsewhere showed diffuse reduction in sensitivity in both eyes. The lids were normal bilaterally. She has mild dry eye bilaterally. The corneas are clear bilaterally. The anterior chamber is deep and quiet bilaterally. Irides appear normal. The lenses show well centered posterior chamber intraocular lenses bilaterally.

Dilated fundus exam shows clear vitreous bilaterally. The optic nerves are normal in size. They both appear to have mild pallor. The optic cups in both eyes are shallow. The cup-to-disc ratio in the right eye is not overtly large, would estimate to be 0.5 to 0.6; however, she does have very thin rim tissue inferotemporally in the right eye. In the left eye, the glaucoma appears to be more advanced to the larger cup-to-disc ratio and a thinner rim tissue.

The macula on the right shows drusen (yellow deposits under the retina) with focal areas of retinal pigment epithelial (RPE) atrophy. I do not see any evidence of neovascularization such as subretinal fluid, lipid or hemorrhage. She does have a punctate area of RPE atrophy which is just adjacent to the fovea of the right eye. In the left eye, she has also several high-risk drusen, but no evidence of neovascularization. The RPE in the left eye does appear to be more diffusely abnormal although these changes do appear somewhat mild. I do not see any dense or focal areas of frank RPE atrophy or hypertrophy.

The peripheral retinas are attached in both eyes.

She has pseudophakia bilaterally which is stable and she is doing well in this regard. She has advanced stage open-angle glaucoma, which likely is worse in the left eye and also likely explains her poor vision in the left eye. The intraocular pressure in the mid-to-high teens in the left eye is probably high for her. She has allergic reaction to penicillin. I will recommend starting latanoprost ophthalmic OS nightly. I think the intraocular pressure in the right eye is acceptable and is probably a stable pressure for her OD. She will need followup at home in the next 1 or 2 months after starting the new medication which is latanoprost.

Regarding the drusen macular degeneration, she has had high-risk changes in both eyes. The vision in the right eye is good, but she does have a very concerning area of RPE atrophy just adjacent to the fovea of the right eye. I strongly recommend that she see a retina specialist as soon as possible to fully discuss prophylactic measures to prevent worsening of her macular degeneration in the right eye.

HISTORY: Problem focused

Setting & patient type

HPI: Brief (2-3)

Chief complaint (CC)

PFSH: Pertinent (1-2)

ROS: Problem focused (None)

EXAMINATION: Detailed

(9+ elements performed and documented)

MEDICAL DECISION MAKING: Moderate Complexity

MDM Data: Ordering or reviewing diagnostic data (Straightforward Data)

MDM Risk: Acute illness with significant risk, Prescription drug management (Moderate Risk)

MDM Management: New presenting problem with strong recommendation for workup (Moderate Management Options

KEY: HPI History of the present illness   ROS Review of systems
PFSH Past, family, and social history   MDM Medical decision making

Figure 43-7 ■ Ophthalmology Encounter. *Source:* © *PB Resources, Inc. Used with permission.*

category **New Patient**. She reads the code description of the first code, which states **requires these 3 key components**. All codes in the category have the same requirements for key components. This tells her that all three key components must meet or exceed the levels listed in the code (3/3).

▶ Next, Megan identifies the level of history.

❑ *What is the level of HPI?* The HPI is **brief** because two elements are documented.

❑ *What is the level of ROS?* The ROS is **problem focused** because no systems are documented.

❑ *What is the level of PFSH?* The PFSH is **pertinent** because two elements are documented.

❑ *Based on these factors, what is the overall level of history?* The level of history is **problem focused** because the lowest of the three factors (HPI, ROS, and PFSH) determines the history level. The HPI and PFSH qualify for an expanded problem-focused history, but the ROS qualifies for only a problem-focused history.

▶ Megan refers to the eye examination in the 1997 DG (Figure 43-6) to abstract information needed to determine the level of the examination.

❑ *What is the level of examination?* The level of examination is **detailed**. Twelve (12) elements of the examination are documented, which exceeds the requirement of one or more bulleted elements for a detailed examination. A comprehensive examination requires that all bulleted items with a shaded border be documented—which they are—plus one bulleted element from a box with an unshaded border, which is not. The DG for the Eye Examination contain only two bulleted elements from a box with an unshaded border. If the physician had examined and documented at least one of these, the criteria for a comprehensive examination would have been met and the encounter would qualify for higher reimbursement.

▶ Megan determines the level of medical decision making. (Refer to Table 31-12 Medical Decision Making Levels.)

❑ *What is the level of complexity of the number of diagnoses or management options based on the presenting problem?* The level is **high** because there is a new presenting problem, with strong recommendation for workup.

❑ *What is the amount and/or complexity of data to be reviewed?* The level is **straightforward** because the physician reviewed the patient's intraocular pressure.

❑ *What is the level of risk of significant complications, morbidity, and/or mortality?* Megan reviews each column in the Table of Risk in the 1997 DG and determines that the level of risk is **moderate**. The patient presents with a new problem that poses a significant risk to the patient (Moderate), no clinical labs are ordered, and prescription drug management is provided (Moderate). The single highest element in the Table of Risk determines the overall risk. The column **Management Options Selected** is the highest level (Moderate).

❑ *Based on these factors, what is the overall level of medical decision making?* The medical decision making is **moderate complexity**. At least two of the three MDM factors are required to qualify for a specific level of MDM. Two of the three MDM factors meet moderate-complexity decision making.

Now Megan is ready to assign the code for the ophthalmology encounter. The exercise that follows guides you through additional abstracting skills and allows you to assign the correct code.

CODING PRACTICE

Exercise 43.5 Evaluation and Management Coding for the Eye

Instructions: Refer to the *1997 Documentation Guidelines for Evaluation and Management Services* (available at www.cms.gov) or Chapter 31 Evaluation and Management Services (99201-99499) (Tables 31-7 to 31-12) in this text. Answer the following questions about the Ophthalmology Encounter (Figure 43-7).

1. a. Which elements of the HPI are documented? Circle all that apply. Location, Quality, Severity, Duration, Timing, Context, Modifying factors, Associated signs and symptoms

    b. How many elements are documented? _____

    c. What is the level of HPI? _____

2. a. Which systems are reviewed in the ROS? Circle all that apply. Constitutional, Allergic/ immunologic, CV, Endocrine, ENT/M, Eyes, GI, GU, Hemic/lymphatic, MS, Neurologic, Psychiatric, Respiratory, Skin/breast

    b. How many systems are documented? _____

    c. What is the level of ROS? _____

3. a. Which PFSH elements are documented? Circle all that apply. Past medical, Family, Social

    b. What is the level of PFSH? _____

    c. What is the overall level of history? (The lowest history factor—HPI, ROS, or PFSH—determines the level of history.) _____

4. Refer to Figure 43-6 (1997 DG for Eye Examination).

    a. Which bulleted items are documented for the examination? (Check off the items documented.)

    b. How many bulleted items in the shaded box are documented? _____

    c. How many bulleted items in the unshaded box are documented? _____

    d. What is the level of the examination? _____

(continued)

CODING PRACTICE (continued)

5. Refer to Table 31-12 Medical Decision Making Levels or the 1997 DG.

   a. What is the MDM level for the number of diagnoses or management options? _____

   b. What is the MDM level for the amount and/or complexity of data to be reviewed? _____

   c. Refer to the Table of Risk in the 1997 DG. Which elements of risk are documented for each risk factor?

      1. Presenting problem: _____

      2. Diagnostic procedures ordered: _____

      3. Management options selected: _____

   d. What is the level of risk? (The highest of the three risk factors determines the overall level of risk.) _____

   e. What is the overall level of MDM? (2/3 MDM factors are needed to determine the overall level.) _____

6. a. What is the setting? _____

   b. What is the patient (or service) type? _____

   c. What is the code range? _____

   d. How many key components are required? _____

   e. What is the level of history? _____

   f. What is the level of examination? _____

   g. What is the level of medical decision making? _____

   h. What is the correct code? _____

   i. Which key component has the greatest impact on code selection for this case, based on the documentation?

      _____

7. Abstract, assign, and arrange (sequence) the diagnosis code(s) that support the E/M code.

   4 ICD-10-CM Code(s) _____

   _____

CHAPTER SUMMARY

In this chapter you learned that:

- Ophthalmologists are MDs who provide medical evaluation of eye conditions and perform surgery to correct eye problems; subspecialties of ophthalmology are cornea and external disease, glaucoma, neuro-ophthalmology, ophthalmic pathology, ophthalmic plastic surgery, pediatric ophthalmology, and vitreoretinal diseases.

- The CPT section/subsection **Eye and Ocular Adnexa (65091-68899)** contains five subheadings that are divided by anatomic site. Within each subheading, codes are further divided by more specific anatomic sites and the type of procedure.

- Although the eye is a small structure compared with other organs, it has numerous specific sites that affect the choice of codes, such as the pars plana, trabecular network, and extraocular muscles.

- To locate codes for eye procedures, search the Index for the Main Term of the anatomic site, then identify the first-level modifying term for the type of procedure or condition. Alternatively, use the procedure name as the Main Term when necessary.

- The NCCI provides direction for when separate procedures should be reported with cataract removal.

- The *1997 Documentation Guidelines for Evaluation and Management Services* (1997 DG), published by CMS, provides requirements for each level of an ophthalmologic E/M examination.

- Special instructions in the Eye and Ocular Adnexa subsection identify services that are bundled with certain codes and also identify codes that should and should not be reported together.

CONCEPT QUIZ

Take a moment to look back at the eye and ocular adnexa and solidify your skills. Try to answer the questions from memory first, then refer to the discussion in this chapter if you need a little extra help.

Completion

Instructions: Write the term that answers each question based on the information you learned in this chapter. Choose from the list at the top of the next page. Some choices may be used more than once and some choices may not be used at all.

DSEK

enucleation

evisceration

exenteration

fistulization

goniotomy

intravitreal

IOL

IOP

iridotomy

ocular implant

phacoemulsification

photocoagulation

PKP

radial keratotomy

recession

trabeculectomy

trabeculotomy

1. A(n) _____ procedure removes the eyeball, including the ocular contents, and may include removal of bone and muscle or a myocutaneous flap.

2. One reason for a(n) _____ injection is to treat diabetic retinopathy.

3. A(n) _____ procedure is flattening the cornea by making a series of incisions in a radial pattern resembling the spokes of a wheel.

4. The _____ procedure, used to treat strabismus, is the cutting of a muscle from the surface of the eye and reattaching it farther back from the front of the eye to weaken or lengthen the muscle.

5. A(n) _____ procedure is removal of the eyeball without removing the ocular contents of the orbit or muscles.

6. A(n) _____ is implanted in the eye during cataract surgery after the cataract has been removed.

7. A(n) _____ is the incision and repair of the trabecular meshwork to improve aqueous humor outflow and reduce intraocular pressure.

8. _____ is the destruction of a natural lens, which is then suctioned out of the eye.

9. _____ is the fluid pressure inside the eye.

10. _____ describes removal of only the corneal endothelium layer and replacement with a cadaver endothelium graft.

Multiple Choice

Instructions: Circle the letter of the best answer to each question based on the information you learned in this chapter.

1. Which eye muscle is a lateral muscle?
   A. Superior rectus
   B. Superior oblique
   C. Medial rectus
   D. Inferior rectus

2. What is the segment in the front of the eye that contains the cornea, anterior chamber, anterior sclera, iris, ciliary body, and lens?
   A. Anterior
   B. Lateral

   C. Ventral
   D. Posterior

3. Where does CPT classify codes for blepharoplasty that involves only the skin of the eyelids?
   A. Eye and Ocular Adnexa
   B. Nervous System
   C. General Surgery
   D. Integumentary System

4. What is the name of the site where the upper and lower eyelids meet?
   A. Lacrimal gland
   B. Sclera
   C. Canthus
   D. Palpebra

5. What is the transparent covering of the anterior portion of the eye and contains the most nerve endings of any site in the body?
   A. Macula
   B. Cornea
   C. Tenon's capsule
   D. Ocular nerve

6. What structure is located behind the iris and produces aqueous humor?
   A. Epithelium
   B. Internal eye
   C. Orbit
   D. Ciliary body

7. What procedure is typically performed by an ocularist?
   A. Ocular implant
   B. Orbital implant
   C. IOL implant
   D. Phacoemulsification

8. What type of eye procedures does CPT classify in codes 92002-92499?
   A. Diagnostic radiology
   B. Laboratory panels
   C. Medical
   D. Injuries

9. What is the tissue that supports the eyelid?
   A. Extraocular muscle
   B. Tarsus
   C. Conjunctiva
   D. Pars plana

10. In what list do the abbreviations OU, OS, and OD appear?
    A. *Do Not Use List*
    B. HCPCS modifiers list
    C. *Latin Abbreviations Accepted for Medical Use* list
    D. *Error-Prone Abbreviations, Symbols, and Dose Designations* list

CODING CHALLENGE

Instructions: Read the mini-medical-record of each patient's encounter, then abstract, assign, and arrange ICD-10-CM diagnosis codes and CPT procedure codes using the appropriate Index and Tabular List. Assign quantities and modifiers where needed. Write the code(s) on the line provided.

---

1. OFFICE Gender: M Age: 42

Preprocedure diagnosis: Metal foreign body of conjunctiva, right eye, initial encounter

Procedure: Removal of metal foreign body embedded in the conjunctiva, right eye. Washed out the eye with sterile saline and identified the location of a small metal fragment. Wiped away FB with a cotton-tipped applicator.

1 ICD-10-CM Code _____

1 CPT Code _____

---

2. EMERGENCY DEPT Gender: M Age: 19

Preprocedure diagnosis: Traumatic perforation of left cornea while playing softball, initial encounter

Procedure: Repair of corneal perforation, left eye

Tip: Assign a diagnosis code to identify the patient's activity at the time of the injury.

2 ICD-10-CM Codes _____

1 CPT Code _____

---

3. OUTPATIENT SURGERY Gender: F Age: 31

Preprocedure diagnosis: Corneal scarring due to corneal herpes simplex, left eye

Procedure: PKP, left eye. Used a trephine to remove the corneal tissue. Removed the entire thickness of the cornea and replaced it with a new disc from the donor eye. Applied running sutures around the corneal disc to secure.

2 ICD-10-CM Codes _____

1 CPT Code _____

---

4. OUTPATIENT SURGERY Gender: F Age: 41

Preprocedure diagnosis: Staphyloma, left eye

Procedure: Repair of sclera of left eye with graft. Made incision in the left conjunctiva and sclera where the uveal tissue was protruding. Identified the staphyloma and excised it. Sutured a scleral graft, administered a topical antibiotic to the eye, and applied an eye pressure patch. Patient tolerated procedure well.

1 ICD-10-CM Code _____

1 CPT Code _____

---

5. OUTPATIENT SURGERY Gender: M Age: 57

Preprocedure diagnosis: Anterior synechiae, right eye; borderline glaucoma with increased IOP, bilateral

Procedure: Trabeculotomy ab externo to decrease IOP; used the same incision to access and sever anterior synechiae of the right eye

2 ICD-10-CM Codes _____

2 CPT Codes _____

---

6. OFFICE Gender: F Age: 67

Preprocedure diagnosis: Neoplasm of uncertain behavior on cornea, left

Procedure: Excision of lesion, left cornea

Postprocedure diagnosis: Malignant melanoma, left cornea

Pathology report: Corneal tissue submitted is consistent with malignant melanoma

1 ICD-10-CM Code _____

1 CPT Code _____

---

7. OFFICE Gender: M Age: 79

Preprocedure diagnosis: Hypermature extracapsular cataracts, bilateral

Procedure: Phacoemulsification of extracapsular cataracts with insertion of anterior IOL, bilateral

Tip: Report a HCPCS code for the IOL.

1 ICD-10-CM Code _____

2 CPT Codes _____

---

8. OUTPATIENT SURGERY Gender: F Age: 57

Preprocedure diagnosis: Retinal detachment, right eye

Procedure: Photocoagulation repair of retinal detachment with drainage of subretinal fluid, right eye

1 ICD-10-CM Code _____

1 CPT Code _____

9. OFFICE   Gender: M   Age: 37

Preprocedure diagnosis: Cyst of the ciliary body, left eye

Procedure: Destruction of ciliary body cyst, left eye

Postprocedure diagnosis: Ciliary body cyst of the pars plana, left eye

1 ICD-10-CM Code _____

1 CPT Code _____

10. OFFICE   Gender: F   Age: 64

Preprocedure diagnosis: Macular degeneration, bilateral

Procedure: Injection of vitreous substitute, right eye

1 ICD-10-CM Code _____

1 CPT Code _____

KEEP ON CODING

Instructions: Read the procedural statement, then use the appropriate Index and Tabular List to assign CPT procedure codes, quantities, and modifiers. Write the code(s) on the line provided.

1. Repair of retina using diathermy without drainage of subretinal fluid, left eye: CPT Code(s) _____

2. Mechanical vitrectomy, pars plana approach, to remove a spontaneous hemorrhage, right eye: CPT Code(s) _____

3. Severing of vitreous face adhesions using a laser, bilateral: CPT Code(s) _____

4. Strabismus correction with surgery on the superior oblique muscle and the inferior rectus muscle, left eye: CPT Code(s) _____

5. Excisional tarsal wedge repair for entropion, right upper eyelid: CPT Code(s) _____

6. Bilateral canthoplasty: CPT Code(s) _____

7. Removal of embedded foreign body of left upper eyelid: CPT Code(s) _____

8. Incision and drainage of abscess of right lacrimal gland: CPT Code(s) _____

9. Conjunctival follicles expressed, bilateral: CPT Code(s) _____

10. Plastic laceration repair of the lacrimal canaliculi, left eye: CPT Code(s) _____

11. Fistulization of sclera to release IOP due to glaucoma, right eye: CPT Code(s) _____

12. Correction of presbyopia by epikeratoplasty, left eye: CPT Code(s) _____

13. Photocoagulative treatment of diabetic retinopathy, two sessions, right eye: CPT Code(s) _____

14. Peripheral excision of iris due to glaucoma, left eye: CPT Code(s) _____

15. Excision of multiple chalazion on both the upper and lower lids of the right eye while under anesthesia: CPT Code(s) _____

16. Suture of laceration of left upper eyelid: CPT Code(s) _____

17. Exenteration of right orbit with myocutaneous graft: CPT Code(s) _____

18. Removal of foreign body from anterior chamber of left eye: CPT Code(s) _____

19. Reconstruction of ocular surface using amniotic membrane transplantation with multiple layers, right cornea: CPT Code(s) _____

20. Paracentesis of anterior chamber of left eye with removal of blood, with irrigation: CPT Code(s) _____

21. Prophylactic photocoagulation of retinal detachment using a laser, bilateral: CPT Code(s) _____

22. Decompression of optic nerve by incision, right: CPT Code(s) _____

23. Tarsorrhaphy with Frost sutures, left eyelids: CPT Code(s) _____

24. Probing and irrigation of nasolacrimal duct, bilateral: CPT Code(s) _____

25. Insertion of ocular implant after right enucleation with muscles attached to implant, secondary procedure: CPT Code(s) _____

Chapter 44

Auditory System (69000-69979) and Operating Microscope Procedures (69990)

Chapter Outline

- **Auditory System Procedure Basics**
- **Coding Overview of Auditory System Procedures**
- **Coding for the Operating Microscope**
- **Abstracting Auditory System Procedures**
- **Assigning Codes for Auditory System Procedures**
- **Arranging Codes for Auditory System Procedures**
- **E/M Coding for Otolaryngology**

Learning Objectives

After completing this chapter, you should have the skills to:

44.1 Spell and define the key words, medical terms, and abbreviations related to auditory system procedures.

44.2 Discuss the types of auditory system procedures.

44.3 Identify the main characteristics of coding for the Auditory System.

44.4 Discuss the CPT coding guidelines for Operating Microscope.

44.5 Abstract procedural information from the medical record for coding Auditory System procedures.

44.6 Assign codes for Auditory System procedures.

44.7 Arrange codes for Auditory System procedures.

44.8 Code evaluation and management services for otolaryngology.

44.9 Discuss the CPT coding guidelines related to the Auditory System.

Key Terms and Abbreviations

AD	middle fossa approach	postauricular	translabyrinthine
AS	operating microscope	transcanal	transmastoid
AU	osseointegrated implant	transcranial	

In addition to the key terms listed here, students should know the terms defined within tables in this chapter.

For updates and corrections, visit our student resource site at

www.pearsonhighered.com/healthprofessionsresources

INTRODUCTION

Advertisements and news constantly overload our sense of hearing to the point that mute buttons are available on television remotes, computers, and phones. Although most people think of the ear as an external structure, the main function of the external ear is to collect and funnel sound waves to the middle and inner ear, where they are transmitted to the brain to create meaningful communication. The ear contains elements of the integumentary, cardiovascular, nervous, lymph, and musculoskeletal systems. In addition to the Auditory System, this chapter also discusses the Operating Microscope.

AUDITORY SYSTEM PROCEDURE BASICS

Otolaryngology is a subspecialty of internal medicine that specializes in the ears and throat. Otolaryngologists, otologists, and neuro-otologists are physicians that perform medical procedures and surgery on the ear. Plastic surgeons perform reconstructive repairs involving the external ear. Audiologists are nonphysician healthcare professionals who specialize in hearing, balance, and related disorders. Speech-language pathologists (SLPs), also known as speech therapists, specialize in the evaluation and treatment of communication disorders and swallowing disorders. They can assist people with hearing disorders with their speech production.

When working with medical terms, first identify the literal meaning of the term based on the meaning of roots, suffixes, and prefixes. Then, interpret the procedure being described within the context of the body system and procedures actually performed. The practical meaning sometimes varies from the literal meaning. Some medical terms with different suffixes are used as synonyms, such as *myringotomy* and *myringostomy*, both of which describe making an incision into the eardrum to drain fluid. *Myringotomy* is the more commonly used term because the incision is temporary. The word roots *myring/o* and *tympan/o* both mean eardrum or tympanic membrane, with the only difference being that *myring/o* is derived from Latin and *tympan/o* is derived from Greek. The terms *myringoplasty* and *tympanoplasty* are used synonymously, but *myringotomy* and *tympanostomy* are different

procedures because of the different suffixes. Myringotomy involves an incision into the ear drum only, whereas tympanostomy includes both an incision into the eardrum and the creation of a longer-term opening with the use of tubes in the tympanic membrane. Coders must refer to the CPT manual and other medical references to understand how the terms are used in any particular situation. Refer to ■ TABLE 44-1 for a refresher on how to build medical terms related to the auditory system.

CODING CAUTION

Be alert for medical terms that are pronounced similarly and have different meanings.

aural (*pertaining to the ear*) and **oral** (*pertaining to the mouth*)

cerumen (*earwax*) and **semen** (*fluid containing sperm*)

cochlea (*a coiled canal in the inner ear*) and **cholera** (*an acute gastrointestinal disease*)

electrocochleography (*recording of electrical activity of the cochlea*) and **electroencephalography** (*recording of electrical activity of the brain*)

Procedures commonly performed on each section of the auditory system are discussed next. Refer to detailed anatomic diagrams of specific parts of the ear when you need to refresh your memory on the location of specific structures or sites. Chapter 17 of this text provides additional information about the anatomy and conditions of the ear.

Procedures of the Auditory System

Procedures commonly performed on the Auditory System are summarized in ■ TABLE 44-2. In particular, coders need to understand the variations of mastoidectomy. *Mastoidectomy* is an example of a single term that can refer to a variety of techniques and requires a verbal modifier, such as simple or complete, to fully describe the procedure (■ TABLE 44-3). A mastoidectomy, which literally means "surgical excision of the mastoid bone," can be described as partial, complete, modified radical, or radical, based on the extent of the bone and surrounding structures

---

Table 44-1 ■ **EXAMPLE OF CONSTRUCTING MEDICAL TERMS FOR AUDITORY SYSTEM PROCEDURES**

Combining Form	Suffix	Complete Medical Term
myring/o (*eardrum, tympanic membrane*)		**myringo + plasty** (*surgical repair of the eardrum*)
		tympano + plasty (*surgical repair of the eardrum*)
tympan/o (*eardrum, tympanic membrane*)	**-plasty** (*surgical repair*) **-ectomy** (*excision*) **-tomy** (*incision*)	**myring + ectomy** (*excision of the eardrum*)
		tympan + ectomy (*excision of the eardrum*)
		myringo + tomy (*incision into the eardrum*)
		tympano + tomy (*incision into the eardrum*)

Source: © PB Resources, Inc. Used with permission.

Table 44-5 ■ LOCATING ICD-10-CM AND ADDITIONAL CPT CODES FOR THE AUDITORY SYSTEM

Type of Code	Codes
ICD-10-CM Auditory System-Related Codes	
Auditory system conditions	H60-H95
Neoplasms	C30, C44.2, C72.4, D02.3, D03.2, D04.2, D16, D22.2, D23.2
Symptoms and signs	R47-R49
Injuries	S00-S09, T20, T33
CPT Auditory System-Related Codes	
Medicine procedures	92502-92700
Radiologic procedures	
• Diagnostic radiology	70010-70559
• Radiologic guidance	77001-77022
• Diagnostic ultrasound	76506-76536
Laboratory organ/disease panels	Not applicable

Source: © PB Resources, Inc. Used with permission. CPT codes only © American Medical Association.

CODING FOR THE OPERATING MICROSCOPE

The CPT subsection **Operating Microscope (69990)** is the final **Surgery** subsection and contains only one code. It is used in conjunction with codes from multiple organ systems.

An **operating microscope** is a microscope that a physician uses to see small structures, such as in eye or ear surgery. Surgeons also use microdissection for blood vessels and nerve repair, including free tissue transfer.

When a surgery requires an operating microscope and the physician cannot perform the surgery without it, the microscope is an integral component of the procedure and should not be coded separately. When it is not an integral component of a procedure, assign code **69990**, which is an add-on code, to report use of the operating microscope. Refer to ■ TABLE 44-6 for guidance in abstracting operating microscope procedures.

To locate the code for use of the operating microscopic, search the Index for the Main Term **Operating Microscope**. One code is provided. Always verify the code in the Tabular List so that you can check the special instructions. Coders who frequently report the operating microscope quickly memorize the code number.

The CPT Tabular List provides instructional notes and special instructions regarding the use of code **69990** throughout the Surgery section, but notes do not appear consistently with all codes for which the operating microscope might

Table 44-6 ■ KEY CRITERIA FOR ABSTRACTING OPERATING MICROSCOPE PROCEDURES

❑ What is the primary procedure performed?

❑ Is use of the operating microscope documented?

❑ Do CPT guidelines or instructional notes indicate that the use of the operating microscope is included in the primary procedure?

For Medicare patients:

❑ Does the NCCI prohibit coding for the operating microscope in conjunction with the primary procedure?

Source: © PB Resources, Inc. Used with permission.

be used. A summary of operating microscope guidelines follows.

• A special instruction before code **69990** in the Tabular List identifies codes for which the operating microscope is an inclusive component. Do not assign code **69990** with any of these codes.

• Instructional notes throughout the Surgery section in the Tabular List sometimes, but not always, appear after the primary procedure code, reminding you not to code the operating microscope separately.

• An instructional note at the beginning of the subsection **Eye and Ocular Adnexa** states **(Do not report code 69990 in addition to codes 65091-68850)**. This instruction applies globally to all procedures in this code range.

• For procedures that do not have instructional notes prohibiting reporting of the operating microscope, report code **69990** when documented.

• CPT provides an instructional note following some procedure codes that states **(For operating microscope, use 69990)**. Assign code **69990** when the operating microscope is used with these procedures because it is not bundled.

Code **69990** reports the work required to set up, calibrate, position, and adjust the operating microscope when it is brought into the surgical field. Therefore, it is reported once per operative session, even if it is used for multiple procedures on the same patient.

Because code **69990** is an add-on code, do not append modifier **-51 Multiple procedures**. It should be sequenced as a secondary code.

CODING CAUTION

The National Correct Coding Initiative (NCCI) prohibits the use of code **69990** for many procedures for Medicare patients, even though it is not excluded by CPT. Be aware of private payers' rules regarding reporting of the operating microscope because they might have more flexible guidelines.

CODING PRACTICE

Exercise 44.2 Coding for the Operating Microscope

Instructions: Read the mini-medical-record of each patient's encounter and use the Key Criteria for Abstracting Operating Microscope Procedures (Table 44-6) to abstract the case. Assign CPT codes, quantities, and modifiers using the Index and Tabular List and arrange the codes as required. Write the code(s) on the line provided.

1. INPATIENT HOSPITAL   Gender: F   Age: 27

Preprocedure diagnosis: *herniated disk, L2-L3*

Procedure: *left hemilaminectomy L2-L3, foraminotomy, with use of operating microscope for microdissection*

a. What is the primary procedure performed? _____

b. Is use of the operating microscope documented? _____

c. Do CPT guidelines or instructional notes indicate that the use of the operating microscope is included in the primary procedure? _____

2 CPT Codes _____

2. OUTPATIENT SURGERY   Gender: F   Age: 54

Preprocedure diagnosis: *congenital bilateral esotropia*

Procedure: *bilateral medial rectus recession with microscopic control, 8 mm, both eyes*

a. What is the primary procedure performed? _____

b. Is use of the operating microscope documented? _____

c. Do CPT guidelines or instructional notes indicate that the use of the operating microscope is included in the primary procedure? _____

2 CPT Codes _____

3. OUTPATIENT SURGERY   Gender: F   Age: 54

Preprocedure diagnosis: *airway compromise; rule out squamous cell carcinoma of the larynx*

Procedure: *direct laryngoscopy with biopsy using a Zeiss operating microscope*

Postprocedure diagnosis: *squamous cell carcinoma of the larynx*

a. What is the primary procedure performed? _____

b. Is use of the operating microscope documented? _____

c. Do CPT guidelines or instructional notes indicate that the use of the operating microscope is included in the primary procedure? _____

1 CPT Code _____

ABSTRACTING AUDITORY SYSTEM PROCEDURES

Laterality is always relevant for ear procedures. Some clinicians might use Latin-based abbreviations to designate the laterality of the ear: **AD** (*auris dexter*) for the right ear; **AS** (*auris sinister*) for the left ear; **AU** (*auris uterque*) for each ear or both ears. These abbreviations are not on The Joint Commission's (TJC) required *Do Not Use List*; however, they are on TJC's supplemental list of abbreviations that it suggests, but does not require, that institutions prohibit through internal policy. The abbreviations also appear on the list *Error-Prone Abbreviations, Symbols, and Dose Designations* published by the Institute for Safe Medication Practices (ISMP). Therefore, it is best not to use these abbreviations, but coders should know what they mean if they encounter them.

The anatomic approach to ear procedures describes the path the surgeon uses to access the middle ear and inner ear. Some of the commonly used approaches include the following:

- **middle fossa approach**—through incision and partial removal of the bone above the ear
- **postauricular**—behind the ear
- **transcanal**—through the ear canal
- **transcranial**—through the skull
- **translabyrinthine**—through the labyrinth
- **transmastoid**—through the mastoid bone

Refer to ■ TABLE 44-7 for guidance on how to abstract procedures on the Auditory System, then work through the detailed example that follows. Remember that the abstracting questions

Table 44-7 ■ **KEY CRITERIA FOR ABSTRACTING AUDITORY SYSTEM PROCEDURES**

❑ What is the procedure?
❑ What part(s) of the ear is affected?
❑ What is the laterality?
❑ What is the surgical approach?
❑ What is the anatomic approach?
❑ What type of anesthesia is used?
❑ What additional procedures are performed during the same operative session?

Source: © PB Resources, Inc. Used with permission.

are a guide and that not every question applies to, or can be answered for, every case. For example, the type of anesthesia affects the coding of some, but not all, Auditory System procedures.

Guided Example of Abstracting Auditory System Procedures

Refer to the following example throughout this chapter to practice skills for abstracting, assigning, and arranging Auditory System codes.

OUTPATIENT SURGERY   Gender: F   Age: 7

Preoperative diagnosis: Recurrent acute suppurative otitis media, bilateral middle ear effusions. Chronic rhinitis. Recurrent adenoiditis with adenoid hypertrophy. Both parents are cigarette smokers.

Procedure: Bilateral myringotomies. Placement of ventilating tubes. Nasal endoscopy. Adenoidectomy. General anesthesia was administered by the CRNA. Inspected ears bilaterally with an operating microscope, which was also used for the procedure. Proceeded with anterior inferior quadrant myringotomy incisions, then evacuated a modest amount of serous and mucoid

---

material. Inserted PE tubes. Instilled antibiotic drops. Examined nasal passageways with endoscope. Acute purulent adenoiditis was evident. Shaved back the adenoids and flushed the area. Some material remained, which we resected, guided by the nasal endoscope. Submitted adenoid tissue to pathology. Patient tolerated procedure well.

Follow along as fictitious coder, Gabriella Javiera, CPC, abstracts the procedure. Check off each step after you complete it.

▶ Gabriella reads through the entire record, paying special attention to the reason for the encounter, the procedure performed, and the postoperative diagnosis. She refers to the Key Criteria for Abstracting Auditory System Procedures (Table 44-7).

❑ She notes several preoperative diagnoses: recurrent acute otitis media, bilateral middle ear effusions, chronic rhinitis, and recurrent adenoiditis with adenoid hypertrophy.

❑ *What is the procedure?* myringotomies, placement of ventilating tubes

❑ *What part(s) of the ear is affected?* middle ear

❑ *What is the laterality?* Bilateral

❑ *What is the surgical approach?* open

❑ *What is the anatomic approach?* anterior

❑ *What type of anesthesia is used?* General anesthesia

❑ *What additional procedures are performed during the same operative session?* Nasal endoscopy, adenoidectomy

▶ At this time, Gabriella does not know which of these procedures may need to be coded, nor how many codes she will end up with. She will learn about this when she moves on to assigning codes.

CODING PRACTICE

Exercise 44.3 Abstracting Auditory System Procedures

Instructions: Read the mini-medical-record of each patient's encounter and answer the abstracting questions. Write the answer on the line provided. Do not assign any codes.

---

1. OFFICE   Gender: F   Age: 2

Preprocedure diagnosis: pea lodged in left ear

Procedure: foreign body removal with forceps, auditory canal, left ear. Local anesthesia was used.

(continued)

---

1. (continued)
a. What is the procedure? _____
b. What part(s) of the ear is affected? _____
c. What is the laterality? _____
d. What is the surgical approach? _____
e. What is the anatomic approach? _____
f. What type of anesthesia is used? _____
g. What additional procedures are performed during the same operative session? _____

2. OUTPATIENT SURGERY Gender: M Age: 13

Preprocedure diagnosis: macrotia

Procedure: under general anesthesia, performed otoplasty to reduce the size of the ears, bilateral

a. What is the procedure? _____

b. What part(s) of the ear is affected? _____

c. What is the laterality? _____

d. What is the surgical approach? _____

e. What is the anatomic approach? _____

f. What type of anesthesia is used? _____

g. What additional procedures are performed during the same operative session? _____

3. OUTPATIENT HOSPITAL Gender: M Age: 43

Preprocedure diagnosis: hearing loss due to otosclerosis of the otic capsule in the right ear

Procedure: right stapedectomy with footplate (*part of the stapes*) drill out. Administered general anesthesia. Made an incision in the posterior ear canal via the ear canal opening and, using microscopic visualization, moved the skin flap and posterior eardrum forward. Created an opening in the thickened footplate and inserted a prosthetic replacement, which was stabilized with a piece of fascia on the incus.

a. What is the procedure? _____

b. What part(s) of the ear is affected? _____

c. What is the laterality? _____

d. What is the surgical approach? _____

e. What is the anatomic approach? _____

f. What type of anesthesia is used? _____

g. What additional procedures are performed during the same operative session? _____

4. OFFICE Gender: M Age: 52

Preprocedure diagnosis: vertigo due to Ménière disease

Procedure: endolymphatic sac exploration with shunt, bilateral. General anesthesia was administered. Made an incision exposing the right mastoid bone. Opened the mastoid and removed the bony cover of the sigmoid sinus. Worked our way down to the inner ear, taking great care to preserve all landmarks. When the endolymphatic sac was exposed, made an incision to drain it. Placed a tube between the endolymphatic sac and the mastoid cavity of the middle ear. Repeated procedure on the left ear with no problems. Patient tolerated procedure well.

a. What is the procedure? _____

b. What part(s) of the ear is affected? _____

c. What is the laterality? _____

d. What is the surgical approach? _____

e. What is the anatomic approach? _____

f. What type of anesthesia is used? _____

g. What additional procedures are performed during the same operative session? _____

ASSIGNING CODES FOR AUDITORY SYSTEM PROCEDURES

To assign codes for Auditory System procedures, search the Index for the Main Term **Ear**; the first-level modifying term for the site within the ear—**External Ear, Inner Ear, Middle Ear**, or **Temporal Bone**; then the second-level modifying term for the type of procedure. Cross-reference notes after the first-level modifying term **Drum** and the entry **External Ear, Tympanic Membrane** redirect you to the Main Term **Tympanic Membrane**. Alternatively, use the name of the procedure as the Main Term.

Assigning Codes for Myringotomy and Tympanostomy

Myringotomy and tympanostomy are among the most commonly performed procedures among children and are used to treat ear infections. In a myringotomy, the physician uses a myringotome to make an incision in the tympanic membrane to drain fluid from the middle ear. In a tympanostomy, a ventilating tube, also called a pressure-equalization (PE) tube, is inserted through the incision to form a permanent opening in the middle ear (■ FIGURE 44-1). The tube usually falls out on its own but in some cases might be surgically removed by the physician.

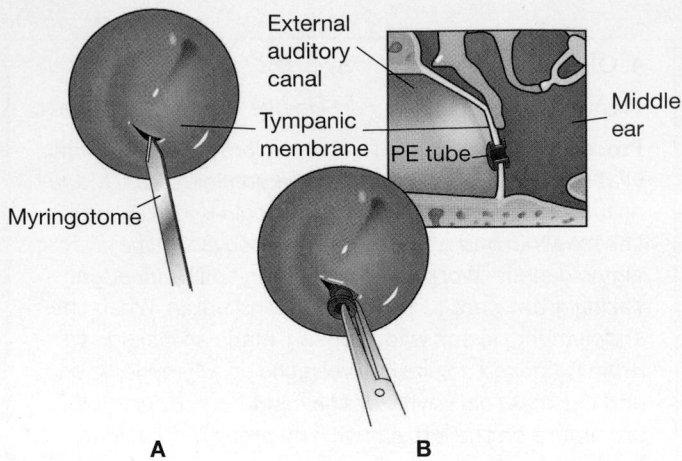

Figure 44-1 ■ Myringotomy (A) and Tympanostomy (B) Procedures

To assign codes for myringotomy or tympanostomy, search the Index for the Main Term that describes the procedure: **Myringotomy** when only drainage is performed and **Tympanostomy** when tubes also are inserted. In the Tabular List, codes for both procedures are divided by whether general anesthesia is provided (■ FIGURE 44-2). However, administration of general anesthesia is not included in codes **69421** or **69436**. The anesthesiologist bills for administration of anesthesia separate from the surgeon's bill for the procedure. When the surgeon administers the anesthesia, append modifier **-47 Anesthesia by surgeon** to the primary procedure code.

Assigning Codes for Removal of Foreign Bodies and Impacted Cerumen

The ear is a common entrance site for foreign bodies, especially among young children. CPT provides codes for removal of a foreign body from the external auditory canal with and without the use of general anesthesia (**69200, 69205**). To locate codes for removal of a foreign body from the ear, search the Index for the Main Term **Ear**, the first-level modifying term **External Ear**, and the second-level modifying term **Removal**, then **Foreign Body**. Refer to the Tabular List to select the appropriate code based on whether general anesthesia is used.

Impacted cerumen is reported with a separate code, not the code for foreign body removal, because it is a natural byproduct, not a foreign object. Report code **69210 Removal impacted cerumen requiring instrumentation, unilateral** only when instrumentation is required. When cerumen is not impacted or can be removed by irrigation, report only the appropriate Evaluation and Management (E/M) code. This guideline is discussed in the instructional note that follows code **69210** in the Tabular List.

Assigning Codes for the Middle and Inner Ear

The category **Other Procedures** under the subheading **Middle Ear** provides codes for hearing devices, such as the implantation, removal, or replacement of an electromagnetic bone-conduction hearing device or an **osseointegrated** (*integrated with bone*) **implant**. These codes represent the professional service. HCPCS codes identify the specific devices implanted (■ FIGURE 44-3) and may be billed by the facility where the procedure is performed, not by the physician. To locate these codes in the HCPCS manual, search the HCPCS Index for the Main Term **Auditory osseointegrated device**, then refer to the Tabular List to select the appropriate code.

The subheading **Inner Ear** includes procedures on the labyrinth, cochlea, vestibular chamber, and semicircular canals. In a cochlear implant procedure the physician implants a receiver into bone, which sends signals to electrodes implanted in the cochlea. The procedure destroys all residual natural hearing in the ear, so it is usually performed in only one ear.

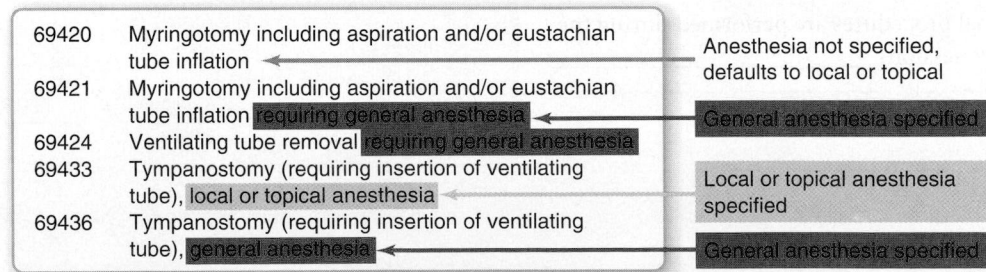

Figure 44-2 ■ CPT Tabular List Entry for Myringotomy and Tympanostomy. *Source: © PB Resources, Inc. Used with permission. CPT codes only © American Medical Association.*

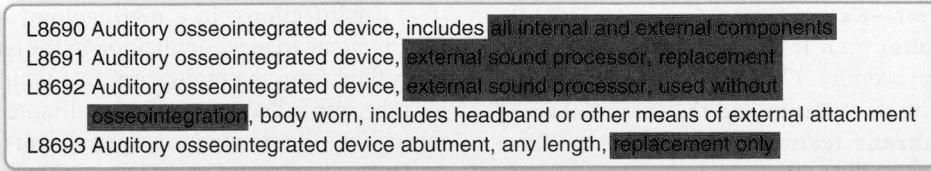

Figure 44-3 ■ HCPCS Tabular List Codes for Osseointegrated Hearing Implants

> Surgeon implants a cochlear device into the patient's right ear. The surgeon also provides the device.

> **69930-RT Cochlear device implantation, with or without mastoidectomy; -RT Right ear**
> **L8614 Cochlear device, includes all internal and external components**

Figure 44-4 ■ Example of Coding for a Cochlear Implant. *Source: © PB Resources, Inc. Used with permission. CPT codes only © American Medical Association.*

The implant device is usually provided by the facility where the procedure is performed, but if the surgeon supplies it, assign the appropriate HCPCS codes. Also remember to identify laterality (■ FIGURE 44-4).

Guided Example of Assigning Auditory System Procedure Codes

To practice skills for assigning codes for the Auditory System, continue with the example from earlier in the chapter about a patient who was seen for myringotomies. Follow along in your CPT manual as Gabriella Javiera, CPC, assigns codes. Check off each step after you complete it.

▶ First, Gabriella confirms the procedures performed: bilateral myringotomies, placement of ventilating tubes, nasal endoscopy, and adenoidectomy.

▶ Gabriella begins by coding the myringotomies. She identifies that because ventilating tubes also were placed, the procedure is coded as a tympanostomy. She searches the Index for the Main Term **Tympanostomy**.

  ❏ She locates the first-level modifying term **General Anesthesia**.

  ❏ She identifies code **69436**.

▶ Gabriella turns to the Tabular List to review, select, and verify the code.

  ❏ She reads the title for code **69436, Tympanostomy (requiring insertion of ventilating tube), general anesthesia** and confirms that this accurately describes the primary procedure.

  ❏ She reads the instructional note following the procedure description that states (**For bilateral procedure, report 69436 with modifier 50**).

▶ Gabriella checks for instructions in the Tabular List.

  ❏ She cross-references the beginning of the subcategory **Incision** and verifies that there are no special instructions.

  ❏ She cross-references the beginning of the subheading **Middle Ear** and verifies that there are no instructional notes.

  ❏ She cross-references the beginning of the subsection **Auditory System**. The only instructional note is a cross-reference to codes for diagnostic services that does not apply to this patient.

▶ Gabriella notices that use of an operating microscope is documented.

  ❏ She turns to the Index and locates the Main Term **Operating Microscope**, which directs her to code **69990 Microsurgical techniques, requiring use of operating microscope**.

  ❏ In the Tabular List, she reads the special instructions under the subsection title **Operating Microscope** and confirms that code **69436** is not listed as a bundled code. She also checks with the patient's payer to confirm that the code is allowed, even though it is excluded from Medicare by NCCI.

▶ Next, Gabriella needs to code for the adenoidectomy. This procedure was performed endoscopically, and a diagnostic nasal endoscopy also was performed. She recognizes that surgical endoscopy includes diagnostic endoscopy, so because both endoscopies used the nasal passage for access, she does not code for the diagnostic nasal endoscopy.

  ❏ She searches the Index for the Main Term **Adenoids** and the first-level modifying term **Excision**. She identifies the code range **42830-42836**.

  ❏ She turns to the Tabular List to review and verify the code selection.

  ❏ She identifies that codes **42830** and **42831** are for a primary adenoidectomy. Codes **42835** and **42836** are for a secondary adenoidectomy. She recalls that a secondary adenoidectomy refers to a follow-up adenoidectomy on the same patient to remove additional tissue that was missed during the original procedure. This is not the situation with this patient, so Gabriella needs a code for primary adenoidectomy.

  ❏ She reviews the codes for primary adenoidectomy and notices that they are divided by patient age: **younger than 12** and **age 12 or over**. She confirms in the medical record that the current patient is 7 years old, so she selects code **42830 Adenoidectomy, primary; younger than age 12**.

  ❏ She checks for instructional notes below the code and for special instructions at the beginning of the category, subheading, and subsection and finds none.

▶ Gabriella reviews the procedure codes she has assigned for this case.

  ❏ **42830 Adenoidectomy, primary; younger than age 12**

  ❏ **69436-50 Tympanostomy (requiring insertion of ventilating tube), general anesthesia**

  ❏ **69990 Microsurgical techniques, requiring use of operating microscope**

▶ Next, Gabriella must determine how to sequence the codes.

CODING PRACTICE

Exercise 44.4 Assigning Codes for Auditory System Procedures

Instructions: Read the mini-medical-record of each patient's encounter. Review the information abstracted in Exercise 44.3 for questions 1 and 2. For questions 3 and 4, abstract the case on your own. Assign CPT codes, quantities, and modifiers using the Index and Tabular List. Write the code(s) on the line provided.

---

1. OFFICE   Gender: F   Age: 2

Preprocedure diagnosis: pea lodged in left ear

Procedure: foreign body removal with forceps, auditory canal, left ear. Local anesthesia was used.

1 CPT Code _____

---

2. OUTPATIENT SURGERY   Gender: M   Age: 13

Preprocedure diagnosis: macrotia

Procedure: under general anesthesia, performed otoplasty to reduce the size of the ears, bilateral

1 CPT Code _____

---

3. OUTPATIENT SURGERY   Gender: F   Age: 51

Preprocedure diagnosis: profound mixed sensorineural conductive hearing loss, right side

Procedure: right middle ear exploration with a Goldenberg TORP reconstruction

1 CPT Code _____

---

4. OUTPATIENT SURGERY   Gender: M   Age: 68

Preprocedure diagnosis: squamous cell carcinoma of right temporal bone/middle ear space

Procedure: right temporal bone resection

1 CPT Code _____

ARRANGING CODES FOR AUDITORY SYSTEM PROCEDURES

The Auditory System does not provide any unique guidelines for sequencing codes. However, coders must be careful not to unbundle procedures that are integral to a code.

Unbundling

Do not assign multiple codes for procedures included in the primary procedure. For example, in a labyrinthotomy procedure the surgeon makes an incision into the labyrinth of the ear, and sometimes injects drugs, to treat Ménière disease. CPT instructional notes state **(Do not report 69801 more than once per day)** and also provide a list of codes that should not be reported together with a labyrinthotomy on the same ear. Vestibular function testing is performed for monitoring during the procedure and should not be reported separately. Diagnostic vestibular function testing is performed on a different date of service before the need for the procedure is determined. Diagnostic testing should not be reported with a labyrinthotomy procedure code on the same date of service.

Procedures that include a mastoidectomy should not be reported with a separate code for mastoidectomy, for example, codes **69910 Labyrinthectomy; with mastoidectomy** or **69530 Petrous apicectomy including radical mastoidectomy**.

-47 Anesthesia by Surgeon

For some procedures, CPT provides separate codes based on whether general anesthesia is provided. When general anesthesia is provided, and is provided by the operating surgeon, append modifier **-47 Anesthesia by surgeon**.

Guided Example of Arranging Auditory System Procedure Codes

To practice skills for arranging codes for procedures on the Auditory System, continue with the example from earlier in the chapter about the patient who was seen for myringotomies. Follow along in your CPT manual as Gabriella Javiera, CPC, arranges the codes. Check off each step after you complete it.

▶ First, Gabriella reviews the procedure codes she has assigned for this case.

❑ **42830 Adenoidectomy, primary; younger than age 12**

❑ **69436-50 Tympanostomy (requiring insertion of ventilating tube), general anesthesia**

❑ **69990 Microsurgical techniques, requiring use of operating microscope**

▶ Gabriella arranges the codes in descending RVU order according to the Medicare Physician Fee Schedule Database (MPFSDB). Although the patient is not covered by Medicare, the payer follows the Medicare RVUs. She uses the facility RVU because the procedure was performed at an outpatient surgery facility, not at the physician's office.

- ❏ **42830** Facility RVU = 6.98
- ❏ **69990** Facility RVU = 6.21
- ❏ **69436** Facility RVU = 4.62

▶ Gabriella examines the need for modifiers. (Refer to Table 30-1 Key Criteria for Abstracting CPT Modifiers or Appendix A in the CPT manual.)

- ❏ Code **42830** does not require modifiers because no special circumstances exist.

- ❏ Code **69990** does not require modifiers because, as an add-on code, it does not accept modifier **-51 Multiple procedures**.

- ❏ Code **69436** requires modifier **-51** because it is not an add-on code. It also requires modifier **-50 Bilateral procedure**.

▶ Gabriella finalizes the procedure codes and sequencing for this case:

(1) **42830 Adenoidectomy, primary; younger than age 12**

(2) **69990 Microsurgical techniques, requiring use of operating microscope**

(3) **69436-51-50 Tympanostomy (requiring insertion of ventilating tube), general anesthesia; -51 Multiple procedures; -50 Bilateral procedure**

▶ Gabriella also assigns and sequences the ICD-10-CM diagnosis codes that support the need for the service.

(1) **H66.003 Acute suppurative otitis media without spontaneous rupture of ear drum, bilateral**

(2) **J35.02 Chronic adenoiditis**

(3) **J31.0 Chronic rhinitis**

(4) **Z77.22 Contact with and (suspected) exposure to environmental tobacco smoke (acute) (chronic)**

CODING PRACTICE

Exercise 44.5   Arranging Codes for Auditory System Procedures

Instructions: Read the mini-medical-record of each patient's encounter. Review the information abstracted in Exercise 44.3 for questions 1 and 2. For questions 3 and 4, abstract the case on your own. Assign CPT codes, quantities, and modifiers using the Index and Tabular List, and arrange the codes in proper sequence. Write the code(s) on the line provided.

1. OUTPATIENT HOSPITAL   Gender: M   Age: 43

Preprocedure diagnosis: *hearing loss due to otosclerosis of the otic capsule in the right ear*

Procedure: *right stapedectomy with footplate (part of the stapes) drill out. Administered general anesthesia. Made an incision in the posterior ear canal via the ear canal opening and, using microscopic visualization, moved the skin flap and posterior eardrum forward. Created an opening in the thickened footplate and inserted a prosthetic replacement, which was stabilized with a piece of fascia on the incus.*

1 CPT Code _____

2. OFFICE   Gender: M   Age: 52

Preprocedure diagnosis: *vertigo due to Ménière disease*

Procedure: *endolymphatic sac exploration with shunt, bilateral. General anesthesia was administered. Made an incision exposing the right mastoid bone. Opened*

(continued)

2. (continued)

the mastoid and removed the bony cover of the sigmoid sinus. Worked our way down to the inner ear, taking great care to preserve all landmarks. When the endolymphatic sac was exposed, made an incision to drain it. Placed a tube between the endolymphatic sac and the mastoid cavity of the middle ear. Repeated procedure on the left ear with no problems. Patient tolerated procedure well.

1 CPT Code _____

3. OUTPATIENT SURGERY   Gender: M   Age: 6

Preprocedure diagnosis: *bilateral chronic otitis media and possible cholesteatoma, left middle ear*

Procedure: *bilateral myringotomy with insertion of tubes; middle ear exploration via myringotomy, left ear. Under general anesthesia, a right anterior inferior myringotomy was performed and a tube placed in the myringotomy site. Two myringotomies were performed on the left: one anterior and one inferior. Anterior view revealed a small mass, which was aspirated in part and sent to pathology. Patient tolerated the procedure well.*

Postprocedure diagnosis: *bilateral chronic otitis media, cholesteatoma, left middle ear*

Tip: Assign the laterality separately for each procedure.

2 CPT Codes _____

(continued)

4. OUTPATIENT SURGERY   Gender: F   Age: 54

Preprocedure diagnosis: chronic eustachian tube dysfunction; dizziness

Procedure: removed the old right pressure-equalizing tube; removed impacted cerumen, right ear canal; myringotomy with placement of a left pressure-

(continued)

4. (continued)

equalizing tube. The old tube on her right side was removed and the cerumen cleaned out. On the left we saw a retracted tympanic membrane and made an inferior anterior incision to place a ventilating tube. The procedure was completed without complication.

2 CPT Codes _____

E/M CODING FOR OTOLARYNGOLOGY

The *1997 Documentation Guidelines for Evaluation and Management Services* (1997 DG), published by CMS, provides requirements for each level of an ear, nose, and throat E/M examination (■ FIGURE 44-5). Otolaryngologists are not limited to using the guidelines for an ear, nose, and throat examination only. They can also use guidelines for a general multiorgan system examination, or any other single organ system examination, based on what is most advantageous for a specific encounter. However, physicians cannot combine elements from more than one type of examination for a given encounter. The ear examination guidelines typically provide the best results when a detailed ear examination is performed.

To determine the appropriate E/M code, coders must review the documentation in detail and identify the specific elements documented.

- To translate the documentation into the E/M requirements for the history, refer back to Chapter 31, Evaluation and Management Services (99201-99499), Tables 31-7 to 31-10, or the 1997 DG.
- To determine the requirements for an examination, refer to Figure 44-5 or to the single organ system examination for an ear, nose, and throat examination in the 1997 DG.
- To determine the levels for medical decision making (MDM), refer to Chapter 31, Table 31-12, and the Table of Risk in the 1997 DG.

Guided Example of E/M Coding for Otolaryngology

Refer to the otolaryngology encounter (■ FIGURE 44-6) to practice skills for abstracting and assigning E/M codes. Follow along as fictitious coder Gabriella Javiera, CPC, abstracts the procedure. Check off each step after you complete it.

▶ First, Gabriella needs to establish the category of service so she can determine the information needed to abstract and assign the code.

❑ *What is the setting?* office

❑ *What is the type of service?* new patient

❑ *What is the code range?* Gabriella refers to the CPT Index and looks up the Main Term **Evaluation and Management** and the subterm **Office and Other Outpatient**. The code range listed is **99201-99215**.

❑ *How many key components are required?* Gabriella refers to the code range in the Tabular List and identifies that the category New Patient comprises codes **99201-99215**. She reads the code description of the first code, which states **requires these 3 key components**. All codes in the category have the same requirements for key components. This tells her that all three key components must meet or exceed the levels listed in the code (3/3).

▶ Next, Gabriella identifies the level of history.

❑ *What is the level of HPI?* The HPI is **Extended** because four or more elements are documented.

❑ *What is the level of ROS?* The ROS is **Extended** because two to nine systems are documented.

❑ *What is the level of PFSH?* The PFSH is **Complete** because three elements are documented.

❑ *Based on these factors, what is the overall level of history?* The level of history is **Detailed** because the lowest of the three factors (HPI, ROS, and PFSH) determines the history level. The PFSH qualifies for a comprehensive history, but the HPI and ROS qualify for only a detailed history.

▶ Gabriella refers to the Ear, Nose, and Throat examination in the 1997 DG (Figure 44-5) to abstract information needed to determine the level of the examination.

❑ *What is the level of examination?* The level of examination is **Expanded problem focused**. Nine (9) elements of the examination are documented, which exceeds the requirement of 6–11 or more bulleted elements for an expanded problem-focused examination. A comprehensive examination requires that every element in each box with a shaded border and at least one element in each box with an unshaded border be documented, which they are not.

▶ Gabriella determines the level of medical decision making. (Refer to Table 31-12 Medical Decision Making Levels.)

❑ *What is the level of complexity of the number of diagnoses or management options, based on the presenting*

System/Body Area	Elements of Ear, Nose, and Throat Examination
Constitutional	❑ Measurement of any **three** of the following seven **vital** signs: • 1) sitting or standing blood pressure, • 2) supine blood pressure, • 3) pulse rate and regularity, • 4) respiration, • 5) temperature, • 6) height, • 7) weight (May be measured and recorded by ancillary staff) ❑ General **appearance** of patient (eg, development, nutrition, body habitus, deformities, attention to grooming) ❑ Assessment of ability to communicate (eg, use of sign language or other communication aids) and quality of voice
Head and Face	❑ Inspection of **head** and **face** (eg, overall appearance, scars, lesions and masses) ❑ Palpation and/or percussion of face with notation of presence or absence of **sinus** tenderness ❑ Examination of **salivary glands** ❑ Assessment of **facial strength**
Eyes	❑ Test ocular motility including primary gaze alignment
Ears, Nose, Mouth and Throat	❑ Otoscopic examination of external **auditory canals** and **tympanic membranes** ❑ Assessment of **hearing** with tuning forks and clinical speech reception thresholds (eg, whispered voice, finger rub) ❑ External **inspection** of ears and nose (eg, overall appearance, scars, lesions, masses) ❑ Inspection of **nasal mucosa, septum** and **turbinates** ❑ Inspection of **lips, teeth** and **gums** ❑ Examination of **oropharynx:** oral mucosa, salivary glands, hard and soft palates, tongue, tonsils and posterior pharynx (eg, asymmetry, lesions, hydration of mucosal surfaces) ❑ Inspection of **pharyngeal walls** and **pyriform sinuses** (eg, pooling of saliva, asymmetry, lesions) ❑ Examination by mirror of **larynx** including the condition of the epiglottis, false vocal cords, true vocal cords and mobility of larynx (Use of mirror not required in children) ❑ Examination by mirror of **nasopharynx** including appearance of the mucosa, adenoids, posterior choanae and eustachian tubes (Use of mirror not required in children)
Neck	❑ Examination of **neck** (eg, masses, overall appearance, symmetry, tracheal position, crepitus) ❑ Examination of **thyroid** (eg, enlargement, tenderness, mass)
Respiratory	❑ Inspection of **chest** including symmetry, expansion and/or assessment of respiratory effort (eg, intercostal retractions, use of accessory muscles, diaphragmatic movement) ❑ Auscultation of **lungs** (eg, breath sounds, adventitious sounds, rubs)
Cardiovascular	❑ **Auscultation** of heart with notation of abnormal sounds and murmurs ❑ Examination of **peripheral vascular system** by observation (eg, swelling, varicosities) and palpation (eg, pulses, temperature, edema, tenderness)
Lymphatic	❑ Palpation of **lymph nodes** in neck, axillae, groin and/or other location
Neurological/ Psychiatric	❑ Test **cranial nerves** with notation of any deficits *Brief assessment of mental status including:* ❑ **Orientation** to time, place and person ❑ **Mood** and affect (eg, depression, anxiety, agitation)

Total # Bullets Performed and Documented →	☐	# of ❑ Elements Performed and Documented	Level of Examination
		1–5	Problem focused
		6–11	Expanded problem focused
		12	Detailed
		ALL	Comprehensive (Document **every** element in each box with a shaded border and at least **one** element in each box with an unshaded border)

Figure 44-5 ■ 1997 DG for Ear, Nose, and Throat Examination. *Source: Centers for Medicare and Medicaid Services, 1997 Documentation Guidelines for Evaluation and Management Services (with formatting adjustments).*

OTOLARYNGOLOGY ENCOUNTER

HISTORY: Detailed

Setting & patient type

PRESENTATION: New patient, 13 years old, comes to the office with his mother complaining about severe ear pain bilaterally. He awoke during the night with severe ear pain, and mom states that this is the third time this year he has had earaches.

Chief complaint (CC)

HPI: Extended (4+)

HISTORY OF PRESENT ILLNESS: Patient reports that he felt good after taking antibiotics with each earache episode and has recently started on the wrestling team. Mom reports that patient has been afebrile with each of the earache episodes, and he has not had upper respiratory symptoms. Patient denies any head trauma associated with wrestling practice.

BIRTH AND DEVELOPMENTAL HISTORY: Patient's mother reports a normal pregnancy with no complications, having received prenatal care from 12 weeks. Vaginal delivery was uneventful with a normal perinatal course. Patient sat alone at 6 months, crawled at 9 months, and walked at 13 months. His verbal and motor developmental milestones were as expected.

FAMILY/SOCIAL HISTORY: Patient lives with both parents and two siblings (brother – age 11 years, sister – age 15 years). He reports enjoying school, remains active in scouts, and is very excited about being on the wrestling team. Mom reports that he has several friends, but she is concerned about the time required for the wrestling team. Patient is in 8th grade this year and an A/B student. Both siblings are healthy. His Dad has hypertension. Mom is healthy and has asthma.

PFSH: Complete (3)

PAST MEDICAL HISTORY: Patient has been seen in the clinic yearly for well child exams. He has had no major illnesses or hospitalizations. He had one emergency room visit 2 years ago for a knee laceration. Patient has been healthy except for the past year when he had two episodes of otitis media not associated with respiratory infections. He received antibiotic therapy (amoxicillin) for the otitis media and both episodes resolved without problems.

ROS: Extended (2-9)

PHYSICAL EXAM:
Height/weight: Patient weighs 109 pounds (60th percentile) and is 69 inches tall (93rd percentile). He is following the growth pattern he established in infancy.
Vital signs: BP 110/60, T 99.2, HR 70, R 16.
General: Alert, cooperative but a bit shy.
Neuro: DTRs symmetric, 2+, negative Romberg, able to perform simple calculations without difficulty, short-term memory intact. He responds appropriately to verbal and visual cues, and movements are smooth and coordinated.
HEENT: Normocephalic, PEERLA, red reflex present, optic disk and ocular vessels normal. TMs deep red, dull, landmarks obscured, full bilaterally. Post auricular and submandibular nodes on left are palpable and slightly tender.
Lungs: CTA, breath sounds equal bilaterally, excursion and chest configuration normal.
Cardiac: S1, S2 split, no murmurs, pulses equal bilaterally.
Abdomen: Soft, rounded, reports no epigastric tenderness. Bowel sounds active in all quadrants. No hepatosplenomegaly or tenderness. No CVA tenderness.
Musculoskeletal: Full range of motion, all extremities. Spine straight, able to perform jumping jacks and duck walk without difficulty.

EXAMINATION:
Expanded Problem Focused

(6-11 bulleted elements)

LABS: Normal CBC and urinalysis.

MEDICAL DECISION MAKING: Moderate Complexity

MDM Data: Ordering or reviewing diagnostic data (Straightforward Data)

ASSESSMENT: Chronic otitis media due to a penicillin resistant organism would be the obvious diagnosis in this case. It is rare for an adolescent to have otitis media with no precipitating factor such as being on a swim team or otherwise exposed to unusual organisms or in an unusual environment. It is certainly unusual for him to have three episodes in 1 year.

MDM Management: Established problem that is worsening (Low Management Options)

PLAN: He was given a prescription for 10 days of Augmentin and a follow-up appointment for 2 weeks if not improved.

MDM Risk: Prescription management (Moderate Risk)

KEY: HPI History of the present illness   ROS Review of systems
                    PFSH Past, family, and social history   MDM Medical decision making

Figure 44-6 ■ Otolaryngology Encounter

problem? The level is **Low** because there is an established problem that is worsening.

❏ *What is the amount and/or complexity of data to be reviewed?* The level is **Straightforward** because clinical labs were ordered.

❏ *What is the level of risk of significant complications, morbidity, and/or mortality?* Gabriella reviews each column in the Table of Risk in the 1997 DG and determines that the level of risk is **Moderate**. The patient presents with a chronic illness with mild exacerbation (Moderate), clinical labs ordered are CBC and urinalysis (Straightforward), and prescription drug management is provided (Moderate). The single highest element in the Table of Risk determines the overall risk. The columns **Presenting Problem** and **Management Options Selected** both are Moderate.

❑ *Based on these factors, what is the overall level of medical decision making?* The medical decision making is **Low complexity**. At least two of the three MDM factors are

required to qualify for a specific level of MDM. Two of the three MDM factors meet or exceed low-level decision making.

Now Gabriella is ready to assign the code for the audiology encounter. The exercise that follows guides you through additional abstracting skills and allows you to assign the correct code.

CODING PRACTICE

Exercise 44.6 E/M Coding for Otolaryngology

Instructions: Refer to the *1997 Documentation Guidelines for Evaluation and Management Services* (available at www.cms.gov) or Chapter 31 Evaluation and Management Services (99201-99499) (Tables 31-7 to 31-12) in this text. Answer the following questions about the otolaryngology encounter (Figure 44-6).

1. a. Which elements of the HPI are documented? Circle all that apply. Location, Quality, Severity, Duration, Timing, Context, Modifying factors, Associated signs and symptoms

   b. How many elements are documented? _____

   c. What is the level of HPI? _____

2. a. Which systems are reviewed in the ROS? Circle all that apply. Constitutional, Allergic/immunologic, CV, Endocrine, ENT/M, Eyes, GI, GU, Hemic/lymphatic, MS, Neurologic, Psychiatric, Respiratory, Skin/breast

   b. How many systems are documented? _____

   c. What is the level of ROS? _____

3. a. Which PFSH elements are documented? Circle all that apply. Past medical, Family, Social

   b. What is the level of PFSH? _____

   c. What is the overall level of history? (The lowest history factor—HPI, ROS, or PFSH—determines the level of history.) _____

4. Refer to Figure 44-5 1997 DG for Ear, Nose, and Throat Examination.

   a. Which bulleted items are documented for the examination? (Check off the items documented.)

   b. How many bulleted items are documented? _____

   c. What is the level of the examination? _____

5. Refer to Table 31-12 Medical Decision Making Levels or the 1997 DG.

   a. What is the MDM level for the number of diagnoses or management options?

   b. What is the MDM level for the amount and/or complexity of data to be reviewed?

   c. Refer to the Table of Risk in the 1997 DG. Which elements of risk are documented for each risk factor?

      1. Presenting problem: _____

      2. Diagnostic procedures ordered: _____

      3. Management options selected: _____

   d. What is the level of risk? (The highest of the three risk factors determines the overall level of risk.) _____

   e. What is the overall level of MDM? (2/3 MDM factors are needed to determine the overall level.) _____

6. a. What is the setting? _____

   b. What is the patient (or service) type? _____

   c. What is the code range? _____

   d. How many key components are required? _____

   e. What is the level of history? _____

   f. What is the level of examination? _____

   g. What is the level of medical decision making? _____

   h. What is the correct code? _____

7. Abstract, assign, and arrange (sequence) the diagnosis code(s) that support the E/M code.

   2 ICD-10-CM Code(s) _____

CHAPTER SUMMARY

In this chapter you learned that:

- When working with medical terms, first identify the literal meaning, then interpret the procedure being described within the context of the body system and procedures performed.

- When a surgery requires an operating microscope and the physician cannot perform the surgery without it, the microscope is an integral component of the procedure and should not be coded separately; when it is not an integral component of a procedure, assign code **69990**.

- The CPT subsection **Auditory System (69000-69970)** contains four subheadings that are divided by anatomic site.

- Laterality is always relevant for ear procedures, but coders should be aware of the abbreviations AD, AS, and AU that providers are discouraged from using.

- To assign codes for Auditory System procedures, search the Index for the Main Term **Ear**, the first-level modifying term for

the site within the ear—**External Ear**, **Inner Ear**, **Middle Ear**, or **Temporal Bone**—then the second-level modifying term for the type of procedure.

- Coders must be careful not to unbundle Auditory System procedures that are integral to a code.

- The *1997 Documentation Guidelines for Evaluation and Management Services* (1997 DG), published by CMS, provides requirements for each level of an ear, nose, and throat E/M examination.

- CPT provides guidelines and instructional notes on the operating microscope. Instructional notes appear throughout the Auditory System Tabular List to alert coders to the need for modifiers, provide cross-references to codes for similar procedures on other sites, identify when additional codes for radiological services might be needed, and highlight resequenced and recently deleted codes.

CONCEPT QUIZ

Take a moment to look back at the Auditory System and solidify your skills. Try to answer the questions from memory first, then refer to the discussion in this chapter if you need a little extra help.

Completion

Instructions: Write the term that answers each question based on the information you learned in this chapter. Choose from the list below. Some choices may be used more than once and some choices may not be used at all.

AD   osseointegrated implant

AS   otologists

AU   postauricular

audiologists   RT

BI   LT

cochlear device implantation   transcranial

middle fossa approach   translabyrinthine

operating microscope   transmastoid

1. The approach conducted through the skull is referred to as
   _____.

2. The use of a(n) _____ is coded separately when it is not an integral component of the procedure.

3. _____ is a procedure where a receiver is implanted into bone, which sends signals to electrodes implanted in the cochlea.

4. The abbreviation for "right ear" is _____.

5. A through incision and partial removal of the bone above the ear is referred to as a(n) _____.

6. The approach conducted through the labyrinth is referred to as
   _____.

7. The approach conducted through the mastoid bone is
   _____.

8. The abbreviation for "left ear" is _____.

9. Nonphysician healthcare professionals who specialize in hearing, balance, and related disorders are _____.

10. The abbreviation used when both ears are referenced is
    _____.

Multiple Choice

Instructions: Circle the letter of the best answer to each question based on the information you learned in this chapter.

1. What procedure is performed to repair the tympanic membrane, involving the drumhead and donor area, usually with a graft of living tissue such as fat or fascia?
   A. Tympanostomy
   B. Stapedectomy
   C. Myringotomy
   D. Myringoplasty

2. What procedure is performed due to Ménière disease, involving an incision into the labyrinth of the ear, and may involve administration/injection of drugs?
   A. Radical mastoidectomy
   B. Labyrinthectomy
   C. Labyrinthotomy
   D. Simple transmastoid antrotomy

3. What procedure is performed when a patient presents with suppurative otitis media?
   A. Simple mastoidectomy
   B. Complete mastoidectomy
   C. Radical mastoidectomy
   D. Modified radical mastoidectomy

4. What procedure is used to treat adhesions or scar tissue where tympanic membrane adhesions are destroyed?
   A. Tympanolysis
   B. Tympanogram
   C. Tympanostomy
   D. Tympanoplasty

5. What procedure is a mastoidectomy with more extensive removal of the mastoid process?
   A. Complete mastoidectomy
   B. Simple mastoidectomy
   C. Total mastoidectomy
   D. Radical mastoidectomy

6. What procedure drains fluid or pus from the eardrum?
   A. Tympanotomy
   B. Myringotomy
   C. Myringectomy
   D. Stapedectomy

7. What procedure includes total mastoidectomy following a prior mastoidectomy that did not resolve the patient's condition?
   A. Revision mastoidectomy
   B. Radical mastoidectomy
   C. Complete mastoidectomy
   D. Simple mastoidectomy

8. What procedure is used to treat impaired mobility of the malleus and includes excision of part of the temporal bone and radical resection of the entire mastoid part of the posterior temporal bone?
   A. Tympanolysis
   B. Tympanostomy
   C. Petrous apicectomy
   D. Radical mastoidectomy

9. What procedure is commonly performed when neoplasms are present in the ear canal?
   A. Petrous apicectomy
   B. Radical mastoidectomy
   C. Tympanolysis
   D. Fenestration semicircular canal

10. What procedure is performed due to otosclerosis and involves an incision into the footplate of the stapes?
    A. Stapedectomy
    B. Fenestration semicircular canal
    C. Myringoplasty/tympanoplasty
    D. Stapedotomy

CODING CHALLENGE

Instructions: Read the mini-medical-record of each patient's encounter, then abstract, assign, and arrange ICD-10-CM diagnosis codes and CPT procedure codes using the appropriate Index and Tabular List. Assign quantities and modifiers where needed. Write the code(s) on the line provided.

1. OUTPATIENT SURGERY   Gender: F   Age: 22

Assessment: chronic suppurative otitis media right ear

Procedure: tympanoplasty with mastoidectomy, with ossicular chain reconstruction

1 ICD-10-CM Code _____

1 CPT Code _____

2. EMERGENCY DEPARTMENT   Gender: M   Age: 2

Reason for encounter: bead in external ear canal

Procedure: removal of foreign body using conscious sedation

1 ICD-10-CM Code _____

1 CPT Code _____

3. OUTPATIENT SURGERY   Gender: F   Age: 45

Reason for encounter: labyrinthitis becoming worse, right ear

Procedure: labyrinthectomy with mastoidectomy, postauricular incision, right ear

1 ICD-10-CM Code _____

1 CPT Code _____

4. OUTPATIENT SURGERY   Gender: F   Age: 21

Reason for encounter: foreign body in right ear

Procedure: removal of foreign body under general anesthesia, subsequent encounter

1 ICD-10-CM Code _____

1 CPT Code _____

(*continued*)

(continued from page 873)

5. OUTPATIENT SURGERY   Gender: M   Age: 53

Assessment: ruptured ear drum

Procedure: repair of tympanic membrane perforation using synthetic patch

1 ICD-10-CM Code _____

1 CPT Code _____

---

6. OUTPATIENT SURGERY   Gender: M   Age: 39

Assessment: cyst, right external ear

Procedure: excision of right external ear cyst

1 ICD-10-CM Code _____

1 CPT Code _____

---

7. OUTPATIENT SURGERY   Gender: M   Age: 71

Assessment: tinnitus

Procedure: exploration of middle ear via postauricular incision, left ear

1 ICD-10-CM Code _____

1 CPT Code _____

---

8. OUTPATIENT SURGERY   Gender: F   Age: 8

Assessment: 80% conductive hearing loss, right ear

Procedure: cochlear implantation

1 ICD-10-CM Code _____

1 CPT Code _____

---

9. OUTPATIENT SURGERY   Gender: M   Age: 11

Reason for encounter: Ears are severely protruding

Procedure: bilateral otoplasty

1 ICD-10-CM Code _____

1 CPT Code _____

---

10. OUTPATIENT SURGERY   Gender: F   Age: 18 months

Assessment: chronic otitis media in left ear

Procedure: myringotomy with tube insertion

1 ICD-10-CM Code _____

1 CPT Code _____

KEEP ON CODING

Instructions: Read the procedural statement, then use the appropriate Index and Tabular List to assign CPT procedure codes, quantities, and modifiers. Write the code(s) on the line provided.

1. Transtympanic eustachian tube catheterization: CPT Code(s) _____

2. Repair oval window fistula: CPT Code(s) _____

3. Revision of stapedotomy: CPT Code(s) _____

4. Ear piercing: CPT Code(s) _____

5. Decompression of internal auditory canal: CPT Code(s) _____

6. Simple mastoidectomy, right ear : CPT Code(s) _____

7. Biopsy of earlobe: CPT Code(s) _____

8. Facial nerve repair, medial/geniculate, left: CPT Code(s) _____

9. Simple incision and drainage of abscess, left external meatus: CPT Code(s) _____

10. Complete mastoidectomy: CPT Code(s) _____

11. Routine cleaning of right mastoid cavity: CPT Code(s) _____

12. Removal of tumor from temporal bone, right side: CPT Code(s) _____

13. Myringoplasty, left: CPT Code(s) _____

14. Bilateral removal of impacted cerumen using forceps: CPT Code(s) _____

15. Semicircular canal fenestration, left ear: CPT Code(s) _____

16. Amputation, left external ear: CPT Code(s) _____

17. Excision, left extratemporal glomus tumor: CPT Code(s) _____

18. Use of operating microscope: CPT Code(s) _____

19. Resection, left temporal bone: CPT Code(s) _____

20. Excision, aural polyp: CPT Code(s) _____

21. Complex debridement of mastoid cavity under general anesthesia: CPT Code(s) _____

22. Excision, external left ear, simple repair: CPT Code(s) _____

23. Mastoidectomy with tympanoplasty, reconstruct left ossicular chain: CPT Code(s) _____

24. Myringotomy with aspiration under general anesthesia: CPT Code(s) _____

25. Inflation/catheterization, left eustachian tube, transnasal approach: CPT Code(s) _____

Chapter 45

Urinary (50010-53899), Male Genital System Procedures (54000-55899), Reproductive System (55920), and Intersex Surgery (55970-55980) Procedures

Chapter Outline

- **Urinary and Male Genital System Procedure Basics**
- **Coding Overview of Urinary System Procedures**
- **Coding Overview of Male Genital System and Other Reproductive Procedures**
- **Abstracting Procedures for the Urinary and Male Genital Systems**
- **Assigning Codes for Urinary and Male Genital System Procedures**
- **Arranging Codes for Urinary and Male Genital System Procedures**
- **E/M Coding for Urology**

Learning Objectives

After completing this chapter, you should have the skills to:

45.1 Spell and define the key words, medical terms, and abbreviations related to urinary and male genital system procedures.

45.2 Discuss the types of procedures on the urinary and male genital systems.

45.3 Identify the main characteristics of coding for the Urinary and Male Genital Systems.

45.4 Abstract procedural information from the medical record for coding the Urinary and Male Genital Systems procedures.

45.5 Assign codes for the Urinary and Male Genital Systems procedures.

45.6 Arrange codes for the Urinary and Male Genital Systems procedures.

45.7 Code evaluation and management services for urology.

45.8 Discuss the CPT coding guidelines related to the Urinary and Male Genital Systems.

Key Terms and Abbreviations

antegrade	obstructive uropathy	retrograde	transpubic
gender data mismatch	ostomy	retroperitoneal	transurethral
ileal conduit	penile	retropubic	transvaginal
indwelling (catheter)	perineum	transcatheter	
nonindwelling (catheter)	perirenal	transperineal	

In addition to the key terms listed here, students should know the terms defined within tables in this chapter.

For updates and corrections, visit our student resource site at

www.pearsonhighered.com/healthprofessionsresources

INTRODUCTION

Advertisements for products and pharmaceuticals related to urinary system problems appear frequently on television and in magazines. These health challenges present tangible limitations on many people's daily functioning.

This chapter discusses several related CPT subsections. The **Urinary System** subsection is discussed under chapter subtitles with the same name. Subtitles for the Male Genital System discuss three CPT subsections: **Male Genital System, Reproductive System Procedures**, and **Intersex Surgery**. The CPT subsections **Female Genital System** and **Maternity Care and Delivery** are discussed in Chapter 46 of this text.

URINARY AND MALE GENITAL SYSTEM PROCEDURE BASICS

Urology is a surgical specialty that deals with diseases of the male and female urinary tract and the male reproductive organs. Although urology is classified as a surgical specialty, a knowledge of internal medicine, pediatrics, gynecology, and other specialties is required because of the wide variety of clinical problems encountered. The American Urological Association recognizes seven subspecialty areas:

- Pediatric urology
- Urologic oncology
- Renal transplantation
- Male infertility
- Calculi
- Female urology—urinary incontinence and pelvic outlet relaxation disorders
- Neurourology—voiding disorders, urodynamic evaluation of patients, and erectile dysfunction or impotence

Refer to ■ TABLE 45-1 for a refresher on how to build medical terms related to the urinary system. Refer to ■ TABLE 45-2 for a refresher on how to build medical terms related to the male genital system.

CODING CAUTION

Be alert for medical words that are spelled similarly and have different meanings.

glomerul/o (*globular tuft [formed by capillaries in the kidney]*) and **globulin** (*a type of protein used by the body*)

pyle/o (*renal pelvis*) and **pylor/o** (*most distal part of the stomach*)

diuresis (*excessive urination*) and **dialysis** (*separation of waste material [from the blood]*)

epididymis (*spermatic duct*) and **epidermis** (*outer layer of the skin*)

perirenal (*surrounding the kidney*) and **perineal** (*surrounding the perineum [the area between the anus and external genitalia]*)

Commonly performed procedures on the urinary and male genital systems are discussed next. Refer to detailed anatomic diagrams when you need to refresh your memory of the relationship of organs and sites to each other. Chapters 22 and 23 of this text provide additional information on the anatomy and conditions of the urinary system and male and female reproductive systems. Procedures commonly performed on the Urinary System are summarized in ■ TABLE 45-3. Procedures commonly performed on the Male Genital System are summarized in ■ TABLE 45-4. In particular, coders need to understand treatment of **obstructive uropathy** (*the inability of urine to flow*), calculi (*stones*), congenital anomalies, and bladder reconstruction.

Obstructive Uropathy

Obstructive uropathy can affect anyone from infants with congenital anomalies to older adults. Surgeons perform a variety of procedures depending on the cause of the problem, such as obstructed posterior urethral valves or obstructed ureteropelvic junction, bladder outlet obstruction, or benign prostatic hyperplasia.

Table 45-1 ■ EXAMPLE OF CONSTRUCTING MEDICAL TERMS FOR URINARY SYSTEM PROCEDURES

Combining Form	Suffix	Complete Medical Term
nephr/o (*kidney*)		nephro + scopy (*visual examination of the kidney*)
		cysto + scopy (*visual examination of the urinary bladder*)
	-scopy (*visual examination*)	uretero + scopy (*visual examination of the ureters*)
	-ectomy (*excision*)	nephr + ectomy (*excision of the kidney*)
cyst/o (*urinary bladder*)		cyst + ectomy (*excision of the bladder*)
		ureter + ectomy (*excision of the ureters*)
ureter/o (*ureter*)		

Table 45-2 ■ EXAMPLE OF CONSTRUCTING MEDICAL TERMS FOR MALE GENITAL SYSTEM PROCEDURES

Combining Form	Suffix	Complete Medical Term
prostat/o (*prostate*)		prostato + tomy (*incision into the prostate*)
	-tomy (*incision into*)	vaso + tomy (*incision into the vas deferens*)
	-ectomy (*excision*)	prostat + ectomy (*excision of the prostate*)
vas/o (*vas deferens*)		vas + ectomy (*excision of the vas deferens*)

Table 45-3 ■ **COMMON PROCEDURES OF THE URINARY SYSTEM**

Procedure Name	Definition	Reason Performe
Aspiration of bladder	Removal of urine using a needle, a trocar, or a catheter	Urinary retention
Cutaneous vesicostomy	Temporary surgical procedure to create an opening in the umbilicus (*lower abdomen*), which allows urine to continuously drain from the bladder	Bladder neck obstruction, hypertonicity of the bladder, congenital atresia and stenosis of the urethra and bladder neck
Cystectomy	Partial or complete excision of the bladder; may also involve other procedures, including removing surrounding lymph nodes	Bladder cancer
Cystolithotomy	Incision of the bladder to remove calculi	Bladder calculi
Cystometrogram	Use of a manometer (*pressure-measuring device*) to evaluate bladder function; the bladder is emptied using a catheter, then filled using a smaller catheter	Voiding dysfunction
Cystostomy	Creation of an opening in the bladder, with possible removal of the bladder neck	Neoplasm
Cystotomy	Incision into the bladder	Cryosurgical lesion destruction, catheter or stent insertion, diverticulum, tumor, or ureterocele
Extracorporeal shock wave lithotripsy (ESWL)	Use of lithotriptor to aim pulsating sound waves at a kidney stone to break it into pieces	Calculi
Nephrectomy	Partial or complete removal of a kidney	Neoplasm, end-stage hydronephrosis
Nephrolithotomy	Incision of the kidney to remove a kidney calculus	Kidney calculi
Nephrorrhaphy	Suture of kidney wound or injury	Laceration
Nephrostomy	Creation of an opening in the kidney with percutaneous catheter insertion, with imaging guidance	Ureter occlusion, such as kidney calculi, neoplasm; tear in the ureter that allows urine to leak
Nephrotomy	Incision into the kidney	Obstruction, hemorrhage, neoplasm
Pelvic exenteration	Excision of the bladder, urethra, ureters, lymph nodes, prostate/vagina, uterus, colon and rectum; may also include a hysterectomy and resecting the rectum and colon	Neoplasm
Pyeloplasty	Repair of the renal pelvis (complicated if it involves a congenital kidney abnormality, a secondary pyeloplasty, solitary kidney, or calycoplasty [*repair of the calyx*])	A ureteropelvic junction obstruction
Pyelotomy	Incision into the renal pelvis	Diagnose disorders; drain urine from the renal pelvis; calculi
Renal endoscopy	Endoscopy through an established nephrostomy, pyelostomy, nephrotomy, or pyelotomy	Biopsy, ureteral catheterization, removal of a foreign body or calculus, or tumor fulguration
Renal transplant	Implantation of a cadaver or living donor kidney to take over the function of the patient's natural kidney. Consists of a donor nephrectomy; backbench work to dissect and remove fat and prepare attached ureters, veins, and arteries for transplantation; and transplantation into the recipient	End-stage renal disease (ESRD)
Transurethral resection of prostate (TURP)	Insertion of a resectoscope via the urethra and removal of a portion of the prostate; may include cystoscopy, meatotomy, and urethral dilation	Benign prostatic hypertrophy (BPH)
Ureterectomy	Excision of the ureter	Neoplasm
Ureterolithotomy	Incision into a ureter	Calculi
Ureteroplasty	Repair of the ureter; may include excision of a portion of the ureter, then anastomosis of the ends that were not removed or grafting of tissue from the bladder	Ureteral stricture
Ureterotomy	Incision into the ureter; may include stent placement	Occlusion, stenosis

Table 45-3   ■   (*continued*)

Procedure Name	Definition	Reason Performe
Urethroneocystostomy	Repair of a defect in the bladder and urethra, with reimplantation of one or both of the ureters into the bladder	Incontinence, stricture
Urodynamic tests	A variety of tests that measure the contraction of the bladder muscle as it fills and empties, ranging from simple visual observation to precise measurements using sophisticated instruments	Lower urinary tract symptoms (LUTSs)
Vesicourethropexy, Marshall-Marchetti-Krantz (MMK) procedure, Burch procedure	Suturing of the vaginal wall to the urethra or bladder neck, with anchoring to the pubic bone or Cooper ligament	Stress urinary incontinence (SUI), cystocele, urethrocele

Source: © PB Resources, Inc. Used with permission.

Calculi

Treatment of kidney stones and bladder stones has benefitted from advances in technology that have eliminated the need for most surgeries to treat these problems. The use of rigid and flexible ureteroscopy enables urologists to extract calculi with forceps or a basket. Management of stones in the kidney has progressed with the introduction of percutaneous methods to disintegrate and extract kidney stones, and extracorporeal shock wave lithotripsy (ESWL) uses shock waves to break a kidney stone into small pieces that can more easily travel through the urinary tract and pass from the body. In addition, urologists can help reduce the risk of stone formation because of advances in the diagnosis and metabolic management of recurrent nephrolithiasis.

Congenital Anomalies

The urinary tract is affected by congenital anomalies more than any other organ system. Conditions range from the relatively common problem of cryptorchidism (*failure of testes to descend*) to the complex area of intersexuality. Most urologists surgically repair many congenital anomalies in children, but the more complex problems are often referred to subspecialists in pediatric urology.

Bladder Reconstruction

According to the National Institutes of Health, bladder cancer is the sixth most common cancer in the United States. Surgical removal of tumors or, in some cases, the entire bladder is often the first step of treatment. Surgeons may reconstruct the bladder using a portion of the intestine and creating an **ileal conduit** (*a channel that joins the ureters to the ileum*). In some cases a cutaneous ostomy (*opening on the skin of the abdomen*) and a collection appliance might be used.

This section provides a general reference to help understand the most common urinary system procedures. Remember to keep standard reference books handy in case you get stuck.

Table 45-4   ■   **COMMON PROCEDURES OF THE MALE GENITAL SYSTEM**

Procedure Name	Definition	Reason Performed
Electroejaculation	Insertion of an electrostimulator probe into the patient's rectum next to the prostate to transmit an electrical current and stimulate ejaculation	In vitro fertilization, paralysis, retrograde ejaculation
Epididymovasostomy	Removal of a portion of the vas deferens and attachment of the vas deferens to the epididymis	Obstruction of spermatic flow
Ligation	Excision or tying off of dilated vein(s) using a laparoscopic approach	Varicocele (*dilated vein in the scrotum*)
Prostatectomy	Removal of the prostate gland, including possible biopsy or removal of the lymph nodes	Prostate cancer or BPH
Vasectomy	Cutting out a piece of the vas deferens and cauterizing or suturing the ends closed	Sterilization
Vesiculectomy	Removal of one of the seminal vesicles	Chronic infection, prostate cancer

Source: © PB Resources, Inc. Used with permission.

CODING PRACTICE

Exercise 45.1 Urinary and Male Genital System Procedure Basics

Instructions: Use your medical terminology skills and resources to define the following procedures related to the urinary and male genital system, then identify the code(s) or code range listed in the CPT Index. Follow these steps:

- Use slash marks "/" to break down each term into its root(s) and suffix.
- Define the meaning of the word based on the meaning of each word part.
- Identify the CPT code(s) or code range listed in the CPT Index.

Example: <u>nephrotomy</u> nephro/tomy   Meaning *making an incision into the kidney*   CPT Code *50040-50045*

1. penis, <u>plethysmography</u>   Meaning _____   CPT Code _____

2. <u>epididymectomy</u>, bilateral   Meaning _____   CPT Code _____

3. <u>ureteroureterostomy</u>   Meaning _____   CPT Code _____

4. <u>vesicourethropexy</u>   Meaning _____   CPT Code _____

5. <u>urethrorrhaphy</u>   Meaning _____   CPT Code _____

6. <u>cystometrogram</u>   Meaning _____   CPT Code _____

7. <u>pyelolithotomy</u>   Meaning _____   CPT Code _____

8. <u>calycoplasty</u>   Meaning _____   CPT Code _____

9. <u>cystourethroscopy</u>, biopsy, brush   Meaning _____   CPT Code _____

10. <u>vesiculectomy</u>   Meaning _____   CPT Code _____

CODING OVERVIEW OF URINARY SYSTEM PROCEDURES

The CPT subsection **Urinary System (50010-53899)** contains three subheadings that are divided by anatomic site (■ TABLE 45-5). Within each anatomic site, codes are divided by the type of procedure, such as incision, excision, introduction, and so on. Review the subheading and category names and code ranges listed in the Urinary System subsection to become familiar with the content and organization. Some editions of the CPT manual provide a summary list of the subheadings and categories at the beginning of the Urinary System subsection, which also displays an asterisk (*) next to categories that contain special coding instructions.

This subsection includes invasive, minimally invasive, and noninvasive surgical procedures on the Urinary System. Codes for diagnostic tests on the urinary system appear in the Medicine section. CPT codes in the Urinary System subsection are frequently supported by diagnosis codes from ICD-10-CM **Chapter 14 Diseases of the Genitourinary System (N00-N99)**, as well as neoplasms, symptoms and signs, and injuries (■ TABLE 45-6). These are the codes most commonly used to support procedures on the Urinary System; however, diagnosis codes from any ICD-10-CM chapter are permissible. CPT codes must always be linked on claims with one or more diagnosis codes to justify the medical necessity of the service.

CPT guidelines for the Surgery section apply to the Urinary System. Special instructions provide definitions and coding guidelines at the beginning of many categories. Special instructions are provided for **Laparoscopy** and **Endoscopy** categories in several places throughout the Urinary System, as well as for **Renal Transplantation (50300-50380)**, **Bladder-Urodynamics (51725-51798)**, and **Bladder-Transurethral Surgery (52320-52356)**.

Instructional notes appear throughout the Tabular List to alert coders to the need for modifiers, provide cross-references to codes for similar procedures on other sites, identify when additional codes for radiological services might be needed, and highlight resequenced and recently deleted codes.

Most codes for the urinary system apply to both males and females, although some are gender-specific, such as those for procedures on the prostate. Due to anatomic differences in the urethra between males and females, some codes for procedures on the urethra are also gender-specific. Such codes are discussed later in this chapter.

Table 45-5 ■ **URINARY SYSTEM SUBHEADINGS**

Subheading	Code Range
Kidney	50010-50135
Ureter	50600-50980
Bladder	51020-52700

Table 45-6 ■ LOCATING ICD-10-CM AND ADDITIONAL CPT CODES FOR THE URINARY AND MALE GENITAL SYSTEM

Type of Code	Codes
ICD-10-CM Urinary and Male Genital System-Related Codes	
Urinary system conditions	N00-N39
Male genital system conditions	N40-N65, Z31
Neoplasms	C50, C60-C63, C64-C68
Symptoms and signs	R30-R39
Injuries	S37-S39
CPT Urinary and Male Genital System-Related Codes	
Medicine procedures	90935-90999, 96040
Radiologic procedures	
• Diagnostic radiology	74400-74485
• Radiologic guidance	77001-77022
• Diagnostic ultrasound	76700-76776
• Nuclear medicine, diagnostic	78700-78799
Laboratory organ/disease panels	80047, 80048, 80050, 80053, 80069

Source: © PB Resources, Inc. Used with permission. CPT codes only © American Medical Association.

Table 45-7 ■ MALE GENITAL SYSTEM SUBHEADINGS

Subheading	Code Range
Penis	54000-54450
Testis	54500-54699
Epididymis	54700-54901
Tunica Vaginalis	55000-55060
Scrotum	55100-55180
Vas Deferens	55200-55450
Spermatic Cord	55500-55559
Seminal Vesicles	55600-55680
Prostate	55700-55899

CODING OVERVIEW OF MALE GENITAL SYSTEM AND OTHER REPRODUCTIVE PROCEDURES

This chapter discusses three CPT subsections that describe the Male Genital System and other reproductive procedures. The first subsection, **Male Genital System (54000-55899)**, contains nine subheadings that are divided by anatomic site (■ TABLE 45-7). Within each anatomic site, codes are divided by the type of procedure, such as incision, excision, introduction, and so on. Review the subheading and category names and code ranges listed in the Male Genital System subsection to become familiar with the content and organization. Special instructions are provided for **Laparoscopy** and **Endoscopy** categories in several places throughout the Male Genital System subsection.

The second subsection, **Reproductive System Procedures (55920)**, contains one code that identifies **Placement of needles or catheters into pelvic organs and/or genitalia (except prostate) for subsequent interstitial radioelement application.**

The third subsection, **Intersex Surgery (55970-55980)**, contains two codes: one for male-to-female intersex surgery and one for female-to-male intersex surgery.

These three CPT subsections are discussed in the remainder of this chapter under the subtitles for the Male Genital System.

This subsection includes invasive, minimally invasive, and noninvasive surgical procedures on the Male Genital System and other reproductive system procedures. Codes for diagnostic tests on the Male Genital System appear in the Medicine section. CPT codes in the Male Genital System subsection are frequently supported by diagnosis codes from ICD-10-CM **Chapter 14 Diseases of the Genitourinary System (N00-N99)**, as well as neoplasms, symptoms and signs, and injuries. These are the codes most commonly used to support procedures on the Male Genital System; however, diagnosis codes from any ICD-10-CM chapter are permissible.

CPT guidelines for the Surgery section apply to the Male Genital System.

Special instructions provide definitions and coding guidelines at the beginning of many categories.

Instructional notes appear throughout the Tabular List to alert coders to the need for modifiers, provide cross-references to codes for similar procedures on other sites, identify when additional codes for radiological services might be needed, and highlight resequenced and recently deleted codes.

Codes for the male genital system are gender-specific and apply only to males.

ABSTRACTING PROCEDURES FOR THE URINARY AND MALE GENITAL SYSTEMS

Abstracting for urinary and male genital system procedures uses similar processes. For both systems, coders must identify the anatomic approach and the patient's gender. Refer to ■ TABLE 45-8 for guidance on how to abstract procedures on the urinary system. Refer to ■ TABLE 45-9 for guidance on how to abstract procedures on the male genital system. A detailed guided example on abstracting skills follows. Remember that the abstracting questions are a guide and that not every question applies to, or can be answered for, every case. For example, anastomosis is not always performed, but when it is, you must identify the structures that are joined.

Abstracting the Anatomic Approach

As is the case with procedures in many body systems, procedures on the urinary and male genital systems often use a specific anatomic approach to access the surgical site. Coders must understand and be able to identify the correct anatomic

Table 45-8 ■ KEY CRITERIA FOR ABSTRACTING URINARY SYSTEM PROCEDURES

- ❑ What is the procedure?
- ❑ What is the patient's gender?
- ❑ What is the anatomic site?
- ❑ What structures outside the urinary system are involved, if any?
- ❑ What is the surgical approach?
- ❑ What is the anatomic approach?
- ❑ What is the laterality?
- ❑ What type of obstruction is treated, if any?
- ❑ What structures are joined in an anastomosis, if performed?
- ❑ Is a stoma created?

Source: © PB Resources, Inc. Used with permission.

approach based on the documentation. Commonly used anatomic approaches include the following:

- **penile**—in or through the penis (male only)
- **perirenal**—in tissues surrounding the kidney
- **retroperitoneal**—behind the peritoneal membrane that covers the abdominal and pelvic organs
- **retropubic**—behind the pubic bone
- **ostomy**—through an existing stoma
- **transcatheter**—through an existing catheter
- **transperineal**—through the **perineum** (*the area between the anus and external genitalia*)
- **transpubic**— through the pubic bone
- **transurethral**—through the urethra
- **transvaginal**—through the vagina (female only)

Table 45-9 ■ KEY CRITERIA FOR ABSTRACTING MALE GENITAL SYSTEM PROCEDURES

- ❑ What is the procedure?
- ❑ What is the patient's gender?
- ❑ What is the anatomic site?
- ❑ What structures outside the male genital system are involved, if any?
- ❑ What is the surgical approach?
- ❑ What is the anatomic approach?
- ❑ What is the laterality?
- ❑ What type of obstruction is treated, if any?
- ❑ What structures are joined in an anastomosis, if performed?

Source: © PB Resources, Inc. Used with permission.

Abstracting Gender

Coders must always be attentive to the patient's gender, especially when abstracting for the urinary and reproductive systems. A **gender data mismatch** occurs when the patient's documented gender is inconsistent with the procedure coded. Obviously, it is impossible to perform a gender-specific procedure on an opposite-sex patient, but a data mismatch can happen. This is most likely to occur with procedures that are gender-specific, such as a prostatectomy, and those that use a gender-specific anatomic approach—such as penile or transvaginal. A gender data mismatch can be caused by data entry errors or confusion of names, so coders must verify the patient's gender against any gender-specific edits for a code. When the gender does not match the procedure described, refer back to any source documents, such as patient registration forms, to confirm the correct information. In most cases, claims that contain a gender data mismatch cannot be transmitted for payment because they are flagged by the electronic claims processing system as containing invalid data. If they are transmitted, they will not be processed by the payer. Either way, the error causes delays and added processing time for the medical office. Sometimes, rejected or unprocessable claims are not corrected immediately but are added to the medical facility's backlog of claims that need to be resubmitted and might be neglected for weeks or months. A quick double check by the coder to verify the patient's gender while abstracting can save significant time and money later in the claims process.

Guided Example of Abstracting Urinary System Procedures

Refer to the following example throughout this chapter to practice skills for abstracting, assigning, and arranging urinary system codes.

> OUTPATIENT HOSPITAL   Gender: M   Age: 40
>
> Preprocedure diagnosis: red, swollen penis
>
> Procedure: ureterography; inserted bilateral ureteral catheter percutaneously through the renal pelvis using imaging guidance, injected contrast medium through catheter using imaging guidance, and viewed both ureters. Provided radiological supervision, reviewed findings, and dictated report for both radiological procedures.
>
> Postprocedure diagnosis: ureteral stricture

Follow along as fictitious coder, Chrystal Crago, CCA, abstracts the procedure. Check off each step after you complete it.

▶ Chrystal reads through the entire record, paying special attention to the reason for the encounter, the procedure performed, and the postprocedure diagnosis. She refers to the Key Criteria for Abstracting Urinary System Procedures (Table 45-8).

  ❑ She notes preoperative diagnosis, red, swollen penis, and the postprocedure diagnosis, ureteral stricture.

❑ *What is the procedure?* ureterography

❑ *What is the patient's gender?* male

❑ *What is the anatomic site?* ureter

❑ *What structures outside the urinary system are involved, if any?* none

❑ *What is the surgical approach?* external

❑ *What is the anatomic approach?* transcatheter

❑ *What is the laterality?* viewed both ureters (bilateral)

❑ *What type of obstruction is treated, if any?* a ureteral stricture was identified as the diagnosis, but it was not treated

❑ *What additional procedure is performed?* inserted a ureteral catheter

❑ *What is the anatomic site?* renal pelvis

❑ *What is the surgical approach?* percutaneous

❑ *What is the laterality?* viewed both ureters (bilateral)

❑ *What additional procedure is performed?* radiological supervision

▶ At this time, Chrystal does not know which of these procedures may need to be coded, nor how many codes she will end up with. She will learn about this when she moves on to assigning codes.

CODING PRACTICE

Exercise 45.2   Abstracting Procedures for the Urinary and Male Genital Systems

Instructions: Read the mini-medical-record of each patient's encounter and answer the abstracting questions. Write the answer on the line provided. Do not assign any codes.

1. INPATIENT HOSPITAL   Gender: M   Age: 69

Preprocedure diagnosis: urinary incontinence

Procedure: Sling operation. Made an incision in the perineum to advance a synthetic sling under the bladder and attached it to the muscles surrounding the urethra.

a. What is the procedure? _____

b. What is the patient's gender? _____

c. What is the anatomic site? _____

d. What structures outside the urinary system are involved, if any? _____

e. What is the surgical approach? _____

f. What is the anatomic approach? _____

g. What is the laterality? _____

h. What type of obstruction is treated, if any? _____

i. What structures are joined in an anastomosis, if performed? _____

j. Is a stoma created? _____

2. OUTPATIENT SURGERY   Gender: M   Age: 29

Preprocedure diagnosis: infected seminal vesicles due to E. coli

Procedure: vesiculotomy; incised both seminal vesicles to drain infection. Complex dissection was required due to scar tissue in the area.

a. What is the procedure? _____

b. What is the patient's gender? _____

c. What is the anatomic site? _____

d. What structures outside the male genital system are involved, if any? _____

e. What is the surgical approach? _____

f. What is the anatomic approach? _____

g. What is the laterality? _____

h. What type of obstruction is treated, if any? _____

i. What structures are joined in an anastomosis, if performed? _____

3. OUTPATIENT SURGERY   Gender: M   Age: 58

Preprocedure diagnosis: residual tissue 60 days post-TURP that was performed by the same surgeon due to BPH

Procedure: TURP to remove residual tissue; advanced flexible cystourethroscope through the external opening of the urethra to the prostate and located the residual prostate tissue that continues to partially obstruct the urethra. Excised tissue using blunt and sharp dissection. A catheter was placed. Patient tolerated procedure well.

a. What is the procedure? _____

(continued)

CODING PRACTICE (continued)

3. (continued)

b. What is the patient's gender? _____

c. What is the anatomic site? _____

d. What structures outside the urinary system are involved, if any? _____

e. What is the surgical approach? _____

f. What is the anatomic approach? _____

g. What is the laterality? _____

h. What type of obstruction is treated, if any? _____

i. Was the procedure provided within the global period of another procedure by the same physician? _____

---

4. INPATIENT HOSPITAL Gender: M Age: 46

Preprocedure diagnosis: bladder cancer; previously removed the bladder and created an ileal conduit (*use of a segment of the ileum to connect the ureters to a stoma on the abdominal wall*)

Procedure: ureteropyelography; injected contrast medium through the existing stoma to view the ureters and ileal conduit. Supervised the radiology procedure and dictated the interpretation report.

Preprocedure diagnosis: ileal conduit was visualized to be functioning properly

a. What is the procedure? _____

b. What is the patient's gender? _____

c. What is the anatomic site? _____

d. What structures outside the urinary system are involved, if any? _____

e. What is the surgical approach? _____

f. What is the anatomic approach? _____

g. What structures are joined in an anastomosis, if performed? _____

h. Is a stoma created? _____

i. Was radiological supervision and interpretation provided by the same physician? _____

---

5. INPATIENT HOSPITAL Gender: M Age: 67

Preprocedure diagnosis: bladder cancer of contiguous sites of the bladder with metastasis to the colon and rectum

Procedure: functioned as a member of a surgical team; completely excised the urinary bladder; created a

(continued)

---

5. (continued)

ureteroileal conduit and intestinal anastomosis; performed bilateral pelvic lymphadenectomy including external iliac, hypogastric, and obturator nodes; performed an open total colectomy with a complete proctectomy

Tip: Code for one surgeon who is working as part of the surgical team.

a. What is the anatomic site? _____

b. What is the first procedure? _____

c. What is the second procedure? _____

d. What is the third procedure? _____

e. What is the fourth procedure? _____

f. What structures outside the urinary system are involved, if any? _____

g. What is the surgical approach? _____

h. What structures are joined in an anastomosis, if performed? _____

i. Is a stoma created? _____

---

6. OFFICE/OUTPATIENT HOSPITAL Gender: M Age: 72

Reason for encounters: new patient with complaints of urinary incontinence

Procedure (Tuesday): conducted a comprehensive history and exam with moderate-complexity medical decision making. Recommended further testing and discussed treatment options with patient.

Procedure (Friday): performed postvoid residual (PVR) ultrasound test to measure the amount of urine left in the bladder after the patient urinates

Plan: incontinence sling surgery

a. What service is provided on Tuesday? _____

b. What is the setting? _____

c. What is the patient type? _____

d. What is the level of history? _____

e. What is the level of examination? _____

f. What is the level of medical decision making? _____

g. What procedure is performed on Friday? _____

h. What is the anatomic site? _____

i. What testing modality is used? _____

j. What is the laterality? _____

k. What is the plan? _____

ASSIGNING CODES FOR URINARY AND MALE GENITAL SYSTEM PROCEDURES

Coders must be aware of gender-specific codes when coding for the Urinary and Male Genital Systems. They must also be familiar with coding for urinary catheterization and radiological guidance and supervision and interpretation (S&I). These skills are discussed next, followed by the continuation of the guided example.

Assigning Gender-Specific Codes

Because of the anatomic differences between the male and female urethra, some procedures are gender-specific. Differences include the longer length of the female urethra and the different types of anatomic approach, such as transvaginal, prostatic, or penile. Gender edits are not identified in the official CPT manual, although some third-party publishers provide enhanced manuals with annotations or symbols. Some encoders and medical billing software programs also provide an alert for gender edits. If you do not have access to these resources, rely on the code description to identify gender-specific codes (■ TABLE 45-10).

Assigning Codes for Urinary Catheterization

Urinary catheters are hollow, flexible tubes used to drain urine from the bladder into an external collection bag. Codes for urinary catheterization are divided based on the type of catheter, the anatomic site of catheter insertion, and, in some cases, the reason for the bladder catheter. The codes differentiate between indwelling and nonindwelling catheters, which are defined as follows:

- **indwelling**—a flexible, hollow tube inserted into the urinary bladder left in short or long term to provide continuous urine flow; may be inserted through the urethra or ureters
- **nonindwelling**—includes two types of catheters that are not left in the bladder: a condom catheter placed outside the body to catch urine or a straight catheter inserted into the bladder only to drain the urine then removed; also called an external catheter

Table 45-10   ■   **EXAMPLES OF GENDER EDITS FOR THE URINARY SYSTEM**

Gender	CPT Code
Male	53410 Urethroplasty, 1-stage reconstruction of male anterior urethra
Male	53415 Urethroplasty, transpubic or perineal, 1-stage, for reconstruction or repair of prostatic or membranous urethra
Female	53430 Urethroplasty, reconstruction of female urethra
Female	53500 Urethrolysis, transvaginal, secondary, open, including cystourethroscopy (eg, postsurgical obstruction, scarring)
Both	52300 Biopsy of urethra
Both	53431 Urethroplasty with tubularization of posterior urethra and/or lower bladder for incontinence (eg, Tenago, Leadbetter procedure)

Source: © PB Resources, Inc. Used with permission. CPT codes only © American Medical Association.

Refer to ■ TABLE 45-11 to learn about the various types of urinary catheters.

Insertion of a urinary bladder catheter is a component of the global surgical package and is not separately reportable when performed at the time of or just prior to the procedure. However, when the catheter is inserted due to unforeseen circumstances after the patient has left the operating room, report the CPT code that identifies the type of catheter inserted. Electronic edit checks for claims processing often automatically deny a catheterization on the same date as a procedure. Insurance companies might request the use of modifier **-59 Distinct procedural service**, a separate diagnosis code, or a special report that clearly identifies the problem necessitating the catheterization.

Table 45-11   ■   **TYPES OF URINARY CATHETERS**

Type of Catheter	Description
Balloon catheter	An urethral catheter with an inflatable balloon near the tip to hold the catheter in place and/or dilate the urethra
Condom catheter	A nonindwelling catheter consisting of a sac that fits over the penis to collect urine and drain it through a tube that leads to a collection bag; is left in place
Coudé catheter	A type of elbowed catheter with a slightly curved tip
Elbowed catheter, prostatic catheter	A urethral catheter with a sharp bend near the intake; used to navigate past obstructions in the urinary tract
Female catheter	A short urethral catheter for passage through the female urethra
Foley catheter	The most commonly used design of indwelling balloon catheter
Nephrostomy catheter	A catheter inserted through an existing nephrostomy
Olive-tip catheter	A ureteral catheter with an olive-shaped end, used to dilate a constricted ureter
Straight catheter	A nonindwelling catheter consisting of a short, rigid tube that is inserted via the urethra to allow for drainage of urine, then removed
Suprapubic catheter	An indwelling catheter inserted into the bladder through a laparotomy incision a few inches below the navel; less likely to harbor infection than indwelling urethral catheters
Ureteral catheter	An indwelling catheter inserted into the ureter, either through the urethra and bladder or posteriorly through the kidney
Urethral catheter	An Indwelling catheter inserted through the urethra into the urinary bladder, percutaneously or through an existing ostomy
Winged catheter	An urethral catheter that is retained in the bladder by winglike projections on the end

Source: © PB Resources, Inc. Used with permission.

To assign codes for urinary catheterization, search the Index for the Main Term **Catheterization**, then locate the first-level modifying term **Bladder**. Refer to the Tabular List to select and verify the correct code. Codes are divided based on the use of a cystotomy (**51045**), suprapubic catheter (**51102**), nonindwelling (**51701**), or indwelling type (**51702**, **51703**). Indwelling catheter codes are divided based on the extent of the procedure as simple or complicated. A complicated catheterization should be documented as such by the physician and may include working with abnormal anatomy, retrieving a fractured (*broken*) catheter or balloon, or treating another complicating circumstance that requires an extensive amount of time to complete.

To locate codes for ureteral catheterization, search the Index for the Main Term **Ureter** and the first-level modifying term **Catheterization**. When a ureteral catheter is inserted *endoscopically*, search the Index for the Main Term **Catheterization**, the first-level modifying term **Ureter**, and the second-level modifying term **Endoscopic**. Although these two coding paths seem similar, they lead to different codes in the CPT Index. Another option is to search the Index for the Main Term **Insertion**, the first-level modifying term **Catheter**, and the second-level modifying terms **Bladder**, **Kidney**, **Ureter**, or **Urethra**. Remember that when you cannot easily locate a code that accurately describes the procedure using your preferred coding path, try searching for a different Main Term.

SUCCESS STEP

A *catheter* is a thin, flexible, hollow tube used in many types of medical procedures. In addition to being used for urinary system procedures, catheters are used in procedures on the heart, vascular system, lung, and brain. When you see a catheter mentioned in documentation, always identify the type and purpose of the catheter being used.

Assigning Codes Requiring Radiologic Guidance

Some urinary system procedures are performed with radiologic guidance, such as fluoroscopy, to project a real-time X-ray image of anatomic structures onto a screen while the surgeon is manipulating instruments. Radiologic guidance can be provided by the same surgeon performing the procedure or by a radiologist, and it is almost always reported as a separate procedure with a code from the Radiology section of CPT. In the Tabular List, codes for procedures that are frequently performed with imaging guidance may be accompanied by an instructional note that directs coders to the corresponding Radiology code. The wording of the instructional note varies. Keep in mind the following information when assigning codes for imaging procedures (■ TABLE 45-12):

- Instructional notes may appear immediately after a code or at the beginning of a range or category.

- The instructional note might list one code or multiple codes.

- Always verify the codes in the Radiology section of the Tabular List.

- Multiple Radiology codes are listed when more than one type of imaging procedure is potentially applicable. Review

Table 45-12 ■ **EXAMPLES OF CODE DESCRIPTIONS AND INSTRUCTIONAL NOTES FOR RADIOLOGICAL SERVICES**

Description	Code Example
Bundled fluoroscopy	50389 Removal of nephrostomy tube, requiring fluoroscopic guidance (eg, with concurrent indwelling ureteral stent) (Removal of nephrostomy tube not requiring fluoroscopic guidance is considered inherent to E/M services. Report the appropriate level of E/M service provided)
Fluoroscopy coded separately	50081 Percutaneous nephrostolithotomy or pyelostolithotomy, with or without dilation, endoscopy, lithotripsy, stenting, or basket extraction; over 2 cm (For fluoroscopic guidance, see 76000, 76001)
Multiple code options for S&I	50390 Aspiration and/or injection of renal cyst or pelvis by needle, percutaneous (For radiological supervision and interpretation, see 74425, 74470, 76942, 77002, 77012, 77021)
Radiologic service not bundled	52010 Cystourethroscopy, with ejaculatory duct catheterization, with or without irrigation, instillation, or duct radiography, exclusive of radiologic service (For radiological supervision and interpretation, use 74440)
Single code option for S&I	53600 Dilation of urethral stricture by passage of sound or urethral dilator, male; initial (For radiological supervision and interpretation, use 74485)
Multiple code options for imaging guidance	55876 Placement of interstitial device(s) for radiation therapy guidance (eg, fiducial markers, dosimeter), prostate (via needle, any approach), single or multiple (For imaging guidance, see 76942, 77002, 77012, 77021)

Source: © PB Resources, Inc. Used with permission.

all codes listed and select the *one* that describes the specific procedure performed. Do not randomly assign a code without confirming that it accurately describes the procedure.

- When the code description of the primary procedure states that imaging guidance is included, do not assign a separate Radiology code.

- Most Radiology codes include a professional component (*physician supervision, interpretation, and written report*) and a technical component (*facility, staffing, and equipment*). The Radiology code may require a modifier based on the service being provided. (Review Chapters 30 and 47 in this text for more information and examples.)

  ▪ When coding for a physician who provides both components, assign the code with no modifiers.

- When coding for a physician who provides only the professional component, append modifier **-26 Professional component** to the Radiology code.
- When coding for a facility that provides only the technical component, append modifier **-TC Technical component** to the Radiology code.

Guided Example of Assigning Urinary System Procedure Codes

To practice skills for assigning codes for the Urinary System, continue with the example from earlier in the chapter about a patient who was seen for urography. Follow along in your CPT manual as Chrystal Crago, CCA, assigns codes. Check off each step after you complete it.

▶ First, Chrystal confirms the procedure: transcatheter ureterography with imaging guidance.

▶ Chrystal searches the Index for the Main Term **Ureterography**.

❑ She locates the first-level modifying term **Injection procedure**.

❑ She identifies the single code listed: **50684**.

▶ Chrystal verifies code **50684** in the Tabular List.

❑ She reads the code title for **50684 Injection procedure for ureterography or ureteropyelography through ureterostomy or indwelling ureteral catheter**.

❑ She notices that the anatomic approach is **through ureterostomy or indwelling ureteral catheter**. She refers to the medical record to verify that a ureterostomy was not performed and an indwelling (previously inserted) catheter was not present. The physician inserted a catheter specifically for the purpose of this procedure. Therefore, she believes that she should code for the catheter insertion.

▶ Chrystal searches the Index for the Main Term **Ureter**.

❑ She locates the first-level modifying term **Insertion**.

❑ She locates the second-level modifying term **Catheter**.

❑ She identifies two codes listed **50393, 51045**.

▶ Chrystal refers to the Tabular List to review and select the code.

❑ First, she locates code **50393** and reads the description: **Introduction of ureteral catheter or stent into ureter through renal pelvis for drainage and/or injection, percutaneous**.

❑ She locates the second code **51045** and reads the description: **Cystotomy, with insertion of ureteral catheter or stent (separate procedure)**.

❑ She determines from the documentation that the catheter was inserted percutaneously through the renal pelvis and that a cystotomy was not performed, so she selects code **50393**.

▶ Chrystal checks for instructions in the Tabular List, beginning with code **50393**.

❑ She reads the instructional note after code **50393** that states **(For radiological supervision and interpretation, see 74480, 76942, 77002, 77012)**.

❑ She refers to the documentation to confirm that the physician provided the radiological supervision and interpretation (S&I) for this procedure, so she reviews the suggested codes.

❑ The code description that identifies the service provided is **74480 Introduction of ureteral catheter or stent into ureter through renal pelvis for drainage and/or injection, percutaneous, radiological supervision and interpretation**.

❑ She further checks the beginning of the category and subheading for code **50393** and finds no special instructions.

▶ Chrystal checks for instructions in the Tabular List for code **50684**.

❑ She reads the instructional note after code **50684** that states **(For radiological supervision and interpretation, use 74425)**.

❑ She refers to the documentation to confirm that the physician provided the radiological supervision and interpretation (S&I) for this procedure, so she reviews code **74425 Urography, antegrade (pyelostogram, nephrostogram, loopogram), radiological supervision and interpretation**. Although an ureterogram is not among the example procedures listed in parentheses, the rest of the description is accurate. In particular, a ureterogram is performed in an **antegrade** (*the normal or forward direction of flow*) manner because the renal pelvis is located above the ureters. This is in contrast to a **retrograde** procedure, which would be performed "upstream" or against the normal direction of flow.

❑ She further checks the beginning of the category and subheading for code **50684** and finds no special instructions.

▶ Chrystal reviews the procedure codes she has assigned for this case.

❑ **50684 Injection procedure for ureterography or ureteropyelography through ureterostomy or indwelling ureteral catheter**

❑ **74425 Urography, antegrade (pyelostogram, nephrostogram, loopogram), radiological supervision and interpretation**

❑ **50393 Introduction of ureteral catheter or stent into ureter through renal pelvis for drainage and/or injection, percutaneous**

❑ **74480 Introduction of ureteral catheter or stent into ureter through renal pelvis for drainage and/or injection, percutaneous, radiological supervision and interpretation**

▶ Next, Chrystal must determine how to sequence the codes.

CODING PRACTICE

Exercise 45.3 Assigning Codes for Urinary and Male Genital System Procedures

Instructions: Read the mini-medical-record of each patient's encounter. Review the information abstracted in Exercise 45.2 for questions 1–3. For questions 4–6, abstract the case on your own. Assign CPT codes, quantities, and modifiers using the Index and Tabular List. Write the code(s) on the line provided.

1. INPATIENT HOSPITAL   Gender: M   Age: 69

Preprocedure diagnosis: urinary incontinence

Procedure: Sling operation. Made an incision in the perineum to advance a synthetic sling under the bladder and attached it to the muscles surrounding the urethra.

1 CPT Code _____

2. OUTPATIENT SURGERY   Gender: M   Age: 29

Preprocedure diagnosis: infected seminal vesicles due to E. coli

Procedure: vesiculotomy; incised both seminal vesicles to drain infection. Complex dissection was required due to scar tissue in the area.

Tip: The documentation of complex dissection qualifies this as a *complicated* procedure.

1 CPT Code _____

3. OUTPATIENT SURGERY   Gender: M   Age: 58

Preprocedure diagnosis: residual tissue 60 days post-TURP that was performed by same surgeon due to BPH

Procedure: TURP to remove residual tissue; advanced flexible cystourethroscope through the external opening of the urethra to the prostate and located the residual prostate tissue that continues to partially obstruct the urethra. Excised tissue using blunt and sharp dissection. A catheter was placed. Patient tolerated procedure well.

Tip: TURP has a 90-day global period.

1 CPT Code _____

4. OUTPATIENT SURGERY   Gender: M   Age: 54

Preprocedure diagnosis: carcinoma of the prostate

Procedure: cryoablation of the prostate. Ultrasound used to assist with cryoprobe placement. A double freeze–thaw cycle was performed, with excellent evidence of freezing obtained. Monitoring probes were withdrawn.

1 CPT Code _____

5. OUTPATIENT SURGERY   Gender: M   Age: 24

Preprocedure diagnosis: phimosis

Procedure: circumcision. Under general anesthesia, heavy scissors used to cut the foreskin and retract over the glans. A cut was made around the glans and penile shaft to excise the foreskin. Hemostasis obtained with cautery. Shaft skin reapproximated. Patient sent to recovery room.

1 CPT Code _____

6. OUTPATIENT SURGERY   Gender: M   Age: 61

Preprocedure diagnosis: bladder mass

Procedure: cystoscopy with transurethral resection of 0.6-cm bladder tumor

Postprocedure diagnosis: cystoscope used to identify the presence of the bladder tumor. Resectoscope inserted into the bladder to resect the tumor off the posterior wall. Hemostasis achieved with cautery. Scope removed and patient taken to recovery.

1 CPT Code _____

ARRANGING CODES FOR URINARY AND MALE GENITAL SYSTEM PROCEDURES

Coders must be familiar with rules for bundling and multiple coding related to endoscopy procedures. Also, be informed about how to apply modifiers for laterality and ESWL. These guidelines are discussed next, followed by the conclusion of the guided example.

Endoscopy Coding

Endoscopy is performed to visualize and treat components of the urinary system. The only natural opening of the urinary system is the urethra, which is too narrow for endoscopic access, so laparoscopic access is required through an abdominal or pelvic incision into the desired site, such as the bladder, ureters, or kidney. Physicians also use an established ostomy access when one is available.

Coders must be familiar with the National Correct Coding Initiative (NCCI) rules and private payer rules regarding endoscopy coding. Review the following NCCI guidelines regarding multiple coding of endoscopies applied to the genitourinary system:

- Surgical endoscopy/laparoscopy always includes a diagnostic endoscopy/laparoscopy performed at the same time using the same access. Report a code only for the surgical endoscopy/laparoscopy.

- When an endoscopic procedure is converted to an open procedure, report only the open procedure.

- When endoscopic visualization of the urinary system involves several regions, such as the kidney, renal pelvis, calyx, and ureter, assign the CPT code based on the anatomic approach, such as nephrostomy, pyelostomy, or ureterostomy. The approach is identified in the CPT code description, as in the following examples:

  - **50551 Renal endoscopy through established nephrostomy or pyelostomy, with or without irrigation, instillation, or ureteropyelography, exclusive of radiologic service**

  - **50951 Ureteral endoscopy through established ureterostomy, with or without irrigation, instillation, or ureteropyelography, exclusive of radiologic service**

- When multiple endoscopic approaches are utilized to attempt the same procedure, report the code for the completed approach.

- When multiple endoscopic approaches are *medically reasonable and necessary* to perform *different* procedures at the same patient encounter, report each separately and append modifier **-51** to the less extensive procedure code. The separate endoscopies may be linked to the same or different diagnosis codes (■ Figure 45-1).

CODING CAUTION

Always check with the patient's payer regarding endoscopy billing rules. The information presented in this chapter reflects the NCCI. Individual payer policies may vary.

Physician performs separate endoscopies due to left kidney cancer. He performs a renal endoscopy of the left kidney through a nephrostomy. He also performs a cystourethroscopy and inserts a suction and irrigation probe to evacuate multiple obstructing clots.

C64.2 Malignant neoplasm of left kidney, except renal pelvis

52001 Cystourethroscopy with irrigation and evacuation of multiple obstructing clots

50551-51-LT Renal endoscopy through established nephrostomy or pyelostomy, with or without irrigation, instillation, or ureteropyelography, exclusive of radiologic service; -51 Multiple procedures; -LT Left side

Figure 45-1 ■ Example of Coding Multiple Endoscopies. *Source: © PB Resources, Inc. Used with permission. CPT codes only © American Medical Association.*

Cystoscopy Procedures

Cystoscopy is a common component of many more complex procedures. CPT code definitions or National Correct Coding Initiative (NCCI) edits often bundle cystoscopy into the codes for more complex procedures. Under some circumstances, you can break the bundles and separately report the cystoscopy performed with another procedure(s). In most cases, a modifier is required. Review the following examples for a patient who had a TURP performed and returns to the physician because of hematuria during the 90-day global period. In each example the physician performs a cystoscopy, but it is billed differently based on the reason it was performed and the diagnosis (■ Figures 45-2 and 45-3).

Laterality Modifiers

Some Urinary System and Male Genital System codes involve paired anatomic sites, such as the kidneys, ureters, testes, and epididymides. Coders must read code descriptions carefully to determine how a code reports laterality and whether a modifier

---

A surgeon performs a cystoscopic examination to evaluate prolonged postoperative bleeding during the 90-day global period of a TURP for BPH.

The cystoscopy is an evaluation of a postoperative complication and not billable for Medicare and many other payers.

R31.9 Hematuria

99024 Postoperative follow-up visit, normally included in the surgical package, to indicate that an evaluation and management service was performed during a postoperative period for a reason(s) related to the original procedure

Figure 45-2 ■ Example of Coding a Bundled Cystoscopy. *Source: © PB Resources, Inc. Used with permission. CPT codes only © American Medical Association.*

Patient presents with complaints of hematuria during the postoperative period of a TURP. The physician performs a problem focused history; a detailed examination; and medical decision making of moderate complexity. She performs a cystoscopic examination and discovers benign bladder tumors.

Report the cystoscopy because this is a separately identifiable problem from the TURP.
R31.9 Hematuria
D30.3 Benign neoplasm of bladder
99214-24-25 Office or other outpatient visit for the evaluation and management of an established patient, which requires at least 2 of these 3 key components: A detailed history; A detailed examination; Medical decision making of moderate complexity; -24 Unrelated E/M service by the same physician or other qualified health care professional during a postoperative period); -25 Significant, separately identifiable E/M service by the same physician or other qualified health care professional on the same day of the procedure or other service
52000-79 Cystourethoscopy (separate procedure); -79 Unrelated procedure or service by the same physician or other qualified health care professional during the postoperative period

On the CMS-1500 or electronic billing system, link the E/M with hematuria and the cystoscopic examination with the tumor.

21. DIAGNOSIS OR NATURE OF ILLNESS OR INJURY Relate A-L to service line below (24E)	ICD Ind. 0	22. RESUBMISSION CODE	ORIGINAL REF. NO.
A. R31.9 B. D30.3 C. D.			
E. F. G. H.		23. PRIOR AUTHORIZATION NUMBER	
I. J. K. L.			

24. A. DATE(S) OF SERVICE		B. PLACE OF SERVICE	C. EMG	D. PROCEDURES, SERVICES, OR SUPPLIES (Explain Unusual Circumstances) CPT/HCPCS MODIFIER	E. DIAGNOSIS POINTER	F. $ CHARGES	G. DAYS OR UNITS	H. EPSDT Family Plan	I. ID. QUAL.	J. RENDERING PROVIDER ID. #
From MM DD YY	To MM DD YY									
1 05 05 YY		11		99214 24 25	A	175 00	01		NPI	99 99999999
2 05 05 YY		11		52000 79	B	277 00	01		NPI	99 99999999

Figure 45-3 ■ Example of Coding a Separate Cystoscopy. *Source: © PB Resources, Inc. Used with permission. CPT codes only © American Medical Association.*

is needed. Review the following variations for reporting laterality based on the code description.

- One CPT code is used regardless of whether the procedure is unilateral or bilateral. Do not append any laterality modifiers.
    - **55250 Vasectomy, unilateral or bilateral (separate procedure), including postoperative semen examination(s)**

- Separate CPT codes are provided for unilateral and bilateral procedures. Report modifier **-RT Right side** or **-LT Left side** for unilateral procedures for informational purposes. Do not report modifier **-50 Bilateral procedure** for bilateral procedures because it is part of the code description and the payment is based on the higher RVUs for the bilateral procedure.
    - **54860 Epididymectomy; unilateral**
    - **54861 Epididymectomy; bilateral**

- The code description identifies a unilateral procedure. Report modifier **-RT** or **-LT** for informational purposes. For bilateral procedures, report the same code and append modifier **-50** as directed in the instructional note that follows the code.
    - **50593 Ablation, renal tumor(s), unilateral, percutaneous, cryotherapy**
    (50593 is a unilateral procedure. For bilateral procedure, report 50593 with modifier 50)

Modifiers for ESWL

ESWL is one of the most frequently performed procedures in urology practices. It is an effective, noninvasive treatment for kidney stones, which may be located in the renal pelvis, the calyx, the ureteropelvic junction, and/or the ureter. These sites are bilateral and the code **50590 Lithotripsy, extracorporeal shock wave** is reported once per side, regardless of how many sites contain stones. When stones are present in multiple locations on one side, assign only one occurrence of code **50590**.

When stones occur bilaterally, each side is often treated separately. One side is treated first, then a second appointment to treat the contralateral side is scheduled for several weeks later. The second appointment usually is preplanned to occur within the 90-day global period of the first procedure, meeting the definition of a staged procedure. The physician must clearly document this prospective planning for a staged procedure in the preoperative note, the medical record, or the operative note for the first procedure. Append the appropriate laterality modifier, **-RT Right side** or **-LT Left side**, to each occurrence of the procedure code **50590**. Append modifier **-58 Staged or related procedure or service by the same physician or other qualified health care professional during the postoperative period** to the second procedure (■ FIGURE 45-4).

In the event that stones are treated on both sides at the same time, append modifier **-50 Bilateral procedure** to code **50590**.

Patient presents with calculi in both kidneys and the left ureter. Physician plans to treat each kidney separately. On March 1, he performs ESWL on the left kidney and ureter. On April 15, he performs ESWL on the right kidney

March 1
N20.2 Calculus of kidney with calculus of ureter
50590-LT Lithotripsy, extracorporeal shock wave; -LT
      Left side
April 15
N20.0 Calculus of kidney
50590-58-RT Lithotripsy, extracorporeal shock wave;
      -58 Staged or related procedure or service by the
      same physician or other qualified health care
      professional during the postoperative period;
      -RT Right side

Figure 45-4 ■ Example of Coding for ESWL. *Source: © PB Resources, Inc. Used with permission. CPT codes only © American Medical Association.*

CODING CAUTION

Remember that ICD-10-CM diagnosis codes justify the medical necessity of a procedure. The most frequently used ICD-10-CM codes are **N20.0 Calculus of kidney, N20.1 Calculus of ureter**, and **N20.2 Calculus of kidney with calculus of ureter**. Diagnosis codes for calculi do not identify laterality.

Guided Example of Arranging Urinary System Procedure Codes

To practice skills for arranging codes for procedures of the Urinary System, continue with the example from earlier in the chapter about a patient who was seen for urography. Follow along in your CPT manual as Chrystal Crago, CCA, arranges the codes. Check off each step after you complete it.

▶ First, Chrystal confirms the codes she assigned.

❑ **50684 Injection procedure for ureterography or ureteropyelography through ureterostomy or indwelling ureteral catheter**

❑ **74425 Urography, antegrade (pyelostogram, nephrostogram, loopogram), radiological supervision and interpretation**

❑ **50393 Introduction of ureteral catheter or stent into ureter through renal pelvis for drainage and/ or injection, percutaneous**

❑ **74480 Introduction of ureteral catheter or stent into ureter through renal pelvis for drainage and/or injection, percutaneous, radiological supervision and interpretation**

▶ Chrystal arranges the codes in descending RVU order according to the MPFSDB that is used by the patient's payer. She uses the facility RVU because the procedure was performed at the hospital, not at the physician's office.

For the radiological procedures, she uses the RVU for the professional component only, not the technical component, because the technical component was provided by the facility.

❑ **50393** Facility RVU = 6.27

❑ **50684** Facility RVU = 1.44

❑ **74480** Facility RVU = 0.76 (professional component)

❑ **74425** Facility RVU = 0.51 (professional component)

▶ Chrystal examines the need for modifiers. (Refer to Table 30-1 Key Criteria for Abstracting CPT Modifiers or Appendix A in the CPT manual.)

❑ Code **50393** requires modifier **-50 Bilateral procedure** because both ureters were catheterized.

❑ Code **50684** requires modifier **-51 Multiple procedures** because it is the second procedure performed. The payer will reimburse 50% of its usual rate for the procedure because of the efficiencies gained when performing two procedures at the same operative session. Modifier **-50** also is required because the ureterography was performed bilaterally. The payer will reimburse 150% of its usual rate for a bilateral procedure (Table 45-10). Multiple payment modifiers can be applied in any order without changing the final calculation (■ TABLE 45-13).

❑ Code **74480** requires modifier **-26 Professional component** because the physician provided the S&I service. Modifier **-51** is not required on this code because the multiple procedure payment reduction does not apply to radiological interpretations.

❑ Code **74425** does not require modifier **-26 Professional component** because the physician provided the S&I service. Modifier **-51** is not required on this code because the multiple procedure payment reduction does not apply to radiological interpretations.

▶ Chrystal finalizes the procedure codes and sequencing for this case:

(1) **50393-50 Introduction of ureteral catheter or stent into ureter through renal pelvis for drainage and/ or injection, percutaneous; -50 Bilateral procedure**

(2) **50684-51-50 Injection procedure for ureterography or ureteropyelography through ureterostomy or**

Table 45-13 ■ EXAMPLE OF REIMBURSEMENT CALCULATIONS FOR MODIFIERS -51 AND -50

Criterion	Value	Example Calculation
Allowed rate (example)— CPT code 50684	$125.00	—
Reduction—modifier -51	50%	$125.00 × 0.50 = $62.50
Bonus—modifier -50	150%	$62.50 × 1.50 = $93.75
Final payment	$93.75	—

Source: © PB Resources, Inc. Used with permission.

indwelling ureteral catheter; -51 Multiple procedures; -50 Bilateral procedure

(3) **74480-26 Introduction of ureteral catheter or stent into ureter through renal pelvis for drainage and/or injection, percutaneous, radiological supervision and interpretation; -26 Professional component**

(4) **74425-26 Urography, antegrade (pyelostogram, nephrostogram, loopogram), radiological supervision and interpretation; -26 Professional component**

▶ Chrystal also assigns and sequences the ICD-10-CM diagnosis code that supports the need for the service.

(1) **N13.5 Crossing vessel and stricture of ureter without hydronephrosis**

CODING PRACTICE

Exercise 45.4 Arranging Codes for Urinary and Male Genital System Procedures

Instructions: Read the mini-medical-record of each patient's encounter. Review the information abstracted in Exercise 45.2 for questions 1–3. For questions 4–6, abstract the case on your own. Assign CPT codes, quantities, and modifiers using the Index and Tabular List, and arrange the codes in proper sequence. Write the code(s) on the line provided.

1. INPATIENT HOSPITAL Gender: M Age: 46

Preprocedure diagnosis: bladder cancer; previously removed the bladder and created an ileal conduit (*use of a segment of the ileum to connect the ureters to a stoma on the abdominal wall*)

Procedure: ureteropyelography; injected contrast medium through the existing stoma to view the ureters and ileal conduit. Supervised the radiology procedure and dictated the interpretation report.

Preprocedure diagnosis: ileal conduit was visualized to be functioning properly

Tip: Read the instructional note following the code for the ureteropyelography to help determine the second code.

2 CPT Codes _____

2. INPATIENT HOSPITAL Gender: M Age: 67

Preprocedure diagnosis: bladder cancer of contiguous sites of the bladder with metastasis to the colon and rectum

Procedure: functioned as a member of a surgical team; completely excised the urinary bladder; created a ureteroileal conduit and intestinal anastomosis; performed bilateral pelvic lymphadenectomy including external iliac, hypogastric, and obturator nodes; performed an open total colectomy with a complete proctectomy

Tip: Code for one surgeon who is working as part of the surgical team and apply the appropriate modifier. Apply other modifiers as needed.

2 CPT Codes _____

3. OFFICE/OUTPATIENT HOSPITAL Gender: M Age: 72

Reason for encounters: new patient with complaints of urinary incontinence

Procedure (Tuesday): conducted a comprehensive history and exam with moderate-complexity medical decision making. Recommended further testing and discussed treatment options with patient.

Procedure (Friday): performed postvoid residual (PVR) ultrasound test to measure the amount of urine left in the bladder after the patient urinates

Plan: incontinence sling surgery

Tip: Assign one code for Tuesday and one code for Friday.

2 CPT Codes (Tuesday) _____
(Friday) _____

4. OUTPATIENT SURGERY Gender: M Age: 54

Preprocedure diagnosis: bladder calculi; urethral calculus

Procedure: cystolitholapaxy; left ureteral stent placement. Cystoscope used to examine the bladder. Telescope inserted through urethra into the bladder. Stones broken using crushing forceps. Next, the ureteral orifice was entered and a left ureteral stent placed. Urine was clear pink at termination of procedure.

2 CPT Codes _____

5. OFFICE Gender: M Age: 55

Preprocedure diagnosis: penoscrotal abscess

Procedure: incision and drainage of abscess sites. The deep open sore on the right side of the penis was opened to allow pus to drain. A second incision and drainage was performed at the proximal scrotum. A tight scrotal Kling was applied.

2 CPT Codes _____

6. OFFICE   Gender: M   Age: 47

Preprocedure diagnosis: *recurrent dysuria, most consistent with interstitial cystitis*

Procedure: *cystourethroscopy, bladder biopsies, bilateral retrograde pyelography. Cystoscope inserted and advanced into the bladder under direct visualization. Submucosal glomerulations on the lateral wall of the bladder were biopsied and sent to pathology. Bilateral retrograde pyelograms were*

(continued)

6. (continued)

obtained using an 8-French cone-tip catheter. The right collecting system was normal based on retrograde pyelography.

Postprocedure diagnosis: *bladder lesions, interstitial cystitis*

Tip: Include the correct modifier for the professional component of the pyelography.

2 CPT Codes _____

E/M CODING FOR UROLOGY

The *1997 Documentation Guidelines for Evaluation and Management Services* (1997 DG), published by CMS, provide requirements for each level of a genitourinary E/M examination (■ FIGURE 45-5). Urologists are not limited to using the guidelines for a genitourinary examination only. They can also use guidelines for a general multiorgan system examination, or any other single organ system examination, based on what is most advantageous for a specific encounter. However, physicians cannot combine elements from more than one type of examination for a given encounter. Typically, the genitourinary examination guidelines provide the best results when a detailed genitourinary examination is performed.

To determine the appropriate E/M code, coders must review the documentation in detail and identify the specific elements documented.

- To translate the documentation into the E/M requirements for the history, refer back to Chapter 31, Evaluation and Management Services (99201-99499), Tables 31-7 to 31-10, or to the 1997 DG.
- To determine the requirements for an examination, refer to Figure 45-5 or to the single organ system examination for Genitourinary in the 1997 DG.
- To determine the levels for medical decision making (MDM), refer to Chapter 31, Table 31-12, and also to the Table of Risk in the 1997 DG.

Guided Example of E/M Coding for Urology

Refer to the urology encounter (■ FIGURE 45-6) to practice skills for abstracting and assigning E/M codes. Follow along as fictitious coder Chrystal Crago, CCA, abstracts the procedure. Check off each step after you complete it.

▶ First, Chrystal needs to establish the category of service so she can determine the information needed to abstract and assign the code.

- ❑ *What is the setting?* emergency department
- ❑ *What is the type of service?* new or established patient
- ❑ *What is the code range?* Chrystal refers to the CPT Index and looks up the Main Term **Evaluation and Manage-**

ment and the subterm **Emergency Department**. The code range listed is **99281-99288**.

- ❑ *How many key components are required?* Chrystal refers to the code range in the Tabular List and reads the code description of the first code, which states **requires these 3 key components**. All codes in the category have the same requirements for key components. This tells her that all three key components must meet or exceed the levels listed in the code (3/3).

▶ Next, Chrystal identifies the level of history.

- ❑ *What is the level of HPI?* The HPI is **Extended** because four elements are documented.
- ❑ *What is the level of ROS?* The ROS is **Complete** because 10 or more systems are documented.
- ❑ *What is the level of PFSH?* The PFSH is **Pertinent** because two elements are documented.
- ❑ *Based on these factors, what is the overall level of history?* The level of history is **Detailed** because the lowest of the three factors (HPI, ROS, and PFSH) determines the history level. The HPI and ROS qualify for a comprehensive history, but the PFSH qualifies for only a detailed history.

▶ Chrystal refers to the genitourinary examination in the 1997 DG (Figure 45-5) to abstract information needed to determine the level of the examination.

- ❑ *What is the level of examination?* The level of examination is **Detailed**. Fourteen (14) elements of the examination are documented, which exceeds the requirement of 12 or more bulleted elements for a genitourinary examination. A comprehensive examination requires that every element in each box with a shaded border and at least one element in each box with an unshaded border be documented, which they are not.

▶ Chrystal determines the level of medical decision making. (Refer to Table 31-12 Medical Decision Making Levels.)

- ❑ *What is the level of complexity of the number of diagnoses or management options based on the presenting problem?*

System/Body Area	Elements of Genitourinary Examination
Constitutional	❑ Measurement of any **three** of the following seven **vital** signs: • 1) sitting or standing blood pressure, • 2) supine blood pressure, • 3) pulse rate and regularity, • 4) respiration, • 5) temperature, • 6) height, • 7) weight (May be measured and recorded by ancillary staff) ❑ General **appearance** of patient (eg, development, nutrition, body habitus, deformities, attention to grooming)
Neck	❑ Examination of **neck** (eg, masses, overall appearance, symmetry, tracheal position, crepitus) ❑ Examination of **thyroid** (eg, enlargement, tenderness, mass)
Respiratory	❑ Assessment of **respiratory effort** (eg, intercostal retractions, use of accessory muscles, diaphragmatic movement) **Auscultation** of lungs (eg, breath sounds, adventitious sounds, rubs)
Cardiovascular	❑ **Auscultation** of heart with notation of abnormal sounds and murmurs ❑ Examination of **peripheral vascular system** by observation (eg, swelling, varicosities) and palpation (e.g. pulses, temperature, edema, tenderness)
Chest (Breasts)	See genitourinary (female)
Gastrointestinal (Abdomen)	❑ Examination of **abdomen** with notation of presence of masses or tenderness ❑ Examination for presence or absence of **hernia** ❑ Examination of **liver** and **spleen** ❑ Obtain **stool sample** for occult blood test when indicated
Genitourinary	**MALE:** ❑ Inspection of **anus** and **perineum** Examination (with or without specimen collection for smears and cultures) of genitalia including: ❑ **Scrotum** (eg, lesions, cysts, rashes) ❑ **Epididymides** (eg, size, symmetry, masses) ❑ **Testes** (eg, size, symmetry, masses) ❑ **Urethral meatus** (eg, size, location, lesions, discharge) ❑ **Penis** (eg, lesions, presence or absence of foreskin, foreskin retractability, plaque, masses, scarring, deformities) **Digital rectal** examination including: ❑ Prostate gland (eg, size, symmetry, nodularity, tenderness) ❑ Seminal vesicles (eg, symmetry, tenderness, masses, enlargement) ❑ Sphincter tone, presence of hemorrhoids, rectal masses **FEMALE:** Includes at least **seven of the following eleven elements** identified by bullets: ❑ Inspection and palpation of **breasts** (eg, masses or lumps, tenderness, symmetry, nipple discharge) ❑ **Digital rectal** examination including sphincter tone, presence of hemorrhoids, rectal masses Pelvic examination (with or without specimen collection for smears and cultures), including: ❑ **External genitalia** (eg, general appearance, hair distribution, lesions) ❑ **Urethral meatus** (eg, size, location, lesions, prolapse) ❑ **Urethra** (eg, masses, tenderness, scarring) ❑ **Bladder** (eg, fullness, masses, tenderness) ❑ **Vagina** (eg, general appearance, estrogen effect, discharge, lesions, pelvic support, cystocele, rectocele) ❑ **Cervix** (eg, general appearance, lesions, discharge) ❑ **Uterus** (eg, size, contour, position, mobility, tenderness, consistency, descent or support) ❑ **Adnexa**/parametria (eg, masses, tenderness, organomegaly, nodularity) ❑ **Anus** and **perineum**
Lymphatic	Palpation of **lymph nodes** in neck, axillae, groin and/or other location
Skin	❑ **Inspection** and/or **palpation** of skin and subcutaneous tissue (eg, rashes, lesions, ulcers)
Neurological/ Psychiatric	*Brief assessment of mental status including:* ❑ **Orientation** to time, place and person ❑ **Mood** and affect (eg, depression, anxiety, agitation, hypomania, lability)

Total # Bullets Performed and Documented →	☐	# of ❑ Elements Performed and Documented	Level of Examination
		1–5	Problem focused
		6–11	Expanded problem focused
		12	Detailed
		ALL	Comprehensive (Perform **all** elements identified by a bullet. Document **every** element in each box with a shaded border and at least **one** element in each box with an unshaded border)

Figure 45-5 ■ 1997 DG for Genitourinary Examination. *Source: Centers for Medicare and Medicaid Services, 1997 Documentation Guidelines for Evaluation and Management Services (with formatting adjustments).*

UROLOGY ENCOUNTER

HISTORY: Detailed

CHIEF COMPLAINT: Blood in urine.

> Chief complaint (CC)

HISTORY OF PRESENT ILLNESS: This is a 78-year-old male who presents to the Emergency Department with blood in his urine since yesterday. He has prostate cancer with metastatic disease to his bladder and several locations throughout the skeletal system including the spine and shoulder. The patient has had problems with hematuria in the past, but states that this episode began yesterday, and today he has been passing principally blood with very little urine. The patient has already completed chemotherapy and is beyond treatment for his cancer at this time. He is receiving radiation therapy targeted to the bones for symptomatic relief of skeletal pain. It is not intended to treat and cure the cancer. The patient is not enlisted in hospice, but the principle around the patient's current treatment management is focusing on comfort care measures.

> Setting & patient type
>
> ROS
>
> HPI: Extended (4+)
>
> MDM Risk
>
> MDM Management

REVIEW OF SYSTEMS: CONSTITUTIONAL: No fever or chills. The patient does report generalized fatigue and weakness over the past several days. HEENT: No headache, no neck pain, no rhinorrhea, no sore throat. CARDIOVASCULAR: No chest pain. RESPIRATIONS: No shortness of breath or cough, although the patient does get easily winded with exertion over these past few days. GASTROINTESTINAL: Denies any abdominal pain. No nausea or vomiting. No changes in the bowel movement. No melena or hematochezia. GENITOURINARY: A gross hematuria since yesterday as previously described. Able to pass urine without difficulty. Denies any groin pain. The patient denies any other changes to the genital region. MUSCULOSKELETAL: The chronic lower back pain which has not changed over these past few days. The patient does have multiple other joints that cause him discomfort, but there have been no recent changes. SKIN: No rashes or lesions. No easy bruising. NEUROLOGIC: No focal weakness or numbness. No incontinence of urine or stool. No saddle paresthesia. No dizziness, syncope or near-syncope. ENDOCRINE: No polyuria or polydipsia. No heat or cold intolerance. HEMATOLOGIC/LYMPHATIC: The patient does not have a history of easy bruising or bleeding, but has had previous episodes of hematuria.

> ROS: Complete (10+)

PAST MEDICAL HISTORY: Prostate cancer with metastatic disease as previously described.

PAST SURGICAL HISTORY: TURP.

> PFSH: Pertinent (2)

CURRENT MEDICATIONS: Morphine, Darvocet, Flomax, Avodart and ibuprofen.

ALLERGIES: VICODIN.

SOCIAL HISTORY: The patient is a nonsmoker. Denies any alcohol or illicit drug use. The patient does live with his family.

EXAMINATION: Detailed

PHYSICAL EXAMINATION: VITAL SIGNS: Temperature is 98.8 oral, blood pressure is 108/65, pulse is 109, respirations 16, oxygen saturation is 97% on room air and interpreted as normal. CONSTITUTIONAL: The patient is well nourished, well developed. The patient appears to be pale, but otherwise looks well. The patient is calm, comfortable. The patient is pleasant and cooperative. HEENT: Eyes normal with clear conjunctivae and corneas. Nose is normal without rhinorrhea or audible congestion. Mouth and oropharynx normal without any sign of infection. Mucous membranes are moist. NECK: Supple. Full range of motion. No JVD. CARDIOVASCULAR: Heart is mildly tachycardic with regular rhythm without murmur, rub or gallop. Peripheral pulses are +2. RESPIRATIONS: Clear to auscultation bilaterally. No shortness of breath. No wheezes, rales or rhonchi. Good air movement bilaterally. GASTROINTESTINAL: Abdomen is soft, nontender, nondistended. No rebound or guarding. No hepatosplenomegaly. Normal bowel sounds. No bruit. No masses or pulsatile masses. GENITOURINARY: The patient has normal male genitalia, uncircumcised. There is no active bleeding from the penis at this time. There is no swelling of the testicles. There are no masses palpated to the testicles, scrotum or the penis. There are no lesions or rashes noted. There is no inguinal lymphadenopathy. Normal male exam. MUSCULOSKELETAL: Back is normal and nontender. There are no abnormalities noted to the arms or legs. The patient has normal use of the extremities. SKIN: The patient appears to be pale, but otherwise the skin is normal. There are no rashes or lesions. NEUROLOGIC: Motor and sensory are intact to the extremities. The patient has normal speech. PSYCHIATRIC: The patient is alert and oriented x4. Normal mood and affect. HEMATOLOGIC/LYMPHATIC: There is no evidence of bruising noted to the body. No lymphadenitis is palpated.

> (12+ bulleted elements)

EMERGENCY DEPARTMENT TESTING: CBC was done, which had a hemoglobin of 7.7 and hematocrit of 22.6. Neutrophils were 81%. The RDW was 18.5, and the rest of the values were all within normal limits and unremarkable. Chemistry had a sodium of 134, a glucose of 132, calcium is 8.2, and rest of the values are unremarkable. Alkaline phosphatase was 770 and albumin was 2.4. Rest of the values all are within normal limits of the LFTs. Urinalysis was grossly bloody with a large amount of blood and greater than 50 RBCs. The patient also had greater than 300 of the protein reading, moderate leukocytes, 30-50 white blood cells, but no bacteria were seen. Coagulation profile study had a PT of 15.9, PTT of 43 and INR of 1.3.

> **MEDICAL DECISION MAKING: High Complexity**
>
> MDM Data: Ordering or reviewing diagnostic data (Straightforward Data)

Figure 45-6 ■ Urology Encounter. *Source: © PB Resources, Inc. Used with permission.*

(continued on page 896)

EMERGENCY DEPARTMENT COURSE: The patient was given normal saline 2 liters over 1 hour without any adverse effect and multiple doses of morphine to maintain his comfort while here in the emergency room without any adverse effect. The morphine did relieve his pain and make him pain free. I spoke with the patient's urologist about most appropriate step for the patient. He said he would be happy to care for the patient in the hospital and do urologic scopes if necessary and surgery if necessary and blood transfusion. It was all a matter of what the patient wished to do given the advanced stage of his cancer. I spoke with the patient and his son about what he would like to do and what the options were from doing nothing from keeping him comfortable with pain medicines to admitting him to the hospital with the possibility of scopes and even surgery being done as well as the blood transfusion. The patient and his son chose a middle ground in which he would be transfused with 2 units of blood here in the emergency room and go home tonight. The patient was transfused 2 units of packed red blood cells after appropriately typed and match. The patient did not have any adverse reaction at any point with his transfusion. There was no fever, no shortness of breath, and at the time of disposition, the patient stated he felt a little better and felt like he had a little more strength. Over the course of the patient's several-hour stay in the emergency room, the patient did end up developing enough problems with clotted blood in his bladder that he had a urinary obstruction. Foley catheter was placed, which produced bloody urine and relieved the developing discomfort of a full bladder. The patient was given a leg bag and the Foley catheter was left in place.

DIAGNOSES
1. HEMATURIA.
2. PROSTATE CANCER WITH BONE AND BLADDER METASTATIC DISEASE.
3. SIGNIFICANT ANEMIA.
4. URINARY OBSTRUCTION.

CONDITION ON DISPOSITION: Fair, but improved.

DISPOSITION: To home with his son.

PLAN: Patient is to follow up with his urologist in 2 days for reevaluation. He was encouraged to drink extra water. I gave discharge instructions on hematuria and asked him to return to the emergency room should he have any worsening of his condition or develop any other problems or symptoms of concern.

> MDM Management:
> New problem with workup (High Management Options)

> MDM Risk:
> Acute/chronic illness that poses risk to patient (High Risk)

KEY: HPI History of the present illness ROS Review of systems
PFSH Past, family, and social history MDM Medical decision making

Figure 45-6 ■ (Continued)

The level is **High** because there is a new presenting problem, with workup.

❑ *What is the amount and/or complexity of data to be reviewed?* The level is **Straightforward** because clinical labs were reviewed.

❑ *What is the level of risk of significant complications, morbidity, and/or mortality?* She reviews each column in the Table of Risk in the 1997 DG and determines that the level of risk is **High**. The patient presents with an acute or chronic illness that poses a risk to a bodily function (High), several clinical labs are ordered and reviewed (Minimal), and the decision to de-escalate care because of a poor prognosis was reconfirmed (High). The single

highest element in the Table of Risk determines the overall risk. Two columns, **Presenting Problem** and **Management Options Selected**, are at the highest level (High).

❑ *Based on these factors, what is the overall level of medical decision making?* The medical decision making is **High complexity**. At least two of the three MDM factors are required to qualify for a specific level of MDM. Two of the three MDM factors meet or exceed high-complexity decision making.

Now Chrystal is ready to assign the code for the urology encounter. The exercise that follows guides you through additional abstracting skills and allows you to assign the correct code.

CODING PRACTICE

Exercise 45.5 Evaluation and Management Coding for Urology

Instructions: Refer to the *1997 Documentation Guidelines for Evaluation and Management Services* (available at www.cms.gov) or Chapter 31 Evaluation and Management Services (99201-99499) (Tables 31-7 to 31-12) in this text. Answer the following questions about the Urology Encounter (Figure 45-6).

1. a. Which elements of the HPI are documented? Circle all that apply. Location, Quality, Severity, Duration, Timing, Context, Modifying factors, Associated signs and symptoms

b. How many elements are documented? _____

c. What is the level of HPI? _____

2. a. Which systems are reviewed in the ROS? Circle all that apply. Constitutional, Allergic/ immunologic, CV, Endocrine, ENT/M, Eyes, GI, GU, Hemic/lymphatic, MS, Neurologic, Psychiatric, Respiratory, Skin/breast

   b. How many systems are documented? _____

   c. What is the level of ROS? _____

3. a. Which PFSH elements are documented? Circle all that apply. Past medical, Family, Social

   b. What is the level of PFSH? _____

   c. What is the overall level of history? (The lowest history factor—HPI, ROS, or PFSH—determines the level of history.) _____

4. Refer to Figure 45-6 Urology Encounter.

   a. Which bulleted items are documented for the examination? (Check off the items documented.)

   b. How many bulleted items are documented? _____

   c. What is the level of the examination? _____

5. Refer to Table 31-12 Medical Decision Making Levels or the 1997 DG.

   a. What is the MDM level for the number of diagnoses or management options?

   b. What is the MDM level for the amount and/or complexity of data to be reviewed?

c. Refer to the Table of Risk in the 1997 DG. Which elements of risk are documented for each risk factor?

   1. Presenting problem: _____

   2. Diagnostic procedures ordered: _____

   3. Management options selected: _____

d. What is the level of risk? (The highest of the three risk factors determines the overall level of risk.) _____

e. What is the overall level of MDM? (2/3 MDM factors are needed to determine the overall level.) _____

6. a. What is the setting? _____

   b. What is the patient (or service) type? _____

   c. What is the code range? _____

   d. How many key components are required? _____

   e. What is the level of history? _____

   f. What is the level of examination? _____

   g. What is the level of medical decision making? _____

   h. What is the correct code? _____

7. Abstract, assign, and arrange (sequence) the diagnosis code(s) that support the E/M code.

   6 ICD-10-CM Code(s) _____
   _____

CHAPTER SUMMARY

In this chapter you learned that:

- Although urology is classified as a surgical specialty, a knowledge of internal medicine, pediatrics, gynecology, and other specialties is required because of the wide variety of clinical problems encountered.

- Coders need to understand treatment of obstructive uropathy, calculi, congenital anomalies, and bladder reconstruction.

- The CPT subsection **Urinary System (50010-53899)** contains three subheadings that are divided by anatomic site.

- The CPT subsection **Male Genital System (54000-55899)** contains nine subheadings that are divided by anatomic site.

- Abstracting for urinary and male genital system procedures uses similar processes. For both systems, coders must identify the anatomic approach and the patient's gender.

- Coders must be aware of gender-specific codes when coding for the Urinary and Male Genital Systems. They must also be familiar with coding for urinary catheterization and radiological guidance and supervision/interpretation.

- Coders must be familiar with rules for bundling and multiple coding related to endoscopy procedures, as well as how to apply modifiers for laterality and ESWL.

- The *1997 Documentation Guidelines for Evaluation and Management Services* (1997 DG), published by CMS, provides requirements for each level of a genitourinary E/M examination.

- CPT special instructions provide definitions and coding guidelines at the beginning of many categories.

CONCEPT QUIZ

Take a moment to look back at Urinary and Male Genital System procedures and solidify your skills. Try to answer the questions from memory first, then refer to the discussion in this chapter if you need a little extra help.

Completion

Instructions: Write the term that answers each question based on the information you learned in this chapter. Choose from the list below. Some choices may be used more than once and some choices may not be used at all.

catheter	pyeloplasty
cystometrogram	resectoscope
electroejaculation	trocar
epididymovasostomy	ureterolithotomy
lithotripter	ureterotomy
manometer	vasectomy
nephrolithotomy	vesicourethropexy
nephrorrhaphy	vesiculectomy

1. A(n) _____ is a pressure-measuring device used to evaluate bladder function.

2. A(n) _____ is used to treat stress urinary incontinence.

3. _____ is removal of one of the seminal vesicles.

4. A(n) _____ is used via the urethra to remove a portion of the prostate.

5. Aspiration of the bladder can be done using a needle, a trocar, or a(n) _____.

6. _____ is a procedure that can be done through an incision to remove a kidney stone.

7. An obstruction of spermatic flow can be treated with a(n) _____.

8. A(n) _____ is removal of a ureteral stone through an incision into the ureter.

9. _____ is the medical term for suturing a laceration of the kidney.

10. A(n) _____ aims pulsating sound waves at a kidney stone to break it into pieces.

Multiple Choice

Instructions: Circle the letter of the best answer to each question based on the information you learned in this chapter.

1. How should a bilateral kidney procedure be coded when the code description specifies a unilateral procedure?
   A. Append both modifiers -RT and -LT.
   B. Append modifier -50 Bilateral procedure.
   C. Append modifier -22 Increased procedural services.
   D. Report the procedure code with the quantity 2.

2. Which of the following categories in the Urinary System has special instructions unique to that section?
   A. Excision
   B. Repair

C. Laparoscopy
D. Introduction

3. What type of catheter is placed in the urethra temporarily to allow the drainage of urine?
   A. Ureteral catheter
   B. Suprapubic catheter
   C. Foley catheter
   D. Straight catheter

4. How should you code a laparoscopic procedure that is converted to an open procedure?
   A. Assign codes for both procedures.
   B. Code and bill the open procedure only.
   C. Append modifier -22 to the open procedure to report it was more extensive than usual.
   D. Append modifier -53 to the laparoscopic procedure to report it was discontinued.

5. What modifier(s) is used when coding for a physician who provides both the professional and technical components of a radiology procedure?
   A. -26
   B. -26, -TC
   C. -59
   D. No modifier is used.

6. Which of the following would be considered an invasive urological procedure?
   A. Pelvic exenteration
   B. Percutaneous nephrolithotomy
   C. Vasectomy
   D. Vesiculectomy

7. What modifier is used for the second procedure when kidney stones occur bilaterally and ESWL is done on the left, followed by ESWL on the right two months later?
   A. -50
   B. -51
   C. -58
   D. -76

8. Which codes are reported when multiple endoscopic approaches are utilized to attempt the same procedure?
   A. A code for the completed approach
   B. A code for the approach that reached the farthest point
   C. A code for each approach attempted
   D. A code for the open procedure only

9. What anatomic approach can be used for urinary and male genital system procedures?
   A. Endoscopic
   B. Laparoscopic
   C. Percutaneous
   D. Retropubic

10. Which of the following modifiers increases the usual reimbursement when appended to a surgical code?
    A. -25
    B. -27
    C. -50
    D. -51

CODING CHALLENGE

Instructions: Read the mini-medical-record of each patient's encounter, then abstract, assign, and arrange ICD-10-CM diagnosis codes and CPT procedure codes using the appropriate Index and Tabular List. Assign quantities and modifiers where needed. Write the code(s) on the line provided.

Urinary System

1. OUTPATIENT SURGERY   Gender: M   Age: 56

Preprocedure diagnosis: right–side renal calculi

Procedure: cystoscope was inserted into the urethra, which was normal. The bladder was free of neoplasm, infection, or calculus. A guidewire was introduced into the right ureteral orifice and advanced to the right renal-collecting system without difficulty. A balloon was used to dilate the ureter and a scope was introduced. The gravel from the stone being fragmented was washed out. The stent was inserted. Patient was transferred to the recovery room in stable condition.

1 ICD-10-CM Code _____

2 CPT Codes _____

2. OFFICE   Gender: M   Age: 32

Preprocedure diagnosis: recurrent bladder tumors of the posterior wall

Procedure: cystoscopy with biopsy and fulguration of the bladder tumors and transurethral incision of vesical neck. The cystourethroscope was used to identify the location of the bladder tumors. A resectoscope was inserted after dilating the urethra and the bladder neck was incised; 0.4-cm and 1.5-cm tumors were biopsied and then fulgurated. A Foley catheter was placed and the patient sent to the recovery room.

1 ICD-10-CM Code _____

2 CPT Codes _____

3. OFFICE   Gender: F   Age: 41

Preprocedure diagnosis: recurrent UTIs possibly related to left ureteral stent placed about 7 weeks ago

Procedure: patient placed in dorsal lithotomy position, given IV pain med. Cystoscopy was performed using graspers. The stent was removed without difficulty and a new stent was inserted. Patient to continue on antibiotics and new stent to remain in place for 3 months.

Tip: Refer to the OGCR for Outpatient Services for help selecting the right code.

1 ICD-10-CM Code _____

1 CPT Code _____

4. OUTPATIENT SURGERY   Gender: M   Age: 65

Preprocedure diagnosis: bladder calculus obstructing prostate

Procedure: holmium laser cystolithotripsy; planned transurethral resection of his prostate was not performed as planned. A 27-French Olympus rectoscope was passed via the urethra into the bladder. He had a large 3.5-cm bladder calculus. Holmium laser with the largest fiber through the continuous flow resectoscope and sheath was used to break up the stone. Most of the chips were able to be irrigated out of the bladder. The TURP was not performed due to the substantial amount of time needed to break up the stone.

1 ICD-10-CM Code _____

1 CPT Code _____

5. INPATIENT HOSPITAL   Gender: M   Age: 56

Preprocedure diagnosis: multi-invasive bladder cancer

Procedure: laparoscopic radical cystectomy with bilateral pelvic lymph node dissections and orthotopic neobladder. After port placement, the bladder was meticulously dissected free and removed. Right and left obturator and pelvic lymph nodes were dissected next. The continent urinary diversion was performed by Dr. Alfred and is reported separately.

Tip: Use a modifier to report that two surgeons performed distinct parts of the procedure.

1 ICD-10-CM Code _____

1 CPT Code _____

6. OUTPATIENT SURGERY   Gender: F   Age: 39

Preprocedure diagnosis: right distal ureteral stone. A stent had been placed two months ago due to a 5-mm ureteral stone. KUB showed stent in place and the stone in the same location as two months ago.

Procedure: right semirigid ureteroscopy with basket stone extraction. The stent was removed and a semirigid scope was placed in the right ureter. Basket was used to retrieve the stone without incident.

Tip: Removal of the stent is bundled with the surgery at the time the stent is inserted.

1 ICD-10-CM Code _____

1 CPT Code _____

(continued)

(continued from page 899)

7. OFFICE Gender: M Age: 51

Preprocedure diagnosis: adenocarcinoma of the prostate

Procedure: implant of I-125 seeds into the prostate. Under fluoroscopic and ultrasound guidance, 19 needles were inserted into the prostate based on a premeasured template. Approximately 70 I-125 seeds were placed into the prostate. The patient tolerated the procedure well.

1 ICD-10-CM Code _____

1 CPT Code _____

Male Genital System

8. OUTPATIENT SURGERY Gender: M Age: 48

Preprocedure diagnosis: normal-volume azoospermia

Procedure: bilateral testis biopsies; bilateral scrotal explorations; bilateral vasograms; right-to-left crossover vasoepididymostomy using the operating microscope. The left vas deferens was transected through a scrotal incision. Vasogram revealed the vas was not patent. Testis biopsy on the left was positive for motile sperm. The same procedure was performed on the right testis; however, the biopsy was negative for motile sperm. At this point the left vas deferens was ligated and, using the operating microscope, a right-to-left crossover vasoepididymostomy performed. The testis and epididymis were placed back in the scrotal sac and the closed. The patient tolerated the procedure well.

1 ICD-10-CM Code _____

5 CPT Codes _____

_____

9. OUTPATIENT SURGERY Gender: M Age: 5

Preprocedure diagnosis: sudden severe testicular pain, possible testicular detorsion on the left

Procedure: left scrotal exploration with detorsion and orchidopexy. With a transverse incision, a dartos pouch was created before opening the tunica vaginalis of the testis. After detorsion of the testis, it was found to be viable, and bilateral orchidopexy was done to prevent future torsion and to preserve fertility.

1 ICD-10-CM Code _____

1 CPT Code _____

10. OUTPATIENT SURGERY Gender: M Age: 37

Preprocedure diagnosis: fractured penis

Procedure: repair of fractured penis; placement of Foley catheter. Patient taken to the OR emergently to repair the tear. An incision was made circumferentially on the ventral aspect of the penis secondary to this being the area of the hematoma. Dissecting along the urethra, we placed a Foley catheter. There was a large amount of bright blood coming from the penis, indicating the point of tear. The tear of the corpus cavernosum was repaired and a leak test showed no extravasation. The Buck fascia was repaired and skin reapproximated, dressing applied.

1 ICD-10-CM Code _____

1 CPT Code _____

KEEP ON CODING

Instructions: Read the procedural statement, then use the appropriate Index and Tabular List to assign CPT procedure codes, quantities, and modifiers. Write the code(s) on the line provided.

Urinary System

1. Cystoscopy for insertion of double-J ureteral stent: CPT Code(s) _____

2. Closure of ureterocutaneous fistula: CPT Code(s) _____

3. Ablation of renal tumor using radiofrequency: CPT Code(s) _____

4. Cryosurgical ablation of the prostate: CPT Code(s) _____

5. Cystometrogram: CPT Code(s) _____

6. Transurethral resection of a 2-cm bladder tumor: CPT Code(s) _____

7. Transurethral ultrasound-guided laser induced prostatectomy (TULIP, noncontact): CPT Code(s) _____

8. Pyeloscopy and biopsy of right renal pelvis: CPT Code(s) _____

9. Takedown of ureteroileal conduit: CPT Code(s) _____

10. Laparoscopic donor nephrectomy: CPT Code(s) _____

11. EMG of urethral sphincter: CPT Code(s) _____

12. Retropubic radical prostatectomy with pelvic lymph node biopsies: CPT Code(s) _____

13. Aspiration of the bladder with insertion of a suprapubic catheter: CPT Code(s) _____

14. Insertion of prosthetic urethral sphincter: CPT Code(s) _____

15. Cystoscopy with dilation of constricted bladder neck under local anesthesia: CPT Code(s) _____

16. Cystotomy with excision of bladder diverticulum: CPT Code(s) _____

17. Bilateral epididymectomy: CPT Code(s) _____

18. Insertion of straight catheter: CPT Code(s) _____

19. Cystourethroscopy, left ureteroscopy with laser lithotripsy: CPT Code(s) _____

20. Extracorporeal shock wave lithotripsy, bladder stone: CPT Code(s) _____

Male Genital System

21. Insertion of a multicomponent, inflatable penile prosthesis: CPT Code(s) _____

22. Removal of previously implanted semirigid penile implant and replacement with new semirigid implant: CPT Code(s) _____

23. Simple bilateral orchiectomy with insertion of prosthesis using scrotal approach: CPT Code(s) _____

24. Revision of circumcision with urethral meatoplasty: CPT Code(s) _____

25. Excision of right spermatocele: CPT Code(s) _____

Table 46-2 ■ **COMMON PROCEDURES OF THE FEMALE GENITAL SYSTEM**

Procedure Name	Definition	Reason Performed
Cerclage (nonobstetrical)	Extensive suturing around the cervix to make the opening smaller	Cervical incompetence (dilated, weakened cervix)
Clitoroplasty	Reduction of the size of an enlarged clitoris	Congenital anomaly
Colpocentesis	Puncture of the posterior vaginal wall with a needle to withdraw fluid from the peritoneal cul-de-sac (*area between the uterus and rectum*)	Abscess
Colpopexy/vaginofixation	Suture of the vagina to another structure, such as the abdominal wall	Vaginal prolapse
Colporrhaphy	Suture of the vagina	Cystocele, rectocele
Colpotomy	Incision into the wall of the vagina; may also include draining an abscess	Lesion, abscess
Conization of cervix	Removal of a cone-shaped piece of tissue from the uterine cervix	Diagnostic testing, precancerous cell removal, cancer
Dilation and curettage (D&C) (nonobstetrical)	Widening of the cervix and scraping of the uterine wall	Biopsy; remove retained products of conception
Endocervical curettage	Scraping tissue from the endocervical canal (which joins the cervix and uterus)	Diagnostic testing
Fallopian tube catheter introduction	Insertion of a catheter through the cervix and uterus into the fallopian tube(s)	Diagnosis and treatment of infertility, repeated miscarriages, dysmenorrhea, tumors, polyps, or fibroids; eliminate a tube occlusion or stricture
Fimbrioplasty	Opening an obstructed fallopian tube to save the function of the fimbriae (*border of the fallopian tube entrance*) for transporting an oocyte	Infertility
Hymenotomy	Incision of the hymen (*the fold of mucous membrane that partially covers the external opening of the vagina*)	Allow for the release of menstrual fluid and sexual intercourse
Hysterectomy	Removal of the uterus and/or related structures, such as the ovaries and fallopian tubes	Cancer, uterine fibroids, endometriosis, abnormal vaginal bleeding, uterine prolapse
Hysteroplasty	Repair of a malformed uterus	Congenital anomaly
Hysterorrhaphy (nonobstetrical)	Suturing the uterus	Perforated or ruptured uterus
Hysterosalpingography	X-ray of the uterus and fallopian tubes after injecting contrast dye	Diagnose blockage or abnormality
Hysteroscopy	Visualization of the cervix and uterus using a hysteroscope, passing it through the vagina into the cervix and uterine cavity	Diagnostic testing, biopsy, polyp removal
In vitro fertilization	Removal of an egg from the female patient, which is manually fertilized with sperm and then returned to the fallopian tube or implanted in the uterus	Infertility; assisted reproductive technology (ART)
Lysis of labial adhesions	Destruction or freeing of adhesions between the labia minor and major	Adhesions, which often occur as a result of fibrous bands of scar tissue; a common pediatric procedure
Marsupialization	To incise a cyst or abscess by cutting a slit into it to drain it and then suturing the edges to surrounding tissue; the surgical formation of a pouch-like sac (marsupialization) on the Bartholin's gland	Creation of a pouch-like sac for continued drainage and healing; prevention of recurrent cysts or infections
Mesh/prosthesis insertion	Repair of tissues that are too weak to be repaired without inserting a mesh or other prosthesis to strengthen them	Pelvic floor defect
Myomectomy	Removal of uterine fibroid tumors without removing healthy uterine tissue	Uterine fibroids
Pereyra procedure	Elevation of the bladder by attaching it to abdominal fascia	Stress urinary incontinence

Table 46-2 ■ *(continued)*

Procedure Name	Definition	Reason Performed
Perineoplasty	Repair of the tissues of the perineum	Tissue damage during childbirth
Pessary insertion/fitting	Evaluation and placement of a rubber, silicone, or plastic device into the vagina to support surrounding structures	Prolapsed uterus or rectum
Plastic repair introitus	Restoration of the vaginal opening to its original size	Vaginal introitus hypertrophy, often due to childbirth
Salpingostomy	Surgical creation of an opening in a fallopian tube to restore its patency	Treatment of infection or inflammation
Sonohysterography	Ultrasound of uterus after a saline solution is infused into the uterus	Fibroids, polyps, lesions
Sperm washing	Separation of the sperm from seminal fluid and removing chemicals that can be harmful to the uterus	Artificial insemination
Trachelectomy/cervicectomy	Removal of the uterine cervix	Cancer
Trachelorrhaphy	Suture of a laceration of the uterine cervix	Laceration
Uterine suspension	Shortening of the ligament that suspends the uterus by plicating (*folding*) and tacking it back in place; may also include presacral sympathectomy (*surgical excision or chemical destruction of the presacral nerve in the sympathetic nervous system; the nerve is anterior to the sacrum at the base of spine*)	Uterine or uterovaginal prolapse; malposition of the uterus; dysmenorrhea
Vulvectomy	Surgical removal of part of the vulva	Cancer

Source: © PB Resources, Inc. Used with permission.

Maternity Care and Delivery Procedures

Common Maternity Care and Delivery procedures are summarized in ■ TABLE 46-3. These procedures are performed on pregnant women specifically. Procedures on an unborn fetus are coded as procedures performed on the mother. After birth, the newborn constitutes a separate patient, so procedures on the newborn are coded separately from the mother using codes from the Surgery subsection for the appropriate body system.

This section provides a general reference to help understand the most common OB/GYN procedures. Remember to keep standard reference books handy in case you get stuck. Refer to Chapter 22 of this text for additional information and anatomic diagrams related to pregnancy and delivery.

Table 46-3 ■ **COMMON MATERNITY CARE AND DELIVERY PROCEDURES**

Procedure Name	Definition	Reason Performed
Abdominal hysterotomy	Surgical incision into the lower portion of the uterus	Abortion; removal of hydatidiform mole (*a grape-like cluster that represents a nonviable fetus*)
Amniocentesis	Surgical puncture into the amniotic sac to remove amniotic fluid	Remove excess amniotic fluid; diagnose fetal disorders
Assisted vaginal delivery (AVD)	The birth of an infant through the vagina, with the use of drugs or techniques to induce labor, and/or with forceps or vacuum extraction to aid in moving the infant through the birth canal	Preferred outcome for pregnancy when delivery cannot be accomplished without assistance
Cephalic version	Turning the fetus so the head is oriented toward the cervix	Malposition of fetus (breech)
Cerclage (obstetrical)	Suturing the cervix closed during pregnancy	Incompetent (weak) cervix; to reduce the risk of miscarriage
Cervical dilator insertion	Transcatheter administration of a substance into the cervix to widen it. Substances used include prostaglandins, a sticky gel, and laminaria, a sterile rod made of kelp, which both expand when placed inside the cervix and help the uterus to contract	Abortion; predelivery cervical ripening (*thinning, softening, and widening*)

(continued)

Table 46-3 ■ (*continued*)

Procedure Name	Definition	Reason Performed
Cesarean delivery	Incision into the abdomen and uterus to deliver an infant	Delivery risks such as obstructed labor, fetal or maternal distress, postterm pregnancy
Chorionic villus sampling (CVS)	Aspiration of fetal tissue under ultrasonic guidance, by catheter through the cervix or by needle through the mother's abdominal and uterine walls into the uterine cavity	Diagnose chromosomal abnormalities and biochemical disorders
Cordocentesis/percutaneous umbilical blood sampling (PUBS)	Use of ultrasound to detect the umbilical cord and removal of a sample of fetal blood from the cord	Diagnose abnormalities
Curettage (obstetrical)	Scraping away the uterine lining	Retained placenta, abortion
Episiotomy (obstetrical)	Surgical incision into the perineum and vagina	Prevention of traumatic tear during delivery
Evacuation	Suctioning the fetus and placenta out of the uterus with a suctioning instrument placed through the vagina, into the cervix, and into the uterus	Abortion
Fetal nonstress test (NST)	Monitoring of the fetal heartbeat and oxygenation	Postterm or high-risk pregnancy
Fetal scalp blood sampling	Obtaining a blood specimen from the scalp of the fetus through the dilated cervix	Diagnose intrapartum fetal hypoxia (*insufficient amount of oxygen to the fetus during labor and delivery*)
Normal spontaneous vaginal delivery (NSVD)	The birth of an infant through the vagina, without the use of drugs or techniques to induce labor, without forceps, vacuum extraction, or cesarean delivery	Preferred outcome for pregnancy
Repeat cesarean	Performing a cesarean delivery for a mother who had a cesarean delivery with a previous pregnancy	Risk of rupturing scar of previous cesarean
Vaginal delivery after cesarean (VBAC)	Performing a vaginal delivery for a mother who had a cesarean delivery with a previous pregnancy	Preferred outcome for pregnancy when there is no risk of rupturing scar of previous cesarean
Vesicocentesis	Prenatal aspiration of fetal urine	Diagnose birth defects; remove excess urine

Source: © PB Resources, Inc. Used with permission.

CODING PRACTICE

Exercise 46.1   OB/GYN Procedure Basics

Instructions: Use your medical terminology skills and resources to define the following OB/GYN procedures, then identify the code(s) or code range listed in the CPT Index. Follow these steps:

• Use slash marks "/" to break down the underlined term into its root(s) and suffix.

• Define the meaning of the underlined word based on the meaning of each word part.

• Use the entire phrase to identify the code or code range shown in the CPT Index.

Example: <u>hysterectomy</u>, abdominal, supracervical

    hyster/ectomy   Meaning *excision of the uterus*   CPT Code *58180*

1. <u>vaginoscopy</u>, biopsy   Meaning _____   CPT Code _____

2. <u>colpoperineorrhaphy</u>   Meaning _____   CPT Code _____

3. fistula, <u>urethrovaginal</u>   Meaning _____   CPT Code _____

4. <u>oophorectomy</u>   Meaning _____   CPT Code _____

5. <u>vulvectomy</u>, simple, complete Meaning _____ CPT Code _____

6. <u>clitoroplasty</u>, intersex state Meaning _____ CPT Code _____

7. <u>ovariolysis</u> Meaning _____ CPT Code _____

8. <u>hysterosalpingography</u>, catheterization Meaning _____ CPT Code _____

9. <u>colpopexy</u>, laparoscopic Meaning _____ CPT Code _____

10. <u>salpingostomy</u> Meaning _____ CPT Code _____

CODING OVERVIEW OF OB/GYN PROCEDURES

The CPT subsection **Female Genital System (56405-58999)** contains seven subheadings that are divided by anatomic site (■ TABLE 46-4). Within each anatomic site, codes are divided by the type of procedure, such as incision, excision, introduction, and so on.

The CPT subsection **Maternity Care and Delivery (59000-59899)** contains nine subheadings that are divided by anatomic site (■ TABLE 46-5). Within each anatomic site, codes are divided by the type of procedure, such as excision, vaginal delivery, cesarean delivery, and so on.

Review the subheading and category names and code ranges listed in each subsection to become familiar with the content and organization. Some editions of the CPT manual provide a summary list of the subheadings and categories at the beginning of each subsection, which also displays an asterisk (*) next to categories that contain special coding instructions. Special instructions are provided for the subheading **Vulva, Perineum, and Introitus** under the Female Genital System, as well as for the **Laparoscopy** and **Endoscopy** categories in several places throughout this subsection. Guidelines are provided at the beginning of the Maternity Care and Delivery subsection and for the category **Delivery After Previous Cesarean Delivery**.

These subsections include invasive, minimally invasive, and noninvasive surgical procedures on the female genital system and obstetrics. Codes for diagnostic tests on these systems appear in the Medicine section. When billing, the medical necessity of procedures must be justified by diagnosis codes. CPT codes in the Female Genital System subsection are frequently supported by diagnosis codes from ICD-10-CM **Chapter 14 Diseases of the Genitourinary System (N00-N99)**, as well as neoplasms, symptoms and signs, and injuries (■ TABLE 46-6). These are the codes used most commonly to support procedures on the **Female Genital System**; however, diagnosis codes from any ICD-10-CM chapter are permissible.

CPT codes in the **Maternity Care and Delivery** subsection are frequently supported by diagnosis codes from ICD-10-CM **Chapter 15 Pregnancy, Childbirth and the Puerperium (O00-O9A)** (Table 46-6). These are the codes used most commonly to support procedures for **Maternity Care and Delivery**; however, diagnosis codes from other ICD-10-CM chapters are used to document the presence of non-obstetric-related conditions.

CPT guidelines for the Surgery section apply to the Female Genital System and Maternity Care and Delivery.

The **Maternity Care and Delivery** subsection provides detailed special instructions regarding the bundling of antepartum, delivery, and postpartum procedures.

Instructional notes appear throughout the Tabular List to alert coders to the need for modifiers, provide cross-references to codes for similar procedures on other sites, identify when additional codes for radiological services might be needed, and highlight resequenced and recently deleted codes.

Table 46-4 ■ **FEMALE GENITAL SYSTEM SUBHEADINGS**

Subheading	Code Range
Vulva, Perineum and Introitus	56405-56821
Vagina	57000-57426
Cervix Uteri	57452-57800
Corpus Uteri	58100-58579
Oviduct/Ovary	58600-58770
Ovary	58800-58960
In Vitro Fertilization	58970-58976
Other Procedures	58999-58999

Table 46-5 ■ **MATERNITY CARE AND DELIVERY SUBHEADINGS**

Subheading	Code Range
Antepartum and Fetal Invasive Services for Maternity Care and Delivery	59000-59076
Excision	59100-59160
Introduction	59200-59200
Repair	59300-59350
Vaginal Delivery, Antepartum and Postpartum Care	59400-59430
Cesarean Delivery	59510-59525
Delivery Procedures After Previous Cesarean Delivery	59610-59622
Abortion Procedures	59812-59857
Other Procedures	59866-59899

Table 46-6 ■ LOCATING ICD-10-CM AND ADDITIONAL CPT CODES FOR OB/GYN

Type of Code	Codes
ICD-10-CM OB/GYN-Related Codes	
Female genital system conditions	N65-N99
Neoplasms	C50, C51-58
Symptoms and signs	R30-R39
Injuries	S37-S39
Maternity Care and Delivery	O00-O9A, Z30-Z39
CPT OB/GYN-Related Codes	
Medicine procedures	None applicable
Radiologic procedures:	
• Diagnostic radiology	74710-74775
• Radiologic guidance	77001-77022
• Diagnostic ultrasound	76700-76776, 76801-76857
• Breast mammography	77051-77063
• Nuclear medicine, diagnostic	78700-78799
Laboratory organ/disease panels	80055

Source: © PB Resources, Inc. Used with permission.

ABSTRACTING OB/GYN PROCEDURES

Coders must abstract anatomic approaches used with OB/GYN procedures. They also must identify the extent of the procedure with regard to the structures affected. Separate abstracting criteria are provided for gynecology procedures and obstetric procedures.

Anatomic Approach

The anatomic approach identifies the physical route used to access the surgical site. Most approaches can be used with either open or laparoscopic procedures. When you encounter an approach description that is unfamiliar, identify the word root to identify the anatomic site, then identify the prefix to identify the direction. Commonly used anatomic approaches for gynecological procedures include the following:

- abdominal—through the abdomen
- **intraperitoneal**—within the peritoneum
- **paravaginal**—adjacent to the vagina or part of the vagina
- **supracervical**—above the cervix uteri
- **transcervical**—through the cervix uteri
- **transperineal**—through the perineum
- vaginal/**transvaginal**—through the vagina

Extent of Procedure

Some procedures are described based on the extent, such as partial or complete, simple or extensive, and so on. When abstracting, always identify the anatomic sites, or portions of sites, treated. Then, when assigning codes, read the code descriptions to learn how a particular code defines the extent.

Table 46-7 ■ KEY CRITERIA FOR ABSTRACTING FEMALE GENITAL SYSTEM PROCEDURES

- ❑ What is the patient's gender?
- ❑ What procedure is performed?
- ❑ What is the anatomic site?
- ❑ What additional sites are treated?
- ❑ What is the surgical approach?
- ❑ What is the anatomic approach?
- ❑ Is the procedure obstetrical or nonobstetrical?
- ❑ What is the extent of the procedure?
- ❑ What is the laterality?
- ❑ What additional procedure(s) are performed?

Source: © PB Resources, Inc. Used with permission.

You can refer back to the medical record to interpret the procedure description in light of the coding manual definitions.

The descriptions and definition of extent vary and are not uniform for all procedures. The definition of extent often appears within the code description or may appear in special instructions at the beginning of the category. When abstracting a procedure for the first time, you may not be aware of the CPT options and definitions for the extent because you have not yet identified the code options.

For example, when abstracting a vulvectomy you may read in the operative note that the physician *excised 70% of the vulvar area*. When you assign the code for vulvectomy in the Tabular List, you will read special instructions before code **56405** that state **A partial procedure is the removal of less than 80% of the vulvar area**. This definition, along with other elements in the code description, will guide you in assigning the correct code.

Refer to ■ TABLE 46-7 for guidance on how to abstract procedures on the Female Genital System and Maternity Care and Delivery. ■ TABLE 46-8 identifies additional abstracting questions for only Maternity Care and Delivery. Remember that the abstracting questions are a guide and that not every question applies to, or can be answered for, every case. For example, not every gynecological procedure is divided by extent and not every obstetrical procedure includes identification of the trimester.

SUCCESS STEP

Although trimester of pregnancy does not have to be abstracted for all obstetrical procedures, the weeks of gestation, and sometimes the trimester, must be abstracted to assign ICD-10-CM diagnosis codes.

Guided Example of Abstracting OB/GYN Procedures

Refer to the following example throughout this chapter to practice skills for abstracting, assigning, and arranging OB/GYN codes.

Table 46-8 ■ KEY CRITERIA FOR ABSTRACTING MATERNITY CARE AND DELIVERY PROCEDURES

These criteria are specific to Maternity Care and Delivery procedures. Also review the criteria for the Female Genital System.

For delivery:

❑ What is the trimester?

❑ How many infants were delivered?

❑ What is the method of delivery for each infant?

❑ Is a vaginal delivery attempted before cesarean delivery is performed?

❑ Has the patient had a previous cesarean delivery?

❑ What services are provided at the time of delivery in addition to the delivery itself?

❑ Is more than one physician involved in the antepartum care, delivery, and postpartum care?

If Yes:

• Which part of the process is provided by the current physician?

• How many antepartum visits were provided by the same physician?

For abortions:

❑ What is the trimester?

❑ Is the abortion induced?

❑ What method is used (evacuation, D&C, or drug administration)?

❑ Is the abortion complete or incomplete?

Source: © PB Resources, Inc. Used with permission.

INPATIENT HOSPITAL   Gender: F   Age: 28

Gravida: 2   Para: 3   EGA: 39

Reason for admission: full-term labor

Assessment: cord entanglement and compression of fetus 2

Delivery: fetus 1 (boy) TBLC NSVD with third-degree tear that required repair, fetus 2 (girl) TBLC

vaginal delivery converted to cesarean d/t cord entanglement

Note: The patient's first delivery was vaginal. The physician provided all antepartum and postpartum care for this patient.

Follow along as fictitious coder, Daphne Wittman, CCS-P, abstracts the procedure. Check off each step after you complete it.

▶ Daphne reads through the entire record, paying special attention to the reason for the encounter, the procedure performed, and the postoperative diagnosis. She refers to the Key Criteria for Abstracting Maternity Care and Delivery Procedures (Table 46-8).

❑ She notes the reason for admission, full-term labor, and identifies that a delivery of twins occurred.

❑ *What is the patient's gender?* She confirms that the medical record shows the correct gender, female.

❑ *What is the trimester?* The EGA of 39 is the third trimester.

❑ *How many infants were delivered?* two

❑ *What is the method of delivery for each infant?* fetus 1 (boy) TBLC NSVD, fetus 2 (girl) TBLC vaginal delivery converted to cesarean

❑ *Is a vaginal delivery attempted before cesarean delivery is performed?* Yes, fetus 2 (girl) TBLC vaginal delivery converted to cesarean

❑ *Has the patient had a previous cesarean delivery?* No, the patient's first delivery was vaginal.

❑ *What services are provided at the time of delivery in addition to the delivery itself?* third-degree tear that required repair

❑ *Is more than one physician involved in the antepartum care, delivery, and postpartum care?* No

▶ At this time, Daphne does not know which of these procedures may need to be coded, nor how many codes she will end up with. She will learn about this when she moves on to assigning codes.

CODING PRACTICE

Exercise 46.2   Abstracting OB/GYN Procedures

Instructions: Read the mini-medical-record of each patient's encounter and answer the abstracting questions. Write the answer on the line provided. Do not assign any codes.

1. INPATIENT HOSPITAL   Gender: F   Age: 84

Preoperative diagnosis: vaginal prolapse and stress incontinence

(continued)

1. (continued)

Procedure: LeForte-type procedure (colpocleisis); after preparing the patient, we used forceps to grasp the cervix and prolapse the vagina. After removing segments of the pubocervical and posterior rectovaginal fascia, we stitched together underlying supporting layers of the fascia with circular stitches. The prolapse was reduced back into the

(continued)

CODING PRACTICE (continued)

1. (continued)

patient's vagina and pelvis. Patient tolerated the procedure well.

a. What is the patient's gender? _____

b. What procedure is performed? _____

c. What is the anatomic site? _____

d. What additional sites are treated? _____

e. What is the surgical approach? _____

f. What is the anatomic approach? _____

g. Is the procedure obstetrical or nonobstetrical?
_____

h. What is the laterality? _____

i. What additional procedure(s) are performed?
_____

2. INPATIENT HOSPITAL   Gender: F   Age: 32

Gravida: 2   Para: 2   EGA: 39

Preprocedure diagnosis: full-term labor

Procedure: attended the delivery and performed routine antepartum and postpartum care

Delivery: NSVD, TBLC, 1 boy, 7 lb., 2 oz.

a. What is the patient's gender? _____

b. Is the procedure obstetrical or nonobstetrical?
_____

c. What is the trimester? _____

d. Is delivery performed? _____

e. What is the method of delivery? _____

f. Is a vaginal delivery attempted before cesarean delivery is performed? _____

g. Has the patient had a previous cesarean delivery?
_____

h. What services are provided at the time of delivery in addition to the delivery itself? _____

i. Is more than one physician involved in the antepartum care, delivery, and postpartum care? _____

j. Which part of the process is provided by the current physician? _____

3. OFFICE   Gender: F   Age: 28

Gravida: 2   Para: 1   EGA: 28

Reason for encounter: prenatal checkup

Assessment: no pregnancy complications

Plan: Patient is moving out of town, where she will continue care with a different physician. This office provided five antepartum visits.

a. What is the patient's gender? _____

b. What service is provided? _____

c. Is the service obstetrical or nonobstetrical?
_____

d. What additional procedure(s) are performed?
_____

e. What is the trimester? _____

f. Is delivery performed? _____

g. Is more than one physician involved in the antepartum care, delivery, and postpartum care? _____

h. Which part of the process is provided by the current physician? _____

i. How many antepartum visits were provided by the same physician? _____

4. OUTPATIENT SURGERY   Gender: F   Age: 38

Preoperative diagnosis: hydatidiform mole; patient also states that she desires no future pregnancies and requests that sterilization be performed at the same time

Procedure: hysterotomy for excision of hydatidiform mole. Made a horizontal incision in the lower abdominal wall and entered the uterus through the lower uterine segment. Identified and removed hydatidiform mole, along with remaining membranes and placenta from the uterine cavity. After hemostasis was achieved, we sutured the uterine incisions. We then turned our attention to the fallopian tubes, using the stapler to divide each tube and then, using a needle, relocated both tube ends in the uterus. Closed the abdominal incision. Patient tolerated procedure well.

Postoperative diagnosis: hydatidiform mole

a. What is the patient's gender? _____

b. What procedure is performed? _____

c. What is the anatomic site? _____

(continued)

4. (continued)

d. What additional sites are treated? _____

e. What is the surgical approach? _____

f. What is the anatomic approach? _____

g. Is the procedure obstetrical or nonobstetrical? _____

h. What additional procedure(s) are performed? _____

5. (continued)

h. What is the extent of the procedure? _____

i. What is the laterality? _____

j. What additional procedure(s) are performed? _____

---

5. OFFICE   Gender: F   Age: 37

Preprocedure diagnosis: vulvar lesions

Procedure: biopsies of three vulvar lesions; used scalpel to excise three lesions with margins from the base of the vulva. Total excised diameters were 0.5 cm, 0.75 cm, and 1.0 cm. Sent to pathology for analysis.

Pathology report: vulvar intraepithelial neoplasia—moderate (VIN II) precancerous abnormal cell growth

Postprocedure diagnosis: VIN II

a. What is the patient's gender? _____

b. What procedure is performed? _____

c. What is the anatomic site? _____

d. What additional sites are treated? _____

e. What is the surgical approach? _____

f. What is the anatomic approach? _____

g. Is the procedure obstetrical or nonobstetrical? _____

(continued)

6. INPATIENT HOSPITAL   Gender: F   Age: 78

Preoperative diagnosis: rectocele

Procedure: posterior colporrhaphy with mesh reinforcement. Inserted speculum into the vagina to hold it open during the procedure. Evaluated the extent of the rectocele. Made an incision in the posterior vaginal wall from the top of the vagina to the levator muscles. Plicated the fascia and approximated the edges together and sutured them, making sure to include the levator muscle in the repair. Unable to repair the perineal muscles due to lack of viable tissue, so we elected to insert a prosthetic graft over the anterior vaginal wall.

a. What is the patient's gender? _____

b. What procedure is performed? _____

c. What is the anatomic site? _____

d. What additional sites are treated? _____

e. What is the surgical approach? _____

f. What is the anatomic approach? _____

g. Is the procedure obstetrical or nonobstetrical? _____

h. What additional procedure(s) are performed? _____

ASSIGNING CODES FOR OB/GYN PROCEDURES

To assign codes for Female Genital System Procedures, search the Index for the anatomic site, such as **Vulva**, and the first-level modifying term for the condition or type of procedure, such as **Lesion** or **Excision**. Alternatively, look up the Main Term for name of the procedure, such as **Vulvectomy**, then read through the first-level modifying terms to locate the one that best describes the procedure performed. Refer to the Tabular List to read any guidelines and instructional notes, and select and verify the code.

Coders also should be familiar with how to assign codes for hysterectomy procedures, the global obstetric package, and multiple births. These skills are discussed next.

Assigning Codes for Hysterectomy

Hysterectomy, the second most common surgical procedure performed in the United States, is the removal of the uterus and sometimes related structures such as the ovaries and fallopian tubes. Physicians perform hysterectomies to treat cancer, uterine fibroid tumors, endometriosis, abnormal vaginal bleeding, and uterine prolapse. CPT provides 19 codes for hysterectomy that are divided based on the following criteria:

- Surgical approach—laparoscopic or open
- Anatomic approach—abdominal, vaginal
- Associated structures removed—ovaries, fallopian tubes, lymph nodes
- Extent—total, subtotal, radical, or partial
- Weight of uterus—for vaginal hysterectomies

To assign codes for a hysterectomy, search the Index for the Main Term **Uterus**, the first-level modifying term **Excision**, and the second-level modifying term for the type of procedure based on approach or extent, such as **Laparoscopic**, **Total**, **Vaginal**,

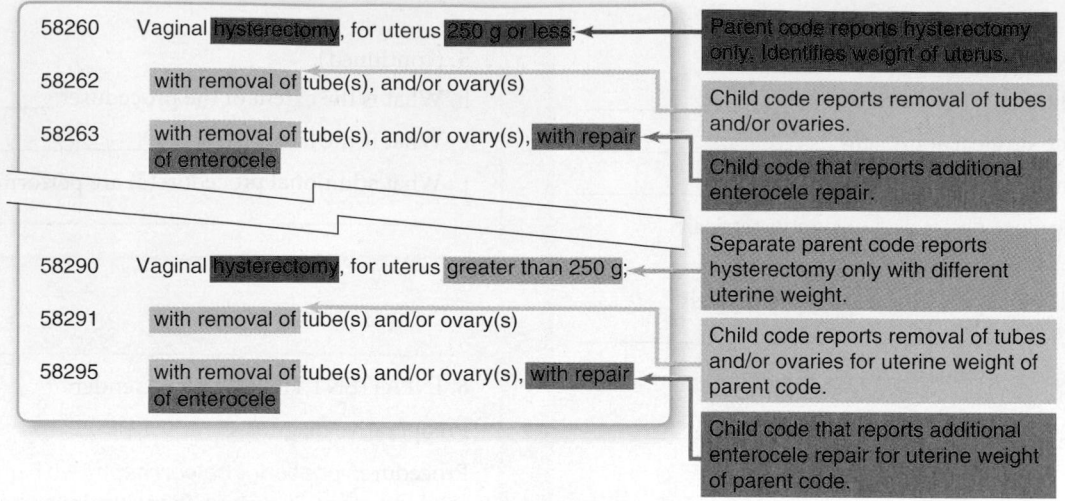

Figure 46-1 ■ CPT Tabular List Entries for Vaginal Hysterectomy. *Source: © PB Resources, Inc. Used with permission. CPT codes only © American Medical Association.*

and so on. In the Tabular List, read code descriptors carefully to identify the specific criteria for each code. Identify any additional procedures listed in code descriptors to ensure that you do not separately code for services already included with the hysterectomy.

For example, code **58150** describes **Total abdominal hysterectomy (corpus and cervix), with or without removal of tube(s), with or without removal of ovary(s)**. The words **with or without** mean the same code is reported regardless of whether the physician removes the fallopian tubes and ovaries.

However, codes for vaginal hysterectomy (**58260-58270, 58275-58285, 58290-58294**) and laparoscopic hysterectomy (**54541-54554**) are divided by whether or not the fallopian tubes and/or ovaries are removed in addition to the uterus. If only the uterus is removed, one code is reported; if either the tubes or ovaries or both are removed, a different code is reported, but the same code reports either structure. Codes for vaginal and laparoscopic hysterectomies are divided based on the weight of the uterus (■ FIGURES 46-1 and 46-2).

Assigning Codes for the Global Obstetric Package

Coders must understand the scope of the **global obstetric package**, which includes routine antepartum, delivery, and postpartum care. When one physician or medical group provides all services within the package, report only the global obstetric package code. When additional or nonroutine

services not part of the global obstetric package are provided, report them with additional codes. ■ TABLE 46-9 identifies the elements included, or bundled, in the global obstetric package and those that can be billed separately. The required modifier, if any, for the additional services is also shown. Report global obstetric package codes at the time of delivery, not during antepartum visits.

To assign codes for the global obstetric package, search the Index for the Main Term **Obstetrical Care** and the first-level modifying term for the type of delivery, such as **Vaginal delivery** or **Cesarean delivery**, and the second-level modifying term **Routine**. Refer to the Tabular List to verify the code or review the code range to select the applicable code. More information is provided in the following paragraphs.

To assign codes for nonroutine obstetric procedures not included in the global package, search the Index for the Main Term that identifies the procedure, such as **Amniocentesis** or **Ultrasound**. Select the first-level modifying term **Obstetrical** when available, or select another appropriate modifying term. For example, the first-level modifying term under **Ultrasound** is **Pregnant uterus**. Verify the code in the Tabular List and review all available codes to select the most specific. Apply the appropriate modifier, if any, as illustrated in Table 46-9.

To assign codes for E/M services not included in the global package, follow the usual procedure for assigning E/M codes. Search the Index for the Main Term **Evaluation and Management** and locate the first-level modifying term for the location of service. Refer to the Tabular List to select the appropriate code based on the three key components of an E/M service or other criteria as specified by the code description. Apply the appropriate modifier, if any, as illustrated in Table 46-9.

CPT provides four codes for the global obstetric package based on the type and circumstances of delivery (**59400, 59510, 59610**, and **59618**). Vaginal and cesarean methods of delivery require different amounts of physician work and skill, so separate codes, with different RVU values, are provided.

> Physician performs a vaginal hysterectomy with removal of both fallopian tubes and the left ovary. The uterus weighs 280 grams.
>
> **58291 Vaginal hysterectomy, for uterus greater than 250 g; with removal of tube(s) and/or ovary(s)**

Figure 46-2 ■ Example of Coding Vaginal Hysterectomy. *Source: © PB Resources, Inc. Used with permission. CPT codes only © American Medical Association.*

Table 46-9 ■ **ELEMENTS OF THE GLOBAL OBSTETRIC PACKAGE**

Global Obstetric Package/Routine Services	Additional/Nonroutine Services
Antepartum Care	
Initial and subsequent history	Venipuncture and lab tests performed, other than routine chemical urinalysis
Physical exams	Procedures for problems related to the pregnancy
Recording weight, blood pressures, fetal heart tones	*Examples:*
Routine chemical urinalysis	• Amniocentesis
Monthly visits up to 28 weeks' gestation	• Chronic villous sampling
Biweekly visits from 29–36 weeks' gestation	• Cordocentesis
Weekly visits from 37 weeks until delivery	• Fetal stress testing
	• Fetal nonstress testing
	• OB ultrasounds (limited or complete)
	• Fetal biophysical profile
	• Fetal electrocardiography
	• Rh immune globulin administration
	E/M for complications of pregnancy
	Examples:
	• Preterm labor (PTL)
	• Decreased fetal movement (FM)
	• Preeclampsia
	• Diabetes
	• Gestational diabetes
	• Hyperemesis
	E/M and/or procedures for conditions unrelated to pregnancy
	Examples:
	• Urinary tract infection
	• Upper respiratory infection
	• Influenza
	• Vaginitis
	• Fractures, sprains
	• Any other medical condition
	Append modifier **-24 Unrelated evaluation and management service by the same physician during the global period** to alert the payer that the E/M service(s) is unrelated to the global OB package
Delivery Care	
Hospital admission	E/M services that occur more than 24 hours before the delivery may be separately reported.
Admission history and physical exam	Report multiple gestation vaginal births, or a combination of vaginal and cesarean births, using additional codes for each infant delivered. (Append modifier **-51 Multiple procedures** to a vaginal delivery code when done with a cesarean. Append modifier **-59 Distinct procedural service** to multiple vaginal deliveries.)
Management of uncomplicated labor	
One delivery, vaginal or cesarean	
Any E/M services provided within 24 hours of delivery	Report one cesarean delivery regardless of the number of infants born because only one incision is made, and append modifier **-22 Increased procedural services** to identify the increased difficulty of the procedure when more than one fetus is delivered by cesarean delivery.
Induction labor using pitocin or oxytocin	
Artificial rupturing of membranes	Treatment of surgical complications of pregnancy, labor, and delivery such as appendectomy, hernia, or ovarian cyst
Insertion of a cervical dilator for vaginal deliveries (on the same date as the delivery)	Additional OB/GYN procedures performed at time of delivery such as hysterectomy or tubal ligation
Delivery of the placenta	
Repair of any minor lacerations (first or second degree)	Insertion of a cervical dilator for vaginal deliveries (on a separate date from the delivery)
Episiotomy, forceps, or vacuum assistance in delivery	

(continued)

work required for the additional delivery(s) and attach a report that explains the circumstances.

When multiple births are mixed—at least one vaginal and one cesarean—report the global obstetric package code for the cesarean delivery because it has a higher RVU. Report vaginal deliveries using code **59409** or **59610** for vaginal delivery only. Sequence the code for the cesarean global package first, even though the cesarean delivery occurs after the vaginal delivery(s) chronologically. Append modifier **-51 Multiple procedures** to the first vaginal delivery. If there is more than one vaginal delivery, append modifier **-59** to the second and subsequent vaginal deliveries.

SUCCESS STEP

General CPT guidelines are discussed here. Individual payers have differing requirements about how to report codes when only a portion of the global obstetric package is provided. Checking with payers before submitting a claim saves time and money.

Guided Example of Assigning Obstetrical Procedure Codes

To practice skills for assigning codes for Maternity Care and Delivery, continue with the example from earlier in the chapter about a patient who was seen for the birth of twins. Follow along in your CPT manual as Daphne Wittman, CCS-P, assigns codes. Check off each step after you complete it.

▶ First, Daphne confirms that a twin birth occurred, one NSVD and one *vaginal delivery converted to cesarean.*

▶ Daphne searches the Index for the Main Term **Cesarean delivery**.

   ❏ She locates the first-level modifying term **Routine Care**. Because a cesarean delivery is more extensive and has a higher RVU than a vaginal delivery, she associates the routine care for the global obstetric package with the cesarean delivery.

   ❏ She identifies the code **59510**.

   ❏ She notices a second-level modifying term, **Unsuccessful attempted vaginal delivery**, and wonders if she should select this code. She notices that it appears under the first-level modifying term **Previous cesarean delivery**. Because this patient's first pregnancy resulted in a vaginal delivery, she does not think this code applies, but makes a note of the code **59618** for routine care so she can check it in the Tabular List.

▶ Daphne verifies code **59510** in the Tabular List.

   ❏ She reads the code title for **59510 Routine obstetric care including antepartum care, cesarean delivery, and postpartum care** and confirms that this accurately describes the principal procedure and that the physician provided all services in the global obstetric package.

   ❏ She also compares code **59618 Routine obstetric care including antepartum care, cesarean delivery,**

and postpartum care, following attempted vaginal delivery after previous cesarean delivery. The code clearly describes a cesarean delivery **following attempted vaginal delivery after previous cesarean delivery**. Although there was an attempted vaginal delivery, it did not occur after a previous cesarean delivery, so **59618** is not an accurate code for this patient.

   ❏ She reads through the descriptions for codes in the **Cesarean Delivery** category, but does not find any others that describe a cesarean following an attempted vaginal delivery. Therefore, she stays with her original choice of code **59510**.

▶ Daphne checks for instructions in the Tabular List.

   ❏ She cross-references the beginning of category **Cesarean Delivery** and verifies that there are no special instructions. There are two instructional notes that provide cross-references to other codes, but they do not apply to this case.

   ❏ She cross-references the beginning of the subsection **Maternity Care and Delivery** and reviews the instructions about bundled services in the global obstetric package.

▶ Next Daphne codes for the vaginal delivery. She searches the Index for the Main Term **Vaginal Delivery**.

   ❏ She locates the first-level modifying term **Delivery Only** because the routine care for the global obstetric package, which consists of antepartum and postpartum care, was included in the code for the cesarean delivery.

   ❏ She identifies the code **59409**.

▶ Daphne verifies code **59409** in the Tabular List.

   ❏ She reads the code title for **59409, Vaginal delivery only (with or without episiotomy and/or forceps)** and confirms that this accurately describes the delivery.

▶ Daphne checks for instructions in the Tabular List.

   ❏ She cross-references the beginning of category **Vaginal Delivery** and verifies that there are no special instructions.

▶ Daphne reviews the medical record and identifies that the patient also sustained a *third-degree tear that required repair.* This service does not require a separate code, but does qualify for a modifier. She makes a note to review this further when she arranges the codes and assigns modifiers.

▶ Daphne reviews the procedure codes she has assigned for this case.

   ❏ **59409 Vaginal delivery only (with or without episiotomy and/or forceps)**

   ❏ **59510 Routine obstetric care including antepartum care, cesarean delivery, and postpartum care**

▶ Next, Daphne must determine how to sequence the codes.

CODING PRACTICE

Exercise 46.3   Assigning Codes for OB/GYN Procedures

Instructions: Read the mini-medical-record of each patient's encounter. Review the information abstracted in Exercise 46.2 for questions 1–3. For questions 4–6, abstract the case on your own. Assign CPT codes, quantities, and modifiers using the Index and Tabular List. Write the code(s) on the line provided.

1. INPATIENT HOSPITAL   Gender: F   Age: 84

Preoperative diagnosis: *vaginal prolapse and stress incontinence*

Procedure: *LeForte-type procedure (colpocleisis); after preparing the patient, we used forceps to grasp the cervix and prolapse the vagina. After removing segments of the pubocervical and posterior rectovaginal fascia, we stitched together underlying supporting layers of the fascia with circular stitches. The prolapse was reduced back into the patient's vagina and pelvis. Patient tolerated the procedure well.*

Tip: The suffix –clesis means closure.

1 CPT Code _____

2. INPATIENT HOSPITAL   Gender: F   Age: 32

Gravida: 2   Para: 2   EGA: 39

Preprocedure diagnosis: *full-term labor*

Procedure: *attended the delivery and performed routine antepartum and postpartum care*

Delivery: *NSVD, TBLC, 1 boy, 7 lb., 2 oz.*

1 CPT Code _____

3. OFFICE   Gender: F   Age: 28

Gravida: 2   Para: 1   EGA: 28

Reason for encounter: *prenatal checkup*

Assessment: *no pregnancy complications*

Plan: *Patient is moving out of town, where she will continue care with a different physician. This office provided five antepartum visits.*

1 CPT Code _____

4. OUTPATIENT HOSPITAL   Gender: F   Age: 33

Gravida: 2   Para: 1   EGA: 37-2/7 weeks

Reason for encounter: *Oxytocin stress test after abnormal nonstress test last week*

Assessment: *IV oxytocin administered in increasing doses until patient had three contractions within 10 minutes lasting longer than 45 seconds. Oxytocin augmented with intermittent nipple stimulation. Monitor applied and fetal heart rate and uterine contractions recorded. No late decelerations.*

Plan: *expect fetus to be able to handle stress of labor and vaginal delivery planned*

1 CPT Code _____

5. HOSPITAL INPATIENT   Gender: F   Age: 33

Preprocedure diagnosis: *desires sterilization*

Procedure: *laparoscopic tubal fulguration. Veress needle inserted through the infraumbilical incision. Abdomen insufflated and laparoscope inserted. Bipolar cautery used to fulgurate the right and left fallopian tubes distal to the uterine crown. A second fulguration completed bilaterally at a point distal to lateral point. Instruments removed, incisions repaired.*

1 CPT Code _____

6. OUTPATIENT SURGERY   Gender: F   Age: 42

Gravida: 4   Para: 0   EGA: 12 weeks

Reason for encounter: *elderly primipara with incomplete miscarriage*

Procedure: *dilation and evacuation of fetal tissue. Visible products of conception removed with forceps. Anterior lip of cervix grasped and suction curettage x2 was completed.*

Plan: *return to the office in two weeks*

1 CPT Code _____

ARRANGING CODES FOR OB/GYN PROCEDURES

Arranging codes for the Female Genital System and Maternity Care and Delivery follows the general CPT rules. Sequence codes in descending RVU order, particularly those that are reported as multiple procedures using modifier **-51**. This helps ensure that the most costly procedure is paid in full and the multiple procedure reduction is applied to less costly procedures.

When sequencing codes for multiple births, sequence them in descending RVU order, not by birth order. For example, a cesarean delivery has a higher RVU value than a vaginal delivery. If infant one is born vaginally and its twin is delivered by cesarean, sequence the cesarean delivery first. If the global obstetric package was provided by the delivering physician, associate the global package with the cesarean delivery and sequence it first.

Modifiers Commonly Used with OB/GYN Codes

CPT does not provide any unique modifiers for use with procedures of the Female Genital System and Maternity Care and Delivery. Use standard CPT modifiers when needed to further describe the circumstances of a procedure or service. In some cases, the literal description of a modifier is interpreted with reference to obstetrics. For example, modifiers pertaining to the postoperative period are understood to refer to the period of the global obstetric package.

Always check with the payer to identify the services covered under a particular modifier, and submit a special report with the claim that describes the circumstances in detail.

In addition to the usual guidelines for using modifiers that apply to all OB/GYN encounters, obstetric encounters also use modifiers for the following purposes.

-22 Increased Procedural Services

Use modifier **-22** when billing for cesarean delivery of multiple fetuses. Because only one surgical incision is made, only one CPT code for the delivery or global obstetric package is reported. Therefore, the modifier identifies the additional work involved in delivering multiple infants via cesarean. Do not use modifier **-22** for multiple vaginal deliveries because each vaginal delivery is assigned a separate CPT code for the delivery or global obstetric package; the second and subsequent vaginal deliveries are reported with modifier **-51** appended.

Modifier **-22** is also used to report excessive antepartum visits beyond those typically included in the global obstetric package and for other complications of pregnancy or delivery.

When the physician repairs a third- or fourth-degree perineal laceration, append modifier **-22** to the delivery code. Do not report a separate repair code. Do not report modifier **-22** for first- or second-degree repairs.

-24 Unrelated E/M During Global Obstetric Period

When the physician supervising the pregnancy and performing the delivery also sees the patient for reasons unrelated to the pregnancy, append modifier **-24** to identify that the visit is not part of the global obstetric package. Examples include abdominal pain, genital tract infection, yeast infection, and pelvic inflammatory disease.

Physician sees a new patient for two antepartum visits, after which the patient decides to seek another physician. The first visit consisted of a detailed history, a detailed examination, and medical decision making of low complexity. The second visit consisted of a problem focused history, an expanded problem focused examination, and low complexity medical decision making.

99203-24 Office or other outpatient visit for the evaluation and management of a new patient, which requires these 3 key components: A detailed history; A detailed examination; Medical decision making of low complexity. -24 Unrelated E/M

99213-24 Office or other outpatient visit for the evaluation and management of an established patient, which requires at least 2 of these 3 key components: An expanded problem focused history; An expanded problem focused examination; Medical decision making of low complexity. -24 Unrelated E/M

Figure 46-5 ■ Example of Coding Antepartum Visits with Modifier -24. *Source: © PB Resources, Inc. Used with permission. CPT codes only © American Medical Association.*

When a physician provides three or fewer antepartum visits, report them with E/M code(s). CPT does not provide separate E/M codes for antepartum visits. Append modifier **-24** to identify that they are not part of a global obstetric package that will be billed at the time of delivery (■ FIGURE 46-5). A special report may also be needed so the payer does not assume that the encounters are part of a global obstetric package.

-51 Multiple Procedures

When multiple births occur with one or more cesarean deliveries and one or more vaginal deliveries with one or more cesarean deliveries at the same time, report the first vaginal birth with modifier **-51** because different CPT codes are used. Report the second and subsequent vaginal births with modifier **-59**.

-52 Reduced Services

When a physician provides all services in the global obstetric package, but provides fewer than seven antepartum visits, report the code for the global package with modifier **-52**. This is more efficient than reporting three separate codes for the antepartum, delivery, and postpartum services.

-59 Distinct Procedural Service

Report multiple vaginal deliveries with modifier **-59** on the second and subsequent deliveries to clarify that the same procedure is not being reported twice. Some payers may require HCPCS modifier **-XS Separate Structure**, instead of **-59**, to identify that the delivery was performed on a separate infant.

When there are multiple vaginal deliveries in addition to one or more cesarean deliveries, apply modifiers as follows:

- One cesarean delivery—no modifier
- Multiple cesarean deliveries—append modifier **-22** to the code for the cesarean delivery

- One vaginal delivery followed by cesarean delivery(ies)
  - append modifier **-51** to the vaginal delivery
  - append modifier **-22** to the cesarean delivery if there are multiple cesarean births
- Multiple vaginal deliveries followed by cesarean delivery(ies)
  - append modifier **-51** to the first vaginal delivery
  - append modifier **-59** to the second and subsequent vaginal deliveries
  - append modifier **-22** to the cesarean delivery if there are multiple cesarean births

-80 Assistant Surgeon

When cesarean deliveries use a primary surgeon and an assistant surgeon, the assistant surgeon bills the code for the delivery only with modifier **-80**. In most circumstances, an assistant surgeon bills the same procedure code as the primary surgeon and appends modifier **-80**. However, in obstetrics, if the primary surgeon reports a code for the global obstetric package, the assistant surgeon should report a code for the delivery only because the assistant surgeon does not provide the global package.

Guided Example of Arranging OB/GYN Procedure Codes

To practice skills for assigning codes for Maternity Care and Delivery, continue with the example from earlier in the chapter about a patient who was seen for the birth of twins. Follow along in your CPT manual as Daphne Wittman, CCS-P, arranges the codes. Check off each step after you complete it.

▶ First, Daphne confirms the procedure codes she assigned:

❑ **59409 Vaginal delivery only (with or without episiotomy and/or forceps)**

❑ **59510 Routine obstetric care including antepartum care, cesarean delivery, and postpartum care**

▶ She sequences code **59510** first because it is the more extensive code, based on the global obstetric package and the

cesarean delivery. She understands that codes for deliveries are not sequenced in chronological order but in descending order according to RVU or price.

▶ Daphne examines the need for modifiers. (Refer to Table 30-1 Key Criteria for Abstracting CPT Modifiers or Appendix A in the CPT manual.)

❑ Code **59510** does not require modifiers because there are no alterations to the service or special circumstances.

❑ Code **59409** requires modifier **-51 Multiple procedures** and will be subject to a 50% reduction in payment because it is the second procedure/delivery reported at the same encounter.

❑ Code **59409** also requires modifier **-22 Increased procedural services** to report the additional work involved in repairing the third-degree perineal laceration. She knows that she needs to assign a diagnosis code to support the need for the modifier and that she will also need to prepare a special report describing the need for the service.

▶ Daphne finalizes the procedure codes and sequencing for this case:

(1) **59510 Routine obstetric care including antepartum care, cesarean delivery, and postpartum care**

(2) **59409-51-22 Vaginal delivery only (with or without episiotomy and/or forceps); -51 Multiple procedures; -22 Increased procedural services**

▶ Daphne also assigns and sequences the ICD-10-CM diagnosis codes that support the need for the service.

(1) **O69.2XX2 (Delivery, complicated by, cord, entanglement, with compression, fetus 2)**

(2) **O30.043 (Pregnancy, twin, dichorionic/diamniotic, third trimester)**

(3) **O70.2 Third degree perineal laceration during delivery**

(4) **Z37.2 (Outcome of delivery, twins, both liveborn)**

(5) **Z3A.39 (Pregnancy, weeks of gestation, 39 weeks)**

CODING PRACTICE

Exercise 46.4   Arranging Codes for OB/GYN Procedures

Instructions: Read the mini-medical-record of each patient's encounter. Review the information abstracted in Exercise 46.2 for questions 1–3. For questions 4–6, abstract the case on your own. Assign CPT codes, quantities, and modifiers using the Index and Tabular List, and arrange the codes in proper sequence. Write the code(s) on the line provided.

1. OUTPATIENT SURGERY   Gender: F   Age: 38

Preoperative diagnosis: hydatidiform mole; patient also states that she desires no future pregnancies and requests that sterilization be performed at the same time

Procedure: hysterotomy for excision of hydatidiform mole. Made a horizontal incision in the lower abdominal wall and entered the uterus through the lower uterine

(*continued*)

1. (continued)

segment. Identified and removed hydatidiform mole, along with remaining membranes and placenta from the uterine cavity. After hemostasis was achieved, we sutured the uterine incisions. We then turned our attention to the fallopian tubes, using the stapler to divide each tube and then, using a needle, relocated both tube ends in the uterus. Closed the abdominal incision. Patient tolerated procedure well.

Postoperative diagnosis: hydatidiform mole

Tip: Tubal ligation is, by definition, a bilateral procedure, so a modifier is not required.

2 CPT Codes _____

2. OFFICE Gender: F Age: 37

Preprocedure diagnosis: vulvar lesions

Procedure: biopsies of three vulvar lesions; used scalpel to excise three lesions with margins from the base of the vulva. Total excised diameters were 0.5 cm, 0.75 cm, and 1.0 cm. Sent to pathology for analysis.

Pathology report: vulvar intraepithelial neoplasia—moderate (VIN II) precancerous abnormal cell growth

Postprocedure diagnosis: VIN II

Tip: Identify the quantity for each code.

2 CPT Codes _____

3. INPATIENT HOSPITAL Gender: F Age: 78

Preoperative diagnosis: rectocele

Procedure: posterior colporrhaphy with mesh reinforcement. Inserted speculum into the vagina to hold it open during the procedure. Evaluated the extent of the rectocele. Made an incision in the posterior vaginal wall from the top of the vagina to the levator muscles. Plicated the fascia and approximated the edges together and sutured them, making sure to include the levator muscle in the repair. Unable to repair the perineal muscles due to lack of viable tissue, so we elected to insert a prosthetic graft over the anterior vaginal wall

2 CPT Codes _____

4. OUTPATIENT SURGERY Gender: F Age: 24

Preprocedure diagnosis: chronic pelvic pain

Procedure: laparoscopic right ovarian, paratubal cystectomy; omentectomy resection of abdominal hematoma. Inspection of the pelvic region revealed a right paratubal ovarian cyst with torsion and a 4- to 5-cm hematoma within the omentum. Omentectomy carried out and the paratubal ovarian cyst excised. Good hemostasis noted before removing instruments.

2 CPT Codes _____

5. INPATIENT HOSPITAL Gender: F Age: 59

Preprocedure diagnosis: symptomatic leiomyomatous uterus; pelvic endometriosis

Procedure: laparoscopic-assisted vaginal hysterectomy of 240-g uterus with right salpingo-oophorectomy; ablation of pelvic endometriosis. Pelvic exam revealed uterine size of 7- to 9-week gestation consistent with fibroid uterus. Under laparoscopic guidance implants of endometriosis were coagulated with the Harmonic scalpel. Our attention turned to the uterus, which was dissected free with care to preserve the ovaries. The specimen was delivered through the vagina. The laparoscopic instruments were removed and incisions closed. There were no complications.

2 CPT Codes _____

6. INPATIENT HOSPITAL Gender: F Age: 38

Gravida: 4 Para: 3 EGA: 36 + 5

Preprocedure diagnosis: previous ultrasound confirmation of fetus in a frank breech position in this multiparous young woman

Procedure: nonstress test completed to document fetal status prior to the version. Tocolytic injection given to relax the uterus and prevent contractions. External cephalic version performed by rolling the fetus to a head-down position. The fetal heart rate was monitored throughout and remained in normal range, with no distress noted.

Postprocedure diagnosis: fetus in cephalic position

2 CPT Codes _____

E/M CODING FOR OB/GYN

The *1997 Documentation Guidelines for Evaluation and Management Services* (1997 DG), published by CMS, provides requirements for each level of a genitourinary E/M examination, with separate criteria for males and females (■ FIGURE 46-6). A separate obstetric examination does not exist. Gynecologists are not limited to using the guidelines for a genitourinary examination only. They can also use guidelines for a general multiorgan system examination, or any other single organ system examination, based on what is most advantageous for a specific encounter. However, physicians cannot combine elements from more than one type of examination for a given encounter. Typically the genitourinary examination guidelines provide the best results when a detailed genitourinary examination is performed.

To determine the appropriate E/M code, coders must review the documentation in detail and identify the specific elements documented.

- To translate the documentation into the E/M requirements for the history, refer back to Chapter 31, Evaluation and Management Services (99201-99499), Tables 31-7 to 31-10, or to the 1997 DG.

- To determine the requirements for an examination, refer to Figure 46-6 or to the single organ system examination for genitourinary in the 1997 DG.

- To determine the levels for medical decision making (MDM), refer to Chapter 31, Table 31-12, and also to the Table of Risk in the 1997 DG.

Guided Example of E/M Coding for Gynecology

Refer to the gynecology encounter (■ FIGURE 46-7) to practice skills for abstracting and assigning E/M codes. Follow along as fictitious coder Daphne Wittman, CCS-P, abstracts the procedure. Check off each step after you complete it.

▶ First, Daphne needs to establish the category of service so she can determine the information needed to abstract and assign the code.

❏ *What is the setting?* Office

❏ *What is the type of service?* This is a consultation because the patient was referred by the primary care physician for an opinion and a report was sent back by the consulting physician.

❏ *What is the code range?* Daphne refers to the CPT Index and looks up the Main Term **Evaluation and Management** and the subterm **Consultation**. The code range listed is **99241-99255**.

❏ *How many key components are required?* Daphne refers to the code range in the Tabular List. The subheading **Consultations** is divided into two categories: **Office or other outpatient consultations** and **Inpatient consultations**. She locates the code rage **99241-99245** for office consultations and reads the code description of the first code, which requires **these 3 key components**. All codes in the category have the same requirements for key components. This tells her that all three key

components must meet or exceed the levels listed in the code (3/3).

▶ Next, Daphne identifies the level of history.

❏ *What is the level of HPI?* The HPI is **Extended** because four or more elements are documented.

❏ *What is the level of ROS?* The ROS is **Extended** because two to nine systems are documented.

❏ *What is the level of PFSH?* The PFSH is **Complete** because two elements are documented.

❏ *Based on these factors, what is the overall level of history?* The level of history is **Detailed** because the lowest of the three factors (HPI, ROS, and PFSH) determines the history level. The PFSH qualifies for a comprehensive history, but the HPI and ROS qualify for only a detailed history.

▶ Daphne refers to the genitourinary examination in the 1997 DG (Figure 46-6) to abstract information needed to determine the level of the examination.

❏ *What is the level of examination?* The level of examination is **Detailed**. Fourteen (14) elements of the examination are documented, which exceeds the requirement of 12 or more bulleted elements for a Detailed examination. A comprehensive examination requires that every element in each box with a shaded border and at least one element in each box with an unshaded border be documented, which they are not.

▶ Daphne determines the level of medical decision making. (Refer to Table 31-12 Medical Decision Making Levels.)

❏ *What is the level of complexity of the number of diagnoses or management options, based on the presenting problem?* The level is **High** because there is a new presenting problem, without workup.

❏ *What is the amount and/or complexity of data to be reviewed?* The level is **Low** because the physician reviewed the patient's past medical record.

❏ *What is the level of risk of significant complications, morbidity, and/or mortality?* She reviews each column in the Table of Risk in the 1997 DG and determines that the level of risk is **Moderate**. The patient presents with an undiagnosed new problem with uncertain prognosis (Moderate), clinical labs are reviewed (Minimal), and a diagnostic endoscopy is performed (Moderate). The single highest element in the Table of Risk determines the overall risk. The columns **Presenting problem** and **Diagnostic procedure(s) ordered** are the highest level (Moderate).

❏ *Based on these factors, what is the overall level of medical decision making?* The medical decision making is **Moderate complexity**. At least two of the three MDM factors are required to qualify for a specific level of MDM. Two of the three MDM factors meet or exceed moderate decision making.

Now Daphne is ready to assign the codes for the gynecology encounter. The exercise that follows guides you through additional abstracting skills and allows you to assign the correct codes.

System/Body Area	Elements of Genitourinary Examination
Constitutional	❑ Measurement of any **three** of the following seven **vital** signs: • 1) sitting or standing blood pressure, • 2) supine blood pressure, • 3) pulse rate and regularity, • 4) respiration, • 5) temperature, • 6) height, • 7) weight (May be measured and recorded by ancillary staff) ❑ General **appearance** of patient (eg, development, nutrition, body habitus, deformities, attention to grooming)
Neck	❑ Examination of **neck** (eg, masses, overall appearance, symmetry, tracheal position, crepitus) ❑ Examination of **thyroid** (eg, enlargement, tenderness, mass)
Respiratory	❑ Assessment of **respiratory effort** (eg, intercostal retractions, use of accessory muscles, diaphragmatic movement) **Auscultation** of lungs (eg, breath sounds, adventitious sounds, rubs)
Cardiovascular	❑ **Auscultation** of heart with notation of abnormal sounds and murmurs ❑ Examination of **peripheral vascular system** by observation (eg, swelling, varicosities) and palpation (e.g. pulses, temperature, edema, tenderness)
Chest (Breasts)	See genitourinary (female)
Gastrointestinal (Abdomen)	❑ Examination of **abdomen** with notation of presence of masses or tenderness ❑ Examination for presence or absence of **hernia** ❑ Examination of **liver** and **spleen** ❑ Obtain **stool sample** for occult blood test when indicated
Genitourinary	**MALE:** ❑ Inspection of **anus** and **perineum** Examination (with or without specimen collection for smears and cultures) of genitalia including: ❑ **Scrotum** (eg, lesions, cysts, rashes) ❑ **Epididymides** (eg, size, symmetry, masses) ❑ **Testes** (eg, size, symmetry, masses) ❑ **Urethral meatus** (eg, size, location, lesions, discharge) ❑ **Penis** (eg, lesions, presence or absence of foreskin, foreskin retractability, plaque, masses, scarring, deformities) **Digital rectal** examination including: ❑ Prostate gland (eg, size, symmetry, nodularity, tenderness) ❑ Seminal vesicles (eg, symmetry, tenderness, masses, enlargement) ❑ Sphincter tone, presence of hemorrhoids, rectal masses **FEMALE:** Includes at least **seven of the following eleven elements** identified by bullets: ❑ Inspection and palpation of **breasts** (eg, masses or lumps, tenderness, symmetry, nipple discharge) ❑ **Digital rectal** examination including sphincter tone, presence of hemorrhoids, rectal masses Pelvic examination (with or without specimen collection for smears and cultures), including ❑ **External genitalia** (eg, general appearance, hair distribution, lesions) ❑ **Urethral meatus** (eg, size, location, lesions, prolapse) ❑ **Urethra** (eg, masses, tenderness, scarring) ❑ **Bladder** (eg, fullness, masses, tenderness) ❑ **Vagina** (eg, general appearance, estrogen effect, discharge, lesions, pelvic support, cystocele, rectocele) ❑ **Cervix** (eg, general appearance, lesions, discharge) ❑ **Uterus** (eg, size, contour, position, mobility, tenderness, consistency, descent or support) ❑ **Adnexa**/parametria (eg, masses, tenderness, organomegaly, nodularity) ❑ **Anus** and **perineum**
Lymphatic	Palpation of **lymph nodes** in neck, axillae, groin and/or other location
Skin	❑ **Inspection** and/or **palpation** of skin and subcutaneous tissue (eg, rashes, lesions, ulcers)
Neurological/ Psychiatric	*Brief assessment of mental status including:* ❑ **Orientation** to time, place and person ❑ **Mood** and affect (eg, depression, anxiety, agitation, hypomania, lability)

Total # Bullets Performed and Documented →	☐	# of ❑ Elements Performed and Documented	Level of Examination
		1–5	Problem focused
		6–11	Expanded problem focused
		12	Detailed
		ALL	Comprehensive (Perform **all** elements identified by a bullet. Document **every** element in each box with a shaded border and at least **one** element in each box with an unshaded border)

Figure 46-6 ■ 1997 DG for Genitourinary Examination. *Source: Centers for Medicare and Medicaid Services, 1997 Documentation Guidelines for Evaluation and Management Services (with formatting adjustments).*

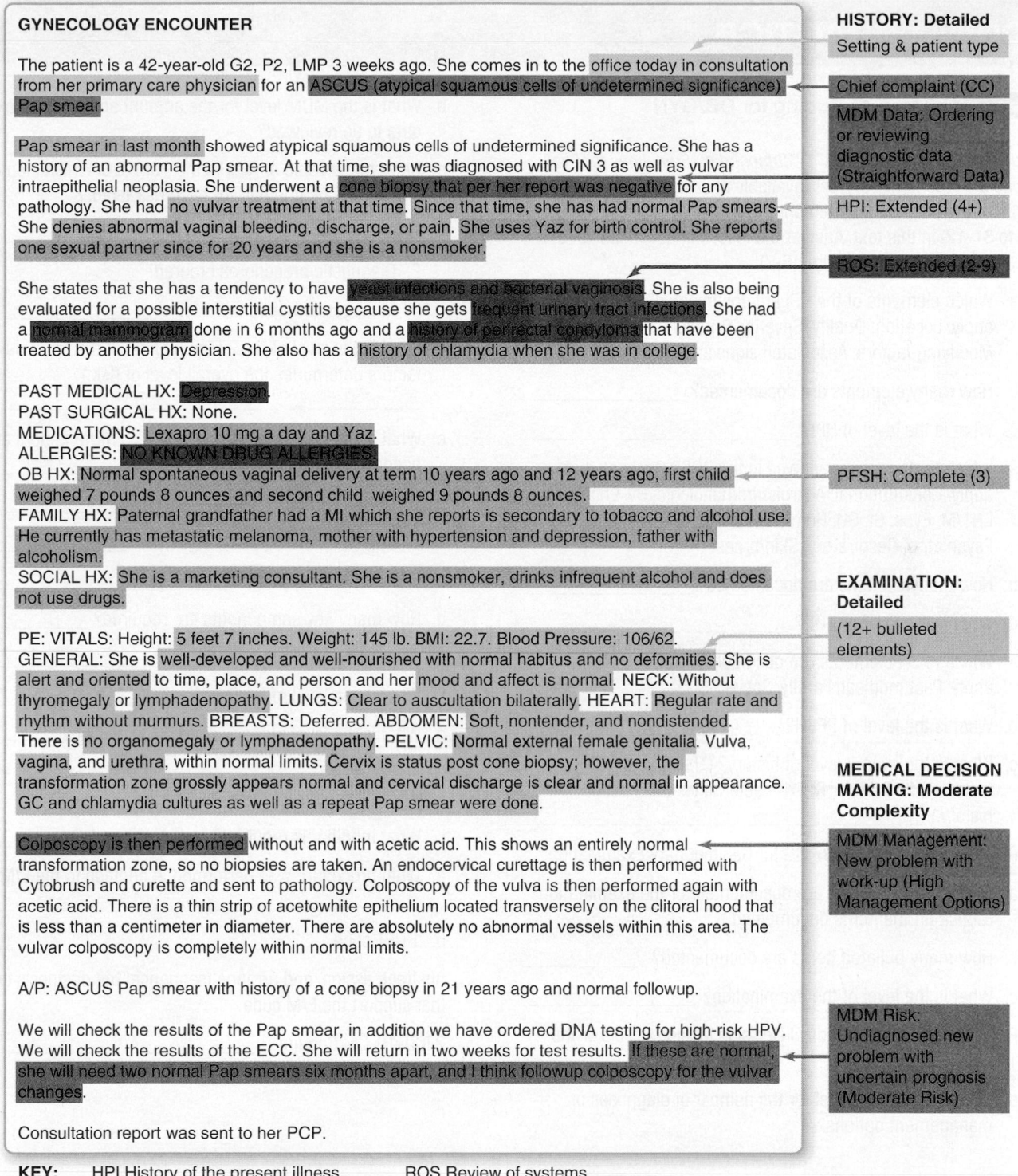

GYNECOLOGY ENCOUNTER

The patient is a 42-year-old G2, P2, LMP 3 weeks ago. She comes in to the office today in consultation from her primary care physician for an ASCUS (atypical squamous cells of undetermined significance) Pap smear.

Pap smear in last month showed atypical squamous cells of undetermined significance. She has a history of an abnormal Pap smear. At that time, she was diagnosed with CIN 3 as well as vulvar intraepithelial neoplasia. She underwent a cone biopsy that per her report was negative for any pathology. She had no vulvar treatment at that time. Since that time, she has had normal Pap smears. She denies abnormal vaginal bleeding, discharge, or pain. She uses Yaz for birth control. She reports one sexual partner since for 20 years and she is a nonsmoker.

She states that she has a tendency to have yeast infections and bacterial vaginosis. She is also being evaluated for a possible interstitial cystitis because she gets frequent urinary tract infections. She had a normal mammogram done in 6 months ago and a history of perirectal condyloma that have been treated by another physician. She also has a history of chlamydia when she was in college.

PAST MEDICAL HX: Depression.
PAST SURGICAL HX: None.
MEDICATIONS: Lexapro 10 mg a day and Yaz.
ALLERGIES: NO KNOWN DRUG ALLERGIES.
OB HX: Normal spontaneous vaginal delivery at term 10 years ago and 12 years ago, first child weighed 7 pounds 8 ounces and second child weighed 9 pounds 8 ounces.
FAMILY HX: Paternal grandfather had a MI which she reports is secondary to tobacco and alcohol use. He currently has metastatic melanoma, mother with hypertension and depression, father with alcoholism.
SOCIAL HX: She is a marketing consultant. She is a nonsmoker, drinks infrequent alcohol and does not use drugs.

PE: VITALS: Height: 5 feet 7 inches. Weight: 145 lb. BMI: 22.7. Blood Pressure: 106/62.
GENERAL: She is well-developed and well-nourished with normal habitus and no deformities. She is alert and oriented to time, place, and person and her mood and affect is normal. NECK: Without thyromegaly or lymphadenopathy. LUNGS: Clear to auscultation bilaterally. HEART: Regular rate and rhythm without murmurs. BREASTS: Deferred. ABDOMEN: Soft, nontender, and nondistended. There is no organomegaly or lymphadenopathy. PELVIC: Normal external female genitalia. Vulva, vagina, and urethra, within normal limits. Cervix is status post cone biopsy; however, the transformation zone grossly appears normal and cervical discharge is clear and normal in appearance. GC and chlamydia cultures as well as a repeat Pap smear were done.

Colposcopy is then performed without and with acetic acid. This shows an entirely normal transformation zone, so no biopsies are taken. An endocervical curettage is then performed with Cytobrush and curette and sent to pathology. Colposcopy of the vulva is then performed again with acetic acid. There is a thin strip of acetowhite epithelium located transversely on the clitoral hood that is less than a centimeter in diameter. There are absolutely no abnormal vessels within this area. The vulvar colposcopy is completely within normal limits.

A/P: ASCUS Pap smear with history of a cone biopsy in 21 years ago and normal followup.

We will check the results of the Pap smear, in addition we have ordered DNA testing for high-risk HPV. We will check the results of the ECC. She will return in two weeks for test results. If these are normal, she will need two normal Pap smears six months apart, and I think followup colposcopy for the vulvar changes.

Consultation report was sent to her PCP.

HISTORY: Detailed
Setting & patient type

Chief complaint (CC)

MDM Data: Ordering or reviewing diagnostic data (Straightforward Data)

HPI: Extended (4+)

ROS: Extended (2-9)

PFSH: Complete (3)

EXAMINATION: Detailed
(12+ bulleted elements)

MEDICAL DECISION MAKING: Moderate Complexity

MDM Management: New problem with work-up (High Management Options)

MDM Risk: Undiagnosed new problem with uncertain prognosis (Moderate Risk)

KEY: HPI History of the present illness   ROS Review of systems
PFSH Past, family, and social history   MDM Medical decision making

Figure 46-7 ■ Gynecology Encounter. *Source: © PB Resources, Inc. Used with permission.*

CODING PRACTICE

Exercise 46.5 E/M Coding for OB/GYN

Instructions: Refer to the *1997 Documentation Guidelines for Evaluation and Management Services* (available at www.cms.gov) or Chapter 31 Evaluation and Management Services (99201-99499) (Tables 31-7 to 31-12) in this text. Answer the following questions about the Genitourinary Encounter (Figure 46-7).

1. a. Which elements of the HPI are documented? Circle all that apply. Location, Quality, Severity, Duration, Timing, Context, Modifying factors, Associated signs and symptoms

   b. How many elements are documented? _____

   c. What is the level of HPI? _____

2. a. Which systems are reviewed in the ROS? Circle all that apply. Constitutional, Allergic/ immunologic, CV, Endocrine, ENT/M, Eyes, GI, GU, Hemic/lymphatic, MS, Neurologic, Psychiatric, Respiratory, Skin/breast

   b. How many systems are documented? _____

   c. What is the level of ROS? _____

3. a. Which PFSH elements are documented? Circle all that apply. Past medical, Family, Social

   b. What is the level of PFSH? _____

   c. What is the overall level of history? (The lowest history factor—HPI, ROS, or PFSH—determines the level of history.) _____

4. Refer to Figure 46-6 1997 DG for Genitourinary Examination.

   a. Which bulleted items are documented for the examination? (Check off the items documented.)

   b. How many bulleted items are documented? _____

   c. What is the level of the examination? _____

5. Refer to Table 31-12 Medical Decision Making Levels or the 1997 DG.

   a. What is the MDM level for the number of diagnoses or management options?

   b. What is the MDM level for the amount and/or complexity of data to be reviewed?

   c. Refer to the Table of Risk in the 1997 DG. Which elements of risk are documented for each risk factor?

      1. Presenting problem: _____

      2. Diagnostic procedures ordered: _____

      3. Management options selected: _____

   d. What is the level of risk? (The highest of the three risk factors determines the overall level of risk.)

      _____

   e. What is the overall level of MDM? (2/3 MDM factors are needed to determine the overall level.) _____

6. a. What is the setting? _____

   b. What is the patient (or service) type? _____

   c. What is the code range? _____

   d. How many key components are required? _____

   e. What is the level of history? _____

   f. What is the level of examination? _____

   g. What is the level of medical decision making?

      _____

   h. What is the correct code? _____

   i. What modifier is required? _____

7. a. What procedure was performed in addition to the E/M?

      _____

   b. 1 CPT code _____

8. Abstract, assign, and arrange (sequence) the diagnosis code(s) that support the E/M code.

   2 ICD-10-CM Code(s) _____

CHAPTER SUMMARY

In this chapter you learned that:

- Most procedures on the Female Genital System are performed on women without regard to their pregnant state, although some procedures, such as cerclage or dilation and curettage, can be performed for obstetrical or nonobstetrical purposes, with different codes assigned based on the purpose.

- Maternity Care and Delivery procedures are performed on pregnant women; procedures on the unborn fetus are coded as procedures performed on the mother.

- The CPT subsection **Female Genital System (56405-58999)** contains seven subheadings that are divided by anatomic site. The CPT subsection **Maternity Care and Delivery (59000-59899)** contains nine subheadings that are divided by anatomic site.

- Coders must abstract anatomic approaches and the extent of the procedure for OB/GYN procedures.

- Coders should be familiar with how to assign codes for hysterectomy procedures and the global obstetric package.

- Use standard CPT modifiers when needed to further describe the circumstances of a procedure or service, but be aware that the literal description of a modifier may be interpreted slightly differently than usual with reference to obstetrics.

- The *1997 Documentation Guidelines for Evaluation and Management Services* (1997 DG), published by CMS, provides requirements for each level of a genitourinary E/M examination, with separate criteria for males and females; a separate obstetric examination does not exist.

- The **Maternity Care and Delivery** subsection provides detailed special instructions regarding the bundling of antepartum, delivery, and postpartum procedures.

CONCEPT QUIZ

Take a moment to look back at OB/GYN and solidify your skills. Try to answer the questions from memory first, then refer to the discussion in this chapter if you need a little extra help.

Completion

Instructions: Write the term that answers each question based on the information you learned in this chapter. Choose from the list below. Some choices may be used more than once and some choices may not be used at all.

amniocentesis	hysteroscopy
cerclage	hysterotomy
colpocentesis	in vitro fertilization
colpocleisis	mesh
colpotomy	myomectomy
conization	sperm washing
cordocentesis	stress test
episiotomy	version

1. The removal of uterine fibroid tumors without removing healthy uterine tissue is called a(n) _____.

2. A uterine polyp can be removed vaginally via _____.

3. _____ is a type of assisted reproductive technology.

4. If surrounding tissues are too weak to be repaired, _____ may be inserted to strengthen the area.

5. A(n) _____ may be done early in the pregnancy to diagnose fetal disorders.

6. Removal of fetal blood from the umbilical cord is called a(n) _____.

7. To prevent injury to the perineum during delivery, a(n) _____ may be done.

8. Precancerous cervical tissue can be removed by _____.

9. It may be necessary to perform a cephalic _____ if the fetus is in an abnormal position.

10. An obstetrical _____ involves closing the cervix with sutures during the pregnancy.

Multiple Choice

Instructions: Circle the letter of the best answer to each question based on the information you learned in this chapter.

1. What procedure is performed to diagnose a blockage or abnormality of the fallopian tubes?
   A. Hysterosalpingography
   B. Salpingostomy
   C. Sonohysterography
   D. Fimbrioplasty

2. How is the oxygen level of the fetus monitored during labor and delivery?
   A. Vesicocentesis
   B. Cordocentesis
   C. Chorionic villus sampling
   D. Fetal scalp blood sampling

3. What procedure can be done to treat a prolapsed uterus or rectum?
   A. Pereyra procedure
   B. Pessary insertion
   C. Perineoplasty
   D. Hysteroscopy

4. What is one of the criteria used in assigning a code for a vaginal hysterectomy?
   A. Age of the patient
   B. Imaging guidance
   C. Uterine weight
   D. Type of anesthesia

5. Which service is not included in the global obstetric package?
   A. Delivery
   B. Forceps
   C. Episiotomy
   D. Amniocentesis

6. What instrument is used for direct visualization of the peritoneal cavity, ovaries, and the outer surfaces of the fallopian tubes and uterus?
   A. Laparoscope
   B. Hysteroscope
   C. Colposalpingoscope
   D. Peritoneoscope

(continued)

(continued from page 925)

7. What type of device is used to treat a uterine prolapse?
   A. Hysteroscope
   B. Pessary
   C. Cerclage
   D. Catheter

8. Which anatomic approach means "through the cervix uteri"?
   A. Supracervical
   B. Transperineal
   C. Transuteri
   D. Transcervical

9. When is an antepartum visit billed using an E/M code?
   A. When it is part of the global obstetric package
   B. When a physician provides one to three antepartum visits
   C. When a physician provides seven or fewer antepartum visits
   D. Never

10. Which modifier would be used to report the cesarean delivery of twins?
    A. -51
    B. -59
    C. -22
    D. -52

CODING CHALLENGE

Instructions: Read the mini-medical-record of each patient's encounter, then abstract, assign, and arrange ICD-10-CM diagnosis codes and CPT procedure codes using the appropriate Index and Tabular List. Assign quantities and modifiers where needed. Write the code(s) on the line provided.

Female Genital System

1. OUTPATIENT SURGERY Gender: F Age: 27

Preprocedure diagnosis: cervical dysplasia

Procedure: loop electrical excision procedure (LEEP). Laser speculum inserted into vagina and colposcopic exam of the vagina and cervix performed. A loop electrical excision was done to remove all of the abnormal tissue on the posterior lip of the cervix consistent with moderate dysplasia. Procedure completed without incident.

1 ICD-10-CM Code _____

2 CPT Codes _____

2. INPATIENT HOSPITAL Gender: F Age: 62

Preprocedure diagnosis: vault prolapse; previous hysterectomy

Procedure: abdominosacrocolpopexy, lysis of adhesions. Significant adhesions encountered from previous surgeries and they were released. Mesh was attached to the vagina and lower part of the spine to pull the vagina into a normal position. Patient taken to PACU in stable condition.

Tip: A status code for the hysterectomy should not be used because the diagnosis code contains this information.

2 ICD-10-CM Codes _____

2 CPT Codes _____

3. INPATIENT HOSPITAL Gender: F Age: 56

Preprocedure diagnosis: left anterior uterine wall fibroid, uterine descensus with cystocele and rectocele

Procedure: hysteroscopy with D&C and endometrial ablation. The uterus and the cervix were sounded and measured 10 cm. Hysteroscopy completed with normal findings. Endocervical and endometrial curettage was carried out with copious curettings obtained. A NovaSure endometrial ablation procedure was then performed without difficulty. The follow-up hysteroscopy showed satisfactory ablation of the endometrium. Patient left the operating room in good condition.

Tip: Read the procedure description carefully to see what it includes.

2 ICD-10-CM Codes _____

1 CPT Code _____

4. OUTPATIENT SURGERY Gender: F Age: 34

Preprocedure diagnosis: infertility caused by adhesions

Procedure: bilateral fimbrioplasty. An incision was made above the pubic hairline and fimbrial adhesions on both sides were lysed. Procedure tolerated well and patient sent to recovery.

2 ICD-10-CM Codes _____

1 CPT Code _____

5. OFFICE   Gender: F   Age: 32

Preprocedure diagnosis: insertion of IUD for contraception

Procedure: IUD placement

Postprocedure diagnosis: vaginal speculum placed, cervix prepped. Uterus was sounded to 6 cm and a Mirena IUD inserted. Threads were trimmed to 4 cm. Patient tolerated the procedure well.

1 ICD-10-CM Code _____

1 CPT Code _____

---

6. OUTPATIENT SURGERY   Gender: F   Age: 24

Gravida: 1   Para: 0   EGA: 19

Preprocedure diagnosis: fetus at 19 weeks with posterior urethral valves resulting in bilateral urinary obstruction; progressive oligohydramnios.

Procedure: vesicoamniotic shunt under spinal anesthesia using ultrasound for guidance. Fetus paralyzed using vecuronium. A vesicoamniotic shunt was placed low into the pelvis of the fetus. This was done in a single attempt, with good placement. Patient taken to recovery in stable condition.

Tip: Report a HCPCS Level II code for in utero surgical repair of the urinary tract obstruction in the fetus.

3 ICD-10-CM Codes _____

_____

1 CPT Code _____

1 HCPCS Code _____

---

7. INPATIENT HOSPITAL   Gender: F   Age: 33

Gravida: 3   Para: 2   EGA: 39 + 1

Preprocedure diagnosis: intrauterine pregnancy at 39-1/7 weeks with breech/breech, dichorionic-diamniotic twin gestation. Patient desires primary low transverse cesarean delivery and bilateral tubal ligation for permanent sterilization.

Procedure: low cervical cesarean delivery; bilateral tubal ligation. A low transverse incision was made in lower uterine segment. Baby A delivered without difficulty, as was Baby B. Cords clamped, infants suctioned and handed off to the pediatricians. Placenta delivered spontaneously. Uterus sutured. Attention turned to the tubal ligation. A 2-cm portion of each fallopian tube was removed and remaining ends

(*continued*)

Maternity Care and Delivery

7. (continued)

cauterized. Uterus returned to the abdomen, fascia closed, skin closed, and patient and infants sent to recovery in stable condition.

Delivery: cesarean delivery, Baby Boy A, complete breech, 4 lb. 7 oz; Baby Boy B, complete breech, 5 lb. 2 oz.

Tip: Remember to code outcome of delivery and weeks of gestation.

6 ICD-10-CM Codes _____

_____

2 CPT Codes _____

---

8. OFFICE   Gender: F   Age: 23

Preprocedure diagnosis: suspected left ectopic pregnancy

Procedure: D&C, left salpingectomy. The cervix was dilated and uterus curetted. Tissue sent for immediate pathology, with no villi found. A laparotomy incision was made on the left. The ectopic pregnancy was excised from the proximal end of the tube and patency of the tube restored. After hemostasis was obtained, the fascia and skin were closed. Patient taken to the recovery room.

Postprocedure diagnosis: ruptured left ectopic pregnancy

1 ICD-10-CM Code _____

2 CPT Codes _____

---

9. INPATIENT HOSPITAL   Gender: F   Age: 27

Gravida: 4   Para: 2   EGA: 38 + 6

Preprocedure diagnosis: postpartum hemorrhage

Procedure: exam under anesthesia; removal of intrauterine clots 36 hours after an NSVD. I was able to remove the clots with my hand. Inspection of the uterus by hand revealed no retained placenta. Curettage was somewhat difficult due to contractions. Her hemoglobin was 9.1 and hematocrit 25.9 upon completion of the procedure.

Tip: Code only for this procedure. Because this procedure is occurring in the postoperative period, a modifier is needed.

1 ICD-10-CM Code _____

1 CPT Code _____

(*continued*)

(continued from page 927)

10. INPATIENT HOSPITAL   Gender: F   Age: 29

Gravida: 1   Para: 0   EGA: 38 + 4

Preprocedure diagnosis: *uterine fetal demise*

Procedure: *normal spontaneous vaginal delivery of an intrauterine fetal demise. After induction of labor, patient was fully dilated and contracting. The female*

(continued)

10. (continued)

infant was delivered over a midline episiotomy. Apgars 0 and 0, weight 5 lb. 14 oz. Episiotomy repaired. Mother and father with infant.

Tip: Use a HCPCS Level III code to report the induction of labor.

3 ICD-10-CM Codes _____

_____

1 CPT Code _____

1 HCPCS Code _____

KEEP ON CODING

Instructions: Read the procedural statement, then use the appropriate Index and Tabular List to assign CPT procedure codes, quantities, and modifiers. Write the code(s) on the line provided.

Female Genital System

1. Laparoscopic fulguration of fallopian tubes: CPT Code(s) _____

2. D&C performed for a patient with dysfunctional bleeding: CPT Code(s) _____

3. Vaginal hysterectomy with salpingo-oophorectomy (uterus weight 250 g): CPT Code(s) _____

4. Biopsy of two lesions, one from labia minora and another from the vaginal orifice: CPT Code(s) _____

5. Incision and drainage of vaginal hematoma, post-trauma: CPT Code(s) _____

6. Endometrial cryoablation with ultrasonic guidance: CPT Code(s) _____

7. Vulvectomy, partial removal of skin and superficial subcutaneous tissues: CPT Code(s) _____

8. Retrieval of oocytes with ultrasound guidance: CPT Code(s) _____

9. Bilateral salpingo-oophorectomy, omentectomy for ovarian malignancy: CPT Code(s) _____

10. Radical abdominal hysterectomy with bladder aspiration and placement of suprapubic catheter: CPT Code(s) _____

11. Cold-knife conization of cervix: CPT Code(s) _____

12. Marsupialization of Bartholin gland cyst: CPT Code(s) _____

13. Laparoscopic abdominal hysterectomy, 230-g uterus: CPT Code(s) _____

14. Uterine suspension: CPT Code(s) _____

15. Intrauterine in vitro fertilization: CPT Code(s) _____

Maternity Care and Delivery

16. Induced abortion with abortifacient: CPT Code(s) _____

17. Antepartum care only, 5 visits: CPT Code(s) _____

18. Vacuum-assisted vaginal delivery: CPT Code(s) _____

19. Fetal contraction stress test: CPT Code(s) _____

20. D&C for postpartum hemorrhage: CPT Code(s) _____

21. Cesarean delivery, delivery only, with total hysterectomy: CPT Code(s) _____

22. Repeat fetal scalp blood sampling by the same PA: CPT Code(s) _____

23. Repeat cesarean delivery after unsuccessful attempt at vaginal delivery: CPT Code(s) _____

24. Successful vaginal birth after cesarean delivery: CPT Code(s) _____

25. Ultrasound-guided amniocentesis: CPT Code(s) _____

Radiology Services (70010-79999)

Chapter 47

Learning Objectives

After completing this chapter, you should have the skills to:

47.1 Spell and define the key words, medical terms, and abbreviations related to radiology procedures.

47.2 Discuss the types of radiology procedures.

47.3 Identify the main characteristics of coding for Radiology.

47.4 Abstract procedural information from the medical record for coding Radiology.

47.5 Assign codes for Radiology procedures.

47.6 Arrange codes for Radiology procedures.

47.7 Discuss the CPT coding guidelines related to Radiology.

Chapter Outline

- **Radiology Procedure Basics**
- **Coding Overview of Radiology Procedures**
- **Abstracting Radiology Procedures**
- **Assigning Codes for Radiology Procedures**
- **Arranging Codes for Radiology Procedures**

Key Terms and Abbreviations

contrast medium	interstitial	intrathecal	radiolucent
endocavity	interventional radiologist	modality	radiopaque
gestational sac	intra-articular	radiation oncologist	radiopharmaceutical
imaging guidance	intracavity	radiology technician	

In addition to the key terms listed here, students should know the terms defined within tables in this chapter.

INTRODUCTION

Digital imaging technology has transformed consumer photography from a complicated hobby that required film, processing, and printing to one that can conveniently capture and store images on a computer chip, where they can be accessed for manipulation, printing, and sharing. In the same way, radiology began as a film-based technology that today uses many forms of digital imaging to record the human body. In addition, radiology techniques are used to diagnose and treat a wide variety of conditions.

RADIOLOGY PROCEDURE BASICS

Radiology is a medical specialty that uses radiation, sound waves, magnetic fields, or radio fields to visualize internal body structures, such as arteries and bones. Radiological procedures can be noninvasive, such as an X-ray or MRI, or minimally invasive, such as fluoroscopy or angiography. Procedures can be performed to assist in diagnosing a condition, for **imaging guidance** (*real-time visualization of body structures during a medical or surgical procedure*), or for therapeutic (*treatment*) purposes.

A radiologist is a physician with specialized training in obtaining and interpreting radiological images to determine a patient's diagnosis and recommend additional testing or treatment. Radiologists can specialize in different areas of medicine, including diagnosing disorders of the cardiovascular system, gastrointestinal system, and breast. A **radiation oncologist** provides cancer treatment through radiation. An **interventional radiologist** performs minimally invasive, image-guided surgeries.

A **radiology technician** is a nonphysician staff member who is trained to operate and adjust imaging equipment, explain procedures to patients and answer questions, position patients for imaging, and ensure that the patient's exposure to radiation is limited. A radiology technician may also operate portable X-ray equipment to obtain images in the emergency room, operating room, or even at the patient's bedside. A registered radiologist assistant (RRA) and a radiology practitioner assistant (RPA) are both radiological technologists with advanced education who perform more complex radiological procedures.

Radi/o is the combining form for X-ray. Radiology is the study of X-rays. Radiography is the process of recording X-rays. A radiograph is the image that results. X-rays or other radiographic images of specific body sites are often described by combining the word root for the anatomic site with the suffix *-graphy*, such as mammography, which means making a recording of the breast. X-ray images may be recorded on traditional film and developed then viewed on a light box, or the images may be captured digitally and viewed on a computer screen.

Refer to ■ TABLE 47-1 for a refresher on how to build medical terms related to Radiology.

Table 47-1 ■ **EXAMPLE OF CONSTRUCTING MEDICAL TERMS FOR RADIOLOGY PROCEDURES**

Combining Form	Suffix	Complete Medical Term
arthr/o (*joint*) bronch/o (*bronchus tube*) sial/o (*salivary duct, gland*) tom/o (*cut or slice*) ur/o (*urinary tract*)	**-graphy** (*process of recording*) **-gram** (*a record or picture*)	**arthro + graphy** (*process of recording a joint*)
		broncho + graphy (*process of recording the bronchus*)
		sialo + graphy (*process of recording the salivary duct*)
		tomo + graphy (*process of recording a slice*)
		uro + graphy (*process of recording the urinary tract*)
		arthro + gram (*a record or picture of a joint*)
		broncho + gram (*a record or picture of the bronchus*)
		sialo + gram (*a record or picture of the salivary duct*)

Source: © PB Resources, Inc. Used with permission.

CODING CAUTION

The suffixes *-graph* and *-gram* can refer to other types of recordings besides X-rays and other radiological images. For example, an electrocardiogram is an electrical recording of the heart and a polysomnogram is a recording of multiple sleep parameters

Be alert for medical word roots that are spelled similarly and have different meanings.

dosimetry (*measurement of a dose*) and **densitometry** (*measurement of density*)

anteroposterior (*from front to back*) and **posteroanterior** (*from back to front*)

density (*mass or substance*) and **dentistry** (*the practice of a dentist*)

Commonly performed radiology procedures are discussed next. Refer to detailed anatomic diagrams of specific parts of the digestive system when you need to refresh your memory of the relationship of organs and sites to each other.

Radiology Procedures

The field of radiology comprises **modalities** (*methods of applying a therapeutic/physical treatment*) that use distinct technology and equipment to obtain images. Radiological modalities include plain radiography, also called X-ray (■ FIGURE 47-1), ultrasound (US), computed tomography (CT) (■ FIGURE 47-2), nuclear medicine (NM), positron emission tomography (PET), and magnetic resonance imaging (MRI) (■ FIGURE 47-3). The physician who orders the procedure determines the modality to be used based on the information needed and the structure(s)

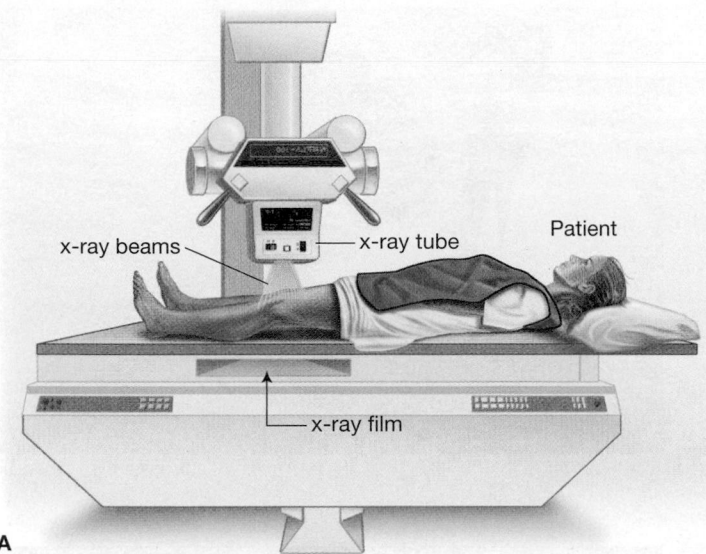

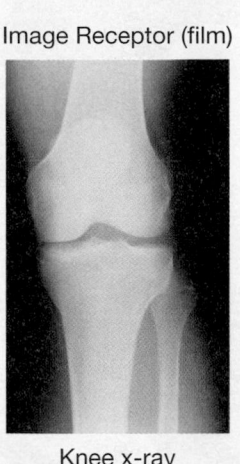

Image Receptor (film)

B   Knee x-ray

A

Figure 47-1 ■ X-ray of Knee: (A) Procedure (B) Image

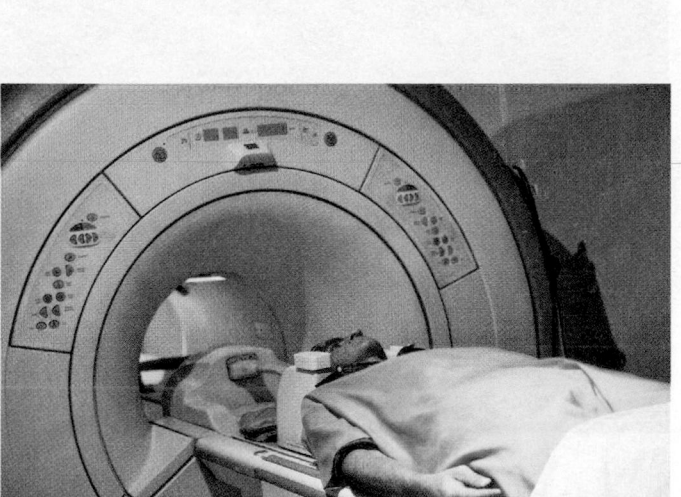

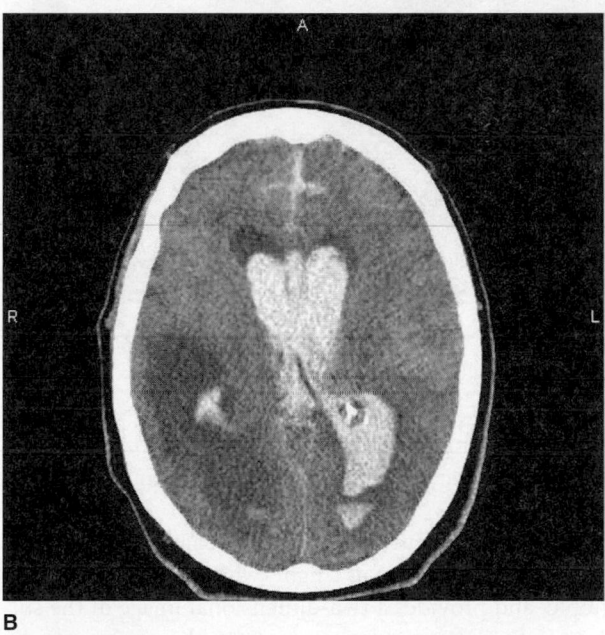

A

B

Figure 47-2 ■ CT Scan of Head: (A) Procedure (B) Image

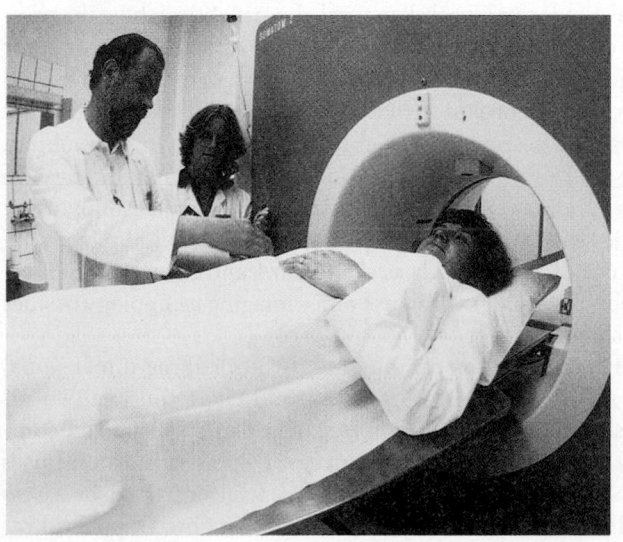

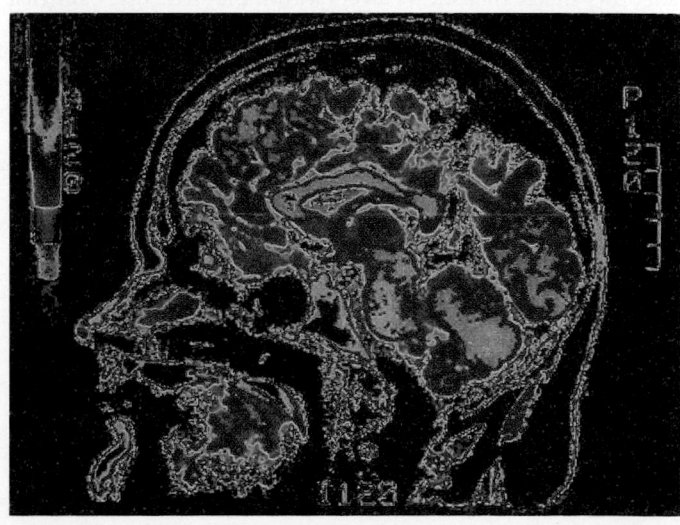

A

B

Figure 47-3 ■ MRI of Head: (A) Procedure (B) Image

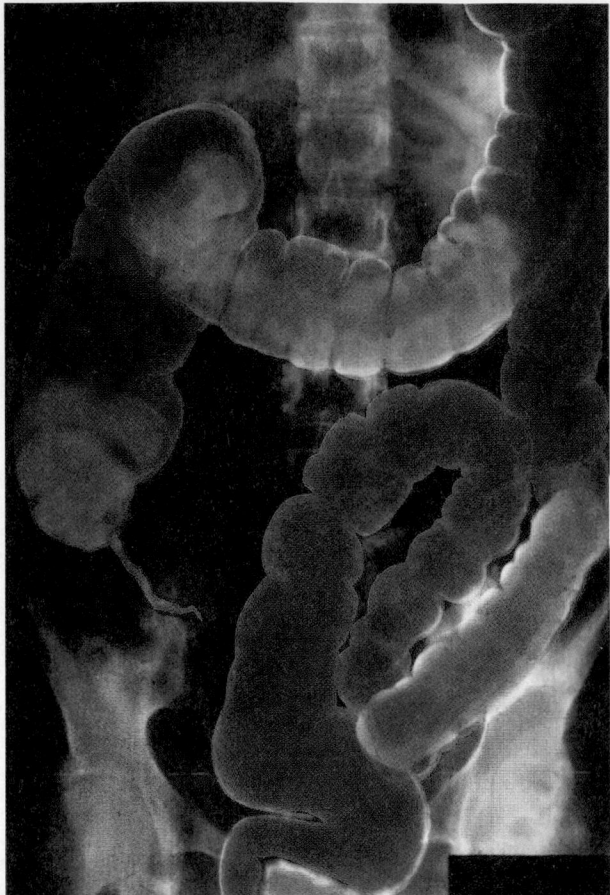

Figure 47-4 ■ X-ray of the Colon Using Contrast Media (Barium Enema)

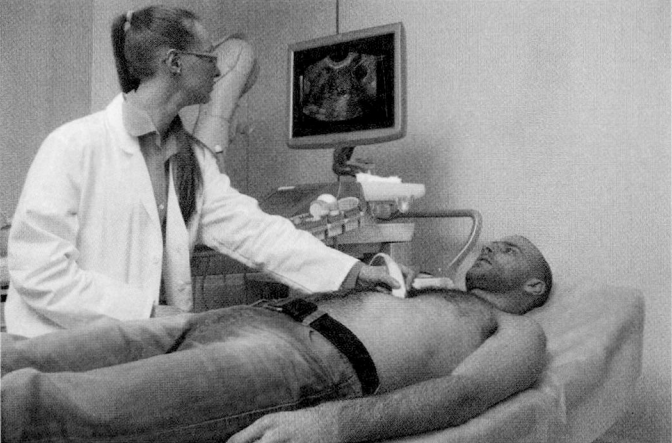

A

B

Figure 47-5 ■ Ultrasound of Abdomen: (A) Procedure (B) Image

to be examined. Some modalities provide clearer images of certain body structures; some are less invasive than others; and some are less costly.

A **radiopaque** structure, such as a bone, allows few X-rays to pass through; it shows up as a light (white) image using plain radiography and provides a two-dimensional image of the surface. A **radiolucent** structure, such as the skin or lungs, permits X-rays to pass into and through it, resulting in a darker, shadowy image that shows layers within the structure. **Contrast medium** (*a radiopaque substance injected or swallowed*) can be used to help visualize other soft tissues that cannot otherwise be seen clearly in an X-ray by making them stand out from surrounding tissues (■ FIGURE 47-4).

Commonly performed Radiology procedures are summarized in ■ TABLE 47-2. Ultrasound and nuclear medicine are discussed in detail next.

Ultrasound

Ultrasound literally means *beyond sound*. Procedures use sound waves whose frequency is beyond human hearing to evaluate a patient's internal organs and structures. Ultrasound can be diagnostic or therapeutic. It is a noninvasive imaging technology that captures an image of echoes from sound bouncing off structures such as the abdomen, pelvis, heart, vessels, muscles, joints, and tendons. Ultrasound images are viewed in real time, showing movements within the body, such

as blood flowing through vessels or a fetus moving in the womb. Ultrasounds can reveal structural abnormalities, show the presence of a lesion and whether it is solid or fluid-filled, monitor the growth of a fetus, and identify disorders of the arteries and veins, such as occlusions (■ FIGURE 47-5). Physicians also use ultrasound to image procedures, such as when they obtain biopsies, or for interventional radiology, a minimally invasive procedure that can be performed anywhere in the body using needles and catheters advanced into arteries, including treating vascular disorders such as embolisms and aneurysms. Interventional radiologists can use other imaging technology besides ultrasound.

Ultrasound scans can be one-, two-, or three-dimensional (3-D) (■ TABLE 47-3). 3-D ultrasound takes multiple two-dimensional scans and combines them using specialized computer software to form 3-D images. Doppler ultrasound uses high-frequency sound to monitor a fetal heartbeat or assess the direction and velocity (*speed*) of blood flow. Doppler ultrasound can be black and white or color.

Table 47-2 ■ **COMMON RADIOLOGY PROCEDURES**

Procedure Name	Definition	Reason Performed
Cineradiography/ videoradiography	The process of making radiographs of moving objects in rapid sequence and quickly projecting them back to simulate a motion picture	Diagnose or evaluate heart or joint conditions
Clinical brachytherapy	Application of small, encapsulated radioactive elements implanted directly into or near a tumor	Malignant tumors
Computed tomography (CT)	Creation of a three-dimensional image of a body structure by computer, using a series of cross-sectional images	Infection, masses and tumors, including cancer, study blood vessels
Computer-aided detection (CAD)	Use of pattern recognition software to help identify suspicious features on a radiological image, to decrease false-negative readings	Mammography, chest CT, chest X-rays
Dual-energy X-ray absorptiometry (DXA/DEXA), bone density study	Measurement of the density or mass of a material is measured by comparing the amounts of material absorbed from X-ray beams of two different energies	Bone density study, osteoporosis screening
Fluoroscopy	Projection of a live X-ray image onto a fluorescent screen	Image-guided procedures, such as venous or arterial catheter placement
Hyperthermia, thermal therapy, thermotherapy	Exposing tissue to high temperatures (up to 113°F)	Damage or kill cancer cells in a localized area
Magnetic resonance angiography (MRA)	Use of a magnetic field and pulses of radio wave energy to visualize the heart, blood vessels, or blood flow in the circulatory system	Arterial aneurysm, aortic coarctation or dissection, carotid artery disease, atherosclerosis of the arms or legs
Magnetic resonance imaging (MRI)	Use of strong magnets and radio waves to produce computerized images of internal body tissues	Tumors, bleeding, infection, arthritis, soft-tissue damage, and many other conditions
Mammary ductogram, galactogram	Use of mammography and contrast material to view the inside of the breast's milk ducts	Lesions causing nipple discharge
Mammography—diagnostic	X-ray image of the male or female breast to determine whether a problem exists or to determine the nature of a problem	Signs or symptoms of breast disease, dense tissue, a personal history of breast cancer or benign breast disease, inconclusive screening mammogram results
Mammography—screening	X-ray image of the breast of a woman without signs or symptoms of breast disease	Early detection of breast cancer or other abnormalities
Proton beam treatment (PBT) delivery	Use of noninvasive electromagnetic radiation to treat both in situ benign and malignant tumors	Inoperable or radiation-resistant tumors
Positron emission tomography (PET)	Use of a positron-emitting radionuclide tracer to show how organs and tissues are working in real time	Check brain function, examine blood flow to the heart, diagnose cancer or metastases
Radiologic guidance/guided imaging	Use of a radiological modality to visualize access to an anatomic site in real time	Direct or guide the placement and/or removal of surgical objects
Radiosurgery	A form of radiation therapy that focuses high-power energy on a small area of the body (e.g., Cyberknife, Gamma Knife)	Treatment of tumors that lie too close to sensitive structures for traditional surgery; treatment of tumors in patients who are too high risk for traditional surgery
Single photon emission computed tomography (SPECT)	Use of photons emitted by a radioactive tracer to create an image of lower quality than PET	Mapping brain function
Stereotactic imaging	Three-dimensional imaging to pinpoint a specific location	Biopsy of breast lesion
Ultrasound	Use of sound waves to capture an image of echoes bouncing off structures showing real-time movements within the body	*Diagnostic:* structural abnormalities, show the presence of a lesion and if it is solid or fluid-filled, monitor the growth of a fetus, and identify disorders of the arteries and veins, such as occlusions

Therapeutic: biopsies, interventional radiology, catheter placement |

Source: © PB Resources, Inc. Used with permission.

Table 47-3 ■ TYPES OF ULTRASOUND

Type of Ultrasound	Definition
A-mode (amplitude)	A one-dimensional ultrasonic measurement
M-mode (motion)	A one-dimensional ultrasonic measurement used to display movement of a structure
B-scan/gray-scale (brightness)	A two-dimensional ultrasonic scan that displays movement of tissues and organs
Real-time scan	A rapid succession of B-mode images producing a moving video; a two-dimensional ultrasonic scan, with displays of both two-dimensional structures and motion with time
3-D ultrasound	Taking and combining multiple two-dimensional scans using specialized computer software to form 3-D images
Doppler	Use of high-frequency sound to monitor a fetal heartbeat or assess the direction and velocity of blood flow

Source: © PB Resources, Inc. Used with permission.

Nuclear Medicine

NM procedures use an extremely small amount of radioactive materials—called **radiopharmaceuticals**, radiotracers, or tracers—to image the body, diagnose, and treat diseases. Radioactive elements are administered to the patient through injection, swallowing, or inhalation. They are attracted to specific organs, bones, or tissues, which allows clinicians to image both structure and function of the anatomy. Not only can the radiologist see what an organ looks like, she can also see how it functions. NM procedures are most often performed to image the thyroid, bone, heart, liver, brain, and lungs and help detect and treat a variety of diseases such as cancer, aneurysms, irregular or inadequate blood flow, and organ disorders (■ FIGURE 47-6).

Therapeutic NM can deliver palliative (*pain-relieving*) or therapeutic doses of radiation to specific tissues or body areas. Procedures help detect or locate tumor cells, kill the cancerous tissue, reduce the size of a tumor, or reduce pain. They can treat an overactive thyroid, thyroid cancer, blood disorders, chronic inflammatory rheumatism, lymphoma, or certain metastatic bone lesions.

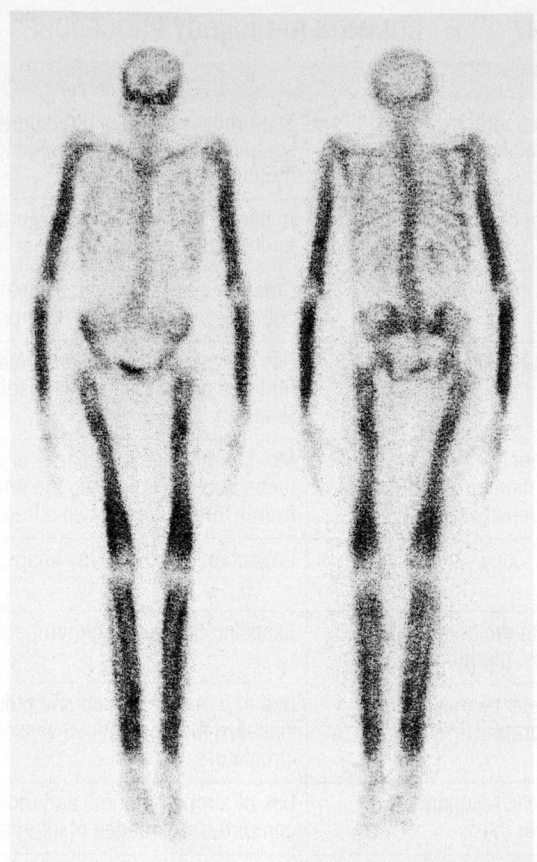

Figure 47-6 ■ Nuclear Medicine Bone Scan Image

Examples of NM radiopharmaceuticals include the following:

- Sodium iodide I-123—for thyroid imaging
- Technetium-99m sestamibi—for various nuclear medicine procedures
- Thallium-201—for myocardial perfusion scans (heart functions)
- Strontium-89—for palliative treatment of pain from metastatic bone cancer

Radiology uses many techniques, equipment, and modalities that require detailed knowledge and are constantly changing because of advances in technology. This section provides a general reference to help understand the most common Radiology procedures. Remember to keep standard reference books handy to locate additional information that may be needed for a specific situation.

CODING PRACTICE

Exercise 47.1 Radiology Procedure Basics

Instructions: Use your medical terminology skills and resources to define the following procedures related to radiology, then identify the code(s) or code range listed in the CPT Index. Follow these steps:

- Use slash marks "/" to break down the underlined term into its root(s) and suffix.
- Define the meaning of the underlined word based on the meaning of each word part.
- Use the entire phrase to identify the code or code range shown in the CPT Index.

Example: <u>laryngography</u> laryngo/graphy   Meaning <u>making a recording of the larynx</u>   CPT Code <u>70373</u>

1. <u>radiopharmaceutical</u> therapy   Meaning _____   CPT Code _____

2. X-ray, spine, <u>thoracolumbar</u>   Meaning _____   CPT Code _____

3. <u>myelography</u>, brain   Meaning _____   CPT Code _____

4. Uterus, <u>sonohysterography</u>   Meaning _____   CPT Code _____

5. <u>echoencephalography</u>, intracranial   Meaning _____   CPT Code _____

6. <u>spectroscopy</u>, magnetic resonance   Meaning _____   CPT Code _____

7. <u>hyperthermia</u> treatment   Meaning _____   CPT Code _____

8. <u>cholangiography</u>, intraoperative   Meaning _____   CPT Code _____

9. <u>pelvimetry</u>   Meaning _____   CPT Code _____

10. <u>mammography</u>   Meaning _____   CPT Code _____

CODING OVERVIEW OF RADIOLOGY PROCEDURES

The CPT section **Radiology (70010-79999)** contains seven subsections that are divided by modality (■ Table 47-4). Within the Diagnostic Radiology and Diagnostic Ultrasound subsections, categories are divided by anatomic region. In the Diagnostic Radiology categories, all modalities—radiography, CT, and MRI—appear sequentially within each anatomic category. CPT does not provide titles to separate these modalities in the Tabular List.

In other subsections, categories are divided by the type of procedure. Review the subheading and category names and code ranges listed in the Radiology section to become familiar with the content and organization. Some editions of the CPT manual provide a summary list of the subheadings and categories at the beginning of the Radiology section, and they also display an asterisk (*) next to categories that contain special coding instructions.

This CPT section includes invasive and minimally invasive radiology procedures. Radiology procedures must be supported by diagnosis codes that justify the medical necessity of the procedure. Because radiology procedures are performed on every organ system and for many different reasons, diagnosis codes from any ICD-10-CM chapter can be used. The ordering physician provides the diagnosis code(s) with the order for the procedure.

Table 47-4 ■ RADIOLOGY SUBHEADINGS

Subheading	Code Range
Diagnostic Radiology (Diagnostic Imaging)	70010–76499
Diagnostic Ultrasound	76506–76999
Radiologic Guidance	77001–77032
Breast Mammography	77051–77063
Bone/Joint Studies	77071–77086
Radiation Oncology	77261–77799
Nuclear Medicine	78012–79999

Radiology Guidelines

CPT provides guidelines for Radiology at the beginning of the section that apply to all codes in the section. In particular, coders need to understand radiological supervision and interpretation, administration of contrast, and written report.

Radiological Supervision and Interpretation (S&I)

Most Radiology codes, except those in the Radiation Oncology subsection, consist of a technical component and professional component. The technical component encompasses the costs of the facility, equipment, staff, and related expenses. Supervision and interpretation (S&I) describes the professional component of a radiological procedure that reports the physician's work. Supervision is the radiologist personally performing the procedure or overseeing radiology clinicians who perform the procedure. Interpretation is the radiologist's analysis of the image(s), or the findings, and writing of a report that documents the findings and provides a diagnosis. The report is sent to the referring physician, who considers the findings and radiological diagnosis, together with other clinical indicators and test results, to establish the patient's final diagnosis.

Many procedures in the CPT Medicine and Surgery sections have a radiology component for guided imaging. The guidelines, instructional notes, or code descriptors may state that imaging guidance is included in the CPT code and should not be reported separately. When this occurs, do not report separate Radiology section codes for imaging guidance or S&I. When the imaging guidance is not bundled with the primary procedure code, assign a Radiology code.

Administration of Contrast Materials

Contrast materials, or contrast agents, are special dyes used to improve the visibility of structures or tissues. Radiation cannot penetrate body structures containing contrast, so contrast makes certain areas stand out more in an X-ray or other image. The patient receives contrast through various methods, such as injection into a vein, artery, or the subarachnoid space of the spinal cord; through the rectum; or by swallowing. The guidelines identify when to report an additional code for the administration of contrast material, which is based on the route of administration:

- Intra-articular—Assign an additional code for the joint injection.
- Intravascular—A Radiology code that includes the phrase **with contrast** includes the injection; do not assign a separate code.
- Intrathecal—Assign **61055** or **62284** in addition to the Radiology code.
- Oral or rectal—This does not qualify as a study with contrast.

Written Report

The physician who provides the S&I must prepare and sign a written report for each procedure. The written report is a legal document outlining the reason for the procedure, the type of procedure, the physician's findings and discussion with the patient and/or family, and the definitive diagnosis. Do not assign a separate code for a written report because it is included in a radiology procedure or interpretation.

Additional Guidelines and Instructions

Special instructions at the beginning of many categories provide definitions and coding guidelines. Instructional notes appear throughout the Tabular List to alert coders to the need for modifiers, provide cross-references to codes for similar procedures on other sites, identify when additional codes for radiological services might be needed, alert you to other codes in CPT that you should not report with specific Radiology codes, and highlight resequenced and recently deleted codes. Be sure to carefully read all coding guidelines, special instructions, and instructional notes before final code assignment.

CODING CAUTION

Although you may think you are familiar with the guidelines for frequently used codes, be sure to check for updates when the new CPT manual is released each January. Guidelines may change even when codes numbers remain the same. Also check for updates from Medicare and other payers throughout the year.

ABSTRACTING RADIOLOGY PROCEDURES

Plain radiographic procedures (X-rays) are described by the number and type of radiographic views—the angle and direction from which the image is taken. The view(s) also determines how the technician must position the patient. Refer to ■ FIGURE 47-7 for examples of common views and body positions. CT scans, MRIs, and other modalities are not described the same way because cross-sectional views, real-time imaging, and functional mapping require different details in the physician orders.

The anatomic approach can refer to how a site is accessed, such as a transabdominal ultrasound, or how a substance or injection is administered, such as intracavity brachytherapy or

intrathecal injection. Commonly used anatomic approaches include the following:

- **endocavity**—within a cavity
- **interstitial**—between tissues
- **intra-articular**—within a joint
- **intracavity**—within a cavity
- **intrathecal**—into the sheath (*outer covering*) of the spinal cord
- **transabdominal**—through the abdomen
- **transvaginal**—through the vagina

Refer to ■ TABLE 47-5 for guidance on how to abstract radiology procedures and ■ TABLE 47-6 for radiation oncology procedures, then work through the detailed example that follows. Remember that the abstracting questions are a guide and that not every question applies to, or can be answered for, every case. For example, the number of views is applicable to plain radiography procedures but not to MRIs or CT scans.

Table 47-5 ■ KEY CRITERIA FOR ABSTRACTING RADIOLOGY PROCEDURES

❑ What is the patient's age?
❑ What is the anatomic site?
❑ What is the type of radiology procedure?
❑ Is the procedure diagnostic or therapeutic?
❑ How many and what views are taken?
❑ What body positions are used?
❑ What is the anatomic approach?
❑ What is the laterality?
❑ Is contrast medium used?
❑ Is the service technical, professional, or global?
❑ Is imaging guidance used to assist in another procedure?
❑ What additional procedures are performed?

Source: © PB Resources, Inc. Used with permission.

Table 47-6 ■ KEY CRITERIA FOR ABSTRACTING RADIATION ONCOLOGY PROCEDURES

❑ Is the service treatment planning or treatment delivery?
❑ Is treatment planning clinical or simulation?
❑ What is the treatment delivery modality (radiation, proton beam, brachytherapy)?
❑ What anatomic site(s) is treated?
❑ How many distinct areas are treated?
❑ How many and what type of ports are used?
❑ How many and what type of blocks are used?
❑ What is the total radiation dose delivered?
❑ How many treatments are given in the period being reported?
❑ Is the service technical, professional, or global?

Source: © PB Resources, Inc. Used with permission.

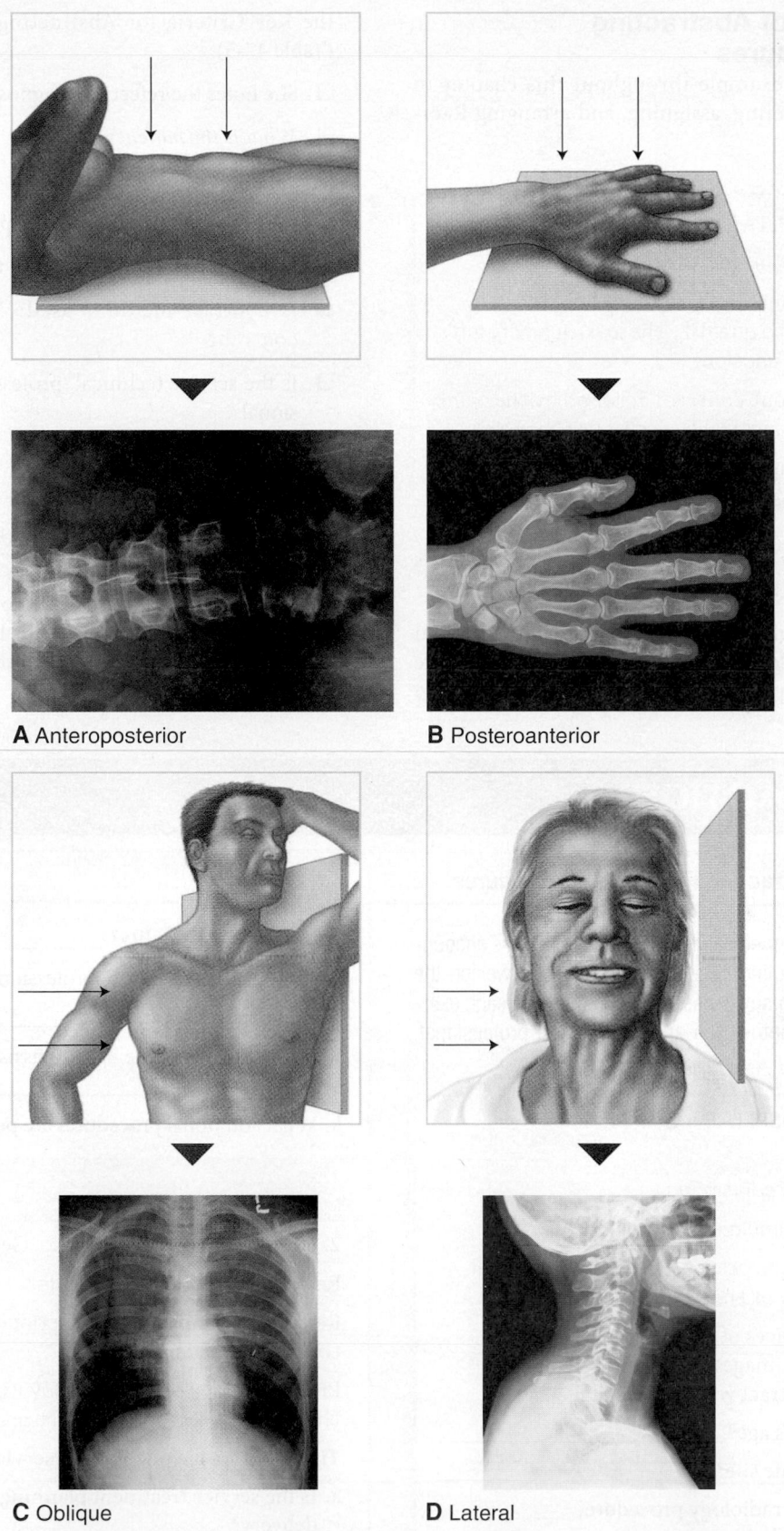

A Anteroposterior

B Posteroanterior

C Oblique

D Lateral

Figure 47-7 ■ Examples of Common X-ray Views (Positions) and Resulting Images

Guided Example of Abstracting Radiology Procedures

Refer to the following example throughout this chapter to practice skills for abstracting, assigning, and arranging Radiology codes.

> OUTPATIENT HOSPITAL   Gender: F   Age: 52
>
> Referring physician: Cardiologist
>
> Referring diagnosis: mitral valve prolapse, evaluate mitral regurgitation to quantify the leak, quantify left ventricular size and function
>
> Procedure: MRI without contrast followed by the same views with contrast, including velocity flow mapping
>
> Note: Code for the supervising radiologist.

Follow along as fictitious coder, Marcy Elwood, CCS, abstracts the procedure. Check off each step after you complete it.

▶ Marcy reads through the entire record, paying special attention to the reason for the encounter, the procedure performed, and the postoperative diagnosis. She refers to the Key Criteria for Abstracting Radiology Procedures (Table 47-5).

- ❑ She notes the referring diagnosis: mitral value prolapse
- ❑ *What is the patient's age?* 52
- ❑ What is the anatomic site? heart/mitral valve
- ❑ What is the type of radiology procedure? MRI
- ❑ Is the procedure diagnostic or therapeutic? diagnostic
- ❑ Is contrast medium used? Yes, without and with contrast
- ❑ Is the service technical, professional, or global? professional
- ❑ Is imaging guidance used to assist in another procedure? No
- ❑ What additional procedures are performed? velocity flow mapping

▶ At this time, Marcy does not know which of these procedures may need to be coded, nor how many codes she will end up with. She will learn about this when she moves on to assigning codes.

CODING PRACTICE

Exercise 47.2   Abstracting Radiology Procedures

Instructions: Read the mini-medical-record of each patient's encounter and answer the abstracting questions. Write the answer on the line provided. Do not assign any codes. Read the tips with each exercise to help determine whether you are coding for a professional, technical, or global service.

1. OUTPATIENT HOSPITAL   Gender: F
Age: 16 months

Referring physician: Pediatrician

Referring diagnosis: limping while walking

Procedure: X-ray of the pelvis (AP), AP and bilateral frog-leg (lateral) view of the hips

Tip: Code for the services of the hospital's radiology department only. The images were interpreted by a radiologist under contract with the hospital.

a. What is the patient's age? _____

b. What is the anatomic site? _____

c. What is the type of radiology procedure? _____

d. How many and what views are taken? _____

e. What body positions are used? _____

f. What is the anatomic approach? _____

(continued)

1. (continued)

g. What is the laterality? _____

h. Is the service technical, professional, or global? _____

i. Is contrast medium used? _____

j. Is imaging guidance used to assist in another procedure? _____

k. What additional procedures are performed? _____

2. OUTPATIENT HOSPITAL   Gender: F   Age: 46

Referring physician: Oncologist

Referring diagnosis: status post-thyroidectomy due to thyroid cancer

Procedure: one session, 3 MeV radiation treatment to the thyroid using a single port and simple block

Tip: Code for the oncologist's services.

a. Is the service treatment planning or treatment delivery? _____

b. Is treatment planning clinical or simulation? _____

c. What is the treatment delivery modality (radiation, proton beam, brachytherapy)? _____

(continued)

2. (continued)

d. What anatomic site(s) is treated? _____

e. How many distinct areas are treated? _____

f. How many and what type of ports are used? _____

g. How many and what type of blocks are used?

_____

h. What is the total radiation dose delivered? _____

i. How many treatments are given in the period being reported?_____

j. Is the service technical, professional, or global?

_____

3. OUTPATIENT HOSPITAL   Gender: M   Age: 81

Referring physician: Pulmonologist

Referring diagnosis: SOB, mild chest pain, hemoptysis

Procedure: ventilation-perfusion scan (V/Q scan)

Postprocedure diagnosis: pulmonary artery thrombosis

Tip: Code for the technical services of the hospital's radiology department.

a. What is the patient's age? _____

b. What is the anatomic site? _____

c. What is the type of radiology procedure? _____

d. How many and what views are taken? _____

e. What body positions are used? _____

f. What is the anatomic approach? _____

g. What is the laterality? _____

h. Is the service technical, professional, or global?

_____

i. Is contrast medium used? _____

j. Is imaging guidance used to assist in another procedure? _____

k. What additional procedures are performed?

_____

4. OUTPATIENT HOSPITAL   Gender: F   Age: 64

Referring physician: Pulmonologist

Referring diagnosis: lifelong smoker, severe cough, hemoptysis

Procedure: AP and lateral chest X-ray, standing. A dense mass in the lower lobe of the left lung is noted.

Findings: Patient's pulmonologist consents to performing a CT scan of the chest without contrast.

Postprocedure diagnosis: carcinoma of the left lower lobe

(continued)

4. (continued)

Tip: Code for the supervising radiologist.

a. What is the patient's age? _____

b. What is the anatomic site? _____

c. What is the type of radiology procedure? _____

d. How many and what views are taken? _____

e. What body positions are used? _____

f. What is the anatomic approach? _____

g. What is the laterality? _____

h. Is the service technical, professional, or global?

_____

i. Is contrast medium used? _____

j. Is imaging guidance used to assist in another procedure? _____

k. What additional procedures are performed?

_____

5. OFFICE   Gender: F   Age: 29

Performing physician: Obstetrician

Preprocedure diagnosis: routine pregnancy, EGA 10 weeks

Procedure: transabdominal ultrasound for fetal and maternal evaluation, supine

Postprocedure diagnosis: twin fetuses

a. What is the patient's age? _____

b. What is the anatomic site? _____

c. What is the type of radiology procedure? _____

d. How many and what views are taken? _____

e. What body positions are used? _____

f. What is the anatomic approach? _____

g. What is the laterality? _____

h. Is the service technical, professional, or global?

_____

i. Is contrast medium used? _____

j. Is imaging guidance used to assist in another procedure? _____

k. What additional procedures are performed? _____

6. OUTPATIENT HOSPITAL   Gender: M   Age: 55

Referring physician: Nephrologist

Diagnosis: ESRD, diabetic nephropathy

Procedure: placed a central venous nontunneled catheter using fluoroscopic guidance for temporary dialysis access

(continued)

6. (continued)

Tip: Code for the service of the interventional radiologist.

a. What is the patient's age? _____

b. What is the anatomic site? _____

c. What is the type of radiology procedure? _____

d. How many and what views are taken? _____

e. What body positions are used? _____

f. What is the anatomic approach? _____

(continued)

6. (continued)

g. What is the laterality? _____

h. Is the service technical, professional, or global?

_____

i. Is contrast medium used? _____

j. Is imaging guidance used to assist in another procedure?_____

k. What additional procedures are performed? _____

ASSIGNING CODES FOR RADIOLOGY PROCEDURES

To assign codes for Radiology services, search the Index for the Main Term of the modality, such as **X-ray**, **CT Scan**, **Ultrasound**, and so on. First-level modifying terms vary based on the modality, so review each Main Term entry carefully to understand how it is organized, then follow the necessary path to identify the anatomic site. For example, under the Main Term **X-ray**, first-level modifying terms identify the anatomic site. Under the Main Term **CT Scan**, most sites appear as second-level modifying terms under the first-level modifying terms **with contrast**, **without and with contrast**, and **without contrast**. Under the Main Term **Ultrasound**, most first-level modifying terms identify the anatomic site, but there are also first-level modifying terms for **3-D Rendering** and **Guidance**.

After locating the code range for the modality and anatomic site, refer to the Tabular List to select and verify the code based on the type of examination, number of views, and other details in the code descriptions.

The following information gives examples of Radiology coding for technical, professional, and global services; ultrasound; mammography; procedures using contrast; and radiation oncology.

CODING CAUTION

When searching a Main Term entry that has multiple levels of modifying terms, be sure to identify the correct first-level modifying term before selecting the anatomic site.

Assigning Codes for Ultrasound

Ultrasound examinations of the pelvis are divided based on whether the procedure is obstetrical or nonobstetrical. Codes for obstetrical ultrasounds include the phrase **pregnant uterus**. Codes are further divided based on the age of fetus as younger than 14 weeks or 14 weeks and older (■ FIGURE 47-8). Codes are also divided for the first fetus, also called the **gestational sac**, and each additional fetus or gestational sac. To assign codes for a pelvic ultrasound procedure, search the Index for

the Main Term **Ultrasound** and the first-level modifying term **Pelvis** for a nonobstetrical procedure or the first-level modifying term **Pregnant uterus** for an obstetrical procedure. Refer to the Tabular List to select and verify the correct code based on the criteria contained in the code descriptions.

Assigning Codes for Mammography

CPT provides three codes for basic mammography, based on whether the procedure is for screening or diagnostic purposes. A screening mammogram is one performed for preventive reasons for a woman with no symptoms. By definition, a screening mammogram (code **77057**) is bilateral and does not require modifier **-50 Bilateral procedure**. A diagnostic mammogram is performed because of symptoms or a suspected problem and can be performed on both men and women. A diagnostic mammogram can be either unilateral (code **77055**) or bilateral (code **77056**). Append the appropriate laterality modifier **-RT Right side** or **-LT Left side** for a unilateral procedure, but do not report modifier **-50** with code **77056**.

Screening and diagnostic mammography are supported by different ICD-10-CM diagnosis codes. In general, report **Z12.31** or **Z12.39** for a screening mammogram (■ FIGURE 47-9). For a diagnostic mammogram, use codes that describe the symptom(s) or condition(s) that caused the physician to order the procedure (■ FIGURE 47-10). Always check with payers for specific coding requirements.

Patient receives a transabdominal ultrasound examination with real-time image documentation and fetal and maternal evaluation. One gestational sac is identified with an estimated gestational age of 12 weeks.

76801 Ultrasound, pregnant uterus, real time with image documentation, fetal and maternal evaluation, first trimester (< 14 weeks 0 days), transabdominal approach; single or first gestation

Figure 47-8 ■ Example of Coding Obstetrical Ultrasound.
Source: © PB Resources, Inc. Used with permission.

Patient was seen for a bilateral screening mammogram with 2 views of each breast.

Z12.31 Encounter for screening mammogram for malignant neoplasm of breast

77057 Screening mammography, bilateral (2-view film study of each breast)

Figure 47-9 ■ Example of Coding for a Screening Mammogram. *Source: © PB Resources, Inc. Used with permission. CPT codes only © American Medical Association.*

Patient was seen for a diagnostic mammogram of the right breast because of a suspicious lump.

N63 Unspecified lump in breast

77055-RT Mammography; unilateral; -RT Right side

Figure 47-10 ■ Example of Coding for a Diagnostic Mammogram. *Source: © PB Resources, Inc. Used with permission. CPT codes only © American Medical Association.*

CODING CAUTION

When a Medicare patient has a screening mammogram followed by a diagnostic mammogram the *same day*, report codes for both procedures and append HCPCS modifier **-GG Performance and payment of a screening mammogram and diagnostic mammogram on the same patient, same day** to the diagnostic mammogram code.

Assigning Codes for With and Without Contrast

A radiologist, radiologic technologist, or nurse may administer contrast media, subject to the requirements of state law. Radiology departments often provide physicians with a reference card that identifies the clinical circumstances under which imaging should be ordered without contrast, with contrast, or both. This enables physicians to obtain the most useful images possible while minimizing patient exposure to radiation or contrast medium. Overexposure to radiation can cause illness, gene mutation, and cancer. Contrast media can cause serious allergic reactions in some people.

The wording of the code description describes whether and how contrast is used. The most common variations are discussed next.

With Contrast

When the Radiology code descriptor includes the phrase **with contrast material(s)**, it means that clinicians performed the test using contrast. The code includes the radiological procedure and the contrast material(s).

Although the Radiology code usually includes the injection procedure when contrast is administered by injection, this is

not always the case. Instructional notes may appear after the code descriptor for the primary procedure stating that a separate code for the injection can be reported. In this situation, assign a minimum of three codes:

- the primary procedure from the Surgery or Medicine section
- the injection procedure from the Surgery section
- the radiology procedure from the Radiology section

Contrast Supplies

When contrast is used but the Radiology code descriptor does not state **with contrast**, assign an additional code for the type of contrast administered, in addition to the procedure codes. Depending on the payer's requirements, report CPT code **99070 Supplies and materials** or a HCPCS code for the specific contrast agent.

Do not assign a code for oral or rectal contrast because these are bundled in the Radiology procedure code.

With or Without Contrast

Some radiology procedures can be performed either with contrast or without contrast, based on the judgment of the physician. These procedures may have two codes: one that states **with contrast** and a second that states **without contrast**. Select the appropriate code based on whether or not contrast was used.

Without Contrast Followed by With Contrast

In some cases, a Radiology procedure might be performed twice at the same encounter: first *without* contrast and then again *with* contrast. This procedure is often done to evaluate tumors, metastases, infection, and hematuria. Different structures and tissues are visible without contrast than when using contrast. Both procedures are bundled into one code, so do not assign two Radiology codes to report the two methods. Look for a code in which the description states **without contrast material(s), followed by contrast material(s)**.

Assigning Codes for Radiation Oncology

Radiation oncology, also called radiation therapy, is a form of cancer treatment that uses high-energy ionizing radiation to shrink or kill malignant neoplasms. It also is used to shrink benign neoplasms or stop their growth. Radiation is usually administered in a precise, calculated dose on a daily basis and over a period of several days to several weeks.

The radiation oncology treatment process is a complex, multidisciplinary service that involves a team of experts including a radiation oncologist physician, radiation therapist, physicist (*a scientist who plans resources and selects equipment to use*), medical dosimetrist (*a healthcare professional who measures and administers radiation*), nurse, and radiotherapy technician.

The Radiation Oncology subsection provides extensive special instructions regarding coding for the stages of radiation oncology treatment, which are summarized in ■ TABLE 47-7. In many categories, codes are divided based on the complexity of the treatment. The special instructions define simple, intermediate, and complex services applicable to each category.

Table 47-7 ■ **SUMMARY OF RADIATION ONCOLOGY CODING**

Phase	Description	Coding Guidelines
Consultation and clinical management	Physician evaluation of patient's condition and recommendation of treatment options	Report codes from E/M, Medicine, and Surgery sections for the specific services provided.
Clinical treatment planning	The process of special testing and interpretation, tumor localization, treatment volume determination, treatment time/dosage determination, choice of treatment modality, determination of number and size of treatment ports, selection of appropriate treatment devices, and other procedures	Codes are divided by simple, intermediate, and complex planning based on the number of treatment areas and ports. Clinical treatment planning is reported once per patient for the entire course of treatment.
Simulation	Determination and testing of treatment field, location, and ports without administering any radiation	Codes are divided by simple, intermediate, and complex planning based on the number of treatment areas and ports. Simulation usually is reported once per patient for the entire course of treatment.
Isodose planning/ dosimetry	Calculation and verification of the amount of radiation to be delivered	Codes are divided by the type and complexity of radiation delivery.
Treatment delivery	Technical-only services of providing radiation treatment according to the established plan	Codes are divided by the type of therapy; simple, intermediate, and complex; and volume of treatment. Treatment delivery is reported once per treatment session.
Treatment management	Physician supervision of the treatment process, including one physical examination and other specified services	Report one code (77427) per five treatments provided. If fewer than five treatments are given to finish out a course of treatment, report 77427 for three to five treatments. For one or two final treatments, do not report a code. CPT guidelines specify services to be provided. Additional codes report short-course treatments and stereotactic radiation therapy.

Source: © PB Resources, Inc. Used with permission.

To locate codes for radiation oncology services, search the Index for the Main Term **Radiation Therapy**; the first-level modifying term for the type of service, such as **Treatment delivery** or **Dose plan**; and the second-level modifying term for the specific service provided. Refer to the Tabular List to review the guidelines and select the appropriate code based on the complexity of the service and other details of the code description.

Refer to ■ FIGURE 47-11 to learn more about coding for both facility and physician services for Radiation Oncology.

Guided Example of Assigning Radiology Procedure Codes

To practice skills for assigning codes for radiology, continue with the example from earlier in the chapter about a patient who was seen for an MRI of the heart. Follow along in your CPT manual as Marcy Elwood, CCS, assigns codes. Check off each step after you complete it.

▶ First, Marcy confirms the procedure: MRI without contrast followed by the same views with contrast, including velocity flow mapping.

▶ Marcy searches the Index for the Main Term **Magnetic Resonance Imaging (MRI)**.

❏ She locates the first-level modifying term **Heart**.

❏ She identifies the code range **75557-75565**.

▶ Marcy turns to the Tabular List to select and verify the codes. She notices that this code range comprises its own category, **Heart**, that has extensive special instructions, so she begins by studying the special instructions. She highlights several important points that may pertain to this case:

❏ Whereas traditional MRI produces static images, cardiac MRI provides a real-time **physiologic evaluation of cardiac function**.

❏ Some codes include contrast and others do not. Some codes include pharmacologic perfusion stress testing and others do not.

❏ **Cardiac MRI for velocity flow mapping can be reported in conjunction with 75557, 75559, 75561, or 75563.**

Patient receives his final nine radiation treatment sessions to end his radiation therapy to treat esophageal cancer. Treatment is greater than 1 MeV, simple.

Facility services:
77402 x 9 Radiation treatment delivery, > than 1 MeV, simple
Physician services:
77427 x 2 Radiation treatment management, 5 treatments

Figure 47-11 ■ Example of Coding for Radiation Oncology.
Source: © PB Resources, Inc. Used with permission. CPT codes only © American Medical Association.

❑ **Only one add-on code for flow velocity can be reported per session**.

❑ This information leads her to believe that she will probably need two codes: one for the MRI without and with contrast and one for the velocity flow mapping.

▶ Marcy reads the code descriptions to locate the code(s) she may need.

❑ Codes **75557** and **75559** are for without contrast, so they do not apply.

❑ Code **75561** describes **Cardiac magnetic resonance imaging for morphology and function without contrast material(s), followed by contrast material(s) and further sequences**. It identifies MRI as well as without and with contrast, so she makes a note of this code.

❑ Code **75563** is the same as **75561** with stress imaging added, but stress imaging was not performed.

❑ She reads the instructional note following code **75563** that states (**75558, 75560, 75564 have been deleted. To report flow velocity, use 75565**). She assumes that the codes listed as deleted must have been used for flow velocity previously, before the introduction of code **75565**.

❑ She reads the description for code **75565** and notes that it is the add-on code for **Cardiac magnetic resonance imaging for velocity flow mapping** discussed in the special instructions.

▪ An instructional note following code **75565** states (**Use 75565 in conjunction with 75557, 75559, 75561, 75563**), which also concurs with the special instructions. She verifies that the MRI code she has tentatively selected, **75561**, appears in the list of allowed codes.

❑ The remaining codes in this category identify computed tomography, so they do not apply.

▶ Marcy reviews the procedure codes she has identified for this case and confirms that they accurately describe the procedures performed.

❑ **75565 Cardiac magnetic resonance imaging for velocity flow mapping**

❑ **75561 Cardiac magnetic resonance imaging for morphology and function without contrast material(s), followed by contrast material(s) and further sequences**

▶ Next, Marcy must determine how to sequence the codes.

CODING PRACTICE

Exercise 47.3   Assigning Codes for Radiology Procedures

Instructions: Read the mini-medical-record of each patient's encounter. Review the information abstracted in Exercise 47.2 for questions 1–3. For questions 4–6, abstract the case on your own. Read the tips with each exercise to help determine whether you are coding for a professional, technical, or global service. Assign CPT codes, quantities, and modifiers using the Index and Tabular List. Write the code(s) on the line provided.

1. OUTPATIENT HOSPITAL   Gender: F
Age: 16 months

Referring physician: Pediatrician

Referring diagnosis: limping while walking

Procedure: X-ray of the pelvis (AP), AP and bilateral frog-leg (lateral) view of the hips

Tip: Code for the services of the hospital's radiology department only. The images were interpreted by a radiologist under contract with the hospital.

1 CPT Code _____

2. OUTPATIENT HOSPITAL   Gender: F   Age: 46

Performing physician: Oncologist

Preprocedure diagnosis: status post-thyroidectomy due to thyroid cancer

Procedure: one session, 3 MeV radiation treatment to the thyroid, using a single port and simple block

Tip: Code for the oncologist's services.

1 CPT Code _____

3. OUTPATIENT HOSPITAL   Gender: M   Age: 81

Referring physician: Pulmonologist

Referring diagnosis: SOB, mild chest pain, hemoptysis

Procedure: ventilation-perfusion scan (V/Q scan)

Impression: pulmonary artery thrombosis

Tip: Code for the technical services of the hospital's radiology department.

1 CPT Code _____

(continued)

CODING PRACTICE (continued)

4. OFFICE Gender: F Age: 47

Referring physician: Primary care

Referring diagnosis: recurring constipation

Procedure: barium enema. Rectal tube inserted and barium instilled with fluoroscopy images of evacuation. Barium seemed to flow with no difficulty through the GI tract.

Impression: normal barium enema

Tip: Code the professional and technical components.

1 CPT Code _____

5. OUTPATIENT HOSPITAL Gender: F Age: 29

Referring physician: Primary care

Referring diagnosis: seizure disorder

Procedure: noncontrast CT of head. No evidence of hemorrhage or infarction. No fluid indicating hydrocephalus. There is no midline shift.

(*continued*)

5. (continued)

Impression: Normal CT; no acute process seen.

Tip: Code the professional component only.

1 CPT Code _____

6. OFFICE Gender: M Age: 68

Performing physician: Cardiologist

Preprocedure diagnosis: CAD with ischemia

Procedure: myocardial perfusion imaging. Following 4 minutes of exercise, the patient was injected with 3013 mCi of Cardiolite technetium-99m sestamibi. Perfusion images obtained to compare to resting images.

Impression: abnormal perfusion imaging with a moderately large-sized defect consistent with anterior wall ischemia.

Tip: Code for the technical and professional components.

1 CPT Code _____

ARRANGING CODES FOR RADIOLOGY PROCEDURES

When multiple Radiology procedures are performed on the same date, sequence codes in descending RVU order. Be aware of how to report codes for radiologic guidance and how to apply modifiers correctly.

Multiple Coding for Radiologic Guidance

Radiologic guidance can be real-time or static. Real-time guidance generates a live image of anatomic structures that the operating physician views on a screen to guide his movements. The combination of laparoscopic surgery and real-time imaging guidance makes minimally invasive procedures more readily available because open incisions to view and access the operative field are needed less often. In most cases, multiple coding is required: one code for the radiological imaging and one code for the surgical procedure. In some cases, a third code for the injection of the contrast medium is required. When the code for the surgical procedure specifies that a radiological procedure is being done at the same time, such as **with cholangiography**, the injection procedure is included in the CPT code for the surgical procedure. However, report the code for radiological S&I in addition to the surgical procedure code. When the Radiology code specifies **radiological supervision and interpretation**, the code identifies only the professional component, so modifier **-26 Professional component** is not required (■ FIGURE 47-12).

Static radiologic guidance involves the placement of a clip or wire, usually during a biopsy, to mark a site that must be treated or operated on at a later time. Multiple coding is required: one code for the placement of the clip or wire and one code for the surgical procedure.

Coders must always identify the physician they are coding for and the services provided by that physician. When a surgeon performs the surgical procedure and an interventional radiologist performs the imaging guidance, do not assign both codes for both providers. Assign a code only for the services rendered by that physician. When one physician performs both the surgery and the radiological guidance, assign both codes for the same physician.

A gastroenterologist, performs a laparoscopic cholecystectomy, with a cholangiogram as part of the procedure. The gastroenterologist also provides radiological supervision and interpretation.

47563 Laparoscopy, surgical; cholecystectomy with cholangiography

74300 Cholangiography and/or pancreatography; intraoperative, radiological supervision and interpretation

Figure 47-12 ■ Example of Coding for Real-Time Radiologic Guidance. *Source:* © *PB Resources, Inc. Used with permission. CPT codes only* © *American Medical Association.*

Modifiers Used with Radiology

Modifiers that are frequently used with Radiology codes include those that identify the professional and technical components, reduced services, and laterality. These are discussed next.

-26 Professional Component

Many Radiology services consist of a professional component that includes physician supervision and interpretation and a technical component that includes space, equipment, and staff. When coding for a physician who provides only the professional component, append modifier **-26** to the Radiology code. The Medicare Physician Fee Schedule Database (MPFSDB) lists the total relative value units (RVUs), as well as the RVUs and pricing for both the professional and technical components. The allocation of cost between the professional and technical components varies by the complexity of a procedure and the amount of equipment and supplies required. Typically, the professional component ranges from 20% to 45% of the total procedure cost.

-TC Technical Component

When coding for a facility that provides only the technical component, append modifier **-TC** to the Radiology code. Typically, the technical component ranges from 55% to 80% of the total procedure cost. When the same provider performs both the professional and technical components, code for a global service without any modifier.

In the workplace, coders have a clear understanding of whether they should code for the professional component, technical component, or global service based on the place of employment and organization of services. Consider the following examples:

- A coder who works for a radiology practice comprised of physicians who provide the S&I component for a facility codes for the professional component only.
- A coder who works for a hospital outpatient department that provides the equipment, facility, and technicians but contracts out all professional services codes for the technical component only.
- A coder who works for a freestanding radiology facility that employs physicians and technical staff and owns all the equipment codes for a global service.

Refer to Chapter 30 of this text for more information and figures on the use of modifiers **-26** and **-TC**.

-52 Reduced Services

Sometimes more than one physician is involved in supervision and interpretation, with one physician supervising the procedure and another interpreting the results. Each physician reports the same procedure code and appends modifier **-52 Reduced services** to show that each physician did not perform a complete service. Submit a report with the claim to explain why the modifier is used. Also report modifier **-26** for codes that have both a technical and professional component.

Laterality

Report laterality modifiers with Radiology services on paired anatomic sites if laterality is not defined in the code. CPT provides two codes for some procedures: one defined as unilateral and one defined as bilateral. Report modifier **-RT** or **-LT** with the unilateral code, but do not report modifier **-50 Bilateral procedure** when the code description specifies that the procedure is bilateral.

Guided Example of Arranging Radiology Procedure Codes

To practice skills for arranging codes for radiology procedures, continue with the example from earlier in the chapter about the patient who was seen for an MRI of the heart. Follow along in your CPT manual as Marcy Elwood, CCS, arranges the codes. Check off each step after you complete it.

▶ First, Marcy confirms the procedure in the medical record: MRI without contrast followed by the same views with contrast, including velocity flow mapping.

▶ Marcy arranges the codes in descending RVU order according to the Medicare Physician Fee Schedule Database (MPFSDB). She uses the facility RVU because the procedure was performed at the hospital, not at the physician's office, and reviews the RVUs for the professional component (modifier **-26**).

❑ **75565 Cardiac magnetic resonance imaging for velocity flow mapping** Facility RVU = 1.57 (modifier -26 = 0.35/modifier –TC = 1.22)

❑ **75561 Cardiac magnetic resonance imaging for morphology and function without contrast material(s), followed by contrast material(s) and further sequences** Facility RVU = 12.20 (modifier -26 = 3.63/modifier -TC = 8.57)

▶ Marcy examines the need for modifiers. (Refer to Table 30-1 Key Criteria for Abstracting CPT Modifiers or Appendix A in the CPT manual.)

❑ Code **75561** requires modifier **-26** because she is coding for the supervising radiologist, so only the professional component was provided.

❑ Code **75565** requires modifier **-26** because she is coding for the supervising radiologist, so only the professional component was provided.

▶ Marcy finalizes the procedure codes and sequencing for this case:

(1) **75561-26 Cardiac magnetic resonance imaging for morphology and function without contrast material(s), followed by contrast material(s) and further sequences; -26 Professional component**

(2) **75565-26 Cardiac magnetic resonance imaging for velocity flow mapping; -26 Professional component**

▶ Marcy also assigns and sequences the ICD-10-CM diagnosis codes that support the need for the service.

(1) **I34.1 Nonrheumatic mitral (valve) prolapse**

CODING PRACTICE

Exercise 47.4 **Arranging Codes for Radiology Procedures**

Instructions: Read the mini-medical-record of each patient's encounter. Review the information abstracted in Exercise 47.2 for questions 1–3. For questions 4–6, abstract the case on your own. Read the tips with each exercise to help determine whether you are coding for a professional, technical, or global service. Assign CPT codes, quantities, and modifiers using the Index and Tabular List, and arrange the codes in proper sequence. Write the code(s) on the line provided.

1. OUTPATIENT HOSPITAL Gender: F Age: 64

Referring physician: Pulmonologist

Referring diagnosis: lifelong smoker, severe cough, hemoptysis

Procedure: AP and lateral chest X-ray, standing. A dense mass in the lower lobe of the left lung is noted.

Findings: Patient's pulmonologist consents to performing a CT scan of the chest without contrast.

Impression: carcinoma of the left lower lobe

Tip: Code for the supervising radiologist.

2 CPT Codes _____

2. OFFICE Gender: F Age: 29

Performing physician: Obstetrician

Preprocedure diagnosis: routine pregnancy, EGA 10 weeks

Procedure: transabdominal ultrasound for fetal and maternal evaluation, supine

Impression: twin fetuses

Tip: Read the Tabular List carefully to determine the second code.

2 CPT Codes _____

3. OUTPATIENT HOSPITAL Gender: M Age: 55

Referring physician: Nephrologist

Diagnosis: ESRD, diabetic nephropathy

Procedure: placed a central venous nontunneled catheter using fluoroscopic guidance for temporary dialysis access

Tip: Code for the service of the interventional radiologist.

2 CPT Codes _____

4. EMERGENCY ROOM Gender: M Age: 71

Referring physician: Emergency Medicine

Referring diagnosis: pain in left hip s/p fall on ice

Procedure: AP pelvis and left hip radiograph performed. There is generalized demineralization of bone. There is an intertrochanteric fracture of the left hip with moderate angulation and displacement present.

Impression: intertrochanteric fracture, left hip

Tip: Code the technical component only.

2 CPT Codes _____

5. INPATIENT HOSPITAL Gender: M Age: 1 Day

Referring physician: Neonatologist

Preprocedure diagnosis: facial mass

Procedure: MRI of orbit/face with and without contrast; MR angiography of the head with contrast. Multiplanar, multisequence images of the head and neck obtained without contrast followed by contrast. The origin of the mass could not be identified. MR angiography of the head with contrast was limited and suboptimal.

Impression: hemangioma should be considered

Tip: Code the professional component only.

2 CPT Codes _____

6. OUTPATIENT HOSPITAL   Gender: F   Age: 10

Referring physician: Pediatrician

Referring diagnosis: recurrent urinary tract infections

Procedure: radiopharmaceutical voiding cystogram. A Foley catheter was inserted through the urethra and

(continued)

6. (continued)

the bladder filled with contrast. The patient was instructed to void and X-ray images were obtained.

Impression: vesicoureteral reflux

2 CPT Codes _____

CHAPTER SUMMARY

In this chapter you learned that:

- Radiology is a medical specialty that uses radiation, sound waves, magnetic fields, or radio fields to visualize internal body structures, such as arteries and bones; each type of technology is referred to as a modality.

- The CPT section **Radiology (70010-79999)** contains seven subsections that are divided by modality.

- Plain radiographic procedures (X-rays) are described by the number and type of radiographic views—the angle and direction from which the image is taken, which also determine how the technician must position the patient.

- To assign codes for Radiology services, search the Index for the Main Term of the modality, then review how the first-level

modifying terms are organized and follow the necessary path to identify the anatomic site.

- In most cases, multiple coding is required for radiological guidance: one code for the radiologic imaging and one code for the surgical procedure.

- CPT provides guidelines for Radiology at the beginning of the section that apply to all codes in the section; in particular, coders need to understand radiological supervision and interpretation, administration of contrast, and written report.

CONCEPT QUIZ

Take a moment to look back at Radiology and solidify your skills. Try to answer the questions from memory first, then refer to the discussion in this chapter if you need a little extra help.

Completion

Instructions: Write the term that answers each question based on the information you learned in this chapter. Choose from the list below. Some choices may be used more than once and some choices may not be used at all.

A-mode

clinical brachytherapy

computed tomography

computer-aided detection

diagnostic

Doppler

DXA

fluoroscopy

hyperthermia

magnetic resonance angiography

magnetic resonance imaging

M-mode

PET

screening

stereotactic imaging

1. _____ is one form of an image-guided procedure using a live X-ray image on a fluorescent screen.

2. A _____ ultrasound uses high-frequency sound to monitor a fetal heartbeat.

3. Pattern recognition software, called _____, is used to decrease false-negative readings of images.

4. The purpose of _____ mammography is to determine the nature of a problem in the breast.

5. During a breast biopsy, _____ may be used to pinpoint a specific location using 3-D imaging.

6. _____ is a one-dimensional ultrasonic measurement used to display movement of a structure.

7. The treatment of malignant tumors by implanting small, encapsulated radioactive elements in a tumor is called

_____.

8. A diagnosis of carotid artery disease can be determined through _____, which shows the blood flow in the artery.

9. The procedure used to expose tissue to high temperatures in order to damage cancer cells is called _____.

10. _____ is used to show how organs and tissues are working in real time using a positron-emitting radionuclide tracer.

Multiple Choice

Instructions: Circle the letter of the best answer to each question based on the information you learned in this chapter.

1. Which type of contrast media injection usually requires an additional code for the injection?
   A. Intra-articular
   B. Intravascular
   C. Intrathecal
   D. Rectal

(continued)

(continued from page 947)

2. Which service is included in radiologic S&I?
   A. Injection
   B. Guided imaging
   C. Written report
   D. Department management

3. When might a physician order an image without contrast, followed by with contrast?
   A. Routine fracture
   B. Tumor
   C. Mammography
   D. Cholangiogram

4. What direction is an AP image taken from?
   A. Back to front
   B. Front to back
   C. Left to right
   D. Top to bottom

5. What anatomic approach means "within a joint"?
   A. Intra-articular
   B. Interstitial
   C. Intrathecal
   D. Intracavity

6. What second-level modifying term directs coders to obstetrical codes for an ultrasound of the pelvis?
   A. Pregnant uterus
   B. Maternity
   C. Obstetrical
   D. Fetus

7. What type of structure permits X-rays to pass into and through it, resulting in a darker, shadowy image that shows layers?
   A. Radiopaque
   B. Translucent
   C. Radiolucent
   D. Medium density

8. What is the correct modifier for a bilateral screening mammogram?
   A. -50
   B. -RT, -LT
   C. -51
   D. None

9. How often should a code for radiation treatment management be reported?
   A. Once per course of treatment
   B. Each treatment
   C. Every five treatments
   D. Once per month

10. What modifier should be reported when the same physician provides both the technical and professional components of a radiology procedure?
    A. -26
    B. -TC
    C. -26 and -TC
    D. No modifier

CODING CHALLENGE

Instructions: Read the mini-medical-record of each patient's encounter, then abstract, assign, and arrange ICD-10-CM diagnosis codes and CPT procedure codes using the appropriate Index and Tabular List. Assign quantities and modifiers where needed. Write the code(s) on the line provided.

1. OUTPATIENT HOSPITAL   Gender: M   Age: 65

Referring physician: Primary care

Referring diagnosis: adenocarcinoma of the prostate, rule out bone metastasis

Procedure: whole-body radionuclide bone scan. The skeleton was imaged in the anterior and posterior position after the IV administration of 26.5 mCi of technetium 99m MDP. The right parietal region of the skull showed abnormal activity. The uptake in the remainder of the skeleton is within normal limits.

Impression: focus of abnormal increased tracer activity overlying the right parietal region of the skull. CT scanning or magnetic resonance imaging of the skull and brain could be done for further assessment if it is clinically indicated.

Tip: Code for the professional component only.

1 ICD-10-CM Code _____

1 CPT Code _____

2. OUTPATIENT SURGERY   Gender: M   Age: 59

Referring physician: Oncologist

Referring diagnosis: pancreatic adenocarcinoma; procedure planned for typing and staging of pancreatic cancer

Procedure: percutaneous biopsy of the pancreas guided by CT scan. Multiple biopsies taken. The scan shows a tumor of the head of the pancreas with invasion of the superior mesenteric artery, making it unresectable.

Impression: Stage III pancreatic cancer

1 ICD-10-CM Code _____

2 CPT Codes _____

3. OFFICE   Gender: F   Age: 23

Performing physician: Gynecologist

Preprocedure diagnosis: pelvic pain

Procedure: transvaginal ultrasound attempted. The patient fainted within the first 60 seconds of the procedure and it had to be discontinued. The procedure was not completed.

(continued)

3. (continued)

Impression: *procedure not completed*

Tip: The attempted procedure is coded using a modifier to report it was discontinued.

1 ICD-10-CM Code _____

1 CPT Code _____

---

4. OFFICE   Gender: M   Age: 91

Performing physician: *Gastroenterologist*

Preprocedure diagnosis: *achalasia of the lower esophageal sphincter*

Procedure: *balloon dilation of the esophagus with fluoroscopic guidance. Scope was passed under direct supervision. Webs were dilated with pneumatic 20-mm-diameter angioplasty balloons x2 for 10 seconds each across the LES. No complications.*

Impression: *the LES successfully dilated, with obliteration of the waist*

Tip: Code the S/I component for the fluoroscopic guidance by the gastroenterologist in addition to the primary procedure.

1 ICD-10-CM Code _____

2 CPT Codes _____

---

5. OFFICE   Gender: F   Age: 68

Performing physician: *Primary care*

Preprocedure diagnosis: *severe shoulder pain on the left*

Procedure: *X-ray of left shoulder, AP view*

Findings: *the bones of the glenohumeral and acromioclavicular joints showed normal alignment and normal bone density. No focal lytic or sclerotic lesion is detected in the visualized bones. Moderate to severe osteoarthritis of the acromioclavicular joint was identified. Normal soft tissues.*

Impression: *moderate to severe osteoarthritis of the acromioclavicular joint.*

Tip: Code both the professional component and technical component.

1 ICD-10-CM Code _____

1 CPT Code _____

---

6. OUTPATIENT HOSPITAL   Gender: M   Age: 63

Referring physician: *Neurologist*

Referring diagnosis: *impaired memory and apraxia, rule out Alzheimer's disease*

(continued)

---

4. (continued)

Procedure: *CT scan of the head without IV contrast*

Findings: *revealed a diffuse, moderately large area of localized atrophy involving the superior-most portion of the left parietal region. There is no other significant abnormality.*

Impression: *findings consistent with early Alzheimer's disease.*

Tip: Code only the technical component of the procedure.

2 ICD-10-CM Codes _____

1 CPT Code _____

---

7. INPATIENT HOSPITAL   Gender: F   Age: 58

Referring physician: *Vascular surgeon*

Referring diagnosis: *patient with HTN, hyperlipidemia, and leg pain who comes for arteriogram evaluation*

Procedure: *magnetic resonance angiography of both lower extremities. One milliliter gadolinium-DTPA injected via cubital vein. On the left, the proximal anterior tibial artery has 90% atherosclerotic occlusion; the right proximal anterior tibial artery has 100% atherosclerotic occlusion.*

Impression: *bilateral obstructive peripheral arterial disease (PAD)*

Tip: Only code the professional component of the procedure.

4 ICD-10-CM Codes _____

_____

1 CPT Code _____

---

8. OUTPATIENT SURGERY   Gender: M   Age: 47

Performing physician: *Anesthesiologist*

Referring diagnosis: *chronic neck and back pain*

Procedure: *epidural injection at L4-5 in a patient with chronic back and leg pain. Fluoroscopic guidance was used for needle placement, and contrast was injected, and it was confirmed that the needle tip was in the epidural space. Steroid injection was performed. The procedure was tolerated well.*

Tip: Code the professional component for the fluoroscopic guidance.

3 ICD-10-CM Codes _____

_____

2 CPT Codes _____

(continued)

(continued from page 949)

9. OFFICE Gender: F Age: 39

Reason for encounter: right knee pain x2 weeks not relieved by NSAIDs. She reports the pain began shortly after her yoga class.

Assessment: patient known to me is seen for complaint of severe knee pain, which is now interfering with activities of daily living. Exam of both knees showed limited movement on the right, normal on the left. Problem-focused history and examination was performed.

Procedure: right knee X-ray, 2 views

Impression: X-ray shows tendinitis

Tip: Do not code the external cause of injury. Do assign an E/M code.

1 ICD-10-CM Code _____

2 CPT Codes _____

10. INPATIENT HOSPITAL Gender: M Age: 75

Referring physician: Neurologist

Referring diagnosis: MRI to rule out brain neoplasm; recurring confusion, increasing in duration over the past month; history of a stroke 10 years ago.

Procedure: MRI brain with and without contrast. Decreased T1 and increased T2 signal in the right temporal lobe. The lesion increased in size and enhances more greatly when compared with the previous MRI exam. There is also edema surrounding the affected area and associated mass effect.

Impression: MRI positive for astrocytoma, left temporal lobe

Tip: Only code the technical component for the procedure.

1 ICD-10-CM Code _____

1 CPT Code _____

KEEP ON CODING

Instructions: Read the procedural statement, then use the appropriate Index and Tabular List to assign CPT procedure codes, quantities, and modifiers. Write the code(s) on the line provided.

1. CT of the abdomen and pelvis with oral contrast, professional component: CPT Code(s) _____

2. Bilateral screening mammogram, technical component: CPT Code(s) _____

3. Supervision and interpretation of transvaginal and complete abdominal ultrasound with real-time imaging: CPT Code(s) _____

4. SPECT kidney imaging, technical component: CPT Code(s) _____

5. Radiological supervision and interpretation for ultrasonic guidance needle biopsy: CPT Code(s) _____

6. Simple simulation-aided field setting for prostate radiation treatment by radiation oncologist: CPT Code(s) _____

7. MRI of the upper abdomen with and without gadolinium, global component: CPT Code(s) _____

8. Thyroid uptake, single, technical component: CPT Code(s) _____

9. MUGA scan with right ventricular ejection fraction by first-pass technique; global component: CPT Code(s) _____

10. Intraoperative cholangiopancreatography, radiologic supervision and interpretation: CPT Code(s) _____

11. Screening mammogram and ultrasound of breasts, global component: CPT Code(s) _____

12. Saline infusion hysterosonography with color flow Doppler, professional component: CPT Code(s) _____

13. Nuclear medicine lymphatic scan, global component: CPT Code(s) _____

14. IVP with KUB, global component: CPT Code(s) _____

15. Bilateral pulmonary angiogram, radiological S/I: CPT Code(s) _____

16. Voiding urethrocystography with contrast, professional component: CPT Code(s) _____

17. Testicular ultrasound, global component: CPT Code(s) _____

18. Lumbosacral myelogram, radiological supervision and interpretation: CPT Code(s) _____

19. Computed tomography, chest; without contrast material, followed by contrast material(s) and further sections, professional component: CPT Code(s) _____

20. X-ray lumbosacral spine, bending views only, 2 views, global component: CPT Code(s) _____

21. 3-D CT evaluation of the heart with contrast, technical component: CPT Code(s) _____

22. Radiation treatment delivery to four separate areas with a rotational beam at 4 MeV, global component: CPT Code(s) _____

23. Nuclear HIDA scan with contrast, technical component: CPT Code(s) _____

24. Ultrasound of the right upper and left upper quadrants of the abdomen, global component: CPT Code(s) _____

25. Review of dosimetry, dose delivery and treatment parameters, five weekly treatments: CPT Code(s) _____

Pathology and Laboratory Services (80047-89398)

Chapter 48

Learning Objectives

After completing this chapter, you should have the skills to:

48.1 Spell and define the key words, medical terms, and abbreviations related to pathology and laboratory procedures.

48.2 Discuss the types of pathology and laboratory procedures.

48.3 Identify the main characteristics of coding for Pathology and Laboratory.

48.4 Abstract procedural information from the medical record for coding Pathology and Laboratory.

48.5 Assign codes for Pathology and Laboratory procedures.

48.6 Arrange codes for Pathology and Laboratory procedures.

48.7 Discuss the CPT coding guidelines related to Pathology and Laboratory.

Chapter Outline

- **Pathology and Laboratory Procedure Basics**
- **Coding Overview of Pathology and Laboratory Procedures**
- **Abstracting Pathology and Laboratory Procedures**
- **Assigning Codes for Pathology and Laboratory Procedures**
- **Arranging Codes for Pathology and Laboratory Procedures**

Key Terms and Abbreviations

analyte
Bethesda System
Certificate of Compliance (COC)
Certificate of Waiver (COW)
Clinical Laboratory Improvement Amendments (CLIA)
conventional Pap test
definitive drug testing
direct optical observation
gross (examination)
lab report
lab requisition
physician office laboratory (POL)
presumptive drug class screening
provider-performed microscopy procedure (PPMP)
qualitative test
quantitative test
rapid strep test (RST)
reference range
specimen
therapeutic drug assay

In addition to the key terms listed here, students should know the terms defined within tables in this chapter.

INTRODUCTION

Any drugstore and many online outlets sell kits for at-home pregnancy testing, glucose testing, stool testing, and a variety of other simple laboratory tests that provide preliminary results for patients. However, these are not a replacement for physician diagnosis and treatment or the detailed analysis and quality control of a professional laboratory.

This chapter discusses the services of the laboratory to process and interpret a test. There are several components to consider when laboratory services are provided. Physician examinations to determine the need for a test are usually included in the examination component of E/M codes or an appropriate procedure code if done as part of a procedure, such as colonoscopy. Specimen collection is reported with the CPT code that describes the method of collection, such as venipuncture or a biopsy. Transfer of the specimen to the laboratory is reported with a separate CPT code. Physician review of the lab results, determination of the final diagnosis, and any other follow-up are included in the medical decision-making component of an E/M code.

PATHOLOGY AND LABORATORY PROCEDURE BASICS

Clinical pathology is a medical specialty that is concerned with the diagnosis of disease based on the laboratory analysis of bodily fluids and tissue. A pathologist is a physician who examines tissues, checks the accuracy of lab tests, and interprets the results. Recognized subspecialties include chemical pathology—also called clinical chemistry—clinical hematology, transfusion medicine, microbiology, cytogenetics, and molecular genetics. The patient's personal physician uses information from laboratory tests and pathology reports to determine the diagnosis and treatment plan.

Medical terms used for laboratory procedures utilize word parts from all body systems, with prefixes and suffixes that identify what action is being performed. Refer to ■ TABLE 48-1 for a refresher on how to build medical terms related to Pathology and Laboratory.

CODING CAUTION

Be alert for medical terms that are spelled similarly and have different meanings.

cyt/o (*cell*) and **cyst/o** (*bladder*)

antigen (*a foreign substance that evokes an immune response and possibly infection*) and **antibody** (*a protein in the blood that creates an immune response against an antigen or other invader*)

The laboratory requisition, testing, and reporting process is discussed next, followed by a discussion of the Clinical Laboratory Improvement Amendments (CLIA). The general types of laboratory procedures are discussed in the next section of this chapter, "Coding Overview of Pathology and Laboratory Procedures."

Overview of the Laboratory Testing Process

The most commonly performed pathology and laboratory services require a specimen to be collected and sent to a lab for processing. The physician must document in the patient's

Table 48-1 ■ **EXAMPLE OF CONSTRUCTING MEDICAL TERMS FOR PATHOLOGY AND LABORATORY PROCEDURES**

Combining Form	Prefix/Suffix	Complete Medical Term
hemat/o (*blood*) bi/o (*life*) cyt/o (*cell*) path/o (*abnormal*)	micro- (*small*)	hemato + logy (*study of the blood*) patho + logy (*study of the abnormal*) cyto + patho + logy (*study of abnormal cells*)
	-scopy (*visual examination*) -logy (*study of*)	micro + bio + logy (*study of small life*) micro + scopy (*visual examination of small things*)

Source: © PB Resources, Inc. Used with permission.

medical record the tests ordered and the medical necessity of each. The lab performs the test and sends a report back to the physician. The ordering physician reviews the test results and determines their implication for the patient's care, including documenting how the findings were used to determine a diagnosis and formulate a treatment plan.

A **specimen** is a sample of any bodily fluid or tissue. An **analyte** is the specific substance within the sample to be examined or tested for. For example, a blood specimen might be tested for a variety of analytes, such as glucose, sodium, or cholesterol.

Specimens can be acquired in the physician's office, during a medical procedure, by the patient at home, or at the lab. Physician offices that perform a limited number of laboratory tests in the office are called a **physician office laboratory** (POL). Tests that cannot be processed in a physician's office are sent to a hospital or a reference laboratory for processing (■ TABLE 48-2).

Table 48-2 ■ **TYPES OF LABORATORY PROVIDERS**

Type of Laboratory	Description
Physician Office Laboratory (POL)	Small laboratory in a physician office that performs a limited number of tests on site, eliminating the need to send them to an outside lab.
Hospital Laboratory	Laboratory located in a hospital facility, used to perform tests needed in emergency situations, tests where STAT results are needed rapidly for patient care, those done in high volume for both inpatients and outpatients.
Independent Clinical Lab/Reference Lab	A Medicare-enrolled laboratory that receives a specimen performs the test(s) for a separate, referring laboratory.
Public Health Lab	Lab operated by state and local health departments to diagnose disease and protect the public from health threats, such as outbreaks of infectious diseases and environmental hazards.

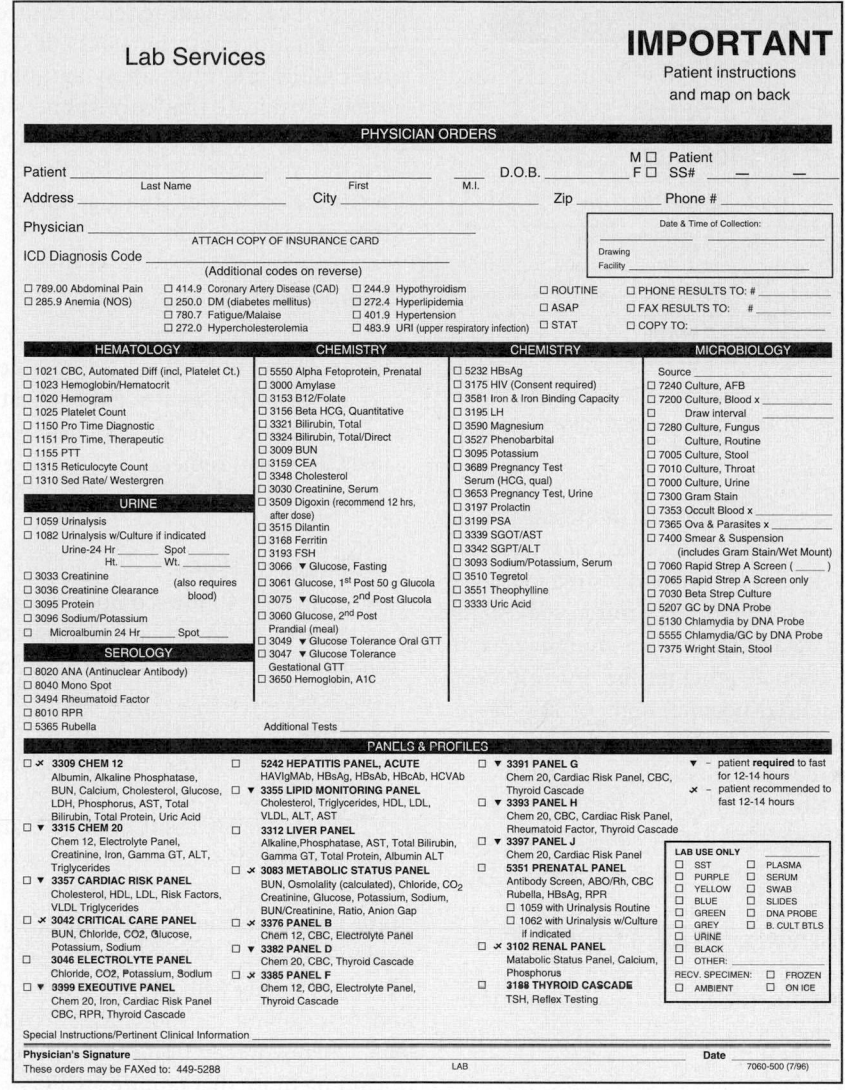

Figure 48-1 ■ Example of a Laboratory Requisition or Order

Specimens that are sent out for processing must be accompanied by a lab requisition or order that describes the test(s) to be performed (■ FIGURE 48-1). A **lab requisition** typically provides the following information:

- Physician's name, address, and phone number
- Patient's name, date of birth, and medical record number
- Diagnosis to justify the lab test
- Type of test to perform
- Date and time the specimen was collected
- Any pertinent past medical history or past lab results that the lab needs to review
- Signature of the physician or clinician who ordered the test(s) (required by some payers)

A **lab report** provides the results of the test and other information useful to the physician in making a diagnosis. The lab report typically contains:

- Patient name and identification number
- Name of laboratory

- Name of physician or practitioner ordering the test
- Date and time the specimen was collected and date and time of receipt
- Reason for an unsatisfactory specimen, if applicable
- Test or evaluation performed
- Result
- Date and time of report

The type of report or test results depends on the type of test performed. Qualitative tests, which include some chemistry and immunology tests, provide a basic *Positive/Negative* or *Present/Absent* answer to questions such as *Is a particular substance* (such as a drug, virus, or bacteria) *present in the sample?*

Quantitative tests, which include most chemistry tests, drug assays, and some immunology tests, provide the concentration of a substance in the sample, such as a glucose test that reports the concentration of glucose in blood plasma. Quantitative tests are usually accompanied by a **reference range**, a numeric range of typical results in the average population and the levels considered to be *High* or *Low*, determined by the

Component	Value	Reference Range	Flag
Sodium	140	137-145 mmol/L	
Potassium	4.4	3.5-5.1 mmol/L	
Glucose	121	74-106 mg/dL	H (High)
Calcium	9.5	8.4-10.4 mg/dL	
Total Protein	6.0	6.3-8.2 g/L	L (Low)
Alkaline Phosphatase	107	38-126 Unit/L	
TSH	2.0	0.5-5.0 mIU/L	

Figure 48-2 ■ Example of Test Results and Reference Ranges. *Source: © PB Resources, Inc. Used with permission.*

statistic calculation of two standard deviations (■ FIGURE 48-2). Reference ranges are not universally standard for many analytes because they are specific to the equipment and testing methods used by the laboratory. Thus, each laboratory must establish its own reference ranges using data from its own equipment and methods. Physicians must evaluate whether the test result for a particular patient is considered normal, high, or low based on that patient's symptoms, medical history, and the reason the physician ordered the test. For some conditions, a physician may be concerned about a lab value that lies within the reference range because of the patient's particular situation. In other cases, a physician may not be concerned about a value flagged as high or low.

Results of microbiology cultures report the concentration and type of organism.

Surgical pathology reports provide a narrative description of the specimen and the pathologist's diagnosis.

Clinical Laboratory Improvement Amendments

Congress passed the **Clinical Laboratory Improvement Amendments (CLIA)** in 1988 to establish quality standards for all laboratory testing to ensure the accuracy, reliability, and timeliness of patient test results regardless of where the test was performed. CLIA is administered by the Centers for Medicare and Medicaid Services (CMS), Survey and Certification Group, Division of Laboratory Services. CLIA requires all facilities that perform even one test for the diagnosis, prevention, or treatment of human disease, including waived tests, to meet certain federal requirements. If a facility performs tests for these purposes, it is considered a laboratory under CLIA and must apply and obtain from the CLIA program a certificate that corresponds to the complexity of tests performed. Five types of certificates are available under CLIA, with the most common being the Certificate of Compliance, Certificate of Waiver, and Certificate for Provider-Performed Microscopy Procedures.

Certificate of Compliance

A **Certificate of Compliance (COC)** is issued to a laboratory that performs nonwaived—moderate and high complexity—testing. The State Department of Health conducts an inspection and determines that the laboratory is compliant with all applicable CLIA requirements. Labs with a CLIA COC are issued an individual CLIA number that identifies the lab.

Certificate of Waiver

Approximately 40 low-complexity lab tests are approved for a CLIA waiver. CLIA-waived lab tests do not require a trained lab technician or technologist to review and analyze them, such as a urine pregnancy test. If the lab or POL performs only waived tests, then it can obtain a CLIA **Certificate of Waiver (COW)** instead of a COC. The POL must complete an application and pay a Certificate of Waiver fee every two years.

The U.S. Department of Health and Human Services publishes the list of CLIA-waived tests on its website. For some waived tests, Medicare requires providers to append modifier **-QW CLIA-waived test** to the CPT code or to the HCPCS code. There are a limited number of HCPCS codes for lab services, beginning with the letter **G**, which Medicare requires providers to submit instead of a CPT code. Refer to the CMS website, where you can find more information about waived tests, including those that require HCPCS codes and modifier **-QW**.

Certificate for Provider-Performed Microscopy Procedures

Provider-performed microscopy procedures (PPMPs) are moderate-complexity tests that require use of a microscope. The test must be performed during a patient visit on a specimen obtained from the provider's patient or a patient of the group practice. Examples include urinalysis with microscopy, pinworm examinations, semen analysis, and nasal smears for eosinophils.

CODING PRACTICE

Exercise 48.1 Pathology and Laboratory Procedure Basics

Instructions: Use your medical terminology skills and resources to define the following procedures, then identify the applicable code or code range. Follow these steps:

- Use slash marks "/" to break down the underlined term into its root(s) and suffix.
- Define the meaning of the underlined word based on the meaning of each word part.
- **Look up the Main Term *Pathology and Laboratory* in the CPT Index.**
- Use the entire phrase as the first- and second-level modifying terms and identify the code or code range shown in the CPT Index.

Meaning *measurement of cells*
(Look up the Main Term *Pathology and Laboratory*,
then the first-level modifying term *flow cytometry*)

Example: flow cytometry cyto/metry   CPT Code *88182-88189*

1. microorganism identification, by virus isolation   Meaning _____   CPT Code _____

2. postmortem   Meaning _____   CPT Code _____

3. spectrometry, mass, qualitative   Meaning _____   CPT Code _____

4. surgical pathology, decalcification procedure   Meaning _____   CPT Code _____

5. chemistry, chromatography   Meaning _____   CPT Code _____

6. radioimmunoassay   Meaning _____   CPT Code _____

7. transfusion medicine, leukocyte transfusion   Meaning _____   CPT Code _____

8. sperm, cryopreservation   Meaning _____   CPT Code _____

9. white blood cell, phagocytosis   Meaning _____   CPT Code _____

10. surgical pathology, immunocytochemistry   Meaning _____   CPT Code _____

CODING OVERVIEW OF PATHOLOGY AND LABORATORY PROCEDURES

The CPT section **Pathology and Laboratory Services (80047-89398)** contains 21 subsections that are divided by the type of procedure (■ TABLE 48-3). Review the subheading and category names and code ranges listed in the Pathology and Laboratory Services section to become familiar with the content and organization. Some editions of the CPT manual provide a summary list of the subheadings and categories at the beginning of the section, and also displays an asterisk (*) next to categories that contain special coding instructions.

On claims, procedures represented by CPT codes in the Pathology and Laboratory section must be linked with diagnosis codes that support the medical necessity of the procedure. Diagnosis codes may come from any ICD-10-CM chapter.

CPT provides brief guidelines at the beginning of the Pathology and Laboratory section that address the provider of services, separate or multiple procedures, unlisted procedures, and special reports. Special instructions provide definitions and coding guidelines at the beginning of many subsections and categories.

Instructional notes appear throughout the Tabular List to alert coders to the need for modifiers, provide cross-references to codes for similar procedures on other sites, identify when additional codes for radiological services might be needed, and highlight resequenced and recently deleted codes.

Diagnosis Coding Based on Laboratory Results

Coders need to understand how to use laboratory results to assign diagnosis codes for the patient's encounter. Although the pathologist who supervises the test and interprets the results provides a diagnosis, the referring or ordering physician must make the final diagnosis based on the full picture of the patient's health history, symptoms, medical conditions, and any other tests or procedures yet to be completed. Coders should not assign diagnosis codes based solely on the lab report, even when the results are clearly stated as abnormal.

The referring or ordering physician must confirm the clinical significance of an abnormal result before it can be assigned as a diagnosis code (ICD-10-CM OGCR III.B).

Diagnosis coding rules differ between inpatient and outpatient. The Uniform Hospital Data Discharge Set (UHDDS) defines the principal diagnosis for inpatient encounters as the one **established after study**, including after all test results are known (OGCR II). Inpatient coders must hold the patient's claim until lab results are released and confirmed to assign the diagnosis.

Outpatient coders can code the claim based on the information known at the time of billing. They can use the symptoms or ordering diagnosis on the claim if lab results are not available at the time of billing. They do not need to provide an update to the insurance company after lab results are available and confirmed (OGCR IV.K).

However, if there is reason to suspect that the claim could be denied or delayed by the payer pending lab results, it is best to wait until after lab results are available to send the outpatient claim. When a malignancy is suspected, outpatient coders should hold the claim until the malignancy is confirmed because some procedures, such as the excision of lesions, have separate CPT codes for malignant and benign lesions, with different payment rates.

When lab results are abnormal and confirmed as such by the ordering physician but a definitive diagnosis cannot be established, assign a code for abnormal test results. To locate the appropriate code, search the ICD-10-CM Index for the Main Term entry **Findings, abnormal, inconclusive, without diagnosis** and a subterm for the type of test or specimen, such as **Papanicolaou cervix** or **urine**. Locate any additional subterms needed to fully describe the result.

When the purpose of the encounter is a routine medical examination, such as those reported with ICD-10-CM categories **Z00** and **Z01**, separate codes for each type of examination are provided based on whether there are abnormal findings. An instructional note directs coders to **Use additional code to identify abnormal findings**.

Table 48-3 ■ **PATHOLOGY AND LABORATORY SUBHEADINGS**

Subsections	Code Range	Description
Organ or Disease-Oriented Panels	80047-80076	A group of tests performed at the same time for the same patient. All tests in the panel must be performed to report the code.
Drug Assay	80300-80377	**Qualitative tests** (*detection of the presence of a substance in the specimen*) and **quantitative tests** (*analysis of the amount of a substance in the specimen*) for drug classes and specific drugs
Therapeutic Drug Assay	80150-80299	Quantitative tests for the amount of a prescribed drug present in the specimen
Evocative/Suppression Testing	80400-80439	Administration of a pharmaceutical agent to test the body's response to the agent compared with normal bodily responses
Consultations (Clinical Pathology)	80500-80502	Analysis of a specimen by a pathologist, based on a request by another physician, including a written report of the pathologist's medical interpretation of the findings
Urinalysis	81000-81099	Tests on a urine specimen to identify abnormalities; may or may not include use of a microscope
Molecular Pathology	81161-81479	Medical laboratory procedures involving analyses of nucleic acid to detect variants in genes that may be indicative of germline (e.g., constitutional disorders) or somatic (e.g., neoplasia) conditions, or to test for histocompatibility antigens. Genes are described using Human Genome Organization (HUGO)–approved gene names and are italicized in the code descriptors.
Multianalyte Assays with Algorithmic Analyses (MAAA)	81500-81599	Procedures that utilize multiple results from assays of various types, and possibly patient information, to perform algorithmic (*structured step-by-step*) analysis that is reported typically as a numeric score or probability about treatment options or disease outcomes
Chemistry	82009-84999	Quantitative tests for numerous analytes on a wide variety of specimens; also includes a limited number of qualitative tests which are described as such
Hematology and Coagulation	85002-85999	Tests to determine the number or behavior of various types of blood cells
Immunology	86000-86849	Qualitative and quantitative tests on antigens, allergens, and antibodies
Transfusion Medicine	86850-86999	Testing, treatment, and separation of blood products in preparation for a blood transfusion
Microbiology	87003-87999	Testing for and identification of bacteria, fungi, parasites, and viruses in various types of specimens
Anatomic Pathology	88000-88099	Autopsy; a postmortem examination of a cadaver to determine the cause of death, the victim's overall health at the time of death, circumstances surrounding the death, and whether medical treatment or neglect contributed to the death
Cytopathology	88104-88199	Examination of cells from anywhere in the body to detect various conditions and determine whether neoplasms are benign or malignant
Cytogenetic Studies	88230-88299	Tests involving the structure and function of cells, such as analysis of chromosomes, which carry genetic material and hereditary traits
Surgical Pathology	88300-88399	**Gross** (*viewing with the naked eye*) and/or microscopic examination of a specimen removed from a patient during a procedure
In Vivo (e.g., Transcutaneous) Laboratory Procedures	88720-88749	Tests to measure bilirubin and hemoglobin transcutaneously (*through unbroken skin*), most often performed on neonates to avoid painful blood draws
Other Procedures	89049-89240	A miscellaneous group of tests not readily classified in other subsections, such as leukocyte assessment on a fecal specimen; nasal smear for eosinophils (*white blood cells*); sweat collection, to assess whether the patient has elevated chloride and sodium ions in the sweat, which indicates cystic fibrosis (CF); and meat fibers in feces, to determine whether the body properly digests food
Reproductive Medicine Procedures	89250-89398	Testing and preparation for in vitro fertilization (IVF) or intrauterine insemination; testing on sperm, semen, oocytes, and embryos to identify disorders; and cryopreservation and thawing.

Source: © PB Resources, Inc. Used with permission. CPT codes only © American Medical Association.

Table 48-4 ■ KEY CRITERIA FOR ABSTRACTING PATHOLOGY AND LABORATORY PROCEDURES

❏ What is the referring or ordering diagnosis?

❏ What specimen is tested or examined?

❏ How many specimens are submitted?

❏ How many tests or examinations are performed?

❏ What type of test(s) or examination(s) is performed?

❏ Is the test qualitative or quantitative?

❏ What type of equipment is used (e.g., microscope, automated, nonautomated)?

❏ Are any panel tests performed? Are all tests in the code description performed?

❏ What testing method is used?

❏ What constituents or analytes are tested?

❏ Is only the professional component provided?

❏ Is the physician billing on behalf of an outside laboratory?

❏ Is the laboratory test repeated on the same day?

❏ Is the service a CLIA-waived test?

Source: © PB Resources, Inc. Used with permission.

ABSTRACTING PROCEDURES FOR PATHOLOGY AND LABORATORY

Abstracting for pathology and laboratory tests varies widely based on the type of test. In informal discussion, people make general references to tests such a glucose test, strep test, or urinalysis. However, each of these has several distinct CPT codes based on the details of how it is performed. Refer to ■ TABLE 48-4 for guidance on how to abstract Pathology and Laboratory procedures, then work through the detailed example that follows. Remember that the abstracting questions are a guide and that not every question applies to, or can be answered for, every case. For example, the type of equipment is not a factor for all tests.

Guided Example of Abstracting Pathology and Laboratory Procedures

Refer to the following example throughout this chapter to practice skills for abstracting, assigning, and arranging Pathology and Laboratory codes.

HOSPITAL LABORATORY   Gender: M   Age: 62

Ordering diagnosis: Previous aldosterone (*a steroid hormone*)/renin ratio (*an enzyme produced by the kidneys*) (ARR) result was high at 30. Probable primary hyperaldosteronism (*overproduction of aldosterone*). Drug-resistant hypertension.

Ordering physician: Endocrinologist

Test ordered: aldosterone suppression evaluation panel performed to confirm primary hyperaldosteronism as the cause for hypertension.

Hospital Lab: Patient was placed in a recumbent position. Specimen was acquired through venipuncture and aldosterone concentration and renin concentrations were performed. Two liters of saline were administered intravenously over 4 hours. A second specimen was acquired through venipuncture after 4 hours (*to determine whether the saline infusion lowered the aldosterone level to a normal level, which makes a diagnosis of primary hyperaldosteronism unlikely. BP and HR monitored throughout*).

Results: 0:00 hr aldosterone 22 ng/dL; 4:00 hr aldosterone 20 ng/dL; not a significant reduction

---

Follow along as fictitious coder, Teresa Lee, CCS, abstracts the procedure. Check off each step after you complete it.

▶ Teresa reads through the entire record, paying special attention to the ordering diagnosis and the lab tests performed. She refers to the Key Criteria for Abstracting Pathology and Laboratory Procedures (Table 48-4).

❏ She determines that the referring diagnosis for the lab test is aldosterone/renin ratio (ARR) result was high. Although probable primary hyperaldosteronism is indicated as the reason the test is ordered, an uncertain or probable diagnosis cannot be used as the first-listed diagnosis on an outpatient claim.

❏ *What specimen is tested or examined?* Blood

❏ *How many specimens are obtained?* Two serum samples are obtained: one for a baseline and a second one after the infusion of the agent (saline).

❏ *How many tests or examinations are performed?* One panel

❏ *What type of test(s) or examination(s) is performed?* aldosterone suppression evaluation panel

❏ *Are any panel tests performed?* Yes. *Are all tests in the code description performed?* Two aldosterone tests and two renin tests are performed. Teresa will need to compare the individual tests to the code description when assigning codes to determine whether all components of the panel were performed.

❏ *What constituents or analytes are tested?* aldosterone and renin

❏ *Is only the professional component provided?* No.

❏ *Is the physician billing on behalf of an outside laboratory?* No.

▶ At this time, Teresa does not know which of these procedures may need to be coded, nor how many codes she will end up with. She will learn about this when she moves on to assigning codes.

CODING PRACTICE

Exercise 48.2 Abstracting Procedures for Pathology and Laboratory

Instructions: Read the mini-medical-record of each patient's encounter and answer the abstracting questions. Write the answer on the line provided. Do not assign any codes.

1. HOSPITAL LABORATORY Gender: F Age: 20

Ordering physician: Primary care

Referring diagnosis: yellowish vaginal discharge with a foul odor

Specimen received: 2 slides with vaginal discharge

Tests: chlamydia culture, *Neisseria* gonorrhea immunoassay with direct optical observation

Results: positive for chlamydia, negative for gonorrhea

a. What is the referring or ordering diagnosis?

_____

b. What specimen is tested or examined?

_____

c. How many specimens are submitted?

_____

d. How many tests or examinations are performed?

_____

e. What type of test(s) or examination(s) is performed?

_____

f. What testing method is used?

_____

g. What constituents or analytes are tested?

_____

2. HOSPITAL LABORATORY Gender: F Age: 37

Ordering physician: Surgical oncologist

Referring diagnosis: lung lesion, smoker, intraoperative frozen section, consultation requested

Specimen received: Lung, wedge biopsy right lower lobe

Gross description: 1-cm-diameter tissue

Microscopic description: invasion of the overlying pleura with free resection margin

Results/findings: Adenocarcinoma, grade 2; called results up to operating suite

a. What is the referring or ordering diagnosis?

_____

b. What specimen is tested or examined?

_____

(continued)

2. (continued)

c. How many specimens are submitted?

_____

d. How many tests or examinations are performed?

_____

e. What type of test(s) or examination(s) is performed?

_____

f. What type of equipment is used?

_____

3. HOSPITAL LABORATORY Gender: M Age: 68

Ordering physician: Cardiologist

Referring diagnosis: HTN, CHF

Specimen received: venous blood

Tests: Therapeutic drug assay for total digoxin level

Results: Value: 0.4 Reference Range: 0.5–0.8 ng/mL Flag: Low

a. What is the referring or ordering diagnosis?

_____

b. What specimen is tested or examined?

_____

c. How many specimens are submitted?

_____

d. How many tests or examinations are performed?

_____

e. What type of test(s) or examination(s) is performed?

_____

f. Is the test qualitative or quantitative?

_____

g. What testing method is used?

_____

h. What constituents or analytes are tested?

_____

4. OFFICE Gender: F Age: 28

Gravida: 1 Para: 0 EGA: 10 weeks

Reason for encounter: prenatal care

Assessment: routine prenatal visit that will be part of the patient's total OB package

Office procedure: venipuncture for OB panel (3 tubes)

(continued)

4. (continued)

Hospital lab procedure: CBC automated; automated differential WBC count; hepatitis B surface antigen (HBsAg); antibody rubella; syphilis test, nontreponemal antibody, qualitative; antibody screen, RBC; blood typing, ABO; blood typing, Rh (D)

a. What is the referring or ordering diagnosis?

_____

b. What specimen is tested or examined?

_____

c. How many specimens are submitted?

_____

d. How many tests or examinations are performed?

_____

e. What type of test(s) or examination(s) is performed?

_____

f. Are any panels performed? _____ Are all tests in the code description performed? _____

g. What antigens are tested for?

_____

h. What antibodies are tested for?

_____

i. Is the physician billing on behalf of an outside laboratory?

_____

5. OFFICE   Gender: F   Age: 71

Diagnosis: atrial fibrillation, long-term use of warfarin

Office procedure: venipuncture for PT/PTT

Hospital lab procedure: Prothrombin time (PT); partial thromboplastin time (PTT) (1 tube)

Results: PT/INR: Value: 2.5 Reference Range: 2.0–3.0 INR Flag: None

PTT: Value: 60 Reference Range: 60–70 seconds Flag: None

a. What is the referring or ordering diagnosis?

_____

b. What specimen is tested or examined?

_____

c. How many specimens are submitted?

_____

d. How many tests or examinations are performed?

_____

e. What type of test(s) or examination(s) is performed?

_____

f. Is the physician billing on behalf of an outside laboratory? _____

6. OFFICE   Gender: F   Age: 25

Reason for encounter: urinary frequency and dysuria

Assessment: expanded problem-focused history, problem-focused examination, and low-complexity medical decision making

Office procedure: urinalysis using the dip stick method, nonautomated, no microscopy

Finding: leukocytes, nitrates, and a small amount of blood are present

Diagnosis: urinary tract infection

a. What is the referring or ordering diagnosis?

_____

b. What specimen is tested or examined?

_____

c. How many specimens are submitted?

_____

d. How many tests or examinations are performed?

_____

e. What type of test(s) or examination(s) is performed?

_____

f. Is the test qualitative or quantitative?

_____

g. What testing method is used?

_____

h. What equipment is used?

_____

i. Is the physician billing on behalf of an outside laboratory? _____

j. Was an E/M service provided at the same encounter?

_____

ASSIGNING CODES FOR PATHOLOGY AND LABORATORY PROCEDURES

Most laboratory procedures can be located in the CPT Index under the Main Term **Pathology and Laboratory**, then a first-level modifying term that corresponds to the Tabular List subsection, such as **Chemistry** or **Cytopathology**, then a second-level modifying term for the type of test. The Index provides numerous cross-references to other Main Terms, such as **Blood Test, Cell Count, See Blood Cell Count.** Many lab tests also can be located by searching the Index for one of the following types of Main Terms:

- Name of the test: blood test, blood cell count, occult blood, drug assay, urinalysis
- Analyte: substance tested for: glucose, lipoprotein, iron, insulin
- Type of specimen: bone marrow smear, tissue culture
- Method of testing: fine-needle aspiration, microbiology

When verifying codes in the Tabular List, confirm not only that the analyte is correct but also that the specimen and method of testing are accurate.

Assigning Codes for Specimen Collection

To assign codes for the collection of specimens, search the Index for the Main Term **Collection and Processing**, then select one of the following first-level modifying terms: **Brushings**, **Specimen**, **Stem Cells**, or **Washings**. Codes for blood specimens, sweat, sputum, tears, duodenum, and stomach appear under the first-level modifying term **Specimen**.

Most codes for specimen collection appear within the CPT Surgery section and the subsection for the body system. For example, codes for blood draws appear in the CPT Surgery section and the Cardiovascular subsection. A few codes for specimen collection, such as those for sputum and sweat, appear in the Pathology and Laboratory section. Codes for specimen collection also can be located by searching the Index for the Main Term of the anatomic site. ■ TABLE 48-5 shows alternative ways to locate codes for blood draws.

Some payers do not reimburse separately for a blood draw when a patient has an E/M service during the same encounter because they bundle the blood draw into the E/M service. To clarify that the blood draw is a separate and distinct service from the E/M service, append modifier **-25 Significant, separately identifiable evaluation and management service by the same physician or other qualified health care professional on the same day of the procedure or other service** to the E/M code.

Offices can also assign code **99000 Handling and/or conveyance of specimen for transfer from the physician's office to a laboratory** to show that they prepared and sent a blood specimen to an outside lab, including labeling and packaging. To locate this code, search the Index for the Main Term **Handling** and the first-level modifying term **Specimen transport.** Some payers do not pay separately for this service and may bundle it into other services the patient receives. Others pay for this service only when the specimen is blood.

Table 48-5 ■ LOCATING CODES FOR COLLECTION OF BLOOD SPECIMENS

Code	Description	Index Entry
36415	Collection of venous blood by venipuncture	Main Term: Venipuncture First-level modifying terms: Child/Adult, Infant, or Routine
36416	Collection of capillary blood specimen (e.g., finger, heel, ear stick)	Main Term: Finger First-level modifying term: Blood specimen, finger stick Main Term: Heel First-level modifying term: Stick, for collection of blood Main Term: Ear First-level modifying term: Collection of blood
36600	Arterial puncture, withdrawal of blood for diagnosis	Main Term: Arterial Puncture First-level modifying term: for Diagnosis Main Term: Puncture Modifying terms: Artery, Diagnosis

Source: © PB Resources, Inc. Used with permission. CPT codes only © American Medical Association.

Assigning Codes for Urinalysis

To assign codes for urinalysis, search the Index for the Main Term **Urinalysis**, then select the appropriate first-level modifying term for the type of procedure. CPT provides four codes for **urinalysis by dipstick or tablet reagent (81000-81003)**. This type of procedure tests for any or all of the constituents bilirubin, glucose, hemoglobin, ketones, leukocytes, nitrite, pH, protein, specific gravity, and urobilinogen. In the Tabular List, these codes are divided based on whether the test is automated or nonautomated and whether microscopy is used. Code **81002** identifies **non-automated, without microscopy** and is often referred to as routine urinalysis.

Assigning Codes for Drug Assays

A drug assay determines the presence (qualitative) and amount (quantitative) of a drug in a specimen such as urine, blood, sputum, or hair. Procedures include presumptive drug class screening, definitive drug testing, and therapeutic drug assays (TDAs). CPT provides extensive guidelines and definitions for these codes, which begin with **80300**. In the Tabular List, codes **80300-80377** appear out of numerical sequence, after code **80076** and before code **80150**.

Presumptive drug class screening procedures are qualitative tests that identify the possible use or nonuse of a drug or drug class. CPT provides two lists of drug classes, **Drug class list A** and **Drug class list B**, which are reported with separate CPT codes for presumptive testing. After the presence of a drug or drug class has been identified with presumptive screening, definitive drug testing can also be performed (■ FIGURE 48-3).

The laboratory performed a presumptive drug class screening for oxycodone, a Drug Class List A substance using a non-TLC method. The test gave a positive result for the presence of the drug, so then a quantitative definitive drug test was performed.

80300 Drug screen, any number of drug classes from Drug Class List A; any number of non-TLC devices or procedures, (eg, immunoassay) capable of being read by direct optical observation, including instrumented-assisted when performed (eg, dipsticks, cups, cards, cartridges), per date of service
80365 Oxycodone

Figure 48-3 ■ Example of Coding Drug Assays. *Source: © PB Resources, Inc. Used with permission. CPT codes only © American Medical Association.*

Definitive drug testing identifies the individual drugs present in the sample using qualitative, quantitative, or semiquantitative methods. Codes are divided by drug class and the number of analytes reported. The Tabular List provides a table, *Definitive Drug Classes Listing*, that identifies the codes, classes, and individual drugs for each. Codes are reported once per date of service.

To locate codes for drug assays, search the Index for the Main Term **Drug Assay** and the first-level modifying term **Drug Procedure**. For presumptive drug class screening, select the third-level modifying term **Presumptive Drug Class**, then **Drug Class List A** or **Drug Class List B** and the name of the drug or drug class. For definitive drug testing, select the third-level modifying term **Definitive Drug Class** and the name of the drug class. Turn to the Tabular List to verify the code and make any additional code selections.

A **therapeutic drug assay** is performed to monitor a known, prescribed medication so the physician can evaluate how it is affecting the patient. Codes are divided by the name of the drug. To locate codes for therapeutic drug assays, search the Index for the Main Term **Therapeutic Drug Assay** and the first-level modifying term for the name of the drug. Verify the code in the Tabular List.

SUCCESS STEP

Always check for the annual code updates. The subsection **Drug Assays** is an example of a CPT subsection that was completely revised and updated in 2015. All existing codes were deleted; new codes with new organization and logic were added. New guidelines, tables, and definitions were added. After such a drastic change, it can take physicians and payers a while to become clear and comfortable about how new codes and guidelines should be implemented.

Assigning Codes for Rapid Strep Tests

Physician offices often perform what is known as a **rapid strep test (RST)**, which produces results within 10 to 20 minutes. This is in contrast to a throat culture, which requires several days to produce a result. An RST detects the group A *Streptococcus* (GAS) antigen from throat swabs and is used as an aid in the diagnosis of GAS infection, which typically causes strep throat, tonsillitis, and scarlet fever. Kits are supplied by several manufacturers. The clinician swabs the throat and tonsils to collect a sample of mucus from the infected area for testing. The mucus sample is then exposed to a reagent containing antibodies that bind specifically to a GAS antigen. Clinicians then use **direct optical observation** (*looking at the results with the naked eye*) to identify a specific feature—such as a color change—that indicates a positive result and the presence of the GAS bacteria. The test is reported with code **87880 Infectious agent antigen detection by immunoassay with direct optical observation; Streptococcus, Group A**.

Rapid stress test is not a Main Term in the CPT Index. To locate the code, search the Index for the Main Term **Pathology and Laboratory**, the first-level modifying term **Streptococcus, Group A**, and the second-level modifying term **Direct optical observation**.

CODING CAUTION

RST is an informal way of referring to a test and is not an official CPT code description. Some offices may use other methods to perform a strep test, so always confirm the exact test that is being performed when the physician reports an RST.

Assigning Codes for Surgical Pathology

Surgical pathology is the gross and microscopic examination of tissue specimens removed during surgery. The purpose is to identify any abnormalities or malignancies to aid in the diagnosis of disease. After examining the specimen, the pathologist writes a report describing the appearance of the tissue and the findings.

To assign codes for surgical pathology, search the Index for the Main Term **Pathology and Laboratory**, the first-level modifying term **Surgical pathology**, and the second-level modifying term **Gross and micro exam**. The third-level modifying terms list codes for **Level II** through **Level VI**. Refer to the second-level modifying term **Gross Exam, Level I, 88300** if the examination was gross, with no microscopic examination. Although experienced coders may know the level needed for a particular specimen, new coders and those coding for less common specimens may not know the level and must refer to the Tabular List to select the appropriate code.

The Tabular List organizes codes **88302-88309** for Level II through Level VI examinations based on the type of specimen, with the higher levels reflecting more difficult examinations. Under each code description, the names of the specimens appear in alphabetical order. Review the list of specimens under each code until you find the correct one. Some specimens appear under more than one level, with an indication of the purpose of the procedure. For example, an appendix from an incidental appendicectomy appears under code **88302 Level II**, whereas an appendix, other than incidental—such as an abscessed appendix—appears under code **88304 Level III**. Until coders are very familiar with the surgical pathology codes, they must review each specimen list under each code to be sure they have identified the correct level of examination.

■ FIGURE 48-4 provides an alphabetical crosswalk of specimens corresponding to the surgical pathology level. This tool is an aid to navigating these codes and understanding how they are organized, but all code choices should be verified in the Tabular List.

Specimen: Level

Abortion, induced: III

Abortion, spontaneous/ missed: IV

Abscess: III

Adrenal, resection: V

Aneurysm, arterial/ventricular: III

Anus, tag: III

Appendix incidental: II

Appendix, not incidental: III

Artery, atheromatous plaque: III

Artery, biopsy: IV

Bartholin's gland cyst: III

Bone, biopsy/curettings: V

Bone, exostosis: IV

Bone, fragment(s), other than
   pathologic fracture: III

Bone, fragment(s), pathologic
   fracture: V

Bone, marrow, biopsy: IV

Bone, resection: VI

Brain, biopsy: V

Brain/meninges, other than for
   tumor: IV

Brain/meninges, tumor: V

Breast, biopsy, not requiring
   microscopic evaluation of surgical
   margins: IV

Breast, excision of lesion, with
   microscopic evaluation of surgical
   margins: V

Breast, mastectomy, partial/simple: V

Breast, mastectomy, with regional
   lymph nodes: VI

Breast, reduction mammoplasty: IV

Bronchus, biopsy: IV

Bursa/synovial cyst: III

Carpal tunnel tissue: III

Cartilage, shavings: III

Cell block, any source: IV

Cervix, biopsy: IV

Cervix, conization: V

Cholesteatoma: III

Colon, biopsy: IV

Colon, colostomy stoma: III

Colon, segmental for tumor: VI

Colon, segmental resection, other than
   for tumor: V

Colon, total resection: VI

Conjunctiva, biopsy/ pterygium: III

Cornea: III

Diverticulum, esophagus/small
   intestine: III

Duodenum, biopsy: IV

Dupuytren contract tissue: III

Endocervix, curettings/biopsy: IV

Endometrium, curettings/ biopsy: IV

Esophagus, biopsy: IV

Esophagus, partial/total: VI

Extremity, amputation, non-traumatic: V

Extremity, amputation, traumatic: IV

Extremity, disarticulation: VI

Eye, enucleation: V

Fallopian tube, biopsy: IV

Fallopian tube, ectopic pregnancy: IV

Fallopian tube, sterilization: II

Femoral head, fracture: IV

Femoral head, other than fracture: III

Fetus, with dissection: VI

Fingers/toes, amputation,
   non-traumatic: IV

Fingers/toes, amputation, traumatic: II

Fissure/fistula: III

Foreskin, newborn: II

Foreskin, not newborn: III

Gallbladder: III

Ganglion cyst: III

Gingiva/oral mucosa, biopsy: IV

Heart valve: IV

Hematoma: III

Hemorrhoids: III

Hernia sac, any location: II

Hydatid of Morgagni: III

Hydrocele sac Nerve: II

Intervertebral disc: III

Joint, loose body: III

Joint, resection: IV

Kidney, biopsy: IV

Kidney, partial/total nephrectomy: V

Larynx, biopsy: IV

Larynx, partial/total, with regional
   lymph nodes: VI

Larynx, partial/total: V

Leiomyoma, uterine, myomec tomy,
   without uterus: IV

Lip, biopsy/wedge: IV

Liver, biopsy, needle/wedge: V

Liver, partial: V

Lung, total/lobe/segment: VI

Lung, transbronchial biopsy: IV

Lung, wedge biopsy: V

Lymph node, biopsy: IV

Lymph nodes, regional: V

Mediastinum, mass: V

Meniscus: III

Mucocele, salivary: III

Muscle, biopsy: IV

Myocardium, biopsy: V

Nasal mucosa, biopsy: IV

Nasopharynx/oropharynx, biopsy: IV

Nerve, biopsy: IV

Neuroma, Morton's/traumatic: III

Odontogenic tumor: V

Odontogenic/dental cyst: IV

Omentum, biopsy: IV

Ovary with or without tube,
   neoplastic: V

Ovary with or without tube,
   non-neoplastic: IV

Ovary, biopsy/wedge: IV

Pancreas, biopsy: V

Pancreas, total/subtotal: VI

Parathyroid gland: IV

Pericardium, biopsy/tissue: IV

Peritoneum, biopsy: IV

Pilonidal cyst/sinus: III

Pituitary tumor: IV

Placenta, other than third trimester: IV

Placenta, third trimester: V

Pleura, biopsy/tissue: IV

Polyp, cervical/endometrial: IV

Polyp, colorectal: IV

Polyp, stomach/small intest: IV

Polyps, inflammatory, nasal/
   sinusoidal: III

Prostate, except radical: V

Prostate, needle biopsy: IV

Prostate, radical: VI

Prostate, TUR: IV

Salivary gland, biopsy: IV

Salivary gland: V

Sentinel lymph node: V

Sinus, paranasal biopsy: IV

Skin, debridement/cyst/tag: III

Skin, not debridement/cyst/ tag/plastic
   repair: IV

Skin, plastic repair: II

Small intestine, biopsy: IV

Small intestine, for tumor: VI

Small intestine, not tumor: V

Soft tissue, debridement: III

Soft tissue, lipoma: III

Soft tissue, mass (except lipoma)
   biopsy/simple excision: V

Soft tissue, other than tumor/ mass/
   lipoma/debridement: IV

Soft tissue, tumor, extensive: VI

Spermatocele: III

Spleen: IV

Stomach, biopsy: IV

Stomach, subtotal/total for tumor: VI

Stomach, subtotal/total, not for tumor: V

Sympathetic ganglion: II

Synovium: IV

Tendon/tendon sheath: III

Testicular appendage: III

Testis, biopsy: V

Testis, castration: II

Testis, other than tumor/ biopsy/
   castration: IV

Testis, tumor: VI

Thrombus or embolus: III

Thymus, tumor: V

Thyroglossal duct/brachial cleft cyst: IV

Thyroid, total/lobe: V

Tongue, biopsy: IV

Tongue/tonsil, for tumor: VI

Tonsil and/or adenoids: III

Tonsil, biopsy: IV

Trachea, biopsy: IV

Ureter, biopsy: IV

Ureter, resection: V

Urethra, biopsy: IV

Urinary bladder, biopsy: IV

Urinary bladder, partial/total: VI

Urinary bladder, TUR: V

Uterus, with or without tubes and
   ovaries, for prolapse: IV

Uterus, with or without tubes and
   ovaries, neoplastic: VI

Uterus, with or without tubes and
   ovaries, other than neoplastic/
   prolapse: V

Vagina, biopsy: IV

Vaginal mucosa: Incidental: II

Varicocele: III

Vas deferens, other than sterilization: III

Vas deferens, sterilization: II

Vein: Varicosity: III

Vulva, total/subtotal: VI

Vulva/labia, biopsy: IV

Figure 48-4 ■ Crosswalk of Specimens to Surgical Pathology Levels. *Source: © PB Resources, Inc. Used with permission.*

The pathologist receives two specimens that are sent to the lab during surgery. The first specimen is tissue from the right breast. The second specimen is the sentinel lymph node. The pathologist freezes both blocks and takes two sections from the breast tissue and one from the node. After examination, he determines that the breast tissue shows evidence of malignancy and the lymph node is clear. This suggests that the disease has not metastasized. The pathologist calls the operating room with the results and prepares a report.

88331 Pathology consultation during surgery; first tissue block, with frozen section(s), single specimen

88332 Pathology consultation during surgery; each additional tissue block with frozen section(s) (List separately in addition to code for primary procedure)

Figure 48-5 ■ Example of Coding an Intraoperative Consultation. *Source:* © PB Resources, Inc. Used with permission. CPT codes only © American Medical Association.

CPT also provides codes for a pathology consultation during surgery (**88329-88334**). The pathologist examines a specimen while the patient is still in surgery to determine whether the surgeon needs to perform additional procedures. The pathologist may be in the lab or be present in the operating room. The intraoperative consult can include the examination of tissue blocks and cytologic examination.

Pathology consults that involve examination of tissue specimens are coded based on the number of specimens or tissue blocks that are received. When a single specimen is frozen and multiple sections or slices are examined, code for one specimen. When multiple tissue blocks of the same or different sites are submitted, assign a code for each specimen. CPT provides add-on code **88332** to report each additional tissue block (■ FIGURE 48-5). Cytologic examinations are coded based on the number of sites examined, with code **88333** for the initial site and an add-on code (**88334**) for each additional site.

Assigning Codes for Pap Smears

CPT provides several series of codes for reporting Pap smears based on the type of screening and reporting performed. To locate codes for Pap smears, search the Index for the Main Term **Pap Smears**, then the first-level modifying term for the type of reporting system, to be discussed next.

Conventional Pap smears involve scraping cells from the cervix and fixing them on a slide to be evaluated by the lab. Codes are divided based on whether the screening is automated or manual and whether results are reported using the Bethesda System:

- **88147-88148** Automated screening and rescreening, regardless of reporting system
- **88150-88154** Conventional Pap smears using non-Bethesda reporting
- **88164-88167** Conventional Pap smears using the Bethesda System of reporting

Table 48-6 ■ BETHESDA SYSTEM CLASSIFICATION OF ABNORMAL PAP RESULTS

Atypical squamous cells of undetermined significance (ASC-US)

Atypical squamous cells—cannot exclude HSIL (ASC-H)

Low-grade squamous intraepithelial lesion (LGSIL or LSIL)

High-grade squamous intraepithelial lesion (HGSIL or HSIL)

Squamous cell carcinoma

Atypical glandular cells not otherwise specified (AGC-NOS)

Atypical glandular cells, suspicious for AIS or cancer (AGC-neoplastic)

Adenocarcinoma in situ (AIS)

Liquid-based Pap smears are reported using codes **88174-88175**.

The **Bethesda System** is a method of reporting findings from Pap tests that includes the following components:

- A statement of the adequacy of the specimen
- A general categorization of the specimen
- A descriptive diagnosis
- Interpretation of abnormalities using specific nomenclature (■ TABLE 48-6)
- A statement of review and any ancillary testing

Pap smear codes are technical services and describe screening for abnormalities. When the lab finds an abnormal Pap test, a pathologist interprets the slide and provides a diagnosis. Report the professional interpretation with code **88141 Cytopathology, cervical or vaginal (any reporting system), requiring interpretation by physician**.

Medicare and some other payers require the use of HCPCS codes to report Pap tests (■ FIGURE 48-6). Screening Paps are reported by different codes than diagnostic Paps. HCPCS provides multiple codes for professional interpretation, so the technical code must be linked to the appropriate professional. Be aware that Medicare has specific guidelines regarding the diagnoses that are acceptable to justify the need for the test, based on the frequency with which it is done and the risk level of a particular patient for developing cancer. Review Medicare billing guidelines to be sure you understand the rules.

SUCCESS STEP

Cytopathology codes for nongynecological procedures (**88104-88112** and **88160-88162**) include both the technical and professional service. Append modifier **-TC Technical component** or **-26 Professional component** to identify that a provider performed only one part of the service.

Billing for Laboratory Tests

There are several types of providers involved in rendering laboratory-related services and several types of services that can potentially be billed. The physician's office may fulfill one of several roles related to laboratory testing:

- Collection of a specimen that is sent to a lab for testing
- Collection of a specimen that is tested in the office
- Collection of a specimen and billing for the lab services for a test performed by the lab

The physician's office bills for any specimen collection and specimen handling and conveyance. Specimen collection usually consists of venipuncture but could include other methods, such as a tissue biopsy or cell scraping. Collection of specimens by the patient, such as urine samples, are not billed. If an E/M service was provided in addition to the specimen collection, the

physician's office also bills for that. When the physician orders the test but does not collect a specimen, bill only the E/M service. When the only service is specimen collection, do not bill an E/M service.

When the physician's office sends a specimen to an outside lab for testing, the lab usually bills for performing the test. However, some payers—but not Medicare—allow the physician's office to bill for the lab test on behalf of the lab. This arrangement might be done as a convenience to the lab. The physician's office charges the payer the exact amount charged by the lab, then pays the lab that amount. No markup is allowed. The CMS-1500 must be completed in a specific way to identify that the physician is billing for a test performed by an outside lab. Complete Item 20 on the

HCPCS Code	Description	HCPCS Interpretation Code	Corresponding CPT Code	Key
P3000	Screening Papanicolaou smear, cervical or vaginal, up to three smears, by technician under physician supervision	P3001	88150	Technical service
P3001	Screening Papanicolaou smear, cervical or vaginal, up to three smears, requiring interpretation by physician		88141	Professional service
G0123	Screening cytopathology, cervical or vaginal (any reporting system), collected in preservative fluid, automated thin layer preparation, screening by cytotechnologist under physician supervision	G0124	88142	Screening method
G0124	Screening cytopathology, cervical or vaginal (any reporting system), collected in preservative fluid, automated thin layer preparation, requiring interpretation by physician		88141	
G0141	Screening cytopathology smears, cervical or vaginal, performed by automated system, with manual rescreening, requiring interpretation by physician		88141	
G0143	Screening cytopathology, cervical or vaginal (any reporting system), collected in preservative fluid, automated thin layer preparation, with manual screening and rescreening by cytotechnologist under physician supervision	G0124	88143	
G0144	Screening cytopathology, cervical or vaginal (any reporting system), collected in preservative fluid, automated thin layer preparation, with screening by automated system, under physician supervision	G0124	88174	
G0145	Screening cytopathology, cervical or vaginal (any reporting system), collected in preservative fluid, automated thin layer preparation, with screening by automated system and manual rescreening under physician supervision	G0124	88175	
G0147	Screening cytopathology smears, cervical or vaginal, performed by automated system under physician supervision	G0141	88147	
G0148	Screening cytopathology smears, cervical or vaginal, performed by automated system with manual rescreening	G0141	88148	

Figure 48-6 ■ HCPCS Codes for Pap Smears. *Source: © PB Resources, Inc. Used with permission.*

| 14. DATE OF CURRENT ILLNESS, INJURY, or PREGNANCY (LMP) MM DD YY QUAL. | 15. OTHER DATE QUAL. MM DD YY | 16. DATES PATIENT UNABLE TO WORK IN CURRENT OCCUPATION MM DD YY MM DD YY FROM TO |

(CMS-1500 claim form — Items 14–24)

14. DATE OF CURRENT ILLNESS, INJURY, or PREGNANCY (LMP) | 15. OTHER DATE | 16. DATES PATIENT UNABLE TO WORK IN CURRENT OCCUPATION

17. NAME OF REFERRING PROVIDER OR OTHER SOURCE — 17a. | 17b. NPI | 18. HOSPITALIZATION DATES RELATED TO CURRENT SERVICES

19. ADDITIONAL CLAIM INFORMATION (Designated by NUCC) | 20. OUTSIDE LAB? [X] YES [ ] NO — $ CHARGES 11 50

21. DIAGNOSIS OR NATURE OF ILLNESS OR INJURY Relate A-L to service line below (24E) — ICD Ind. 0
A. Z00.00 B. C. D. E. F. G. H. I. J. K. L.
22. RESUBMISSION CODE — ORIGINAL REF. NO.
23. PRIOR AUTHORIZATION NUMBER

24. A. DATE(S) OF SERVICE From MM DD YY To MM DD YY	B. PLACE OF SERVICE	C. EMG	D. PROCEDURES, SERVICES, OR SUPPLIES CPT/HCPCS MODIFIER	E. DIAGNOSIS POINTER	F. $ CHARGES	G. DAYS OR UNITS	H. EPSDT Family Plan	I. ID. QUAL.	J. RENDERING PROVIDER ID. #
1 06 06 YY	11		99396	A	125 00	01		NPI	99 99999999
2 06 06 YY	81		80047 90	A	11 50	01		NPI	99 11111111

Figure 48-7 ■ Example of Completing the CMS-1500 When Physician Office Bills for the Outside Laboratory Service

CMS-1500 (■ FIGURE 48-7) by marking YES and entering the lab charge for the test in the Charges portion. In Item 24, enter the date of service, CPT code, charge, and other information normally required for a charge. In addition, enter charges for any services provided directly by the physician's office.

When the laboratory also collects the specimen, as occurs when the patient travels to a lab collection site for a blood draw, the lab bills for the venipuncture.

When a POL collects the specimen and performs the test, it bills for both services. Enter the date of service, CPT code, charge, and other information in Item 24. Do not complete Item 20.

The supervising pathologist bills for professional supervision and interpretation and, in most cases, appends modifier **-26 Professional component** to the laboratory code.

Refer to ■ TABLE 48-7 for a summary of the services billed by various types of providers.

Table 48-7 ■ LABORATORY-RELATED SERVICES BILLED BY VARIOUS PROVIDER TYPES

Provider Type	Services Billed
Physician office (not billing for an outside laboratory)	E/M service (when provided and separate from the lab draw)
	Venipuncture or other specimen collection
	Handling and conveyance
Physician office laboratory (POL)	E/M service (when provided and separate from the lab draw)
	Venipuncture or other specimen collection
	Conducting the test
Physician office billing for an outside laboratory	E/M service (when provided and separate from the lab draw)
	Venipuncture or other specimen collection
	Handling and conveyance
	Laboratory charges
Laboratory	Conducting the test
Pathologist	Supervision and interpretation of the laboratory test

Source: © PB Resources, Inc. Used with permission.

CODING CAUTION

Always check with payer policies regarding the billing for specimen collection and handling and conveyance. Some payers disallow one or both of these services, especially when provided in conjunction with an E/M service.

Guided Example of Assigning Pathology and Laboratory Procedure Codes

To practice skills for assigning codes for Pathology and Laboratory, continue with the example from earlier in the chapter about a patient who was seen for an aldosterone suppression evaluation panel. Follow along in your CPT manual as Teresa Lee, CCS, assigns codes. Check off each step after you complete it.

▶ First, Teresa confirms the procedure: *aldosterone suppression evaluation panel*.

▶ Teresa searches the Index for the Main Term **Aldosterone**.

❑ She locates the first-level modifying term **Suppression evaluation**.

❑ She identifies the code **80408**.

▶ Teresa verifies code **80408** in the Tabular List.

❑ She reads the code title for **80408: Aldosterone suppression evaluation panel (eg, saline infusion). This panel must include the following: Aldosterone (82088 × 2) Renin (84244 × 2)**.

❑ She identifies that the panel includes four tests, aldosterone ×2 and renin ×2. She confirms in the patient's record that all tests were performed. The first instance of each test was performed as a baseline. After administration of the saline suppression agent, both tests were administered a second time.

▶ Teresa checks for instructions in the Tabular List.

❑ She looks for instructional notes after the code entry and finds none.

❏ She cross-references the beginning of the subsection **Evocative/Suppression Testing** and reads the guidelines. She notices the instructions that state **For the administration of the evocative or suppressive agents, see Hydration, Therapeutic, Prophylactic, Diagnostic Injections and Infusions, and Chemotherapy and Other Highly Complex Drug or Highly Complex Biologic Agent Administration (eg, 96365, 96366, 96367, 96368, 96372, 96374, 96375, 96376).**

❏ This information tells her that because the lab administered a saline infusion, she should code for that in addition to the test.

❏ She cross-references the beginning of the **Pathology and Laboratory** section and verifies that there are no additional guidelines that apply.

▶ Teresa turns to codes **96365** and following in the Tabular List, as indicated in the subsection guidelines, to identify the code for the service Saline IV infusion was administered for 4 hours.

❏ She reads the description for code **96365 Intravenous infusion, for therapy, prophylaxis, or diagnosis (specify substance or drug); initial, up to 1 hour.**

❏ This seems to describe the service provided, but she notices that it reports only one hour, whereas infusion was provided for four hours.

❏ She reads the description for code **96366**, which is an indented add-on code that reports **each additional hour** of IV infusion. She makes a note that she needs to report three occurrences of this code in addition to one occurrence of code **96365** to report the full four hours of infusion.

❏ Codes **96367** and **96368** describe additional time and additional substances, so they do not apply.

❏ Codes **96369-96371** describe subcutaneous infusion, so they do not apply.

❏ Codes **96372-96376** describe injections, so they do not apply.

▶ Next, Teresa assigns a HCPCS code for the saline product.

❏ In the HCPCS manual, she turns to the *Table of Drugs and Biologicals*, then locates the entry for **Saline Solution, Sterile** in the first column.

❏ In the second column, she identifies the unit to be **500 mL** and in the third column, the route as **IV**. She confirms the amount documented in the patient's record to be 2 liters of saline. This means that 4 units were administered because 1 liter is 500 mL, so 500 × 4 = 2000 mL or 2 liters.

❏ She identifies the code listed in the fourth column of the table, **J7040**, and verifies it in the HCPCS Tabular List. The code description states **Infusion, normal saline solution, sterile (500 ml=1 unit).**

▶ Finally, Teresa needs to code for the venipuncture procedures.

❏ She searches the Index for the Main Term **Venipuncture** and the first-level modifying term **Routine**.

❏ She identifies code **36415** and verifies it in the Tabular List. The code description states **Collection of venous blood by venipuncture.**

▶ Teresa reviews the procedure codes she has assigned for this case.

❏ **80408 Aldosterone suppression evaluation panel**

❏ **36415 Collection of venous blood by venipuncture**

❏ **J7040 Infusion, normal saline solution, sterile (500 ml=1 unit)**

❏ **96365 Intravenous infusion, for therapy, prophylaxis, or diagnosis (specify substance or drug); initial, up to 1 hour**

❏ **96366 Intravenous infusion, for therapy, prophylaxis, or diagnosis (specify substance or drug); each additional hour**

▶ Next, Teresa must determine how to sequence the codes.

CODING PRACTICE

Exercise 48.3 Assigning Codes for Pathology and Laboratory Procedures

Instructions: Read the mini-medical-record of each patient's encounter. Review the information abstracted in Exercise 48.2 for questions 1–3. For questions 4–6, abstract the case on your own. Assign CPT codes, quantities, and modifiers using the Index and Tabular List. Write the code(s) on the line provided.

1. HOSPITAL LABORATORY Gender: F Age: 20
Ordering physician: Primary care
(continued)

1. (continued)
Referring diagnosis: yellowish vaginal discharge with a foul odor

Specimen received: 2 slides with vaginal discharge

Tests: chlamydia culture, *Neisseria* gonorrhea immunoassay with direct optical observation

Results: positive for chlamydia, negative for gonorrhea

Tip: The chlamydia culture is a higher-priced test than the *Neisseria* gonorrhea immunoassay.

2 CPT Codes _____

2. HOSPITAL LABORATORY   Gender: F   Age: 37

Ordering physician: Surgical oncologist

Referring diagnosis: lung lesion, smoker, intraoperative frozen section, consultation requested

Specimen received: Lung, wedge biopsy right lower lobe

Gross description: 1-cm-diameter tissue

Microscopic description: invasion of the overlying pleura with free resection margin

Results/findings: Adenocarcinoma, grade 2; called results up to operating suite

Tip: This service is surgical pathology.

1 CPT Code _____

3. HOSPITAL LABORATORY   Gender: M   Age: 68

Ordering physician: Cardiologist

Referring diagnosis: HTN, CHF

Specimen received: blood

Tests: Therapeutic drug assay for total digoxin level

Results: Value: 0.4 Reference Range: 0.5–0.8 ng/mL Flag: Low

1 CPT Code _____

4. HOSPITAL LABORATORY   Gender: F   Age: 18

Ordering physician: Emergency medicine

Referring diagnosis: intoxication

Specimen received: blood

Tests: blood alcohol level by chromatography

Results: reportable at 0.020 g/dL (%)

1 CPT Code _____

5. HOSPITAL LABORATORY   Gender: F   Age: 39

Ordering physician: Gynecologist

Referring diagnosis: vaginal chancres

Specimen received: blood

Test: VDRL, qualitative and quantitative

Results: nonreactive

1 CPT Code _____

6. PATHOLOGY LABORATORY   Gender: F   Age: 62

Ordering physician: Dermatologist

Referring diagnosis: Grover disease

Specimen received: skin of the chest, punch biopsy

Gross description: specimen is 0.4 × 0.4 cm with a depth of 0.6 cm. Submitted in one cassette for microscopic examination.

Microscopic description: focal areas of suprabasal clefting and a few acantholytic cells are seen

Results/findings: Corps ronds and grains are present, consistent with Grover disease.

Tip: Code for the pathologist service.

1 CPT Code _____

ARRANGING CODES FOR PATHOLOGY AND LABORATORY PROCEDURES

In general, codes for laboratory tests are sequenced in descending price or RVU order. Laboratory billing systems sequence codes automatically. When physician offices bill for laboratory tests they are sequenced after any E/M codes and other services because they are usually the lowest-priced service. Codes for lab tests should not be intermixed with codes that require modifier **-51 Multiple procedures** because the multiple procedure payment reduction does not apply. List the lab codes after any services that take modifier **-51** so that the payer does not accidentally apply a payment reduction.

Modifiers

Three unique modifiers are used only for laboratory services: **-90**, **-91**, and HCPCS modifier **-QW**. In addition, modifiers for the professional and technical components, as well as separate procedures, apply to lab services. Some modifiers are discussed earlier in this chapter, so the following information is a summary.

-90 Outside Laboratory

When a physician's office bills for services provided by an outside laboratory, append modifier **-90** to the codes for the lab tests performed by the lab. Do not apply this modifier to any code other than a code for lab tests performed by an outside lab. Do not use this modifier when the physician's office collects the

> Patient presents to the Emergency Department with a headache, nausea and vomiting, and confusion. The physician diagnoses dehydration and orders electrolyte panel, which shows hyponatremia and hypokalemia. Fluids, as well as sodium and potassium, are administered. Later in the day, the physician orders a second electrolyte panel, which confirms that all components have returned to normal levels.
>
> **80051 x 1 Electrolyte panel**
> **80051-91 x 1 Electrolyte panel; -91 Repeat clinical laboratory test**

Figure 48-8 ■ Example of Using Modifier -91. *Source: © PB Resources, Inc. Used with permission. CPT codes only © American Medical Association.*

specimen, sends it to the lab, and the lab bills for the test or when the POL conducts the test.

Remember to complete Item 20 on the CMS-1500 when billing for outside lab services.

-91 Repeat Clinical Laboratory Test

Report modifier **-91 Repeat clinical laboratory test** when the physician orders that the same laboratory test be repeated on the same patient and same day to monitor or manage treatment (■ FIGURE 48-8). The key to using this modifier is the *clinical need* to repeat the test to obtain subsequent results as determined by the physician. Do not use modifier **-91** in the following situations:

- Tests rerun by the lab to confirm initial results
- Testing problems with specimens or equipment
- Any time a normal, one-time, reportable result is all that is required
- Other codes describe a series of test results (e.g., glucose tolerance tests, evocative/suppression testing)

-92 Alternative Laboratory Platform Testing

Modifier **-92 Alternative laboratory platform testing** identifies the use of a kit or transportable instrument that employs a single-use, disposable analytical chamber. This modifier is used with only four codes for HIV testing: **86701, 86702, 86703,** and **87389**. Because the test does not require permanent dedicated space, it can be hand carried or transported to the patient's location. However, the location of the testing does not determine the use of this modifier. Append the modifier to the laboratory procedure code.

-QW CLIA-Waived Test

When billing Medicare, physician offices with a COW must append modifier **-QW** to CLIA-waived tests, including PPM, performed in the office. Refer to the discussion on CLIA earlier in this chapter for details.

-26 Professional Component and -TC Technical Component

A limited number of lab codes, such as surgical pathology and some cytopathology codes, contain both professional and technical components. Append modifier **-26** or **-TC** to identify the component of the service provided by the billing entity. Codes for chemistry, drug assays, microbiology, immunology, evocation/suppression testing, and molecular pathology generally do not separate components. Refer to the Medicare Physician Fee Schedule Database (MPFSDB) to identify codes that accept these modifiers.

-XS Separate Structure and -XU Nonoverlapping Service

Modifier **-XS Separate structure** identifies the same laboratory procedure performed on more than one body site. Examples of this are wound cultures from separate parts of the body or skin biopsies from multiple sites.

Apply modifier **-XU Unusual non-overlapping service** when the same CPT code is used for separate procedures. For example, code **86003 Allergen specific IgE; quantitative or semiquantitative, each allergen** reports allergen testing on multiple allergens. The code description specifies that each occurrence of the code reports one allergen. When multiple allergens are tested—for example, nuts, milk, eggs, and grass—report code **86003** once for each allergen and append modifier **-XU** to the second and subsequent tests.

Guided Example of Arranging Pathology and Laboratory Procedure Codes

To practice skills for arranging codes for Pathology and Laboratory procedures, continue with the example from earlier in the chapter about the patient who was seen for an aldosterone suppression evaluation panel. Follow along in your CPT manual as Teresa Lee, CCS, arranges the codes. Check off each step after you complete it.

▶ First, Teresa confirms the lab test performed: *aldosterone suppression evaluation panel*.

▶ Teresa reviews the procedure codes she has assigned for this case.

❑ **80408 Aldosterone suppression evaluation panel**

❑ **36415 Collection of venous blood by venipuncture**

❑ **J7040 Infusion, normal saline solution, sterile (500 ml=1 unit)**

❑ **96365 Intravenous infusion, for therapy, prophylaxis, or diagnosis (specify substance or drug); initial, up to 1 hour**

❑ **96366 Intravenous infusion, for therapy, prophylaxis, or diagnosis (specify substance or drug); each additional hour**

▶ Teresa determines the quantity for each code.

❑ Although four tests were performed, they are all bundled into one code for aldosterone suppression evaluation panel, so code **80408** is a quantity of 1.

❑ She notes that venipuncture was performed twice, so she assigns a quantity of 2 to code **36415**.

❑ One unit of code **J7040** is 500 mL, and 2 L were administered, so she reports a quantity of 4.

❑ Code **96365** identifies up to one hour of infusion, so the unit of reporting for this code is 1 because less than one hour was required.

▶ Teresa arranges the codes in descending price order according to the payer's fee schedule. No modifiers apply.

▶ Teresa finalizes the procedure codes and sequencing for this case:

(1) **80408 × 1 Aldosterone suppression evaluation panel**

(2) **96365 × 1 Intravenous infusion, for therapy, prophylaxis, or diagnosis (specify substance or drug); initial, up to 1 hour**

(3) **96366 × 3 Intravenous infusion, for therapy, prophylaxis, or diagnosis (specify substance or drug); each additional hour**

(4) **36415 × 2 Collection of venous blood by venipuncture**

(5) **J7040 × 4 Infusion, normal saline solution, sterile (500 ml=1 unit)**

▶ Teresa also assigns and sequences the ICD-10-CM diagnosis codes from the lab requisition that support the need for the service.

(1) **R79.89 Other specified abnormal findings of blood chemistry**

(2) **I10 Essential (primary) hypertension**

CODING PRACTICE

Exercise 48.4 Arranging Codes for Pathology and Laboratory Procedures

Instructions: Read the mini-medical-record of each patient's encounter. Review the information abstracted in Exercise 48.2 for questions 1–3. For questions 4–6, abstract the case on your own. Assign CPT codes, quantities, and modifiers using the Index and Tabular List, and arrange the codes in proper sequence. Write the code(s) on the line provided.

---

1. OFFICE   Gender: F   Age: 28

Gravida: 1   Para: 0   EGA: 10 weeks

Reason for encounter: prenatal care

Assessment: routine prenatal visit that will be part of the patient's total OB package

Office Procedure: venipuncture for OB panel (3 tubes)

Hospital Lab Procedure: CBC automated; automated differential WBC count; hepatitis B surface antigen (HBsAg); antibody rubella; syphilis test, nontreponemal antibody, qualitative; antibody screen, RBC; blood typing, ABO; blood typing, Rh (D)

Tip: Assign codes for the physician's office and the laboratory.

Physician office: 2 CPT Codes _____

Laboratory: 1 CPT Code _____

---

2. OFFICE   Gender: F   Age: 71

Diagnosis: atrial fibrillation, long-term use of warfarin

Office procedure: venipuncture for PT/PTT (1 tube)

Hospital lab procedure: Prothrombin time (PT); partial thromboplastin time (PTT)

(continued)

---

2. (continued)

Results: PT/INR: Value: 2.5 Reference Range: 2.0–3.0 INR Flag: None

PTT: Value: 60 Reference Range: 60–70 seconds Flag: None

Tip: Assign codes for the physician's office and the laboratory. The PTT test is a higher-priced code than the PT test.

Physician office: 2 CPT Codes _____

Laboratory: 2 CPT Codes _____

---

3. OFFICE   Gender: F   Age: 25

Reason for encounter: urinary frequency and dysuria, established patient

Assessment: expanded problem-focused history, problem-focused examination, and low-complexity medical decision making

Office procedure: urinalysis using the dip stick method, nonautomated, no microscopy

Finding: leukocytes, nitrates, and a small amount of blood are present

Diagnosis: urinary tract infection

Tip: Assign an E/M code with the appropriate modifier to indicate that the E/M was provided on the same day as another service or procedure.

2 CPT Codes _____

(continued)

CODING PRACTICE (continued)

4. HOSPITAL LABORATORY Gender: M Age: 2 weeks

Ordering physician: Pediatrician

Referring diagnosis: positive newborn screen for cystic fibrosis

Specimen received: sweat

Tests: sweat stimulation, sweat collection by iontophoresis, and sweat chloride analysis

Results: borderline results at 50 mEq/L

Tip: Sweat specimens are collected in duplicate from two different sites.

2 CPT Codes _____

---

5. HOSPITAL LABORATORY Gender: F Age: 24

Ordering physician: Neurologist

Referring diagnosis: headache, neck stiffness, fever, and altered mental status. Workup for possible bacterial meningitis.

Specimen received: cerebrospinal fluid

Tests: cell count (and differential count) and culture

2 CPT Codes _____

---

6. OUTPATIENT LABORATORY Gender: F Age: 2

Ordering physician: Pediatrician

Referring diagnosis: sickle cell trait

Specimen received: blood

Tests: hemoglobinopathy (Hb) electrophoresis, peripheral blood smear with manual differential

Results: HbA_1: 95%, HbA_2: 2%, HbF: <2%, HbC Absent, HbS Absent. Within normal limits.

2 CPT Codes _____

CHAPTER SUMMARY

In this chapter you learned that:

- Clinical pathology is a medical specialty that is concerned with the diagnosis of disease based on the laboratory analysis of bodily fluids and tissue.

- The CPT section **Pathology and Laboratory Services (80047–89398)** contains 21 subsections that are divided by the type of procedure.

- Abstracting for pathology and laboratory tests varies widely based on the type of test. In informal discussion, people make general references to tests such as a glucose test, strep test, or urinalysis; however, each of these has several distinct CPT codes based on the details of how it is performed.

- Most laboratory procedures can be located in the CPT Index under the Main Term **Pathology and Laboratory**, then a first-level modifying term that corresponds to the Tabular List subsection, such as **Chemistry** or **Cytopathology**, then a second-level modifying term for the type of test. Most procedures are also indexed by the name of the test, analyte, specimen, or testing method.

- Three unique modifiers are used only for laboratory services: -90, -91, and HCPC modifier -QW. In addition, modifiers for the professional and technical components, as well as separate procedures, apply to lab services.

- CPT provides brief guidelines at the beginning of the Pathology and Laboratory section that address the provider of services, separate or multiple procedures, unlisted procedures, and special reports. Special instructions provide definitions and coding guidelines at the beginning of many subsections and categories.

CONCEPT QUIZ

Take a moment to look back at Pathology and Laboratory and solidify your skills. Try to answer the questions from memory first, then refer to the discussion in this chapter if you need a little extra help.

Completion

Instructions: Write the term that answers each question based on the information you learned in this chapter. Choose from the list below. Some choices may be used more than once and some choices may not be used at all.

analyte	immunology
anatomic	in vivo
autopsy	microbiology
chemistry	microscope
cytogenic studies	molecular
cytopathology	qualitative
evocative/suppression testing	quantitative
gross	surgical

1. The _____ description of a pathology report is limited to what can be seen with the naked eye.

2. _____ pathology procedures involve the analysis of nucleic acid to detect variants in genes.

3. _____ is the administration of a pharmaceutical agent to test the body's response to the agent compared with normal bodily responses.

4. A(n) _____ may be used to identify abnormalities in a urine specimen.

5. Tests for identification of bacteria are found in the _____ section of CPT.

6. The _____ portion of a drug assay detects the presence of a substance in the specimen.

7. A(n) _____ is another term for a postmortem exam to determine the cause of death.

8. _____ is the area of laboratory medicine that includes qualitative and quantitative tests on antigens.

9. _____ involves examination of cells from anywhere in the body to determine whether neoplasms are benign or malignant.

10. Both qualitative and quantitative tests on a wide variety of specimens are found in the _____ section of CPT.

Multiple Choice

Instructions: Circle the letter of the best answer to each question based on the information you learned in this chapter.

1. When should modifier –90 be reported?
   A. When the lab test is performed in the office
   B. When the specimen is sent to an outside lab
   C. When the physician office bills for a test sent to an outside lab
   D. When the specimen is collected by the lab

2. Who is eligible for a COW?
   A. Labs that perform moderate- and high-complexity tests
   B. Labs that perform CLIA-waived tests only
   C. Labs that perform only microscopy
   D. Reference labs

3. What modifier should be appended to an E/M code when a venipuncture is performed during the encounter?
   A. –25
   B. –51
   C. –90
   D. –QW

4. How should a lab panel be reported if one test in the panel is not performed?
   A. Report each test code individually
   B. Report the panel code with no modifier
   C. Report the panel code with modifier –52
   D. Do not report any code

5. What Main Term in the CPT Index can be used to locate most lab tests?
   A. Pathology
   B. Laboratory
   C. Test
   D. Findings

6. What is a qualitative test that identifies the possible use or nonuse of a drug or drug class?
   A. Therapeutic drug assay
   B. Presumptive drug class screening
   C. Cytopathology
   D. Definitive drug testing

7. How many units of code *J7040 Infusion, normal saline solution, sterile (500 ml=1 unit)* should be reported for two liters of saline?
   A. 1
   B. 2
   C. 3
   D. 4

8. What is the Bethesda System?
   A. A format required by Medicare for reporting lab results
   B. A testing procedure for abnormal Pap smears
   C. A process for evocation/suppression testing
   D. A method of reporting findings from Pap tests

9. What level of surgical pathology is reported for an abscessed appendix?
   A. Level I
   B. Level II
   C. Level III
   D. Level IV

10. How many tests must be performed to report code *80408 Aldosterone suppression evaluation panel*?
   A. 1
   B. 2
   C. 3
   D. 4

CODING CHALLENGE

Instructions: Read the mini-medical-record of each patient's encounter, then abstract, assign, and arrange ICD-10-CM diagnosis codes, CPT procedure codes, and HCPCS codes using the appropriate Index and Tabular List. Assign quantities and modifiers where needed. Pay special attention to whether you are coding for the physician's office, the pathologist, or the laboratory facility. Write the code(s) on the line provided.

---

1. OFFICE   Gender: F   Age: 24

Reason for encounter: routine prenatal visit of primipara at 26 weeks, 4 days

Assessment: test performed at the office; results within normal limits

Office procedure: glucose tolerance test, three specimens of blood drawn

2 ICD-10-CM Codes _____

1 CPT Code _____

---

2. OUTPATIENT LABORATORY   Gender: M   Age: 89

Ordering physician: Primary care

Referring diagnosis: blood in urine; under treatment for prostate cancer with metastasis to the bladder and spine

Tests: hemoglobin and hematocrit, microscopic urinalysis, coagulation profile (PT, PTT, INR)

Tip: Follow the outpatient coding guidelines for patients receiving diagnostic services only.

4 ICD-10-CM Codes _____
_____

5 CPT Codes _____
_____

---

3. OFFICE   Gender: M   Age: 70

Reason for encounter: bloody stools, weight loss, constipation, and abdominal pain for the past two weeks. Patient is otherwise in good health for his age.

Assessment: positive result for fecal occult blood. Referred to gastroenterologist for colonoscopy.

Office procedure: stool guaiac test

4 ICD-10-CM Codes _____
_____

1 CPT Code _____

---

4. OFFICE   Gender: F   Age: 53

Reason for encounter: complaint of vertigo/generalized dizziness for the past two weeks. This is not usually precipitated by change in position from supine to upright. History of hypertension and paroxysmal atrial fibrillation.

Office procedure: blood drawn to be sent out for TSH level, lipid profile, LFTs, B12 level, and folic acid level

Outpatient laboratory procedure: TSH level, lipid profile, LFTs, B12 level, and folic acid level

Plan: obtain carotid ultrasound and refer to a neurologist

3 ICD-10-CM Codes _____
_____

Physician office: 2 CPT Codes _____

Laboratory: 4 CPT Codes _____
_____

---

5. OUTPATIENT LABORATORY   Gender: M   Age: 21

Ordering physician: General surgeon

Referring diagnosis: nonhealing surgical wound with abscess. The wound is malodorous and has purulent drainage.

Test(s): wound culture to isolate bacteria; culture negative

1 ICD-10-CM Code _____

1 CPT Code _____

---

6. OUTPATIENT LABORATORY   Gender: F   Age: 39

Ordering physician: Rheumatologist

Referring diagnosis: persistent pain and discomfort with swelling of joints of both hands/fingers. Maternal grandmother has rheumatoid arthritis.

Tests: antinuclear antibody (ANA), rheumatoid factor, anti–cyclic citrullinated peptide (anti-CCP) antibodies, C-reactive protein (CRP), erythrocyte sedimentation rate, automated (ESR, or sed rate)

5 ICD-10-CM Codes _____
_____

5 CPT Codes _____
_____

7. PATHOLOGY LABORATORY Gender: M Age: 49

Clinical history: low-density soft-tissue lesion at the nasolabial region seen on CT scan

Specimen received: soft-tissue lesion

Gross description: received in container labeled "nasolabial cyst" is an ovoid, yellowish cyst, measuring 1 cm × 1.8 cm in diameter

Microscopic description: yellowish cyst consistent with an epidermal inclusion cyst

Diagnosis: epidermal inclusion cyst of the nasolabial fold

Tip: Code for the pathologist service.

1 ICD-10-CM Code _____

1 CPT Code _____

8. PATHOLOGY LABORATORY Gender: M Age: 53

Clinical history: patient has chronic hepatitis B. A liver biopsy is being done to determine the stage of fibrosis and grade of inflammation.

Specimen received: liver biopsy

Gross description: the specimen is received in a container labeled "liver biopsy," retrieved with a percutaneous needle. The specimen is 1.5 cm in length and 1 mm in width.

Microscopic description: hematoxylin stain shows stage 4 fibrosis (i.e., cirrhosis). Moderate portal inflammation and lymphocytic necrosis involving all portal tracts, with noticeable lobular inflammation and hepatocellular change consistent with grade 3 liver damage.

Diagnosis: fibrosis (cirrhosis) of the liver due to chronic hepatitis B

Tip: Code for the pathologist service.

2 ICD-10-CM Codes _____

1 CPT Code _____

9. OFFICE Gender: M Age: 45

Reason for Encounter: new patient visit of a 45-year-old male for his annual wellness exam

Assessment: the patient states that he has had multiple sexual partners, both male and female. The rapid HIV test was negative.

Office procedure: rapid HIV-1 immunoassay using a single-use disposable analytical chamber; venipuncture for CBC and BMP for transport to hospital outpatient laboratory

Laboratory procedure: CBC and BMP automated analysis

Tip: This is a new patient being seen for an initial comprehensive preventive medicine visit. Use the appropriate modifier to indicate that the E/M was provided on the same day as another service or procedure. Use of a kit for the immunoassay requires a modifier for alternative laboratory platform testing. Include the HCPCS code for the rapid HIV test kit.

3 ICD-10-CM Codes _____

_____

Physician office: 4 CPT Codes _____

_____

1 HCPCS Code: _____

Laboratory: 2 CPT Codes _____

10. OFFICE Gender: F Age: 45

Reason for encounter: jaundiced appearance and complaint of sluggishness. The patient last seen one year ago.

Assessment: a problem-focused history with straightforward medical decision making and a problem-focused exam were completed

Office procedure: blood specimen drawn and packaged for HBsAb (hepatitis B surface antibody) to be done at the hospital outpatient laboratory

Plan: return to office in 2 weeks to review lab results

2 ICD-10-CM Codes _____

Physician office: 3 CPT Codes _____

_____

Laboratory: 1 CPT Code _____

KEEP ON CODING

Instructions: Read the procedural statement, then use the appropriate Index and Tabular List to assign CPT procedure codes, quantities, and modifiers. Write the code(s) on the line provided.

1. Gross and microscopic examination of left mastectomy with regional lymph nodes: CPT Code(s) _____

2. Lipid panel: total serum cholesterol, HDL, and triglycerides; electrolyte panel: carbon dioxide, chloride, potassium, and sodium: CPT Code(s) _____

3. Nonautomated urinalysis (dip stick), without microscopy: CPT Code(s) _____

4. Quantitative screen for mercury and lead: CPT Code(s) _____

5. Hospital blood bank irradiates two units of leukoreduced red cells: CPT Code(s) _____

6. Physician orders part of a hepatic function panel: serum albumin, total bilirubin, and direct bilirubin: CPT Code(s) _____

7. Pathologist consultation and report on referred slides prepared elsewhere for evaluation of multiple myeloma: CPT Code(s) _____

8. Vancomycin peak and trough levels: CPT Code(s) _____

9. Basic metabolic panel and renal profile, blood sample: CPT Code(s) _____

10. Urine culture and susceptibility with negative urine culture (reflex testing): CPT Code(s) _____

11. Gross and microscopic examination of three lung biopsy tissue samples: CPT Code(s) _____

12. Urine drug screen for cannabis: CPT Code(s) _____

13. Comprehensive metabolic panel: CPT Code(s) _____

14. PT with INR, PTT: CPT Code(s) _____

15. Automated CBC with differential WBC: CPT Code(s) _____

16. Patient underwent two lab tests to determine total bilirubin levels. The first specimen was obtained during the morning and the second in the afternoon on the same day.: CPT Code(s) _____

17. Heel stick of newborn for thyroid-stimulating hormone (TSH): CPT Code(s) _____

18. Preoperative collection of blood for autotransfusion: CPT Code(s) _____

19. Thawing of cryopreserved embryos: CPT Code(s) _____

20. CRP (C-reactive protein test for systemic inflammation) and ANA (antinuclear antibodies): CPT Code(s) _____

21. Analysis of a Pap smear using the Bethesda System; manual screening under physician supervision was performed: CPT Code(s)

_____

22. Amitriptyline level: CPT Code(s) _____

23. Interpretation of bone marrow smear: CPT Code(s) _____

24. Arterial blood gas analysis including pH, PCO_2, PO_2, O_2 saturation, base-excess, bicarbonate, total CO_2, and ventilation status: CPT Code(s) _____

25. Sperm count and motility: CPT Code(s) _____

SECTION FIVE

ICD-10-PCS Procedure Coding

Section Five: ICD-10-PCS Procedure Coding guides you through the steps of hospital procedure coding for each type of procedure. You will learn how to apply the three skills of an "Ace" coder—abstract, assign, and arrange—for a broad variety of patient encounters.

PROFESSIONAL PROFILE

MEET...

Karen Weiss, RHIA, Lead Coder
Avera Queen of Peace Hospital and Health Services

I have been in coding for over 30 years. When I started, healthcare was just rolling out ICD-9-CM. Now, here we are again, rolling out ICD-10-CM/PCS. Hopefully the industry will be able to use what it learned when implementing ICD-9-CM to create a more successful transition to ICD-10-CM/PCS.

My education includes a B.S. in health information administration, and my first coding position began after a one-month management internship with Marion Health Center in Sioux City, Iowa. After learning all of the basic processes and work flow in the department, I was educated in the management of those processes and other departmental responsibilities. Upon receiving my degree, I accepted a coding and abstracting position with Marion Health Center while my husband finished his course studies. Six months later, I accepted a position as Medical Record (Health Information) Department Director at a 120-bed acute care hospital.

In my current position as a Lead Coder, I am responsible for staffing, work flow analysis, auditing, and education. I also assist with inpatient and emergency department coding. I enjoy the variety in coding, because no two patients are alike. I feel like I am helping the patient by being thorough in recording their health history; helping the physician by meeting documentation standards; and helping the hospital by obtaining the maximum accurate reimbursement. The challenges are staying abreast of the multitude of changes in the healthcare industry, educating physicians, and feeling like hospital administration does not always truly understand coders' role and the true impact coders have on facility reimbursement.

My advice to coding students is to learn the Official Guidelines for Coding and Reporting (OGCR); they are the foundation of the coding classification and reimbursement systems. Be able to cite, apply, and communicate those guidelines to other professionals to ensure appropriate documentation to support reimbursement.

The transition to ICD-10-CM/PCS will be difficult and very expensive for hospitals and all affiliated providers. The expense is not only the cost of training and software, but also the loss of productivity. Studies from other countries, which implemented less complex versions of ICD-10 than the United States, reveal that productivity took a significant downturn after implementation and did not return to the same level, even five years later.

This is similar to what we experienced after ICD-9-CM was implemented in 1980, which was followed by the implementation of the inpatient prospective payment system (IPPS) and diagnosis related groups (DRGs) in 1983. The codes were new to us; coding as a profession was not as well defined as it is today; and many coders were not fully trained. Consequently, the data used for rate setting was not accurate and payment rates for inpatient hospital services were severely impacted. It took nearly five years after implementation to get the reimbursement calculations reset to more appropriate levels so that providers were accurately reimbursed for their services. Using what we learned from the previous experience, CMS, AHIMA, and AAPC are guiding providers to undertake appropriate planning and training for ICD-10-CM/PCS well in advance in order to minimize the impacts on productivity and reimbursement.

Chapter 49

Introduction to ICD-10-PCS Procedure Coding

Chapter Outline

- **The Purpose of ICD-10-PCS**
- **ICD-10-PCS Coding Manual Organization**
- **ICD-10-PCS Code Structure**
- **ICD-10-PCS Coding Guidelines**
- **Introduction to the Steps of ICD-10-PCS Procedure Coding**

Learning Objectives

After completing this chapter, you should have the skills to:

49.1 Spell and define the key words, medical terms, and abbreviations related to ICD-10-PCS coding.

49.2 Identify the purpose of ICD-10-PCS.

49.3 Outline the organization of the ICD-10-PCS manual.

49.4 Explain the ICD-10-PCS code structure.

49.5 Discuss ICD-10-PCS Official Guidelines for Coding and Reporting.

49.6 Describe the basic ICD-10-PCS procedure coding process.

Key Terms and Abbreviations

837I
Approach
Body Part
Body System
case-based
character
charge capture
charge description master (CDM)
clinical documentation improvement (CDI)

Completeness
Device
Diagnosis related group (DRG)
DRG grouper
expandability
granular
ICD-10-PCS Official Guidelines for Coding and Reporting (PCS OGCR)

Medicare Severity-adjusted DRGs (MS-DRGs)
multiaxial nature
National Uniform Billing Committee (NUBC)
principal procedure
prospective payment system (PPS)
Qualifier
revenue code

Root Operation
Section
significant procedure
standardized terminology
structural integrity
Table
UB-04
value

In addition to the key terms listed here, students should know the terms defined within tables in this chapter.

For updates and corrections, visit our student resource site at

www.pearsonhighered.com/healthprofessionsresources

INTRODUCTION

When a new interchange opens on a road you are familiar with, it can be confusing and frustrating. The old road got you where you wanted to go, and you probably wish they had left it alone. Now you have to think about a trip that once was automatic. Coding is much the same way. While ICD-10-CM diagnosis coding represents a new interchange, ICD-10-PCS procedure coding is an entirely new road, from the dirt, to the substrate, to the top coat. It is also different from every other coding system that new coders learn, including ICD-10-CM diagnosis coding and CPT coding. However, just as you eventually realize that a new road or new interchange is efficient and faster, you will also appreciate the new procedure coding system's ease, consistency, and logic.

In this chapter, you will learn about why a new inpatient procedure coding system was developed, how it is structured, and how to use it. Most importantly, you will practice locating basic information in the ICD-10-PCS coding manual.

THE PURPOSE OF ICD-10-PCS

ICD-10-PCS (referred to as PCS in this text) is a new coding system used by hospitals for coding inpatient procedures. Unlike ICD-10-CM, which parallels ICD-9-CM in its overall structure, ICD-10-PCS is an entirely new system, designed from scratch, for use in the United States. It was developed to overcome the limitations of other coding systems, with specific goals and usability criteria.

History of the ICD-10-PCS Code Set

Because procedural technology has advanced considerably since ICD-9-CM procedure codes were adopted in 1979, procedure codes are now extremely outdated. In addition, the four-digit format of ICD-9-CM procedure codes limited the total number of codes that could exist and, consequently, limited the ability to add new codes as technology progressed. As a result, in 1992 CMS funded a project to design a complete replacement for ICD-9-CM Volume 3. In 1995, CMS awarded a three-year contract to 3M Health Information Systems (3M) to develop a new inpatient procedure coding system, which was completed in 1998. CMS updates the system annually to incorporate new technologies and procedures. ICD-10-PCS was developed by the United States solely for use in the United States. ICD-10-PCS is not used by other countries.

Characteristics of ICD-10-PCS

The goal in developing ICD-10-PCS was to incorporate several specific attributes (characteristics): completeness, unique definitions, expandability, multiaxial nature, standardized terminology, and structural integrity. Understanding these characteristics helps coders appreciate the benefits of the system.

Completeness

Completeness means that there should be a unique code for every procedure that is significantly different in body part, approach, or method. In ICD-9-CM Volume 3, the same code is sometimes used to describe procedures on different body parts, with different approaches, or different methods, which created confusion due to lack of detail.

Unique Definitions

ICD-10-PCS codes are constructed of seven **characters**, or positions, each with a distinct purpose and meaning. The description of a code is based on the meaning of each value in the code, so the description is unique and cannot change. New codes are created by adding a new value for one of the positions. By design, an entire code cannot be redefined, reused, or resequenced, as can happen in other medical coding systems.

Expandability

Expandability means that the structure of the code set allows new procedures to be easily incorporated. In ICD-9-CM Volume 3, sometimes all of the codes in a specific numeric grouping have already been used, making it impossible to add a new code for a new procedure in the same grouping. New codes were often added in an illogical place, with unrelated codes.

Multiaxial Nature

The **multiaxial nature** of PCS codes means that each position or character within a code number has a designated meaning or purpose. Each position is defined to be used for that meaning for all related codes and, to the extent possible, for all codes in the manual. For example, in the Medical and Surgical Section, the fourth character of the code represents the body part on which the physician performed the procedure. So regardless of the procedure done, or the body system, the fourth character identifies the body part.

Standardized Terminology

Standardized terminology means that the code set includes definitions of the terminology it uses; each term must have only one meaning. This is in contrast to the use, in other coding systems, of eponyms and Latin-based medical terms, both of which can be interpreted with a wide range of meanings. ICD-10-PCS includes English definitions for 31 different types of medical and surgical procedures to ensure consistent reporting. Examples of the benefits of this approach include the following:

- ICD-10-PCS defines the specific meaning of each procedure so that all users apply it in the same way. In CPT and ICD-9-CM, a Latin-based medical term, such as *arthroplasty*, can refer to the repair of a joint, replacement of part of a joint, or replacement of the entire joint. ICD-10-PCS uses common English words to describe procedures, such as **Repair** or **Replacement**, and each has a specific definition. **Repair** is officially defined as *restoring a body part to its normal structure*. **Replacement** is officially defined as *putting in a device that replaces a body part*. Every user of ICD-10-PCS applies these definitions.

- ICD-10-PCS eliminates the use of eponyms to describe procedures. For example, the Whipple procedure, a pancreaticoduodenectomy, is a complex surgical procedure that involves the pancreas, as well as portions of the stomach, duodenum, common bile duct, and gallbladder. The specific organs, and portions of the organs, removed depend on the patient's needs and the surgeon. ICD-9-CM provided one code for the Whipple procedure, regardless of what was done, and CPT provides a limited number of

Table 49-1 ■ **COMPARISON OF ICD-10-PCS AND ICD-10-CM CODE SYSTEMS**

Characteristic	ICD-10-PCS	ICD-10-CM
Developed by	CMS/3M	WHO/CDC
Used by	Inpatient hospitals	All HIPAA entities
Code length	Always 7, no decimal	3 to 7, decimal after 3rd character
7th character requirement	Always required	Sometimes required
7th character name	Qualifier	7th character
Body system characters	Characters are unique to this system. Occupy 2nd character Example: Gastrointestinal = D	Letters are unique to this system. Occupy 1st character Example: Digestive = K
Laterality	Always reported Occupies 4th character	Sometimes reported Occupies 5th or 6th character
Letters not used	O, I	U
Placeholder	Z	X
Combination codes	Not used	Many
Eponyms	Not used	Used

Source: © PB Resources, Inc. Used with permission.

codes. ICD-10-PCS breaks the procedure down into its component parts, with each organ receiving its own code, resulting in as many as five codes to report the procedure. This detail provides accurate and consistent reporting.

- ICD-10-PCS limits the use of combination codes, which describe two or more procedures with a single code. Instead, separate codes are reported for each separate procedure performed. This gives a full and accurate report of exactly what was done for each patient.

Structural Integrity

Structural integrity means that ICD-10-PCS can be expanded easily without disrupting the structure of the system. The values of the seven characters that make up a code can be assigned as needed. The system can evolve as medical technology and clinical practice progress, with much greater room for expansion than other medical coding systems. For example, in CPT, some sections of the book are running out of numbers, requiring that numbers be borrowed from other sections and then be resequenced out of numerical order. This cannot happen in ICD-10-PCS.

A coding system that is internally consistent, logically constructed, and adaptable to new technology enables coders to use it more consistently, resulting in data that is more **granular** (*specific*), reliable (*reported in the same way by all users*), and valid (*accurately describes what it is intended to describe*).

ICD-10-PCS Compared with ICD-10-CM and CPT

Because coders learn and use several coding systems, they must understand the specific differences between them so they can use each system accurately. This is especially important when learning a system such as ICD-10-PCS, which is completely new to the healthcare industry.

ICD-10-CM

Although ICD-10-CM and ICD-10-PCS both carry the name *ICD-10* and have the same implementation date in the United States, the two systems share no features or similarities. ICD-10-CM is used for diagnosis coding and is based on the World Health Organization's ICD-10, which is used internationally, whereas ICD-10-PCS was developed by CMS for hospital inpatient procedure coding and is not based on another system. Both systems use alphanumeric codes, but each has a unique organization, code structure, and guidelines. Refer to ■ Table 49-1 for a summary of differences.

CPT

Although CPT and ICD-10-PCS are both procedure coding systems, they share no features or similarities. CPT was developed by the American Medical Association (AMA) for physician coding, whereas ICD-10-PCS was developed by CMS for hospital inpatient procedure coding. All procedures performed in an inpatient hospital setting are coded in both systems; physicians code and bill their services using CPT, and hospitals code and bill their services related to the procedure using ICD-10-PCS. However, CPT and ICD-10-PCS share no similarities. Each has a unique organization, code structure, terminology, and guidelines. Refer to ■ Table 49-2 for a summary of differences.

Physician Documentation for PCS

Inpatient hospital coding is based on physician documentation of the procedures performed. The accuracy of coding impacts the accuracy of reimbursement. This presents a unique challenge for hospitals because their reimbursement is ultimately based on documentation they do not generate. When physician documentation is incomplete, inpatient coders might not be able to assign codes with the specificity required by payers, or

Table 49-2 ■ **COMPARISON OF ICD-10-PCS AND CPT CODE SYSTEMS**

Characteristic	ICD-10-PCS	CPT
Developed by	CMS/3M	AMA
Used by	Inpatient hospitals	Physicians
Number of codes	72,000	9,000
Length	7 alphanumeric	5 digits (except T and F codes, 5 alphanumeric)
Modifiers	None	CPT, HCPCS modifiers
Body systems	31 systems (Med/Surg)	Traditional organ systems
Laterality	4th character	Modifiers -RT, -LT, –50
Code structure	Multiaxial	Undefined
Combination codes	Not used	Yes
Eponyms	Not used	Yes
E/M codes	Not used	Yes
Indented (dependent) and add-on codes	Not used	Yes
General Equivalency Mapping (GEMS) to other code sets	ICD-9-CM, Volume 3	None

Source: © PB Resources, Inc. Used with permission.

they might need to spend significant amounts of time following up with and querying physicians regarding the necessary details of a procedure. Examples of details needed for PCS coding that physicians might not be accustomed to documenting include laterality, anatomic site with the specificity needed for coders to assign the Body Part, and procedural details with the specificity needed for coders to assign the Root Operation.

Clinical documentation improvement (CDI) is a program implemented by many hospitals that educates physicians and helps them achieve complete documentation that accurately reflects the care patients receive. CDI specialists review patients' charts concurrently (while the patient is in the hospital) and retrospectively (after the patient is discharged) to identify missing or inadequate documentation and query the physician for clarification when needed. They also provide ongoing education to help physicians better understand and comply with documentation requirements for ICD-10-CM/PCS.

Inpatient Hospital Billing

According to the Uniform Hospital Data Discharge Set (UHDDS), inpatient hospitals must report all **significant procedures**. Significant procedures are those that are surgical in nature, carry a procedural risk, carry an anesthetic risk, or require specialized training.

The **principal procedure** is one that was performed for definitive treatment, rather than one performed for diagnostic or exploratory purposes, or was necessary to take care of a complication. If there appear to be two procedures that meet these criteria, then the one most related to the principal diagnosis should be selected as the principal procedure.

Hospitals use ICD-10-PCS procedure codes to identify the resources hospitals use in performing procedures when billing the patient's insurance. Hospital resources include the following:

- hospital staff, such as nurses, surgical technicians, nurse aides, and ancillary personnel
- space, equipment, and supplies, such as operating rooms, surgical instruments, X-ray, MRI, and CT equipment, surgical supplies, and linens
- overhead, such as utilities, operating expenses, and general administration

Hospital resources do not include the physician. In most cases, physicians own their own practices or are members of a group practice. The hospital does not employ them. The physician's practice bills the patient's insurance for the professional service performed by the physician. The hospital bills the patient's insurance for resources the hospital used.

SUCCESS STEP

PCS is used only when a hospital or other inpatient facility bills for inpatient services. Hospital outpatient services and physicians use CPT and HCPCS codes. However, some states may require that ICD-10-PCS codes be included when reporting statistics for outpatient hospital services.

Billing for inpatient hospital services requires more information and a different format than that used by physicians. The process is more complicated because charges must be collected from multiple departments for services that usually occur over a period of several days or longer. Charges are captured throughout the hospital stay; assigning the diagnosis and procedure codes is the final step that releases the bill to the payer. A summary of information about hospital charges, diagnosis-related groups, and claims follows to provide an introduction to hospital billing. For more comprehensive information, refer to professional resource books.

Charge Capture

ICD-10-PCS codes report procedures performed, not every supply item and resource used by the hospital. **Charge capture** is the process of entering the nonprocedural services provided throughout the patient stay, which is best done through a computer at the time the service is provided. For example, when a lab test is processed, the laboratory staff enter or scan an internal code that identifies the service provided. The services are listed in the facility's **charge description master (CDM)** and linked to the financial charge. For ancillary services such as laboratory and radiology, the service also is linked to the CPT or HCPCS code. The CDM assigns the charge to a **revenue code**, a four-digit code that identifies a general category of service, such as accommodation (*room charge*), type of ancillary service, pharmacy, or supplies. Revenue codes are used to summarize charges on the final inpatient bill.

Diagnosis Related Groups

Diagnosis related groups (DRGs) are a payment system that categorizes patients who are medically related with respect to diagnosis and treatment and statistically have similar lengths of stay. Consequently, they also tend to have similar costs and charges associated with the hospitalization. Several DRG systems have been developed, with the best known being **Medicare Severity-adjusted DRGs (MS-DRGs)** used by Medicare. MS-DRGs consist of approximately 500 DRG classifications that aggregate the thousands of diagnoses and procedures available in the coding manuals. DRGs are a case-based **prospective payment system (PPS)**. **Case-based** means that the rate is determined per case, or per inpatient admission, rather than on a per diem (daily) basis or a fee-for-service basis. Prospective payment means that a standard payment rate is predetermined based on the average amount of staff, supplies, and other resources typically used and assigned to each DRG. The hospital is paid the same amount for all patients classified to a particular DRG, regardless of the actual costs incurred. Each hospital receives a unique reimbursement rate per DRG based on its geographic location and other factors. This reimbursement method places the risk of cost-effectively managing the patient's stay on the hospital rather than the payer.

Cost outliers are unusual cases in which the cost is above or below a standard threshold amount established for the DRG. High cost outliers can qualify for additional payment; low cost outliers can be paid a lower-than-usual rate. Reasons for outliers are unique combinations of diagnoses and surgeries causing high costs, very rare conditions, long lengths stay, deaths, and cases admitted and discharged on the same day. Examples of comorbidities that may contribute to high cost outliers are alcoholism, diabetes mellitus, and renal failure. Outlier payments for high cost outliers help protect the hospital against extraordinary costs incurred from extremely ill patients. Payment reductions for low cost inliers help protect the insurance company against overpaying.

A **DRG grouper** is software that considers several clinical and demographic characteristics of a patient. After a patient's diagnoses are coded, the case is assigned to a Major Diagnostic Category (MDC) then classified into a DRG based on seven variables:

- Principal diagnosis
- Secondary diagnoses
- Surgical procedure(s)
- Comorbidities and complications (CC)
- Age and gender
- Discharge status
- Trim points (*the typical high and low length of stay for a diagnosis*)

Other payment systems used for hospital reimbursement include per diem (*an all-inclusive flat charge per day*) and a fee-for-service discount (*a negotiated reduction of usual charges*).

Hospital Claims

According to the American Hospital Association, over 80% of hospital claims are submitted electronically. The electronic billing format for institutions is the 837I. The standard hospital billing form is the UB-04, also known as the CMS-1450. The UB-04 is maintained by the **National Uniform Billing Committee (NUBC)**, which is chaired by the American Hospital Association and consists of representatives from more than 15 healthcare industry groups. The 837 and UB-04 have the same data requirements, which appear in a completed UB-04 form (■ FIGURE 49-1). The UB-04 has 81 Form Locators (FLs) divided into the following sections:

- 1–41 Patient information
- 42–49 Billing information
- 50–65 Payer information
- 66–81 Diagnosis information

Some fields require unique two-digit indicators called occurrence codes, condition codes, and value codes to communicate information to the payer. These are informational codes that appear in the instructions for completing the UB-04 form; they are not billing codes and do not appear in the coding manuals. Use of these codes allows flexibility in how certain form locators are used. They make a shorter form than would be possible if every potential data point occupied a dedicated field.

Condition codes identify certain events or circumstances related to a patient. For example, if a condition is employment-related, the biller enters condition code **02** in the first available field of FL 18–28. The code **02** informs the payer that the condition is employment-related.

Occurrence codes and occurrence span codes are used to identify a significant event that could affect payer processing. For example, if an accident or injury caused the condition being treated, the biller enters occurrence code **01** and the date of the accident in the first available field of FL 31–34. The code **01** informs the payer that an accident or injury occurred and the date it happened.

Value codes are entered in FL 39–41 and identify the number and dollar amount of certain services provided. For example, if a patient has physical therapy visits, the biller enters the value code **50** in the Code column on the left side of FL 39a and the actual number of physical therapy visits in the Amount column for FL 39, for example, **5** for five visits. The code **50** informs the payer that physical therapy services were provided, and the number **5** informs the payer that there were five visits.

Revenue codes are entered in FL 42, lines 1 to 22, with related service and charge information in FL 43–48. This information summarizes charges by department. An itemized bill showing each individual charge item is submitted with the claim.

FL 66 is used to identify the coding system being used on the claim, such as **9** for ICD-9-CM or **0** for ICD-10-CM.

The patient's principal diagnosis is entered in FL 67, with additional diagnoses in FL 67A–67Q. The admitting diagnosis appears in FL 69.

The principal procedure is entered in FL 74 and additional procedures in FL 74a–74d.

For detailed instructions on how to complete the UB-04, refer to **www.cms.gov** or **www.nubc.org**.

INPATIENT

1 Any Hospital	2 Any Hospital	3a PAT CNTL # 1234	4 TYPE OF BILL
123 Any Street	456 Any Street	b MED REC # 98765	0111
Philadelphia PA 19103	Philadelphia PA 19103	5 FED. TAX. NO. 221234567	6 STATEMENT COVERS PERIOD FROM 11 03 06 THROUGH 11 04 06	7 RESERVED

| 8 PATIENT NAME a Patient ID if different from Sub | 9 PATIENT ADDRESS a 1234 Main Street | | |
| b Doe, John | b Philadelphia | c PA d 19111 | Country code if other than USA |

| 10 BIRTHDATE | 11 SEX | 12 DATE | ADMISSION 13 HR | 14 TYPE | 15 SRC | 16 DHR | 17 STAT | 18 | 19 | 20 | 21 | CONDITION CODES 22 | 23 | 24 | 25 | 26 | 27 | 28 | 29 ACDT STATE | 30 |
| 03 20 1971 | M | 11 03 06 | 08 | 3 | 3 | 12 | 01 | Condition Codes Required Identifying Events | | | | | | | | | | | PA | RESERVED |

31 OCCURRENCE CODE DATE	32 OCCURRENCE CODE DATE	33 OCCURRENCE CODE DATE	34 OCCURRENCE CODE DATE	35 OCCURRENCE SPAN CODE FROM THROUGH	36 OCCURRENCE SPAN CODE FROM THROUGH	37
a Occurrence and Occurrence Span Codes may be used to define a significant event that may affect payer processing						FUTURE USE
b						

38		39 VALUE CODES CODE AMOUNT	40 VALUE CODES CODE AMOUNT	41 VALUE CODES CODE AMOUNT
John Doe 1234 Main Street Philadelphia, PA 19111		a A1 952 00		
		b Value Codes and amounts required when necessary to process claim		
		c		
		d		

	42 REV.CD.	43 DESCRIPTION	44 HCPCS/RATE/HPPS CODE	45 SERV. DATE	46 SERV. UNIT	47 TOTAL CHARGES	48 NON-COVERED CHARGES	49
1	0129	Semi-Private	200.00		2	400 00	0 00	Future Use	1
2	0250	Pharmacy			1	50 00	0 00		2
3	0360	OR Services				100 00	0 00		3
4									4
5									5
6									6
7									7
8									8
9									9
10									10
11									11
12									12
13									13
14									14
15									15
16									16
17									17
18									18
19									19
20									20
21									21
22									22
23	PAGE _1_ OF _1_		CREATION DATE		TOTALS ▶	550 00	0 00		23

50 PAYER NAME	51 HEALTH PLAN ID	52 REL INFO	53 ASG BEN.	54 PRIOR PAYMENTS	55 EST. AMOUNT DUE	56 NPI 2222222222	
A Independence Blue Cross	Report HIPAA National	Y	Y	Required when indicated payer has paid amount to Provider	Amount estimated to be due	57 OTHER PRV. ID	1234567890	A
B Secondary Payer	Health Plan Identifier						Secondary	B
C Tertiary Payer	when mendatory						Tertiary	C

58 INSURED'S NAME	59	60 INSURED'S UNIQUE ID	61 GROUP NAME	62 INSURANCE GROUP NO.	
A Doe, John	18	ABC12345678900	Watch Repair, Inc.	1234	A
B Secondary					B
C Tertiary					C

63 TREATMENT AUTHORIZATION CODES	64 DOCUMENT CONTROL NUMBER	65 EMPLOYER NAME	
A 02468	491234	Watch Repair, Inc.	A
B Secondary			B
C Tertiary			C

| 66 K50115 | A Use A through Q to report "Other Diagnosis" if applicable | E | F | G | H | 68 Reserved |
| 0 | I | J | K | L | M | N | O | P | Q | |

| 69 ADMIT DX K50115 | 70 PATIENT REASON DX May be used to report reason for visit | 71 PPS CODE DRS | 72 ECI May be used to report external cause of injury | 73 Reserved |

74 PRINCIPAL PROCEDURE CODE DATE	a OTHER PROCEDURE CODE DATE	b OTHER PROCEDURE CODE DATE	75	76 ATTENDING NPI 2222222222 QUAL 16 1234569822
0D1B0Z4 08 26 YY			Reserved	LAST Smith FIRST David
c OTHER PROCEDURE CODE DATE	d OTHER PROCEDURE CODE DATE	e OTHER PROCEDURE CODE DATE		77 OPERATING NPI QUAL
				LAST FIRST

80 REMARKS	81CC a B3 292N00000X	78 OTHER NPI QUAL
May be used to report additional	b Secondary	LAST FIRST
information.	c Tertiary	79 OTHER NPI QUAL
	d	LAST FIRST

UB-04 CMS-1450   APPROVED OMB NO.   **NUBC**™ National Uniform Billing Committee   THE CERTIFICATIONS ON THE REVERSE APPLY TO THIS BILL AND ARE MADE A PART HEREOF.

Red = Required
Black = Situational/Required, if applicable/Reserved

Figure 49-1 ■ Example of a Completed Inpatient UB-04 Form

Guided Example of the Use of ICD-10-PCS

Refer to the following example throughout this chapter to learn about ICD-10-PCS codes.

Date of procedure: 8/26/yy Location: *Branton Medical Center* Surgeon: *Tanya Schmitt, MD*

Anesthesiologist: *Reginald Pincus, MD*

Patient: *Michael Longo* Gender: M Age: *52*

Preprocedure diagnosis: *Crohn's disease with abscess*

Procedure description: *Temporary loop ileostomy. Made incision in right abdominal wall. Opened anterior wall of ileum loop and brought through to the skin, then closed the wound around the exposed ileum. Patient tolerated px (procedure) well.*

Postprocedure diagnosis: *Crohn's disease of large intestine with abscess*

Follow this patient's surgical procedure and bill through the hospital, physician's office, and anesthesiologist's office to understand the difference between inpatient procedure codes and physician procedure codes.

▶ Tanya Schmitt, MD, who is part of Branton Professional Group, uses the operating rooms, surgical instruments, equipment, supplies, and nursing staff at Branton Medical Center to perform the procedure.

▶ Reginald Pincus, MD, who is part of Branton Anesthesiology Providers, administers the anesthesia using Branton Medical Center's anesthesia equipment and supplies; monitors the patient during and after the procedure; and ensures that the patient wakes up without complications.

▶ After surgery, Mr. Longo is transferred to a medical-surgical floor. Dr. Schmitt checks on Mr. Longo each day and discharges him six days after surgery.

▶ Mr. Longo's insurance will receive three separate bills for services from the following organizations, for the amounts listed:
   1. Branton Medical Center, $12,500.00
   2. Branton Professional Group, $1,027.00
   3. Branton Anesthesiology Providers, $485.00

▶ Review the information outlined below to better understand why there are three bills.
   1. **Branton Medical Center** bills Mr. Longo's insurance for his entire length of stay, including room and board, the technical component of laboratory tests, and operating room resources. The cost is $12,500.00.
      - Branton Medical Center's coder, Marcy Elwood, CCS, assigns the ICD-10-CM diagnosis code **K50.114 Crohn's disease of large intestine with abscess** as the principal diagnosis. The coder assigns an ICD-10-PCS procedure code, **0D1B0Z4 Bypass Ileum to Cuta-**neous, **Open Approach**, as the principal procedure. (You will learn how to assign PCS codes in the next chapter.)
      - The hospital's biller prepares the UB-04 form. The biller enters the principal diagnosis, ICD-10-CM code **K50.115** in FL 67; the principal procedure, ICD-10-PCS code **0D1B0Z4**, in the left side of FL 74; and the date of the procedure, 8/26/YY, in the right side of FL 74. In FL 77, the block for operating physician, Dr. Schmitt's name and National Provider Identifier (NPI) are entered. Total charges are entered as $12,500.00 in FL 47, line 23. The facility is Branton Medical Center. Payment will be made to Branton Medical Center.

2. **Branton Professional Group** bills Mr. Longo's insurance for Dr. Schmitt's services, which include admitting him, performing the procedure, making the follow-up visits, and discharging him. The surgeon's fee is $1,027.00.
   - Branton Professional Group's coder, Chrystal Crago, CCA, assigns the same ICD-10-CM diagnosis code, **K50.114,** that the hospital did, but assigns a CPT surgical code (**44310 Ileostomy or jejunostomy, non-tube**) for the procedure.
   - Branton Professional Group's biller prepares a claim on the CMS-1500 form (*the standard physician billing form*) or its electronic equivalent, the 837P. The biller lists the ICD-10-CM code **K50.114** in the diagnosis block (21), the date of the procedure, 8/26/YY, CPT surgical code **44310** in the services block (24). The charge for the surgeon is $1,027.00. Branton Medical Center is listed as the service facility. The billing provider is Branton Professional Group. Payment will be made to Branton Professional Group.

3. **Branton Anesthesiology Providers** bills Mr. Longo's insurance for the anesthesia management by Dr. Pincus. The anesthesiologist's fee is $485.00.
   - Branton Anesthesiology Providers' coder, Lance Staiger, CPC, assigns the same ICD-10-CM diagnosis code, **K50.114**, but assigns a CPT anesthesia code (**00840-P1 Anesthesia for intraperitoneal procedures in lower abdomen including laparoscopy; not otherwise specified; -P1 a Normal healthy patient**) for the anesthesiologist's services.
   - The Branton Anesthesiology Providers' biller prepares a claim on the CMS-1500 form or its electronic equivalent. The biller enters the ICD-10-CM code **K50.114** as the diagnosis, the date of the procedure, 8/26/YY, and the CPT anesthesia code **00840-P1** in the services block. The charge for the anesthesiologist is $485.00. Branton Medical Center is listed as the service facility. The billing provider is Branton Anesthesiology Providers. Payment will be made to Branton Anesthesiology Providers.

CODING PRACTICE

Exercise 49.1 The Purpose of ICD-10-PCS

Instructions: Fill in each blank with the correct term(s) from this section of the chapter.

1. _____ means that there should be a unique code for every procedure that is significantly different in body part, approach, or methods.

2. _____ means that each position or character within a code number has a designated meaning or purpose and should be used for that meaning for all related codes.

3. _____ means that the code set includes definitions of the terminology it uses and each term must have only one meaning.

4. Data that is granular is _____.

5. _____ are those that are surgical in nature, carry a procedural risk, carry an anesthetic risk, or require specialized training.

6. The _____ is one that was performed for definitive treatment, rather than one performed for diagnostic or exploratory purposes or was necessary to take care of a complication.

7. Hospitals use ICD-10-PCS procedure codes to describe and bill the patient's insurance for the _____ hospital's use in performing procedures.

8. What are the three entities who will submit bills after a patient has an inpatient hospital surgical procedure performed?

   _____

   _____

   _____

9. Of the three entities listed in question 8, which one(s) bill using ICD-10-CM diagnosis codes? _____

10. Of the three entities listed in question 8, which one(s) bill using ICD-10-PCS procedure codes?

   _____

ICD-10-PCS CODING MANUAL ORGANIZATION

Open the ICD-10-PCS manual and follow along with the information outlined next, which describes the overall organization of the manual. The ICD-10-PCS manual has the following major sections:

- **Introduction**—The Introduction describes the history of ICD-10-PCS and gives detailed instructions on how to use the manual. It provides reference material that lists the character definitions and values for each section of the manual.

- **ICD-10-PCS Official Guidelines for Coding and Reporting (OGCR)**—This section consists of A. Conventions, B. Medical and Surgical Section Guidelines, and C. Obstetrics Section Guidelines.

- **Index**—This section is an alphabetical listing of procedures, which identifies the correct reference table to use to build the code.

- **Tables**—This section contains reference tables or grids used to build each ICD-10-PCS code. Tables appear in alphanumeric order based on the first three characters of the code (■ FIGURE 49-2).

- **Appendices**—This section contains several appendices with additional reference material (■ TABLE 49-3). Coders should become familiar with the appendices because they contain valuable information that makes coding easier and more accurate.

Section	0	Medical and Surgical
Body System	F	Hepatobiliary System and Pancreas
Operation	9	Drainage Taking or letting out fluids and/or gases from a body part

Body Part Character 4	Approach Character 5	Device Character 6	Qualifier Character 7
0 Liver 1 Liver, Right Lobe 2 Liver, Left Lobe 4 Gallbladder G Pancreas	0 Open 3 Percutaneous 4 Percutaneous Endoscopic	0 Drainage Device	Z No Qualifier
0 Liver 1 Liver, Right Lobe 2 Liver, Left Lobe 4 Gallbladder G Pancreas	0 Open 3 Percutaneous 4 Percutaneous Endoscopic	Z No Device	X Diagnostic Z No Qualifier

Figure 49-2 ■ Example of a PCS Table

Table 49-3 ■ **ICD-10-PCS CODING MANUAL APPENDICES**

Appendix Title	Contents	Use
Body Part Key	Crosswalk between anatomic terms and the PCS Body Part description.	Determine what Body Part value corresponds with a specific anatomic site, such as a blood vessel, tendon, or nerve.
Character Meanings	Lists all possible values and meanings for Character 3 through Character 7. Organized by Section, then Body System, in the same order as the Tables.	Interpret the meaning of codes already assigned.
Comparison of Medical and Surgical Root Operations	Organizes Medical and Surgical Root Operations into nine groups with similar objectives.	Help determine the appropriate Root Operation.
Components of the Medical and Surgical Approach Definitions	Defines all Approaches (Character 5) for the Medical and Surgical Section.	Identify the official definition of surgical Approaches.
Device Aggregation Table	Defines the operation, body system, and general Device value for each specific device.	Determine the appropriate operations, body systems, and PCS device value for each class of devices.
Device Key	Crosswalk from device brand names and common names to the PCS Device description.	Determine what Device value to use for a specific product.
Root Operation Definitions	Defines all Root Operations in Sections 0 Medical and Surgical, and Sections 1 through 9, Medical and Surgical-Related. Organized by Section.	Identify the official definition of Root Operations.
Type and Type Qualifier Definitions Sections B–H	Defines all Types (Character 3) and Type Qualifiers (Character 5) for Ancillary Sections, B through H. Organized by Character and Section.	Identify the official definition of Types and Type Qualifiers.

SUCCESS STEP

The order of the sections and specific content may vary based on the manual's publisher or based on yearly updates, so it is helpful to review the organization of your particular manual. Apply self-adhesive tabs on the pages to identify each appendix.

In addition to the supplemental information contained within the ICD-10-PCS coding manual, CMS also publishes a separate electronic *ICD-10-PCS Reference Manual* (■ TABLE 49-4). The Reference Manual is updated annually and can be downloaded from the CMS website free of charge. This document provides detailed background on ICD-10-PCS, explanations of all Sections and Root Operations, tables of all character values, and many case examples.

Table 49-4 ■ **ICD-10-PCS REFERENCE MANUAL CONTENTS**

Chapter	Title	Contents
1	Overview	Includes a general introduction to ICD-10-PCS, a brief history of its development, and a presentation of the code structure, organization, and characteristics. The first part of the overview contains basic information; the second and third parts discuss structure, characteristics, and applications in more detail.
2	Procedures in the Medical and Surgical Section	Provides reference material for each root operation in the Medical and Surgical section (0), with the full definition, additional explanation as needed, a code example, and coding exercises for each root operation.
3	Procedures in the Medical and Surgical-Related Sections	Provides reference material for each of the Medical and Surgical-related sections (1 through 9), with definitions, additional explanation as needed, a code example, and coding exercises for each section.
4	Procedures in the Ancillary Sections	Provides reference material for each of the ancillary sections (B through H), with definitions, additional explanation as needed, a code example, and coding exercises for each section.
Appendix A	ICD-10-PCS Definitions	Tables listing the full definitions of all root operations and approaches in the Medical and Surgical section.
Appendix B	ICD-10-PCS Device and Substance Classification	Discusses the distinguishing features of device, substance, and equipment as classified in ICD-10-PCS.

The ICD-10-PCS Reference Manual can be downloaded from the current ICD-10 page at www.cms.gov.

CODING PRACTICE

Exercise 49.2 ICD-10-PCS Coding
Manual Organization

Instructions: Fill in each blank with the correct term(s) from this section of the chapter.

Part A

Name the section of the ICD-10-PCS coding manual coders use to locate the following information:

1. Conventions _____

2. An alphabetical listing of procedures that identifies the correct reference table to use to build the code _____

3. Reference material that lists the character definitions and values for each section of the manual _____

Part B

Refer to Table 49-3 and name the title of the appendix in the ICD-10-PCS coding manual coders use to locate the following information:

4. Identify the official definition of Root Operations

_____

5. Determine what Body Part value corresponds with a specific anatomic site _____

6. Determine what Device value to use for a specific product

_____

7. The electronic *ICD-10-PCS Reference Manual* can be downloaded free from what organization's website?

_____

Part C

Name the chapter of the *ICD-10-PCS Reference Manual* coders use to locate the following information:

8. Definitions, additional explanation as needed, a code example, and coding exercises for the ancillary Sections B through H

_____

9. A general introduction to ICD-10-PCS, a brief history of its development, and a presentation of the code structure, organization, and characteristics _____

10. Reference material for each root operation in the Medical and Surgical section (0) _____

ICD-10-PCS CODE STRUCTURE

ICD-10-PCS codes have a logical, consistent structure that contains seven alphanumeric positions, called characters. An ICD-10-PCS code is best understood as the result of a process in which coders assign, or build, a code. The process consists of assigning values to each character based on specific characteristics of the procedure the physician performs. The ICD-10-PCS manual uses **Tables**, which are reference grids used to select the body part, operative approach, and other characteristics of the procedure.

ICD-10-PCS codes consist of seven positions or characters, each with a designated purpose, which creates consistency across codes. Coders select individual letters and numbers, called **values**, in a standard order to occupy the seven characters of the code. Each character represents a specific aspect of the procedure and can have up to 34 different values, consisting of the 10 digits, 0 to 9, and 24 letters, A to H, J to N, and P to Z. Not every character uses all 34 values. For some sections and some characters, only a few values are used while in others, most of the values are used. Each Section of the manual designates how each character of the code is used within that Section. The definition of each value, for example, **1** or **A**, is based on the position it occupies. Examples are provided in the discussion that follows.

The options and values for a character vary based on the first character of the code, which identifies the Section. The largest Section is Medical and Surgical, which is used as an example to introduce PCS codes in the remainder of this chapter.

Characters in the Medical and Surgical Section are defined as follows:

- Character 1 defines the **Section**, or broad procedure category where the code is found.
- Character 2 defines the **Body System** in which the procedure is performed.
- Character 3 defines the **Root Operation**, or the objective of the procedure.
- Character 4 defines the **Body Part**, or specific anatomic site where the physician performed the procedure.
- Character 5 defines the **Approach**, or the surgical technique used to reach the procedure site.
- Character 6 defines the **Device** left in place at the end of the procedure.
- Character 7 defines a **Qualifier** for the code, which describes additional information about the procedure.

The Introduction in the ICD-10-PCS coding manual identifies the character meanings for each Section. An appendix in most ICD-10-PCS manuals provides a complete listing of all the Characters for all Sections. Refer to the Introduction and the appendix Character Meanings to become familiar with information needed to fully understand and assign ICD-10-PCS codes.

The following discussion identifies the purpose of each character and gives examples of how it is used. The next several chapters of this text discuss how to use the Index and Tables to arrive at a code.

Table 49-5 ■ **CHARACTER 1: SECTION**

Value	Section Name
0	Medical and Surgical
Medical and Surgical-<u>Related</u> Procedures	
1	Obstetrics
2	Placement
3	Administration
4	Measurement and Monitoring
5	Extracorporeal Assistance and Performance
6	Extracorporeal Therapies
7	Osteopathic
8	Other Procedures
9	Chiropractic
Ancillary Procedures	
B	Imaging
C	Nuclear Medicine
D	Radiation Oncology
F	Physical Rehabilitation and Diagnostic Audiology
G	Mental Health
H	Substance Abuse Treatment
New Technology	
X	New Technology

Character 1: Section

The first character in all PCS codes describes the Section, or the broad procedure category, where the code is found (■ TABLE 49-5). The largest Section is Medical and Surgical. Other Sections classify medical and surgical-<u>related</u> procedures, such as Obstetrics or Chiropractic, ancillary services, such as Nuclear Medicine or Mental Health, and new technology.

Character 2: Body System

The second character in the Medical and Surgical Section identifies the Body System, the general physiological system or anatomic region involved, such as central nervous system or endocrine system. The Medical and Surgical Section has 31 possible values for the Body System. The Body System values do not always correlate to the commonly defined organ systems. Large systems may have multiple values in Character 2. For example, the skeletal system has five Body System values, each referring to a specific component (■ TABLE 49-6). Because within each PCS Body System there can be up to 34 values for Body Part, codes can be more specific when large systems are divided into multiple values. This enables the skeletal system, for example, to have up to 170 Body Part values. If the Skeletal System were defined with only one value, then the number of Body Part values would be limited to 34.

Table 49-6 ■ **BODY SYSTEM VALUES FOR THE SKELETAL SYSTEM**

Value	Description
N	Head and Facial Bones
P	Upper Bones
Q	Lower Bones
R	Upper Joints
S	Lower Joints

Many Sections other than Medical and Surgical also use Character 2 to describe Body System, but may also use it for other purposes. The Placement Section (Section value 2) uses Character 2 for Anatomical Orifice. The Physical Rehabilitation and Diagnostic Audiology Section (Section value F) uses Character 2 for Section Qualifier, which is a broad type of service such as Rehabilitation.

Character 3: Root Operation

The third character in the Medical and Surgical Section, and most other Sections, defines the Root Operation, which describes the objective of the procedure (excision, destruction, extraction). The options and values for Character 3 vary from one Section to the next and from one Body Part value to the next within a Section. Root Operations are Main Terms in the Index, so coders must be familiar with their names and definitions. The names and definitions of Character 3 appear at the top of each Table in the ICD-10-PCS manual. In addition, an appendix in most ICD-10-PCS manuals defines all the Root Operations for the Medical and Surgical Section, provides expanded explanations, and gives examples.

For example, a Latin-based medical term such as *gastrectomy* can mean removing all or part of the stomach. The definitions of the words *excision* and *resection* are sometimes used interchangeably in common medical usage, such as stomach excision or stomach resection, and can mean that either all of the stomach or part of the stomach is removed. Without referring to the operative report, the extent of the procedure is unclear. ICD-10-PCS defines these terms in specific ways. **Excision** is defined as *cutting off a <u>portion</u> of a body part without replacement* while **Resection** is defined as *cutting off <u>all</u> of a body part without replacement*. Therefore, cutting out a portion of the stomach is coded as the Root Operation **Excision** (value **B**), while cutting out all of the stomach is coded as the Root Operation **Resection** (value **T**).

The 31 Medical and Surgical Root Operations are organized into nine groups based on the overall objective of the

CODING CAUTION

Coders are required to follow the definitions in the ICD-10-PCS manual, but physicians are not expected to change the words they use in documentation. Regardless of what word the physician uses to describe a procedure, coders are required to assign the Root Operation based on the official ICD-10-PCS definition (PCS OGCR A11).

Table 49-7 ■ EXAMPLE OF MULTIPLE BODY PART VALUES FOR A SINGLE ORGAN: THE LARGE INTESTINE

Excerpt from Table OBD, Excision, Gastrointestinal System: Character 4, Body Part	
Value	Description
E	Large Intestine
F	Large Intestine, Right
G	Large Intestine, Left
H	Cecum
J	Appendix
K	Ascending Colon
L	Transverse Colon
M	Descending Colon
N	Sigmoid Colon
P	Rectum

procedure. An appendix in most ICD-10-PCS manuals provides a useful breakdown of the nine groups, which makes it easier to locate a desired Root Operation. The nine groups are not part of the final code; they are simply an organizational tool for coders.

Character 4: Body Part

The fourth character in the Medical and Surgical Section identifies the Body Part, or specific anatomic site, where the physician performed the procedure. The Body System (Character 2) provides a general indication of the procedure location. The Body Part and Body System values together provide a precise description of the procedure site.

Most Sections use Character 2 for Body System and Character 4 for Body Part. However, some Sections use Character 2 for a different purpose. Sections that do not define Body System in Character 2 may use Character 4 for Body System.

The definition of each Body Part value in the Medical and Surgical Section is unique to each Body System. For example, in Character 2 (Body System), value **5** identifies the upper veins and the Body Part value of **B** refers to the **right basilic vein**. When the Character 2 (Body System) value is **7** for the

lymphatic and hemic systems, the Body Part Value **B** refers to the mesenteric lymphatic system. Review the appendix to see how the same value represents different information in different Body System tables.

When selecting the Body Part for a particular Root Operation, coders must refer to the appropriate Table and identify how that Table defines Body Part. Some organs and anatomic areas are divided into multiple Body Parts for coding purposes. For example, the large intestine is a single organ, but ICD-10-PCS assigns multiple Body Part values (■ TABLE 49-7). Coders should match the most specific Body Part value with the most specific Root Operation value. For example, when surgeons cut out the entire descending colon, they are taking out *part* of the organ, the large intestine, but *all* of the PCS Body Part value **M Descending Colon**. Therefore, coders select the Root Operation **T Resection**, defined as *cutting out, without replacement, all of a body part* and match it with the Body Part value **M Descending Colon**. Do not assign the Root Operation **B Excision**, which is defined as *cutting out, without replacement, a portion of a body part*, and match it with the less specific Body Part value **E Large Intestine** (■ FIGURE 49-3).

Character 5: Approach

The fifth character in the Medical and Surgical Section defines the Approach, or the surgical technique used to reach the procedure site, such as open, endoscopic, or external. Each Table in the ICD-10-PCS manual lists the acceptable Approaches for each Root Operation value and Body Part value. Definitions for each Approach appear in the appendix and are further discussed in later chapters.

Sections other than Medical and Surgical use Character 5 for a wide range of purposes. For example, the Extracorporeal Therapies Section (Section value 6) uses Character 5 for Duration and the Imaging Section (Section value **B**) uses Character 5 for **Contrast**.

Character 6: Device

The sixth character in the Medical and Surgical Section defines the Device left in place at the end of the procedure for those procedures that involve a device. Device values fall into four basic categories: grafts and prostheses, implants, simple or mechanical appliances, electronic appliances. Each Table in the ICD-10-PCS manual lists the acceptable devices for each Root Operation value and Device value.

Procedure description: *Partial colectomy. Excised the entire descending colon.*

CORRECT
Root Operation: **T - Resection,** *cutting out, without replacement, all of a body part*
Body Part: **M - Descending Colon**

INCORRECT
Root Operation: **B - Excision,** *cutting out, without replacement, a portion of a body part*
Body Part: **E - Large Intestine**
Explanation: Select the most specific Body Part value (**Descending Colon (M)**) and match it with the most specific Root Operation (**Resection (T)**). Also notice that you should not select the Root Operation **Excision (B)** based on the physician's use of the word "excised." Select the Root Operation based on the PCS definition.

Figure 49-3 ■ Example of Matching the Root Operation with the Body Part

Sections other than Medical and Surgical use Character 6 for a variety of purposes, including **Method** (Osteopathic section) and **Isotope** (Radiation Oncology section). When no device applies, the Table lists the value **Z No Device** for Character 6.

Character 7: Qualifier

The seventh character in the Medical and Surgical Section defines a Qualifier for the code. A Qualifier specifies an additional attribute of the procedure, if applicable. Examples of Medical and Surgical Qualifiers are the type of adhesive used on a replacement joint, such as cemented or uncemented, and the direction of the surgical approach, such as anterior or posterior. Each Table in the ICD-10-PCS manual lists the acceptable Qualifier values for each Approach value. When no qualifier applies, the Table lists the value **Z No Qualifier** for Character 7.

Guided Example of Building a PCS Code

Continue with the example of Michael Longo, who had an ileostomy, to learn the meaning of an ICD-10-PCS code.

Follow along as Marcy Elwood, CCS, the coder at Branton Medical Center, assigns the ICD-10-PCS code **0D1B0Z4**.

▶ Refer to ■ TABLE 49-8 to understand how a PCS code is structured. You will learn how Marcy used the Index and Tables to arrive at this code in the following chapters of this text.

❏ The value **0** for Character 1 identifies that the procedure is from the Medical and Surgical Section.

❏ The value **D** for Character 2 identifies that the Body System is **Gastrointestinal**.

❏ The value **1** for Character 3 identifies that the Root Operation is **Bypass**. PCS defines **Bypass** as *altering*

Table 49-8 ■ **CODE 0D1B0Z4 BYPASS ILEUM TO CUTANEOUS, OPEN APPROACH**

Character (Position)	Name	Value	Description
1	Section	0	Medical and Surgical
2	Body System	D	Gastrointestinal
3	Root Operation	1	Bypass
4	Body Part	B	Ileum
5	Approach	0	Open
6	Device	Z	No Device
7	Qualifier	4	Cutaneous

the route of passage of the contents of a tubular body part.

❏ The value **B** for Character 4 identifies that the Body Part is **Ileum**.

❏ The value **0** for Character 5 identifies that the Approach is **Open**.

❏ The value **Z** for Character 6 identifies that the Device is **No Device** because the PCS Table does not provide any options for this character.

❏ The value **4** for Character 7 identifies that the Qualifier is **Cutaneous** because in the Root Operation **Bypass**, PCS uses the Qualifier to identify the end site of the bypass.

▶ Now you can see the entire meaning of the code **0D1B0Z4 Bypass Ileum to Cutaneous, Open Approach**. You will learn how to use the Index and Tables to arrive at this code in later chapters of this text.

CODING PRACTICE

Exercise 49.3 ICD-10-PCS Code Structure

Instructions: Fill in each blank with the correct term(s) from this section of the chapter.

1. _____ are reference grids used to select the body part, operative approach, and other characteristics of the procedure.

2. Coders select individual letters and numbers, called _____, in a standard order to occupy the seven characters of the code.

3. ICD-10-PCS values do not use the letters _____ and _____ in order to avoid confusion with numbers.

Provide the Character number (1 through 7) and name for the following:

4. Character _____, called the _____, has the value of 0 for all Medical and Surgical procedures.

5. Character _____, called the _____, identifies the technique used to reach the procedure site in the Medical and Surgical Section.

6. Character _____, called the _____, identifies the specific anatomic site where the physician performed the procedure, in the Medical and Surgical Section.

7. Resection is an example of Character _____, called the _____, in the Medical and Surgical Section.

8. The direction of the surgical approach, such as anterior or posterior, is an example of Character _____, called the _____, in the Medical and Surgical Section.

9. Character _____, called the _____, identifies the general physiological system or anatomic region

involved, such as central nervous system or endocrine system in the Medical and Surgical Section.

10. Values for Character _____, called the _____, fall into four basic categories: grafts and prostheses, implants, simple or mechanical appliances, electronic appliances.

ICD-10-PCS CODING GUIDELINES

ICD-10-PCS provides Official Guidelines for Coding and Reporting (OGCR) at the front of the ICD-10-PCS manual. OGCR are also available as a separate document that can be downloaded from **www.cms.gov** or **www.cdc.gov**. ICD-10-PCS OGCR are a separate document from ICD-10-CM OGCR. Guidelines are divided into three sections: A-Conventions; B-Medical and Surgical Section Guidelines; C-Obstetric Section Guidelines, and D-New Technology Section Guidelines. Throughout this text, information from the ICD-10-PCS OGCR will be referenced as PCS OGCR, followed by the specific reference number, such as PCS OGCR A6 or PCS OGCR B3.6a. Follow along in the ICD-10-PCS manual to become acquainted with each section of the OGCR.

A—Conventions

Conventions describe how ICD-10-PCS codes are constructed and the basic rules of using ICD-10-PCS. Examples are presented for many specific guidelines. The most important guidelines to memorize while learning PCS include the following. This provides an overview. The details will be discussed later in this chapter and other PCS chapters.

- A6. The purpose of the alphabetic index is to locate the appropriate table that contains all information necessary to construct a procedure code. The PCS Tables should always be consulted to find the most appropriate valid code.

- A8. All seven characters must be specified to be a valid code. If the documentation is incomplete for coding purposes, query the physician for the necessary information.

- A9. Within a PCS table, valid codes include all combinations of choices in Characters 4 through 7 contained in the <u>same row</u> of the table.

- A11. Many of the terms used to construct PCS codes are defined within the system. It is the coder's responsibility to determine what the documentation in the medical record equates to in the PCS definitions.

B—Medical and Surgical Section Guidelines (Section 0)

Medical and Surgical Section Guidelines apply specifically to ICD-10-PCS in the Medical and Surgical Section (value **0**). The organization of this section correlates with each character in the Medical and Surgical Codes, as follows:

- B2. Body System
- B3. Root Operation
- B4. Body Part
- B5. Approach
- B6. Device
- B7. Qualifier

Each of these subsections contains *General guidelines*, which apply to the Medical and Surgical Section as a whole, and also provides additional guidelines that apply to specific Root Operations, Approaches, and other elements. Specific guidelines from this section will be discussed later in this text.

C—Obstetrics and D-New Technology

Specific guidelines for Obstetrics (Section 0) are discussed in Chapter 57 of this text. Guidelines for New Technology (Section X) are discussed in Chapter 58 of this text.

CODING PRACTICE

Exercise 49.4 ICD-10-PCS Official Guidelines for Coding and Reporting

Instructions: Fill in each blank with the correct term(s) from this section of the chapter.

1. _____ describe how ICD-10-PCS codes are constructed and the basic rules of using ICD-10-PCS.

2. PCS OGCR _____ states that all seven characters must be specified to be a valid code.

3. Within a PCS table, valid codes include all combinations of choices in Characters 4 through 7 contained in the same _____ the table.

4. Who is responsible to determine what the documentation in the medical record equates to in the PCS definitions? _____.

5. _____ is the only Section besides Medical and Surgical that has specific guidelines.

INTRODUCTION TO THE STEPS OF ICD-10-PCS PROCEDURE CODING

The three skills of an ace coder apply to coding procedures, but the mechanics are unique to this code set. Follow these steps:

1. **Abstract** procedures from the medical record, beginning with PCS definitions of the Root Operation.

2. **Assign**, or build, the PCS code values using the Index and Tables.

3. **Arrange**, or sequence, PCS codes based on the definition of the principal procedure.

An overview of these skills is provided next. The next several chapters of this text discuss these skills in detail and provide examples.

Abstract Procedures from the Medical Record

The key to accurate abstracting in PCS is to read the information provided in the procedure report and interpret it in a manner consistent with ICD-10-PCS definitions of the Root Operation or Root Type. The Root Operation or Root Type also functions as the Main Term in the Index and directs coders to the correct Table. The Introduction of the ICD-10-PCS manual provides the definition for each Root Operation and Root Type, which are divided by Section.

SUCCESS STEP

The appendix provides Root Operation definitions for Section **0**, Medical and Surgical, and Sections **1** through **9**, Medical and Surgical-Related. The appendix also provides Root Type definitions for Sections **B** through **H**, Ancillary.

Coders must read the procedure report and *interpret* what was done based on the definitions of the Root Operations or Root Types. Physicians are not required or expected to document using ICD-10-PCS definitions, but may document using the terminology they are most comfortable and familiar with.

Coders will not find Root Operations described in the procedure report using the exact PCS words (■ FIGURE 49-4). Even when physicians use words that are similar to Root Operations, such as *excision*, *resection*, or *removal*, the coder is obligated to interpret the physician's description in light of the PCS definitions. PCS OCGR A11 states the following:

> **Many of the terms used to construct PCS codes are defined within the system. It is the coder's responsibility to determine what the documentation in the medical record equates to in the PCS definitions. The physician is not expected to use the terms used in PCS code descriptions, nor is the coder required to query the physician when the correlation between the documentation and the defined PCS terms is clear.**

SUCCESS STEP

Although you do not need to memorize specific codes or character values, you should plan to memorize the *definitions* of the most commonly used Root Operations and Root Types. While in the learning stage, ALWAYS verify the definition of the Root Operation in the PCS manual.

Assign ICD-10-PCS Codes

Assigning PCS codes requires coders to locate the Root Operation in the Index then refer to a Table to build the code.

ICD-10-PCS Index

The Index uses two types of Main Terms for the Medical and Surgical Section:

- the name of the Root Operation, such as Excision

- the common procedure name, excluding eponyms, such as appendectomy

Under the Main Term are indented subterms that describe the anatomic sites or other variations of the Root Operation. Following the subterm is the partial code, which provides the

---

Procedure description: *Appendectomy. Removed entire appendix laparoscopically.*

CORRECT
Root Operation: **T - Resection** *cutting off all of a body part, without replacement*

INCORRECT
Root Operation: **P - Removal** *taking out or off a device from a body part*

Explanation: Even though the documentation uses the word *removed*, do not use the Root Operation **Removal** because the PCS definition does not describe the procedure performed. The Root Operation **Removal** identifies taking devices out of the body. The Root Operation **Resection** describes cutting off a body part, such as the appendix.

Figure 49-4 ■ Example of Abstracting a Root Operation

first three to five characters of the code. The first *three* characters of the partial code identify the appropriate Table to use.

ICD-10-PCS Tables

After locating the appropriate procedure in the Index and identifying the first three characters of the partial code, cross-reference the appropriate Table to build the rest of the code. Follow three steps to look up a PCS code in the tables:

1. Locate the Table using the first three characters of the partial code provided in the Index.

2. Build the code by locating the row in the Table that contains the appropriate Body Part value for Character 4. Then select the appropriate values for Characters 4, 5, 6, and 7 from within the same row of the Table.

3. Verify the character values by comparing the values selected against the documentation.

Arrange ICD-10-PCS Codes

Sequencing procedure codes is generally easier than sequencing diagnosis codes because there are fewer sequencing rules. When multiple procedures are performed, follow these general sequencing guidelines:

- Sequence as the first procedure the one most closely related to the principal diagnosis.

- When a procedure is required to care for a complication, sequence it before other procedures.

- When a diagnostic or exploratory procedure is followed by a definitive treatment, sequence the definitive procedure first and the diagnostic or exploratory procedure second.

ICD-10-PCS Medical and Surgical Section Guidelines provide guidance on coding multiple procedures. The PCS OGCR are discussed further in later chapters of this text.

CODING PRACTICE

Exercise 49.5 Introduction to the Steps of PCS Procedure Coding

Instructions: Fill in each blank with the correct term(s) from this section of the chapter.

1. The _____ functions as the Main Term in the Index and directs coders to the correct Table.

2. Coders _____ find Root Operations described in the procedure report using the exact PCS words.

3. Coders must read the procedure report and _____ what was done based on the definitions of the Root Operations.

4. Coders should plan to memorize the _____ of the most commonly used Root Operations and Root Types.

5. In the Medical and Surgical Section, the Index uses what two types of Main Terms? _____

6. The anatomic site is a _____ in the Index.

7. The first _____ characters of the partial code identify the appropriate Table to use.

8. Build the code by locating the row in the Table that contains _____.

9. Select the appropriate values for Characters _____ from within the same row of the Table.

10. The first sequenced procedure should be one most closely related to the _____.

CHAPTER SUMMARY

In this chapter you learned that:

- ICD-10-PCS is a new coding system to be used by hospitals for coding inpatient procedures.

- The ICD-10-PCS manual contains the Introduction, ICD-10-PCS Official Guidelines for Coding and Reporting (OGCR), Index, Tables, and Appendices.

- ICD-10-PCS codes have a logical, consistent structure that contains seven alphanumeric positions, called characters.

- ICD-10-PCS OGCR are divided into three sections: Conventions, which are labeled beginning with the letter A; Medical and Surgical Section Guidelines, which are labeled beginning with the letter B; and Obstetric Section Guidelines, which are labeled beginning with the letter C.

- The three skills of an ace coder—abstract, assign, and arrange—apply to coding procedures in ICD-10-PCS, but the mechanics are unique to this code set.

CONCEPT QUIZ

Take a moment to look back at your trip through ICD-10-PCS and solidify your skills. This is your opportunity to pull together everything you have learned.

Completion

Instructions: Write the term that answers each question based on the information you learned in this chapter. Choose from the list below. Some choices may be used more than once and some choices may not be used at all. Refer to the discussion in this chapter and the Glossary at the end of this book if you need a little extra help.

Approach(es)	Body System(s)
Body Part(s)	Character(s)
Device(s)	Root Operation(s)
expandability	Section(s)
multiaxial	standardized terminology
Qualifier(s)	value(s)

1. ICD-10-PCS codes are constructed of seven _____ or positions, each with a distinct purpose and meaning.

2. _____ means that the structure of the code set allows new procedures to be easily incorporated.

3. _____ means that the code set includes definitions of the terminology it uses and each term must have only one meaning.

4. To build a PCS code, coders assign _____ to each character, based on specific characteristics of the procedure the physician performs.

5. Each Section of the manual designates how each _____ of the code is used within that Section.

6. The Medical and Surgical Section has 31 possible values for the _____.

7. P, Upper Bones, is a(n) _____ value with the skeletal system.

8. The _____ describes the objective of the procedure.

9. Character 5 in the Medical and Surgical Section provides definitions for the _____.

10. Assign value Z when there is no _____.

Multiple Choice

Instructions: Circle the letter of the best answer to each question based on the information you learned in this chapter. Refer to the discussion in this chapter and the Glossary at the end of this book if you need a little extra help.

1. What feature is NOT part of ICD-10-PCS?
   A. Eponyms
   B. Standardized terminology
   C. Definitions
   D. Granularity

2. Where are hospital services and financial charges listed?
   A. Revenue code listing
   B. Charge description master
   C. ICD-10-PCS manual
   D. DRG grouper

3. What services are billed using ICD-10-PCS?
   A. Physician services
   B. Hospital outpatient services
   C. Hospital inpatient services
   D. All of the above

4. Which characters of a code are used to identify a PCS Table?
   A. The first character
   B. The first two characters
   C. The first three characters
   D. The first four characters

5. What Root Operation is defined as *cutting off a portion of a body part without replacement*?
   A. Excision
   B. Resection
   C. Removal
   D. Bypass

6. What Root Operation is ileostomy an example of?
   A. Excision
   B. Resection
   C. Removal
   D. Bypass

7. What is the Body Part when coding an ileostomy?
   A. Gastrointestinal
   B. Small intestine
   C. Ilium
   D. Ileum

8. What PCS definitions are the starting point for abstracting?
   A. Body System
   B. Root Operation
   C. Body Part
   D. Approach

9. What part of the PCS manual is used to assign code values?
   A. Only the Index
   B. The Index and Tables
   C. The appendix
   D. Section descriptors

10. What feature is characteristic of ICD-10-PCS but not CPT?
    A. Modifiers are often required.
    B. Combination codes identify procedures commonly performed together.
    C. Laterality is identified in the 4th character.
    D. Eponyms are a Main Term in the Index.

CODING CHALLENGE

Part A

Instructions: Using the PCS Index, look up the Root Operation and subterms listed. Write the partial code provided in the Index in the space provided.

> Example: Alteration, Abdominal Wall
>
> Partial Code: *0W0F*
>
> 1. Bypass, Duct, Hepatic, Left: Partial Code
>
> _____
>
> 2. Excision, Disc, Lumbosacral: Partial Code
>
> _____
>
> 3. Fusion, Metacarpophalangeal, Right: Partial Code
>
> _____
>
> 4. Release, Pulmonary Trunk: Partial Code
>
> _____
>
> 5. Supplement, Tendon, Foot, Left: Partial Code
>
> _____

Part B

Instructions: Look up the Table represented by the three-character partial code. Write out the values represented by the Section, Body System, and Root Operation.

> Example: Table **021**
>
> Character 1, Section: *0 Medical and Surgical*
>
> Character 2, Body System: *2 Heart and Great Vessels*
>
> Character 3, Root Operation: *1 Bypass*
>
> (*continued*)

> (continued)
>
> 6. Table **B51**
>
>   Character 1, Section: _____
>
>   Character 2, Body System: _____
>
>   Character 3, Root Operation: _____
>
> 7. Table **0H9**
>
>   Character 1, Section: _____
>
>   Character 2, Body System: _____
>
>   Character 3, Root Operation: _____
>
> 8. Table **0KS**
>
>   Character 1, Section: _____
>
>   Character 2, Body System: _____
>
>   Character 3, Root Operation: _____
>
> 9. Table **07L**
>
>   Character 1, Section: _____
>
>   Character 2, Body System: _____
>
>   Character 3, Root Operation: _____
>
> 10. Table **04R**
>
>   Character 1, Section: _____
>
>   Character 2, Body System: _____
>
>   Character 3, Root Operation: _____

KEEP ON CODING

Part A

Instructions: Using the PCS Index, look up the Root Operation and subterms listed. Write the partial code provided in the Index in the space provided.

> Example: Alteration, Abdominal Wall: Partial Code *0W0F*

1. Alteration, Nose: Partial Code _____

2. Change Diaphragm: Partial Code _____

3. Creation, Male: Partial Code _____

4. Destruction, Cervix: Partial Code _____

5. Dilation, Esophagus: Partial Code _____

6. Extirpation, Anus: Partial Code _____

(*continued*)

(continued from page 993)

7. Fragmentation, Trachea: Partial Code _____

8. Inspection, Fallopian Tube: Partial Code _____

9. Map, Brain: Partial Code _____

10. Occlusion, Urethra: Partial Code _____

11. Reattachment, Tooth, Upper: Partial Code _____

12. Release, Nerve, Trigeminal: Partial Code _____

13. Repair, Jejunum: Partial Code _____

14. Supplement, Larynx: Partial Code _____

15. Transfer, Tendon, Head and Neck: Partial Code _____

Part B

Instructions: Look up the Table represented by the three-character partial code. Write out the values represented by the Section, Body System, and Root Operation.

Example: Table **021**

Character 1, Section: *O Medical and Surgical*

Character 2, Body System: *2 Heart and Great Vessels*

Character 3, Root Operation: *1 Bypass*

16. Table **OCR**

Character 1, Section: _____

Character 2, Body System: _____

Character 3, Root Operation: _____

17. Table **OJH**

Character 1, Section: _____

Character 2, Body System: _____

Character 3, Root Operation: _____

18. Table **ON9**

Character 1, Section: _____

Character 2, Body System: _____

Character 3, Root Operation: _____

19. Table **OPT**

Character 1, Section: _____

Character 2, Body System: _____

Character 3, Root Operation: _____

20. Table **10E**

Character 1, Section: _____

Character 2, Body System: _____

Character 3, Root Operation: _____

21. Table **2W3**

    Character 1, Section: _____

    Character 2, Anatomical Region: _____

    Character 3, Root Operation: _____

22. Table **BV2**

    Character 1, Section: _____

    Character 2, Body System: _____

    Character 3, Root Type: _____

23. Table **F07**

    Character 1, Section: _____

    Character 2, Section Qualifier: _____

    Character 3, Root Type: _____

24. Table **GZJ**

    Character 1, Section: _____

    Character 2, Body System: _____

    Character 3, Root Type: _____

25. Table **HZ4**

    Character 1, Section: _____

    Character 2, Body System: _____

    Character 3, Root Type: _____

Chapter 50

Overview of Medical and Surgical Procedures (Section 0)

Chapter Outline

- **Medical and Surgical Basics**
- **The Characters of Medical and Surgical Codes**

Learning Objectives

After completing this chapter, you should have the skills to:

50.1 Spell and define the key words, medical terms, and abbreviations related to medical and surgical procedures.

50.2 Discuss common Medical and Surgical procedures.

50.3 Identify the seven characters and definitions of an ICD-10-PCS Medical and Surgical code.

50.4 Discuss PCS guidelines for Medical and Surgical procedures.

Key Terms and Abbreviations

Device
diagnostic procedure
divided
External

Open
Percutaneous
Percutaneous Endoscopic
surgical approach

therapeutic procedure
Via Natural or Artificial Opening
Via Natural or Artificial Opening Endoscopic

Via Natural or Artificial Opening Endoscopic with Percutaneous Endoscopic Assistance

In addition to the key terms listed here, students should know the terms defined within tables in this chapter.

For updates and corrections, visit our student resource site at
www.pearsonhighered.com/healthprofessionsresources

INTRODUCTION

In your preliminary tour of the PCS Medical and Surgical Section in this chapter, you will become familiar with the largest section in the PCS manual, how it is structured, and how to use it. Most importantly, you learn many of the definitions that are the cornerstone of ICD-10-PCS and are essential to accurate code assignment. Later chapters provide more detailed information.

MEDICAL AND SURGICAL BASICS

Physicians perform a wide range of procedures on any body part. Because no coder can be familiar with every possible procedure, it is important to apply medical terminology skills to combine familiar word roots, prefixes, and suffixes to define new procedural terms. Procedural terms combine the word root(s) for one or more body parts, such as *gastr/o*, with a suffix that describes the type of procedure, such as *-ectomy*.

Although PCS establishes its own terminology and definitions of Root Operations, physicians will continue to use traditional Latin-based medical terms, such as *gastrectomy*, and eponyms, such as the Whipple procedure, which is one type of gastrectomy. Latin-based medical terms appear in the PCS Index and redirect coders to the most likely Root Operations. There is no direct correlation between medical terms and Root Operation definitions. Coders must read the operative report to determine exactly what was done and interpret this information in light of the Root Operations.

Coders need to know the difference between a treatment and a diagnostic procedure; they also need to know the types of surgical approaches to a procedure.

Treatment and Diagnostic Procedures

Physicians may order procedures for either therapeutic or diagnostic purposes. A **therapeutic procedure** is performed in order to treat a disease or condition. Examples are a cholecystectomy due to gallbladder disease, a coronary artery bypass to treat atherosclerosis, or removal of a skin lesion that is cancerous. A **diagnostic procedure** is performed to obtain information needed to make a diagnosis and treatment plan. Examples are performing a biopsy of a tumor in order to determine whether it is malignant or performing amniocentesis to determine whether a fetus has chromosomal abnormalities.

Surgical Approaches

The **surgical approach** describes how the surgeon accessed the operative site. A variety of methods may be used for most procedures. The surgeon's decision is based on the reason the procedure is being done, the circumstances of the patient, the proven effectiveness of one approach over others, and other factors.

In some cases, the surgeon may plan to use one approach then need to change to another approach due to complicating factors. For example, the surgeon may plan to perform an endoscopic cholecystectomy, but due to adhesions must change to an open approach. PCS definitions of the Approach character follow. These terms and definitions may differ slightly from those used in CPT.

Open

An **Open** procedure is one in which an incision is made through the skin and subcutaneous tissue. Fascia and muscles are divided (*separated*) and the organ, body cavity, or region is directly visualized with the naked eye by the surgeon. All steps to access the procedure site, including the initial incision on the skin, subsequent divisions to reach the surgical site, and layered closure, are part of the procedure. An open approach is the most invasive and carries the highest risk to the patient. Surgeons will generally opt for a less invasive approach whenever possible. Examples of the open approach are an abdominal hysterectomy and an open coronary artery bypass graft (CABG).

Percutaneous

In a **Percutaneous** procedure, the skin is punctured or a very small incision is made to access the site, but a full-length incision is not made. An example is a needle biopsy of any joint or organ.

Percutaneous Endoscopic

In a **Percutaneous Endoscopic** procedure, the surgeon makes several, usually two to four, small incisions, approximately one-half to one inch in length. A fiber optic camera is inserted through one incision and surgical instruments are inserted through the other openings. The camera transmits an image of the operative site to a television monitor. Examples of the percutaneous endoscopic approach are a laparoscopic cholecystectomy and arthroscopic repair of a joint.

SUCCESS STEP

Endoscopy is a generic name for any procedure using a fiber optic viewing scope. The procedure may also carry the name of the site accessed, such as colonoscopy, laparoscopy, or gastroscopy.

Via Natural or Artificial Opening

In the approach **Via Natural or Artificial Opening**, the surgeon accesses the surgical site through a body opening that already exists, such as the mouth, nose, ear, anus, or vagina. Artificially made openings, such as a tracheotomy or colostomy mouth, may also be used. In either situation, a new incision is not required. Examples are insertion of an endotracheal tube through the oral cavity and placement of a Foley catheter through the urinary tract.

Via Natural or Artificial Opening Endoscopic

In the approach **Via Natural or Artificial Opening Endoscopic**, the surgeon inserts an endoscope through an existing natural or artificial opening. Examples are a colonoscopy, in which the endoscope is inserted through the anus, and an endoscopic examination of the esophagus, in which the endoscope is inserted through the mouth.

Via Natural or Artificial Opening Endoscopic <u>with</u> Percutaneous Endoscopic Assistance

In the approach **Via Natural or Artificial Opening Endoscopic with Percutaneous Endoscopic Assistance**, two endoscopes are used: one through a natural or artificial opening and the second one through percutaneous access. Surgeons choose this approach when they cannot perform the entire procedure through the natural or artificial opening. An example is vaginal hysterectomy performed with laparoscopic assistance (LAVH).

External

When the entire treatment is performed on the skin or mucous membranes, the approach is **External**. Examples of the external approach are a tonsillectomy and removal of a skin lesion. Another method for an external approach is applying direct or indirect pressure. An example is a closed fracture reduction.

The surgical approach is always documented in the procedure note, but it is not necessarily stated with the PCS terms. For example, when using an open approach, the surgeon describes the initial incision, each subsequent division, and the layered closure but may not use the word *open*. When accessing the site through a natural or artificial opening, the documentation names the opening, such as vagina, but does not state "via natural opening." Coders are responsible for interpreting the documentation and assigning the correct PCS value based on PCS definitions.

In addition to the surgical approach, some procedures also identify the directional approach. For example, procedures on the spine may be performed from a posterior or anterior approach and, in some cases, both. When the directional approach is not explicitly stated, the coder can determine it based on the location of the incision.

CODING PRACTICE

Exercise 50.1 Medical and Surgical Basics

Instructions: Use your medical terminology skills and resources to define the following terms, then look them up in the ICD-10-PCS Index. Follow these steps:

- Use slash marks "/" to break down each term into its root(s) and suffix.
- Define the meaning of the word based on the meaning of each word part.
- Look up the term in the ICD-10-PCS Index, and write down the **name(s)** of Root Operation(s) the Index cross-references you to and the Table(s), if provided.
- Do not assign any codes.

Example: gastrectomy gastr/ectomy   Meaning: *excision of the stomach*   Root Operation(s): *Excision, Resection*

1. angioplasty   Meaning _____   Root Operation(s) _____
2. hysterectomy   Meaning _____   Root Operation(s) _____
3. ovariocentesis   Meaning _____   Root Operation(s) _____
4. arthrodesis   Meaning _____   Root Operation(s) _____
5. herniorrhaphy   Meaning _____   Root Operation(s) _____
6. adhesiolysis   Meaning _____   Root Operation(s) _____
7. colostomy   Meaning _____   Root Operation(s) _____
8. tracheotomy   Meaning _____   Root Operation(s) _____
9. esophagoplication   Meaning _____   Root Operation(s) _____
10. cholecystopexy   Meaning _____   Root Operation(s) _____

THE CHARACTERS OF MEDICAL AND SURGICAL CODES

The Medical and Surgical Section is the largest Section of ICD-10-PCS, containing 31 Body Systems and 31 Root Operations. ICD-10-PCS provides guidelines for Medical and Surgical codes in section B of the PCS OGCR. Six subdivisions of the guidelines, B2 through B7, correspond to each character within a Medical and Surgical code.

CODING CAUTION

If you are already familiar with CPT coding for physicians, be careful to not confuse CPT guidelines with PCS guidelines. The two are not comparable and, sometimes, are contradictory.

The Section value for Medical and Surgical is **0**. The characters of Medical and Surgical procedure codes are shown in ■ TABLE 50-1. In the following sections, coding requirements for Characters 2 through 7 are highlighted.

Character 2: Medical and Surgical Body System

The second character in the Medical and Surgical Section defines the Body System, the general physiological system or anatomic region. PCS divides most organ systems into multiple Body System values in order to achieve greater granularity (■ TABLE 50-2).

Table 50-1 ■ **SEVEN CHARACTERS OF MEDICAL AND SURGICAL PROCEDURES**

1	2	3	4	5	6	7
Section 0	Body System	Root Operation	Body Part	Approach	Device	Qualifier

Table 50-2 ■ **MEDICAL AND SURGICAL CHARACTER 2: BODY SYSTEM VALUES WITH ORGAN SYSTEM**

Value	PCS Body System Description	Organ System
0	Central Nervous System	Nervous system
1	Peripheral Nervous System	
2	Heart and Great Vessels	
3	Upper Arteries	
4	Lower Arteries	Cardiovascular system
5	Upper Veins	
6	Lower Veins	
7	Lymphatic and Hemic System	Blood and immune system
8	Eye	Special senses
9	Ear, Nose, Sinus	Special senses (Ear) and Respiratory system
B	Respiratory System	
C	Mouth and Throat	
D	Gastrointestinal System	Digestive system
F	Hepatobiliary System and Pancreas	
G	Endocrine System	Endocrine system
H	Skin and Breast	Integumentary system
J	Subcutaneous Tissue and Fascia	
K	Muscles	
L	Tendons	Muscular system
M	Bursae and Ligaments	
N	Head and Facial Bones	
P	Upper Bones	
Q	Lower Bones	Skeletal system
R	Upper Joints	
S	Lower Joints	
T	Urinary System	
U	Female Reproductive System	Genitourinary system
V	Male Reproductive System	
W	Anatomical Regions, General	
X	Anatomical Regions, Upper Extremities	Body areas
Y	Anatomical Regions, Lower Extremities	

Adapted from: Department of Health and Human Services, Centers for Medicare and Medicaid Services, ICD-10-PCS Coding Manual.

Values **W**, **X**, and **Y** describe Anatomic Regions, which are used when a procedure is performed on an area that is larger than a specific Body Part (PCS OGCR B2.1a). Examples include the following types of procedures:

- control of postprocedural bleeding in an extremity
- amputation of all or part of an extremity
- drainage of a body cavity

The Index is organized by Root Operation, with the first-level subterm often being the Body System. Coders must select the most specific Body System value available. Search for a subterm that identifies the specific Body System before selecting a subterm for an anatomic region.

Character 3: Medical and Surgical Root Operation

The Medical and Surgical Section has 31 Root Operations, the most of any Section. Root Operations are the core of PCS coding because they serve as Main Terms in the Index. Coders cannot assign a Root Operation based on the common meaning of a word such as *removal* or *excision*; they must apply the full definition that PCS provides in the Tables (PCS OGCR B3.1a).

The PCS definition of all Root Operations appears in the appendix of most ICD-10-PCS coding manuals. Root Operations are divided into groups of procedures with similar objectives (■ TABLE 50-3). These groupings also appear in a PCS appendix and are discussed in the following chapters of this text.

> ### SUCCESS STEP
>
> PCS is unique among medical coding systems because it provides standard, official definitions for each character of the code. Although it may feel intimidating to memorize definitions, this feature makes the system user-friendly and logical.

Table 50-3 ■ **ROOT OPERATION GROUPS, WITH PROCEDURE OBJECTIVE, SITE, AND EXAMPLES**

Root Operations That Take Out Some or All of a Body Part				
Root Operation	**Value**	**Objective of Procedure**	**Procedure Site**	**Example**
Excision	B	Cutting out/off without replacement	Some of a body part	Breast lumpectomy
Resection	T	Cutting out/off without replacement	All of a body part	Total mastectomy
Detachment	6	Cutting out/off without replacement	Extremity only, any level	Amputation above elbow
Destruction	5	Eradicating without replacement	Some/all of a body part	Fulguration of endometrium
Extraction	D	Pulling out/off without replacement	Some/all of a body part	Suction D&C

Root Operations That Take Out Solids/Fluids/Gases from a Body Part				
Root Operation	**Value**	**Objective of Procedure**	**Procedure Site**	**Example**
Drainage	9	Taking/letting out fluids/gases	Within a body part	Incision and drainage
Extirpation	C	Taking/cutting out solid matter	Within a body part	Thrombectomy
Fragmentation	F	Breaking solid matter into pieces	Within a body part	Lithotripsy

Root Operations Involving Cutting or Separation Only				
Root Operation	**Value**	**Objective of Procedure**	**Procedure Site**	**Example**
Division	8	Cutting into/separating a body part	Within a body part	Neurotomy
Release	N	Freeing a body part from constraint	Around a body part	Adhesiolysis

Root Operations That Put In/Put Back or Move Some/All of a Body Part				
Root Operation	**Value**	**Objective of Procedure**	**Procedure Site**	**Example**
Transplantation	Y	Putting in a living body part from a person/animal	Some/all of a body part	Kidney transplant
Reattachment	M	Putting back a detached body part	Some/all of a body part	Reattach finger
Transfer	X	Moving a body part to function for a similar body part	Some/all of a body part	Skin transfer flap
Reposition	S	Moving a body part to normal or other suitable location	Some/all of a body part	Move undescended testicle

Table 50-3 ■ (*continued*)

Root Operations That Alter the Diameter/Route of a Tubular Body Part

Root Operation	Value	Objective of Procedure	Procedure Site	Example
Restriction	V	Partially closing orifice/lumen	Tubular body part	Gastroesophageal fundoplication
Occlusion	L	Completely closing orifice/lumen	Tubular body part	Fallopian tube ligation
Dilation	7	Expanding orifice/lumen	Tubular body part	Percutaneous transluminal coronary angioplasty (PTCA)
Bypass	1	Altering route of passage	Tubular body part	Coronary artery bypass graft (CABG)

Root Operations That Always Involve a Device

Root Operation	Value	Objective of Procedure	Procedure Site	Example
Insertion	H	Putting in nonbiological device	In/on a body part	Central line insertion
Replacement	R	Putting in device that replaces a body part	Some/all of a body part	Total hip replacement
Supplement	U	Putting in device that reinforces or augments a body part	In/on a body part	Abdominal wall herniorrhaphy using mesh
Change	2	Exchanging device without cutting/puncturing	In/on a body part	Drainage tube change

Root Operations That Always Involve a Device

Root Operation	Value	Objective of Procedure	Procedure Site	Example
Removal	P	Taking out device	In/on a body part	Central line removal
Revision	W	Correcting a malfunctioning/displaced device	In/on a body part	Revision of pacemaker insertion

Root Operations Involving Examination Only

Root Operation	Value	Objective of Procedure	Procedure Site	Example
Inspection	J	Visual/manual exploration	Some/all of a body part	Diagnostic cystoscopy
Map	K	Locating electrical impulses/functional areas	Brain/cardiac conduction mechanism	Cardiac electro-physiological study

Root Operations That Define Other Repairs

Root Operation	Value	Objective of Procedure	Procedure Site	Example
Control	3	Stopping/attempting to stop postprocedural bleed	Anatomic region	Post-prostatectomy bleeding control
Repair	Q	Restoring body part to its normal structure	Some/all of a body part	Suture laceration

Root Operations That Define Other Objectives

Root Operation	Value	Objective of Procedure	Procedure Site	Example
Fusion	G	Rendering joint immobile	Joint	Spinal fusion
Alteration	0	Modifying body part for cosmetic purposes without affecting function	Some/all of a body part	Face lift
Creation	4	Making new structure for sex change operation	Perineum	Artificial vagina/penis

Source: Department of Health and Human Services, Centers for Medicare and Medicaid Services, ICD-10-PCS Reference Manual.

Character 4: Medical and Surgical Body Part

The fourth character in the Medical and Surgical Section defines the Body Part, or specific anatomic site, where the physician performed the procedure. The definition of each Body Part value in the Medical and Surgical Section is unique to each Body System. For example, in Body System **8 Eye**, the Body Part value **1** is **Left Eye**. In Body System **L Tendons**, the Body Part value **1** is **Right Shoulder Tendon**. Body Parts appear as first- or second-level subterms in the Index. In most cases, the partial code in the Index directs coders not only to the correct Table, but also to the correct Character 4 value.

The challenge for coders is matching the documented anatomic site to the most specific PCS Body System and Body Part value. For example, under the Root Operation **Reposition**, PCS provides Body System and Body Part values for the following sites in the upper arm:

- muscles of the upper arm
- tendons of the upper arm
- head of the humerus
- shaft of the humerus
- acromioclavicular joint

Each of these is a separate Index entry (■ FIGURE 50-1) under Root Operation **Reposition (S)**. The Body System and Body Part values differ. It would be easy to miss the entry, **humeral head**, and focus instead on the entry for **upper arm** without noticing the previous-level subterm, which identifies the Body System as **Muscle**, **Tendon**, or **Joint**.

Another challenge with Body Parts is that the site documented in the medical record may be more specific, or use a different term, than what PCS provides. PCS OGCR B4 specifies how to code Body Parts for various Body Systems. Assign a code for the closest body part, branch, or region for which PCS provides a value.

The Index includes entries for many anatomic sites that direct coders to the PCS Body Part to use. Anatomic site entries do not provide a partial code or Table number; they simply identify the PCS Body Part (■ FIGURE 50-2). Coders still need to locate the corresponding Root Operation as an Index Main Term in order to identify the correct Table, as follows:

1. Identify the anatomic site documented.
2. Locate the anatomic term in the Index.
3. Identify the corresponding PCS Body Part description, which appears after the word *use*.
4. Use the PCS description to select the Body Part value from the Table corresponding to the Root Operation and Body System.

The Body Part Key appendix of the PCS manual provides a helpful table that cross-references specific anatomic terms to the PCS Body Part (■ TABLE 50-4). If an anatomic site cannot be located in the Index, also refer to this appendix. Use the Body Part Key as follows (■ FIGURE 50-3):

1. Identify the anatomic site documented.
2. Locate the anatomic term in the first column.

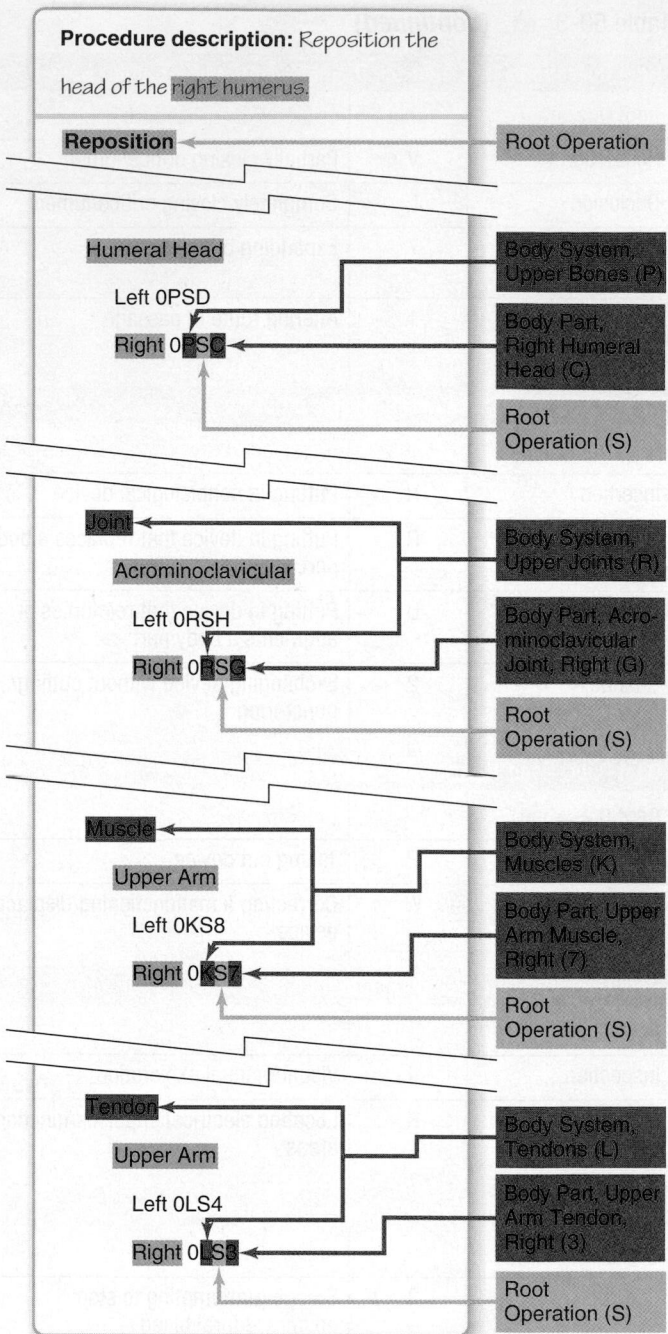

Figure 50-1 ■ Example of Locating the Correct Body Part in the Index

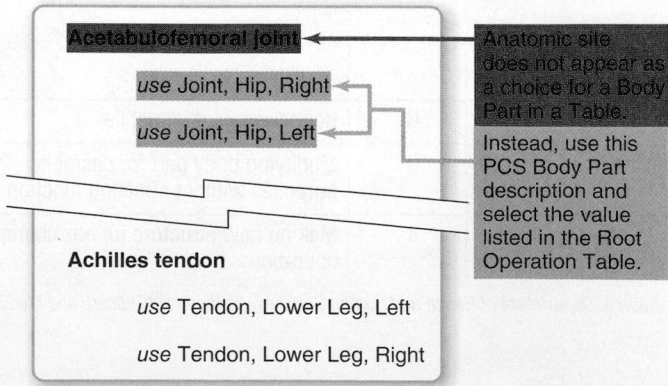

Figure 50-2 ■ Index Entry for an Anatomic Site with Cross-Reference to PCS Body Part

Table 50-4 ■ **EXCERPT FROM PCS BODY PART KEY APPENDIX**

Anatomic Term	PCS Description
Acetabulofemoral joint	Hip Joint, Right
	Hip Joint, Left
Achilles tendon	Lower Leg Tendon, Right
	Lower Leg Tendon, Left
Alveolar process of maxilla	Maxilla, Right
	Maxilla, Left
Aortic intercostal artery	Thoracic Aorta

Source: Department of Health and Human Services, Centers for Medicare and Medicaid Services, ICD-10-PCS Coding Manual.

3. Identify the corresponding PCS description in the second column.

4. Use the PCS description to locate a subterm in the Index, or select the Body Part value from the Table corresponding to the Root Operation and Body System.

Character 5: Medical and Surgical Approach

The Medical and Surgical Section uses seven different values to define the Approach (■ TABLE 50-5). An appendix in most ICD-10-PCS manuals defines each Approach, which were also defined earlier in this chapter of the text. PCS OGCR B5 discusses specific coding situations related to an open approach with percutaneous endoscopic assistance, the external approach,

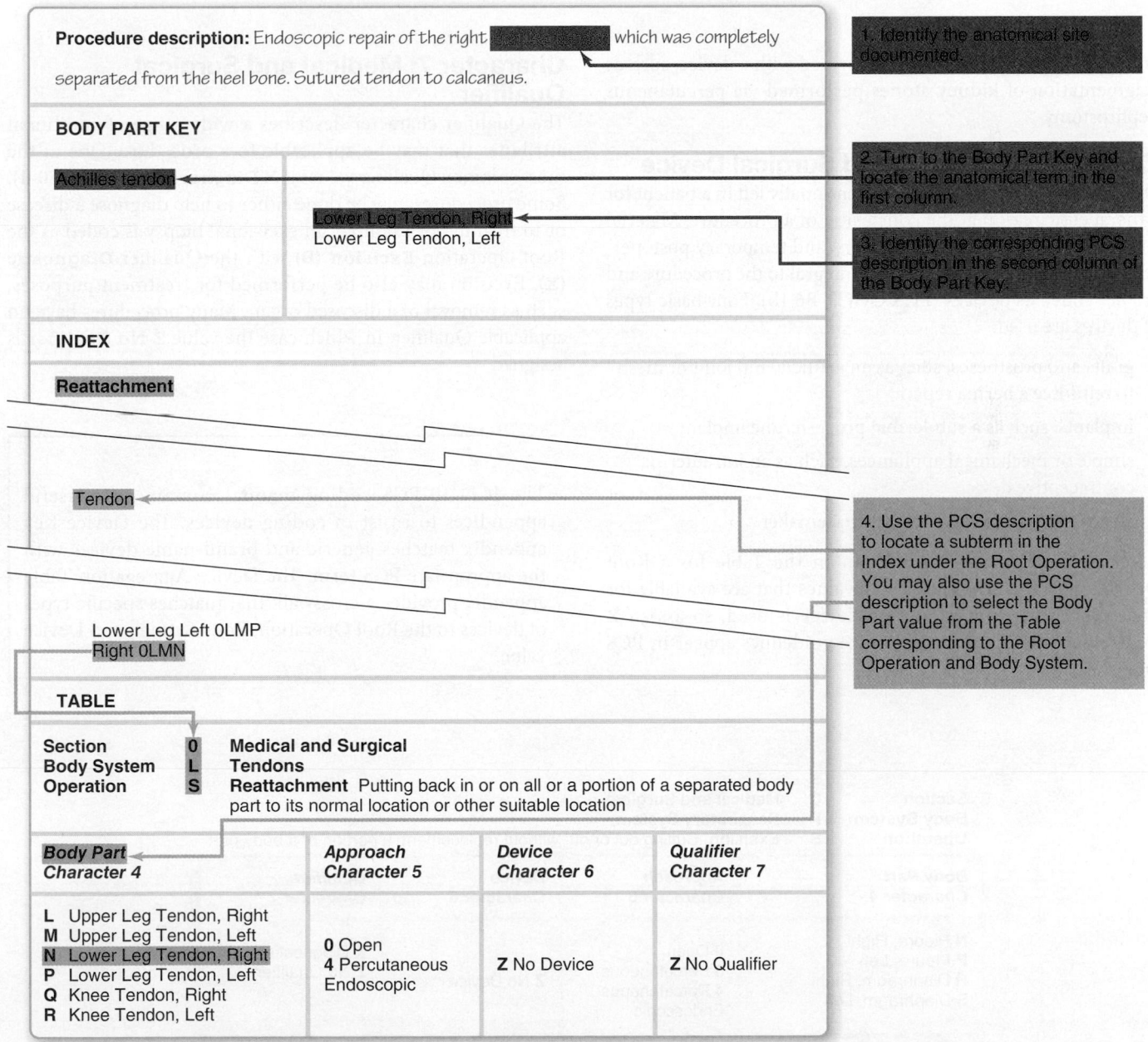

Figure 50-3 ■ Example of Using the Body Part Key Appendix to PCS Body Part

Table 50-5 ■ **VALUES FOR MEDICAL AND SURGICAL APPROACH**

Value	Approach
0	Open
3	Percutaneous
4	Percutaneous Endoscopic
7	Via Natural or Artificial Opening
8	Via Natural or Artificial Opening Endoscopic
F	Via Natural or Artificial Opening Endoscopic with Percutaneous Endoscopic Assistance
X	External

Source: Department of Health and Human Services, Centers for Medicare and Medicaid Services, ICD-10-PCS Reference Manual.

and percutaneous procedures performed with a device, such as fragmentation of kidney stones performed via percutaneous nephrostomy.

Character 6: Medical and Surgical Device

Device refers to material that is intentionally left in a patient for a therapeutic reason at the conclusion of a procedure. Material such as sutures, radiological markers, and temporary postoperative wound drains are considered integral to the procedure and are *not* coded as devices (PCS OGCR B6.1b). Four basic types of devices are used:

- grafts and prostheses, such as an artificial hip joint or mesh to reinforce a hernia repair
- implants, such as a subdermal progesterone implant
- simple or mechanical appliances, such as an intrauterine contraceptive device
- electronic appliances, such as a pacemaker

Refer to the Character 6 column in the Table for a Root Operation to identify the Device values that are available for each procedure. Frequently, no device is used, so assign **Z No Device** for Character 6. Device guidelines appear in PCS OGCR B6.

Character 7: Medical and Surgical Qualifier

The Qualifier character describes a wide range of additional attributes that may be applicable to a procedure. One of the most common Qualifier values is **X Diagnostic** (■ FIGURE 50-4). Some procedures may be done either to help diagnose a disease or to treat it. For example, an excisional biopsy is coded as the Root Operation **Excision (B)** with the Qualifier **Diagnostic (X)**. Excision may also be performed for treatment purposes, such as removal of a diseased organ. Many procedures have no applicable Qualifier, in which case the value **Z No Qualifier** is assigned.

SUCCESS STEP

The ICD-10-PCS coding manual contains two useful appendices to assist in coding devices. The Device Key appendix matches generic and brand-name devices with the appropriate PCS term. The Device Aggregation Table appendix provides a crosswalk that matches specific types of devices to the Root Operation, Body System, and Device value.

Section	0	Medical and Surgical
Body System	P	Respiratory System
Operation	S	Excision Cutting out or off, without replacement, a portion of a body part

Body Part Character 4	Approach Character 5	Device Character 6	Qualifier Character 7
N Pleura, Right P Pleura, Left R Diaphragm, Right S Diaphragm, Left	0 Open 3 Percutaneous 4 Percutaneous Endoscopic	Z No Device	X Diagnostic Z No Qualifier

Figure 50-4 ■ Example of a Diagnostic Qualifier

CODING PRACTICE

Exercise 50.2   The Characters of Medical and Surgical Codes

Instructions: Refer to Table 50-3. Locate the name of the Root Operation in the first column of the table, then write your answer to the question in the space provided.

1. What procedure is an example of the Root Operation Extirpation? _____

2. What Root Operation group does the Root Operation Division belong to? _____

   (*Tip*: Root Operation groups are the subheadings or sections of Table 50-3.)

3. What is the objective of the procedure for the Root Operation Restriction? _____

4. What is the objective of the procedure for the Root Operation Removal? _____

5. What is the procedure site for the Root Operation Fusion? _____

6. What is the value for the Root Operation Transplantation? _____

7. What procedure is an example of the Root Operation Map? _____

8. What Root Operation group does the Root Operation Supplement belong to? _____

9. What is the procedure site for the Root Operation Detachment? _____

10. What is the value of the Root Operation Repair? _____

CHAPTER SUMMARY

In this chapter you learned that:

- Coders need to understand the difference between treatments and diagnostic procedures as well as the description of various surgical approaches.

- The Medical and Surgical Section is the largest Section of ICD-10-PCS, containing 31 Body Systems and 31 Root Operations.

- The seven characters of a Medical and Surgical Procedure are (1) Section, (2) Body System, (3) Root Operation, (4) Body Part, (5) Approach, (6) Device, and (7) Qualifier.

- ICD-10-PCS provides guidelines for Medical and Surgical codes in section B of the PCS OGCR, which contains six subdivisions, one corresponding to each character within a Medical and Surgical code.

CONCEPT QUIZ

Completion

Instructions: Use the Body Part Key appendix in the ICD-10-PCS manual to identify the PCS description for each anatomic term. Search for the anatomic term in the left column of the Body Part Key, then write down the PCS description from the right column of the Body Part Key. PCS descriptions will come from the following list, but you must use the Body Part Key to identify the correct answer. Some choices may be used more than once and some choices may not be used at all. Refer to the discussion in this chapter if you need a little extra help.

Example: Achilles tendon *Lower Leg Tendon*

Ampulla of Vater	Pancreatic Duct
Basal Ganglia	Pelvic Bone
Colic Vein	Pons
Common Bile Duct	Prepuce
External Iliac Artery	Pulmonary Artery, Left
Facial Muscle	Small Intestine
Greater Omentum	Trigeminal Nerve
Greater Saphenous Vein	Uterine Supporting Structure
Intracranial Vein	Vas Deferens

1. Anterior cerebral vein _____
2. Duct of Wirsung _____
3. Gasserian ganglion _____
4. Basis pontis _____
5. Broad ligament _____
6. Hepatopancreatic ampulla _____
7. Botallo's duct _____
8. Glans penis _____
9. External pudendal vein _____
10. Iliac crest _____

(*continued*)

(continued from page 1005)

Multiple Choice

Instructions: Circle the letter of the best answer to each question based on the information you learned in this chapter. Refer to tables in the chapter for assistance.

1. What Approach is used for a procedure in which an incision is made through the skin and subcutaneous tissue?
   A. Open
   B. Percutaneous
   C. Percutaneous Endoscopic
   D. External

2. What Approach is used for a procedure in which the endoscope is inserted through the anus?
   A. Percutaneous Endoscopic
   B. Via Natural or Artificial Opening
   C. External
   D. Via Natural or Artificial Opening Endoscopic

3. Which of the following is a Body System in ICD-10-PCS?
   A. Digestive System
   B. Skeletal System
   C. Upper Bones
   D. Cardiovascular System

4. Which Root Operation is lithotripsy an example of?
   A. Excision
   B. Destruction
   C. Fragmentation
   D. Removal

5. Which Root Operation is fallopian tube ligation an example of?
   A. Resection
   B. Occlusion
   C. Destruction
   D. Restriction

6. What Root Operation is used when the procedure involves cutting out the left upper lobe of the lung?
   A. Repair
   B. Resection
   C. Removal
   D. Excision

7. What is one of the most common Qualifier values?
   A. T Therapeutic
   B. X Diagnostic
   C. 0 Open
   D. R Bilateral

8. What type of procedure, by definition, leaves a drainage device in the patient?
   A. Therapeutic
   B. Diagnostic
   C. Exploratory
   D. Supplemental

9. How many PCS Body Systems are used for the muscular system?
   A. 1
   B. 2
   C. 3
   D. 5

10. Which of the following Root Operations always involves a device?
    A. Change
    B. Drainage
    C. Occlusion
    D. Reposition

CODING CHALLENGE

Instructions: Refer to Table 50-3. For each Root Operation group listed below, write down the **names** and **values** of all Root Operations in the group.

Example: Root Operations that define other objectives

Fusion G, Alteration 0, Creation 4

1. Root Operations involving examination only

   _____

   _____

2. Root Operations that always involve a device

   _____

   _____

3. Root Operations involving cutting or separation only

   _____

   _____

4. Root Operations that put in/put back or move some/all of a body part _____

   _____

5. Root Operations that take out solids/fluids/gases from a body part _____

   _____

KEEP ON CODING

Instructions: Refer to Table 50-3. Provide an example of each Root Operation.

Example: Change *Drainage tube change*

1. Supplement _____

2. Excision _____

3. Extraction _____

4. Restriction _____

5. Revision _____

6. Resection _____

7. Reposition _____

8. Release _____

9. Reattachment _____

10. Dilation _____

Chapter 51

Coding for Medical and Surgical Procedures (Section 0)

Chapter Outline

- **Abstracting Medical and Surgical Procedures**
- **Assigning Medical and Surgical Procedure Codes**
- **Arranging Medical and Surgical Procedure Codes**

Learning Objectives

After completing this chapter, you should have the skills to:

51.1 Spell and define the key words, medical terms, and abbreviations related to Medical and Surgical procedure coding.

51.2 Abstract information from the medical record for Medical and Surgical Root Operations and procedures.

51.3 Assign codes for Medical and Surgical procedures.

51.4 Arrange codes for Medical and Surgical procedures.

51.5 Discuss PCS guidelines for Medical and Surgical procedures.

Key Terms and Abbreviations

operative report
procedure report

In addition to the key terms listed here, students should know the terms defined within tables in this chapter.

For updates and corrections, visit our student resource site at
www.pearsonhighered.com/healthprofessionsresources

INTRODUCTION

After you get the lay of the land in a large sightseeing venue, you are better equipped to enjoy specific parts of it that are most appealing. In your continuing tour of the PCS Medical and Surgical section in this chapter, you will have the opportunity to become more acquainted with the details. You will learn how the three skills of an ace coder—abstracting, arranging, and assigning—apply to PCS Medical and Surgical codes.

ABSTRACTING MEDICAL AND SURGICAL PROCEDURES

Because identifying the correct Root Operation is the basis of ICD-10-PCS coding, coders must learn the differences between similar Root Operations. This enables them to abstract appropriately. Physicians are not expected to use PCS terminology when documenting. Coders must read what physicians document and equate it to the definitions provided by PCS (PCS OGCR A11). Refer to PCS OGCR B3, which provides further details on Root Operations. Then, follow key criteria for abstracting Medical and Surgical procedures to identify the correct Root Operation.

Key Criteria for Abstracting Medical and Surgical Procedures

To abstract for Medical and Surgical procedures, coders need to determine what procedures were performed and what approach was used. After reading the procedure report, use the abstracting table (■ Table 51-1, page 1010) as follows:

1. Answer the General Questions to get a basic understanding of the procedure.
2. Answer the Root Operation Questions. One question should be answered *Yes*, the rest should be answered *No*.
3. For the Root Operation Question that was answered *Yes*, refer to the right-hand column to identify the Root Operations that could apply.

4. Look up the definition of each of the applicable Root Operations in the ICD-10-PCS coding manual appendix, Root Operation Definitions, or Comparison of Medical and Surgical Root Operations (■ Table 51-2, pages 1011–1013).
5. Identify the one Root Operation that matches the procedure documented. This Root Operation will be the Main Term when you use the Index.
6. Repeat the abstracting process for each procedure that was performed.

Abstracting criteria for Medical and Surgical-<u>Related</u> procedures and Ancillary procedures are presented in later chapters.

Abstracting Procedure Reports

After completing a procedure, physicians prepare a **procedure report** or **operative report** that describes the details of what was done. The format varies with each physician or hospital but must include the following information:

- date of procedure
- name of procedure performed
- names of the surgeon and all assistants
- preprocedure or provisional diagnosis
- a detailed description of the procedure, such as patient preparation, anesthesia, instruments and supplies used, incisions made, visualized structures, findings, alterations performed, tissue removed, estimated blood loss, closing process, and patient status
- postprocedure diagnosis

The procedure report may be dictated, then transcribed, or entered directly into an electronic health record (EHR). The procedure report is maintained in a designated section of the patient's overall medical record. The mini-medical-record used for procedure cases in this text provides a limited snapshot of the most pertinent information. Refer to ■ Figure 51-1 to learn how to interpret the mini-medical-record used for procedure reports.

(*Text continued on page 1013.*)

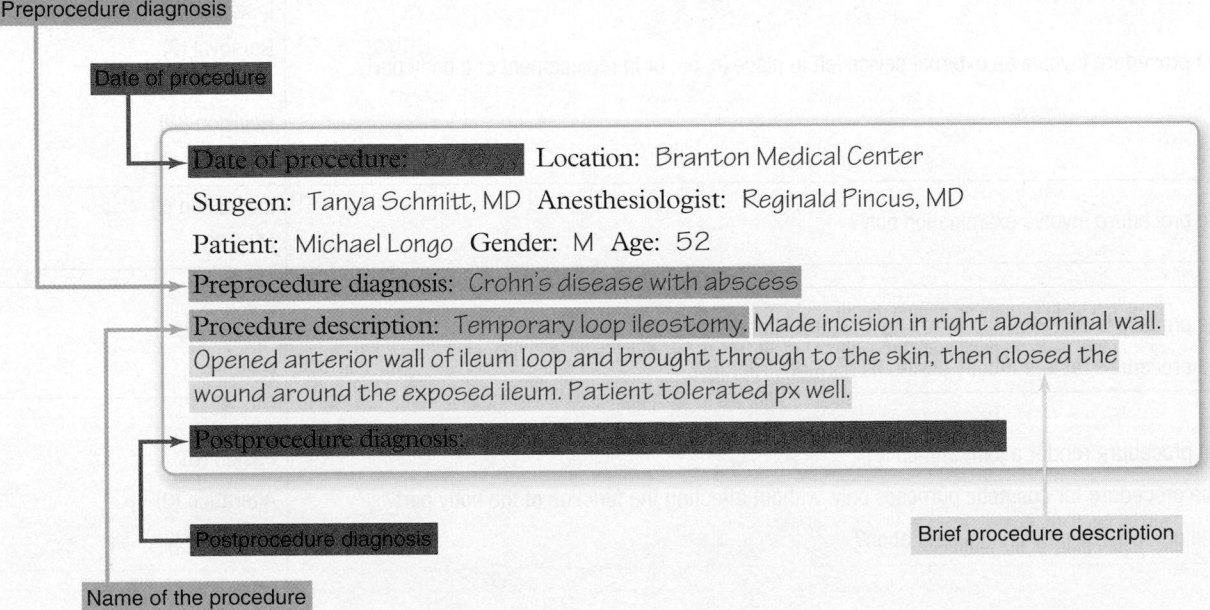

Preprocedure diagnosis

Date of procedure

Date of procedure: Location: Branton Medical Center

Surgeon: Tanya Schmitt, MD Anesthesiologist: Reginald Pincus, MD

Patient: Michael Longo Gender: M Age: 52

Preprocedure diagnosis: Crohn's disease with abscess

Procedure description: Temporary loop ileostomy. Made incision in right abdominal wall. Opened anterior wall of ileum loop and brought through to the skin, then closed the wound around the exposed ileum. Patient tolerated px well.

Postprocedure diagnosis:

Postprocedure diagnosis

Name of the procedure

Brief procedure description

Figure 51-1 ■ Key to Interpreting the Procedure Report Mini-Medical-Record

Table 51-1 ■ **KEY CRITERIA FOR ABSTRACTING MEDICAL AND SURGICAL PROCEDURES**

General Questions
❑ What is the stated procedure?
❑ What organ or body part is involved?
❑ How many sites are treated?
❑ What is the laterality (if applicable)?
❑ Is the procedure description what you would expect based on the name of the procedure?
❑ What surgical approach is used?
❑ Was more than one procedure, or a combined procedure, performed?

Root Operation Questions	Root Operation (Value)
❑ Did the procedure take out some or all of a body part without replacement?	Destruction (5) Detachment (6) Excision (B) Extraction (D) Resection (T)
❑ Did the procedure take out solids, fluids, or gases from a body part?	Drainage (9) Extirpation (C) Fragmentation (F)
❑ Did the procedure involve cutting or separation only, within or around a body part?	Division (8) Release (N)
❑ Did the procedure put in, put back, or move some or all of a body part?	Reattachment (M) Reposition (S) Transfer (X) Transplantation (Y)
❑ Did the procedure alter the diameter or route of a tubular body part?	Bypass (1) Dilation (7) Occlusion (L) Restriction (V)
❑ Did the procedure involve an external device left in place in, on, or in replacement of a body part?	Change (2) Insertion (H) Removal (P) Replacement (R) Revision (W) Supplement (U)
❑ Did the procedure involve examination only?	Inspection (J) Map (K)
Operations Involving Other Repairs	
❑ Did the procedure stop or attempt to stop postprocedural bleeding?	Control (3)
❑ Did the procedure restore a body part to its normal structure?	Repair (Q)
Operations Involving Other Objectives	
❑ Did the procedure render a joint immobile?	Fusion (G)
❑ Was the procedure for cosmetic purposes only, without affecting the function of the body part?	Alteration (0)
❑ Was the procedure a sex change operation?	Creation (4)

Table 51-2 ■ **ROOT OPERATION DEFINITIONS IN ALPHABETICAL ORDER, WITH EXPLANATIONS AND EXAMPLES**

Value	Root Operation	Description
0	Alteration	**Definition:** Modifying the anatomic structure of a body part without affecting the function of the body part. **Explanation:** Principal purpose is to improve appearance. **Includes/Examples:** Face lift, breast augmentation
1	Bypass	**Definition:** Altering the route of passage of the contents of a tubular body part. **Explanation:** Rerouting contents of a body part to a downstream area of the normal route, to a similar route and body part, or to an abnormal route and dissimilar body part. Includes one or more anastomoses, with or without the use of a device. **Includes/Examples:** Coronary artery bypass, colostomy formation
2	Change	**Definition:** Taking out or off a device from a body part and putting back an identical or similar device in or on the same body part without cutting or puncturing the skin or a mucous membrane. **Explanation:** All Change procedures are coded using the approach External. **Includes/Examples:** Urinary catheter change, gastrostomy tube change
3	Control	**Definition:** Stopping, or attempting to stop, postprocedural bleeding. **Explanation:** The site of the bleeding is coded as an anatomic region and not to a specific body part. **Includes/Examples:** Control of post-prostatectomy hemorrhage, control of post-tonsillectomy hemorrhage
4	Creation	**Definition:** Making a new genital structure that does not take over the function of a body part. **Explanation:** Used only for sex change operations. **Includes/Examples:** Creation of vagina in a male, creation of penis in a female
5	Destruction	**Definition:** Physical eradication of all or a portion of a body part by the direct use of energy, force, or a destructive agent. **Explanation:** None of the body part is physically taken out. **Includes/Examples:** Fulguration of rectal polyp, cautery of skin lesion
6	Detachment	**Definition:** Cutting off all or a portion of the upper or lower extremities. **Explanation:** The body part value is the site of the detachment, with a qualifier if applicable to further specify the level where the extremity was detached. **Includes/Examples:** Below-knee amputation, disarticulation of shoulder
7	Dilation	**Definition:** Expanding an orifice or the lumen of a tubular body part. **Explanation:** The orifice can be a natural orifice or an artificially created orifice. Accomplished by stretching a tubular body part using intraluminal pressure or by cutting part of the orifice or wall of the tubular body part. **Includes/Examples:** Percutaneous transluminal angioplasty, pyloromyotomy
8	Division	**Definition:** Cutting into a body part without draining fluids and/or gases from the body part in order to separate or transect a body part. **Explanation:** All or a portion of the body part is separated into two or more portions. **Includes/Examples:** Spinal cordotomy, osteotomy
9	Drainage	**Definition:** Taking or letting out fluids and/or gases from a body part. **Explanation:** The qualifier Diagnostic is used to identify drainage procedures that are biopsies. **Includes/Examples:** Thoracentesis, incision and drainage
B	Excision	**Definition:** Cutting out or off, without replacement, a portion of a body part. **Explanation:** The qualifier Diagnostic is used to identify excision procedures that are biopsies. **Includes/Examples:** Partial nephrectomy, liver biopsy
C	Extirpation	**Definition:** Taking or cutting out solid matter from a body part. **Explanation:** The solid matter may be an abnormal byproduct of a biological function or a foreign body; it may be imbedded in a body part or in the lumen of a tubular body part. The solid matter may or may not have been previously broken into pieces. **Includes/Examples:** Thrombectomy, choledocholithotomy

(continued)

Table 51-2 ■ **(continued)**

Value	Root Operation	Description
D	Extraction	**Definition:** Pulling or stripping out or off all or a portion of a body part by the use of force. **Explanation:** The qualifier Diagnostic is used to identify extraction procedures that are biopsies. **Includes/Examples:** Dilation and curettage, vein stripping
F	Fragmentation	**Definition:** Breaking solid matter in a body part into pieces. **Explanation:** Physical force (e.g., manual, ultrasonic) applied directly or indirectly is used to break the solid matter into pieces. The solid matter may be an abnormal byproduct of a biological function or a foreign body. The pieces of solid matter are not taken out. **Includes/Examples:** Extracorporeal shockwave lithotripsy, transurethral lithotripsy
G	Fusion	**Definition:** Joining together portions of an articular body part, rendering the articular body part immobile. **Explanation:** The body part is joined together by fixation device, bone graft, or other means. **Includes/Examples:** Spinal fusion, ankle arthrodesis
H	Insertion	**Definition:** Putting in a nonbiological appliance that monitors, assists, performs, or prevents a physiological function but does not physically take the place of a body part. **Includes/Examples:** Insertion of radioactive implant, insertion of central venous catheter
J	Inspection	**Definition:** Visually and/or manually exploring a body part. **Explanation:** Visual exploration may be performed with or without optical instrumentation. Manual exploration may be performed directly or through intervening body layers. **Includes/Examples:** Diagnostic arthroscopy, exploratory laparotomy
K	Map	**Definition:** Locating the route of passage of electrical impulses and/or locating functional areas in a body part. **Explanation:** Applicable only to the cardiac conduction mechanism and the central nervous system. **Includes/Examples:** Cardiac mapping, cortical mapping
L	Occlusion	**Definition:** Completely closing an orifice or the lumen of a tubular body part. **Explanation:** The orifice can be a natural orifice or an artificially created orifice. **Includes/Examples:** Fallopian tube ligation, ligation of inferior vena cava
M	Reattachment	**Definition:** Putting back in or on all or a portion of a separated body part to its normal location or other suitable location. **Explanation:** Vascular circulation and nervous pathways may or may not be reestablished. **Includes/Examples:** Reattachment of hand, reattachment of avulsed kidney
N	Release	**Definition:** Freeing a body part from an abnormal physical constraint by cutting or by the use of force. **Explanation:** Some of the restraining tissue may be taken out, but none of the body part is taken out. **Includes/Examples:** Adhesiolysis, carpal tunnel release
P	Removal	**Definition:** Taking out or off a device from a body part. **Explanation:** If a device is taken out and a similar device put in without cutting or puncturing the skin or mucous membrane, the procedure is coded to the root operation Change. Otherwise, the procedure for taking out a device is coded to the root operation Removal. **Includes/Examples:** Drainage tube removal, cardiac pacemaker removal
Q	Repair	**Definition:** Restoring, to the extent possible, a body part to its normal anatomic structure and function. **Explanation:** Used only when the method to accomplish the repair is not one of the other root operations. **Includes/Examples:** Colostomy takedown, suture of laceration
R	Replacement	**Definition:** Putting in or on biological or synthetic material that physically takes the place and/or function of all or a portion of a body part. **Explanation:** The body part may have been taken out or replaced, or may be taken out, physically eradicated, or rendered nonfunctional during the Replacement procedure. A Removal procedure is coded for taking out the device used in a previous replacement procedure. **Includes/Examples:** Total hip replacement, bone graft, free skin graft
S	Reposition	**Definition:** Moving to its normal location, or other suitable location, all or a portion of a body part. **Explanation:** The body part is moved to a new location from an abnormal location or from a normal location where it is not functioning correctly. The body part may or may not be cut out or off to be moved to the new location. **Includes/Examples:** Reposition of undescended testicle, fracture reduction

Table 51-2 ■ *(continued)*

Value	Root Operation	Description
T	Resection	**Definition:** Cutting out or off, without replacement, all of a body part. **Includes/Examples:** Total nephrectomy, total lobectomy of lung
V	Restriction	**Definition:** Partially closing an orifice or the lumen of a tubular body part. **Explanation:** The orifice can be a natural orifice or an artificially created orifice. **Includes/Examples:** Esophagogastric fundoplication, cervical cerclage
W	Revision	**Definition:** Correcting, to the extent possible, a portion of a malfunctioning device or the position of a displaced device. **Explanation:** Revision can include correcting a malfunctioning or displaced device by taking out or putting in components of the device, such as a screw or pin. **Includes/Examples:** Adjustment of position of pacemaker lead, recementing of hip prosthesis
U	Supplement	**Definition:** Putting in or on biological or synthetic material that physically reinforces and/or augments the function of a portion of a body part. **Explanation:** The biological material is nonliving or is living and from the same individual. The body part may have been previously replaced, and the Supplement procedure is performed to physically reinforce and/or augment the function of the replaced body part. **Includes/Examples:** Herniorrhaphy using mesh, free nerve graft, mitral valve ring annuloplasty, put a new acetabular liner in a previous hip replacement
X	Transfer	**Definition:** Moving, without taking out, all or a portion of a body part to another location to take over the function of all or a portion of a body part. **Explanation:** The body part transferred remains connected to its vascular and nervous supply. **Includes/Examples:** Tendon transfer, skin pedicle flap transfer
Y	Transplantation	**Definition:** Putting in or on all or a portion of a living body part taken from another individual or animal to physically take the place and/or function of all or a portion of a similar body part. **Explanation:** The native body part may or may not be taken out, and the transplanted body part may take over all or a portion of its function. **Includes/Examples:** Kidney transplant, heart transplant

Source: Department of Health and Human Services, Centers for Medicare and Medicaid Services, ICD-10-PCS Coding Manual

(Text continued from page 1009)

CODING CAUTION

To assign a Root Operation, its full definition in the PCS manual must be applied (PCS OGCR B3.1a). If the full definition is not applicable, continue searching for another Root Operation.

SUCCESS STEP

Each of the Root Operation questions in Table 51-1 correlates with one of the nine Root Operation groups in the Comparison of Medical and Surgical Root Operations appendix of the ICD-10-PCS manual. The first question relates to the first group in this appendix, the second question relates to the second group in this appendix, and so forth.

Guided Example of Abstracting PCS Procedures

To practice skills for abstracting procedures, refer to the following example of Michael Longo, who had an ileostomy at Branton Medical Center, which will be used throughout this chapter. Marcy Elwood, CCS, is the fictitious coder at the hospital who guides you through the coding process.

Date of procedure: *8/26/yy*   Location: *Branton Medical Center*   Surgeon: *Tanya Schmitt, MD*

Anesthesiologist: *Reginald Pincus, MD*

Patient: *Michael Longo*   Gender: *M*   Age: *52*

Preprocedure diagnosis: *Crohn's disease with abscess*

Procedure description: *Temporary loop ileostomy. Made incision in right abdominal wall. Opened anterior wall of ileum loop and brought through to the skin, then closed the wound around the exposed ileum. Patient tolerated px (procedure) well.*

Postprocedure diagnosis: *Crohn's disease of large intestine with abscess*

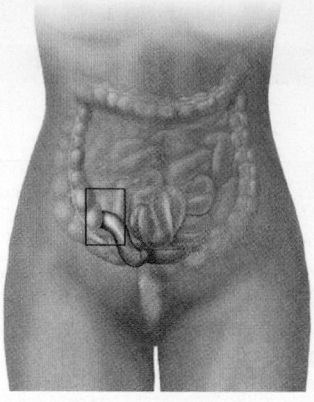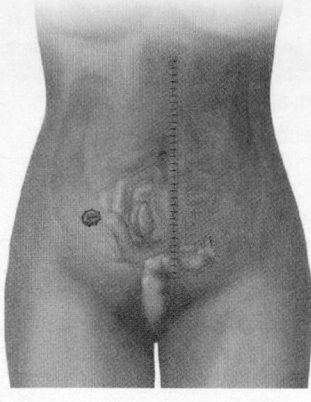

Figure 51-2 ■ A loop ileostomy reroutes the contents of the small intestine in order to bypass the large intestine

Follow along as Marcy Elwood, CCS, abstracts the Root Operation from the medical record. (*Questions from the Key Criteria table appear in italics.* Verbiage taken directly from the medical record appears in this special font. Any other comments or observations appear in a normal font.) Check off each step after you complete it.

▶ Marcy reads through the procedure report, with special attention to the preprocedure diagnosis, the procedure name and description, and the postprocedure diagnosis.

▶ Marcy refers to Key Criteria for Abstracting Medical and Surgical Procedures (Table 51-1).

❑ *What is the procedure?* temporary loop ileostomy (■ Figure 51-2)

❑ *What organ or body part is involved?* the ileum

❑ *Is the procedure description what you would expect based on the name of the procedure?* Yes, the ileum was divided

and the free end was brought through the right abdominal wall to the skin. This created a new route to evacuate the contents of the small intestine.

❑ *What surgical approach is used?* open

❑ *Was more than one procedure, or a combined procedure, performed?* No

❑ She reads the abstracting questions and answers **Yes** to the question, *Did the procedure alter the diameter or route of a tubular body part?*

▶ The Key Criteria for Abstracting Medical and Surgical Procedures directs Marcy to review the definitions of four Root Operations.

▶ She turns to the appendix Comparison of Medical and Surgical Root Operations in the ICD-10-PCS coding manual.

❑ She locates the group titled Procedures That Alter the Diameter/Route of a Tubular Body Part and reads the definition of each Root Operation.

❑ After reading the definitions, she believes that **Bypass (1)** best describes the ileostomy.

▶ Next, Marcy turns to the appendix Root Operation Definitions in the ICD-10-PCS manual.

❑ She locates the entry for **1 Bypass**.

❑ She reads the Definition, Explanation, and Examples listed and concludes that **Bypass** is the correct Root Operation because this operation altered the route of a tubular body part, the ileum.

▶ At this time, Marcy has abstracted the procedure and determined that the Root Operation is **Bypass**. Next, she will build the PCS code.

CODING PRACTICE

Exercise 51.1   Abstracting Medical and Surgical Procedures

Instructions: Read the mini-medical-record of each patient's encounter and answer the abstracting questions. Write the answer on the line provided. Do not assign any codes.

1. INPATIENT HOSPITAL   Gender: F   Age: 83

Preprocedure diagnosis: pressure ulcer, left hip

Procedure description: Open excisional debridement of left hip. Used scissors to cut out necrosis and devitalized tissue, through full epidermis and subcutaneous tissue, 1 cm beyond the wound margin.

Postprocedure diagnosis: healing stage III pressure ulcer, left hip

(continued)

1. (continued)

a. What is the stated procedure? _____

_____

b. What organ or body part is involved? _____

_____

c. Is the procedure description what you would expect based on the name of the procedure? _____

_____

d. What surgical approach is used? _____

_____

e. Was more than one procedure, or a combined procedure, performed? _____

_____

(continued)

1. (continued)

f. Review the Root Operation Questions. To which question did you answer yes? _____ _____

g. Review the definitions of the Root Operations that answer this question. Which Root Operation correctly describes this procedure? _____ _____

2. INPATIENT HOSPITAL Gender: F Age: 48

Preprocedure diagnosis: *mass in left breast*

Procedure description: *Needle biopsy. Using a needle, took out a tissue sample from the left breast that was previously marked with a wire.*

Postprocedure diagnosis: *benign neoplasm, breast per pathology report*

a. What is the stated procedure? _____ _____

b. What organ or body part is involved? _____

c. Is the procedure description what you would expect based on the name of the procedure? _____ _____

d. What surgical approach is used? _____ _____

e. Was more than one procedure, or a combined procedure, performed? _____ _____

f. Review the Root Operation Questions. To which question did you answer yes? _____ _____

g. Review the definitions of the Root Operations that answer this question. Which Root Operation correctly describes this procedure? _____ _____

h. Was the procedure diagnostic or therapeutic? _____ _____

3. INPATIENT HOSPITAL Gender: M Age: 15

Preprocedure assessment: *presented to ED with vomiting, acute abdominal pain, RLQ tenderness, T 101 degrees*

Procedure description: *Appendectomy. Made three small umbilical incisions and placed laparoscope. Expanded abdominal cavity with carbon dioxide to aid visualization. Grasped appendix and divided with*

(*continued*)

3. (continued)

stapler. Cauterized appendiceal stump. Removed appendix, irrigated and suctioned abdominal cavity. Removed instruments and closed incision. Patient tolerated procedure well, no complications.

Postprocedure diagnosis: *acute appendicitis with rupture*

a. What is the stated procedure? _____

b. What organ or body part is involved? _____ _____

c. Is the procedure description what you would expect based on the name of the procedure? _____ _____

d. What surgical approach is used? _____ _____

e. Was more than one procedure, or a combined procedure, performed? _____

f. Review the Root Operation Questions. To which question did you answer yes? _____ _____

g. Review the definitions of the Root Operations that answer this question. Which Root Operation correctly describes this procedure? _____ _____

4. INPATIENT HOSPITAL Gender: F Age: 61

Preprocedure diagnosis: *gangrene in left great toe due to nonhealing plantar (sole of foot) ulcer*

Procedure description: *midlevel amputation of L great toe at interphalangeal joint*

Postprocedure diagnosis: *diabetes with gangrene*

a. What is the stated procedure? _____ _____

b. What organ or body part is involved? _____ _____

c. Is the procedure description what you would expect based on the name of the procedure? _____ _____

d. What surgical approach is used? _____ _____

e. Was more than one procedure, or a combined procedure, performed? _____ _____

(*continued*)

CODING PRACTICE *(continued)*

4. (continued)

f. Review the Root Operation Questions. To which question did you answer yes? _____

_____

g. Review the definitions of the Root Operations that answer this question. Which Root Operation correctly describes this procedure? _____

_____

5. INPATIENT HOSPITAL Gender: F Age: 23

Preprocedure: hypermenorrhea

Procedure description: Transvaginal dilation and curettage. Inserted speculum to hold the vagina open. Progressively dilated cervix and uterus with os dilator. Inserted curette and scraped endometrial wall. Tissue sent to lab for analysis.

Postprocedure diagnosis: hypermenorrhea

Tip: Scraping (curretage) is classified as removal by force.

a. What is the stated procedure? _____

_____

b. What organ or body part is involved? _____

_____

c. Is the procedure description what you would expect based on the name of the procedure? _____

_____

d. What surgical approach is used? _____

e. Was more than one procedure, or a combined procedure, performed? _____

_____

f. Review the Root Operation Questions. To which question did you answer yes? _____

_____

g. Review the definitions of the Root Operations that answer this question. Which Root Operation correctly describes this procedure? _____

_____

h. Was the procedure diagnostic or therapeutic?

_____

6. INPATIENT HOSPITAL Gender: F Age: 52

Preprocedure diagnosis: endometriosis

Procedure description: Ablation of ovaries and endometrium. Inserted the endoscope through the

(continued)

6. (continued)

vagina into the uterus to cauterize the endometrium (*lining of uterus*). When that was successfully completed, withdrew the scope, applied a new tip. Made three incisions on the lower abdomen and inserted endoscope to treat each ovary.

Postprocedure diagnosis: endometriosis

Tip: Code multiple procedures when the same root operation is performed on different Body Parts as defined by distinct values of the Body Part character (PCS OGCR B3.2a).

a. What is the stated procedure? _____

_____

b. What organ or body part is involved? _____

_____

c. Is the procedure description what you would expect based on the name of the procedure? _____

_____

d. What surgical approach is used? _____

_____

e. Was more than one procedure, or a combined procedure, performed? _____

_____

f. Review the Root Operation Questions. To which question did you answer yes? _____

_____

g. Review the definitions of the Root Operations that answer this question. Which Root Operation correctly describes this procedure? _____

_____

h. Repeat the abstracting process for each procedure that was performed.

7. INPATIENT HOSPITAL Gender: F Age: 52

Preprocedure diagnosis: pain RUQ, T 102 degrees, vomiting, acute cholecystitis with calculi in the common bile duct, causing obstruction. Extensive known abdominal adhesions prevent a laparoscopic approach.

Procedure description: Cholecystectomy. Made subcostal incision and isolated gallbladder from surrounding structures with laparotomy packs. Excised entire gallbladder and common bile duct. Hemostasis was achieved. Closed operative wound. Patient tolerated procedure well.

(continued)

7. (continued)

Postprocedure diagnosis: *acute cholecystitis with calculi in the common bile duct, causing obstruction*

Tip: Code multiple procedures when the same root operation is performed on different Body Parts as defined by distinct values of the Body Part character (PCS OGCR B3.2a).

a. What is the stated procedure? _____
_____

b. What organ or body part is involved? _____
_____

c. Is the procedure description what you would expect based on the name of the procedure? _____
_____

d. What surgical approach is used? _____
_____

e. Was more than one procedure, or a combined procedure, performed? _____
_____

f. Review the Root Operation Questions. To which question did you answer yes? _____
_____

g. Review the definitions of the Root Operations that answer this question. Which Root Operation correctly describes this procedure? _____
_____

h. Repeat the abstracting process for each procedure that was performed.

8. INPATIENT HOSPITAL   Gender: M   Age: 43

Preprocedure diagnosis: *detached R retina*

Procedure description: *Trans pars plana vitrectomy (TPPV) with synthetic scleral buckle. Made incision in pars plana and used vitreous cutter to suction out all vitreous. Injected balanced saline solution (BSS) to replace vitreous. Sutured scleral buckle, which effectively closed the break. Pt tolerated px well.*

Postprocedure diagnosis: *detached R retina*

a. What is the stated procedure? _____
_____

b. What organ or body part is involved? _____
_____

c. Is the procedure description what you would expect based on the name of the procedure? _____
_____

d. What surgical approach is used? _____
_____

(*continued*)

8. (continued)

e. Was more than one procedure, or a combined procedure, performed? _____
_____

f. Review the Root Operation Questions. To which question did you answer yes? _____
_____

g. Review the definitions of the Root Operations that answer this question. Which Root Operation correctly describes this procedure? _____
_____

h. Repeat the abstracting process for each procedure that was performed.

9. INPATIENT HOSPITAL   Gender: M   Age: 75

Preprocedure diagnosis: *blepharoptosis obscuring vision*

Procedure description: *Bilateral upper blepharoplasty. Cut out a crescent of skin and subcutaneous tissue from fold of R eyelid, sutured to restore normal position of eyelid. Repeated on left side.*

Postprocedure diagnosis: *blepharoptosis obscuring vision*

a. What is the stated procedure? _____
_____

b. What organ or body part is involved? _____
_____

c. Is the procedure description what you would expect based on the name of the procedure? _____
_____

d. What surgical approach is used? _____
_____

e. Was more than one procedure, or a combined procedure, performed? _____
_____

f. Review the Root Operation Questions. To which question did you answer yes? _____
_____

g. Review the definitions of the Root Operations that answer this question. Which Root Operation correctly describes this procedure? _____
_____

h. Repeat the abstracting process for each procedure that was performed.

(*continued*)

CODING PRACTICE *(continued)*

10. INPATIENT HOSPITAL   Gender: F   Age: 23

Preprocedure diagnosis: fractured R tibia and R humerus

Procedure description: Open reduction, R tibia with internal fixation device. Closed reduction, percutaneous internal fixation. Applied cast to right humerus.

Postprocedure diagnosis: fractured R tibia, fractured R humerus shaft

a. What is the stated procedure? _____

b. What organ or body part is involved? _____

c. Is the procedure description what you would expect based on the name of the procedure? _____

(continued)

10. *(continued)*

d. What surgical approach is used? _____

e. Was more than one procedure, or a combined procedure, performed? _____

f. Review the Root Operation Questions. To which question did you answer yes? _____

g. Review the definitions of the Root Operations that answer this question. Which Root Operation correctly describes this procedure? _____

h. Repeat the abstracting process for each procedure that was performed.

ASSIGNING MEDICAL AND SURGICAL PROCEDURE CODES

Assigning PCS codes requires coders to locate the Root Operation in the Index, then refer to a Table to build the code. PCS does not contain any modifiers. The Tables do not contain any instructional notes.

ICD-10-PCS Index

The Index uses two types of Main Terms for the Medical and Surgical Section:

- the name of the Root Operation
- the common procedure name

ICD-10-PCS does *not* use eponyms as Main Terms or procedure names. The most direct way to locate a code is to use the Root Operation. However, when the Root Operation is difficult to determine, locate a Main Term for the common procedure name, such as *colectomy*, then follow the cross-references to the appropriate Main Term(s) and Table(s) (■ Figure 51-3). The Index may provide more than one cross-reference because

the common procedure names can be ambiguous. For example, a colectomy may involve any of the following procedures:

- cutting out the entire colon, which is a **Resection**
- cutting out one complete segment of the colon, which is also a **Resection**, because each segment has a separate Body Part value
- cutting out a portion of one segment, which is an **Excision**, because a portion of a defined Body Part is cut out

Under the Main Term are indented subterms that describe the anatomic site or other variation of the Root Operation. Following the subterm is the partial code, which provides the first three to five characters of the code. The first *three* characters of the partial code identify the appropriate Table to use.

CODING CAUTION

When the Index provides more than one cross-reference, it does NOT mean that you can use any of the options listed for any procedure. It is your responsibility as a coder to determine which specific Root Operation accurately describes the procedure you are coding.

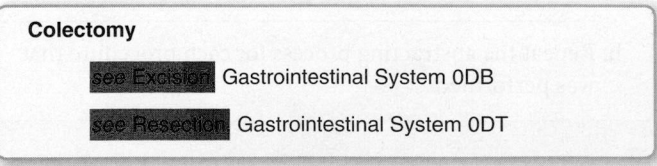

Colectomy

    see Excision Gastrointestinal System 0DB

    see Resection Gastrointestinal System 0DT

Figure 51-3 ■ Example of Index Entry for a Common Procedure Name, with Cross-References to Multiple Root Operations

Guided Example of Using the PCS Index

To practice skills for using the PCS Index, continue with the example from earlier in the chapter of Michael Longo, who had an ileostomy at Branton Medical Center.

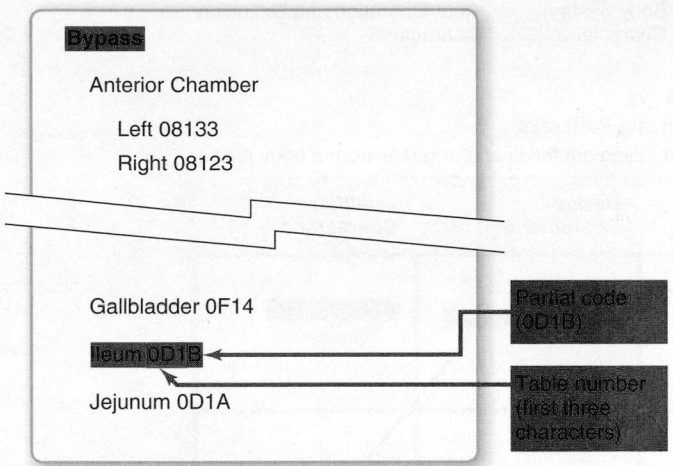

Figure 51-4 ■ Index Entry for Main Term Bypass and Subterm Ileum

Follow along as Marcy Elwood, CCS, searches the Index for the Root Operation. Check off each step after you complete it.

▶ First, Marcy confirms the procedure and Root Operation she abstracted.

❑ The Root Operation is **Bypass (1)**.

❑ The anatomic site is the ileum.

❑ The procedure is ileostomy.

▶ Marcy searches the Index for the Main Term **Bypass** and locates it (■ FIGURE 51-4).

❑ She locates the subterm **Ileum 0D1B**.

❑ She notes **0D1B** is the partial code.

❑ She determines that she needs Table **0D1**, which is the first three letters of the partial code.

▶ Marcy demonstrates an alternative way to locate the code, in case you are unsure of the Root Operation.

❑ She locates the Main Term **Ileostomy**.

❑ Under **Ileostomy**, the Index provides two subterm entries with cross-references to the Root Operations (■ FIGURE 51-5).

■ *see* **Bypass, Ileum 0D1B**

■ *see* **Drainage, Ileum 0D9B**

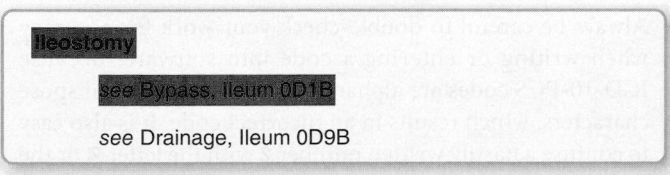

Figure 51-5 ■ Index Entry for Main Term Ileostomy

❑ These cross-references direct her to two possible Root Operations.

■ She reviews the PCS definition of each Root Operation and determines that **Bypass** is the correct Root Operation based on the objective of the procedure.

▶ Next, Marcy will locate the Table and build the code.

ICD-10-PCS Tables

After locating the appropriate procedure in the Index and identifying the first three characters of the partial code, cross-reference the appropriate Table to build the rest of the code. Follow three steps to look up a PCS code in the tables:

1. Locate the Table.
2. Build the code.
3. Verify the character values.

CODING CAUTION

Never assign a code based on the Index alone. You must always refer to the Table to build all seven characters of the code. The Index rarely lists more than three or four characters. Even when the Index provides a seven-character code, you must still verify the values using the Table to be certain it accurately describes the documented procedure.

1. Locate the Table

Locate the Table that matches the first *three* letters of the partial code. The Tables are organized in alphanumeric order by the Section, the first character of a code. Tables beginning with numbers **0** through **9** appear first, followed by Tables beginning with a letter, **B** through **Z**. Within each Section, Tables are sequentially arranged according to the value of the second character, Body System.

For example, Tables that begin with **001** through **09Z** appear before Tables that begin with **0B1** through **0ZZ**. The first three letters of the code and the definition of each letter are listed at the top of the Table.

SUCCESS STEP

To locate Tables quickly, use small adhesive tabs. Within the Medical and Surgical Section, create tabs for the first two characters of the Table numbers, such as 00, 01, and so on, through 0Y.

2. Build the Code

The three characters of the partial code that identify the Table are the first three characters of the code, representing the Section (**0** for Medical and Surgical), the Body System, and the Root Operation. The Table consists of a grid that lists the available options for characters 4 through 7 (■ FIGURE 51-6). To build the rest of the code, select one value from each column to describe the procedure. The first column of the grid is for Body Part (Character 4); the second column is for Approach (Character 5); the third column is for Device (Character 6); and the

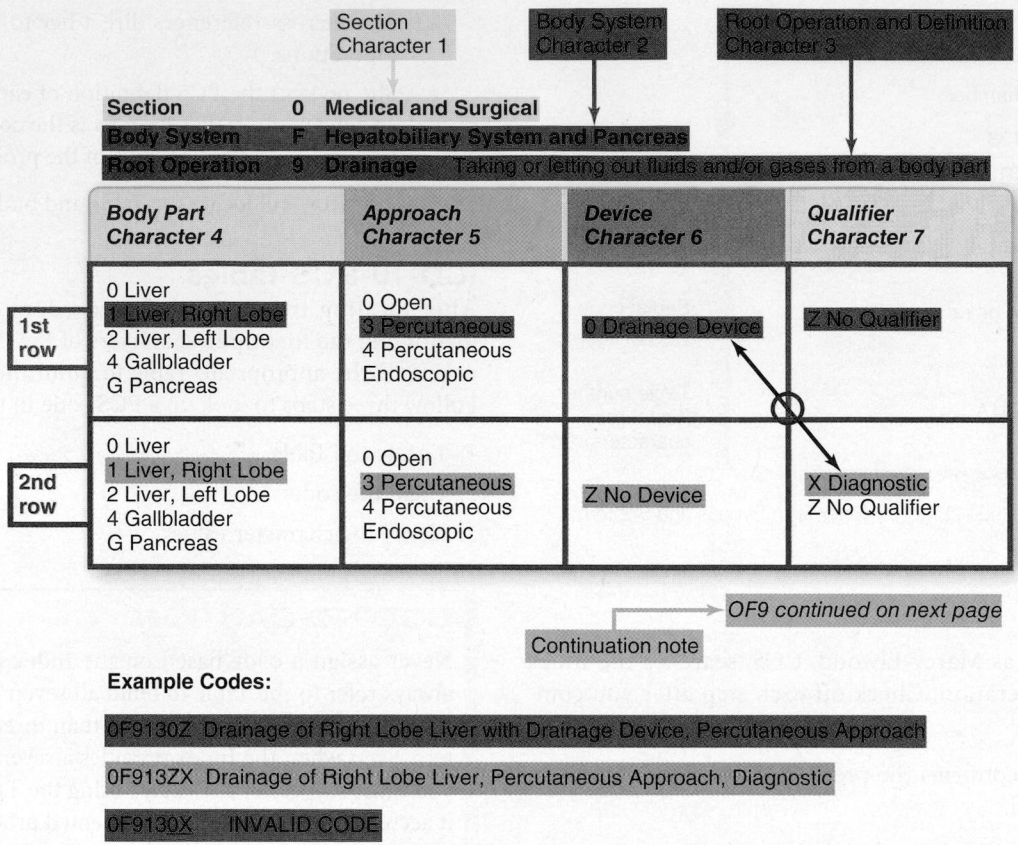

Figure 51-6 ■ Annotated PCS Table

final column is for Qualifier (Character 7). Select one, and only one, value from each column, staying within the same row.

Each row is mutually exclusive of other rows in the same Table. All values for a code must be taken from the *same* boxed row within the Table. Review the sample codes shown at the bottom of Figure 51-6 and note the following:

- Code **0F9130Z** is a valid code that is built from values in the first row of the table.
- Code **0F913ZX** is a valid code that is built from values in the second row of the table.
- Code **0F9130X** is NOT a valid code because it mixes a value from the first row for Character 6 with a value from the second row for Character 7.

The differences between the first and second rows of this Table are as follows:

- The first row contains a value for Character 6 for **0 Drainage Device** and the second row does not.
- The second row contains a value for Character 7 for **X Diagnostic** and the first row does not.

A procedure that leaves a drainage device in the patient is therapeutic by definition, not diagnostic. Therefore the values for Character 6, Device, **0 Drainage**, and Character 7, Qualifier, **X Diagnostic,** are mutually exclusive and cannot be used together. By choosing all character values from the same row of the Table, coders are able to construct valid codes.

SUCCESS STEP

If it seems that the row you are working from does not list the value choices you need, review the rest of the Table to see if another row applies. Sometimes, the values in the first column, Character 4, Body Part, are repeated in multiple rows, with other rows providing a different set of values for Characters 5 through 7. In the example Table (Figure 51-6), Characters 4 and 5 are exactly the same in both rows, but Characters 6 and 7 are different.

3. Verify the Character Values

After building a valid code from values within the same row of the Table, review the final choices for accuracy. Double-check the value of each character of the code to verify that it accurately describes the documented procedure. Identify a statement in the documentation that supports each value chosen for the code.

CODING CAUTION

Always be careful to double-check your work for accuracy when writing or entering a code into software. Because ICD-10-PCS codes are alphanumeric, it is easy to transpose characters, which results in an incorrect code. It is also easy to confuse a hastily written number **2** with the letter **Z** or the number **5** with the letter **S**.

Tips for Using Tables

Certain formatting and layout elements of a Table affect the ability to build an accurate code. Be alert for the following items:

- Pages may contain more than one grid. Be careful to select the grid that *exactly* matches the first three code characters listed in the Index.

- Tables may be subdivided into rows, which are separated with solid lines. To build a valid code, all values must come from the same row within the Table. Do not combine values from different rows or different Tables. Doing so will result in an invalid code.

- Long Tables may span more than one page. If you cannot find what you need, even though you are confident that you have selected the correct three-character Table, look to see if it continues on the next page. When a Table is continued on the next page, a note stating ***continued on next page*** appears below the Table.

SUCCESS STEP

Due to the large number of ICD-10-PCS codes, the ICD-10-PCS manual does not provide a complete description for the final code. However, CMS does post a searchable electronic file with short and long code descriptions for all valid codes. You can download the file from the ICD-10 page on www.cms.gov. The file name is Code Descriptions-Long and Abbreviated Titles. The associated README files also are useful.

Bypass Procedures

When coding procedures for the Root Operation **Bypass (1)**, identify both the site bypassed *from* and the site bypassed *to*. The Index Main Term is the Root Operation **Bypass**. The sub-term is the site bypassed *from*. Locate the correct Table, then assign characters 4 through 7 as follows (PCS OGCR B3.6a):

- Character 4, Body Part: Identify the anatomic site bypassed *from*.

- Character 5, Approach.

- Character 6, Device: Identify the material used for the bypass. If existing material is used, select **Z No Device**.

- Character 7, Qualifier: Identify the anatomic site bypassed *to*.

CODING CAUTION

Coding coronary artery bypass grafts (CABGs) follows a different protocol than coding bypass procedures on other parts of the body (PCS OGCR B3.6b). For CABGs, Character 4 identifies the *number* of sites; Character 7 identifies the site bypassed *from*.

Guided Example of Using PCS Tables

To practice skills for building a code using the PCS Tables, continue with the example from earlier in the chapter of Michael Longo, who had an ileostomy at Branton Medical Center.

Follow along as Marcy Elwood, CCS, builds the code for the ileostomy. Check off each step after you complete it.

▶ Marcy searches the Tables for Table **0D1** (■ FIGURE 51-7).

❑ She verifies the identifying information at the top of the Table to be certain she has the correct Table.

- Section **0 Medical and Surgical**
- Body System **D Gastrointestinal System**
- Operation **1 Bypass**: Altering the route of passage of the contents of a tubular body part

❑ She notes that **0D1** are the first three characters of the code.

▶ Marcy now needs to assign the value for Character 4, Body Part.

❑ She searches the first column of the Table until she locates the entry for **B Ileum**.

❑ **Ileum** occupies only one row of the Table, so she determines that this is the correct row to use.

❑ The value for Character 4 is **B**.

❑ The code is now **0D1B**, which matches the partial code that was in the Index.

▶ Next, Marcy needs to assign the value for Character 5, Approach.

❑ She rereads the procedure description in the medical record and identifies that the surgeon used an open approach.

❑ In row **B Ileum** of the Table, she reads the values in the second column for Approach.

❑ She locates the entry for **0 Open** and determines that it is consistent with the documentation.

❑ Marcy now has five characters in the code: **0D1B0**.

▶ Next, Marcy needs to assign the value for Character 6, Device.

❑ She rereads the procedure description in the medical record and determines that no device was used.

❑ In row **B Ileum** of the Table, she reads the values in the third column for Device.

❑ She locates the entry for **Z No Device** and determines that it is consistent with the documentation.

❑ Marcy now has six characters in the code: **0D1B0Z**.

▶ Finally, Marcy needs to assign the value for Character 7, Qualifier.

❑ She refers to PCS OGCR B3.6a, which states: **Bypass procedures are coded by identifying the body part bypassed 'from' and the body part bypassed 'to.' The fourth character body part specifies the body part bypassed from, and the <u>qualifier specifies the body part bypassed to</u>.**

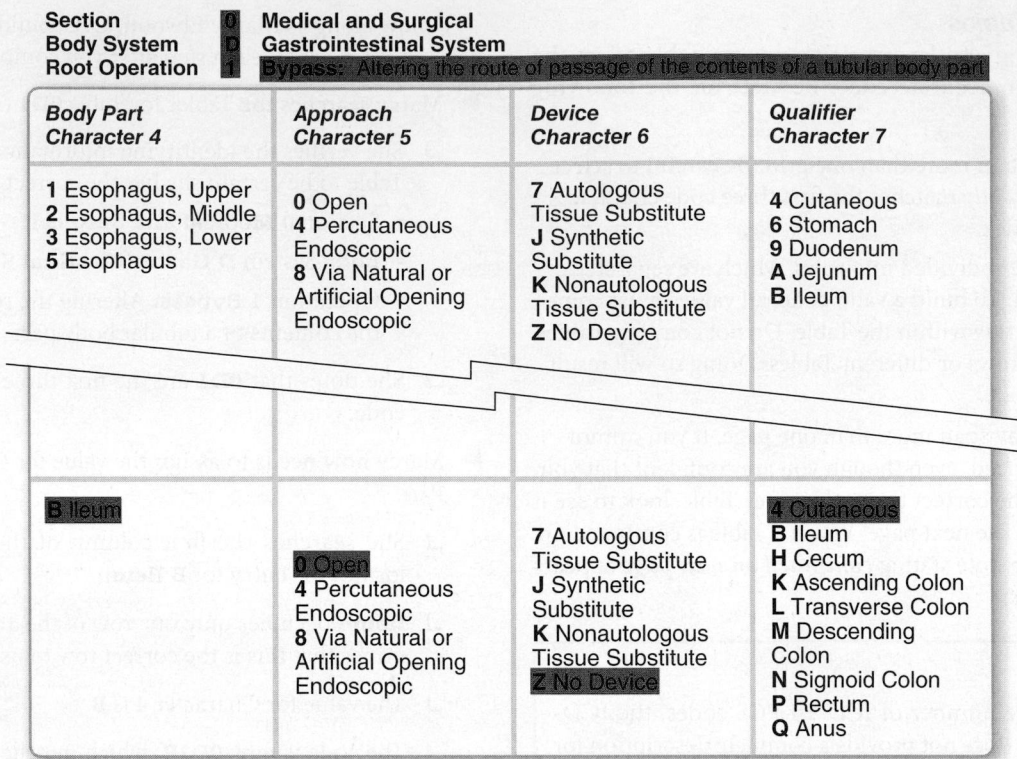

Figure 51-7 ■ Table 0D1, Code 0D1B0Z4

❏ She rereads the procedure description in the medical record and determines that the body part bypassed *to* was the skin.

❏ In row **B Ileum** of the Table, she reads the values in the fourth column for Qualifier.

❏ She locates the entry for **4 Cutaneous** and determines that it is consistent with the documentation.

❏ Marcy now has all seven characters in the code: **0D1B0Z4**.

▶ Marcy double-checks each value in the code for accuracy.

❏ She writes each code value into her Build-A-Code table (■ TABLE 51-3).

❏ She compares each value with the documentation and identifies the specific statement in the document to support each value.

▶ Marcy's final code is **0D1B0Z4**, which means **Bypass Ileum to Cutaneous, Open Approach**.

Table 51-3 ■ **CHARACTER VALUES FOR CODE 0D1B0Z4**

Character (Position)	Name	Value	Description
1	Section	0	Medical and Surgical
2	Body System	D	Gastrointestinal
3	Root Operation	1	Bypass
4	Body Part	B	Ileum
5	Approach	0	Open
6	Device	Z	No Device
7	Qualifier	4	Cutaneous

CODING PRACTICE

Exercise 51.2 Assigning Medical and Surgical Procedure Codes

Instruction: Read the mini-medical-record of each patient's encounter. Review the information abstracted in Exercise 51.1, then assign ICD-10-PCS procedure codes using the Index and Tables.

1. INPATIENT HOSPITAL   Gender: F   Age: 83

Preprocedure diagnosis: pressure ulcer, left hip

Procedure description: Open excisional debridement of left hip. Used scissors to cut out necrosis and devitalized tissue, through full epidermis and subcutaneous tissue, 1 cm beyond the wound margin.

Postprocedure diagnosis: healing stage III pressure ulcer, left hip

Tip: Use the Body Part Key appendix of the ICD-10-PCS manual to determine how to classify the hip.

1 PCS Code _____

2. INPATIENT HOSPITAL   Gender: F   Age: 48

Preprocedure diagnosis: mass in left breast

Procedure description: Needle biopsy. Using a needle, took out a tissue sample from the left breast that was previously marked with a wire.

Postprocedure diagnosis: benign neoplasm, breast per pathology report

1 PCS Code _____

3. INPATIENT HOSPITAL   Gender: M   Age: 15

Preprocedure assessment: presented to ED with vomiting, acute abdominal pain, RLQ tenderness, T 101 degrees

Procedure description: Appendectomy. Made three small umbilical incisions and placed laparoscope.

(continued)

3. (continued)

Expanded abdominal cavity with carbon dioxide to aid visualization. Grasped appendix and divided with stapler. Cauterized appendiceal stump. Removed appendix, irrigated and suctioned abdominal cavity. Removed instruments and closed incision. Patient tolerated procedure well, no complications.

Postprocedure diagnosis: acute appendicitis with rupture

1 PCS Code _____

4. INPATIENT HOSPITAL   Gender: F   Age: 61

Preprocedure diagnosis: gangrene in left great toe, due to nonhealing plantar (*sole of foot*) ulcer

Procedure description: midlevel amputation of L great toe at interphalangeal joint

Postprocedure diagnosis: diabetes with gangrene

1 PCS Code _____

5. INPATIENT HOSPITAL   Gender: F   Age: 23

Preprocedure: hypermenorrhea

Procedure description: Transvaginal dilation and curettage. Inserted speculum to hold the vagina open. Progressively dilated cervix and uterus with os dilator. Inserted curette and scraped endometrial wall. Tissue sent to lab for analysis.

Postprocedure diagnosis: hypermenorrhea

Tip: Hypermenorrhea is abnormally heavy menstrual flow. Dilation is a procedural step necessary to reach the operative site (uterus), so it does not get a separate code (PCS OGCR B3.1b).

1 PCS Code _____

ARRANGING MEDICAL AND SURGICAL PROCEDURE CODES

PCS OGCR B3.2 provides specific information about coding multiple procedures. Additional guidelines within B3 provide further direction relating to specific Root Operations. A summary of multiple procedure guidelines follows.

Components of a Procedure

Do not assign separate codes to integral components of a Root Operation (PCS OGCR B3.1b). The procedural steps required to open the operative field, reach the operative site, and close the operative wound are included in the Root Operation and are not coded separately (■ FIGURE 51-8). A Root Operation definition that includes multiple steps should be assigned a single code (■ FIGURE 51-9).

Multiple Body Parts

When the same Root Operation is performed on different Body Parts with distinct values, assign separate codes for each Body Part character (PCS OGCR B3.2a). Sequence first the procedure

Surgeon performed a laparotomy to reach the site of an open liver biopsy, excised tissue from the right lobe of the liver, and performed a layered closure

0FB10ZX Excision of Right Lobe Liver, Open Approach, Diagnostic

Figure 51-8 ■ Example of a Single Code That Includes the Incision, Excision, and Layered Closure

Surgeon performed a laparoscopic repair of a left inguinal hernia and inserted a mesh panel for reinforcement.

0YU64JZ Supplement Left Inguinal Region with Synthetic Substitute, Percutaneous Endoscopic Approach

Figure 51-9 ■ Example of a Single Code That Includes Multiple Components

most closely related to the principal diagnosis. If both procedures are equally related to the principal diagnosis, either may be sequenced first (■ FIGURE 51-10).

Multiple Body Sites with the Same Body Part Value

When the same Root Operation is performed on two different sites, but they both share the same Body Part value, assign a separate code for each procedure (PCS OGCR B3.2b). Both codes will be exactly the same (■ FIGURE 51-11).

SUCCESS STEP

ICD-10-PCS does NOT require any modifiers to indicate that multiple procedures were performed.

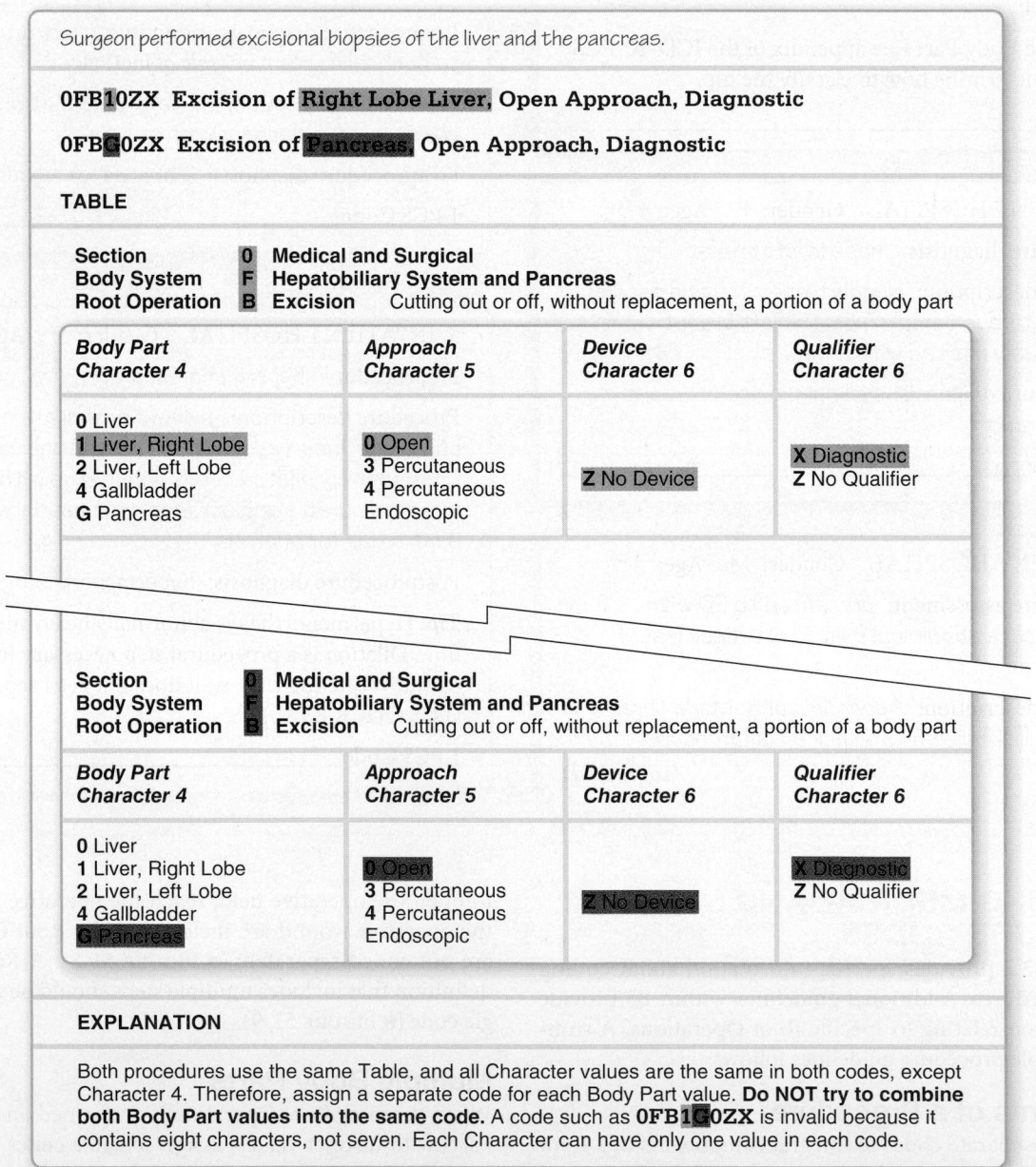

Surgeon performed excisional biopsies of the liver and the pancreas.

0FB10ZX Excision of Right Lobe Liver, Open Approach, Diagnostic

0FBG0ZX Excision of Pancreas, Open Approach, Diagnostic

TABLE

Section · **0** · Medical and Surgical
Body System · **F** · Hepatobiliary System and Pancreas
Root Operation · **B** · Excision · Cutting out or off, without replacement, a portion of a body part

Body Part Character 4	Approach Character 5	Device Character 6	Qualifier Character 6
0 Liver **1** Liver, Right Lobe **2** Liver, Left Lobe **4** Gallbladder **G** Pancreas	**0** Open **3** Percutaneous **4** Percutaneous Endoscopic	**Z** No Device	**X** Diagnostic **Z** No Qualifier

Section · **0** · Medical and Surgical
Body System · **F** · Hepatobiliary System and Pancreas
Root Operation · **B** · Excision · Cutting out or off, without replacement, a portion of a body part

Body Part Character 4	Approach Character 5	Device Character 6	Qualifier Character 6
0 Liver **1** Liver, Right Lobe **2** Liver, Left Lobe **4** Gallbladder **G** Pancreas	**0** Open **3** Percutaneous **4** Percutaneous Endoscopic	**Z** No Device	**X** Diagnostic **Z** No Qualifier

EXPLANATION

Both procedures use the same Table, and all Character values are the same in both codes, except Character 4. Therefore, assign a separate code for each Body Part value. **Do NOT try to combine both Body Part values into the same code.** A code such as **0FB1G0ZX** is invalid because it contains eight characters, not seven. Each Character can have only one value in each code.

Figure 51-10 ■ Example of Multiple Coding of the Same Root Operation and Different Body Part Values

Surgeon performed percutaneous excisional biopsies on the sartorius muscle and gracilis muscle of

the right leg.

BODY PART KEY

Anatomical Site	PCS Description
Gracilis muscle	Upper Leg Muscle, Right
	Upper Leg Muscle, Left
Sartorius muscle	Upper Leg Muscle, Right
	Upper Leg Muscle, Left

0KBQ3ZX Excision of Right Upper Leg Muscle, Percutaneous Approach, Diagnostic

0KBQ3ZX Excision of Right Upper Leg Muscle, Percutaneous Approach, Diagnostic

Figure 51-11 ■ Example of Multiple Coding for Separate Sites with the Same Body Part Value

Multiple Root Operations on the Same Body Part

When more than one Root Operation, each with a distinct objective, is performed on the same Body Part, assign a separate code to each procedure. Use a separate Root Operation Table for each procedure (PCS OGCR 2b.3c). For example, assign separate codes for **Destruction** of sigmoid lesion (Table **0D5**) and **Bypass** of sigmoid colon (Table **0D1**) performed at the same operative session.

Root Operation Is Converted

When an intended Root Operation is attempted using one Approach but is converted to a different approach, assign separate codes for each approach (PCS OGCR 2b.3d). For example, when a laparoscopic cholecystectomy is converted to an open cholecystectomy, code the laparoscopic approach as percutaneous endoscopic **Inspection (0FJ44ZZ)** because **Inspection** describes the first procedure that was performed using the percutaneous endoscopic approach. Code the open procedure as open **Resection (0FT40ZZ)** because the cutting out of the body part was performed using the open approach. Sequence the code for the approach that was converted *to* (**Resection**) first and the approach that was converted *from* (**Inspection**) second.

Discontinued Procedures

When the intended procedure is discontinued, code the procedure to the Root Operation performed (PCS OGCR B3.3). If a procedure is discontinued before any other Root Operation is performed, code the root operation **Inspection (J)** of the body part or anatomic region inspected. For example, a planned aortic valve replacement procedure is discontinued after the initial thoracotomy and before any incision is made in the heart muscle, when the patient becomes hemodynamically unstable. This procedure is coded as an open **Inspection** of the mediastinum (**0WJC0ZZ**).

Biopsy Followed by More Definitive Treatment

Biopsies and therapeutic treatments may use the same Root Operations. When the procedure is stated to be diagnostic, assign Character 7 Qualifier as **X Diagnostic**. When a diagnostic **Excision (B)**, **Extraction (D)**, or **Drainage (9)** is followed by a definitive treatment, such as **Destruction (5)**, **Excision (B)**, or **Resection (T)** at the same procedure site, code *both* the biopsy and the definitive treatment (PCS OGCR B3.4) (■ FIGURE 51-12). The definitive treatment is the procedure most closely related to the principal diagnosis, so sequence the definitive procedure first, followed by the diagnostic procedure.

Surgeon performed a needle biopsy from a suspicious area of the left breast and sent to pathology for an intraoperative frozen section. The pathologist called back that the tissue was malignant, so an open partial mastectomy was performed.

(1) **0HBU0ZZ Excision of Left Breast, Open Approach**
(2) **0HBU3ZX Excision of Left Breast, Percutaneous Approach, Diagnostic**

Figure 51-12 ■ Example of Coding Biopsy Followed by Definitive Treatment

CODING PRACTICE

Exercise 51.3 Arranging Medical and Surgical Procedure Codes

Instructions: Read the mini-medical-record of each patient's encounter. Review the information abstracted in Exercise 51.1, then assign ICD-10-PCS procedure codes using the Index and Tables, and arrange them correctly.

1. INPATIENT HOSPITAL Gender: F Age: 52

Preprocedure diagnosis: *endometriosis*

Procedure description: *Ablation of ovaries and endometrium. Inserted the endoscope through the vagina into the uterus to cauterize the endometrium (lining of uterus). When that was successfully completed, withdrew the scope, applied a new tip. Made three incisions on the lower abdomen and inserted endoscope to treat each ovary.*

Postprocedure diagnosis: *endometriosis*

Tip: This procedure describes endoscopic ablation of endometriosis in the endometrium and ovaries. Assign one code for each site.

2 PCS Codes _____

2. INPATIENT HOSPITAL Gender: F Age: 52

Preprocedure diagnosis: *Pain RUQ, T 102 degrees, vomiting, acute cholecystitis with calculi in the common bile duct causing obstruction. Extensive known abdominal adhesions prevent a laparoscopic approach.*

Procedure description: *Cholecystectomy. Made subcostal incision and isolated gallbladder from surrounding structures with laparotomy packs. Excised entire gallbladder and common bile duct. Hemostasis was achieved. Closed operative wound. Patient tolerated procedure well.*

Postprocedure diagnosis: *acute cholecystitis with calculi in the common bile duct causing obstruction*

2 PCS Codes _____

3. INPATIENT HOSPITAL Gender: M Age: 43

Preprocedure diagnosis: *detached R retina*

Procedure description: *Trans pars plana vitrectomy (TPPV) with synthetic scleral buckle. Made incision in pars plana and used vitreous cutter to suction out all vitreous. Injected balanced saline solution (BSS) to replace vitreous. Sutured scleral buckle, which effectively closed the break. Pt tolerated px well.*

Postprocedure diagnosis: *detached R retina*

2 PCS Codes _____

4. INPATIENT HOSPITAL Gender: M Age: 75

Preprocedure diagnosis: *blepharoptosis obscuring vision*

Procedure description: *Bilateral upper blepharoplasty. Cut out a crescent of skin and subcutaneous tissue from fold of R eyelid, sutured to restore normal position of eyelid. Repeated on left side.*

Postprocedure diagnosis: *blepharoptosis obscuring vision*

2 PCS Codes _____

5. INPATIENT HOSPITAL Gender: F Age: 23

Preprocedure diagnosis: *fractured R tibia and R humerus*

Procedure description: *Open reduction, R tibia with internal fixations device. Closed reduction, percutaneous internal fixation. Applied cast to right humerus*

Postprocedure diagnosis: *fractured R tibia, fractured R humerus shaft*

Tip: Refer to PCS OGCR B3.15.

2 PCS Codes _____

CHAPTER SUMMARY

In this chapter you learned that:

- Because identifying the correct Root Operation is the basis of ICD-10-PCS coding, coders must learn the differences between similar Root Operations in order to abstract appropriately.

- Assigning PCS codes requires coders to locate the Root Operation in the Index, then refer to a Table to build the code.
- PCS OGCR discuss when multiple PCS codes are required.

CONCEPT QUIZ

Take a moment to look back at your trip through Medical and Surgical procedures and solidify your skills. This is your opportunity to pull together everything you have learned.

Completion

Instructions: Write the term that answers each question based on the information you learned in this chapter. Choose from the list below. Some choices may be used more than once and some choices may not be used at all. Refer to the discussion in this chapter if you need a little extra help. When the question provides a pair of terms in parentheses, choose the correct answer from one of the two word choices.

does	Removal
does NOT	Resection
Excision	to
from	two
one	

1. When coding an ileostomy, Character 7 identifies the site bypassed (to/from) _____.

2. When a diagnostic procedure is followed by a definitive treatment at the same procedure site, assign _____ code(s).

3. ICD-10-PCS (does/does NOT) _____ require modifiers to indicate that multiple procedures were performed.

4. When coding CABG, Character 7 identifies the site bypassed (to/from) _____.

5. When dilation is a procedural step necessary to reach the operative site, it (does/does NOT) _____ get a separate code.

6. Endoscopic ablation of endometriosis in the endometrium and ovaries is assigned _____ code(s).

7. Taking out a lymph node chain is assigned to the Root Operation _____.

8. A PCS Table (does/does NOT) _____ contain instructional notes.

9. When coding a colostomy, Character 4 identifies the site bypassed (to/from) _____.

10. When the Index provides more than one cross-reference, it (does/does NOT) _____ mean that you can choose any of the options listed for any procedure.

Multiple Choice

Instructions: Circle the letter of the best answer to each question based on the information you learned in this chapter. Refer to the discussion in this chapter and the Glossary at the end of this book if you need a little extra help.

1. How should coders interpret physician documentation?
   A. Assign codes that use the exact same words.
   B. Refer to ICD-10-PCS manual Body Part Key appendix to identify the Root Operation.
   C. Locate the Approach as the Main Term in the Index.
   D. Equate documentation to the definitions provided by PCS.

2. Which PCS code Character must be correctly identified as the basis of PCS coding?
   A. Section
   B. Root Operation
   C. Approach
   D. Qualifier

3. Which Root Operation should NOT be used when the procedure takes out some or all of a body part without replacement?
   A. Removal (P)
   B. Destruction (5)
   C. Extraction (D)
   D. Resection (T)

4. Which Root Operation SHOULD be used when the procedure restores a body part to its normal structure?
   A. Resection (T)
   B. Revision (W)
   C. Alteration (0)
   D. Repair (Q)

5. Which Root Operation should NOT be used when the procedure alters the diameter or route of a tubular body part?
   A. Bypass (1)
   B. Change (2)
   C. Dilation (7)
   D. Restriction (V)

6. Which of the following items does NOT normally appear on a procedure report?
   A. Date of admission
   B. Date of procedure
   C. Estimated blood loss
   D. Postprocedure diagnosis

(continued)

(continued from page 1027)

7. Which of the following procedures does NOT qualify as a colectomy?
   A. Cutting out the entire colon
   B. Cutting out one complete segment of the colon
   C. Cutting out a portion of one segment
   D. Creating a new outlet for the colon contents

8. Which of the following Tables appears first in the ICD-10-PCS manual?
   A. 09Z
   B. 0D1
   C. 102
   D. B00

9. Which is a characteristic of PCS Tables?
   A. Each page contains one Table.
   B. Tables may contain more than one Root Operation.

C. Tables may be subdivided into rows.
D. No Table is longer than one page.

10. What Root Operation(s) should be reported for a laparoscopic cholecystectomy converted to an open cholecystectomy?
   A. Assign the Root Operation Conversion to report both procedures.
   B. Assign the Root Operation Inspection for the laparoscopic cholecystectomy and the Root Operation Resection for the open procedure.
   C. Assign the Root Operation Resection to report the open procedure only.
   D. Assign the Root Operation Removal to report both procedures.

CODING CHALLENGE

Instructions: Look up the PCS Table represented by the first three characters of the code. Refer to the Table to identify the values for each Character in the code. Write your answer on the line provided.

Example: 08B43ZX

Character 2 Body System: Value _8_ Definition _Eye_

Character 3 Root Operation: Value _B_ Definition _Excision_

Character 4 Body Part: Value _4_ Definition _Vitreous, Right_

Character 5 Approach: Value _3_ Definition _Percutaneous_

Character 6 Device: Value _Z_ Definition _No Device_

Character 7 Qualifier: Value _X_ Definition _Diagnostic_

1. 00C00ZZ

   Character 2 Body System: Value _____ Definition _____

   Character 4 Body Part: Value _____ Definition _____

   Character 5 Approach: Value _____ Definition _____

   Character 6 Device: Value _____ Definition _____

   Character 7 Qualifier: Value _____ Definition _____

2. 0BBB8ZX

   Character 2 Body System: Value _____ Definition _____

   Character 3 Root Operation: Value _____ Definition _____

   Character 4 Body Part: Value _____ Definition _____

   Character 5 Approach: Value _____ Definition _____

   Character 6 Device: Value _____ Definition _____

   Character 7 Qualifier: Value _____ Definition _____

3. 0HQXXZZ

   Character 2 Body System: Value _____ Definition _____

   Character 3 Root Operation: Value _____ Definition _____

Character 4 Body Part: Value _____ Definition _____

Character 5 Approach: Value _____ Definition _____

Character 6 Device: Value _____ Definition _____

Character 7 Qualifier: Value _____ Definition _____

4. 0QHK38Z

   Character 2 Body System: Value _____ Definition _____

   Character 3 Root Operation: Value _____ Definition _____

   Character 4 Body Part: Value _____ Definition _____

   Character 5 Approach: Value _____ Definition _____

   Character 6 Device: Value _____ Definition _____

   Character 7 Qualifier: Value _____ Definition _____

5. 0T784DZ

   Character 2 Body System: Value _____ Definition _____

   Character 3 Root Operation: Value _____ Definition _____

   Character 4 Body Part: Value _____ Definition _____

   Character 5 Approach: Value _____ Definition _____

   Character 6 Device: Value _____ Definition _____

   Character 7 Qualifier: Value _____ Definition _____

6. 0212493

   Character 2 Body System: Value _____ Definition _____

   Character 3 Root Operation: Value _____ Definition _____

   Character 4 Body Part: Value _____ Definition _____

   Character 5 Approach: Value _____ Definition _____

   Character 6 Device: Value _____ Definition _____

   Character 7 Qualifier: Value _____ Definition _____

7. 0KHX4MZ

Character 2 Body System: Value _____ Definition _____

Character 3 Root Operation: Value _____ Definition _____

Character 4 Body Part: Value _____ Definition _____

Character 5 Approach: Value _____ Definition _____

Character 6 Device: Value _____ Definition _____

Character 7 Qualifier: Value _____ Definition _____

8. 0ULG7DZ

Character 2 Body System: Value _____ Definition _____

Character 3 Root Operation: Value _____ Definition _____

Character 4 Body Part: Value _____ Definition _____

Character 5 Approach: Value _____ Definition _____

Character 6 Device: Value _____ Definition _____

Character 7 Qualifier: Value _____ Definition _____

9. 0DUC4JZ

Character 2 Body System: Value _____ Definition _____

Character 3 Root Operation: Value _____ Definition _____

Character 4 Body Part: Value _____ Definition _____

Character 5 Approach: Value _____ Definition _____

Character 6 Device: Value _____ Definition _____

Character 7 Qualifier: Value _____ Definition _____

10. 0M9G40Z

Character 2 Body System: Value _____ Definition _____

Character 3 Root Operation: Value _____ Definition _____

Character 4 Body Part: Value _____ Definition _____

Character 5 Approach: Value _____ Definition _____

Character 6 Device: Value _____ Definition _____

Character 7 Qualifier: Value _____ Definition _____

KEEP ON CODING

Instructions: Write down the definition of each Root Operation. Refer to Table 51-2 or the ICD-10-PCS Appendix.

Example: Drainage *Taking or letting out fluids and/or gases from a body part*

1. Bypass _____

2. Excision _____

3. Extraction _____

4. Removal _____

5. Control _____

6. Release _____

7. Supplement _____

8. Extirpation _____

9. Division _____

10. Resection _____

CODING PRACTICE

Exercise 52.1 Basics of Procedures That Take Out Some or All of a Body Part

Instructions: Use your medical terminology skills and resources to define the following procedures that take out some or all of a Body Part, then identify the code(s) or code range listed in the ICD-10-PCS Index. Follow these steps:

- Use slash marks "/" to break down each underlined term into its root(s) and suffix.
- Define the meaning of the word based on the meaning of each word part.
- Look up the phrase in the ICD-10-PCS Index, and write down the name(s) and of Root Operation(s) the Index cross references you to and the Table(s), if provided.
- Do not assign any codes.

Example: <u>fasciectomy</u> fasci/ectomy   Meaning *excision of the fascia*   PCS Root Operation(s)/Table(s) *Excision 0JB*

1. <u>cryoablation</u>   Meaning _____   PCS Root Operation(s)/Table(s) _____
2. <u>phacoemulsification</u>, lens   Meaning _____   PCS Root Operation(s)/Table(s) _____
3. <u>polypectomy</u>, gastrointestinal   Meaning _____   PCS Root Operation(s)/Table(s) _____
4. <u>electrocautery</u>   Meaning _____   PCS Root Operation(s)/Table(s) _____
5. <u>phlebectomy</u>   Meaning _____   PCS Root Operation(s)/Table(s) _____
6. <u>adenoidectomy</u>   Meaning _____   PCS Root Operation(s)/Table(s) _____
7. <u>disarticulation</u>   Meaning _____   PCS Root Operation(s)/Table(s) _____
8. <u>chondrectomy</u>   Meaning _____   PCS Root Operation(s)/Table(s) _____
9. <u>phrenicoexeresis</u>   Meaning _____   PCS Root Operation(s)/Table(s) _____
10. <u>arteriectomy</u>   Meaning _____   PCS Root Operation(s)/Table(s) _____

CODING OVERVIEW OF ROOT OPERATIONS B, T, 6, 5, AND D

PCS OGCR section B provides guidelines for the Medical and Surgical Section (0), organized by the Characters of the PCS code:

- B2 Body System
- B3 Root Operation
- B4 Body Part
- B5 Approach
- B6 Device

Within the guidelines for each Character, general guidelines appear first, followed by those for specific Root Operations. Information about specific Qualifiers appears throughout the guidelines, but there is not a separate section with guidelines for Character 7 Qualifier.

Guidelines for Coding Multiple Procedures

General guidelines related to coding multiple procedures include the following. These guidelines apply to all Root Operations. Refer to the PCS OGCR for clinical examples of each. ■ TABLE 52-3 summarizes the criteria for identifying when multiple codes might be needed.

- Procedural components—The Root Operation definition includes all components of the procedure, which should not be coded separately. Procedural steps necessary to reach the operative site and close the operative site, including

anastomosis of a tubular body part, are not coded separately (PCS OGCR B3.1b).

- Multiple Body Parts—When the same Root Operation is performed on different Body Part values defined in Character 4, assign separate codes for each Body Part value (PCS OGCR B3.2.a).
- Multiple anatomic sites—When the same Root Operation is repeated at different anatomic sites that are included in the same Body Part value, assign separate codes for each site using the same Body Part value (PCS OGCR B3.2.b).
- Multiple Root Operations—When multiple Root Operations with distinct objectives are performed on the same Body Part, assign separate codes for each Root Operation (PCS OGCR B3.2.c).
- Multiple Approaches—When the intended Root Operation is attempted using one Approach (Character 5) but is converted to a different Approach, assign separate codes for each Approach value (PCS OGCR B3.2.d).
- Discontinued procedures—When the intended procedure is discontinued, assign one code for the Root Operation that is completed. If a procedure is discontinued and no other Root Operation is performed, code the Root Operation Inspection of the Body Part or Anatomical Region inspected (PCS OGCR B3.3). (Note: The Root Operation Inspection is discussed in Chapter 55 of this text.)

Table 52-3 ■ KEY CRITERIA FOR CODING MULTIPLE PROCEDURES

- ❏ Which components are included in the Root Operation (Character 3) or procedural steps?
- ❏ Is the same Root Operation (Character 3) performed on multiple Body Parts (Character 4)?
- ❏ Is the same Root Operation (Character 3) performed on multiple anatomic sites with the same Body Part (Character 4) value?
- ❏ Are multiple Root Operations (Character 3) with distinct objectives performed on the same Body Part (Character 4)?
- ❏ Is a Root Operation (Character 3) attempted with one Approach (Character 5) then converted to a different Approach?
- ❏ Is the initial Root Operation (Character 3) discontinued and a different Root Operation completed?
- ❏ Are a biopsy and a definitive procedure performed at the same operative session?
- ❏ Is an autograft harvested from a distinct anatomic site?

Source: © PB Resources, Inc. Used with permission.

Guidelines for Root Operations B, T, 6, 5, and D

Guidelines specific to the Root Operations B, T, 6, 5, and D include the following. Refer to the PCS OGCR for clinical examples of each guideline.

- Biopsy procedures—Code biopsy procedures using the Root Operations Excision, Extraction, or Drainage and the qualifier Diagnostic (X) (PCS OGCR B3.4a). (Note: The Root Operation Drainage is discussed in Chapter 55 of this text.)
- Biopsy followed by more definitive treatment—When biopsy is followed by a more definitive procedure, such as Excision or Resection, at the same procedure site, code both the biopsy and the more definitive treatment (PCS OGCR B3.4b). PCS uses the term **definitive treatment** similarly to therapeutic treatment—a treatment intended to cure, eliminate, improve, or reduce the effects of a condition.
- Excision and Resection—Use the most specific Body Part to assign the Root Operation. Assign Resection of the specific Body Part whenever all of the Body Part is cut out or off, rather than coding Excision of a less specific Body Part (PCS OGCR B3.8).
- Excision for graft—When an autograft is harvested from a different site to complete the objective of the procedure, assign separate codes for harvesting the graft and performing the primary procedure (PCS OGCR B3.9).

SUCCESS STEP

The PCS OGCR are not as extensive as those for ICD-10-CM or CPT, so you should try to memorize as many guidelines as possible. It is especially helpful to memorize the guidelines regarding multiple coding. Doing so will make the coding process faster and more accurate.

ABSTRACTING FOR ROOT OPERATIONS B, T, 6, 5, AND D

Abstracting for PCS focuses on identifying the correct Root Operation, which involves reading the operative report and interpreting it in light of Root Operation definitions. When reading the operative report, remember to focus on the objective of the procedure and the activities performed, not the specific medical terms the surgeon uses to describe the procedure. Many times the Root Operation can be determined conclusively during abstracting. Other times, the Root Operation can be narrowed down to two options, which must be differentiated based on other Characters that are assigned from the PCS Tables. This occurs frequently with the Root Operations Excision and Resection. The Root Operation definition is a combination of the functional objective of the procedure and the anatomic site. The following information summarizes the objective, definition, unique features, and examples of Root Operations B, T, 6, 5, and D.

Abstracting for Excision (B)

The objective of the Root Operation Excision is cutting out or off without replacement. The site of the procedure is some of a Body Part as defined by PCS. The Body Part definition may be more or less specific than the physical structure. For example, PCS divides the colon into 10 Body Part values for the Root Operation Excision but only one Body Part value for the Root Operation Revision. Therefore, when abstracting the Root Operation, you may be able to narrow it down to only two options—Excision or Resection—until you refer to the Table to identify how Body Parts are divided. This process will be discussed later in this chapter under "Assigning Characters 4–7 for Root Operations B, T, 6, 5, and D."

Assign the Root Operation Excision only when the Body Part is not replaced, supplemented, reinforced, moved, repaired, or performed as part of a procedure with a more specific objective. Biopsies obtained through cutting are coded to the Root Operation Excision, but biopsies obtained through other methods are coded to the Root Operation that describes the method used, such as Drainage, used for needle aspiration, or Extraction, used for pulling or scraping. Examples of Excision are a breast lumpectomy or excision of a single lymph node (■ TABLE 52-4).

Abstracting for Resection (T)

The objective of the Root Operation Resection is cutting out or off without replacement. The site of the procedure is all of a Body Part as defined by PCS. The only difference between the Root Operations Excision and Resection is whether the PCS Body Part is partially or completely removed. This determination can be made only after consulting the PCS Table. As you become more proficient with PCS coding, you will learn how Body Parts are defined for various organ systems, and determining which Root Operation is applicable in a given situation will be easier.

As with Excision, assign the Root Operation Resection only when the Body Part is not replaced, supplemented, reinforced, moved, repaired, or performed as part of a procedure with a more specific objective. Examples of Resection are a total mastectomy or excision of an entire lymph chain (■ TABLE 52-5).

Table 52-4 ■ EXAMPLES OF THE ROOT OPERATION EXCISION (B)

Organ System	Procedural Examples
Blood and Immune	Harvesting of saphenous vein for grafting, lymph node excision
Cardiovascular	Open endarterectomy of an artery
Digestive	EGD with biopsy
Endocrine	Thyroid biopsy
Genitourinary	Partial nephrectomy
Hepatobiliary	Liver biopsy, excision of tail of pancreas
Integumentary	Breast lumpectomy, excision of cyst or lesion
Lymphatic and Hemic	Excision of a single lymph node
Musculoskeletal	Muscle biopsy, partial discectomy (*removal of disc fragments*)
Nervous	Brain biopsy
Respiratory	Biopsy of lung, excision of partial lobe of lung
Special Senses (Ear, Eye)	Biopsy of eye

Source: © PB Resources, Inc. Used with permission.

SUCCESS STEP

When an entire lymph node chain is cut out, the appropriate root operation is Resection. When a lymph node(s) is cut out, the root operation is Excision. *ICD-10-PCS Reference Manual* (2015), page 42.

Table 52-5 ■ EXAMPLES OF THE ROOT OPERATION RESECTION (T)

Organ System	Procedural Examples
Blood and Immune	Lymph chain excision
Digestive	Sigmoidectomy
Endocrine	Total excision of left lobe of thyroid
Genitourinary	Total nephrectomy, vaginal hysterectomy
Hepatobiliary	Cholecystectomy
Integumentary	Total mastectomy
Lymphatic and Hemic	Excision of an entire lymph chain
Musculoskeletal	Excision of entire disc
Respiratory	Excision of entire lobe of lung
Special Senses (Ear, Eye)	Enucleation of eyeball

Source: © PB Resources, Inc. Used with permission.

Table 52-6 ■ EXAMPLES OF THE ROOT OPERATION DETACHMENT (6)

Organ System	Procedural Examples
Musculoskeletal	Amputation above elbow, disarticulation of shoulder, below-knee amputation

Source: © PB Resources, Inc. Used with permission.

Abstracting for Detachment (6)

The objective of the Root Operation Detachment is cutting out or off without replacement. The site of the procedure is all or part of any extremity—arms, legs, hands, feet, fingers, or toes. Assign the Root Operation Detachment only when the Body Part is not replaced, supplemented, reinforced, moved, repaired, or performed as part of a procedure with a more specific objective. Examples of Detachment are amputation of the foot or part of a finger (■ TABLE 52-6).

Abstracting for Destruction (5)

The objective of the Root Operation Destruction is eradicating without replacement. The site of the procedure is some or all of a Body Part. There is not a distinction between eradicating some of a Body Part compared with all of a Body Part, as there is with Excision and Resection. Physical eradication involves the direct use of energy, force, or a destructive agent on an anatomic Body Part. None of the Body Part is physically taken out.

Destruction "takes out" a Body Part in the sense that it obliterates the Body Part so it is no longer there. This Root Operation defines a broad range of common procedures and can be used anywhere in the body to treat a variety of conditions, including warts, polyps, lesions, and varices.

Assign the Root Operation Destruction only when the Body Part is not replaced, supplemented, reinforced, moved, repaired, or performed as part of a procedure with a more specific objective. Examples of Destruction are fulguration of a rectal polyp and cautery of a skin lesion.

Destruction can be confused with the Root Operation Fragmentation (F), which is discussed in Chapter 55 of this text. Fragmentation is breaking solid matter in a Body Part, such as a foreign body or an abnormal byproduct, into pieces, whereas Destruction is the eradication of the Body Part itself or abnormal tissue in the Body Part. The most common example of Fragmentation is destruction of calculus, which can be accomplished using a number of different methods, such as ultrasound, a laser beam, and extracorporeal shock wave technology (■ TABLE 52-7).

Abstracting for Extraction (D)

The objective of the Root Operation Extraction is pulling out or off without replacement. The site of the procedure is some or all of a Body Part. There is not a distinction between pulling out or off some of a Body Part compared with all of a Body Part. Extraction is coded when the method used to take out the Body Part is pulling or stripping. Minor cutting, such as that used in vein stripping procedures, is included in Extraction if the objective of the procedure is met by pulling or stripping and is not coded separately. When a biopsy is obtained through pulling or stripping, as occurs with an endometrial biopsy, the Root Operation is Extraction, not Excision.

Table 52-7 ■ EXAMPLES OF THE ROOT OPERATION DESTRUCTION (5)

Organ System	Procedural Examples
Cardiovascular	Vein stripping, ablation of arrhythmogenic focus
Digestive	Fulguration of rectal polyp
Endocrine	Radioablation of parathyroid gland
Genitourinary	Fulguration of endometrium, conization of cervix by cryotherapy
Hepatobiliary	Ablation of tumor in cystic duct
Integumentary	Cautery of skin lesion, cryotherapy of wart
Nervous	Sclerotherapy of nerve lesion, radiofrequency destruction of a nerve
Respiratory	Cautery of nosebleed
Special Senses (Ear, Eye)	Laser coagulation of retinal hemorrhage

Source: © PB Resources, Inc. Used with permission.

Assign the Root Operation Extraction only when the Body Part is not replaced, supplemented, reinforced, moved, repaired, or performed as part of a procedure with a more specific objective. Examples of Extraction are a suction dilation and curettage and phacoemulsification without implantation of an intraocular lens (■ TABLE 52-8).

Key Criteria for Abstracting

Refer to Table 51-1 for general guidance on abstracting PCS procedures and Root Operation groups. Then refer to ■ TABLE 52-9 for more specific guidance on how to abstract and distinguish among procedures in the Root Operation group *Procedures that Take Out Some or All of a Body Part*. Answer the questions in the left-hand column, then refer to the suggested Root Operation(s) in the right-hand column. The first three questions help verify that you have identified the correct Root

Table 52-8 ■ EXAMPLES OF THE ROOT OPERATION EXTRACTION (D)

Organ System	Procedural Examples
Cardiovascular	Microincisional phlebectomy of varicose veins, vein stripping and ligation
Digestive	Tooth extraction
Genitourinary	Suction dilation and curettage, endometrial biopsy
Integumentary	Nail removal, liposuction for medical reasons
Musculoskeletal	Bone marrow biopsy
Nervous	Extraction of hypoglossal nerve
Respiratory	Extraction of the pleura
Special Senses (Ear, Eye)	Cataract phacoemulsification without intraocular lens implant

Source: © PB Resources, Inc. Used with permission.

Table 52-9 ■ KEY CRITERIA FOR ABSTRACTING ROOT OPERATIONS THAT TAKE OUT SOME OR ALL OF A BODY PART

Question	Root Operation (Value)
❏ Was a body part or abnormal tissue growth (such as a lesion or tumor) removed?	If *Yes*, continue below to Root Operations B, T, 6, 5, D.
❏ Was a foreign object or abnormal material (such as calculus) removed?	If *Yes*, do not use Root Operations B, T, 6, 5, or D.
❏ Was the body part replaced with a natural or synthetic substitute?	If *Yes*, do not use Root Operations B, T, 6, 5, or D.
Answer the following questions to help distinguish Root Operations B, T, 6, 5, and D:	
❏ Was removal performed by cutting?	Excision (B)
	Resection (T)
❏ Was removal performed through physical eradication, such as energy, force, or a destructive agent?	Destruction (5)
❏ Was an extremity removed?	Detachment (6)
❏ Was removal performed through the use of force, such as pulling or stripping?	Extraction (D)

Source: © PB Resources, Inc. Used with permission.

Operation Groups. The remaining questions help identify the correct Root Operation within the group.

Coders must use good judgment and critical thinking when answering the questions and applying Root Operation definitions. There may be overlap between some questions, in which case you must refer to the Root Operation definitions to determine the correct procedure. For example, when an amputation is performed, two questions are answered *Yes*:

- Was removal performed by cutting?
- Was an extremity removed?

The only correct Root Operation for an amputation is Detachment (D)—cutting off all or a portion of the upper or lower extremities—because it is more specific than Excision (B) or Resection (T).

Cutting might be performed as a component of the surgical process and followed by another method, such as stripping or suction, to accomplish the objective of the procedure. In this situation, cutting is not coded or considered as part of the Root Operation. Use only the stripping or suction method to determine the Root Operation.

In some cases you may not be able to determine the final Root Operation during abstracting. For example, you may not be able to distinguish between Excision and Resection until you refer to PCS Tables when assigning codes. A guided example of abstracting for the Root Operations Excision and Resection follows.

Guided Example of Abstracting for Excision and Resection

Refer to the following example throughout this chapter to practice skills for abstracting, assigning, and arranging codes for the Root Operations Excision and Resection. Similar principles apply to working with other Root Operations that take out some or all of a Body Part.

INPATIENT HOSPITAL   Gender: F   Age: 48

Preoperative diagnosis: metastatic breast cancer

Procedure: Lymphadenectomy. Open left lymphadenectomy of entire axillary chain and percutaneous left cervical lymphadenectomy of the first node only.

Postoperative diagnosis: left breast cancer with metastasis to lymph nodes

---

Follow along as fictitious coder, Marcy Elwood, CCS, abstracts the procedure. Check off each step after you complete it.

▶ Marcy reads through the entire record, paying special attention to the reason for the encounter, the procedure performed, and the postoperative diagnosis. She refers to the Key Criteria for Abstracting (Table 52-9) and Key Criteria for Coding Multiple Procedures (Table 52-3).

❑ She notes the preoperative diagnosis: metastatic breast cancer.

❑ *What is the stated procedure?* Lymphadenectomy

❑ *What organ or body part is involved?* axillary chain, left cervical node

❑ *Is the procedure description what you would expect based on the name of the procedure?* Yes

❑ *What surgical approach(es) is used?* Open and percutaneous

❑ *Was more than one procedure, or a combined procedure, performed?* Yes, the first procedure is open left lymphadenectomy of entire axillary chain; the second procedure is percutaneous left cervical lymphadenectomy of the first node.

❑ *Did the procedure take out some or all of a Body Part without replacement?* Yes

❑ *Was a body part or abnormal tissue growth (such as a lesion or tumor) removed?* Yes, a cancerous tumor or lesion was removed.

❑ *Was a foreign object or abnormal material (such as calculus) removed?* No

❑ *Was the body part replaced with a natural or synthetic substitute?* No

❑ *Was removal performed by cutting?* No

❑ *Was removal performed through physical eradication, such as energy, force, or a destructive agent?* No

❑ *Was an extremity removed?* No

❑ *Was removal performed through the use of force, such as pulling or stripping?* No

▶ At this time, Marcy believes that she will use the Root Operations Excision and/or Resection and anticipates that she will need two codes, one for each procedure. She will verify this information when she refers to the PCS Tables to assign codes.

CODING PRACTICE

Exercise 52.2 Abstracting for Root Operations B, T, 6, 5, and D

Instructions: Read the mini-medical-record of each patient's encounter and answer the abstracting questions. Write the answer on the line provided. Do not assign any codes.

---

1. INPATIENT HOSPITAL   Gender: F   Age: 26

Preprocedure diagnosis: polycystic ovaries

Procedure: Oophorectomy. Approached transvaginally with laparoscopic assistance. Located and removed entirety of both ovaries.

Postprocedure diagnosis: polycystic ovaries

(continued)

---

1. (continued)

a. What is the stated procedure? _____

b. What organ or body part is involved? _____

c. What is the laterality? _____

d. Is the procedure description what you would expect based on the name of the procedure? _____

e. What surgical approach is used? _____

f. Was more than one procedure, or a combined procedure, performed? _____

g. Did the procedure take out some or all of a body part without replacement? _____

h. Was a body part or abnormal tissue growth (such as a lesion or tumor) removed? _____

(continued)

1. (continued)

i. Was a foreign object or abnormal material (such as calculus) removed? _____

j. Was the body part replaced with a natural or synthetic substitute? _____

k. Was removal performed by cutting? _____

l. Was removal performed through physical eradication, such as energy, force, or a destructive agent? _____

m. Was an extremity removed? _____

n. Was removal performed through the use of force, such as pulling or stripping? _____

o. Which Root Operation(s) should be considered for this procedure? _____ Why? _____

2. (continued)

n. Was removal performed through the use of force, such as pulling or stripping? _____

o. Which Root Operation(s) should be considered for this procedure? _____ Why? _____

2. INPATIENT HOSPITAL   Gender: F   Age: 47

Preprocedure diagnosis: star cataract, right eye

Procedure: extracapsular cataract phacoemulsification without intraocular lens implantation, right eye. Performed phacoemulsification using hydrodissection to separate the lens nucleus by injecting fluid into the capsule (percutaneously), then suctioned out the lens and fluid.

Postprocedure diagnosis: star cataract, right eye

a. What is the stated procedure? _____

b. What organ or body part is involved? _____

c. What is the laterality? _____

d. Is the procedure description what you would expect based on the name of the procedure? _____

e. What surgical approach is used? _____

f. Was more than one procedure, or a combined procedure, performed? _____

g. Did the procedure take out some or all of a body part without replacement? _____

h. Was a body part or abnormal tissue growth (such as a lesion or tumor) removed? _____

i. Was a foreign object or abnormal material (such as calculus) removed? _____

j. Was the body part replaced with a natural or synthetic substitute? _____

k. Was removal performed by cutting? _____

l. Was removal performed through physical eradication, such as energy, force, or a destructive agent? _____

m. Was an extremity removed? _____

(continued)

3. INPATIENT HOSPITAL   Gender: F   Age: 36

Preprocedure diagnosis: varicose veins

Procedure: Vein stripping of left greater saphenous vein to the level of the knee. Small incisions were made in the groin area and below the vein, then a wire was threaded up the vein to the first incision, and the vein was grasped and removed.

Postprocedure diagnosis: varicose veins

Tip: Ligation is the surgical tying off of a vein; stripping is the removal of the vein through incisions. In a percutaneous approach, small incisions are made through which instruments are inserted. In an open approach, the entire operative field is opened up with a large incision.

a. What is the stated procedure? _____

b. What organ or body part is involved? _____

c. What is the laterality? _____

d. Is the procedure description what you would expect based on the name of the procedure? _____

e. What surgical approach is used? _____

f. Was more than one procedure, or a combined procedure, performed? _____

g. Did the procedure take out some or all of a body part without replacement? _____

h. Was a body part or abnormal tissue growth (such as a lesion or tumor) removed? _____

i. Was a foreign object or abnormal material (such as calculus) removed? _____

j. Was the body part replaced with a natural or synthetic substitute? _____

k. Was removal performed by cutting? _____

l. Was removal performed through physical eradication, such as energy, force, or a destructive agent? _____

m. Was an extremity removed? _____

n. Was removal performed through the use of force, such as pulling or stripping? _____

o. Which Root Operation(s) should be considered for this procedure? _____ Why? _____

(continued)

CODING PRACTICE (continued)

4. INPATIENT HOSPITAL Gender: M Age: 18

Preprocedure diagnosis: spinal cord lesions

Procedure: Electrocauterization. Made two 1.5-cm incisions at T7 and inserted endoscope and electrocautery device. Cauterized single lesion. Withdrew instruments and closed wounds. Proceeded to make two 1.5-cm incisions at L3 and inserted endoscope and electrocautery device. Cauterized two lesions. Withdrew instruments and closed wounds.

Postprocedure diagnosis: benign neoplasm, spinal cord, lumbar and thoracic

a. What is the stated procedure? _____

b. What organ or body part is involved? _____

c. How many and which sites are treated? _____

d. Is the procedure description what you would expect based on the name of the procedure? _____

e. What surgical approach is used? _____

f. Did the procedure take out some or all of a body part without replacement? _____

g. Was a body part or abnormal tissue growth (such as a lesion or tumor) removed? _____

h. Was a foreign object or abnormal material (such as calculus) removed? _____

i. Was the body part replaced with a natural or synthetic substitute? _____

j. Was removal performed by cutting? _____

k. Was removal performed through physical eradication, such as energy, force, or a destructive agent? _____

l. Was an extremity removed? _____

m. Was removal performed through the use of force, such as pulling or stripping? _____

n. Which Root Operation(s) should be considered for this procedure? _____ Why? _____

---

5. INPATIENT HOSPITAL Gender: M Age: 61

Preprocedure diagnosis: cholecystitis with gallstones

Procedure: laparoscopic cholecystectomy and CBD removal; wedge biopsy, liver. Created 3 ports to access RUQ and examined the area with laparoscope. Identified gall bladder inflammation and gall stones in the common bile duct. Dissected the gall bladder and common bile duct. Visualized a nodule on the right lobe of liver and obtained a wedge biopsy that was sent to pathology with the gall bladder.

(continued)

---

5. (continued)

Postprocedure diagnosis: acute cholecystitis with cholelithiasis, adenoma of liver

a. What is the stated procedure? _____

b. What organ or body part is involved? _____

c. What is the laterality? _____

d. Is the procedure description what you would expect based on the name of the procedure? _____

e. What surgical approach is used? _____

f. Was more than one procedure, or a combined procedure, performed? _____

g. Did the procedure take out some or all of a body part without replacement? _____

h. Was a body part or abnormal tissue growth (such as a lesion or tumor) removed? _____

i. Was a foreign object or abnormal material (such as calculus) removed? _____

j. Was the body part replaced with a natural or synthetic substitute? _____

k. Was removal performed by cutting? _____

l. Was removal performed through physical eradication, such as energy, force, or a destructive agent? _____

m. Was an extremity removed? _____

n. Was removal performed through the use of force, such as pulling or stripping? _____

o. Which Root Operation(s) should be considered for this procedure? _____ Why? _____

---

6. INPATIENT HOSPITAL Gender: M Age: 26

Preprocedure diagnosis: necrosis and spreading infection after injury 1 month ago, with potential for sepsis

Procedure: Amputation. Removed 4th phalanges and entire metacarpal, right hand, and 5th phalanges and entire metacarpal, right hand

Postprocedure diagnosis: infection, subcutaneous tissue, right hand, organism unknown

a. What is the stated procedure? _____

b. What organ or body part is involved? _____

c. How many sites are treated? _____

d. What is the laterality? _____

(continued)

6. (continued)

e. Is the procedure description what you would expect based on the name of the procedure? _____

f. What surgical approach is used? _____

g. Was more than one procedure, or a combined procedure, performed? _____

h. Did the procedure take out some or all of a body part without replacement? _____

i. Was a body part or abnormal tissue growth (such as a lesion or tumor) removed? _____

j. Was a foreign object or abnormal material (such as calculus) removed? _____

(continued)

6. (continued)

k. Was the body part replaced with a natural or synthetic substitute? _____

l. Was removal performed by cutting? _____

m. Was removal performed through physical eradication, such as energy, force, or a destructive agent? _____

n. Was an extremity removed? _____

o. Was removal performed through the use of force, such as pulling or stripping? _____

p. Which Root Operation(s) should be considered for this procedure? _____ Why? _____

ASSIGNING CHARACTERS 4–7 FOR ROOT OPERATIONS B, T, 6, 5, AND D

To assign codes after the Root Operation is determined, search the PCS Index for the name of the Root Operation as the Main Term. Locate the subterm(s) for the correct anatomic site and identify the PCS Table. When you locate the PCS Table, verify the first three characters of the code, then locate the row with the Body Part needed. Assign the remaining characters from each respective column of the Table. The following information summarizes and highlights unique information for working with the Tables for each Root Operation B, T, 6, 5, and D. Each Root Operation has one Table in each applicable PCS Body System. Because of the differences between organ systems, Table details vary.

Character 4: Body Part

Every PCS code must contain a valid value for Character 4, Body Part. *None* is never an option. PCS lists the Body Part values separately for each Body System value and each Root Operation. A Body System might not contain the same Body Part values for each Root Operation, so refer to the appropriate PCS Table to identify the Body Part options for the combination of the applicable Body System and Root Operation.

For example, in Table **09B** (Ear, Nose, Sinus Excision) the Body Part values include **0 External Ear, Right**, **1 External Ear, Left**, and **K Nose**. In Table **09D** (Ear, Nose, Sinus Extraction), the Body Part values do not include the external ear or nose because the Root Operation Extraction does not apply to these sites.

Body Parts for Excision and Resection

Identifying the Body Part values is the key to distinguishing between the Root Operations Excision and Resection. Because Excision is cutting off a portion of a Body Part and Resection is cutting off all of a Body Part, the Root Operation cannot be assigned until the level of specificity of the Body Part values is known. This may require that the coder review both the Table for Excision and the Table for Resection for a given Body System (PCS OGCR B3.8).

Sometimes Body Part values overlap, in which case you need to select the most specific Body Part value applicable to the procedure. The Root Operation Excision must be assigned only when a portion of a body part, as identified by the smallest Body Part value, is removed.

PCS provides nine Body Part values for lungs, although they comprise one organ. Body Part values range from the most general—**M Lungs, Bilateral**—to each side right (**K**) and left (**L**), and then to each lobe and the lingula (*a tongue-like projection of the upper left lobe*). Select the most specific Body Part value applicable to the Root Operation Resection. When one entire lobe is cut out, use Resection to identify that the entire lobe was removed. Do not use Excision to describe that a portion of the entire organ (the lung) was removed because a more specific Body Part is provided (■ FIGURE 52-1). When a portion of a lobe is removed, code the Root Operation Excision because no smaller Body Part value is available.

By contrast, the stomach has only two PCS Body Part values: Stomach, Pylorus (7) and Stomach (6). When the pylorus or the entire stomach is removed, code Resection. When any portion of the stomach is removed, code Excision.

> ## SUCCESS STEP
>
> When a colectomy is performed, PCS requires only the Root Operation Excision or Resection. The type of anastomosis—such as end to side or side to side—is not reported with a Character value or a separate code.

Body Parts for Detachment

The Root Operation Detachment does not appear under Tables for individual PCS Body Systems, such as Skeletal, but under the Body System values **W Anatomical Regions, General**, **X Anatomical Regions, Upper Extremities**, and **Y Anatomical Regions, Lower Extremities**. Refer to Tables **06W**, **06X**, and **06Y**.

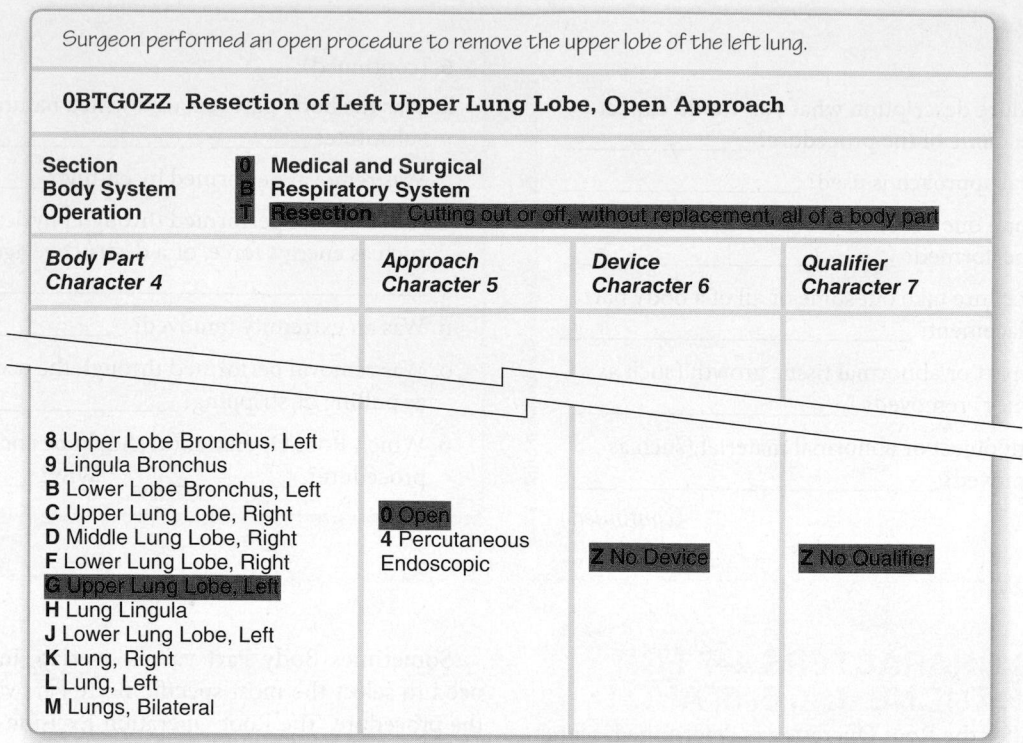

Figure 52-1 ■ Example of Coding Resection Instead of Excision

Character 5: Approach

Every PCS code must contain a valid value for Character 5, Approach. *None* is never an option.

Assign the value for Character 5, Approach, based on the surgical approach used. Remember to refer to PCS Approach definitions in the ICD-10-PCS coding manual Introduction or the PCS Appendix *Components of the Medical and Surgical Approach Definitions.* The Approach comprises three components: the access location, method, and type of instrumentation.

Access location, referred to elsewhere in this text as the anatomic approach, refers to the anatomic site through which the target site for the procedure is reached. The two general types of access locations are the skin/mucous membranes and an external orifice. The skin or mucous membranes can be punctured or incised to reach the procedure site and is the access location for all percutaneous and open procedures. An external orifice may be natural— such as the nose, mouth, rectum, or vagina— or artificial, such as a colostomy stoma. An endoscopic procedure can be performed percutaneously or through an external orifice. The external approach identifies procedures performed directly on the skin or mucous membranes, such as the excision of a skin lesion, and those performed indirectly through the application of force, such as closed reduction of a fracture. (Note: Procedures performed indirectly through the use of force are not coded to Root Operations B, T, 6, 5, and D and are discussed elsewhere in this text.)

Method identifies how the access location is entered to reach an internal body part. An open procedure involves cutting through the skin or mucous membrane and subcutaneous layers to reach the procedure site. When instrumentation, such as an endoscope, is used, the method identifies whether the

instrumentation is introduced percutaneously or through an external orifice. The incisions during a percutaneous procedure are part of that method and are not identified or coded separately.

Instrumentation is specialized equipment used to reach an internal body part, such as an endoscope or needle. (Note: Procedures using needles as the primary instrument are not coded to Root Operations B, T, 6, 5, and D and are discussed elsewhere in this text.)

When an Approach value does not apply to all Body Parts, the PCS Table is divided into two or more rows. Be sure to read all rows in the Table before assigning the code because all values for a code must come from the same row in the Table. For example, in Table **0BB Medical and Surgical, Respiratory System, Excision**, two rows appear because the Approach values **7 Via Natural or Artificial Opening** and **8 Via Natural or Artificial Opening Endoscopic** do not apply to Body Part values for the diaphragm and pleura (■ FIGURE 52-2).

Character 6: Device

None of the Root Operations in this group, *Procedures that Take Out Some or All of Body Part,* use Character 6, Device. The value is always **Z No Device**. Temporary devices such as postoperative drains are considered part of the procedure and are not coded separately. When a permanent device is put in place, a different Root Operation is required.

Character 7: Qualifier

Character 7, Qualifier, is used for Root Operations in this group primarily to identify biopsies, the level of an amputation, and the number of teeth extracted. When no Qualifier applies, assign **Z No qualifier** as the value for Character 7.

Section	0	Medical and Surgical
Body System	B	Respiratory System
Operation	B	Excision: Cutting out or off, without replacement, a portion of a body part

Body Part Character 4	Approach Character 5	Device Character 6	Qualifier Character 7
1 Trachea 2 Carina 3 Main Bronchus, Right 4 Upper Lobe Bronchus, Right 5 Middle Lobe Bronchus, Right 6 Lower Lobe Bronchus, Right 7 Main Bronchus, Left 8 Upper Lobe Bronchus, Left 9 Lingula Bronchus B Lower Lobe Bronchus, Left C Upper Lung Lobe, Right D Middle Lung Lobe, Right F Lower Lung Lobe, Right G Upper Lung Lobe, Left H Lung Lingula J Lower Lung Lobe, Left K Lung, Right L Lung, Left M Lungs, Bilateral	0 Open 3 Percutaneous 4 Percutaneous Endoscopic 7 Via Natural or Artificial Opening 8 Via Natural or Artificial Opening Endoscopic	Z No Device	X Diagnostic Z No Qualifier
N Pleura, Right P Pleura, Left R Diaphragm, Right S Diaphragm, Left	0 Open 3 Percutaneous 4 Percutaneous Endoscopic	Z No Device	X Diagnostic Z No Qualifier

Figure 52-2 ■ Example of Two Rows in PCS Table with Different Approach Values

Biopsy

A biopsy is performed for diagnostic reasons as opposed to therapeutic or treatment reasons. Biopsies take out only a portion of an organ or structure, so biopsies involving cutting are almost always coded to Excision (B). Biopsies using other methods, such as needle aspiration, are coded to other Root Operations. When a biopsy is performed, assign the Character 7 Qualifier value **X Diagnostic**.

Detachment Qualifiers

The specific qualifiers used for the Root Operation Detachment (6) are dependent on the Body Part value in the upper and lower extremities body systems. ■ TABLE 52-10 defines the meaning of the qualifiers used in both the upper and lower extremities.

Extraction Qualifiers

For the Root Operation Extraction (D) and Body Parts Upper Tooth (W) and Lower Tooth (X), the Qualifier identifies the number of teeth extracted:

- **0 Single**
- **1 Multiple**
- **2 All**

Guided Example of Assigning Characters 4–7 for Excision and Resection

To practice skills for assigning codes for Excision and Resection, continue with the example from earlier in the chapter about a patient who was seen for a lymphadenectomy. Follow along in your ICD-10-PCS manual as Marcy Elwood, CCS, assigns codes. Check off each step after you complete it.

▶ First, Marcy confirms the procedures: open left lymphadenectomy of entire axillary chain and percutaneous left cervical lymphadenectomy of the first node only.

❑ She confirms that the Root Operations are Excision and/or Resection, depending on how Body Part values are identified in the PCS Table.

▶ Marcy searches the Index for the Main Term **Excision**.

❑ She locates the first-level subterm **Lymphatic**.

❑ She locates the second-level subterm **Axillary**.

❑ She locates the third-level subterm **Left**.

❑ She identifies the Table: **07B6**.

❑ She then locates another second-level subterm **Neck** for the cervical lymph node.

❑ She locates the third-level subterm **Left**.

❑ She identifies the Table: **07B2**.

❑ The first three letters of each partial code, **07B**, refer her to the PCS Table for the Lymphatic system, Root Operation Excision. The fourth character identifies the Body Part.

Table 52-10 ■ **CHARACTER 7 QUALIFIER VALUES FOR THE ROOT OPERATION DETACHMENT**

Value	Meaning	Definition
Upper Arm and Upper Leg		
1	High	Amputation at the proximal portion of the shaft of the humerus or femur
2	Mid	Amputation at the middle portion of the shaft of the humerus or femur
3	Low	Amputation at the distal portion of the shaft of the humerus or femur
Hand and Foot		
0	Complete	Amputation through the carpometacarpal joint of the hand or through the tarsal-metatarsal joint of the foot
4	Complete 1st Ray	
5	Complete 2nd Ray	
6	Complete 3rd Ray	
7	Complete 4th Ray	
8	Complete 5th Ray	
9	Partial 1st Ray	Partial: Amputation anywhere along the shaft or head of the metacarpal bone of the hand or of the metatarsal bone of the foot
B	Partial 2nd Ray	
C	Partial 3rd Ray	
D	Partial 4th Ray	
F	Partial 5th Ray	
Thumb, Finger, or Toe		
0	Complete	Amputation at the metacarpophalangeal/metatarsal-phalangeal joint
1	High	Amputation anywhere along the proximal phalanx
2	Mid	Amputation through the proximal interphalangeal joint or anywhere along the middle phalanx
3	Low	Amputation through the distal interphalangeal joint or anywhere along the distal phalanx

Source: © PB Resources, Inc. Used with permission.

▶ Then, Marcy searches the Index for the Main Term **Resection** because she does not know which Root Operation is needed for each procedure.

❑ She locates the first-level subterm **Lymphatic**.

❑ She locates the second-level subterm **Axillary**.

❑ She locates the third-level subterm **Left**.

❑ She identifies the Table: **07T6**.

❑ She then locates another second-level subterm **Neck** for the cervical lymph node.

❑ She locates the third-level subterm **Left**.

❑ She identifies the Table: **07T2**.

❑ The first three letters of each partial code, **07T**, refer her to the PCS Table for the Lymphatic system, Root

Operation Resection. The fourth character identifies the Body Part.

▶ To confirm her choices, Marcy searches the Index for the Main Term **Lymphadenectomy**. She reads the cross-reference notes that appear below the Main Term.

❑ *see* **Excision, Lymphatic and Hemic Systems 07B**

❑ *see* **Resection, Lymphatic and Hemic Systems 07T**

▶ Marcy turns to Table **07B** for the Root Operation Excision.

❑ She reads the Table title **07B, Section 0 Medical and Surgical, Body System 7 Lymphatic and Hemic Systems, Root Operation B Excision** and confirms that this accurately describes the Body System and Root Operation. She reads the Root Operation definition **Cutting out or off, without replacement, a portion** of a body part and confirms that the definition is what she expected.

▶ Marcy reads the values for Character 4, Body Part, to identify how the Body Parts are defined.

❑ The value **6** identifies **Lymphatic, Left Axillary**, referring to the entire lymph chain. The *entire* left axillary chain was removed, so the Root Operation Excision does not apply because Excision describes removing only a portion of the Body Part. She will need to refer to the Root Operation Resection for removal of the entire lymph chain.

❑ The value **2** identifies **Lymphatic, Left Neck** and does not specify individual lymph nodes. Because only one cervical lymph node was removed, the Root Operation Excision applies because a *portion* of the lymph chain, that is, a single node, was removed. She will assign the remainder of the code for the cervical lymph node removal from the Excision Table.

▶ Marcy assigns the value for Character 5, Approach.

❑ She refers to the operative report, which documents *percutaneous left cervical lymphadenectomy.*

❑ She assigns the value **3 Percutaneous** for the Approach.

▶ Marcy assigns the value for Character 6, Device.

❑ The Table provides only one option: **Z No Device.**

▶ Marcy assigns the value for Character 7, Qualifier.

❑ She refers to the operative report and confirms that the procedure was not a biopsy, which would require **X Diagnostic.**

❑ She assigns the value **Z No Qualifier.**

❑ She reviews the code she has assigned for the *percutaneous left cervical lymphadenectomy:* **07B23ZZ** (■ Figure 52-3).

▶ Next, Marcy turns to Table **07T** for the Root Operation Resection to assign the code for *open left lymphadenectomy of entire axillary chain.*

❑ She reads the Table title **07T, Section 0 Medical and Surgical, Body System 7 Lymphatic and Hemic Systems, Root Operation T Resection** and confirms that this accurately describes the Body System and Root Operation. She reads the Root Operation definition **Cutting out or off, without replacement, all of a body part** and confirms that the definition is what she expected.

▶ Marcy reads the values for Character 4, Body Part.

❑ The value **6** identifies **Lymphatic Left Axillary**, referring to the entire lymph chain. The *entire* left axillary chain was removed, so the Root Operation Resection applies.

▶ Marcy assigns the value for Character 5, Approach.

❑ She refers to the operative report, which documents *open left lymphadenectomy.*

❑ She assigns the value **0 Open** for the Approach.

▶ Marcy assigns the value for Character 6, Device.

❑ The Table provides only one option: **Z No Device.**

▶ Marcy assigns the value for Character 7, Qualifier.

❑ The Table provides only one option: **Z No Qualifier.**

❑ She reviews the code she has assigned for the *open left lymphadenectomy of entire axillary chain:* **07T60ZZ** (■ Figure 52-4).

▶ Next, Marcy must determine how to sequence the codes.

Section	0	Medical and Surgical
Body System	7	Lymphatic and Hemic Systems
Operation	B	Excision: Cutting out or off, without replacement, a portion of a body part

Body Part Character 4	Approach Character 5	Device Character 6	Qualifier Character 7
0 Lymphatic, Head **1** Lymphatic, Right Neck **2** Lymphatic, Left Neck **3** Lymphatic, Right Upper Extremity **4** Lymphatic, Left Upper Extremity	**0** Open **3** Percutaneous **4** Percutaneous Endoscopic	**Z** No Device	**X** Diagnostic **Z** No Qualifier

Figure 52-3 ■ Assigning Code 07B23ZZ. *Source: Annotation © PB Resources, Inc. Used with permission.*

Section	0	**Medical and Surgical**
Body System	7	**Lymphatic and Hemic Systems**
Operation	T	**Resection:** Cutting out or off, without replacement, all of a body part

Body Part Character 4	Approach Character 5	Device Character 6	Qualifier Character 7
0 Lymphatic, Head **1** Lymphatic, Right Neck **2** Lymphatic, Left Neck **3** Lymphatic, Right Upper Extremity **4** Lymphatic, Left Upper Extremity **5** Lymphatic, Right Axillary **6** Lymphatic, Left Axillary **7** Lymphatic, Thorax	**0** Open **4** Percutaneous Endoscopic	**Z** No Device	**Z** No Qualifier

Figure 52-4 ■ Assigning Code 07T60ZZ. *Source: Annotation © PB Resources, Inc. Used with permission.*

CODING PRACTICE

Exercise 52.3 Assigning Characters 4–7 for Root Operations B, T, 6, 5, and D

Instructions: Read the mini-medical-record of each patient's encounter. Review the information abstracted in Exercise 52.2 for questions 1–3. For questions 4–6, abstract the case on your own. Assign PCS codes using the Index and Tables. Write the code(s) on the line provided.

1. INPATIENT HOSPITAL Gender: F Age: 26

Preprocedure diagnosis: polycystic ovaries

Procedure: Oophorectomy. Approached transvaginally with laparoscopic assistance. Located and removed entirety of both ovaries.

Postprocedure diagnosis: polycystic ovaries

Tip: Ovary is defined as a distinct Body Part. All of the ovary was removed.

1 PCS Code _____

2. INPATIENT HOSPITAL Gender: F Age: 47

Preprocedure diagnosis: star cataract, right eye

Procedure: extracapsular cataract phacoemulsification without intraocular lens implantation, right eye. Performed phacoemulsification using hydrodissection to separate the lens nucleus by injecting fluid into the capsule, then suctioned out the lens and fluid.

Postprocedure diagnosis: star cataract, right eye

1 PCS Code _____

3. INPATIENT HOSPITAL Gender: F Age: 36

Preprocedure diagnosis: varicose veins

Procedure: Vein stripping of left greater saphenous vein to the level of the knee. Small incisions were made in the groin area and below the vein, then a wire was threaded up the vein to the first incision, and the vein was grasped and removed.

Postprocedure diagnosis: varicose veins

Tip: Ligation is the surgical tying off of a vein; stripping is the removal of the vein through incisions. In a percutaneous approach, small incisions are made through which instruments are inserted. In an open approach, the entire operative field is opened up with a large incision.

1 PCS Code _____

4. INPATIENT HOSPITAL Gender: F Age: 62

Preprocedure diagnosis: hallux abductovalgus with bunion deformity

Procedure: Keller bunionectomy, right. Incision made over 1st metatarsal head. Exostosis removed and head remodeled. Excellent capillary refill after tourniquet release.

Postprocedure diagnosis: hallux abductovalgus with bunion deformity

Tip: A bunion is an enlargement of the joint at the base of the big toe composed of bone and soft tissue.

1 PCS Code _____

5. INPATIENT HOSPITAL   Gender: M **Age:** 44

Preprocedure diagnosis: myasthenia gravis, thymoma

Procedure: transthoracic thymectomy. Made a lengthwise incision in the chest slightly left of the midline. Explored the chest and excised the entire thymus gland. No adjacent structures were disturbed. Inspected the surgical field to ensure no residual thymic tissue. Closed surgical wound and transferred patient to the postoperative area in stable condition.

Postprocedure diagnosis: thymoma

Tip: The entire thymus (body part) was removed.

1 PCS Code _____

6. INPATIENT HOSPITAL   Gender: M   **Age:** 28

Preprocedure diagnosis: uncontrolled bilateral epistaxis

Procedure: limited cautery of nasal hemorrhage. Used nasal speculum to locate site of bleeding in the right anterior nasal passage, cleaned, and applied silver nitrate stick to cauterize. Repeated on the left anterior passage. Hemostasis was achieved.

Postprocedure diagnosis: epistaxis

Tip: Read the definitions for destruction and repair carefully.

1 PCS Code _____

ARRANGING CODES FOR ROOT OPERATIONS B, T, 6, 5, AND D

When more than one procedure is performed during an inpatient admission, hospitals must determine the **principal procedure**. The principal procedure impacts the diagnosis-related groups (DRGs) to which the patient is assigned for reimbursement purposes. Selection of the principal procedure is directly related to the principal diagnosis. The principal diagnosis, as defined by the Uniform Hospital Data Discharge Set (UHDDS), is "that condition established after study to be chiefly responsible for occasioning the admission of the patient to the hospital for care." Refer to ICD-10-CM OGCR Section II to review the guidelines for establishing the principal diagnosis.

The principal procedure is entered in FL 74 on the UB-04; secondary procedures are entered in FL 74a–74e. The principal and additional diagnoses are entered in FL 67–67M (■ FIGURE 52-5).

The PCS OGCR section "Selection of the Principal Procedure" provides instructions on how to select the principal procedure. These guidelines apply to all Root Operations. The general sequencing priorities for PCS codes are as follows:

1. Definitive procedure related to principal diagnosis

2. Diagnostic procedure related to principal diagnosis

3. Definitive procedure related to secondary diagnosis

4. Diagnostic procedure related to secondary diagnosis

When more than one definitive procedure equally relates to the principal diagnosis, sequence the most extensive procedure as the principal procedure. Various types of procedure combinations are discussed in PCS OGCR and are summarized next.

- The principal procedure is the procedure performed for definitive treatment most related to principal diagnosis. Sequence procedures related to the secondary diagnoses as subsequent procedures (■ FIGURE 52-6).

- When a diagnostic procedure and a procedure for definitive treatment are performed for both the principal and secondary diagnoses, the principal procedure is the procedure performed for definitive treatment most related to the principal diagnosis. Diagnostic procedures related to the principal diagnosis are sequenced as secondary procedures. All procedures related to the secondary diagnoses are sequenced as secondary procedures (■ FIGURE 52-7).

- When a diagnostic procedure is performed for the principal diagnosis and definitive treatment is provided for the secondary diagnosis, the diagnostic procedure is the principal procedure because it is most related to the principal diagnosis (■ FIGURE 52-8).

Surgeon removed the descending colon due to cancer, using endoscopic access through the anus. A percutaneous biopsy was taken of the pelvic lymph nodes, which were positive for metastases, so a percutaneous endoscopic pelvic lymphadenectomy also was performed to remove several, but not all, nodes.

C18.6 Malignant neoplasm of descending colon
C77.5 Secondary and unspecified malignant neoplasm
of intrapelvic lymph nodes
0DTM8ZZ Resection, Descending colon, Via natural or
artificial opening endoscopic, No device,
No qualifier
07BC4ZZ Excision, Lymphatic pelvis, Percutaneous
endoscopic, No device, No qualifier
07BC3ZX Excision, Lymphatic pelvis, Percutaneous,
No device, Diagnostic

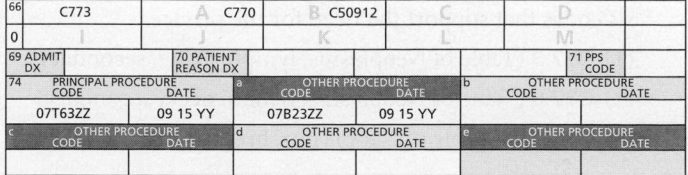

66		C773	A	C770	B	C50912	C		D		
0		I		J		K		L	M		
69 ADMIT DX			70 PATIENT REASON DX						71 PPS CODE		
74 PRINCIPAL PROCEDURE CODE	DATE	a	OTHER PROCEDURE CODE	DATE	b	OTHER PROCEDURE CODE	DATE				
07T63ZZ	09 15 YY		07B23ZZ	09 15 YY							
c	OTHER PROCEDURE CODE	DATE	d	OTHER PROCEDURE CODE	DATE	e	OTHER PROCEDURE CODE	DATE			

Figure 52-5 ■ UB-04 Example of Principal Diagnosis and Principal Procedure. *Source: Annotations © PB Resources, Inc. Used with permission.*

Figure 52-6 ■ Example of Sequencing Procedures for the Principal and Secondary Diagnoses. *Source: © PB Resources, Inc. Used with permission.*

Surgeon performs an endometrial biopsy using a speculum through the vaginal opening. The biopsy is found to be cancerous, so a vaginal hysterectomy is performed.

C54.1 Malignant neoplasm of endometrium
0UT97ZZ Resection, Uterus, Via natural or artificial opening, No device, No qualifier
0UDB7ZX Extraction, Endometrium, Via natural or artificial opening, No device, Diagnostic

Figure 52-7 ■ Example of Sequencing Definitive and Diagnostic Procedures. *Source: © PB Resources, Inc. Used with permission.*

Patient was admitted for alcoholic cirrhosis of the liver. An endoscopic excisional biopsy was performed of the left lobe of the liver. During additional workup, a rectal polyp was found which was removed endoscopically using fulguration.

K70.30 Alcoholic cirrhosis of liver without ascites
K62.1 Rectal polyp
0FB24ZX Excision, Liver left lobe, Percutaneous endoscopic, No device, Diagnostic
0D5P8ZZ Destruction, Rectum, Via natural or artificial opening endoscopic, No device, No qualifier

Figure 52-8 ■ Example of Sequencing a Diagnostic Procedure for the Principal Procedure. *Source: © PB Resources, Inc. Used with permission.*

- When the only procedure(s) performed relate to the secondary diagnosis, the principal procedure is the one performed for definitive treatment of the secondary diagnosis. Sequence diagnostic procedures related to the secondary diagnosis as secondary procedures. Because there are no procedures related to the principal diagnosis, a procedure related to the secondary diagnosis must be the principal procedure (■ FIGURE 52-9).

SUCCESS STEP

The *AHA Coding Clinic*, published quarterly by the American Hospital Association (AHA), provides definitive guidance, clarification, and examples regarding inpatient coding issues. Inpatient hospitals also develop internal coding guidelines to direct coders in specific situations.

Guided Example of Arranging Codes for Excision and Resection

To practice skills for arranging codes for procedures of the Root Operations **Excision** and **Resection**, continue with the example from earlier in the chapter about the patient who was seen for a lymphadenectomy. Follow along in your ICD-10-PCS manual as Marcy Elwood, CCS, arranges the codes. Check off each step after you complete it.

▶ First, Marcy confirms the codes she assigned:

❏ **07B23ZZ Excision, Lymphatic left neck, Percutaneous, No device, No qualifier**

Patient was admitted because of weakness due to hyponatremia and dehydration. Medical treatment was provided. During the admission, the patient developed a nosebleed, which was treated with electrocautery through the nasal opening.

E87.1 Hypo-osmolality and hyponatremia
E86.0 Dehydration
R04.0 Epistaxis
095KXZZ Destruction, Ear nose sinus, Nose, External, No device, No qualifier

Figure 52-9 ■ Example of Sequencing a Principal Procedure for the Secondary Procedure. *Source: © PB Resources, Inc. Used with permission.*

❏ **07T60ZZ Resection, Lymphatic left axillary, Open, No device, No qualifier**

▶ Marcy reviews the diagnoses for this case: left breast cancer with metastasis to lymph nodes.

❏ Metastasis to the lymph nodes is the reason for the hospital admission and the services provided.

❏ In the ICD-10-CM Table of Neoplasms, diagnosis codes for lymph node metastases are divided by site. Both the cervical node and axillary chain equally meet the criteria for principal diagnosis.

- Marcy sequences the axillary chain as the principal diagnosis because it is the predominant, or larger, site.

- Marcy sequences metastasis to the single cervical node as a secondary diagnosis.

❏ Marcy sequences left breast cancer as secondary diagnosis because it was not treated during this admission.

▶ Next, Marcy arranges the procedure codes.

❏ Resection of the left axillary lymph chain is a definitive procedure related to the principal diagnosis, so she sequences it as the principal procedure.

❏ Excision of the cervical lymph node is a definitive procedure related to a secondary diagnosis, so she sequences it as a secondary procedure.

▶ Marcy finalizes the procedure codes and sequencing for this case:

(1) **07T60ZZ Resection, Lymphatic left axillary, Open, No device, No qualifier**

(2) **07B23ZZ Excision, Lymphatic left neck, Percutaneous, No device, No qualifier**

▶ Marcy also assigns and sequences the ICD-10-CM diagnosis codes that support the need for the service.

(1) **C77.3** (Table of Neoplasms, lymph, axilla, secondary)

(2) **C77.0** (Table of Neoplasms, lymph, neck, secondary)

(3) **C50.912** (Table of Neoplasms, breast, primary, left)

▶ Figure 52-5 shows the completion of the UB-04 for these diagnoses and procedures.

CODING PRACTICE

Exercise 52.4 **Arranging Codes for Root Operations B, T, 6, 5, and D**

Instructions: Read the mini-medical-record of each patient's encounter. Review the information abstracted in Exercise 52.2 for questions 1–3. For questions 4–6, abstract the case on your own. Assign PCS codes using the Index and Tables, and arrange the codes in proper sequence. Write the code(s) on the line provided.

---

1. INPATIENT HOSPITAL   Gender: M   Age: 18

Preprocedure diagnosis: spinal cord lesions

Procedure: Electrocauterization. Made two 1.5-cm incisions at T7 and inserted endoscope and electrocautery device. Cauterized single lesion. Withdrew instruments and closed wounds. Proceeded to make two 1.5-cm incisions at L3 and inserted endoscope and electrocautery device. Cauterized two lesions. Withdrew instruments and closed wounds.

Postprocedure diagnosis: benign neoplasm, spinal cord, lumbar and thoracic

Tip: When the same Root Operation is performed at two distinct Body Part sites, assign separate codes (PCS OGCR B3.2a).

2 PCS Codes _____

---

2. INPATIENT HOSPITAL   Gender: M   Age: 61

Preprocedure diagnosis: cholecystitis with gallstones

Procedure: laparoscopic cholecystectomy and CBD removal; wedge biopsy, liver. Created 3 ports to access RUQ and examined the area with laparoscope. Identified gall bladder inflammation and gall stones in the common bile duct. Dissected the gall bladder and common bile duct. Visualized a nodule on the right lobe of liver and obtained a wedge biopsy that was sent to pathology with the gall bladder.

Postprocedure diagnosis: acute cholecystitis with cholelithiasis, adenoma of liver

Tip: A biopsy is diagnostic.

3 PCS Codes _____

_____

---

3. INPATIENT HOSPITAL   Gender: M   Age: 26

Preprocedure diagnosis: necrosis and spreading infection after injury 1 month ago, with potential for sepsis

Procedure: Amputation. Removed 4th phalanges and entire metacarpal, right hand, and 5th phalanges at the interphalangeal joint, right hand

Postprocedure diagnosis: infection, subcutaneous tissue, right hand, organism unknown

Tip: Assign the Qualifier based on the extent of the amputation. Refer to Table 52-10.

2 PCS Codes _____

---

4. INPATIENT HOSPITAL   Gender: M   Age: 56

Preprocedure diagnosis: multi-invasive bladder cancer

Procedure: laparoscopic radical cystectomy with bilateral pelvic lymph node dissections and orthotopic neobladder. After port placement, the bladder was meticulously dissected free and removed. Right and left obturator and pelvic lymph nodes were dissected next. The continent urinary diversion was performed by Dr. Alfred and is reported separately.

Tip: Code only the procedures for the first surgeon, not Dr. Alfred.

2 PCS Codes _____

---

5. INPATIENT HOSPITAL   Gender: F   Age: 34

Preprocedure diagnosis: painful enlarged navicula, right foot; osteochondroma of right fifth metatarsal

Procedure: partial tarsectomy navicular and partial metatarsectomy, fifth metatarsal right foot. The enlarged portion of the navicular bone was removed. Osteochondroma removed from the fifth metatarsal neck. Tourniquet released with good capillary refill.

Tip: A portion of the tarsal and metatarsal bones were removed on the same foot.

2 PCS Codes _____

(continued)

CODING PRACTICE (continued)

6. INPATIENT HOSPITAL Gender: M Age: 63

Preprocedure diagnosis: *carious teeth and periodontal disease affecting all remaining teeth*

Procedure: *extraction of remaining teeth numbers 2, 3, 4, 5, 7, 8, 9, 10, 11, 12, 13, 14, 15, 16, 17, 18, 19, 20, 21, 22, 23, 24, 25, 26, 27, 28, 29, 30, 31, and 32. Routine forceps extraction of teeth was*

(continued)

6. (continued)

begun on the upper left quadrant followed by the lower left quadrant. Attention turned to extraction of teeth on the upper right quadrant and right lower quadrant.

Postprocedure diagnosis: *carious teeth and periodontal disease*

Tip: Report the number of teeth removed using the Qualifier.

2 PCS Codes _____

CHAPTER SUMMARY

In this chapter you learned that:

- The Root Operation group *Procedures that Take Out Some or All of a Body Part* includes five Root Operations: Excision (B), Resection (T), Detachment (6), Destruction (5), and Extraction (D).

- The Root Operation Excision (B) is cutting out or off, without replacement, a portion of a PCS Body Part.

- The Root Operation Resection (T) is cutting out or off, without replacement, all of a PCS Body Part.

- The Root Operation Detachment (6) is cutting off all or a portion of the upper or lower extremities.

- The Root Operation Destruction (5) is physical eradication of all or a portion of a Body Part by the direct use of energy, force, or a destructive agent.

- The Root Operation Extraction (D) is pulling or stripping out or off all or a portion of a Body Part by the use of force.

- Abstracting for PCS focuses on identifying the correct Root Operation, which involves reading the operative report and interpreting it in light of Root Operation definitions.

- Identifying the Body Part values is the key to distinguishing between the Root Operations Excision and Resection.

- When an Approach value does not apply to all Body Parts, the PCS Table is divided into two or more rows.

- None of the Root Operations in this group use Character 6, Device.

- Character 7, Qualifier, is used for Root Operations in this group primarily to identify biopsies, the level of an amputation, and the number of teeth extracted.

- The PCS OGCR section "Selection of the Principal Procedure" provides instructions on how to select the principal procedure.

- PCS OGCR section B provides guidelines for the Medical and Surgical Section (0), organized by the Characters of the PCS code. Specific guidelines are provided for biopsy procedures, biopsy followed by more definitive treatment, comparison of Excision and Resection, and Excision for a graft.

CONCEPT QUIZ

Take a moment to look back at Root Operations that take out some or all of a Body Part and solidify your skills. Try to answer the questions from memory first, then refer to the discussion in this chapter if you need a little extra help.

Completion

Instructions: Write the term that answers each question based on the information you learned in this chapter. Choose from the list below. Some choices may be used more than once and some choices may not be used at all.

Destruction   Extraction

Detachment   Resection

Excision

1. The root operation for traumatic amputation of the hand is

   _____.

2. _____ is the main term for a nonobstetric suction curettage.

3. To code enucleation of the eyeball, search for the Main Term

   _____.

4. An amputation of the leg above the knee is the Root Operation

   _____

5. A biopsy can be found under the Main Term Drainage or
   _____.

6. A cholecystectomy is indexed under the Root Operation for
   _____.

7. Cautery of a nose bleed is an example of the Root Operation
   for _____.

8. To find the root operation for a bone marrow biopsy, search for
   the Main Term _____.

9. _____ is the Root Operation for cryotherapy of a wart.

10. A partial discectomy is indexed under the Root Operation for
    _____.

Multiple Choice

Instructions: Circle the letter of the best answer to each question
based on the information you learned in this chapter.

1. How is the principal procedure determined when a diagnostic
   procedure is related to the principal diagnosis and a definitive
   procedure is related to a secondary diagnosis?
   A. Date of procedure
   B. Procedure most related to the principal diagnosis
   C. More extensive procedure
   D. Definitive procedure is always the principal procedure

2. What qualifier is used to report an amputation anywhere along
   the proximal phalanx?
   A. Complete
   B. High
   C. Mid
   D. Low

3. Which of the following is coded to the Root Operation Excision?
   A. Fine-needle aspiration biopsy of the lung
   B. Bone marrow biopsy
   C. Lymph node sampling with biopsy
   D. Endometrial biopsy

4. What should the coder do if the physician documents "partial
   resection of the descending colon"?
   A. Query the physician
   B. Code to root operation Resection, qualifier of partial

C. Code to root operation Extraction
D. Code to root operation Excision

5. Which of the following is a surgical approach?
   A. Open
   B. Subcutaneous
   C. Intravenous
   D. Evacuation

6. What is the anatomic site through which the target site for the
   procedure is reached?
   A. External approach
   B. Method
   C. Access location
   D. Instrumentation

7. Which approach can be used to remove a prostate?
   A. Open
   B. Percutaneous
   C. Via natural opening
   D. All of the above

8. Consult the 0BB Table. Which of these is an incorrect ICD-10-
   PCS code?
   A. 0BB10ZZ
   B. 0BBR7ZZ
   C. 0BBC8ZZ
   D. 0BBN4ZZ

9. What root operation applies to removal of disc fragments?
   A. Excision
   B. Resection
   C. Destruction
   D. Extraction

10. Which character value is the key to distinguishing between the
    Root Operations Excision and Resection?
    A. Approach
    B. Device
    C. Body Part
    D. Qualifier

CODING CHALLENGE

Instructions: Read the mini-medical-record of each patient's encounter, then abstract, assign, and arrange ICD-10-CM diagnosis codes
and PCS procedure codes using the appropriate Index and Tables.
Write the code(s) on the line provided.

---

1. INPATIENT HOSPITAL   Gender: F   Age: 26

Preprocedure diagnosis: menorrhagia

Procedure: endometrial ablation. Uterus sounded to
10 cm and a NovaSure balloon inserted into the
uterine cavity. Full cycle of 8 minutes with pressure of
170 completed. Balloon deflated and withdrawn.

(continued)

---

1. (continued)

Postprocedure diagnosis: menorrhagia

Tip: Ablation is removal of material from the surface of
an object by vaporization, chipping, or other erosive
processes.

1 ICD-10-CM Code _____

1 ICD-10-PCS Code _____

(continued)

(continued from page 1049)

2. INPATIENT HOSPITAL   Gender: M **Age:** 6

Preprocedure diagnosis: multiple warts on the left foot

Procedure: cryotherapy of 2 warts on left great toe and 3 warts on left heel. Using a cotton swab, liquid nitrogen was applied to the warts until a white margin was evident, approximately 60 seconds.

Postprocedure diagnosis: verruca plantaris of left great toe and left heel

Tip: If a body system does not contain a separate body part value for toes, procedures performed on the toes are coded to the body part value for the foot. Assume that this procedure was performed during an inpatient stay for another reason because by itself it would not require an inpatient admission.

1 ICD-10-CM Code _____

1 ICD-10-PCS Code _____

---

3. INPATIENT HOSPITAL   Gender: M **Age:** 18

Preprocedure diagnosis: chronic ethmoidal sinusitis, nasal polyposis

Procedure: endoscopic sinus surgery, bilateral total ethmoidectomy, bilateral ethmoid polypectomy. Sinus endoscopy confirmed gross ethmoidal polypoid disease. The tissue of the anterior ethmoid was very thickened and polypoid.

2 ICD-10-CM Codes _____

4 ICD-10-PCS Codes _____

_____

---

4. INPATIENT HOSPITAL   Gender: F **Age:** 56

Preprocedure diagnosis: submucous leiomyoma of the uterus, postmenopausal bleeding

Procedure: total abdominal hysterectomy and bilateral salpingo-oophorectomy. Upon entering the peritoneal cavity the uterus and bilateral tubes and ovaries were freed and removed from the cavity. Fascia and skin were closed. Patient tolerated the procedure well.

Tip: Three procedure codes are required because of the specificity of body part values. For the tubes and ovaries, there is a code for bilateral.

2 ICD-10-CM Codes _____

3 ICD-10- PCS Codes _____

_____

---

5. INPATIENT HOSPITAL   Gender: M **Age:** 56

Preprocedure diagnosis: squamous cell carcinoma of the supraglottis; 2 pack per day cigarette smoker

Procedure: total laryngectomy; bilateral modified radical neck dissection. A hemi-apron incision was made and a level 2, 3, 4 neck dissection was performed. A partial laryngectomy could not be performed due to invasion of the tumor into the cricoid cartilage.

Postprocedure diagnosis: squamous cell carcinoma of the supraglottis with invasion to the cricoid cartilage; cervical lymphatic metastases

Tip: Follow the instruction at the diagnosis category in the tabular list to identify one of the second diagnosis codes.

4 ICD-10-CM Codes _____

3 ICD-10-PCS Codes _____

_____

---

6. INPATIENT HOSPITAL   Gender: F **Age:** 20

Preprocedure diagnosis: increasing fatigue and lethargy

Procedure: bone marrow biopsy. After making a small incision, an 11-gauge Jamshidi biopsy needle was used to obtain a core bone marrow biopsy sample from the right posterior iliac crest.

Postprocedure diagnosis: acute lymphoblastic leukemia

1 ICD-10-CM Code _____

1 ICD-10-PCS Code _____

---

7. INPATIENT HOSPITAL   Gender: M **Age:** 48

Preprocedure diagnosis: normal-volume azoospermia

Procedure: bilateral testis biopsies. Percutaneous testis biopsy on the left positive for motile sperm. The same procedure was performed on the right testis; however, the biopsy was negative for motile sperm. The patient tolerated the procedure well.

Postprocedure diagnosis: azoospermia

Tip: Assume that this procedure was performed during an inpatient stay for another reason because by itself it would not require an inpatient admission.

1 ICD-10-CM Code _____

1 ICD-10-PCS Code _____

8. INPATIENT HOSPITAL   Gender: F   Age: 17

Preprocedure diagnosis: *hyperhidrosis involving the soles of the feet, hands, and underarms*

Procedure: *bilateral endoscopic thoracic sympathectomy under general anesthesia. After making a small incision under the armpit, the endoscope was inserted. Sympathetic nerves were divided and the instrument withdrawn. No drains left in place.*

Postprocedure diagnosis: *hyperhidrosis involving the soles of the feet, hands, and underarms*

3 ICD-10-CM Codes _____

_____

1 ICD-10-PCS Code _____

9. INPATIENT HOSPITAL   Gender: F   Age: 28

Preprocedure diagnosis: *moderately atypical melanocytic nevus, abdomen*

Procedure: *excision of atypical melanocytic nevus, abdomen, and complex repair approximately 3 cm. A 15 blade was used to excise a specimen through skin and superficial subcutaneous tissue.*

Postprocedure diagnosis: *moderately atypical melanocytic nevus proliferation, abdomen*

Tip: Assume that this procedure was performed during an inpatient stay for another reason because by itself it would not require an inpatient admission.

1 ICD-10-CM Code _____

1 ICD-10-PCS Code _____

10. INPATIENT HOSPITAL   Gender: M   Age: 66

Preprocedure diagnosis: *chronic diabetic ulcer of left midfoot with muscle necrosis*

Procedure: *below-the-knee amputation at the distal portion, left leg. After inflation of the tourniquet, skin incised. The tibia and fibula were divided using an oscillating saw and hand-held bone cutter. An amputation knife was used to complete the amputation. Bleeding controlled with cautery.*

Postprocedure diagnosis: *diabetic ulcer of plantar surface of the left midfoot with muscle necrosis*

Tip: Assume that this procedure was performed during an inpatient stay for another reason because by itself it would not require an inpatient admission.

2 ICD-10-CM Codes _____

1 ICD-10-PCS Code _____

KEEP ON CODING

Instructions: Read the procedural statement, then use the appropriate Index and Tables to assign PCS procedure codes. Write the code(s) on the line provided.

1. Open biopsy of left extraocular muscle: ICD-10-PCS Code(s) _____

2. Laparoscopic excision of the sigmoid colon through the anus and rectum: ICD-10-PCS Code(s) _____

3. Left first toe amputation, complete: ICD-10-PCS Code(s) _____

4. Removal of wart from epidermis using nitrous oxide, right hand: ICD-10-PCS Code(s) _____

5. Diagnostic dilation and curettage (D&C): ICD-10-PCS Code(s) _____

6. Endoscopic polypectomy, right nares: ICD-10-PCS Code(s) _____

7. Right lobe thyroidectomy: ICD-10-PCS Code(s) _____

8. Cataract extraction, right eye: ICD-10-PCS Code(s) _____

9. Amputation of left thumb at the midproximal phalangeal joint: ICD-10-PCS Code(s) _____

(*continued*)

(continued from page 1051)

10. Cystoscopy with fulguration of bladder polyp: ICD-10-PCS Code(s) _____

11. Upper gingivectomy: ICD-10-PCS Code(s) _____

12. Nephrectomy, left kidney: ICD-10-PCS Code(s) _____

13. Bone marrow biopsy, iliac crest: ICD-10-PCS Code(s) _____

14. Complete amputation of little right toe: ICD-10-PCS Code(s) _____

15. Cauterization of skin of right upper leg: ICD-10-PCS Code(s) _____

16. Left breast percutaneous lumpectomy: ICD-10-PCS Code(s) _____

17. Total excision of pituitary gland: ICD-10-PCS Code(s) _____

18. Phacoemulsification of left eye lens without intraocular implant: ICD-10-PCS Code(s) _____

19. Midlevel BKA, right leg: ICD-10-PCS Code(s) _____

20. Percutaneous sialectomy, partial left sublingual gland: ICD-10-PCS Code(s) _____

21. Endoscopic cauterization of esophageal varices: ICD-10-PCS Code(s) _____

22. Splenectomy: ICD-10-PCS Code(s) _____

23. Percutaneous lesser saphenous vein stripping, left leg: ICD-10-PCS Code(s) _____

24. Cryoablation of cervix: ICD-10-PCS Code(s) _____

25. Transmetacarpal amputation of left hand at index finger: ICD-10-PCS Code(s) _____

Section 0: Root Operations Y, M, X, S

Procedures That Put in/Put Back or Move Some/All of a Body Part

Chapter 53

Learning Objectives

After completing this chapter, you should have the skills to:

53.1 Spell and define the key words, medical terms, and abbreviations related to procedures that put in/put back or move some/all of a Body Part.

53.2 Discuss the types of procedures that put in/put back or move some/all of a Body Part.

53.3 Identify the main characteristics of coding for the Root Operations Transplantation, Reattachment, Transfer, and Reposition.

53.4 Abstract procedural information from the medical record for coding for the Root Operations Y, M, X, and S.

53.5 Assign codes for the Root Operations Y, M, X, and S.

53.6 Arrange codes for the Root Operations Y, M, X, and S.

53.7 Discuss the ICD-10-PCS coding guidelines related to Root Operations Y, M, X, and S.

Chapter Outline

- **Basics of Procedures That Put in/Put Back or Move Some/All of a Body Part**
- **Coding Overview of Root Operations Y, M, X, and S**
- **Abstracting for Root Operations Y, M, X, and S**
- **Assigning Characters 4–7 for Root Operations Y, M, X, and S**
- **Arranging Codes for Root Operations Y, M, X, and S**

Key Terms and Abbreviations

avulsed
forequarter
musculocutaneous
United Network for Organ Sharing (UNOS)

In addition to the key terms listed here, students should know the terms defined within tables in this chapter.

INTRODUCTION

Traffic engineers sometimes need to reconfigure an intersection to make traffic flow more smoothly. This might involve reinstalling detached lines or cables to a traffic signal, replacing a malfunctioning traffic signal, or moving an exit ramp to a new location. Surgeons might need to perform similar procedures for malfunctioning body parts.

This chapter discusses the Medical and Surgical Root Operations in the group *Procedures that Put in/Put Back or Move Some/All of a Body Part*: Transplantation, Reattachment, Transfer, and Reposition. Although the Root Operations share a common purpose—putting back or moving some or all of a body part—each has a unique aspect that makes it different from the other procedures in this group. Pay careful attention to the differences between each Root Operation so that you can use each confidently and accurately.

BASICS OF PROCEDURES THAT PUT IN/PUT BACK OR MOVE SOME/ALL OF A BODY PART

Root Operations in the group *Procedures that Put in/Put Back or Move Some/All of a Body Part* includes five Root Operations. ■ TABLE 53-1 provides the definitions of Root Operations in

Table 53-1 ■ ROOT OPERATIONS THAT PUT IN/PUT BACK OR MOVE SOME/ALL OF A BODY PART

Root Operation	Value	Definition	Terms
Transplantation	Y	Putting in or on all or a portion of a living body part taken from another individual or animal to physically take the place and/or function of all or a portion of a similar Body Part	Transplant
Reattachment	M	Putting back in or on all or a portion of a separated Body Part to its normal location or other suitable location	Reattachment, replantation
Transfer	X	Moving, without taking out, all or a portion of a Body Part to another location to take over the function of all or a portion of a Body Part	Transfer, move
Reposition	S	Moving to its normal location, or other suitable location, all or a portion of a Body Part	Reposition, reduction, move, relocate

Table 53-2 ■ EXAMPLE OF CONSTRUCTING MEDICAL TERMS FOR PROCEDURES THAT PUT IN/PUT BACK OR MOVE SOME/ALL OF A BODY PART

Combining Form	Suffix	Complete Medical Term
col/o (*colon*)	-pexy (*surgical fixation*) -plasty (*repair*)	colo + pexy (*surgical fixation of the colon*)
colp/o (*vagina*)		colpo + pexy (*surgical fixation of the vagina*)
choledoch/o (*common bile duct*)		choledocho + plasty (*repair of the common bile duct*)
conjunctiv/o (*conjunctiva*)		conjunctivo + plasty (*repair of the conjunctiva*)

Source: © PB Resources, Inc. Used with permission.

this group and identifies procedural terms frequently associated with each. Some procedural terms, such as transfer or reposition, can be associated with more than one Root Operation. There is not a direct match between a specific procedural term and a Root Operation because some medical terms can be associated with more than one Root Operation. For example, the suffix -*plasty* can be used for several Root Operations, including Repair, Replacement, Reposition, and Supplement. Root Operations are assigned based on the content of the operative report regarding what was actually performed, not on the terms used by the physician in documentation. Refer to ■ TABLE 53-2 for a refresher on how to build medical terms related to procedures that put in/put back or move some/all of a Body Part.

Refer to detailed anatomic diagrams of specific organ systems in Chapters 9 through 48 of this text, or in external references, when you need to refresh your memory of human anatomy.

CODING CAUTION

Be alert for Root Operations that have similar English meanings but different PCS definitions.

Transfer (X) (*Moving, without taking out, all or a portion of a body part <u>to another location to take over the function</u> of all or a portion of a body part*) and **Reposition (S)** (*Moving <u>to its normal location</u>, or other suitable location, all or a portion of a body part*)

Reattachment (M) (*Putting back in or on all or a portion of a <u>separated body part</u> to its normal location or other suitable location*) and **Fusion (G)** (*<u>Joining together portions of an articular body part</u> rendering the articular body part <u>immobile</u>*)

CODING PRACTICE

Exercise 53.1 Basics of Procedures That Put in/Put Back or Move Some/All of a Body Part

Instructions: Use your medical terminology skills and resources to define the following procedures that take out some or all of a body part, then identify the code(s) or code range listed in the ICD-10-PCS Index. Follow these steps:

- Use slash marks "/" to break down each term into its root(s) and suffix.
- Define the meaning of the underlined word based on the meaning of each word part.
- Look up the term in the ICD-10-PCS Index, and write down the name(s) of Root Operation(s) the Index cross-references you to and the Table(s), if provided.
- Do not assign any codes.

Example: <u>pneumonopexy</u>

pneumono/pexy   Meaning *fixation of the lung*   PCS Root Operation(s)/Table(s) *Repair OBQ Reposition OBS*

1. <u>arthropexy</u>   Meaning _____   PCS Root Operation(s)/Table(s) _____

2. <u>transposition</u>   Meaning _____   PCS Root Operation(s)/Table(s) _____

3. <u>patellapexy</u>   Meaning _____   PCS Root Operation(s)/Table(s) _____

4. <u>blepharoplasty</u>   Meaning _____   PCS Root Operation(s)/Table(s) _____

5. <u>reimplantation</u>   Meaning _____   PCS Root Operation(s)/Table(s) _____

6. <u>ileopexy</u>   Meaning _____   PCS Root Operation(s)/Table(s) _____

7. <u>cecopexy</u>   Meaning _____   PCS Root Operation(s)/Table(s) _____

8. <u>autotransplant</u>   Meaning _____   PCS Root Operation(s)/Table(s) _____

9. <u>detorsion</u>   Meaning _____   PCS Root Operation(s)/Table(s) _____

10. pedicled <u>TRAM</u> (transverse rectus abdominis <u>myocutaneous</u>) flap reconstruction   Meaning _____   PCS Root Operation(s)/Table(s) _____

CODING OVERVIEW OF ROOT OPERATIONS Y, M, X, AND S

Root Operations in this group involve putting in, putting back, or moving some or all of a Body Part. These procedures do not include repair or removal of a Body Part.

Guidelines specific to the Root Operations Y, M, X, and S include the following. Refer to the PCS OGCR for clinical examples of each guideline.

- Reposition for fracture treatment—Reduction of a displaced fracture is coded to the root operation Reposition (S) (PCS OGCR B3.15). The application of a cast or splint in conjunction with the Reposition procedure is not coded separately. For example, reduction and casting of a displaced fracture is coded to the Root Operation Reposition. Treatment of a nondisplaced fracture is coded to the procedure performed. For example, casting of a nondisplaced fracture is coded to the Root Operation Immobilization (3) in the Placement (2) Section.

- Transplantation vs. Administration—The Root Operation Transplantation (Y) is putting in a mature and functioning living body part taken from another individual or animal (PCS OGCR 3.16), such as transplantation of a kidney or lung. Root Operations in the Administration (3) Section report putting in autologous or nonautologous cells. For example, putting in autologous or nonautologous bone marrow, pancreatic islet cells, or stem cells is coded to the Root Operation Transfusion (2). Procedures in the Administration Section are discussed in Chapter 57 of this text.

- Devices—A device is coded only if a device remains after the procedure is completed. If no device remains, the device value No Device is coded (PCS OGCR B6.1a). The Root Operation Reposition uses Character 6, Device, to identify the type of internal or external fixation devices left in place. Assigning values for the Device is discussed later in this chapter.

ABSTRACTING FOR ROOT OPERATIONS Y, M, X, AND S

The Root Operation definition is a combination of the functional objective of the procedure and the anatomic site. The following information summarizes the objectives, definitions, unique features, and examples of Root Operations Y, M, X, and S.

Abstracting for Transplantation (Y)

The objective of the Root Operation Transplantation is putting in a living body part from a person or animal. The site of the procedure is some or all of a Body Part. The Body Part can be an organ, part of an organ, or tissue.

Transplantation includes a small number of procedures because a limited number of organs can be transplanted. The Root Operation includes only the procedure on the Body Part(s) being transplanted. The native organ may or may not be taken out, and the transplanted organ may take over all or a portion of its function. Harvesting of the donor organ and any other procedures necessary to complete the transplant, such as cardiopulmonary bypass, are coded separately.

Examples of Transplantation are a kidney transplant and heart transplant (■ TABLE 53-3).

The **United Network for Organ Sharing (UNOS)** is a nonprofit organization that administers the United States' Organ Procurement and Transplantation Network, including the organ transplant waiting list. UNOS deals with six major organs: the heart, kidney, lung, pancreas, liver, and intestine. The kidney is the most commonly transplanted single organ, and the least common is the intestine. A double transplant is the transplantation of two related organs, such as the heart and lung or kidney and pancreas.

CODING CAUTION

Bone marrow transplant procedures are coded with the Root Operation Transfusion (3), which is part of PCS Section 3, Administration.

Table 53-3 ■ EXAMPLES OF THE ROOT OPERATION TRANSPLANTATION (Y)

Organ System	Procedural Examples
Cardiovascular	Heart transplant
Digestive	Stomach, esophagus, intestine transplant
Endocrine	Thymus, spleen transplant
Genitourinary	Kidney, ovary transplant
Hepatobiliary	Liver, pancreas transplant
Respiratory	Lung transplant
Special Senses (Ear, Eye)	Cornea transplant

Source: © PB Resources, Inc. Used with permission.

Table 53-4 ■ EXAMPLES OF THE ROOT OPERATION REATTACHMENT (M)

Organ System	Procedural Examples
Digestive	Replantation of avulsed teeth, tongue, lip, intestine
Endocrine	Reattachment of thyroid, parathyroid, or adrenal gland(s)
Genitourinary	Reattachment of severed testes, kidney, ureter, bladder, ovary, vulva
Hepatobiliary	Replantation of liver or pancreas
Integumentary	Replantation of avulsed scalp, skin from any location, or breast
Musculoskeletal	Reattachment of muscle, tendon, or ligament avulsion; reattachment of severed extremity
Respiratory	Replantation of lung, bronchus, or trachea
Special Senses (Ear, Eye)	Reattachment of severed ear or eyelid

Source: © PB Resources, Inc. Used with permission.

Abstracting for Reattachment (M)

The objective of the Root Operation Reattachment is putting back a detached Body Part. The site of the procedure is some or all of a Body Part.

Procedures coded to Reattachment include putting back a body part that has been cut off or **avulsed** (*ripped or torn away*). Nerves and blood vessels may or may not be reconnected in a Reattachment procedure, and such reconnection is not coded separately.

Examples of Reattachment are reattachment of the hand and reattachment of an avulsed kidney (■ TABLE 53-4).

Abstracting for Transfer (X)

The objective of the Root Operation Transfer is moving a Body Part to function for a similar Body Part. The site of the procedure is some or all of a Body Part.

The body part transferred remains connected to its vascular and nervous supply. The Root Operation Transfer is used to identify procedures where a body part is moved to another location without disrupting its vascular and nervous supply. In the Body Systems that classify the subcutaneous tissue, fascia, and muscle Body Parts, Character 7, Qualifier, can be used to specify when more than one tissue layer was used in the transfer procedure, such as a **musculocutaneous** (*pertaining to both muscles and skin*) flap transfer.

Examples of Transfer are a tendon transfer and skin pedicle flap transfer (■ TABLE 53-5).

Abstracting for Reposition (S)

The objective of the Root Operation Reposition is moving a Body Part to its normal or another suitable location. The site of the procedure is some or all of a Body Part.

Table 53-5 ■ EXAMPLES OF THE ROOT OPERATION TRANSFER (X)

Organ System	Procedural Examples
Digestive	Lip, gingiva, stomach, small or large intestine
Integumentary	Skin flap
Musculoskeletal	Muscle, tendon, or ligament transfer
Nervous	Nerve transfer
Special Senses (Ear, Eye)	Extraocular muscle transfer

Source: © PB Resources, Inc. Used with permission.

The body part is moved to a new location from an abnormal location to its normal location or from a normal location where it is not functioning correctly to a new location to enhance its ability to function. The body part may or may not be cut out or off to be moved to the new location.

Examples of Reposition are the reposition of an undescended testicle and fracture reduction (■ TABLE 53-6).

Key Criteria for Abstracting

Refer to Table 51-1 for general guidance on abstracting PCS procedures and Root Operation groups. Then refer to ■ TABLE 53-7 for more specific guidance on how to abstract procedures that Put in/Put Back or Move Some/All of a Body Part and distinguish among Root Operations in this group. A guided example

Table 53-6 ■ EXAMPLES OF THE ROOT OPERATION REPOSITION (S)

Organ System	Procedural Examples
Blood and Immune	Reposition of thymus or spleen
Cardiovascular	Reposition of thoracic aorta, pulmonary artery, pulmonary vein, or peripheral arteries or veins
Digestive	Gastropexy for malrotation; reposition of a portion of the large or small intestine
Endocrine	Reposition of thyroid, parathyroid, or adrenal glands
Genitourinary	Orchiopexy; reposition of kidney, ureter, bladder, or urethra, ovary, uterus, vagina
Hepatobiliary	Reposition of the liver, gallbladder, pancreas, or related duct(s)
Integumentary	Reposition of hair, breast, or nipple
Musculoskeletal	Reposition of muscle, tendon, ligament, or bone; fracture reduction (open or closed, with or without fixation device)
Nervous	Transposition of nerve
Respiratory	Reposition of bronchus, lung, diaphragm
Special Senses (Ear, Eye)	Reposition of ocular muscles, vessels, or eyelid; reposition of external ear, nose, nasal septum, tympanic membrane

Source: © PB Resources, Inc. Used with permission.

of abstracting for the Root Operation Reposition follows. Remember that the abstracting questions are a guide and that not every question applies to, or can be answered for, every case.

Guided Example of Abstracting for Reposition

Refer to the following example throughout this chapter to practice skills for abstracting, assigning, and arranging codes for the Root Operation Reposition. Similar principles apply to working with other Root Operations that put in/put back or move some/all of a Body Part.

INPATIENT HOSPITAL   Gender: F   Age: 23

Preoperative diagnosis: fractured R tibia and R humerus

Procedure: Open reduction, R tibia, with internal fixation device. Closed reduction, R humerus, percutaneous external fixation using a monoplanar device.

Preoperative diagnosis: displaced fracture R tibia, displaced fracture R humerus shaft

---

Table 53-7 ■ KEY CRITERIA FOR ABSTRACTING ROOT OPERATIONS THAT PUT IN/PUT BACK OR MOVE SOME/ALL OF A BODY PART

Question	Root Operation (Value)
❏ Was a body part reattached, replaced, or moved?	
❏ Was a body part replaced with a human or animal substitute?	
❏ Was a body part replaced with a synthetic substitute?	Do not use root operations Y, M, X, or S.
Answer *Yes* to one of the following questions to help distinguish Root Operations Y, M, X, and S:	
❏ Was an organ or part of an organ replaced (transplanted) with a human or animal substitute?	Transplantation (Y)
❏ Was a severed or avulsed body part or extremity reattached?	Reattachment (M)
❏ Was a body part moved, without disrupting its nervous or blood supply, to serve a similar function in a new location?	Transfer (M)
❏ Was a body part moved to a new location from an abnormal location to improve its function, with or without detaching it?	Reposition (S)
❏ Was a body part moved to a new location from its normal location where it was not functioning properly to improve its function, with or without detaching it?	

Source: © PB Resources, Inc. Used with permission.

Follow along as fictitious coder, Marcy Elwood, CCS, abstracts the procedure. Check off each step after you complete it.

▶ Marcy reads through the entire record, paying special attention to the reason for the encounter, the procedure performed, and the postoperative diagnosis. She refers to the Key Criteria for Abstracting (Table 53-7).

❑ She notes preoperative diagnosis: displaced fracture R tibia and R humerus.

❑ *What are the stated procedures?* reduction of two fractures

❑ *What organ or body part(s) is involved?* R tibia, R humerus

❑ *Is the procedure description what you would expect based on the name of the procedure?* yes

❑ *What surgical approach is used for the first procedure (right tibia)?* Open

❑ *Was more than one procedure, or a combined procedure, performed?* Yes, internal fixation was used.

❑ *What surgical approach is used for the second procedure (right humerus)?* Closed

❑ *Was more than one procedure, or a combined procedure, performed?* Yes, external fixation was used.

❑ *Did the procedure put in/put back or move some/all of a body part?* Yes

❑ *Was a body part reattached, replaced, or moved?* Yes, both body parts were moved.

❑ *Was a body part replaced with a human or animal substitute?* No

❑ *Was a body part replaced with a synthetic substitute?* No

❑ *Was an organ or part of an organ replaced with a human or animal substitute?* No

❑ *Was a severed or avulsed body part or extremity reattached?* No

❑ *Was a body part moved, without disrupting its nervous or blood supply, to serve a similar function in a new location?* No

❑ *Was a body part moved to a new location from an abnormal location to improve its function, with or without detaching it?* No

❑ *Was a body part moved to a new location from its normal location where it was not functioning properly to improve its function, with or without detaching it?* Yes

▶ At this time, Marcy believes that she will use the Root Operation Reposition (PCS OGCR B3.15). She anticipates that she will need two codes because the same Root Operation was performed on two distinct sites (PCS OGCR B3.2a). She will verify this information when she refers to the PCS Tables to assign codes.

CODING PRACTICE

Exercise 53.2 Abstracting for Root Operations Y, M, X, and S

Instructions: Read the mini-medical-record of each patient's encounter and answer the abstracting questions. Write the answer on the line provided. Do not assign any codes.

1. INPATIENT HOSPITAL   Gender: M
Age: 15 months

Preprocedure diagnosis: undescended testicles in inguinal canal

Procedure: orchiopexy; an inguinal incision was made in the left groin and carried through the subcutaneous tissues to the anterior fascia. The fascia was opened, exposing the testicle, which lay high in the canal. The testicle was located in a superficial pouch of the inguinal canal and there was adequate length on the spermatic cord to reposition it without problem. The testicle was freed with dissection and moved to its normal location. Procedure was repeated on right side.

(continued)

1. (continued)

Patient tolerated procedure well. No other abnormalities were found.

Postprocedure diagnosis: bilateral undescended testicles

a. What is the stated procedure? _____

b. What organ or body part is involved? _____

c. What is the laterality? _____

d. Is the procedure description what you would expect based on the name of the procedure? _____

e. What surgical approach is used? _____

f. Was more than one procedure, or a combined procedure, performed? _____

g. Was a body part reattached, replaced, or moved?

_____

h. Was a body part replaced with a human or animal substitute? _____

i. Was a body part replaced with a synthetic substitute?

_____

(continued)

1. (continued)

j. Was an organ or part of an organ replaced (transplanted) with a human or animal substitute? _____

k. Was a severed or avulsed body part or extremity reattached? _____

l. Was a body part moved, without disrupting its nervous or blood supply, to serve a similar function in a new location? _____

m. Was a body part moved to a new location from an abnormal location to improve its function, with or without detaching it? _____

n. Was a body part moved to a new location from its normal location where it was not functioning properly to improve its function, with or without detaching it? _____

o. What is the root operation? _____

2. INPATIENT HOSPITAL   Gender: F   Age: 52

Preprocedure diagnosis: hyperparathyroidism

Procedure: parathyroid autotransplantation; endoscopic transthoracic parathyroidectomy ×4 with mediastinal exploration and parathyroid autotransplantation to left forearm

a. What is the stated procedure? _____

b. What organ or body part is involved? _____

c. What is the laterality? _____

d. Is the procedure description what you would expect based on the name of the procedure? _____

e. What surgical approach is used? _____

f. Was more than one procedure, or a combined procedure, performed? _____

g. Was a body part reattached, replaced, or moved? _____

h. Was a body part replaced with a human or animal substitute? _____

i. Was a body part replaced with a synthetic substitute? _____

j. Was an organ or part of an organ replaced (transplanted) with a human or animal substitute? _____

k. Was a severed or avulsed body part or extremity reattached? _____

l. Was a body part moved, without disrupting its nervous or blood supply, to serve a similar function in a new location? _____

(continued)

2. (continued)

m. Was a body part moved to a new location from an abnormal location to improve its function, with or without detaching it? _____

n. Was a body part moved to a new location from its normal location where it was not functioning properly to improve its function, with or without detaching it? _____

o. What is the root operation? _____

3. INPATIENT HOSPITAL   Gender: F   Age: 23

Preprocedure diagnosis: fractured R ulna

Procedure: open reduction, R ulna with clamp and rod internal fixation (CRIF)

a. What is the stated procedure? _____

b. What organ or body part is involved? _____

c. What is the laterality? _____

d. Is the procedure description what you would expect based on the name of the procedure? _____

e. What surgical approach is used? _____

f. Was more than one procedure, or a combined procedure, performed? _____

g. Was a body part reattached, replaced, or moved? _____

h. Was a body part replaced with a human or animal substitute? _____

i. Was a body part replaced with a synthetic substitute? _____

j. Was an organ or part of an organ replaced (transplanted) with a human or animal substitute? _____

k. Was a severed or avulsed body part or extremity reattached? _____

l. Was a body part moved, without disrupting its nervous or blood supply, to serve a similar function in a new location? _____

m. Was a body part moved to a new location from an abnormal location to improve its function, with or without detaching it? _____

n. Was a body part moved to a new location from its normal location where it was not functioning properly to improve its function, with or without detaching it? _____

o. What is the root operation? _____

(continued)

4. INPATIENT HOSPITAL   Gender: M   Age: 27

Preprocedure diagnosis: traumatic amputation of distal segment of little finger and two segments of the ring finger on left hand while using a table saw in home workshop

Procedure: replantation of distal segments of the little finger and ring finger on the left hand

a. What is the stated procedure? _____

b. What organ or body part is involved? _____

c. What is the laterality? _____

d. Is the procedure description what you would expect based on the name of the procedure? _____

e. What surgical approach is used? _____

f. Was more than one procedure, or a combined procedure, performed? _____

g. Was a body part reattached, replaced, or moved? _____

h. Was a body part replaced with a human or animal substitute? _____

i. Was a body part replaced with a synthetic substitute? _____

j. Was an organ or part of an organ replaced (transplanted) with a human or animal substitute? _____

k. Was a severed or avulsed body part or extremity reattached? _____

l. Was a body part moved, without disrupting its nervous or blood supply, to serve a similar function in a new location? _____

m. Was a body part moved to a new location from an abnormal location to improve its function, with or without detaching it? _____

n. Was a body part moved to a new location from its normal location where it was not functioning properly to improve its function, with or without detaching it? _____

o. What is the root operation? _____

5. INPATIENT HOSPITAL   Gender: F   Age: 36

Preprocedure diagnosis: type 1 diabetes mellitus, unresponsive to treatment

Procedure: Simultaneous kidney–pancreas transplantation. The donor kidney came from the patient's sister. The donor pancreas came from a cadaver. Patient's left kidney was removed and replaced.

a. What is the stated procedure? _____

b. What organ or body part is involved? _____

c. What is the laterality? _____

d. Is the procedure description what you would expect based on the name of the procedure? _____

e. What surgical approach is used? _____

f. Was more than one procedure, or a combined procedure, performed? _____

g. Was a body part reattached, replaced, or moved? _____

h. Was a body part replaced with a human or animal substitute? _____

i. Was a body part replaced with a synthetic substitute? _____

j. Was an organ or part of an organ replaced (transplanted) with a human or animal substitute? _____

k. Was a severed or avulsed body part or extremity reattached? _____

l. Was a body part moved, without disrupting its nervous or blood supply, to serve a similar function in a new location? _____

m. Was a body part moved to a new location from an abnormal location to improve its function, with or without detaching it? _____

n. Was a body part moved to a new location from its normal location where it was not functioning properly to improve its function, with or without detaching it? _____

o. What is the root operation? _____

6. INPATIENT HOSPITAL   Gender: F   Age: 43

Preprocedure diagnosis: low radial nerve palsy, right arm

Procedure: Tendon transfer, open. Rerouted the belly and insertion point of palmaris longus tendon to the extensor pollicis longus (EPL) muscle, leaving the blood and nerve supply intact. Rerouted belly and insertion point of the pronator teres tendon to the abductor pollicis longus (APL) muscle, leaving the blood and nerve supply intact.

a. What is the stated procedure? _____

b. What organ or body part is involved?

_____

c. What is the laterality? _____

d. Is the procedure description what you would expect based on the name of the procedure?

_____

e. What surgical approach is used? _____

f. Was more than one procedure, or a combined procedure, performed? _____

g. Was a body part reattached, replaced, or moved?

_____

(*continued*)

6. (continued)

h. Was a body part replaced with a human or animal substitute? _____

i. Was a body part replaced with a synthetic substitute?

_____

j. Was an organ or part of an organ replaced (transplanted) with a human or animal substitute?

_____

k. Was a severed or avulsed body part or extremity reattached? _____

l. Was a body part moved, without disrupting its nervous or blood supply, to serve a similar function in a new location? _____

m. Was a body part moved to a new location from an abnormal location to improve its function, with or without detaching it? _____

n. Was a body part moved to a new location from its normal location where it was not functioning properly to improve its function, with or without detaching it?

_____

o. What is the root operation? _____

ASSIGNING CHARACTERS 4–7 FOR ROOT OPERATIONS Y, M, X, AND S

To assign codes after the Root Operation is determined, search the PCS Index for the name of the Root Operation as the Main Term. Locate the subterm(s) for the correct anatomic site and identify the PCS Table. When you locate the PCS Table, verify the first three characters of the code, then locate the row with the Body Part needed. Assign the remaining characters from each respective column of the Table. The following information summarizes and highlights unique information for working with the Tables for each Root Operation Y, M, X, and S. Each Root Operation has one Table in each applicable PCS Body System. Because of the differences between organ systems, Table details vary.

Character 4: Body Part

The Body Part identifies the anatomic site treated in the Root Operation, such as the organ transplanted and the structure reattached, transferred, or repositioned. Use the most specific Body Part value provided in the Table being used. For example, in Table 0BY, Respiratory System Transplantation, select the most specific part of the lung applicable. When only one lobe of the lung is transplanted, select the Body Part value for the appropriate lobe. When the entire lung is transplanted, assign **K Lung, Right** or **L Lung, Left**. When both lungs are transplanted, assign **M Lungs, Bilateral**.

For the Root Operations Transfer and Reposition, identify the site that is moved, not the location to which it is moved.

Reattachment of the extremities is reported with the Body System Anatomical Regions, not Upper Bones or Lower Bones, because the entire limb, not just the bone(s), is reattached. The Body Part values identify various segments and the laterality of each extremity (■ TABLE 53-8).

SUCCESS STEP

The Body Part **forequarter** refers to the extremity and all or part of the adjoining structure, such as the arm, shoulder joint, and all or part of the scapula and clavicle or the leg, hip joint, and all or part of the pelvic girdle.

Character 5: Approach

The Approach for Transplantation is always Open. The Approach for Reattachment is Open, Percutaneous Endoscopic, or External. Reattachment, Transfer, and Reposition procedures for the Skin and Breast always use the Approach External.

Character 6: Device

The Root Operation Reposition uses Device to identify the type of internal or external skeletal fixation device applied

Table 53-8 ■ CHARACTER 4, BODY PART VALUES FOR TABLE 0XM: BODY SYSTEM ANATOMICAL REGIONS, UPPER EXTREMITIES (X) AND ROOT OPERATION REATTACHMENT (M)

Value	Body Part
0	Forequarter, Right
1	Forequarter, Left
2	Shoulder Region, Right
3	Shoulder Region, Left
4	Axilla, Right
5	Axilla, Left
6	Upper Extremity, Right
7	Upper Extremity, Left
8	Upper Arm, Right
9	Upper Arm, Left
B	Elbow Region, Right
C	Elbow Region, Left
D	Lower Arm, Right
F	Lower Arm, Left
G	Wrist Region, Right
H	Wrist Region, Left
J	Hand, Right
K	Hand, Left
L	Thumb, Right
M	Thumb, Left
N	Index Finger, Right
P	Index Finger, Left
Q	Middle Finger, Right
R	Middle Finger, Left
S	Ring Finger, Right
T	Ring Finger, Left
V	Little Finger, Right
W	Little Finger, Left

Table 53-9 ■ TYPES OF SKELETAL FIXATION DEVICES

External Fixation Devices

Delta frame external fixator

Ilizarov external fixator

Monoplanar (uniplanar) external fixator

Sheffield hybrid external fixator

Sheffield ring external fixator

Internal Fixation Devices

Bone screw (interlocking, lag, pedicle, recessed)

Clamp and rod internal fixation system (CRIF)

Fusion screw (compression, lag, locking)

Intramedullary (IM) rod (nail)

Intramedullary skeletal kinetic distractor (ISKD)

Joint fixation plate

Kirschner wire (K-wire)

Kuntscher nail

Neutralization plate

Titanium sternal fixation system (TSFS)

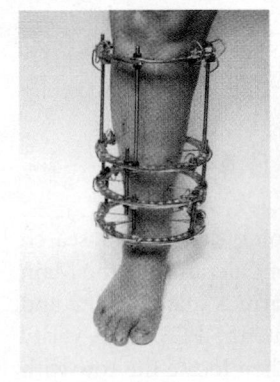
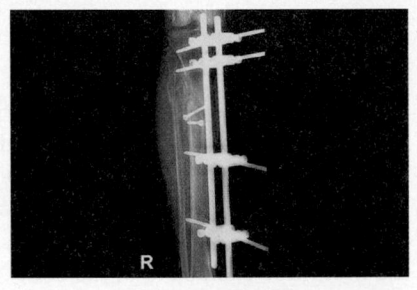
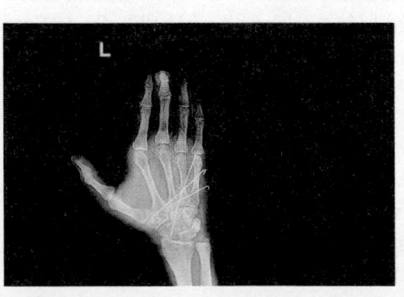
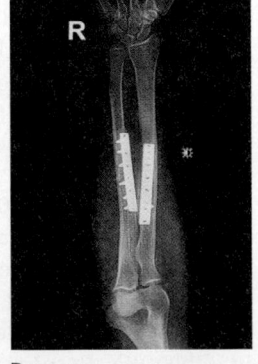

A B

C D

Figure 53-1 ■ Images of Fixation Devices. (A) Ilizarov Ring External Fixation (*Source: Shutterstock © sima*); (B) Monoplanar External Fixation (*Source: Shutterstock © Praisaeng*); (C) Kirschner Wire (K-Wire) External Fixation (*Source: Shutterstock © Praisaeng*); (D) Plate and Screw Internal Fixation (*Source: Shutterstock © Praisaeng*).

(■ TABLE 53-9 and ■ FIGURE 53-1). PCS provides specific values for fixation devices based on the Body Systems and Body Part because not all fixation devices are used on all anatomic sites (■ FIGURE 53-2). The type of fixation is documented in the operative report, so the coder must identify the specific device used and convert it to the appropriate PCS value. If the correct PCS value is not immediately obvious, refer to the Device Key Appendix in the ICD-10-PCS manual, which provides a crosswalk between the specific device and the PCS value (■ FIGURE 53-3).

Section	0	Medical and Surgical
Body System	P	Upper Bones
Operation	S	Reposition: Moving to its normal location, or other suitable location, all or a portion of a body part

Body Part Character 4	Approach Character 5	Device Character 6	Qualifier Character 7
C Humeral Head, Right D Humeral Head, Left F Humeral Shaft, Right G Humeral Shaft, Left H Radius, Right J Radius, Left K Ulna, Right L Ulna, Left	0 Open 3 Percutaneous 4 Percutaneous Endoscopic	4 Internal Fixation Device 5 External Fixation Device 6 Internal Fixation Device, Intramedullary B External Fixation Device, Monoplanar C External Fixation Device, Ring D External Fixation Device, Hybrid Z No Device	Z No Qualifier

Figure 53-2 ■ Example of Character 6 Device Values for Skeletal Fixation Devices

Joint fixation plate	Use: Internal Fixation Device in Upper Joints Internal Fixation Device in Lower Joints
Kirschner wire (K-wire)	Use: Internal Fixation Device in Head and Facial Bones Internal Fixation Device in Upper Bones Internal Fixation Device in Lower Bones Internal Fixation Device in Upper Joints Internal Fixation Device in Lower Joints

Figure 53-3 ■ Example of the PCS Device Key Appendix

Fixation devices are used with the following Body Systems:

- Mouth and Throat (C)
- Head and Facial Bones (N)
- Upper Bones (P)
- Lower Bones (Q)
- Upper Joints (R)
- Lower Joints (S)

The Root Operations Transfer, Reattachment, Transplantation always have a value of **Z No Device**.

Character 7: Qualifier

Character 7, Qualifier, is used for a variety of purposes for the Root Operations in this group. The use depends on the specific Root Operation.

Transplantation

For the Root Operation Transplantation, Qualifier values specify the genetic compatibility of the body part transplanted:

- 0 Allogeneic
- 1 Syngeneic
- 2 Zooplastic

Transfer

For the Root Operation Transfer, the Qualifier provides additional details about the procedure. For procedures involving transfer of tissue layers such as skin, fascia, and muscle, the Body System value identifies the deepest tissue layer in the flap. The Qualifier identifies the other tissue layers being transferred when the tissue transferred is composed of more than one tissue

---

> Surgeon performed an open fasciocutaneous flap closure of left thigh.

0JXM0ZC Medical and Surgical, Subcutaneous tissue and fascia, Transfer, Subcutaneous tissue and fascia left upper leg, Open, No device, Skin subcutaneous tissue and fascia

Figure 53-4 ■ Example of Coding a Tissue Flap Transfer. *Source: © PB Resources, Inc. Used with permission.*

layer (■ FIGURE 53-4). When only one tissue layer is transferred, assign **Z No qualifier**.

For Transfer procedures classified to other body systems, such as peripheral nervous system, the Body Part value specifies the body part that is the source of the transfer (*from*). The Qualifier specifies the destination of the transfer (*to*) (■ FIGURE 53-5).

Reposition and Reattachment

For the Root Operations Reposition and Reattachment and the Body System **C Mouth and Throat**, the Qualifier identifies the number of teeth being repositioned or reattached. Refer to PCS Table 0CS.

Guided Example of Assigning Characters 4–7 for Reposition

To practice skills for assigning codes for the Root Operation Reposition, continue with the example from earlier in the chapter about a patient who was seen for fracture reduction and fixation. Follow along in your ICD-10-PCS manual as Marcy Elwood, CCS, assigns codes. Check off each step after you complete it.

> Surgeon performed a percutaneous endoscopic transfer of the trigeminal nerve to the facial nerve.

00XK4ZM Medical and Surgical, Central nervous system, Transfer, Trigeminal nerve, Percutaneous endoscopic, No device, Facial nerve

Figure 53-5 ■ Example of Coding a Nerve Transfer. *Source: © PB Resources, Inc. Used with permission.*

▶ First, Marcy confirms the procedures.

❑ The Root Operation for the first procedure, open reduction of the right tibia, is Reposition.

❑ The Root Operation for the second procedure, closed reduction of the right humerus, is Reposition.

▶ Marcy searches the Index for the Main Term **Reposition**.

❑ She locates the first-level subterm **Tibia**.

❑ She locates the second-level subterm **Right**.

❑ She identifies the Table **0QS** for reduction of the right tibia.

▶ Under the same Main Term for **Reposition** she searches for the entry for the humerus. She notices there are two subterms: **Humeral head** and **Humeral shaft**. She refers to the documentation to confirm the site as R humerus shaft.

❑ She locates the second-level subterm **Humeral shaft** and the third-level subterm **Right**.

❑ She identifies the Table **0PS** for reduction of the right humerus.

▶ Marcy turns to Table **0QS** to assign the code for reduction of the right tibia.

❑ She reads the Table title **0QS, Medical and Surgical, Lower Bones, Reposition** and confirms that this accurately describes the Body System and Root Operation.

▶ Marcy assigns the value for Character 4, Body Part.

❑ She notices that Table **0QS** contains several rows and searches for the one that contains the tibia.

❑ She locates tibia and notices there are two rows that contain a value for the tibia. She reads the entire row and identifies that one row provides multiple options for Character 5, Approach, and Character 6, Device.

The other row provides only one option, **X External**, for Character 5, Approach, and only one option, **Z No device**, for Character 6, Device. Because a fixation device was used, she selects the row that provides multiple options for Character 6, Device.

❑ She returns to the column for Character 4, Body Part, and selects **G Tibia, Right**. This value is consistent with the partial code 0QSG provided in the Index.

▶ Marcy assigns the value for Character 5, Approach.

❑ She refers to the documentation and confirms the approach is open reduction.

❑ She selects **0 Open** for the Approach value.

▶ Marcy assigns the value for Character 6, Device.

❑ She refers to the documentation and confirms the device is internal fixation.

❑ She selects **4 Internal Fixation Device** for the Device value.

▶ Marcy assigns the value for Character 7, Qualifier.

❑ The Table provides only one option, **Z No qualifier**.

▶ She reviews the code she has assigned for the open reduction, R tibia with internal fixation device: **0QSG04Z** (■ Figure 53-6).

▶ Marcy turns to Table **0PS** to assign the code for reduction of the right humerus.

❑ She reads the Table title **0PS, Medical and Surgical, Lower Bones, Reposition** and confirms that this accurately describes the Body System and Root Operation for reduction of the humerus.

▶ Marcy assigns the value for Character 4, Body Part.

❑ She locates the row of the table that contains Body Part values for the humerus.

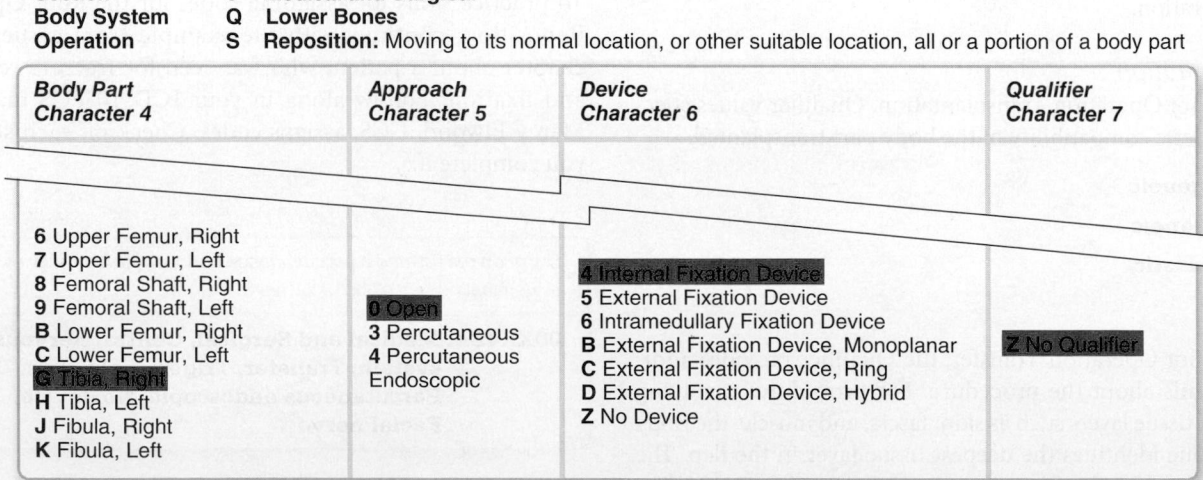

Section	0	Medical and Surgical
Body System	Q	Lower Bones
Operation	S	Reposition: Moving to its normal location, or other suitable location, all or a portion of a body part

Body Part Character 4	Approach Character 5	Device Character 6	Qualifier Character 7
6 Upper Femur, Right 7 Upper Femur, Left 8 Femoral Shaft, Right 9 Femoral Shaft, Left B Lower Femur, Right C Lower Femur, Left **G Tibia, Right** H Tibia, Left J Fibula, Right K Fibula, Left	**0 Open** 3 Percutaneous 4 Percutaneous Endoscopic	**4 Internal Fixation Device** 5 External Fixation Device 6 Intramedullary Fixation Device B External Fixation Device, Monoplanar C External Fixation Device, Ring D External Fixation Device, Hybrid Z No Device	**Z No Qualifier**

Figure 53-6 ■ Assigning Code 0QSG04Z. *Source: Annotation © PB Resources, Inc. Used with permission.*

Section 0 Medical and Surgical
Body System P Upper Bones
Operation S Reposition: Moving to its normal location, or other suitable location, all or a portion of a body part

Body Part Character 4	Approach Character 5	Device Character 6	Qualifier Character 7
C Humeral Head, Right D Humeral Head, Left F Humeral Shaft, Right G Humeral Shaft, Left H Radius, Right J Radius, Left K Ulna, Right L Ulna, Left	0 Open 3 Percutaneous 4 Percutaneous Endoscopic	4 Internal Fixation Device 5 External Fixation Device 6 Internal Fixation Device, Intramedullary B External Fixation Device, Monoplanar C External Fixation Device, Ring D External Fixation Device, Hybrid Z No Device	Z No Qualifier

Figure 53-7 ■ Assigning Code 0PSF3BZ. *Source: Annotation © PB Resources, Inc. Used with permission.*

❑ She notices that she must select either **Humeral head** or **Humeral shaft**, so she refers to the documentation and confirms that the humeral shaft was involved.

❑ She also must select laterality and identifies Body Part value **F Humeral shaft, right**.

▶ Marcy assigns the value for Character 5, Approach.

❑ She refers to the documentation and confirms the approach is *closed reduction, percutaneous external fixation*.

❑ She selects **3 Percutaneous** for the Approach value.

▶ Marcy assigns the value for Character 6, Device.

❑ She notices that there are several options for an external fixation device. She refers to the documentation to confirm that the type of device is *monoplanar*.

❑ She assigns **B External Fixation Device, Monoplanar**.

▶ Marcy assigns the value for Character 7, Qualifier.

❑ She assigns the only choice, **Z No Qualifier**.

▶ Marcy reviews the code she assigned for *closed reduction, R humerus, percutaneous external fixation using a monoplanar device*: **0PSF3BZ** (■ FIGURE 53-7).

▶ Marcy reviews the procedure codes she has assigned for this case.

❑ **0QSG04Z Reposition, Lower Bones, Tibia Right, Open, Internal Fixation Device, No Qualifier**

❑ **0PSF3BZ Reposition, Upper Bones, Humeral Shaft Right, Percutaneous, External Fixation Device, Monoplanar, No Qualifier**

▶ Next, Marcy must determine how to sequence the codes.

CODING PRACTICE

Exercise 53.3 Assigning Characters 4–7 for Root Operations Y, M, X, and S

Instructions: Read the mini-medical-record of each patient's encounter. Review the information abstracted in Exercise 53.2 for questions 1–3. For questions 4–6, abstract the case on your own. Assign PCS codes using the Index and Tables. Write the code(s) on the line provided.

1. INPATIENT HOSPITAL   Gender: M   Age: 15 months

Preprocedure diagnosis: *undescended testicles in inguinal canal*

Procedure: *orchiopexy; an inguinal incision was made in the left groin and carried through the subcutaneous*

(continued)

1. (continued)

tissues to the anterior fascia. The fascia was opened, exposing the testicle, which lay high in the canal. The testicle was located in a superficial pouch of the inguinal canal and there was adequate length on the spermatic cord to reposition it without problem. The testicle was freed with dissection and moved to its normal location. Procedure was repeated on right side. Patient tolerated procedure well. No other abnormalities were found.

Postprocedure diagnosis: *bilateral undescended testicles*

1 PCS Code _____

(continued)

2. INPATIENT HOSPITAL　Gender: F　Age: 52

Preprocedure diagnosis: hyperparathyroidism

Procedure: parathyroid autotransplantation; endoscopic transthoracic parathyroidectomy x4 with mediastinal exploration and parathyroid autotransplantation to left forearm

1 PCS Code _____

3. INPATIENT HOSPITAL　Gender: F　Age: 23

Preprocedure diagnosis: fractured R ulna

Procedure: open reduction, R ulna with clamp and rod internal fixation (CRIF)

1 PCS Code _____

4. INPATIENT HOSPITAL　Gender: F　Age: 34

Preprocedure diagnosis: complete tear of the patellar tendon, right knee

Procedure: arthroscopic repair of the patellar tendon. Using three suture anchors, the tendon was sewn to the bottom of the patella. Fixation was tested and no pull-out occurred. Hemostasis was obtained with electrocautery.

1 PCS Code _____

5. INPATIENT HOSPITAL　Gender: M　Age: 44

Preprocedure diagnosis: deltoid muscle paralysis, left shoulder

Procedure: trapezius muscle transfer. Fascia over trapezius muscle incised and trapezius detached from insertion. Deltoid muscle was exposed. The detached trapezius muscle was transferred and sutured as close as possible to the insertion of the deltoid muscle. Highest possible tension was achieved in the transferred muscle.

1 PCS Code _____

6. INPATIENT HOSPITAL　Gender: F　Age: 34

Preprocedure diagnosis: previous bilateral tubal ligation desiring reversal

Procedure: endoscopic tubal reanastomosis. Using the laparoscope, we obtained access to the fallopian tubes. The ends of the left fallopian tube were incised to open the lumen and reattached with use of the operating microscope. The procedure was repeated on the right. Methylene blue was used to ensure tubal patency.

Tip: If the identical procedure is performed on contralateral body parts, and a bilateral body part value exists for that body part, a single procedure is coded using the bilateral body part value. PCS OGCR B4.3.

1 PCS Code _____

ARRANGING CODES FOR ROOT OPERATIONS Y, M, X, AND S

Multiple coding is required more often with PCS than with ICD-9-CM Volume 3 or with CPT. Refer to PCS OGCR and Chapter 52 of this text for guidance on situations when multiple coding may be required. In addition to this general guidance, specific situations for Root Operations Y, M, X, and S that require multiple coding include the following:

- Transplantation: Root Operation Y identifies only transplantation of the organ or tissue. Assign separate codes for harvesting of the donor organ and any other procedures necessary to complete the transplant, such as cardiopulmonary bypass. When more than one organ is transplanted during the same operation, assign a separate code for each organ. The organ transplant should be sequenced as the principal procedure and the associated procedures should be sequenced as secondary.

- Laterality: Most Body Part values associated with Transfer, Reposition, and Reattachment procedures are unilateral. When the procedure is performed bilaterally, assign separate codes for each side if no bilateral Body Part value is available. Typically, either side can be sequenced as the principal procedure.

Guided Example of Arranging Codes for Reposition

To practice skills for arranging codes for procedures of the Root Operation Reposition, continue with the example from earlier in the chapter about the patient who was seen for fracture reduction and fixation. Follow along in your ICD-10-PCS manual as Marcy Elwood, CCS, arranges the codes. Check off each step after you complete it.

▶ First, Marcy confirms the procedures: open reduction of the right tibia and closed reduction of the right humerus.

► Marcy reviews the codes she assigned:

❑ **0QSG04Z Reposition, Lower Bones, Tibia Right, Open, Internal Fixation Device, No Qualifier**

❑ **0PSF3BZ Reposition, Upper Bones, Humeral Shaft Right, Percutaneous, External Fixation Device, Monoplanar, No Qualifier**

► Both procedures equally meet the PCS OGCR criteria for the principal procedure:

❑ **Sequence procedure performed for definitive treatment most related to principal diagnosis as principal procedure.**

❑ She chooses to sequence the open reduction of the right tibia first because it is the more extensive procedure.

► Marcy finalizes the procedure codes and sequencing for this case:

(1) **0QSG04Z Reposition, Lower Bones, Tibia Right, Open, Internal Fixation Device, No Qualifier**

(2) **0PSF3BZ Reposition, Upper Bones, Humeral Shaft Right, Percutaneous, External Fixation Device, Monoplanar, No Qualifier**

► Marcy also assigns and sequences the ICD-10-CM diagnosis codes that support the need for the service.

(1) **S82.201A Unspecified fracture of shaft of right tibia, initial encounter for closed fracture**

(2) **S42.301A Unspecified fracture of shaft of humerus, right arm, initial encounter for closed fracture**

► ICD-10-CM codes for the external cause of injury, if known, can also be assigned.

CODING PRACTICE

Exercise 53.4   Arranging Codes for Root Operations Y, M, X, and S

Instructions: Read the mini-medical-record of each patient's encounter. Review the information abstracted in Exercise 53.2 for questions 1–3. For questions 4–6, abstract the case on your own. Assign PCS codes using the Index and Tables, and arrange the codes in proper sequence. Write the code(s) on the line provided.

1. INPATIENT HOSPITAL   Gender: M   Age: 27

Preprocedure diagnosis: traumatic amputation of distal segment of little finger and two segments of the ring finger on left hand while using a table saw in home workshop

Procedure: replantation of distal segments of the little finger and ring finger on the left hand

2 PCS Codes _____

2. INPATIENT HOSPITAL   Gender: F   Age: 36

Preprocedure diagnosis: type 1 diabetes mellitus, unresponsive to treatment

Procedure: Simultaneous kidney–pancreas transplantation. The donor kidney came from the patient's sister. The donor pancreas came from a cadaver. Patient's left kidney was removed and replaced.

2 PCS Codes _____

3. INPATIENT HOSPITAL   Gender: F   Age: 43

Preprocedure diagnosis: low radial nerve palsy, right arm

Procedure: Tendon transfer, open. Rerouted the palmaris longus tendon to the extensor pollicis longus (EPL) muscle. Rerouted the pronator teres tendon to the abductor pollicis longus (APL) muscle.

Tip: Refer to PCS OGCR B3.2.b Multiple Procedures.

2 PCS Codes _____

4. INPATIENT HOSPITAL   Gender: M   Age: 44

Preprocedure diagnosis: left angle and right body mandible fractures

Procedure: closed reduction of mandible fractures with Erich arch bars and elastic fixation. Arch bars placed on the maxillary and mandibular dentition and secured with 25-gauge wire. Elastic fixation was placed on the arch bars; patient awakened.

Tip: If no bilateral body part value exists, each procedure is coded separately using the appropriate body part value. PCS OGCR B4.3.

2 PCS Codes _____

(continued)

5. INPATIENT HOSPITAL   Gender: M   Age: 54

Preprocedure diagnosis: *right tibiotalar subluxation; right distal tibiofibular fracture*

Procedure: *application of spanning external fixator to reduce tibiotalar subluxation; open reduction and internal fixation with arthroscopic-assisted tibial plafond fixation. A series of 0.062 K-wires and 2-mm K-wires were used to reduce the posterior impaction. Medial malleolar fixation was then performed with two medial malleolar screws, inserting and reducing the medial malleolar articular surface.*

Tip: The spanning external fixator is used to prevent ankle dislocation. The distal tibiofibular joint comprises the convex distal aspect of the fibula and the concave lateral aspect of the distal end of the tibia.

2 PCS Codes _____

6. INPATIENT HOSPITAL   Gender: M   Age: 44

Preprocedure diagnosis: *blepharoptosis, both eyes, obstructing the field of vision*

Procedure: *levator aponeurosis resection and advancement of both upper eyelids using an external approach. The desired level of lid elevation achieved by advancing the superior aspect of the tarsus to the inferior margin of the tarsus. Careful hemostasis obtained and skin closed with 6-0 Prolene.*

2 PCS Codes _____

CHAPTER SUMMARY

In this chapter you learned that:

- The Medical and Surgical Root Operations in the group *Procedures that Put in/Put Back or Move Some/All of a Body Part:* Transplantation (Y), Reattachment (M), Transfer (X), and Reposition (S).

- The Root Operation Transplantation (Y) is putting in or on all or a portion of a living body part taken from another individual or animal to physically take the place and/or function of all or a portion of a similar Body Part.

- The Root Operation Reattachment (M) is putting back in or on all or a portion of a separated Body Part to its normal location or other suitable location.

- The Root Operation Transfer (X) is moving, without taking out, all or a portion of a Body Part to another location to take over the function of all or a portion of a Body Part.

- The Root Operation Reposition (S) is moving to its normal location, or another suitable location, all or a portion of a Body Part.

- The Root Operation definition is a combination of the functional objective of the procedure and the anatomic site.

- For the Root Operations Transfer and Reposition, identify the site that is moved, not the location to which it is moved.

- The Root Operation Reposition uses Device to identify the type of internal or external skeletal fixation device applied.

- For the Root Operation Transfer, the Qualifier can identify the deepest tissue layer in a flap or the site that is the destination of the transfer.

- When a Transfer, Reposition, or Reattachment procedure is performed bilaterally, assign separate codes for each side if no bilateral Body Part value is available.

- PCS provides guidelines for Reposition of a fracture and the use of the Root Operations Transplantation and Administration.

CONCEPT QUIZ

Take a moment to look back at Root Operations that put in/put back or move some or all of a Body Part (Y, M, X, and S) and solidify your skills. Try to answer the questions from memory first, then refer to the discussion in this chapter if you need a little extra help.

Completion

Instructions: Write the term that answers each question based on the information you learned in this chapter. Choose from the list below. Some choices may be used more than once and some choices may not be used at all.

animal	orchiopexy
external	reattachment
fixation	replantation
flap graft	reposition
internal	synthetic
kidney	transfer
lung	transplantation
open	

1. The Root Operation _____ includes closed reduction of a dislocated shoulder.

2. The _____ is the most commonly transplanted organ.

3. A common type of procedure reported with the Root Operation Transfer is a(n) _____

4. A(n) _____ procedure may or may not include reconnection of nerves and blood vessels.

5. _____ is another term used for the root operation reattachment.

6. A K-wire is an example of a(n) _____ fixation device.

7. When a Body Part is replaced with a(n) _____ substitute, do not use root operations Y, M, X, or S.

8. There are a small number of procedures in the Root Operation _____.

9. The 6th character of code 0SSGX5Z indicates a(n) _____ fixation device.

10. The Root Operation _____ identifies the site that is moved, not the location to which it is moved.

Multiple Choice

Instructions: Circle the letter of the best answer to each question based on the information you learned in this chapter.

1. Which Root Operation is used to report fracture reduction?
   A. Transplantation
   B. Reattachment
   C. Transfer
   D. Reposition

2. Which procedure is not coded to the Root Operation Transplant?
   A. Bone marrow transplant
   B. Heart transplant
   C. Cornea transplant
   D. Ovary transplant

3. What Root Operation reports a Body Part that may or may not be cut out or off to be moved to the new location?
   A. Transplantation
   B. Reattachment
   C. Transfer
   D. Reposition

4. What Body Part is identified in ICD-10-PCS code 0LX80ZZ?
   A. Tendons
   B. Left hand tendon
   C. Upper tendon
   D. Lower tendon

5. Which Root Operation classifies a rectopexy?
   A. Reposition
   B. Transfer
   C. Reattachment
   D. Transplantation

6. What Approach is reported in ICD-10-PCS code 09SKXZZ?
   A. Open
   B. Percutaneous
   C. Percutaneous endoscopic
   D. External

7. What is the Root Operation for the procedure to treat an avulsed kidney?
   A. Transplantation
   B. Reattachment
   C. Transfer
   D. Reposition

8. Which of the following is an example of a procedure with the Root Operation Transfer?
   A. Gastropexy
   B. Free graft
   C. Pedicle graft
   D. Ulnar nerve transposition

9. What Qualifier is identified in ICD-10-PCS code 0JX00ZC?
   A. No qualifier
   B. Skin and subcutaneous tissue
   C. Skin and fascia
   D. Skin, subcutaneous tissue, and fascia

10. What is the Approach for all transplants?
   A. Closed
   B. External
   C. Open
   D. Percutaneous

CODING CHALLENGE

Instructions: Read the mini-medical-record of each patient's encounter, then abstract, assign, and arrange ICD-10-CM diagnosis codes and PCS procedure codes using the appropriate Index and Tables. Write the code(s) on the line provided.

1. INPATIENT HOSPITAL Gender: M Age: 38

Preprocedure diagnosis: right shoulder, rotator cuff repair

Procedure: rotator cuff repair. Complete tear of rotator cuff repaired by arthroscopic reattachment of the tendon. A synovectomy of the shoulder was also done through the arthroscope due to significant tenosynovitis.

Postprocedure diagnosis: complete tear of right shoulder rotator cuff, tenosynovitis

2 ICD-10-CM Codes _____

2 ICD-10-PCS Codes _____

2. INPATIENT HOSPITAL Gender: M Age: 26

Preprocedure diagnosis: cubital tunnel syndrome, left arm

Procedure: subcutaneous left ulnar nerve transposition. The nerve was transposed anteriorly to the medial epicondyle, lying under the skin and fat but on top of the muscle. Flexor-pronator fascia was used to prevent the nerve from relocating.

Tip: Refer to the definitions to select the correct approach character.

1 ICD-10-CM Code _____

1 ICD-10-PCS Code _____

3. INPATIENT HOSPITAL Gender: F Age: 17

Preprocedure diagnosis: acute traumatic nasal bone fracture with obstruction as a result of being hit with a baseball; severe orbital bruising, bilateral

Procedure: closed reduction of nasal bone fracture with stabilization. The nose was manually refractured and repositioned to its normal anatomic position. A thermoplastic cast was placed externally to stabilize the fracture.

Tip: Application of a cast or splint in conjunction with the reposition procedure is not coded separately. PCS OGCR B3.15.

3 ICD-10-CM Codes _____

1 ICD-10-PCS Code _____

4. INPATIENT HOSPITAL Gender: F Age: 21

Preprocedure diagnosis: right ear was torn off during pit bull attack

Procedure: severed pinna of right ear reattached. Using a microscope and extremely delicate tools the ear was reattached. I found a tiny artery only 0.3 millimeters in diameter and reattached the vessel to the woman's blood supply with three microscopic stitches. We were unable to find any viable veins and will use leech therapy to allow the veins to regenerate.

Tip: Assign an ICD-10-CM external cause code.

2 ICD-10-CM Codes _____

1 ICD-10-PCS Code _____

5. INPATIENT HOSPITAL Gender: F Age: 55

Preprocedure diagnosis: prolapse of vaginal vault status post hysterectomy 6 years prior

Procedure: Da Vinci laparoscopic sacrocolpopexy. After ports were placed the robot was docked. The posterior and anterior vaginal walls were dissected from the peritoneum. GyneMesh was used to lift the vagina into the pelvic cavity and secured with Gore-Tex suture. All instruments were removed; excellent hemostasis.

1 ICD-10-CM Code _____

2 ICD-10-PCS Codes _____

6. INPATIENT HOSPITAL Gender: M Age: 64

Preprocedure diagnosis: end-stage renal disease with need for a long-term hemodialysis access.

Procedure: right basilic vein transposition. Incision made along the medial aspect of the arm to expose the vein. Sharp dissection used to free the entire vein. Excellent flow through the vein with a palpable thrill.

Tip: End-stage renal disease (kidney failure) is when your kidneys stop working well enough for you to live without dialysis or a kidney transplant.

2 ICD-10-CM Codes _____

1 ICD-10-PCS Code _____

7. INPATIENT HOSPITAL   Gender: F   Age: 49

Preprocedure diagnosis: right hamstring avulsion

Procedure: reattachment of right hamstring to the ischial tuberosity. A vertical incision was made under the gluteal fold, and after identification and neurolysis of the sciatic nerve, transosseous tendon reinsertion to the pelvis was performed with four resorbable suture anchors.

Tip: The hamstring is a group of three muscles that run along the back of the thigh.

1 ICD-10-CM Code _____

1 ICD-10-PCS Code _____

8. INPATIENT HOSPITAL   Gender: M   Age: 16

Preprocedure diagnosis: involved in a fist fight; the lateral and central incisors of the lower jaw were knocked out

Procedure: closed replantation of two avulsed permanent teeth, lower jaw

Postprocedure diagnosis: under local anesthesia, the lateral incisor alveolar socket was irrigated with saline solution. Using slight digital pressure, the tooth was slowly replanted. This was repeated for the central incisor. X-ray confirmed normal position of teeth. A flexible splint was applied to be worn for two weeks.

Tip: Assign an ICD-10-CM external cause code.

2 ICD-10-CM Codes _____

1 ICD-10-PCS Code _____

9. INPATIENT HOSPITAL   Gender: F   Age: 8

Preprocedure diagnosis: right elbow fracture

Procedure: closed reduction of oblique fracture of the right distal humerus. Using conscious sedation, gentle traction applied to distal elbow and force applied to the olecranon to reduce the fracture. Long-arm fiberglass splint applied.

1 ICD-10-CM Code _____

1 ICD-10-PCS Code _____

10. INPATIENT HOSPITAL   Gender: M   Age: 73

Preprocedure diagnosis: acquired defect of left nose following Mohs procedure yesterday for basal cell carcinoma

Procedure: local cheek advancement and full-thickness skin graft measuring 1 cm x 3 cm. The area on the nose was debrided to remove necrotic tissue. A subcutaneous incision was made over the check and the flap advanced to the defect of the nose. Flap secured and a tie-over bolster used to secure the graft.

1 ICD-10-CM Code _____

2 ICD-10-PCS Codes _____

KEEP ON CODING

Instructions: Read the procedural statement, then use the appropriate Index and Tables to assign PCS procedure codes. Write the code(s) on the line provided.

1. Open pancreas transplant from organ donation: ICD-10-PCS Code(s) _____

2. Reattachment of right index finger: ICD-10-PCS Code(s) _____

3. Endoscopic facial nerve transfer: ICD-10-PCS Code(s) _____

4. Open reduction internal fixation (ORIF) of left humeral head: ICD-10-PCS Code(s) _____

5. Heart transplantation from organ donation: ICD-10-PCS Code(s) _____

6. Reattachment of the nose: ICD-10-PCS Code(s) _____

7. Open radial to median nerve transfer: ICD-10-PCS Code(s) _____

8. Reposition of intraocular lens (IOL) of left eye: ICD-10-PCS Code(s) _____

(continued)

(continued from page 1071)

9. Glossopexy of tongue: ICD-10-PCS Code(s) _____

10. Right kidney transplantation from organ donation: ICD-10-PCS Code(s) _____

11. Reattachment of left thumb: ICD-10-PCS Code(s) _____

12. Adjacent skin transfer of forehead: ICD-10-PCS Code(s) _____

13. Orchiopexy of left undescended testicle via endoscopy: ICD-10-PCS Code(s) _____

14. Transfer of subcutaneous tissue of anterior neck: ICD-10-PCS Code(s) _____

15. Liver transplantation from organ donation: ICD-10-PCS Code(s) _____

16. Open reduction internal fixation (ORIF) of tibial fracture of left leg: ICD-10-PCS Code(s) _____

17. Endoscopic colpopexy of vagina: ICD-10-PCS Code(s) _____

18. Reattachment of 5th left toe: ICD-10-PCS Code(s) _____

19. Endoscopic reattachment of the right tunica vaginalis: ICD-10-PCS Code(s) _____

20. Open detorsion of transverse colon: ICD-10-PCS Code(s) _____

21. Reattachment of left testicle: ICD-10-PCS Code(s) _____

22. Bilateral endoscopic salpingopexy: ICD-10-PCS Code(s) _____

23. Left kidney transplantation from organ donation: ICD-10-PCS Code(s) _____

24. Adjacent tissue transfer of scalp to repair 3 sq. cm deficit: ICD-10-PCS Code(s) _____

25. Percutaneous reposition left kidney: ICD-10-PCS Code(s) _____

Section 0: Root Operations V, L, 7, 1

Procedures That Alter the Diameter/Route of a Tubular Body Part

Chapter 54

Learning Objectives

After completing this chapter, you should have the skills to:

54.1 Spell and define the key words, medical terms, and abbreviations related to procedures that alter the diameter/route of a tubular Body Part.

54.2 Discuss the types of procedures that alter the diameter/route of a tubular Body Part.

54.3 Identify the main characteristics of coding for the Root Operations Restriction, Occlusion, Dilation, and Bypass.

54.4 Abstract procedural information from the medical record for coding for the Root Operations V, L, 7, and 1.

54.5 Assign codes for the Root Operations V, L, 7, and 1.

54.6 Arrange codes for the Root Operations V, L, 7, and 1.

54.7 Discuss the ICD-10-PCS coding guidelines related to Root Operations V, L, 7, and 1.

Chapter Outline

- **Basics of Procedures That Alter the Diameter/Route of a Tubular Body Part**
- **Coding Overview of Root Operations V, L, 7, and 1**
- **Abstracting for Root Operations V, L, 7, and 1**
- **Assigning Characters 4–7 for Root Operations V, L, 7, and 1**
- **Arranging Codes for Root Operations V, L, 7, and 1**

Key Terms and Abbreviations

extraluminal
intraluminal
orifice

In addition to the key terms listed here, students should know the terms defined within tables in this chapter.

For updates and corrections, visit our student resource site at
www.pearsonhighered.com/healthprofessionsresources

INTRODUCTION

Most urban areas have one or more bypass highways that reroute traffic around a congested area to improve traffic flow. The PCS Root Operation Bypass reroutes the contents of a tubular Body Part around a problem area of the anatomy to improve functioning.

This chapter discusses the five Medical and Surgical Root Operations in the group *Procedures that Alter the Diameter/Route of a Tubular Body Part*: Restriction, Occlusion, Dilation, and Bypass. Although the Root Operations share a common purpose—altering the diameter or route of a Body Part—each has a unique aspect that makes it different from the other procedures in this group. Pay careful attention to the differences between each Root Operation so that you can use each confidently and accurately.

BASICS OF PROCEDURES THAT ALTER THE DIAMETER/ROUTE OF A TUBULAR BODY PART

■ TABLE 54-1 defines Root Operations in this group and identifies procedural terms frequently associated with each. Some terms, such as *embolization*, can be associated with more than one Root Operation. There is not a direct match between a specific procedural term and a Root Operation because some medical terms, such as *embolization*, can be associated with more than one Root Operation. Root Operations are assigned based on the content of the operative report regarding what was actually performed, not on the terms used by the physician in documentation.

Refer to detailed anatomic diagrams of specific organ systems in Chapters 9 through 48 of this text, or in external references, when you need to refresh your memory of human anatomy.

Examples of Root Operations that alter the diameter/route of a tubular Body Part appear later in this chapter in Table 54-3 through Table 54-6. This section provides a general reference to help understand the most common procedures that alter the diameter/route of a tubular Body Part.

Table 54-2 ■ **EXAMPLE OF CONSTRUCTING MEDICAL TERMS FOR PROCEDURES THAT ALTER THE DIAMETER/ROUTE OF A TUBULAR BODY PART**

Combining Form	Suffix	Complete Medical Term
trache/o (*trachea*)	-stomy (*new opening/mouth*) -plication (*folding*) -plasty (*repair*)	tracheo + stomy (*creation of a new opening in the trachea*)
gastr/o (*stomach*)		gastro + plication (*folding of the stomach*)
angi/o (*vessel*)		angio + plasty (*repair of a vessel*)

Source: © PB Resources, Inc. Used with permission.

Remember to keep standard reference books handy in case you get stuck.

Refer to ■ TABLE 54-2 for a refresher on how to build medical terms related to procedures that alter the diameter/route of a tubular Body Part. Medical terms for these procedures sometimes use a separate word, such as *bypass* or *dilation*, rather than a word part to describe the procedure.

CODING CAUTION

Be alert for Root Operations that have similar English meanings but different PCS definitions.

Restriction (V) (*Partially* closing a tubular PCS Body Part) and **Occlusion (L)** (*Completely* closing a tubular PCS Body Part)

Bypass (1) (*Rerouting* the contents of a *tubular* PCS Body Part) and **Transfer (F)** (*Moving*, without taking out, all or a portion of a Body Part *to another location to take over the function* of all or a portion of a Body Part)

Table 54-1 ■ **ROOT OPERATIONS THAT ALTER THE DIAMETER/ROUTE OF A TUBULAR BODY PART**

Root Operation	Value	Definition	Terms
Restriction	V	Partially closing an orifice or the lumen of a tubular Body Part	Restriction, cerclage, banding, clipping, embolization
Occlusion	L	Completely closing an orifice or the lumen of a tubular Body Part	Occlusion, ligation, embolization
Dilation	7	Expanding an orifice or the lumen of a tubular Body Part	Dilation, balloon dilation, intraluminal dilation, angioplasty
Bypass	1	Altering the route of passage of the contents of a tubular Body Part	Bypass, shunt, stoma, diversion

CODING PRACTICE

Exercise 54.1   Basics of Procedures That Alter the Diameter/Route of a Tubular Body Part

Instructions: Use your medical terminology skills and resources to define the following procedures that take out some or all of a Body Part, then identify the code(s) or code range listed in the ICD-10-PCS Index. Follow these steps:

- Use slash marks "/" to break down each underlined term into its root(s) and suffix.
- Define the meaning of the underlined word based on the meaning of each word part.
- Look up the term in the ICD-10-PCS Index, and write down the name(s) of Root Operation(s) the Index cross references you to and the Table(s), if provided.
- Do not assign any codes.

Example: <u>angioplasty</u> angio/plasty   Meaning *repair of a vessel*   PCS Root Operation(s)/Table(s) *Dilation 027, 047, 037*

1. <u>pyelostomy</u>   Meaning _____   PCS Root Operation(s)/Table(s) _____

2. <u>ligation</u>, hemorrhoid   Meaning _____   PCS Root Operation(s)/Table(s) _____

3. <u>cannulation</u>   Meaning _____   PCS Root Operation(s)/Table(s) _____

4. <u>catheterization</u>   Meaning _____   PCS Root Operation(s)/Table(s) _____

5. <u>embolization</u>   Meaning _____   PCS Root Operation(s)/Table(s) _____

6. <u>anastomosis</u>   Meaning _____   PCS Root Operation(s)/Table(s) _____

7. closure   Meaning (word parts not required)   PCS Root Operation(s)/Table(s) _____

8. <u>cecocolostomy</u>   Meaning _____   PCS Root Operation(s)/Table(s) _____

9. <u>pylorodiosis</u>   Meaning _____   PCS Root Operation(s)/Table(s) _____

10. <u>ureteroplication</u>   Meaning _____   PCS Root Operation(s)/Table(s) _____

CODING OVERVIEW OF ROOT OPERATIONS V, L, 7, AND 1

The PCS OGCR specific to the Root Operations V, L, 7, and 1 clarifies the difference between the Root Operations Occlusion and Restriction. It also discusses the use of Character 4 and Character 7 with the Root Operation Bypass. These are discussed next. Refer to the PCS OGCR for additional details and clinical examples of each guideline.

Occlusion and Restriction

A vessel embolization procedure might be performed to completely close a vessel, as is done with a tumor embolization, or to narrow the diameter but not completely close it, as is done with an aneurysm. When the objective is to completely close the vessel, code the Root Operation Occlusion. When the objective is to narrow it, code the Root Operation Restriction (PCS OGCR B3.12).

Bypass

Bypass procedures identify the Body Part bypassed *from* and the Body Part bypassed *to*. Character 4, Body Part, specifies the Body Part bypassed from, and Character 7, Qualifier, specifies the Body Part bypassed to (PCS OGCR B3.6a) (■ FIGURE 54-1).

> Surgeon performs a percutaneous endoscopic bypass from the stomach to the jejunum, using autologous tissue.

> **0D1647A Medical and Surgical, Gastrointestinal, Stomach, Percutaneous Endoscopic, Autologous Tissue Substitute, Jejunum**

Figure 54-1 ■ Example of Guideline for Coding a Bypass Procedure. *Source:* © *PB Resources, Inc. Used with permission.*

Coronary artery bypass procedures are coded differently than other bypass procedures. Coronary arteries are classified by the number of distinct sites treated, rather than the number of coronary arteries or the anatomic name of a coronary artery, such as left anterior descending. Character 4, Body Part, identifies the *number* of coronary artery sites bypassed *to*, and Character 7, Qualifier, specifies the *vessel* bypassed *from* (PCS OGCR B3.6b) (■ FIGURE 54-2).

When multiple coronary artery sites are bypassed, code a separate procedure for each coronary artery site that uses a different Device and/or Qualifier value (PCS OGCR B3.6b). For example, when an aortocoronary artery bypass and internal mammary coronary artery bypass are both performed, assign two codes.

Surgeon performs an aortocoronary artery bypass of one site on the left anterior descending coronary artery and one site on the obtuse marginal coronary artery. The greater saphenous vein was used for both sites.

021109W Medical and Surgical, Heart and Great Vessels, Bypass, Coronary artery two sites, Open, Autologous venous tissue, Aorta

Figure 54-2 ■ Example of Guideline for Coding Coronary Artery Bypass. *Source: © PB Resources, Inc. Used with permission.*

CODING CAUTION

It is helpful to memorize PCS OGCR B3.6a–c about the Root Operation Bypass because PCS Tables simply list the Body Part and Qualifier values; they do not contain instructions on how to assign the values. Without knowing or referring to the OGCR, you may not know how to assign the characters of the code.

ABSTRACTING FOR ROOT OPERATIONS V, L, 7, AND 1

Abstracting for PCS focuses on identifying the correct Root Operation, which involves reading the operative report and interpreting it in light of Root Operation definitions. When reading the operative report, remember to focus on the objective of the procedure and the activities performed, not the specific medical terms the surgeon uses to describe the procedure. Many times the Root Operation can be determined conclusively during abstracting. Other times, the Root Operation can be narrowed down to two options, which must be differentiated based on other Characters that are assigned from the PCS Tables. The Root Operation definition is a combination of the functional objective of the procedure and the anatomic site. The following information summarizes the objectives, definitions, unique features, and examples of Root Operations V, L, 7, and 1.

Root Operations in this group treat a tubular Body Part. Examples include arteries, veins, and vessels; organs of the digestive system, such as the esophagus, stomach, small intestine, and large intestine; urethra and ureters; vagina, uterus, fallopian tubes; and many others. Body systems that do not contain tubular Body Parts, such as the integumentary and musculoskeletal systems, do not use Root Operations in this group.

Abstracting for Restriction (V)

The objective of the Root Operation Restriction is partially closing an orifice (*opening*) or lumen. The site of the procedure is a tubular Body Part. The orifice can be a natural orifice or an artificially created orifice such as a stoma. The Root Operation Restriction is coded when the objective of the procedure is to narrow the diameter of a tubular Body Part or orifice. Restriction includes both **intraluminal** (*from within the vessel*) or **extraluminal** (*from outside the vessel*) methods for narrowing the diameter.

Examples of Restriction are esophagogastric fundoplication and cervical cerclage (■ TABLE 54-3).

Table 54-3 ■ **EXAMPLES OF THE ROOT OPERATION RESTRICTION (V)**

Organ System	Procedural Examples
Blood and Immune	Restriction of thoracic lymphatic duct
Cardiovascular	Banding of pulmonary artery, clipping of cerebral aneurysm
Digestive	Esophagogastric fundoplication
Genitourinary	Cervical cerclage
Special Senses (Ear, Eye)	Stent placement in right lacrimal duct

Source: © PB Resources, Inc. Used with permission.

Abstracting for Occlusion (L)

The objective of the Root Operation Occlusion is completely closing an orifice/lumen. The site of the procedure is a tubular Body Part.

The Root Operation Occlusion is coded when the objective of the procedure is to close off a tubular Body Part or orifice. Division of the tubular Body Part before closing it is an integral part of the Occlusion procedure. Occlusion includes both intraluminal or extraluminal methods of closing off the Body Part, such as a clip either inside or outside of the vessel. Coders must read the operative report to determine the method used because different occlusive methods are reported with different Device values in Character 6.

The term *ligation* might be used to describe a procedure coded to Occlusion. However, the method of ligation must be determined from the operative report before determining the Root Operation. Ligation performed with clips, sutures, or rings is coded as Occlusion, but ligation performed with cauterization or electrocoagulation is coded to the Root Operation Destruction (5). The Root Operation Destruction is discussed in Chapter 52 of this text.

Examples of Occlusion are fallopian tube ligation and uterine artery embolization (■ TABLE 54-4).

Abstracting for Dilation (7)

The objective of the Root Operation Dilation is expanding an orifice/lumen. The site of the procedure is a tubular Body Part.

The Root Operation Dilation is coded when the objective of the procedure is to enlarge the diameter of a tubular Body Part or orifice. The orifice can be a natural orifice or artificially created. Dilation is accomplished by stretching a tubular Body Part using intraluminal pressure or by cutting part of the orifice or

Table 54-4 ■ **EXAMPLES OF THE ROOT OPERATION OCCLUSION (L)**

Organ System	Procedural Examples
Cardiovascular	Ligation of a vein, suture ligation of failed arteriovenous graft
Genitourinary	Uterine artery embolization, fallopian tube ligation (clipping), vasectomy (clipping or sealing)

Source: © PB Resources, Inc. Used with permission.

Table 54-5 ■ EXAMPLES OF THE ROOT OPERATION DILATION (7)

Organ System	Procedural Examples
Cardiovascular	Percutaneous transluminal coronary angioplasty (PTCA), dilation of old anastomosis
Digestive	Pyloromyotomy, balloon dilation of common bile duct, dilation of upper esophageal stricture
Genitourinary	Intraluminal dilation of bladder neck stricture, balloon dilation of fallopian tubes
Respiratory	Dilation of tracheal stenosis
Special Senses (Ear, Eye)	Transnasal dilation and stent placement in right lacrimal duct

Source: © PB Resources, Inc. Used with permission.

wall of the tubular Body Part and includes both intraluminal or extraluminal methods of enlarging the diameter. A device that is placed to maintain the new diameter is an integral part of the Dilation procedure and is coded to Character 6, Device.

Examples of Dilation are percutaneous transluminal coronary angioplasty (PTCA) and pyloromyotomy (■ TABLE 54-5).

Abstracting for Bypass (1)

The objective of the Root Operation Bypass is altering route of passage. The site of the procedure is a tubular Body Part.

Contents of a Body Part are rerouted to a downstream area of the normal route, to a similar route and Body Part, or to an abnormal route and dissimilar Body Part. The procedure includes one or more anastomoses, with or without the use of a device.

Examples of Bypass are coronary artery bypass graft (CABG) and colostomy formation (■ TABLE 54-6).

Key Criteria for Abstracting

Refer to Table 51-1 for general guidance on abstracting PCS procedures and Root Operation groups. Then refer to ■ TABLE 54-7 for more specific guidance on how to abstract procedures that alter the diameter/route of a tubular Body Part and distinguish among Root Operations in this group. A guided example of abstracting for the Root Operation Bypass follows. Remember that the abstracting questions are a guide and that not every question applies to, or can be answered for, every case.

Table 54-6 ■ EXAMPLES OF THE ROOT OPERATION BYPASS (1)

Organ System	Procedural Examples
Cardiovascular	Femoral-popliteal artery bypass
Digestive	Gastric bypass, colostomy formation
Genitourinary	Urinary diversion
Nervous	Placement of ventriculoperitoneal shunt
Respiratory	Tracheostomy formation with tracheostomy tube placement

Source: © PB Resources, Inc. Used with permission.

Table 54-7 ■ KEY CRITERIA FOR ABSTRACTING ROOT OPERATIONS THAT ALTER THE DIAMETER/ROUTE OF A TUBULAR BODY PART

Question	Root Operation (Value)
❑ What tubular Body Part was treated?	(If a tubular Body Part was not treated, do not use Root Operations V, L, 7, or 1.)

Answer *Yes* to one of the following questions to help distinguish Root Operations V, L, 7, and 1:

❑ Was an orifice or lumen partially closed?	Restriction (V)
❑ Was an orifice or lumen completely closed?	Occlusion (L)
❑ Was an orifice or lumen expanded?	Dilation (7)
❑ Were the contents of a tubular Body Part rerouted?	Bypass (1)

Source: © PB Resources, Inc. Used with permission.

Guided Example of Abstracting for Bypass

Refer to the following example throughout this chapter to practice skills for abstracting, assigning, and arranging codes for the Root Operation Bypass. Similar principles apply to working with other Root Operations that alter the diameter/route of a tubular Body Part.

INPATIENT HOSPITAL   Gender: M   Age: 67

Preoperative diagnosis: chronic unstable angina, acute STEMI involving the anterior wall and left anterior descending (LAD) coronary artery

Procedure: Coronary artery bypass grafting (CABG) ×2. The sternotomy was performed, the heart was physically stabilized, and the pericardium was entered. Total cardiopulmonary bypass (CPB) was initiated. Used the left internal mammary artery (LIMA) to LAD. The LIMA was clipped distally, divided, and spatulated (*spread open*) for anastomosis. The LAD was identified and opened. End-to-side anastomosis was performed through the LIMA. The right greater saphenous vein (GSV) was harvested laparoscopically and grafted from the aorta to the obtuse marginal (OM) coronary artery. The OM was identified, opened, and anastomosed in an end-to-side fashion to the reversed autologous GSV. An aortotomy was made and the vein was cut to fit and sutured in place. The patient was fully warmed and weaned from CPB. Good hemostasis was noted. A single mediastinal and left pleural chest tube was placed. The sternum was closed with interrupted wire, and the linea alba, sternal fascia, and subcutaneous tissue were closed. The patient tolerated the procedure well and was transferred to PACU in stable condition.

(continued)

(continued)

Postoperative diagnosis: Acute STEMI LAD; atherosclerotic heart disease with 90% blockage in LAD and 80% blockage in the OM. Unstable angina due to 50 years' continuous cigarette nicotine dependence.

Follow along as fictitious coder, Marcy Elwood, CCS, abstracts the procedure. Check off each step after you complete it.

▶ Marcy reads through the entire record, paying special attention to the reason for the encounter, the procedure performed, and the postoperative diagnosis. She refers to the Key Criteria for Abstracting Root Operations That Alter the Diameter/Route of a Tubular Body Part (Table 54-7).

❏ She notes preoperative diagnosis: chronic unstable angina, acute STEMI.

❏ *What is the stated procedure?* Coronary artery bypass grafting (CABG) ×2

❏ *What organ or Body Part is involved?* coronary arteries (LAD and OM)

❏ *Is the procedure description what you would expect based on the name of the procedure?* yes

❏ *What surgical approach is used?* open

❏ *Was more than one procedure, or a combined procedure, performed?* Two sites were bypassed using different tissue substitutes. Cardiopulmonary bypass equipment also was used.

❏ *Did the procedure alter the diameter/route of a tubular Body Part?* Yes

❏ *What tubular Body Part was treated?* Coronary arteries

❏ *Was an orifice or lumen partially closed?* No

❏ *Was an orifice or lumen completely closed?* No

❏ *Was an orifice or lumen expanded?* No

❏ *Were the contents of a tubular Body Part rerouted?* Yes

▶ At this time, Marcy believes that she will use the Root Operation Bypass and anticipates that she will need two codes for the CABG because each site was treated with a separate type of tissue and each bypass began in a distinct location. She will verify this information when she refers to the PCS Tables to assign codes. (Note: Mary also needs to assign codes for the cardiopulmonary bypass equipment, which is discussed in Chapter 57 of this text.)

CODING PRACTICE

Exercise 54.2 **Abstracting for Root Operations V, L, 7, and 1**

Instructions: Read the mini-medical-record of each patient's encounter and answer the abstracting questions. Write the answer on the line provided. Do not assign any codes.

1. INPATIENT HOSPITAL Gender: F Age: 55

Preprocedure diagnosis: epiphora (*overflow of tears*)

Procedure: Transnasal placement of stent to partially close left lacrimal duct

a. What is the stated procedure? _____

b. What organ or body part is involved? _____

c. What is the laterality? _____

d. Is the procedure description what you would expect based on the name of the procedure? _____

e. What surgical approach is used? _____

f. Was more than one procedure, or a combined procedure, performed? _____

g. What tubular Body Part was treated? _____

(continued)

1. (continued)

h. Was an orifice or lumen partially closed? _____

i. Was an orifice or lumen completely closed? _____

j. Was an orifice or lumen expanded? _____

k. Were the contents of a tubular Body Part rerouted? _____

l. What is the Root Operation(s)? _____

2. INPATIENT HOSPITAL Gender: M Age: 61

Preprocedure diagnosis: esophageal varices, portal hypertension due to cirrhosis

Procedure: ligation of esophageal vein. Passed endoscope through the mouth down the esophagus and visualized the varices. Snared the varices and placed rubber bands around the veins to tie them off. Patient tolerated procedure well.

a. What is the stated procedure? _____

b. What organ or body part is involved? _____

c. What is the laterality? _____

(continued)

2. (continued)

d. Is the procedure description what you would expect based on the name of the procedure? _____

e. What surgical approach is used? _____

f. Was more than one procedure, or a combined procedure, performed? _____

g. What tubular Body Part was treated? _____

h. Was an orifice or lumen partially closed? _____

i. Was an orifice or lumen completely closed? _____

j. Was an orifice or lumen expanded? _____

k. Were the contents of a tubular Body Part rerouted? _____

l. What is the Root Operation(s)? _____

---

3. INPATIENT HOSPITAL   Gender: F   Age: 57

Preprocedure diagnosis: occlusive disease, right iliac artery

Procedure: Fem-fem bypass from left femoral artery to right femoral artery due to a blocked right iliac artery. Made bilateral longitudinal incisions to expose both femoral arteries. Carried out subcutaneous tunneling, paying careful attention to the geometry of the graft to avoid kinking. Passed the Dacron graft through the tunnel in a C shape and completed end-to-side anastomoses on both sides.

a. What is the stated procedure? _____

b. What organ or body part is involved? _____

c. What is the laterality? _____

d. Is the procedure description what you would expect based on the name of the procedure? _____

e. What surgical approach is used? _____

f. Was more than one procedure, or a combined procedure, performed? _____

g. What tubular Body Part was treated? _____

h. Was an orifice or lumen partially closed? _____

i. Was an orifice or lumen completely closed? _____

j. Was an orifice or lumen expanded? _____

k. Were the contents of a tubular Body Part rerouted? _____

l. What is the Root Operation(s)? _____

---

4. INPATIENT HOSPITAL   Gender: M   Age: 66

Preprocedure diagnosis: atherosclerosis with 50% blockage of LAD and 30% blockage of RCA

Procedure: PTCA of two coronary arteries, LAD with stent placement, RCA with no stent

a. What is the stated procedure? _____

b. What organ or body part is involved? _____

c. What is the laterality? _____

d. Is the procedure description what you would expect based on the name of the procedure? _____

e. What surgical approach is used? _____

f. Was more than one procedure, or a combined procedure, performed? _____

g. What tubular Body Part was treated? _____

h. Was an orifice or lumen partially closed? _____

i. Was an orifice or lumen completely closed? _____

j. Was an orifice or lumen expanded? _____

k. Were the contents of a tubular Body Part rerouted? _____

l. What is the Root Operation(s)? _____

---

5. INPATIENT HOSPITAL   Gender: F   Age: 43

Preprocedure diagnosis: uterine fibroids

Procedure: Uterine artery embolization using intraluminal coils. Accessed the right internal iliac artery with a needle puncture. Introduced sheath and guidewire into the artery and guided it to the right uterine artery under fluoroscopic guidance. Placed coil within the vessel. Then accessed the left internal iliac artery in the same manner and placed a coil in the left uterine artery.

a. What is the stated procedure? _____

b. What organ or body part is involved? _____

c. What is the laterality? _____

d. Is the procedure description what you would expect based on the name of the procedure? _____

e. What surgical approach is used? _____

f. Was more than one procedure, or a combined procedure, performed? _____

g. What tubular Body Part was treated? _____

h. Was an orifice or lumen partially closed? _____

i. Was an orifice or lumen completely closed? _____

j. Was an orifice or lumen expanded? _____

k. Were the contents of a tubular Body Part rerouted? _____

l. What is the Root Operation(s)? _____

(continued)

CODING PRACTICE (continued)

6. INPATIENT HOSPITAL Gender: M Age: 72

Preprocedure diagnosis: intracranial cerebral aneurysm, left internal carotid aneurysm

Procedure: Craniotomy with clipping of cerebral aneurysm in an intracranial artery. A clip was placed lengthwise around the outside of the widened portion of the vessel. Using a percutaneous approach, placed an intraluminal bioactive stent in the left internal carotid artery.

a. What is the stated procedure? _____

b. What organ or body part is involved? _____

c. What is the laterality? _____

d. Is the procedure description what you would expect based on the name of the procedure? _____

(continued)

6. (continued)

e. What surgical approach is used? _____

f. Was more than one procedure, or a combined procedure, performed? _____

g. What tubular Body Part was treated? _____

h. Was an orifice or lumen partially closed? _____

i. Was an orifice or lumen completely closed? _____

j. Was an orifice or lumen expanded? _____

k. Were the contents of a tubular Body Part rerouted? _____

l. What is the Root Operation(s)? _____

ASSIGNING CHARACTERS 4–7 FOR ROOT OPERATIONS V, L, 7, AND 1

To assign codes after the Root Operation is determined, search the PCS Index for the name of the Root Operation as the Main Term. Locate the subterm(s) for the correct anatomic site and identify the PCS Table. When you locate the PCS Table, verify the first three characters of the code, then locate the row with the Body Part needed. Assign the remaining characters from each respective column of the Table. The following information summarizes and highlights unique information for working with the Tables for each Root Operation V, L, 7, and 1. Each Root Operation has one Table in each applicable PCS Body System. Because of the differences between organ systems, Table details vary.

Character 4: Body Part

As discussed earlier in this chapter, the Root Operation Bypass uses Body Part to identify the site bypassed from. In the event of a coronary artery bypass, Character 4 identifies the number of sites treated.

The coronary arteries are classified as a single Body Part that is further identified by number of sites treated and not by name or number of arteries. Sometimes multiple sites on one artery are treated with grafts or stents. When this occurs, report the number of sites, not the number of arteries. Separate Body Part values identify the number of sites treated, such as one, two, three, or four sites, when the same procedure is performed on multiple sites in the coronary arteries (PCS OGCR B4.4) (■ FIGURE 54-3).

PCS provides no Body Part value and no modifiers to identify the names of the coronary arteries treated. When reporting Bypass or Dilation of other arteries and veins, the Body Part value identifies the name and laterality of the vessel.

Surgeon performs percutaneous angioplasty of two distinct sites in the left anterior descending coronary artery, one with an intraluminal stent and one without.

02704DZ Medical and Surgical, Heart and great vessels, Dilation, Coronary artery one site, Percutaneous endoscopic, Intraluminal Device, No qualifier

02704ZZ Medical and Surgical, Heart and great vessels, Dilation, Coronary artery one site, Percutaneous endoscopic, No device, No qualifier

Figure 54-3 ■ Example of Coding Angioplasty on Coronary Arteries. *Source: © PB Resources, Inc. Used with permission.*

SUCCESS STEP

When searching the Index, remember that the Main Term is the Root Operation and the subterms are Character 4 Body Part values. Under the Main Term Bypass, the subterm for a coronary artery procedure is the number of sites, whereas the subterm for other bypass procedures is the Body Part bypassed from.

Character 5: Approach

All Approaches except External can be used for Root Operations in this group. Restriction, Occlusion, and Dilation procedures on vessels are often performed using the Percutaneous or Percutaneous Endoscopic Approach. Procedures on the Gastrointestinal and Respiratory systems might be performed Via Natural or Artificial Opening or Via Natural or Artificial Opening

Endoscopic. Bypass procedures are more likely to use an Open Approach but can also use a Percutaneous or Percutaneous Endoscopic Approach. Read the documentation carefully to identify the correct Approach.

CODING CAUTION

Because PCS is a new system and not yet fully tested in the field, occasionally you might encounter situations for which the PCS Tables provide inadequate information. Table 06L Occlusion, Lower Veins, is used for banding of esophageal varices, but Character 5, Approach, does not provide a value for Via Natural or Artificial Opening Endoscopic, a commonly used method. According to the American Hospital Association's *Coding Clinic*, select the next best available option, Percutaneous Endoscopic.

Character 6: Device

The Root Operations Restriction, Occlusion, and Dilation use Device to identify the type of device left in place. Options vary by procedure and might include either intraluminal or extraluminal, drug-eluting, radioactive, or other characteristics of the stent.

The Root Operation Bypass uses the Device to identify the type of tissue or tissue substitute used for the bypass procedure. It also identifies any intraluminal device left in place and whether it is drug-eluting.

Coronary artery bypass procedures often use the internal mammary artery (IMA) for the bypass. The right and left IMAs, also called internal thoracic arteries, begin at the subclavian artery and run to the anterior thoracic wall and breasts. Because of the location of the IMA, the vessel does not need to be harvested as do those from distant sites, such as the greater saphenous vein (GSV). Instead, the proximal end of the IMA remains connected to the subclavian artery and the distal end is freed and grafted to the destination site on a coronary artery (■ FIGURE 54-4). Therefore, use of the IMA is coded as **Z No Device** because no tissue substitute is used. The IMA is identified in Character 7 as the vessel bypassed from.

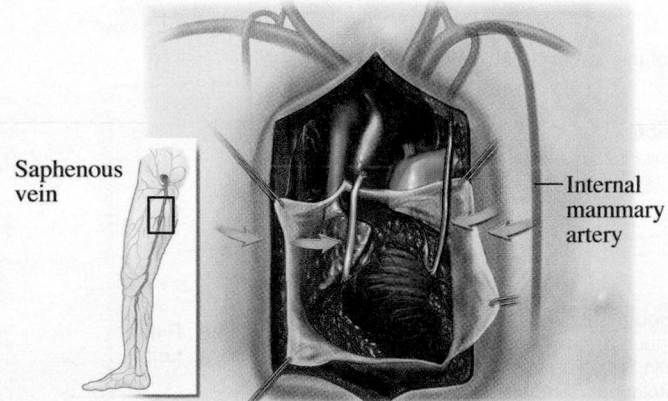

Figure 54-4 ■ Use of the Internal Mammary Artery and Greater Saphenous Vein for Coronary Artery Bypass. © *Nucleus Medical Art Inc/ Alamy*.

When an autologous vein such as the GSV is harvested and used for the graft, select Device value **9 Autologous Venous Tissue**. When an autologous artery such as the radial artery is harvested and used for the graft, select Device value **A Autologous Arterial Tissue**. Select other Device values for Synthetic (J) or Nonautologous Tissue (K) substitutes as appropriate.

Character 7: Qualifier

The Root Operation Restriction uses the Qualifier to identify a temporary procedure for the Abdominal Aorta (Table 04V).

The Root Operation Occlusion uses the Qualifier for the Body System Heart and Great Vessels (Table 02L) to identify the Left Atrial Appendage (K) and Ductus Arteriosus (T).

As discussed earlier in this chapter, the Root Operation Bypass uses the Qualifier to identify the Body Part bypassed to.

For coronary artery bypass procedures, Character 7 identifies the vessel bypassed from. This includes the IMA when used:

- **8 Internal Mammary, Right**
- **9 Internal Mammary, Left**

Guided Example of Assigning Characters 4–7 for Bypass

To practice skills for assigning codes for the Root Operation Bypass, continue with the example from earlier in the chapter about a patient who was seen for CABG ×2. Follow along in your ICD-10-PCS manual as Marcy Elwood, CCS, assigns codes. Check off each step after you complete it.

▶ First, Marcy confirms the procedure *CABG ×2, LIMA to LAD and aorta to OM*.

   ❑ The Root Operation for both procedures is Bypass, but separate codes are assigned because each site was treated with a separate type of tissue and each bypass began in a distinct location.

▶ Marcy searches the Index for the Main Term **Bypass**.

   ❑ She locates the first-level subterm **Artery**.

   ❑ She locates the second-level subterm **Coronary**.

   ❑ She locates the third-level subterm **One Site**.

   ❑ She identifies the Table: **021**.

   ❑ She also reviews the second-level modifying term for Two Sites and notices that it leads to the same table, but the fourth Character is different. She will refer to the Table to determine the details of how many codes are needed.

▶ Marcy turns to Table **021** to assign the codes.

   ❑ She reads the Table title **021, Medical and Surgical, Heart and Great Vessels, Bypass** and confirms that this accurately describes the Body System and Root Operation.

▶ Marcy assigns the value for Character 4, Body Part, for the bypass of the LIMA to the LAD.

   ❑ She selects **0 Coronary Artery, One Site**.

   ❑ The Table contains several rows with this Body Part value. She notices that Characters 5 through 7 provide different values in each row.

► Marcy assigns the value for Character 5, Approach.

   ❑ She knows the Approach is **0 Open** because the operative report identifies that a sternotomy was performed.

   ❑ The Table provides two rows that contain the value **0 Open** for Approach. Marcy will need to determine which row to use as she continues through each Character of the code.

► Marcy assigns the value for Character 6, Device.

   ❑ Because the LIMA was used, the vessel was not harvested. The proximal end of the LIMA was freed and reconnected to the LDA, and the distal end remained intact.

   ❑ She selects the row that contains **Z No Device** because no tissue substitute was used.

► Marcy assigns the value for Character 7, Qualifier.

   ❑ For Bypass procedures, Character 7 identifies the site bypassed from.

   ❑ She selects **9 Internal Mammary, Left**.

► She reviews the code she has assigned for the *CABG LIMA to LAD*: **02100Z9** (■ FIGURE 54-5).

► Marcy remains in Table 021 to assign the code for *CABG aorta to OM using the GSV*.

► Marcy assigns the value for Character 4, Body Part.

   ❑ She selects **0 Coronary Artery, One Site**.

► Marcy assigns the value for Character 5, Approach.

   ❑ The Approach is the same as for the previous procedure, **0 Open**.

► Marcy assigns the value for Character 6, Device.

   ❑ The GSV is **9 Autologous Venous Tissue**.

   ❑ The value for the Device is in a different row of the Table than the one used for the previous procedure, so this is the reason she needs two codes, each with the Body Part value **0 Coronary Artery, One Site**.

► Marcy assigns the value for Character 7, Qualifier.

   ❑ She selects **W Aorta** as the site bypassed from.

► She reviews the code she has assigned for the *CABG aorta to OM using the GSV*: **021009W** (■ FIGURE 54-6).

► Marcy reviews the procedure codes she has assigned for this case.

   ❑ **02100Z9** Medical and Surgical, Heart and great vessels, Bypass, Coronary artery one site, Open, No device, Internal mammary left

   ❑ **021009W** Medical and Surgical, Heart and great vessels, Bypass, Coronary artery one site, Open, Autologous venous tissue, Aorta

► Next, Marcy must determine how to sequence the codes.

Section	0	Medical and Surgical
Body System	2	Heart and Great Vessels
Operation	1	Bypass: Altering the route of passage of the contents of a tubular body part

Body Part Character 4	Approach Character 5	Device Character 6	Qualifier Character 7
0 Coronary Artery, One Site 1 Coronary Artery, Two Sites 2 Coronary Artery, Three Sites 3 Coronary Artery, Four or More Sites	**0 Open**	**Z No Device**	3 Coronary Artery 8 Internal Mammary, Right **9 Internal Mammary, Left** C Thoracic Artery F Abdominal Artery

Figure 54-5 ■ Assigning Code 02100Z9. *Source: Annotation © PB Resources, Inc. Used with permission.*

Section	0	Medical and Surgical
Body System	2	Heart and Great Vessels
Operation	1	Bypass: Altering the route of passage of the contents of a tubular body part

Body Part Character 4	Approach Character 5	Device Character 6	Qualifier Character 7
0 Coronary Artery, One Site 1 Coronary Artery, Two Sites 2 Coronary Artery, Three Sites 3 Coronary Artery, Four or More Sites	**0 Open**	**9 Autologous Venous Tissue** A Autologous Arterial Tissue J Synthetic Substitute K Nonautologous Tissue Substitute	3 Coronary Artery 8 Internal Mammary, Right 9 Internal Mammary, Left C Thoracic Artery F Abdominal Artery **W Aorta**

Figure 54-6 ■ Assigning Code 021009W. *Source: Annotation © PB Resources, Inc. Used with permission.*

CODING PRACTICE

Exercise 54.3   Assigning Characters 4–7 for Root Operations V, L, 7, and 1

Instructions: Read the mini-medical-record of each patient's encounter. Review the information abstracted in Exercise 54.2 for questions 1–3. For questions 4–6, abstract the case on your own. Assign PCS codes using the Index and Tables. Write the code(s) on the line provided.

1. INPATIENT HOSPITAL   Gender: F   Age: 55

Preprocedure diagnosis: epiphora (*overflow of tears*)

Procedure: Transnasal placement of stent to partially close left lacrimal duct

1 PCS Code _____

2. INPATIENT HOSPITAL   Gender: M   Age: 61

Preprocedure diagnosis: esophageal varices, portal hypertension due to cirrhosis

Procedure: ligation of esophageal vein. Passed endoscope through the mouth down the esophagus and visualized the varices. Snared the varices and placed rubber bands around the veins to tie them off. Patient tolerated procedure well.

1 PCS Code _____

3. INPATIENT HOSPITAL   Gender: F   Age: 57

Preprocedure diagnosis: occlusive disease, right iliac artery

Procedure: Fem-fem bypass from left femoral artery to right femoral artery due to a blocked right iliac artery. Made bilateral longitudinal incisions to expose both femoral arteries. Carried out subcutaneous tunneling, paying careful attention to the geometry of the graft to avoid kinking. Passed the Dacron graft through the tunnel in a C shape and completed end-to-side anastomoses on both sides.

Tip: Refer to PCS OGCR B3.6a to identify the use of Characters 4 and 7.

1 PCS Code _____

4. INPATIENT HOSPITAL   Gender: F   Age: 50

Preprocedure diagnosis: GERD

Procedure: Nissen fundoplication. Entrance to the abdomen gained via laparoscope. The fundus of the stomach was wrapped around the esophagus and sewn into place. The lower portion of the esophagus was passed through a stomach muscle tunnel to strengthen the lower esophageal sphincter. Patient tolerated the procedure well with no complications.

1 PCS Code _____

5. INPATIENT HOSPITAL   Gender: M   Age: 44

Preprocedure diagnosis: right subclavian artery steal syndrome

Procedure: right common carotid artery to subclavian artery bypass. The common carotid artery was exposed and dissected free. The right subclavian artery was exposed. An arteriotomy incision was made and a Dacron 8-mm graft used for the bypass in an end-to-end fashion.

1 PCS Code _____

6. INPATIENT HOSPITAL   Gender: F   Age: 2 weeks

Preprocedure diagnosis: patent ductus arteriosus, severe prematurity, operative weight less than 4 kg (600 grams)

Procedure: ligation (clip interruption) of patent ductus arteriosus. A posterolateral thoracotomy incision was performed and the ductus arteriosus was interrupted with a medium titanium clip. There was good pulsatile flow and palpable bilateral femoral pulses were noted.

1 PCS Code _____

ARRANGING CODES FOR ROOT OPERATIONS V, L, 7, AND 1

In addition to general guidance provided by PCS OGCR on assigning and sequencing multiple codes, specific situations for Root Operations V, L, 7, and 1 may require multiple coding.

The Body Part values for the coronary arteries are identified by the number of sites treated for the Root Operations Bypass and Dilation, so that multiple sites can be reported with a single code. However, separate codes must be assigned for each site with a unique combination of Device (Character 6) and Qualifier

Cardiologist performed percutaneous transluminal coronary angioplasty on three sites. An intraluminal drug-eluting stent was inserted into the LAD and non-drug eluting stents were inserted into the RCA and OM of the left circumflex artery.

027034Z Medical and Surgical, Heart and great vessels, Dilation, Coronary artery one site, Percutaneous, Intraluminal device drug-eluting, No qualifier

02713DZ Medical and Surgical, Heart and great vessels, Dilation, Coronary artery two sites, Percutaneous, Intraluminal device, No qualifier

Figure 54-7 ■ Example of Multiple Coding for Coronary Arteries. *Source: © PB Resources, Inc. Used with permission.*

(Character 7). For example, if three sites are treated but there are multiple Device or Qualifier values, do not use Body Part value **2 Coronary Artery, Three Sites.** Instead, assign separate codes for each combination of values (■ FIGURE 54-7).

CABG procedures require multiple codes for different treatments of multiple sites, graft harvesting, cardiopulmonary bypass, catheterization, and so on.

Guided Example of Arranging Codes for Bypass

To practice skills for arranging codes for procedures of the Root Operation Bypass, continue with the example from earlier in the chapter about the patient who was seen for CABG ×2. Follow along in your ICD-10-PCS manual as Marcy Elwood, CCS, arranges the codes. Check off each step after you complete it.

▶ First, Marcy confirms the procedure *CABG ×2, LIMA to LAD and aorta to OM.*

▶ Marcy reviews the procedure codes she has assigned for this case.

❑ **02100Z9 Medical and Surgical, Heart and great vessels, Bypass, Coronary artery one site, Open, No device, Internal mammary left**

❑ **021009W Medical and Surgical, Heart and great vessels, Bypass, Coronary artery one site, Open, Autologous venous tissue, Aorta**

▶ Marcy arranges the codes following the definition of the principal procedure contained in PCS OGCR and the Uniform Hospital Data Discharge Set (UHDDS).

❑ The principal diagnosis is *acute STEMI LAD.*

❑ CABG of the LIMA to LAD is the procedure most directly related to the principal diagnosis, so she sequences code **02100Z9** first.

▶ Marcy finalizes the procedure codes and sequencing for this case:

(1) **02100Z9 Medical and Surgical, Heart and Great Vessels, Bypass, Coronary artery one site, Open approach, No device, Internal mammary artery left**

(2) **0210293 Medical and Surgical, Heart and Great Vessels, Bypass, Coronary artery one site, Open approach, Autologous venous tissue, Coronary artery**

▶ A separate code is assigned for harvesting of the GSV.

(3) **06BP4ZZ Medical and Surgical, Lower veins, Excision, Greater saphenous vein right, Percutaneous endoscopic approach, No device, No qualifier**

▶ Codes for use of cardiopulmonary bypass equipment are assigned from PCS Section 5 Extracorporeal Assistance and Performance. These codes are discussed in Chapter 57 of this text.

(4) **5A1221Z Extracorporeal assistance and performance, Physiological systems, Performance, Cardiac, continuous, Output, No qualifier**

(5) **5A1935Z Extracorporeal Assistance and Performance, Physiological Systems, Performance, Respiratory, Less than 24 consecutive hours, Ventilation, No qualifier**

▶ Marcy also assigns and sequences the ICD-10-CM diagnosis codes that support the need for the service.

(1) **I21.02 ST elevation (STEMI) myocardial infarction involving left anterior descending coronary artery**

(2) **I25.110 Atherosclerotic heart disease of native coronary artery with unstable angina pectoris**

(3) **F17.218 Nicotine dependence, cigarettes, with other nicotine-induced disorders**

CODING PRACTICE

Exercise 54.4 Arranging Codes for Root Operations V, L, 7, and 1

Instructions: Read the mini-medical-record of each patient's encounter. Review the information abstracted in Exercise 54.2 for questions 1–3. For questions 4–6, abstract the case on your own. Assign PCS codes using the Index and Tables, and arrange the codes in proper sequence. Write the code(s) on the line provided.

1. INPATIENT HOSPITAL   Gender: M   Age: 66

Preprocedure diagnosis: atherosclerosis with 50% blockage of LAD and 30% blockage RCA

Procedure: PTCA of two coronary arteries, LAD with stent placement, RCA with no stent

2 PCS Codes _____

2. INPATIENT HOSPITAL   Gender: F   Age: 43

Preprocedure diagnosis: uterine fibroids

Procedure: Uterine artery embolization using intraluminal coils. Accessed the right internal iliac artery with a needle puncture. Introduced sheath and guidewire into the artery and guided it to the right uterine artery under fluoroscopic guidance. Placed coil within the vessel. Then accessed the left internal iliac artery in the same manner and placed a coil in the left uterine artery.

Tip: Do not code the fluoroscopy for this exercise.

2 PCS Codes _____

3. INPATIENT HOSPITAL   Gender: M   Age: 72

Preprocedure diagnosis: intracranial cerebral aneurysm, left internal carotid aneurysm

Procedure: Craniotomy with clipping of cerebral aneurysm in an intracranial artery. A clip was placed lengthwise around the outside of the widened portion of the vessel. Using a percutaneous approach, placed an intraluminal bioactive stent in the left internal carotid artery.

2 PCS Codes _____

4. INPATIENT HOSPITAL   Gender: F   Age: 59

Preprocedure diagnosis: angina, coronary artery bypass graft one year ago

Procedure: left heart catheterization; percutaneous transluminal coronary angioplasty and stenting with Cypher drug-eluting stent. Using the right femoral

(continued)

4. (continued)

artery, catheters were used for left ventriculography and selective coronary angiography. The LAD was 60% stenosed in the mid vessel and a balloon was deployed with minimal pressure ×2 with reduction to 0% stenosis. The proximal RCA was 80% occluded and a Cypher drug-eluting stent was deployed with reduction to 0%.

Tip: Refer to PCS OGCR B4.4.

2 PCS Codes _____

5. INPATIENT HOSPITAL   Gender: M   Age: 54

Preprocedure diagnosis: ureteropelvic obstruction, bilateral

Procedure: endoscopic ureteral stent on the right and balloon dilation on the left. Cystoscope was passed without difficulty. A small incision was made at the blocked portion of the right ureter and a stent was inserted. We then turned our attention to the left ureter, where we deployed a balloon. With minimal pressure, the ureter opened nicely and the balloon was removed. There was good flow of urine upon completion.

Tip: Refer to the PCS OGCR B3.2.

2 PCS Codes _____

6. INPATIENT HOSPITAL   Gender: M   Age: 3 weeks

Preprocedure diagnosis: infantile hypertrophic pyloric stenosis

Procedure: laparoscopic pyloromyotomy converted to open. Using the laparoscope we attempted a 1.5-cm incision in the pylorus. Because of the pyloric thickness I wasn't confident of the depth of the incision and elected to open the patient with a right semicircular umbilical incision. As suspected the incision was incomplete, which I corrected and enlarged to a 2-cm incision.

Tip: Refer to PCS OGCR B3.2. Code the laparoscopic procedure using the Root Operation Inspection because the laparoscopic procedure was converted to an open procedure. The Root Operation Inspection is discussed in Chapter 55 of this text.

2 PCS Codes _____

CHAPTER SUMMARY

In this chapter you learned that:

- The Medical and Surgical Root Operations in the group *Procedures that Alter the Diameter/Route of a Tubular Body Part* are Restriction, Occlusion, Dilation, and Bypass.

- The Root Operation Restriction (V) is partially closing an orifice or the lumen of a tubular Body Part.

- The Root Operation Occlusion (L) is completely closing an orifice or the lumen of a tubular Body Part.

- The Root Operation Dilation (7) is expanding an orifice or the lumen of a tubular Body Part.

- The Root Operation Bypass (1) is altering the route of passage of the contents of a tubular Body Part.

- Root Operations in this group treat a tubular Body Part, such as arteries, veins, and vessels; organs of the digestive system; urethra and ureters; and many others.

- The Root Operation Bypass uses Character 4, Body Part, to identify the site bypassed from. In the event of a coronary artery bypass, Character 4 identifies the number of sites treated.

- The Root Operations Restriction, Occlusion, and Dilation use Character 6, Device, to identify the type of device left in place.

- Character 7, Qualifier, is used for limited purposes in this group except for the Root Operation Bypass, which uses it to identify the site bypassed to or, for coronary artery bypass, the vessel bypassed from.

- PCS provides guidelines for Occlusion versus Restriction and for Bypass.

CONCEPT QUIZ

Take a moment to look back at Root Operations that alter the diameter/route of a tubular Body Part (V, L, 7, and 1) and solidify your skills. Try to answer the questions from memory first, then refer to the discussion in this chapter if you need a little extra help.

Completion

Instructions: Write the term that answers each question based on the information you learned in this chapter. Choose from the list below. Some choices may be used more than once and some choices may not be used at all.

Restriction   Dilation

Occlusion   Bypass

1. Balloon angioplasty is an example of the Root Operation _____.

2. The Root Operation _____ is altering the route of passage of the contents of a tubular Body Part.

3. Vasectomy using clips is an example of the Root Operation _____.

4. _____ is partially closing an orifice or the lumen of a tubular Body Part.

5. Urinary diversion is an example of the Root Operation _____.

6. The Root Operation _____ is completely closing an orifice or the lumen of a tubular Body Part.

7. Esophagogastric fundoplication is an example of the Root Operation _____.

8. The Root Operation _____ is expanding an orifice or the lumen of a tubular Body Part.

9. Placement of a ventriculoperitoneal shunt is an example of the Root Operation _____.

10. Clipping of cerebral aneurysm is an example of the Root Operation _____.

Multiple Choice

Instructions: Circle the letter of the best answer to each question based on the information you learned in this chapter.

1. What is the criterion for assigning the Body Part value for Coronary Artery?
   A. The name of the artery
   B. The number of arteries treated
   C. The number of sites treated
   D. The number of branches treated

2. Which Body System does NOT contain tubular Body Parts?
   A. Special senses (Eye, Ear)
   B. Hepatobiliary
   C. Musculoskeletal
   D. Nervous

3. What does Character 4 identify in a Bypass procedure?
   A. The site bypassed from
   B. The site bypassed to
   C. The approach
   D. The type of anastomosis

4. What Device value for Character 6 is used to identify the internal mammary artery when used for a coronary artery bypass?
   A. Autologous arterial tissue
   B. Autologous venous tissue
   C. Native artery
   D. No device

5. Which Body System is most likely to use the Approach Via Natural or Artificial Opening Endoscopic?
   - A. Heart and Great Vessels
   - B. Endocrine
   - C. Nervous
   - D. Gastrointestinal

6. What is the term for a Device placed around the outside of a Body Part?
   - A. Extraluminal
   - B. External
   - C. Intraluminal
   - D. No device

7. What does Character 7 identify in a coronary bypass procedure?
   - A. The number of sites treated
   - B. The vessel bypassed from
   - C. The vessel bypassed to
   - D. The type of stent

8. What Root Operation is usually used for formation of a stoma?
   - A. Bypass
   - B. Dilation
   - C. Resection
   - D. Restriction

9. What Root Operation is used for ligation performed with clips, sutures, or rings?
   - A. Destruction
   - B. Occlusion
   - C. Restriction
   - D. Ligation

10. Which procedure should be coded separately when a CABG is performed?
   - A. Sternotomy
   - B. Harvesting of the graft
   - C. STEMI
   - D. Anastomosis

CODING CHALLENGE

Instructions: Read the mini-medical-record of each patient's encounter, then abstract, assign, and arrange ICD-10-CM diagnosis codes and PCS procedure codes using the appropriate Index and Tables. Write the code(s) on the line provided.

---

1. INPATIENT HOSPITAL   Gender: F   Age: 59

Preprocedure diagnosis: elevated liver function study; dilated CBD on ultrasound

Procedure: ERCP with balloon dilation of common bile duct. The endoscope was inserted in the esophagus and advanced into the descending duodenum. Cholangiogram showed filling defects and so a balloon was advanced and dragged through the common bile duct, removing sludge but no stones. No strictures seen and the scope was withdrawn.

Tip: Only code the dilation.

2 ICD-10-CM Codes _____

1 ICD-10-PCS Code _____

---

2. INPATIENT HOSPITAL   Gender: F   Age: 59

Preprocedure diagnosis: peripheral arterial disease, left leg, with disabling intermittent claudication, ASHD

Procedure: femoral-tibial bypass with a polytetrafluoroethylene (PTFE) graft. An incision was made in the groin and thigh to expose the affected artery above the blockage and another incision to expose the artery below the blockage. The arteries were blocked off with vascular clamps. The PTFE graft

(continued)

---

2. (continued)

was sutured into an opening in the side of the femoral artery and then into the side of the posterior tibial artery. The clamps were removed, with good blood flow through the bypass.

2 ICD-10-CM Codes _____

1 ICD-10-PCS Code _____

---

3. INPATIENT HOSPITAL   Gender: M   Age: 19

Preprocedure diagnosis: recurrent stenosis of left arteriovenous fistula, end-stage renal disease, on dialysis

Procedure: left arm fistula/cephalic vein balloon angioplasty. Fistulogram showed a stenosis of about 75% at the arterial anastomosis. The fistula was accessed percutaneously with guidewire threaded toward the wrist. Balloon angioplasty was completed with a 6–mm-diameter × 4-cm balloon up to 8 atmospheres for two minutes. Fistulogram showed the vein now well dilated.

Tip: Only code the angioplasty.

3 ICD-10-CM Codes _____

_____

1 ICD-10-PCS Code _____

(continued)

(continued from page 1087)

4. INPATIENT HOSPITAL   Gender: F   Age: 41

Preprocedure diagnosis: grade II bleeding internal hemorrhoids

Procedure: endoscopic band ligation of two prolapsed internal rectal hemorrhoids. After inserting the anoscope into the anus, the right posterior hemorrhoid was grasped and a rubber band placed tightly around the base of it. The same procedure was repeated for the right anterior hemorrhoid.

Tip: Code the rubber band as a Device.

1 ICD-10-CM Code _____

1 ICD-10-PCS Code _____

5. INPATIENT HOSPITAL   Gender: M   Age: 70

Preprocedure diagnosis: severe segmental arteriosclerotic stenosis of the distal abdominal aorta, COPD, alcoholic cirrhosis

Procedure: aortobifemoral bypass graft using 19 × 8 Gelsoft Vascutek bifurcated graft. Both groins and the retroperitoneum were opened. The bifurcated graft from the aorta was tunneled down to the groin and the graft sutured to the right and then the left femoral artery. Flow was restored to both lower extremities and there were palpable femoral and dorsalis pedis pulses bilaterally.

3 ICD-10-CM Codes _____

_____

1 ICD-10-PCS Code _____

6. INPATIENT HOSPITAL   Gender: M   Age: 63

Preprocedure diagnosis: esophageal stricture from reflux of stomach acid, dysphagia

Procedure: esophageal dilation. The endoscope was passed through the mouth and into the esophagus. A 15- to 18-mm balloon was used to dilate the mild ring at the lower esophageal sphincter. The patient tolerated the procedure well.

2 ICD-10-CM Codes _____

1 ICD-10-PCS Code _____

7. INPATIENT HOSPITAL   Gender: F   Age: 29

Preprocedure diagnosis: two second-trimester miscarriages, high risk for premature birth, cervical incompetence at 12 weeks

Procedure: transvaginal intraluminal cervical cerclage using the Shirodkar technique. The cervix was exposed at the level of the internal os and a curved Allis clamp was used to grasp the lateral edges of the anterior and posterior aspects of the transverse incisions and some paracervical tissue. A suture was then placed anteriorly and tied posteriorly using a 5-mm tape suture with a double blunt needle at each end.

3 ICD-10-CM Codes _____

_____

1 ICD-10-PCS Code _____

8. INPATIENT HOSPITAL   Gender: F   Age: 46

Preprocedure diagnosis: clotted arteriovenous graft of left upper arm, stage 4 chronic kidney disease on dialysis

Procedure: removal of AV graft, left upper arm, and repair of brachial artery with end-to-end anastomosis. Old arterial incision opened and the graft artery anastomosis was excised, leaving an end-to-end portion of the artery for reanastomosis, which was done without difficulty. Wounds closed with a mid-portion of the graft left open for drainage.

3 ICD-10-CM Codes _____

_____

1 ICD-10-PCS Code _____

9. INPATIENT HOSPITAL   Gender: M   Age: 66

Preprocedure diagnosis: subglottic upper tracheal stenosis, former 2 ppd smoker ten years ago

Procedure: direct laryngoscopy, rigid bronchoscopy, and dilation of subglottic upper tracheal stenosis. A rigid bronchoscope showed a narrowing in the upper trachea. The area was dilated and the remainder of the bronchi evaluated. A bronchoscope was then used for further dilation. Tolerated well without complication.

2 ICD-10-CM Codes _____

1 ICD-10-PCS Code _____

10. INPATIENT HOSPITAL   Gender: F   Age: 50

Preprocedure diagnosis: cerebral aneurysm, hypertension

Procedure: craniotomy with clipping of a cerebral aneurysm. Small burr holes were made and, using a microscope, the right middle cerebral artery was

(continued)

10. (continued)

isolated. The clip was placed on the neck of the aneurysm, effectively stopping any flow.

Tip: Clips are made of titanium and remain on the artery permanently.

2 ICD-10-CM Codes _____

1 ICD-10-PCS Code _____

KEEP ON CODING

Instructions: Read the procedural statement, then use the appropriate Index and Tables to assign PCS procedure codes. Write the code(s) on the line provided.

1. Open clipping of aneurysm of the right vertebral artery: ICD-10-PCS Code(s) _____

2. Endoscopic bilateral vasectomy with clips: ICD-10-PCS Code(s) _____

3. Endoscopic dilation of ileocecal valve: ICD-10-PCS Code(s) _____

4. Bypass ileum to skin, open: ICD-10-PCS Code(s) _____

5. Dilation of urethral stricture by passage of urethral dilator without visualization.

   Tip: No device was left in the patient.: ICD-10-PCS Code(s) _____

6. Open bypass Gore-Tex graft, venous, right femoral-popliteal: ICD-10-PCS Code(s) _____

7. Percutaneous tumor embolization of right temporal artery: ICD-10-PCS Code(s) _____

8. Percutaneous revascularization of the left anterior descending artery using XIENCE Alpine Everolimus Eluting Coronary Stent:

   ICD-10-PCS Code(s) _____

9. Percutaneous endoscopic ligation of esophageal varices: ICD-10-PCS Code(s) _____

10. Embolization of a bleeding maxillary arteriovenous malformation: ICD-10-PCS Code(s) _____

11. Open splenorenal shunt to right renal vein: ICD-10-PCS Code(s) _____

12. Open suture ligation of failed arteriovenous hemodialysis graft, left brachial artery: ICD-10-PCS Code(s) _____

13. Laparoscopic bilateral tubal ligation using extraluminal clips: ICD-10-PCS Code(s) _____

14. Ventriculoperitoneal shunting with synthetic substitute to peritoneal cavity: ICD-10-PCS Code(s) _____

15. Hysteroscopy with dilation of fallopian tubes, bilateral: ICD-10-PCS Code(s) _____

16. Open occlusion of left atrial appendage (*a small, ear-shaped sac in the muscle wall of the left atrium*), using extraluminal pressure clips:

    ICD-10-PCS Code(s) _____

17. Percutaneous revascularization of the left common iliac artery using the Absolute Pro Vascular Self-Expanding Stent:

    ICD-10-PCS Code(s) _____

18. Endoscopic placement of restrictive stent in left parotid duct: ICD-10-PCS Code(s) _____

19. Percutaneous endoscopic ligation of portal vein: ICD-10-PCS Code(s) _____

20. Percutaneous transluminal coronary angioplasty (PTCA) of left anterior descending artery with placement of two drug-eluting stents:

    ICD-10-PCS Code(s) _____

21. Percutaneous transvenous intrahepatic portosystemic shunt (TIPS): ICD-10-PCS Code(s) _____

22. Percutaneous ligation of left brachial artery: ICD-10-PCS Code(s) _____

23. Percutaneous endoscopic occlusion of mesenteric lymphatic duct: ICD-10-PCS Code(s) _____

24. Open gastric bypass with Roux-en-Y limb to ileum: ICD-10-PCS Code(s) _____

25. Percutaneous transluminal angioplasty, left renal artery: ICD-10-PCS Code(s) _____

Chapter 55

Section 0: Root Operations 9, C, F, 8, N, J, and K

Procedures that Take Out Solids/Fluids/Gases from a Body Part (9, C, F)

Procedures Involving Cutting or Separation Only (8, N)

Procedures Involving Examination Only (J, K)

Chapter Outline

- **Basics of Procedures 9, C, F, 8, N, J, and K**
- **Coding Overview of Root Operations 9, C, F, 8, N, J, and K**
- **Abstracting for Root Operations 9, C, F, 8, N, J, and K**
- **Assigning Characters 4–7 for Root Operations 9, C, F, 8, N, J, and K**
- **Arranging Codes for Root Operations 9, C, F, 8, N, J, and K**

Learning Objectives

After completing this chapter, you should have the skills to:

55.1 Spell and define the key words, medical terms, and abbreviations related to procedures that take out solids/fluids/gases from a Body Part, involving cutting or separation only, or involving examination only.

55.2 Discuss the types of procedures that take out solids/fluids/gases from a Body Part, involving cutting or separation only, or involving examination only.

55.3 Identify the main characteristics of coding for the Root Operations Drainage, Extirpation, Fragmentation, Release, Division, Inspection, and Map.

55.4 Abstract procedural information from the medical record for coding for the Root Operations 9, C, F, 8, N, J, and K.

55.5 Assign codes for the Root Operations 9, C, F, 8, N, J, and K.

55.6 Arrange codes for the Root Operations 9, C, F, 8, N, J, and K.

55.7 Discuss the ICD-10-PCS coding guidelines related to Root Operations 9, C, F, 8, N, J, and K.

Key Terms and Abbreviations

rhizotomy
solid matter (PCS)

In addition to the key terms listed here, students should know the terms defined within tables in this chapter.

For updates and corrections, visit our student resource site at
www.pearsonhighered.com/healthprofessionsresources

INTRODUCTION

An electronic or paper map shows common features as well as highlights and hazards you might want to be aware of during your trip. PCS provides a Root Operation Map to identify procedures that generate electronic images of the brain or conduction system. The Root Operation Map is one of two Root Operations involving examination only.

This chapter discusses three groups of Medical and Surgical Root Operations:

- Procedures that Take Out Solids/Fluids/Gases from a Body Part (9, C, F)
- Procedures Involving Cutting or Separation Only (8, N)
- Procedures Involving Examination Only (J, K)

Although the Root Operations in each group share a common purpose, each has a unique aspect that makes it different from the other procedures in this group. Sometimes only a few words distinguish one Root Operation from a similar one. Pay careful attention to the differences between Root Operations so that you can use each confidently and accurately.

BASICS OF PROCEDURES 9, C, F, 8, N, J, AND K

This section introduces each Root Operation group and provides definitions and examples of each Root Operation. Details will be discussed as you progress through this chapter.

Basics of Procedures that Take Out Solids/Fluids/Gases from a Body Part (9, C, F)

Procedures that take out solids, fluids, or gases from a Body Part focus on the removal of the unwanted substance and not on removal of the Body Part itself. Solid matter refers to a nonnative solid that may result from biological processes, such as calculi or a clot, or may be a nonbiological solid, such as a foreign body. Fluids can include any bodily fluid such as urine, blood, water, or a nonnative fluid introduced into the body. Air is the most common gas treated. Refer to ■ TABLE 55-1

Table 55-1 ■ ROOT OPERATIONS THAT TAKE OUT SOLIDS/FLUIDS/GASES FROM A BODY PART

Root Operation	Value	Definition	Terms
Drainage	9	Taking or letting out fluids and/or gases from a Body Part	Drainage, centesis, placement, aspiration
Extirpation	C	Taking or cutting out solid matter from a Body Part	Removal, excision
Fragmentation	F	Breaking solid matter in a Body Part into pieces	Lithotripsy, crushing, fragmentation

Table 55-2 ■ ROOT OPERATIONS INVOLVING CUTTING OR SEPARATION ONLY

Root Operation	Value	Definition	Terms
Division	8	Cutting into a Body Part, without draining fluids and/or gases from the Body Part, to separate or transect a Body Part	Separation, division
Release	N	Freeing a Body Part from an abnormal physical constraint by cutting or by the use of force	Lysis, release, freeing

for the definitions and terms commonly used with the Root Operations Drainage (9), Extirpation (C), and Fragmentation (F).

Basics of Procedures Involving Cutting or Separation Only (8, N)

Procedures involving cutting or separation focus only on separating, transecting, or freeing a Body Part *without removing* the Body Part itself and *without draining* fluids or gases from the Body Part. Separation can be accomplished through cutting or other use of force. Refer to ■ TABLE 55-2 for the definitions and terms commonly used with the Root Operations Division (8) and Release (N).

Basics of Procedures Involving Examination Only (J, K)

Procedures involving examination only focus on visualizing, exploring, or mapping a Body Part for diagnostic purposes. The Body Part is *not treated* in these Root Operations. When the Body Part is treated, assign the appropriate Root Operation that describes the work done. Refer to ■ TABLE 55-3 for the definitions and terms commonly used with the Root Operations Inspection (J) and Map (K).

Table 55-3 ■ ROOT OPERATIONS INVOLVING EXAMINATION ONLY

Root Operation	Value	Definition	Terms
Inspection	J	Visually and/or manually exploring a Body Part	Endoscopy, laparoscopy, diagnostic, exploration
Map	K	Locating the route of passage of electrical impulses and/or locating functional areas in a Body Part	Mapping

Table 55-4 ■ **EXAMPLE OF CONSTRUCTING MEDICAL TERMS FOR PROCEDURES 9, C, F, 8, N, J, AND K**

Combining Form	Suffix	Complete Medical Term
esophag/o (*esophagus*)	**-scopy** (*visual examination*)	**esophago + gastro + duodeno + scopy** (*visual examination of the esophagus, stomach, and duodenum*)
gastr/o (*stomach*)	**-ectomy** (*excision*)	**esophag + ectomy** (*excision of the esophagus*)
duoden/o (*duodenum*)		**gastr + ectomy** (*excision of the stomach*)
		duoden + ectomy (*excision of the duodenum*)

Source: © PB Resources, Inc. Used with permission.

■ TABLE 55-4 provides a refresher on how to build medical terms related to procedures that are discussed in this chapter. Some suffixes, such as *-ectomy*, *-tomy*, and *-scopy*, can be associated with more than one Root Operation. There is not a direct match between a specific procedural term and a Root Operation because some medical terms, such as excision and endoscopy, can be associated with more than one Root Operation. Root Operations are assigned based on the content of the operative report regarding what was actually performed, not on the terms used by the physician in documentation or by the surgical approach.

Refer to detailed anatomic diagrams of specific organ systems in Chapters 9 through 48 of this text, or in external references, when you need to refresh your memory of human anatomy.

CODING CAUTION

Be alert for Root Operations that have similar English meanings but different PCS definitions.

Extirpation (C) (*Taking or cutting out <u>abnormal solid matter</u> from within a PCS Body Part*) and **Extraction (D)** (*Pulling out or off without replacement <u>a portion</u> of a PCS Body Part*)

Release (N) (*<u>Freeing a Body Part</u> from an <u>abnormal physical constraint</u> by cutting or by the use of force*) and **Detachment (6)** (*Cutting an <u>extremity</u> out/off without replacement*)

CODING PRACTICE

Exercise 55.1 Basics of Procedures 9, C, F, 8, N, J, and K

Instructions: Use your medical terminology skills and resources to define the following procedures 9, C, F, 8, N, J, and K, then identify the code(s) or code range listed in the PCS Index. Follow these steps:

- Use slash marks "/" to break down each term into its root(s) and suffix.
- Define the meaning of the word based on the meaning of each word part.
- Look up the term in the ICD-10-PCS Index, and write down the name(s) of the Root Operation(s) the Index cross-references you to and the Table(s), if provided.
- Do not assign any codes.

Example: thoracotomy
thoraco/tomy   Meaning *incision into the chest*   PCS Root Operation(s)/Table(s) *Drainage 0W9*

1. oophorotomy   Meaning _____   PCS Root Operation(s)/Table(s) _____
2. cholecystostomy   Meaning _____   PCS Root Operation(s)/Table(s) _____
3. lithotripsy   Meaning _____   PCS Root Operation(s)/Table(s) _____
4. colopuncture   Meaning _____   PCS Root Operation(s)/Table(s) _____
5. laminotomy   Meaning _____   PCS Root Operation(s)/Table(s) _____
6. arthrolysis   Meaning _____   PCS Root Operation(s)/Table(s) _____
7. thrombectomy   Meaning _____   PCS Root Operation(s)/Table(s) _____
8. laparoscopy   Meaning _____   PCS Root Operation(s)/Table(s) _____
9. thoracocentesis   Meaning _____   PCS Root Operation(s)/Table(s) _____
10. lobotomy   Meaning _____   PCS Root Operation(s)/Table(s) _____

CODING OVERVIEW OF ROOT OPERATIONS 9, C, F, 8, N, J, AND K

The PCS OGCR specific to the Root Operations in these groups provide several criteria for the Root Operation Inspection. General guidelines related to coding multiple procedures using Inspection are discussed below, and those specific to Characters 4 through 7 are discussed later in this chapter. PCS OGCR provide a guideline regarding coding biopsies using the Root Operation Drainage and also clarify the difference between the Root Operation Release and Division. These are discussed next. Refer to the PCS OGCR for additional details and clinical examples of each guideline.

Guidelines for Inspection

When the intended Root Operation is attempted using one Approach but is converted to a different Approach, assign separate procedure codes for each Approach. A laparoscopic procedure converted to an open procedure is coded as a percutaneous endoscopic Inspection; the open procedure is coded as an Excision or Resection (PCS OGCR B3.2.d) (■ FIGURE 55-1).

When a procedure is begun but discontinued before any other Root Operation is performed, code the Root Operation Inspection of the Body Part or anatomic region inspected (PCS OGCR B3.3) (■ FIGURE 55-2). A second code is not required because no other procedure was performed.

CODING CAUTION

In CPT, modifier **-53** is appended to a code to identify a discontinued procedure. PCS does not use modifiers.

Surgeon made 4 abdominal incisions for a laparoscopic cholecystectomy. Due to the level of inflammation, the procedure was converted to an open approach and completed.

0FT40ZZ [Medical and Surgical, Hepatobiliary System and Pancreas] Resection, Gall bladder, Open, No device, No qualifier

0FJ44ZZ [Medical and Surgical, Hepatobiliary System and Pancreas] Inspection, Gall bladder, Percutaneous endoscopic, No device, No qualifier

Figure 55-1 ■ Example of Coding a Laparoscopic Procedure Converted to Open Approach. *Source: © PB Resources, Inc. Used with permission.*

Surgeon made the initial thoracotomy incision for aortic valve replacement procedure. The patient became hemodynamically unstable so the procedure was discontinued before the heart muscle was incised.

0WJC0ZZ [Medical and Surgical, Anatomical regions general] Inspection, Mediastinum, Open, No device, No qualifier

Figure 55-2 ■ Example of Coding Inspection for a Discontinued Procedure. *Source: © PB Resources, Inc. Used with permission.*

Guidelines for Drainage

Drainage procedures can be done for diagnostic or therapeutic purposes. A physician may aspirate fluid to sample it and determine a diagnosis before creating a treatment plan. When a diagnostic Drainage, Excision, or Resection procedure (biopsy) is followed by a more definitive procedure, such as Destruction, Excision, or Resection, at the same procedure site, code *both* the biopsy and the more definitive treatment (PCS OGCR B3.4b).

Guidelines for Release and Division

Use the Root Operation Release when the sole objective of the procedure is freeing a Body Part *without* cutting the Body Part. Use the Root Operation Division when the sole objective of the procedure is separating or transecting a Body Part (PCS OGCR B3.14). For example, freeing a nerve root from surrounding scar tissue to relieve pain is coded to the Root Operation Release. Severing a nerve root to relieve pain is coded to the Root Operation Division.

ABSTRACTING FOR ROOT OPERATIONS 9, C, F, 8, N, J, AND K

Abstracting for PCS focuses on identifying the correct Root Operation, which involves reading the operative report and interpreting it in light of Root Operation definitions. When reading the operative report, remember to focus on the objective of the procedure and the activities performed, not the specific medical terms the surgeon uses to describe the procedure. Many times the Root Operation can be determined conclusively during abstracting. Other times the Root Operation can be narrowed down to two options, which must be differentiated based on other Characters that are assigned from the PCS Tables. The following information summarizes the Root Operations in each of the groups discussed in this chapter. Refer to Table 51-1 for general guidance on abstracting PCS procedures and Root Operation groups, then refer to the Key Criteria for Abstracting Root Operations in each of the following sections. This information is followed by a Guided Example of Abstracting Inspection, Release, and Resection.

Abstracting for Procedures That Take Out Solids, Fluids, or Gases from a Body Part

The following information summarizes the objective, definition, unique features, examples, and Key Criteria for Abstracting Root Operations for procedures that take out solids, fluids, or gases from a Body Part.

Abstracting for Drainage (9)

The objective of the Root Operation Drainage is taking or letting out fluids or gases. The site of the procedure is within a Body Part.

The Root Operation Drainage is coded for both diagnostic and therapeutic drainage procedures. When drainage is accomplished by putting in a catheter, assign the value Drainage Device for Character 6, Device. When the purpose is diagnostic, assign the value Diagnostic (X) for Character 7, Qualifier.

Examples of Drainage are thoracentesis and incision and drainage (I&D), which is performed in multiple Body Systems (■ TABLE 55-5).

Table 55-5 ■ EXAMPLES OF THE ROOT OPERATION DRAINAGE (9)

Organ System	Procedural Examples
Cardiovascular	Thoracentesis
Digestive	Incision and drainage of external perianal abscess, percutaneous drainage of ascites
Genitourinary	Urinary nephrostomy catheter placement, routine Foley catheter placement, ovarian cystotomy and drainage
Hepatobiliary	Drain placement for liver abscess
Musculoskeletal	Arthrotomy with drain placement
Nervous	Ventricular CSF drainage catheter placement
Respiratory	Chest tube placement for right pneumothorax, sinus drainage, pleurocentesis

Source: © PB Resources, Inc. Used with permission.

Abstracting for Extirpation (C)

The objective of the Root Operation Extirpation is taking or cutting out solid matter. The site of the procedure is within a Body Part.

Extirpation represents a range of procedures where the Body Part itself is not the focus of the procedure. Instead, the objective is to remove nonnative solid matter such as a foreign body, thrombus, or calculus from the Body Part. The solid matter may be an abnormal byproduct of a biological function and it may be imbedded in a Body Part or in the lumen of a tubular Body Part. The solid matter may or may not have been previously broken into pieces. Extirpation is not used to identify removal of the Body Part itself.

Examples of Extirpation are a thrombectomy and choledocholithotomy (■ TABLE 55-6).

> ### CODING CAUTION
>
> Removal of a tumor or lesion is coded to the Root Operation Excision, which was discussed in Chapter 52 of this text.

Table 55-6 ■ EXAMPLES OF THE ROOT OPERATION EXTIRPATION (C)

Organ System	Procedural Examples
Cardiovascular	Declotting of AV dialysis graft, mechanical thrombectomy, endarterectomy
Digestive	Removal of bezoar from stomach
Genitourinary	Removal of bladder stone
Integumentary	Foreign body removal, skin of left thumb
Respiratory	Removal of foreign body in right nostril
Special Senses (Ear, Eye)	Removal of foreign body from cornea

Source: © PB Resources, Inc. Used with permission.

> Surgeon made the initial thoracotomy incision for aortic valve replacement procedure. The patient became hemodynamically unstable so the procedure was discontinued before the heart muscle was incised.
>
> **0WJC0ZZ [Medical and Surgical, Anatomical regions general] Inspection, Mediastinum, Open, No device, No qualifier**

Figure 55-3 ■ Extracorporeal Shockwave Lithtripsy (ESWL) for Kidney Stones. *Source: Shutterstock © Designua*

Abstracting for Fragmentation (F)

The objective of the Root Operation Fragmentation is breaking solid matter into pieces. The site of the procedure is within a Body Part. The solid matter is nonnative material such as calculus.

Physical force, including manual and ultrasonic, is applied directly or indirectly to break the solid matter into pieces. The solid matter may be an abnormal byproduct of a biological function or a foreign body. The pieces of solid matter are *not* taken out. Fragmentation is coded for procedures to break up, but not remove, solid material such as a calculus or foreign body. This Root Operation includes both direct and extracorporeal Fragmentation procedures (■ FIGURE 55-3).

Fragmentation differs from the Root Operation Destruction (5), which was discussed in Chapter 52 of this text, in that the focus of Fragmentation is nonnative solid matter, whereas the focus of Destruction is the Body Part itself, such as fulguration of a polyp or cauterization of a skin lesion.

Examples of Fragmentation are extracorporeal shockwave lithotripsy and transurethral lithotripsy (■ TABLE 55-7).

> ### CODING CAUTION
>
> Fragmentation and Extirpation should not be used together for the same procedure. When solid matter is broken up, then removed by force, assign only the Root Operation Extirpation, which includes removal of the fragments. When the solid matter is broken up but not removed, assign the Root Operation Fragmentation.

Table 55-7 ■ EXAMPLES OF THE ROOT OPERATION FRAGMENTATION (F)

Organ System	Procedural Examples
Cardiovascular	Thoracotomy with crushing of pericardial calcifications
Genitourinary	Extracorporeal shockwave lithotripsy (ESWL) of kidney, intraluminal lithotripsy of fallopian tube calcification
Hepatobiliary	Endoscopic retrograde cholangiopancreatography (ERCP) with lithotripsy of common bile duct stone

Source: © PB Resources, Inc. Used with permission.

Table 55-8 ■ **KEY CRITERIA FOR ABSTRACTING ROOT OPERATIONS THAT TAKE OUT SOLIDS, FLUIDS, OR GASES FROM A BODY PART**

Question	Root Operation (Value)
Answer *Yes* to one of the following questions to help distinguish Root Operations 9, C, and F:	
❏ Were gases or fluids let out from within a Body Part?	Drainage (9)
❏ Was nonnative solid matter taken out of a Body Part?	Extirpation (C)
❏ Was nonnative solid matter within a Body Part broken into pieces?	Fragmentation (F)

Source: © PB Resources, Inc. Used with permission.

Key Criteria for Abstracting Root Operations 9, C, and F

Refer to ■ Table 55-8 for more specific guidance on how to abstract procedures that Take Out Solids/Fluids/Gases from a Body Part and distinguish among Root Operations in this group.

Abstracting for Procedures Involving Cutting or Separation Only

The following information summarizes the objective, definition, unique features, examples, and Key Criteria for Abstracting Root Operations for procedures involving cutting or separation only.

Abstracting for Division (8)

The objective of the Root Operation Division is cutting into or separating a Body Part. The site of the procedure is within a Body Part. All or a portion of the Body Part is separated into two or more portions. The Root Operation Division is coded when the objective of the procedure is to *cut into*, transect, or otherwise separate all or a portion of a Body Part. If the Body Part itself is not cut or separated into portions, do not assign this Root Operation.

Examples of Division are a spinal cordotomy and an osteotomy (■ Table 55-9).

Abstracting for Release (N)

The objective of the Root Operation Release is freeing a Body Part from constraint. The site of the procedure is around a Body Part.

The objective of procedures represented in the Root Operation Release is to free a Body Part from abnormal constraint. Release

Table 55-9 ■ **EXAMPLES OF THE ROOT OPERATION DIVISION (8)**

Organ System	Procedural Examples
Cardiovascular	Division of bundle of His
Digestive	Anal sphincterotomy, EGD with esophagotomy of esophagogastric junction
Musculoskeletal	Division of tendon, osteotomy
Nervous	spinal cordotomy, sacral nerve rhizotomy (*interruption of a cranial or spinal nerve root*)

Source: © PB Resources, Inc. Used with permission.

Table 55-10 ■ **EXAMPLES OF THE ROOT OPERATION RELEASE (N)**

Organ System	Procedural Examples
Cardiovascular	Mitral valvulotomy for release of fused leaflets
Digestive	Frenulotomy, lysis of peritoneal adhesions
Genitourinary	Adhesiolysis of ureter
Integumentary	Incision of scar contracture
Musculoskeletal	Ligament release, tendon release
Nervous	Carpal tunnel release

Source: © PB Resources, Inc. Used with permission.

procedures are coded to the Body Part *being freed*, not sites causing the constraint that might be cut as part of the procedure. The procedure can be performed on the area around a Body Part, on the attachments to a Body Part, or between subdivisions of a Body Part that are causing the abnormal constraint. Assign Release when the objective is to cut or separate the area *around* a Body Part, the attachments to a Body Part, or between subdivisions of a Body Part that are causing abnormal constraint. Some of the restraining tissue may be taken out but none of the Body Part is taken out.

Examples of Release are adhesiolysis, which can be performed in multiple Body Systems, and carpal tunnel release (■ Table 55-10).

> ## SUCCESS STEP
>
> Keep the ultimate objective of the procedure in mind. When one Body Part is cut to free another Body Part being constrained, the ultimate objective is freeing of the second Body Part. For example, in the procedure commonly referred to as carpal tunnel release, the transverse carpal ligament is cut to release pressure on the median nerve. Assign the Root Operation Release and the Body Part value for the median nerve.

Key Criteria for Abstracting Root Operations 8 and N

Refer to ■ Table 55-11 for more specific guidance on how to abstract procedures Involving Cutting or Separation Only and distinguish among Root Operations in this group.

Table 55-11 ■ **KEY CRITERIA FOR ABSTRACTING ROOT OPERATIONS INVOLVING CUTTING OR SEPARATION ONLY**

Question	Root Operation (Value)
Answer *Yes* to one of the following questions to help distinguish Root Operations 8 and N:	
❏ Was a Body Part cut into to separate or transect it, without draining fluids and/or gases?	Division (8)
❏ Was a Body Part freed of abnormal constraint by loosening or removing an attachment or constraint around the Body Part?	Release (N)

Source: © PB Resources, Inc. Used with permission.

Table 55-12 ■ **EXAMPLES OF THE ROOT OPERATION INSPECTION (J)**

Organ System	Procedural Examples
Digestive	Colonoscopy, esophagogastroduodenoscopy (EGD), digital rectal exam (DRE)
Genitourinary	colposcopy, transurethral diagnostic cystoscopy
Hepatobiliary	Laparotomy with palpation of liver
Musculoskeletal	Exploratory arthrotomy
Respiratory	Diagnostic laryngoscopy, sinus endoscopy

Source: © PB Resources, Inc. Used with permission.

Abstracting for Procedures Involving Examination Only

The following information summarizes the objective, definition, unique features, examples, and Key Criteria for Abstracting Root Operations for procedures involving examination only.

Abstracting for Inspection (J)

The objective of the Root Operation Inspection is visual or manual exploration. The site of the procedure is some or all of a Body Part.

Visual exploration may be performed with or without optical instrumentation. Manual exploration may be performed directly or through intervening body layers. The Root Operation Inspection represents procedures where the *sole objective* is to examine a Body Part. When examination is integral to a more definitive procedure, code only the more definitive procedure. Procedures that are discontinued without any other Root Operation being performed also are coded to Inspection.

Examples of Inspection are a diagnostic arthroscopy or exploratory laparotomy (■ TABLE 55-12).

Abstracting for Map (K)

The objective of the Root Operation Map is locating electrical impulses and/or functional areas. The site of the procedure is the brain or cardiac conduction mechanism.

Map represents a very narrow range of procedures. The Root Operation Map is applicable only to the cardiac conduction mechanism and the central nervous system.

Examples of Map are cardiac mapping and cortical mapping (■ TABLE 55-13).

Table 55-13 ■ **EXAMPLES OF THE ROOT OPERATION MAP (K)**

Organ System	Procedural Examples
Cardiovascular	Cardiac mapping during heart catheterization or open heart surgery
Nervous	Cortical mapping, mapping of basal ganglia, intraoperative whole-brain mapping

Source: © PB Resources, Inc. Used with permission.

Table 55-14 ■ **KEY CRITERIA FOR ABSTRACTING ROOT OPERATIONS INVOLVING EXAMINATION ONLY**

Question	Root Operation (Value)
Answer *Yes* to one of the following questions to help distinguish Root Operations J and K:	
❑ Was some or all of a Body Part visually or manually examined or explored?	Inspection (J)
❑ Was a brain or cardiac conduction mechanism mapped to locate electrical impulses or functional areas?	Map (K)

Source: © PB Resources, Inc. Used with permission.

Key Criteria for Abstracting Root Operations J and K

Refer to ■ TABLE 55-14 for more specific guidance on how to abstract procedures Involving Examination Only and distinguish among Root Operations in this group.

Guided Example of Abstracting for Inspection, Release, and Resection

Refer to the following example throughout this chapter to practice skills for abstracting, assigning, and arranging codes for multiple Root Operations from different groups. In this example, two Root Operations discussed in this chapter are used and one Root Operation from Chapter 52 is used.

INPATIENT HOSPITAL   Gender: F   Age: 37

Preoperative diagnosis: *acute appendicitis*

Procedure: *laparoscopic appendectomy converted to open due to extensive adhesions in abdominal cavity, requiring an additional 30 minutes to lyse. A periumbilical incision was made and the fascia was incised. The peritoneal cavity entered bluntly. A 10-mm trocar and scope was passed. Peritoneal cavity was insufflated. Five-millimeter ports placed in left lower and hypogastric areas. We were unable to visualize the appendix or most of the right lower quadrant because of extensive adhesions to the colon and peritoneum. These are likely the result of scarring after multiple surgeries 10 years ago following an automobile accident. We worked on freeing the adhesions laparoscopically until we made no further progress, then, after careful consideration, converted to an open procedure. After making a McBurney incision, we spent another 30 minutes dissecting the adhesions from the peritoneum and the right side of the large intestine until we were able to visualize and access the appendix. We proceeded to take the mesoappendix down to the base, and once the base was free, we performed simple ligation with 2-0 plain Vicryl, tying off the base twice, and removed the appendix through the wound. The wound was copiously irrigated and a layered closure was performed. Patient tolerated procedure well.*

Postoperative diagnosis: *acute appendicitis, peritoneal and intestinal adhesions*

Follow along as fictitious coder, Marcy Elwood, CCS, abstracts the procedure. Check off each step after you complete it.

▶ Marcy reads through the entire record, paying special attention to the reason for the encounter, the procedure performed, and the postoperative diagnosis. She refers to several tables of Key Criteria for Abstracting because multiple procedures are performed.

❑ She notes preoperative diagnosis: acute appendicitis.

❑ *What is the stated procedure?* appendectomy

❑ *What organ or Body Part is involved?* appendix

❑ *Is the procedure description what you would expect based on the name of the procedure?* yes

❑ *What surgical approach is used?* laparoscopic converted to open

❑ *Was more than one procedure, or a combined procedure, performed?* Yes, laparoscopic access, open appendectomy, and extensive lysis of adhesions.

❑ First, Marcy abstracts for the open appendectomy (Table 52-9).

  ▪ *Did the procedure take out some or all of a Body Part without replacement?* Yes

  ▪ *Was removal performed by cutting?* Yes

  ▪ *Was all of body part or only a portion of a body part removed?* The entire appendix was removed, and Marcy believes this will equate to all of a PCS Body Part. She will need to verify this when she refers to the PCS Tables.

  ▪ *What is the most likely Root Operation?* Resection. (Refer to Chapter 52 of this text for more information on Resection procedures.)

❑ Next, Marcy abstracts for the lysis of adhesions (Table 55-11). She believes that she can code for this procedure in addition to the appendectomy because it required substantial additional time, documented as an additional 30 minutes, and was the reason that conversion to an open procedure was necessary.

  ▪ *Did the procedure involve cutting or separation only?* Yes

  ▪ *Was a Body Part cut into to separate or transect it, without draining fluids and/or gases?* No

  ▪ *Was a Body Part freed of abnormal constraint by loosening or removing an attachment or constraint around the Body Part?* Yes

  ▪ *What is the most likely Root Operation?* Release

❑ Marcy is unsure how to code for the initial laparoscopic procedure, or whether it should be coded at all. She refers to PCS OGCR B3.2.d, which confirms that a laparoscopic procedure converted to an open procedure is coded as a percutaneous endoscopic Inspection. She verifies that this is consistent with the abstracting question for Inspection (Table 55-14).

  ▪ *Was some or all of a Body Part visually or manually examined or explored?* Yes, the peritoneal cavity was examined laparoscopically.

▶ At this time, Marcy believes that she will need three codes and use the Root Operations Inspection, Release, and Resection. She will verify this information when she refers to the PCS Tables to assign codes.

CODING PRACTICE

Exercise 55.2   Abstracting for Root Operations 9, C, F, 8, N, J, and K

Instructions: Read the mini-medical-record of each patient's encounter and answer the abstracting questions. Write the answer on the line provided. Do not assign any codes.

1. INPATIENT HOSPITAL   Gender: F   Age: 62

Preprocedure diagnosis: acute urinary retention

Procedure: Inserted Foley catheter. After prepping the patient, we identified the urinary meatus and guided the tube until urine was observed. We inflated the balloon and connected the catheter to the drainage system.

a. What is the stated procedure? _____

b. What organ or body part is involved? _____

(continued)

1. (continued)

c. What is the laterality? _____

d. Is the procedure description what you would expect based on the name of the procedure? _____

e. What surgical approach is used? _____

f. Was more than one procedure, or a combined procedure, performed? _____

g. Were gases or fluids let out from within a Body Part? _____

h. Was nonnative solid matter taken out of a Body Part? _____

i. Was nonnative solid matter within a Body Part broken into pieces? _____

j. What is the Root Operation? _____

(continued)

CODING PRACTICE (continued)

2. INPATIENT HOSPITAL   Gender: M   Age: 48

Preprocedure diagnosis: clotted AV graft

Procedure: Made a transverse incision 1 cm below the elbow crease on the right arm. The venous limb of the graft was dissected free up to the venous anastomosis.

A small incision on the graft was performed. Then a catheter was passed on the venous side. The cephalic vein was found to be obstructed about 4 cm proximal to the anastomosis. A large number of clots were extracted. After the embolectomy a good back flow from the venous side was obtained. Then the embolectomy was performed throughout the limb on the arterial side of the cephalic vein. More clots were extracted and a good arterial flow was obtained.

a. What is the stated procedure? _____

b. What organ or body part is involved? _____

c. What is the laterality? _____

d. Is the procedure description what you would expect based on the name of the procedure? _____

e. What surgical approach is used? _____

f. Was more than one procedure, or a combined procedure, performed? _____

g. Were gases or fluids let out from within a Body Part? _____

h. Was nonnative solid matter taken out of a Body Part? _____

i. Was nonnative solid matter within a Body Part broken into pieces? _____

j. What is the Root Operation? _____

3. INPATIENT HOSPITAL   Gender: F   Age: 33

Preprocedure diagnosis: carpal tunnel syndrome

Procedure: carpal tunnel release. A small incision was made over the right palm and wrist. We cut through the palmar fascia and exposed the carpal ligament. The ligament was surgically divided to release pressure on the median nerve. Care was taken to ensure safety of the median nerve and the tendons surrounding it. A layered closure was performed.

a. What is the stated procedure? _____

b. What organ or body part is involved? _____

(continued)

3. (continued)

c. What is the laterality? _____

d. Is the procedure description what you would expect based on the name of the procedure? _____

e. What surgical approach is used? _____

f. Was more than one procedure, or a combined procedure, performed? _____

g. Was a Body Part cut into in order to separate or transect it, without draining fluids and/or gases? _____

h. Was a Body Part freed of abnormal constraint by loosening or removing an attachment or constraint around the Body Part? _____

i. What is the Root Operation? _____

4. INPATIENT HOSPITAL   Gender: M   Age: 68

Preprocedure diagnosis: atrial arrhythmia

Procedure: During open heart surgery, divided the bundle of His using sharp division of the atrial septum at its attachment to the right fibrous trigone. Also performed intraoperative cardiac mapping.

a. What is the stated procedure? _____

b. What organ or body part is involved? _____

c. What is the laterality? _____

d. Is the procedure description what you would expect based on the name of the procedure? _____

e. What surgical approach is used? _____

f. Was more than one procedure, or a combined procedure, performed? _____

g. Was some or all of a Body Part visually or manually examined or explored? _____

h. Was a brain or cardiac conduction mechanism mapped to locate electrical impulses or functional areas? _____

i. Was a Body Part cut into in order to separate or transect it, without draining fluids and/or gases? _____

j. Was a Body Part freed of abnormal constraint by loosening or removing an attachment or constraint around the Body Part? _____

k. What are the Root Operations? _____

5. INPATIENT HOSPITAL   Gender: M   Age: 52

Preprocedure diagnosis: renal calculi

Procedure: ESWL. The patient was placed on a fluid-filled cushion on the treatment table. Located the calculi in both the left and right renal pelvis using fluoroscopic guidance. Directed ultrasound shock waves at the stones through the water medium, breaking up the calculi into small fragments. Patient tolerated procedure well.

a. What is the stated procedure? _____

b. What organ or body part is involved? _____

c. What is the laterality? _____

d. Is the procedure description what you would expect based on the name of the procedure? _____

e. What surgical approach is used? _____

f. Was more than one procedure, or a combined procedure, performed? _____

g. Were gases or fluids let out from within a Body Part? _____

h. Was nonnative solid matter taken out of a Body Part? _____

i. Was nonnative solid matter within a Body Part broken into pieces? _____

j. What is the Root Operation? _____

6. INPATIENT HOSPITAL   Gender: F   Age: 41

Preprocedure diagnosis: Mass in liver

Procedure: Diagnostic laparoscopy with palpation of liver, followed by open procedure to cut out a tumor from right lobe.

(continued)

6. (continued)

Postprocedure diagnosis: Focal nodular hyperplasia (FNH)

a. What is the stated procedure? _____

b. What organ or body part is involved? _____

c. What is the laterality? _____

d. Is the procedure description what you would expect based on the name of the procedure? _____

e. What surgical approach is used? _____

f. Was more than one procedure, or a combined procedure, performed? _____

g. Was some or all of a Body Part visually or manually examined or explored? _____

h. Was a brain or cardiac conduction mechanism mapped to locate electrical impulses or functional areas? _____

i. Were gases or fluids let out from within a Body Part? _____

j. Was nonnative solid matter taken out of a Body Part? _____

k. Was nonnative solid matter within a Body Part broken into pieces? _____

l. Did the procedure take out some or all of a Body Part without replacement? _____

m. Was removal performed by cutting? _____

n. Was all of body part or only a portion of a body part removed? _____

o. What are the Root Operations? _____

Tip: This scenario requires a Root Operation discussed in a previous chapter of this text.

ASSIGNING CHARACTERS 4–7 FOR ROOT OPERATIONS 9, C, F, 8, N, J, AND K

To assign codes after the Root Operation is determined, search the PCS Index for the name of the Root Operation as the Main Term. Locate the subterm(s) for the correct anatomic site and identify the PCS Table. When you locate the PCS Table, verify the first three characters of the code, then locate the row with the appropriate Body Part. Assign the remaining characters from each respective column of the Table. The following information summarizes and highlights unique information for working with the Tables for the Root Operations discussed in this chapter. Each Root Operation has one Table in each applicable PCS Body System. Because of the differences between organ systems, Table details vary.

Character 4: Body Part

Character 4, Body Part, is usually identified in the Index, but it is important to verify it in the PCS Table as well. PCS OGCR provide guidelines for reporting of the Body Part for the Root Operations Inspection, Release, and Division. Some Body Parts may appear in more than one row of a Table, in which case Characters 5 to 7 must also be reviewed to select the correct row. For example, in some Tables, certain combinations of Character 6 and Character 7 cannot be used in the same code, so the valid combinations for these characters appear in different rows, but with the same Body Part values for Character 4. This occurs with the Root Operation Drainage because a drainage procedure can have a drainage device (Character 6) or be diagnostic in nature (Character 7), but one procedure cannot meet both criteria. (Refer back to Figure 51-6 for an example.)

Inspection Procedures

When the Root Operations Inspection, Excision, or Repair are performed on overlapping layers of the musculoskeletal system, code the Body Part that identifies the deepest layer (PCS OGCR B3.5).

When a Body Part is inspected as part of a larger procedure with a specific objective, the inspection—usually endoscopy—is included in the broader procedure and is not coded separately (PCS OGCR B3.11a). For example, when fiber-optic bronchoscopy is performed for irrigation of bronchus, code only the irrigation procedure with the Approach value Via natural or artificial opening endoscopic. Do not assign a separate code for the Root Operation Inspection.

When multiple tubular Body Parts are inspected, code the most distal Body Part inspected (PCS OGCR B3.11b). For example, a cystoureteroscopy with inspection of bladder and ureters is coded to the Body Part value for the ureter. This requires anatomic knowledge of the relationship of the bladder and ureters. When multiple nontubular Body Parts in a region are inspected, code the Body Part that specifies the entire area inspected. This may require use of the one of the Body System values for Anatomical Regions (W, X, or Y), rather than a specific organ system.

> **SUCCESS STEP**
>
> An exploratory laparotomy with examination of the general abdominal contents is coded to the Root Operation Inspection and the Body Part value Peritoneal Cavity (G). This Body Part belongs to the Body System Anatomical Regions, General (W).

Release Procedures

In the Root Operation Release, assign the Body Part value for the Body Part being freed, not the tissue being manipulated or cut to free the Body Part (PCS OGCR B3.13). For example, lysis of intestinal adhesions uses the Body Part value for the intestine.

Character 5: Approach

PCS OGCR provide guidelines for using Character 5, Approach, with Root Operations in this chapter.

- Procedures performed percutaneously via a device placed for the procedure are coded to the Approach Percutaneous (PCS OGCR B5.4) (■ FIGURE 55-4).

- Both an Inspection procedure and another procedure might be performed on the same Body Part during the same operative episode. Code the Inspection procedure separately when it is performed using a different Approach than the other procedure (PCS OGCR B3.11c) (■ FIGURE 55-5).

> Surgeon places a percutaneous nephrostomy tube into the left kidney to crush calculi.
>
> **0TF43ZZ [Medical and Surgical, Urinary System], Fragmentation, Kidney pelvis left, Percutaneous, No device, No qualifier**

Figure 55-4 ■ Example of Coding Percutaneous Device Placement. *Source:* © *PB Resources, Inc. Used with permission.*

> Surgeon performs a duodenoscopy followed by an open excision of a portion of the duodenum.
>
> **0DB90ZZ [Medical and Surgical, Gastrointestinal System], Excision, Duodenum, Open, No device, No qualifier**
> **0WJP8ZZ [Medical and Surgical, Anatomical Regions General], Inspection, Gastrointestinal tract, Via natural or artificial opening endoscopic, No device, No qualifier**

Figure 55-5 ■ Example of Coding Inspection Followed by Excision. *Source:* © *PB Resources, Inc. Used with permission.*

Character 6: Device

When a separate procedure is performed to put in a drainage device, assign the Root Operation Drainage with the value Drainage Device for Character 6 (PCS OGCR B6.2).

The Root Operations Division, Release, Map, Inspection, Extirpation, and Fragmentation do not use Character 6 Device.

Character 7: Qualifier

The Root Operations Release and Extirpation use the Qualifier with the Body System Mouth and Throat to identify the number of teeth treated.

The Root Operation Drainage uses the qualifier Diagnostic (X) to identify Drainage procedures that are biopsies (PCS OGCR B3.4a) (■ FIGURE 55-6).

The Root Operations Division, Map, Inspection, and Fragmentation do not use Character 7 Qualifier.

> **CODING CAUTION**
>
> A Drainage procedure can have a Drainage Device (0) for Character 6 or a Diagnostic (X) qualifier for Character 7, but not both. These values appear in separate rows of the PCS Table, so be sure to locate the correct row.

Guided Example of Assigning Characters 4–7 for Inspection, Release, and Resection

To practice skills for assigning codes for the Root Operations Inspection, Release, and Resection, continue with the example from earlier in the chapter about the patient who was seen for an appendectomy. Follow along in your ICD-10-PCS manual as Marcy Elwood, CCS, assigns codes. Check off each step after you complete it.

> Surgeon performs a diagnostic fine needle aspiration of the upper lobe of the right lung.
>
> **0B9C3ZX [Medical and Surgical, Respiratory System], Drainage, Upper lung lobe right, Percutaneous, No device, Diagnostic**

Figure 55-6 ■ Example of Coding a Diagnostic Drainage Procedure. *Source:* © *PB Resources, Inc. Used with permission.*

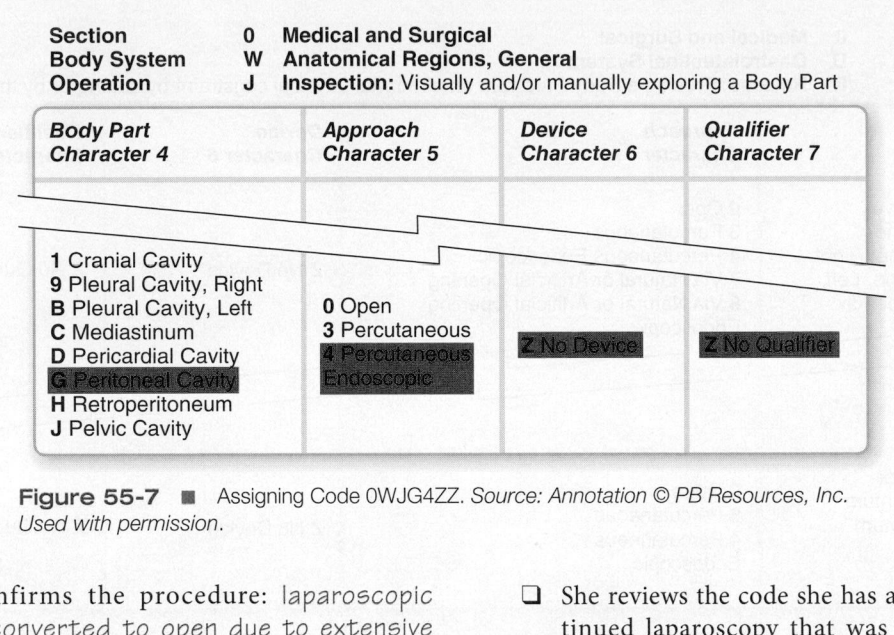

Section	0	Medical and Surgical
Body System	W	Anatomical Regions, General
Operation	J	Inspection: Visually and/or manually exploring a Body Part

Body Part Character 4	Approach Character 5	Device Character 6	Qualifier Character 7
1 Cranial Cavity 9 Pleural Cavity, Right B Pleural Cavity, Left C Mediastinum D Pericardial Cavity G Peritoneal Cavity H Retroperitoneum J Pelvic Cavity	0 Open 3 Percutaneous 4 Percutaneous Endoscopic	Z No Device	Z No Qualifier

Figure 55-7 ■ Assigning Code 0WJG4ZZ. *Source: Annotation © PB Resources, Inc. Used with permission.*

▶ First, Marcy confirms the procedure: laparoscopic appendectomy converted to open due to extensive adhesions.

❑ The Root Operation for the laparoscopic access is Inspection.

❑ The Root Operation for the adhesiolysis is Release.

❑ The Root Operation for the open appendectomy is Resection. If only a portion of a PCS Body Part was removed, she would use the Root Operation Excision.

▶ Marcy searches the Index for the Main Term **Inspection** for the laparoscopic access.

❑ She locates first-level subterm for **Abdominal Wall** but not *abdominal cavity*. The site inspected is not the abdominal wall, so she searches further and locates a first-level subterm for **Peritoneal Cavity**.

❑ She identifies the Table **0WJ** and partial code **0WJG**.

▶ Marcy turns to Table **0WJ** to assign the code for Inspection of the peritoneal cavity.

❑ She reads the Table title **0WJ, Medical and Surgical, Anatomical Regions General, Inspection** and confirms that this accurately describes the Body System and Root Operation.

❑ Marcy assigns the value for Character 4, Body Part.

▪ She reviews the values provided and confirms that **G Peritoneal cavity**, which was part of the partial code **0WJG** provided in the Index, is correct.

❑ Marcy assigns the value for Character 5, Approach.

▪ The Root Operation Inspection is used to identify the initial laparoscopic approach that was discontinued, so she assigns **4 Percutaneous endoscopic**.

❑ Marcy assigns the value **Z No device** for Character 6, Device.

❑ Marcy assigns the value **Z No qualifier** for Character 7, Qualifier.

❑ She reviews the code she has assigned for the discontinued laparoscopy that was converted: **0WJG4ZZ** (■ FIGURE 55-7).

▶ Marcy searches the Index for the Main Term **Release** for adhesiolysis.

❑ She refers to the documentation to confirm that two sites were documented for the adhesions, *extensive adhesions to the right side of the colon and peritoneum,* so she will need to locate subterms and assign codes for each site. If the adhesions had been documented as adhered to the appendix only, she would have selected a subterm for the appendix.

❑ She locates the first-level subterm **Peritoneum**.

❑ She identifies the Table **0DN** and partial code **0DNW**.

❑ She locates the first-level subterm **Large Intestine, Right**.

❑ She identifies the Table **0DN** and partial code **0DNF**.

▶ Marcy turns to Table **0DN** to assign the code for adhesiolysis.

❑ She reads the Table title **0DN, Medical and Surgical, Gastrointestinal System, Release: Freeing a Body Part from an abnormal physical constraint by cutting or by the use of force** and confirms that this accurately describes the Body System and Root Operation.

❑ She assigns the value **W Peritoneum** for Character 4, Body Part, which is consistent with the partial code **0DNW** provided in the Index.

❑ She assigns the value **0 Open** for Character 5, Approach. Although some lysis was performed laparoscopically, the significant portion was performed after the open procedure was initiated.

❑ She assigns the value **Z No device** for Character 6, Device.

❑ She assigns the value **Z No qualifier** for Character 7, Qualifier.

Section	0	Medical and Surgical
Body System	D	Gastrointestinal System
Operation	N	Release: Freeing a Body Part from an abnormal physical constraint by cutting or by the use of force

Body Part Character 4	Approach Character 5	Device Character 6	Qualifier Character 7
C Ileocecal Valve E Large Intestine F Large Intestine, Right G Large Intestine, Left H Cecum J Appendix	0 Open 3 Percutaneous 4 Percutaneous Endoscopic 7 Via Natural or Artificial Opening 8 Via Natural or Artificial Opening Endoscopic	Z No Device	Z No Qualifier
R Anal Sphincter S Greater Omentum T Lesser Omentum V Mesentery W Peritoneum	0 Open 3 Percutaneous 4 Percutaneous Endoscopic	Z No Device	Z No Qualifier

Figure 55-8 ■ Assigning Codes 0DNF0ZZ and 0DNW0ZZ. *Source: Annotation © PB Resources, Inc. Used with permission.*

❑ She reviews the code she has assigned for adhesiolysis of the peritoneum: **0DNW0ZZ** (■ FIGURE 55-8, lower row).

▶ Marcy uses the same table to assign the code for lysis of the intestinal adhesions.

❑ She assigns the value **F Large Intestine, Right** for Character 4, Body Part, which is consistent with the partial code **0DNF** provided in the Index.

  ■ She notices that this Body Part value appears in a different row of the Table than the value for the peritoneum. She determines this is because the procedures for the Body Parts in this row can be performed by Approaches not available in the row with the peritoneum. Specifically, the Body Parts in this row can be accessed using Via Natural or Artificial Opening (7) or Via Natural or Artificial Opening Endoscopic (8).

❑ The other values of the code are the same as those for the peritoneal adhesiolysis:

  ■ **0 Open** for Character 5, Approach

  ■ **Z No device** for Character 6, Device

  ■ **Z No qualifier** for Character 7, Qualifier

❑ She reviews the code she has assigned for adhesiolysis of the large intestine: **0DNF0ZZ** (Figure 55-8, upper row).

▶ Marcy searches the Index for the Main Term **Resection** for the open appendectomy.

❑ She locates the first-level subterm **Appendix**.

❑ She identifies the Table **0DT** and partial code **0DTJ**.

▶ Marcy turns to Table **0DT** to assign the code for the open appendectomy.

❑ She reads the Table title **0DT, Medical and Surgical, Gastrointestinal System, Resection: Cutting out or off, without replacement, all of a Body Part** and

confirms that this accurately describes the Body System and Root Operation.

❑ Marcy assigns the value **J Appendix** for Character 4, Body Part.

  ■ If only a portion of a Body Part had been removed, she would need to use the Root Operation Excision. However, the entire appendix was removed and it would be extremely rare for only part of the appendix to be removed.

❑ Marcy assigns the value **0 Open** for Character 5, Approach, because the Resection was performed after the procedure was converted to an open approach.

❑ Marcy assigns the value **Z No device** for Character 6, Device.

❑ Marcy assigns the value **Z No qualifier** for Character 7, Qualifier.

❑ She reviews the code she has assigned for the open appendectomy: **0DTJ0ZZ** (■ FIGURE 55-9).

▶ Marcy reviews the procedure codes she has assigned for this case.

❑ **0DNW0ZZ** Medical and Surgical, Gastrointestinal system, Release, Peritoneum, Open, No device, No qualifier

❑ **0DNF0ZZ** Medical and Surgical, Gastrointestinal system, Release, Large intestine right, Open, No device, No qualifier

❑ **0WJG4ZZ** Medical and Surgical, Anatomical regions, General, Inspection, Peritoneal cavity, Percutaneous endoscopic, No device, No qualifier

❑ **0DTJ0ZZ** Medical and Surgical, Gastrointestinal system, Resection, Appendix, Open, No device, No qualifier

▶ Next, Marcy must determine how to sequence the codes.

Section	0	Medical and Surgical
Body System	D	Gastrointestinal System
Operation	T	Resection: Cutting out or off, without replacement, all of a Body Part

Body Part Character 4	Approach Character 5	Device Character 6	Qualifier Character 7
F Large Intestine, Right G Large Intestine, Left H Cecum J Appendix K Ascending Colon L Transverse Colon M Descending Colon N Sigmoid Colon P Rectum Q Anus	0 Open 3 Percutaneous 4 Percutaneous Endoscopic 7 Via Natural or Artificial Opening 8 Via Natural or Artificial Opening Endoscopic	Z No Device	Z No Qualifier

Figure 55-9 ■ Assigning Code 0DTJ0ZZ. *Source: Annotation © PB Resources, Inc. Used with permission.*

CODING PRACTICE

Exercise 55.3 Assigning Characters 4–7 for Root Operations 9, C, F, 8, N, J, and K

Instructions: Read the mini-medical-record of each patient's encounter. Review the information abstracted in Exercise 55.2 for questions 1–3. For questions 4–6, abstract the case on your own. Assign PCS codes using the Index and Tables. Write the code(s) on the line provided.

---

1. INPATIENT HOSPITAL Gender: F Age: 62

Preprocedure diagnosis: acute urinary retention

Procedure: Inserted Foley catheter. After prepping the patient, we identified the urinary meatus and guided the tube until urine was observed. We inflated the balloon and connected the catheter to the drainage system.

1 PCS Code _____

---

2. INPATIENT HOSPITAL Gender: M Age: 48

Preprocedure diagnosis: clotted AV graft

Procedure: Made a transverse incision 1 cm below the elbow crease on the right arm. The venous limb of the graft was dissected free up to the venous anastomosis.

(continued)

---

2. (continued)

A small incision on the graft was performed. Then a catheter was passed on the venous side. The cephalic vein was found obstructed about 4 cm proximal to the anastomosis. A large number of clots were extracted. After the embolectomy a good back flow from the venous side was obtained. Then the embolectomy was performed throughout the limb on the arterial side of the cephalic vein. More clots were extracted and a good arterial flow was obtained.

1 PCS Code _____

---

3. INPATIENT HOSPITAL Gender: F Age: 33

Preprocedure diagnosis: carpal tunnel syndrome

Procedure: carpal tunnel release. A small incision was made over the right palm and wrist. We cut through the palmar fascia and exposed the carpal ligament. The ligament was surgically divided to release pressure on the median nerve. Care was taken to ensure safety of the median nerve and the tendons surrounding it. A layered closure was performed.

Tip: The Body Part value identifies the structure released, not the structure cut to obtain the release.

1 PCS Code _____

(continued)

CODING PRACTICE (continued)

4. INPATIENT HOSPITAL Gender: F Age: 54

Preprocedure diagnosis: *chronic plantar fasciitis*

Procedure: *open plantar fasciotomy, right foot. Blunt dissection was carried out to expose the deep fascia and the medial plantar fascial band. Transection of the medial two-thirds of the plantar fascia band began at the junction of the deep fascia of the abductor hallucis muscle belly and medial plantar fascial band, extending to the lateral two-thirds of the band. Visualization and finger probe confirmed adequate transection.*

1 PCS Code _____

5. INPATIENT HOSPITAL Gender: F Age: 4

Preprocedure diagnosis: *father noticed child placing an object into her nose*

(continued)

5. (continued)

Procedure: *removal of foreign body in right nostril. Under mild sedation, a pebble was removed from her nasal passage.*

1 PCS Code _____

6. INPATIENT HOSPITAL Gender: F Age: 34

Preprocedure diagnosis: *recurrent right lower extremity soft-tissue infection, diabetes*

Procedure: *incision and drainage of right lower extremity soft-tissue abscess. The old incision was elongated. Loculations of fibrous tissue were broken up. Seropurulent, somewhat bloody fluid was noted. The infection appeared contained to a golf ball–sized area in the subcutaneous tissues above the fascia. The area was cleaned and the wound packed.*

1 PCS Code _____

ARRANGING CODES FOR ROOT OPERATIONS 9, C, F, 8, N, J, AND K

When arranging PCS codes, remember to sequence codes based on the Uniform Hospital Data Discharge Set (UHDDS) definition of the principal procedure, not on the order in which the procedures were performed. Consider the following situations discussed earlier in this chapter:

- When a laparoscopic procedure is converted to an open procedure, sequence the open procedure first because it is most directly related to the principal diagnosis.

- When multiple procedures are performed at the same operative session, sequence the principal procedure as the one most related to the principal diagnosis. In this chapter, procedures such as those classified by the Root Operation Map might be secondary procedures in addition to the principal procedure.

- Division of the bundle of His during open heart surgery could be a principal or secondary procedure, depending on the principal diagnosis and the reason the open heart surgery is performed. However, it is unlikely that open heart surgery is performed primarily to divide the bundle of His because it can also be done using a Percutaneous Endoscopic Approach.

- When a biopsy is followed by a more definitive procedure, sequence the more definitive treatment as the principal diagnosis.

- Adhesiolysis is often performed to reach an organ for a definitive procedure, so when this occurs, sequence adhesiolysis as a secondary procedure.

Also keep in mind when multiple procedures should *not* be coded:

- A procedure, such as endoscopy, is done as part of the objective of a more definitive procedure.

- Fragmentation and Extirpation of the same solid matter should not be coded together because they are mutually exclusive. For example, if calculi are crushed, then extracted, code only Extirpation, not Fragmentation. Code Fragmentation only when the solid matter remains in the body after the procedure.

- Code only the deepest tissue layer when multiple layers are accessed in one operation.

Guided Example of Arranging Codes for Inspection, Release, and Resection

To practice skills for arranging codes for the Root Operations Inspection, Release, and Resection, continue with the example from earlier in the chapter about the patient who was seen for an appendectomy. Follow along in your ICD-10-PCS manual as Marcy Elwood, CCS, arranges the codes. Check off each step after you complete it.

▶ First, Marcy confirms laparoscopic appendectomy converted to open due to extensive adhesions and reviews the codes she has assigned.

❑ **0DNW0ZZ Medical and Surgical, Gastrointestinal system, Release, Peritoneum, Open, No device, No qualifier**

❑ **0DNF0ZZ** Medical and Surgical, Gastrointestinal system, Release, Large intestine right, Open, No device, No qualifier

❑ **0WJG4ZZ** Medical and Surgical, Anatomical regions, General, Inspection, Peritoneal cavity, Percutaneous endoscopic, No device, No qualifier

❑ **0DTJ0ZZ** Medical and Surgical, Gastrointestinal system, Resection, Appendix, Open, No device, No qualifier

▶ The principal procedure must be the one most closely related to the principal diagnosis, *acute appendicitis*, so Marcy sequences code **0DTJ0ZZ** for Resection of the appendix first.

▶ Marcy sequences codes **0DNW0ZZ** and **0DNF0ZZ** for Release of the adhesions second and third because they are related to the secondary diagnosis and are the reason the procedure was converted from laparoscopic to open. It does not matter which of these codes appears before the other.

▶ Marcy sequences code **0WJG4ZZ** for Inspection of the peritoneal cavity fourth.

▶ Marcy finalizes the procedure codes and sequencing for this case:

(1) **0DTJ0ZZ** Medical and Surgical, Gastrointestinal system, Resection, Appendix, Open, No device, No qualifier

(2) **0DNW0ZZ** Medical and Surgical, Gastrointestinal system, Release, Peritoneum, Open, No device, No qualifier

(3) **0DNF0ZZ** Medical and Surgical, Gastrointestinal system, Release, Large intestine right, Open, No device, No qualifier

(4) **0WJG4ZZ** Medical and Surgical, Anatomical regions, General, Inspection, Peritoneal cavity, Percutaneous endoscopic, No device, No qualifier

▶ Marcy also assigns and sequences the ICD-10-CM diagnosis codes that support the need for the service.

(1) **K35.80** Unspecified acute appendicitis

(2) **K66.0** Peritoneal adhesions (postprocedural) (postinfection)

CODING PRACTICE

Exercise 55.4 Arranging Codes for Root Operations 9, C, F, 8, N, J, and K

Instructions: Read the mini-medical-record of each patient's encounter. Review the information abstracted in Exercise 55.2 for questions 1–3. For questions 4–6, abstract the case on your own. Assign PCS codes using the Index and Tables, and arrange the codes in proper sequence. Write the code(s) on the line provided.

1. INPATIENT HOSPITAL Gender: M Age: 68

Preprocedure diagnosis: atrial arrhythmia

Procedure: During open heart surgery, divided the bundle of His using sharp division of the atrial septum at its attachment to the right fibrous trigone. Also performed intraoperative cardiac mapping.

Tip: The bundle of His is a conduction mechanism.

2 PCS Codes _____

2. INPATIENT HOSPITAL Gender: M Age: 52

Preprocedure diagnosis: renal calculi

Procedure: ESWL. The patient was placed on a fluid-filled cushion on the treatment table. Located the calculi in both the left and right renal pelvis using fluoroscopic guidance. Directed ultrasound shock waves at the stones through the water medium, breaking up the calculi into small fragments. Patient tolerated procedure well.

2 PCS Codes _____

3. INPATIENT HOSPITAL Gender: F Age: 41

Preprocedure diagnosis: Mass in liver

Procedure: Diagnostic laparoscopy with palpation of liver, followed by open procedure to cut out a tumor from right lobe.

Postprocedure diagnosis: Focal nodular hyperplasia (FNH)

2 PCS Codes _____

(continued)

CODING PRACTICE *(continued)*

4. INPATIENT HOSPITAL Gender: M Age: 44

Preprocedure diagnosis: chronic subcutaneous abscess of a midline wound, large left thigh lipoma.

Procedure: excision of chronic abscess pocket in the subxiphoid region of the epigastrium; excision of left thigh lipoma. Incision was made at the level of the skin around the chronic abscess cavity. Dissection was carried down to the subcutaneous tissue. The abscess cavity appeared to have been excised in its entirety. We decided to leave a drain in this time to see if it would prevent recurrence. Following this a skin incision was made overlying the lipoma. Dissection was carried down the subcutaneous tissue and the lipoma excised intact.

2 PCS Codes _____

5. INPATIENT HOSPITAL Gender: M Age: 54

Preprocedure diagnosis: proximal interphalangeal (PIP) joint flexion contracture of 30°, right little finger; metacarpophalangeal (MCP) joint contracture of 50°, right ring finger.

(continued)

5. (continued)

Procedure: PIP joint release, right little finger, followed by MCP joint release, right ring finger. The palmar fascia was exposed and carefully separated from nerves, arteries, and tendons. Special care was taken not to damage the nearby nerves and blood vessels. The fibrous tissue was dissected free at the PIP joint of the little finger and the MCP joint of the ring finger.

2 PCS Codes _____

6. INPATIENT HOSPITAL Gender: M Age: 44

Preprocedure diagnosis: ureteral calculi, bilateral

Procedure: ESWL bilateral ureters. The patient was treated at a power setting of 7 and 8 for total of 2500 shocks delivered to all areas of the stone in the right ureter. The procedure was repeated on the left. There appeared to be good fragmentation of the stone.

Tip: Refer to PCS OGCR B3.2, multiple procedures, for guidance.

2 PCS Codes _____

CHAPTER SUMMARY

In this chapter you learned that:

- The Medical and Surgical Root Operations in the group *Procedures that Take Out Solids/Fluids/Gases from a Body Part* are Root Operations Drainage (9), Extirpation (C), and Fragmentation (F).

- The Root Operation Drainage (9) is taking or letting out fluids and/or gases from a Body Part.

- The Root Operation Extirpation (C) is taking or cutting out solid matter from a Body Part.

- The Root Operation Fragmentation (F) is breaking solid matter in a Body Part into pieces.

- The Medical and Surgical Root Operations in the group *Procedures Involving Cutting or Separation Only* are Division (8) and Release (N).

- The Root Operation Division (8) is cutting into a Body Part, without draining fluids and/or gases from the Body Part, in order to separate or transect a Body Part.

- The Root Operation Release (N) is freeing a Body Part from an abnormal physical constraint by cutting or by the use of force.

- The Medical and Surgical Root Operations in the group *Procedures Involving Examination Only* are Inspection (J) and Map (K).

- The Root Operation Inspection (J) is visually and/or manually exploring a Body Part.

- The Root Operation Map (K) is locating the route of passage of electrical impulses and/or locating functional areas in a Body Part.

- When a Body Part is inspected as part of a larger procedure with a specific objective, the inspection is included in the broader procedure and is not coded separately.

- In the Root Operation Release, assign the Body Part value for the Body Part being freed, not the tissue being manipulated or cut to free the Body Part.

- When an Inspection procedure and another procedure are performed on the same Body Part during the same operative episode, assign a separate code for the Inspection procedure when it is performed using a different Approach.

- PCS provides guidelines regarding coding biopsies using the Root Operation Drainage and also clarifies the difference between the Root Operation Release and Division. Other references to Root Operation in this chapter appear throughout PCS OGCR.

CONCEPT QUIZ

Take a moment to look back at Root Operations 9, C, F, N, 8, J, and K and solidify your skills. Try to answer the questions from memory first, then refer to the discussion in this chapter if you need a little extra help.

Completion

Instructions: Write the term that answers each question based on the information you learned in this chapter. Choose from the list below. Some choices may be used more than once and some choices may not be used at all.

Division	Fragmentation
Drainage	Inspection
Extirpation	Release

1. The Root Operation _____ is taking or letting out fluids and/or gases from a Body Part.

2. The Root Operation _____ is visually and/or manually exploring a Body Part.

3. The Root Operation _____ is cutting into a Body Part, without draining fluids and/or gases from the Body Part, in order to separate or transect a Body Part.

4. The Root Operation _____ is sometimes described by the suffix *-lysis.*

5. The Root Operation _____ is taking or cutting out solid matter from a Body Part.

6. The Root Operation _____ is sometimes described by the suffix *-centesis.*

7. The Root Operation _____ Is sometImes described by the medical term *lithotripsy.*

8. The Root Operation _____ is breaking solid matter in a Body Part into pieces.

9. The Root Operation _____ is locating the route of passage of electrical impulses and/or locating functional areas in a Body Part.

10. The Root Operation _____ is freeing a Body Part from an abnormal physical constraint by cutting or by the use of force.

Multiple Choice

Instructions: Circle the letter of the best answer to each question based on the information you learned in this chapter.

1. Which Root Operation discussed in this chapter uses the Qualifier Diagnostic (X) for biopsies?
   A. Drainage
   B. Inspection
   C. Extirpation
   D. Release

2. What code(s) should be assigned when the intended Root Operation is attempted using one Approach but is discontinued and converted to a different Approach?

A. Assign only a code for the procedure completed.
B. Assign only a code for the procedure intended.
C. Assign separate procedure codes for each Approach.
D. Assign a code for the procedure completed and Character 7, Qualifier, to identify the discontinued procedure.

3. What Body Part value is assigned for an exploratory laparotomy with examination of the general abdominal contents?
   A. Abdominal wall
   B. Peritoneal cavity
   C. Thoracic cavity
   D. Abdominal cavity

4. Which Root Operation discussed in this chapter uses Character 6, Device?
   A. Fragmentation
   B. Drainage
   C. Extirpation
   D. Inspection

5. Which Root Operation discussed in this chapter uses the Qualifier with the Body System Mouth and Throat to identify the number of teeth treated?
   A. Extirpation
   B. Fragmentation
   C. Inspection
   D. Division

6. What Root Operation is assigned when a procedure is begun but discontinued before any other Root Operation is performed?
   A. Extirpation
   B. Discontinuation
   C. Map
   D. Inspection

7. What anatomic site determines the Body Part value in the Root Operation Release?
   A. The site removed
   B. The site causing constraint
   C. The site cut or transected
   D. The site being freed

8. Which two Root Operations are mutually exclusive and should not be coded together?
   A. Inspection and Extirpation
   B. Map and Inspection
   C. Fragmentation and Extirpation
   D. Extirpation and Division

9. Which Root Operation is used to report removal of a tumor?
   A. Excision
   B. Release
   C. Extirpation
   D. Fragmentation

(continued)

(continued from page 1107)

10. What Body Part value should be assigned when the Root Operation Inspection is performed on overlapping layers of the musculoskeletal system?

A. Assign a Body Part value for multiple sites.

B. Assign separate codes with different Body Part values for each layer accessed.

C. Assign a Body Part value for the first layer accessed.

D. Assign a Body Part value for the deepest layer reached.

CODING CHALLENGE

Instructions: Read the mini-medical-record of each patient's encounter, then abstract, assign, and arrange ICD-10-CM diagnosis codes and PCS procedure codes using the appropriate Index and Tables. Write the code(s) on the line provided.

---

1. INPATIENT HOSPITAL   Gender: M   Age: 52

Preprocedure diagnosis: left patellar chondromalacia, bilateral osteoarthritis of hips

Procedure: left knee arthroscopy with lateral capsular release. After inflation of the tourniquet, ports were placed. Visualization of patellofemoral joint revealed type 2 chondromalacia with slight lateral subluxation. The anteromedial portal was used to identify the lateral capsule and it was released using the Excise PDW Plasma Wand. Instruments were removed, portals closed, and the tourniquet released.

2 ICD-10-CM Codes _____

1 ICD-10-PCS Code _____

---

2. INPATIENT HOSPITAL   Gender: F   Age: 74

Preprocedure diagnosis: left malignant pleural effusion secondary to a left lung adenocarcinoma

Procedure: thoracentesis at bedside. After infiltrating the skin with an anesthetic, an incision was made below the 6th rib and meticulously dissected to the pleural space. A serosanguineous effusion was encountered and a Yankauer suction tip used to drain the fluid. A portable chest X-ray showed a significant decrease in the effusion.

2 ICD-10-CM Codes _____

1 ICD-10-PCS Code _____

---

3. INPATIENT HOSPITAL   Gender: F   Age: 59

Preprocedure diagnosis: streptococcal cellulitis, left foot, status post left foot incision and drainage, status post left foot Austin bunionectomy

(continued)

---

3. (continued)

Procedure: left foot, incision and drainage and delayed primary closure. The two sutures at the previous incision site were removed and the site opened. The incision was deepened and frank purulence noted at the fascia level. This was drained and the incision irrigated. We decided to leave the wound open to try clear this infection up.

3 ICD-10-CM Codes _____

_____

1 ICD-10-PCS Code _____

---

4. INPATIENT HOSPITAL   Gender: M   Age: 70

Preprocedure diagnosis: carotid artery stenosis, 80% on right and 50% on left, ASHD, hypertension

Procedure: right common carotid artery endarterectomy. Incision made on the right side of the neck to expose the carotid artery. The artery was clamped above the blocked area and the area incised. The plaque was removed from the artery and the artery closed. Clamp released, showing excellent flow. The neck incision was closed and the patient taken to the recovery room.

3 ICD-10-CM Codes _____

_____

1 ICD-10-PCS Code _____

---

5. INPATIENT HOSPITAL   Gender: F   Age: 53

Preprocedure diagnosis: surveillance EGD for history of esophageal cancer, surveillance colonoscopy for history of adenomatous colonic polyps

Procedure: esophagogastroduodenoscopy, colonoscopy with polypectomy. The endoscope was passed through the oral cavity under direct visualization and advanced to the second portion of the duodenum. Findings are consistent with esophagectomy colonic transposition. The patient was turned and an Olympus colonoscope was passed through the anal verge under direct

(continued)

5. (continued)

visualization. Cecum, ascending and descending colon revealed melanosis coli. Two sessile polyps of the transverse colon were removed by cold forceps and sent to pathology.

Postprocedure diagnosis: diffuse melanosis coli, transverse colon polyps, no abnormal findings on EGD

Tip: Select the principal procedure using the PCS OGCR D.

5 ICD-10-CM Codes _____

_____

2 ICD-10-PCS Codes _____

---

6. INPATIENT HOSPITAL   Gender: F   Age: 9

Preprocedure diagnosis: chronic adenotonsillitis and ankyloglossia

Procedure: adenoidectomy and tonsillectomy, lingual frenotomy. Metzenbaum scissors were used to free the lingual frenulum. The right tonsil was freed from the anterior pillar and posterior pillar and amputated at the same plane as the tongue base. An adenoid curet was used to remove the adenoid tissue. The same procedure was repeated on the left. Hemostasis was achieved and patient was extubated.

Tip: Combination codes are coded separately.

2 ICD-10-CM Codes _____

3 ICD-10-PCS Codes _____

_____

---

7. INPATIENT HOSPITAL   Gender: F   Age: 60

Preprocedure diagnosis: acquired chronic subglottic stenosis from endotracheal intubation

Procedure: fiberoptic bronchoscopy. The bronchoscope was inserted orally and we could see scar tissue and narrowing of the upper trachea just below the vocal cords in the subglottic area. No abnormalities seen of the carina, right upper, middle and lower lobe bronchi; left main stem bronchus and upper and lower lobe bronchi. No specimens were collected. Patient tolerated the procedure well.

1 ICD-10-CM Code _____

1 ICD-10-PCS Code _____

---

8. INPATIENT HOSPITAL   Gender: F   Age: 27

Preprocedure diagnosis: chronic anal fissure with persistent pain and bleeding, old anal sphincter tear

Procedure: lateral internal sphincterotomy. A linear incision was made from the dentate line to just beyond the anal verge. The dissection was carried out until the internal sphincter and a few fibers of the external sphincter were exposed. Under direct vision, the full thickness of the internal sphincter was divided from the level of the dentate line distally. The incision was closed with a 3-0 chromic catgut suture.

2 ICD-10-CM Codes _____

1 ICD-10-PCS Code _____

---

9. INPATIENT HOSPITAL   Gender: M   Age: 8

Preprocedure diagnosis: spastic cerebral palsy, dysarthria

Procedure: selective dorsal rhizotomy. The spinous processes and a portion of the lamina were removed to expose the spinal cord and spinal nerves at L1. The sensory nerves were exposed and tested with EMG. The severely abnormal roots were cut between L1 and S1/S2. The dura was closed and tissue layers closed up to the skin, which was closed with glue.

Tip: Procedural steps necessary to reach the operative site are not coded separately (PCS OGCR B3.1b).

2 ICD-10-CM Codes _____

1 ICD-10-PCS Code _____

---

10. INPATIENT HOSPITAL   Gender: M   Age: 3

Preprocedure diagnosis: esophageal foreign body; patient swallowed a quarter, which lodged in his esophagus, and is having difficulty breathing

Procedure: esophagoscopy with removal of foreign body. A flexible EGD was performed under general anesthesia. The quarter was seen at the mid esophagus and removed with a grasper. The patient tolerated the procedure well.

1 ICD-10-CM Code _____

1 ICD-10-PCS Code _____

KEEP ON CODING

Instructions: Read the procedural statement, then use the appropriate Index and Tables to assign PCS procedure codes. Write the code(s) on the line provided.

1. Drainage of right knee fluid, percutaneous: ICD-10-PCS Code(s) _____

2. Endoscopic left internal carotid endarterectomy: ICD-10-PCS Code(s) _____

3. Extracorporeal shockwave lithotripsy (ESWL) of calculus in right ureter: ICD-10-PCS Code(s) _____

4. Tarsal tunnel release, right, endoscopic: ICD-10-PCS Code(s) _____

5. Open trigeminal neurotomy: ICD-10-PCS Code(s) _____

6. Arthroscopic examination of left ankle: ICD-10-PCS Code(s) _____

7. Craniotomy with brain mapping: ICD-10-PCS Code(s) _____

8. Percutaneous drainage of left knee bursa: ICD-10-PCS Code(s) _____

9. Cystoscopy with left ureteral stone basketing of ureteral calculi: ICD-10-PCS Code(s) _____

10. Endoscopic lithotripsy of common bile duct stone with access through the upper GI tract: ICD-10-PCS Code(s) _____

11. Frenulotomy of buccal mucosa via oral cavity: ICD-10-PCS Code(s) _____

12. Open division of median nerve: ICD-10-PCS Code(s) _____

13. Exploratory laparotomy of the retroperitoneum: ICD-10-PCS Code(s) _____

14. Bundle of His Mapping, percutaneous: ICD-10-PCS Code(s) _____

15. Drainage of peritoneum via percutaneous Jackson-Pratt drain: ICD-10-PCS Code(s) _____

16. Removal of rusted nail from sole of left foot: ICD-10-PCS Code(s) _____

17. Percutaneous fragmentation of calculus of right parotid duct: ICD-10-PCS Code(s) _____

18. Percutaneous endoscopic right hand carpal tunnel release: ICD-10-PCS Code(s) _____

19. Drainage of neck abscess: ICD-10-PCS Code(s) _____

20. Percutaneous endoscopic hemilaminotomy of phrenic nerve: ICD-10-PCS Code(s) _____

21. Arthroscopy of right shoulder: ICD-10-PCS Code(s) _____

22. Division of chordae tendineae, percutaneous endoscopic: ICD-10-PCS Code(s) _____

23. Removal of popcorn kernel from right nostril: ICD-10-PCS Code(s) _____

24. Arthroscopy of left knee: ICD-10-PCS Code(s) _____

25. Gastrolysis, open: ICD-10-PCS Code(s) _____

Section 0: Root Operations H, R, U, 2, P, W, 3, Q, G, 0, 4

Chapter 56

Procedures That Always Involve a Device (H, R, U, 2, P, W)

Procedures That Define Other Repairs (3, Q)

Procedures That Define Other Objectives (G, 0, 4)

Learning Objectives

After completing this chapter, you should have the skills to:

56.1 Spell and define the key words, medical terms, and abbreviations related to procedures H, R, U, 2, P, W, 3, Q, G, 0, and 4.

56.2 Discuss the types of procedures that always involve a device, that define other repairs, and that define other objectives.

56.3 Identify the main characteristics of coding for the Root Operations Insertion, Replacement, Supplement, Change, Removal, Revision, Control, Repair, Fusion, Alteration, and Creation.

56.4 Abstract procedural information from the medical record for coding for the Root Operations H, R, U, 2, P, W, 3, Q, G, 0, and 4.

56.5 Assign codes for the Root Operations H, R, U, 2, P, W, 3, Q, G, 0, and 4.

56.6 Arrange codes for the Root Operations H, R, U, 2, P, W, 3, Q, G, 0, and 4.

56.7 Discuss the ICD-10-PCS coding guidelines related to Root Operations H, R, U, 2, P, W, 3, Q, G, 0, and 4.

Chapter Outline

- **Basics of Procedures H, R, U, 2, P, W, 3, Q, G, 0, and 4**
- **Coding Overview of Root Operations H, R, U, 2, P, W, 3, Q, G, 0, and 4**
- **Abstracting for Root Operations H, R, U, 2, P, W, 3, Q, G, 0, and 4**
- **Assigning Characters 4–7 for Root Operations H, R, U, 2, P, W, 3, Q, G, 0, and 4**
- **Arranging Codes for Root Operations H, R, U, 2, P, W, 3, Q, G, 0, and 4**

Key Term and Abbreviation

postprocedural bleeding

In addition to the key term listed here, students should know the terms defined within tables in this chapter.

INTRODUCTION

When repairing a car, sometimes a part must be removed and replaced with an identical one, and other times modifications or repairs can be made to the original part so it functions properly. Mechanical devices frequently are used to take the place of or augment a Body Part. The Root Operations discussed in this chapter include procedures that always involve a device.

This chapter discusses three groups of Medical and Surgical Root Operations:

- Procedures That Always Involve a Device (H, R, U, 2, P, W)
- Procedures That Define Other Repairs (3, Q)
- Procedures That Define Other Objectives (G, 0, 4)

Although the Root Operations within each group share a common purpose each has a unique aspect that makes it different from the other procedures in the same group. Pay careful attention to the differences between each Root Operation so that you can use each confidently and accurately.

BASICS OF PROCEDURES H, R, U, 2, P, W, 3, Q, G, 0, AND 4

This section introduces each Root Operation group and provides definitions and examples of each Root Operation. Details are discussed as you progress through this chapter. Some terms, such as removal and repair, can be associated with more than one Root Operation. There is not a direct match between a specific procedural term and a Root Operation because some medical terms, such as excision and removal, can be associated with more than one Root Operation. Root Operations are assigned based on the content of the operative report regarding what was actually performed, not on the terms used by the physician in documentation.

Refer to detailed anatomic diagrams of specific organ systems in Chapters 9 through 48 of this text, or in external references, when you need to refresh your memory of human anatomy.

Basics of Procedures That Always Involve a Device

Procedures that always involve a medical device in or on a Body Part do not involve changes to the Body Part itself. When the Body Part is treated in addition to the procedure related to the device, assign an additional code(s) to identify the type of treatment. The Root Operations in this group *always* involve a device, by definition. This differs from the use of Character 6, Device, with other Root Operations in that other Root Operations do not always involve a device. For example, insertion, replacement, or repair of a pacemaker, by definition, always involves a device—a pacemaker. By contrast, the reduction of a fracture might or might not involve a fixation device, so when a fixation device is used, Character 6 identifies the type of device.

Refer to ■ TABLE 56-1 for the definitions and procedural terms commonly used with the Root Operations Insertion (H), Replacement (R), Supplement (U), Change (2), Removal (P), and Revision (W).

Table 56-1 ■ **ROOT OPERATIONS THAT ALWAYS INVOLVE A DEVICE**

Root Operation	Value	Definition	Terms
Insertion	H	Putting in a nonbiological appliance that monitors, assists, performs, or prevents a physiological function but does not physically take the place of a Body Part	Insert, install, place
Replacement	R	Putting in or on biological or synthetic material that physically takes the place and/or function of all or a portion of a Body Part	Joint replacement, arthroplasty, replace, exchange
Supplement	U	Putting in or on biological or synthetic material that physically reinforces and/or augments the function of a portion of a Body Part	Reinforce, supplement
Change	2	Taking out or off a device from a Body Part and putting back an identical or similar device in or on the same Body Part without cutting or puncturing the skin or a mucous membrane	Replace, exchange
Removal	P	Taking out or off a device from a Body Part	Remove, take out
Revision	W	Correcting, to the extent possible, a portion of a malfunctioning device or the position of a displaced device	Revise, correct, replace

Basics of Procedures That Define Other Repairs

Two Root Operations in this group identify unrelated repair procedures that are not described by other Root Operation groups (■ TABLE 56-2).

Table 56-2 ■ **ROOT OPERATIONS THAT DEFINE OTHER REPAIRS**

Root Operation	Value	Definition	Terms
Control	3	Stopping, or attempting to stop, postprocedural bleeding	Control
Repair	Q	Restoring, to the extent possible, a Body Part to its normal anatomic structure and function	Repair, suture

Table 56-3 ■ **ROOT OPERATIONS THAT DEFINE OTHER OBJECTIVES**

Root Operation	Value	Definition	Terms
Fusion	G	Joining together portions of an articular Body Part, rendering the articular Body Part immobile	Arthrodesis, fusion
Alteration	0	Modifying the anatomic structure of a Body Part without affecting the function of the Body Part	Liposuction, face lift
Creation	4	Making a new genital structure that does not take over the function of a Body Part	Transgender operation

Table 56-4 ■ **EXAMPLE OF CONSTRUCTING MEDICAL TERMS FOR PROCEDURES H, R, U, 2, P, W, 3, Q, G, 0, AND 4**

Combining Form	Suffix	Complete Medical Term
stomat/o (*mouth*)		**stomato + rrhaphy** (*suturing of the mouth*)
		tendono + rrhaphy (*suturing of a tendon*)
		spleno + rrhaphy (*suturing of the spleen*)
tendon /o (*tendon*)	**-rrhaphy** (*suturing*) **-plasty** (*surgical repair*)	**stomato + plasty** (*surgical repair of the mouth*)
		tendono + plasty (*surgical repair of a tendon*)
splen/o (*spleen*)		**spleno + plasty** (*surgical repair of the spleen*)

Source: © PB Resources, Inc. Used with permission.

Basics of Procedures That Define Other Objectives

Three Root Operations in this group identify unrelated procedures that are described by the objectives of other Root Operation groups (■ TABLE 56-3).

When reading medical terms related to procedures in this chapter, remember that the same suffix can describe a wide variety of procedures and multiple Root Operations. Although terms ending with *-ectomy* most often identify procedures coded with the Root Operation Excision or Resection, they could also identify procedures coded with Extirpation, Extraction, Destruction, or Alteration. The suffix *-plasty* can identify procedures coded with the Root Operations Repair, Replacement, Supplement, Reposition, Alteration, and Excision. Refer to ■ TABLE 56-4 for a refresher on how to build medical terms related to procedures discussed in this chapter.

This section provides a general reference to help understand the most common procedures that always involve a device, as well as procedures that define other repairs and other objectives. Remember to keep standard reference books handy in case you get stuck.

> ### CODING CAUTION
> Be alert for Root Operations that have similar English meanings but different PCS definitions.
>
> **Insertion (H)** (*Putting in a nonbiological appliance that <u>monitors, assists, performs, or prevents</u> a physiological function but does not physically take the place of a Body Part*) and **Supplement (U)** (*Putting in or on biological or synthetic material that <u>physically reinforces and/or augments</u> the function of a portion of a Body Part*)
>
> **Removal (P)** (*Taking out or off <u>a device from</u> a Body Part*) and **Resection (T)** (*<u>Cutting out</u> or off without replacement <u>all of a Body Part</u>*)

CODING PRACTICE

Exercise 56.1   Basics of Procedures H, R, U, 2, P, W, 3, Q, G, 0, and 4

Instructions: Use your medical terminology skills and resources to define the following procedures, then identify the code(s) or code range listed in the PCS Index. Follow these steps:

- Use slash marks "/" to break down the underlined term into its root(s) and suffix.
- Define the meaning of the word based on the meaning of each word part.
- Look up the phrase in the ICD-10-PCS Index, and write down the name(s) of the Root Operation(s) the Index cross-references you to and the Table(s), if provided.
- Do not assign any codes.

(continued)

CODING PRACTICE (continued)

Example: <u>conjunctivoplasty</u>
conjunctivo/plasty

Meaning <u>*surgical repair of the lining*</u>
<u>*of the eyelids*</u>

PCS Root Operation(s)/Table(s) <u>*Repair 08Q,*</u>
<u>*Replacement 08R*</u>

1. <u>epididymorrhaphy</u> — Meaning _____ — PCS Root Operation(s)/Table(s) _____

2. <u>acromioplasty</u> — Meaning _____ — PCS Root Operation(s)/Table(s) _____

3. <u>diaphragmatic</u> pacemaker lead — Meaning _____ — PCS Root Operation(s)/Table(s) _____

4. <u>neurostimulator</u> generator — Meaning _____ — PCS Root Operation(s)/Table(s) _____

5. <u>epiphysiodesis</u> — Meaning _____ — PCS Root Operation(s)/Table(s) _____

6. <u>genioplasty</u> — Meaning _____ — PCS Root Operation(s)/Table(s) _____

7. <u>canthorrhaphy</u> — Meaning _____ — PCS Root Operation(s)/Table(s) _____

8. <u>costosternoplasty</u> — Meaning _____ — PCS Root Operation(s)/Table(s) _____

9. <u>esophagocoloplasty</u> — Meaning _____ — PCS Root Operation(s)/Table(s) _____

10. intraluminal device, <u>endotracheal</u> airway — Meaning _____ — PCS Root Operation(s)/Table(s) _____

CODING OVERVIEW OF ROOT OPERATIONS H, R, U, 2, P, W, 3, Q, G, 0, AND 4

The PCS OGCR provide several guidelines specific to the Root Operations discussed in this chapter. A general guideline related to the Root Operation Control is discussed below. Those specific to Characters 4 through 7 are discussed later in this chapter. Refer to the PCS OGCR for additional details and clinical examples of each guideline.

The definition of the Root Operation Control is *stopping, or attempting to stop, postprocedural bleeding.* **Postprocedural bleeding**, also called postoperative bleeding or hemorrhage, is bleeding that occurs after a surgical procedure. It may occur immediately or be delayed. Common causes are a deficient clotting mechanism in the blood or loose clips or ties around blood vessels. An initial attempt to control postoperative bleeding might be unsuccessful and require that a more definitive Root Operation—such as Bypass, Detachment, Excision, Extraction, Reposition, Replacement, or Resection—be performed. In this situation, code only the more definitive Root Operation. Assign the Root Operation Control only when a more definitive procedure is not performed (PCS OGCR B3.7).

ABSTRACTING FOR ROOT OPERATIONS H, R, U, 2, P, W, 3, Q, G, 0, AND 4

Abstracting for PCS focuses on identifying the correct Root Operation, which involves reading the operative report and interpreting it in light of Root Operation definitions. When reading the operative report, remember to focus on the objective of the procedure and the activities performed, not the specific medical terms the surgeon uses to describe the procedure. Many times the Root Operation can be determined conclusively during abstracting. Other times the Root Operation can be narrowed down to two options, which must be differentiated based on other Characters that are assigned from the PCS Tables. The Root Operation definition is a combination of the functional objective of the procedure and the anatomic site. The following information summarizes the objectives, definitions, unique features, and examples of Root Operations discussed in this chapter.

A table that outlines the Key Criteria to Abstracting Root Operations appears for each Root Operation group to help distinguish among procedures in the group. Refer to Table 51-1 for general guidance on abstracting PCS procedures and Root Operation groups. A guided example of abstracting for the Root Operations Fusion, Insertion, and Resection follows. Refer to Chapter 52 of this text for a refresher on the Root Operation Resection.

Abstracting for Procedures That Always Involve a Device

The following information summarizes the objectives, definitions, unique features, examples, and Key Criteria for Abstracting Root Operations for procedures that always involve a device. Differences among Root Operations in this group include whether the device is put in, taken out, or repaired and whether the device augments the function of a Body Part or replaces it entirely.

Abstracting for Insertion (H)

The objective of the Root Operation Insertion is putting in a nonbiological device. The site of the procedure is in or on a Body Part.

The Root Operation Insertion represents those procedures where the sole objective is to put in a device without doing anything else to a Body Part. Procedures typical of those coded to Insertion include putting in a vascular catheter, a pacemaker lead, or a tissue expander. Imaging guidance done to assist in the performance of a procedure can be coded separately in the Imaging section (Section B).

Table 56-5 ■ **EXAMPLES OF THE ROOT OPERATION INSERTION (H)**

Organ System	Procedural Examples
Cardiovascular	Insertion of central venous catheter, pacemaker insertion, percutaneous replacement of broken pacemaker lead in left atrium
Genitourinary	Insertion of urinary catheter, placement of brachytherapy seeds in prostate gland
Integumentary	Percutaneous placement of intrathecal infusion pump in the subcutaneous tissue of the back for pain management
Musculoskeletal	Placement of bone growth stimulator
Nervous	Insertion of spinal neurostimulator generator to replace old neurostimulator
Respiratory	Insertion of brachytherapy seeds in bronchus
Special Senses (Ear, Eye)	Insertion of multiple-channel cochlear implant

Source: © PB Resources, Inc. Used with permission.

Examples of Insertion are insertion of radioactive implant or central venous catheter (■ Table 56-5).

Abstracting for Replacement (R)

The objective of the Root Operation Replacement is putting in a device that replaces a Body Part. The site of the procedure is some/all of a Body Part. The Body Part may have been taken out or replaced previously, or may be taken out, physically eradicated, or rendered nonfunctional during the Replacement procedure. When a device that was put in during a previous encounter is taken out, assign the Root Operation Removal.

Replacement encompasses a wide range of procedures, from joint replacements to grafts of all kinds. Examples of Replacement are a total hip replacement, bone graft, and free skin graft (■ Table 56-6).

Table 56-6 ■ **EXAMPLES OF THE ROOT OPERATION REPLACEMENT (R)**

Organ System	Procedural Examples
Cardiovascular	Excision of abdominal aorta with Gore-Tex graft replacement, mitral valve replacement
Integumentary	Free skin graft, mastectomy with insertion of saline breast implants, mastectomy with free TRAM flap reconstruction
Musculoskeletal	Joint replacement, excision of diseased bone with bone graft
Special Senses (Ear, Eye)	Prosthetic lens implantation

Source: © PB Resources, Inc. Used with permission.

Table 56-7 ■ **EXAMPLES OF THE ROOT OPERATION SUPPLEMENT (U)**

Organ System	Procedural Examples
Cardiovascular	Mitral valve ring annuloplasty
Genitourinary	Colporrhaphy with Gynemesh
Musculoskeletal	Hernia with Marlex plug, resurfacing procedure on femoral head, replacement of joint liner in previous joint replacement
Nervous	Free nerve graft

Source: © PB Resources, Inc. Used with permission.

Abstracting for Supplement (U)

The objective of the Root Operation Supplement is putting in a device that reinforces or augments a Body Part. The site of the procedure is in or on a Body Part.

The biological material is nonliving or is living and from the same individual. The Body Part may have been previously replaced, with the Supplement procedure being performed to physically reinforce or augment the function of the replaced Body Part.

Examples of Supplement are a herniorrhaphy using mesh and putting a new acetabular liner in a previous hip replacement (■ Table 56-7).

Abstracting for Change (2)

The objective of the Root Operation Change is exchanging a device *without cutting* or puncturing. The site of the procedure is in or on a Body Part. The Approach is always External. When any other Approach is used, assign a Root Operation that identifies what was done. For example, when the skin is cut or punctured to take out a device and put in a new one, assign the Root Operations Removal and Replacement.

Examples of Change are urinary catheter change and drainage tube change (■ Table 56-8).

Abstracting for Removal (P)

The objective of the Root Operation Removal is taking out a device. The site of the procedure is in or on a Body Part. When the device is taken out by cutting or puncturing the skin, or taken out and not replaced, assign the Root Operation Removal. Assign the Root Operation Replacement when the device is replaced. When a device is taken out and a similar device put in *without cutting* or puncturing the skin or mucous membrane, assign the Root Operation Change.

Table 56-8 ■ **EXAMPLES OF THE ROOT OPERATION CHANGE (2)**

Organ System	Procedural Examples
Digestive	Gastrostomy tube change
Genitourinary	Foley catheter exchange
Musculoskeletal	Exchange of drainage tube in a joint
Respiratory	Tracheostomy tube exchange, change chest tube for left pneumothorax

Source: © PB Resources, Inc. Used with permission.

Table 56-9 ■ EXAMPLES OF THE ROOT OPERATION REMOVAL (P)

Organ System	Procedural Examples
Cardiovascular	Removal of a broken pacemaker lead, removal of cardiac pacemaker, nonincisional removal of Swan-Ganz catheter
Digestive	Nonincisional PEG tube removal
Genitourinary	Transvaginal removal of brachytherapy seeds, endoscopic retrieval of ureteral stent
Musculoskeletal	Removal of arm or leg external fixation device, incision with removal of K-wire fixation
Nervous	Removal of an old neurostimulator generator
Respiratory	Extubation of endotracheal tube, removal of nasogastric drainage tube

Source: © PB Resources, Inc. Used with permission.

Examples of Removal are drainage tube removal and cardiac pacemaker removal (■ TABLE 56-9).

Abstracting for Revision (W)

The objective of the Root Operation Revision is correcting a malfunctioning or displaced device. The site of the procedure is in or on a Body Part.

Revision can include correcting a malfunctioning or displaced device by taking out or putting in components of the device such as a screw or pin.

Examples of Revision are adjusting the position of pacemaker lead and recementing of a hip prosthesis (■ TABLE 56-10).

Key Criteria for Abstracting Root Operations H, R, U, 2, P, and W

Refer to ■ TABLE 56-11 for more specific guidance on how to abstract procedures that Always Take Out a Device and distinguish among Root Operations in this group.

Abstracting for Procedures That Define Other Repairs

The Root Operation group *Procedures that Define Other Repairs* consists of procedures that do not fit in any of the other Root

Table 56-10 ■ EXAMPLES OF THE ROOT OPERATION REVISION (W)

Organ System	Procedural Examples
Cardiovascular	Adjusting the position of pacemaker lead, repositioning of Swan-Ganz catheter
Musculoskeletal	Recementing of joint prosthesis, replacement of screw in a fracture plate

Source: © PB Resources, Inc. Used with permission.

Table 56-11 ■ KEY CRITERIA FOR ABSTRACTING ROOT OPERATIONS THAT ALWAYS TAKE OUT A DEVICE

Question	Root Operation (Value)
Did the procedure involve an external device left in place in, on, or in replacement of a Body Part?	
Answer *Yes* to one of the following questions to help distinguish Root Operations H, R, U, 2, P, and W:	
❑ Was a nonbiological device put in or on a Body Part?	Insertion (H)
❑ Was a device put in to replace a Body Part?	Replacement (R)
❑ Was a device put in to reinforce or augment a Body Part?	Supplement (U)
❑ Was a device exchanged without cutting or puncturing the skin?	Change (2)
❑ Was a device taken out and not replaced? ❑ Was a device taken out by cutting or puncturing the skin?	Removal (P)
❑ Was a malfunctioning or displaced device corrected?	Revision (W)

Source: © PB Resources, Inc. Used with permission.

Operation groups. The Root Operation Control is very specific and is used in a narrow range of circumstances. The other Root Operation in this group, Repair, is very general and is used similarly to code for not elsewhere classified (NEC) or unspecified procedures in other coding systems.

Abstracting for Control (3)

The objective of the Root Operation Control is stopping or attempting to stop postprocedural bleeding. The site of the procedure is an anatomic region rather than a specific Body Part. Control is used to represent a small range of procedures performed to treat postprocedural bleeding. Control is not coded separately when another Root Operation is required to stop the bleeding, such as Bypass, Detachment, Excision, Extraction, Reposition, Replacement, or Resection.

Examples of Control are control of postprostatectomy hemorrhage, control of posttonsillectomy hemorrhage (■ TABLE 56-12). Examples reflect the organ system in which the original procedure was performed. The Root Operation Control is always coded to one of the PCS Body Systems labeled Anatomical Regions. Use procedure codes in Body Systems for general Anatomical Regions when the procedure is performed on an anatomic region rather than a specific Body Part or on the rare occasion when no information is available to support assignment of a code to a specific Body Part (PCS OGCR B2.1a).

Abstracting for Repair (Q)

The objective of the Root Operation Repair is Restoring a Body Part to its normal structure. The site of the procedure is some or all of a Body Part.

Use the Root Operation Repair only when the method to accomplish the repair is not defined by another Root Operation.

Table 56-12 ■ **EXAMPLES OF THE ROOT OPERATION CONTROL (3)**

Organ System	Procedural Examples
Cardiovascular	Control of postop hemopericardium
Endocrine	Control of posttonsillectomy hemorrhage
Genitourinary	Control of postprostatectomy hemorrhage, cautery of posthysterectomy oozing and evacuation of clot
Musculoskeletal	Exploration and ligation of postop arterial bleeder in arm, drainage of hemarthrosis at previous operative site

Source: © PB Resources, Inc. Used with permission.

The Root Operation Repair represents a broad range of procedures for restoring the anatomic structure of a Body Part, such as suture of lacerations. Repair also functions as the "not elsewhere classified (NEC)" Root Operation, to be used when the procedure performed does not meet the definition of one of the other Root Operations.

Examples of Repair are herniorrhaphy (without mesh or other supplement) and suture of a laceration (■ TABLE 56-13).

Key Criteria for Abstracting Root Operations 3 and Q

Refer to ■ TABLE 56-14 for more specific guidance on how to abstract procedures that Define Other Repairs and distinguish among Root Operations in this group.

Abstracting for Procedures That Define Other Objectives

The Root Operation group *Procedures that Define Other Objectives* is a collection of three Root Operations that are not related to each other. Each Root Operation is used in very limited and specific situations.

Abstracting for Fusion (G)

The objective of the Root Operation Fusion is rendering a joint immobile. The site of the procedure is a joint.

The Body Part is joined together by fixation device, bone graft, or other means. A limited range of procedures is represented in the Root Operation Fusion because fusion procedures are by definition only performed on the joints.

Table 56-13 ■ **EXAMPLES OF THE ROOT OPERATION REPAIR (Q)**

Organ System	Procedural Examples
Digestive	Colostomy takedown
Genitourinary	Perineoplasty with repair of old obstetric laceration
Musculoskeletal	Suture repair of right biceps tendon laceration, closure of abdominal wall stab wound, herniorrhaphy
Nervous	Repair of nerve laceration

Source: © PB Resources, Inc. Used with permission.

Table 56-14 ■ **KEY CRITERIA FOR ABSTRACTING ROOT OPERATIONS THAT DEFINE OTHER REPAIRS**

Question	Root Operation (Value)
Answer *Yes* to one of the following questions to help distinguish Root Operations 3 and Q:	
❑ Did the procedure stop or attempt to stop postprocedural bleeding?	Control (3)
❑ Was another Root Operation performed to stop postprocedural bleeding?	Assign a Root Operation other than Control.
❑ Did the procedure restore a Body Part to its normal structure?	Repair (Q)
❑ Is the procedure more specifically identified by another Root Operation?	Assign a Root Operation other than Repair.

Source: © PB Resources, Inc. Used with permission.

Table 56-15 ■ **EXAMPLES OF THE ROOT OPERATION FUSION (G)**

Organ System	Procedural Examples
Musculoskeletal	Vertebral fusion, hand fusion, interphalangeal fusion

Source: © PB Resources, Inc. Used with permission.

Examples of Fusion are spinal fusion and ankle arthrodesis (■ TABLE 56-15).

Abstracting for Alteration (0)

The objective of the Root Operation Alteration is modifying a Body Part for *cosmetic* purposes without affecting function. The site of the procedure is some or all of a Body Part.

The principal purpose is to improve appearance. Alteration is coded for all procedures performed solely to improve appearance. All methods, approaches, and devices used for the objective of improving appearance are coded here. Because some surgical procedures can be performed for either medical or cosmetic purposes, coding for Alteration requires diagnostic confirmation that the surgery is in fact performed to improve appearance.

Examples of Alteration are face lift and breast augmentation (■ TABLE 56-16).

Table 56-16 ■ **EXAMPLES OF THE ROOT OPERATION ALTERATION (0)**

Organ System	Procedural Examples
Integumentary	Cosmetic liposuction, breast augmentation, face lift
Respiratory	Cosmetic rhinoplasty
Special Senses (Ear, Eye)	Cosmetic blepharoplasty

Source: © PB Resources, Inc. Used with permission.

Table 56-17 ■ **EXAMPLES OF THE ROOT OPERATION CREATION (4)**

Organ System	Procedural Examples
Genitourinary	Creation of vagina in a male, creation of penis in a female

Source: © PB Resources, Inc. Used with permission.

Abstracting for Creation (4)

The objective of the Root Operation Creation is making a new genital structure that does not physically take the place of a Body Part. The site of the procedure is the perineum.

This Root Operation represents only two procedures: creation of a vagina in a male and creation of a penis in a female (■ TABLE 56-17). Only the procedures performed for sex change operations are included here. When a separate procedure is performed to harvest autograft tissue, assign the appropriate Root Operation that describes the work performed in addition to the primary procedure for the sex change operation.

Key Criteria for Abstracting Root Operations G, 0, and 4

Refer to ■ TABLE 56-18 for more specific guidance on how to abstract procedures that Define Other Objectives and distinguish among Root Operations in this group.

Guided Example of Abstracting for Fusion, Insertion, and Resection

Refer to the following example throughout this chapter to practice skills for abstracting, assigning, and arranging codes for the Root Operations Fusion, Insertion, and Resection. Similar principles apply to working with other Root Operations that always involve a device, define other repairs, or define other objectives.

INPATIENT HOSPITAL   Gender: M   Age: 27

Preoperative diagnosis: Degenerative disc disease

Procedure: Discectomy with spinal arthrodesis. A vertical incision 11 cm in length was made over L4-L5. The interspace was visualized. All disc material was excised and the area was irrigated. Applied a synthetic bone substitute to the posterior column using the same incision. Fixation plate and screws also were installed through the same incision. Hemostasis was achieved and the incision was closed. Patient was transferred to PACU in stable condition.

Follow along as fictitious coder, Marcy Elwood, CCS, abstracts the procedure. Check off each step after you complete it.

▶ Marcy reads through the entire record, paying special attention to the reason for the encounter, the procedure performed, and the postoperative diagnosis.

   ❑ She notes the preoperative diagnosis, *degenerative disc disease.*

Table 56-18 ■ **KEY CRITERIA FOR ABSTRACTING ROOT OPERATIONS THAT DEFINE OTHER OBJECTIVES**

Question	Root Operation (Value)
Answer *Yes* to one of the following questions to help distinguish Root Operations G, 0, and 4:	
❑ Did the procedure render a joint immobile?	Fusion (G)
❑ Was the procedure for cosmetic purposes only, without affecting the function of a Body Part?	Alteration (0)
❑ Was the procedure a sex change operation?	Creation (4)

Source: © PB Resources, Inc. Used with permission.

❑ *What is the stated procedure?* discectomy with spinal arthrodesis

❑ *What organ or Body Part is involved?* L4-L5 disc

❑ *Is the procedure description what you would expect based on the name of the procedure?* Yes, but some of the details are not known, including the number and type of devices.

❑ *What surgical approach is used?* Open

❑ *Was more than one procedure, or a combined procedure, performed?* Yes, discectomy, arthrodesis, and insertion of fixation device.

❑ First, Marcy abstracts for the arthrodesis (Table 56-14).

   ▪ *Did the procedure render a joint immobile?* Yes

   ▪ *Was the procedure for cosmetic purposes only, without affecting the function of a Body Part?* No

❑ Next, Marcy abstracts for installation of the plate and screws (Table 56-11).

   ▪ *Did the procedure involve an external device left in place in, on, or in replacement of a Body Part?* Yes

   ▪ *Was a nonbiological device put in or on a Body Part?* Yes

   ▪ *Was a device put in to replace a Body Part?* No

   ▪ *Was a device put it to reinforce or augment a Body Part?* No

   ▪ *Was a device exchanged without cutting or puncturing the skin?* No

   ▪ *Was a device taken out and not replaced?* No

   ▪ *Was a device taken out by cutting or puncturing the skin?* No

   ▪ *Was a malfunctioning or displaced device corrected?* No

   ▪ *What is the most likely Root Operation?* Insertion

❑ Next, Marcy abstracts for the discectomy (Table 52-9).

   ▪ *Did the procedure take out some or all of a Body Part without replacement?* Yes

   ▪ *Was removal performed by cutting?* Yes

- *Was all of Body Part or only a portion of a Body Part removed?* The entire disc was removed, and Marcy believes this will equate to all of a PCS Body Part. She will need to verify this when she refers to the PCS Tables.

- *What is the most likely Root Operation?* Resection

▶ At this time, Marcy believes that she will use the Root Operations Fusion, Insertion, and Resection and/or Excision and anticipates that she will need three codes. She will verify this information when she refers to the PCS Tables to assign codes.

CODING PRACTICE

Exercise 56.2   **Abstracting for Root Operations H, R, U, 2, P, W, 3, Q, G, 0, and 4**

Instructions: Read the mini-medical-record of each patient's encounter and answer the abstracting questions. Write the answer on the line provided. Do not assign any codes.

1. INPATIENT HOSPITAL   Gender: F   Age: 81

Preprocedure diagnosis: status post-arthroplasty

Procedure: exchange of drainage tube from right hip joint following total hip replacement

a. What is the stated procedure? _____

b. What Body Part is involved? _____

c. What is the laterality? _____

d. Is the procedure description what you would expect based on the name of the procedure? _____

e. What surgical approach is used? _____

f. Was more than one procedure, or a combined procedure, performed? _____

g. Did the procedure involve an external device left in place in, on, or in replacement of a Body Part?
_____

h. Was a nonbiological device put in or on a Body Part?
_____

i. Was a device put in to replace a Body Part?
_____

j. Was a device put in to reinforce or augment a Body Part? _____

k. Was a device exchanged without cutting or puncturing the skin? _____

l. Was a device taken out and not replaced? _____

m. Was a device taken out by cutting or puncturing the skin? _____

n. Was a malfunctioning or displaced device corrected?
_____

o. Which Root Operation(s) should be considered for this procedure? _____ Why? _____

2. INPATIENT HOSPITAL   Gender: M   Age: 75

Preprocedure diagnosis: sick sinus syndrome, displaced pacemaker lead

Procedure: percutaneous adjustment of position of left pacemaker lead in left atrium

a. What is the stated procedure? _____

b. What Body Part is involved? _____

c. What is the laterality? _____

d. Is the procedure description what you would expect based on the name of the procedure? _____

e. What surgical approach is used? _____

f. Was more than one procedure, or a combined procedure, performed? _____

g. Did the procedure involve an external device left in place in, on, or in replacement of a Body Part?
_____

h. Was a nonbiological device put in or on a Body Part?
_____

i. Was a device put in to replace a Body Part? _____

j. Was a device put in to reinforce or augment a Body Part? _____

k. Was a device exchanged without cutting or puncturing the skin? _____

l. Was a device taken out and not replaced? _____

m. Was a device taken out by cutting or puncturing the skin? _____

n. Was a malfunctioning or displaced device corrected?
_____

o. Which Root Operation(s) should be considered for this procedure? _____ Why? _____

(continued)

CODING PRACTICE (continued)

3. INPATIENT HOSPITAL Gender: F Age: 36

Preprocedure diagnosis: drooping right upper eyelid affects patient's perception of appearance but does not interfere with vision

Procedure: cosmetic blepharoplasty. Cut out a crescent of skin and subcutaneous tissue from fold of R eyelid, sutured to restore normal position of eyelid.

a. What is the stated procedure? _____

b. What Body Part is involved? _____

c. What is the laterality? _____

d. Is the procedure description what you would expect based on the name of the procedure? _____

e. What surgical approach is used? _____

f. Was more than one procedure, or a combined procedure, performed? _____

g. Was the procedure for cosmetic purposes only, without affecting the function of a Body Part? _____

h. Which Root Operation(s) should be considered for this procedure? _____ Why? _____

4. INPATIENT HOSPITAL Gender: M Age: 72

Preprocedure diagnosis: blepharoptosis obscuring vision

Procedure: Bilateral upper blepharoplasty. Cut out a crescent of skin and subcutaneous tissue from fold of R eyelid, sutured to restore normal position of eyelid. Repeated on left side.

a. What is the stated procedure? _____

b. What Body Part is involved? _____

c. What is the laterality? _____

d. Is the procedure description what you would expect based on the name of the procedure? _____

e. What surgical approach is used? _____

f. Was more than one procedure, or a combined procedure, performed? _____

g. Did the procedure restore a Body Part to its normal structure? _____

h. Is the procedure more specifically identified by another Root Operation? _____

i. Which Root Operation(s) should be considered for this procedure? _____ Why? _____

5. INPATIENT HOSPITAL Gender: M Age: 53

Preprocedure diagnosis: detached R retina

Procedure: Trans pars plana vitrectomy (TPPV) with synthetic scleral buckle. Made incision in pars plana and used vitreous cutter to remove all vitreous. Injected balanced saline solution (BSS) to replace vitreous. Sutured scleral buckle, which effectively closed the retinal break. Pt tolerated px well.

a. What is the stated procedure? _____

b. What Body Part is involved? _____

c. What is the laterality? _____

d. Is the procedure description what you would expect based on the name of the procedure? _____

e. What surgical approach is used? _____

f. Was more than one procedure, or a combined procedure, performed? _____

g. Did the first procedure (vitrectomy) take out some or all of a Body Part without replacement? _____

h. Was a Body Part or abnormal tissue growth (such as a lesion or tumor) removed? _____

i. Was a foreign object or abnormal material (such as calculus) removed? _____

j. Was the Body Part replaced with a natural or synthetic substitute? _____

k. Was removal performed by cutting? _____

l. Was removal performed through physical eradication, such as energy, force, or a destructive agent? _____

m. Was removal performed through the use of force, such as pulling or stripping? _____

n. Which Root Operation(s) should be considered for the first procedure? _____ Why? _____

o. Did the second procedure (application of scleral buckle) involve an external device left in place in, on, or in replacement of a Body Part? _____

p. Was a nonbiological device put in or on a Body Part?

q. Was a device put in to replace a Body Part? _____

r. Was a device put in to reinforce or augment a Body Part? _____

s. Was a device exchanged without cutting or puncturing the skin? _____

t. Was a device taken out and not replaced? _____

(continued)

5. (continued)

u. Was a device taken out by cutting or puncturing the skin? _____

v. Was a malfunctioning or displaced device corrected?

_____

w. Which Root Operation(s) should be considered for the second procedure? _____ Why? _____

---

6. INPATIENT HOSPITAL   Gender: F   Age: 68

Preprocedure diagnosis: bradycardia, malfunctioning pacemaker lead

Procedure: percutaneous exchange of a malfunctioning pacemaker lead in the left atrium with a new one

a. What is the stated procedure? _____

b. What Body Part is involved? _____

c. What is the laterality? _____

d. Is the procedure description what you would expect based on the name of the procedure? _____

(continued)

---

6. (continued)

e. What surgical approach is used? _____

f. Was more than one procedure, or a combined procedure, performed? _____

g. Did the procedure involve an external device left in place in, on, or in replacement of a Body Part? _____

h. Was a nonbiological device put in or on a Body Part?

_____

i. Was a device put in to replace a Body Part? _____

j. Was a device put in to reinforce or augment a Body Part? _____

k. Was a device exchanged without cutting or puncturing the skin? _____

l. Was a device taken out and not replaced? _____

m. Was a device taken out by cutting or puncturing the skin? _____

n. Was a malfunctioning or displaced device corrected?

_____

o. Which Root Operation(s) should be considered for this procedure? _____ Why? _____

ASSIGNING CHARACTERS 4–7 FOR ROOT OPERATIONS H, R, U, 2, P, W, 3, Q, G, 0, AND 4

To assign codes after the Root Operation is determined, search the PCS Index for the name of the Root Operation as the Main Term. Locate the subterm(s) for the correct anatomic site and identify the PCS Table. When you locate the PCS Table, verify the first three characters of the code, then locate the row with the Body Part needed. Assign the remaining characters from each respective column of the Table. The following information summarizes and highlights unique information for working with the Tables for each Root Operation H, R, U, 2, P, W, 3, Q, G, 0, and 4. Each Root Operation has one Table in each applicable PCS Body System. Because of the differences between organ systems, Table details vary.

The Index Main Term entries for the Root Operations Insertion, Removal, and Revision include the phrase **of device in** or **of device from** to clarify that the procedure is performed on a device and not a Body Part. The Index also provides the standalone Main Term entries **Insertion** and **Removal**. These standalone entries lead to procedures other than Medical and Surgical procedures dealing with a device. For example, the standalone Main Term **Removal** leads to procedures in Section 2 Placement. Although the Root Operation Removal is assigned to the code, it uses a different value for the Root Operation and also uses only the Body Systems belonging to one of the Anatomical Regions (W, X, Y) (■ FIGURE 56-1). The Placement section is discussed in Chapter 57 of this text.

Character 4: Body Part

PCS OGCR provide guidelines for assigning Body Part values when coding the Root Operations Control, Change/Revision/Removal, and Fusion. These are discussed next.

Control Procedures

Code the site of the bleeding as an Anatomical Region (W, X, Y) and not a specific Body Part.

Change, Revision, and Removal Procedures

A PCS Table might not always provide a specific Body Part value for the exact anatomic site treated. Assign a general Body

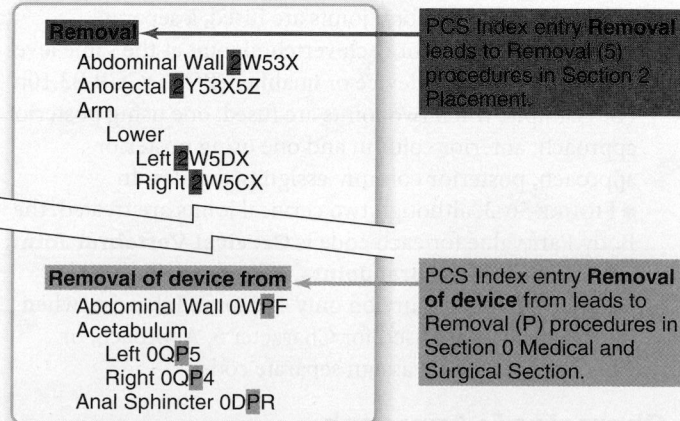

Figure 56-1 ■ PCS Index Entries for Removal Procedures.
Source: © PB Resources, Inc. Used with permission.

Surgeon removed a feeding gastrostomy tube and replaced it with a new one using the existing stoma in the ████████.

0D20XUZ [Medical and Surgical, Gastrointestinal System], Change, Upper intestinal tract, External, Feeding device, No qualifier

Figure 56-2 ■ Example of Assigning a General Body Part Value. *Source: © PB Resources, Inc. Used with permission.*

Part value when the specific Body Part value is not in the Table. For example, in the Gastrointestinal (D) body system, the general Body Part values **Upper Intestinal Tract** and **Lower Intestinal Tract** are provided as options for the Root Operations Change, Removal, and Revision. The upper intestinal tract includes from the esophagus down to and including the duodenum. The lower intestinal tract includes from the jejunum down to and including the rectum and anus (PCS OGCR B4.8). ■ FIGURE 56-2 demonstrates how to code the general Body Part value **0 Upper Intestinal Tract** because Table 0D2 does not provide a specific value for the stomach.

SUCCESS STEP

PCS OGCR B4.8 also applies to the Root Operation Inspection (J), which was discussed in Chapter 55 of this text.

Fusion Procedures

In documentation, a vertebral joint is named based on the vertebra joined, such as C4-C5 for the fusion of the fourth and fifth cervical vertebra. PCS Tables for the Root Operation Fusion do not identify the specific vertebral segments but, rather, the overall level of the spine: cervical, thoracic, lumbar, sacral. Follow these PCS OGCR when assigning Body Part values for Fusion procedures.

- Assign the Body Part value that identifies the level of the spine rendered immobile (PCS OGCR B3.10a). PCS Tables provide distinct Body Part values for a single vertebral joint and multiple vertebral joints at each spinal level. Tables also provide values for joints that link sections of the spine, such as cervicothoracic and sacrococcygeal.

- When multiple vertebral joints are fused, a separate procedure is coded for each vertebral joint at the same level that uses a different device or qualifier (PCS OGCR B3.10b). For example, when two joints are fused, one using posterior approach, anterior column and one using posterior approach, posterior column, assign two codes. In ■ FIGURE 56-3, although two cervical joints are treated, the Body Part value for each code is **Cervical Vertebral Joint**, not **Cervical Vertebral Joints, 2 or more**. Each code describes the procedure on only one joint. Likewise, when different values are used for Character 5, Approach, or Character 6, Device, assign separate codes.

Character 5: Approach

The Root Operations Change and Fusion have special considerations regarding Character 5.

Surgeon performed spinal fusion on C3-C4 using an open posterior approach, anterior column and C4-C5 using an open posterior approach, posterior column. Autologous tissue was used for both procedures.

0RG107J [Medical and Surgical, Upper Joints], Fusion, Cervical Vertebral Joint, Open, Autologous tissue substitute, Posterior approach, anterior column
0RG107 [Medical and Surgical, Upper Joints], Fusion, Cervical Vertebral Joint, Open, Autologous tissue substitute, Posterior approach, posterior column

Figure 56-3 ■ Example of Coding Multiple Fusion Procedures at the Same Level. *Source: © PB Resources, Inc. Used with permission.*

The Root Operation Change always uses the Approach External because the definition of the procedure is **Taking out or off a device from a Body Part and putting back an identical or similar device in or on the same Body Part <u>without cutting or puncturing the skin or a mucous membrane</u>**. When the exchange of a device requires cutting or puncturing, assign two Root Operations: Removal and Insertion.

In the Root Operation Fusion, Character 5 describes the surgical Approach as open, percutaneous, and so on, as it does in other PCS codes. Character 7, Qualifier, describes the directional approach—from the back, a posterior approach, or from the front, an anterior approach—and the anatomic site on the spinal column, that is, the posterior or anterior side of the vertebra. Refer to Chapter 38 of this text for a refresher on the approaches for spinal procedures.

Character 6: Device

Six of the Root Operations discussed in this chapter always involve a device, so Character 6 is used frequently to identify the specific device, or type of device, involved (■ TABLE 56-19).

Table 56-19 ■ EXAMPLES OF DEVICES IDENTIFIED BY CHARACTER 6

Artificial sphincter
Autologous tissue substitute
Contraceptive device
Feeding device
Hearing device, single-channel cochlear prosthesis
Infusion device
Internal fixation device
Intraluminal device, pessary
Monitoring device
Monitoring electrode
Neurostimulator lead
Pacemaker, single-chamber rate responsive
Radioactive element
Spacer
Spinal stabilization device, interspinous process
Tissue expander
Tracheostomy device

Source: © PB Resources, Inc. Used with permission.

The Root Operations Change, Removal, and Revision describe procedures performed on a device only and not on a Body Part. Code the procedure on the device to the appropriate Root Operation based on the definition of each Root Operation (PCS OGCR B6.1c).

CODING CAUTION

Character values, including Device values, can vary among PCS Tables for different Root Operations and Body Systems. Although many letter and number values have consistent meanings across most Tables in the Medical and Surgical Section, they can have different meanings in different tables. For example, the value **4** for Character 6, Device, identifies a single chamber pacemaker in Table 0JH, a bone conduction hearing device in Table 09H, and an autologous tissue substitute in Table 0QP.

Fusion Devices

The Root Operation Fusion uses Character 6 to identify the type of tissue or tissue substitute used to render a vertebral joint immobile. PCS OGCR B3.10c provides the following guidance regarding how to assign Character 6 when combinations of devices and materials are used on the same vertebral joint:

- Interbody fusion device—When an interbody fusion device is used to render the joint immobile, alone or in combination with another material such as a bone graft, use the Device value **Interbody Fusion Device**.
- Bone graft—When bone graft is the only device used to render the joint immobile, assign device value **Nonautologous Tissue Substitute** or **Autologous Tissue Substitute** as appropriate.
- Mixture of tissue substitutes—Code a combination of autologous and nonautologous bone graft used to render the joint immobile with the Device value **Autologous Tissue Substitute**. Code the use of both autologous bone graft and bone bank bone graft with the Device value **Autologous Tissue Substitute**.

- Bone dowel interbody fusion device—Code fusion of a vertebral joint using a bone dowel interbody fusion device made of cadaver bone and packed with a mixture of local morsellized bone and demineralized bone matrix with the Device value **Interbody Fusion Device**.

Insertion, Reposition, and Replacement Devices

Although some PCS Device values are very specific, in other cases they are more general, representing an entire family of devices. A device can have a specific value in a Table for one Root Operation and Body System and a more general value in the Table for another Root Operation or Body System. For example, in PCS Table 02P, a cardiac pacemaker lead has the Device value J and a cardiac defibrillator lead has the Device value K. However, in the PCS Table 02H, the Device value **M Cardiac Lead** identifies any type of cardiac lead, including both a pacemaker lead and a defibrillator lead. The Device Aggregation Table, located in the PCS coding manual appendix, identifies when this situation occurs. It provides a crosswalk of the specific device type to the more general Character 6 Device value needed in some PCS Tables (■ Figure 56-4).

SUCCESS STEP

When the documentation specifies a brand name device that you are uncertain how to code, you often can look up the brand name in the Index to obtain a cross-reference to the correct Character 6 Device value. You also can use the Device Key appendix in the PCS coding manual to crosswalk the device term to the PCS description.

Character 7: Qualifier

As discussed earlier in this chapter, the Root Operation Fusion uses Character 7 to specify whether a vertebral joint fusion uses an anterior or posterior approach and whether the anterior or posterior column of the spine is fused. Other uses of the

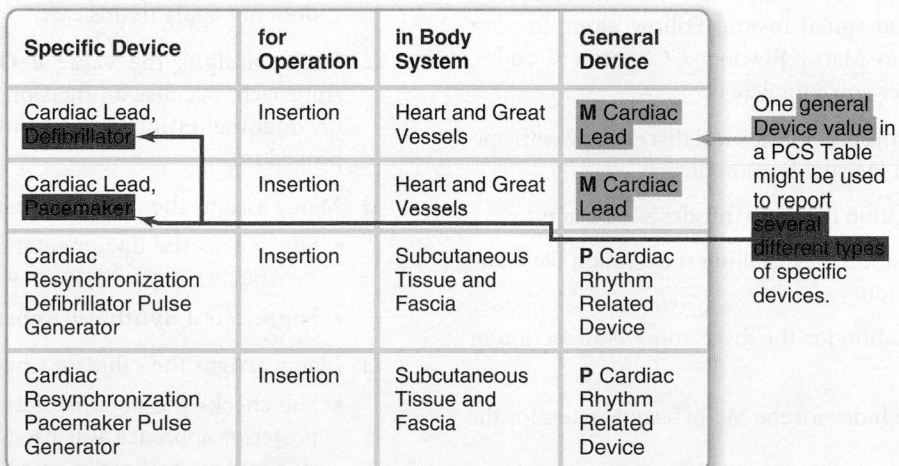

Specific Device	for Operation	in Body System	General Device
Cardiac Lead, Defibrillator	Insertion	Heart and Great Vessels	**M** Cardiac Lead
Cardiac Lead, Pacemaker	Insertion	Heart and Great Vessels	**M** Cardiac Lead
Cardiac Resynchronization Defibrillator Pulse Generator	Insertion	Subcutaneous Tissue and Fascia	**P** Cardiac Rhythm Related Device
Cardiac Resynchronization Pacemaker Pulse Generator	Insertion	Subcutaneous Tissue and Fascia	**P** Cardiac Rhythm Related Device

One general Device value in a PCS Table might be used to report several different types of specific devices.

Figure 56-4 ■ Example of PCS Device Aggregation Table. *Source: Annotations ©PB Resources, Inc. Used with permission.*

Section	0	**Medical and Surgical**
Body System	H	**Skin and Breast**
Operation	R	**Replacement:** Putting in or on biological or synthetic material that physically takes the place and/or function of all or a portion of a Body Part

Body Part Character 4	Approach Character 5	Device Character 6	Qualifier Character 7
T Breast, Right **U** Breast, Left **V** Breast, Bilateral	**0** Open	**7** Autologous Tissue Substitute	**5** Latissimus Dorsi Myocutaneous Flap **6** Transverse Rectus Abdominis Myocutaneous Flap **7** Deep Inferior Epigastric Artery Perforator Flap **8** Superficial Inferior Epigastric Artery Flap **9** Gluteal Artery Perforator Flap **Z** No Qualifier

Figure 56-5 ■ Example of Character 7 Used to Identify the Source of Autologous Tissue

Qualifier with Root Operations discussed in this chapter include the following:

- Identify the source of autologous tissue in a graft or fusion procedure (■ FIGURE 56-5)
- Distinguish whether a prosthetic joint is cemented or uncemented
- Indicate the use of a partial- or full-thickness graft in skin graft procedures
- Provide greater specificity of the anatomic site

Guided Example of Assigning Characters 4–7 for Fusion, Insertion, and Resection

To practice skills for assigning codes for the Root Operations Fusion, Insertion, and Resection, continue with the example from earlier in the chapter about a patient who was seen for a lumbar discectomy and spinal fusion. Follow along in your ICD-10-PCS manual as Marcy Elwood, CCS, assigns codes. Check off each step after you complete it.

▶ First, Marcy confirms the procedures: discectomy with spinal arthrodesis and internal fixation device.

❑ The Root Operation for the arthrodesis is Fusion.

❑ The Root Operation for installing the fixation plate and screws is Insertion.

❑ The Root Operation for the discectomy is Resection or Excision.

▶ Marcy searches the Index for the Main Term **Fusion** for the arthrodesis.

❑ She locates the first-level subterm **Lumbar vertebral**.

❑ She identifies the Table **0SG** and partial code **0SG0**.

▶ Marcy turns to Table **0SG** to assign the code for arthrodesis.

❑ She reads the Table title **0SG, Medical and Surgical, Lower Joints, Fusion** and confirms that this accurately describes the Body System and Root Operation.

❑ Marcy assigns the value for Character 4, Body Part.

■ She reviews the values provided and confirms that **0 Lumbar vertebral**, which was part of the partial code **0SG0** provided in the Index, is correct.

■ The second value for the lumbar spine is **Lumbar vertebral joints, 2 or more**. L4 and L5 comprise one joint, which is the joint being fused. If the fusion was L4-L5 and L5-L6, the value for two or more joints would be used.

■ There is also an option for Lumbosacral joint, which does not apply to this case.

❑ Marcy assigns the value **0 Open** for Character 5, Approach, because an incision was made and there is no documentation of a percutaneous or endoscopic procedure.

❑ Marcy assigns the value for Character 6, Device.

■ She checks the documentation and identifies that a synthetic bone substitute was used.

■ She selects **J Synthetic Substitute** as the Device.

❑ Marcy assigns the value for Character 7, Qualifier.

■ She checks the documentation and identifies that a posterior approach was used because an 11-cm incision was made directly over L4-L5.

■ She checks the documentation and identifies that the posterior column was treated.

Section	0	Medical and Surgical
Body System	S	Lower Joints
Operation	G	**Fusion:** Joining together portions of an articular Body Part rendering the articular Body Part immobile

Body Part Character 4	Approach Character 5	Device Character 6	Qualifier Character 7
0 Lumbar Vertebral Joint 1 Lumbar Vertebral Joints, 2 or more 3 Lumbosacral Joint	**0 Open** 3 Percutaneous 4 Percutaneous Endoscopic	7 Autologous Tissue Substitute A Interbody Fusion Device **J Synthetic Substitute** K Nonautologous Tissue Substitute Z No Device	0 Anterior Approach, Anterior Column **1 Posterior Approach, Posterior Column** J Posterior Approach, Anterior Column

Figure 56-6 ■ Assigning Code 0SG00J1. *Source: Annotation © PB Resources, Inc. Used with permission.*

- She selects **1 Posterior Approach, Posterior Column** as the Qualifier.

❑ She reviews the code she has assigned for the spinal arthrodesis: **0SG00J1** (■ FIGURE 56-6).

▶ Marcy searches the Index for the Main Term **Insertion** for installation of the fixation plate and screws. This procedure is in addition to the Fusion and requires a separate code.

❑ She locates the first-level subterm **Spinal stabilization device**.

❑ She locates the second-level subterm *see* **Insertion of device in, Lower Joints 0SH**. This instruction cross-references her to the next Main Term, **Insertion of device in**, which has several columns of entries.

❑ She locates the first-level subterm under this Main Term, **Joint**.

❑ She locates the second-level subterm **Lumbar vertebral**.

❑ She identifies the Table **0SH** and partial code **0SH0**.

▶ Marcy turns to Table **0SH** to assign the code for installation of the fixation plate and screws.

❑ She reads the Table title **0SH, Medical and Surgical, Lower Joints, Insertion** and confirms that this accurately describes the Body System and Root Operation.

❑ Marcy assigns the value **0 Lumbar Vertebral Joint** for Character 4, Body Part.

❑ Marcy assigns the value **0 Open** for Character 5, Approach.

❑ Marcy assigns the value **4 Internal Fixation Device** for Character 6, Device, because it identifies the use of the plate and screws.

❑ Marcy assigns the value **Z No Qualifier** for Character 7, Qualifier.

❑ She reviews the code she has assigned for the fixation plate and screws: **0SH004Z** (■ FIGURE 56-7)

▶ Marcy searches the Index for the Main Term **Resection** for the discectomy. Because the documentation specifies all disc material, and not just a portion of the disc, was removed, she can use the Root Operation **Resection** rather than **Excision**.

❑ She locates the first-level subterm **Disc**.

❑ She locates the second-level subterm **Lumbar Vertebral**.

❑ She identifies Table **0ST** and partial code **0ST20ZZ**. Although this appears to be a complete seven-character code, she knows she cannot assign the code from the Index and must refer to the PCS Table to verify all the characters.

▶ Marcy turns to Table **0ST** to assign the code for the discectomy.

❑ She reads the Table title **0ST, Medical and Surgical, Lower Joints, Resection** and confirms that this accurately describes the Body System and Root Operation.

Section	0	Medical and Surgical
Body System	S	Lower Joints
Operation	H	**Insertion:** Putting in a nonbiological appliance that monitors, assists, performs, or prevents a physiological function but does not physically take the place of a Body Part

Body Part Character 4	Approach Character 5	Device Character 6	Qualifier Character 7
0 Lumbar Vertebral Joint 3 Lumbosacral Joint	**0 Open** 5 Percutaneous 6 Percutaneous Endoscopic	3 Infusion Device **4 Internal Fixation Device** 8 Spacer B Spinal Stabilization Device, Interspinous Process C Spinal Stabilization Device, Pedicle-Based D Spinal Stabilization Device, Facet Replacement	**Z No Qualifier**

Figure 56-7 ■ Assigning Code 0SH004Z. *Source: Annotation © PB Resources, Inc. Used with permission.*

Section	0	Medical and Surgical
Body System	S	Lower Joints
Operation	T	Resection: Cutting out or off, without replacement, all of a Body Part

Body Part Character 4	Approach Character 5	Device Character 6	Qualifier Character 7
2 Lumbar Vertebral Disc	0 Open	Z No Device	Z No Qualifier
4 Lumbosacral Disc	3 Percutaneous		
5 Sacrococcygeal Joint	4 Percutaneous Endoscopic		
6 Coccygeal Joint	7 Via Natural or Artificial Opening		
7 Sacroiliac Joint, Right	8 Via Natural or Artificial Opening Endoscopic		
8 Sacroiliac Joint, Left			

Figure 56-8 ■ Assigning Code 0ST20ZZ. *Source: Annotation © PB Resources, Inc. Used with permission.*

❑ Marcy assigns the value **2 Lumbar Vertebral Disc** for Character 4, Body Part.

❑ Marcy assigns the value **0 Open** for Character 5, Approach, which is the only choice.

❑ Marcy assigns the value **Z No Device** for Character 6, Device, which is the only choice.

❑ Marcy assigns the value **Z No Qualifier** for Character 7, Qualifier, which is the only choice.

❑ She reviews the code she has assigned for the *discectomy*: **0ST20ZZ** (■ FIGURE 56-8).

▶ Marcy reviews the procedure codes she has assigned for this case:

❑ **0SG00J1** [Medical and Surgical, Lower Joints], Fusion, Lumbar vertebral joint, Open, Synthetic substitute, Posterior approach posterior column

❑ **0SH004Z** [Medical and Surgical, Lower Joints], Insertion, Lumbar vertebral joint, Open, Internal fixation device, No qualifier

❑ **0ST20ZZ** [Medical and Surgical, Lower Joints], Resection, Lumbar vertebral disc, Open, No device, No qualifier

▶ Next, Marcy must determine how to sequence the codes.

CODING PRACTICE

Exercise 56.3 Assigning Characters 4–7 for Root Operations H, R, U, 2, P, W, 3, Q, G, 0, and 4

Instructions: Read the mini-medical-record of each patient's encounter. Review the information abstracted in Exercise 56.2 for questions 1–3. For questions 4–6, abstract the case on your own. Assign PCS codes using the Index and Tables. Write the code(s) on the line provided.

1. INPATIENT HOSPITAL Gender: F Age: 81

Preprocedure diagnosis: status post-arthroplasty

Procedure: exchange of drainage tube from right hip joint following total hip replacement

Tip: The skin was not pierced to replace the drainage tube.

1 PCS Code _____

2. INPATIENT HOSPITAL Gender: M Age: 75

Preprocedure diagnosis: sick sinus syndrome, displaced pacemaker lead

Procedure: percutaneous adjustment of position of left pacemaker lead in left atrium

1 PCS Code _____

3. INPATIENT HOSPITAL Gender: F Age: 36

Preprocedure diagnosis: drooping right upper eyelid affects patient's perception of appearance but does not interfere with vision

Procedure: cosmetic blepharoplasty. Cut out a crescent of skin and subcutaneous tissue from fold of R eyelid, sutured to restore normal position of eyelid.

Tip: Review the purpose of the procedure to determine the Root Operation.

1 PCS Code _____

4. INPATIENT HOSPITAL   Gender: M   Age: 25

Preprocedure diagnosis: *puncture wound from knife, left lower arm surface*

Procedure: *suture of 2-cm laceration, depth of 0.6 cm into the dermis. Wound irrigated. Deep sutures 4/0 PDS with 5-0 nylon running suture used to realign the skin. Antibiotic ointment and compression bandage applied.*

Tip: Lacerations most often affect the skin, but any tissue may be lacerated, including deeper layers of subcutaneous fat, tendon, muscle, or bone.

1 PCS Code _____

5. INPATIENT HOSPITAL   Gender: F   Age: 35

Preprocedure diagnosis: *central venous pressure measurement, septic shock*

(continued)

5. (continued)

Procedure: *emergency internal jugular central venous catheter insertion, left side. An 8.5 French CV quad-lumen catheter was advanced into the internal jugular vein and secured in place with the tip of the catheter in the superior vena cava.*

Tip: The CVP is inserted for hemodynamic monitoring.

1 PCS Code _____

6. INPATIENT HOSPITAL   Gender: F   Age: 42

Preprocedure diagnosis: *bleeding postop hysterectomy.*

Procedure: *control of postop hemorrhage and evacuation of clot via hysteroscope. Bleeders cauterized and blood clot evacuated. No further bleeding noted.*

Tip: The only objective of the procedure is to stop hemorrhaging after the procedure.

1 PCS Code _____

ARRANGING CODES FOR ROOT OPERATIONS H, R, U, 2, P, W, 3, Q, G, 0, AND 4

In addition to the general PCS OGCR for multiple coding, coders should be alert for specific situations related to the Root Operations discussed in this chapter when multiple coding might be required.

Multiple codes with multiple Root Operations are required with Insertion procedures when:

- a device is placed during another procedure and the more definitive procedure does not provide a Character 6 Device value. Sequence the more definitive procedure as the principal procedure because it is most related to the principal diagnosis.

- an existing device is taken out and replaced with a new one, requiring an Approach other than External. Code the Root Operation Insertion for placement of the new device. Recall that the Root Operation Change is used for an exchange procedure only when the skin or mucous membrane is not punctured or cut.

Multiple codes with multiple Root Operations are required with Removal procedures when:

- an existing device is taken out and replaced with a new one, requiring an Approach other than External. Code the Root Operation Removal for taking out the existing device.

Multiple codes using the Root Operation Fusion are required when:

- multiple vertebral segments within the same spinal region use different surgical approaches, anatomic approaches, or devices.

Guided Example of Arranging Codes for Fusion, Insertion, and Resection

To practice skills for arranging codes for the Root Operations Fusion, Insertion, and Resection, continue with the example from earlier in the chapter about a patient who was seen for a lumbar discectomy and spinal fusion. Follow along in your ICD-10-PCS manual as Marcy Elwood, CCS, arranges the codes. Check off each step after you complete it.

▶ First, Marcy confirms the procedures *discectomy with spinal arthrodesis* and *fixation plate and screws* and reviews the codes she has assigned.

❑ **0SG00J1 [Medical and Surgical, Lower Joints], Fusion, Lumbar vertebral joint, Open, Synthetic substitute, Posterior approach posterior column**

❑ **0SH004Z [Medical and Surgical, Lower Joints], Insertion, Lumbar vertebral joint, Open, Internal fixation device, No qualifier**

❑ **0ST20ZZ [Medical and Surgical, Lower Joints], Resection, Lumbar vertebral disc, Open, No device, No qualifier**

▶ The principal procedure must be the one most closely related to the principal diagnosis, *degenerative disc disease*. All the procedures are directly related to the principal diagnosis, so because there was a specific problem with the L4-L5 disc, she sequences code **0ST20ZZ** for Resection of the disc first.

▶ Marcy sequences code **0SG00J1** for the arthrodesis second and **0SH004Z** for installation of the internal fixation device third.

▶ Marcy finalizes the procedure codes and sequencing for this case:

(1) **0ST20ZZ [Medical and Surgical, Lower Joints], Resection, Lumbar vertebral disc, Open, No device, No qualifier**

(2) **0SG00J1 [Medical and Surgical, Lower Joints], Fusion, Lumbar vertebral joint, Open, Synthetic substitute, Posterior approach posterior column**

(3) **0SH004Z [Medical and Surgical, Lower Joints], Insertion, Lumbar vertebral joint, Open, Internal fixation device, No qualifier**

▶ Marcy also assigns and sequences the ICD-10-CM diagnosis code that supports the need for the service.

(1) **M51.36 Other intervertebral disc degeneration, lumbar region**

CODING PRACTICE

Exercise 56.4 Arranging Codes for Root Operations H, R, U, 2, P, W, 3, Q, G, 0, and 4

Instructions: Read the mini-medical-record of each patient's encounter. Review the information abstracted in Exercise 56.2 for questions 1–3. For questions 4–6, abstract the case on your own. Assign PCS codes using the Index and Tables, and arrange the codes in proper sequence. Write the code(s) on the line provided.

1. INPATIENT HOSPITAL   Gender: M   Age: 72

Preprocedure diagnosis: blepharoptosis obscuring vision

Procedure: Bilateral upper blepharoplasty. Cut out a crescent of skin and subcutaneous tissue from fold of R eyelid, sutured to restore normal position of eyelid. Repeated on left side.

Tip: Review the purpose of the procedure to determine the Root Operation.

2 PCS Codes _____

2. INPATIENT HOSPITAL   Gender: M   Age: 53

Preprocedure diagnosis: detached R retina

Procedure: Trans pars plana vitrectomy (TPPV) with synthetic scleral buckle. Made incision in pars plana and used vitreous cutter to remove all vitreous. Injected balanced saline solution (BSS) to replace vitreous. Sutured scleral buckle, which effectively closed the retinal break. Pt tolerated px well.

Tip: Injection of BSS is part of the procedure and is not coded separately.

2 PCS Codes _____

3. INPATIENT HOSPITAL   Gender: F   Age: 68

Preprocedure diagnosis: bradycardia, malfunctioning pacemaker lead

Procedure: percutaneous exchange of a malfunctioning pacemaker lead in the left atrium with a new one

Tip: The PCS Tables for each Root Operation provide different Body Part and Device values.

2 PCS Codes _____

4. INPATIENT HOSPITAL   Gender: F   Age: 59

Preprocedure diagnosis: adenocarcinoma of the right breast

Procedure: right modified radical mastectomy with immediate breast reconstruction with tissue expander. The breast was removed, including the skin, breast tissue, areola, and nipple, and most of the lymph nodes under the arm. The pectoralis major muscle was spared for reconstruction. The expander was placed and the pectoralis muscle reapproximated for total muscle coverage. Wounds were closed and skin flap appeared healthy.

2 PCS Codes _____

5. INPATIENT HOSPITAL   Gender: M   Age: 57

Preprocedure diagnosis: metastatic glossal carcinoma, needing chemotherapy and a port

Procedure: open exploration of the left subclavian/axillary vein; insertion of a double lumen port through the left femoral vein, radiological guidance. The subclavian vein was identified and we were unable to subcutaneously cannulate it due to sclerosis. Decision was made to insert the port through the left femoral vein. Femoral vein cannulated without difficulty and double lumen port inserted.

Tip: If the intended procedure is discontinued, code the procedure to the root operation performed. PCS OGCR B3.3.

2 PCS Codes _____

6. INPATIENT HOSPITAL   Gender: M   Age: 13 months

Preprocedure diagnosis: involutional entropion, right and left lower eyelids

Procedure: tightening of the eyelid was achieved via the lateral tarsal strip procedure. The tarsal plate (*cartilage in the lower lid*) was shortened and used as the tendon to suspend to the orbital bone. The procedure was performed on both sides.

2 PCS Codes _____

CHAPTER SUMMARY

In this chapter you learned that:

- The Medical and Surgical Root Operations in the group *Procedures that Always Involve a Device* are Insertion (H), Replacement (R), Supplement (U), Change (2), Removal (P), and Revision (W).

- The Root Operation Insertion (H) is putting in a nonbiological appliance that monitors, assists, performs, or prevents a physiological function but does not physically take the place of a Body Part.

- The Root Operation Replacement (R) is putting in or on biological or synthetic material that physically takes the place and/or function of all or a portion of a Body Part.

- The Root Operation Supplement (U) is putting in or on biological or synthetic material that physically reinforces and/or augments the function of a portion of a Body Part.

- The Root Operation Change (2) is taking out or off a device from a Body Part and putting back an identical or similar device in or on the same Body Part without cutting or puncturing the skin or a mucous membrane.

- The Root Operation Removal (P) is taking out or off a device from a Body Part.

- The Root Operation Revision (W) is correcting, to the extent possible, a portion of a malfunctioning device or the position of a displaced device.

- The Medical and Surgical Root Operations in the group *Procedures that Define Other Repairs* are Control (3) and Repair (Q).

- The Root Operation Control (3) is stopping, or attempting to stop, postprocedural bleeding.

- The Root Operation Repair (Q) is restoring, to the extent possible, a Body Part to its normal anatomic structure and function.

- The Medical and Surgical Root Operations in the group *Procedures that Define Other Objectives* are Fusion (G), Alteration (0), and Creation (4).

- The Root Operation Fusion (G) is joining together portions of an articular Body Part, rendering the articular Body Part immobile.

- The Root Operation Alteration (0) is modifying the anatomic structure of a Body Part without affecting the function of the Body Part.

- The Root Operation Creation (4) is making a new genital structure that does not take over the function of a Body Part.

- Assign a general Body Part value when the specific Body Part value is not in a PCS Table.

- PCS Tables for the Root Operation Fusion do not identify the specific vertebral segments but, rather, the overall level of the spine: cervical, thoracic, lumbar, sacral.

- The Root Operation Change always uses the Approach External.

- The Root Operation Fusion uses Character 6 to identify the type of tissue or tissue substitute used to render a vertebral joint immobile.

- The PCS Device Aggregation Table, located in the PCS coding manual appendix, provides a crosswalk of a specific device type to a more general Character 6 Device value needed in some PCS Tables.

- PCS provides guidelines related to the Root Operations Change, Control, Fusion. It also provides guidance regarding the use of Character 4, Body Part, and Character 6, Device, related to Root Operations discussed in this chapter.

CONCEPT QUIZ

Take a moment to look back at Root Operations discussed in this chapter and solidify your skills. Try to answer the questions from memory first, then refer to the discussion in this chapter if you need a little extra help.

Completion

Instructions: Write the term that answers each question based on the information you learned in this chapter. Choose from the list below. Some choices may be used more than once and some choices may not be used at all.

Alteration	Removal
Change	Repair
Control	Replacement
Creation	Revision
Fusion	Supplement
Insertion	

1. The Root Operation _____ is joining together portions of an articular Body Part, rendering the articular Body Part immobile.

2. The Root Operation _____ is making a new genital structure that does not take over the function of a Body Part.

3. The Root Operation _____ is restoring, to the extent possible, a Body Part to its normal anatomic structure and function.

4. The Root Operation _____ is putting in or on biological or synthetic material that physically takes the place and/or function of all or a portion of a Body Part.

(continued)

(continued from page 1129)

5. The Root Operation _____ is putting in or on biological or synthetic material that physically reinforces and/or augments the function of a portion of a Body Part.

6. The Root Operation _____ is modifying the anatomic structure of a Body Part without affecting the function of the Body Part.

7. The Root Operation _____ is putting in a nonbiological appliance that monitors, assists, performs, or prevents a physiological function but does not physically take the place of a Body Part.

8. The Root Operation _____ is correcting, to the extent possible, a portion of a malfunctioning device or the position of a displaced device.

9. The Root Operation _____ is taking out or off a device from a Body Part and putting back an identical or similar device in or on the same Body Part without cutting or puncturing the skin or a mucous membrane.

10. The Root Operation _____ is taking out or off a device from a Body Part.

Multiple Choice

Instructions: Circle the letter of the best answer to each question based on the information you learned in this chapter.

1. What Root Operation always uses the Approach External?
   A. Removal (P)
   B. Control (3)
   C. Alteration (0)
   D. Change (2)

2. Which procedure is an example of the Root Operation Supplement (U)?
   A. Prosthetic lens implantation
   B. Placement of bone growth stimulator
   C. Mitral valve ring annuloplasty
   D. Vertebral arthrodesis

3. What PCS coding manual appendix provides a crosswalk of a specific device type to a more general Character 6 Device value needed in some PCS Tables?
   A. Device Combination Crosswalk
   B. Device Conversion Guide
   C. Device Key
   D. Device Aggregation Table

4. What Root Operation uses Character 6 to identify the type of tissue or tissue substitute used to render a vertebral joint immobile?
   A. Fusion (G)
   B. Control (3)
   C. Repair (Q)
   D. Revision (W)

5. Which Root Operation is coded for all procedures performed solely to improve appearance?
   A. Supplement (U)
   B. Alteration (0)
   C. Revision (W)
   D. Creation (4)

6. Which Root Operation is typically used to code putting in a multiple-channel cochlear implant?
   A. Supplement (U)
   B. Replacement (R)
   C. Insertion (H)
   D. Repair (Q)

7. Which of the following situations requires multiple codes?
   A. Multiple vertebral segments within the same spinal region use different devices.
   B. An attempt to control postprocedural bleeding is unsuccessful, so a resection procedure must be performed.
   C. An existing device is taken out and replaced with a new one using the External Approach.
   D. A combination of autologous and nonautologous bone graft tissue is used to render a joint immobile.

8. Which PCS Character is used to distinguish whether a prosthetic joint is cemented or uncemented?
   A. 4
   B. 5
   C. 6
   D. 7

9. Which Root Operation contains only two procedure codes, used for sex change operations?
   A. Change (2)
   B. Creation (4)
   C. Revision (W)
   D. Replacement (R)

10. What PCS coding manual appendix provides a crosswalk from brand name devices to the PCS Description?
   A. Device Key
   B. Device Brand Crosswalk
   C. Device Aggregation Table
   D. Manufacturer's Brand Guide to PCS

CODING CHALLENGE

Instructions: Read the mini-medical-record of each patient's encounter, then abstract, assign, and arrange ICD-10-CM diagnosis codes and PCS procedure codes using the appropriate Index and Tables. Write the code(s) on the line provided.

1. INPATIENT HOSPITAL   Gender: F   Age: 68

Preprocedure diagnosis: primary degenerative osteoarthritis localized to the knee, extreme difficulty walking

Procedure: total L knee replacement. Made midline incision 10 cm above L patella, entered joint capsule medially, and exposed tibiofemoral joint. Resected tibia and femur, then sized for prosthetic. Inserted synthetic knee prosthesis, cemented in place, and closed operative wound. Minimal blood loss. Patient tolerated procedure well.

1 ICD-10-CM Code _____

1 ICD-10-PCS Code _____

2. INPATIENT HOSPITAL   Gender: F   Age: 74

Preprocedure diagnosis: macular edema, right eye

Procedure: insertion of radioactive plaque, right eye with lateral canthotomy. The plaque was positioned on the scleral surface immediately behind the macula and secured with two sutures of 5-0 Dacron. The placement was confirmed with indirect ophthalmoscopy.

1 ICD-10-CM Code _____

1 ICD-10-PCS Code _____

3. INPATIENT HOSPITAL   Gender: M   Age: 26

Preprocedure diagnosis: left ventral hernia

Procedure: left ventral hernia repair with Marlex mesh via laparoscope. Ports placed in the abdomen and a stab incision made overlying the skin and hernia. Marlex mesh introduced and secured in position overlying the hernia. Ports removed and incisions closed.

1 ICD-10-CM Code _____

1 ICD-10-PCS Code _____

4. INPATIENT HOSPITAL   Gender: F   Age: 68

Preprocedure diagnosis: abdominal aortic aneurysm (AAA)

Procedure: EVAR (endovascular aneurysm repair) with synthetic graft. Made incision into the femoral artery. With fluoroscopic guidance, guided delivery catheter with compressed graft into abdominal aorta to site of aneurysm. Inflated balloon to expand graft and affix it to vessel wall. Withdrew catheter and closed incision.

Tip: An endovascular graft is placed inside the vessel and physically takes over the function, rendering the original vessel nonfunctional. Do not assign an additional code for the fluoroscopy portion because it is not a Medical and Surgical procedure from Section 0.

1 ICD-10-CM Code _____

1 ICD-10-PCS Code _____

5. INPATIENT HOSPITAL   Gender: F   Age: 17

Preprocedure diagnosis: second debridement for extensive burns on both arms

Procedure: excisional debridement and graft. Cut out necrotic subcutaneous tissue and fascia and applied autologous skin substitute on both lower arms and nonautologous tissue substitute on both upper arms.

Postprocedure diagnosis: second- and third-degree burns to anterior and posterior of right and left upper and lower arms, 18% TBSA (total body surface area) with burns, 9% TBSA third-degree burns.

Tip: Each portion (upper and lower) of each arm is coded as a separate body area for the diagnosis and procedure. Refer to OGCR I.C.19.a to review the use of ICD-10-CM code extensions. Do not code external cause, source, or intent of burns.

5 ICD-10-CM Codes _____

_____

4 ICD-10-PCS Codes _____

_____

6. INPATIENT HOSPITAL   Gender: F   Age: 6

Preprocedure diagnosis: congenital cleft earlobe defect, left ear

Procedure: open cosmetic plastic repair of deformed left ear lobe. The skin of the cleft was completely excised and a flap along the cleft made at the posterior side of the lobe. The wound was closed with simple stitches on both anterior and posterior sides of the lobe.

1 ICD-10-CM Code _____

1 ICD-10-PCS Code _____

(continued)

(continued from page 1131)

7. INPATIENT HOSPITAL   Gender: M   Age: 4

Preprocedure diagnosis: *congenital myotonic muscular dystrophy with bilateral planovalgus feet*

Procedure: *bilateral Crawford subtalar arthrodesis with open Achilles Z-lengthening and bilateral long-leg cast. Incision was made over the left lateral aspect of the hind foot. A ⅞-inch staple was placed across the sinus tarsi to maintain the desired reduction. The incision was extended posteriorly to allow for visualization of the Achilles, which was Z-lengthened with the release of the lateral distal half. Wounds closed and dressing applied. The procedure was performed on both the right and left side without complication.*

2 ICD-10-CM Codes _____

4 ICD-10-PCS Codes _____

_____

8. INPATIENT HOSPITAL   Gender: M   Age: 22

Preprocedure diagnosis: *epistaxis, left nasal passage, following sinus endoscopy six hours prior*

Procedure: *endoscopic left anterior ethmoid artery cauterization, sphenopalatine artery cauterization. No obvious bleeding site seen endoscopically. Incision carried down to ethmoid artery, which was cauterized, and incision closed. Attention turned to the nose; the sphenopalatine artery identified and cauterized using suction cautery. Hemostasis obtained and the area packed with Metrogel.*

2 ICD-10-CM Codes _____

1 ICD-10-PCS Code _____

9. INPATIENT HOSPITAL   Gender: F   Age: 10

Preprocedure diagnosis: *dislodged G tube, inserted 12 hours prior; spastic cerebral palsy*

Procedure: *gastrostomy tube change. The G tube inserted earlier today was removed. The tract was assessed; new G tube lubricated and slid easily into the tract. Tube secured and placement verified by X-ray.*

Tip: The device was removed and a similar device immediately inserted without making an incision or puncturing the skin or mucous membrane.

2 ICD-10-CM Codes _____

1 ICD-10-PCS Code _____

10. INPATIENT HOSPITAL   Gender: F   Age: 25

Preprocedure diagnosis: *menorrhagia; dyspareunia*

Procedure: *intrauterine device extraction. IUD strings identified and grasped with the ring forceps. Steady gentle outward traction was applied and the IUD easily appeared in the vagina and was removed.*

2 ICD-10-CM Codes _____

1 ICD-10-PCS Code _____

KEEP ON CODING

Instructions: Read the procedural statement, then use the appropriate Index and Tables to assign PCS procedure codes. Write the code(s) on the line provided.

1. Central line insertion, percutaneous, right subclavian vein for infusion therapy: ICD-10-PCS Code(s) _____

2. Right total knee replacement with cemented implant: ICD-10-PCS Code(s) _____

3. Right inguinal herniorrhaphy with mesh: ICD-10-PCS Code(s) _____

4. PEG tube change: ICD-10-PCS Code(s) _____

5. Removal of drainage tube from gallbladder: ICD-10-PCS Code(s) _____

6. Open revision of left hip replacement liner: ICD-10-PCS Code(s) _____

7. Control of postoperative tonsillectomy bleeding: ICD-10-PCS Code(s) _____

8. Suture of laceration of skin of back: ICD-10-PCS Code(s) _____

9. Open fusion of right finger phalangeal joint with internal fixation: ICD-10-PCS Code(s) _____

10. Bilateral breast augmentation with Corning silicone implants: ICD-10-PCS Code(s) _____

11. Gender alteration of male with creation of vagina using synthetic material: ICD-10-PCS Code(s) _____

12. Insertion of Vaxcel Plus dialysis catheter in the right internal jugular vein, percutaneous: ICD-10-PCS Code(s) _____

13. Aortic valve replacement with Medtronic mechanical valve: ICD-10-PCS Code(s) _____

14. Remove subclavian cardiac output central line: ICD-10-PCS Code(s) _____

15. Percutaneous Vaxcel port implantation for central access chemotherapy via the left internal jugular (LIJ): ICD-10-PCS Code(s)

_____

16. Remove PEG tube: ICD-10-PCS Code(s) _____

17. Cosmetic supplemental rhinoplasty of nasal septum with synthetic substitute: ICD-10-PCS Code(s) _____

18. Change chest tube (for right hemothorax): ICD-10-PCS Code(s) _____

19. Anterior spinal fusion of C3-C4 with cadaver bone graft: ICD-10-PCS Code(s) _____

20. Percutaneous reposition of pacemaker lead in left atrium: ICD-10-PCS Code(s) _____

21. Laparoscopic control of perineum bleeding, posthysterectomy: ICD-10-PCS Code(s) _____

22. Percutaneous endoscopic tympanoplasty, or right ruptured tympanic membrane: ICD-10-PCS Code(s) _____

23. Endoscopic posterior spinal fusion L3-L4, posterior column, using cadaver bone graft: ICD-10-PCS Code(s) _____

24. PICC (peripherally inserted central catheter) into the left cephalic vein for antibiotic therapy: ICD-10-PCS Code(s) _____

25. Percutaneous revision of left breast tissue expander: ICD-10-PCS Code(s) _____

Chapter Outline

- **Basics of Medical and Surgical-<u>Related</u> Procedures**
- **Coding Overview of Medical and Surgical-<u>Related</u> Procedures**
- **Abstracting for Medical and Surgical-<u>Related</u> Procedures**
- **Assigning Characters 4–7 for Medical and Surgical-<u>Related</u> Procedures**
- **Arranging Codes for Medical and Surgical-<u>Related</u> Procedures**

Learning Objectives

After completing this chapter, you should have the skills to:

57.1 Spell and define the key words, medical terms, and abbreviations used with Medical and Surgical-<u>Related</u> procedures.

57.2 Discuss the types of procedures covered by Medical and Surgical-<u>Related</u> Procedures.

57.3 Identify the main characteristics of coding for the Root Operations for Medical and Surgical-<u>Related</u> procedures.

57.4 Abstract procedural information from the medical record for coding for Medical and Surgical-<u>Related</u> procedures.

57.5 Assign codes for the Root Operations for Medical and Surgical-<u>Related</u> procedures.

57.6 Arrange codes for the Root Operations for Medical and Surgical-<u>Related</u> procedures.

57.7 Discuss the ICD-10-PCS coding guidelines associated with Medical and Surgical-<u>Related</u> procedures.

Key Terms and Abbreviations

abortifacient	cardiopulmonary bypass (CPB)	doctor of osteopathy (DO)	hyperbaric oxygen treatment (HBOT)
allopathic	chiropractic manipulation	extracorporeal	product of conception

In addition to the key terms listed here, students should know the terms defined within tables in this chapter.

For updates and corrections, visit our student resource site at

www.pearsonhighered.com/healthprofessionsresources

INTRODUCTION

If you are an avid traveler, going to new places does not intimidate you. After you learn how to get around a few towns or even a few backcountry areas, you learn certain strategies and techniques that you can use anywhere you go. Thus you are able to quickly adapt to a new environment and begin seeing what it has to offer. PCS coding is similar. After you understand the structure of a PCS code and develop the skills for navigating the Medical and Surgical Section, you can apply those skills to learn how to code procedures in other Sections.

This chapter discusses PCS Sections 1 through 9, referred to as Medical and Surgical-<u>Related</u> procedures. Note the presence of the word <u>Related</u> in the Section title to avoid potential confusion with PCS Section 0, Medical and Surgical procedures, which has a similar name. You will learn how codes in these Sections are structured, how Root Operations are defined, and other unique characteristics. As with the Medical and Surgical Section, pay careful attention to the differences between each Root Operation so that you can use each confidently and accurately.

BASICS OF MEDICAL AND SURGICAL-RELATED PROCEDURES

"Medical and Surgical-<u>Related</u> procedures" is a descriptive title that summarizes nine PCS Sections, but it does not occupy a Character within the code itself. ■ TABLE 57-1 summarizes the value, name, and purpose of each Section. Although there are many Sections and some new Root Operations, Medical and Surgical-<u>Related</u> Sections contain approximately 2,500 codes, or 4% of PCS, compared with over 62,000 codes (86%) in the Medical and Surgical (0) Section.

Medical and Surgical-<u>Related</u> procedure codes have seven Characters, but in some Sections the purpose of a Character is different than in the Medical and Surgical (0) Section (■ TABLE 57-2). In the Obstetrics (1) and Placement (2) Sections,

Table 57-1 ■ CHARACTER 1: SECTION NAMES AND PURPOSE OF MEDICAL AND SURGICAL-<u>RELATED</u> PROCEDURES

Value	Section Name	Purpose
1	Obstetrics	Procedures on an embryo, fetus, or unborn child
2	Placement	Procedures involving devices and materials that are performed without making an incision or a puncture
3	Administration	Procedures in which a diagnostic or therapeutic substance is given to the patient
4	Measurement and Monitoring	Procedures that take a single or series of readings of physiologic levels, such as temperature or heart rate
5	Extracorporeal Assistance and Performance	Procedures in which equipment outside the body is used to assist or perform a physiological function
6	Extracorporeal Therapies	Use of equipment outside the body for a therapeutic purpose that does not involve the assistance or performance of a physiological function.
7	Osteopathic	Osteopathic manipulation procedures
8	Other Procedures	Miscellaneous procedures not included in other Medical and Surgical-<u>Related</u> Sections
9	Chiropractic	Chiropractic manipulation procedures

Table 57-2 ■ SEVEN CHARACTERS OF MEDICAL AND SURGICAL-<u>RELATED</u> PROCEDURES

	Character					
1	2	3	4	5	6	7
Obstetrics **1**	Body System	Root Operation	Body Part	Approach	Device	Qualifier
Placement **2**	Body System	Root Operation	Body Region	Approach	Device	Qualifier
Administration **3**	Body System	Root Operation	Body Region	Approach	Substance	Qualifier
Measurement and Monitoring **4**	Body System	Root Operation	Body Region	Approach	Function	Qualifier
Extracorporeal Assistance and Performance **5**	Body System	Root Operation	Body System	Duration	Function	Qualifier
Extracorporeal Therapies **6**	Body System	Root Operation	Body System	Duration	Qualifier	Qualifier
Osteopathic **7**	Body System	Root Operation	Body Region	Approach	Method	Qualifier
Other Procedures **8**	Body System	Root Operation	Body Region	Approach	Method	Qualifier
Chiropractic **9**	Body System	Root Operation	Body Region	Approach	Method	Qualifier

Table 57-3 ■ **EXAMPLE OF CONSTRUCTING MEDICAL TERMS FOR MEDICAL AND SURGICAL-RELATED PROCEDURES**

Combining Form	Suffix	Complete Medical Term
amni/o (*amnion [sac surrounding the embryo]*)	**-scopy** (*visual examination*)	**amnio + scopy** (*visual examination of the amnion*)
	-centesis (*surgical puncture to remove fluid*)	**amnio + centesis** (*surgical puncture to remove fluid from the amnion*)
	-tomy (*incision into*)	**amnio + tomy** (*incision into the amnion*)
	-infusion (*introducing a substance*)	**amnio + infusion** (*introducing a substance into the amnion*)
electr/o (*electrical*) **cardi/o** (*heart*) **encephal/o** (*brain*) **cyst/o** (*bladder*) **metr/o** (*measurement*)	**-graphy** (*the process of making a recording*) **-gram** (*a visual record or recording*)	**electro + cardio + graphy** (*the process of making a recording of the electrical activity of the heart*) **electro + encephalo + graphy** (*the process of making a recording of the electrical activity of the brain*) **cysto + metro + gram** *a visual record or recording of measurement [of pressure] in the bladder*)

Source: © PB Resources, Inc. Used with permission.

all seven Characters are defined in the same way as they are in the Medical and Surgical Section. In Sections 3 through 9, Character 6 is used for new purposes as follows:

- Section **3 Administration** defines Character 6 as **Substance**.

- Section **4 Measurement and Monitoring** and **5 Extracorporeal Assistance and Performance** define Character 6 as **Function**.

- Sections **7 Osteopathic**, **8 Other Procedures**, and **9 Chiropractic** define Character 6 as **Method**.

Details of how to abstract, assign, and arrange codes for each Section are discussed in the remainder of this chapter.

Medical terms for Medical and Surgical-Related procedures sometimes use different suffixes than those in the Medical and Surgical Section. Familiar suffixes such as -*ectomy* and -*plasty* do not appear because procedures in these Sections do not cut out or repair Body Parts. The exception is the Obstetrics (1) Section, which does classify invasive procedures. Some procedure names do not use Latin forms at all. There is not a direct match between a specific procedural term and a Root

Operation. Root Operations are assigned based on the content of the operative report regarding what was actually performed, not on the terms used by the physician in documentation. Refer to ■ TABLE 57-3 for a refresher on how to build terms related to Medical and Surgical-Related procedures.

CODING CAUTION

Be alert for Root Operations that have similar English meanings but different PCS definitions.

Immobilization (3) (*Limiting or preventing* motion of a body region by external methods and devices) and **Fusion (G)** (*Joining together portions* of an articular body part, rendering the articular body part immobile)

Introduction (5) (*Putting in or on a* *therapeutic, diagnostic, nutritional, physiological, or prophylactic substance* except blood or blood products) and **Insertion (H)** (*Putting in a* *nonbiological appliance that monitors, assists, performs, or prevents* a physiological function but does not physically take the place of a body part)

CODING PRACTICE

Exercise 57.1 Basics of Medical and Surgical-Related Procedures

Instructions: Use your medical terminology skills and resources to define the following Medical and Surgical-Related procedures, then identify the code(s) or code range listed in the PCS Index. Follow these steps:

- Use slash marks "/" to break down the underlined term into its root(s) and suffix.
- *Do not attempt to break down words or abbreviations marked with an *.
- Define the meaning of the word based on the meaning of each word part or letter in the abbreviation.
- Look up the phrase in the ICD-10-PCS Index, and write down the name(s) of Root Operation(s) the Index cross-references you to and the Table(s), if provided. If the Index lists only a code and not the Root Operation, list only the Table characters.
- Do not assign any codes.

Example: peritoneal dialysis
  peritone/al   Meaning *pertaining to the peritoneum*   PCS Root Operation(s)/Table(s) *3E1*

1. chemoembolization   Meaning _____   PCS Root Operation(s)/Table(s) _____

2. electromyogram   Meaning _____   PCS Root Operation(s)/Table(s) _____

3. leukopheresis, therapeutic   Meaning _____   PCS Root Operation(s)/Table(s) _____

4. measurement, olfactory acuity   Meaning _____   PCS Root Operation(s)/Table(s) _____

5. pleurodesis   Meaning _____   PCS Root Operation(s)/Table(s) _____

6. near infrared spectroscopy, circulatory system   Meaning _____   PCS Root Operation(s)/Table(s) _____

7. oximetry, fetal pulse   Meaning _____   PCS Root Operation(s)/Table(s) _____

8. neurophysiologic monitoring   Meaning _____   PCS Root Operation(s)/Table(s) _____

9. ECMO*   Meaning _____   PCS Root Operation(s)/Table(s) _____

10. IPPB*   Meaning _____   PCS Root Operation(s)/Table(s) _____

CODING OVERVIEW OF MEDICAL AND SURGICAL-RELATED PROCEDURES

Obstetrics is the only Section besides Medical and Surgical that has guidelines, which appear in section C of the PCS OGCR. The guidelines help clarify the types of procedures to be coded from the Obstetrics (1) Section and those to be coded from the Medical and Surgical (0) Section.

- The Obstetrics Section classifies procedures performed on the Body Part Products of Conception only (PCS OGCR C1). For example, therapeutic amniocentesis is coded using the Root Operation Drainage and the Body Part Products of Conception in the Obstetrics Section, resulting in the code **10903ZC**.

- Procedures performed on the pregnant female, other than the products of conception, are coded with the appropriate Root Operation in the Medical and Surgical Section. For example, repair of an obstetric urethral laceration is coded using the Root Operation Repair and the Body Part Urethra in the Medical and Surgical section, resulting in a code such as **0TQD8ZZ**, depending on the Approach.

- Procedures performed following a delivery or abortion for curettage of the endometrium or evacuation of retained products of conception are coded in the Obstetrics Section (PCS OGCR C2). Assign the Root Operation Extraction and the Body Part Products of Conception, Retained, resulting in a code such as **10D18ZZ**, depending on the Approach.

- Diagnostic or therapeutic dilation and curettage performed during times other than the postpartum or postabortion period are coded in the Medical and Surgical Section using the Root Operation Extraction and the Body Part Endometrium, resulting in a code such as **0UDB7ZZ**, depending on the Approach and purpose of the procedure.

ABSTRACTING FOR MEDICAL AND SURGICAL-RELATED PROCEDURES

Medical and Surgical-Related procedures in Sections 1 through 9 are usually performed in conjunction with Medical and Surgical (Section 0) procedures but are not operative procedures in and of themselves. Abstracting for Medical and Surgical-Related procedures is similar to abstracting Medical and Surgical (0) procedures and focuses on reading the procedure report and interpreting it in light of Root Operation definitions. Remember to focus on the objective of the procedure and the activities performed, not the specific medical terms used to describe the procedure.

The following information highlights the definitions and unique criteria for Sections 1 through 9 and provides a Key Criteria for Abstracting table to identify the Root Operations in each Section. After reading the procedure report, use the abstracting table as follows:

1. Answer the General Questions to get a basic understanding of the procedure (■ TABLE 57-4).

2. Answer the Root Operation Questions. One question should be answered *Yes*; the rest should be answered *No*.

3. For the Root Operation Question that was answered *Yes*, refer to the Section identified in the second column and review the Root Operations available in that Section. Refer to the tables for Key Criteria for Abstracting each Section that appear in this chapter.

4. Look up the definition of each of the applicable Root Operations in the appendix of the ICD-10-PCS coding manual.

5. Identify the one Root Operation that matches the procedure documented. This Root Operation will be the Main Term when you use the Index.

6. Repeat the abstracting process for each procedure that was performed.

Because some of these sections are relatively short with few codes, brief information on assigning codes is presented with some Sections or Root Operations discussed below, rather than dividing the information into separate topics in this chapter. Procedures with more extensive information about assigning codes are discussed later in the chapter under the topic "Assigning Characters 4–7 for Medical and Surgical-Related Procedures."

Table 57-4 ■ KEY CRITERIA FOR ABSTRACTING MEDICAL AND SURGICAL-<u>RELATED</u> SECTIONS

General Questions

❑ What is the stated procedure?
❑ What body region or body part is involved?
❑ How many sites are treated?
❑ What is the laterality (if applicable)?
❑ What approach is used?
❑ Is the procedure description what you would expect based on the name of the procedure?
❑ Was more than one procedure, or a combined procedure, performed?

Section Questions (Answer *Yes* to one question)	Refer to Root Operations in This Section
❑ Does the procedure involve a fetus?	Section 1 Obstetrics
❑ Does the procedure place an object in or on the patient without cutting or puncturing the skin or mucous membrane?	Section 2 Placement
❑ Is a diagnostic or therapeutic substance given to the patient?	Section 3 Administration
❑ Does the procedure involve measurement or monitoring?	Section 4 Measurement and Monitoring
❑ Does the procedure use equipment outside the body to assist or perform a physiological function?	Section 5 Extracorporeal Assistance and Performance
❑ Does the procedure use equipment outside the body for a therapeutic purpose that does not involve the assistance or performance of a physiological function?	Section 6 Extracorporeal Therapies
❑ Is osteopathic or chiropractic manipulation provided?	Section 7 Osteopathic or Section 9 Chiropractic
❑ Does the procedure involve another methodology in attempt to remediate or cure a disorder or disease?	Section 8 Other Procedures

Source: © PB Resources, Inc. Used with permission.

CODING CAUTION

Root Operation values are independent between Sections, so the same alphanumeric value can be reused for Root Operations in different Sections. For example, you will find that several Sections use the values 0, 1, 2, and so on for different Root Operations. Always refer to the values listed in a specific PCS Table to determine the meaning of an alphanumeric character.

Abstracting for Obstetrics (Section 1)

The Obstetrics Section classifies procedures performed on the **products of conception**, which encompasses all components of pregnancy, including the embryo, fetus, amnion, placenta, and umbilical cord. Examples of procedures are vaginal and cesarean delivery, abortion, amniocentesis, and transfusions. Procedures performed on the pregnant female are coded with the appropriate Root Operation from the Medical and Surgical or other PCS Sections.

Obstetrics has only one value for Character 2, Body System—Pregnancy (0)—and only three Character 4 Body Part values, as follows:

- Products of Conception (0)
- Products of Conception, Retained (1)
- Products of Conception, Ectopic (2)

Table 57-5 ■ UNIQUE ROOT OPERATIONS IN THE OBSTETRICS SECTION

Root Operation	Value	Definition	Examples
Abortion	A	Artificially terminating a pregnancy	Mechanical abortion, surgical abortion, use of **abortifacient** (*an agent that causes abortion*)
Delivery	E	Assisting the passage of the Products of Conception from the genital canal	Vaginal delivery, cesarean delivery, manually assisted delivery, spontaneous delivery, forceps-assisted delivery

Source: © PB Resources, Inc. Used with permission.

The Obstetrics Section has 12 Root Operations. Ten of these are also used in the Medical and Surgical (0) Section and carry the same values and definitions in this Section. Two Root Operations are unique to Obstetrics and are defined in ■ TABLE 57-5. The Root Operations in the Obstetrics Section are:

- Change (2)
- Drainage (9)
- Abortion (A)

- Extraction (D)
- Delivery (E)
- Insertion (H)
- Inspection (J)
- Removal (P)
- Repair (Q)
- Reposition (S)
- Resection (T)
- Transplantation (Y)

To abstract for Obstetrics procedures, first identify that the procedure is performed on the Products of Conception, then apply abstracting questions for each potential Root Operation. Abstracting criteria for Root Operations shared with the Medical and Surgical Section are the same as those presented in previous chapters of this text, with the added specificity that the procedure is performed on the Products of Conception (■ TABLE 57-6).

Some procedures on the Products of Conception are coded from Sections other than Obstetrics. For example, fetal heart rate monitoring is coded from Section 4, Measurement and

Monitoring. Follow the guidance in the Index when coding such procedures.

SUCCESS STEP

When coding procedures performed for pregnant women, use ICD-10-PCS procedure codes from any Section of the manual, based on the Root Operation performed. This differs from coding diagnoses for pregnant women because you must always assign a code from the ICD-10-CM obstetrics chapter, even if the condition was not caused by the pregnancy, such as preexisting diabetes or hypertension. You then assign additional diagnosis codes from other ICD-10-CM chapters when needed to fully describe the condition.

Abstracting for the Placement (2), Administration (3), and Measurement and Monitoring (4) Sections

The next three sections are Placement (2), Administration (3), and Measurement and Monitoring (4). Each section has separate purposes and separate Root Operations.

Table 57-6 ■ KEY CRITERIA FOR ABSTRACTING OBSTETRICS PROCEDURES

Section Question	
❑ Is the procedure performed on the products of conception?	If *No*, do not use Obstetrics codes.

Root Operation Questions	Root Operation (Value)
Answer *Yes* to one of the following questions to help distinguish Root Operations in the Obstetrics (1) Section.	
❑ Does the procedure take a device out or off from a Body Part on the fetus and put back an identical or similar device in or on the same Body Part without cutting or puncturing the skin or a mucous membrane?	Change (2)
❑ Does the procedure take or let fluids and/or gases from a Body Part on the fetus?	Drainage (9)
❑ Is a pregnancy artificially terminated?	Abortion (A)
❑ Does the procedure pull or strip out or off all or a portion of a Body Part on the fetus by the use of force?	Extraction (D)
❑ Does the procedure assist a fetus, embryo, or unborn child pass through the genital canal?	Delivery (E)
❑ Was a nonbiological appliance put in the fetus that monitors, assists, performs, or prevents a physiological function but does not physically take the place of a Body Part?	Insertion (H)
❑ Is all or part of a Body Part of the fetus visually and/or manually explored?	Inspection (J)
❑ Is a device taken off from a body part, region, or orifice on the fetus?	Removal (P)
❑ Is a Body Part of the fetus restored to its normal anatomic structure and function to the extent possible?	Repair (Q)
❑ Is all or a portion of a Body Part of the fetus moved to its normal location, or other suitable location?	Reposition (S)
❑ Is a Body Part of the fetus cut out or off, without replacement?	Resection (T)
❑ Does the procedure put in or on all or a portion of a living Body Part taken from another individual or animal to physically take the place and/or function of all or a portion of a similar Body Part on the fetus?	Transplantation (Y)

Source: © PB Resources, Inc. Used with permission.

Table 57-7 ■ UNIQUE ROOT OPERATIONS IN THE PLACEMENT SECTION

Root Operation	Value	Definition	Examples
Compression	1	Putting pressure on a body region	Placement of intermittent pressure device
Dressing	2	Putting material on a body region for protection	Application of sterile dressing to wound
Immobilization	3	Limiting or preventing motion of a body region	Neck brace, arm cast
Packing	4	Putting material in a body region or orifice	Nasal packing, packing of wound
Traction	6	Exerting a pulling force on a body region in a distal direction	Mechanical traction of arm or leg

Source: © PB Resources, Inc. Used with permission.

Placement (Section 2) Root Operations

The Placement Section has seven Root Operations. Two of these, Change and Removal, also are used in the Medical and Surgical (0) Section and carry the same definitions but have *different values for the Root Operations in Character 3.* Five Root Operations are unique to Placement and are defined in ■ TABLE 57-7. The Root Operations in the Placement Section are:

- Change (0)
- Removal (5)
- Compression (1)
- Dressing (2)
- Immobilization (3)
- Packing (4)
- Traction (6)

Placement Section procedures use two values for Character 2, Body System:

- Anatomical Regions (W)
- Anatomical Orifices (Y)

To abstract for Placement procedures, apply abstracting questions for each potential Root Operation (■ TABLE 57-8). Abstracting criteria for Root Operations shared with the Medical and Surgical Section are the same as those presented in previous chapters of this text.

Coders need to make distinctions between certain procedures in Section 2 Placement compared to Section F Physical Rehabilitation and Diagnostic Audiology. The Root Operation Immobilization (3) in the Placement Section applies to the fitting of devices, such as splints and braces, in *inpatient settings other than rehabilitation* (■ FIGURE 57-1). When these services are provided in a rehabilitation setting, use the Root Operation Device Fitting (D) in Section F

Table 57-8 ■ KEY CRITERIA FOR ABSTRACTING PLACEMENT PROCEDURES

Section Question	
Is the procedure performed on an anatomic region or natural orifice without making an incision or puncture?	If *No*, do not use Placement codes.

Root Operation Questions	Root Operation (Value)

Answer *Yes* to one of the following questions to help distinguish Root Operations in the Placement (2) Section.

❑ Does the procedure take a device out or off of a Body Part and put back an identical or similar device in or on the same Body Part without cutting or puncturing the skin or a mucous membrane?	Change (0)
❑ Is pressure applied on a body region?	Compression (1)
❑ Is material put on a body region for protection?	Dressing (2)
❑ Does the procedure limit or prevent the movement of a body region?	Immobilization (3)
❑ Is material put in a body region or orifice?	Packing (4)
❑ Is a device taken off from a body part, region, or orifice?	Removal (5)
❑ Is a force pulling in a distal direction exerted on a body region?	Traction (6)

Source: © PB Resources, Inc. Used with permission.

Physical Rehabilitation and Diagnostic Audiology. Section F is part of Ancillary Procedures, discussed in Chapter 58 of this text.

The Root Operation Traction (6) in the Placement Section applies to the use of a mechanical traction apparatus. When manual traction is performed by a physical therapist or physician, use Section F Physical Rehabilitation and Diagnostic Audiology, Root Type Motor Treatment (7) and the Type Qualifier Manual Therapy Techniques (7) (■ FIGURE 57-2).

Devices coded in Section 2 are manufactured and ready to use without extensive fabrication or fitting. Custom-fabricated devices or those requiring extensive fitting are coded in Section F of Ancillary procedures, Physical Rehabilitation and Diagnostic Audiology.

Physician places a cast on the left forearm of a hospital inpatient.

2W3DX2Z [Placement, Anatomical Regions], Immobilization, Lower arm left, External, Cast, No qualifier

Figure 57-1 ■ Example of Coding from the Placement Section for a Hospital Inpatient. *Source:* © *PB Resources, Inc. Used with permission.*

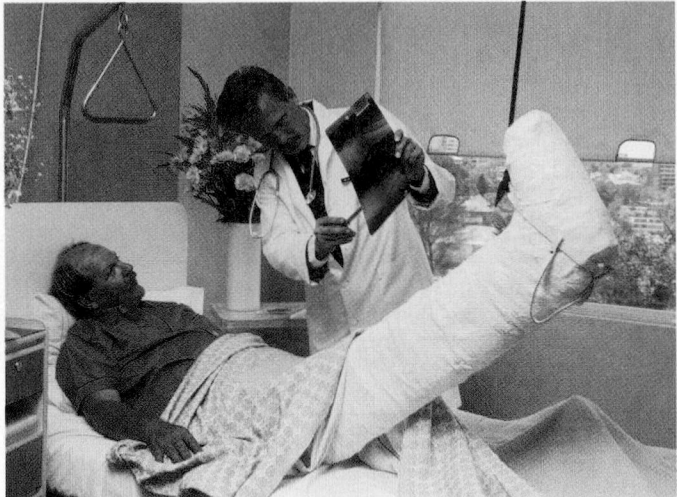

A

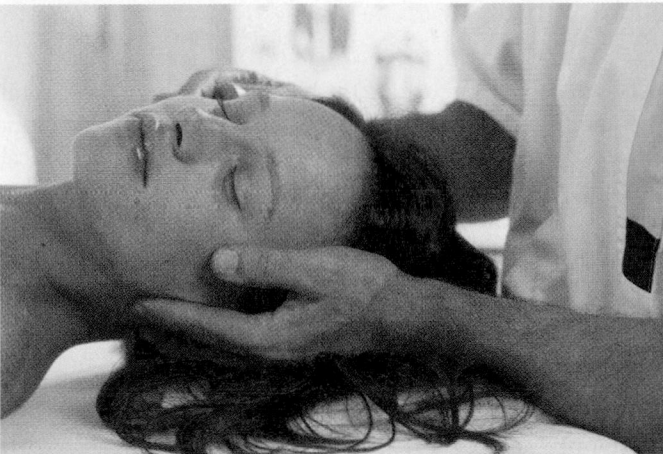

B

Figure 57-2 ■ Types of Traction (A) Mechanical traction uses equipment to apply a pulling force. *Source:* © ClassicStock/Alamy. (B) Manual traction is performed with the hands. *Source:* Getty Images/ Credit: BSIP/UIG.

Administration (Section 3) Root Operations

The Administration Section classifies procedures in which a therapeutic, prophylactic, protective, diagnostic, nutritional, or physiological substance is given to the patient. It includes infusions, injections, and transfusions, as well as other related procedures, such as irrigation and tattooing.

The Administration Section has three Root Operations, all unique to this Section, which are classified according to the broad category of substance administered (■ TABLE 57-9). Use the Root Operation Transfusion when a blood product is given. Use the Root Operation Irrigation when a cleansing substance is administered. Use the Root Operation Introduction for all other substances administered, such as antineoplastic substances.

Character 2, Body System, uses three values:

- Circulatory (0)
- Indwelling Device (C)
- Physiological Systems and Anatomical Regions (E)

Character 5, Approach, uses values from the Medical and Surgical Section. Assign the Approach Percutaneous (3) for all

Table 57-9 ■ **UNIQUE ROOT OPERATIONS IN THE ADMINISTRATION SECTION**

Root Operation	Value	Definition	Examples
Introduction	0	Putting in or on a therapeutic, diagnostic, nutritional, physiological, or prophylactic substance except blood or blood products	Nerve block injection, transabdominal in vitro fertilization
Irrigation	1	Putting in or on a cleansing substance	Flushing of the eye, peritoneal dialysis using indwelling catheter
Transfusion	2	Putting in blood or blood products	Blood transfusion, bone marrow transplant

Source: © PB Resources, Inc. Used with permission.

Table 57-10 ■ **KEY CRITERIA FOR ABSTRACTING ADMINISTRATION PROCEDURES**

Section Question	
❑ Is a diagnostic or therapeutic substance given to the patient?	If *No*, do not use Administration codes.

Root Operation Questions	Root Operation (Value)
Answer *Yes* to one of the following questions to help distinguish Root Operations in the Administration (3) Section.	
❑ Is a cleansing substance put in or administered to the patient?	Irrigation (1)
❑ Is blood or blood products put in or administered to the patient?	Transfusion (2)
❑ Is a therapeutic, diagnostic, nutritional, physiological, or prophylactic substance except blood or blood products put in or administered to the patient?	Introduction (0)

Source: © PB Resources, Inc. Used with permission.

injections, regardless of whether they are administered using an intradermal, subcutaneous, or intramuscular route.

To abstract for Administration procedures, apply abstracting questions for each potential Root Operation (■ TABLE 57-10). Abstracting criteria for Root Operations shared with the Medical and Surgical Section are the same as those presented in previous chapters of this text.

SUCCESS STEP

For the Root Operation Introduction (0), Character 4, Body Part, identifies the site where the procedure occurs, although the substance introduced might affect a different site. For the Root Operation Irrigation (1), Character 4, Body Part, identifies the site that is irrigated.

Table 57-11 ■ UNIQUE ROOT OPERATIONS IN THE MEASUREMENT AND MONITORING SECTION

Root Operation	Value	Definition	Examples
Measurement	0	Determining the level of a physiological or physical function at a point in time	Routine ECG, venous pulse single measurement
Monitoring	1	Determining the level of a physiological or physical function repetitively over a period of time	Holter monitoring, fetal heart monitoring

Source: © PB Resources, Inc. Used with permission.

Table 57-12 ■ KEY CRITERIA FOR ABSTRACTING MEASUREMENT AND MONITORING PROCEDURES

Section Question	
❏ Does the procedure measure the level of a physiological or physical function?	If *No*, do not use Measurement and Monitoring codes.

Root Operation Questions	Root Operation (Value)
Answer *Yes* to one of the following questions to help distinguish Root Operations in the Measurement and Monitoring (4) Section.	
❏ Does the procedure take a single reading at a point in time?	Measurement (0)
❏ Are multiple readings of the same function taken repetitively over a period of time?	Monitoring (1)

Source: © PB Resources, Inc. Used with permission.

Measurement and Monitoring (Section 4) Root Operations

The Measurement and Monitoring Section classifies procedures that measure the level of a physiological or physical function, such as temperature, visual mobility, or urinary pressure. This Section has two Root Operations, Measurement (0) and Monitoring (1), both unique to this Section (■ TABLE 57-11).

Be aware that overlap exists between the name of the Section and the names of the two Root Operations. The Section Measurement and Monitoring has a Character 1 value of **4**. The Root Operation Measurement has a Character 3 value of **0**, and the Root Operation Monitoring has a Character 3 value of **1**.

Character 2, Body System, uses two values:

- Physiological Systems (A), used with the Root Operation Measurement and Monitoring
- Physiological Devices (B), used with the Root Operation Measurement

When abstracting for procedures in this Section, keep in mind the definitions of the Root Operations. The Root Operations Measurement and Monitoring both record levels of the same physiological and physical functions. The Root Operation Measurement takes a single reading at a point in time, whereas the Root Operation Monitoring takes multiple readings at intervals over a period of time. The number of measurements is the only criteria that distinguishes between these two Root Operations (■ TABLE 57-12).

Character 6, Function/Device, identifies the physiological function being tested, such as conductivity, pressure, or temperature.

Abstracting for the Extracorporeal (5) (6) Procedures Sections

PCS provides two Sections of Root Operations for **extracorporeal** procedures and processes, which are those that take place outside of the body. Each of these sections is discussed next.

Extracorporeal Assistance and Performance (Section 5) Root Operations

Procedures in the Section Extracorporeal Assistance and Performance (5) use equipment to support a physiological function, such as breathing, circulating the blood, or restoring the natural rhythm of the heart. Procedures include those performed in a critical care setting but are not restricted to a designated critical care unit. An operating room or emergency department also qualifies as a critical care setting. Examples of critical care procedures are mechanical ventilation and cardioversion. Other procedures in this Section are hemodialysis and **hyperbaric oxygen treatment (HBOT)** (*breathing 100% oxygen under increased atmospheric pressure*).

The Section Extracorporeal Assistance and Performance has three Root Operations, all of which are unique to this Section (■ TABLE 57-13). The Root Operations Assistance (0) and Performance (1) describe similar types of procedures. They vary only in the degree of control exercised over the physiological

Table 57-13 ■ UNIQUE ROOT OPERATIONS IN THE EXTRACORPOREAL ASSISTANCE AND PERFORMANCE SECTION

Root Operation	Value	Definition	Examples
Assistance	0	Taking over a portion of a physiological function by extracorporeal means	Hyperbaric oxygenation of wound, continuous intra-aortic balloon pump (IABP),
Performance	1	Completely taking over a physiological function by extracorporeal means	Cardiopulmonary bypass, hemodialysis encounter, continuous mechanical ventilation
Restoration	2	Returning, or attempting to return, a physiological function to its original state by extracorporeal means	External cardioversion, defibrillation

Source: © PB Resources, Inc. Used with permission.

Table 57-14 ■ UNIQUE ROOT OPERATIONS IN THE EXTRACORPOREAL THERAPIES SECTION

Root Operation	Value	Definition
Atmospheric Control	0	Extracorporeal control of atmospheric pressure and composition
Decompression	1	Extracorporeal elimination of undissolved gas from body fluids
Electromagnetic Therapy	2	Extracorporeal treatment by electromagnetic rays
Hyperthermia	3	Extracorporeal raising of body temperature
Hypothermia	4	Extracorporeal lowering of body temperature
Pheresis	5	Extracorporeal separation of blood products
Phototherapy	6	Extracorporeal treatment by light rays
Ultrasound Therapy	7	Extracorporeal treatment by ultrasound
Ultraviolet Light Therapy	8	Extracorporeal treatment by ultraviolet light
Shock Wave Therapy	9	Extracorporeal treatment by shock waves

Source: © PB Resources, Inc. Used with permission.

Table 57-15 ■ KEY CRITERIA FOR ABSTRACTING EXTRACORPOREAL PROCEDURES

Section Question	
❏ Does the procedure use equipment to support a physiological function?	If *No*, do not use Extracorporeal Assistance and Performance codes.

Root Operation Questions	Root Operation (Value)
Answer *Yes* to one of the following questions to help distinguish Root Operations in the Extracorporeal Assistance and Performance (5) Section.	
❏ Does the procedure take over a portion of a physiological function by extracorporeal means?	Assistance (0)
❏ Does the procedure completely take over a portion of a physiological function by extracorporeal means?	Performance (1)
❏ Does the procedure return, or attempt to return, a failed physiological function to its original state by extracorporeal means?	Restoration (2)
❏ Does the procedure use other methods, such as light, heat, cold, electromagnetic force, or similar, to support a physiological function?	Review and select the appropriate Root Operation from Section 6, Extracorporeal Therapies.

Source: © PB Resources, Inc. Used with permission.

function. Assistance classifies procedures that *support* a physiological function but do not take complete control of it, such as an intra-aortic balloon pump used to support cardiac output and hyperbaric oxygen treatment. Performance classifies procedures where *complete control* is exercised over a physiological function, such as total mechanical ventilation, cardiac pacing, and cardiopulmonary bypass.

Character 5 is Duration and Character 6 is Function. These characters describe the duration of the procedure and the body function being acted on, rather than the Approach and Device, as is the case in the Medical and Surgical (0) Section.

Extracorporeal Therapies (Section 6) Root Operations

The Section Extracorporeal Therapies describes other extracorporeal procedures that are not defined by Section 5 Assistance and Performance. Examples are Bili-lite phototherapy, apheresis, and whole-body hypothermia.

The Extracorporeal Therapies Section has 10 Root Operations, all unique to this Section (■ Table 57-14).

Character 2, Body System, provides one choice, Physiological Systems. Character 6 is defined as a Qualifier but contains no specific qualifier values. Character 7, Qualifier, identifies various blood components separated out in pheresis procedures.

Refer to ■ Table 57-15 for assistance in abstracting Extracorporeal procedures. The table encompasses both Sections 5 and 6. To avoid redundancy, the definitions of Section 6 Root Operations are not repeated in the abstracting table.

Although the definitions of most Root Operations in this Section are consistent with terms used in the medical community, coders should still refer to the PCS definition of each procedure. For example, the Root Operations Decompression (1)

and Hyperthermia (4) have more specialized meanings in PCS than in the medical community in general. Decompression describes treatment for decompression sickness (the bends) in a hyperbaric chamber. Hyperthermia is the intentional lowering of body temperature to treat temperature imbalance.

Pheresis is used to treat diseases where too much of a blood component is produced, such as leukemia, or to remove a blood product such as platelets from a donor for transfusion into a patient who needs them.

Phototherapy to the circulatory system means exposing the blood to light rays outside the body, using a machine that recirculates the blood and returns it to the body after phototherapy.

Abstracting for the Osteopathic (7), Chiropractic (9), and Other Procedures (8) Sections

The final three Sections of Medical and Surgical-Related procedures are the short sections for osteopathic and chiropractic services and a grouping of miscellaneous procedures not classified in other Sections. Refer to Table 57-4 to abstract for procedures in these Sections.

Osteopathic (Section 7) Root Operations

Section 7, Osteopathic, consists of a single Body System, Anatomical Regions, and a single Root Operation, Treatment, which is unique to this Section (■ Table 57-16, page 1144). Osteopathic manipulative treatment (OMT) uses the hands to

Table 57-16 ■ UNIQUE ROOT OPERATIONS IN THE OSTEOPATHIC SECTION

Root Operation	Value	Definition
Treatment	0	Manual treatment to eliminate or alleviate somatic dysfunction and related disorders

Source: © PB Resources, Inc. Used with permission.

diagnose, treat, and prevent illness or injury. The physician moves muscles and joints using techniques such as stretching, gentle pressure, and resistance. A **doctor of osteopathy (DO)** is a licensed physician who has the same licensing, training, and qualifications as a doctor of medicine (MD), also called **allopathic** physicians. Osteopathic physicians receive an additional 300 to 500 hours in the study of the musculoskeletal system and hands-on manual manipulation. The codes in this Section are specifically for osteopathic manual manipulation. Assign codes from any PCS section for other services provided by an osteopath.

Character 4, Body Region, identifies the regions of the spine, extremities, and trunk. Character 5, Approach, is always **X External**. Character 6 is Method of treatment, such as Lymphatic Pump and Fascial Release. The definitions of methods rely on the standard definitions as used in this specialty and are not explicitly defined in PCS. ■ TABLE 57-17 provides a summary of commonly used osteopathic methods. Character 7, Qualifier, is always **Z None**.

Table 57-17 ■ OSTEOPATHIC TREATMENT METHODS

Method	Description
Articulatory-raising	Rotation of rib heads through direct application of force
Counterstrain or indirect	Positioning of a patient to passively release tenderness on a specific point
General mobilization	Movement of joints and tissues to release tension
High velocity-low amplitude (HVLA) or thrust technique	Use of a brief, rapid force that engages and releases a restrictive barrier within a joint's anatomic range of motion
Low velocity-high amplitude	Large-scale mobilization to relieve tension
Lymphatic pump treatment (LPT)	Application of manual force to the thoracic cage, abdomen, pelvis, and other areas to stimulate lymph flow
Muscle energy—isotonic	Application of resistance against the patient's motion
Muscle energy—isometric	Application of equal force against the patient's motion
Myofascial release or fascial release	Application of manual pressure to trigger points to relax contracted muscles, stimulate the stretch reflex, and increase circulation and lymphatic drainage

Source: © PB Resources, Inc. Used with permission.

Table 57-18 ■ UNIQUE ROOT OPERATIONS IN THE CHIROPRACTIC SECTION

Root Operation	Value	Definition
Manipulation	B	Manual procedure that involves a directed thrust to move a joint past the physiological range of motion, without exceeding the anatomic limit

Source: © PB Resources, Inc. Used with permission.

Chiropractic (Section 9) Root Operations

The Chiropractic Section consists of a single body system, Anatomical Regions, and a single root operation, Manipulation (■ TABLE 57-18).

Chiropractic focuses on disorders of the musculoskeletal and nervous system and the effects of these disorders on general health. **Chiropractic manipulation** or adjustment uses direct manual force or an instrument to manipulate the joints of the body, most commonly the spine, to restore or enhance joint function. Treatment focuses on neuromusculoskeletal complaints, such as pain in the back, neck, and joints, and headaches. Doctors of Chiropractic (DC) are trained in chiropractic colleges and have broad diagnostic skills. They also are qualified to recommend therapeutic and rehabilitative exercises, as well as to provide nutritional, dietary, and lifestyle counseling.

Character 4, Body Region, identifies the regions of the spine, extremities, and trunk. Character 5, Approach, is always **X External**. Character 6 is Method of treatment, such as nonmanual and mechanically assisted. The definitions of methods rely on the standard usage in the chiropractic specialty and are not explicitly defined in PCS. ■ TABLE 57-19 provides a summary of commonly used chiropractic methods. Character 7, Qualifier, is always **Z None**.

Table 57-19 ■ CHIROPRACTIC TREATMENT METHODS

Method	Description
Direct visceral	Treatment of internal organ dysfunction, adhesions, or tension by direct pressure to mobilize the organ
Extra-articular	Manipulation of areas other than joints
Indirect visceral	Treatment of internal organ dysfunction by stretching or mobilizing areas adjacent to the organ
Long- and short-lever-specific contact	A combination of direct spinal thrusts and long lever contact (femur, head, or pelvis)
Long-lever-specific contact	Manipulation of the femur, head, or pelvis to adjust the spine
Mechanically assisted	Use of an instrument to aid in manipulation
Nonmanual	Heat, ice, ultrasound, electrical stimulation, therapeutic exercise
Short-lever-specific contact	Direct thrusts applied to the spine

Source: © PB Resources, Inc. Used with permission.

Table 57-20 ■ UNIQUE ROOT OPERATIONS IN THE OTHER PROCEDURES SECTION

Root Operation	Value	Definition
Other Procedures	0	Methodologies that attempt to remediate or cure a disorder or disease

Source: © PB Resources, Inc. Used with permission.

Other Procedures (Section 8) Root Operations

The Other Procedures section contains codes for procedures not included in the other medical and surgical-related sections. This section has one Root Operation, Other Procedures (0) (■ TABLE 57-20). Character 2 is Body System and has two values:

- Indwelling Device (C)
- Physiological Systems and Anatomical Regions (E)

There are relatively few procedure codes in this section, for nontraditional, whole-body therapies including acupuncture and meditation. There is also a code for the fertilization portion of an in vitro fertilization procedure.

Character 6 is Method and identifies the method or technique used in the procedure. Examples include the following:

- Robotic Assisted Procedure (C)
- Computer Assisted Procedure (B)
- Acupuncture (0)
- Therapeutic Massage (1)

Guided Example of Abstracting for Medical and Surgical-Related Procedures

Refer to the following example throughout this chapter to practice skills for abstracting, assigning, and arranging codes for Medical and Surgical-Related procedures. Two services are using Root Operation in Medical and Surgical-Related Sections. Three services are coded from the Medical and Surgical (0) Section and were discussed in the Guided Example in Chapter 54 of this text. Refer to Chapter 54 for details of abstracting and assigning codes for these procedures.

> INPATIENT HOSPITAL   Gender: M   Age: 72
>
> Reason for admission: angina, SOB
>
> Procedures: Cardiac stress test of total activity, single measurement. CABG x2 with CP bypass, LIMA to LAD, OM with GSV.
>
> Discharge diagnosis: atherosclerotic heart disease with 90% blockage in LAD and 80% blockage in the OM with unstable angina pectoris

Follow along as fictitious coder, Marcy Elwood, CCS, abstracts the procedure. Check off each step after you complete it.

▶ Marcy reads through the entire record, paying special attention to the reason for admission, the procedure performed, and the principal diagnosis. She refers to the Key Criteria for Abstracting Medical and Surgical-Related Sections (Table 57-4).

❑ She notes the reason for admission: angina, SOB.

❑ She also notes the discharge diagnosis: atherosclerotic heart disease with 90% blockage in LAD and 80% blockage in the OM with unstable angina pectoris.

❑ *What services were provided during the inpatient stay?*
  - Cardiac stress test
  - CABG x2
  - CP bypass

▶ First, Marcy abstracts for the cardiac stress test. She refers to Table 57-4 Key Criteria for Abstracting Medical and Surgical-Related Sections.

❑ *What is the stated procedure?* Cardiac stress test

❑ *What body region or body part is involved?* Heart

❑ She reviews the abstracting questions and answers *Yes* to one question:
  - *Does the procedure involve measurement or monitoring?* Refer to the Measurement and Monitoring (4) Section.

❑ Marcy reviews the Root Types for the Measurement and Monitoring Section. To select the Root Operation she must determine whether the measurement was taken at a point in time or was a series of readings over a period of time.
  - The documentation states single measurement, so she selects the definition that describes the procedure: Measurement (0): Determining the level of a physiological or physical function at a point in time.

▶ Next, Marcy abstracts for CP bypass. She again refers to Table 57-4.

❑ *What is the stated procedure?* Cardiopulmonary bypass during open heart surgery

❑ *What body region or body part is involved?* Heart and lungs

❑ She reviews the abstracting questions and answers *Yes* to one question:
  - *Is a procedure performed in a critical care setting to support a physiological function(s)?* Refer to the Extracorporeal Assistance and Performance (5) Section.

❑ Marcy reviews the Root Types for the Extracorporeal Assistance and Performance Section and selects the one definition that describes the procedure:
  - Performance (1): Completely taking over a physiological function by extracorporeal means.

▶ At this time, Marcy believes that she will need five codes: two for the CABG (abstracted in Chapter 54 of this text), one for harvesting the GSV (also abstracted in Chapter 54), one for the cardiac stress test, and one for cardiopulmonary bypass. She believes that she will use the Root Operation Measurement for the cardiac stress test and the Root Operation Performance for cardiopulmonary bypass. She will verify this information when she refers to the PCS Tables to assign codes.

CODING PRACTICE

Exercise 57.2 Abstracting for Medical and Surgical-
Related Procedures

Instructions: Read the mini-medical-record of each patient's encounter and answer the abstracting questions. Write the answer on the line provided. Do not assign any codes.

1. INPATIENT HOSPITAL   Gender: F   Age: 22

Gravida: 2   Para: 2   EGA: 33 + 2

Reason for admission: *premature rupture of membranes*

Assessment: *severe preeclampsia requires C/S*

Delivery: *low C/S, PTBLC, 1 girl*

Tip: PTBLC (Preterm birth, live child)

a. What is the stated procedure? _____

b. What body region or body part is involved? _____

c. What approach is used? _____

d. Was more than one procedure, or a combined procedure, performed? _____

e. Does the procedure involve a fetus? _____

f. Does the procedure place an object in or on the patient without cutting or puncturing the skin or a mucous membrane? _____

g. Is a diagnostic or therapeutic substance given to the patient? _____

h. Does the procedure involve measurement or monitoring? _____

i. Does the procedure use equipment outside the body to assist or perform a physiological function? _____

j. Does the procedure use equipment outside the body for a therapeutic purpose that does not involve the assistance or performance of a physiological function? _____

k. Is osteopathic or chiropractic manipulation provided? _____

l. What PCS Section should be used? _____

m. Review the Root Operations in the Section selected. What is the most likely Root Operation? _____

2. INPATIENT HOSPITAL   Gender: M   Age: 32

Preprocedure diagnosis: *peripheral neuritis, left arm*

Procedure: *nerve block injection to the median nerve using a regional anesthetic*

a. What is the stated procedure? _____

b. What body region or body part is involved? _____

c. What approach is used? _____

d. Was more than one procedure, or a combined procedure, performed? _____

(continued)

2. (continued)

e. Does the procedure involve a fetus? _____

f. Does the procedure place an object in or on the patient without cutting or puncturing the skin or a mucous membrane? _____

g. Is a diagnostic or therapeutic substance given to the patient? _____

h. Does the procedure involve measurement or monitoring? _____

i. Does the procedure use equipment outside the body to assist or perform a physiological function? _____

j. Does the procedure use equipment outside the body for a therapeutic purpose that does not involve the assistance or performance of a physiological function? _____

k. Is osteopathic or chiropractic manipulation provided? _____

l. What PCS Section should be used? _____

m. Review the Root Operations in the Section selected. What is the most likely Root Operation? _____

3. INPATIENT HOSPITAL   Gender: M   Age: 17

Preprocedure diagnosis: *aplastic anemia*

Procedure: *bone marrow transplant via central venous line using donor marrow from his identical twin*

a. What is the stated procedure? _____

b. What body region or body part is involved? _____

c. What approach is used? _____

d. Was more than one procedure, or a combined procedure, performed? _____

e. Does the procedure involve a fetus? _____

f. Does the procedure place an object in or on the patient without cutting or puncturing the skin or a mucous membrane? _____

g. Is a diagnostic or therapeutic substance given to the patient? _____

h. Does the procedure involve measurement or monitoring? _____

i. Does the procedure use equipment outside the body to assist or perform a physiological function? _____

j. Does the procedure use equipment outside the body for a therapeutic purpose that does not involve the assistance or performance of a physiological function? _____

k. Is osteopathic or chiropractic manipulation provided? _____

l. What PCS Section should be used? _____

m. Review the Root Operations in the Section selected. What is the most likely Root Operation? _____

4. INPATIENT HOSPITAL   Gender: F   **Age:** 15

Preprocedure diagnosis: displaced fracture R tibia

Procedure: closed reduction of fracture with percutaneous insertion of internal fixation device. Applied leg cast and initiated mechanical traction of lower R leg

a. What is the stated procedure? _____

b. What body region or body part is involved? _____

c. What approach is used? _____

d. Was more than one procedure, or a combined procedure, performed? _____

e. Does the procedure involve a fetus? _____

f. Does the procedure place an object in or on the patient without cutting or puncturing the skin or a mucous membrane? _____

g. Is a diagnostic or therapeutic substance given to the patient? _____

h. Does the procedure involve measurement or monitoring? _____

i. Does the procedure use equipment outside the body to assist or perform a physiological function? _____

j. Does the procedure use equipment outside the body for a therapeutic purpose that does not involve the assistance or performance of a physiological function? _____

k. Is osteopathic or chiropractic manipulation provided? _____

l. What PCS Section(s) should be used? _____

m. Review the Root Operations in the Section selected. What is the most likely Root Operation(s)? _____

5. INPATIENT HOSPITAL   Gender: F   **Age:** 33

Gravida: 2   Para: 2   EGA: 39 + 1

Assessment: fetal bradycardia

Procedure: mid forceps delivery with repair of perineal laceration

Delivery: TBLC, 1 girl

Tip: TBLC (Term birth, live child)

a. What is the stated procedure? _____

b. What body region or body part is involved? _____

c. What approach is used? _____

d. Was more than one procedure, or a combined procedure, performed? _____

e. Does the procedure involve a fetus? _____

f. Does the procedure place an object in or on the patient without cutting or puncturing the skin or a mucous membrane? _____

(*continued*)

5. (continued)

g. Is a diagnostic or therapeutic substance given to the patient? _____

h. Does the procedure involve measurement or monitoring? _____

i. Does the procedure use equipment outside the body to assist or perform a physiological function? _____

j. Does the procedure use equipment outside the body for a therapeutic purpose that does not involve the assistance or performance of a physiological function? _____

k. Is osteopathic or chiropractic manipulation provided? _____

l. What PCS Section(s) should be used? _____

m. Review the Root Operations in the Section selected. What is the most likely Root Operation(s)? _____

6. INPATIENT HOSPITAL   Gender: F   **Age:** 75

Preprocedure diagnosis: cardiac arrhythmia

Procedure: 24-hour ambulatory Holter monitoring followed by external measurement of cardiac output

a. What is the stated procedure? _____

b. What body region or body part is involved? _____

c. What approach is used? _____

d. Was more than one procedure, or a combined procedure, performed? _____

e. Does the procedure involve a fetus? _____

f. Does the procedure place an object in or on the patient without cutting or puncturing the skin or a mucous membrane? _____

g. Is a diagnostic or therapeutic substance given to the patient? _____

h. Does the procedure involve measurement or monitoring? _____

i. Does the procedure use equipment outside the body to assist or perform a physiological function? _____

j. Does the procedure use equipment outside the body for a therapeutic purpose that does not involve the assistance or performance of a physiological function? _____

k. Is osteopathic or chiropractic manipulation provided? _____

l. What PCS Section(s) should be used? _____

m. Review the Root Operations in the Section selected. What is the most likely Root Operation(s)? _____

ASSIGNING CHARACTERS 4–7 FOR MEDICAL AND SURGICAL-<u>RELATED</u> PROCEDURES

To assign codes after the Root Operation is determined, search the PCS Index for the name of the Root Operation as the Main Term. Locate the subterm(s) for the correct anatomic site and identify the PCS Table. When you locate the PCS Table, verify the first three characters of the code, then locate the row with the Body Part needed. Assign the remaining characters from each respective column of the Table.

For many procedures, you also can look up the common name of the procedure, such as **Cardioversion**, or an abbreviation, such as **EEG**, in the Index. This method might give you a partial or full code. Other times, the Index lists an instruction that cross-references you to one or more possible Root Operations. If you have difficulty locating a code using one Main Term or method, try a different one.

As discussed earlier in this chapter, the meaning of Characters 4 through 7 varies based on the Section, so it is important to review the Character meanings in each PCS Table. Special considerations for the use of Characters 4 through 7 were discussed with the individual Sections or Root Operations in the "Abstracting" section of this chapter. Additional information regarding Obstetrics procedures is discussed next.

> ### CODING CAUTION
>
> When a full code is listed in the Index, you must also refer to the PCS Table to verify the code. Never code directly from the Index.

Assigning Codes for Obstetrics (1)

The type of delivery is described by Character 3, Root Operation, as follows:

- Use the Root Operation Extraction (D) for cesarean section deliveries and forceps-assisted vaginal deliveries (■ FIGURE 57-3).
- Use the Root Operation Delivery (E) for manually assisted vaginal deliveries.

For procedures performed following a delivery or abortion involving curettage of the endometrium or evacuation of retained products of conception, use the Root Operation Extraction (D) and the Body Part Products of Conception, Retained (0).

For diagnostic or therapeutic dilation and curettage performed during times *other* than the postpartum or postabortion

period, use Section 0 Medical and Surgical, Root Operation D Extraction, and the Body Part B Endometrium (PCS OGCR C2).

For the Root Operation Abortion (Table 10A), Qualifier values identify whether an additional device such as a laminaria or abortifacient is used, or whether the abortion is performed by mechanical means. When a laminaria or abortifacient is used, the Approach is Via Natural or Artificial Opening and the Qualifier identifies the method or device. All other abortion procedures are performed by mechanical means because the products of conception are physically removed using instrumentation. Mechanical abortions are coded from a separate row in Table 10A. A choice of Approaches is provided; Device is always No Device (Z); Qualifier is always No Qualifier (Z).

Guided Example of Assigning Characters 4–7 for Medical and Surgical-<u>Related</u> Procedures

To practice skills for assigning codes for Medical and Surgical-<u>Related</u> procedures, continue with the example from earlier in the chapter about a patient who was seen for a cardiac stress test and CABG. Follow along in your ICD-10-PCS manual as Marcy Elwood, CCS, assigns codes. Check off each step after you complete it.

▶ First, Marcy confirms the services provided and the Root Operations she abstracted:

❑ The Root Operation for the *cardiac stress test of total activity, single measurement*, is Measurement (0) from the Measurement and Monitoring (4) Section.

❑ The Root Operation for *CP bypass* is Performance (1) from the Extracorporeal Assistance and Performance (5) Section.

▶ Marcy searches the Index for the Main Term **Stress** for the cardiac stress test.

❑ She locates two codes, **4A02XM4** and **4A12XM4**.

❑ She recognizes that the codes are exactly the same except for Character 3, Root Operation.

❑ She identifies that she must consult and compare two Tables: **4A0** and **4A1**.

❑ Alternatively, Marcy could search the Index for the Main Term of the Root Operation **Measurement** and the subterms **Cardiac** and **Total Activity**. This path also leads to code **4A02XM4**, Table **4A0**.

▶ Marcy turns to Table **4A0** to assign the code for cardiac stress test.

❑ She reads the Table title **4A0, Measurement and Monitoring, Physiological Systems, Measurement** and confirms that this accurately describes the Body System and Root Operation Measurement.

❑ As a confirmation, she also checks Table **4A1, Measurement and Monitoring, Physiological Systems, Monitoring**. She determines this Table is not correct because the procedure was a *single measurement*, not monitoring.

> Surgeon delivers one liveborn infant with a low cervical cesarean delivery.
>
> **10D00Z1 [Medical and Surgical-Related, Obstetrics], Extraction, Products of conception, Open, No device, Low cervical**

Figure 57-3 ■ Example of Coding for the Obstetrics Section, Root Operation Extraction. *Source: © PB Resources, Inc. Used with permission.*

Section   4   **Measurement and Monitoring**
Body System   A   **Physiological Systems**
Operation   0   **Measurement:** Determining the level of a physiological
                  or physical function at a point in time

Body System Character 4	Approach Character 5	Function/Device Character 6	Qualifier Character 7
2 Cardiac	X External	M Total Activity	4 Stress

Figure 57-4 ■ Assigning Code 4A02XM4. *Source: Annotation © PB Resources, Inc. Used with permission.*

❑ Marcy verifies the value for Character 4, Body System: **2 Cardiac**.

❑ Marcy verifies the value for Character 5, Approach: **X External**.

❑ Marcy assigns the value for Character 6, Function/Device: **M Total Activity**.

❑ Marcy assigns the value for Character 7, Qualifier: **4 Stress**.

❑ She reviews the code she has assigned for the *cardiac stress test, single measurement:* **4A02XM4** (■ FIGURE 57-4).

▪ **4A02XM4 Measurement and monitoring, Physiological systems, Measurement, Cardiac, External, Total activity, Stress**

▶ Marcy searches the Index for the Main Term **Performance** for cardiopulmonary bypass. She does not use the Main Term Bypass because it would lead to Tables for the Root Operation Bypass (1) in the Medical and Surgical (0) Section, defined as *altering the route of passage of the contents of a tubular Body Part.* **Cardiopulmonary bypass (CPB)** refers to the equipment that takes over the function of the heart and lungs, maintaining the circulation of blood and the oxygen content of the body.

❑ She locates the first-level subterm **Cardiac**.

❑ She locates the second-level subterm **Continuous**.

❑ She locates the third-level subterm **Output**.

❑ She identifies the Table **5A1** and code **5A1221Z**.

▪ Although a full seven-character code is listed, Marcy knows that she cannot assign a code from the Index and must verify the code in the PCS Table.

▶ Marcy turns to Table **5A1** to assign the code for the cardiopulmonary bypass.

❑ She reads the Table title **5A1, Extracorporeal Assistance and Performance, Physiological Systems, Performance** and confirms that this accurately describes the Body System and Root Operation.

❑ Marcy verifies the value for Character 4, Body System: **2 Cardiac**.

❑ Marcy verifies the value for Character 5, Duration: **2 Continuous**.

❑ Marcy verifies the value for Character 6, Function: **1 Output**.

❑ Marcy verifies the value for Character 7, Qualifier: **Z No Qualifier**.

Section   5   **Extracorporeal Assistance and Performance**
Body System   A   **Physiological Systems**
Operation   1   **Performance:** Completely taking over a physiological
                  function by extracorporeal means

Body System Character 4	Duration Character 5	Function Character 6	Qualifier Character 7
2 Cardiac	2 Continuous	1 Output 3 Pacing	Z No Qualifier

Figure 57-5 ■ Assigning Code 5A1221Z. *Source: Annotation © PB Resources, Inc. Used with permission.*

❏ She reviews the code she has assigned for the *cardiopul-monary bypass*: **5A1221Z** (■ FIGURE 57-5).

- **5A1221Z Extracorporeal assistance and performance, Physiological systems, Performance, Cardiac, Continuous, Output, No qualifier**

▶ Marcy reviews the procedure codes she has assigned for this case.

❏ **4A02XM4 Measurement and monitoring, Physiological systems, Measurement, Cardiac, External, Total activity, Stress**

❏ **5A1221Z Extracorporeal assistance and performance, Physiological systems, Performance, Cardiac, Continuous, Output, No qualifier**

▶ Next, Marcy must determine how to sequence the codes.

CODING PRACTICE

Exercise 57.3 Assigning Characters 4–7 for Medical and Surgical-Related Procedures

Instructions: Read the mini-medical-record of each patient's encounter. Review the information abstracted in Exercise 57.2 for questions 1–3. For questions 4–6, abstract the case on your own. Assign PCS codes using the Index and Tables. Write the code(s) on the line provided.

1. INPATIENT HOSPITAL   Gender: F   Age: 22

Gravida: 2   Para: 2   EGA: 33 + 2

Reason for admission: *premature rupture of membranes*

Assessment: *severe preeclampsia requires C/S*

Delivery: *low C/S, PTBLC, 1 girl*

Tip: PTBLC (Preterm birth, live child)

1 PCS Code _____

2. INPATIENT HOSPITAL   Gender: M   Age: 32

Preprocedure diagnosis: *peripheral neuritis, left arm*

Procedure: *nerve block injection to the median nerve using a regional anesthetic*

Tip: The median nerve is in the arm.

1 PCS Code _____

3. INPATIENT HOSPITAL   Gender: M   Age: 17

Preprocedure diagnosis: *aplastic anemia*

Procedure: *bone marrow transplant via central venous line using donor marrow from his identical twin*

1 PCS Code _____

4. INPATIENT HOSPITAL   Gender: F   Age: 15

Preprocedure diagnosis: *fractured R radius*

Procedure: *application of three layers of fiberglass short arm cast. Cast was molded to arm.*

Tip: The Root Operation Immobilization (3) in Section 2 Placement applies to the fitting of devices in inpatient settings other than rehabilitation.

1 PCS Code _____

5. INPATIENT HOSPITAL   Gender: F   Age: 19

Preprocedure diagnosis: *3rd-degree burn to left groin*

Procedure: *sterile dressing placement to left groin region. The old dressing was removed and the burned area was washed with mild soap and water. A clean sterile dressing was applied and held in place by wrapping a sterile gauze roll over the dressings, securing the ends with tape.*

1 PCS Code _____

6. INPATIENT HOSPITAL   Gender: M   Age: 53

Preprocedure diagnosis: *achalasia*

Procedure: *esophagogastroscopy with Botox injection into esophageal sphincter. Under endoscopic guidance, I injected 20 units BT-A, diluted in 1 mL of saline, in each of the 4 lower esophageal sphincter quadrants approximately 1 cm above the Z-line into the bulging muscle.*

Tip: Botulinum toxin is a paralyzing agent with temporary effects; it does not sclerose or destroy the nerve.

1 PCS Code _____

ARRANGING CODES FOR MEDICAL AND SURGICAL-<u>RELATED</u> PROCEDURES

Procedures from the Obstetrics Section are usually sequenced as the principal procedure because delivery is commonly the reason for admission and the services provided during the inpatient admission. By contrast, many Medical and Surgical-<u>Related</u> procedures are not sequenced as the principal procedure because they are performed in addition to a more definitive procedure. Refer to ■ Figure 57-6 for an example in which the Root Operation Reposition (S) from the Medical and Surgical (0) Section is sequenced as the principal diagnosis, followed by the Root Operations Immobilization (3) and Traction (6) from the Placement (2) Section. In this example, Reposition is the definitive procedure.

SUCCESS STEP

Many Medical and Surgical-<u>Related</u> procedures also are performed as standalone outpatient procedures, but they are reported with CPT codes because PCS is used only by inpatient facilities.

Guided Example of Arranging Codes for Medical and Surgical-<u>Related</u> Procedures

To practice skills for arranging codes for Medical and Surgical-<u>Related</u> procedures, continue with the example from earlier in the chapter about the patient who was seen for a cardiac stress test and CABG. Follow along in your ICD-10-PCS manual as Marcy Elwood, CCS, arranges the codes. Check off each step after you complete it.

▶ First, Marcy confirms the procedures performed:

❑ Cardiac stress test

❑ Cardiopulmonary bypass

❑ CABG ×2 of LIMA to LAD, OM with GSV

❑ Harvesting of the GSV

Patient was admitted with a displaced fracture of the left femoral shaft and a fractured left radius. Open reduction with internal fixation was performed on the femur and a short arm cast was applied. Following surgery, the femur was placed in mechanical traction.

0QS904Z [Medical and surgical, Lower bones], Reposition, Femoral shaft left, Open, Internal fixation device, No qualifier
2W3DX2Z [Medical and surgical, Anatomical regions], Immobilization, Lower arm left, External, Cast, No qualifier
2W6PX0Z [Medical and surgical, Anatomical regions], Traction, Upper leg left, External, Traction apparatus, No qualifier

Figure 57-6 ■ Example of Arranging Medical and Surgical-<u>Related</u> Procedure Codes. *Source: © PB Resources, Inc. Used with permission.*

▶ Marcy reviews the diagnoses and determines the principal diagnosis:

❑ *atherosclerotic heart disease with 90% blockage in LAD and 80% blockage in the OM with unstable angina pectoris*

❑ She also identifies the definitive procedure as the CABG.

▶ Marcy reviews the procedure codes assigned:

❑ **4A02XM4 Measurement and monitoring, Physiological systems, Measurement, Cardiac, External, Total activity, Stress**

❑ **5A1221Z Extracorporeal assistance and performance, Physiological systems, Performance, Cardiac, Continuous, Output, No qualifier**

❑ **0210293 Medical and surgical, Heart and great vessels, Bypass, Coronary artery one site, Open approach, Autologous venous tissue, Coronary artery** (Chapter 54)

❑ **02100Z9 Medical and surgical, Heart and great vessel, Bypass, Coronary artery one site, Open approach, No device, Internal mammary artery left** (Chapter 54)

❑ **06BP4ZZ Medical and surgical, Lower veins, Excision, Greater saphenous vein right, Percutaneous endoscopic approach, No device, No qualifier** (Chapter 54)

▶ Marcy determines that the principal procedure is the CABG. The principal diagnosis determines the sequencing order because the principal procedure must be the one most closely related to the principal diagnosis. The CABG is the definitive procedure, so the codes for Bypass are sequenced first.

▶ Marcy finalizes the procedure codes and sequencing for this case:

(1) **0210293 Medical and surgical, Heart and great vessels, Bypass, Coronary artery one site, Open approach, Autologous venous tissue, Coronary artery**

(2) **02100Z9 Medical and surgical, Heart and great vessels, Bypass, Coronary artery one site, Open approach, No device, Internal mammary artery left**

(3) **06BP4ZZ Medical and surgical, Lower veins, Excision, Greater saphenous vein right, Percutaneous endoscopic approach, No device, No qualifier**

(4) **5A1221Z Extracorporeal assistance and performance, Physiological systems, Performance, Cardiac, Continuous, Output, No qualifier**

(5) **4A02XM4 Measurement and monitoring, Physiological systems, Measurement, Cardiac, External, Total activity, Stress**

▶ Marcy also assigns the ICD-10-CM diagnosis code that supports the need for the service.

(1) **I25.110 Atherosclerotic heart disease of native coronary artery with unstable angina pectoris**

CODING PRACTICE

Exercise 57.4 Arranging Codes for Medical and Surgical-<u>Related</u> Procedures

Instructions: Read the mini-medical-record of each patient's encounter. Review the information abstracted in Exercise 57.2 for questions 1–3. For questions 4–6, abstract the case on your own. Assign PCS codes using the Index and Tables, and arrange the codes in proper sequence. Write the code(s) on the line provided.

1. INPATIENT HOSPITAL Gender: F Age: 15

Preprocedure diagnosis: displaced fracture R tibia

Procedure: closed reduction of fracture with percutaneous insertion of internal fixation device. Applied leg cast and initiated mechanical traction of lower R leg

Tip: The Root Operation Immobilization (3) in Section 2 Placement applies to the fitting of devices in inpatient settings other than rehabilitation.

3 PCS Codes _____

_____

2. INPATIENT HOSPITAL Gender: F Age: 33

Gravida: 2 Para: 2 EGA: 39 + 1

Assessment: fetal bradycardia

Procedure: mid forceps delivery with repair of perineal laceration

Delivery: TBLC, 1 girl

Tip: TBLC (Term birth, live child)

2 PCS Codes _____

3. INPATIENT HOSPITAL Gender: F Age: 75

Preprocedure diagnosis: cardiac arrhythmia

Procedure: 24-hour ambulatory Holter monitoring followed by external measurement of cardiac output

2 PCS Codes _____

4. INPATIENT HOSPITAL Gender: F Age: 78

Preprocedure diagnosis: left hip fracture following a fall

Procedure: placement of intermittent pneumatic compression (IPC) device covering both calves to prevent deep venous thrombosis (DVT)

2 PCS Codes _____

5. INPATIENT HOSPITAL Gender: F Age: 39

Preprocedure diagnosis: primigravida at term, 39 weeks 4 days, in labor

Procedure: NSVD of term newborn; fetal heart rate monitoring, transvaginal. Patient in active labor, fetal heart monitor applied to monitor any variability. Patient delivered a healthy 7 lb. 2 oz female via manually assisted delivery.

Tip: For internal monitoring, a sensor is attached to the thigh of the mother. An electrode from the sensor is inserted transvaginally into the uterus and the electrode is attached to the baby's scalp.

2 PCS Codes _____

6. INPATIENT HOSPITAL Gender: M Age: 62

Preprocedure diagnosis: angina

Procedure: cardiac exercise stress test, Bruce protocol; cardiac countershock. At the conclusion of the stress portion of the test, the patient went into cardiac arrest. He was successfully converted to sinus rhythm.

2 PCS Codes _____

CHAPTER SUMMARY

In this chapter you learned that:

- The Medical and Surgical-<u>Related</u> Sections are Obstetrics (1), Placement (2), Administration (3), Measurement and Monitoring (4), Extracorporeal Assistance and Performance (5), Extracorporeal Therapies (6), Osteopathic (7), Other Procedures (8), and Chiropractic (9).

- The Section Obstetrics (1) is procedures on an embryo, fetus, or unborn child and has 12 Root Operations, two of which are unique to this Section.

- The Section Placement (2) is procedures involving devices and materials that are performed without making an incision or a puncture and has seven Root Operations, five of which are unique to this Section.

- The Section Administration (3) is procedures in which a diagnostic or therapeutic substance is given to the patient and has three Root Operations, all unique to this Section.

- The Section Measurement and Monitoring (4) is procedures that take a single or series of readings of physiologic levels, such as temperature or heart rate, and has two Root Operations, both unique to this Section.

- The Section Extracorporeal Assistance and Performance (5) is procedures performed in a critical care setting to support physiological functions and has three Root Operations, all unique to this Section.

- The Section Extracorporeal Therapies (6) is other extracorporeal procedures not described in Section 5 and has 10 Root Operations, all unique to this Section.

- The Section Osteopathic (7) is osteopathic manipulation procedures and has one Root Operation, which is unique to this Section.

- The Section Other Procedures (8) is miscellaneous procedures not included in other Medical and Surgical-<u>Related</u> Sections and has one Root Operation, which is unique to this Section.

- The Section Chiropractic (9) is chiropractic manipulation procedures and has one Root Operation, which is unique to this Section.

- The meaning of Characters 4 through 7 varies based on the Section, so it is important to review the Character meanings in each PCS Table.

- Many Medical and Surgical-<u>Related</u> procedures are not sequenced as the principal procedure because they are performed in addition to a more definitive procedure.

- PCS provides guidelines for the Obstetrics Section, which clarify the types of procedures to be coded from the Obstetrics Section and those to be coded from the Medical and Surgical (0) Section.

CONCEPT QUIZ

Take a moment to look back at Medical and Surgical-<u>Related</u> Procedures and solidify your skills. Try to answer the questions from memory first, then refer to the discussion in this chapter if you need a little extra help.

Completion

Instructions: Write the Root Operation that matches the definition based on the information you learned in this chapter. Choose from the list below. Some choices may be used more than once and some choices may not be used at all.

Administration (3)

Assistance (0)

Chiropractic (9)

Dressing (2)

Extracorporeal Assistance and Performance (5)

Extracorporeal Therapies (6)

Hyperthermia (3)

Hypothermia (4)

Immobilization (3)

Introduction (0)

Irrigation (1)

Measurement and Monitoring (4)

Monitoring (1)

Obstetrics (1)

Osteopathic (7)

Other Procedures (8)

Packing (4)

Pheresis (5)

Placement (2)

Restoration (2)

Traction (6)

Treatment (0)

1. The Root Operation _____ from the _____ Section is putting in or on a cleansing substance.

2. The Root Operation _____ from the _____ Section is returning, or attempting to return, a physiological function to its original state by extracorporeal means.

3. The Root Operation _____ from the _____ Section is limiting or preventing motion of a body region.

4. The Root Operation _____ from the _____ Section is putting in or on a therapeutic, diagnostic, nutritional, physiological, or prophylactic substance except blood or blood products.

5. The Root Operation _____ from the _____ Section is determining the level of a physiological or physical function repetitively over a period of time.

(continued)

(continued from page 1153)

6. The Root Operation _____ from the _____ Section is Extracorporeal separation of blood products

7. The Root Operation _____ from the _____ Section is manual treatment to eliminate or alleviate somatic dysfunction and related disorders.

8. The Root Operation _____ from the _____ Section is putting material on a body region for protection.

9. The Root Operation _____ from the _____ Section is taking over a portion of a physiological function by extracorporeal means.

10. The Root Operation _____ from the _____ Section is extracorporeal raising of body temperature.

Multiple Choice

Instructions: Circle the letter of the best answer to each question based on the information you learned in this chapter.

1. Which Section classifies procedures in which a diagnostic or therapeutic substance is given to the patient?
   A. Placement (2)
   B. Extracorporeal Therapies (6)
   C. Other Procedures (8)
   D. Administration (3)

2. Which Root Operation is unique to the Placement (2) Section?
   A. Change
   B. Compression
   C. Treatment
   D. Removal

3. What Section defines Character 6 as Substance?
   A. Extracorporeal Therapies (6)
   B. Obstetrics (1)
   C. Other Procedures (8)
   D. Administration (3)

4. What Character identifies the anatomic site that is irrigated in the Root Operation Irrigation (1)?
   A. Character 4, Body Part
   B. Character 5, Approach
   C. Character 6, Device
   D. Character 7, Qualifier

5. Which Medical and Surgical-Related Section has guidelines in PCS OGCR?
   A. Obstetrics (1)
   B. Placement (2)
   C. Administration (3)
   D. Extracorporeal Therapies (6)

6. Which Section defines Character 6 as Function?
   A. Other Procedures (8)
   B. Administration (1)
   C. Placement (2)
   D. Extracorporeal Assistance and Performance (5)

7. Which Section classifies procedures that use equipment to support a physiological function in a critical care setting?
   A. Administration (3)
   B. Extracorporeal Assistance and Performance (5)
   C. Placement (2)
   D. Measurement and Monitoring (4)

8. What is the only Body Part value in the Obstetrics (1) Section?
   A. Products of Conception
   B. Fetus
   C. Uterus
   D. Birth Canal

9. What Section uses the Character 2 Body System value Indwelling Device (C)?
   A. Placement (2)
   B. Measurement and Monitoring (4)
   C. Extracorporeal Assistance and Performance (5)
   D. Other Procedures (8)

10. What Section defines Character 6 as Method?
   A. Obstetrics (1)
   B. Measurement and Monitoring (4)
   C. Chiropractic (9)
   D. Extracorporeal Assistance and Performance (5)

CODING CHALLENGE

Instructions: Read the mini-medical-record of each patient's encounter, then abstract, assign, and arrange ICD-10-CM diagnosis codes and PCS procedure codes using the appropriate Index and Tables. Write the code(s) on the line provided.

---

1. INPATIENT HOSPITAL   Gender: F   Age: 42

Preprocedure diagnosis: *nosebleed, status post rhinoplasty 30 days prior*

Procedure: *both nostrils packed with a 7.5-cm Rhino Rocket. During this procedure the patient became unresponsive for about 45 seconds and was resuscitated with a liter bolus of normal saline.*

(continued)

---

1. (continued)

Postprocedure diagnosis: *epistaxis, transient loss of consciousness*

Tip: Patient had a loss of consciousness but not a loss of cardiac or respiratory function.

2 ICD-10-CM Codes _____

2 ICD-10-PCS Codes _____

2. INPATIENT HOSPITAL   Gender: F   Age: 50

Preprocedure diagnosis: suspected ventricular tachycardia following an episode of syncope. Transient heart arrhythmias and transient cardiac ischemia.

Procedure: 24-hour Holter monitor

Postprocedure diagnosis: ventricular tachycardia confirmed

1 ICD-10-CM Code _____

1 ICD-10-PCS Code _____

3. INPATIENT HOSPITAL   Gender: F   Age: 37

Preprocedure diagnosis: plantar fasciitis, right and left foot

Procedure: extracorporeal shock wave therapy directed at the plantar fascia on the right and left. Patient tolerated the procedure with minimal discomfort.

Tip: Identify the repeated nature of this procedure in Character 5, Duration, with the value Multiple.

1 ICD-10-CM Code _____

1 ICD-10-PCS Code _____

4. INPATIENT HOSPITAL   Gender: F   Age: 25

Preprocedure diagnosis: active labor, 40 weeks, 3 days

Procedure: placement of epidural catheter with continuous infusion of 0.2% ropivacaine with 1.5 mL of fentanyl at 10 mL per hour. The catheter was placed at the level of L3-4 without incident. Patient experienced immediate pain relief.

Tip: An epidural catheter is a plastic catheter placed through the skin into the epidural space within the spinal canal.

2 ICD-10-CM Codes _____

2 ICD-10-PCS Codes _____

5. INPATIENT HOSPITAL   Gender: F   Age: 27

Preprocedure diagnosis: full-term labor, EGA 37 + 5

Procedure: spontaneous vaginal delivery of one liveborn female

3 ICD-10-CM Codes _____

_____

1 ICD-10-PCS Code _____

6. INPATIENT HOSPITAL   Gender: M   Age: 31

Preprocedure diagnosis: postpolio syndrome (PPS). Severe neck pain and weakness. Had polio at age 5 when living overseas.

Procedure: osteopathic myofascial release of the neck. Pressure was applied to release the trigger points of the cervical area.

2 ICD-10-CM Codes _____

1 ICD-10-PCS Code _____

7. INPATIENT HOSPITAL   Gender: F   Age: 40

Preprocedure diagnosis: cervical spinal stenosis status post decompression, opioid dependence, long-standing low-back pain radiating into the right leg.

Procedure: needle EMG, nerve conduction study. Needle EMG was performed on the right leg and lumbosacral paraspinal muscles using a disposable concentric needle. It revealed the spontaneous activity in right peroneus longus and gastrocnemius medialis muscles as well as the right lower lumbosacral paraspinal muscles. There is evidence of denervation in right gastrocnemius medialis muscle.

Postprocedure diagnosis: no evidence of left lower extremity radiculopathy, peripheral neuropathy, or entrapment neuropathy.

Tip: Refer to ICD-10-CM OGCR I.C.6.b.(ii) for diagnosis sequencing instructions. Two codes for the EMG procedure are needed: one for the nervous system and one for the musculoskeletal system.

3 ICD-10-CM Codes _____

_____

2 ICD-10-PCS Codes _____

8. INPATIENT HOSPITAL   Gender: F   Age: 32

Preprocedure diagnosis: intrauterine fetal demise at 34 weeks' gestation

Procedure: preterm induced vaginal delivery of intrauterine fetal demise. IV Pitocin initiated and labor progressed to complete dilation after AROM. A stillborn fetus was delivered vaginally without incident.

Tip: Products of Conception refer to all components of pregnancy, including the fetus, embryo, amnion, umbilical cord, and placenta.

3 ICD-10-CM Codes _____

_____

3 ICD-10-PCS Codes _____

(continued)

(continued from page 1155)

9. INPATIENT HOSPITAL   Gender: M   Age: 3 days

Preprocedure diagnosis: NSVD of newborn now with jaundice and hyperbilirubinemia

Procedure: phototherapy with Bili light ×2 days. Baby was placed under the Bili light with soft eye patches and a diaper. After two days of therapy bilirubin returned to normal.

2 ICD-10-CM Codes _____

1 ICD-10-PCS Code _____

10. INPATIENT HOSPITAL   Gender: M   Age: 57

Preprocedure diagnosis: angina pectoris

Procedure: cardiac stress test to measure total activity, single measurement, followed by catheterization of left and right heart to obtain sampling and pressure.

Tip: Heart catheterization by definition uses a percutaneous approach.

1 ICD-10-CM Code _____

2 ICD-10-PCS Codes _____

KEEP ON CODING

Instructions: Read the procedural statement, then use the appropriate Index and Tables to assign PCS procedure codes. Write the code(s) on the line provided.

1. Abortion using laminaria: ICD-10-PCS Code(s) _____

2. Pain nerve block injection in the spine: ICD-10-PCS Code(s) _____

3. Traction for fracture of right upper leg: ICD-10-PCS Code(s) _____

4. Esophageal motility study, via endoscope: ICD-10-PCS Code(s) _____

5. Splinting of left hand: ICD-10-PCS -10-PCS Code(s) _____

6. Classical cesarean delivery: ICD-10-PCS Code(s) _____

7. Transfusion of nonautologous frozen red blood cells via peripheral vein: ICD-10-PCS Code(s) _____

8. Electroencephalogram (EEG): ICD-10-PCS Code(s) _____

9. Intermittent positive airway pressure (IPAP) respiratory ventilation for 36 hours: ICD-10-PCS Code(s) _____

10. Basal metabolic rate (BMR): ICD-10-PCS Code(s) _____

11. Transfusion of 2 units of fresh RBCs via peripheral vein: ICD-10-PCS Code(s) _____

12. Osteopathic treatment of the neck using general mobilization: ICD-10-PCS Code(s) _____

13. Collection of sperm for fertility study: ICD-10-PCS Code(s) _____

14. Chiropractic manipulation of the lumbar spine using mechanically assisted technique: ICD-10-PCS Code(s) _____

15. Continuous hyperbaric oxygen treatment for nonhealing ulcer, left ankle: ICD-10-PCS Code(s) _____

16. Peritoneal dialysis via Port-a-Cath: ICD-10-PCS Code(s) _____

17. Saline irrigation of nasopharynx: ICD-10-PCS Code(s) _____

18. Cortisone injection in right ankle: ICD-10-PCS Code(s) _____

19. Robotic-assisted endoscopic right knee arthroplasty: ICD-10-PCS Code(s) _____

20. Whole-body hyperthermia: ICD-10-PCS Code(s) _____

21. Musculoskeletal shock wave therapy, multiple: ICD-10-PCS Code(s) _____

22. Sandbag compression for hematoma at right femoral catheter insertion site: ICD-10-PCS Code(s) _____

23. Manually assisted vaginal delivery: ICD-10-PCS Code(s) _____

24. Endoscopic bronchial alveolar lavage, right main bronchus, for diagnostic specimen: ICD-10-PCS Code(s) _____

25. Hemodialysis, single session: ICD-10-PCS Code(s) _____

Learning Objectives

After completing this chapter, you should have the skills to:

58.1 Spell and define the key words, medical terms, and abbreviations related to Ancillary procedures.

58.2 Discuss the types of Ancillary procedures.

58.3 Identify the main characteristics of coding for the Root Types for Ancillary procedures.

58.4 Abstract information from the medical record for coding Ancillary procedures.

58.5 Assign codes for the Root Types for Ancillary procedures.

58.6 Arrange codes for the Root Types for Ancillary procedures.

58.7 Abstract and assign codes for New Technology.

58.8 Discuss the ICD-10-PCS coding guidelines related to Ancillary procedures and New Technology.

Chapter Outline

- **Basics of Ancillary Procedures**
- **Coding Overview of Ancillary Procedures**
- **Abstracting for Ancillary Procedures**
- **Assigning Characters 4–7 for Ancillary Procedures**
- **Arranging Codes for Ancillary Procedures**
- **New Technology (Section X)**

Key Terms and Abbreviations

activities of daily living (ADLs)	assessment (PCS Section F)	orthosis	radiopharmaceutical
anatomic imaging	functional imaging	prosthesis	treatment (PCS Section F)

In addition to the key terms listed here, students should know the terms defined within tables in this chapter.

For updates and corrections, visit our student resource site at

www.pearsonhighered.com/healthprofessionsresources

INTRODUCTION

Visual images of a trip can be either still or motion. Likewise, physicians use a variety of imaging technologies to better understand the human body. Radiographic imaging is one of several types of procedures classified in the PCS Ancillary Sections.

This chapter discusses PCS Sections B, C, D, F, G, and H, referred to as Ancillary procedures and Section X, New Technology. (There is no section E.) You will learn how codes in these Sections are structured, how Root Types are defined, and other unique characteristics. As with other PCS Sections, pay careful attention to the differences between each Root Type so that you can use each confidently and accurately.

BASICS OF ANCILLARY PROCEDURES

"Ancillary procedures" is a descriptive title that summarizes nine PCS Sections, but it does not occupy a Character within the code itself. ■ TABLE 58-1 summarizes the value, name, and purpose of each Section. Ancillary Sections contain approximately 7,500 codes and compose 10% of PCS. All Root Types are unique to Sections in this portion of PCS.

Ancillary procedure codes have seven Characters, but the purpose of many Characters is different than in the Medical and Surgical (0) Section (■ TABLE 58-2). Some of the differences include the following:

- In the Section Physical Rehabilitation and Diagnostic Audiology (F), Character 2 is the Section Qualifier that distinguishes between the two types of service reported in this section: Physical Rehabilitation (0) or Diagnostic Audiology (1).
- All Sections except Radiation Therapy (D) define Character 3 as Root Type rather than Root Operation because no operations are performed. Radiation Therapy defines Character 3 as Modality.
- The Section Imaging (B) defines Character 5 as Contrast and Character 6 as Qualifier.
- The Section Nuclear Medicine (C) defines Character 5 as Radionuclide.
- The Section Radiation Therapy (D) defines Character 4 as Treatment Site, Character 5 as Modality Qualifier, and Character 6 as Isotope.

Table 58-1 ■ CHARACTER 1: SECTION NAMES AND PURPOSE FOR ANCILLARY PROCEDURES

Value	Section Name	Purpose
B	Imaging	Creating a visual representation of internal body structures to diagnose conditions
C	Nuclear Medicine	Introduction of radioactive materials into the body to capture images, diagnose diseases, or treat abnormalities
D	Radiation Therapy	Use of radiation to treat malignancies
F	Physical Rehabilitation and Diagnostic Audiology	Procedures and therapy to help patients regain body functions lost due to medical conditions or injury; procedures to diagnose hearing-related conditions
G	Mental Health	A variety of methods to diagnose and treat psychiatric and mental disorders
H	Substance Abuse Treatment	Procedures to treat disorders related to substance abuse

- Physical Rehabilitation and Diagnostic Audiology defines Character 4 as Body System and Region, rather than Body Part. It defines Character 5 as Type Qualifier and Character 6 as Equipment.
- The Sections Mental Health (G) and Substance Abuse Treatment (H) define Characters 4 through 7 as Qualifier. These Characters always have the value None (Z).

CODING CAUTION

Character names and values used in Ancillary procedures frequently are unique to a particular Table, so take time to review the Character definitions when coding from this portion of PCS to avoid confusion.

Medical terms for Ancillary procedures often contain a suffix that describes the type of procedure performed, such as making a recording or providing therapy, and a root that identifies the specific method, such as radiation or sound waves.

Table 58-2 ■ SEVEN CHARACTERS OF ANCILLARY PROCEDURES

		Character				
1	**2**	**3**	**4**	**5**	**6**	**7**
Imaging **B**	Body System	Root Type	Body Part	Contrast	Qualifier	Qualifier
Nuclear Medicine **C**	Body System	Root Type	Body Part	Radionuclide	Qualifier	Qualifier
Radiation Therapy **D**	Body System	Modality	Treatment Site	Modality Qualifier	Isotope	Qualifier
Physical Rehabilitation and Diagnostic Audiology **F**	Section Qualifier	Root Type	Body System/ Region	Type Qualifier	Equipment	Qualifier
Mental Health **G**	Body System	Root Type	Type Qualifier	Qualifier	Qualifier	Qualifier
Substance Abuse Treatment **H**	Body System	Root Type	Type Qualifier	Qualifier	Qualifier	Qualifier

Table 58-3 ■ EXAMPLE OF CONSTRUCTING MEDICAL TERMS FOR ANCILLARY PROCEDURES

Combining Form	Suffix	Complete Medical Term
radi/o (*radiation*) **son/o** (*sound*) **tom/o** (*cut, slice*)	**-graph/-gram** (*record*)	**radio + graph** (*a record made with radiation*)
		sono + gram (*a record made with sound*)
		tomo + graph (*a record made with [visual] slices*)
	-therapy (*treatment*)	**radio + therapy** (*treatment with radiation*)
psych/o (*mind*) **ultra/sound** (*high-frequency sound*)		**ultrasound + therapy** (*treatment with high-frequency sound waves*)
		psycho + therapy (*treatment of the mind*)

Source: © PB Resources, Inc. Used with permission.

Procedure names can combine the medical term for the procedure with additional terms for the anatomic site and isotope, contrast agent, or other pharmaceutical used. Be sure to review documentation thoroughly to locate all modifying terms that describe the procedure. Refer to ■ TABLE 58-3 for a refresher on how to build medical terms related to Ancillary procedures. Refer to detailed anatomic diagrams of specific organ systems in Chapters 9 through 48 of this text, or in external references, when you need to refresh your memory of human anatomy.

CODING CAUTION

Be alert for Root Types that are spelled similarly but have different PCS definitions.

Computerized Tomography (2) (Section B) (*Computer reformatted digital display* of multiplanar images developed from the capture of multiple exposures of *external ionizing radiation*) and **Tomographic (Tomo) Nuclear Medicine Imaging (2) (Section C)** (*Introduction of radioactive materials into the body* for three-dimensional display of images developed from the capture of radioactive emissions)

Ultrasonography (4) (Section B) (*Real-time display of images* of anatomy or flow information developed from the capture of reflected and attenuated high-frequency sound waves) and **Ultrasound Therapy (7) (Section F)** (*Extracorporeal treatment* by high-frequency sound waves [ultrasound])

CODING PRACTICE

Exercise 58.1 Basics of Ancillary Procedures

Instructions: Use your medical terminology skills and resources to define the following Ancillary procedures, then identify the code(s) or code range listed in the PCS Index. Follow these steps:

- Use slash marks "/" to break down the underlined term into its root(s) and suffix.
- *Do not attempt to break down words or abbreviations marked with an *.
- Define the meaning of the word based on the meaning of each word part.
- Look up the phrase in the ICD-10-PCS Index, and write down the name(s) and of Root Type(s) or Modality(ies) the Index cross-references you to and the Table(s), if provided.
- Do not assign any codes.

Example: discography, bones   Meaning: *make a recording of an*   PCS Root Type(s)/Table(s): *Plain Radiography BR0,*
disco/graphy   *intervertebral disc*   *Fluoroscopy BR1*

1. audiometry   Meaning _____   PCS Root Type(s)/Table(s) _____

2. pyelography   Meaning _____   PCS Root Type(s)/Table(s) _____

3. pharmacotherapy for substance abuse   Meaning _____   PCS Root Type(s)/Table(s) _____

4. tonometry   Meaning _____   PCS Root Type(s)/Table(s) _____

5. cholangiogram   Meaning _____   PCS Root Type(s)/Table(s) _____

6. KUB* X-ray   Meaning _____   PCS Root Type(s)/Table(s) _____

7. myelogram   Meaning _____   PCS Root Type(s)/Table(s) _____

8. electroconvulsive therapy   Meaning _____   PCS Root Type(s)/Table(s) _____

9. venography   Meaning _____   PCS Root Type(s)/Table(s) _____

10. laser interstitial thermal therapy, brain stem   Meaning _____   PCS Root Type(s)/Table(s) _____

CODING OVERVIEW OF ANCILLARY PROCEDURES

PCS OGCR provide no guidelines for Ancillary procedures. The appendix in the PCS coding manual "Type and Type Qualifier Definitions, Sections B–H," provides official definitions of many of the terms used in the Ancillary Sections (■ FIGURE 58-1). The Sections and Characters for which definitions are provided are as follows:

- Section B, Imaging
  - Character 3, Root Type
- Section C, Nuclear Medicine
  - Character 3, Root Type
- Section F, Physical Rehabilitation and Diagnostic Audiology
  - Character 3, Root Type
  - Character 5, Type Qualifier
- Section G, Mental Health
  - Character 3, Root Type
  - Character 4, Type Qualifier
- Section H, Substance Abuse
  - Character 3, Root Type

Use the appendix as follows when assigning codes in PCS Sections B through H:

1. Locate the desired Section name in the appendix.
2. Confirm the Character position and name.
3. If the Section defines values for more than one Character, locate the segment for the correct character.
4. Locate the Character value(s) needed, read the definition, and confirm whether it accurately describes the service to be coded.
5. If the definition is not accurate, review other definitions to find the appropriate one.

ABSTRACTING FOR ANCILLARY PROCEDURES

The following information highlights the definitions and unique criteria for Sections B, C, D, F, G, and H. Because of the brief and specialized nature of these sections, guidance about Characters 4 through 7 is incorporated into the following discussion. General information about assigning codes is presented in the "Assigning" section of this chapter. A Key Criteria for Abstracting to help determine the appropriate PCS Section is provided. Individual abstracting tables for each Section are not provided because the appropriate Root Types can generally be determined by reviewing the PCS definitions.

Key Criteria for Abstracting Ancillary Procedures

Key abstracting criteria aid in identifying the Section of Root Types that should be used (■ TABLE 58-4). After reading the procedure report, use the abstracting table as follows:

1. Answer the General Questions to get a basic understanding of the procedure.
2. Answer the Section Questions. One question should be answered *Yes*; the rest should be answered *No*.
3. For the Section Question that was answered *Yes*, refer to the Section identified to review the Root Types that could apply.
4. Look up the definition of each of the applicable Root Types in the appendix of the ICD-10-PCS coding manual.
5. Identify the one Root Type or Modality that matches the procedure documented. This will be the Main Term when you use the Index.
6. Repeat the abstracting process for each procedure performed.

Section F: Physical Rehabilitation and Diagnostic Audiology Character 3: Root Type	
Value	**Definition**
Activities of Daily Living Assessment	Measurement of functional level for activities of daily living
Activities of Daily Living Treatment	Exercise or activities to facilitate functional competence for activities of daily living
Caregiver Training	Training in activities to support patient's optimal level of function
Cochlear Implant Treatment	Application of techniques to improve the communication abilities of individuals with cochlear implant

Figure 58-1 ■ Example of PCS Appendix "Type and Type Qualifier Definitions, Sections B–H."

Table 58-4 ■ KEY CRITERIA FOR ABSTRACTING ANCILLARY PROCEDURES

General Questions

- ❑ What is the stated procedure?
- ❑ What body region or body part is involved?
- ❑ What method is used?
- ❑ Is the procedure description what you would expect based on the name of the procedure?
- ❑ Was more than one procedure, or a combined procedure, performed?

Section Questions (Answer *Yes* to one question)	Refer to Root Types in This Section
❑ Does the procedure involve imaging/radiography?	Section B Imaging
❑ Does the procedure involve nuclear medicine?	Section C Nuclear Medicine
❑ Does the procedure involve radiation treatment for a malignancy?	Section D Radiation Therapy
❑ Does the procedure involve physical rehabilitation or diagnostic audiology?	Section F Physical Rehabilitation and Diagnostic Audiology
❑ Are mental health services provided?	Section G Mental Health
❑ Is substance abuse treatment provided?	Section 6 Substance Abuse Treatment

Source: © PB Resources, Inc. Used with permission.

Abstracting for Radiology Procedures (Sections B, C, and D)

Ancillary procedures include three classes of radiology procedures, each with a separate PCS Section: Imaging (B), Nuclear Medicine (C), and Radiation Therapy (D). The Root Types within each Section identify various techniques and modalities.

Imaging (Section B) Root Types

The Imaging (B) Section includes diagnostic radiology and its branches, each of which is a Root Type (■ TABLE 58-5), for a total of five Root Types. This section classifies anatomic imaging, which captures a static image of an anatomic part. ■ FIGURE 58-2

Table 58-5 ■ ROOT TYPES IN THE IMAGING (B) SECTION

Value	Description	Definition
0	Plain Radiography	Planar (*flat, single plane*) display of an image developed from the capture of external ionizing radiation on photographic or photoconductive plate
1	Fluoroscopy	Single plane or biplane real-time display of an image developed from the capture of external ionizing radiation on a fluorescent screen; may also be stored by either digital or analog means
2	Computerized Tomography (CT scan)	Computer-reformatted digital display of multiplanar images developed from the capture of multiple exposures of external ionizing radiation
3	Magnetic Resonance Imaging (MRI)	Computer-reformatted digital display of multiplanar images developed from the capture of radiofrequency signals emitted by nuclei in a body site excited within a magnetic field
4	Ultrasonography	Real-time display of images of anatomy or flow information developed from the capture of reflected and attenuated high-frequency sound waves

shows images creating by various imaging methods. Characters are defined as follows:

- Character 4, Body System, provides values for the major body systems, as well as Anatomical Regions (W) and Fetus and Obstetrical (Y). The skeletal system is identified by the following values, which differ from the classical divisions of axial skeleton and appendicular skeleton:

  - Skull and Facial Bones (N)
  - Axial Skeletal System, Except Skull and Facial Bones (R), which includes the vertebral column, pelvis, and sternum
  - Non-axial Upper Bones (P), which includes the shoulders, ribs, arms, and hands
  - Non-axial Lower Bones (Q), which includes the legs and feet

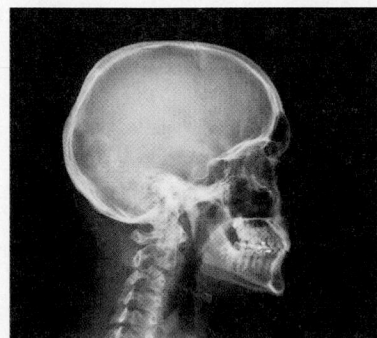

A Plain Radiography

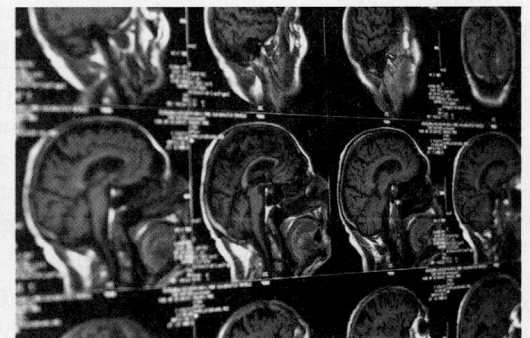

B Computed Tomography (CT)

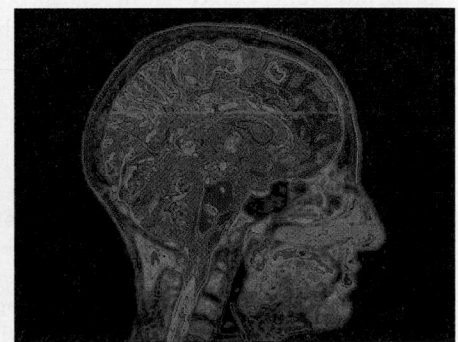

C Magnetic Resonance Imaging (MRI)

Figure 58-2 ■ Examples of Imaging Methods. (A) Plain Radiography. *Source: Shutterstock © itsmejust.* (B) Computed Tomography (CT). *Source: Shutterstock.* (C) Magnetic Resonance Imaging (MRI). *Source: Shutterstock © SpeedKingz.*

- Character 5, Contrast, identifies the type of contrast medium used, if any. Because X-ray beams pass through soft tissue, the use of a contrast dye makes soft structures more readily visible. Examples of Contrast values are High Osmolar and Low Osmolar.

- Character 6, Qualifier value Unenhanced and Enhanced (0), identifies an image taken without contrast followed by one with contrast. When no contrast medium is used, assign the value None (Z).

- Character 7, Qualifier, has only one value, None (Z), which should be assigned for all codes.

The Root Type Plain Radiography (0) is traditionally referred to as X-ray and also includes mammography.

Operative procedures sometimes use imaging guidance to assist in visualizing the procedure with the use of fluoroscopy or ultrasound. Code the operative procedure as the definitive procedure, usually from the Medical and Surgical (0) Section, then assign an additional code from the Imaging Section for the imaging guidance. Use the Character 7 Qualifier value for Guidance (A) (■ FIGURE 58-3).

SUCCESS STEP

Ultrasound is energy created by high-frequency sound waves, which can be used for therapy, such as stimulating muscle and nerve tissue, or for imaging purposes. When you see a reference to ultrasound, remember to determine whether it is therapeutic ultrasound or ultrasound imaging, also called ultrasonography or sonogram, so you can select the correct Root Type (■ FIGURE 58-4).

Nuclear Medicine (Section C) Root Types

Root Types for Nuclear Medicine (C) identify the methods used (■ TABLE 58-6). Nuclear medicine is a specialized branch of radiology that provides **functional imaging**, which allows the physician to observe organ function in real time. Patients take a very small amount of radioactive material, also called a **radiopharmaceutical**, internally. The radiopharmaceutical emits gamma rays that are detected by equipment to create the resulting image.

The Nuclear Medicine Section uses Characters 5 through 7 as follows:

- Character 5, Radionuclide, identifies the radiation source used in the procedure. Choices are dependent on the procedure described by the Root Type. Examples are Carbon 11 and Fluorine.

Radiologist provided fluoroscopic guidance with high osmolar contrast for a percutaneous thrombectomy in the right popliteal vein.

06CY3ZZ [Medical and surgical, Lower veins], Extirpation, Pericardial cavity, Percutaneous, No device, No qualifier
B51B0ZA [Imaging, Veins], Fluoroscopic, Lower extremity veins right, High osmolar, Guidance

Figure 58-3 ■ Example of Coding for Imaging Guidance.
Source: © PB Resources, Inc. Used with permission.

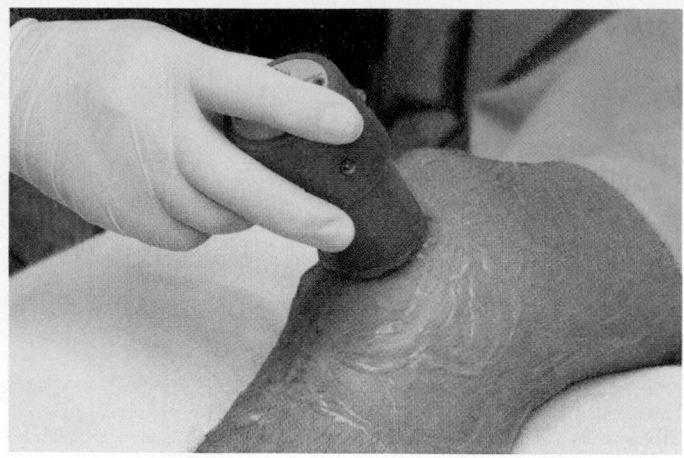

A

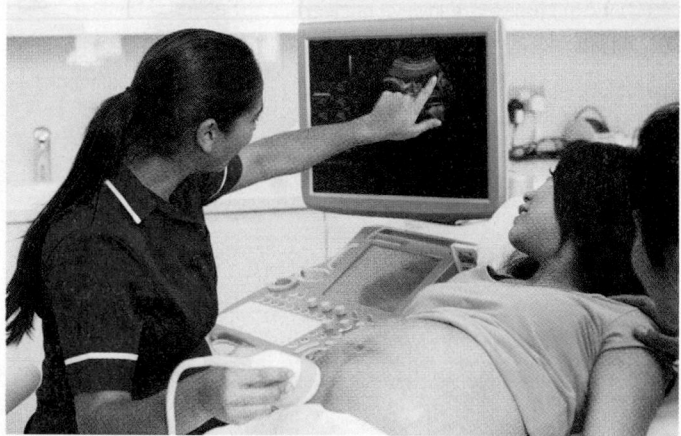

B

Figure 58-4 ■ (A) Ultrasound Therapy (Ultrasonography) Uses Sound Waves to Stimulate Tissue. *Source: Shutterstock © Praisaeng.* (B) Ultrasound Imaging Uses Sound Waves to Create an Image. *Source: Shutterstock © Monkey Business Images.*

- Character 6, Qualifier, and Character 7, Qualifier, have only one value, None (Z), which should be assigned in both positions for all codes.

Radiation Therapy (Section D) Modalities

The Radiation Therapy (D) Section contains therapeutic radiology procedures performed for cancer treatment. Character meanings are described below.

- Character 3 is Modality rather than Root Type. Modality definitions are based on standard usage within the specialty (■ TABLE 58-7) and are not provided within the PCS system.

- Character 4, Treatment Site, is the site targeted by the radiation treatment.

- Character 5, Modality Qualifier, further specifies treatment modality, such as the type or dose of radiation. Examples for Beam Radiation (0) are Photons <1 MeV, Photons 1–10 MeV, and so on. Values for Brachytherapy (1) are High Dose Rate and Low Dose Rate.

Table 58-6 ■ **ROOT TYPES IN THE NUCLEAR MEDICINE (C) SECTION**

Value	Description	Definition
1	Planar Nuclear Medicine Imaging	Introduction of radioactive materials into the body for single-plane display of images developed from the capture of radioactive emissions
2	Tomographic (Tomo) Nuclear Medicine Imaging	Introduction of radioactive materials into the body for three-dimensional display of images developed from the capture of radioactive emissions
3	Positron Emission Tomography (PET)	Introduction of radioactive materials into the body for three-dimensional display of images developed from the simultaneous capture, 180 degrees apart, of radioactive emissions
4	Nonimaging Nuclear Medicine Uptake	Introduction of radioactive materials into the body for measurements of organ function, from the detection of radioactive emissions
5	Nonimaging Nuclear Medicine Probe	Introduction of radioactive materials into the body for the study of distribution and fate of certain substances by the detection of radioactive emissions from an external source
6	Nonimaging Nuclear Medicine Assay	Introduction of radioactive materials into the body for the study of body fluids and blood elements by the detection of radioactive emissions
7	Systemic Nuclear Medicine Therapy	Introduction of unsealed radioactive materials into the body for treatment

- Character 6, Isotope, defines the radioactive isotope used, if applicable. This Character is used in Brachytherapy (1). Examples are Cesium 137 and Iridium 192.
- Character 7, Qualifier, has only one value, None (Z), which should be assigned for all codes.

Abstracting for Sections F, G, and H

The remaining PCS Sections classify physical rehabilitation, diagnostic audiology, mental health, and substance abuse. These are discussed next.

Table 58-7 ■ **MODALITIES IN THE RADIATION THERAPY (D) SECTION**

Value	Description	Definition
0	Beam radiation	Aiming radiation beams at a small target area to destroy tissue
1	Brachytherapy	Insertion of radioactive implants directly into body tissue
2	Stereotactic radiosurgery	Delivery of high doses of radiation to a target area with minimal exposure to the surrounding healthy tissue
V	Other radiation	Modalities not identified by other values

Source: © PB Resources, Inc. Used with permission.

Physical Rehabilitation and Diagnostic Audiology (Section F) Root Types

This Section classifies two general types of procedures that are not related: physical rehabilitation and diagnostic audiology. Physical rehabilitation includes physical, occupational, and speech therapy services. Diagnostic audiology includes services to diagnose hearing conditions. Character 2, Section Qualifier, distinguishes between these two types of services. Values for Characters 3 through 7 are dependent on the Character 2 value.

The Character definitions in this Section are distinct from other PCS Sections, as follows:

- Character 2 is Section Qualifier, rather than Body System, and specifies whether the procedure is Rehabilitation (0) or Diagnostic Audiology (1).
- Character 3, Root Type, defines the general type of procedure (■ TABLE 58-8).
- Character 4, Body System and Region, defines the body system and body region combined, where applicable.
- Character 5, Type Qualifier, further specifies the procedure type beyond what is specified in Character 3.
- Character 6, Equipment, specifies the equipment used, if any.
- Character 7, Qualifier, has only one value, None (Z), which should be assigned for all codes.

In this Section, the term **treatment** consists of a wide variety of activities typically associated with rehabilitation, such as swallowing dysfunction exercises, bathing and showering techniques, wound management, and gait training. **Assessments** are procedures to diagnose a condition and are classified into more than 100 tests and methods. The majority of these focus on hearing and speech, but others focus on various aspects of body function and on the patient's quality of life, such as muscle performance, neuromotor development, and reintegration skills.

Character 5 of the Root Type Device Fitting (D) describes the device being fitted, not the method used to fit the device. PCS provides definitions for some devices, located in the definitions appendix of the PCS coding manual, under Section F, Character 5. For example, for the Root Type Vestibular Treatment (C), the Type Qualifier identifies the type of treatment, such as Postural Control (3), Vestibular (0), Perceptual Processing (1), or Visual Motor Integration (2). This Root Type is for use by inpatient rehabilitation facilities only and can include highly customized devices (■ FIGURE 58-5). All other inpatient facilities should assign codes for the Root Operation Immobilization (3) from the Placement (2) Section.

Physician places a cast on the left forearm of an inpatient in a rehabilitation facility.

F0DZ7EZ [Physical rehabilitation and diagnostic audiology, Rehabilitation], Device fitting, None, Static orthosis, Orthosis, None

---

Figure 58-5 ■ Example of Coding the Root Type Device Fitting (3) for a Rehabilitation Facility Patient. *Source:* © PB Resources, Inc. Used with permission.

Table 58-8 ■ **ROOT TYPES IN THE PHYSICAL REHABILITATION AND DIAGNOSTIC AUDIOLOGY (F) SECTION**

Value	Description	Definition
0	Speech Assessment	Measurement of speech and related functions
1	Motor and/or Nerve Function Assessment	Measurement of motor, nerve, and related functions
2	Activities of Daily Living Assessment	Measurement of functional level for activities of daily living
3	Hearing Assessment	Measurement of hearing and related functions
4	Hearing Aid Assessment	Measurement of the appropriateness and/or effectiveness of a hearing device
5	Vestibular Assessment	Measurement of the vestibular system and related functions
6	Speech Treatment	Application of techniques to improve, augment, or compensate for speech and related functional impairment
7	Motor Treatment	Exercise or activities to increase or facilitate motor function
8	Activities of Daily Living Treatment	Exercise or activities to facilitate functional competence for activities of daily living
9	Hearing Treatment	Application of techniques to improve, augment, or compensate for hearing and related functional impairment
B	Hearing Aid Treatment	Application of techniques to improve the communication abilities of individuals with cochlear implant
C	Vestibular Treatment	Application of techniques to improve, augment, or compensate for vestibular and related functional impairment
D	Device Fitting	Fitting of a device designed to facilitate or support achievement of a higher level of function
F	Caregiver Training	Training in activities to support patient's optimal level of function

The Root Type Caregiver Training (F) is divided into 18 different broad subjects taught to help a caregiver provide proper patient care. Character 5, Type Qualifier, identifies the specific type of training. Character 6, Equipment, identifies any equipment used (■ FIGURE 58-6).

The mother of a child with club foot was trained how to apply a solid bar abduction brace.

F0FZFEZ [Physical Rehabilitation and Diagnostic Audiology, Rehabilitation], Caregiver training, None, Application proper use and care of orthoses, Orthoses, None

Figure 58-6 ■ Example of Coding for Caregiver Training. *Source:* © PB Resources, Inc. Used with permission.

Coders must use their knowledge of medical equipment to select the correct value for Character 6, Equipment, because PCS does not provide official definitions. The value can be specific, such as Audiometer (1), or general, such as Assistive, Adaptive, Supportive, or Protective (F). An **orthosis** is an orthopedic appliance or apparatus used to support, align, prevent, or correct deformities or to improve the function of movable parts of the body. A **prosthesis** is an artificial substitute for a missing body part. An assistive, adaptive, supportive, or protective device aids or protects a patient while performing **activities of daily living (ADLs)** (*daily self-care activities such as bathing, dressing, grooming, eating, and leisure*). Examples of such devices are wheelchairs, walkers, bath chairs, and special beds, chairs, and tables.

SUCCESS STEP

The Root Type Motor Treatment includes a wide variety of activities typically associated with physical therapy, such as therapeutic exercise, wheelchair training, and gait training.

Mental Health (Section G) Root Types

Section G Mental Health uses Character 3, Root Type (■ TABLE 58-9), and Character 4, Type Qualifier. Characters 2, 5, 6, and 7 are placeholders only and should be assigned the value None (Z) for all codes.

Substance Abuse Treatment (Section H) Root Types

The Substance Abuse Treatment (H) Section is organized similarly to Mental Health and has seven Root Types (■ TABLE 58-10). The Root Type Detoxification Services (2) does not provide values for Characters 4 through 7. Root Types 3 through 6 use Character 4 for Type Qualifier, which describes the type of counseling provided. Root Types Medication Management (8) and Pharmacotherapy (9) use Character 4 to identify the medication. The Root Type Medication Management appears both in this Section with the value **8** and in the Mental Health (G) Section with the value **3** and a different definition.

Guided Example of Abstracting for Ancillary Procedures

Refer to the following example throughout this chapter to practice skills for abstracting, assigning, and arranging codes for Ancillary Procedures. The Guided Example uses two Root Types from the Ancillary Sections and one Root Operation from the Medical and Surgical Section (0). The principles discussed here also apply to other Ancillary Root Types.

INPATIENT HOSPITAL   Gender: M   Age: 84

Reason for admission: hip pain and inability to bear weight following fall on the stairs in her single-family home

Procedures performed: X-ray of the acetabulofemoral joint with low osmolar contrast medium, total left hip arthroplasty with an uncemented metal on polyethylene prosthesis, gait training with walker

Discharge diagnosis: fractured left hip at the base of the femoral neck

Table 58-9 ■ ROOT TYPES IN THE MENTAL HEALTH (G) SECTION

Value	Description	Definition
1	Psychological Tests	The administration and interpretation of standardized psychological tests and measurement instruments for the assessment of psychological function
2	Crisis Intervention	Treatment of a traumatized, acutely disturbed or distressed individual for the purpose of short-term stabilization
3	Medication Management	Monitoring and adjusting the use of medications for the treatment of a mental health disorder
5	Individual Psychotherapy	Treatment of an individual with a mental health disorder by behavioral, cognitive, psychoanalytic, psychodynamic, or psychophysiological means to improve functioning or well-being
6	Counseling	The application of psychological methods to treat an individual with normal developmental issues and psychological problems in order to increase function, improve well-being, alleviate distress, address maladjustment, or resolve crises
7	Family Psychotherapy	Treatment that includes one or more family members of an individual with a mental health disorder by behavioral, cognitive, psychoanalytic, psychodynamic, or psychophysiological means to improve functioning or well-being
B	Electroconvulsive Therapy	The application of controlled electrical voltages to treat a mental health disorder
C	Biofeedback	Provision of information from the monitoring and regulating of physiological processes in conjunction with cognitive-behavioral techniques to improve patient functioning or well-being
F	Hypnosis	Induction of a state of heightened suggestibility by auditory, visual, and tactile techniques to elicit an emotional or behavioral response
G	Narcosynthesis	Administration of intravenous barbiturates in order to release suppressed or repressed thoughts
H	Group Therapy	Treatment of two or more individuals with a mental health disorder by behavioral, cognitive, psychoanalytic, psychodynamic, or psychophysiological means to improve functioning or well-being
J	Light Therapy	Application of specialized light treatments to improve functioning or well-being

Table 58-10 ■ ROOT TYPES IN THE SUBSTANCE ABUSE TREATMENT (H) SECTION

Value	Description	Definition
2	Detoxification Services	Detoxification from alcohol and/or drugs
3	Individual Counseling	The application of psychological methods to treat an individual with addictive behavior
4	Group Counseling	The application of psychological methods to treat two or more individuals with addictive behavior
5	Individual Psychotherapy	Treatment of an individual with addictive behavior by behavioral, cognitive, psychoanalytic, psychodynamic, or psychophysiological means
6	Family Counseling	The application of psychological methods that includes one or more family members to treat an individual with addictive behavior
8	Medication Management	Monitoring and adjusting the use of replacement medications for the treatment of addiction
9	Pharmacotherapy	The use of replacement medications for the treatment of addiction

Follow along as fictitious coder, Marcy Elwood, CCS, abstracts the procedure. Check off each step after you complete it.

▶ Marcy reads through the entire record, paying special attention to the reason for the admission, the procedures performed, and the final diagnosis.

❑ She notes the reason for admission: hip pain and inability to bear weight following fall on the stairs in her single-family home.

❑ She also notes the discharge diagnosis: fractured left hip at the base of the femoral neck.

❑ *What services were provided during the inpatient stay?*
- X-ray of the acetabulofemoral joint
- total left hip arthroplasty
- gait training with walker

▶ First, Marcy abstracts for the surgical procedure, total left hip arthroplasty. She refers to Table 51-1 Key Criteria for Abstracting Medical and Surgical Procedures.

❑ *What organ or body part is involved?* left hip

❑ *Did the procedure involve an external device left in place in, on, or in replacement of a body part?* Yes. The abstracting table refers the coder to the Root Operations Change (2), Insertion (H), Removal (P), Replacement (R), Revision (W), and Supplement (U).

❑ To abstract the correct Root Operation, Marcy refers to Table 56-11 Key Criteria for Abstracting Root Operations That Always Take Out a Device.

- She reviews the abstracting questions and answers *Yes* to one question:
  - *Was a device put in to replace a Body Part?* Refer to the Root Operation Replacement (R).

▶ Next, Marcy abstracts for X-ray of the acetabulofemoral joint. She refers to the Key Criteria for Abstracting Ancillary Procedures (Table 58-4).

- ❑ *What is the stated procedure?* X-ray
- ❑ *What body region or body part is involved?* acetabulo-femoral joint
- ❑ *What method is used?* low osmolar contrast medium
- ❑ She reviews the abstracting questions and answers *Yes* to one question:
  - *Does the procedure involve imaging/radiography?* Refer to the Imaging (B) Section.
- ❑ Marcy reviews the Root Types for the Imaging Section and selects the one definition that describes the procedure:
  - Plain Radiography (0): Planar display of an image developed from the capture of external ionizing radiation on photographic or photoconductive plate.

▶ Next, Marcy abstracts for gait training with walker. She again refers to Table 58-4.

- ❑ *What is the stated procedure?* Gait training
- ❑ *What equipment is used?* walker
- ❑ She reviews the abstracting questions and answers *Yes* to one question:
  - *Does the procedure involve physical rehabilitation or diagnostic audiology?* Refer to the Section Physical Rehabilitation and Diagnostic Audiology (F).
- ❑ Marcy reviews the Root Types for the Physical Rehabilitation and Diagnostic Audiology Section and selects the one definition that describes the procedure:
  - Motor Treatment (7): Exercise or activities to increase or facilitate motor function.

▶ At this time, Marcy anticipates that she will need three codes, one for each service. She believes that she will use the Root Operation Replacement for the hip arthroplasty, the Root Type Plain Radiography for the X-ray, and the Root Type Motor Training for the gait training. She will verify this information when she refers to the PCS Tables to assign codes.

CODING PRACTICE

Exercise 58.2 Abstracting for Ancillary Procedures

Instructions: Read the mini-medical-record of each patient's encounter and answer the abstracting questions. Write the answer on the line provided. Do not assign any codes.

---

1. INPATIENT HOSPITAL   Gender: M   Age: 57

Preprocedure diagnosis: cirrhosis, rule out hepatocellular carcinoma

Procedure: CT scan of liver with and without contrast (high osmolar)

Findings: enlarged liver as expected but no tumors identified

a. What is the stated procedure? _____

b. What body region or body part is involved? _____

c. What method is used? _____

d. Was more than one procedure, or a combined procedure, performed? _____

e. Does the procedure involve imaging/radiography? _____

f. Does the procedure involve nuclear medicine? _____

g. Does the procedure involve radiation treatment for a malignancy? _____

(continued)

---

1. (continued)

h. Does the procedure involve physical rehabilitation or diagnostic audiology? _____

i. Are mental health services provided? _____

j. Is substance abuse treatment provided? _____

k. What PCS Section should be used? _____

l. Review the Root Types in the Section selected. What is the most likely Root Type? _____

---

2. INPATIENT HOSPITAL   Gender: M   Age: 61

Preprocedure diagnosis: prostate cancer

Procedure: low dose rate (LDR) brachytherapy of prostate using Iridium 192

a. What is the stated procedure? _____

b. What body region or body part is involved? _____

c. What method is used? _____

d. Was more than one procedure, or a combined procedure, performed? _____

e. Does the procedure involve imaging/radiography? _____

(continued)

2. (continued)

f. Does the procedure involve nuclear medicine? _____

g. Does the procedure involve radiation treatment for a malignancy? _____

h. Does the procedure involve physical rehabilitation or diagnostic audiology? _____

i. Are mental health services provided? _____

j. Is substance abuse treatment provided? _____

k. What PCS Section should be used? _____

l. Review the Root Types or Modalities in the Section selected. What is the most likely Root Type or Modality? _____

---

3. INPATIENT HOSPITAL   Gender: F   Age: 81

Preprocedure diagnosis: *status post–hip replacement, left hip*

Procedure: *range of motion and joint mobility exercises for the left hip with walker*

a. What is the stated procedure? _____

b. What body region or body part is involved? _____

c. What method or equipment is used? _____

d. Was more than one procedure, or a combined procedure, performed? _____

e. Does the procedure involve imaging/radiography? _____

f. Does the procedure involve nuclear medicine? _____

g. Does the procedure involve radiation treatment for a malignancy? _____

h. Does the procedure involve physical rehabilitation or diagnostic audiology? _____

i. Are mental health services provided? _____

j. Is substance abuse treatment provided? _____

k. What PCS Section should be used? _____

l. Review the Root Types or Modalities in the Section selected. What is the most likely Root Type or Modality? _____

---

4. INPATIENT HOSPITAL   Gender: M   Age: 18

Preprocedure diagnosis: *injured left leg, multiple sites*

Procedure: *X-ray of left femur, tibia, and fibula, MRI pelvis unenhanced and enhanced with contrast*

(continued)

---

4. (continued)

Postprocedure diagnosis: *fractures of the left femur, tibia, and pelvis*

a. What is the stated procedure? _____

b. What body region or body part is involved? _____

c. What method is used? _____

d. Was more than one procedure, or a combined procedure, performed? _____

e. Does the procedure involve imaging/radiography? _____

f. Does the procedure involve nuclear medicine? _____

g. Does the procedure involve radiation treatment for a malignancy? _____

h. Does the procedure involve physical rehabilitation or diagnostic audiology? _____

i. Are mental health services provided? _____

j. Is substance abuse treatment provided? _____

k. What PCS Section should be used? _____

l. Review the Root Types in the Section selected. What is the most likely Root Type? _____

---

5. INPATIENT HOSPITAL   Gender: M   Age: 47

Preprocedure diagnosis: *peripheral artery disease*

Procedure: *intraoperative percutaneous transluminal angioplasty (PTA) of left common femoral artery with laser fluoroscopic guidance, low osmolar contrast. Placed an intraluminal drug-eluting stent.*

a. What is the stated procedure? _____

b. What body region or body part is involved? _____

c. What method is used? _____

d. Was more than one procedure, or a combined procedure, performed? _____

e. Does the procedure involve imaging/radiography? _____

f. Does the procedure involve nuclear medicine? _____

g. Does the procedure involve radiation treatment for a malignancy? _____

h. Does the procedure involve physical rehabilitation or diagnostic audiology? _____

i. Are mental health services provided? _____

j. Is substance abuse treatment provided? _____

k. What PCS Section(s) should be used? _____

l. Review the Root Operation(s) and Root Type(s) in the Section(s) selected. What are the most likely Root Operation(s) and Root Type(s)? _____

(continued)

6. INPATIENT HOSPITAL Gender: M Age: 47

Preprocedure diagnosis: angina pectoris

Procedure: cardiac stress test to measure total activity, single measurement, followed by ECC of the right and left heart

a. What is the stated procedure? _____

b. What body region or body part is involved? _____

c. What method is used? _____

d. Was more than one procedure, or a combined procedure, performed? _____

e. Does the procedure involve imaging/radiography? _____

(continued)

6. (continued)

f. Does the procedure involve nuclear medicine? _____

g. Does the procedure involve radiation treatment for a malignancy? _____

h. Does the procedure involve physical rehabilitation or diagnostic audiology? _____

i. Are mental health services provided? _____

j. Is substance abuse treatment provided? _____

k. What PCS Section(s) should be used? _____

l. Review the Root Operation(s) and Root Type(s) in the Section selected. What is the most likely Root Operation(s) and Root Type(s)? _____

ASSIGNING CHARACTERS 4–7 FOR ANCILLARY PROCEDURES

To assign codes after the Root Type is determined, search the PCS Index for the name of the Root Type as the Main Term. Locate the subterm(s) for the correct anatomic site and identify the PCS Table. For many Ancillary procedures, the Root Type is also the common name of the procedure, such as **Fluoroscopy**, or a slight variation of the common name, such as speech therapy, which is classified under the Root Type and Main Term **Speech Treatment**. Other times, the Index lists an instruction that cross-references you to one or more possible Root Types. If you have difficulty locating a code using one Main Term or method, try a different one.

When you locate the PCS Table, verify the first three characters of the code, then locate the row with the Body Part needed. Assign the remaining characters from each respective column of the Table.

Each Section of Ancillary procedures introduces characters and definitions unique to its procedures that were discussed earlier in this chapter. When a particular character is not used for a specific purpose, it is labeled as a Qualifier with the default value **Z None**. All codes must contain seven characters. Refer to the PCS coding manual appendix "Type and Type Qualifier Definitions, Sections B–H" for detailed definitions used in these Sections.

SUCCESS STEP

X-ray procedures are coded to the Root Type Plain Radiography. The Index entry for **X-ray** provides an instructional note that cross-references you to the Main Term **Plain Radiography**.

Guided Example of Assigning Characters 4–7 for Ancillary Procedures

To practice skills for assigning codes for Ancillary procedures, continue with the example from earlier in the chapter about the patient who was seen for a total hip replacement, with X-ray and gait training. Follow along in your ICD-10-PCS manual as Marcy Elwood, CCS, assigns codes. Check off each step after you complete it.

▶ First, Marcy confirms the services provided and the Root Operations and Root Types she abstracted.

❏ The Root Operation for the total left hip arthroplasty is Replacement (R) in the Medical and Surgical (0) Section.

❏ The Root Type for X-ray of the acetabulofemoral joint is Plain Radiography (0) in the Imaging (B) Section.

❏ The Root Type for gait training is Motor Training (7) in the Physical Rehabilitation and Diagnostic Audiology (F) Section.

▶ Marcy assigns the code for the total hip arthroplasty procedure (■ FIGURE 58-7). Refer to Chapter 56 of this text for more information about assigning codes for the Root Operation Replacement.

❏ **0SRB02A Medical and Surgical, Lower Joints, Replacement, Synthetic Substitute, Metal on Polyethylene, Uncemented**

▶ Marcy assigns the code for X-ray of the acetabulofemoral joint.

❏ She searches the Index for the Main Term for the Root Type **Plain Radiography**.

Section	0	**Medical and Surgical**
Body System	S	**Lower Joints**
Operation	R	**Replacement:** Putting in or on biological or synthetic material that physically takes the place and/or function of all or a portion of a body part

Body Part Character 4	Approach Character 5	Device Character 6	Qualifier Character 7
9 Hip Joint, Right **B** Hip Joint, Left	**0** Open	**1** Synthetic Substitute, Metal **2** Synthetic Substitute, Metal on Polyethylene **3** Synthetic Substitute, Ceramic **4** Synthetic Substitute, Ceramic on Polyethylene **J** Synthetic Substitute	**9** Cemented **A** Uncemented **Z** No Qualifier

Figure 58-7 ■ Assigning Code 0SRB02A. *Source: Annotation © PB Resources, Inc. Used with permission.*

- ❑ She does not locate a subterm for *acetabulofemoral joint* and is unsure whether it should be coded to the hip, the femur, or another value.
  - ▪ She refers to the Body Part Key in the Appendix of the PCS coding manual.
  - ▪ She locates an entry for **acetabulofemoral joint**, which refers her to the PCS Body Part **Hip Joint**.
- ❑ In the Index, she locates the first-level subterm **Hip** under the Main Term **Plain Radiography**.
- ❑ She verifies the laterality in the documentation and locates the second-level subterm **Left**.
- ❑ She sees a third-level subterm **Densitometry**, but this is not the procedure performed, so she does not use it.
- ❑ She identifies the Table **BQ0** and partial code **BQ01**.

▶ Marcy turns to Table **BQ0** to assign the code for the X-ray.

- ❑ She reads the Table title **BQ0, Imaging, Non-Axial Lower Bones, Plain Radiography** and confirms that this accurately describes the Body System and Root Type.
- ❑ Marcy assigns the value for Character 4, Body Part.
  - ▪ She verifies the laterality in the documentation and assigns **1 Hip, Left**.

- ❑ Marcy assigns the value for Character 5, Contrast.
  - ▪ She verifies the type of contrast in the documentation and assigns **1 Low Osmolar**.
- ❑ Marcy assigns the value for Character 6, Qualifier, **Z None**.
- ❑ Marcy assigns the value for Character 7, Qualifier, **Z None**.
- ❑ She reviews the code she has assigned for the X-ray of the acetabulofemoral joint: **BQ011ZZ** (■ FIGURE 58-8)
  - ▪ **BQ011ZZ Imaging, Non-Axial Lower Bones, Plain radiography, Hip left, Low osmolar, None, None**

▶ Marcy searches the Index for the Main Term **Gait Training** for *gait training with walker*.

- ❑ She reads the instructional note with a cross-reference that states *see Motor Treatment, Rehabilitation F07*.

▶ Marcy turns to Table **F07** to assign the code for gait training.

- ❑ She reads the Table title **F07, Physical Rehabilitation and Diagnostic Audiology, Rehabilitation, Motor Treatment** and confirms that this accurately describes the Body System and Root Type.
- ❑ Marcy assigns the value for Character 4, Body System/Region, **Z None**.

Section	B	**Imaging**
Body System	Q	**Non-Axial Lower Bones**
Type	0	**Plain Radiography:** Planar display of an image developed from the capture of external ionizing radiation on photographic or photoconductive plate

Body Part Character 4	Contrast Character 5	Qualifier Character 6	Qualifier Character 7
0 Hip, Right **1** Hip, Left	**0** High Osmolar **1** Low Osmolar **Y** Other Contrast	**Z** None	**Z** None

Figure 58-8 ■ Assigning Code BQ011ZZ. *Source: Annotation © PB Resources, Inc. Used with permission.*

Section	F	Physical Rehabilitation and Diagnostic Audiology
Section Qualifier	0	Rehabilitation
Type	7	Motor Treatment: Exercise or activities to increase or facilitate motor function

Body System/Region Character 4	Type Qualifier Character 5	Equipment Character 6	Qualifier Character 7
Z None	9 Gait Training/Functional Ambulation	C Mechanical D Electrotherapeutic E Orthosis F Assistive, Adaptive, Supportive or Protective G Aerobic Endurance and Conditioning U Prosthesis Y Other Equipment Z None	Z None

Figure 58-9 ■ Assigning Code F07Z9FZ. *Source: Annotation © PB Resources, Inc. Used with permission.*

❑ Marcy assigns the value for Character 5, Type Qualifier.

- She must search through several rows of the Table to locate the entry for gait training and assigns the only value, **9 Gait Training/Functional Ambulation**.

❑ Marcy assigns the value for Character 6, Equipment.

- A walker is assistive equipment, so she assigns **F Assistive, Adaptive, Supportive or Protective**.

❑ Marcy assigns the value for Character 7, Qualifier, **Z None**.

❑ She reviews the code she has assigned for *gait training with walker*: **F07Z9FZ** (■ FIGURE 58-9).

- **F07Z9FZ** Physical Rehabilitation and Diagnostic Audiology, Rehabilitation, Motor treatment, None, Gait training/functional ambulation, Assistive adaptive supportive or protective, None

▶ Marcy reviews all the procedure codes she has assigned for this case.

❑ **0SRB02A** Medical and surgical, Lower joints, Replacement, Synthetic substitute metal on polyethylene, Uncemented

❑ **BQ011ZZ** Imaging, Non-axial lower bones, Plain radiography, Hip left, Low osmolar, None, None

❑ **F07Z9FZ** Physical rehabilitation and diagnostic audiology, rehabilitation, Motor treatment, None, Gait training/functional ambulation, Assistive adaptive supportive or protective, None

▶ Next, Marcy must determine how to sequence the codes.

CODING PRACTICE

Exercise 58.3 Assigning Characters 4–7 for Ancillary Procedures

Instructions: Read the mini-medical-record of each patient's encounter. Review the information abstracted in Exercise 58.2 for questions 1–3. For questions 4–6, abstract the case on your own. Assign PCS codes using the Index and Tables. Write the code(s) on the line provided.

1. INPATIENT HOSPITAL Gender: M Age: 57

Preprocedure diagnosis: *cirrhosis, rule out hepatocellular carcinoma*

Procedure: *CT scan of liver with and without contrast (high osmolar)*

Findings: *enlarged liver as expected but no tumors identified*

1 PCS Code _____

2. INPATIENT HOSPITAL Gender: M Age: 61

Preprocedure diagnosis: *prostate cancer*

Procedure: *low dose rate (LDR) brachytherapy of prostate using Iridium 192*

Tip: Iridium 192 is the isotope used.

1 PCS Code _____

3. INPATIENT HOSPITAL Gender: F Age: 81

Preprocedure diagnosis: *status post–hip replacement, left hip*

Procedure: *range of motion and joint mobility exercises for the left hip with walker*

Tip: A walker is assistive equipment.

1 PCS Code _____

4. INPATIENT HOSPITAL   Gender: M   Age: 26

Preprocedure diagnosis: *severe depression*

Procedure: *electroconvulsive therapy (ECT) bilateral, single seizure, done under general anesthesia*

Tip: The aim of ECT is to induce a therapeutic seizure in which the person loses consciousness and has convulsions lasting for at least 15 seconds.

1 PCS Code _____

---

5. INPATIENT HOSPITAL   Gender: M   Age: 46

Preprocedure diagnosis: *bladder cancer; previously removed the bladder and created an ileal conduit (use of a segment of the ileum to connect the ureters to a stoma on the abdominal wall)*

(continued)

---

5. (continued)

Procedure: *ureteropyelography; injected high osmolar contrast medium through the existing stoma to view the ureters and ileal conduit. Ileal conduit was visualized to be functioning properly.*

1 PCS Code _____

---

6. INPATIENT HOSPITAL   Gender: M   Age: 57

Preprocedure diagnosis: *cirrhosis, r/o hepatocellular carcinoma*

Procedure: *CT scan of pelvis, without contrast and with nonionic low osmolar contrast.*

Postprocedure diagnosis: *enlarged liver as expected but no tumors identified*

Tip: Contrast dye is used to help certain areas show up better.

1 PCS Code _____

ARRANGING CODES FOR ANCILLARY PROCEDURES

Ancillary procedures often are performed in addition to a more definitive procedure while a patient is hospitalized, so they might not qualify as a principal procedure. Be sure to review the documentation carefully to ensure that all services are identified and coded. Failure to code and report ancillary services can result in revenue loss to the hospital.

SUCCESS STEP

When services reported in the Ancillary Sections are performed as standalone outpatient procedures, they are reported with CPT codes because PCS is used only by inpatient facilities.

Guided Example of Arranging Codes for Ancillary Procedures

To practice skills for arranging codes for Ancillary procedures, continue with the example from earlier in the chapter about the patient who was seen for a total hip replacement, with X-ray and gait training. Follow along in your ICD-10-PCS manual as Marcy Elwood, CCS, arranges the codes. Check off each step after you complete it.

▶ First, Marcy confirms the procedures performed:

❑ X-ray of the acetabulofemoral joint

❑ Total left hip arthroplasty

❑ Gait training with walker

▶ Marcy reviews the diagnoses and determines the principal diagnosis. The Uniform Hospital Discharge Data Set (UHDDS) defines the principal diagnosis as "that condition established after study to be chiefly responsible for occasioning the admission of the patient to the hospital for care."

❑ Fractured left hip at the base of the femoral neck

▶ Marcy reviews the procedure codes assigned:

❑ **0SRB02A Medical and surgical, Lower joints, Replacement, Synthetic substitute metal on polyethylene, Uncemented**

❑ **BQ011ZZ Imaging, Non-axial lower bones, Plain radiography, Hip left, Low osmolar, None, None**

❑ **F07Z9FZ Physical rehabilitation and diagnostic audiology, Rehabilitation, Motor treatment, Non, Gait training/functional ambulation, Assistive adaptive supportive or protective, None**

▶ Marcy determines that the principal procedure is the surgical procedure of the hip replacement. The principal diagnosis determines the sequencing order because the principal procedure must be the one most closely related to the principal diagnosis.

▶ Marcy finalizes the procedure codes and sequencing for this case:

(1) **0SRB02A Medical and surgical, Lower joints, Replacement, Synthetic substitute metal on polyethylene, Uncemented**

(2) **BQ011ZZ Imaging, Non-axial lower bones, Plain radiography, Hip left, Low osmolar, None, None**

(3) **F07Z9FZ Physical rehabilitation and diagnostic audiology, Rehabilitation, Motor treatment, Non, Gait training/functional ambulation, Assistive adaptive supportive or protective, None**

▶ Marcy also assigns and sequences the ICD-10-CM diagnosis codes that support the need for the services.

(1) **S72.045A Displaced fracture of base of neck of left femur, initial encounter for closed fracture**

(2) **W10.9XXA Fall (on) (from) unspecified stairs and steps, initial encounter**

(3) **Y92.019 Unspecified place in single-family (private) house as the place of occurrence of the external cause**

CODING PRACTICE

Exercise 58.4 Arranging Codes for Ancillary Procedures

Instructions: Read the mini-medical-record of each patient's encounter. Review the information abstracted in Exercise 58.2 for questions 1–3. For questions 4–6, abstract the case on your own. Assign PCS codes using the Index and Tables, and arrange the codes in proper sequence. Write the code(s) on the line provided.

---

1. INPATIENT HOSPITAL   Gender: M   Age: 18

Preprocedure diagnosis: injured left leg, multiple sites

Procedure: X-ray of left femur, tibia, and fibula, MRI pelvis unenhanced and enhanced with contrast

Postprocedure diagnosis: fractures of the left femur, tibia, and pelvis

2 PCS Codes _____

---

2. INPATIENT HOSPITAL   Gender: M   Age: 47

Preprocedure diagnosis: peripheral artery disease

Procedure: intraoperative percutaneous transluminal angioplasty (PTA) of left common femoral artery with laser fluoroscopic guidance, low osmolar contrast. Placed an intraluminal drug-eluting stent.

2 PCS Codes _____

---

3. INPATIENT HOSPITAL   Gender: M   Age: 47

Preprocedure diagnosis: angina pectoris

Procedure: cardiac stress test to measure total activity, single measurement, followed by ECC of the right and left heart

2 PCS Codes _____

---

4. INPATIENT HOSPITAL   Gender: F   Age: 68

Preprocedure diagnosis: locally advanced colorectal carcinoma

Procedure: sigmoid colectomy with IORT (intraoperative radiation therapy) of colon, 3 ports. A midline incision was made and the colon wall divided with a stapler. Dissection continued to the distal margin, where the colon was resected. Following removal of the sigmoid colon, a single IORT dose of 20.0 Gy was delivered to the excised tumor area.

2 PCS Codes _____

---

5. INPATIENT HOSPITAL   Gender: M   Age: 46

Preprocedure diagnosis: carotid artery occlusive disease; peripheral vascular disease

Procedure: bilateral internal carotid artery angiogram; right femoral-popliteal angiogram. The right carotid artery showed no significant disease. The intracranial portion of the left carotid artery showed a 40–50% stenosis. Visualization of the right lower extremity femoral and popliteal arteries under fluoroscopic guidance showed no significant disease.

2 PCS Codes _____

---

6. INPATIENT HOSPITAL   Gender: F   Age: 54

Preprocedure diagnosis: alcohol withdrawal and dependence; marital and family conflict due to alcohol dependence

Procedure: group counseling through Alcoholics Anonymous; marital counseling

2 PCS Codes _____

NEW TECHONOLOGY (SECTION X)

Section **X, New Technology**, classifies procedures requested through the Centers for Medicare and Medicaid Services (CMS) new technology application process, as well as new technologies not otherwise classified in PCS. CMS' new technology application process allows hospitals to request add-on payments for new medical services and technologies demonstrated to be inadequately paid under the diagnosis related group (DRG) reimbursement system.

Section X is a separate location in the PCS coding manual for selected new technology procedures. It was implemented in the 2016 coding manual because users did not support adding new technology codes to the other sections of ICD-10-PCS. Section X does not introduce any new coding concepts or unusual guidelines for correct coding.

Codes identify a broad range of new technology procedures including medical and surgical, medical and surgical-related, and ancillary. Examples are infusion of new technology drugs, orbital atherectomy technology used to treat coronary artery disease, and an intraoperative knee replacement sensor used for soft tissue balancing in total knee arthroplasty.

The Section value for New Technology is **X**. The characters of New Technology codes are summarized as follows (■ Table 58-11):

- Character 2: Body System– Character 2 combines the uses of Body System, Body Region, and Physiological System as specified in other PCS Sections, resulting in broader values than elsewhere in the code set. Body Part values can be as general or specific as they need to be to efficiently represent the application of a new technology.

- Character 3: Root Operation–Root Operations use the same values and same definitions as in other PCS Sections.

- Character 4: Body Part–Body Parts use the same values as their closest counterparts in other PCS Sections.

- Character 5: Approach–Approach uses the same values and definitions as in other PCS Sections.

- Character 6: Device/Substance/Technology— Character 6 provides a general description of the key feature of the new technology, such as the name of the drug.

- Character 7: Qualifier—Character 7 identifies the New Technology Group, a value that is updated each year. For example, Section X codes added for the first year have the

Table 58-12 ■ **CODE XW03321 INFUSION OF CEFTAZIDIME VIA PERIPHERAL VENOUS CATHETER**

Character	Name	Value	Description
1	Section	X	New Technology
2	Body System	W	Anatomical Regions
3	Root Operation	0	Introduction
4	Body Part	3	Peripheral Vein
5	Approach	3	Percutaneous
6	Device/Substance/ Technology	2	Ceftazidime-Avibactam Anti-infective
7	Qualifier	1	New Technology Group 1

seventh character value **1, New Technology Group 1**, and the next year that Section X codes are added, they have the seventh character value **2, New Technology Group 2**, and so on. The updating of the seventh character allows the PCS system to reuse values in Characters 3, 4, and 5 as needed and still retain unique codes for each procedure. This process maximizes the flexibility of Section X, allowing it evolve as medical technology evolves and not run out of codes.

New Technology codes can be located in the Index in the following ways:

1. Search for the Main Term **New Technology** and a subterm for the name of the technology, such as **Ceftazidime-Avibactam Anti-infective**.

2. Search for the name of the technology as the Main Term, such as **Ceftazidime-Avibactam Anti-infective**.

3. Search for the Root Operation as the Main Term, such as **Introduction** and a subterm for the technology.

Regardless of the Main Term selected, always identify the Table listed in the Index, then refer to the Table to assign and verify all characters of the code (■ Table 58-12).

PCS OGCR D discusses the use of Section X codes and clarifies that they are standalone codes. When a Section X code fully describes the procedure being done, it is not necessary to report an additional less specific code from another PCS Section.

Table 58-11 ■ **SEVEN CHARACTERS OF NEW TECHNOLOGY PROCEDURES**

1	2	3	4	5	6	7
Section X	Body System	Root Operation	Body Part	Approach	Device/Substance/ Technology	Qualifier

CODING PRACTICE

Exercise 58.5 New Technology (Section X)

Instructions: Read the procedural statement, then use the Index and Tables to assign the PCS procedure code. Write the code on the line provided.

1. Infusion of blinatumomab antineoplastic immunotherapy via central catheter.
   1 ICD-10-PCS Code: _____

2. Monitoring of soft tissue balancing during a total left knee arthroplasty using an intraoperative knee replacement sensor.
   1 ICD-10-PCS Code: _____

3. Use of an orbital atherectomy system to clear a severely calcified lesion in the RCA.
   1 ICD-10-PCS Code: _____

CHAPTER SUMMARY

In this chapter you learned that:

- The Ancillary Sections are Imaging (B), Nuclear Medicine (C), Radiation Therapy (D), Physical Rehabilitation and Diagnostic Audiology (F), Mental Health (G), and Substance Abuse Treatment (H).

- The Section Imaging (B) is creating a visual representation of internal body structures to diagnose conditions and has five Root Types.

- The Section Nuclear Medicine (C) is the introduction of radioactive materials into the body to capture images, diagnose diseases, or treat abnormalities and has seven Root Types.

- The Section Radiation Therapy (D) is the use of radiation to treat malignancies and has four Root Types.

- The Section Physical Rehabilitation and Diagnostic Audiology (F) is procedures and therapy to help patients regain body functions lost due to medical conditions or injury, and to diagnose hearing-related conditions. It has 14 Root Types.

- The Section Mental Health (G) consists of a variety of methods to diagnose and treat psychiatric and mental disorders and has 13 Root Types.

- The Section Substance Abuse Treatment (H) is procedures to treat disorders related to substance abuse and has 8 Root Types.

- The meaning of Characters 4 through 7 varies based on the Section, so it is important to review the Character meanings in each PCS Table Root Types.

- Many Ancillary procedures are not sequenced as the principal procedure because they are performed in addition to a more definitive procedure Root Types.

- Section **X, New Technology**, classifies procedures requested through the Centers for Medicare and Medicaid Services (CMS) new technology application process, as well as new technologies not otherwise classified in PCS.

- PCS does not provide guidelines for any Ancillary procedures.

CONCEPT QUIZ

Take a moment to look back at Ancillary procedures and solidify your skills. Try to answer the questions from memory first, then refer to the discussion in this chapter if you need a little extra help.

Completion

Instructions: Write the term that answers each question based on the information you learned in this chapter. Choose from the list below. Some choices may be used more than once and some choices may not be used at all.

Brachytherapy (1)

Computerized Tomography (2)

Fluoroscopy (1)

Imaging (B)

Magnetic Resonance Imaging (3)

Medication Management (3)

Medication Management (8)

Mental Health (G)

Motor and/or Nerve Function Assessment (1)

Motor Treatment (7)

Narcosynthesis (G)

Nonimaging Nuclear Medicine Uptake (4)

Nuclear Medicine (C)

Pharmacotherapy (9)

Physical Rehabilitation and Diagnostic Audiology (F)

Plain Radiography (0)

Positron Emission Tomography (PET) (3)

Radiation Therapy (D)

Speech Assessment (0)

Speech Treatment (6)

Substance Abuse Treatment (H)

Systemic Nuclear Medicine Therapy (7)

Tomographic Nuclear Medicine Imaging (2)

1. The Root Type _____ from the _____ Section is the introduction of unsealed radioactive materials into the body for treatment.

2. The Root Type _____ from the _____ Section is exercise or activities to increase or facilitate motor function.

3. The Root Type _____ from the _____ Section is the computer-reformatted digital display of multiplanar images developed from the capture of multiple exposures of external ionizing radiation.

4. The Root Type _____ from the _____ Section is the introduction of radioactive materials into the body for three-dimensional display of images developed from the capture of radioactive emissions.

5. The Root Type _____ from the _____ Section is the application of techniques to improve, augment, or compensate for speech and related functional impairment.

6. The Root Type _____ from the _____ Section is the planar display of an image developed from the capture of external ionizing radiation on a photographic or photoconductive plate.

7. The Root Type _____ from the _____ Section is the single plane or biplane real-time display of an image developed from the capture of external ionizing radiation on a fluorescent screen.

8. The Modality _____ from the _____ Section is the insertion of radioactive implants directly into body tissue.

9. The Root Type _____ from the _____ Section is the administration of intravenous barbiturates in order to release suppressed or repressed thoughts.

10. The Root Type _____ from the _____ Section is monitoring and adjusting the use of replacement medications for the treatment of addiction.

Multiple Choice

Instructions: Circle the letter of the best answer to each question based on the information you learned in this chapter.

1. What type of service is classified in the Nuclear Medicine (C) Section?
   A. Functional imaging
   B. Planar imaging
   C. Anatomic imaging
   D. Radioactive implant imaging

2. What is the value Cesium 137 an example of?
   A. Modality
   B. Modality Qualifier
   C. Isotope
   D. Radionuclide

3. Where are definitions of Ancillary Root Type and Type Qualifier definitions located?
   A. PCS OGCR
   B. PCS Tables
   C. PCS coding manual appendix
   D. PCS coding manual introduction

4. Which character in Section F identifies whether the procedure is Rehabilitation or Diagnostic Audiology?
   A. Character 2, Section Qualifier
   B. Character 3, Root Type
   C. Character 4, Body System
   D. Character 5, Qualifier

5. What information is identified by Character 5 in the Imaging (B) Section?
   A. Isotope
   B. Contrast
   C. Approach
   D. Type Qualifier

6. What is an orthopedic appliance or apparatus used to support, align, prevent, or correct deformities or to improve the function of movable parts of the body?
   A. Orthopedic
   B. Arthrodesis
   C. Prosthesis
   D. Orthosis

7. What PCS Body Part is the acetabulofemoral joint coded to?
   A. Femur
   B. Hip
   C. Pelvis
   D. Acetabulum

8. What Character 6 Qualifier value identifies an image taken without contrast followed by one with contrast in the Imaging (B) Section?
   A. Contrast
   B. Both
   C. With and Without
   D. Unenhanced and Enhanced

9. What Character in the Nuclear Medicine (C) section identifies the radiation source used in the procedure?
   A. Character 4, Source
   B. Character 5, Radionuclide
   C. Character 6, Isotope
   D. Character 7, Qualifier

10. Which Section classifies ultrasound therapy provided to a patient?
    A. Imaging (B)
    B. Nuclear Medicine (C)
    C. Administration (3)
    D. Physical Rehabilitation and Diagnostic Audiology (F)

CODING CHALLENGE

Instructions: Read the mini-medical-record of each patient's encounter, then abstract, assign, and arrange ICD-10-CM diagnosis codes and PCS procedure codes using the appropriate Index and Tables. Write the code(s) on the line provided.

1. INPATIENT HOSPITAL   Gender: F   Age: 4 weeks

Diagnosis: congenital biliary atresia

Procedure: cholangiogram and laparoscopic cholecystojejunostomy. Infant was admitted with obstructive jaundice due to biliary atresia. A cholangiocatheter was threaded to the gallbladder, bile ducts, and pancreatic ducts. Low osmolar contrast was injected and fluoroscopic images obtained. After that, a hepatobiliary-pancreatic bypass was performed and anastomosis of the gallbladder and jejunum was performed.

1 ICD-10-CM Code _____

2 ICD-10-PCS Codes _____

2. INPATIENT HOSPITAL   Gender: F   Age: 18

Preprocedure diagnosis: AAA

Procedure: EVAR (endovascular aneurysm repair) with synthetic graft. Made incision into femoral artery. With low osmolar fluoroscopic guidance, guided delivery catheter with compressed graft into abdominal aorta to site of aneurysm. Inflated balloon to expand graft and affix it to vessel wall. Withdrew catheter and closed incision.

Tip: You previously coded the repair and the graft. Now code the entire procedure, including the fluoroscopy.

1 ICD-10-CM Code _____

2 ICD-10-PCS Codes _____

3. INPATIENT HOSPITAL   Gender: M   Age: 52

Diagnosis: Unabated angina; left ventricular failure

Procedure: PET scan of myocardium using Fluorine 18 to assess myocardial viability and patient's capacity for a revascularization procedure.

Findings: Viable heart muscle. Schedule transmyocardial revascularization (TMR) using laser to produce channels directly into the heart muscle.

1 ICD-10-CM Code _____

1 ICD-10-PCS Code _____

4. INPATIENT HOSPITAL   Gender: F   Age: 48

Diagnosis: pancreatic cancer with liver metastases

Procedure: photon beam radiation >10 MeV treatment of pancreas and heavy-particle radiation treatment of liver

Tip: "10 MeV" describes the strength of the radiation.

2 ICD-10-CM Codes _____

2 ICD-10-PCS Codes _____

5. INPATIENT HOSPITAL   Gender: M   Age: 25

Diagnosis: patient found running naked down the street in the night. Previously diagnosed with bipolar personality disorder. Parents report that he recently stopped his meds because he "felt cured."

Procedure: crisis intervention. Placed on 72-hour hold, lithium (gluconate) resumed plus antipsychotic meds.

Plan: begin psychotherapy and medication regimen to stabilize patient. Family session scheduled to discuss OP tx plan and medication review.

Tip: Assign external cause codes for stopping the medications using the Table of Drugs and Chemicals.

3 ICD-10-CM Codes _____

_____

1 ICD-10-PCS Code _____

6. INPATIENT HOSPITAL   Gender: M   Age: 57

Diagnosis: alcohol addiction with delirium tremens

Procedure: Antabuse therapy

Plan: continue detox with a stimulus-free environment, liver function tests. Admit to inpatient alcohol rehab.

1 ICD-10-CM Code _____

1 ICD-10-PCS Code _____

7. INPATIENT HOSPITAL   Gender: F   Age: 35

Reason for encounter: multigravida with twin gestation of 16 weeks, 2 days; spotting

Procedure: fetal ultrasound, twin gestation

Findings: fetal movement recorded, fetus A: 12 oz, fetus B: 11.5 oz, cardiac heart rate noted. Mother on bed rest; monitor cervix with vaginal ultrasound.

4 ICD-10-CM Codes _____

_____

1 ICD-10-PCS Code _____

8. INPATIENT HOSPITAL   Gender: F Age: 32

Diagnosis: traumatic brain injury, cervical musculoskeletal strain

Procedure: neuromuscular reeducation including therapeutic conditioning exercise to improve range of motion, strength, and coordination; home management

Plan: patient did not reach goal because he has been admitted to inpatient rehabilitation

2 ICD-10-CM Codes _____

2 ICD-10-PCS Codes _____

9. INPATIENT HOSPITAL   Gender: M   Age: 59

Diagnosis: atrial fibrillation, persistent, with rapid ventricular rate

Procedure: transesophageal echocardiogram (TEE) and direct current cardioversion. Transesophageal probe was placed in the esophagus, and views of the right and left heart were then obtained. Following this, direct current cardioversion performed. Unsuccessful conversion to sinus rhythm; remained in atrial fibrillation.

Findings: preserved left ventricular systolic function; dilated left atrium; moderate mitral regurgitation; aortic valve sclerosis with mild to moderate aortic insufficiency; left atrial appendage is free of clots.

2 ICD-10-CM Codes _____

2 ICD-10-PCS Codes _____

10. INPATIENT HOSPITAL   Gender: F Age: 76

Diagnosis: dementia of Alzheimer type with primary parietooccipital involvement

Procedure: MRI brain showed mild generalized atrophy, more severe in the occipital-parietal regions. An FDG-PET scan revealed decreased uptake in the right posterior temporal-parietal and lateral occipital regions.

Findings: unchanged from MRI and PET scan 12 months ago

Tip: Fluorodeoxyglucose (FDG) is the most commonly used radioactive drug (tracer) used in PET scanning.

2 ICD-10-CM Codes _____

2 ICD-10-PCS Codes _____

KEEP ON CODING

Instructions: Read the procedural statement, then use the appropriate Index and Tables to assign PCS procedure codes. Write the code(s) on the line provided.

1. Magnetic resonance imaging (MRI) of the brain without contrast: ICD-10-PCS Code(s) _____

2. Whole-body positron emission tomography (PET) scan of heart: ICD-10-PCS Code(s) _____

3. Stereotactic radiosurgery of the prostate using gamma beam: ICD-10-PCS Code(s) _____

4. Fitting of left prosthetic leg: ICD-10-PCS Code(s) _____

5. Biofeedback: ICD-10-PCS Code(s) _____

6. Ultrasound of the gallbladder: ICD-10-PCS Code(s) _____

7. Alcohol detoxification: ICD-10-PCS Code(s) _____

8. Fluoroscopic imaging of right internal mammary bypass graft, low osmolar: ICD-10-PCS Code(s) _____

9. Individual interpersonal mental health services: ICD-10-PCS Code(s) _____

10. Hearing screening assessment in a sound booth: ICD-10-PCS Code(s) _____

11. Individual interactive mental health psychotherapy services: ICD-10-PCS Code(s) _____

(*continued*)

(continued from page 1177)

12. Methadone maintenance for heroin addiction: ICD-10-PCS Code(s) _____

13. Technetium 99m myocardial nuclear imaging: ICD-10-PCS Code(s) _____

14. Intraoperative 6-MeV photonic beam radiation of the thymus: ICD-10-PCS Code(s) _____

15. Mobility training using a wheelchair: ICD-10-PCS Code(s) _____

16. Technetium 99m nuclear imaging of the thyroid gland: ICD-10-PCS Code(s) _____

17. Electroconvulsive therapy (ECT), bilateral-multiple seizures: ICD-10-PCS Code(s) _____

18. Group 12-step substance abuse counseling: ICD-10-PCS Code(s) _____

19. Annual hearing screening of a commercial airline pilot: ICD-10-PCS Code(s) _____

20. Chest wall radiation therapy, 8 MeV: ICD-10-PCS Code(s) _____

21. Positron emission tomographic (PET) imaging of myocardium using Fluorine 18: ICD-10-PCS Code(s) _____

22. High-dose Cesium 137 brachytherapy of the bladder: ICD-10-PCS Code(s) _____

23. Electrophysiologic motor function test of facial nerves: ICD-10-PCS Code(s) _____

24. Clonidine management for substance abuse: ICD-10-PCS Code(s) _____

25. Light therapy: ICD-10-PCS Code(s) _____

Glossary

The glossary provides definition for key terms, supplemental terms, terms defined in tables, and abbreviations. The number in brackets [ ] indicates the chapter in which the term is introduced.

3-D ultrasound taking and combining multiple two-dimensional scans using specialized computer software to form three-dimensional images [47]

837I electronic billing format for institutions [49]

837P electronic equivalent of the CMS-1500 form; used by physicians to report CPT procedure codes [28]

A

AAPC a professional organization for coders founded in 1988, formerly known as the American Academy of Professional Coders [1]

abdominal hysterectomy surgical incision into the lower portion of the uterus [46]

abnormal finding in which the readings are not within the normal average range established for that particular test [6]

abnormal clinical finding evidence of a disease or condition discovered through physical examination or testing [6]

abnormal development embryonic development of a structure that occurred on schedule but took on an uncommon physical variation or development in the womb [25]

abnormal laboratory test result of a chemistry test, blood test, or biological culture that is outside of (higher or lower than) the normal numerical range, or a microscopic specimen examination that differs from the standard visual features [6]

abortifacient an agent that causes abortion [57]

Abortion (ICD-10-PCS) the Root Operation that identifies artificially terminating a pregnancy [57]

abortion artificially terminating a pregnancy [57]

absence seizure a seizure characterized by muscle twitching or jerking for several seconds [17]

abstract to read the medical record and determine which elements of the encounter require codes [1, 4]

abuse (financial) mistakenly accepting payment for items or services that should not be paid for by Medicare; due to improper coding and billing practices [2]

abuse (personal) physical, emotional, or sexual mistreatment of one person by another [13]

abuse (substance) using a substance in a quantity or frequency that creates legal, employment, social, or family problems, or places the individual at physical risk, without causing physical *dependence* [18]

access location the anatomic site through which the target site for a procedure is reached [52]

accessory organ an organ that assists an organ system carry out its functions but does not fulfill a major function of the system [9]

accessory sinus an air-filled chamber, or space, inside the skull and face bones; also called paranasal sinus [41]

Accredited Standards Committee (ASC) X12N Version 4010 electronic transaction standard used by the healthcare industry before ICD-10-CM/PCS [3]

Accredited Standards Committee (ASC) X12N Version 5010 the revised set of HIPAA transaction standards adopted to replace the current Version 4010 standards [3]

acquired immunodeficiency syndrome (AIDS) a disease caused by the human immunodeficiency virus, which weakens and paralyzes the immune system [21]

actinic keratosis a precancerous lesion [11]

activities of daily living (ADL) daily self-care activities such as bathing, dressing, grooming, eating, and leisure activities [58]

Activities of Daily Living Assessment (ICD-10-PCS) the Root Type that identifies the measurement of functional level for activities of daily living [58]

Activities of Daily Living Treatment (ICD-10-PCS) the Root Type that identifies exercise or activities to facilitate functional competence for activities of daily living [58]

activity describes what a person was doing when an injury occurred, such as running, playing sports, or preparing food [8]

acute exacerbation a sudden increase in the intensity or type of symptoms, such as shortness of breath, wheezing, and chest tightness [16]

acute kidney failure the rapid loss of kidney function over a period of days or weeks [22]

acute myocardial infarction (AMI) a myocardial infarction (heart attack) that occurred within the past four weeks; also called a current myocardial infarction [14]

acute respiratory distress syndrome (ARDS) acute respiratory failure that results in widespread injury to the endothelium in the lung caused by sepsis, massive blood transfusion, aspiration of gastric contents, or pneumonia [16]

acute respiratory failure (ARF) insufficient oxygen passing from the lungs to the blood due to hypercapnia, hypoxemia, or both

acute rhinitis common cold [16]

acute tubular necrosis damage to the renal tubules due to reduced blood flow or toxins in the urine [22]

AD Alzheimer's disease [17]; *auris dexter* (right ear) [44]

addiction a usage pattern that involves compulsive reliance on a substance to the extent that is physically or psychologically difficult to stop, despite the significant problems it creates; also called dependence [18]

additional diagnosis any diagnosis that is not the principal or first-listed diagnosis; also called secondary diagnosis [4]

add-on code a CPT code marked with a + in the CPT manual that must be reported with an additional procedure code [28]

adenocarcinoma cancerous tumor of a gland [5]

adenoma tumor of a gland [5]

adhesiolysis use of a scalpel or electric current to destroy or cut free adhesions [35]

adjacent tissue transfer/rearrangement (ATT/R) transfer of a section of skin or flap from that immediately next to the damaged skin, which can be moved without completely detaching it [37]

adjustment disorder an abnormal difficulty in responding to life changes [18]

adjuvant therapy additional treatments when more than one type of treatment is used [5]

admitting privileges an agreement between a physician and hospital that gives the physician authority to admit a patient to the hospital [1]

adnexa the associated anatomic structures of the eye, which includes the ocular muscles, eyelids, and conjunctiva [19]

adrenalectomy surgical removal of all or most of an adrenal gland(s) [36]

advanced-level job a job obtained after several years of experience that may include management of others or focus on a specialized area of technical expertise [1]

adverse effect a negative physical reaction [8]

aerosol therapy medication suspended in a mist that is inhaled [16]

AHIMA American Health Information Management Association

airway obstruction a reduction in the amount of air inhaled during each breath, most commonly caused by a reduction in the diameter of the bronchioles due to inflammation [16]

alimentary canal a continuous tube, approximately 30 feet long, that begins at the mouth; continues through the esophagus, stomach, small intestine, large intestine; and exits the body at the rectum and anus [9]

allergen immunotherapy treatment that exposes a patient to allergenic extracts or insect venoms to decrease his sensitivity to the allergen, a process called desensitization [32]

allergenic extract a concentration of components from an allergen, such as grass or pollen [32]

allergic rhinitis hay fever [16]

allergy testing a skin or inhalation test to expose a patient to an allergen to determine whether it causes an allergic response [32]

allogeneic from a different person [40]

allograft a skin substitute, where the skin comes from another person [11, 37, 40]

allopathic method of treating disease with remedies such as medicine or surgery that produce effects different from those caused by the disease [57]

allotransplantation receiving an organ from another person [35]

alopecia baldness [11]

Alteration (ICD-10-PCS) the Root Operation that identifies modifying the anatomic structure of a Body Part without affecting the function of the Body Part [51, 56]

alveolus the small air sac where the bronchioles end [16]

Alzheimer's disease (AD) a progressive degenerative brain disease that doubles in prevalence with every five years of age [17]

ambulatory payment classification (APC) groups of CPT codes that describe similar procedures [28]

ambulatory surgery a surgical procedure that does not require an overnight stay in the hospital [1]

amend to add information to [1]

American Health Information Management Association (AHIMA) a professional organization of coders founded in 1928 [1]

AMI acute myocardial infarction [14]

amnesia condition of lack of memory [34]

amniocentesis surgical puncture into the amniotic sac to remove fluid from the amnion [46, 57]

amnioinfusion introducing a substance into the amnion [57]

amnion see *amniotic sac* [23]

amnionitis an infection or inflammation of the amniotic sac [24]

amnioscopy visual examination of the amnion [57]

amniotic sac a membrane that surrounds the embryo; also called the amnion [23]

amniotomy incision into the amnion [57]

A-mode (amplitude) ultrasound a one-dimensional ultrasonic measurement [47]

amyotrophic lateral sclerosis (ALS) a chronic, terminal neurological disease characterized by a progressive loss of motor neurons and muscle atrophy; also called Lou Gehrig disease [17]

analgesia condition of lack of pain [34]

analyte the specific substance within a sample to be examined or tested for [48]

anastomosis a surgical connection between two (usually tubular) structures such as the organs in the digestive tract or blood vessels [35]

anatomic imaging captures a static image of an anatomic part [58]

ancillary provided in addition to medical care, such as laboratory, radiology, or physical therapy services [1]

ancillary reports narrative reports or copies of reports from additional services such as ECGs or imaging [2]

anemia a blood disorder characterized by a reduction in the number of red blood cells, which results in less oxygen reaching the tissues [15]

anencephaly lack of part of the brain [25]

anesthesia a temporary state, induced by drugs, of unconsciousness, loss of memory, lack of pain, and/or muscle relaxation [34]

anesthesia code package a group of services represented in an anesthesia code that includes preoperative visits, administration of anesthesia, intraoperative monitoring [34]

anesthesia conversion factor a dollar value, adjusted for geographic differences in cost, that Medicare (and other payers) assigns to one base unit of anesthesia [34]

anesthesia time the elapsed time that begins when the anesthesia provider starts to prepare the patient for the induction of anesthesia and ends when the anesthesia provider is no longer in personal attendance and the patient can be safely placed under postoperative supervision [34]

anesthesiologist a physician who specializes in providing perioperative care, developing anesthesia plans, and administrating anesthetics [34]

aneurysm a bulge in the wall of an artery due to weakening, most commonly occurring in the abdominal aorta and cerebral arteries [14]

angina intense pain and spasms [14]

angiogram a recording of the heart vessels [14]

angiography an X-ray taken after an opaque dye is injected into a blood vessel [14]

angioplasty insertion into a blood vessel of an inflatable catheter that expands to compress plaque against the walls of the vessel [14, 54]

annulus fibrosus a fibrocartilaginous ring that comprises the outside of a disc and holds the nucleus pulposus in place [42]

anomaly a permanent abnormal shape of an organ or body region, resulting from arrested,

delayed, or abnormal development of the embryo; also called a malformation [25]

antegrade the normal or forward direction of flow [45]

antenatal see *prenatal* [23]

antepartum see *prenatal* [23]

anterior cruciate ligament (ACL) reconstruction replacement of the ACL with a graft [38]

anteroposterior from front to back [47]

antibody a protein in the blood that creates an immune response against an antigen or other invader [48]

antigen any natural or artificial substance that produces an immune response [32]

antrectomy a procedure in which the distal portion of the stomach is excised [35]

anxiety disorder abnormal anxiety that interferes with normal activities [18]

aorta the first artery leading out of the heart to the body, which then repeatedly subdivides into smaller arteries that lead to each body region and anatomic site [14]

aortic coarctation a narrowing of the aorta [25]

aortic valve the valve that controls blood flow from the left ventricle to the aorta [14]

APC ambulatory payment classification [28]

Apgar score an evaluation of a newborn's physical condition that is performed 1 and 5 minutes after birth to determine any immediate need for extra medical or emergency care [24]

aphagia lack of ability to swallow [42]

aphasia lack of ability to speak [42]

aplastic anemia anemia due to loss of or lack of production of red bone marrow [15]

appendectomy surgical removal of the appendix [35]

appendicitis inflammation and possible rupture of the appendix [9]

appendicular skeleton the part of the skeleton consisting of the arms, shoulders, wrists, hands, legs, hips, ankles, and feet; contains 126 bones [12]

Appendix A (CPT manual) an appendix of the CPT manual that provides a full definition of all modifiers [30]

Approach (ICD-10-PCS) Character 5 in an ICD-10-PCS code; defines the surgical technique used to reach the procedure site [49]

approach procedure (skull base) a procedure performed to access or expose a lesion [42]

appropriate for gestational age (AGA) a fetus or newborn infant whose size is within the normal range for his or her gestational age [24]

approximate mapping refers to when codes in both code sets (ICD-9-CM and ICD-10-CM) are similar but not exactly the same [27]

apraxia the inability to perform motor tasks [42]

ARDS acute respiratory distress syndrome [16]

area measurement the space inside a boundary; used to classify the amount of skin treated in a tissue repair or skin graft [37]

ARF acute respiratory failure [16]

arrange to place codes in the order dictated by the OGCR and instructional notes [1, 4]

arrested development embryonic development of a structure that stopped before it should have [25]

arrhythmia an irregular heartbeat [14]

arteriole a small artery [14]

arteriosclerotic heart disease (ASHD) the formation of plaque in the coronary arteries; also called ischemic heart disease and coronary heart disease (CHD) [14]

arteriotomy an incision into an artery [39]

arteriovenous (AV) fistula creation creation of a connection between an artery and a vein [39]

arteriovenous (AV) fistula repair closure of an abnormal connection between two vessels [39]

arteriovenous malformation (AVM) an abnormal connection between arteries and veins, usually congenital [42]

artery any blood vessel that carries blood from the heart to the body tissues [14]

arthralgia a pain in a joint [12]

arthrectomy surgical excision of a joint [38]

arthritis damage to or inflammation of a joint [12]

arthrocentesis aspiration of a small joint or bursa, or collection of synovial fluid from a joint with a needle [38]

arthrodesis surgical fusion of a joint [38]

arthrogram a record or picture of a joint [47]

arthrography the process of recording a joint [47]

arthrotomy cutting into a joint [38, 39]

AS *auris sinister* (left ear) [44]

ASHD arteriosclerotic heart disease [14]

aspiration of bladder the removal of urine using a needle, a trocar, or a catheter [45]

assessment (ICD-10-PCS Section F) a Physical Rehabilitation and Diagnostic Audiology procedure to diagnose a condition; classified into more than 100 tests and methods [58]

assessment a diagnostic statement; the process of a provider asking questions to arrive at a conclusion [2, 32]

assign to determine codes that accurately describe a patient's condition, reflect the highest level of specificity possible, and contain the correct number of characters for that code [1, 5]

Assistance (ICD-10-PCS) the Root Operation that identifies taking over a portion of a physiological function by extracorporeal means [57]

assistance taking over a portion of a physiological function by extracorporeal means [57]

assisted delivery a delivery of a fetus using mechanical, pharmacologic, or medical assistance [23]

assisted vaginal delivery (AVD) birth of an infant through the vagina, with the use of drugs or techniques to induce labor and/or with forceps or vacuum extraction to aid in moving the infant through the birth canal [46]

asthma a chronic lung disease that affects the bronchi and is characterized by inflammation of the airway, a reversible obstruction, and reshaping of the airway [16]

astrocytoma a tumor of the brain or spinal cord that is composed of astrocytes [24]

asymptomatic having no symptoms [21]

ataxia a lack of coordination [42]

atelectasis the collapse of a lung, preventing the exchange of oxygen and carbon dioxide [16]

atherectomy a procedure in which a catheter that has a rotating shaver on its tip is threaded through the veins to cut away plaque from the artery [39]

Atmospheric control (ICD-10-PCS) the Root Operation that identifies extracorporeal control of atmospheric pressure and composition [57]

atmospheric control extracorporeal control of atmospheric pressure and composition [57]

atonic (seizure) a seizure characterized by a sudden loss of consciousness and falling down; affects the entire brain [17]

atopic asthma due to allergens [16]

atresia lack of an opening to an orifice or passage in the body [25]

atrial fibrillation (A-fib) an irregular heartbeat in the atria characterized by an abnormal quivering of heart fibers [14]

atrioventricular (AV) node an electrical relay station between the atria and the ventricles [14]

atrioventricular (AV) valve a valve that controls the flow of blood from the atria to the ventricles [14]

atrioventricular bundle (bundle of His) a group of cardiac muscle fibers that connect the atria with the ventricles [14]

atrium two of the four chambers of the heart that receive blood from the body and the lungs [14]

ATT/R adjacent tissue transfer/rearrangement [37]

attending physician a physician who oversees and coordinates all aspects of a patient's inpatient care [1]

AU *auris uterque* (each ear) [44]

audit an investigation of a provider's billing and coding practices [2]

auditory canal the part of the external ear that funnels sound waves [20]

aura a sensation of hearing voices or seeing colored light [17]

aural pertaining to the ear [44]

auricle the visible part of the ear, which collects sound waves; also called the pinna [20]

autograft the use of a patient's own tissue from one site to replace damaged tissue at another site [11, 37]

autoimmune a condition in which the body's immune system attacks and destroys healthy body tissue [10]

autologous from the same patient [14, 40]

autologous islet cell transplantation a procedure in which the pancreas is surgically removed and the islet cells are isolated then injected into the portal vein [35]

automatic adjudication a process in which a computer automatically determines which procedure codes are covered, calculates how much the insurance company is obligated to pay, then triggers the payment [2]

autonomic nervous system the system that controls sensory impulses from the blood vessels, the heart, and organs in the chest, abdomen, and pelvis, through nerves, to the brain [14]

AV atrioventricular [14]

AV node atrioventricular node [14]

AV valve atrioventricular valve [14]

AVD assisted vaginal delivery [46]

AVM arteriovenous malformation [42]

avulsed ripped or torn away [53]

avulsion forceful tearing of the nail plate [37]

axial skeleton 80 bones that are basically stationary and make up the skull, sternum, ribs, and vertebrae [12]

B

BAC blood alcohol concentration [18]

bacteria one-celled germs that multiply quickly and may release toxins that create illness [21]

bacterial infection an infection caused by bacteria and treatable with antibiotics [11]

BAL blood alcohol level [18]

balloon catheter a urethral catheter with an inflatable balloon near the tip to hold the catheter in place and/or dilate the urethra [45]

barium enema the injection of a chalky substance into the colon through the anus and viewing the organs on an X-ray; also called a lower GI series [9]

Barlow syndrome an eponym for *mitral valve prolapse (MVP)* [14]

Bartholin's gland a gland that secretes mucus [22]

basal cell carcinoma (BCC) a cancer appearing in the lowest layer of the epidermis; accounts for 75% of new skin cancer cases [11]

base unit (B) a number that represents the complexity of an anesthesia, the risk to a patient, and the skills needed by an anesthesia provider to render services for each CPT Anesthesia code [34]

basilar skull fracture a linear fracture in the anterior or middle skull base or the posterior fossa [42]

BBB blood–brain barrier [17]; bundle branch block [14]

BCC basal cell carcinoma [11]

Beam Radiation (ICD-10-PCS) the Modality that identifies aiming radiation beams at a small target area to destroy tissue [58]

beam radiation aiming radiation beams at a small target area to destroy tissue [58]

behavior (tumor) malignant or benign [5]

behavioral disorder the manifestation of a mental disturbance that results in extreme or disruptive conduct, such as rage, withdrawal, or substance abuse [18]

behavioral disturbance an action that includes aggression, wandering, depression, delusion or hallucinations, sleep disturbances, or poor eating habits [18]

Bell's palsy the inflammation of the seventh (VII) cranial nerve, which is the facial nerve [17]

beneficiary the recipient of services [2]

benign not life-threatening [5]

benign prostatic hypertrophy (BPH) the abnormal growth of epithelial cells of the prostate, causing compression or obstruction of the urethra; also called enlarged prostate (EP) or hyperplasia [22]

Bethesda System a method of reporting findings from Pap tests that includes a statement of adequacy of the specimen; a general categorization of the specimen; a descriptive diagnosis; interpretation of abnormalities using specific nomenclature; and a statement of review and any ancillary testing [48]

Billroth I a procedure in which the pylorus is removed and the proximal stomach is anastomosed directly to the duodenum in an end-to-end manner [35]

Billroth II a procedure in which the greater curvature of the stomach is connected to the first part of the jejunum in a side-to-side manner [35]

bilobectomy the surgical excision of two lobes [41]

Biofeedback (ICD-10-PCS) the Root Type that identifies the provision of information from the monitoring and regulating of physiological processes in conjunction with cognitive-behavioral techniques to improve patient functioning or well-being [58]

biopsy the scraping, punching, or cutting of a piece of skin and examining it under a microscope [11]

birth trauma any physical injury to an infant during delivery [24]

blepharitis the inflammation and infection of hair follicles and glands at the margins of the eyelids, due to virus, bacteria, allergic response, or exposure to irritants [19]

block (ICD-10-CM) a contiguous range of codes within a chapter [4]

block/section (ICD-9-CM) a subset of three-digit categories within a chapter that represents related conditions [26]

blood the bodily fluid that transports and passes nutrients, oxygen, carbon dioxide, water, proteins, and hormones to cells and transports waste products to excrete oxygen; also called the hemic system [15]

blood alcohol concentration (BAC) see *blood alcohol level (BAL)* [18]

blood alcohol content see *blood alcohol level (BAL)* [18]

blood alcohol level (BAL) a measurement of the amount of alcohol present in the blood; also called blood alcohol content or blood alcohol concentration (BAC) [18]

blood–brain barrier (BBB) a naturally occurring barrier of vessels and capillaries that filters blood flowing to the brain and prevents certain toxic substances from infiltrating brain tissue and the central nervous system [17]

blood creatinine a blood test used to determine the amount of creatinine present; an abnormal result suggests renal dysfunction [22]

body the main portion of a muscle [12]

Body Part Character 4 in an ICD-10-PCS code; defines the specific anatomic site where a physician performed a procedure [49]

Body System Character 2 in an ICD-10-PCS code; defines where a procedure is performed [49]

bone marrow connective tissue in the cavities of bones [15, 40]

Brachytherapy (ICD-10-PCS) the Modality that identifies the insertion of radioactive implants directly into body tissue [58]

brachytherapy insertion of radioactive implants directly into body tissue [58]

brackets [ ] (ICD-9-CM) a convention in the Volume 3 Index to indicate that a synchronous procedure should be coded along with the main procedure [26]

bradycardia a slow heart rate [24]

bradypnea slow breathing [24]

brain the organ that governs perception of the senses, emotions, consciousness, memory, and voluntary movements [17]

breast engorgement the temporary enlargement of breasts on female or male newborns, due to high levels of maternal hormones in the infant's blood [24]

bronchial tree the configuration of bronchi subdividing into smaller and smaller branches [16]

bronchiectasis the condition of a dilated bronchus [16]

bronchiole the smallest bronchus in the bronchial tree; does not contain rings of cartilage [16]

bronchiolitis inflammation of a bronchiole [16]

bronchitis inflammation of the bronchus [16]

bronchodilator a medication that relaxes muscle spasms in bronchial tubes [16]

bronchogenic of bronchial origin [16]

bronchogram a record or picture of the bronchus [47]

bronchography the process of recording the bronchus [47]

bronchoscope the instrument used to view the bronchus [16]

bronchospasm a contraction of smooth muscle in the walls of the bronchi and bronchioles, causing narrowing of the lumen [16]

bronchus the air tube that begins at the end of the trachea and leads to the lungs [16]

B-scan/gray-scale (brightness) ultrasound a two-dimensional ultrasonic scan that displays the movement of tissues and organs [47]

bulbourethral gland the gland that provides a mucous secretion before ejaculation, which becomes part of the semen [22]

bulla a blister [11]

bundle branch a division of the bundle of His [14]

bundle branch block (BBB) a blockage of the conduction of electrical impulses through the branches of the atrioventricular bundle [14]

bundling edit a coding restriction frequently triggered by the words *includes* and *not separately reportable* that indicates that multiple services are included in a single code [28]

Burch's procedure an eponym for vesicourethropexy [45]

burn damage to the skin by heat, electricity, or radiation [13]

bursitis the inflammation of fluid around a joint [12]

by report based on a report submitted by a physician [35]

Bypass (ICD-10-PCS) the Root Operation that identifies altering the route of passage of the contents of a tubular Body Part [51, 54]

bypass graft the creation of a new route around a blockage in a blood vessel using a vessel from another part of the body, another person, or a synthetic substitute [14, 39]

C

CA carcinoma, cancer [5]

CA in situ cells that have begun to change but are contained within the epithelial layer [5]

CABG coronary artery bypass graft [14]

CAD computer-aided detection [47]; coronary artery disease [14]

calculi hard balls of cholesterol (fat), also called stones, that may accumulate in the kidneys, bladder, or ureters [9, 22]

Caldwell-Luc procedure an incision through the gum and bone to create an opening to the maxillary sinus [41]

cancer (CA) a malignant tumor of epithelial cells, which line body cavities and organs; synonymous with carcinoma [5]

Candida a yeast fungi [21]

cannulation of thoracic duct the insertion of a tube (cannulation) into the thoracic duct to collect lymph [40]

capillary the very thin-walled membrane at the end of arterioles that allows blood to diffuse into body tissues and receives waste products from the tissues to send back into the bloodstream [14]

capsule endoscopy a technology in which patients swallow a capsule the size of a large pill that contains a video microchip, light bulb, battery, and radio transmitter [35]

capsulectomy cutting into or the surgical excision of a joint capsule [38]

capsulodesis the surgical fusion of a joint capsule [38]

carbuncle a skin infection that involves a group of hair follicles [11]

carcinoid a benign or malignant tumor arising from the mucosa of the gastrointestinal tract [10]

carcinoid syndrome a collection of symptoms caused by carcinoid tumors, characterized by flushing, cyanosis, abdominal cramps, diarrhea, and heart valve disease; see also *carcinoid* [10]

carcinoma (CA) a malignant tumor of epithelial cells, which line body cavities and organs [5]

carcinoma of unknown primary (CUP) a neoplasm diagnosed at a late stage after it has metastasized and for which a physician is unable to determine the site of origin [5]

cardiac catheterization the passage of a thin tube through a blood vessel to the heart to visualize the structure, collect blood samples, and determine the blood pressure of the heart [14]

cardiac function test a measurement of the capacity of the heart in real time; tests include cardiac catheterization, electrocardiography, Holter monitor testing, and stress testing [14]

cardiac scan a scan of the heart after a patient receives radioactive thallium intravenously [14]

cardiac sphincter the valve between the esophagus and the stomach [9]

cardiology lab a testing center used to evaluate heart problems [1]

cardiopulmonary bypass (CPB) a heart–lung machine that takes over the function of the heart and lungs, maintaining the circulation of blood and the oxygen content of the body [39, 57]

cardiovascular (CV) system the body system that distributes blood throughout the body and includes the heart and blood vessels; also called the circulatory system [14]

career path the progression of jobs and responsibilities throughout one's working life [1]

Caregiver Training (ICD-10-PCS) the Root Type that identifies the training in activities to support a patient's optimal level of function [58]

carpal tunnel release cutting of the transverse carpal ligament to release pressure on the median nerve [42]

cartilage the fibrous tissue found at the ends of bones [12]

case production the number of cases a coder codes each day while maintaining high accuracy [1]

case-based a reimbursement amount (rate) determined per case, or per inpatient admission, rather than on a per diem (daily) basis or a fee-for-service basis [49]

cataract a cloudiness of the lens of the eye that usually develops slowly over time due to aging [19]

category (CPT) a subdivision of CPT Category I codes that shows specific methods for completing procedures [28]

category (ICD-10-CM) three characters in length [4]

category (ICD-9-CM) a three-digit number that represents the type of condition [26]

Category I a group of permanent CPT codes, numbered 00100 to 99607, to report widely used services and procedures approved by the FDA [28]

Category II a group of optional CPT codes used to collect and track data for performance measurement [28]

Category III a group of temporary CPT codes for data collection and for tracking the use of emerging technology, services, and procedures [28]

catheter a small, flexible tube inserted through a narrow opening into a body cavity to remove fluid or inject medication [32]

catheter ablation/radiofrequency ablation the use of a fluoroscopy-guided catheter at the exact site of arrhythmia in the heart to emit radiofrequency energy that destroys heart muscle cells in a very small area (about one-fifth of an inch) [39]

catheter procedures the implantation, revision, or repositioning of a tunneled intrathecal or epidural catheter [42]

causal event an event or action that results in an injury [8]

causal relationship one disease being caused by another [10]

cause an event or action that results in an injury [8]

CC chief complaint [2, 31]

CDI clinical documentation improvement [49]

CDM charge-description master [49]

celiac disease an abnormal immune reaction to gluten and poor absorption of nutrients [9]

cell type the characteristics or appearance of a cell [5]

cellulitis inflammation under the skin [11]

Centers for Medicare and Medicaid Services (CMS) the division of the Department of Health and Human Services (HHS) that administers Medicare

central nervous system (CNS) the control center for the nervous system, which processes information and provides short-term control over other organ systems; consists of the brain and spinal cord [17]

cephalic version turning of a fetus so the head is oriented toward the cervix [46]

cephalopelvic disproportion (CPD) a cause of obstructed labor due to a mismatch between the size of the fetal head and the mother's pelvic brim; also called fetopelvic disproportion [23]

cerclage (nonobstetrical) extensive suturing around the cervix to make the opening smaller [46]

cerclage (obstetrical) a closed cervix during pregnancy [46]

cerebellum the portion of the brain located below and behind the cerebrum [17]

cerebral an object located within the brain [14]

cerebral palsy a functional disorder of the brain manifested by motor impairment [17]

cerebrospinal fluid (CSF) shunt the creation, removal, or reprogramming of a shunt and the replacement or irrigation of a catheter that transports fluid from one area of the body to another [42]

cerebrovascular accident (CVA) a sudden decrease in blood supplied to the brain; also called stroke [14]

cerebrum the largest structure of the brain that controls sensory and motor activity [17]

Certificate of Compliance (COC) a certificate issued to a laboratory that performs nonwaived—moderate and high complexity— testing [48]

Certificate of Waiver (COW) a certificate issued to a laboratory that performs only CLIA-waived tests [48]

certification a voluntary achievement that documents that a coder has attained a certain level of proficiency by passing a rigorous examination [1]

certified registered nurse anesthetist (CRNA) a registered nurse with advanced education and training in the field of anesthesia [34]

cerumen the earwax that protects and lubricates the ear [20]

cervical approach the performance of a procedure through an incision in the neck [36]

cervical dilator insertion the transcatheter administration of a substance into the cervix to widen it [46]

cervical dysplasia abnormal changes in the cells on the surface of the cervix that may lead to cancer if not treated [22]

cervical intraepithelial neoplasia (CIN) cervical dysplasia seen on a cervical biopsy, classified as mild dysplasia (CIN I), moderate to marked dysplasia (CIN II), and severe dysplasia to cancer in situ (CIN III) [22]

cervicectomy see *trachelectomy*

cesarean delivery the delivery of a fetus by making a surgical incision into the abdominal wall and uterus; also called abdominal delivery [23, 46]

chalazion a small, hard cyst on the eyelid caused by the blockage of a gland on the eyelid [19]

Change (ICD-10-PCS) the Root Operation that identifies taking out or off a device from a Body Part and putting back an identical or similar device in or on the same Body Part, without cutting or puncturing the skin or a mucous membrane [51, 56]

chapter (ICD-10-CM) a subdivision of ICD-10-CM that includes codes for a body system or related conditions [4]

chapter (ICD-9-CM) a range of three-digit categories that include conditions for the same body system [26]

character one of seven positions in an ICD-10-PCS code with an alphanumeric value; each has a distinct purpose and meaning [49]

charge capture the process of entering nonprocedural services provided throughout a patient's stay [49]

charge description master (CDM) a list of the nonprocedural services provided by a hospital throughout a patient's stay [49]

CHD coronary heart disease [14]

chemocauterization the destruction of tissue using chemicals [43]

chemodenervation the injection of a substance into a muscle group or gland(s) to stop overactivity [42]

chemosurgery the use of a chemical agent to destroy tissue [37]

chemotherapy treatment using drugs [32]

CHF congestive heart failure [14]

chief complaint (CC) a concise statement that describes a patient's symptom(s), problem, condition, diagnosis, or history of present illness [31]

childbirth the period of true labor and active delivery; also called parturition [23]

Children's Health Insurance Program (CHIP) a program established in 1997 by the federal government to provide health insurance to children in families with incomes below 200% of the federal poverty level [2]

chiropractic manipulation the use of direct manual force or an instrument to manipulate the joints of the body, mostly commonly the spine, to restore or enhance joint function; also called chiropractic adjustment [57]

cholecystectomy surgical removal of the gall bladder [35]

cholecystitis inflammation of the gall bladder [9]

choledochocystectomy excision of the common bile duct [35]

choledocholithiasis the condition of calculi in the common bile duct [9]

choledochoplasty repair of the common bile duct [53]

cholelithiasis the condition of calculi in the gall bladder [9]

cholera an acute gastrointestinal disease [44]

chondroplasty the reshaping and cleaning of cartilage in a joint to remove uneven surfaces and fragments [38]

chorion the outer membrane that surrounds the amnion [23]

chorionic villus sampling (CVS) the aspiration of fetal tissue under ultrasonic guidance, using a catheter through the cervix or a needle through the mother's abdominal and uterine walls into the uterine cavity, for genetic analysis [23, 46]

choroid the opaque middle layer of the eyeball that supplies blood to the eye [19]

choroiditis inflammation of the vascular coating of the eye [19]

chromosomal abnormality any of a wide range of disorders in which a fetus has an abnormal number of chromosomes or a structural abnormality in one or more chromosomes [23]

chronic bronchitis an inflammation of the bronchi with a productive cough for three months in two consecutive years [16]

chronic kidney disease (CKD) the gradual loss of kidney function over a period of months or years [22]

chronic obstructive pulmonary disease (COPD) the combination of chronic bronchitis and emphysema as comorbidities [16]

chronic pain syndrome (CPS) a collection of pain conditions lasting more than six months and that are unresponsive to treatment [17]

cineradiography the process of making radiographs of moving objects in rapid sequence and quickly projecting them back to simulate a motion picture; also called videoradiography [47]

circulatory system the body system that distributes blood throughout the body and includes the heart, and blood vessels; also called the cardiovascular (CV) system [14]

circumstances of admission the facts, signs, and symptoms that require an admission [4, 13]

cirrhosis the scarring of liver tissue that blocks the normal flow of blood through the liver [9]

cisternal puncture the withdrawal of CSF from the cisterna magna [42]

CKD chronic kidney disease [22]

clavicle the collar bone [13]

clean claim a claim that passes the front-end edit checks and has no missing or invalid information [2]

cleft lip/cleft palate a notch or division of the upper lip or roof of the mouth [25]

cleft lip/cleft palate repair the procedure in which abnormally oriented and attached muscles are repositioned to repair the functionality of the soft palate musculature [35]

CLIA Clinical Laboratory Improvement Amendments [48]

click murmur syndrome see *mitral valve prolapse (MVP)* [14]

clinical brachytherapy the application of small, encapsulated radioactive elements implanted directly into or near a tumor [47]

clinical documentation improvement (CDI) a program implemented by many hospitals that educates physicians and helps them achieve complete documentation that accurately reflects the care patients receive [49]

Clinical Laboratory Improvement Amendments (CLIA) regulations passed by Congress in 1988 to establish quality standards for all laboratory testing to ensure the accuracy, reliability, and timeliness of patient test results regardless of where the test was performed [48]

clinically significant conditions those conditions defined by the Uniform Hospital Data Discharge set (UHDDS) as "all conditions that coexist at the time of admission, that develop subsequently, or that affect the treatment received and/or the length of stay. Diagnoses that relate to an earlier episode which have no bearing on the current hospital stay are to be excluded." [4]

clitoris a small sensitive protrusion that is part of the female genital system [22]

clitoroplasty a reduction of the size of an enlarged clitoris [46]

clonic (seizure) a type of seizure characterized by a series of muscle contractions and relaxations on both sides of the body [17]

closed (fracture) a type of fracture in which the bone does not break the skin [13]

cluster headache a unilateral pain in the eye or temple [17]

CNS central nervous system [17]

COC Certificate of Compliance [48]

cochlea a snail-shaped organ that makes hearing possible [20]

cochlear device implantation the implantation of a receiver into bone, which sends signals to electrodes implanted in the cochlea [44]

code (ICD-10-CM) the final level of subdivision [4]

code set a distinct system of medical codes [1]

Codes on Dental Procedures and Nomenclature (CDT®) the HIPAA-mandated code set for dental services (occupies section D of the HCPCS codes) [1]

coding path the sequence of Main Terms and subterms a coder must search in the Index in order to locate the code [4]

coding the process of accurately assigning codes to verbal descriptions of patients' conditions and the healthcare services provided to treat those conditions [1]

cognitive disorder a failure to develop or the deterioration of mental comprehension [18]

colectomy the surgical removal of all or a part of the large intestine [35]

colloid a gelatin-like or mucous substance found in tissues [19]

colonoscopy the use of an endoscope to view the colon [35]

colopexy surgical fixation of the colon [53]

colorrhaphy suturing of the colon [46]

colostomy division of the colon, bringing the proximal end out through a stoma in the abdominal wall, bypassing the rectum and anus [35]

colpocentesis the puncturing of the posterior vaginal wall with a needle to withdraw fluid from the peritoneal cul-de-sac [46]

colpopexy/vaginofixation the suturing of the vagina to another structure, such as the abdominal wall [46, 53]

colporrhaphy the suturing of the vagina [46]

colpotomy a procedure creating an incision into the wall of the vagina; may also include draining an abscess [46]

Column 1 NNCI data that contain a list of all payable CPT codes

Column 2 NCCI data that contain the code that is not payable with a particular Column 1 code unless a modifier is permitted and submitted [33]

combination code two or more conditions described by a single code [4]

common bile duct (CBD) exploration the injection of a dye into the duct, visualization on an X-ray, removal of calculi, and introduction of a drainage bag when necessary [35]

common descriptor the shared portion of a code before the semicolon [28]

comorbidity two diseases occurring together [9]

complete mastoidectomy a simple mastoidectomy with more extensive removal of the mastoid process [44]

completeness (ICD-10-PCS) the ICD-10-PCS characteristic whereby there should be a unique code for every procedure that is significantly different in body part, approach, or method [48]

complex partial (seizure) a seizure associated with both sides of the cerebrum; causes a change in or loss of consciousness [17]

complex regional pain syndrome see *reflex sympathetic dystrophy (RSD)* [17]

compliance following the rules [2]

complication an abnormal medical reaction that results from a medical or surgical procedure [8]

complications of care the unanticipated results of a medical or surgical procedure [13]

Compression (ICD-10-PCS) the Root Operation that identifies putting pressure on a body region [57]

computed tomography (CT) the creation of a three-dimensional image of a body structure by computer, using a series of cross-sectional images [47]

computer-aided detection (CAD) the use of pattern recognition software to help identify suspicious features on a radiological image, to decrease false-negative readings [47]

Computerized tomography (CT) scan (ICD-10-PCS) the Root Type that identifies the computer-reformatted digital display of multiplanar images developed from the capture of multiple exposures of external ionizing radiation [58]

computerized tomography (CT) scan the computer-reformatted digital display of multiplanar images developed from the capture of multiple exposures of external ionizing radiation [58]

conception the fertilization of the female ova by the male sperm [23]

concurrent care care that occurs when more than one physician treats a patient at the same time for different conditions or different aspects of the same condition [31]

condom catheter a nonindwelling catheter consisting of a sac that fits over the penis to collect urine and drain it through a tube that leads to a collection bag; is left in place [45]

cone a photoreceptor cell of the retina that is sensitive to bright light and color vision [19]

confirmed a diagnostic statement that the physician is confident of [6]

congenital a condition that appears at birth [10]

congenital abnormality a specific type of perinatal condition that originates during pregnancy or the first 28 days of life [25]

congestive heart failure (CHF) the inability of the heart to maintain circulation [14]

conization of cervix the removal of a cone-shaped piece of tissue from the uterine cervix [46]

conjunctiva the membrane that lines the eyelids [19]

conjunctivectomy excision of the conjunctiva [43]

conjunctivitis a viral or bacterial inflammation and infection of the conjunctiva [19]

conjunctivoplasty repair of the conjunctiva [43, 53]

constant attendance modality a physical therapy treatment that requires constant one-to-one contact with the patient by the provider [32]

consultation an evaluation of a patient requested by another physician to obtain a professional opinion on a specific problem [31]

consulting physician the provider who receives a request from a referring physician to see a patient regarding a specific problem; also called consultant [31]

content of service requirements guidelines that define the work done during the patient encounter; also referred to as key components [31]

contralateral an examination on the opposite side from which catheterization was performed [39]

contralateral lobectomy the excision of part of the opposite or second lobe in addition to a partial, subtotal, or total lobectomy of the first lobe [36]

contrast medium a radiopaque substance that is injected or swallowed [47]

Control (ICD-10-PCS) the Root Operation that identifies stopping, or attempting to stop, postprocedural bleeding [51, 56]

controlled hypotension a technique that lowers the mean arterial blood pressure (MAP) by 30% during surgery, with the goal of reducing intraoperative blood loss and minimizing the risk of fluid overload; also called induced hypotension or hypotensive anesthesia [34]

contusion a bruise [13]

convention the use of symbols, typeface, and layout features to succinctly convey interpretive information [4]

conventional Pap test involves scraping cells from the cervix and fixing them on a slide to be evaluated by a lab [48]

conversion factor a constant dollar value multiplied by the relative value unit to determine the price of individual services [28]

Coordination and Maintenance Committee the group that oversees all changes, which must be consistent with WHO's ICD-10 [4]

COPD chronic obstructive pulmonary disease [16]

cordocentesis the use of ultrasound to detect the umbilical cord and removal of a sample of fetal blood from the cord; also called percutaneous umbilical blood sampling (PUBS) [46]

cornea the clear, hard portion of the sclera that protects the lens [19]

coronary artery bypass graft (CABG) openheart surgery to create a bypass around a blocked coronary artery, usually using the internal mammary artery (IMA) or a vein in the leg [14]

coronary artery disease (CAD) an insufficient blood supply to the heart due to an obstruction of one or more coronary arteries [14]

coronary circulation blood flow that occurs within the heart; carries blood from the aorta to the tissues of the heart to maintain the function of the heart itself [14]

coronary heart disease (CHD) see *arteriosclerotic heart disease (ASHD)* [14]

corrosion damage to the skin due to chemicals [13]

cosmetic relating to aesthetics or appearance [37]

coudé catheter a type of elbowed catheter with a slightly curved tip [45]

Counseling (ICD-10-PCS) the Root Type that identifies the application of psychological methods to treat an individual with normal developmental issues and psychological problems in order to increase function, improve well-being, alleviate distress, address maladjustment, or resolve crises [58]

COW Certificate of Waiver [948]

CPS chronic pain syndrome [17]

CPT Current Procedural Terminology [28]

CPT surgical package the services included in a procedure code in addition to the operative procedure [33]

craniectomy excision of part of the skull [42]

cranioplasty repair of part of the skull [42]

craniostomy procedure in which a physician drills or cuts into the skull to drain a hematoma or abscess or to remove part of the bone of the skull to gain access to perform further surgery [42]

craniotomy incision into the skull [42]

Creation (ICD-10-PCS) the Root Operation that identifies making a new genital structure that does not take over the function of a Body Part [51, 56]

cricoid split an incision of the cricoid cartilage to open the airway [41]

Crisis Intervention (ICD-10-PCS) the Root Type that identifies the treatment of a traumatized, acutely disturbed, or distressed individual for the purpose of short-term stabilization [58]

CRNA certified registered nurse anesthetist [34]

Crohn's disease an inflammatory bowel disease (IBD) with inflammation and ulcers in the alimentary tract characterized by a thickening of the mucous membrane [9]

cryosurgery surgery using cold [52]

cryotherapy the use of liquid nitrogen to destroy tissue [37]

CSF fistula an abnormal connection between the subarachnoid space around the brain and either the sinuses or the ear that allows the passage of CSF [42]

culture and sensitivity a lab test of secretions, such as sputum, to observe bacterial growth and determine antibiotic effectiveness [16]

culture performing a test to identify the microorganism that is causing an infection [11]

curettage (obstetrical) scraping away of the uterine lining [46]

curettement see *paring*

current MI a myocardial infarction (MI) that has occurred within the past four weeks [14]

Current Procedural Terminology (CPT) a listing of five-character alphanumeric codes and descriptions that report outpatient medical services and procedures [28]

cutaneous vesicostomy a temporary surgical procedure to create an opening in the umbilicus (lower abdomen), which allows urine to continuously drain from the bladder [45]

CV system cardiovascular system [14]

CVA cerebrovascular accident [14]

CVS chorionic villus sampling [46]

cyclectomy a partial excision of the ciliary body [43]

cystectomy a partial or complete excision of the bladder; may also involve other procedures, including removing surrounding lymph nodes [45]

cystitis a bacterial infection of the urinary bladder; also called urinary tract infection (UTI) [22]

cystolithotomy incision of the bladder to remove calculi [45]

cystometrography the use of a manometer (pressure-measuring device) to evaluate bladder function; the bladder is emptied using a catheter, then filled using a smaller catheter [45]

cystoscopy visual examination of the urinary bladder [45]

cystostomy the creation of an opening in the bladder, with possible removal of the bladder neck [45]

cytopathology the study of abnormal cells [48]

D

DBS deep brain stimulation [42]

DDH developmental dysplasia of the hip [25]

Decompression (ICD-10-PCS) the Root Operation that identifies extracorporeal elimination of undissolved gas from body fluids [57]

decompression cutting into a body site to relieve pressure or provide drainage [38, 42]

decubitus ulcer a breakdown of the skin, usually over bony parts of the body, caused by continuous pressure, friction, moistness, and heat; also referred to as pressure ulcer or bed sore [11]

deep brain simulation (DBS) the implantation of electrodes into a patient's brain to provide electrical stimulation to specific locations in the brain and reduce or eliminate involuntary movements [42]

deep inferior epigastric perforator (DIEP) flap the use of blood vessels called deep inferior epigastric perforators (DIEPs), and the skin and connected fat, or skin only (but no muscle), from the wall of the lower belly to rebuild the breast [37]

deep vein thrombosis (DVT) the formation of a thrombus within a deep vein, usually in the leg or pelvis [14]

default code (ICD-10-CM) a code that may represent a condition most commonly associated with a Main Term, or it may represent the unspecified code for a condition, which usually ends in 9 [4]

definitive drug testing a testing procedure that identifies the individual drugs present in a sample using qualitative, quantitative, or semiquantitative methods [48]

definitive procedure (skull base) performing the repair, biopsy, resection, or excision of a lesion [42]

definitive treatment a treatment intended to cure, eliminate, improve, or reduce the effects of a condition [52]

deformation a change in the size or shape of a normal structure due to physical forces [24]

degeneration the breakdown of bone or tissue [12]

degenerative neural disease a class of diseases marked by degeneration of nerves and brain tissue, resulting in abnormalities in muscle and sensory functions [17]

degree the depth of a burn or corrosion [13]

delayed development the embryonic development of a structure that is started late or progresses slowly [25]

delayed the status of a patient who has waited to seek care [12]

delirium a state of confusion, restlessness, and incoherence [18]

Delivery (ICD-10-PCS) the Root Operation that identifies assisting the passage of the Products of Conception from the genital canal [57]

delivery the expulsion of the fetus and placenta from the uterus [23]

delusion a false belief that hinders the ability to function [18]

dementia a progressive loss of brain function that affects memory, thinking, language, judgment, and behavior [17]

denied a claim that was processed and found to be ineligible for payment [2]

densitometry the measurement of density [47]

density a mass or substance [47]

dentistry the practice of a dentist [47]

Department of Health and Human Services (HHS) the federal government's principal agency for protecting the health and well-being of all Americans [2]

dependence (substance) see *addiction* [18]

dermatitis a flat or raised eruption that can be caused by irritation, allergy, or infection [11]

dermolysis surgical loosening of the skin [37]

dermomycosis a skin condition related to fungus [11]

dermoplasty surgical removal of the skin [37]

dermoplasty surgical repair of the skin [11]

Descemet's stripping endothelial keratoplasty (DSEK) the removal of only the corneal endothelium layer and replacement with a donor (cadaver) endothelial graft [43]

Destruction (ICD-10-PCS) the Root Operation that identifies the physical eradication of all or a portion of a Body Part by the direct use of energy, force, or a destructive agent [51, 52]

Detachment (ICD-10-PCS) the Root Operation that identifies cutting off all or a portion of the upper or lower extremities [51, 52]

Detoxification Services (ICD-10-PCS) the Root Type that identifies detoxification from alcohol and/or drugs

developmental dysplasia of the hip (DDH) a disruption in the normal relationship between the head of the femur and the acetabulum (hip socket) [25]

Device Character 6 in an ICD-10-PCS code; refers to material that is intentionally left in place for a therapeutic reason at the end of a procedure [49, 50]

Device Fitting (ICD-10-PCS) the Root Type that identifies the fitting of a device designed to facilitate or support achievement of a higher level of function [58]

DG documentation guidelines [31]

diabetes mellitus (DM) a common disease of the endocrine system resulting in elevated glucose concentrations over an extended period of time and excess excretion of urine, usually due to malfunction of the pancreas [10]

diabetic ketoacidosis (DKA) the condition of a high concentration of ketones that has accumulated in the blood and turns acidic [10]

diabetic nephropathy the condition of accumulated damage to the glomerulus capillaries due to chronic high blood glucose [22]

diabetic retinopathy the abnormal expression of blood vessels and hemorrhaging in the vessels of the retina; caused by diabetes [19]

diagnosis a patient illness, disease, condition, injury, or other reason for seeking healthcare services [1]

diagnosis-related group (DRG) a payment system that categorizes patients who are medically related with respect to diagnosis and treatment and statistically have similar lengths of stay [49]

diagnostic procedure a procedure performed to obtain information needed to make a diagnosis and treatment plan [33, 50]

diagnostic radiology imaging services used to evaluate or diagnose a health problem [1]

dialysis a treatment that filters the blood to remove waste, excess salt, and water [22, 32, 45]

dialysis-related amyloidosis (DRA) a deposit of the starchy substance amyloid in the joints due to dialysis [22]

diaphragm a muscle shaped like half of a dome that is located between the thoracic and abdominal cavities [40]

diaphysis the long, narrow part of a long bone [12]

diastole the time during the heart cycle when the chamber relaxes as it fills with blood [14]

dichorionic-diamniotic (DiDi) two embryos developed from separate zygotes, resulting in each embryo having its own amnion and chorion [23]

DiDi dichorionic-diamniotic [23]

DIEP deep inferior epigastric perforator

digestive system the body system that receives nutrients, breaks them down, absorbs them into the blood to be used by the body, and eliminates solid waste products; also called the gastrointestinal (GI) system [9]

Dilation (ICD-10-PCS) the Root Operation that identifies expanding an orifice or the lumen of a tubular Body Part [51, 54]

dilation and curettage (D&C) (nonobstetrical) the widening of the cervix and scraping of the uterine wall [46]

direct optical observation the process of looking at results with the naked eye [48]

discectomy the removal of all or part of an intervertebral disc [42]

dislocation a condition in which two bones are out of place at the joint [12]

displaced a condition in which fragments of bone move out of alignment due to a traumatic fracture [13]

displacement therapy (Proetz type) the irrigation of sinuses with a saline solution that is then suctioned out [41]

dissociative disorder a disruption in consciousness, memory, identity, or perception [18]

distal epiphysis the rounded end of a bone farthest from the trunk [12]

distributed (seizure) a seizure that is the result of abnormal activity on both sides of the brain; also called a generalized seizure [17]

diuresis excessive urination [45]

diverticula pouches formed when the lining of the intestine pushes through the intestinal muscle layer [9]

diverticular disease the presence and/or inflammation of diverticula [9]

diverticulitis a bacterial infection of diverticula [9]

divided separated [50]

Division (ICD-10-PCS) the Root Operation that identifies cutting into a Body Part, without draining fluids and/or gases from the Body Part, to separate or transect a Body Part [51, 55]

DM diabetes mellitus [10]

DO doctor of osteopathy [57]

doctor of osteopathy (DO) a licensed physician who has the same licensing, training, and qualifications as a doctor of medicine (MD); also called allopathic physician [57]

document the act of recording the reason a physician saw a patient, the diagnostic techniques used, tests or treatments planned, and the overall assessment of the patient [1]

documentation guidelines (DG) criteria developed by the Centers for Medicare and Medicaid Services and the American Medical Association for Evaluation and Management services that outline general principles of medical documentation and guidelines for documenting the history, examination, and medical decision-making components of E/M services [31]

documentation the written or electronic record of medical care and services provided [2]

dominance the side of the body an individual favors, such as being left-handed or right-handed [17]

Doppler ultrasonography/ultrasound an image created by measuring sound-wave echoes off of tissues and organs [14, 47]

dorsal approach the performance of a procedure through an incision in the midback [36]

dosimetry the measurement of a dose [47]

Down syndrome a genetic condition in which a person has 47 chromosomes instead of the usual 46; also called trisomy 21 [25]

Drainage (ICD-10-PCS) the Root Operation that identifies taking out or letting out fluids and/or gases from a Body Part [51, 55]

Dressing (ICD-10-PCS) the Root Operation that identifies putting material on a body region for protection [57]

DRG diagnosis-related group [49]

DRG grouper software that considers several clinical and demographic characteristics of a patient [49]

drug withdrawal syndrome a collection of symptoms of drug withdrawal in an infant who was exposed to narcotics in the uterus; also called neonatal abstinence syndrome (NAS) [24]

DSEK Descemet's stripping endothelial keratoplasty [43]

dual-energy X-ray absorptiometry (DXA/DEXA) bone density study the measurement of the density or mass of a material by comparing the amounts of material absorbed from X-ray beams of two different energies [47]

ductal (cancer) a cancer that starts in the milk ducts of the breast [22]

duodenectomy the excision of the duodenum [35, 55]

duodenoscopy visual examination of the duodenum [35]

DVT deep vein thrombosis [14]

dysphonia difficulty speaking [16]

dyspnea difficulty breathing [16, 23, 24]

dysrhythmia an abnormal heart beat [24]

dystocia difficult labor [23]

dystonia erratic jerky movements due to improperly functioning muscle tension [17]

E

E codes (ICD-9-CM) codes that classify causes of injury and poisoning; begin with the letter E and range from E800 to E899 [26]

E/M Evaluation and Management [31]

eardrum a membrane that separates the external ear from the middle ear; also called the tympanic membrane or tympanum [20]

early onset (Alzheimer disease) Alzheimer disease that is diagnosed before age 65 [17]

eating disorder a serious disturbance in eating behavior [18]

EBD endoscopic balloon dilation [35]

ECC echocardiogram [14, 32]

ECG electrocardiography [14]

echocardiogram (ECC) a recording of the sounds of the heart [14, 32]

echocardiography the use of noninvasive ultrasound to visualize internal cardiac structures [14]

eclampsia convulsions occurring during pregnancy or the puerperium, associated with preeclampsia [23]

ectopic outside of the uterus [23]

EDD estimated date of delivery [23]

edit a specific coding and billing criterion that is checked for accuracy based on predetermined rules [28]

EEG electroencephalogram [17, 32]

EGA estimated gestational age [23]

EGD esophagogastroduodenoscopy [35]

EKG electrocardiography [14]

elbowed catheter a urethral catheter with a sharp bend near the intake; used to navigate past obstructions in the urinary tract; also called prosthetic catheter [45]

ELBW extremely low birth weight [24]

elective surgery nonemergency surgery that is medically necessary but can be delayed at least 24 hours [33]

electrocardiogram an electrical recording of the heart [14]

electrocardiography (ECG, EKG) the graphical recording of the electrical activity of the heart [14, 57]

electrocauterization the use of a hot instrument to destroy tissue [37]

electrocochleography the process of recording the electrical activity of the cochlea [44]

Electroconvulsive Therapy (ICD-10-PCS) the Root Type that identifies the application of controlled electrical voltages to treat a mental health disorder [58]

electroconvulsive therapy a procedure in which electric currents are deliberately passed through the brain, triggering a brief seizure; can reverse symptoms of certain mental illnesses [18, 32]

electrocorticography the implantation of electrodes on the brain to record electrical impulses and identify areas to surgically remove [42]

electrodessication destruction using electrical energy [52]

electroejaculation the insertion of an electrostimulator probe into a patient's rectum next to the prostate to transmit an electrical current and stimulate ejaculation [45]

electroencephalogram (EEG) a recording of the electrical activity of the heart [17, 32]

electroencephalography the process of recording the electrical activity of the brain [44, 57]

electrolysis surgical destruction using electricity [37]

electrolyte a chemical compound that separates into charged particles in a solution [22]

Electromagnetic therapy (ICD-10-PCS) the Root Operation that identifies extracorporeal treatment by electromagnetic rays [57]

electromagnetic therapy extracorporeal treatment by electromagnetic rays [57]

electromyogram (EMG) a recording of the electrical activity of a muscle [32]

electrosurgery surgery using electrical energy [52]

embolectomy the removal of a clot from a blood vessel [14]

embolus an abnormal particle circulating in the blood, such as an air bubble or thrombus that has broken loose from its point of origin [14]

emergency department an organized department of an acute care hospital that provides treatment of an injury or health problem that cannot be delayed without harm to the patient [1]

emergency surgery surgery that must be performed immediately to save a life or prevent a disability, such as loss of a limb [33]

emphysema the enlargement and rupture of alveolar sacs at the end of the bronchioles, causing an abnormal accumulation of air in the tissue [16]

empyema pus in a body cavity [16]

encephalitis a viral inflammation of the brain and meninges [17]

encephalocele a hernia in the brain [25]

encounter a specific interaction between a patient and a healthcare provider [1]

endarterectomy excision of the lining of a vessel [14, 39]

endocarditis an inflammation in the lining of the heart or valves, due to bacteria or another disease [14]

endocardium the smooth inner layer that reduces friction as blood flows through the heart [14]

endocavity within a cavity [47]

endocervical curettage scraping tissue from the endocervical canal [46]

endocrine system the body system that produces, stores, and releases hormones [10]

endometriosis the growth of endometrial tissue in any area other than the uterus [22]

endoscopic balloon dilation (EBD) a procedure in which through-the-scope (TTS) balloon dilators or plastic dilators are moved over a guide wire to stretch the esophagus, pyloric valve, or duodenum [35]

endoscopic retrograde cholangiopancreatography (ERCP) the injection of contrast medium into the bile ducts via a tube through the ampulla of Vater to visualize the entire biliary tree [35]

endoscopic sclerotherapy a procedure in which a solution that causes inflammation and scarring is injected into a vein to close it off [35]

endotracheal intubation placement of a tube through the mouth and glottis into the trachea to create a viable airway [16]

endovascular aneurysm repair (EVAR) replacement of a weak section of an artery or heart wall with a patch, stent, or graft [39]

endovascular therapy treatment that involves inserting microcatheters into blood vessels to treat aneurysms, lesions, and neoplasms, including intracranial tumors [42]

enlarged prostate (EP) the abnormal growth of epithelial cells of the prostate, causing compression or obstruction of the urethra; also called benign prostatic hypertrophy or hyperplasia (BPH) [22]

enteral nutrition providing nutrients to patients in the nose using a nasogastric (NG) tube, in the stomach using a gastrostomy (G) tube, or in the small intestine using a jejunostomy (J) tube [29]

enterectomy excision of the intestine [39]

entitlement program a health benefit plan funded by federal or state governments that pays for 47% of healthcare services [2]

entry-level job a job performed upon graduation in order to gain basic skills, become familiar with the healthcare field, and establish excellent work habits [1]

enucleation removal of the eyeball without removing the ocular contents of the orbit or muscles [43]

EP enlarged prostate [22]

EP established patient [31]

epicardium the inner layer of the pericardium; also called visceral pericardium [14]

epidermis the outer layer of the skin [45]

epididymis spermatic duct [45]

epididymovasostomy the removal of a portion of the vas deferens and attachment of the vas deferens to the epididymis [45]

epikeratoplasty the transplantation of donor corneal epithelium onto a patient's cornea [43]

epilepsy a brain disorder in which neurons signal abnormally, causing seizures and/or unconsciousness [17]

episiotomy (obstetrical) a surgical incision into the perineum and vagina [46]

eponym named after a person [4]

equilibrium sense of balance [20]

ERCP endoscopic retrograde cholangiopancreatography [35]

erectile dysfunction (ED) the chronic inability to achieve or maintain a penile erection until ejaculation; also called impotence [22]

erythema multiforme red fluid-filled lesions that can cause layers of skin to fall off [11]

erythema redness [40]

erythremia polycythemia; a circulatory disorder [40]

erythroblastosis fetalis a blood disorder that occurs when the blood types of a mother and baby are incompatible; also called hemolytic disease of the newborn (HDN) [24]

erythrocyte a red blood cell [15, 40]

erythrocytopenia a lack of red blood cells [15]

erythroderma red skin [11]

erythropoiesis the process of the formation of red blood cells [15]

Escherichia coli (E. coli) a bacterium that can cause serious food poisoning [21]

esophageal ring an abnormal ring of tissue around the esophagus [25]

esophagectomy a procedure in which all or part of the esophagus is surgically removed [35, 55]

esophagitis irritation of the esophagus caused by acid reflux and a weak cardiac sphincter [9]

esophagogastroduodenoscopy (EGD) a procedure in which an endoscope is inserted through the mouth and moved down the throat into the esophagus, stomach, and duodenum [35, 55]

esophagoscopy visual examination of the esophagus [35]

established patient (EP) a patient who has received professional services from the same physician, or another physician in the group of the same specialty and subspecialty, within the previous three years [31]

estimated date of delivery (EDD) the anticipated due date of a pregnant woman determined by counting 40 weeks from the last menstrual period (LMP) [23]

estimated gestational age (EGA) the number of weeks and days since the last menstrual period [23]

ESWL extracorporeal shock wave lithotripsy [45]

ethmoid sinus a sinus located between the eyes and nose [41]

ethmoidectomy the process of opening the ethmoid sinus cavity [41]

etiology cause [4]

eustachian tube the connection between the ear and the nasopharynx [22]

evacuation suctioning the fetus and placenta out of the uterus with a suctioning instrument placed through the vagina, into the cervix, and into the uterus [46]

Evaluation and Management (E/M) CPT codes that describe patient encounters with a physician for the evaluation and management of a health problem [31]

EVAR endovascular aneurysm repair [39]

evisceration removal of the ocular contents and removal of the cornea; the sclera and extraocular muscles are not removed [43]

exact mapping refers to when codes in both code sets (ICD-9-CM and ICD-10-CM) have exactly the same definition [27]

examination performing a visual and physical inspection, with or without the assistance of instruments, to arrive at a conclusion [32]

exceptionally large newborn a newborn with a birth weight more than 4,500 grams (9 pounds, 15 ounces) [24]

exchange the process of obtaining oxygen from the air and delivering it to the lungs and blood for distribution to tissue cells, and removing the gaseous waste product, carbon dioxide, from the blood and lungs and expelling it [16]

Excision (ICD-10-PCS) the Root Operation that identifies cutting out or off, without replacement, a portion of a Body Part [51, 52]

excision the use of scissors, scalpel, or other sharp instrument to cut out tissue [37]

excisional embolectomy see *thrombectomy*

Excludes2 a convention indicating the condition excluded is not part of the condition represented by the code, but the patient may have both conditions at the same time [4]

exenteration removal of the eyeball, including the ocular contents; may include removal of bone and muscle [43]

exfoliation falling off in scales or layers [11]

exocrine a secretion externally via a duct [10]

expandability (ICD-10-PCS) the characteristic of ICD-10-PCS whereby the structure of the code set allows new procedures to be easily incorporated [49]

explanation of benefits a statement that lists all the services the provider billed, which ones were accepted for payment, how much the insurance company will pay, how much the patient owes, and how much will not be paid [2]

External (ICD-10-PCS) the Approach that identifies the entire treatment is performed on the skin or mucous membranes [50]

external approach the performance of a procedure of the nose through the skin on the outside of the nasal structure [41]

external cause an event such as an accident, force of nature, assault, or situation that causes an injury or adverse effect [8]

external ear a section of the ear that consists of the auricle or pinna, the auditory canal, and the tympanic membrane [20]

external fixation the installation of a rigid device, external to the body, attached to the bone with pins and screws to stabilize it [38]

external radiotherapy a treatment that directs precise doses of X-ray beams at specific sites in order to kill or shrink tumors and cancerous cells [5]

Extirpation (ICD-10-PCS) the Root Operation that identifies taking out or cutting out abnormal solid matter from a Body Part [51, 55]

extracapsular cataract extraction removal of the lens of the eye while leaving the elastic capsule that covers the lens partially intact to allow implantation of an intraocular lens (IOL) [43]

extracorporeal outside of the body [57]

extracorporeal shock wave lithotripsy (ESWL) the use of a lithotripter to aim pulsating sound waves at a kidney stone to break it into pieces [45]

Extraction (ICD-10-PCS) the Root Operation that identifies pulling or stripping out or off all or a portion of a Body Part by the use of force [51, 52, 55]

extraluminal from outside a vessel [54]

extremely low birth weight (ELBW) a birth weight of less than 1,000 grams (2 pounds, 3 ounces) [24]

extrinsic (asthma) asthma due to allergens; also called atopic [16]

F

facet the flat surface on the edge of the spinous process that forms the connection between vertebrae [42]

facetectomy the excision of the vertebral facet [42]

facility fee the fee charged by hospitals or other medical facilities for resources such as nursing and support staff, supplies, medication administration, social services, and the cost of space [31]

failure to thrive (FTT) inadequate physical growth marked by child's weight for age below the fifth percentile of the standard growth chart [24]

fallopian tube catheter introduction the insertion of a catheter through the cervix and uterus into the fallopian tube(s) [46]

fallopian tube the tube through which eggs are transported for fertilization and implantation in the uterus [22]

False Claims Act (FCA) a federal law that imposes penalties on individuals and companies who defraud government programs [2]

Family Counseling (ICD-10-PCS) the Root Type that identifies the application of psychological methods that includes one or more family members to treat an individual with addictive behavior [48]

family history the condition(s) that a patient's family member had in the past or currently has that causes the patient to be at higher risk of also contracting or developing the disease [5]

Family Psychotherapy (ICD-10-PCS) the Root Type that identifies the treatment that includes one or more family members of an individual with a mental health disorder by behavioral, cognitive, psychoanalytic, psychodynamic, or psychophysiological means to improve functioning or well-being [58]

family psychotherapy a method of psychotherapy whereby family members meet with a clinician to discuss the patient's condition and how to help the patient [32]

fascia the fibrous tissue that connects muscle to muscle [12]

fasciotomy cutting into the fascia to relieve pressure or tension [38]

fatigue fracture a fracture of a bone that has been subjected to repeated use or impact [12]

FBR foreign body removal [35]

Federal Register the official daily publication for rules, proposed rules, and notices of federal agencies and organizations, as well as executive orders and other presidential documents [3]

female catheter a short urethral catheter for passage through the female urethra [45]

female factor infertility a problem in the female genital system that diminishes reproduction, such as scarring or obstruction of the fallopian tubes or abnormal interaction between sperm and the mucous membrane in the cervix [22]

femur thigh bone [12]

fenestrated endovascular aneurysm repair (FEVAR) reinforcement of a weak section of the aorta with a stent that has holes customized to accommodate arterial branches [39]

fenestration semicircular canal the creation of an opening in the semicircular canal [44]

fetal nonstress test (NST) testing of the fetal heartbeat and oxygenation [46]

fetal scalp blood sampling a blood specimen from the scalp of a fetus through the dilated cervix [46]

fetopelvic disproportion see *cephalopelvic disproportion (CPD)* [23]

FEVAR fenestrated endovascular aneurysm repair [39]

fibrocystic breast disease a condition of lumps of benign fibrous tissue in the breast [22]

fimbrioplasty a procedure that obstructs a fallopian tube to save the function of the fimbriae [46]

final rule a legally required notice of final regulations, which is published in the *Federal Register* [3]

fine-needle aspiration (FNAB, FNA, NAB) a procedure in which a physician inserts a fine (thin), hollow needle under the skin to obtain aspirate, a small sample of cells, tissue, or fluid [33]

first trimester the time during a pregnancy when the gestational age is less than 14 weeks, 0 days [23]

first-listed diagnosis the diagnosis, condition, problem, or other reason for an encounter shown in the medical record to be chiefly responsible for the services provided [4]

fistulization the creation of a passageway, or opening, in the sclera by incising the iris and allowing the aqueous humor to drain [43]

flap a procedure whereby the blood supply remains intact, or a physician removes the skin and blood vessels and connects them to the recipient site; flaps can also involve subcutaneous tissue, muscle, fascia, and bone [37]

flap transfer moving a section of skin and subcutaneous tissue (sometimes including muscle, fascia, and bone), with blood vessels intact, from one site to another, with anastomosis to vessels at the recipient site [37]

flexible endoscope an instrument used for endoscopy procedures that consists of a soft tube with fiber-optic bundles that transmit an image [41]

Fluoroscopy (ICD-10-PCS) the Root Type that identifies the single plane or biplane real-time display of an image developed from the capture of external ionizing radiation on a fluorescent screen; may also be stored by either digital or analog means [47, 58]

fluoroscopy the single plane or biplane real-time display of an image developed from the capture of external ionizing radiation on a fluorescent screen; may also be stored by either digital or analog means [47, 58]

focal (seizure) a type of seizure that occurs in one part of the brain [17]

Foley catheter the most commonly used design of indwelling balloon catheter [45]

folic acid deficiency anemia an anemia due to a lack of folic acid [15]

folliculitis the inflammation of space around the hair root [11]

foramen an opening in the vertebra that surrounds the spinal cord [42]

forceps delivery the extraction of a fetus from the birth canal by grasping the head with forceps (tongs) [23]

foreign body an object that does not belong in the body [13]

foreign body removal (FBR) a procedure in which an object is retrieved from within the body [35]

forequarter an extremity and all or part of the adjoining structure, such as the arm, shoulder joint, and all or part of the scapula and clavicle, or the leg, hip joint, and all or part of the pelvic girdle [53]

formed element a blood cell [15]

four cooperating parties a federal interdepartmental committee that oversees all ICD-10-changes; comprises representatives from the Centers for Medicare and Medicaid Services (CMS), the National Center for Health Statistics (NCHS; part of the Centers for Disease Control and Prevention [CDC]), the American Hospital Association (AHA), and the American Health Information Management Association (AHIMA) [4]

fracture broken bone [12]

fracture reduction (manipulation) the use of force to move parts of a bone into normal alignment [38]

fragility fracture a broken bone caused by disease rather than trauma [12]

Fragmentation (ICD-10-PCS) the Root Operation that identifies breaking solid matter in a Body Part into pieces [51, 55]

fraud knowingly billing for services that were never given or billing for a service that has a higher reimbursement than the service produced [2]

frontal sinus a sinus located above the eyes [41]

front-end edit check a computerized scan of insurance claims for valid data, performed by the payer [2]

FTSG full-thickness skin graft [37]

full-thickness burn a burn that causes damage to the entire depth of the dermis [11]

full-term pregnancy 37 weeks, 1 day of gestation to 40 weeks, 7 days of gestation [23]

full-thickness skin graft (FTSG) a skin graft consisting of the epidermis and the full depth of the dermis [37]

function study visualizing a physiologic function in real time to observe the processes at work [32]

functional imaging a type of radiology that allows a physician to observe organ function in real time [57]

fungus a primitive vegetable that reproduces through spores [21]

furuncle a skin infection involving an entire hair follicle and the surrounding skin tissue [11]

Fusion (ICD-10-PCS) the Root Operation that identifies joining together portions of an articular Body Part, rendering the articular Body Part immobile [51, 53, 56, 57]

G

galactogram see *mammary ductogram*

gangrene the decay or death of tissue in the body caused by a lack of blood supply [10]

gastrectomy excision of the stomach [33, 35, 52, 55]

gastric bypass a procedure in which the stomach is divided to create a small pouch and causes food to bypass part of the small intestine [35]

gastritis the inflammation of the stomach lining [9]

gastroenteritis a bacterial or viral infection of the stomach and intestines [9]

gastroesophageal reflux disease (GERD) the backward flow of stomach contents into the esophagus [9]

gastrointestinal (GI) system the digestive system [9]

gastroplasty surgical repair of the stomach [33]

gastroplication folding of the stomach [54]

gastrorrhaphy suture of the stomach [33]

gastroscopy visual examination of the stomach [33, 35]

GEMs General Equivalency Mappings [27]

gender data mismatch an error that occurs when the patient's documented gender is inconsistent with the procedure coded [45]

general anesthesia a type of anesthesia that affects the whole body, including the brain, and in which patient feels nothing and has no memory of the procedure afterward [34]

General Equivalency Mappings (GEMs) a set of four data files created by the Centers for Disease Control and Prevention (CDC) to be the authoritative source for comparing codes between ICD-9-CM and ICD-10-CM [3, 27]

generalized (seizure) see *distributed (seizure)* [17]

genital prolapse the downward displacement of the uterus or vagina to an abnormal position [22]

genitourinary (GU) system the body system that includes the urinary and genital systems [22]

geographic practice cost index (GPCI) the Medicare system of adjusting fees based on the region of the country and/or zip code in which the healthcare provider practices [28]

GERD gastroesophageal reflux disease [9]

gestational condition a condition that is first diagnosed during pregnancy [23]

gestational diabetes a type of diabetes that develops during pregnancy in a woman who did not previously have diabetes [23]

gestational diabetes mellitus (GDM) a condition in which elevated glucose concentrations are diagnosed during pregnancy in women with no history of diabetes [10]

gestational hypertension the development of hypertension after 20 weeks' gestation in a woman who previously was not diagnosed with hypertension; also called pregnancy-induced hypertension (PIH) [23]

gestational sac a synonym for a fetus [47]

giant-cell bone tumor a rare, aggressive, benign tumor generally occurring in adults between the ages of 20 and 40 years [42]

Giardia the parasite that causes giardiasis, an intestinal tract infection [21]

glaucoma an increased fluid pressure within the eye that damages the optic nerve and can cause blindness [19]

global obstetric package (CPT) the services of routine antepartum, delivery, and postpartum care provided for a single patient [46]

global period (CPT) the number of days during which a provider must render all services related to a surgery [33]

globin a byproduct of hemoglobin [40]

globulin a protein molecule that comprises immunoglobulins [40, 45]

glomerular filtration rate (GFR) a method used to measure kidney function and to determine the stage of kidney disease [22]

glomerulonephritis inflammation of the glomerulus of the kidney, allowing protein and blood into the urine [22]

glomerulus a cluster of capillaries that separates the urinary space from the blood [22]

glucose tolerance test (GTT) a diagnostic measure to evaluate how the body breaks down sugar [10]

glycouria a condition of sugar in the urine [10]

goiter an enlargement of the thyroid gland that is not cancer [10]

goniotomy placement of a goniolens (gonioscope) on a patient's cornea to view the iris and cornea; allows a physician to see and open the trabecular meshwork to drain aqueous humor and reduce intraocular pressure (IOP) [43]

GPCI geographic practice cost index [28]

grand mal (seizure) a seizure characterized by a sudden loss of consciousness and falling down; affects the entire brain [17]

grand multipara a woman who has had five or more previous pregnancies resulting in a viable fetus [23]

granular detailed; specific [3, 49]

Graves disease overproduction of hormones by the thyroid gland due to an autoimmune condition in which autoantibodies are directed against the thyroid-stimulating hormone (TSH) receptor [10]

gravida (G) the number of pregnancies a woman has had [23]

gross (examination) viewing with the naked eye [48]

Group Counseling (ICD-10-PCS) the Root Type that identifies the application of psychological methods to treat an individual with addictive behavior

group health plan insurance coverage offered through an employer or union [2]

group psychotherapy a method of psychotherapy whereby a group of patients with the same disorder meets with a clinician to share information to help one another change their behaviors [32]

Group Therapy (ICD-10-PCS) the Root Type that identifies the treatment of two or more individuals with a mental health disorder by behavioral, cognitive, psychoanalytic, psychodynamic, or psychophysiological means to improve functioning or well-being [58]

GTT glucose tolerance test [10]

guided imagery see *radiologic guidance*

guidelines (CPT) instructions that appear at the beginning of each of the six sections and apply to all codes in that section [28]

gustatory the sense of taste [17]

Gustilo classification system the classification of open fractures of long bones into three major categories depending on the method of injury, soft-tissue damage, and degree of skeletal involvement [13]

H

hallucination false visual, auditory, olfactory, or tactile perception [18]

Hb hemoglobin [15]

HbA1c a blood test that measures the glucose attached to hemoglobin [10]

HBW high birth weight [24]

HCPCS Health Care Common Procedure Coding System [1]

HCPCS Index an alphabetical listing of services and supplies organized by Main Terms and subterms [29]

HCPCS modifier additional characters added to a code, either alphanumeric or two letters long, ranging from **A1** to **VP**, that can be used with both HCPCS and CPT codes; provides additional information about a service, item, or procedure and encompasses more situations than a CPT modifier does [29]

HCPCS Table of Drugs a table that organizes HCPCS codes for generic and brand name drugs [29]

HCPCS Tabular List the section of the HCPCS manual that arranges codes in alphanumeric order, beginning with codes that start with the letter A, followed by four numbers [29]

HDN hemolytic disease of the newborn [24]

Health Insurance Portability and Accountability Act (HIPAA) a federal law passed in 1996 that has numerous provisions relating to consumer health insurance and electronic health transactions [1]

healthcare administrator an individual in a healthcare organization who is responsible for managing the organization, including the transition to ICD-10-CM/PCS [3]

Healthcare Common Procedure Coding System (HCPCS) the HIPAA-mandated code set for supplies, items, and services not covered by CPT, physician, and nonphysician services [1]

Hearing Aid Assessment (ICD-10-PCS) the Root Type that identifies the measurement of the appropriateness and/or effectiveness of a hearing device [58]

Hearing Aid Treatment (ICD-10-PCS) the Root Type that identifies the application of techniques to improve the communication abilities of individuals with cochlear implant [58]

Hearing Assessment (ICD-10-PCS) the Root Type that identifies the measurement of hearing and related functions [58]

Hearing Treatment (ICD-10-PCS) the Root Type that identifies the application of techniques to improve, augment, or compensate for hearing and related functional impairment [58]

heart transplant replacement of a diseased heart with a healthy heart from a deceased donor [39]

Helicobacter pylori (H. pylori) the bacterium that causes ulcers [9]

Heller myotomy a procedure in which the esophageal sphincter muscle is cut [35]

HELLP syndrome a severe form of preeclampsia with hemolysis, elevated liver enzymes, and low platelet count [23]

helminth a plant or animal that lives in or on another living organism, or host, and often causes damage to the host; also called a parasite [21]

hemapheresis removal of blood [40]

hematology study of blood [48]

hematopoiesis formation of blood [15, 40]

hematuria the condition of blood in the urine [22]

hemiarthroplasty a procedure requiring only one component of a joint be replaced; also called a partial joint replacement [38]

hemic related to blood [40]

hemic system the method to transport and pass nutrients, oxygen, carbon dioxide, water, proteins, and hormones to cells and transport waste products to excretory oxygen; also called blood [15]

hemilaminectomy the partial removal of the lamina; also called laminotomy [42]

hemiplegia paralysis of one side of the body [17]

hemispherectomy excision of one of the two cerebral hemispheres [42]

hemodialysis (HD) a method for removing waste from the blood in which blood is processed through a machine when the kidneys cease to function [22, 32]

hemoglobin (Hb) the oxygen-carrying component of erythrocytes [15]

hemolytic anemia anemia due to excessive loss of erythrocytes [15]

hemolytic disease of the newborn (HDN) see *erythroblastosis fetalis* [24]

hemophilia a genetic disorder in which blood takes too long to clot [15]

hemostasis the stoppage of bleeding or hemorrhage [15]

hepatectomy the surgical removal of all or part of the liver [35]

hepatitis inflammation of the liver due to viruses named A, B, or C [9]

hernia the protrusion of an organ through a weakened area in a muscle [9]

hernia repair the surgical correction of a hernia through the use of manual manipulation, sutures, or mesh [35]

herpes the shingles virus [21]

HHNS hyperosmolarity hyperglycemic nonketotic syndrome [10]

high birth weight (HBW) birth weight greater than 4,000 grams (8 pounds, 13 ounces) [24]

histology type of tissue [5]

history of present illness (HPI) an interview of a patient regarding symptoms related to the chief complaint and how the problem has progressed [2, 31]

Holter monitor a portable ECG machine worn by a patient for an extended period of hours or days to measure heart activity in a variety of situations [14]

homeostasis the maintenance of a stable internal physical state [15, 17]

hordeolum the bacterial inflammation of a sebaceous gland on the edge or lining of the eyelid; also called a stye [19]

hormones chemical messengers that regulate many body functions including growth, development, metabolism, sexual function, reproduction, and mood [10]

hospital-acquired condition (HAC) a serious condition that develops after admission [16]

hospital laboratory a laboratory located in a hospital facility, used to perform tests needed in emergency situations, tests where STAT results are needed rapidly for patient care, and those done in high volume for both inpatients and outpatients [48]

HPI history of present illness [2, 31]

HTN hypertension [14]

human immunodeficiency virus (HIV) a virus that infects and destroys helper T cells of the immune system and causes AIDS [21]

Huntington chorea an inherited progressive, degenerative disease involving loss of muscle control and personality changes [17]

hydrocele a fluid-filled sack in the scrotum caused by abnormal fetal development, injury, hernia, or blockages [22, 25]

hydrocephalus an excess of cerebrospinal fluid trapped in the brain [17, 25]

hydrocephaly water or fluid in the head/brain [25]

hydronephrosis distention of the renal pelvis due to excessive urine collection in the kidney, often due to ureteral obstruction [22]

hymenotomy incision of the hymen [46]

hyperbaric oxygen treatment (HBOT) breathing 100% oxygen under increased atmospheric pressure [57]

hyperbilirubinemia high concentrations of bilirubin in the blood, which causes an infant's skin and sclera to turn yellow [24]

hypercapnia a high carbon dioxide concentration [16]

hyperglycemia a severely elevated blood glucose concentration due to a lack or deficiency of insulin [10]

hyperosmolarity hyperglycemic nonketotic syndrome (HHNS) an elevated glucose concentration without ketoacidosis, usually occurring in elderly type 2 diabetics with other conditions [10]

hypertension (HTN) an abnormally high arterial blood pressure [14]

Hyperthermia (ICD-10-PCS) the Root Operation that identifies extracorporeal raising of body temperature [57]

hyperthermia extracorporeal raising of body temperature [57]

hyperthyroidism inappropriately elevated thyroid function [10]

Hypnosis (ICD-10-PCS) the Root Type that identifies the induction of a state of heightened suggestibility by auditory, visual, and tactile techniques to elicit an emotional or behavioral response [58]

hypogammaglobulinemia a deficiency of gamma globulins and antibodies in the blood [15]

hypoglycemia an abnormally low blood glucose concentration often due to excessive use of insulin or other glucose-lowering medications [10]

hypospadias a congenital condition in which the opening of the urethra is on the underside, rather than the end, of the penile shaft, and may be located as far down as the scrotum or perineum [25]

Hypothermia (ICD-10-PCS) the Root Operation that identifies extracorporeal lowering of body temperature [57]

hypothermia extracorporeal lowering of body temperature [57]

hypothyroidism a deficiency of thyroid hormone, usually due to lack of production by the thyroid or inadequate secretion of hormones by the pituitary gland or hypothalamus [10]

hypoxemia low oxygen concentration [16]

hysterectomy removal of the uterus and/or related structures, such as the ovaries and fallopian tubes [46]

hysteroophorosalpingectomy excision of the uterus, ovary, and fallopian tube [46]

hysteroplasty the repair of a malformed uterus [46]

hysterorrhaphy (nonobstetrical) suturing of the uterus [46]

hysterosalpingography X-ray of the uterus and fallopian tubes after injecting contrast dye [46]

hysteroscopy visualization of the cervix and uterus using a hysteroscope that is passed through the vagina into the cervix and uterine cavity [46]

I

IBD inflammatory bowel disease [9]

IBS irritable bowel syndrome [9]

ICD-10 International Classification of Diseases, 10th Revision [3]

ICD-10-CM International Classification of Diseases, 9th Revision, Clinical Modification [3]

ICD-10-PCS International Classification of Diseases, 10th Revision, Procedure Classification System (ICD-10-PCS) [3]

ICD-10-PCS Official Guidelines for Coding and Reporting (PCS OGCR) consists of A. Conventions, B. Medical and Surgical Section Guidelines, and C. Obstetrics Section Guidelines [49]

idiopathic of unknown cause [17]

ileal conduit a channel that joins the ureters to the ileum [45]

ileostomy division of the ileum that brings the proximal end out to a stoma in the abdominal wall, bypassing the colon, rectum, and anus [35]

ileum small intestine [9]

ileus a condition in which the bowel does not work correctly but there is no structural problem [9, 13]

ilium pelvic bone [12]

IMA internal mammary artery [14]

imaging guidance real-time visualization of body structures during a medical or surgical procedure [47]

imbrication of the diaphragm repair of the diaphragm to resemble normal anatomy [40]

Immobilization (ICD-10-PCS) the Root Operation that identifies limiting or preventing motion of a body region by external methods and devices [57]

immobilization limiting or preventing motion of a body region by external methods and devices [57]

immune globulin a substance that provides passive immunity and consists of serum globulins or recombinant immune globulins [32]

immunization history date and type of past vaccinations and titers (blood tests proving immunity to a specific disease) [2]

immunization administration of a vaccine (virus) or toxoid (bacteria) that provides active immunity [32]

immunodeficiency the result of a body's immune system failure or reduction in function [32]

impairment the degree to which an individual's normal abilities are limited [18]

impotence the chronic inability to achieve or maintain a penile erection until ejaculation [22]

impression an effect produced on the mind by outside stimuli [6]

impulse-control disorder an extreme difficulty in controlling impulses, despite the negative consequences [18]

in remission (substance use) a history of past drug or alcohol dependence documented by the physician [18]

in vitro fertilization the removal of an egg from a female patient, which is manually fertilized with sperm and then returned to the fallopian tube or implanted in the uterus [23, 46]

incidental appendectomy the removal of the appendix as a preventive measure during another procedure [35]

incision site the anatomic location at which a surgeon cuts through the skin and subcutaneous tissue [33]

inconclusive HIV a test result that means the antibody test was neither positive nor negative; also called indeterminate HIV [21]

incontinence the inability to control bladder muscles [22]

incubator a medical device that allows a newborn to be in an environment where the temperature, humidity, and oxygen concentration can be controlled [24]

incus the anvil-shaped bone in the middle ear that receives vibrations from the malleus and transmits them to the stapes [20]

indented code description indented three spaces and beginning with a lowercase letter, this description is the unique descriptor for a specific code number [28]

independent clinical lab a Medicare-enrolled laboratory that receives a specimen and performs a test(s) for a separate, referring laboratory; also called referring lab [48]

indeterminate HIV see *inconclusive HIV* [21]

Individual Counseling (ICD-10-PCS) the Root Type that identifies the application of psychological methods to treat an individual with addictive behavior

individual health insurance a plan that people purchase directly from a health insurance company, such as those who are self-employed or do not have benefits through an employer or government program [2]

Individual Psychotherapy (ICD-10-PCS) the Root Type that identifies the treatment of an individual with a mental health disorder by behavioral, cognitive, psychoanalytic, psychodynamic, or psychophysiological means to improve functioning or well-being [58]

Light Therapy (ICD-10-PCS) the Root Type that identifies the application of specialized light treatments to improve functioning or well-being [58]

indwelling (catheter) a flexible, hollow tube inserted into the urinary bladder and left in short or long term to provide continuous urine flow; may be inserted through the urethra or ureters [45]

infant of diabetic mother (IDM) an infant born to a woman who has diabetes [24]

infection inflammation due to an infectious agent [12]

inferior vena cava the largest veins that carry deoxygenated blood back to the right ventricle [14]

inflammatory bowel disease (IBD) a group of disorders in which the intestines become red and swollen, probably as a result of an immune reaction of the body against its own intestinal tissue; includes Crohn's disease and ulcerative colitis [9]

influenza an acute respiratory infection with sudden onset caused by a virus and characterized by fever, chills, headache, muscle aches, cough, and sore throat [16]

infusion technique a slow, steady rate of release of medication over a long period of time [32]

initial encounter (CPT) the first encounter by the admitting physician during the current admission [31]

initial encounter (ICD-10-CM) active treatment [4]

initial episode identifies that the patient received active treatment for an injury during the encounter [8]

injection the administration of a medication using a needle [38]

inner ear see *labyrinth* [20]

inpatient encounter physician interaction with a patient who has been formally admitted to a healthcare facility, such as an acute-care hospital, long-term care facility, or rehabilitation facility [1]

Insertion (ICD-10-PCS) the Root Operation that identifies putting in a nonbiological appliance that monitors, assists, performs, or prevents a physiological function but does not physically take the place of a Body Part [51, 56, 57]

insertion the position where a muscle attaches to a bone that moves [12]

Inspection (ICD-10-PCS) the Root Operation that identifies visually and/or manually exploring a Body Part [51, 55]

instructional note (CPT) text that appears in parentheses after a code description; directs the user to alternative codes for closely related procedures or to codes that must or must not be used together [28]

instructional note (ICD-10-CM) official coding directions throughout the ICD-10-CM manual [4]

instrumentation specialized equipment, such as an endoscope or needle, used to reach an internal Body Part [52]

insulin pump a small, implantable device that dispenses small doses of rapid-acting insulin [10]

integral component a task that is part of the intraoperative service and is not coded or billed separately [33]

integral routine [6]

integumentary pertaining to a covering [11]

intellectual disability the modern term for mental retardation [18]

intent a term describing whether an event was accidental or intentional [8]

interactive complexity a component of psychiatry services that is used when communication is challenging because of the involvement of third parties in addition to the patient [32]

internal approach the performance of procedure of the nose from within the nasal passage or through the mucous membrane inside the nasal passage [41]

internal fixation the use of special implants, such as plates, screws, nails, rods, and/or wires, applied directly to the bone(s) [38]

internal mammary artery (IMA) the blood vessel located on the inside of the chest cavity, which is resistant to cholesterol buildup; often used in a coronary artery bypass graft [14]

internal radiotherapy the use of radioactive pellets or containers within a body cavity to target a malignant area [5]

International Classification of Diseases, 10th Revision (ICD-10) a worldwide reporting system developed by WHO for classifying epidemiological and mortality data [3]

International Classification of Diseases, 10th Revision, Clinical Modification (ICD-10-CM) a HIPAA-mandated code set for diagnosis coding (replacement system for ICD-9-CM) [1]

International Classification of Diseases, 10th Revision, Procedure Classification System (ICD-10-PCS) a HIPAA-mandated code set for hospital inpatient procedure coding (replacement system for ICD-9-CM, Volume 3) [1]

International Classification of Diseases, 9th Revision, Clinical Modification (ICD-9-CM) a hospital inpatient procedure coding system implemented in 1979 (replaced by ICD-10-PCS)

interspace the space between two vertebrae; identified by the vertebrae above and below [38]

interstitial between tissues [47]

interventional radiologist a physician who performs minimally invasive, image-guided surgeries [47]

intervertebral disc a plate that exists between each pair of vertebrae to provide flexibility and movement to the spine; consists of the nucleus pulposus and annulus fibrosus [42]

intestinal obstruction a physical blockage of the intestine that prevents waste from passing through [9]

intoxication a state of impaired function that occurs when more of a substance is consumed than a person can physically tolerate, resulting in behavioral or physical abnormalities [18]

intra-articular within a joint [47]

intracavity within a cavity [47]

intractable (migraine) a migraine that is resistant to treatment; may also be called pharmaco-resistant or refractory [17]

intradermal pertaining to within the skin [11]

intralesional injection the injection of a drug, such as a corticosteroid, into a skin lesion [37]

intraluminal from within a vessel [54]

intraocular lens (IOL) an artificial lens inserted into the lens capsule of the eye [43]

intraocular pressure (IOP) the pressure of fluid within the eye [43]

intrapartum fetal hypoxia an insufficient amount of oxygen provided to the fetus during labor and delivery [46]

intraperitoneal within the peritoneum [46]

intrathecal into the sheath of the spinal cord [47]

intrauterine growth restriction (IUGR) the poor growth of a baby while in the mother's womb during pregnancy; specifically, the developing baby weighs less than 90% of other babies at the same gestational age [24]

intraventricular hemorrhage (IVH) bleeding in the brain in very-low-birth-weight premature babies that usually resolves within a few days [24]

intravitreal injection the injection of medication into the vitreous body [43]

intrinsic (asthma) asthma that is not due to allergens; also called nonatopic [16]

Introduction (ICD-10-PCS) the Root Operation that identifies putting in or on a therapeutic, diagnostic, nutritional, physiological, or prophylactic substance except blood or blood products [57]

introduction putting in or on a therapeutic, diagnostic, nutritional, physiological, or prophylactic substance except blood or blood products [57]

involuntary (muscles) muscles that are controlled by a subconscious part of the brain [12]

IOL intraocular lens [43]

IOP intraocular pressure [43]

ipsilateral the examination of circulation on the same side on which catheterization was performed [39]

iridectomy excision of the iris [43]

iridencleisis implantation of part of the iris in the cornea [43]

iridoplasty repair of the iris [43]

iridotasis stretching of the iris [43]

iridotomy incision of the iris to drain aqueous humor; can include transfixion for iris bombé [43]

iron deficiency anemia an anemia due to insufficient iron to manufacture hemoglobin [15]

Irrigation (ICD-10-PCS) the Root Operation that identifies putting in or on a cleaning substance [57]

irrigation putting in or on a cleaning substance [57]

irritable bowel syndrome (IBS) a combination of symptoms such as cramping, abdominal pain, bloating, constipation, and diarrhea [9]

ischemia deficient blood supply to a local area due to obstruction of the arterial blood flow, usually due to narrowing of the arteries; also called coronary heart disease or arteriosclerotic heart disease when it affects the heart [14]

IUGR intrauterine growth restriction [24]

IVH intraventricular hemorrhage [24]

J

jaundice a condition due to high bilirubin that causes the skin and parts of the eyes to turn a yellow color [24]

joint replacement the removal of a natural joint and insertion of an artificial ball and cup made of metal, ceramic, polyurethane, or other artificial material [38]

joint the location where two or more bones meet [12]

K

keratectomy excision of the cornea [43]

keratin horny tissues found in the epidermis, hair, and nails [19]

keratitis inflammation and ulceration of the surface of the cornea [19]

keratomileusis a form of keratoplasty in which a slice of the cornea is removed, reshaped (often with a laser), and placed back onto the cornea [43]

keratophakia the reshaping and transplantation of donor corneal tissue onto a patient's cornea [43]

keratoplasty repair of the cornea [43]

keratosis overgrowth of horny tissue [11]

key components (KCs) history, examination, and medical decision making; also referred to as content of service requirements [31]

kidney the part of the urinary system that produces urine and regulates the level of electrolytes and body fluid [22]

L

lab report a report that provides the results of specimen testing and other information useful to a physician in making a diagnosis [48]

lab requisition a form that describes specimen testing to be performed [48]

lab test/pathology results reports from lab tests; report from pathology regarding specimen testing [2]

LABG laparoscopically adjustable gastric banding [35]

labia major the folds of flesh that surround and protect the opening to the vagina [22]

labia minor the fold of flesh that surrounds and protects the urethra [22]

laboratory a department or organization that analyzes biological specimens [1]

labyrinth a fluid-filled cavity in the temporal bone that contains the cochlea; also called the inner ear [20]

labyrinthotomy surgical incision into the labyrinth of the ear, sometimes with the administration/injection of drugs [44]

laceration a torn or jagged wound [13]

lamellar keratoplasty partial-thickness transplantation involving a graft of only specific corneal layers [43]

lamina a thin layer of bone that forms part of the vertebral arch [42]

laminectomy the complete removal of the lamina [42]

laminoplasty repair of the lamina [42]

laminotomy the partial removal of the lamina; also called hemilaminectomy [42]

laparoscopically adjustable gastric banding (LABG) a procedure in which an inflatable silicone device is placed around the top portion of the stomach to divide it into a smaller pouch and a larger pouch [35]

laparoscopy visual examination of the abdomen [35]

laparotomy cutting into the abdomen [35]

large for gestational age (LGA) a fetus or newborn infant who is larger in size than normal for the baby's sex and gestational age [24]

laryngeal reinnervation by neuromuscular pedicle the use of a neuromuscular pedicle to restore nerves [41]

laryngectomy excision of all or part of the larynx [41]

laryngitis inflammation of the larynx, resulting in hoarseness [16]

laryngoscopy (direct) the use of a laryngoscope inserted through the mouth or nose to view the larynx and hypolarynx/subglottis [41]

laryngoscopy (indirect) the use of a mirror to view the base of the tongue, larynx, and hypolarynx [41]

larynx the voice box [16]

last menstrual period (LMP) the last menstrual period that a woman has before becoming pregnant, which is used to determine the estimated date of delivery (EDD) [23]

late effect a problem that occurs after active healing is completed [4]

late onset Alzheimer disease that is diagnosed after age 65 [17]

lateral rhinotomy the creation of an incision along the nose from the inner eyebrow to the nasolabial fold [41]

laterality an indication of the side of the body that a condition affects, such as right, left, or bilateral sides [30]

latissimus dorsi (LD) flap the use of a latissimus dorsi muscle flap, often combined with a tissue expander or implant, to reconstruct the breast [37]

lavage irrigation of the maxillary or sphenoid sinus by puncturing the antrum or creating an ostium [41]

LBW low birth weight [24]

left atrium the upper left chamber of the heart, which receives blood from the lungs [14]

left ventricle the lower left chamber of the heart, which ejects blood to the body [14]

legacy system a coding system used for historical purposes [26]

lens the clear part of the front of the eye that focuses light rays on the retina [19]

leukemia a malignant disease of the blood-forming organs; does not produce tumors [5]

leukocyte white blood cell [15]

leukopenia a lack of white blood cells [15]

level (spinal) a vertebra of the spine [38]

Level I (HCPCS) Current Procedural Terminology, Fourth Edition (CPT) codes [29]

Level II (HCPCS) National Healthcare Common Procedure Coding System codes [29]

level of service in evaluation and management coding, the complexity or duration of a service provided based on the nature of the presenting problem, the history, the examination, and the medical decision making [31]

Lewy body disease a condition in which patients have abnormal protein structures in certain areas of the brain [18]

LGA large for gestational age [24]

lichen an eruption of flat papules [11]

ligament fibrous tissue that connects bones to bones [12]

ligation the excision or tying off of dilated vein(s) using a laparoscopic approach [45]

ligature the tying off a skin tag at its base with thread, eliminating blood flow to the skin tag; it eventually dies and falls off [37]

limited lymphadenectomy the removal of lymph nodes [40]

linear measurement a measurement that identifies the distance between two points and is used to classify the length and the diameter of wound repairs [37]

lipolysis surgical destruction of fat [37]

lithoplasty surgical formation of fat [37]

lithotripsy of gallstones the use of high-frequency sound waves to break up gallstones [35]

liver biopsy the surgical removal of a small piece of the liver [35]

liver transplant the surgical removal of a diseased liver and replacement with some or all of a healthy liver from another person [35]

LMP last menstrual period [23]

lobar pneumonia a bacterial pneumonia that primarily affects one lobe of the lung [16]

lobe a segment of a lung [16]

lobectomy the surgical excision of one lobe of an organ [36, 41, 42]

lobular a breast cancer that starts in the lobules that produce milk [22]

lobular pneumonia a pneumonia that primarily affects the bronchi and lobules; also called bronchopneumonia [16]

local anesthesia numbs a small area of a body part; patient is awake and alert [34]

localized (seizure) see *focal (seizure)* [17]

localized an infection that primarily affects a single organ or body system, such as pneumonia or pharyngitis [21]

low birth weight (LBW) a birth weight less than 2,500 grams (5 pounds, 8 ounces) [24]

lower respiratory tract consists of the trachea, bronchi, and lungs [16]

lower urinary tract symptom (LUTS) a symptom relating to urine storage and voiding disturbances [22]

Lund-Browder classification a system used by physicians to estimate the extent, depth, and percentage of burns [37]

lung a respiratory organ composed of the spongy tissue that receives deoxygenated blood from the heart through the pulmonary artery, re-oxygenates it, and sends it back to the heart through the pulmonary vein [16]

lymph a clear fluid containing proteins, salts, organic substances, and water [40]

lymph chain a sequential grouping of lymph nodes in a localized area along lymph vessels, occurring in sites where the body is most vulnerable to infection [40]

lymph node a small mass of tissue that ranges from the size of a pinhead to about one inch in diameter and is located along the lymph vessels [40]

lymphadenectomy the surgical excision of a lymph gland [40]

lymphangiography a radiology procedure where contrast medium is injected into a patient to visualize lymph nodes and lymph circulation [40]

lymphangiotomy incision into a vessel of the lymphatic system [40]

lysis of labial adhesions the destruction or freeing of adhesions between the labia minor and labia major [46]

M

MAC monitored anesthesia care [34]

macular degeneration the gradual loss of central vision due to aging, with no cure [19]

magnetic resonance angiography (MRA) the use of a magnetic field and pulses of radio wave energy to visualize the heart, blood vessels, or blood flow in the circulatory system [47]

Magnetic resonance imaging (MRI) (ICD-10-PCS) the Root Operation that identifies computer-reformatted digital display of multiplanar images developed from the capture of radiofrequency signals emitted by nuclei in a body site excited within a magnetic field [58]

Magnetic Resonance Imaging (MRI) (ICD-10-PCS) the Root Type that identifies the computer-reformatted digital display of multiplanar images developed from the capture of radiofrequency signals emitted by nuclei in a body site excited within a magnetic field [58]

magnetic resonance imaging (MRI) the use of strong magnets and radio waves to produce computerized images of internal body tissues [47]

Main Term the primary index entry [4]

male factor infertility a problem in the male genital system that diminishes reproduction, such as inability to ejaculate, lack of sperm production, or lack of live sperm [22]

malformation a permanent abnormal shape of an organ or body region, resulting from arrested, delayed, or abnormal development of an embryo [24]

malignant life-threatening [5]

Mallampati score a score that rates the potential difficulty of endotracheal intubation on a scale of I through IV [34]

malleus the hammer-shaped bone in the middle ear that transmits vibrations to the incus [20]

malposition of fetus any presentation of a fetus other than occipitoanterior (OA) [23]

malunion a condition when the ends of fractured bone segments do not heal with proper alignment [12]

mammary ductogram the use of mammography and contrast material to view the inside of a breast's milk ducts [47]

mammography (screening) X-ray imaging of the breast of a woman who has no signs or symptoms of breast disease [47]

mammography (diagnostic) X-ray imaging of the male or female breast to determine whether a problem exists or to determine the nature of a problem [47]

mammoplasty the repair or reconstruction of a breast [37]

managed care plan a company that attempts to control the cost of healthcare while providing better outcomes [2]

manifestation a sign or symptom [4]

manipulation the realignment of bone fragments or segments; also called reduction [38]

manometry a procedure that evaluates muscular activity of the esophagus at rest and during swallowing to diagnose esophageal disorders involving motility or causes of heartburn; also called motility study [32]

manual review a review done by hand instead of through an automatic process [2]

many-to-one mapping the General Equivalency Map (GEM) designation when several codes in ICD-10-CM are combined into a single equivalent code in ICD-9-CM or vice versa [27]

Map (ICD-10-PCS) the Root Operation that identifies locating the route of passage of electrical impulses and/or locating functional areas in a Body Part [51, 55]

march fracture the fracture of a bone that has been subjected to repeated use or impact [12]

Marfan syndrome a genetic disorder of connective tissue characterized by elongated bones and ocular and circulatory defects [25]

Marshall-Marchetti-Krantz (MMK) procedure an eponym for vesicourethropexy [45]

marsupialization to incise a cyst or abscess by cutting a slit into it to drain it and then suturing the edges to surrounding tissue; the surgical formation of a pouch-like sac (marsupialization) on the Bartholin's gland [46]

MAS meconium aspiration syndrome [24]

mastalgia breast pain [23]

mastitis inflammation of the breast [23]

mastoid process the portion of the temporal bone of the skull that juts forward behind the ear [20]

mastopexy a skin reduction with removal or reduction of underlying breast muscles to reorient the breasts into a higher position [37]

mastostomy the incision and drainage of a breast abscess [37]

maxillary sinus a sinus located below the eyes [41]

maxillectomy the removal of all or part of the upper jaw bone [41]

maze surgery the creation of new paths for the heart's electrical signals to travel through [39]

MBD metastatic bone disease [12]

Measurement (ICD-10-PCS) determining the level of a physiological or physical function at a point in time [57]

Measurement (ICD-10-PCS) the Root Operation that identifies determining the level of a physiological or physical function at a point in time [57]

measurement the use of equipment or tools to quantify the body's response, reflex, or perception [32]

mechanical thrombectomy a transcatheter procedure that uses a thrombolytic agent, radiological guidance, and a small blade or water jet to fragment, then suction out, a clot from an artery or vein [39]

Meckel diverticulum a congenital bulge in the intestine caused by a remnant of the embryonic yolk stalk [25]

meconium aspiration syndrome (MAS) a condition in which a newborn breathes a mixture of meconium and amniotic fluid into the lungs before or during delivery [24]

meconium peritonitis an infection of the peritoneal cavity due to perforation of the bowel and leakage of meconium [24]

mediastinotomy incision into the mediastinum [40]

mediastinum located in the thorax and surrounded by connective tissue, an area that separates the lungs and contains the esophagus, heart, and superior and inferior vena cava and aorta [40]

Medicaid a program for low-income families that is funded jointly by the federal government and state governments [2]

medical necessity establishing the medical need for services [2]

medical payment a payment made by automobile insurance policies to pay for medical expenses incurred during an automobile accident; also called med pay [2]

medical record the comprehensive collection of all information on a patient at a particular facility [2]

medical review an investigation conducted by a nurse, physician, or other clinician [2]

Medicare a federal government program that pays for healthcare services for most people age 65 and older or people of any age with end-stage renal disease (ESRD) [2]

Medicare Administrative Contractor (MAC) a private company that processes Medicare Part A and Part B claims [2]

Medicare Advantage the optional replacement of Part A and Part B that is offered by private health insurance companies [2]

Medicare global surgical package a group, or package, of services that all relate to a single surgery and are covered by a single insurance payment, including preoperative, intraoperative, and postoperative services

Medicare Physician Fee Schedule (MPFS) a listing of CPT codes and Medicare-allowable fees published by the Centers for Medicare and Medicaid Services [33]

Medicare Physician Fee Schedule Database (MPFSDB) a listing of CPT codes, Medicare-allowable fees, and related information published by the Centers for Medicare and Medicaid Services [28, 33]

Medicare severity-adjusted DRGs (MS-DRGs) a DRG system developed and used by Medicare consisting of approximately 500 DRG classifications that aggregate the thousands of diagnoses and procedures available in the coding manuals [49]

Medication Management (ICD-10-PCS) the Root Type that identifies the monitoring and adjustment of the use of medications for the treatment of a mental health disorder [58]

Medication Management (ICD-10-PCS) the Root Type that identifies the application of psychological methods that includes one or more family members to treat an individual with addictive behavior

Medigap a Medicare supplement insurance policy sold by private insurance companies to fill gaps in Part A and Part B coverage [2]

melanoma a tumor of melanocytes [11]

meningitis a contagious, acute inflammation of the pia mater and the arachnoid mater in the brain [17]

meniscectomy shaving, debriding, or excising all of the meniscus [38]

mental disorder a psychological or physical condition that disrupts an individual's personality, mind, and emotions in such a way that it affects the ability to function and interact with others [18]

mesh prosthesis/insertion the repair of weak tissues by inserting a mesh or other prosthesis to strengthen them [46]

metabolism the processes of digestion, elimination, breathing, blood circulation, and maintaining body temperature [10]

metastasize to spread and invade organs other than that of origin [5]

metastatic bone disease (MBD) the invasion of a bone by cancer that begins in another organ [12]

method (ICD-10-PCS Approach) identifies how the access location is entered to reach an internal body part [52]

MI myocardial infarction [14]

microcephaly having a small head [25]

microscopy the visual examination of small things [48]

middle ear a small, air-filled cavity in the temporal bone that contains the ossicles, three small bones that are critical to the hearing process [20]

middle fossa approach through the incision and partial removal of the bone above the ear [44]

mid-level job a job obtained after two or three years of experience [1]

migraine headache a severe, debilitating headache caused by vasodilation [17]

millicurie the unit of measurement for radiopharmaceutical drugs [29]

minimally invasive (procedure) a procedure performed using only natural body openings, needles, or small incisions [32]

misadventure an error during a medical or surgical procedure [8]

miscellaneous code a code that allows providers to immediately bill insurances for a service or item as soon as the FDA approves its use, even though there is no permanent or temporary code that describes it [29]

mitral valve prolapse (MVP) a disorder in which the two leaflets that compose the valve fall backward into the left atrium, resulting in regurgitation; also called click murmur syndrome or Barlow's syndrome [14]

mitral valve the valve that controls blood flow from the left atrium to the left ventricle [14]

mitral valve stenosis a narrowing of the valve opening, which may be caused by calcification, as often occurs with the aortic valve, or rheumatic fever, which often occurs with the mitral valve [14]

M-mode (motion) ultrasound a one-dimensional ultrasonic measurement used to display the movement of a structure [47]

MMR measles, mumps, and rubella vaccine [14]

modality the method of applying a therapeutic/physical treatment [47]

moderate (conscious) sedation use of a mild sedative to relax a patient and pain medicine to relieve pain; the patient stays awake but may not remember the procedure afterward [34]

modified radical mastectomy a simple mastectomy plus removal of axillary lymph nodes but not the pectoralis major muscle [37]

modified radical mastoidectomy a mastoidectomy that includes reconstruction of the eardrum and leaves a few middle ear bones intact [44]

modifier (CPT) a two-digit alphanumeric suffix appended to CPT codes to further describe circumstances [28]

modifier a word that limits the meaning of another [6]

modifying term a descriptive word in the Index that appears indented under the Main Term to further describe a service or procedure; also called subterm [28]

modifying unit (M) a value assigned to each physical status modifier and each qualifying circumstance code to represent the added difficulty of the procedure [34]

Moh's micrographic surgery a multistage procedure in which a malignant lesion is excised in microscopic layers [37]

monitored anesthesia care (MAC) a planned procedure during which a patient undergoes local anesthesia together with sedation and analgesia [34]

Monitoring (ICD-10-PCS) the Root Operation that identifies determining the level of a physiological or physical function repetitively over a period of time [57]

monitoring determining the level of a physiological or physical function repetitively over a period of time [57]

monoamniotic multiple fetuses sharing the same amnion [23]

monochorionic multiple fetuses sharing the same chorion [23]

monoplegia paralysis of one limb [17]

mood disorder an instability of mood; also called affective disorder [18]

morbidity a cause of disease and illness [3]

mortality a cause of death [3]

motility study a study evaluating muscular activity of the esophagus at rest and during swallowing to diagnose esophageal disorders involving motility or causes of heartburn; also called manometry [32]

Motor and/or Nerve Function Assessment (ICD-10-PCS) the Root Type that identifies the measurement of motor, nerve, and related functions [58]

Motor Treatment (ICD-10-PCS) the Root Type that identifies the exercise or activities to increase or facilitate motor function [58]

MPFS Medicare Physician Fee Schedule [28, 33]

MPFSDB Medicare Physician Fee Schedule Database [28, 33]

MRA magnetic resonance angiography [47]

MRI magnetic resonance imaging [47]

MS-DRGs Medicare Severity-adjusted DRGs

multiaxial nature (ICD-10-PCS) the characteristic of ICD-10-PCS whereby each position or character within a code has a designated meaning or purpose [49]

multiplane fixator a fixation device that has a ring-shaped frame that surrounds the treatment site [38]

multiple coding the use of two or more codes that are needed to fully describe a condition [4]

multiple endoscopy rule explains how to assign endoscopy codes when more than one procedure is performed during the same session; states that when two codes from the same code family are reported, 100% is allowed on the first procedure and the allowed amount for second procedure is the *difference* in price between the second code and the endoscopic base code [35, 38]

multiple gestation a pregnancy that involves more than one fetus [23]

multiple organ dysfunction the altered function of more than one organ at the same time requiring medical intervention to stabilize the patient [21]

multiple sclerosis a chronic, progressive disorder of the CNS characterized by muscle impairment due to patches of hardened tissue in the brain or spinal cord [17]

multiple-family group psychotherapy a method of psychotherapy whereby a group of families who share the same problems meets to discuss the issues they are having [32]

muscular system provides for movement of the body as well as the operation of individual organs, maintenance of body posture, and production of heat [12]

musculocutaneous pertaining to both muscles and skin [53]

musculoskeletal (MS) system the skeletal and muscular systems of the body that support the body, protect internal organs, produce blood cells, store minerals, provide movement to the body, maintain body posture, and produce heat [12]

MVP mitral valve prolapse [14]

myalgia a muscle pain [12]

myasthenia a weakness in a muscle [12]

myocardial infarction (MI) the death of heart tissue caused by an interruption to the blood supply; commonly known as a heart attack [14]

myocarditis inflammation of the heart muscle [14]

myocardium the thick, muscular inner layers that contract to pump blood [14]

myoclonic (seizure) a seizure characterized by jerking and twitching in the upper body, arms, or legs [17]

myomectomy removal of uterine fibroid tumors without removing healthy uterine tissue [46]

myosarcoma a malignant tumor in a muscle [12]

myositis inflammation of a muscle [12]

myringectomy excision of the eardrum [44]

myringoplasty repair of the tympanic membrane, involving the drumhead and donor area, usually with a graft of living tissue such as fat or fascia; also called tympanoplasty [44]

myringotomy drainage of fluid or pus from the eardrum [44]

N

narcolepsy a condition characterized by brief, sudden attacks of deep sleep [17]

Narcosynthesis (ICD-10-PCS) the Root Type that identifies the administration of intravenous barbiturates in order to release suppressed or repressed thoughts [58]

National Center for Health Statistics (NCHS) the organization that adapted ICD-10 for use in the United States [3]

National Correct Coding Initiative (NCCI) a set of coding rules published by the Centers for Medicare and Medicaid Services that identifies pairs of codes that normally cannot be reported together; implemented to control improper coding leading to inappropriate payment [33]

national drug codes (NDCs) a code set that identifies the manufacturer, product, and package size of all drugs and biologics recognized by the Food and Drug Administration (FDA) [1]

National Uniform Billing Committee (NUBC) the entity that maintains the UB-04 and is chaired by the American Hospital Association, consisting of representatives from more than 15 healthcare industry groups [49]

native (vessel) a patient's original blood vessel [14]

NCCI National Correct Coding Initiative [33]

neck (of bone) area between the proximal epiphysis and the shaft [12]

neck dissection excising lymph nodes and surrounding tissue from the neck during a thyroidectomy [36]

neonatal intensive care unit (NICU) a section of a hospital that treats newborns with serious conditions [24]

neonatal mortality death before 29 days of age [24]

neonate an infant during the first 28 days of life; also called a newborn [24]

neoplasm an abnormal growth of new tissue [5]

neoplastic fracture a fragility fracture due to a neoplastic disease [12]

nephrectomy the partial or complete removal of a kidney [33, 45]

nephritic syndrome a collection of disorders affecting the kidneys, characterized by nonpurulent inflammatory glomerular disorders that allow proteins and red blood cells to pass into the urine, resulting in proteinuria and hematuria (*blood in the urine*) [22]

nephrolithotomy incision of the kidney to remove a calculus [45]

nephron the functioning part of each kidney that filters waste from the blood [22]

nephropathy disease of the kidneys [10]

nephroplasty surgical repair of a kidney [33]

nephroptosis downward placement of a kidney from its normal location [22]

nephrorrhaphy suture of a kidney wound or injury [33]

nephroscopy visual examination of a kidney with an endoscope [33, 45]

nephrostomy catheter a catheter inserted through an existing nephrostomy [45]

nephrostomy the creation of an opening in a kidney with percutaneous catheter insertion, with imaging guidance [45]

nephrotic syndrome a collection of disorders affecting the kidneys, characterized by proteinuria but not hematuria [22]

nephrotomy incision into a kidney [33]

nerve block the introduction or injection of an anesthetic agent [42]

nervous system the body system that directs the body's response to internal and external stimuli and coordinates the activities of other organ systems [17]

neurectomy the excision of a nerve [42, 52]

neurodevelopmental disorder a condition that results from impaired development of the nervous system during infancy or childhood [18]

neuroendoscopy the use of an endoscope to visualize the CNS [42]

neurofibroma a benign tumor of nerve fibers and connective tissue [42]

neuron a cluster of nerve cells [17]

neuropathy a disease of the nerves [10]

neuroplasty any of a variety of surgical procedures to repair or alter a nerve [42]

neuroplegia the paralysis of a nerve [17]

neurostimulator procedures the implantation of electrodes under the skin; the removal or revision of spinal electrodes, plates, or paddles; the insertion, replacement, revision, or removal of a spinal pulse generator or receiver [42]

neurotomy incision into a nerve [42]

neutropenia a decrease in neutrophils [15]

new patient (NP) a patient who has not previously received services from a particular physician or group of physicians in the same specialty or subspecialty [31]

newborn ABO incompatibility an infant with blood type A or B affected by comingling of blood from a mother with blood type O [24]

newborn apnea a condition in which an infant stops breathing [24]

newborn birth status a code that identifies the location of a birth, the delivery method, and the number of multiples [24]

newborn clinically significant condition a condition of newborns that requires clinical evaluation, therapeutic treatment, diagnostic procedures, extended length of hospital stay (LOS), and increased nursing care or monitoring or presents implications for future healthcare needs [24]

newborn Rh incompatibility an Rh-positive infant affected by comingling of blood with an Rh-negative mother [24]

newborn see *neonate* [24]

NF nursing facility [31]

Nissen fundoplication a procedure in which the upper part of the stomach is wrapped around the lower esophageal sphincter [35]

nonatopic (asthma) asthma that is not due to allergens [16]

nonautologous from a source other than a patient, such as cadaver or animal [14]

nonbiological a grafted vessel from a synthetic source [14]

nondisplaced (fracture) a traumatic fracture in which the fragments of bone remain properly aligned [13]

nonessential modifier (ICD-10-CM) a word included in the default description of a code and does not need to be present in the medical record in order to use the code [4]

Nonimaging Nuclear Medicine Assay (ICD-10-PCS) the Root Type that identifies the introduction of radioactive materials into the body for the study of body fluids and blood elements by the detection of radioactive emissions [58]

nonimaging nuclear medicine assay the introduction of radioactive materials into the body for the study of body fluids and blood elements by the detection of radioactive emissions [58]

Nonimaging Nuclear Medicine Probe (ICD-10-PCS) the Root Type that identifies the introduction of radioactive materials into the body for the study of distribution and fate of certain substances by the detection of radioactive emissions from an external source [58]

nonimaging nuclear medicine probe the introduction of radioactive materials into the body for the study of distribution and fate of certain substances by the detection of radioactive emissions from an external source [58]

Nonimaging Nuclear Medicine Uptake (ICD-10-PCS) the Root Type that identifies the introduction of radioactive materials into the body for measurements of organ function, from the detection of radioactive emissions [58]

nonimaging nuclear medicine uptake the introduction of radioactive materials into the body for measurements of organ function, from the detection of radioactive emissions [58]

nonindwelling (catheter) includes two types of catheters that are not left in the bladder: a condom catheter placed outside the body to catch urine or a straight catheter inserted into the bladder only to drain the urine then removed; also called an external catheter [45]

noninvasive (procedure) a procedure performed without puncturing the skin [32]

nonpressure ulcer a breakdown of skin that is not the result of prolonged pressure [11]

nonselective catheter placement the insertion of a catheter that remains in the accessed vessel or the aorta [39]

non-ST elevation MI (NSTEMI) a myocardial infarction in which the ST segment on an EKG is not elevated, indicating that a vessel is only partially blocked [14]

nontoxic goiter an enlargement of the thyroid that is not associated with overproduction of thyroid hormone or malignancy [10]

nontransmural see *subendocardial (infarction)* [14]

nonunion the failure of the ends of fractured bone segments to reunite [12]

normal birth weight a birth weight of 2,500 grams (5 pounds, 8 ounces) to 4,000 grams (8 pounds, 13 ounces) [24]

normal spontaneous vaginal birth (NSVB) a vaginal delivery without mechanical, pharmacologic, or medical assistance [23]

normal spontaneous vaginal delivery the birth of an infant through the vagina, without the use of drugs or techniques to induce labor, without forceps, vacuum extraction, or cesarean delivery [46]

novel influenza A a class of viruses that normally circulate in animals and may infect humans, such as avian flu and H1N1 [16]

NST nonstress test [46]

NSTEMI non-ST elevation myocardial infarction [14]

NSVB normal spontaneous vaginal birth [23]

NUBC National Uniform Billing Committee [49]

nuchal cord the condition of the umbilical cord becoming wrapped around the neck of a fetus [23]

nucleus pulposus a gelatinous substance that comprises the center of a disc and provides cushioning [42]

nursing facility (NF) a residential facility that provides professional medical and nursing care; formerly known as a skilled nursing facility (SNF)

nutritional anemia an anemia due to malabsorption or poor dietary intake of iron, folate, and/or vitamin B$_{12}$ [15]

O

observation extended monitoring that may require an overnight stay but does not meet the requirements for a formal inpatient admission [1]

obstetric history prior pregnancies, complications, and their outcomes [2]

obstructed labor a labor in which the fetus cannot progress into the birth canal, despite adequate uterine contractions, due to a physical blockage [23]

obstructive uropathy the inability of urine to flow [45]

occipitoanterior (OA) the presentation of a fetus in which the back of the baby's head is slightly off center in the pelvis, with the back of the head toward the mother's left thigh [23]

Occlusion (ICD-10-PCS) the Root Operation that identifies completely closing an orifice or the lumen of a tubular Body Part [51]

occlusion a blockage [14]

occlusive disease a buildup of plaque or a blood clot [32]

ocular globe the eyeball [19]

ocular implant the insertion of a small sphere into the orbit where the natural eye used to be [43]

OD *oculus dexter* (right eye) [43]

Office of the Inspector General (OIG) a department within the federal government that investigates cases of fraud and imposes monetary penalties on providers who are found guilty [2]

Official Guidelines for Coding and Reporting (OGCR) rules that provide information and direction in identifying the ICD-9-CM and ICD-10-CM diagnoses and ICD-10-PCS procedures to be reported [4]

old (healed) MI an MI more than four weeks old, as defined by ICD-10-CM [14]

olfactory the sense of smell [17]

olive-tip catheter a ureteral catheter with an olive-shaped end, used to dilate a constricted ureter [45]

omental flap the removal of part of the omentum with blood vessel supply intact [35]

omit code (ICD-9-CM, Volume 3) an instruction that appears in the Index to indicate when a code should *not* be used because it is included in another, more definitive procedure [26]

omphalitis an infection of the umbilical stump in a newborn, usually presenting as superficial cellulitis [24]

oncologist a physician who specializes in the diagnosis and treatment of tumors [5]

one-to-many mapping a single code in ICD-9-CM has several possible equivalents in ICD-10-CM or vice versa [27]

oophorectomy the excision of an ovary [46]

oophoroscopy the visual examination of an ovary [46]

open (fracture) a fracture in which the bone breaks through the skin [13]

Open (ICD-10-PCS) the Approach that identifies an incision is made through the skin and subcutaneous tissue [50]

open heart surgery involves exposing the heart through a 30-cm (6 to 8 inches) incision in the chest wall that requires cutting through the sternum [39]

open wound a wound in which the underlying tissue is exposed to the air [13]

operating endoscope a scope equipped with irrigation and suction channels, as well as channels for inserting special instruments, such as biopsy forceps, to obtain tissue samples [41]

operating microscope a specially designed microscope used to assist in the performance of delicate microsurgical procedures, such as operations on the eye, middle ear, or nerve [43, 44]

operative report a detailed narrative description prepared by a physician after completing a procedure, which describes the details of what was done; also called a procedure report [33, 51]

opportunistic infection a disease that attacks those with weakened immune systems but does not develop in those with healthy immune systems [21]

OPPS outpatient prospective payment system [28]

optic nerve cranial nerve II [19]

optional surgery a type of surgery that provides a personal benefit but provides no medical benefit, such as a cosmetic face lift or breast augmentation; rarely covered by insurance [33]

oral pertaining to the mouth [44]

orbital cavity the bony structure around the eye, commonly known as the eye socket [19]

orbital implant the insertion of glass, plastic, or acrylic under an ocular implant [43]

orbital tumor a benign or malignant tumor in the eye socket or tissues that surround the eyeball; sometimes originates from the surrounding paranasal sinuses, brain, or nasal cavity [42]

orifice an opening [54]

origin the point at which a muscle is attached [12]

Original Medicare hospital insurance that covers a specific list of services for inpatient hospital care, skilled nursing facilities, hospice, and home healthcare; also called Part A [2]

orthosis an orthopedic appliance or apparatus used to support, align, prevent, or correct deformities or to improve the function of movable parts of the body [58]

OS *oculus sinister* (left eye) [43]

osseointegrated implant a hearing implant that is integrated with bone [44]

osseous pertaining to a bone [12]

ossicles a part of the middle ear that amplifies vibrations and transmits them to the inner ear [20]

osteoarthritis an inflammation of a bone and joint [12]

osteoporosis the thinning of bone tissue and loss of bone density [12]

osteoporotic fracture a fragility fracture in a person with osteoporosis [12]

osteosarcoma a malignant tumor in a bone [12]

ostomy an artificial opening between a hollow organ and the skin [7]

other fracture a fragility fracture caused by a disease other than osteoporosis or neoplasm; any other type of pathological fracture [12]

Other Procedures (ICD-10-PCS) the Root Operation that identifies methodologies that attempt to remediate or cure a disorder or disease [57]

Other Radiation (ICD-10-PCS) the Modality that identifies radiation therapy modalities not otherwise identified [58]

otitis media (OM) an infection of the middle ear [20]

otorhinolaryngological pertaining to the ear, nose, and throat [32]

OU *oculus uterque* (each eye) [43]

outpatient encounter an interaction with a patient who has not been formally admitted to a healthcare institution [1]

outpatient prospective payment system (OPPS) Medicare's payment system for outpatient hospitals, which pays a set amount for a service or procedure based on a specific classification [28]

oval window a thin membrane that covers the opening to the inner ear and passes vibrations to the cochlea [20]

ovary the gland in which eggs are produced in females [22]

overcoding coding for a more complex diagnosis or procedure than is documented [2]

overlapping lesion contiguous sites where a tumor continues from one site to an adjacent one without interruption [5]

P

pacemaker a small electronic device that is implanted in the chest to correct arrhythmia by speeding up, slowing down, smoothing out, or coordinating the heartbeat [14]

pacemaker insertion placement under the skin of the chest or abdomen a small device with wires connected to the heart chambers that transmit low-energy electrical pulses to control heart rhythm [39]

Packing (ICD-10-PCS) the Root Operation that identifies putting material in a body region or orifice [57]

packing putting material in a body region or orifice [57]

PACU postoperative anesthesia care unit [34]

PAD peripheral artery disease [10]

pancreatectomy the surgical removal of all or part of the pancreas [35]

pancreaticoduodenectomy the surgical removal of parts of the pancreas, duodenum, common bile duct, and, if required, portions of the stomach [35]

pancreatitis inflammation of the pancreas [9]

pancytopenia an abnormal reduction in the number of all types of blood cells: red, white, and platelets [15]

pandemic a disease outbreak that spreads to multiple continents [21]

papilla a small vascular protrusion of connective tissue or skin [43]

papulosquamous disorders papules and scales [11]

para (P) the number of pregnancies resulting in a fetus of viable gestational age (20 weeks), regardless of whether the fetus was alive at birth [23]

paracentesis a surgical puncture of a body cavity to remove ascites [35]

paraesophageal hernia repair a procedure in which the diaphragm is repaired using sutures or mesh; part of the stomach may be wrapped around the esophagus [35]

paranasal sinus an air-filled chamber, or space, inside the skull and face bones; also called accessory sinus [41]

paranoia a mental condition of delusions of persecution [18]

parasite a plant or animal that lives in or on another living organism, or host, and often causes damage to the host; also called helminth [21]

parathyroid autotransplantation the surgical removal of the four parathyroid glands and their transplantation into a muscle in the neck or forearm [36]

parathyroidectomy the surgical removal of all or part of the parathyroid glands [36]

paravaginal adjacent to the vagina or part of the vagina [46]

parent code a code whose description is left-justified and begins with a capital letter; also called standalone code [28]

parenteral nutrition providing nutrients intravenously because the body is unable to take in nutrients orally or by other methods [29]

parietal pericardium the outer layer of the pericardium [14]

paring the use of a scalpel, blade, or curette to scrape away tissue; also referred to as cutting or curettement [37]

Parkinson disease (PD) a degenerative disease that affects muscle control and coordination, usually occurring in midlife [17]

parkinsonian see *parkinsonism* [17]

parkinsonism a combination of conditions in which dementia is diagnosed first, followed later by an additional diagnosis of Parkinson disease; also called parkinsonian dementia [17]

Part A (Medicare) hospital insurance that covers a specific list of services for inpatient hospital care, skilled nursing facilities, hospice, and home healthcare; also called Original Medicare [2]

Part B (Medicare) the portion of Medicare that covers a specific list of physician services, outpatient hospital care, and home healthcare [2]

Part C (Medicare) an optional replacement of Part A and Part B that is offered by private health insurance companies; also called Medicare Advantage [2]

Part D (Medicare) prescription drug coverage offered by private insurance companies through contracts with Medicare; provides limited benefits for prescription drugs [2]

partial (seizure) see *focal (seizure)* [17]

partial mastectomy (lumpectomy, tylectomy) the removal of only enough breast tissue to ensure that the margins of the specimen are free of malignant cells [37]

partial thickness burn a burn that causes damage to the epidermis and part of the dermis [11]

partial thyroid lobectomy the excision of less than two-thirds of one lobe of the thyroid gland [36]

partum birth [23]

parturition see *childbirth* [23]

past, family, and social history (PFSH) a review of a patient's past experience with illness, injury, treatment, and operations; a review of a patient's family's medical history; and a review of a patient's social history, including current and past activities

patch testing applying an allergen to the skin to observe the reaction [11]

patent foramen ovale an opening in the septum between the two atria of the heart [25]

pathologic fracture a fracture caused by disease rather than trauma [12]

pathologist a physician who identifies diseases by studying cells under a microscope [5]

pathology the study of the abnormal [48]

patient type describes whether the patient is new or established [30]

patient-controlled analgesia (PCA) a method of pain control that patients can administer in response to the level of pain experienced [34]

payers insurance companies or public programs that pay for healthcare services [1]

PBT proton beam treatment [47]

PCA patient-controlled analgesia [34]

PCS OGCR PCS Official Guidelines for Coding and Reporting [49]

PCS Procedure Coding System; used in this text as shorthand for ICD-10-PCS [3]

PD Parkinson disease [17]; peritoneal dialysis [22, 32]

PE physical examination [2]

PEG percutaneous endoscopic gastrostomy [35]

pelvic exenteration excision of the bladder, urethra, ureters, lymph nodes, prostate/vagina, uterus, colon, and rectum; may also include a hysterectomy and resecting the rectum and colon [45]

pelvic girdle pain (PGP) a pain at the back of the pelvis [23]

pelvic inflammatory disease (PID) inflammation of the female reproductive tract above the cervix [22]

pemphigus an autoimmune disease that erupts in blisters [11]

penetrating keratoplasty (PKP) the removal of the entire cornea and transplantation of a full-thickness cornea [43]

penetrating wound see *puncture wound* [13]

penile in or through the penis [45]

penis the external male organ that carries urine and semen out of the body [22]

perceptual disturbance the misinterpretation of surroundings or events [18]

Percutaneous (ICD-10-PCS) the Approach that identifies the skin is punctured or a very small incision is made to access a site, but a full-length incision is not made [50]

Percutaneous Endoscopic (ICD-10-PCS) the Approach that identifies a surgeon makes several, usually two to four, small incisions, approximately one-half to one inch in length, and accesses the operative site with an endoscope [50]

percutaneous endoscopic gastrostomy (PEG) a procedure in which a tube is passed into a patient's stomach through the abdominal wall [35]

percutaneous umbilical blood sampling (PUBS) see *cordocentesis*

Pereyra procedure elevation of the bladder by attaching it to abdominal fascia [46]

perforation the cutting or puncturing of the wall or membrane of an internal organ or structure [13]

Performance (ICD-10-PCS) the Root Operation that identifies completely taking over a physiological function by extracorporeal means [57]

performance completely taking over a physiological function by extracorporeal means [57]

pericarditis an inflammation of the pericardial sac that surrounds the heart [14]

pericardium a double-walled sac filled with fluid, which is the outer layer [14]

perinatal condition a condition that develops before birth or during the first 28 days after birth, but excludes malformations, deformations, and chromosomal abnormalities [24]

perinatal period the time before birth that continues through the 28th day following birth [24]

perinatal relating to the time period before birth that continues through the 28th day following birth [23]

perineal surrounding the perineum

perineoplasty repair of the tissues of the perineum [46]

perineum the area between the anus and external genitalia [45]

peripartum the period comprising the last month of pregnancy to five months' postpartum [23]

peripheral artery disease the damage to arteries outside the heart resulting in decreased blood flow to the limbs [10, 14]

peripheral nervous system (PNS) consists of the 12 nerves that radiate out from the brain and the 31 pairs of nerves that radiate from the spinal cord to all other areas of the body [17]

periprosthetic capsulectomy the removal of a breast implant and the entire contracture capsule surrounding the breast implant [37]

perirenal relating to tissues surrounding the kidney [45]

peritoneal dialysis (PD) a type of dialysis in which the peritoneal membrane is used to filter the blood [22, 32]

peritoneal membrane the lining of the abdomen [22]

permanent national code a code that all U.S. providers and insurances can use for billing and statistical purposes [29]

pernicious anemia an anemia due to insufficient absorption of vitamin B_{12} [15]

personal history a condition a patient had in the past, was removed or resolved, and is no longer being treated, but has the potential for recurrence and therefore may require continued monitoring [5]

personal injury protection (PIP) a payment made by automobile insurance policies to pay for medical expenses incurred during an automobile accident [2]

personality disorder persistent, inflexible patterns of behavior that affect interpersonal relationships [18]

pessary insertion/fitting the evaluation and placement of a rubber, silicone, or plastic device into the vagina to support surrounding structures [46]

PET positron emission tomography [47]

petit mal (seizure) a type of seizure characterized by muscle twitching or jerking for several seconds [17]

petrous apicectomy excision of the petrous, including radical resection of the entire mastoid part of the posterior temporal bone [44]

PFSH past, family, and social history [31]

phacoemulsification destruction, usually with ultrasound, of a natural lens, which is then suctioned out of the eye [43]

pharmacoresistant resistant to medication [17]

Pharmacotherapy (ICD-10-PCS) the Root Type that identifies the use of replacement medications for the treatment of addiction

pharyngitis sore throat; inflammation of the throat [16]

pharynx the throat [16]

Pheresis (ICD-10-PCS) the Root Operation that identifies extracorporeal separation of blood products [57]

pheresis extracorporeal separation of blood products [57]

photochemotherapy treatment using drugs and light [32]

photocoagulation the use of a laser to seal tears [43]

Phototherapy (ICD-10-PCS) the Root Operation that identifies extracorporeal treatment by light rays [57]

phototherapy extracorporeal treatment by light rays [57]

physical examination (PE) a hands-on evaluation of a patient's vital signs, physical functions, and organ systems relevant to the chief complaint [2]

physical status score a value that identifies a patient's health status at the time anesthesia begins, on a scale of 1 through 5 [34]

physical therapy noninvasive treatment to correct a musculoskeletal problem [1]

physician office an outpatient clinic at which physicians evaluate and manage new or existing health problems and provide preventive care services [1]

physician office laboratory (POL) a physician office that performs a limited number of laboratory tests in the office [48]

physis the growth plate near the end of a long bone [13]

pigmentation disorder damage to unhealthy melanin cells that give color to the skin [11]

PIH pregnancy-induced hypertension [23]

pinna the visible part of the ear, which collects sound waves; also called auricle [20]

pituitary tumor an abnormal growth in the pituitary gland that is usually benign [42]

pityriasis rough, dry scales [11]

PKP penetrating keratoplasty [43]

place of occurrence (ICD-9-CM, ICD-10-CM) a category of external cause codes that describe where an injury occurred, such as a public street or a single-family home [8]

place of service (POS) the location of the facility where a physician provides an evaluation and management service, such as an office, hospital, or nursing facility [31]

placenta previa a condition in which the placenta partially or fully covers the cervix, posing a risk that it may separate from the wall of the uterus during labor [23]

placenta the organ that allows for the exchange of oxygen, nutrients, and waste between the fetus and mother [23]

placental infarction a scarring of the placenta due to an inadequate blood supply [23]

Plain Radiography (ICD-10-PCS) the Root Type that identifies the planar (flat, single plane) display of an image developed from the capture of external ionizing radiation on a photographic or photoconductive plate [58]

plain radiography the planar (flat, single plane) display of an image developed from the capture of external ionizing radiation on a photographic or photoconductive plate [58]

plan the treatment that was or will be provided to address a patient's symptoms [2]

Planar Nuclear Medicine Imaging (ICD-10-PCS) the Root Type that identifies the introduction of radioactive materials into the body for single-plane display of images developed from the capture of radioactive emissions [58]

planar nuclear medicine imaging the introduction of radioactive materials into the body for single-plane display of images developed from the capture of radioactive emissions [58]

plaque a buildup of cholesterol inside the wall of blood vessels [14]

plasma clear fluid [15]

plastic repair introitus restoration of the vaginal opening to its original size [46]

plethysmography recording of volume [32]

pleuracentesis the withdrawal of fluid from the pleural cavity/thoracic cavity [40]

pleural effusion an abnormal amount of fluid around the lung [16]

pleural tap the withdrawal of air or fluid from the pleural space using a needle or tube [41]

pleurisy inflammation of the lining of the lungs and thoracic cavity with oozing of fluid or fibrinous material into the pleural cavity [16]

pleurodesis the use of an irritant to create inflammation within the pleural space to cause the two pleura to adhere together [41]

pleurotomy an incision into the pleural cavity/thoracic cavity [40]

pneumocentesis the withdrawal of fluid from a lung [40]

pneumoconiosis an abnormal condition of the lung caused by the inhalation of dust particles, such as coal dust (anthracosis), asbestos (asbestosis), iron dust (siderosis), or quartz (silicosis) [16]

pneumonectomy the surgical excision of an entire lung [41]

pneumonia an inflammatory condition of the lung in which the alveoli and air spaces fill with fluid; caused by a bacteria, virus, fungus, or chemical irritant [16]

pneumonolysis the separation of the parietal pleura from the fascia of the chest wall [41]

pneumothorax a collection of air between the chest wall and lungs, which may cause the lung to collapse [16, 41]

pneumotomy an incision into the lung [40]

PNS peripheral nervous system [17]

poisoning the improper use of a substance that causes an undesired physical response [13]

polycystic kidney disease a condition in which numerous cysts occupy much of the kidney tissue [22]

polycythemia an abnormal increase in the number of circulating red blood cells [15]

polydactyly the presence of many fingers or toes [25]

polynephritis an acute or chronic infection of the renal medulla and upper urinary tract as a result of untreated cystitis; also called pyelonephritis [22]

polypectomy the surgical removal of a polyp(s) [35]

polysomnography multiple recordings of sleep [32]

POS place of service [31]

position (patient) the position in which a patient is arranged for surgery (e.g., supine, dorsal recumbent, prone) [33]

Positron Emission Tomography (PET) (ICD-10-PCS) the Root Type that identifies the introduction of radioactive materials into the body for three-dimensional display of images developed from the simultaneous capture, 180 degrees apart, of radioactive emissions [58]

positron emission tomography (PET) the introduction of radioactive materials into the body for three-dimensional display of images developed from the simultaneous capture, 180 degrees apart, of radioactive emissions [47, 58]

postauricular behind the ear [44]

posteroanterior from back to front [47]

postnatal after birth [23]

postoperative anesthesia care unit (PACU) an area where a patient is taken after surgery is complete to recover from the surgical procedure and the effects of anesthesia [34]

postpartum depression a moderate to severe depression after giving birth [23]

postpartum hemorrhage (PPH) an excessive amount of bleeding following delivery [23]

postpartum psychosis the sudden dramatic onset of psychotic symptoms after giving birth, often occurring in patients with bipolar disorder [23]

postpartum see *puerperium* [23]

postpartum wound infection a bacterial infection of a cesarean delivery wound [23]

postprocedural bleeding bleeding that occurs after a surgical procedure; also called postoperative bleeding or hemorrhage [56]

postterm pregnancy a pregnancy with between 40 and 42 completed weeks of gestation [23]

PPH postpartum hemorrhage [23]

PPMP provider-performed microscopy procedure [48]

PPS prospective payment system [49]

Prader-Willi syndrome a genetic disorder due to a deletion of paternal chromosome 15; characterized by short stature, mental retardation, muscle weakness, abnormally small hands and feet, nonfunctioning gonads, and uncontrolled appetite, leading to extreme obesity [25]

preauthorization prior authorization or approval of elective surgery by an insurance company [33]

precerebral located outside of the brain [14]

prediabetes blood glucose concentrations are higher than normal but not yet high enough to be diagnosed as diabetes [10]

preeclampsia a metabolic disorder of pregnancy that develops after the 20th week and involves gestational hypertension and proteinuria [23]

preexisting diabetes diabetes that is diagnosed in a woman before she becomes pregnant [23]

preexisting hypertension hypertension that is diagnosed in a woman before she becomes pregnant [23]

preferred provider an exclusive network of private health insurance companies and self-insured plans [2]

pregnancy a normal, temporary condition that occurs in the female body, beginning at the time of conception and ending with the birth of a fetus [23]

pregnancy-induced hypertension (PIH) see *gestational hypertension* [23]

premature rupture of membranes (PROM) the rupture of the amniotic sac and chorion more than an hour before the onset of labor; may also be called prelabor rupture of membranes [23]

prenatal the time period from conception to the beginning of labor; also called the prepartum, antepartum, or antenatal period [23]

prepartum see *prenatal* [23]

prepayment edit a set of claims processing rules in which claims are electronically scanned for compliance before the payer accepts them into the claims processing system [28, 33]

presumptive drug class screening a qualitative test that identifies the possible use or nonuse of a drug or drug class [48]

preterm pregnancy, delivery, or labor a pregnancy with less than 37 completed weeks of gestation [23]

primary (malignant neoplasm) a tumor in which malignant cells break through the epithelial membrane into an organ [5]

primary intention healing wound closure performed with sutures, staples, or adhesive tape or glue [37]

principal diagnosis as defined by the Uniform Hospital Data Discharge Set (UHDDS), the "condition established after study to be chiefly responsible for occasioning the admission of the patient to the hospital for care" [4]

principal procedure a procedure that was performed for definitive treatment most related to the principal diagnosis, rather than one performed for diagnostic or exploratory purposes, or was necessary to take care of a complication [49, 52]

private health insurance coverage for healthcare services offered by private corporations [2]

procedure a service that healthcare professionals provide to patients [1]

procedure report a report prepared by a physician after completing a procedure that describes the details of what was done; also called an operative report [51]

process a nodule or projection of a bone [42]

productive cough a cough with sputum [16]

products of conception encompasses all components of pregnancy, including the embryo, fetus, amnion, placenta, and umbilical cord [57]

professional component part of a radiology code; covers the cost of a radiologist supervising a technician and interpreting the results [30]

prognosis future knowledge; the expected course of the disease [5]

progress note the record of a specific patient encounter [2]

prolonged pregnancy a pregnancy with more than 42 completed weeks of gestation [23]

PROM premature rupture of membranes [23]

prompt pay a law that requires insurance companies to process claims within a specific period of time, such as 30 or 45 days [2]

prophylactic prevention of the spread of disease or infection [7]

prospective payment system (PPS) a standard payment rate is predetermined based on the average amount of staff, supplies, and other resources typically used and assigned to each DRG [49]

prostate the part of the male genital system that secretes fluid to nourish the sperm [22]

prostatectomy removal of the prostate gland, including possible biopsy or removal of the lymph nodes [45]

prostate-specific antigen (PSA) a blood test used to screen for prostate cancer [22]

prostatic intraepithelial neoplasia (PIN) neoplastic changes in the epithelial cells of the prostate ducts showing some features of cancer, but is not invasive; a potential precursor of carcinoma or adenocarcinoma [22]

prostatomy an incision into the prostate [45]

prosthesis an artificial substitute for a missing body part [58]

prosthetic catheter a urethral catheter with a sharp bend near the intake; used to navigate past obstructions in the urinary tract; also called elbowed catheter [45]

protection helps prevent invasion by pathogens, mechanical harm, and loss of fluids and electrolytes [11]

proteinemia protein in the blood [10]

proteinuria protein in the urine [10]

proton beam treatment (PBT) delivery the use of noninvasive electromagnetic radiation to treat both in situ benign and malignant tumors [47]

protozoa one-celled organisms, more complex than bacteria, that use other living things as a source of food and a place to live [21]

provider-performed microscopy procedure (PPMP) moderate-complexity tests that require use of a microscope [48]

proximal epiphysis the rounded end of a bone that is closest to the trunk [12]

proximal toward the center of the body [35]

Pseudomonas aeruginosa (P. aeruginosa) the most common Gram-negative bacterium that can cause disease in humans and animals

psoriasis round, red patches covered with white scales [11]

psychiatric diagnostic interview an interview with a patient whereby the provider assesses the patient's mental status by reviewing the patient's medical history, asking the patient a series of questions, and communicating with family members and other providers involved in the patient's care to determine the patient's diagnosis [32]

psychoactive substance a substance that has the ability to alter behavior, impair judgment, or create medical problems [18]

Psychological Tests (ICD-10-PCS) the Root Type that identifies the administration and interpretation of standardized psychological tests and measurement instruments for the assessment of psychological function [58]

psychometry measurement/testing of the mind [32]

psychomotor (seizure) see *complex partial (seizure)* [17]

psychotherapy a method of using nonphysical techniques, such as talking, interpreting, listening, rewarding, and role playing, to treat disorders [18, 32]

psychotic disorders delusions and hallucinations [18]

public health lab a lab operated by state and local health departments to diagnose disease and protect the public from health threats, such as outbreaks of infectious diseases and environmental hazards [48]

PUBS percutaneous umbilical blood sampling [46]

puerperal mastitis the inflammation or infection of the mammary gland in the breast during the postpartum period [23]

puerperal see *puerperium* [23]

puerperium the six-week period following childbirth in which the female reproductive organs return to the prepregnant state; also called puerperal or postpartum [23]

pull-through process whereby a surgeon removes the diseased portion of an organ and connects the healthy segment to the adjacent organ [35]

pulmonary circulation occurs between the heart and the lungs; carries deoxygenated blood from the heart to the lungs, where it is replenished with oxygen, then back to the heart [14]

pulmonary edema an abnormal accumulation of fluid in the lungs, especially the alveoli, resulting in dyspnea [16]

pulmonary function test a diagnostic test that measures air flow into and out of the lungs, lung volumes, and gas exchange between the lungs and blood [16]

pulmonary valve the valve that controls the blood flow from the right ventricle to the pulmonary artery [14]

puncture wound a wound caused by a sharply pointed object passing through the skin into the

underlying tissues; also called penetrating wound [13]

pupil the opening in the iris that dilates and constricts [43]

Purkinje fiber the cardiac muscle that rapidly transmits impulses from the atrioventricular node to the ventricles [14]

purpura small hemorrhages in the skin [15]

purulent otitis media an infection of the middle ear, usually bacterial, involving the discharge of pus [20]

push technique a one-time, rapid injection of medication into the bloodstream [32]

pyelonephritis the acute or chronic infection of the renal medulla and upper urinary tract as a result of untreated cystitis, also called polynephritis [22]

pyeloplasty repair of the renal pelvis [45]

pyelotomy an incision into the renal pelvis [45]

pyogenic arthritis an infectious arthritis in which pus is formed during the disease process [12]

pyothorax pus in the chest [16]

Q

quadriplegia paralysis of all limbs [17]

qualified a diagnosis that is limited or uncertain [6]

Qualifier Character 7 in an ICD-10-PCS code; describes additional information about the procedure [49]

qualifier a word that limits the meaning of another [6]

qualitative test a test performed to detect the presence of a substance in a specimen [48]

query to ask [1]

Qui Tam a provision of the FCA that mandates a financial reward to whistleblowers, those who turn in violators [2]

R

RAC Recovery Audit Contractor [2]

radial keratotomy the flattening of the cornea by making a series of incisions in a radial pattern, resembling the spokes of a wheel [43]

radiation disorders damage to the skin resulting from exposure to radiation [11]

radiation oncologist a physician who provides cancer treatment through radiation [47]

radical lymphadenectomy removal of lymph nodes and nearby structures [40]

radical mastectomy removal of the breast, pectoralis major and minor muscles, axillary lymph nodes, and associated skin and subcutaneous tissue [37]

radical mastoidectomy removal of the entire mastoid, tympanum, middle ear, and possibly the mastoid part of the posterior temporal bone [44]

radiologic guidance use of a radiological modality to visualize access to an anatomic site in real time; also called guided imagery [47]

radiology technician a nonphysician staff member who is trained to operate and adjust imaging equipment, explain procedures to patients and answer questions, position patients for imaging, and ensure that a patient's exposure to radiation is limited [47]

radiolucent permits X-rays to pass into and through it, resulting in a darker, shadowy image that shows layers within a structure [47]

radiopaque allows few X-rays to pass through; shows up as a light (white) image using plain radiography and provides a two-dimensional image of the surface [47]

radiopharmaceutical a radioactive material used for therapeutic or diagnostic purposes [47, 58]

radiosurgery a form of radiation therapy that focuses high-power energy on a small area of the body (e.g., Cyberknife, Gamma Knife) [47]

radiotherapy treatment with radiation [58]

rapid strep test (RST) a strep test that produces results within 10 to 20 minutes [48]

RBRVS resource-based relative value scale [28]

RDS respiratory distress syndrome [24]

real-time scan a rapid succession of B-mode images producing a moving video; a two-dimensional ultrasonic scan, with displays of both two-dimensional structures and motion with time [47]

Reattachment (ICD-10-PCS) the Root Operation that identifies putting back in or on all or a portion of a separated Body Part to its normal location or other suitable location [51, 53]

recession cutting muscle from the surface of the eye and reattaching it farther back from the front of the eye to weaken or lengthen the muscle [43]

reconcile comparison of the EOB to the original bill to verify that each service billed was paid in the amount expected [2]

reconstruction a procedure whereby original tissue is replaced with grafted tissue to create a new structure [38]

reconstructive relating to restoring normal function or appearance [37]

recording creating an image of a structure or process [32]

Recovery Audit Contractor (RAC) uses independent contractors to identify improper Medicare payments to healthcare providers and suppliers made on claims of healthcare services provided to Medicare beneficiaries [2]

reducible a hernia that can be corrected by a physician by pushing the tissue back into place [35]

reduction the realignment of bone fragments or segments; also called manipulation [38]

reference lab see *independent clinical lab*

reference range numeric range of typical results in the average population and the levels considered to be high or low, determined by the statistic calculation of two standard deviations [48]

referring physician a provider who requests a consultation for a patient with another physician [31]

reflex sympathetic dystrophy (RSD) a chronic pain syndrome in which an extremity experiences intense burning pain and changes in skin texture and temperature [17]

reflux nephropathy a disease of the kidneys that results from a backward flow of urine into the kidneys [22]

refractory resistant to treatment [17]

regional anesthesia epidural, spinal, and peripheral nerve blocks; blocks pain in an area of the body, such as an arm or leg, and patient feels nothing in that area of the body [34]

regulation the body function that increases and decreases body temperature through constriction and dilation of blood vessels and sweat glands [11]

regurgitation the backward leakage of blood through the opening of the left atrium [14]

rejected claim a claim that is not accepted into an insurance company's computer system for processing due to missing or invalid data [2]

relapse the return of disease after remission [15]

related a symptom, finding, or sign that is connected to a disease but is not integral to it [6]

relative value unit (RVU) a value that identifies the amount of work and expense involved in providing a particular service [28]

Release (ICD-10-PCS) the Root Operation that identifies freeing a Body Part from an abnormal physical constraint by cutting or by the use of force [51, 55]

release a type of soft-tissue repair/reconstruction whereby the tissue is freed from surrounding adhesions so that it can move freely within the tendon sheath [38]

relevant as defined by UHDDS, "all conditions that coexist at the time of admission, that develop subsequently, or that affect the treatment received and/or the length of stay. Diagnoses that relate to an earlier episode which have no bearing on the current hospital stay are to be excluded." [4]

remission blood counts return to normal and bone marrow samples show no sign of disease [15]

remittance advice (RA) a statement that lists all the services the provider billed, which ones were accepted for payment, how much the insurance company will pay, how much the patient owes, and how much will not be paid [2]

Removal (ICD-10-PCS) the Root Operation that identifies taking out or off a device from a Body Part [51, 56]

renal endoscopy endoscopy through an established nephrostomy, pyelostomy, nephrotomy, or pyelotomy [45]

renal pelvis the portion of a kidney where urine collects [22]

renal pertaining to the kidney [43]

renal transplant the implantation of a cadaver or living donor kidney to take over the function of a patient's natural kidney [45]

Repair (ICD-10-PCS) the Root Operation that identifies restoring, to the extent possible, a Body Part to its normal anatomic structure and function [51, 56]

repair a procedure whereby torn or damaged tissue, such as a muscle, is sewn together [38]

repair of oval window or round window closure of an opening with soft tissue such as fat or fascia [44]

repeat cesarean performing a cesarean delivery for a mother who had a cesarean delivery with a previous pregnancy [46]

Replacement (ICD-10-PCS) the Root Operation that identifies putting in or on biological or synthetic material that physically takes the place and/or function of all or a portion of a Body Part [51, 56]

replantation the reattachment of an amputated body member

Reposition (ICD-10-PCS) the Root Operation that identifies moving to its normal location, or other suitable location, all or a portion of a Body Part [51, 53]

reproductive duct a part of the internal genital organs of the male reproductive system [22]

Resection (ICD-10-PCS) the Root Operation that identifies cutting out or off without replacement all of a Body Part [51, 52, 56]

resequenced code (CPT) a code that does not appear in numerical order; identified with the symbol # [28]

reservoir/pump implantation the replacement, implantation, or removal of a subcutaneous reservoir or pump; electronic analysis of programmable implanted pump [42]

resource-based relative value scale (RBRVS) the scale used by Medicare to establish physician reimbursement rates, which are published in the Medicare Physician Fee Schedule (MPFS) [28]

respiratory distress syndrome (RDS) a condition in which the alveolar sacs collapse due to lack of surfactant [24]

respiratory system the system that obtains oxygen from the air and delivers it to the lungs and blood for distribution to tissue cells and removes the gaseous waste product carbon dioxide from the blood and lungs and expels it [16]

Restoration (ICD-10-PCS) the Root Operation that identifies returning, or attempting to return, a physiological function to its original state by extracorporeal means [57]

restoration returning, or attempting to return, a physiological function to its original state by extracorporeal means [57]

Restriction (ICD-10-PCS) the Root Operation that identifies partially closing an orifice or the lumen of a tubular Body Part [51, 54]

retina the innermost layer that contains sensory receptor cells [19]

retinal detachment the separation of the retina from the choroid layer of the eye [19]

retinal pertaining to the retina [43]

retinopathy of prematurity (ROP) the abnormal growth of blood vessels in the eye that can lead to vision loss [24]

retroperitoneal behind the peritoneal membrane that covers the abdominal and pelvic organs [45]

retropubic behind the pubic bone [45]

revascularization the restoration of flow to the coronary vessels that have been obstructed, usually due to occlusive disease [32]

revenue code a four-digit code reported on the UB-04 that identifies a general category of service, such as accommodation, type of ancillary service, pharmacy, or supplies [49]

review of systems (ROS) a list of questions, arranged by organ system, used by physicians to complete a system-by-system review of body functions with a patient [31]

Revision (ICD-10-PCS) the Root Operation that identifies correcting, to the extent possible, a portion of a malfunctioning device or the position of a displaced device [51, 56]

revision mastoidectomy a total mastoidectomy following a previous mastoidectomy that failed to resolve a patient's condition [44]

Rhesus (Rh) incompatibility a condition in which the mother is Rh negative and develops antibodies against a fetus who is Rh positive [23]

rhinoplasty (primary) surgical repair of the nose [41]

rhinoplasty (secondary) a second rhinoplasty that may be more complex than the primary one, including grafts of cartilage, bone, or tissue to reconstruct the nose or repair the nasal septum [41]

rhizotomy interruption of a cranial or spinal nerve root [55]

right atrium the right upper chamber of the heart, which receives blood from the body [14]

right ventricle the right lower chamber of the heart, which ejects blood to the lungs [14]

rigid endoscope an instrument used for endoscopy procedures that consists of a hard tube with a series of prisms and lenses that reflect the image [41]

rod a light-sensitive receptor cell in the retina [19]

Root Operation Character 3 of an ICD-10-PCS code; defines the objective of a procedure [49]

ROP retinopathy of prematurity [24]

ROS review of systems [31]

rotational deformity an abnormal position of the femur or tibia [25]

Roux-en-Y (RNY) a procedure in which the stomach and small bowel are joined using an end-to-side anastomosis [35]

RSD reflex sympathetic dystrophy [17]

RST rapid strep test [48]

RTO return to office [7]

Rule of Nines the division of the body into areas, each of which comprises 9% of the total body surface area [13]

RVU relative value unit [28]

S

SA sinoatrial [14]

saccule a membranous pouch containing serum fluid of the inner ear [20]

salpingectomy excision of a fallopian tube [46]

salpingoscopy visual examination of a fallopian tube [46]

salpingostomy the surgical creation of an opening in a fallopian tube to restore its patency [46]

Salter-Harris classification a system that classifies epiphysis fractures to identify involvement of the growth plate and estimate the prognosis and potential for growth disturbance [13]

sarcoidosis the formation of nodules in the lymph nodes, lungs, bone, and skin [15]

SCC squamous cell carcinoma [11]

schizoaffective disorder a condition characterized by an extended period in which schizophrenia is accompanied by major depressive, manic, or mixed episodes [18]

schizoid of childhood a condition characterized by severe and sustained impairment in social interactions and restricted, repetitive patterns of behaviors, interests, and activities; also called Asperger syndrome [18]

schizoid personality disorder a condition characterized by a persistent withdrawal from social relationships and lack of emotional responsiveness in most situations [18]

schizophrenia a condition characterized by the inability to distinguish between thoughts and reality, think logically, and have normal emotional and social relationships [18]

schizophreniform disorder a condition that is identical to schizophrenia except that the total duration is greater than one month but less than six months; impaired social or occupational functioning may not be apparent [18]

schizothymia a tendency toward being severely introverted [18]

schizotypal personality disorder a condition characterized by trouble with relationships and disturbances in thought patterns, appearance, and behavior [18]

sclera the tough, white outer layer of the eyeball [19]

screening procedure a procedure performed to determine whether an abnormality exists in a person showing no signs or symptoms of disease [32]

sebaceous pertaining to oil [11]

second trimester the time in a pregnancy when the gestational age is between 14 weeks, 0 days and less than 28 weeks, 0 days [23]

secondary (malignant neoplasm) the site or metastasis where a neoplasm spreads to [5]

secondary diabetes mellitus a condition in which glucose concentrations are elevated due to an external factor, such as medication, surgery, pancreatic disease, or other illness [10]

secondary diagnosis any diagnosis that is not the principal or first-listed; also called additional diagnosis [4]

secondary intention healing an extended process in which a wound is not closed with sutures but left open to granulate [37]

secondary parkinsonism Parkinson-type abnormal movements that are caused by medication or another condition [17]

secondary thyroidectomy a second operation to excise remaining thyroid tissue following a previous thyroidectomy; also called complete thyroidectomy [36]

secretion the release of perspiration to control temperature and sebum to protect from dehydration and penetration by harmful substances [11]

section (CPT) the first level of classification of CPT Category I codes [28]

Section (ICD-10-PCS) Character 1 in an ICD-10-PCS code; defines the broad procedure category in which the code is found [49]

segmentectomy the surgical excision of tissue from part of one lobe of a lung; also called wedge excision [41]

selective catheter placement inserting a catheter into a vessel, moving it to the aorta, then moving it through one or more arteries that branch off the aorta to reach a specific vessel needing treatment [39]

self-insured health plan a plan offered by large employers or unions who, rather than purchasing group health insurance, set aside money in a reserve fund and pay for employees' medical expenses from the fund [2]

semen fluid containing sperm [44]

semicircular canal the superior, posterior, and inferior canals in the ear that contain endolymph [20]

semicolon (CPT) a convention used in the CPT manual to conserve space and avoid having to repeat common terminology [28]

sensation contains sensory receptors for pain, touch, heat, cold, and pressure [11]

sentinel lymph node the first node or group of nodes in a chain [40]

septoplasty surgical repair of the nasal septum, with or without cartilage scoring (incising), contouring, or replacement with graft [41]

sequela (ICD-10-CM) a late effect or problem after active healing is completed [4]

sequela episode identifies an encounter at which a patient is treated for a complication after the healing phase is complete [8]

sequence the placement of codes in the order dictated by the guidelines and instructional notes [1, 4]

serology a blood test used to diagnose diseases [21]

serum assay a lab test that measures the presence and quantity of a substance in the blood [10]

setting the location where a service is provided, such as office/outpatient, hospital, emergency department, or nursing facility; also called place of service [31]

sexual disorder a repetitive and prolonged sexual activity and sexual dysfunction that interferes with normal relationships or daily activities [18]

SGA small for gestational age [24]

shaft the long, narrow part of a bone [12]

shaving use of a sharp instrument [37]

Shock Wave Therapy (ICD-10-PCS) the Root Operation that identifies extracorporeal treatment by shock waves [57]

shock wave therapy extracorporeal treatment by shock waves [57]

Shone syndrome a set of four congenital heart defects: a supravalve mitral membrane, parachute mitral valve, subaortic stenosis, and coarctation of the aorta [25]

sialogram a record or picture of the salivary duct [47]

sialography the process of recording the salivary duct [47]

sialolithotomy a procedure in which calculus is removed from the salivary gland(s) [35]

sickle cell anemia a genetic disorder in which red blood cells take on a sickle shape and lead to hemolytic anemia [15]

sickle cell crisis pain caused because blood vessels have become blocked or defective red blood cells damage organs in the body [15]

sign objective evidence of a disease or condition that can be observed by a physician [6]

significant procedure a procedure that is surgical in nature, carries a procedural risk, carries an anesthetic risk, or requires specialized training [49]

SIL squamous intraepithelial lesion [22]

simple complete mastectomy the removal of only breast tissue, the nipple, and a small portion of the overlying skin; also called simple mastectomy and total mastectomy [37]

simple mastoidectomy incision into the mastoid with dissection of the mastoid process; also called transmastoid antrotomy [44]

simple partial (seizure) a seizure that affects only a small region of the brain and does not cause loss of consciousness [17]

single photon emission computed tomography (SPECT) the use of photons emitted by a radioactive tracer to create an image of lower quality than PET [47]

single quantity a code for which one unit is reported for each service performed [37]

singleton a pregnancy with one fetus [23]

sinoatrial (SA) node the pacemaker of the heart [14]

sinusitis sinus infection [16]

site of origin the anatomic site where a growth begins [5]

skeletal system the system that supports the body, protects internal organs, produces blood cells, stores minerals, and serves as a point of attachment for the skeletal muscles [12]

skeletal traction placing pins and/or wires through broken bones and connecting them to stirrups, ropes, pulleys, and weights outside the body to secure bones in place until they heal [38]

skin appendages nails, hair, sweat glands [11]

skin replacement the use of skin from the patient's own body or a donor to replace damaged skin that cannot be repaired with sutures alone [37]

skin substitute the use of synthetic material to replace damaged skin [37]

skull traction applying cranial tongs or calipers to the head and attaching them to ropes and weights on the outside, which secure the spine in place [38]

sleeping disorder an abnormal sleep problem [18]

small-bowel transplant the surgical removal of a diseased small intestine and replacement with some or all of a small intestine from a healthy person [35]

small for gestational age (SGA) a fetus or newborn infant who is smaller in size than normal for the baby's sex and gestational age [24]

smallpox an infectious disease with the last known case in 1977 [21]

social history education, occupation, religious affiliation, natural support network, lifestyle habits (e.g., tobacco use, alcohol use, illicit drug use, sexual activity) [2]

solid matter (PCS) a nonnative solid that may result from biological processes, such as calculi or a clot, or may be a nonbiological solid, such as a foreign body [55]

somatoform a physical symptom that is not explained by a medical condition(s) [18]

sonohysterography ultrasound of the uterus after a saline solution is infused into the uterus [46]

special instructions (CPT) directions within each section describing specific rules and definitions for use of codes within a particular category or subcategory [28]

specimen a sample of any bodily fluid or tissue [48]

SPECT single photon emission computed tomography [47]

Speech Assessment (ICD-10-PCS) the Root Type that identifies the measurement of speech and related functions [58]

Speech Treatment (ICD-10-PCS) the Root Type that identifies the application of techniques to improve, augment, or compensate for speech and related functional impairment [58]

sperm washing separation of the sperm from seminal fluid and removal of chemicals that can be harmful to the uterus [46]

spermatocele the benign cystic swelling of sperm in the ducts of the epididymis [22]

sphenoid sinus the sinus located at the center of the base of the skull, at the back of the nose [41]

spina bifida a congenital neural tube defect in which vertebrae do not fuse [17]

spinal cord (seizure) see *complex partial (seizure)* [17]

spinal tap or puncture insertion of a needle into the lumbar back to collect a sample of CSF [42]

splenectomy the total or partial excision of the spleen [40]

splenoplasty surgical repair of the spleen [56]

splenorrhaphy repair of a ruptured spleen, with or without partial splenectomy [40]

split-thickness skin graft (STSG) a skin graft consisting of the epidermis and a portion of dermis or a mucosal graft consisting of only a partial thickness of mucosa [37]

sprain the overstretching, bruising, or tearing of a ligament [12]

squamous cell carcinoma (SCC) cancer that occurs in flat squamous cells [11]

squamous intraepithelial disease (SIL) cervical dysplasia seen on a Pap test, graded as low-grade (LSIL), high-grade (HSIL), and possibly cancerous or malignant [22]

ST elevation MI (STEMI) a myocardial infarction in which the ST segment of an EKG is elevated, indicating that the MI completely occludes a vessel [14]

stabilization immobilizing a fracture site to prevent further injury and allow for healing [38]

stage 1 pressure ulcer skin redness due to prolonged pressure that does not go away [11]

stage 2 pressure ulcer damage to the epidermis due to prolonged pressure that extends into the dermis [11]

stage 3 pressure ulcer damage through the full thickness of the dermis and into the subcutaneous tissue due to prolonged pressure [11]

stage 4 pressure ulcer skin damage extending into the muscle, tendon, or bone due to prolonged pressure [11]

staging the process of determining how far a cancer has spread [5]

standalone code the code whose description is left-justified and begins with a capital letter; also called parent code [28]

standardized terminology (ICD-10-PCS) the characteristic of ICD-10-PCS whereby a code set includes definitions of the terminology it uses, with each term having only one meaning [49]

stapedectomy excision of the stapes bone [44]

stapedotomy incision into the footplate of the stapes; may also involve inserting a prosthesis for hearing loss [44]

stapes the stirrup-shaped bone in the middle ear that receives vibrations from the incus [20]

status (ICD-9-CM, ICD-10-CM) the external cause code that describes a person's employment status in relation to the event that caused an injury [8]

status asthmaticus an acute exacerbation that does not respond to the standard medical treatments with bronchodilators and steroids [16]

status epilepticus an epileptic seizure that lasts more than 30 minutes or is a near-constant state of seizures [17]

status migrainosus a migraine that lasts more than 72 hours [17]

STEMI ST elevation myocardial infarction [14]

stenosis a narrowing of a valve or vessel [14]

stent insertion placement of a mesh tube in a blood vessel to keep it open; necessary in atherosclerosis [14]

stereotactic imaging three-dimensional imaging to pinpoint a specific location [47]

Stereotactic radiosurgery (ICD-10-PCS) the Modality that identifies delivery of high doses of radiation to a target area with minimal exposure to the surrounding healthy tissue

stereotactic radiosurgery the use of narrow beams of radiation with three-dimensional guidance to target lesions in difficult-to-treat areas [42]

steroid a type of medication used to reduce inflammation [16]

stomatitis redness, ulcers, and/or bleeding of the mouth due to bacteria, viruses, or fungi [9]

stomatoplasty surgical repair of the mouth [56]

stomatorrhaphy suturing of the mouth [56]

straight catheter a nonindwelling catheter consisting of a short, rigid tube that is inserted via the urethra to allow for drainage of urine, then removed [45]

strain the overstretching, bruising, or tearing of a bone or tendon [12]

stress fracture a fracture of a bone that has been subjected to repeated use or impact; also called March fracture or fatigue fracture [12]

stress testing measuring EKG and oxygen concentrations as a patient performs an increasing level of exercise on a treadmill or stationary bicycle [14]

structural integrity (ICD-10-PCS) the characteristic of ICD-10-PCS whereby the code set can be expanded easily without disrupting the structure of the system [49]

STSG split-thickness skin graft [37]

subcategory (CPT) a further division of some categories of CPT Category I codes that provides more specific information about a procedure or service [28]

subcategory (ICD-10-CM) each level of subdivision after a category and before a code; either four or five characters [4]

subcategory (ICD-9-CM) a four-digit number providing further details of a category, such as variations of a condition or a specific anatomic site [26]

subchapter (ICD-10-CM) a contiguous range of codes within a chapter [4]

subclassification (ICD-9-CM) a five-digit code that further describes a diagnosis and anatomic site [26]

subcutaneous mastectomy excision of breast tissue but not the overlying skin, nipple, and areola, making it possible for the breast form to be reconstructed [37]

subcutaneous under the skin [11]

subdermal pertaining to under the skin [11]

subdural tap withdrawal of CSF through a fontanelle [42]

subendocardial (infarction) the death of heart tissue that affects only a small portion of the heart wall, usually due to a decreased, but not totally occluded, blood supply; also called nontransmural infarction [14]

subheading (CPT) a division of CPT Category I codes that groups procedures by location within a body system [28]

subluxation the partial dislocation of bones in a joint [12]

subsection (CPT) a division of CPT Category I codes that breaks down sections by type and/or anatomic sites [28]

subsequent encounter (CPT) the second or later encounter by the admitting provider during the current admission and to all encounters by other than the admitting physician [31]

subsequent encounter (ICD-10-CM) treatment during the healing phase [4]

subsequent episode (ICD-10-CM) treatment during the healing phase [8]

subsequent MI an MI that occurs within four weeks of a previous AMI [14]

substance disorder drug and alcohol use, abuse, and addiction [18]

subterm a word indented under each Main Term that further describes the Main Term in greater detail, such as an anatomic location or other disease variation [4]

subtotal thyroid lobectomy excision of more than two-thirds of one lobe but less than the entire lobe [36]

sudoriferous pertaining to sweat [11]

superficial burn a burn that causes damage to the epidermis [11]

superficial injury an injury to the surface of the skin, such as an abrasion, blister, contusion, constriction, insect bite, or superficial foreign body [13]

superior vena cava one of the largest veins that carry deoxygenated blood back to the right ventricle [14]

supervised modality a physical therapy treatment that does not require continuous one-on-one contact with a patient by a provider [32]

Supplement (ICD-10-PCS) the Root Operation that identifies putting in or on biological or synthetic material that physically reinforces and/or augments the function of a portion of a Body Part [51, 56]

supracervical above the cervix uteri [46]

suprapubic catheter an indwelling catheter inserted into the bladder through a laparotomy incision a few inches below the navel; less likely to harbor infection than an indwelling urethral catheter [45]

surgical approach the method used by a surgeon to access the operative site [33, 50]

surgical destruction the obliteration of tissue using electrosurgery, cryosurgery, laser, or chemical treatment; also called lysis [33]

surgical facility the setting or location in which surgery is performed [33]

surgical history the date and type of past operations; operative reports (a narrative of exactly how the surgeon performed the procedure) [2]

suspended temporarily held from moving forward [2]

symptom subjective evidence of a disease or condition, usually reported by a patient [6]

syndactyly the presence of webbed fingers or toes [25]

synovectomy surgical removal of the synovial membrane [38]

synthetic manmade; not natural [11]

systemic a class of diseases that affect the entire body [21]

systemic circulation the section of the circulatory system that occurs between the heart and the rest of the body [14]

Systemic Nuclear Medicine Therapy (ICD-10-PCS) the Root Type that identifies the introduction of unsealed radioactive materials into the body for treatment [58]

systemic nuclear medicine therapy the introduction of unsealed radioactive materials into the body for treatment [58]

systole the time during the heart cycle when the chamber contracts as it ejects blood [14]

T

Table (ICD-10-PCS) a reference grid used to select the Body Part, operative approach, and other characteristics of a procedure [49]

tachycardia rapid heart rate [24]

tachypnea rapid breathing [24]

TAH total artificial heart [39]

target organ an organ receiving hormones or treatment [10]

tattooing injection of a colored pigment into the skin [37]

TBSA total body surface area [13]

technical component (CPT) part of a radiology code that covers the cost of staffing and equipment [30]

temporary national code (CPT) a code used for a service or supply that does not have a permanent code [29]

tendon fibrous tissue that connects bones to muscles [12]

tendon repair sewing together the damaged or torn ends of a tendon [38]

tendonitis the inflammation of a tendon [12]

tendonoplasty the surgical repair of a tendon [56]

tendonorrhaphy suturing of a tendon [56]

terrorism an event involving weapons of mass destruction or specific terrorism-related offenses [8]

tertiary intention healing delayed primary closure; wound is initially cleaned, debrided, and left open for observation for several days before closure [37]

testis the part of the male genital system that provides the male sex hormone testosterone [22]

tetralogy of Fallot a congenital heart defect consisting of four malformations: pulmonary stenosis, ventricle septal defect, dextraposition of the overriding aorta, and hypertrophy of the right ventricle [25]

thalassemia a genetic disorder that results in defective formation of hemoglobin [15]

therapeutic drug assay testing performed to monitor a known, prescribed medication so a physician can evaluate how it is affecting a patient [48]

therapeutic procedure a procedure performed to treat a disease or condition [33, 50]

therapeutic radiology treatment using radiation [1]

thermocauterization the destruction of tissue by applying heat [43]

therosclerosis the formation of plaque on the inner walls of arteries in the heart [14]

third trimester the time in a pregnancy when the gestational age is between 28 weeks, 0 days and delivery [23]

third-party administrator (TPA) a private company that processes claims for self-insured health plans [2]

third-party payer an entity other than a patient or physician who pays for healthcare services; they reimburse physicians and hospitals for 86% of all healthcare services in the United States [2]

thoracentesis surgical puncture of the chest wall to remove fluids [16]

thoracoscopy the insertion of an endoscope through a small incision in the chest wall [41]

thoracostomy creation of an opening through the chest to place a chest tube or intercostal catheter in the pleural space [41]

thoracotomy incision into the pleural space [41]

thrombectomy incision into a vein or artery and removal of a clot [39]

thrombocyte a platelet [15]

thrombophilia a tendency to create blood clots [15]

thrombus a clot of blood formed within a blood vessel that remains attached to its point of origin [14]

thymectomy surgical removal of all or most of the thymus gland [36]

thyroglossal pertaining to the thyroid and the tongue [36]

thyroidectomy surgical removal of all or most of the thyroid gland [36]

thyroidectomy, substernal surgical removal of an enlarged thyroid that has grown behind the sternum [36]

thyrotomy cutting into the thyroglossal duct [36]

thyrotoxicosis an excessive quantity of circulating thyroid hormone due to overproduction by the thyroid gland originating from outside the thyroid, or from loss of storage function and leakage from the gland; also referred to as thyroid storm [10]

TIA transient ischemic attack [14]

time units (T) the total minutes of anesthesia service provided for all procedures divided by 15 [34]

tissue expander a temporary inflatable or saline implant placed under the skin to stretch it and allow growth of new skin cells [37]

T-lymphocyte a white blood cell that protects against viruses and bacteria [40]

TMR transmyocardial revascularization [39]

tolerate the ability of a patient to absorb a substance before experiencing behavioral or physical abnormalities [18]

Tomographic (Tomo) Nuclear Medicine Imaging (ICD-10-PCS) the Root Type that identifies the introduction of radioactive materials into the body for three-dimensional display of images developed from the capture of radioactive emissions [58]

tomographic (tomo) nuclear medicine imaging the introduction of radioactive materials into the body for three-dimensional display of images developed from the capture of radioactive emissions [58]

tongue tie a condition in which the bottom of the tongue is attached to the floor of the mouth by a band of tissue called the lingual frenulum [25]

tonic (seizure) a seizure characterized by prolonged muscle contractions or stiffening [17]

tonic-clonic (seizure) a seizure characterized by a sudden loss of consciousness and falling to the floor; affects the entire brain [17]

tonsillectomy/adenoidectomy (T&A) a procedure in which the tonsils and adenoids are surgically removed [35]

tonsillitis inflammation of the tonsils [16]

topical anesthesia a type of anesthesia that numbs the surface area of a body part [34]

topography the anatomic site where a growth begins [5]

total artificial heart (TAH) implementation the insertion of a device that replaces the ventricles [39]

total body surface area (TBSA) the total surface area of the human body, used in a calculation when classifying burns of the skin [13]

total thyroid lobectomy the excision of one entire lobe of the thyroid gland [36]

total/complete thyroidectomy a second operation to excise remaining thyroid tissue following a previous thyroidectomy; also called completion thyroidectomy [36]

total-body hypothermia a technique that lowers the core body temperature below 35°C (95°F) during surgery, with the goal of protecting neurons from injury or degeneration; also called induced hypothermia or hypothermic anesthesia [34]

Tourette syndrome a condition that causes people to make repeated, quick movements or sounds, which they have no control over [17]

toxic effect a harmful substance that is ingested or comes into contact with a person and causes an undesired physical response [13]

toxoid immunization that contains bacteria that are nontoxic so that the immune system will produce antibodies but the individual will not become ill [32]

toxoplasmosis an infection due to the parasite *Toxoplasma gondii*, usually affecting the brain, lung, heart, eyes, or liver [9]

TPA third-party administrator [2]

TPAL a description of parity that identifies the number of term births (T), preterm births (P), spontaneous or induced abortions (A), and living children (L) [23]

trabeculectomy surgical excision of a small portion of the trabecular tissue lying between the anterior chamber of the eye and the canal of Schlemm [43]

trabeculoplasty see *trabeculotomy* [43]

trabeculotomy incision into and repair of the trabecular meshwork to improve aqueous humor outflow and reduce IOP [43]

trachea the windpipe [10, 16]

tracheal cartilage the part of the body that keeps the trachea and bronchi open [16]

trachelectomy removal of the uterine cervix; also called cervicectomy [46]

trachelorrhaphy suture of a laceration of the uterine cervix [46]

tracheobronchoscopy the insertion of an endoscope through an established tracheostomy incision to view the trachea and bronchi [41]

tracheostomy the creation of an opening in the trachea through which a breathing tube is inserted [41, 54]

tracheostomy tube a surgical opening in the neck leading to the trachea [16]

tracheotomy creation of a surgical incision through the neck into the trachea [41]

Traction (ICD-10-PCS) the Root Operation that identifies exerting a pulling force on a body region in a distal direction [57]

traction exerting a pulling force on a body region in a distal direction [57]

tractotomy incision of a nerve tract in the brain stem or spinal cord [42]

TRAM transverse rectus abdominis myocutaneous [37]

transabdominal approach the performance of a procedure through an incision in the abdomen [36]

transabdominal pertaining to across the abdomen [36]

transaction standards programming specifications [3]

transcanal through the ear canal [44]

transcatheter through an existing catheter [45]

transcervical through the cervix uteri [46]

transcranial through the skull [44]

Transfer (ICD-10-PCS) the Root Operation that identifies moving, without taking out, all or a portion of a Body Part to another location to take over the function of all or a portion of a Body Part [51, 53, 54]

transfer of care occurs when a consulting physician assumes management of a patient's care for one or more problems or conditions [31]

Transfusion (ICD-10-PCS) the Root Operation that identifies putting in blood or blood products [57]

transfusion putting in blood or blood products [57]

transient ischemic attack (TIA) a brief episode of cerebral ischemia [14]

transient tachypnea of the newborn (TTN) a short-term condition of rapid breathing due to retained lung fluid that occurs shortly after birth in full-term or near-term newborns [24]

transitory temporary [24]

translabyrinthine through the labyrinth [44]

transmastoid antrotomy see *simple mastoidectomy* [44]

transmastoid through the mastoid bone [44]

transmural MI the death of heart tissue that extends through the entire thickness of the heart muscle [14]

transmyocardial revascularization (TMR) the use of lasers to make small channels through the heart muscle and into the left ventricle [39]

transnasal through the nose [35, 41]

transoral through the oral cavity [35, 41]

transorbital through an incision in the orbit of the eye [41]

transperineal through the perineum [45, 46]

Transplantation (ICD-10-PCS) the Root Operation that identifies putting in or on all or a portion of a living Body Part taken from another individual or animal to physically take the place and/or function of all or a portion of a similar Body Part [51, 53]

transposition of the great vessels a congenital heart defect in which the aorta and pulmonary artery are switched, preventing pulmonary circulation [25]

transpubic through the pubic bone [45]

transthoracic approach the performance of a procedure through an incision in the chest [36]

transurethral resection of prostate (TURP) the insertion of a resectoscope via the urethra and removal of a portion of the prostate; may include cystoscopy, meatotomy, and urethral dilation [45]

transurethral through the urethra [45]

transvaginal through the vagina [45, 46]

transverse rectus abdominis myocutaneous (TRAM) flap the use of transverse rectus abdominis myocutaneous tissue to reconstruct the breast [37]

traumatic an acute current injury that results from an accident [12]

traumatic amputation the accidental severing of a body part [13]

Treatment (ICD-10-PCS) the Root Operation that identifies manual treatment to eliminate or alleviate somatic dysfunction and related disorders [57]

treatment (PCS Section F) a wide variety of activities typically associated with rehabilitation, such as swallowing dysfunction exercises, bathing and showering techniques, wound management, and gait training [58]

Tricare (TC) federal health insurance coverage for family members of active-duty personnel and for retired military personnel and their families [2]

trichiasis turning inward of the eyelashes [43]

trichinosis a disease caused by trichinae parasites [43]

tricuspid valve the valve that controls blood flow from the right atrium to the right ventricle [14]

trisomy a genetic disorder in which a person has three copies, rather than two, of genetic material [25]

true labor the period during which the uterine contracts and the cervix dilates [23]

TTN transient tachypnea of the newborn [24]

TURP transurethral resection of prostate [45]

tympanectomy excision of the eardrum [44]

tympanic membrane perforation (TMP) a hole or break in the eardrum; also called ruptured tympanic membrane [20]

tympanic membrane the eardrum; separates the external ear from the middle ear; also called tympanum [20]

tympanolysis destruction of tympanic membrane adhesions, granulation tissue, or scar tissue [44]

tympanometry measurement of the eardrum [32]

tympanoplasty see *myringoplasty* [44]

tympanostomy the creation of an opening in the eardrum to insert a plastic or metal ventilating tube to drain fluid from the middle ear [44]

tympanotomy incision into the eardrum [44]

tympanum the part of the external ear that separates it from the middle ear; also called tympanic membrane or eardrum [16, 20]

type 1 diabetes a condition in which the body's immune system attacks pancreatic beta cells so that the pancreas does not produce insulin; previously called insulin-dependent diabetes mellitus (IDDM) or juvenile-onset diabetes [10]

type 2 diabetes a condition in which the pancreas produces insulin, but the body does not use it properly; previously called non-insulin-dependent diabetes mellitus (NIDDM) or adult-onset diabetes [10]

U

UB-04 a standard hospital billing form; also known as the CMS-1450 [49]

UHDDS Uniform Hospital Data Discharge Set [4]

ulcer a sore on the lining of the stomach (gastric ulcer) or duodenum (peptic ulcer) [9]

ulcerative colitis an inflammatory bowel disease (IBD) with inflammation and sores, called ulcers, in the lining of the rectum and colon [9]

Ultrasonography (ICD-10-PCS) the Root Type that identifies the real-time display of images of anatomy or flow information developed from the capture of reflected and attenuated high-frequency sound waves [58]

ultrasonography the real-time display of images of anatomy or flow information developed from the capture of reflected and attenuated high-frequency sound waves [58]

Ultrasound Therapy (ICD-10-PCS) the Root Operation that identifies extracorporeal treatment by high-frequency sound waves [57]

ultrasound therapy extracorporeal treatment by high-frequency sound waves [58]

ultrasound the use of sound waves to capture an image of echoes bouncing off structures, showing real-time movements within the body [47]

Ultraviolet Light Therapy (ICD-10-PCS) the Root Operation that identifies extracorporeal treatment by ultraviolet light [57]

ultraviolet therapy extracorporeal treatment by ultraviolet light [57]

uncertain diagnosis diagnoses preceded by the words *probable, possible, suspected, questionable, rule out, working diagnosis,* or a similar word [4]

underdosing taking less of a medication than is prescribed by a provider or a manufacturer's instruction [3, 13]

Uniform Hospital Data Discharge Set (UHDDS) a list of data elements and definitions prepared by the Centers for Disease Control and Prevention and used by hospitals for inpatient discharge data collection [4]

uniplane fixator a fixation device that has a single external rod that runs parallel to a long bone and is used almost exclusively on fractures of the shaft [38]

United Network for Organ Sharing (UNOS) a nonprofit organization that administers the United States' Organ Procurement and Transplantation Network, including the organ transplant waiting list [53]

unlisted procedure (CPT) a procedure or service for which there is no specific CPT code; generally ends with the two digits 99 and appear at the end of the category or subdivision to which they apply [28]

unrelated a symptom, sign, or abnormal finding not connected to a disease [6]

unstable lie repeated changes in the fetal position during or after the 36th week of pregnancy [23]

unstageable pressure ulcer an ulcer covered with dead cells, eschar, or wound exudate that cannot be visually assessed [11]

upper respiratory tract a part of the respiratory system that consists of the nose, pharynx, and larynx [16]

uremia a toxic blood condition due to the inability of the kidneys to remove nitrogenous substances from the blood [22]

ureter a tube that drains each kidney [22]

ureteral catheter an indwelling catheter inserted into the ureter, either through the urethra and bladder or posteriorly through the kidney [45]

ureterectomy excision of the ureters [45]

ureterolithotomy incision into a ureter [45]

ureteroplasty repair of a ureter; may include excision of a portion of the ureter, then anastomosis of the ends that were not removed or grafting of tissue from the bladder [45]

ureterotomy incision into the ureter; may include stent placement [45]

urethra a tube that carries urine out of the body [22]

urethral catheter an indwelling catheter inserted through the urethra into the urinary bladder, percutaneously or through an existing ostomy [45]

urethroneocystostomy repair of a defect in the bladder and urethra, with reimplantation of one or both of the ureters into the bladder [45]

urinary bladder a muscular sac that holds urine until it is expelled through the urethra [22]

urinary tract infection (UTI) a bacterial infection of the urinary bladder; also called cystitis [22]

urodynamic tests a variety of tests that measure the contraction of the bladder muscle as it fills and empties, ranging from simple visual observation to precise measurements using sophisticated instruments [45]

urticaria hives [11]

use (substance) consuming a substance in moderate amounts that do not create significant legal, social, employment, family, or medical problems [18]

uterine suspension the shortening of the ligament that suspends the uterus by plicating and tacking it back in place; may also include presacral sympathectomy [46]

uteroscopy visual examination of the ureters [45]

uterus a hollow muscular organ in females that provides for the development of a fetus; also called the womb [22]

utricle a small, saclike structure of the labyrinth of the inner ear [20]

uvea the middle layer of the eye consisting of the iris, ciliary body, and choroid [19]

uvula a pendant fleshy lobe, most commonly referred to as one in the back of the mouth [19]

V

V codes (ICD-9-CM) values that classify the reason for care, other than an active illness; begin with the letter V and range from V01 to V91 [26]

vaccine immunization that contains antigens from a weakened strain of a virus so that the body will produce antibodies to fight it, but the person will not become ill [32]

VAD ventricular assistive device [39]

vagina the birth canal [22]

vaginal birth after cesarean (VBAC) delivery through the vagina after having a cesarean delivery in a previous pregnancy [23]

vaginal birth the delivery of a fetus from the uterus through the cervix to the vagina (birth canal) [23]

vaginal delivery after cesarean (VBAC) performing a vaginal delivery for a mother who had a cesarean delivery with a previous pregnancy [46]

vaginotomy making an incision into the vagina [46]

vagotomy a procedure in which a portion of the vagus nerve in the stomach is excised [35]

value an individual letter or number in an ICD-10-PCS code

valve repair the correction of a physical defect of the heart [14]

valve replacement the replacement of a heart valve with a synthetic or porcine [pig] valve [14]

valvular disorder a condition characterized by damage to or a defect in one of the four heart valves [14]

VAP ventilator-assisted pneumonia [16]

varicella the chicken pox virus [21]

vascular dementia a form of dementia due to many small strokes [18]

vascular family a network of vessels branching off the same primary vessel [39]

vasectomy cutting out a piece of the vas deferens and cauterizing or suturing the ends closed [45]

vasodilation enlargement of blood vessels [17]

vasoocclusive crisis a form of sickle cell crisis in which the patient experiences severe pain due to infarctions, which may occur in nearly any location [15]

vasotomy incision into the vans deferens [45]

VATS video-assisted thoracoscopic surgery

VBAC vaginal birth after cesarean [23]

vein a tube that carries blood from the capillaries back to the heart in successively larger veins leading to the superior vena cava and inferior vena cava [14]

venography X-ray of veins by tracing the venous pulse [14]

ventilation-perfusion scan a nuclear medicine test useful in identifying pulmonary emboli by showing whether blood is flowing to all parts of a lung [16]

ventilator a machine that assists with breathing [16]

ventilator-associated pneumonia (VAP) pneumonia that develops 48 hours or more after mechanical ventilation is initiated [16]

ventricle one of the lower heart chambers that ejects blood to the lungs and the body [14]

ventricular assist device (VAD) implantation the insertion of a mechanical pump used to support heart function and blood flow [39]

ventricular fibrillation (V-fib) an irregular heartbeat in the ventricles characterized by an abnormal quivering of heart fibers [14]

ventricular puncture the withdrawal of CSF from the ventricles of the brain by drilling a hole in the skull [42]

venule a small vein [14]

vertebra a bony segment of the spine [12]

vertebral body the main anterior bony part of a vertebra [42]

vertebral segment a vertebra [38]

very low birth weight (VLBW) a birth weight less than 1,500 grams (3 pounds, 4 ounces) [24]

vesicocentesis prenatal aspiration of fetal urine [46]

vesicourethropexy suturing of the vaginal wall to the urethra or bladder neck, with anchoring to the pubic bone or Cooper ligament; also referred to as the Marshall-Marchetti-Krantz (MMK) procedure or Burch procedure [45]

vesiculectomy the removal of one of the seminal vesicles [45]

Vestibular Assessment (ICD-10-PCS) the Root Type that identifies the measurement of the vestibular system and related functions [58]

Vestibular Treatment (ICD-10-PCS) the Root Type that identifies the application of techniques to improve, augment, or compensate for vestibular and related functional impairment [58]

vestibulocochlear nerve cranial nerve VIII; the ear makes hearing possible by collecting sound waves from the external world and converting them into impulses that are transmitted to the brain through the vestibulocochlear nerve [20]

Veterans Health Administration (VHA) an integrated healthcare delivery system with more than 1,400 sites of care, including hospitals, community clinics, community living centers, and various other facilities to provide health services to veterans with service-related disabilities [2]

Via Natural or Artificial Opening Endoscopic (ICD-10-PCS) the Approach that identifies the surgeon inserts an endoscope through an existing natural or artificial opening [50]

Via Natural or Artificial Opening Endoscopic with Percutaneous Endoscopic Assistance (ICD-10-PCS) the Approach that identifies two endoscopes are used: one through a natural or artificial opening and the second one through percutaneous access [50]

Via Natural or Artificial Opening (ICD-10-PCS) the Approach that identifies the surgeon accesses the surgical site through a body opening that already exists, such as the mouth, nose, ear, anus, or vagina [50]

video-assisted thoracoscopic surgery (VATS) the use of an endoscope and video camera to perform procedures traditionally performed using a thoracotomy [41]

videoradiography see *cineradiography* [47]

virus a capsule that contains genetic material and uses the body's own cells to multiply [21]

visceral pericardium see *epicardium* [14]

vitiligo a loss of pigmentation [11]

vitreous body the transparent jelly that fills the eyeball and is surrounded by a membrane [19]

VLBW very low birth weight [24]

Volume 1 (ICD-9-CM) Tabular List of Diseases [26]

Volume 2 (ICD-9-CM) Index to Diseases and Injuries [26]

Volume 3 (ICD-9-CM) Inpatient Procedures [26]

voluntary (muscle) a muscle a person can choose to contract and relax [12]

volvulus the twisting of a portion of the small or large intestine or stomach into a loop, which obstructs the passage of digestive material [9]

Von Willebrand disease a genetic disorder marked by bleeding of the mucosa [15]

vulvectomy surgical removal of part of the vulva [46]

vulvovaginitis inflammation of the vulva and vagina due to yeast, bacteria, viruses, parasites, or skin care products [22]

W

wedge excision surgical excision of tissue from part of one lobe of the lung; also called segmentectomy [41]

whistleblower someone who turns in violators [2]

white blood cell disorder a condition that diminishes the body's immune response and increases the risk of infection [15]

winged catheter a urethral catheter that is retained in the bladder by winglike projections on the end [45]

workers' compensation (WC) a plan that pays for medical costs due to employment-related injuries or illnesses; each state establishes its own requirements for WC insurance but must comply with federal minimums [2]

wound a cut or opening in the skin or mucous membrane [13]

wound exploration the enlargement, dissection, and examination of a wound to determine the wound depth or perform a procedure [38]

wound repair, complex a layered closure that also requires scar revision, debridement, extensive undermining, stents, or retention sutures [37]

wound repair, intermediate the layered closure of one or more of the deeper layers of subcutaneous tissue and superficial fascia, in addition to the skin closure; also includes extensive cleaning/decontamination of wounds otherwise requiring single-layer closure [37]

wound repair, simple a one-layer closure of epidermis, dermis, or subcutaneous tissue without significant involvement of deeper structures; includes local anesthesia and electrocauterization, when used [37]

X

xenograft a skin substitute in which the skin comes from another species, such as a pig, or a synthetic substitute [11, 37]

Z

Z codes (ICD-10-CM) codes that represent reasons for encounters; may be used in any healthcare setting when the reason for the encounter is not a disease, injury, or external cause that is classified in the preceding ICD-10-CM chapters for body systems (A00 to Y99) [7]

zygote a fertilized egg [23]

Index